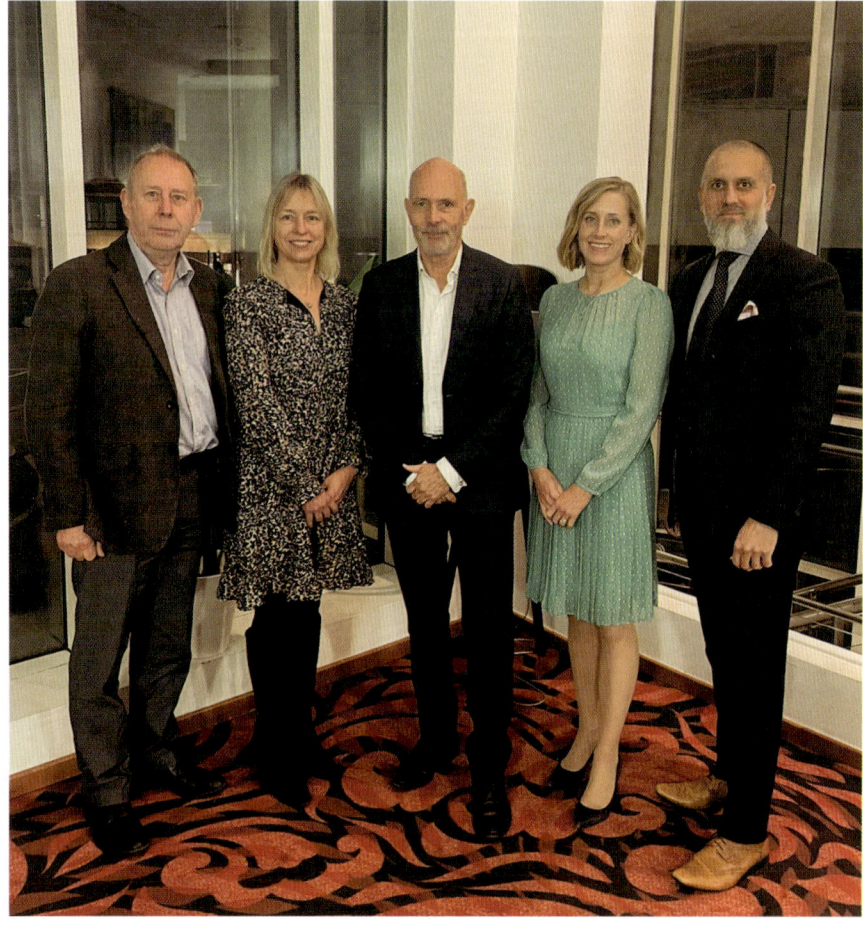

The Editors
From left to right: Jonathan Barker, Tanya Bleiker, Christopher Griffiths, Rosalind Simpson, Walayat Hussain

Rook's
Textbook of Dermatology

TENTH EDITION

EDITED BY

Christopher Griffiths OBE, MD, FMedSci

Emeritus Professor of Dermatology
The University of Manchester
Manchester, UK

Adjunct Professor & Consultant Dermatologist
King's College London
London, UK

Jonathan Barker MD, FRCP

Professor of Medical Dermatology
St John's Institute of Dermatology
Faculty of Life Sciences and Medicine
King's College London
London, UK

Tanya Bleiker FRCP

Consultant Dermatologist
University Hospitals of Derby and Burton NHS Foundation Trust
Derby, UK

Walayat Hussain FRACP

Consultant Dermatological & Mohs Micrographic Surgeon
Dermatology Surgical & Laser Unit
Chapel Allerton Hospital
Leeds, UK

Rosalind Simpson MRCP, PhD

Associate Professor and Consultant Dermatologist
Centre of Evidence Based Dermatology
University of Nottingham
Nottingham, UK

IN FOUR VOLUMES

VOLUME 3

WILEY Blackwell

Contents

PART 8
Skin Disorders Associated with Specific Cutaneous Structures

CHAPTER 86

Acquired Pigmentary Disorders

Nanja van Geel and Reinhart Speeckaert

Department of Dermatology, Ghent University Hospital, Ghent, Belgium

PART 8: SPECIFIC CUTANEOUS STRUCTURES

SKIN PIGMENTATION AND THE MELANOCYTE

The colour of the skin [1,2–7]

Normal skin colour is determined by a number of chromophores, the most important of which is melanin. Besides melanin, haemoglobin (in both the oxygenatedand reduced state) and carotenoids both contribute significantly to skin colour. Racial and ethnic differences in skin colour are related to the number, size, shape, distribution and degradation of melanin-laden organelles called melanosomes. These are produced by melanocytes (Figure 86.1) and are transferred to the surrounding epidermal keratinocytes. Two types of melanin pigmentation occur in humans [1]. The first is *constitutive* skin colour, which is the amount of melanin pigmentation that is

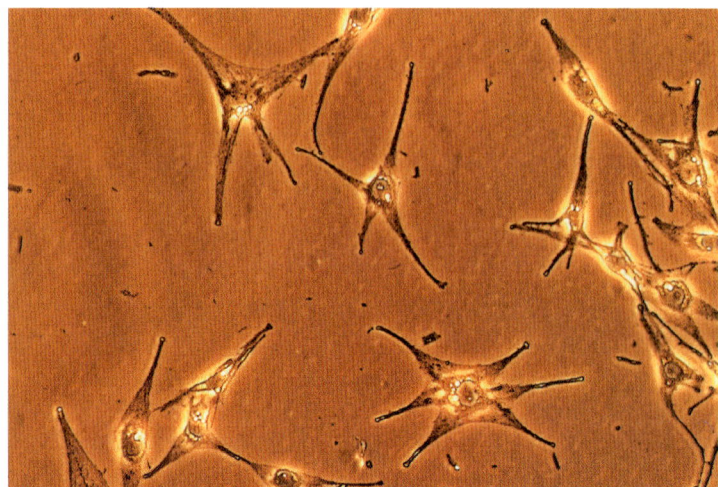

Figure 86.1 Melanocytes in culture.

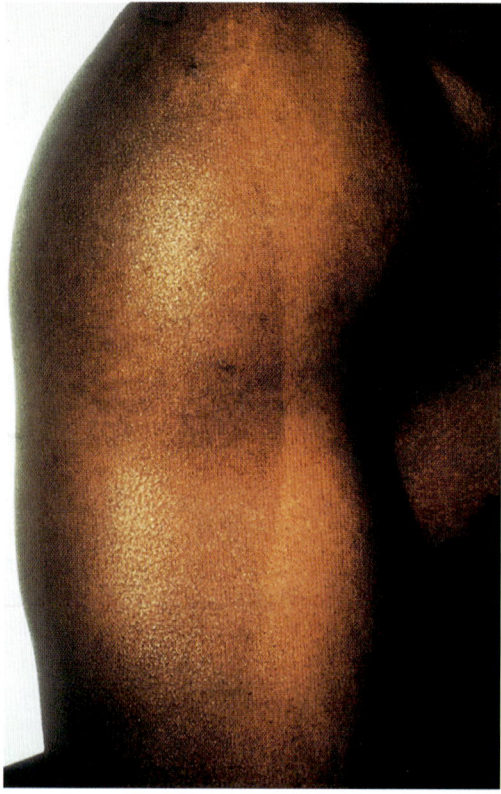

Figure 86.2 Voigt–Futcher lines. Courtesy of the late Dr R.R.M. Harman.

genetically determined in the absence of sun exposure and other influences. The other is *facultative* (inducible) skin colour or 'tan', which results from sun exposure. Increased pigmentation can also be due to endocrine, paracrine and autocrine factors [1,2].

The least pigmented human subjects are almost white and have a skin colour similar to that of an albino. In contrast, the most deeply pigmented human subjects are dark brown or black-brown in colour. Most peoples of the world fall between these two extremes and are moderate brown or yellow-brown in colour. The white peoples of Europe exhibit a light brown colour that can be enhanced by exposure to sunlight. The ability to tan is marked in Mediterranean and Middle Eastern peoples. In contrast, some people from the western parts of northern Europe have fair skin, red hair and a tendency to develop red-brown freckles after exposure to sunlight. The definitive method for the objective measurement of skin colour uses the recording spectrophotometer adapted for reflectance readings [3]. Application of reflectance chromameters in clinical practice includes the measurement of skin colour, the measurement of ultraviolet (UV)-induced pigmentation and the quantification of the bleaching effect of depigmenting agents [3].

In some ethnic groups, a sharply demarcated linear border is seen between more and less pigmented skin [4]. This has been studied most extensively in the Japanese and in black Americans, and is most frequently observed in darkly pigmented individuals (Figure 86.2). Six major forms (designated A–F) of natural pigmentary demarcation boundaries in the skin have been described [4]. These are summarised in Box 86.1.

A blue colour is seen in the congenital pigmentation termed 'Mongolian spot', a form of dermal melanocytosis that can occur on any part of the body, although it is most commonly found in the sacral region [5,6]. These patches fade after birth but can persist in certain sites as in the naevus of Ota (Chapter 131). Blue naevus is an example of acquired blue pigmentation of the skin. The blue coloration of the skin in both of these disorders is due to an optical effect that alters the perceived colour of brown pigment in the dermis. The melanin dispersed in the dermis absorbs incident visible light such that the diffuse reflectance in the longer (red) wavelengths is reduced, giving the pigmented sites a blue appearance.

Box 86.1 Pigmentary demarcation lines (designated A–F)

- **A**: Located on the anterolateral portion of the upper arm (Voigt–Futcher line) (Figure 86.2)
- **B**: Posteromedial portion of the leg
- **C**: Hypopigmented linear bands on the mid chest in the pre- or parasternal region
- **D**: A vertical line in the posteromedial area of the spine
- **E**: Hypopigmented macules located on the chest extending from the clavicle to the periareolar skin
- **F**: Lines on the face

Adapted from [4].

Carotenoids are lipid-soluble yellow to orange-red pigments that are exogenously produced and can be obtained only from plants such as carrots and tomatoes in the diet. Carotenoids serve a photoprotective role in green plants, but their photoprotective effect in humans is small, even when taken in excess [7]. Carotenoids are found in the epidermis as well as the subcutaneous fat. When present in excess, carotenoids impart a yellowish hue to the skin which may sometimes be prominent [7].

The melanocyte [1–3]

Epidermal melanin unit
The estimated mass of all pigment cells within the body is about 1.5 g. Most of these are melanocytes within the epidermis [1].

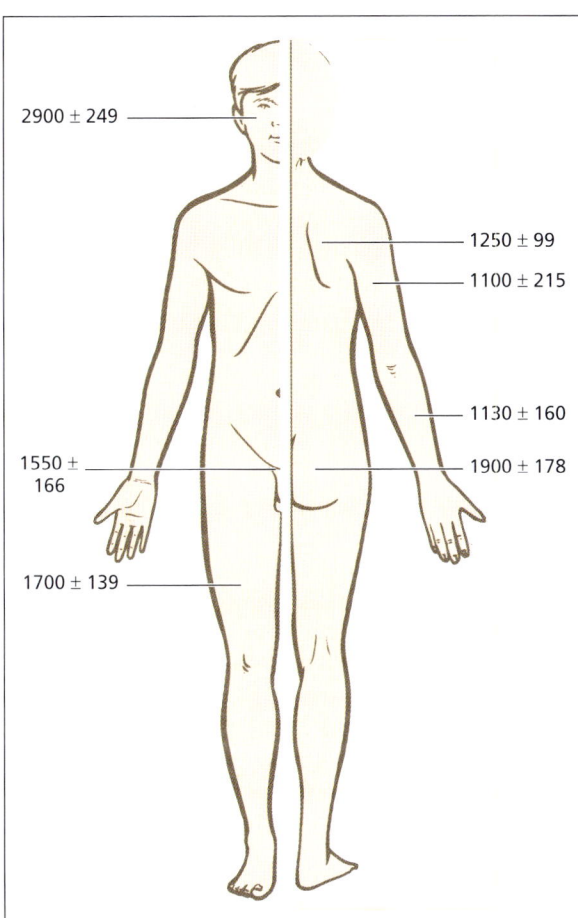

Figure 86.3 Regional variation in the distribution of epidermal melanocytes. The figures are mean values per mm² ± standard error of the mean. Reproduced from Rosdahl and Rorsman 1983 [1] with permission of Elsevier.

The process of melanin production within these melanocytes is a three-stage process, which involves not only the production of melanosomes within the melanocyte, termed melanogenesis, but also the trafficking and transfer of these pigment granules via long arborising dendrites to surrounding epidermal keratinocytes. Each epidermal melanocyte together with the epidermal cells that it serves comprises an 'epidermal melanin unit', as first described by Fitzpatrick and Breathnach in 1963 [2,3]. Although the number of active epidermal melanin units varies considerably in the different regions of the body (Figure 86.3), the number of keratinocytes served by each melanocyte remains constant. It is estimated that a single melanocyte supplies melanosomes to a group of about 36 viable keratinocytes. The number of melanocytes in the skin varies according to the body location [4]. The intricate interface between melanocytes and their keratinocytes is essential for skin pigmentation. Adequate pigmentation of the skin is as dependent on successful transport and transfer of melanosomes to keratinocytes as it is on the formation of the organelle itself.

Distribution of melanocytes [1–3]
Melanocytes are situated in the basal epidermis (Figure 86.4). The number of melanocytes within the skin shows little variation between different races or between the sexes. However, the capacity of melanocytes to synthesise melanin, both in the basal state (constitutive colour) and after stimulation (facultative colour) by

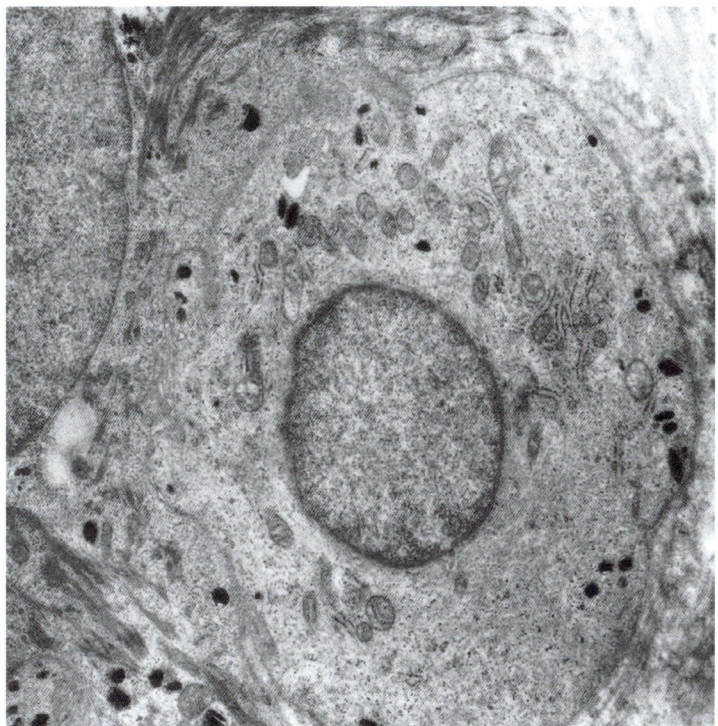

Figure 86.4 Melanocyte in the basal layer of the epidermis.

sunlight, shows great variation. Melanocytes in those with dark skin or with the facility to tan darkly have a great capacity to synthesise melanin and to transfer it to surrounding keratinocytes. In contrast, those with fair skin and lack of tanning facility have very limited capacity. Melanocytes are found in nearly every tissue but are most numerous in the epidermis, hair follicles and the eye [1,2]. A reduction in the number of melanocytes occurs with ageing, with a decrease in melanocyte density of about 6–8% per decade [3]. The density of melanocytes is about twofold higher in exposed than in non-exposed skin [2].

Melanoblast migration and differentiation
Pigment cells arise from the neural crest [1], a region of the embryonic ectoderm that originates from the margins of the neural plate at the time when it sinks in to form the tubular central nervous system. The developmental potential of neural crest cells has been studied by a variety of means including clonal analysis, cell grafting experiments and lineage-specific marker studies. Collectively, these studies indicate that most early neural crest cells are multipotent and become fate-restricted over time [2–4]. Melanoblasts originate in the neural crest and migrate laterally, first to the dermis and then to the basal lamina of the epidermis. Immunocytochemical marker studies with the melanocyte-specific HMB-45 antibody have revealed that melanoblasts appear in the epidermis by 7 weeks' gestation, with a cell density of about 50% of that observed at birth [4]. Ultrastructural studies on early human embryos have demonstrated the presence of melanocytes containing melanosomes showing early melanisation [5]. HMB-45 staining has revealed an approximately twofold increase in melanocyte numbers between gestation weeks 10 and 14, possibly due to mitosis of cells already *in situ* rather than due to additional cell migration. Melanocytes associated with hair

follicles arrive at their final location by following the downgrowth of epidermal cells in developing hair follicles [6].

Studies in mice have demonstrated that melanocyte lineage segregation starts early in neural crest development, with melanoblasts specified prior to or coincident with their emigration from the neural tube [7]. Initial segregation of melanocyte lineage involves the Wnt/β-catenin pathway [8]. The transcription factor *mi* is relatively specific for melanocyte differentiation, as was first identified in the microphthalmia (*mi*) mutant. *Mi* encodes the transcription factor Mitf, which regulates several melanocyte-specific genes [9,10]. In humans, mutations in *mi* are associated with Waardenburg syndrome type 2A, an autosomal dominant condition characterised by deafness and patchy abnormal pigmentation [11]. *Sox10* and *Pax3* are two other genes associated with Waardenburg syndrome, probably through regulation of expression of Mitf protein [12]. *Pax3* appears to prime cells for differentiation, whereas *Wnt* signalling allows cells to proceed along this route [13].

Much of our knowledge about melanocyte development in humans has been derived from studies on mouse pigment mutants [11]. To summarise this body of work in broad terms, mouse coat colour mutants arise from three main groups: those that affect the subcellular structure of melanocytes, those that disrupt the normal synthesis of melanin and those that alter development and differentiation of normal melanocytes. Where possible in this chapter, molecular and biochemical mechanisms for pigmentary abnormalities in humans with genetic disorders will be highlighted.

Melanosome transport [1–10]

The melanosomes are transported in melanocytes from the cell centre to the periphery. Melanosome transport depends upon effective dendrite formation by melanocytes. UV radiation and melanocyte-stimulating hormone (MSH) are both known to stimulate this process [1]. Melanocyte dendrite formation requires actin polymerisation, which in turn is controlled by the activity of the small guanosine triphosphate (GTP)-binding proteins Rac and Rho [2–4]. These are themselves controlled by regulatory associated proteins. Direct visualisation of melanosome trafficking by video microscopy has revealed evidence to suggest that transfer of melanosomes along dendrites occurs on microtubules [5,6], a process driven by dynein (a minus end microtubule motor) and kinesin (a plus end microtubule motor) [7,8]. Dynein binds microtubules and adenosine triphosphate and produces forces which move the dynein and melanosome complex along the microtubule. Both dynein and kinesin remain bound to the melanosomes and their regulation modifies the direction of melanosome movement along the microtubules [9]. Once the melanosomes arrive at the cortical regions of the melanocyte, three individual proteins work together in the final stages of melanosome trafficking. One of these, myosin Va (Myo5a), functions to facilitate the 'capture' of melanosomes at the actin-rich tip of the dendrite [7]. Another, Rab protein Rab27A, associates with the membrane of melanocytes and then forms a complex with myosin Va and a third protein, melanophylin (Mlph). The ability of melanophylin to bind actin, in addition to its ability to link with Rab27A and myosin Va, has led to the hypothesis that transfer of melanosomes from microtubules to actin filaments at the tip of melanocyte dendrites is the final part of the transport process prior to melanosome transfer [10]. The protein–protein interactions between the members of

the Rab27a-Mlph-Myo5a tripartite complex have been extensively investigated and mutations in one of these genes result in genetic pigmentation disorders (e.g. Griscelli syndrome) [11,12].

Melanosome transfer to keratinocytes [1–7]

The successful synthesis of a melanosome, and its transport to the tip of a dendrite, is followed by transfer of the melanosome to the keratinocyte. Both UV radiation and the hormone MSH stimulate this transfer, while niacinamide has been shown to suppress it [1]. However, the exact mechanism by which the melanosome is transferred to the keratinocyte remains unclear. One possibility is exocytosis of melanosomes from the tips of dendrites with subsequent keratinocyte uptake by endocytosis. In support of this, the exocytosis-associated proteins soluble *N*-ethylmaleimide-sensitive factor attachment protein receptor (SNARE) and Rab3a have both been identified on melanosomes [2–4]. Furthermore, *in vivo* high-resolution time-lapse digital images of this process have identified long dynamic filopedia arising from the melanocyte dendrite tips packed with melanosomes [4]. The filopedia have been observed to attach and detach from the keratinocyte membrane: melanocytes have been observed travelling in both directions within the filopedia [4]. Work from several groups has revealed that lectins and their glycosolated ligands may function as receptor–ligand pairs in these melanocyte–keratinocyte interactions [5–7]. Recently, electron microscopy analysis has provided additional evidence for exocytosis and endocytosis as the predominant mechanism of melanin transfer. Nonetheless, other hypotheses still exist [8]. In the theory of cytophagocytosis, melanosome-laden protrusions from the dendritic tips of the melanocyte breach the cell membrane of the keratinocyte. Subsequently, these protrusions are engulfed by the closure of the cell membrane of the keratinocyte. This results in the uptake of melanin granules by keratinocytes. The fusion hypothesis consists of the formation of connecting pores or channels between the membrane of melanocytes and keratinocytes facilitating the transport of melanosomes. A final theory suggests the formation of membrane vesicles containing melanosome globules which are released from the melanocytes [9]. This is followed by the fusion of these particles with the keratinocyte cell membrane or by phagocytosis. However, until now, none of these modes of transfer has been fully confirmed [10].

Melanocyte culture [1–8]

Melanocytes fail to grow and usually die in culture media used for skin fibroblasts or keratinocytes. In contrast to many other cell types, melanocytes do not produce any of the growth factors that are known to stimulate them [1]. Following an intensive search, the first highly effective natural melanocyte mitogen was identified as basic fibroblast growth factor (now termed FGF2) [2]. As more mitogens for melanocytes emerged, it was apparent that a combination of synergistic growth factors was required to stimulate quiescent or moribund melanocytes in culture [1,3]. Additional stimulatory peptides include mast cell growth factor/stem cell factor (M/SCF, also known as Kit ligand and Steel factor), hepatocyte growth factor/scatter factor (HGF/SF), endothelins and, to a lesser degree, MSH. In the presence of FGF2, phorbol ester and cyclic adenosine monophosphate these peptides act synergistically on melanocytes in culture [1,4]. A more recent addition to the list of melanocyte mitogens is leukaemia inhibitory factor (LIF) [5]. With the exception of FGF2, most of these factors also promote melanocyte differentiation [6,7]. Endothelin 1 (ET1) can also sustain the viability of human melanocytes in the absence of other growth factors and stimulate the formation and elongation of dendrites [4,8].

Biochemistry of melanogenesis [1–3,4,5]

Melanins are usually classified into two main groups: the brown to black insoluble eumelanins, and the yellow to reddish-brown alkali-soluble phaeomelanins (Box 86.2). Both pigments are derived from dopaquinone, which is formed by the oxidation of the common amino acid L-tyrosine by tyrosinase. These two types of melanin are different in size, shape and packaging of their granules. Eumelanosomes have a more elliptical form, while phaeomelanin has a rounded contour. Whether eumelanin or phaeomelanin is produced is determined primarily by the melanocortin 1 receptor, which is itself under the control of α-MSH and agouti signal protein [1,2].

Eumelanin formation

Dopaquinone is a highly reactive intermediate and in the absence of sulfhydryl compounds it forms cyclodopa. The redox exchange between cyclodopa and dopaquinone then gives rise to the red intermediate, dopachrome and dopa. Dopachrome then rearranges to 5,6-dihydroxyindole (DHI) and to a lesser extent to 5,6-dihydroxyindole carboxylic acid (DHICA). Finally, DHI and DHICA are oxidised and polymerised to produce eumelanins. Dopachrome tautomerase and Tryp1 (DHICA oxidase) are now both recognised as having a role alongside tyrosinase in the regulation and promotion of eumelanogenesis [3].

Box 86.2 Main types of epidermal melanin pigments

Eumelanins
- Brown or black nitrogenous pigments, insoluble in all solvents, which arise by oxidative polymerisation of 5,6-dihydroxyindoles derived biogenetically from tyrosine

Phaeomelanins
- Alkali-soluble pigments, ranging from yellow to reddish-brown; most of them contain sulphur in addition to nitrogen and arise by oxidative polymerisation of cysteinyl-dopa via 1,4-benzothiazine intermediates

Trichochromes
- A variety of sulphur-containing phaeomelanic pigments with a well-defined structure, characterised by a $\Delta^{2,2'}$-bi(1,4-benzothiazine) chromophore

Reproduced from Prota 1988 [4] with permission of John Wiley & Sons.

Phaeomelanin formation

In contrast to eumelanins, phaeomelanins contain sulphur in addition to nitrogen and are formed from cysteinyldopa (Figure 86.5). Further oxidation of the thiol adducts leads to the formation of phaeomelanin via benzothiazine intermediates. Most melanin pigments in skin are mixtures or copolymers of eumelanins and phaeomelanins. However, the situation is complicated by the fact that some phaeomelanin-like pigments may be structural variants of eumelanins [4]. Thus, in the presence of metal ions, black insoluble eumelanin may be oxidised chemically or photochemically to a soluble form (melanin-free acid), which is light in colour [5,6].

Trichochromes

A further complication is that red human hair contains, in addition to phaeomelanins, small amounts of intensely coloured pigments known as trichochromes [5,7]. Originally isolated from the red feathers of New Hampshire hens, trichochromes are sulphur-containing pigments of a well-defined structure, of which six variants have so far been identified (Figure 86.6).

Regulation of human pigmentation by UV light and by endocrine, paracrine and autocrine factors

Regulation of human melanocytes is complex: in addition to a direct stimulatory effect of UV radiation, there are also effects mediated by endocrine, paracrine and autocrine factors. Constitutive melanin content is determined by the rate of synthesis by melanocytes and by the rate and mode of melanosome delivery to keratinocytes. The response of cultured melanocytes to UV radiation involves growth arrest in conjunction with increased melanogenesis. A differential response is observed between melanocytes derived from individuals of skin types I or II and those from skin types V or IV, with the former showing more prolonged growth arrest, more cyclobutane pyrimidine dimers and less melanogenesis. Exposure of human skin to UV radiation induces a number of epidermal cytokines and growth factors which in turn induce proliferation of melanocytes and/or melanogenesis. Many devoted sun-worshippers know that by deliberately overdosing on sun exposure, the inflammatory sunburn that ensues is more effective at inducing tanning than a more patient, non-burning approach.

Melanocyte response to UV radiation

Skin exposed to sunlight is associated with an increased number of active melanocytes when compared with skin protected from the sun within the same individual. Friedmann and Gilchrest [1] were the first to demonstrate this direct responsiveness in cultured melanocytes by showing that irradiation with solar-simulated UV light resulted in a dose-dependent decrease in proliferation and an increase in pigment production. More recently, research using sublethal doses of UVB showed inhibition of melanocyte proliferation as a result of arrest in the G_2 phase of the cell cycle, and an increased tyrosinase activity and melanin content [2]. Melanocytes derived from different skin types all showed a similar pattern of response [2]. Subsequent research has confirmed that this UV-induced growth arrest of melanocytes is related to increased levels of the tumour suppressor gene product p53, with lightly pigmented melanocytes experiencing a more prolonged growth arrest and a more sustained increase in the p53 protein than occurs in darkly pigmented melanocytes [3]. Furthermore, lightly pigmented melanocytes show more cyclobutane pyrimidine dimers (a reliable marker for UV-induced DNA damage) after UV irradiation

PART 8: SPECIFIC
CUTANEOUS STRUCTURES

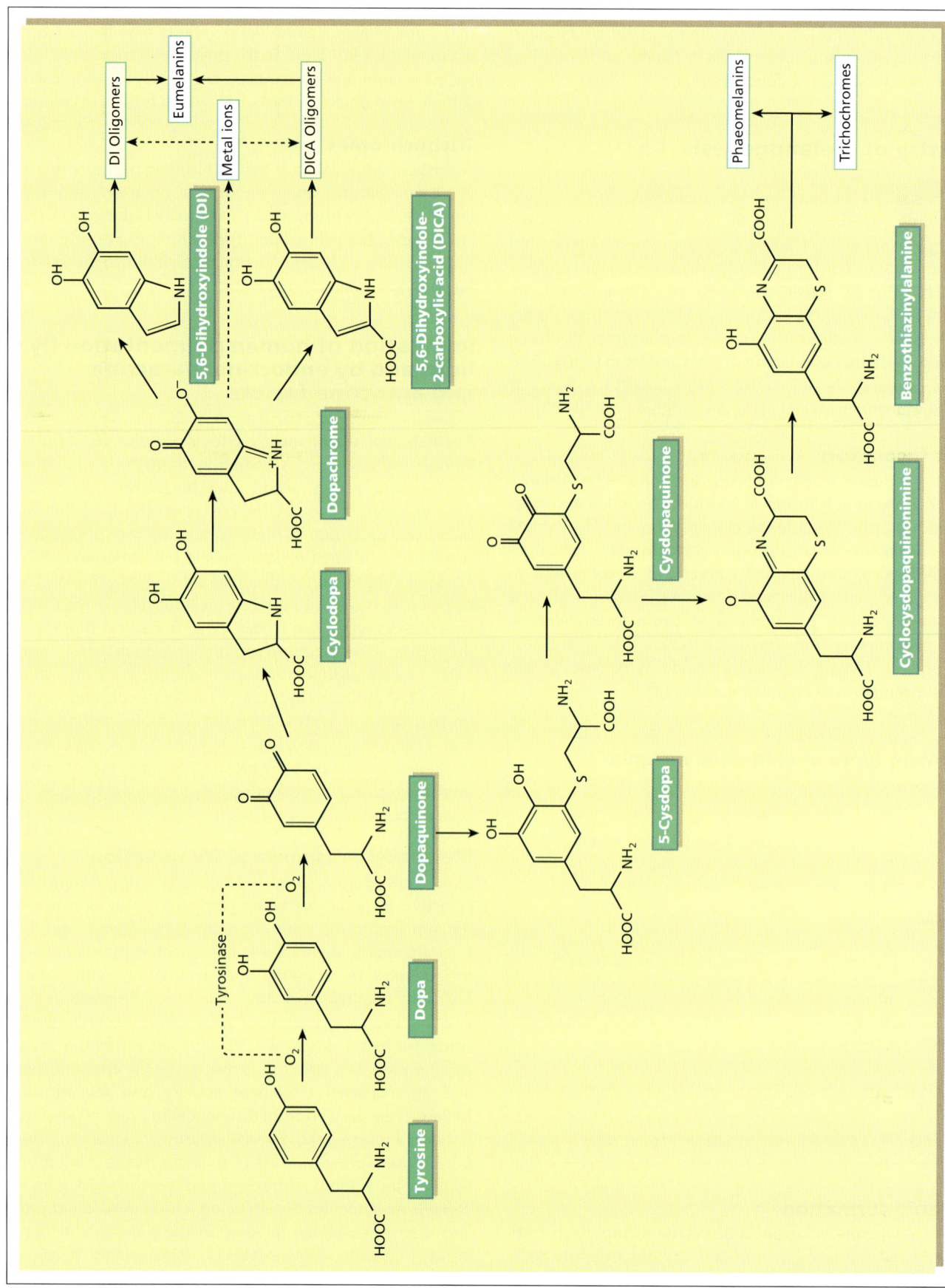

Figure 86.5 A simplified overview of the major metabolic pathways in the synthesis of melanins and trichochromes. Reproduced from Prota 1988 [4] with permission of John Wiley & Sons.

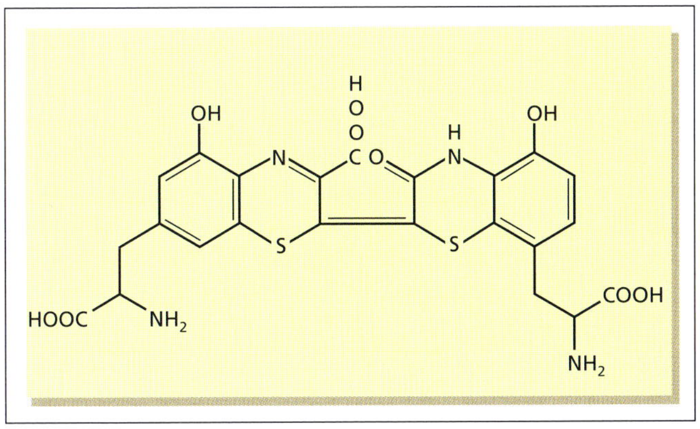

Figure 86.6 Structure of trichochrome B, one of six trichochromes so far identified.

than occurs in heavily pigmented melanocytes [3]. In addition to increased activity of melanocyte tyrosinase, sun exposure leads to elongation and branching of melanocyte dendrites, and an increase in the number and size of melanosomes.

Melanocyte regulation by endocrine factors

The effects of oestrogens on cutaneous pigmentation have been recognised for more than 60 years [4,5]. High levels of oestrogens during pregnancy are implicated in the increased pigmentation that occurs on the face, areola, lower central abdomen and genitalia. Melanocytes express oestrogen receptors and increased levels of oestradiol stimulate enzymes involved in melanogenesis (e.g. tyrosinase, tyrosinase-related protein 1 and tyrosinase-related protein 2) [6].

In Addison disease, the diffuse brown hyperpigmentation results from the melanogenic action of melanocortins derived from the pituitary. The melanocortins are all derived from a precursor molecule, pro-opiomelanocortin. Other melanocortins released from the pituitary in increased quantities in Addison disease include adrenocorticotropin hormone (ACTH), β-lipotropin, α-MSH, β-MSH and γ-MSH. These peptides all have a stimulatory effect on melanocytes [7] and, in the absence of negative feedback to inhibit their secretion, the hyperpigmentation produced is insidious and progressive (Figure 86.7) [8]. A similar mechanism takes place in Cushing syndrome, in which the hyperpigmentation is caused by an overproduction of ACTH from a corticotrophic adenoma or an ectopic non-pituitary tumour [9]. Human melanocytes express the melanocortin 1 receptor (MC1R) that binds α-MSH and ACTH with the same affinity [10]. α-MSH causes a small rise in cyclic adenosine monophosphate (cAMP) but has no effect on basal or UV-stimulated melanogenesis in human melanocytes [11].

Melanocyte regulation by paracrine and autocrine factors

Postinflammatory hyperpigmentation is believed to be mediated by immune inflammatory mediators including interleukin (IL)-1α, IL-1β, IL-6 and tumour necrosis factor (TNF)-α [12]. Human melanocytes have also been demonstrated to respond to and to synthesise IL-1α and IL-1β, which suggests an autocrine as well as a paracrine regulatory role [13]. Other inflammatory mediators that act on human melanocytes include eicosanoids, metabolites of arachidonic acid. Melanocytes respond to prostaglandin E_2 (PGE_2)

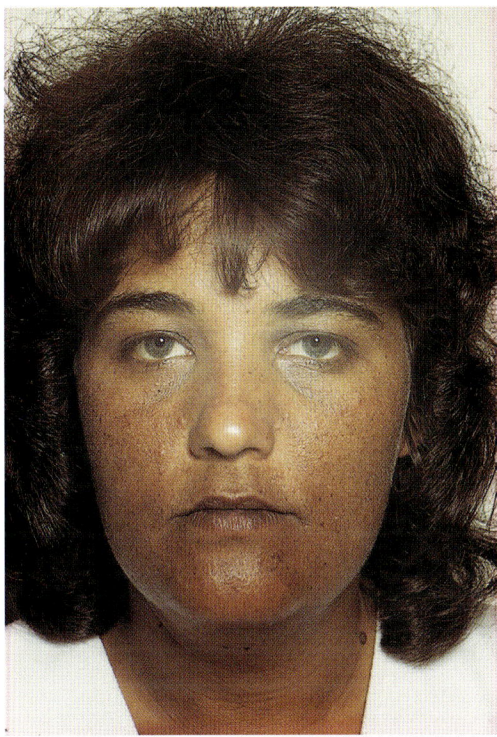

Figure 86.7 Diffuse hyperpigmentation with darkening of the hair and mucous membranes in a woman with Nelson syndrome following bilateral adrenalectomy.

with increased melanogenesis and dendrite formation [14]. Scott *et al.* demonstrated an increase in dendricity of human melanocytes in response to PGE_2 and $PGF_{2\alpha}$ [15]. Prostaglandins, leukotrienes and thromboxanes are the main inducers of tyrosinase [16]. Basic fibroblast growth factor was the first paracrine factor for human melanocytes to be identified. It exerts its effect by binding to a tyrosine kinase receptor that is expressed on human melanocytes [17]. In contrast to IL-1α, IL-1β, IL-6 and TNF-α and the eicosanoids, basic fibroblast growth factor is not secreted by keratinocytes: direct contact between melanocytes and keratinocytes is required for its biological effects [18]. Additionally, leukotrienes C_4 and D_4 have been shown to act as potent mitogens on cultured human neonatal melanocytes [19].

Endothelins are a further important group of peptides that act upon melanocytes in a paracrine manner [20]. ET1 is both mitogenic and melanogenic for human melanocytes that express ET1 receptors [21]. ET1 acts synergistically with α-MSH and basic fibroblast growth factor to stimulate human melanocyte proliferation [22]. ET3 has similar effects to ET1: both peptides bind the endothelin receptor on melanocytes with equal affinity [23]. Furthermore, endothelins appear to have a role in protecting melanocytes: Kadekaro *et al.* demonstrated that treatment of human melanocytes with ET1 reduced UVR-induced apoptosis and prolonged melanocyte survival [24].

Biological significance of melanin

The major biological function of melanin is generally assumed to be protection of the lower layers of the skin against UV light. If human pigment has such adaptive significance, we might expect to find that, among the races of the world, pigment is geographically distributed in relation to solar intensity. It appears to be generally true that pigmentation is greatest in the tropics and reduced in temperate zones, reappearing to some extent in northern races subjected to prolonged snow glare [1]. However, there are exceptions, for example Native Americans, whose skin colour varies little between polar and tropical regions, and Tasmanians, who are dark even though they live in a temperate climate.

The damaging role of UV light is well illustrated by the high incidence of epidermal carcinoma in Europeans exposed to excess sun. The evolutionary usefulness of pigmentation may be twofold. On the one hand, it protects against damage by sunburn. On the other, since it efficiently absorbs UV radiation and is readily activated to a free radical by incident light, it may serve to eliminate genetically damaged cells by a phototoxic mechanism.

Not all the effects of pigmentation are advantageous. Melanin has been demonstrated to react with DNA and produce reactive oxygen species after UVA radiation [2]. There is no doubt that pigmentation increases the heat load in hot climates, so that black people absorb 30% more heat from sunlight than white people, although this factor may be offset by more profuse sweating [3,4]. In addition, in cold climates, pale skin has the advantage that heat loss by radiation is reduced.

A further disadvantage of pigmentation is that it hinders synthesis of vitamin D, so that in areas where nutrition is poor and sun exposure limited black children are more liable to rickets than white children. Thus, loss of pigmentation may facilitate vitamin D synthesis in temperate climates. It might be presumed that the retention of pigment in Arctic latitudes, while providing a protection against snow glare, is only permitted by natural selection because of the high-fat diet in these regions.

Since pigmentation appears to be not entirely advantageous to life in the tropics, other hypotheses about its biological significance have been advanced. For example, Wassermann [5,6] suggested that the major adaptation of black people to tropical Africa is in the ability to survive malaria, multiple parasites and tropical diseases under the hazards of intense solar radiation and, more often than not, poor nutrition. He suggests that diseases, not climatic conditions, are the primary selective factors, and lists evidence that black Africans, in comparison with white people, show increased reticuloendothelial activity and increased serum γ-globulin fractions. These features are inversely related to the size and activity of the adrenal cortex, suggesting that the increased secretion of MSH and ACTH by black people and the consequent enhanced melanogenesis and pigmentation might be secondary to a relative adrenocortical insufficiency.

Classification of disorders of melanin pigmentation

Disorders of melanin pigmentation can be divided on morphological grounds into two types. The first is hypermelanosis, where there is an increased amount of melanin in the skin. This excess may be confined to the epidermis, when the skin appears browner than normal, or it may be present in the dermis, producing a slaty-grey or blue appearance. The second type is hypomelanosis, where there is a lack of pigment in the skin, which therefore appears white or lighter than the normal colour. Amelanosis is the term applied

when there is a total lack of melanin in the skin. Hypermelanosis and hypomelanosis can be generalised and diffuse, or may be localised and circumscribed. Sometimes, localised areas may have a segmental or dermatomal pattern. The term 'depigmentation' is used to describe a loss of pre-existing pigment from the skin. Leukoderma is a white skin that may be congenital or acquired and can be due to a variety of aetiological factors. Examination of the skin with a source of long-wave UV light, for example Wood's light, is often helpful in localising abnormal variations in melanin pigmentation in the skin and as an aid to the diagnosis of various disorders [1].

Changes in pigmentation can arise in a number of ways and can be due to a variety of genetic and environmental factors. It is also pertinent to consider non-melanin pigmentation as a cause of cutaneous colour changes, as discussed at the end of this chapter.

Hypermelanosis similarly can be due to many factors, both genetic and acquired. It can be due to an increased number of melanocytes in the skin such as occurs in the dermal melanocytoses: the naevus of Ota, the naevus of Ito and the Mongolian spot. Many of the hypermelanotic disorders are due to an increase in melanogenesis due to genetic factors. Some may be induced by UV light, hormones and chemical compounds. Finally, the degradation of melanosomes may vary in different disorders of pigmentation.

Constitutive pigmentation, human pigmentation and the response to sun exposure

Genetic factors play the primary role in determining the degree of pigmentation that is normal for the individual. Variation in skin pigmentation is not due to differences in the number of melanocytes but is explained by differences in melanocyte structure and function; melanogenic activity, the size and number of melanosomes, the type of melanin deposited onto melanosomes, and the donation of mature melanosomes to adjacent keratinocytes all contribute to the resulting colour of the skin and are genetically determined [1]. Thus, constitutive skin colour as well as how the colour changes in response to exposure to sunlight are both genetically determined and show relatively little variation within different racial groups. There is, however, marked variation in human skin colour between the main racial groupings ranging from white (previously known as 'Caucasoid'), through lightly pigmented (Asian and Oriental) to black (previously known as 'Negroid' and 'Australoid' and some Asian races). Racial differences in melanocyte morphology and function are apparent, but there is little interracial variation in the density of melanocytes at a particular skin site. Ultrastructural studies have shown that melanosomes in white skin are small and tend to be in membrane-bound complexes of three or more within the keratinocyte [2]. The ellipsoidal melanosomes of indigenous Australians and black people are larger, about 1 μm in length, and tend to be distributed as singlets rather than being aggregated. These larger melanosomes can be found intact in the stratum corneum. The melanosome complexes present in white people show degradative changes even in the basal layer of the epidermis and are presumably broken up by lysosomal enzymes [3]. Whether melanosomes are individually dispersed or aggregated in melanosomal complexes appears to depend on the size of the melanosome [2].

Table 86.1 Classification of sun-reactive skin types.

Skin type	Sun sensitivity	Pigmentary response
I	Very sensitive, always burn easily	Little or no tan
II	Very sensitive, always burn	Minimal tan
III	Sensitive, burn moderately	Tan gradually (light brown)
IV	Moderately sensitive, burn minimally	Tan easily (brown)
V	Minimally sensitive, rarely burn	Tan darkly (dark brown)
VI	Insensitive, never burn	Deeply pigmented (black)

Melanin in the skin exerts its photoprotective effect by reducing the penetration of UV light through the epidermis and by quenching the reactive oxygen radicals that contribute to sun-induced DNA damage [4]. The superior photoprotection of the black epidermis is due not only to its increased melanin content but also to melanogenic activity, the size and number of melanosomes, the type of melanin deposited into melanosomes and the donation of mature melanosomes to adjacent keratinocytes. A classification of sun-reactive skin types based on sunburn and tanning history has been in widespread use since its introduction (Table 86.1) [5]. Two types of pigmentation of the skin in humans occur in response to sun exposure. The first is immediate pigment darkening (IPD), sometimes also referred to as the Meirowsky phenomenon. This is best observed in those with hyperpigmented skins and is most effectively induced by long-wave UV light (UVA). It is transient and, although rapidly induced, soon fades. The second is the increased pigmentation that follows the erythemal response. This is the delayed tanning reaction and can be seen 48–72 h after skin exposure to UV light.

ACQUIRED HYPERMELANOSIS

Physiological hypermelanosis (tanning in response to UV radiation)

Introduction and general description

Tanning is the term used to describe the pigmentary response of the skin following exposure to UV radiation. Tanning occurs in three distinct phases: IPD, persistent pigment darkening (PPD) and delayed tanning. IPD occurs in response to low doses of UVA and manifests as grey-brown pigmentation. It appears within minutes of UV exposure and typically fades within 10–20 min. IPD is believed to result from oxidation and redistribution of pre-existing melanin. Higher doses of UVA induce PPD which persists for 2–24 h. This pigmentation is brown and is also caused by oxidation and redistribution of pre-existing melanin. Delayed tanning involves the formation of new melanin due to an increase in the number of melanocytes and increased melanocyte activity. Both UVA and UVB are able to induce delayed tanning, but UVB is more effective. Delayed tanning becomes visible about 72 h after UV exposure and persists for 1–2 weeks before gradually fading as keratinocytes are shed from the skin surface.

Tanning and DNA damage are closely associated. Repeated suberythemal doses of UV light induce tanning but have also been shown to induce DNA damage [1]. Tanning salon exposure has also been demonstrated to induce cyclobutane pyrimidine dimers and p53 protein expression in epidermal keratinocytes, changes linked with the early stages of cutaneous carcinogenesis [2]. It is widely believed by laypeople that a tan provides good protection against sunburn [3]. However, tanned skin has been shown to be less effective against formation of DNA photoproducts than constitutive pigmentation [3] and has a sun protection factor of 3–5 at best. Population-based surveys reveal that tanning remains popular, particularly with the young, and that episodes of sunburn remain common [4,5].

Facial melanoses

Hypermelanosis involving predominantly the face and neck is relatively common and often presents a complex diagnostic problem. Several more or less well-defined clinical syndromes can be recognised, but many transitional forms defy classification. The causes of the pigmentation are often obscure.

Genetic and racial factors are important, the increased pigmentation occurring more frequently in those with dark skins, especially those of Middle Eastern or Asian descent. Endocrine factors play a major role in melasma and are implicated to some degree in other melanoses. External agents (light and photodynamic chemicals) are essential factors in the occupational melanoses but are also implicated in photocontact dermatitis (Riehl melanosis), and erythromelanosis and poikiloderma of Civatte. Other unknown factors are certainly involved and wide individual variation in susceptibility must be postulated.

Cosmetics may occasionally cause facial melanosis. Facial melanosis is also a conspicuous feature of addisonian pigmentation.

Melasma

Definition and nomenclature

Melasma is the most common cause of facial melanosis and is manifested by hyperpigmented macules on the face that become more pronounced after sun exposure (Figure 86.8) [1,2].

> **Synonyms and inclusions**
> - Mask of pregnancy
> - Chloasma

Epidemiology
Incidence and prevalence

Common. Increased pigmentation is almost invariable in pregnancy and is most marked in brunettes (skin types III–V) [3]. Melasma is frequently seen in women on oral contraceptives.

Age

Mostly starts between the ages of 20 and 40 years. Dependent on pregnancy or use of oral contraceptives [4,5].

Sex

Females are more affected than males. Up to 10% of cases of melasma occur in men (Figure 86.9).

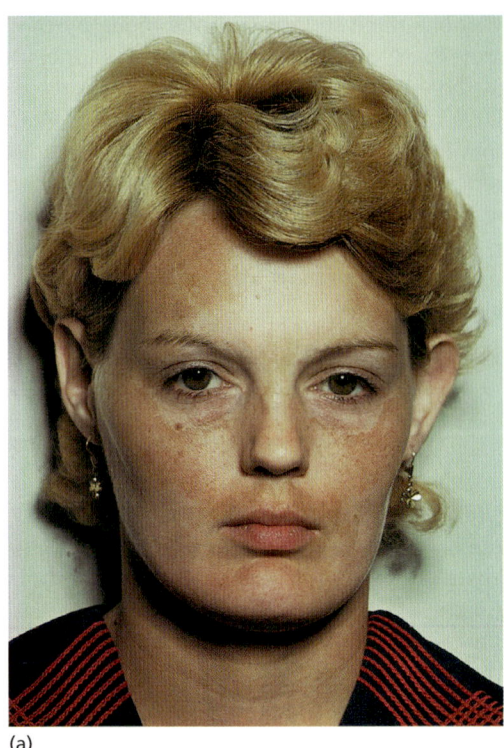

(a)

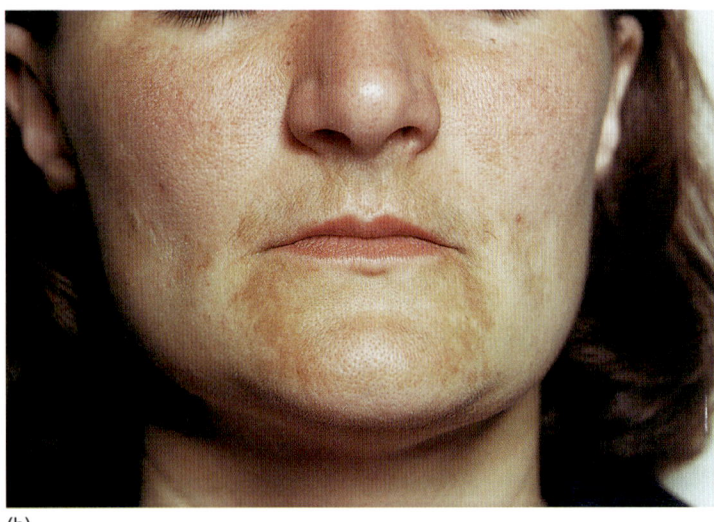

(b)

Figure 86.8 (a, b) Melasma in two female patients.

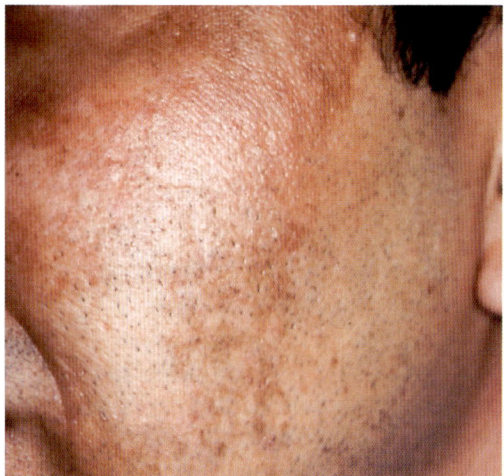

Figure 86.9 Melasma in an adult male from the Indian subcontinent.

Ethnicity

More common in light brown skin types, particularly Latin American people and those from the Middle East or Asia. There is an important geographic and racial difference illustrated by a prevalence of 8.8% in Latino females in the southern USA and up to 40% in South Asia [3].

Pathophysiology
Predisposing factors

Several factors have been linked to melasma, among which UV exposure and hormonal factors appear to be the most significant. Local or diffuse hyperpigmentation can be seen in a subset of women, probably due to these hormonal factors. Pregnancy and oral contraceptives have been linked to increased skin pigmentation. It has been speculated that this is due to increased levels of oestrogen and progesterone stimulating the activity of melanocytes [6]. Melasma is common in the third trimester of pregnancy when levels of oestrogen, progesterone and MSH are elevated.

Many cases are attributed to pregnancy or the combined oral contraceptive pill [4,5]. In the context of pregnancy, melasma is regarded as a normal physiological change, along with darkening of the nipples and linea nigra. It is not uncommon during the years of reproductive activity and has been attributed, without acceptable proof, to a variety of ovarian disorders. The rarity of melasma in postmenopausal women on oestrogen-containing hormone replacement therapy and the fact that men are occasionally affected suggest that oestrogen alone is not the causative agent.

Pathology

The mechanism is not fully elucidated, and although MSH may be involved, it plays a minor part. The plasma concentration of MSH is normal both in patients with idiopathic melasma [7] and in those with melasma attributable to oral contraceptives [8]. Oestrogens and progesterone are involved in the increased pigmentation but other factors are also implicated [9]. The number of melanocytes is not increased but they become enlarged and more dendritic, suggesting a hypermetabolic state. This is reflected by increased melanin deposition in the epidermis and dermis [9,10].

Despite light microscopic, ultrastructural and immunofluorescence studies, the condition remains an enigma [1]. An endocrine mechanism is postulated but the cause of melasma is unknown. A vascular component has also been studied after successful results were observed using tranexamic acid and laser/light therapy targeting the skin vasculature [11]. Endothelin-1 produced by microvascular endothelial cells induces microphthalmia-associated transcription factor phosphorylation and increases tyrosinase activity, stimulating melanogenesis [12].

Genetics

No specific genes have as yet been identified but a family history is common (around 30%). The clinical manifestations are the same in sporadic and familial cases and are seen particularly in those who tan readily when exposed to bright sunlight [13].

Environmental factors

Exacerbated by sun exposure, combined oral contraceptives and other hormone treatments.

Clinical features

Presentation

Melasma is seen predominantly in women. Hypermelanosis affects mainly the upper lip, the malar regions, forehead and chin and may be associated with darkening of the nipples, the linea alba to form the linea nigra, and anogenital skin. Affected skin is brown in colour. The pigmentary changes are usually bilateral and are frequently symmetrical.

Differential diagnosis

See Box 86.3.

Box 86.3 Differential diagnosis of acquired hyperpigmentation

(a) Acquired diffuse hyperpigmentation
- Endocrinopathies
- Metabolic conditions
- Metal-induced non-melanin pigmentation
- Neoplastic or tumoral conditions
- Nutritional conditions
- Physical agents
- Progressive systemic sclerosis
- Toxin- or drug-induced

(b) Acquired localised hyperpigmentation
- Ephelides[a,b]
- Erythromelanosis follicularis faciei et colli[a]
- Exogenous ochronosis[a]
- Fixed drug eruption[a]
- Frictional melanosis[a] (Figure 86.10)
- Iatrogenic[a]
- Lentiginosis[a]
- Melasma[a]
- Poikiloderma of Civatte[a]
- Riehl melanosis[a]

(c) Secondary hyperpigmentation (postinfectious, postinflammatory, post-traumatic)
- Eczema[a,b]
- Lichen planus[a,b]
- Lupus erythematosus[a,b]
- Macular amyloidosis[b]
- Morphoea[a]
- Erythema dyschronicum persistans[b]
- Pityriasis versicolor[b]

(d) Disseminated
- Endogenous ochronosis[a,b]
- Idiopathic eruptive macular pigmentation[b]
- Lichen planus pigmentosus[b]
- Mastocytoses[a,b]
- Phytophotodermatitis[a]

[a] Limited surface areas affected.
[b] Larger surface areas can be affected.

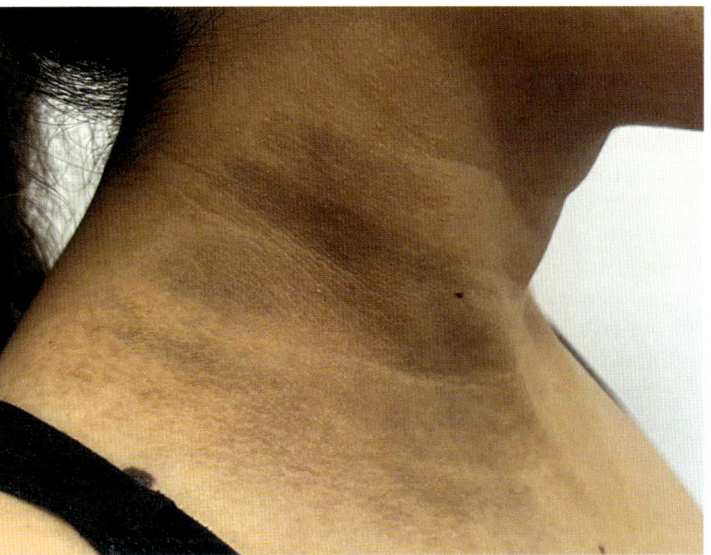

Figure 86.10 Frictional hypermelanosis affecting the neck of a Mexican woman. Courtesy of Dr Julio Salas.

Classification of severity

Cosmetic problem.

Disease course and prognosis

Variable. The pigmentation usually fades after parturition but may persist for months or years. It is noted by some women to be more obvious just prior to menstruation [14]. The pigmentation takes a long time to fade after discontinuing oral contraception and, as after pregnancy, it may never fade completely.

Investigations

No investigations necessary.

Wood's light examination can be helpful to identify the depth of the melanin pigmentation and determine the type of melasma (epidermal, dermal or mixed). Epidermal melasma normally appears light brown and shows enhanced colour contrast with Wood's light examination. Dermal melasma often appears slightly grey or bluish on gross examination and shows less colour contrast with Wood's light. Categorisation of the type of melasma is useful because it may help guide treatment options and patient expectations since dermal melasma is generally less responsive to therapy, especially to topical modalities [1].

Management

Treatment of melasma can be difficult due to the refractory and recurrent nature of the condition. Daily application of sunscreen and avoidance of strong sun exposure are the cornerstones of long-term melasma treatment.

Different skin depigmentation formulations can be used and contain one or several active compounds. Hydroquinone is the most extensively studied depigmenting agent for the treatment of melasma. It inhibits tyrosinase, an enzyme critical to the pigment producing pathway in melanocytes. Topical retinoid therapy has also been used as monotherapy for melasma but with only moderate efficacy [15,**16**].

Triple combination therapy, composed of hydroquinone, a retinoid and a corticosteroid, is a highly effective and safe treatment for melasma. A corticosteroid was introduced to this treatment to reduce inflammation as it is a side effect of both hydroquinone and tretinoin. In addition to this advantage, it also inhibits melanocyte metabolism [16].

Pregnancy-related melasma tends to improve spontaneously postpartum and treatment may not be necessary.

First line
A variety of topical treatments are effective at lightening melasma. Triple therapy with topical hydroquinone, tretinoin and corticosteroid (e.g. hydroquinone 4%, fluocinolone acetonide 0.01% and tretinoin 0.05%) is preferred [16,17]. Alternative, dual therapy (e.g. hydroquinone 2% plus glycolic acid 10%) may be used but can cause severe irritation [16]. Response to monotherapy is generally disappointing and continuous long-term hydroquinone therapy (>1 year) should be avoided because of the risk of exogenous ochronosis [18].

Treatment ladder for melasma

First line
- Sun protection/broad spectrum sunscreen (SPF >30), preferably also blocking visible light
- Change oral contraceptive to an alternative low-oestrogen preparation or change to a different form of contraception
- Avoidance of scented cosmetic products and phototoxic drugs
- Triple therapy with topical hydroquinone, tretinoin and corticosteroid compound cream

Second line
- Chemical peels (e.g. glycolic acid), alone or in combination with topical treatment [15,16]
- Azelaic acid (15–20%) in monotherapy or combination of azelaic acid 20% and tretinoin 0.05% [17,18]
- Topical (2–5%) or intradermal injected tranexamic acid [19]
- Oral tranexamic acid (500–1500 mg/day; most commonly 250 mg twice daily) after excluding risk factors for thromboembolic disease [19]

Third line
- Laser therapy [20]
- Intense pulsed light therapy, adjuvant to topical treatment
- Dermabrasion
- Topical liquiritin [21]
- Topical rucinol [22]
- Kojic acid, in monotherapy or in combination with hydroquinone [23,24]

Resources

Patient resources
Patient information leaflet: https://cdn.bad.org.uk/uploads/2021/12/29200258/Melasma-Updated-March-2018-Lay-Reviewed-March-2018.pdf (last accessed March 2023).

Photocontact facial melanosis

Definition and nomenclature
Facial melanosis attributable to phototoxic reaction to skin contact with photoactive agents.

Synonyms and inclusions
- Riehl melanosis
- Melanodermatitis toxica
- Pigmented cosmetic dermatitis

Epidemiology
Age
Middle age.

Sex
The condition is more frequent in women.

Predisposing factors
Fragrances and tar derivatives are suspected to be the cause [1]. An outbreak of photocontact facial melanosis in Japan was attributed to contact dermatitis to cosmetic ingredients and prompted the term 'pigmented cosmetic dermatitis' for this condition [2].

Pathology
In the early stages, there is liquefaction degeneration of the basal layer of the epidermis and a perivascular or band-like dermal infiltrate with pigmentary incontinence. Later, the epidermis appears normal but many melanophages are present in the upper dermis [3]. Ultrastructural studies show intercellular and intracellular oedema of keratinocytes and a multilayered basal lamina, as well as many melanophages in the dermis [3].

Environmental factors
Cosmetic and textile materials.

Clinical features
History
A distinctive pattern of grey-brown facial pigmentation was first described by Riehl in Vienna between 1916 and 1920 [4]. Riehl attributed this pigmentation to contact with noxious substances or to wartime living conditions. It was subsequently seen in Europe and Asia during and after the Second World War and has also occurred in Argentina [5] and in the South African Bantu [6].

Presentation
Brownish-grey pigmentation develops quite rapidly over the greater part of the face but is more intense on the forehead and temples. Smaller pigmented macules, often perifollicular, lie beyond the indefinite margin. The pigmentation may extend to the chest, neck and scalp, and occasionally involves the hands and forearms. Horny plugs fill the follicles and there may be some scaling.

Differential diagnosis
See Box 86.3.

PART 8: SPECIFIC CUTANEOUS STRUCTURES

Disease course and prognosis

Gradual improvement if the causal substance is avoided.

Investigations

Patch testing.

Treatment ladder for photocontact facial melanosis

First line

- Where a contact cause can be identified and avoided, there follows a slow improvement over many months
- Sun protection

Second line

- Slow improvement may be expected with the use of hydroquinone 2–5% plus tretinoin or glycolic acid [7]

Third line

- Intense pulsed light [8]

Poikiloderma of Civatte

Definition and nomenclature

Poikiloderma of Civatte presents as mottled pigmentation (atrophy, telangiectasia, hyper- and hypopigmentation) which typically appears on the sides of the face and neck and on the upper anterior chest after years of repeated UV exposure (Figure 86.11) [1].

Synonyms and inclusions

- Erythromelanosis interfollicularis colli

Epidemiology

Incidence and prevalence

Unclear as mild cases are underreported.

Age

Age 30–50 years.

Sex

Female predominance.

Ethnicity

Predominance in fair-skinned individuals.

Predisposing factors

Exposure to light and photodynamic substances in cosmetics are influencing factors [2].

Pathology

Poikiloderma of Civatte is histopathologically characterised by thinning of the spinous layer, hydropic degeneration of the basal cell layer, presence of melanophages in the papillary dermis and

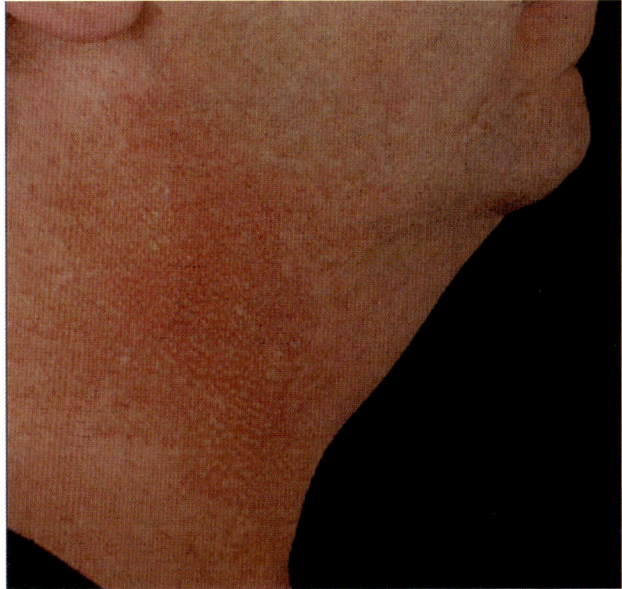

(a)

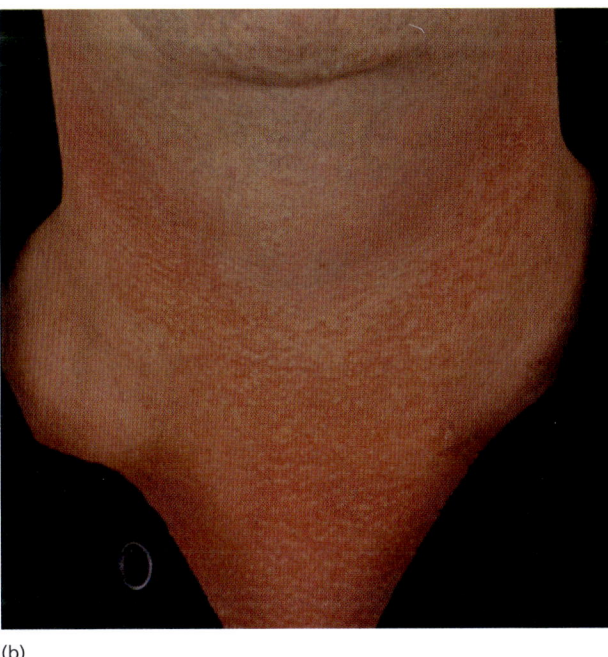

(b)

Figure 86.11 (a, b) Poikiloderma of Civatte: showing submental and submandibular sparing on the neck of a 43-year-old man.

dilatation of the papillary dermal capillaries. These findings are common to any case of poikiloderma [3].

Environmental factors

- Solar radiation.
- Phototoxic or photoallergic reactions to chemicals in fragrances or cosmetics.

Clinical features

History

This characteristic pattern of reticulate hyperpigmentation of the face and neck was first reported in 1923 by Civatte [1].

PART 8: SPECIFIC CUTANEOUS STRUCTURES

Presentation

Poikilodermatous changes develop symmetrically on the sides of the face, neck and upper aspect of the chest with hyperpigmentation, telangiectasia and dermal atrophy. The submandibular and submental areas are spared thus implicating sunlight in the pathogenesis of this condition (Figure 86.11b). Milder forms are common and few patients seek medical advice. The condition is mostly asymptomatic, although some patients experience itching, burning and flushing.

Differential diagnosis

- Erythromelanosis follicularis faciei et colli.
- Melasma.

Classification of severity

Cosmetic problem.

Disease course and prognosis

Slowly progressive and irreversible.

Investigations

Patch testing can be useful if induction by allergen is suspected [3,4].

Treatment ladder for poikiloderma of Civatte

First line
- Photoprotection with a high SPF sunscreen
- Avoiding perfumes

Second line
- Intense pulsed light [5]
- Laser therapy with the tunable dye laser [6]

Erythromelanosis follicularis of the face and neck

Definition and nomenclature

Erythromelanosis follicularis of the face and neck presents with a reddish-brown discoloration affecting the preauricular and maxillary regions, in some cases spreading to the temples and lateral sides of the neck and trunk, with symmetrical distribution and sharp demarcation from normal skin.

Synonyms and inclusions
- Erythromelanosis follicularis faciei et colli

Epidemiology

Incidence and prevalence

Unclear as mild cases are underrecognised and underreported.

Age

Peak age of onset in the second decade of life.

Sex

Affects both sexes, but with male predominance.

Ethnicity

Affects all races, but more frequent in Asians.

Associated diseases

May be associated with keratosis pilaris.

Pathophysiology

Pathology

Histologically, there is slight hyperkeratosis and hyperpigmentation of the basal layer. The hair follicles are enlarged and contain lamellar horny masses. The sebaceous glands are also enlarged. The epidermis overlying the affected follicle is flattened and contains excess melanin. In the dermis, an inconspicuous lymphocytic infiltrate surrounds dilated vessels.

Genetics

Few familial reports.

Clinical features

History

This syndrome, of unknown origin, was originally described in Japan by Kitamura *et al.* in 1960 [1].

Presentation

The clinical picture is distinctive, characterised by a triad of hyperpigmentation, follicular plugging and erythema with or without telangiectasia, affecting the lateral aspects of the cheeks and in some cases the neck (Figure 86.12) [1–5]. It has been suggested that it is a subtype of keratosis pilaris [7]. A background of reddish-brown pigmentation and telangiectasia is studded with pale follicular papules. The hairs are lost from the majority of affected vellus hair follicles but terminal hair follicles of the scalp and beard are less conspicuously affected. The pigmentation involves the skin in front of, beneath and behind the ear, extending to the side of the neck. It spreads slowly, is persistent and is not influenced by treatment. The distribution and lack of clinical follicular keratosis or scarring readily distinguish erythromelanosis from other forms of keratosis pilaris and from other facial melanoses.

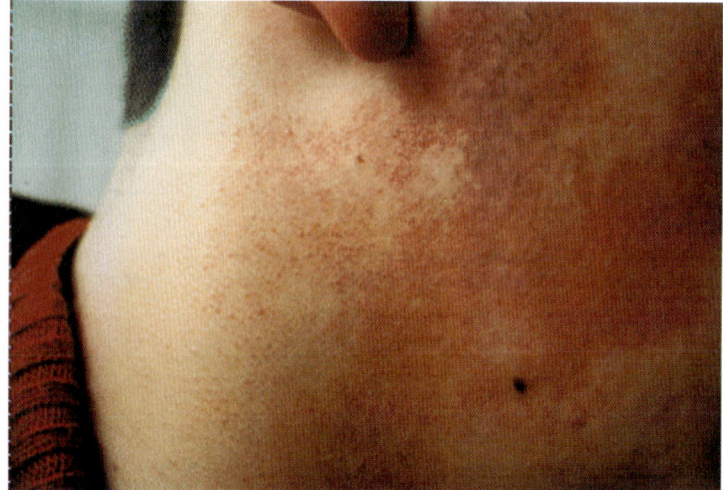

Figure 86.12 Erythromelanosis follicularis of the face and neck. Reproduced from Ermertcan *et al.* 2006 [6] with permission of John Wiley & Sons.

Differential diagnosis

- Keratosis pilaris and its variants (Chapter 85).
- Keratosis pilaris rubra.
- Melasma.
- Poikiloderma of Civatte.
- Corticosteroid-induced rosacea.
- Actinic telangiectasia.

Response to therapy is generally poor and prone to relapse.

Treatment ladder for erythromelanosis follicularis of the face and neck

First line
- A variety of topical keratolytic therapeutics have been advocated, including urea cream (10–20%), ammonium lactate lotion (12%) and tretinoin cream (0.05–0.1%) [5,8]

Second line
- Salicylic acid peels and glycolic acid peels

Third line
- Isotretinoin (0.1–1 mg/kg/day)
- Laser treatment of the background erythema or hyperpigmentation
- Topical tacalcitol [9]

Peribuccal pigmentation of Brocq

Definition and nomenclature

Peribuccal pigmentation of Brocq is a diffuse brownish-red pigmentation around the mouth but sparing a narrow perioral ring [1–3].

Synonyms and inclusions
- Pigmented perioral erythema
- Erythrosis pigmentosa mediofacialis

Epidemiology

Age

Middle age.

Sex

This condition occurs predominantly in middle-aged women and has only rarely been reported in men.

Predisposing factors

A photodynamic substance in cosmetics is probably responsible.

Clinical features

History

It was Brocq in 1923 who first reported a case of perioral hyperpigmentation in a clinical pattern that now bears his name [1].

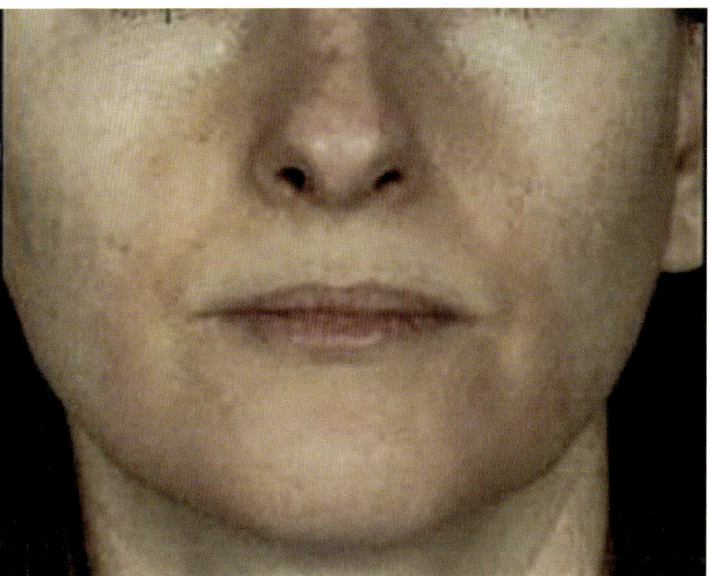

Figure 86.13 Peribuccal pigmentation of Brocq. Courtesy of Dr Luciano Schiazza.

Presentation

Diffuse brownish-red pigmentation develops symmetrically around the mouth but spares a narrow perioral ring. It may extend up the centre of the face to the forehead and in some cases there are well-defined patches of pigmentation over the angles of the jaw and the temples (Figure 86.13).

Differential diagnosis

A similar postinflammatory hyperpigmentation is seen in some patients with perioral dermatitis and may be the result of topical steroid therapy [2].

Classification of severity

Cosmetic problem.

Disease course and prognosis

The erythematous component, and hence the intensity of the pigmentation, may fluctuate over short periods. The pigmentation is usually persistent but tends to fade gradually if the cause is eliminated.

Ephelides

Synonyms and inclusions
- Freckles

Freckles or ephelides are very common and first appear at about the age of 5 years as light-brown pigmented macules on the light-exposed skin of fair-skinned individuals, typically of Celtic (Scottish, Irish, Welsh) origin with red or blond hair, fair skin and blue eyes (Figure 86.14) [1]. Freckling is significantly associated with certain polymorphisms of the melanocortin 1 receptor gene [2,3] and is transmitted in an autosomal dominant fashion without

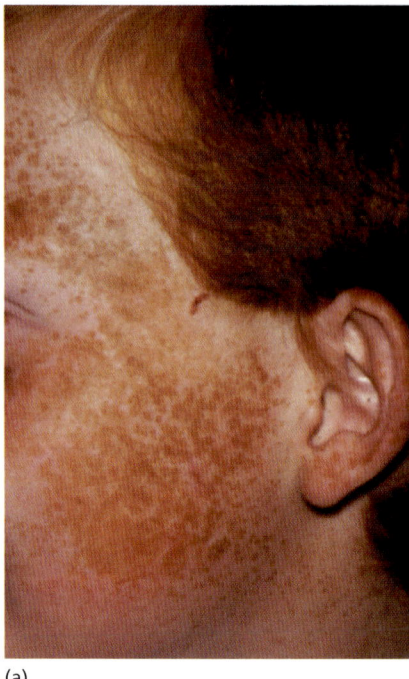

(a)

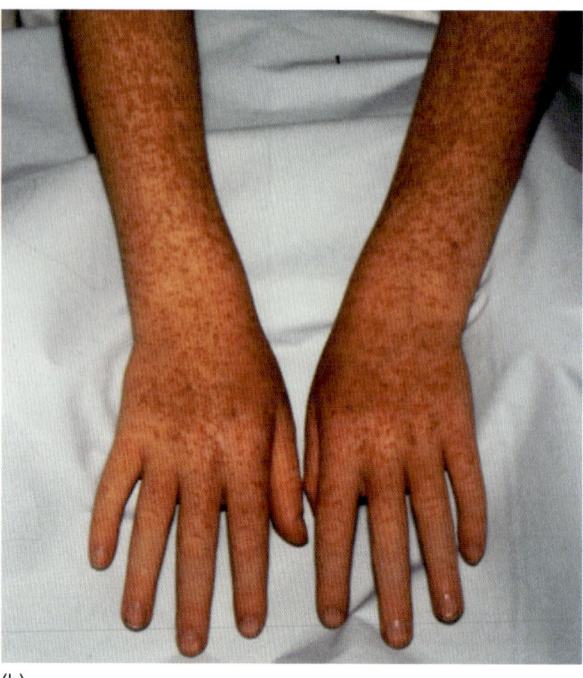

(b)

Figure 86.14 (a, b) Freckles in an 11-year-old boy.

associated abnormalities. Several pigmented skin disorders are, however, associated with freckles, including hereditary symmetrical dyschromatosis, xeroderma pigmentosum and cutaneous malignant melanoma [4].

Freckles are a feature of a number of inherited and acquired disorders. These include xeroderma pigmentosum [5], neurofibromatosis and progeria. The lesions in the various forms of lentiginosis (see later) must also be differentiated. Their distribution and the lack of relationship to light exposure should be noted. They are discussed in more detail in Chapter 131.

Treatment ladder for ephelides

First line
• Broad spectrum sunscreen

Lentiginosis

The histological and clinical features of lentigo, together with other lesions in which the number of melanocytes is increased, are fully described in Chapter 131. A lentigo is a benign pigmented macule in which there is an increased number of melanocytes. The term 'lentiginosis' is applied either when lentigines are present in exceptionally large numbers or when they occur in a distinctive distribution. Genetic syndromes of which lentiginosis is a component are described in Chapter 68. The following isolated or sporadic forms of lentiginosis are recognised.

Generalised lentiginosis

Lentigines are commonly multiple but appear singly or in small crops at irregular intervals from infancy onwards. Their pathogenesis is unknown and in the great majority of cases no genetic factor is demonstrable.

Unilateral lentiginosis (segmental lentiginosis, zosteriform lentiginosis)

Unilateral lentigines occur on one side of the body in specific patterns [1]. In contrast to naevus spilus, uniteral lentiginosis lacks the underlying café-au-lait macule. Cases have been reported with and without associated neurological abnormalities [2–4]. The lentigines can be zosteriform and occur in a dermatome-like or Blaschkolinear distribution [5–8]. These cases are usually without central nervous system abnormalities and are naevoid. Lentigines have also been reported within naevoid hypopigmentation [9]. Treatment can be challenging although successful laser treatment (e.g. QS Nd:YAG laser) has been reported [10].

Inherited patterned lentiginosis in black people [1]

O'Neill and James reported generalised lentiginosis in 10 adult black patients, with onset in childhood; seven showed familial clustering, suggesting autosomal dominant inheritance [1]. Distribution of the lentigines included the face, lips, extremities, buttocks, palms and soles, but not mucosal surfaces. The condition is extremely common in light-skinned black people, especially in combination with reddish-brown hair [2]. There are no known associated abnormalities.

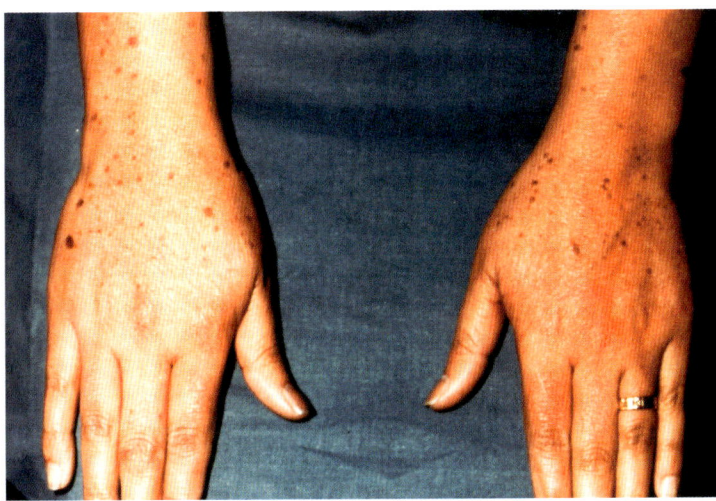

Figure 86.15 Eruptive lentiginosis: 4-month history of widespread eruption of lentigines over the neck, trunk and limbs in a healthy 49-year-old female. Note lentigines in different stages of evolution, particularly on the right wrist and the forearm.

Eruptive lentiginoses [1,2]

Widespread occurrence of very large numbers of lentigines that develop rapidly over the course of a few months to years is typical of eruptive lentiginosis (Figure 86.15). It is well recognised in adolescents and young adults who show no evidence of systemic abnormalities but has also been linked to treatment with cancer chemotherapeutic agents and to immunosuppression, particularly in transplant recipients. In 1956, Degos and Carteaud described telangiectatic papules that darkened and evolved into depressed scaly lentigines [1]. In spite of the misleading title of their report, Eady *et al.* reported two patients in whom very large numbers of lentigines developed over 2 years: histology and electron microscopy confirmed the diagnosis of eruptive lentiginosis [2].

PUVA lentigines [1–5]

These pigmented macules are a common complication of PUVA (psoralen and UVA) therapy occurring on treatment-exposed skin [1–3]. They are discussed in detail in Chapter 131. There is a dose effect with a tendency to a greater number of lentigines in those who have had more therapy [3]. They vary in appearance and may be numerous in number and small in size. Occasionally, larger irregular lentigines are seen, some with a stellate configuration [3] (Figure 131.7). PUVA lentigines are usually permanent and show little tendency to remit. A less common clinical pattern is localisation of lentigines to sites previously affected by psoriasis, creating an appearance not unlike a naevus spilus [2]. The histology is that of a lentigo. The melanocytes are hypertrophic and some may be cytologically atypical [3]. Similar melanocytic macules have been reported following use of a sunbed [4]. PUVA lentigines can sometimes look quite alarming and should be differentiated from melanoma. Melanomas, however, tend to have more variation in colour density within the lesion than in lentigo. PUVA has also been reported to cause hyperpigmentation of the nails [5].

Hypermelanosis due to endocrine disorders

For a full discussion of the effects of endocrine disorders on the skin see Chapter 150. Endocrine disorders which may induce hypermelanosis are described briefly here.

Addison disease

Introduction and general description
Hyperpigmentation may be a cutaneous manifestation of Addison disease. The discoloration in Addison disease is typically diffuse with accentuation in sun-exposed areas (Figure 86.16) [1–4].

Pathophysiology
Pathology
The hypermelanosis is the result of increased secretion of melanotrophic hormones by the pituitary. Affected patients have elevated plasma levels of β-MSH-like immunoreactivity [6]. Absence of hypermelanosis in Addison disease was explained in a single case by a high degree of melanosome degradation in secondary lysosomes [1].

Clinical features
History
Addison disease was first described by Thomas Addison in 1855.

Presentation
Increased pigmentation is such a well-known feature of Addison disease that its absence may significantly delay diagnosis and endanger life [1,2]. When present, the hyperpigmentation of Addison disease is typically diffuse and is most intense on areas exposed to light [3]. It is also accentuated in the flexures, at sites of pressure and friction, and in the creases of palms and soles [3]. Normally pigmented areas, such as the nipples and genital skin, darken. Pigmentation of the buccal mucous membrane is often present, and the conjunctival and vaginal mucous membranes may also be involved [3]. However, less distinctive patterns of pigmentation are not exceptional and, in any unexplained cases of hypermelanosis, adrenal function should be carefully evaluated. Similarly, patients without hyperpigmentation but with other features suggesting Addison disease should have adrenal function assessed. Addison disease may be associated with generalised vitiligo [3,7].

Differential diagnosis
- Acquired diffuse hyperpigmentation: see Box 86.3a.
- Acquired pigmentary disorders of oral mucosa.
- Iatrogenic.
- Irritative (e.g. smokers' melanosis).
- Hyperplastic or neoplastic processes.

Resources

Patient resources
https://www.addisons.org.uk (last accessed March 2023).

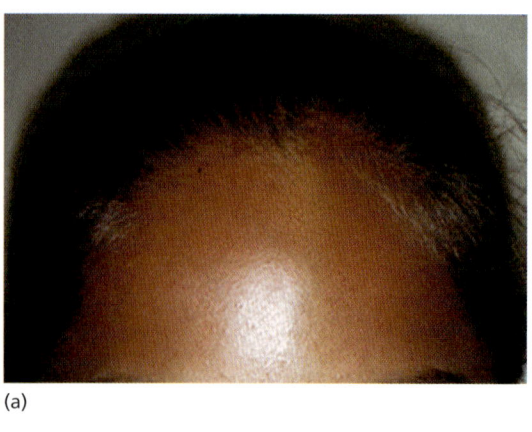
(a)

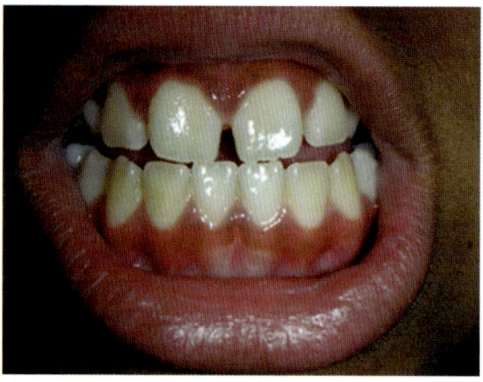
(b)

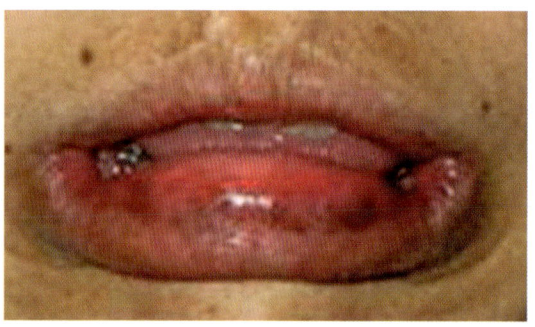
(c)

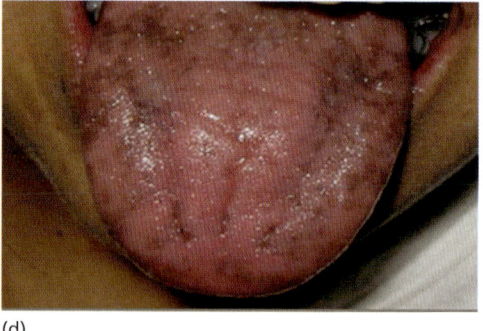
(d)

Figure 86.16 Addison disease: diffuse hypermelanosis of the skin (a) and gingivae (b) in a 13-year-old girl and of the labial mucosa (c) and tongue (d) of a 15-year-old girl. Both girls presented with fatigue, malaise, nausea and weight loss [7]. Reproduced from Burk *et al.* [5] with permission of John Wiley & Sons.

PART 8: SPECIFIC CUTANEOUS STRUCTURES

Acromegaly

Definition

Acromegaly is an acquired condition caused by excessive growth hormone production leading to gradual body disfigurement.

Clinical features

Pigmentation of an addisonian pattern is present in some cases of acromegaly and may be a striking feature [1,2].

Differential diagnosis

Acquired diffuse hyperpigmentation: see Box 86.3a.

Management

Cutaneous signs rapidly respond to hormonal control, with partial regression.

Topical therapy including tretinoin and adapalene creams can be used to ameliorate the cutaneous manifestations.

Resources

Patient resources

http://www.acromegalycommunity.com (last accessed March 2023).

Cushing syndrome

Definition

Cushing syndrome is caused by excessive amounts of cortisol leading to obesity, a moon-shaped face and increased fat deposition in the neck area. If caused by endogenous hypersecretion of cortisol it is known as Cushing disease.

Pathophysiology
Pathology

Cushing syndrome is the overproduction of ACTH by a pituitary corticotrophic adenoma or an ectopic non-pituitary tumour.

Environmental factors

Excessive corticoid intake.

Clinical features
Presentation

Pigmentation of an addisonian pattern has been noted in about 10% of reported patients with Cushing syndrome. It is an indication of secretion of ACTH and β-MSH by the pituitary and suggests the presence of a pituitary tumour. After adrenalectomy, progressive hypermelanosis develops in a proportion of patients (about 10%), in spite of adequate hormone replacement therapy. Only in half of these patients is the sella turcica enlarged [1,2]. These patients with Nelson syndrome (= post adrenalectomy syndrome) [3] show marked hypermelanosis (Figures 86.7 and 86.17), with the mucous membranes also being involved. The hair is often darker and there are sometimes multiple lentigines and longitudinal pigmented bands in the nails. High levels of both β-MSH and ACTH are found in the plasma, with a degree of clinical hyperpigmentation correlating well with the quantity of β-MSH in the plasma [4].

Differential diagnosis

Acquired diffuse hyperpigmentation: see Box 86.3a.

ACTH administration

A small proportion of patients treated with ACTH in high dosages (120 units/day) develop pigmentation of addisonian pattern [1,2].

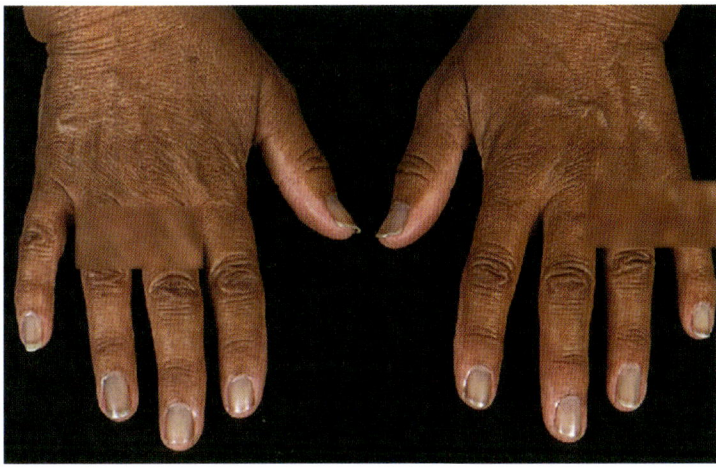

(a)

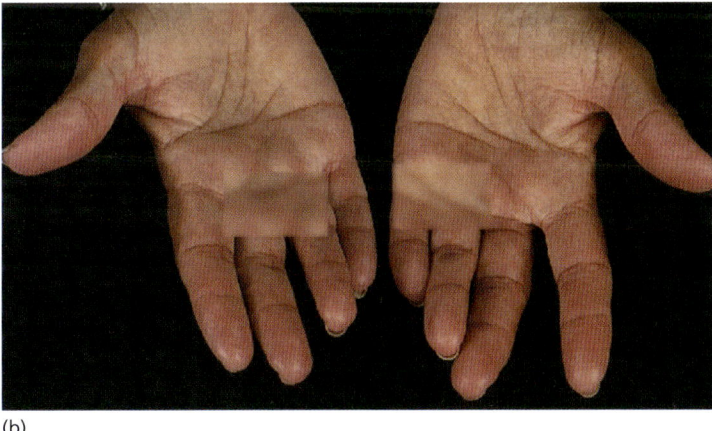

(b)

Figure 86.17 Nelson syndrome: hypermelanosis of the dorsa of the hands and of the palmar creases.

The pigmentation, which is accompanied by a combination of addisonian and cushingoid manifestations, fades when the dose is reduced. The incidence of melanosis appears to be rather higher in patients treated with tetracosactrin [2].

Hyperthyroidism

Definition
Hyperthyroidism is the excessive production of thyroid gland hormones.

Epidemiology
Incidence and prevalence
Pigmentation due to hyperthyroidism is present in up to 40% of patients with hyperthyroidism [1–3].

Pathophysiology
Pathology
It is speculated that the skin discoloration in hyperthyroidism may be due to increased release of pituitary ACTH, compensating for accelerated cortisol degradation [4].

Clinical features
Presentation
Pigmentation occurs in about 10% of patients with primary thyrotoxicosis [1]. It is usually diffuse and is broadly of addisonian pattern, although involvement of the mucous membranes is uncommon and pigmentation of the nipples and genital skin is less striking. The eyelids are occasionally conspicuously pigmented (the Jellinek sign). Some patients show melasma-like rather than diffuse pigmentation. The incidence of vitiligo is increased. Diffuse pigmentation was present at birth in the infant of a thyrotoxic mother [2]. Response of hyperpigmentation to therapy is poor.

Differential diagnosis
Acquired diffuse hyperpigmentation: see Box 86.3a.

Hypermelanosis in other systemic disorders

Neoplastic diseases

Definition
Increased pigmentation is an inconstant feature of a wide variety of systemic disorders and may be associated with malignant disease [1]. In most instances, the mechanism is obscure although, in some, elevated levels of β-MSH-like immunoreactivity are found. A genetic predisposition may be present in those affected. The hypermelanosis may be diffuse or localised. It may be confined to the epidermis, when the skin appears brown in colour, or it may be in the dermis, when often the skin is a slate-grey or blue colour. Pigments other than melanins may also be present.

Solid malignant tumours. ACTH-like peptides secreted typically from oat cell carcinoma of the bronchus may result in widespread hypermelanosis [2]. Diffuse cutaneous melanosis is a rare complication of metastatic melanoma [3,4,5].

Carcinoid syndrome. Spectrum of neuroendocrine tumours, most frequently originating in the digestive tract. Symptoms of flushing, diarrhoea, heart failure and bronchoconstriction developing due to excessive secretion of hormones such as serotonin from carcinoid tumours (Chapter 104) [6].

Lymphoma. Spectrum of malignant neoplasms derived from mature B or T cells, B- or T-cell progenitors or natural killer cells (Chapter 139).

Phaeochromocytoma. Neuroendocrine tumour of the adrenal glands or extra-adrenal chromaffin tissue secreting high levels of catecholamines.

Epidemiology
Incidence and prevalence
Solid malignant neoplasms. Rare.

Carcinoid tumour. Chapter 104.

Lymphomas. Pigmentation is an uncommon manifestation of lymphomas, occurring in 10% of cases of Hodgkin disease and in 1% or 2% of cases of non-Hodgkin lymphoma and lymphatic leukaemia.

Phaeochromocytomas. Rare.

Pathophysiology
Pathology
Solid malignant neoplasms. The mechanism is uncertain. In ectopic ACTH syndrome, which may occur in patients with oat cell carcinoma of the bronchus, pigmentation is usual. The tumour has been shown to produce a distinct MSH-like compound [2]. Diffuse melanosis is a rare complication of metastatic melanoma and is usually associated with widespread visceral metastases. It is thought that free melanin is released into the circulation from the cytolytic breakdown of melanoma metastases and is deposited extracellularly around dermal blood vessels before being taken up by dermal melanophages [3].

Carcinoid syndrome. Unknown.

Lymphoma. Unknown.

Phaeochromocytoma. Pigmentation possibly due to MSH-like activity of ectopic secretion of ACTH and its precursors. Release of α-MSH or analogues that bind on melanocortin 1 receptors.

Genetics
About one-third of phaeochromocytomas arise as part of a genetic syndrome.

Clinical features
Presentation
Solid malignant neoplasms. In cachectic states, there may be diffuse hyperpigmentation of the skin as in Addison disease. In adults, acquired acanthosis nigricans may rarely be associated with internal malignancy, almost invariably an adenocarcinoma. The hypermelanosis affects the axillae, nipples and umbilicus, which also show a warty papillomatosis. These skin changes may later become generalised. The mucous membranes are frequently involved. A diffuse dermal melanosis, having a slaty-blue colour, can occur in patients with advanced melanoma and may be associated with melanuria [3,4,5].

Carcinoid syndrome. Flushing of the face, neck and upper trunk frequently occurs. Diffuse hyperpigmentation of the skin has been noted in a number of patients with this syndrome [6]. A pellagra-like dermatitis on sun-exposed skin may also be observed.

Lymphomas. The pigmentation is of addisonian type, but allegedly without involvement of the mucous membranes. Malnutrition may be a factor and postinflammatory pigmentation after scratching may modify the clinical pattern. Diffuse progressive hyperpigmentation can also be a manifestation of mycosis fungoides [7,8].

Phaeochromocytoma. Pigmentation of addisonian pattern occurs in some cases of malignant phaeochromocytoma. Pallor of the face due to vasoconstriction may also occur. Hypertension, headaches, profuse sweating, palpitations and apprehension will suggest the diagnosis, which is established by the abnormal plasma catecholamines.

Differential diagnosis
Acquired diffuse hyperpigmentation: see Box 86.3a.

Hyperpigmentation in rheumatic diseases (Chapter 155)

Hypermelanosis is occasionally observed in rheumatoid arthritis and is a more frequent feature of Still disease. Most cases of hyperpigmentation in rheumatoid arthritis patients are, however, due to medications such as minocycline [1]. Hyperpigmentation has been reported with methotrexate in a patient with rheumatoid arthritis [2]. For differential diagnosis see Box 86.3a.

Systemic sclerosis and morphoea

Definition
Systemic sclerosis and morphoea (Chapters 54 and 55) comprise a spectrum of autoimmune-mediated diseases of unknown aetiology affecting the connective tissue. Systemic sclerosis may also affect the internal organs, including the heart, lungs, kidneys and gastrointestinal tract.

Pathophysiology
Predisposing factors
Hyperpigmentation in systemic sclerosis is seen most commonly in patients with pigmented skin and is less common in white people [1].

Pathology
Keratinocyte endothelin 1 production has been implicated as playing a central role in the pathogenesis of cutaneous hyperpigmentation in systemic sclerosis [2], as have local expression and systemic release of a stem cell factor [3]. Levels of soluble cell surface L-selectin are elevated in systemic sclerosis with diffuse hyperpigmentation [4].

Clinical features
Presentation
Generalised pigmentation in systemic sclerosis and morphoea may be intense and diffuse or of addisonian type, often with an accentuation in sun-exposed skin and areas of pressure, but without mucous membrane involvement. It may involve predominantly the face and limbs but is often far more extensive than the scleroderma itself (Figure 86.18). A mixture of hyper- and hypomelanosis may also occur in areas of chronic sclerosis.

Pigmentation may also be a conspicuous feature of morphoea [5,6] and is occasionally the presenting symptom (Figure 86.19). Hyperpigmentation is sometimes a feature of atrophoderma of Pasini and Pierini [7], and has also been reported in the linear atrophoderma of Moulin [8].

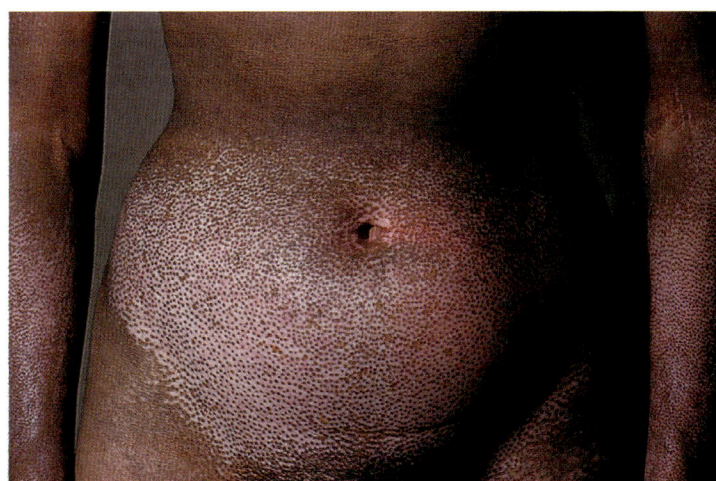

Figure 86.18 Generalised pigmentation in a woman aged 33 years with systemic sclerosis exhibiting also areas of salt and pepper depigmentation on the abdomen and arms.

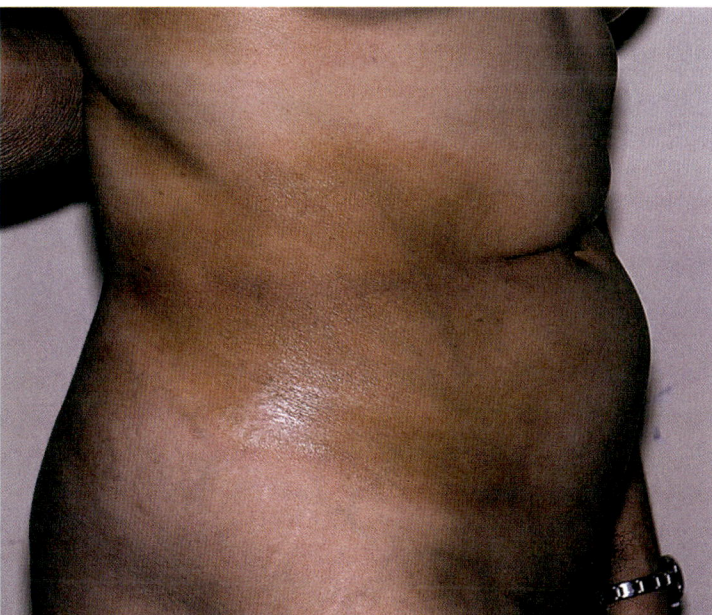

Figure 86.19 Morphoea. Hyperpigmentation was the presenting symptom.

Differential diagnosis
- Acquired diffuse hyperpigmentation: see Box 86.3a.
- Acquired localised hyperpigmentation: see Box 86.3b.

Dermatomyositis and lupus erythematosus

Definition
Dermatomyositis is an idiopathic inflammatory myopathy characterised by proximal muscle weakness and a cutaneous eruption.

Lupus erythematosus is a chronic idiopathic inflammatory disease affecting multiple organs including the skin.

Clinical features
Presentation
In both dermatomyositis and lupus erythematosus, diffuse pigmentation may accompany or follow the cutaneous lesions of dermatomyositis [1]. Acanthosis nigricans has also been reported in association with dermatomyositis [2]. In systemic lupus erythematosus, diffuse pigmentation of light-exposed skin occurs in about 10% of cases. Longitudinal melanonychia may occasionally be a feature of systemic lupus erythematosus [3]. Hyperpigmentation may also be secondary to treatment with antimalarials in systemic lupus erythematosus.

Differential diagnosis
Acquired diffuse hyperpigmentation: see Box 86.3a.

Disease course and prognosis
In systemic lupus erythematosus, the skin may gradually darken even though the disease is controlled by treatment.

Neurological disorders

Definition
Pigmentation, usually conforming to the addisonian pattern, occurs in some diseases of the nervous system, particularly those involving the diencephalon and the substantia nigra. Intense pigmentation is a feature of Schilder disease [1] but some increase in pigmentation is not uncommon in hepatolenticular degeneration [2] and in ependymomas. It is occasionally noted in chronic schizophrenia. In post-encephalitic parkinsonism, it may be diffuse but may be melasma-like. Pigmentation may sometimes develop after intense and prolonged emotional stress [3].

Clinical features
Presentation
Mostly diffuse hyperpigmentation conforming to the addisonian pattern.

Differential diagnosis
Acquired diffuse hyperpigmentation: see Box 86.3a.

Multiple organ failure, renal failure and primary biliary cirrhosis

Introduction and general description
Multiple organ failure. Patients with multiple organ failure who survive for long periods are susceptible to hyperpigmentation. Renal failure, hepatic failure and polypharmacy may all contribute to this. An unusual case of intense green colour in a patient with multiple organ failure was attributed to dyes in the liquid tube feeds [1].

Renal failure. Chronic renal disease with nitrogen retention is frequently accompanied by increased pigmentation of the skin. This hypermelanosis is diffuse and brown in colour. It is most intense on sun-exposed skin, including the hands and face. Hyperpigmented macules are common on the palms and soles [1].

Elevated levels of β-MSH are found in the plasma of these patients [2,3] and cause the excess production of melanin in the skin. The increased levels of β-MSH-like immunoreactivity are due to slow clearance by the kidneys rather than increased production by the pituitary. Lipochromes and carotenoids deposited in the skin may also play a part. Paradoxically, hypopigmentation with acquired lightening of the hair is sometimes a feature of chronic renal failure [4].

Primary biliary cirrhosis. A diffuse hypermelanosis is seen in patients with cirrhosis due to many aetiological factors and is particularly striking in patients with primary biliary cirrhosis [1,2]. The hyperpigmentation is particularly striking on sun-exposed sites. The excess melanin is dispersed widely in the epidermis [1]. No significant difference from normal controls is observed in the levels of MSH-like peptides [1].

Disease course and prognosis
Dermatological manifestations increase with increasing duration and severity of renal disease.

Haemochromatosis

Definition
Haemochromatosis is a hereditary disorder due to excessive intestinal absorption of iron. The commonest and mildest form, accounting for some 90% of cases, is autosomal recessive and due to mutations in the *HFE* gene (*HFE*-related hereditary haemochromatosis). It manifests in the skin as diffuse pigmentation.

Introduction and general description
Haemochromatosis is a hereditary disorder due to excessive intestinal absorption of iron, resulting in gradual deposition of iron in the tissues throughout life [1,2]. The commonest and mildest form, accounting for some 90% of cases, is autosomal recessive and due to mutations in the *HFE* gene (*HFE*-related hereditary haemochromatosis) [3]. It is asymptomatic in 75% of cases, not usually presenting clinically until the fifth decade of life or later. It manifests in the skin as diffuse bronze pigmentation. Other clinical manifestations include hepatic cirrhosis, diabetes, cardiac failure, impotence and arthritis.

Epidemiology
Incidence and prevalence
It is estimated that 1 : 200 to 1 : 300 white people have homozygous *HFE* mutations [4], though only 50% of affected individuals show clinical features of the disease [4].

Age
Fifth decade onwards.

Sex
It is more common in males.

Ethnicity
Most frequent in white people.

Associated diseases
Excessive alcohol consumption accelerates the development of hepatic cirrhosis [5].

Pathophysiology
The common form of haemochromatosis is due to mutations of the *HFE* gene [6].

Clinical features
History
The disease haemochromatosis was first described by Troisier, Hanot and Chauffard in 1865 [1]. The term 'haemochromatosis' was subsequently coined by von Recklinghausen in 1899 in recognition that the skin pigmentation originated from the blood [1].

Presentation
Pigmentation, bronzed or bluish-grey in colour, initially involves exposed sites but later becomes generalised (Figure 86.20) [7,8]. It is present in most cases [9] but may be subtle. Hyperpigmentation of mucous membranes and conjunctivae occurs in 15–20%. The diagnosis should be suspected when pigmentation of this pattern occurs in middle-aged men in association with an enlarged liver and diabetes [10].

Differential diagnosis
Acquired diffuse hyperpigmentation: see Box 86.3a.

Investigations
Fasting transferrin saturation: if >45% arrange gene analysis for *HFE* mutations.

Management
Hyperpigmentation is reversible with phlebotomy [11].

Cutaneous amyloidosis

Definition
Cutaneous pigmentation is a common feature of cutaneous amyloidosis [1,2], which is discussed in detail in Chapter 56.

Pathophysiology
Pathology
Melanophages are found in the papillary dermis. The melanin contained in these dermal cells is derived from degenerating basal keratinocytes and melanocytes [1,3].

Clinical features
Presentation
Localised pigmentation, often symmetrical, and located on the upper back and anterior thighs and forearms, is seen in both lichen amyloidosis and macular amyloidosis [1,2].

Clinical variants
Macular amyloidosis is seen most commonly on the upper back (interscapular areas), chest, buttocks, forearms and shins.

Differential diagnosis
The macular type of amyloidosis may be mistaken for postinflammatory hyperpigmentation, but the lesions usually have a distinctive 'ripple' pattern (Figure 86.21), and microscopic studies reveal the presence of amyloid (Box 86.3a).

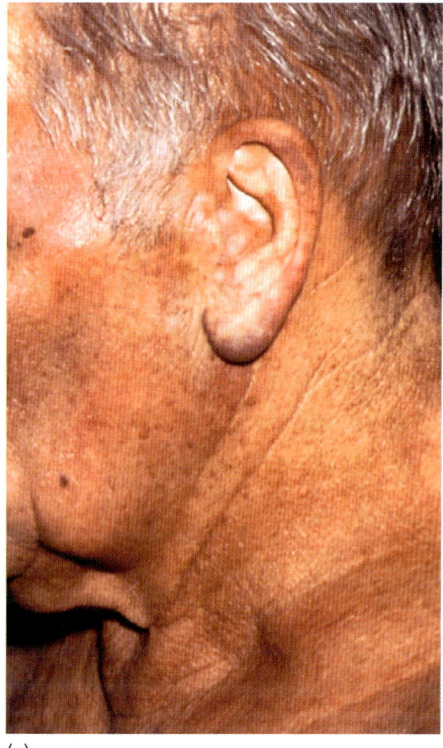
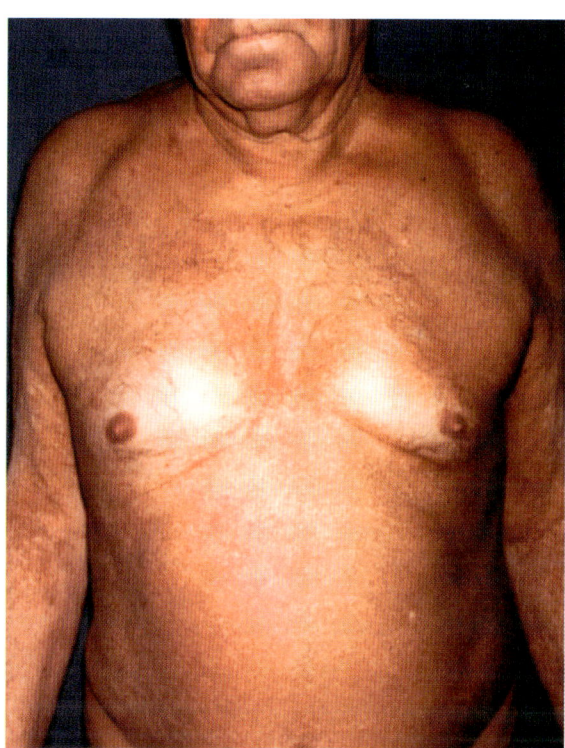

Figure 86.20 (a, b) Haemochromatosis: a 74-year-old male with gradual increase in skin pigmentation for 5 years. Extensive stippled skin pigmentation becoming confluent with marked iron deposition in addition to hypermelanosis on histology. Note gynaecomastia (b).

(a)   (b)

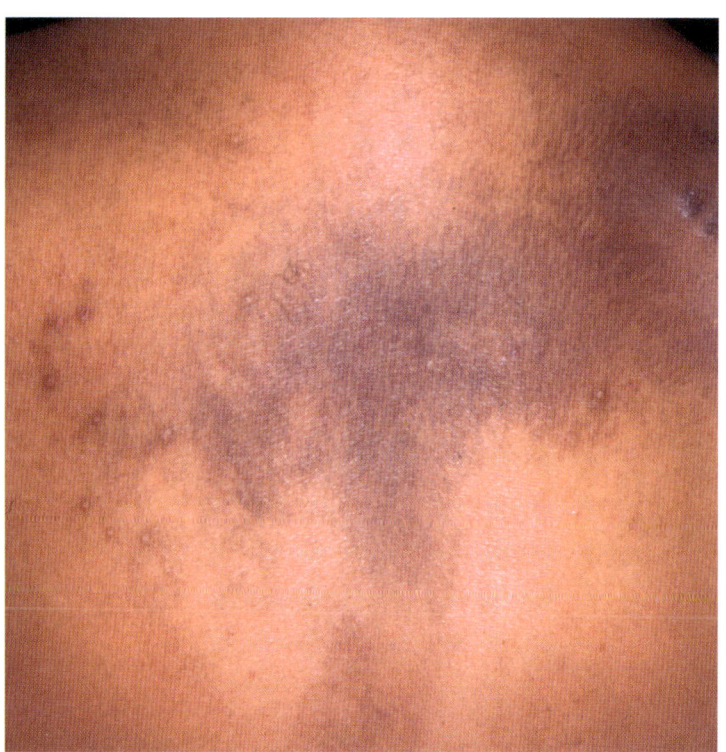

Figure 86.21 Macular amyloidosis: typical rippled hypermelanosis on the upper back of a 40-year-old Indian woman.

Nutritional deficiencies

Definition
The effects of nutritional deficiencies on the skin are addressed in detail in Chapter 61. Those that are associated with pigmentary change are briefly discussed here.

Malabsorption syndromes
Vitamin A deficiency. Most frequently due to inadequate dietary intake.

Vitamin B₁₂ deficiency. Most frequently caused by inadequate absorption.

Folate deficiency. Usually dietary with increased risk in pregnancy.

Pellagra. The classical clinical manifestation of nicotinic acid (vitamin B₃) deficiency.

Vagabonds' disease. Skin disorder typically occurring in older patients with poor diet, lack of personal hygiene and infestation with *Pediculus humanus*.

Epidemiology
Incidence and prevalence
In malabsorption syndromes, such as tropical sprue and Whipple disease (Chapter 153), pigmentation is a common occurrence and may sometimes be prominent [1–3].

Pathophysiology
Vitamin B₁₂. The exact mechanism of hyperpigmentation in vitamin B_{12} deficiency is still unknown. The lack of vitamin B_{12} may lead to lower intracellular glutathione levels, causing a decrease in its inhibitory function on tyrosinase activity in melanogenesis, and inducing an increase in melanogenesis. Another hypothesis is that vitamin B_{12} deficiency is associated with a defect in melanin transport and the incorporation of melanin into keratinocytes, causing incontinence of pigment [4].

PART 8: SPECIFIC CUTANEOUS STRUCTURES

Pellagra. It is due to a cellular deficiency of niacin (vitamin B₃, nicotinic acid) from an inadequate dietary supply of tryptophan. It used to be endemic where diets were based on maize with little animal protein [5]. Although the condition has been recognised since the 17th century, it was not until the early 20th century that it was recognised by Goldberger to be due to a nutritional deficiency [6], which was subsequently shown by Elvehjem to be niacin [7].

Vagabonds' disease. Classically, this occurs in those in whom poor diet is combined with lack of cleanliness and heavy infestation with lice [8,9].

Presentation

General. Hyperpigmentation caused by nutritional deficiencies may be of addisonian type but without involvement of the mucous membranes, or may occur in well-defined patches on the face and neck and occasionally on the trunk [1]. The scaly inflammatory plaques that may develop in these syndromes are usually followed by intense pigmentation (Chapter 61).

Vitamin A deficiency. Patients with severe vitamin A deficiency are often deficient in other vitamins as well. They have ocular and cutaneous abnormalities, of which xerophthalmia and phrynoderma (Chapter 85) are the most characteristic, particularly in children: these may be associated with hyperpigmentation of the face and limbs. In adults, there is dryness and scaling of the skin with desquamation and generalised hyperpigmentation. Conjunctival pigmentation has been noted particularly in oriental races and may be striking, especially in the lower fornix and bulbar conjunctiva.

Vitamin B₁₂ deficiency. The pigmentation seen in association with B₁₂ deficiency often has a rather dappled and mottled appearance; it particularly affects the face and the dorsum of the hands and feet [10–12] but may be limited to the fingertips and nails [13] or, rarely, may be generalised (Figure 86.22) [4,14,15]. Ill-defined hyperpigmentation of the mucosal surfaces and hypopigmentation of the hair may also occur.

Folate deficiency. A diffuse brown pigmentation is also seen occasionally in patients with megaloblastic anaemia due to folic acid deficiency, particularly during pregnancy [16,17].

Pellagra. Affected skin becomes hard, dry and cracked and in extreme cases is black in colour [5]. The sites of involvement are the sun-exposed skin of the face, neck, dorsa of the hands and feet, and sometimes the forearms. Mucosal sites are also affected [18,19]. Also seen in pellagra are dermatitis, diarrhoea and dementia (the three 'D's).

Vagabonds' disease. The pigmentation is basically of addisonian pattern and the mucous membranes may be involved. The pathogenesis is uncertain, but the hypermelanosis is probably postinflammatory and related to the scratching from the pediculosis infestation. Areas of hypomelanosis occur and there is a decrease in the number of melanocytes that show degenerative changes [1]. Adrenal function is in most cases normal [8,9].

Differential diagnosis

Acquired diffuse hyperpigmentation. See Box 86.3a.

Acquired pigmentary disorders of oral mucosa. These include the following:
- Iatrogenic.
- Irritative (e.g. smokers' melanosis).
- Hyperplastic or neoplastic processes.

Disease course and prognosis

Generally, normalisation of pigmentation occurs with treatment of the deficiency.

POEMS syndrome

Definition

Hypermelanosis, along with acrocyanosis, hypertrichosis and skin thickening, is one of the cutaneous manifestations of this complex syndrome. The name POEMS syndrome derives from its principal characteristics, namely *p*olyneuropathy, *o*rganomegaly, *e*ndocrinopathy, *m*onoclonal gammopathy and *s*kin changes. It is discussed in detail in Chapter 149.

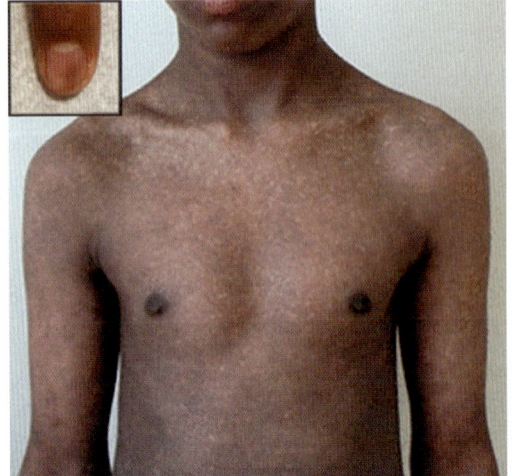

(a)

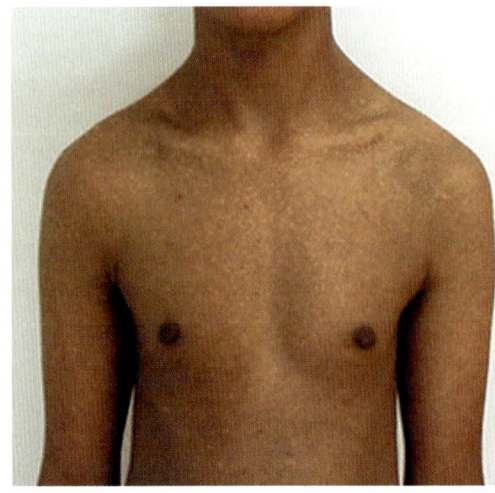

(b)

Figure 86.22 Vitamin B₁₂ deficiency: (a) generalised mottled hypermelanosis as presenting feature of pernicious anaemia in a 16-year-old boy with a 4-year history of progressive darkening of the skin and streaked pigmentation of the nails (inset); (b) marked reduction in pigmentation 9 months after initiation of vitamin B₁₂ therapy. Reproduced from Diamantino *et al.* 2012 [4] with permission of John Wiley & Sons.

Presentation

Hyperpigmentation is reported to be a common cutaneous manifestation of POEMS syndrome, affecting the extremities, torso, areolae, head and neck. Hyperpigmentation may also be generalised [1].

Hypermelanosis of drug origin

Drug-induced hyperpigmentation

Definition

Localised or generalised hyperpigmentation can be caused by a wide range of medications and chemicals.

Introduction and general description

Skin pigmentation may be induced by a wide variety of drugs [1,2,3]. Several mechanisms are involved in drug-induced changes of pigmentation of the skin. These include increased melanin synthesis, increased lipofuscin synthesis, deposition of drug-related material and postinflammatory hyperpigmentation. For example, the phenothiazines, particularly chlorpromazine, react with melanin to form drug–pigment complexes. In contrast to melanin, the chlorpromazine–melanin complexes are not metabolised by the body. Many drugs induce hypermelanosis as a non-specific postinflammatory change in predisposed subjects. The pigmentation following fixed drug eruptions is of this type. Other drugs induce pigmentation more directly; in the case of arsenic, it is believed that it combines avidly with sulphydryl groups in the epidermal cells and promotes the action of tyrosinase. A postinflammatory hyperpigmentation of the skin is seen following the resolution of drug-induced lichenoid reactions. Oestrogens stimulate melanin production, and drug-induced hyperpigmentation may be seen with the combined oral contraceptive. Hyperpigmentation in AIDS patients may occur as a complication of drug therapy, most notably with zidovudine, which causes pigmentation of the nails, skin and oral mucosa.

Amiodarone

Amiodarone is used in the treatment of ventricular and supraventricular tachycardia. Amiodarone has been reported to cause photosensitive and phototoxic reactions in more than 50% of patients [1–3]. Fewer than 5% of patients develop drug-induced discoloration of the skin, characterised by a slate-gray or purple discoloration of mainly the sun-exposed skin, especially the face, with prominent involvement of the nose and sometimes the ears (Figure 86.23) [4–6]. Non-exposed skin may also be affected. The discoloration is caused by UV accumulation of amiodarone and lipofuscin in dermal macrophages. Skin type I patients are more prone to the development of this discoloration. The hyperpigmentation is related to the daily dosage (high risk with dosages >800 mg/day) and duration of treatment.

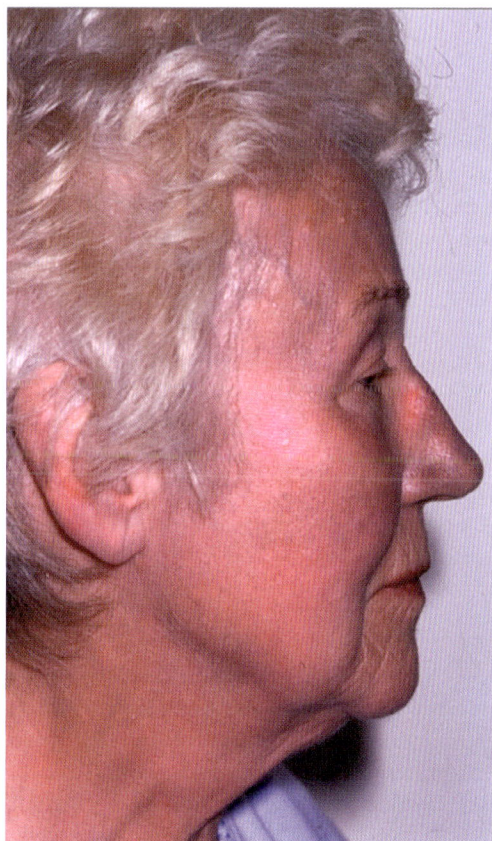
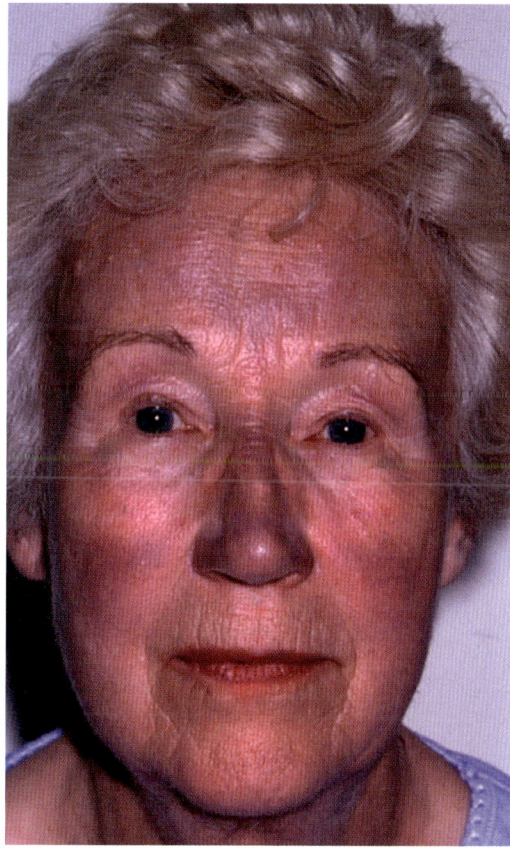

Figure 86.23 (a, b) Amiodarone pigmentation after 5 years of therapy: note slaty-blue dyspigmentation of the forehead, nose, cheeks and earlobe.

(a)   (b)

PART 8: SPECIFIC CUTANEOUS STRUCTURES

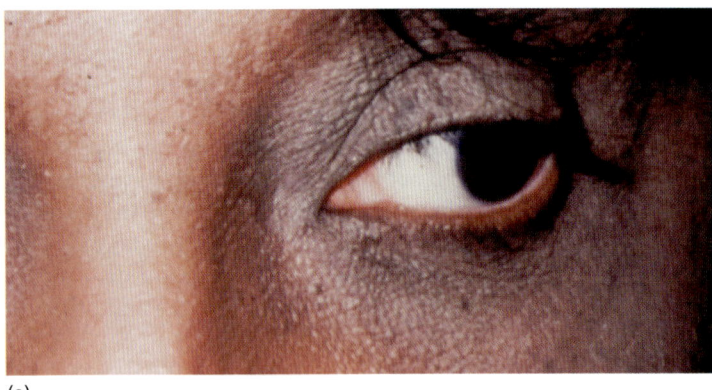

(a)

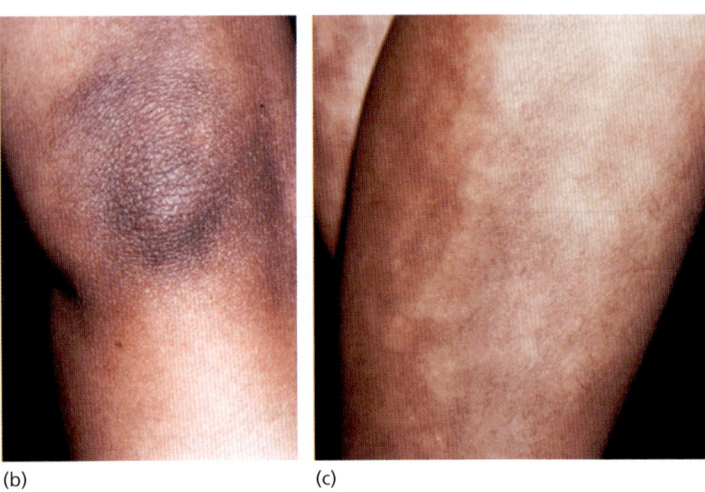

(b)   (c)

Figure 86.24 (a–c) Chloroquine pigmentation: patient received chloroquine for 9 years for rheumatoid arthritis and had developed increasing pigmentation of the periorbital skin and extremities for 4–5 years.

Antimalarial drugs

Chloroquine has been shown to have an affinity for dermal melanin [1]. A yellowish pigmentation of the skin is common with mepacrine [2]. Pigmentation appears to result from complexes of melanin, haemosiderin and mepacrine, in combination with sulphur [3]. Quinine and quinidine may also produce a generalised pigmentation [2,4].

Bluish-grey pigmentation appears mainly on sun-exposed areas, including the face, neck and anterior side of the legs and forearms (Figure 86.24). The nail beds may be affected diffusely or in transverse bands and the hard palate may be bluish-grey. The oral mucosa, especially the hard palate, may also be affected. Bleaching of the colour of the hair occurs and when associated with pigmentation of the skin should suggest the diagnosis [5]. The pigmentation manifests initially as isolated oval macules, which then progressively spread and merge into large patches or diffuse pigmentation [2–5].

Clofazimine

This synthetic riminophenazine dye used in the treatment of leprosy produces an initial redness of the skin due to an accumulation of the drug. Later, with prolonged treatment, a violaceous brown colour develops that is most noticeable in lesional skin [1]. Reddish-blue pigmentation has been reported within scarred areas of lupus erythematosus in one patient [2]. Histochemical studies indicate a ceroid-lipofuscin pigment as well as clofazimine inside macrophage phagolysosomes [2,3].

Cytotoxic drugs

Hyperpigmentation is a common side effect of antitumour agents used in cancer treatment. The skin discoloration may develop in a wide variable interval of time, ranging from 1 week to several months after initiation of the treatment. The hyperpigmentation can be either localised or diffuse, and may affect all parts of the tegument, including the mucous membranes, hair and nails [1].

Long-term administration of busulfan (busulphan) produces a diffuse brown pigmentation, particularly in non-white people with a dark complexion. Less commonly, Addison disease is simulated [2,3]. Light and electron microscopy studies suggest that busulfan has both a stimulatory and a toxic effect on melanocytes [4]. Both busulfan and doxorubicin cause mucous membrane pigmentation. Other cytostatic drugs that may produce hyperpigmentation of skin include cyclophosphamide, bleomycin, fluorouracil, hydroxyurea, daunorubicin, methotrexate, mithramycin, mitomycin, thiotepa and adriamycin [5,6]. Pigmentation of the nails can be caused by many cytotoxic agents, including cisplatin, doxorubicin, idarubicin, fluorouracil, bleomycin, docetaxel, dacarbazine and hydroxyurea. Topical cytostatic drugs that produce localised hyperpigmentation include carmustine, mechlorethamine and fluorouracil. Hair pigmentation may be induced by methotrexate and pigmentation of the teeth may be seen with cyclophosphamide.

Hydantoin

Phenytoin (diphenylhydantoin) is the prototype of the hydantoin derivatives. It has been suggested that hydantoin exerts a direct action on the melanocytes inducing dispersion of melanin granules in the cutis, in addition to increased pigmentation of the basal epidermis. A patient on this drug developed pigmentation of addisonian type and other evidence of hypoadrenalism [1].

Anticonvulsants such as hydantoin, phenytoin and barbiturates may induce skin pigmentation with a pattern of melasma for hydantoins or a diffuse brown, post-exanthematous discoloration for barbiturates [1,2].

Psychotropic drugs (e.g. trifluoperazine, imipramine)

The mechanism is uncertain, but probably involves drug–melanin complexes. There is extensive deposition of melanin-like material throughout the reticuloendothelial system and in parenchymal cells of internal organs. The pigment found in the cells of the dermis stains as for melanin [1,2]. Electron microscopy studies [3] show increased melanin in the epidermis and perivascular macrophages in the dermis that contain electron-dense particles. Radioactively labelled chlorpromazine is found to localise in tissues containing melanin [4]. It is believed that this drug or some metabolite is bound to melanin in the tissues [5]. The level of immunoreactive β-MSH in the plasma of these patients is within the normal range [6]. A blue-grey pigmentation of the sun-exposed areas of the skin has also been reported with trifluoperazine and imipramine [7,8].

Blue-grey pigmentation of the sun-exposed areas of the skin is seen in a small percentage of patients receiving high doses of chlorpromazine for long periods (Figure 86.25) [1,2]. The pigmentation

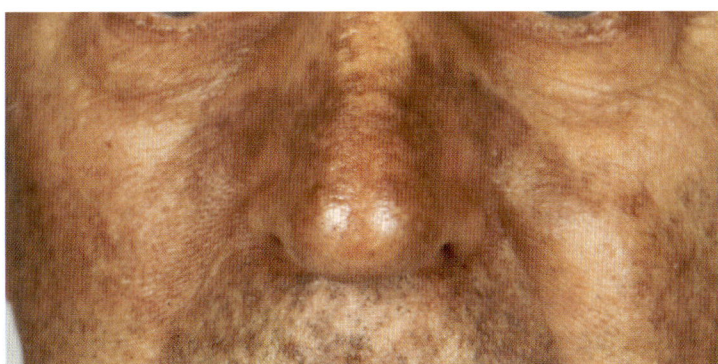

Figure 86.25 Chlorpromazine pigmentation: patchy bands of muddy pigmentation extending across the nose to the paranasal and preauricular skin in an elderly male receiving long-term therapy.

is cumulative and some develop a purplish tint. Related phenothiazines may cause a similar effect, but chlorpromazine is usually implicated [9]. Some of those affected also develop cataracts, corneal opacities and pigmentation of the conjunctivae [10]. The nail beds are also affected in severe cases [2].

Tetracyclines

The pathomechanism of the discoloration is still uncertain. An isomorphic response with hyperproduction of melanin, particularly in inflammatory or sun-exposed zones, by a direct effect of the drug on melanocytes may be involved. Minocycline-induced hyperpigmentation types I and II are believed to be caused by minocycline-iron chelation products. Type III is believed to be caused by either minocycline-induced melanisation or a minocycline–melanin complex, and type IV is due to either a calcium–minocycline or melanin–minocycline complex [1,2].

Tetracycline-induced skin discoloration although uncommon has been mainly reported with minocycline, and only rarely with doxycycline or first-generation molecules [1,2]. Minocycline-induced hyperpigmentation can affect various anatomical locations, including the skin, nails, oral cavity, sclera and conjunctiva, skeleton and cartilage, as well as viscera and body fluids. The risk of pigmentation is higher with longer duration of treatment or high cumulative dose (Figure 86.26), although cutaneous or oral pigmentation can occur regardless of dose or duration of therapy [3].

Four unique patterns of cutaneous minocycline-induced discoloration have been described [4–6]. They share a similar morphology, with well-circumscribed blue-grey macules located respectively in areas of acne scars (type I), at sites of previous inflammation distant from sites of inflammation or infection and mostly affecting sun-exposed areas including the shins, ankles and arms (type II), or on the vermilion of the lower lip (type IV). Type III is known as the 'muddy skin syndrome' and is characterised by diffuse symmetrical brown-grey discoloration with a tendency to photoaggravation.

Electron microscopy reveals electron-dense material in dermal macrophages and X-ray microanalysis confirms the presence of iron [7]. Partial resolution of the pigmentation occurs after the drug is stopped [8]. Similar blue-black pigmentation of the legs has resulted from treatment with the 4-quinolone antibiotic pefloxacin [9] and the tetracycline antibiotic methacycline [10].

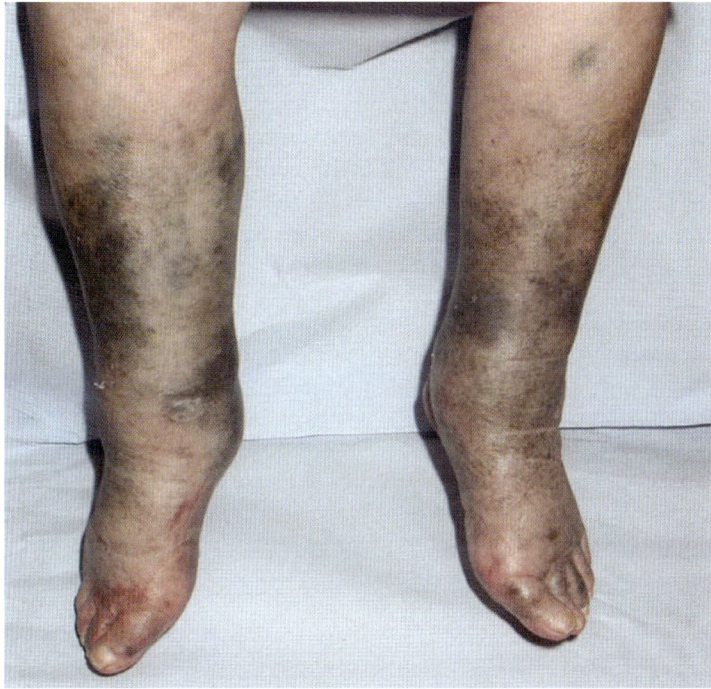

Figure 86.26 Minocycline pigmentation: marked dyspigmentation of the lower legs resulting from minocycline therapy commenced 2 years earlier as adjunctive therapy for control of bullous pemphigoid.

Epidemiology
Incidence and prevalence
Drug-induced hyperpigmentation accounts for 10–20% of all cases of acquired hyperpigmentation.

Antimalarial drugs. About 25% of patients receiving one of the four most commonly used antimalarials (chloroquine, hydroxychloroquine, mepacrine (quinacrine) and mefloquine) for at least 4 months will develop a discoloration of the skin.

Hydantoin. Some 10% of patients receiving hydantoin preparations develop pigmentation of the face and neck, resembling chloasma, which fades in a few months when the drug is stopped.

Tetracyclines. Minocycline-induced hyperpigmentation may affect up to 15% of patients receiving minocycline, particularly in long-duration treatments, with the bones of the oral cavity the most frequently affected sites of pigmentation. Overall incidence is estimated between 3% and 5%.

Clinical features
Differential diagnosis
See Box 86.3a.

Disease course and prognosis
Discoloration is mostly reversible after discontinuation of the causative drug. In a small number of patients, the hyperpigmentation persists even after long-term discontinuation.

Amiodarone. In most cases, the pigmentation is slowly reversible and fades over months to years after discontinuation of the drug.

Dose reduction or withdrawal of amiodarone can lead to complete disappearance of the pigmentation.

Antimalarial drugs. Discoloration slowly fades after discontinuation of treatment, but may take several months to disappear, and rarely resolves completely. With continued therapy, the areas darken, particularly oval patches on the shins, which increase in size. A blue-black colour may develop. Also, these patches are more pigmented in light-exposed areas.

Cytotoxic drugs. After discontinuation of the causative agent, the pigmentation usually fades, at least partially, but may persist for a long time after discontinuation of the treatment (e.g. bleomycin). Rarely, hyperpigmentation can be irreversible.

Tetracyclines. Complete resolution of minocycline-induced hyperpigmentation can be expected in types I and II, but can take several months to years after discontinuation of treatment. Types III and IV seem not to disappear over time.

Treatment ladder for drug-induced hyperpigmentation

First line
- Discontinuation of the causative drug (if possible)
- Sun avoidance/sun protection

Second line
- Laser therapy (e.g. Q-switched laser in minocycline-induced hyperpigmentation [1])

Fixed drug eruption

Definition
Fixed drug eruption is one of the most common forms of drug-induced exanthems. The acute eruption characteristically settles leaving residual hyperpigmentation, especially in those with darker skin types [1,2]. The topic is discussed in detail in Chapter 117.

Pathophysiology
Immunohistological findings suggest that the characteristic same-site recurrence may be induced by prolonged intercellular adhesion molecule 1 (ICAM-1) expression in the lesional keratinocytes correlated with the degree of residing epidermal T-suppressor cytotoxic cells. It is suggested that the eruption may be mediated by a type IV hypersensitivity, although the results of skin tests have been inconsistent and influenced by a range of factors including the causative drug [3].

Predisposing factors
Fixed eruptions are particularly frequent in black people.

Pathology
The slate-brown colour in fixed drug eruption is due to pigmentary incontinence with melanophages in the upper dermis [4].

Environmental factors
A great variety of causative drugs are known to be related with fixed drug eruptions. Most frequently reported drugs include tetracyclines, non-steroidal anti-inflammatory drugs, sulfonamides and sedatives.

Clinical features
Presentation
Well-circumscribed areas of slate-brown pigmentation commonly follow the erythematous and bullous stages of fixed eruptions (Chapter 117) but almost universal brown pigmentation has followed the long-continued ingestion of phenolphthalein [5]. More or less symmetrical, discrete patches are usually seen but the melanosis may be diffuse or melasma-like, and the mucous membranes may be involved [6,7]. The genitalia and perianal area are often affected, although the eruption can appear anywhere on the skin surface. The characteristic course is recurrence of lesions at the same sites with development of new areas of involvement with repeated exposure to the causative agent.

Clinical variants
Rarely, fixed eruptions may be triggered by foods or UV light [8].

Differential diagnosis
See Box 86.3b.

Disease course and prognosis
The lesions may increase in size and/or number with continuation of the causative drug, leaving ever deeper residual pigmentation (Figure 86.27).

Pigmentation resulting from acute photodynamic and phototoxic reactions

Definition and nomenclature
Drugs and other chemicals with photodynamic and phototoxic activity have the potential to induce skin hyperpigmentation (see Photocontact facial melanosis earlier). If the photodynamic agent is applied directly to the skin, the intensity of the pigmentary response is greatly enhanced as in the two conditions described here:
1 Phytophotodermatitis: an inflammatory and pigmentary reaction of the skin to light, potentiated by furocoumarins in plants (Figure 86.28) [1–5].
2 Berloque dermatitis: skin pigmentation due to phototoxic reaction to perfumes applied to the skin (Figure 86.29) [6–9].

Synonyms and inclusions
- Phytophotodermatitis: meadow dermatitis, strimmer dermatitis, weed-wacker dermatitis
- Berloque dermatitis: phototoxic reaction to fragrance

Epidemiology
Incidence and prevalence
Not exactly established, although relatively common in the summer months.

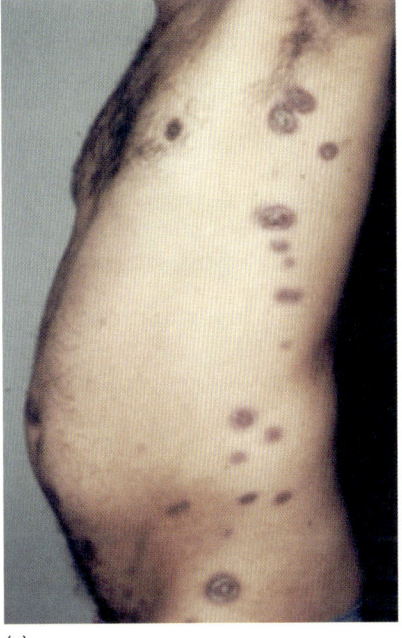
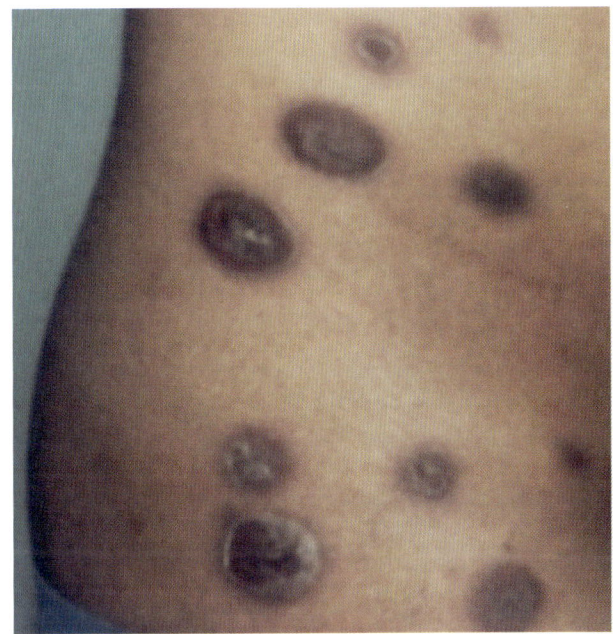

Figure 86.27 (a, b) Pigmented fixed drug eruption: extensive eruption following repeated courses of tetracycline.

(a)   (b)

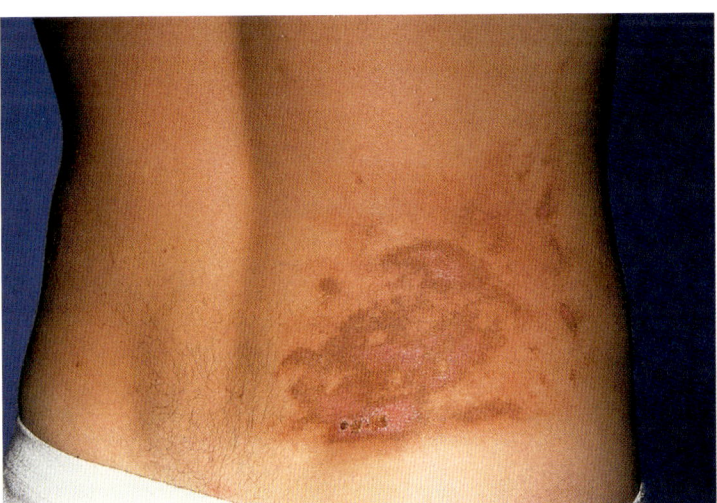

Figure 86.28 Phytophotodermatitis. Linear, streaky pigmentation following an acute blistering reaction caused by giant hogweed and sunlight.

Age
Any age.

Sex
Males and females are equally affected.

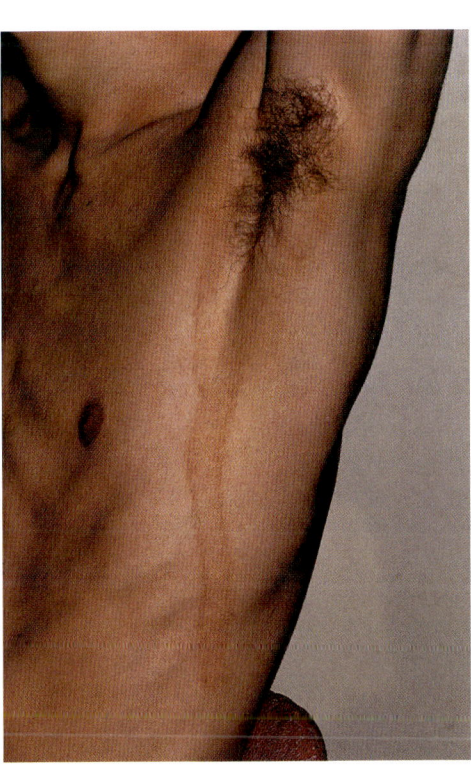

Figure 86.29 Berloque dermatitis.

Ethnicity
No racial predominance.

Susceptibility
Phytophotodermatitis. There is some individual variation in susceptibility but with adequate exposure most will react [1,2].

Berloque dermatitis. There is wide variation in susceptibility, with the reaction occurring in only a small proportion of those exposed [6]. This variation depends on the readiness with which the bergapten is absorbed, the quantity applied, and the intensity and duration of exposure to UV light. Susceptibility is increased by stripping the horny layer. Hot humid conditions favour absorption. The pigmentation occurs in susceptible subjects who have been exposed to light after the application of perfume [7,8].

Pathophysiology
Phytophotodermatitis. All the plants reliably recorded as inducing this reaction in humans have been shown to contain furocoumarins:

they include cow parsley (*Anthriscus sylvestris*) and giant hogweed (*Heracleum sphondylium*) [1,2]. The reaction occurs in those exposed to sunlight after skin contact with these plants, especially if they have been crushed.

Berloque dermatitis. Berloque dermatitis results from the potentiation of UV-stimulated melanogenesis by 5-methoxypsoralen (bergapten) in perfumes containing bergamot oil.

Clinical features
Presentation
Hypermelanosis may sometimes be heavy and persistent following photodynamic and phototoxic reactions. Phytophotodermatitis [1–5] and Berloque dermatitis [6–9] are two distinctive clinical syndromes. If the inflammatory phase is severe, bullae are formed [4,5]. Milder cases show pigmentary changes without inflammation.

Phytophotodermatitis. Initially, intensely pruritic papulovesicular lesions with irregular shapes and criss-crossing linear streaks may be present. Multiple irregular large bullae may form (Figure 86.30). Typically, the lesions rapidly evolve into darkly pigmented macules (Figure 86.28).

Common clinical patterns for phytophotodermatitis include a bizarre network of pigmented streaks on the legs or arms (meadow dermatitis), and much finer spots and small streaks on the forearms and legs from contact with plant material during strimming (strimmer dermatitis). Squeezing limes outside when preparing cold drinks can cause blistering of the hands if carried out on sunny days. Handling celery either at harvest or when it is sold can cause phytophotodermatitis of the fingertips if it takes place in direct sunlight [4]. Handling giant hogweed in sunny weather is a particular hazard (Figure 86.30).

Berloque dermatitis. The distribution of the lesions is therefore variable but their configuration is usually distinctive. Deep-brown pigmentation follows the pattern formed by the trickle of the droplets of perfume over the skin from their points of application (Figure 86.29). The pigmentation fades after weeks or months. The

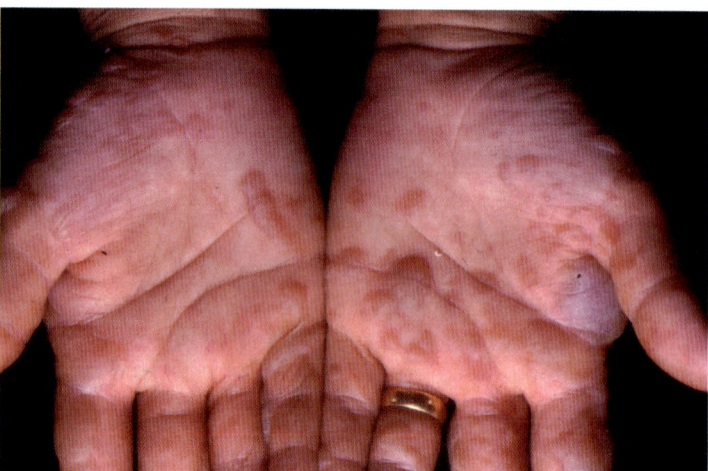

Figure 86.30 Phytophotodermatitis: acute irregular blisters across the palms after grasping giant hogweed.

condition is now much less frequent, although it is a continuing cosmetic problem [9].

Differential diagnosis (Box 86.3b)
- Allergic photocontact dermatitis.
- Drug-induced phototoxicity – photosensitivity.

Disease course and prognosis
Favourable prognosis if the causing agent is avoided.

Investigations
Serial dilutions of psoralens may, in exceptional cases, be needed to distinguish photoallergy from phototoxicity [3].

Treatment ladder for pigmentation resulting from acute photodynamic and phototoxic reactions

First line
- Prevention: avoidance of photodynamic or phototoxic drugs, plants and perfumes
- Oral antihistamines
- Parenterally administered epinephrine in case of anaphylactic reactions

---

Postinflammatory hypermelanosis

Definition
Postinflammatory hypermelanosis is residual macular pigmentation resulting from prior skin inflammation.

Epidemiology
Incidence and prevalence
Common.

Age
Can develop at any age.

Sex
Males and females are equally affected.

Ethnicity
More common in deeply pigmented skin.

Pathophysiology
Predisposing factors
The intensity and persistence of the hypermelanosis are greater in dark-skinned subjects.

Pathology
Hypermelanosis commonly follows acute or chronic inflammatory processes in the skin. Disorders where there is disruption of the basal layer of the epidermis, such as in lichen planus or lupus erythematosus, frequently develop areas of slate-brown hypermelanosis. Similarly, in fixed drug eruptions, hyperpigmentation

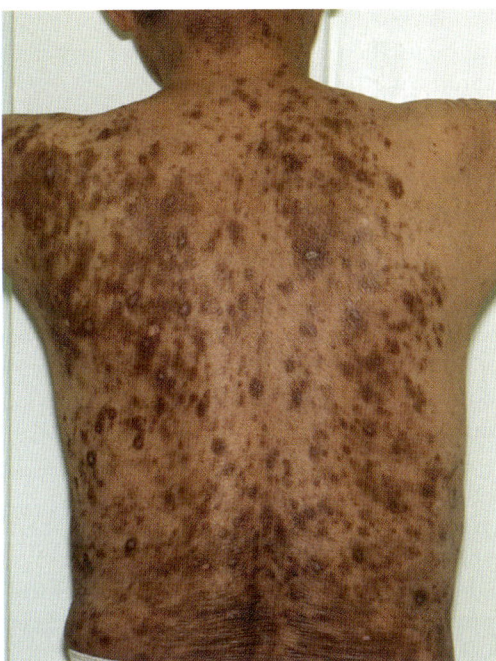

Figure 86.31 Post-inflammatory hypermelanosis on the back following propranolol-provoked lichenoid drug reaction.

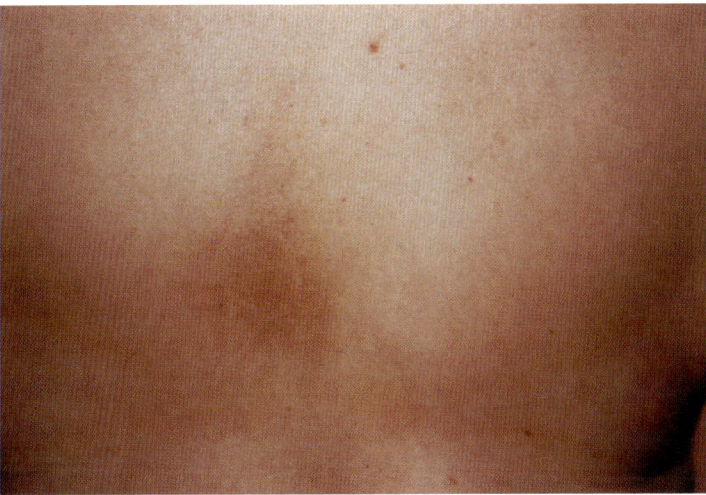

Figure 86.32 Notalgia paraesthetica: note the circumscribed area of hypermelanosis near the base of the left scapula.

occurs due to damage of cells in the basal layer. There is pigmentary incontinence with melanophages in the upper dermis [1]. In the late phase of chronic graft-versus-host reaction, there is a poikilodermatous appearance with hyperpigmentation [2,3].

Hypermelanosis of the epidermis may also occur because of cutaneous inflammation, but more frequently there is reduced epidermal melanin pigmentation. This can be explained by an increased mitotic rate of keratinocytes, diminished transfer of melanosomes from the melanocyte to keratinocyte and a reduced transit time of the latter from the basal layer to the skin surface. Very frequently in inflammatory skin disease, hypermelanosis and hypomelanosis occur together, often with a slaty-blue colour due to the presence of melanophages in the upper dermis. There may be an associated loss of functional melanocytes in the skin [4].

The cause of the pigmentation is usually obvious, although the preceding lesions have sometimes not been noticed by the patient or have been transitory or clinically imperceptible.

Clinical features
Presentation
The pattern and distribution of the pigmentation will sometimes allow a retrospective diagnosis, as in lichen planus, herpes zoster, dermatitis herpetiformis and papular urticaria. Pigmentation is often conspicuous after lichenoid drug eruptions (Figure 86.31). The circumscribed nature and the location at the base of the scapula are characteristic of the pigmentation which typically accompanies notalgia paraesthetica, a sensory neuropathy of dorsal spinal nerves which presents as intense localised pruritus or paraesthesiae (Chapter 83): the pigmentation may be due to chronic rubbing and scratching (Figure 86.32) [5]. Reticulate pigmentation corresponding to the underlying vascular network is seen in erythema ab igne (Chapter 125), a more recently described cause of which is heat from laptop computers rather than open fires or hot water bottles [6].

Infective causes include late secondary syphilis, in which diffuse hypermelanosis of the sides and back of the neck and the shoulders may develop (leukoderma colli syphiliticum) (Chapter 29) [7] and late pinta in which slaty-blue dyspigmentation may be seen (Chapter 26). Postinflammatory hyperpigmentation may also occur following trauma to the skin, including procedures such as dermabrasion, particularly in darker skin types.

Differential diagnosis
Acquired diffuse hyperpigmentation: see Box 86.3a.

Classification of severity
The degree of inflammation appears to be of less significance in determining the pigmentary response than the nature of the dermatosis, for it may be frequent and severe after some conditions and slight after others.

Disease course and prognosis
The skin lightens slowly over time spontaneously or with therapy. This is usually 6–12 months but may take several years.

Treatment ladder for postinflammatory hypermelanosis

First line
- Prevention of the inflammation, regardless of aetiology
- Treatment of underlying cause
- Sun protection

Second line
- A variety of topical treatments may be effective, including hydroquinone 2–4%, retinoids, azelaic acid and α-hydroxy acid, preferably in combination therapy

Third line
- Laser therapy (Q-switched ruby, alexandrite, Nd:YAG) but results are limited. Complete clearance of pigment is rare, and recurrence within 6–12 months is reported [8]

Ashy dermatosis and erythema dyschromicum perstans

Definition and nomenclature

A spectrum of cutaneous pigmentary disorders of uncertain aetiology characterised by the development of persistent grey-blue hypermelanotic cutaneous macules [1,2–5] for which no specific cause can be identified. It has been proposed that ashy dermatosis be used for all such cases but that erythema chronicum perstans be limited to those cases in which an inflammatory phase with redness has been observed [1].

Synonyms and inclusions

- Ashy dermatosis of Ramirez
- Dermatosis cenicienta
- Erythema dyschromicum perstans
- Erythema chronicum figuratum melanodermicum
- Idiopathic eruptive macular pigmentation

Epidemiology

Incidence and prevalence

Dependent on the geographic region.

Age

From childhood to old age, most frequently in young adults.

Sex

It occurs in both sexes, but females more than males.

Ethnicity

Mainly observed in intermediate skin types. Most published cases have been from Central and South America or East Asia [4,5].

Pathophysiology

The underlying cause of ashy dermatosis is unknown and is likely to be heterogeneous. Those cases in which redness is present share many features with lichen planus including lichenoid inflammation histopathologically with basement membrane zone damage and infiltration of T lymphocytes [6,7]. Exocytosis of cutaneous lymphocyte antigen (CLA)+ cells has been observed in areas of basement membrane zone damage, suggesting that response to antigenic stimulation may play a role in its development [7].

Pathology

The active border in cases of erythema chronicum perstans shows vacuolar degeneration of the basal cells. The epidermis contains much pigment and there is pigmentary incontinence; the dermal vessels are sleeved with an infiltrate of lymphocytes and histiocytes, and there are many melanophages [6]. Ultrastructural studies show vacuoles within the cytoplasm of basal and suprabasal keratinocytes that contain many melanosome complexes.

Genetics

In a Mexican population, HLA-DR4 has been associated with erythema dyschromicum perstans [8].

Clinical features

History

This clinical syndrome of unknown origin was first reported by Ramirez of El Salvador in 1957 under the term 'los cenicientos' (the ashy ones) due to the ashy discoloration of the skin. A further case series was reported by Convit, Kerdel-Vegas and Rodriguez from Venezuela in 1961 who commented on the presence of raised red borders in the early stages and proposed the term 'erythema dyschromicum perstans' [3]. Initial inflammation is not, however, always apparent either clinically or histologically [1].

Presentation

Clinically, ashy dermatosis is characterised by numerous macules of varying shades of grey (Figure 86.33); there may initially be signs of inflammation with a red, slightly raised and palpably infiltrated margin (erythema dyschromicum perstans). In a recent review of 68 patients from Korea, less than a fifth were observed to have peripheral red borders to their lesions [5]. In this study, the trunk was affected in two-thirds and the face, neck and upper limbs each in just over one-third of patients; one-quarter had lower limb involvement. The macules vary in size and tend to coalesce over extensive areas of the trunk, limbs and face. Against the general greyish background are macules of hypomelanosis or hypermelanosis. The condition is persistent and slowly extends. The lesions are mostly asymptomatic, although some patients may experience mild pruritus. Mucous membranes are spared.

Differential diagnosis (Box 86.3b)

- Lichen planus pigmentosus.
- Postinflammatory hypermelanosis secondary to identifiable cause.
- Late pinta, which should be excluded in endemic areas.

Disease course and prognosis

The initial erythematous phase tends to settle after several months [1]. The pigmentation is persistent with a tendency to extend gradually over years.

Treatment ladder for ashy dermatosis and erythema dyschromicum perstans

- There is no consistently effective treatment

First line

- Cosmetic: camouflage creams and make-up
- Clofazimine 100 mg/day for 3 months in inflammatory cases (response rate of 66–87%)

Second line

- Dapsone 100 mg/day for 3 months
- Oral corticosteroid therapy
- UV therapy

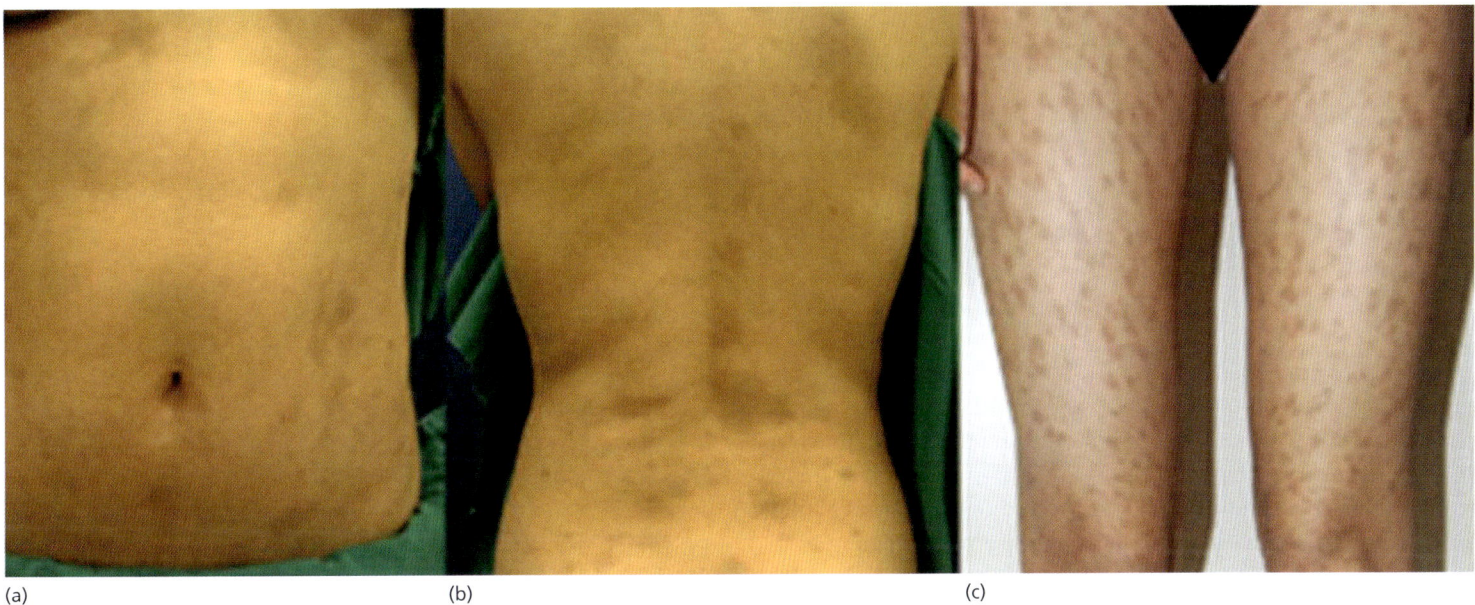

(a)   (b)   (c)

Figure 86.33 Ashy dermatosis: views of two females aged 31 years (a, b) and 15 years (c) with multiple muddy grey non-inflamed macules on the skin. Reproduced from Cheng *et al.* 2015 [5] with permission of John Wiley & Sons.

Treatment of hypermelanosis

Hypermelanosis, particularly affecting areas on the face, can be the cause of marked cosmetic disability and give rise to much mental distress. Treatment depends essentially on establishing the cause and if possible reversing the conditions that have given rise to the hypermelanosis. Because in many cases exposure to sunlight intensifies the pigmentation and lesions can be aggravated by UVA and UVB, a photoprotective preparation should be prescribed and applied during sunny weather. Cosmetic camouflage may also be indicated. In the majority of cases, topical therapy has no place, although some who are perturbed about their cosmetic disability will demand treatment with a skin-bleaching preparation.

A number of compounds have been used in skin-bleaching preparations. The most well-studied hypopigmenting agent used to treat melasma and other hypermelanotic conditions is hydroquinone. Topical hydroquinone is mostly used in a concentration of 4%, included in cold cream or a hydroalcoholic base. Acute side effects associated with hydroquinone include infrequent allergic reactions, postinflammatory hyperpigmentation and transient hypopigmentation [1]. It can be applied alone or in the widely used triple combination cream consisting of hydroquinone 4%, a retinoid and a corticosteroid. Topical hydroquinone and this triple combination cream are highly effective and safe and can be considered as first line agents in the treatment of melasma. Because of concern about steroid-induced facial atrophy, telangiectasia and rosacea-like acneiform eruptions, the use of triple combination cream has been limited to no more than twice daily for 6 months, disqualifying it as a maintenance therapy for melasma [1,2]. Topical hydroquinone and tretinoin are also effective in the treatment of postinflammatory hyperpigmentation but require prolonged treatment [3]. The monobenzylether of hydroquinone has been used only to bleach away the remaining pigmented areas

in patients with extensive vitiligo [4]. Several other substituted phenols, such as 4-isopropylcatechol, can produce cutaneous depigmentation; however, this compound and others are irritant and may sensitise [5].

In cases of pigmentary disorders such as melasma that are refractory to topical medication, combination with procedures such as peels or laser can be considered.

Chemical peels with glycolic acid or salicylic acid can be a useful adjunct to those topical treatments, although the therapeutic response is often unsatisfactory and a universally effective chemical peeling has not yet been discovered [1]. Due to the adverse effects associated with these chemical peels, such as burning, bleeding and an increased risk of hyperpigmentation, they are considered second line agents in the treatment of melasma and should be limited to cases refractory to topical treatment and used cautiously in dark-skinned patients who are at a higher risk of postinflammatory hyperpigmentation [6].

In cases where an underlying vascular component is present in melasma, topical, intradermal or systemic tranexamic acid or vascular light/laser treatments can be considered [7].

Laser or light therapy for the treatment of melasma has become increasingly popular. As with chemical peels, they carry an increased risk of side effects due to direct damage to the skin. Despite the risks, some promising results are seen in randomised trials using laser or light therapy [3,8]. Serial treatments with intense pulsed light (IPL) therapy have been shown to be effective in the treatment of melasma and may be indicated in selected cases. Treatment of melasma with a Q-switched (QS) Nd:YAG laser has produced variable results and a high rate of relapse following treatment. The relatively limited experience and the common adverse effects of laser therapy call for more research to assess the safety and efficacy of this treatment. Lasers are considered third line agents for the treatment of melasma and should be used cautiously, especially in dark-skinned patients [2,6].

PART 8: SPECIFIC CUTANEOUS STRUCTURES

ACQUIRED HYPOMELANOSIS (Figure 86.34)

Vitiligo

Definition

Vitiligo is a common form of localised depigmentation. It is an acquired condition resulting from the progressive loss of melanocytes. It is characterised by milky-white sharply demarcated macules [1].

Vitiligo has in general been classified into two major forms: segmental vitiligo (typically unilateral maculae in a segmental/band-shaped distribution) and non-segmental vitiligo (bilateral maculae, often distributed in an acrofacial pattern or scattered symmetrically over the entire body). According to a recent Vitiligo Global Issue Consensus Conference, the term 'vitiligo' can be used as an umbrella term for all non-segmental forms of vitiligo (including several variants: acrofacial, mucosal, generalised, universal, mixed and rare variants of vitiligo) [2]. Segmental vitiligo (uni-, bi-, or plurisegmental) is classified separately. Focal lesions (small isolated depigmented lesions that are not segmentally distributed and have not evolved into non-segmental vitiligo after 1–2 years) and isolated mucosal lesions on one site are considered as undetermined/unclassified vitiligo.

Epidemiology

Incidence and prevalence

It is stated that vitiligo affects 0.5–1% of the world's population [2].

Age

Vitiligo can begin at any age but in the majority of cases becomes apparent between the ages of 20 and 30 years.

Sex

The prevalence is most probably the same in both sexes [2], although in some series based on outpatient attendances a female preponderance was noted.

Ethnicity

Vitiligo affects all races.

Associated diseases

Conditions associated with vitiligo are listed in Box 86.4.

Among autoimmune diseases, the strongest association is with thyroid disease. The association between vitiligo and halo naevi

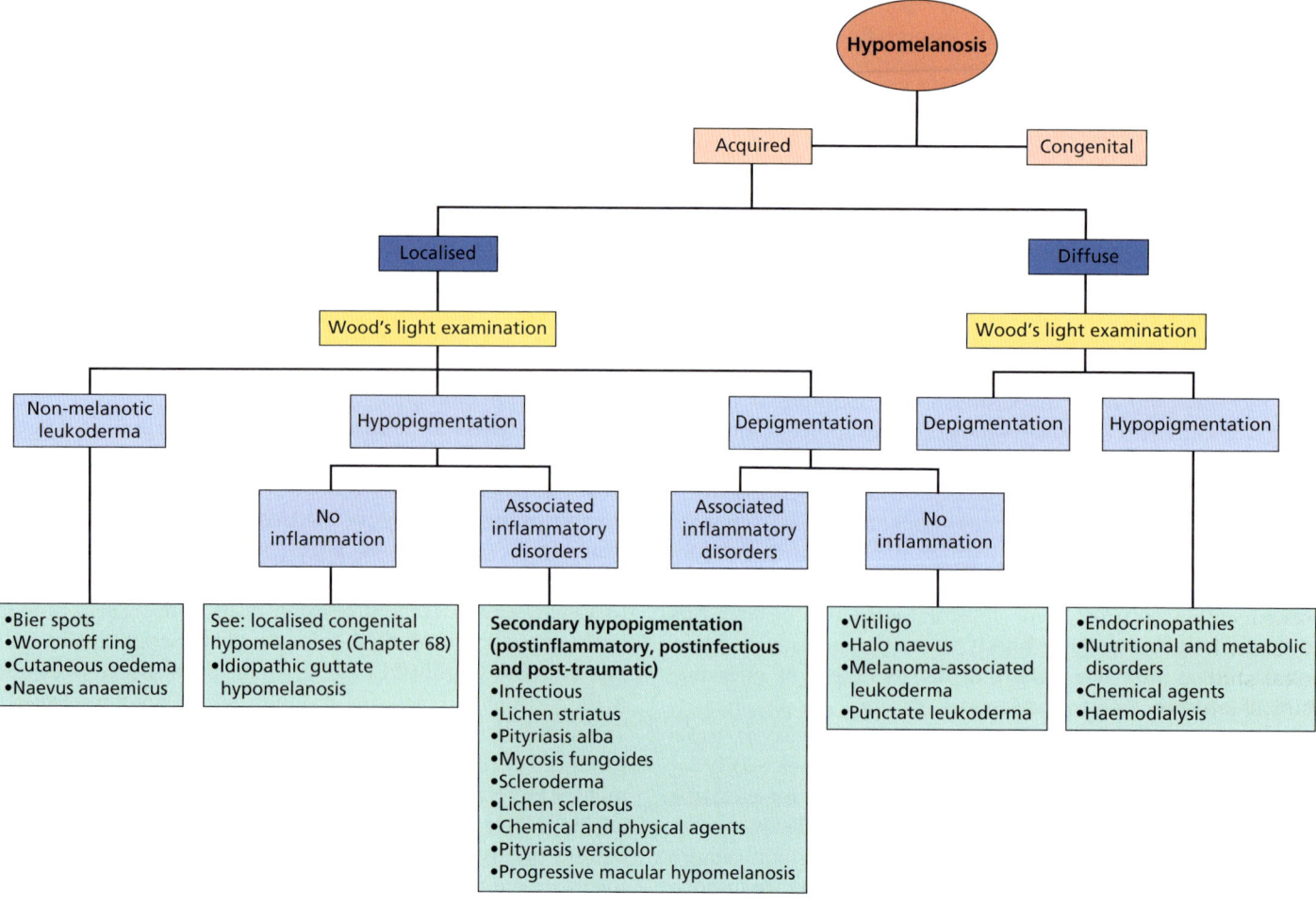

Figure 86.34 Algorithm for the differential diagnosis of hypomelanosis.

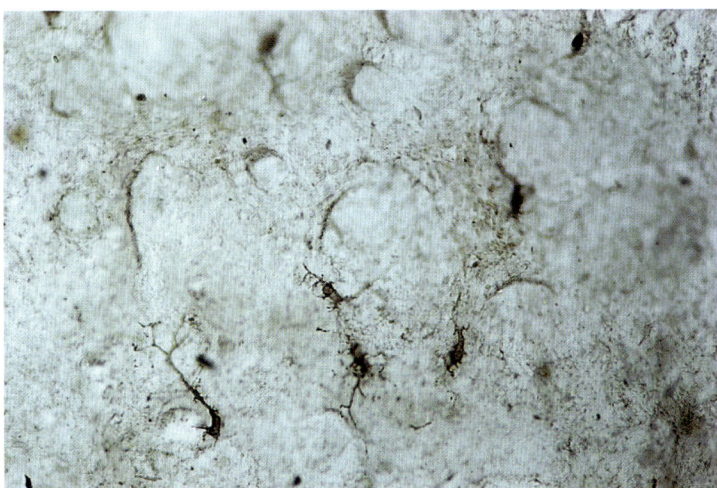

Figure 86.35 Vitiligo. Epidermal sheet of marginal depigmented area showing marked reduction in the number of melanocytes.

is well established: several reports have documented the onset of vitiligo at the same time as or shortly after the appearance of a halo naevus and, in a recent study, halo naevi were present in 31.1% of all vitiligo patients [3]. Areas of depigmentation sometimes develop in patients with melanoma [3]: these may be local or distant. Vitiligo with uveitis, central nervous system involvement and premature greying of the hair occurs in the Vogt–Koyanagi–Harada syndrome (see later).

Box 86.4 Disorders associated with vitiligo

- Thyroid disease[a] (hyperthyroidism and hypothyroidism [7])
- Pernicious anaemia[a]
- Addison disease[a] [8]
- Diabetes[a] [9]
- Hypoparathyroidism[a]
- Myasthenia gravis[a]
- Alopecia areata
- Morphoea and lichen sclerosus
- Halo naevus[a]
- Malignant melanoma[a] [10]

[a] Autoantibodies demonstrable.

Pathophysiology
Pathology

Histochemical studies [4] show a lack of dopa-positive melanocytes in the basal layer of the epidermis (Figure 86.35). Immunohistochemical studies with a large panel of antibodies show only an occasional melanocyte in lesional skin [5]. Electron microscopy studies [6,7] confirm the loss of melanocytes. In the epidermis of areas around the margins of vitiligo, abnormalities of keratinocytes [8,9] as well as degenerating melanocytes are reported. In inflammatory vitiligo, where there is a raised erythematous border, there is an infiltrate of lymphocytes and histiocytes. This infiltrate is also found in the marginal areas of some biopsies, mainly in an active stage of the disease [7].

Causative organisms

Various theories have been suggested for the aetiology of vitiligo; the same mechanism may not apply to all cases. Moreover, the loss of melanocytes in vitiligo may also be the result of different pathogenetic mechanisms working together ('convergence' or 'integrated' theory) [8,9].

- The autoimmune/autoinflammatory theory is currently the leading hypothesis and is supported by strong evidence. It is based on the clinical association of vitiligo with a number of disorders also considered to be autoimmune or autoinflammatory (Box 86.4). The association with vitiligo has demonstrated a shared underlying genetic susceptibility to other autoimmune diseases [10].
- A combination of deregulated innate and adaptive immune responses has been proposed in vitiligo. Interestingly, several components of the innate immune system have been found to be associated with vitiligo (e.g. NLRP-1, XBP-1). Furthermore, an important role of heat shock protein 70 (hsp70) and LL37 (which is released after cell injury) has been suggested [**11**,**12**,13].
- It has also been proposed that increased oxidative stress may trigger the process of 'haptenation' by increasing the levels of surrogate substrates of tyrosinase resulting in the formation of highly immunogenic neoantigens in vitiligo [14].
- Antibodies to normal human melanocytes have been detected using a specific immunoprecipitation assay [15,16], and may have a cytolytic effect on melanocytes [17]. The presence of these melanocyte antibodies has been linked to disease activity [18]. It is currently unclear if these antibodies play an initiating role in the development of vitiligo or are a secondary result of the disease [19].
- Accumulating evidence supports a major aetiological role for melanocyte-specific cytotoxic T cells in coordinating the targeted autoimmune tissue destruction of melanocytes in progressive vitiligo [20,21]. Both helper and cytotoxic T cells from progressing margins generate predominantly type 1 cytokines. This theory is supported by the fact that various effective treatment options in vitiligo have an immunosuppressive effect on the activation and maturation of T cells (e.g. local steroids and topical immunomodulators).

Many other hypotheses have been put forward. The self-destruction theory of Lerner suggested that melanocytes destroyed themselves due to a defect in a natural protective mechanism that removed toxic melanin precursors [22]. This hypothesis was based on the clinical features of vitiligo and on experimental studies of cutaneous depigmentation by chemical compounds that have a selective lethal effect on functional melanocytes [23]: these compounds can produce a leukoderma indistinguishable from idiopathic vitiligo. Other proposed mechanisms for vitiligo include defective keratinocyte metabolism with low catalase levels in the epidermis [24], defective tetrahydrobiopterin and catecholamine biosynthesis [25], and loss of melanocytes through inhibition of their adhesion to fibronectin by extracellular matrix molecules [26]. *In vivo*, repeated frictional trauma to perilesional skin in non-segmental vitiligo has been shown to induce detachment and death of melanocytes ('melanocytorrhagy') [27]. Additionally, a neurogenic mechanism has been suggested whereby it has been hypothesised that a compound released at peripheral nerve endings in the skin could have a toxic effect on melanocytes. Findings from

Figure 86.36 Isomorphic or Koebner phenomenon at site of a scratch in a patient with vitiligo.

a small number of studies on neuropeptide and neuronal markers in vitiligo suggest that neuropeptide Y may play a role [28]. So far there is, however, little support for this hypothesis.

Genetics

A genetic factor is undoubtedly involved in vitiligo. Inheritance has been suggested to be polygenic. Approximately 30% of patients have a positive family history [22] and vitiligo has been reported in monozygotic twins [29].

Genome-wide association studies have identified several susceptibility loci for generalised vitiligo, each responsible for a small part of the genetic risk. Nearly all of the genes identified at these loci encode components of the immune system. The exception is *TYR* [30], which encodes the enzyme tyrosinase, which is not a component of the immune system but catalyses melanin biosynthesis within the melanocyte and is a major autoantigen in generalised vitiligo.

Environmental factors

The Koebner phenomenon is a well-known phenomenon in vitiligo (also called isomorphic response) (Figure 86.36). It has been defined as the development of lesions at sites of trauma to uninvolved skin of patients with cutaneous diseases [11]. To create a universally acceptable specific system for the evaluation of Koebner phenomenon in vitiligo, the Vitiligo European Task Force (VETF) group introduced a new assessment and classification method [11]. It has been suggested that the Koebner phenomenon may function as a clinical parameter to assess and predict the clinical profile and course of vitiligo [31].

Clinical features

Presentation [22] (Figures 86.37 and 86.38)

The amelanotic macules in vitiligo are found particularly in areas of repeated friction, chronic pressure or trauma, for example the hips, dorsa of the hands/fingers, feet, elbows, knees (Figure 86.39) and ankles [11]. The lesions are also prone to sunburn; rarely, itching may be present without previous sun exposure or sunburn. The distribution of the lesions is usually symmetrical, although in the segmental subtype it is usually unilateral and band shaped (Figure 86.40). Rarely, there is complete vitiligo (universalis), although most often a few pigmented areas remain indefinitely (Figure 86.41). The pigment loss may be partial or complete, or both may occur in the same areas (trichrome vitiligo) (Figure 86.42). The macules usually have a convex outline, increase irregularly in size and fuse with neighbouring lesions to form complex patterns. The hairs in the patches can

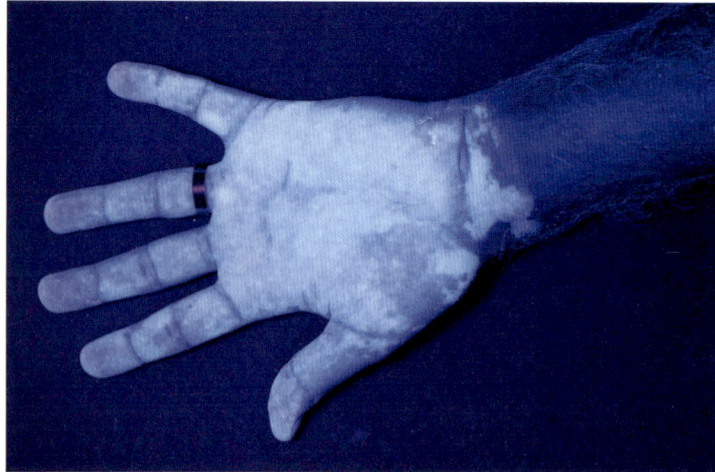

Figure 86.37 Typical distribution of vitiligo on the wrist and volar surface of the hand seen under Wood's light.

remain normally pigmented but can also depigment after a certain period of time (poliosis/leukotrichia). The margins of the lesions may become hyperpigmented. The main symptom is the cosmetic disability, although some patients present because of sunburn in the amelanotic areas. Additionally, psychological symptoms such as anxiety and depression are frequent in patients with vitiligo [32]. Vitiligo can also start in children, who are more likely to show segmental vitiligo [33]. Active vitiligo can be recognised by the presence of hypopigmented borders, confetti-like depigmentations (grouped small/pinpoint-sized hypo- and depigmented macules) and presence of Koebner phenomenon [34].

Clinical variants

Mixed vitiligo. The coexistence of non-segmental and segmental vitiligo in one patient is called mixed vitiligo and is classified as a subgroup of vitiligo (NSV) [2].

Halo naevi-associated leukoderma. This is a form of hypomelanosis analogous to melanoma-associated leukoderma, where discrete areas of depigmentation develop in skin distant from the halo naevi (see later), particularly in individuals with large numbers of them [35]. This phenomenon differs from classical vitiligo in that the depigmented macules are often more limited and not as clearly demarcated from normal skin as in vitiligo and often do not progress. The disorder probably results from a temporary autoimmune process directly linked to the halo phenomenon [35].

Differential diagnosis [36]

- Halo naevi.
- Naevus depigmentosus (Figure 86.43).
- Naevus anaemicus.
- Inherited or genetically induced hypomelanosis (usually present at birth):
  - Piebaldism.
  - Waardenburg syndrome.
  - Tuberous sclerosis.
  - Pigmentary mosaicism (hypomelanosis of Ito).
- Progressive macular hypomelanosis.

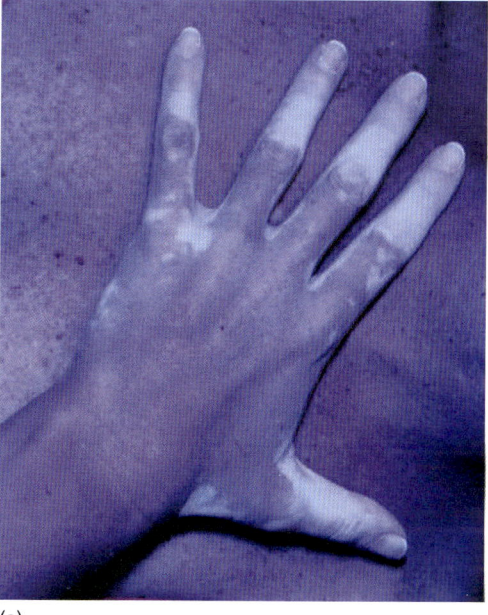
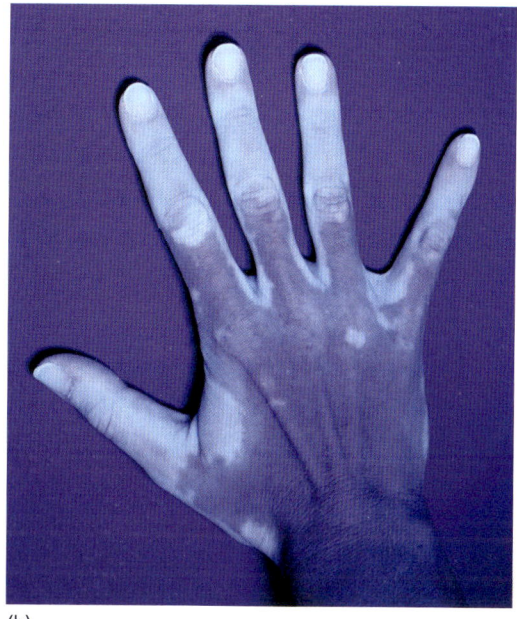

Figure 86.38 (a, b) Typical distribution of vitiligo on dorsum of the hand seen under Wood's light.

(a)   (b)

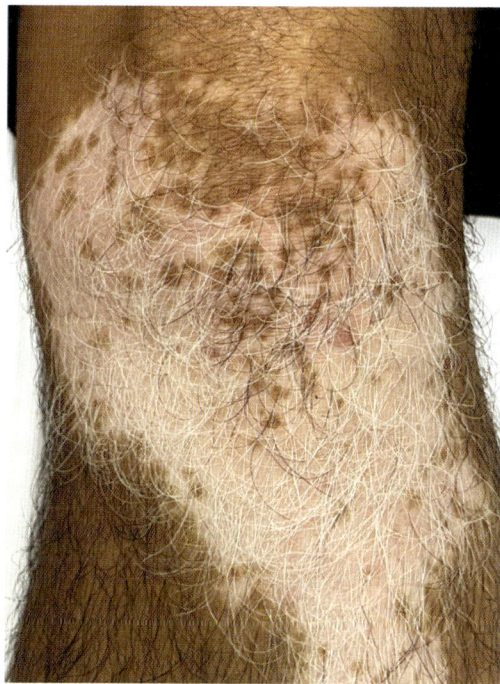

Figure 86.39 Vitiligo on the knee of a patient with skin of colour. Note depigmentation of hairs within the area of vitiligo. Courtesy of Dr Julio Salas.

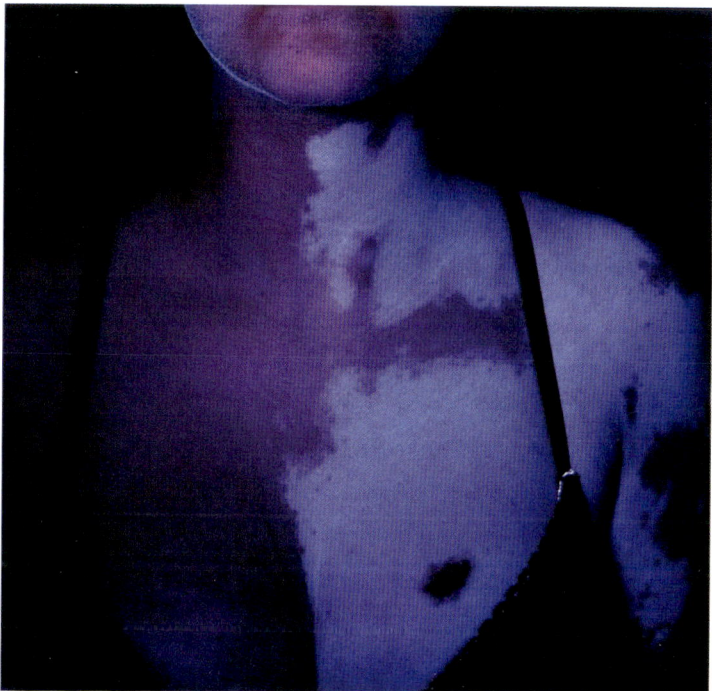

Figure 86.40 Segmental vitiligo on the trunk seen under Wood's light. Note regressing congenital naevus in the centre of the affected area.

- Secondary hypomelanosis:
  - Postinflammatory hypomelanosis (e.g. pityriasis alba, lichen sclerosus, morphoea).
  - Post-traumatic hypomelanosis.
  - Postinfectious hypomelanosis (e.g. pityriasis versicolor, leprosy).
  - Cutaneous lymphoma.

Classification of severity
The affected body surface area is often used to score the severity of the disease [37,38]. The extent of vitiligo can be measured by validated instruments such as the Vitiligo Extent Score (VES) and Vitiligo Area Severity Index (VASI).

Complications and comorbidities
See associated diseases.

Disease course and prognosis
Most frequently, vitiligo is gradually progressive, sometimes extending rapidly over a period of several months and then remaining quiescent for many years. Spontaneous repigmentation can

PART 8: SPECIFIC CUTANEOUS STRUCTURES

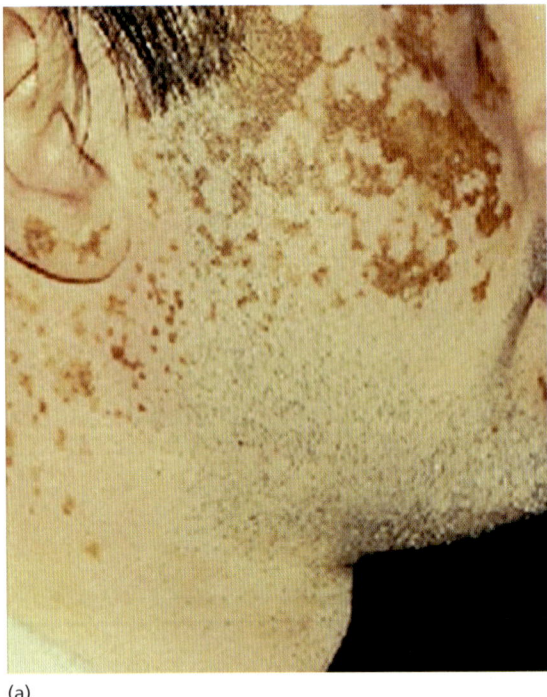

(a)

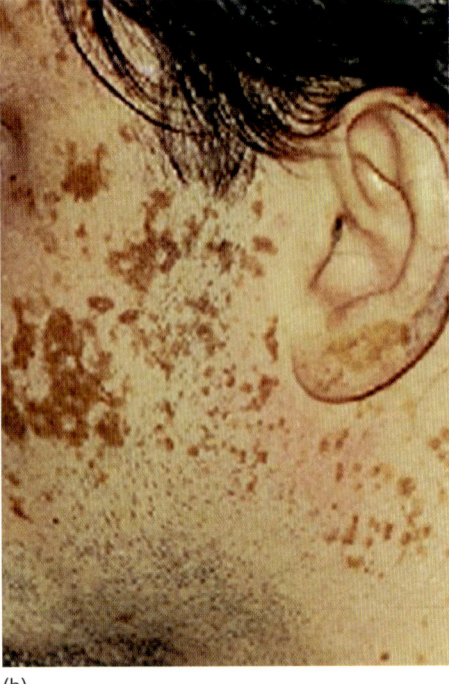

(b)

Figure 86.41 (a, b) Extensive vitiligo in a South Asian man: view of the sides of the face showing the convex expanding margins of the vitiliginous skin 'eating into' the few residual areas of normal pigmentation. Note that pigmentation of the scalp and beard hair is unaffected.

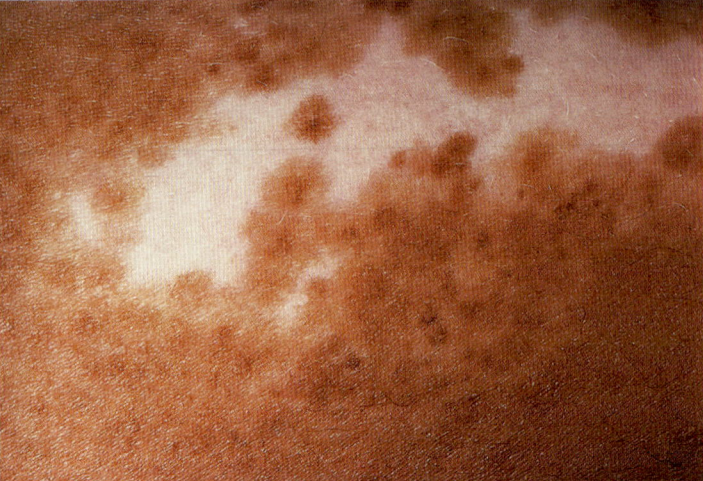

Figure 86.42 Trichrome vitiligo.

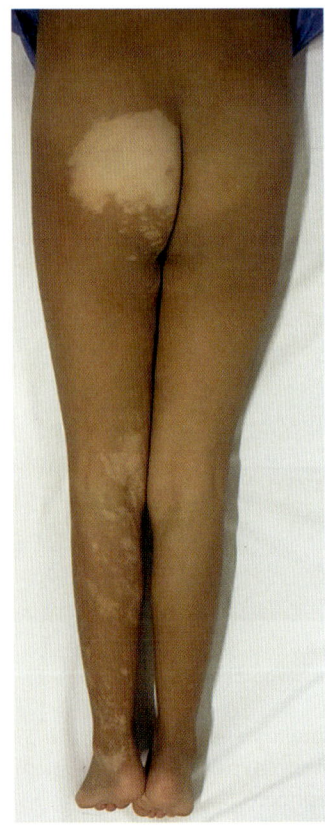

Figure 86.43 Naevus depigmentosus. Courtesy of Dr Julio Salas.

sometimes be noted in sun-exposed areas and can have a typical perifollicular appearance [22]. Segmental vitiligo generally starts earlier in life than non-segmental vitiligo and often stabilises within the first year of onset [33].

Investigations

The diagnosis of vitiligo is based essentially on clinical examination, because the lesions have a typical appearance. However, if the lesions are not distributed in the pattern of classical vitiligo, confusion with other hypomelanotic disorders can arise. Inspection with the aid of a Wood's light can then be helpful. The presence of a family history of vitiligo, the Koebner phenomenon, leukotrichia or associated autoimmune disorders such as thyroid disease can help to support a clinical diagnosis of vitiligo [36].

Management

Response to treatment of vitiligo varies between individuals but is often unsatisfactory, especially for acral lesions. Patients are best advised to seek effective cosmetic camouflage (Figure 86.44) and to use sunscreen. Furthermore, the risk of koebnerisation resulting

PART 8: SPECIFIC CUTANEOUS STRUCTURES

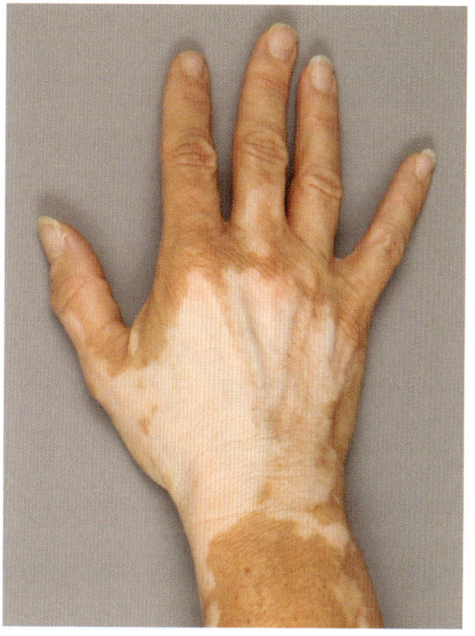 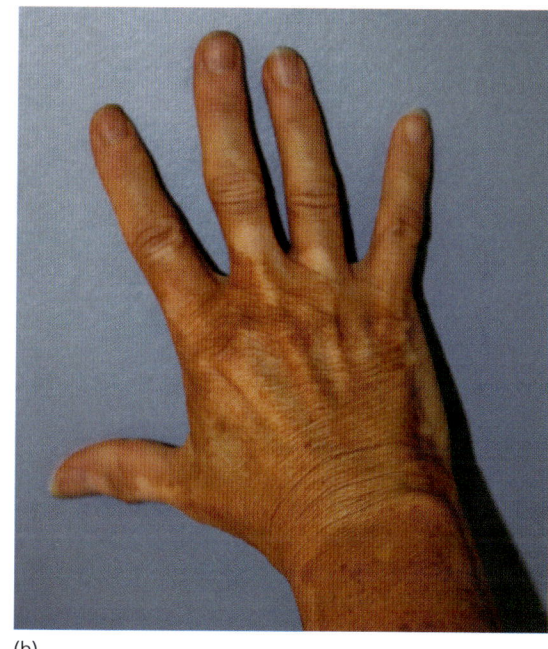

Figure 86.44 (a, b) Vitiligo: before and after camouflage of the hands.

(a)   (b)

from everyday activities should be explained to patients. Some authors suggest that successful repigmentation is mostly the result of combinations of various interventions including light, indicating this is an effective, though not necessarily permanent, treatment for generalised vitiligo. Providing ways of coping with vitiligo could also be of benefit to patients [**39**].

First line

In some patients, once-daily application of potent topical corticosteroid preparations (e.g. 0.1% betamethasone valerate or 0.05% clobetasol propionate) is effective at inducing stabilisation or repigmentation of areas of vitiligo. It is preferable to use an intermittent regimen (e.g. 15 days per month for 6 months) to avoid local side effects (skin atrophy, telangiectasia, striae, hypertrichosis and acneiform eruptions) [**40**]. Topical calcineurin inhibitors (pimecrolimus, tacrolimus) are good alternatives, mainly for lesions on the face and neck [**40**]: twice-daily applications are recommended, initially for 6 months. Topical JAK inhibitors (e.g. ruxolitinib) are promising alternatives displaying excellent efficacy especially in vitiligo on the face [**41,42**].

Second line

UVB therapy can also be used to induce repigmentation and localised targeted phototherapy devices (excimer lamp or lasers with a peak at 308 nm) are attractive alternatives [**39**]. There is no consensus as to the optimum treatment duration of phototherapy. Most often irradiation will be stopped if no repigmentation occurs within the first 3 months of treatment, although slow responders have been reported [**43**].

Treatment with systemic psoralen photochemotherapy (PUVA) is effective but in general narrow-band UVB is preferred because of the much higher risk for skin cancer [**39**]. Guidance on treatment regimens is given in Chapter 21 and in the recommendations of the Vitiligo Working Group [**44**]. The use of topical applications of psoralens is more hazardous and may result in untoward blistering of the skin. Alternative photosensitisers including khellin have been advocated but there are concerns over hepatotoxicity and it has not been widely adopted [**45**].

Third line

Grafting techniques [**40,46**]. Surgical methods have been proposed as a therapeutic option in patients with stable vitiligo (e.g. stable segmental vitiligo). Regardless of the technique used, the stability of the lesions is the main determining factor for a successful treatment. These surgical techniques are based on a common basic principle: to transplant autologous melanocytes from a normal pigmented area to the affected depigmented skin. Different surgical techniques for repigmenting vitiligo have been gradually devised and include tissue grafts (full-thickness punch grafts, split-thickness grafts, suction blister grafts) and cellular grafts (cultured melanocytes, cultured epithelial sheet grafts and non-cultured epidermal cellular grafts). Lately, the use of hair follicle outer root sheath cells has been introduced [**47**]. The three tissue grafting methods (full-thickness punch grafts, split-thickness grafts, suction blister grafts) seem to have comparable success rates in inducing repigmentation. Cellular grafting techniques were in general found to be nearly as effective, although the percentages of patients in whom repigmentation was achieved were slightly lower than with the tissue grafting techniques [**48**]. However, cellular grafting can be used to treat larger areas and has in general better cosmetic results compared with tissue grafts (Figure 86.45) [**49**]. Furthermore, adverse events seem to be less frequent with cellular grafts than with punch or split-skin grafts.

Systemic treatments. Oral corticoid mini-pulse treatment can be used in patients with progressive vitiligo. A dosage of 2.5–5 mg dexamethasone on two consecutive days in a week is able to arrest disease activity in the majority of patients although combination with UVB exposure is in most cases necessary to induce satisfactory repigmentation. Alternative immunomodulators such as methotrexate and even minocycline have also been reported to

PART 8: SPECIFIC CUTANEOUS STRUCTURES

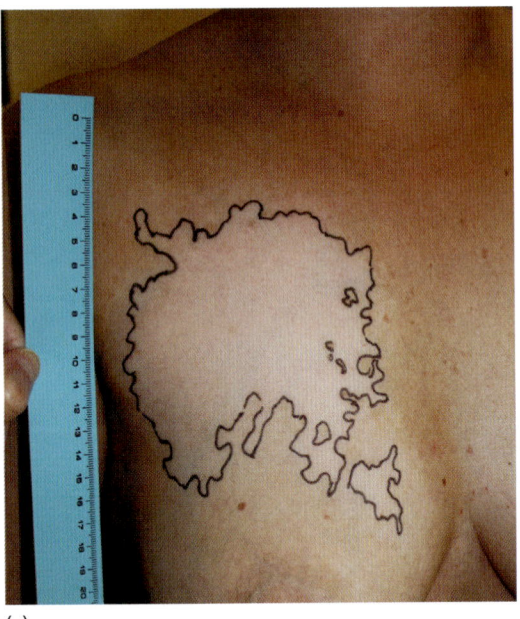

(a)

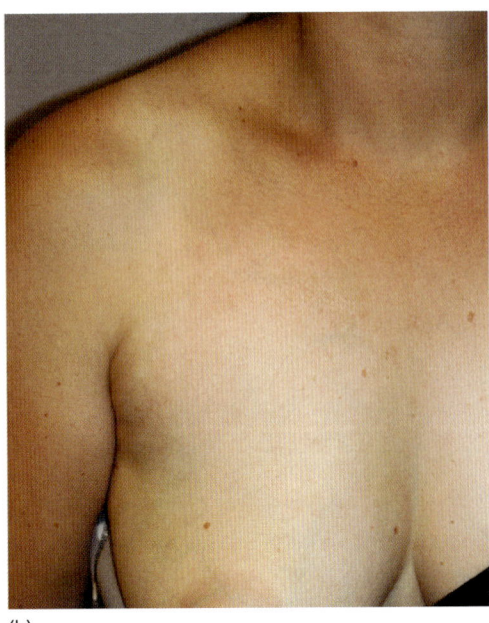

(b)

Figure 86.45 (a,b) Segmental vitiligo (a) before and (b) after treatment with non-cultured epidermal cell transplantation.

prevent further disease spreading [50]. More recently, systemic JAK inhibitors (e.g. tofacitinib, ruxolitinib) have shown promising results. Nonetheless, studies have demonstrated that concomitant UV exposure seems needed for sufficient repigmentation [51].

Antioxidants. A variety of studies has been published on the use of antioxidants in vitiligo although confirmatory results remain scarce. There is some evidence for the use of oral antioxidants (e.g. polypodium leucotomos) in combination with NB-UVB [50].

Depigmenting treatment. In those patients with extensive vitiligo and only a few residual areas of pigmentation, skin bleaching with laser therapy (e.g. Q-switched alexandrite 755 nm, Q-switched ruby 694 nm), cryotherapy or creams (e.g. 20% monobenzylether of hydroquinone) may be used [52].

Treatment ladder for vitiligo

First line
- Topical corticosteroids, topical calcineurin inhibitors [40]

Second line
- Phototherapy

Third line
- Grafting techniques
- Systemic treatment (e.g. corticoid mini-pulse)
- Antioxidants
- Depigmentation

Resources

Further information
Guidelines: references [40] and [48].

Halo naevus

Synonyms and inclusions
- Sutton naevus
- Leukoderma acquisitum centrifugum

Introduction and general description
Leukoderma acquisitum centrifugum designates the development of a halo of hypomelanosis around a central cutaneous tumour [1–10]. This tumour is usually a benign melanocytic naevus but may be a neuroid naevus, blue naevus, neurofibroma, or primary or secondary malignant melanoma [1].

Epidemiology
Incidence and prevalence
The prevalence of halo naevi has been estimated to be approximately 1% in the white population [9].

Age
Halo naevi can be seen at all ages but are usually seen in young people.

Sex
Either sex.

Ethnicity
Not known.

Associated diseases

Halo naevi occur with increased frequency in patients with vitiligo (see earlier) [9]. An immunological and clinical association of halo naevus with cutaneous malignant melanoma has been described. Antibodies against the cytoplasm of malignant melanoma cells are found in the serum of patients with halo naevi [3]. The prevalence of halo naevi was found to be 18% in a study of 72 patients with Turner syndrome compared with 1% in controls; the authors speculated that growth hormone therapy might have played a role [10].

Pathophysiology
Pathology

Most halo naevi are compound naevi, although a junctional or dermal naevoid pattern is also possible. Both congenital and acquired naevi can be affected. There is frequently a lymphocytic infiltration of the naevus and the constituent cells may show damage. Ultrastructural studies show the apposition of mononuclear cells with naevus cells that show cytotoxic changes [5]. In the depigmented halo, there is an absence of melanocytes, but Langerhans cells may be present [6]. Melanophages can be present in the dermis [1,7].

Causative organisms

Usually, no triggering factors are present, although the occurrence of halo naevi has occasionally been mentioned to be associated with sun exposure and sunburn. However, a causal relation has never been confirmed.

Genetics

Not known.

Clinical features
History

Vitiligo can be present in the personal or family history.

Presentation

Circular areas of hypomelanosis occur around pigmented naevi, particularly on the trunk, less commonly on the head and rarely on the limbs. Multiple lesions are common, the halos being about 0.5–2.0 cm wide and developing simultaneously or at intervals around several, but not all, naevi (Figure 86.46).

Clinical variants

A hypomelanotic halo may develop around a melanoma in a manner analogous to halo naevus (Figure 86.46c).

Differential diagnosis (Box 86.5)

Vitiligo.

Complications and comorbidities

Halo naevi can be present with or without associated vitiligo lesions.

Disease course and prognosis

The naevus tends to flatten and may disappear completely (Figure 86.47). The depigmented areas often persist but may pigment after many years.

Investigations

Excision of the naevus may be indicated in case of doubt about its benign character.

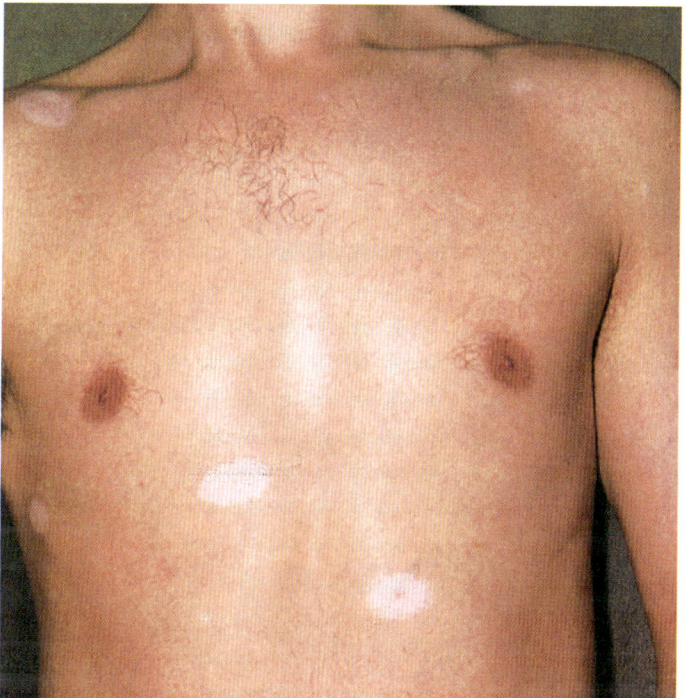

(a)

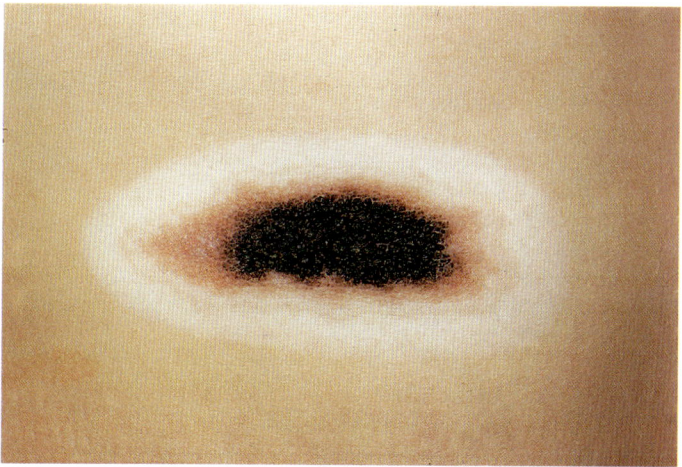

(b)

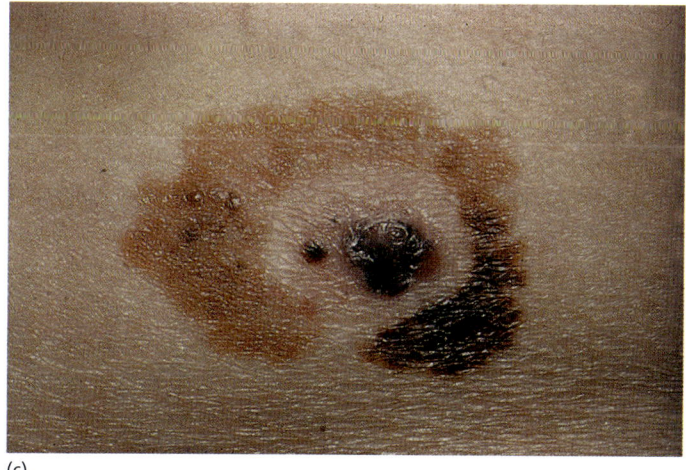

(c)

Figure 86.46 (a) Multiple halo naevi in a young man who also had vitiligo. (b) Unusually large halo naevus. (c) Halo phenomenon developing within a malignant melanoma that later proved fatal.

Box 86.5 Differential diagnosis of acquired hypo- and depigmentation

(a) Acquired diffuse hypo- or depigmentation
- Depigmentation
  - Vitiligo
- Hypopigmentation
  - Chemical-induced hypopigmentation
  - Endocrinopathies
  - Nutritional conditions
  - Postinflammatory
- Non-melanotic leukoderma
  - Anaemia

(b) Acquired localised hypo- or depigmentation
- Depigmentation
  - Vitiligo[a,b]
  - Halo naevi[a]
  - Punctate leukoderma[b]
  - Melanoma-associated leukoderma[a,b]
- Hypopigmentation
  - Progressive macular hypomelanosis[b]
- Idiopathic guttate hypomelanosis[b]
- Secondary hypopigmentation (postinfectious, postinflammatory, post-traumatic)
  - Lichen planus[a,b]
  - Lichen sclerosus[a]
  - Lichen striatus[a]
  - Lupus erythematosus[a,b]
  - Morphoea[a]
  - Pityriasis alba[a]
  - Pityriasis lichenoides chronica[b]
  - Pityriasis versicolor[a,b]
  - Psoriasis[a,b]
  - Sarcoidosis[a,b]
- Non-melanotic leukoderma
  - Bier spots[b]

[a] Limited surface areas affected.
[b] Larger surface areas can be affected.

Management

Normally none is required. The usual diagnostic criteria must be applied if there is any possibility that the central tumour is malignant. It should be remembered that a halo around a benign naevus is relatively common, whereas malignant melanoma is rare, and a melanoma surrounded by a halo is extremely rare. Mutilating surgery must never be undertaken without preliminary histological examination by an experienced pathologist.

Acquired syndromic hypomelanosis

Vogt–Koyanagi–Harada syndrome

In 1906, Vogt reported a patient with atraumatic, idiopathic uveitis, poliosis and alopecia, a syndrome that in time would be associated with his name [1]. In 1926, Harada reported five cases of bilateral posterior uveitis and retinal detachment [2]. In 1929, Koyanagi reported 16 patients with headache, fever, dysacousia, vitiligo, poliosis, alopecia, bilateral anterior uveitis with occasional exudative retinal detachment [3]. Various combinations of synonym have been used for this disorder, which is now generally referred to with the above three names and abbreviated to VKHS.

Pathophysiology

The aetiology of VKHS has yet to be established. An abnormal response to a virus and immunological mechanisms have both been postulated.

Pathology

Electron microscopy of depigmented skin shows an absence of melanocytes as in vitiligo [4]. Colloid-amyloid bodies are also found at the dermal-epidermal junction [5]. Inflammatory skin lesions are characterised by a chronic mixed inflammatory cell infiltrate [6].

Clinical features [7,8]

VKHS mainly affects dark-skinned people or white people with dark pigmentation. It is rare but widely distributed. Most cases occur in the third and fourth decades but children may be affected. It affects the skin, eyes, inner ears and meninges.

Criteria for diagnosis are as follows:
- No history of ocular trauma or surgery preceding the initial onset of uveitis.
- No clinical or laboratory evidence suggestive of ocular disease entities.
- Bilateral ocular involvement: an early sign is diffuse choroiditis; a late sign is ocular depigmentation.
- Neurological and auditory findings: meningismus, tinnitus, cerebrospinal fluid pleocytosis.
- Skin and hair changes: alopecia, vitiligo, poliosis.

Typically, this condition is first diagnosed by ophthalmologists as the uveitis starts the march of symptoms and signs.

Diagnosis

The association of vitiligo with loss of pigment in the brows and lashes and with the residual ocular defects should clearly differentiate this syndrome from any other.

Alezzandrini syndrome [1–4]

Alezzandrini was involved in three papers describing the syndrome that now bears his name in the late 1950s and early 1960s [1–3].

Aetiology

The aetiology of this syndrome is unknown.

Clinical features

Alezzandrini syndrome has only been reported in a small number of cases [1–4]. It is characterised by unilateral, facial vitiligo associated with unilateral retinal degeneration, white hair, poliosis and deafness. There are similarities with VKHS in which skin, eye and auditory changes are also observed.

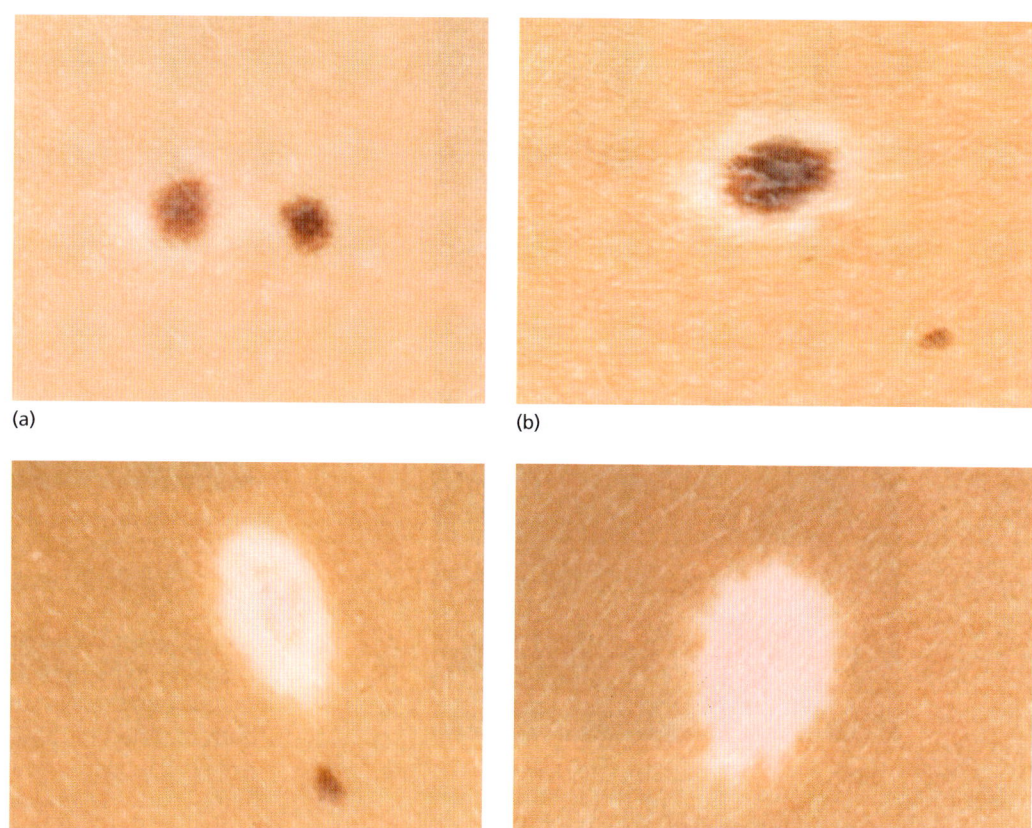

(a)

(b)

(c)

(d)

Figure 86.47 Halo naevi in different stages of evolution concurrently in a 13-year-old girl: (a) early depigmentation; (b) established halo naevus; (c) faint pink residuum of naevus just visible in the centre of the hypomelanotic macule; and (d) residual hypomelanotic macule following complete destruction of the naevus.

Postinflammatory hypomelanosis [1–17]

> **Synonyms and inclusions**
> - Postinflammatory/secondary hypopigmentation

Introduction and general description

Hypomelanotic areas occur following the resolution of areas of eczema and psoriasis (Figure 86.48). Hypomelanosis is also seen in pityriasis lichenoides and cutaneous T-cell lymphoma [1].

The superficial eczema known as pityriasis alba (Chapter 39) commonly presents with white, somewhat scaly, and not so well-defined areas of skin, which are most noticeable on the cheeks of racially pigmented children (Figure 86.49).

Hypopigmented macules also occur in the superficial fungal infection pityriasis versicolor, a condition frequently mistaken for vitiligo (Figure 86.50). Hyperpigmented areas can also be present. In a number of other inflammatory disorders of the skin, there are areas of hypomelanosis and in these there may be a loss of functional melanocytes. This loss is seen in lupus erythematosus and lichen planus. Hypomelanosis is also seen in sarcoidosis [7,8], lichen striatus, leprosy [9] and can occur in syphilis.

Epidemiology
Sex
Males and females are equally predisposed.

Pathophysiology

The hypopigmentation can be a consequence of an impaired transfer of melanin to the keratinocytes secondary to the inflammatory process or the result of application of potent topical steroids. In a number of other inflammatory disorders of the skin, there may be a loss of functional melanocytes (e.g. lupus erythematosus and lichen planus) due to destruction of the epidermal basal layer.

Pityriasis versicolor is one of the most common yeast infections associated with pigmentary changes. It is caused by dimorphic, lipophilic organisms in the genus *Malassezia* [3,4]. Eleven species are recognised within this classification of yeasts, of which *Malassezia globosa*, *Malassezia sympodialis* and *Malassezia sloffiae* are the predominant species isolated in pityriasis versicolor [4]. These yeasts are part of the normal skin flora and seborrhoeic areas in humans (scalp, face, and the back and frontal aspect of the trunk) are always colonised by one or several species of this genus. They can cause disease when they convert to their pathogenic hyphal form. Factors that lead to this conversion include genetic predisposition, warm and humid environments, immunosuppression and malnutrition [4,5].

Environmental factors
See causative organisms.

Clinical features
Presentation
Postinflammatory hypomelanosis usually presents as moderately to well-demarcated areas of pigment loss.

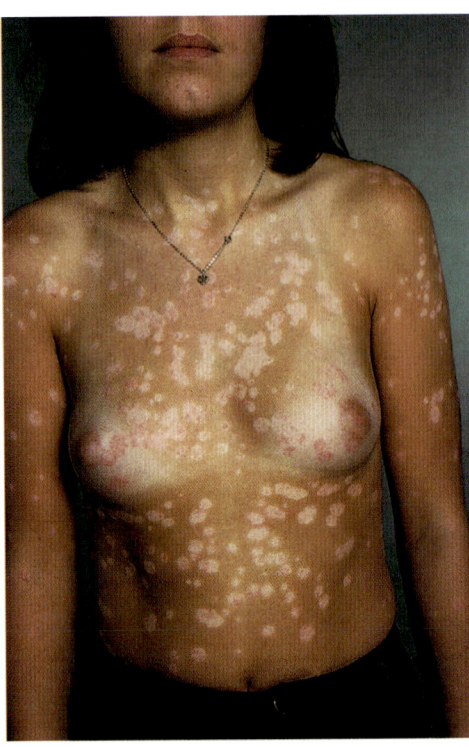

Figure 86.48 Hypopigmentation in a girl with resolving psoriasis.

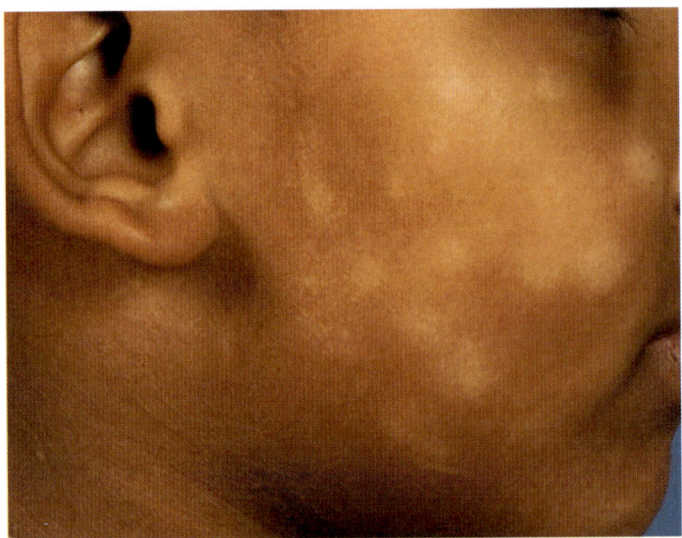

Figure 86.49 Pityriasis alba.

Pityriasis alba is characterised by hypopigmentation, presenting with pale white, well to moderately defined, very slightly scaling plaques. The lesions typically occur on the face and upper arms [1,2].

Cutaneous T-cell lymphoma may sometimes show prominent hypopigmentation. In poikilodermatous mycosis fungoides, clinical lesions are characterised by widespread poikiloderma rather than plaques or nodules. On clinical examination, there is alternating increase and decrease in pigmentation associated with epidermal atrophy. Hypopigmented mycosis fungoides tends to present in dark-skinned individuals: the areas of hypopigmentation are more prominent than in poikilodermatous mycosis fungoides [1,2].

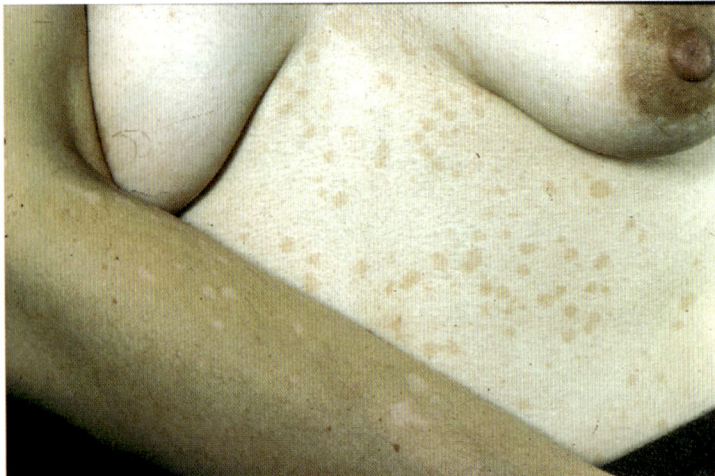

Figure 86.50 Hypomelanotic macules on a sun-exposed arm compared with tan-coloured macules on the trunk of the sun-protected abdominal skin of a woman with pityriasis versicolor.

In *pityriasis versicolor*, well-demarcated finely scaling patches, hyper- or hypopigmentations are found on clinical examination.

Lichen striatus is an asymptomatic linear dermatosis and has been reported to follow the lines of Blaschko. The primary lesions (small, flat, skin-coloured to pink papules) can disappear spontaneously after several months or years, often leaving a linear macular hypopigmentation (postinflammatory) [3].

Differential diagnosis
See Box 86.5b.

Complications and comorbidities
These are related to the underlying cause.

Disease course and prognosis
Postinflammatory hypomelanosis is in general reversible if melanin production and transfer to the keratinocytes can be restored.

Investigations
A skin biopsy can be helpful in investigating possible underlying causes, particularly if mycosis fungoides is suspected. In suspected pityriasis versicolor, demonstrating a yellow-green fluorescence on Wood's light may help confirm the diagnosis.

Progressive macular hypomelanosis

Definition
Progressive macular hypomelanosis (PMH) is a common acquired dermatosis characterised by ill-defined nummular macules, mainly affecting the trunk.

Epidemiology
Incidence and prevalence
The true prevalence of PMH is unknown, but it is a common skin disorder that is often misdiagnosed.

Age
Mostly in adolescents and young adults.

Ethnicity

Although PMH is described in people of mixed racial ancestry (known as 'Creole dyschromia'), it is seen in all races.

Pathophysiology
Causative organisms

It has been postulated that different subtypes of *Cutibacterium* (formerly *Propionibacterium*) species might be responsible for PMH [2,3].

Clinical features
Presentation

PMH is an entity that affects the trunk with ill-defined nummular hypopigmented non-scaly macules. The condition typically affects areas rich in sebaceous glands. The lesions often converge in and around the midline (Figure 86.51). Rarely, the proximal extremities, head and neck may be involved.

Differential diagnosis

See Box 86.5b.

Disease course and prognosis

PMH may be stable or slowly progressive over time. Spontaneous regression is rare, but possible.

Investigations

Wood's light examination: orange-red fluorescence can be observed in a subset of patients, although its absence does not exclude the diagnosis of PMH.

Management

In a recent study of 45 patients with intraperson comparison of two treatment strategies, 5% benzoyl peroxide hydrogel/1% clindamycin lotion in combination with UVA irradiation versus 0.05% fluticasone propionate cream in combination with UVA irradiation, the antibacterial treatment was found to be superior

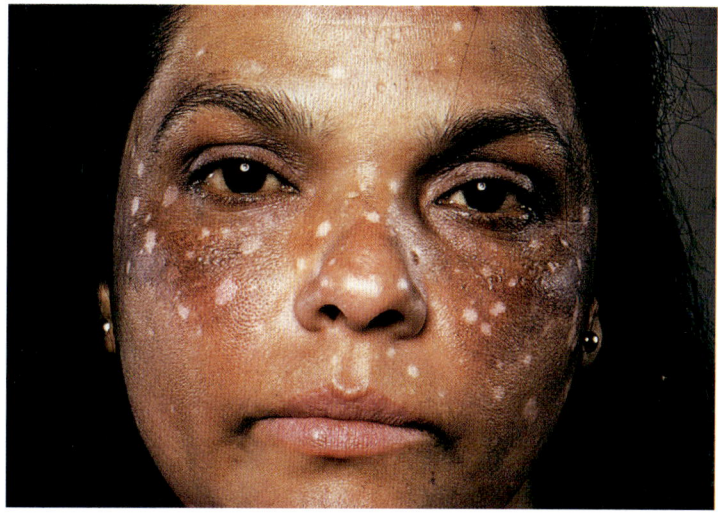

Figure 86.52 Depigmentation on the face following treatment of melasma with monobenzylether of hydroquinone. Courtesy of St John's Institute of Dermatology.

(photometric measurements, patient assessment and dermatologist assessment) [3]. PUVA und UVB therapy was reported to achieve improvement [2,4], at least transiently, in a few cases. PMH may regress spontaneously within a few years.

Chemical depigmentation

A number of chemicals can produce cutaneous depigmentation when applied to the skin [1,2]. Several substituted phenols produce an occupational leukoderma in workers coming into contact with them (Chapter 129). Of these, *p*-tertiarybutylphenol is the most important [2,3,4]. Occupational leukoderma occurs in workers in contact with the monobenzylether of hydroquinone [5]; this compound is used in the treatment of hypermelanosis and can produce confetti-like areas of depigmentation in the treated areas [6] (Figure 86.52). The monomethylether of hydroquinone can induce a similar leukoderma [7]. Several phenolic germicidal preparations can produce depigmentation of the skin [4]. 4-Tertiary-butylcatechol is also a cause of occupational leukoderma [8], and this may follow contact sensitisation [9]. The areas most likely to be affected in occupational leukoderma are the dorsa of the hands (Figure 86.53), but other areas may also be involved, not necessarily in contact with the chemicals. The depigmented areas frequently enlarge and new ones appear even after the patient is no longer in contact. The areas may or may not repigment. Treatment with psoralens is usually ineffective. In the hypomelanotic and amelanotic areas, there is often an almost complete absence of melanocytes [3,4]. Experimental studies [1,10] indicate that these substituted phenols have a selective lethal effect on functional melanocytes.

Idiopathic guttate hypomelanosis

Definition and nomenclature

Idiopathic guttate hypomelanosis (IGH) is an acquired leukoderma with discrete round to oval porcelain-white macules approximately 2–5 mm in diameter increasing in number with age [1–6].

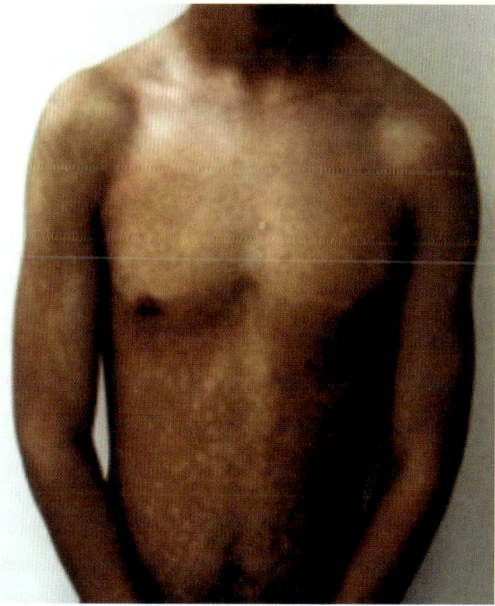

Figure 86.51 Progressive macular hypomelanosis in an 18-year-old man. Reproduced from Relyveld *et al.* (2007) [5] with permission of Springer Nature.

Synonyms and inclusions
- Disseminate lenticular leukoderma

PART 8: SPECIFIC CUTANEOUS STRUCTURES

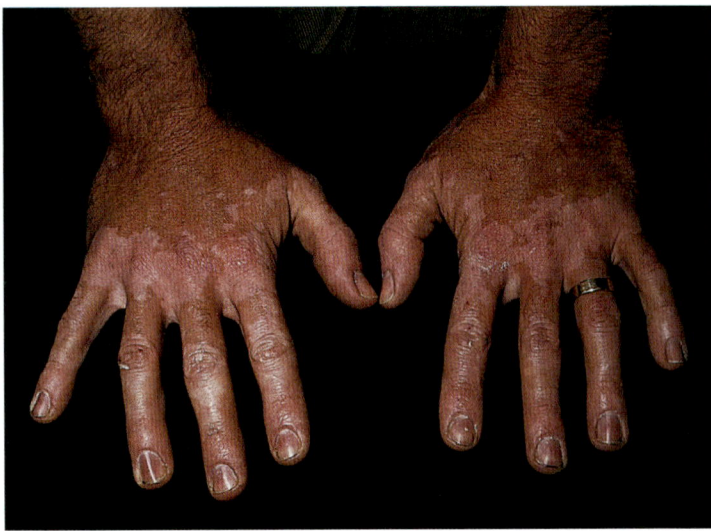

Figure 86.53 Occupational vitiligo due to 4-tertiary-butylphenol.

Epidemiology
Incidence and prevalence
Common; seen in up to 80% of patients over the age of 70 years.

Age
Numbers increase with age.

Sex
Although females are reported to be more affected than males, both sexes are most likely equally affected because IGH may be more reported by women because of the subjective perception of cosmetic disfigurement.

Ethnicity
Most in people with light skin colour.

Pathophysiology
Pathology
Histologically, IGH lesions are characterised by slight basket-weave hyperkeratosis with epidermal atrophy and flattening of the rete pegs. Histochemical and ultrastructural studies show a decrease in melanocytes and melanin content of the affected epidermis and pigment granules are irregularly distributed [5,6].

Causative organisms
IGH has been hypothesised to be UV induced, although controversy exists. Some suggest that IGH may reflect the normal ageing or photoageing process.

Environmental factors
The lesions in white people most frequently occur in sun-exposed areas of the limbs. Solar damage is a factor in these cases.

Clinical features
Presentation
Clinically, the lesions are porcelain-white macules, usually 2–6 mm in size but sometimes much larger (Figure 86.54). The borders are sharply defined, often angular and irregular. The skin markings are normal.

Susceptible locations include the pretibial side of the legs and the forearms. Other chronic sun-exposed sites, including the face, neck and shoulders, may be affected. Non-actinic lesions occur in black people and may be located on the trunk in unexposed areas [1].

Differential diagnosis
See Box 86.5.

Complications and comorbidities
These may be an indication of UV-damaged skin.

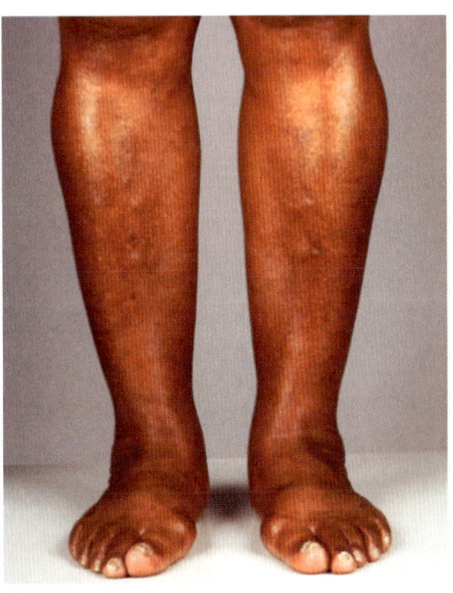
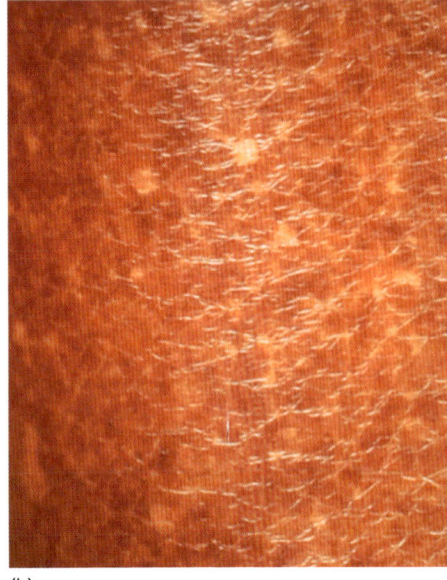
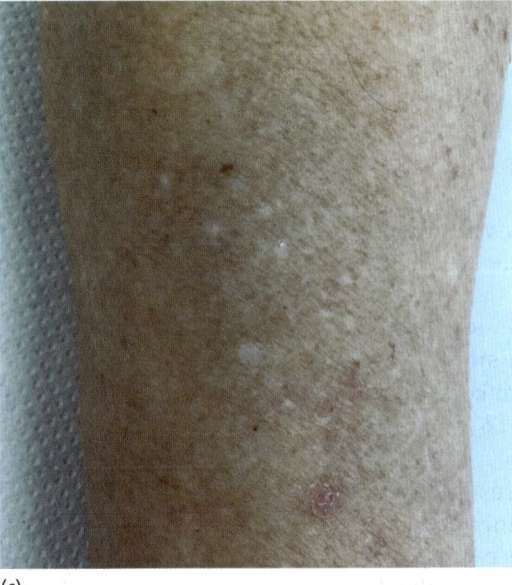

(a)   (b)   (c)

Figure 86.54 Typical appearances on the shins of a 57-year-old Afro-Caribbean woman (a) with close-up view illustrating discrete guttate hypomelanotic macules (b). Appearance on forearm of white British female patient (c). (c) Courtesy of Dr Rosalind Simpson.

Disease course and prognosis

The number increases with age. No spontaneous repigmentation occurs.

Management

Treatment is not usually required. A variety of therapies have been advocated for IGH, including systemic and topical retinoids, topical steroids, cryotherapy, topical tacrolimus and superficial dermabrasion (e.g. carbon dioxide laser). None is predictably successful [7–9].

Punctate leukoderma

Definition and nomenclature

Punctate leukoderma was first described in patients who developed multiple punctiform hypopigmented and achromic spots after several months of PUVA treatment [1]. Later, similar cases were described after UVB therapy for psoriasis and after topical and systemic PUVA for segmental vitiligo [2–4].

Synonyms and inclusions

- Leukoderma punctata
- Symmetrical progressive leukopathy

Epidemiology
Age
Punctate leukoderma develops in young adults.

Ethnicity

This has been reported from Japan and Brazil, where it is relatively common.

Pathophysiology
Pathology
Ultrastructurally, punctate leukoderma demonstrates slight to severe damage of keratinocytes and melanocytes not reported in IGH.

Causative organisms

It has been suggested that phototoxicity damage to keratinocytes and melanocytes is the aetiological factor.

Environmental factors
Sun exposure, UV therapy.

Clinical features
History
Leukoderma punctatum was first reported by Falabella *et al.* in 1988 [5].

Presentation

Multiple round or oval small sharply demarcated punctate macules measuring 0.5–1.5 mm in diameter are found symmetrically on the fronts of the shins and on the extensor aspects of the arms; less often they are also found on the abdomen and interscapular region. The macules are not related to hair follicles.

Differential diagnosis (Box 86.5)

IGH: punctate leukoderma is considered to be distinct from IGH on the basis of its clinical and histological features – the macules are smaller and repigmentation may occur.

Disease course and prognosis

Persistent although spontaneous repigmentation has been observed [5].

NON-MELANIN PIGMENTATION

Endogenous non-melanin pigmentation

A variety of normal constituents of the body may give rise to alterations in skin colour if present in excess or in an abnormal form or site. Substances formed as a result of metabolic defects may also produce pigmentary changes. Special stains of histological specimens, or techniques such as spectroscopy, may help to identify the nature of exogenous and other non-melanin pigments.

Cutaneous haemosiderosis

Definition and nomenclature

Brownish pigmentation resulting from deposition of the iron-containing pigment haemosiderin in the skin. Haemosiderin stimulates melanogenesis and much of the dyspigmentation associated with haemosiderosis may in fact be due to melanin rather than haemosiderin. The most common causes include repetitive minor trauma and venous insufficiency.

Synonyms and inclusions

- Haemosiderin pigmentation

Introduction and general description

Haemosiderin is a brown iron-binding pigment which is found predominantly within macrocytes. The deposition of haemosiderin is commonly the result of the local destruction of red blood cells, but also occurs in haemochromatosis (see earlier) [1]. The presence of haemosiderin stimulates melanogenesis. The accumulation of haemosiderin in the dermis and consequent hypermelanosis results in a brown or coppery discoloration of the skin. In addition to haemosiderin and epidermal melanin, the clinical picture may be due in part to dermal melanin resulting from pigment incontinence and even from dermal melanocytes [2].

Cutaneous haemosiderosis may arise through a number of different mechanisms of which the most important are as follows:

- Trauma: particularly repeated ecchymoses from minor trauma to the lower limbs (Figure 86.55).
- Hypostatic haemosiderosis: associated with chronic lower limb venous hypertension (Figure 86.56).
- Capillaritis (pigmented purpura) (Figure 86.57).

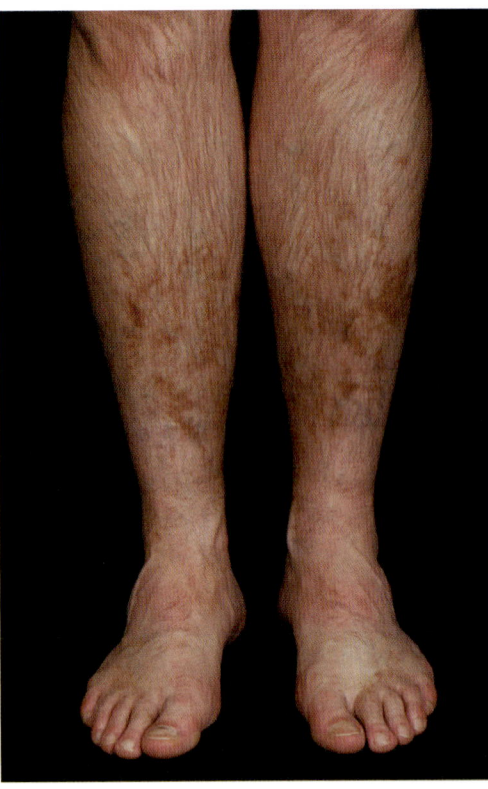

Figure 86.55 Haemosiderin staining on the shins of a 41-year-old rugby football player resulting from repeated minor trauma.

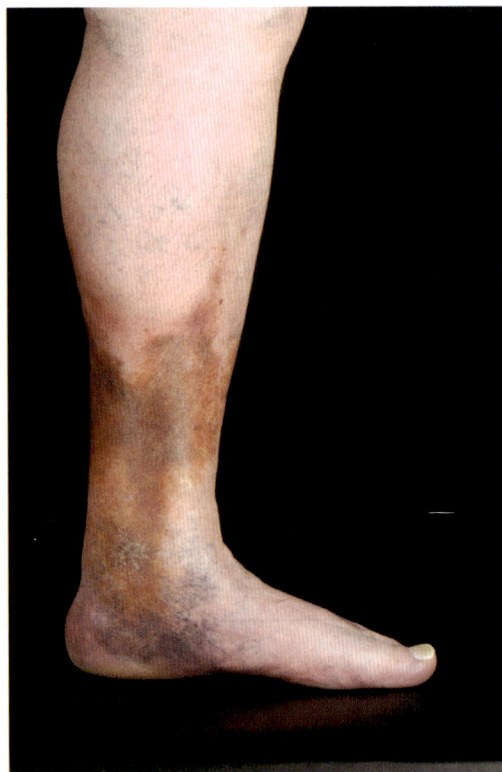

Figure 86.56 Haemosiderosis of the gaiter area in a 98-year-old man with longstanding venous insufficiency: note atrophie blanche above the medial malleolus.

- Congenital haemolytic anaemias: this includes a variety of conditions associated with haemolysis, including sickle cell anaemia.
- Haemochromatosis: this may also be deposited in the skin as the result of repeated episodes of purpura from any other cause, e.g. following clothing- or drug-induced dermatitis.

Clinical features
Clinical variants

Hypostatic haemosiderosis (Chapter 101). In chronic venous hypertension, there is leakage of blood cells from small blood vessels into the tissues. Extravasated erythrocytes are broken down by tissue macrophages and the iron thus released is incorporated into haemosiderin, which remains predominantly intracellular within the macrocyte. Recently involved areas show grouped points of reddish pigment, but recurrent extravasation of red cells combined with increasing hypermelanosis soon produces a more or less uniform deep brown or coppery colour (Figure 86.55).

The relative contributions of haemosiderin and melanin to the dyspigmentation seen in chronic venous insufficiency have been investigated by taking biopsies of pigmented and non-pigmented leg skin from patients with venous hypertension undergoing varicose vein surgery. Control biopsies were taken from patients undergoing orthopaedic surgery. Unsurprisingly, all samples from pigmented skin showed a higher melanin content than those from unpigmented skin. Haemosiderin, however, was detected in only the most deeply pigmented skin. This suggests that hypermelanosis may be provoked by chronic venous insufficiency itself without

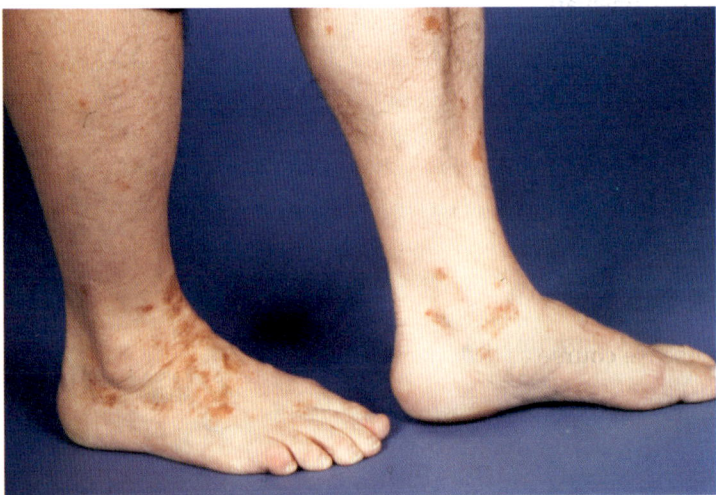

Figure 86.57 Haemosiderosis secondary to capillaritis which first erupted 6 months previously in a 57-year-old male.

the requirement for extravascular erythrocyte destruction and haemosiderin [3].

Interestingly, in a study of 46 patients with various types of leg ulcer it was shown that haemosiderin could be detected in skin biopsies from all patients but that urinary haemosiderin, which was absent from all patients with ischaemic ulcers, could be detected in 22 of 24 patients with venous ulcers [4]. There was, however, no correlation between the amounts deposited in the skin and the amount detected in urine.

Capillaritis (pigmented purpura) (Chapter 99). Haemosiderosis without clinically evident hypermelanosis is seen in Schamberg capillaritis [4]. Reddish-brown plaques with cayenne-pepper points beyond their margins are present on the legs and thighs and sometimes on the arms (Figure 86.57).

Congenital haemolytic anaemia. Conspicuous pigmentation of the lower leg in the third decade or earlier may develop in patients with sickle cell anaemia.

Haemochromatosis. The presence of haemosiderin stimulates melanogenesis, and hypermelanosis may dominate the clinical and histological picture, as in haemochromatosis (see earlier).

Dermatitis. Haemosiderosis of the trunk is a feature of some reactions to textiles. Small patches of haemosiderosis, most numerous on the lower legs but progressively involving the thighs and buttocks, are characteristic of drug reactions to anticonvulsants with a ureide structure, a property common to the majority of them.

Pathophysiology
Environmental factors
May occasionally be secondary to drug reactions or contact dermatitis due to clothing.

Clinical features
Presentation
The pigmentation is orange-red at first, later fading through ochre and tawny shades. It is distributed according to the underlying cause, i.e. either locally as in hydrostatic haemochromatosis or generally as in haemochromatosis.

Capillaritis initially presents with punctate bright red purpuric macules which may evolve into irregular plaques of orange or brown pigmentation. The lesions are chronic and persistent [3].

Differential diagnosis
See Box 86.3.

Disease course and prognosis
Hypostatic haemosiderosis. The pigmentation usually persists even if the venous insufficiency is relieved. In a single case report an IPL device was used apparently successfully to treat this condition [5].

Capillaritis. A chronic condition, this may clear spontaneously over a period from months to years, although recurrences are possible and not uncommon.

Haemochromatosis. See earlier.

Other. For other causes of secondary haemosiderin deposition, the prognosis depends on the successful management of the primary cause.

Management
Treatment of the underlying cause if possible.

Jaundice and bronze baby syndrome

Definition and nomenclature
Jaundice. Yellowish discoloration of the skin, eyes and mucous membranes due to deposition of bile pigments [1].

Bronze baby syndrome. Brown-bronze discoloration of the skin, mucous membranes and urine after phototherapy in children with clinical jaundice [2–4,**5**].

Synonyms and inclusions
- Jaundice: icterus

Pathophysiology
Pathology
Jaundice. This results from the deposition of bilirubin in the tissues. Clinically, it is often first noticed in the sclerae, because bilirubin has affinity for elastic tissue. The range of yellow shades produced by bilirubin may be modified by the presence of biliverdin, which adds a greenish hue. Bronzing is the effect of added melanin pigmentation and is often seen in jaundice of long duration.

Bronze baby syndrome. The nature and origin of the pigment are uncertain. The discoloration may be caused by an abnormal accumulation of a photoisomer of bilirubin, abnormal hepatic function leading to a copper–porphyrin complex which is photodestroyed or accumulation of biliverdin.

Clinical features
Presentation
Jaundice. Range of yellow shades with a greenish hue.

Bronze baby syndrome. This striking grey-brown discoloration of the skin of neonates follows phototherapy for hyperbilirubinaemia and is often associated with evidence of liver dysfunction. The serum is also brownish.

Differential diagnosis (Box 86.3a)
- Carotenaemia.
- Grey baby syndrome (after high doses of chloramphenicol).

Disease course and prognosis
Jaundice. Outcome depends on the management of the underlying disease.

Bronze baby syndrome. The changes are reversible unless there is some chronic underlying liver disease.

Management
Treatment of underlying cause.

Bronze baby syndrome. No treatment is required as pigmentation is reversible after discontinuation of phototherapy.

Treatment ladder for jaundice and bronze baby syndrome

First line
- Neonatal jaundice is routinely treated with 460–490 nm visible light [6].

Carotenoderma

Definition and nomenclature
Carotenoderma is a benign yellowish coloration of the skin due to elevated blood carotene levels [1]. This may be primary due to diet, or secondary due to for example hepatic disease.

Synonyms and inclusions
- Hypercarotenaemia
- Carotenaemia

Pathophysiology
Predisposing factors
Primary carotenoderma is seen most obviously in food faddists who consume large quantities of oranges or carrots. However, it is now more commonly seen in young women drastically reducing their weight and eating foodstuffs with high carotene content [2,3].

Iatrogenic hypercarotenaemia occurs in patients on oral supplements of β-carotene as a photoprotective agent in erythropoietic protoporphyria [4,5] with or without canthaxanthine. Carotenoderma typically occurs when β-carotene concentrations exceed 250 μg/dL or when daily ingestion exceeds 30 mg of β-carotene [6].

In secondary hypercarotenaemia, some increased yellowness is seen in conditions with hyperlipaemia, diabetes, nephritis or hypothyroidism. It may also occur if conversion of carotene to vitamin A is impaired by an inborn metabolic error [7] or by hepatic disease.

Pathology
Carotene, a lipochrome, contributes a yellow component to the colour of normal skin. In the presence of excessive blood carotene levels, this yellow component is increased.

Clinical features
Presentation
The yellow colour is most conspicuous where the horny layer is thick on the palms and soles (Figure 86.58). The sclerae are not discoloured.

Differential diagnosis
See Box 86.3a.

Disease course and prognosis
A diet low in carotene leads to resolution of the signs.

Treatment ladder for carotenoderma
First line
- Treatment of underlying cause
- Diet low in carotene

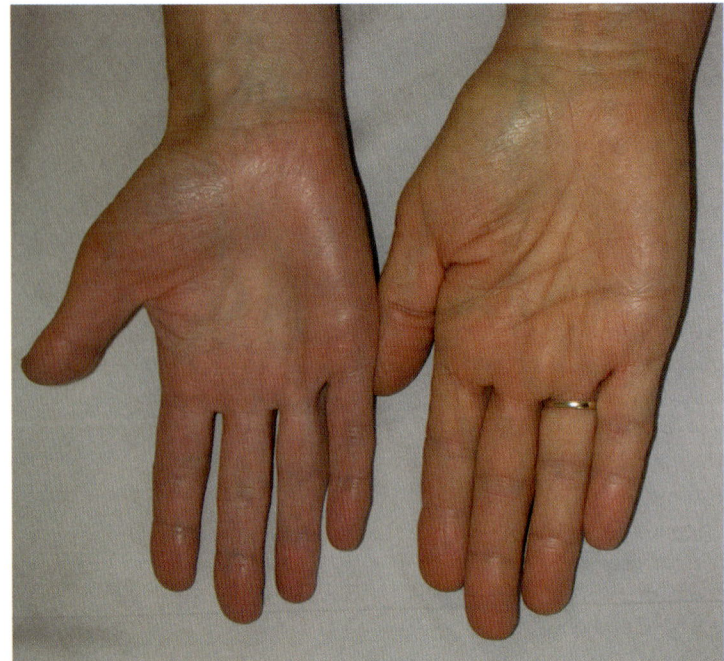

Figure 86.58 Carotenoderma: note yellowish hue of the palm on the right compared with the normal palm on the left. Courtesy of Professor Barbara Leppard, University of Southampton, UK.

Ochronosis

Definition
Endogenous ochronosis. This is the term used to describe the pigmentary changes that occur in connective tissue in patients with alkaptonuria [1].

Exogenous ochronosis. Discoloration of the skin after topical use primarily of hydroquinone, but may also be caused by the use of phenol or resorcinol [2].

Epidemiology
Incidence and prevalence
Endogenous ochronosis. This is present in about 75% of patients with alkaptonuria (Chapter 79).

Exogenous ochronosis. Exact incidence is unknown.

Age
Alkaptonuria: congenital (Chapter 79).

Sex
Males and females are equally affected.

Ethnicity
Alkaptonuria. All races, although more frequent in certain countries such as Slovakia and the Dominican Republic.

Exogenous ochronosis. Seen in populations with widespread use of hydroquinine or phenol/resorcinol. High rates have been reported from South Africa.

Pathophysiology
Predisposing factors
- Exogenous ochronosis: often associated with the use of skin-lightening cosmetics.
- Most frequently reported in heavily pigmented skin, although it can occur in all phototypes.

Pathology
Histopathological examination of both endogenous and exogenous ochronosis is characterised by comma- or banana-shaped ochronotic collagen bundles. Histopathological differentiation between the two forms is not possible [2].

In alkaptonuria, a deficiency in homogentisic acid oxidase causes accumulation of homogentisic acid throughout the body [3].

In exogenous ochronosis, it may be caused by inhibition of homogentisic oxidase and accumulation of homogentisic acid (an intermediate in L-phenylalanine and L-tyrosine catabolism) which polymerises to form ochre (brownish-yellow) pigment in the papillary dermis [2]. Microscopically, deposition of ochre-coloured pigment is seen [2].

Genetics
Alkaptonuria is an autosomal recessive disease.

Environmental factors
- Exogenous ochronosis: sun exposure.
- Use of hydroquinone at concentrations higher than 3% for prolonged periods of time (>6 months). Discoloration is, however, also reported with the use of hydroquinone at concentrations of 2% and less.

Clinical features
History
The term was coined by Virchow in 1866 for the ochre-like (pale yellow) colour of the connective tissue when viewed down a microscope.

Presentation
Endogenous ochronosis. Most frequent is darkening of the ear cartilages and of the sclerae and conjunctivae. Less often the axillary skin is pigmented and there is brown mottled pigmentation of the face (sometimes in a butterfly distribution), neck and trunk. Rarely, pigmentation of the palmar and plantar skin is seen [4].

Exogenous ochronosis. Grey-brown or blue-black macules in the skin in contact with hydroquinone, normally the face, neck, back and the extensor surfaces of the limbs. No hyperpigmentation of cartilage, sclerae or conjunctivae occurs [2,5].

Differential diagnosis
Facial melanosis. As follows:
- Endocrinopathies: Addison disease, Cushing syndrome, hyperthyroidism.
- Metabolic conditions: porphyria cutanea tarda, haemochromatosis.
- Poikiloderma of Civatte.

- Postinflammatory hyperpigmentation.
- Toxin- and drug-induced hyperpigmentation or discoloration (e.g. amiodarone, doxycycline).

Investigations
Alkaptonuria may be identified by urine organic acid analysis, whereas exogenous ochronosis is identified by the patient history.

Management
First line
Alkaptonuria. No definitive treatment exists; nitisinone, ascorbic acid 1 g/day in divided doses and a protein-restricted diet (1.3 g/kg/day) may be beneficial.

Exogenous ochronosis. Discontinuation of hydroquinone use; strict sun protection/avoidance.

Treatment of discoloration is difficult. The use of trichloroacetic acid and cryotherapy has been shown not to be helpful. Some improvement may occur with the use of retinoid acid, although transient hyperpigmentation may also occur. Topical low-potency corticosteroids may be of benefit in combination with photoprotection [2].

Second line
Exogenous ochronosis. Although results are not uniform, superficial dermabrasion using carbon dioxide laser, glycolic acid peelings or Q-switched laser may improve the skin discoloration [2].

Exogenous pigmentation

A wide variety of chemicals, from either occupational or medicinal exposure, can produce discoloration of the skin. Some of these may not only produce an alteration of pigmentation by being deposited in the dermis but may also result in an increase in the amount of melanin in the skin. Of importance are the metals silver, gold, mercury and bismuth, which are cumulatively deposited in the dermis and can produce permanent disfiguring pigmentation. A number of drugs can discolour the skin which leads often to a bluish-grey discoloration especially on the legs. These include the antimalarials, the phenothiazines, clofazimine and minocycline. Of less importance is the transient staining of the skin produced by picric acid, dinitrophenol and chemical dyes.

Metals

Introduction and general description
Argyria
This may develop as a result of systemic absorption or from external contact with silver [1,2]. The silver may be deposited in the skin either as a result of medication containing silver salts [3,4,5] or from industrial exposure [2]. Localised argyria is most commonly caused by mechanical impregnation related to occupational exposure [2].

Most reported cases of generalised argyria occur following ingestion of colloidal silver, which is widely marketed as a folk remedy

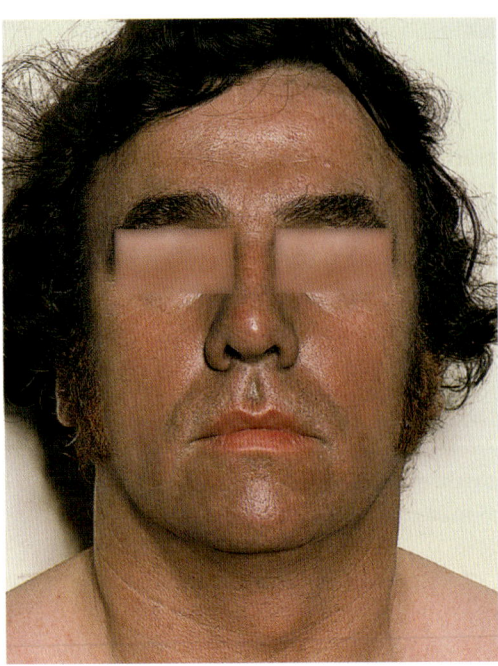

Figure 86.59 Occupational argyria.

for various conditions, including diabetes, AIDS, cancers and infections: a cumulative dose of 4–5 g is required to produce clinical signs [6]. Light and electron microscopy studies [1,2,7–9] show silver granules in the dermis that are most numerous in relation to the basal lamina of the eccrine sweat glands, and in the dermal elastic fibres. Furthermore, silver particles may be seen lying free within the cell cytoplasm of epithelial cells of the secretory segment of eccrine sweat glands and in mast cells [9,10]. Silver granules are readily visible with dark-field illumination. X-ray-dispersive microanalysis confirms that the granules contain silver [2,10]. Silver is widely deposited in the tissues as well as in the skin. The diagnosis of argyria is established by skin biopsy.

The pigmentation is usually a slate-grey colour and may be clinically apparent after a few months, but usually takes many years to develop and depends on the degree of exposure. The hyperpigmentation is most apparent in sun-exposed areas of the skin, especially the forehead, nose and hands (Figure 86.59). In some patients, the entire skin has a slate blue-grey colour. The sclerae, nails and mucous membranes may additionally become hyperpigmented.

Blue macules have appeared at the sites of acupuncture needles [6]. Cases have followed the use of silver salts for the irrigation of nasal, oral and urethral mucous membranes and the excessive use of an oral smoking remedy containing silver acetate [1,10]. 'Food supplements' may also contain colloidal silver [8].

The pigmentation is usually permanent: treatment with depigmenting agents is not effective. Sun protection can limit further pigmentary changes [9].

Arsenic

Prolonged ingestion of inorganic arsenic may result in diffuse pigmentation, most intense on the trunk. The hyperpigmentation is characterised by macular areas of depigmentation within areas of hyperpigmentation that produce the distinctive 'raindrop' appearance, diffuse dark brown spots or diffuse darkening of the skin on the limbs and trunk [1,2]. Many cases also show arsenical keratoses,

usually appearing as bilateral thickening of the palms and soles. Nodular keratosis may also occur as multiple raised keratotic lesions on the palm and soles [2].

Bismuth

The administration of bismuth at regular intervals over a period of years has often been practised, yet generalised pigmentation is extremely rare. The diffuse grey pigmentation resembles that of argyria and involves also the sclera and the oral and sometimes the vaginal mucous membrane [1]. A distinctive blue-black line occurs at the gingival margin. This is due to deposition of bismuth that reacts with hydrogen sulphide formed by bacteria in the mouth [2].

Chrysiasis and chrysoderma

These are terms used to describe permanent pigmentation of the skin due to parenteral administration of gold salts.

Excessive administration of gold leads to its deposition in connective tissue. The diagnosis is confirmed histologically on microscopy with dark-field illumination and on electron microscopy with electron probe microanalysis [1]. The granules of gold are larger and more irregular than those of silver.

Chrysiasis has not been observed in any patient who has received fewer than 50 mg/kg of gold thiosulphate, and appears to be inevitable in any patient receiving more than 150 mg/kg. It may develop after a few months or after a longer latent period. The pigmentation is blue-grey or may show a purplish hue, and is limited to light-exposed skin and to the sclerae (Figure 86.60) [2]. The oral mucous membrane is not affected. The discoloration is permanent.

Mercury

Repeated applications of mercury-containing compounds can produce localised hyperpigmentation of the treated areas [1,2,3]. The pigment is observed in the upper dermis around capillaries and associated with collagen and elastic fibres. Electron microscopy shows an increase in melanin pigmentation and the metal is present as granules in dermal macrophages [1,3].

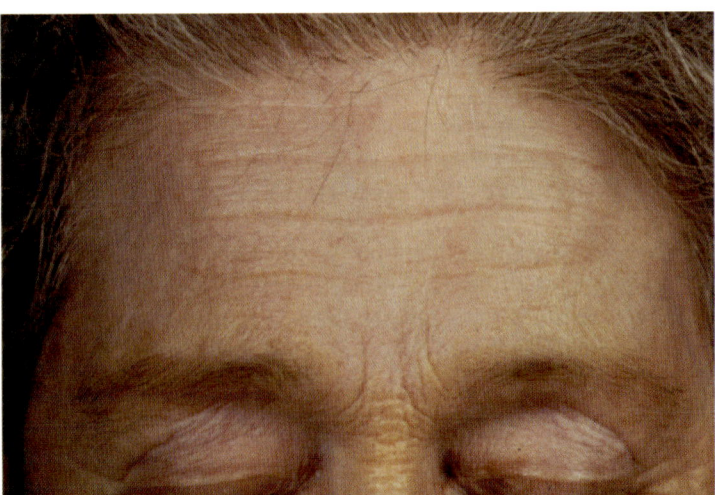

Figure 86.60 Chrysiasis: mild lilac discoloration on the forehead and eyelids contrasting with the yellow of the elastotic skin on the bridge of the nose and eyebrows in a 64-year-old woman with rheumatoid arthritis who 8 years earlier had been treated with parenteral gold for over 2 years.

Systemic administration of mercury results in gingival hyperpigmentation. A case report of homicidal subcutaneous injection of metallic mercury resulted in widespread skin lesions, remote from the radiologically visible mercury; these appeared at 40 days and began to clear at 6 months [4].

Differential diagnosis
See Box 86.3a.

Medication

See Drug-induced hyperpigmentation.

Tattoos

Accidental tattoos
Pigmented particles may be accidentally introduced as contaminants of wounds or may, at high velocity, penetrate previously intact skin.

Superficial abrasions contaminated with chemically inert particles may be followed by disfiguring tattoos. Such irregularly spattered pigmentation is quite commonly seen after road accidents and blast injuries. Some particles may eventually be extruded, but the disfigurement is often permanent. These tattoos often respond well to the Q-switched Nd:YAG laser (Figure 86.61) [1]. Small lesions may also be excised.

Colliers' stripes
These are a very distinctive occupational mark in coalminers [2]. The bluish grey, linear or angular stripes develop at the sites of abrasions. The commonest sites are the forehead, bridge of the nose, wrists and elbows. Histologically, particles of coal dust up to 100 μm in diameter are seen at all levels in the dermis. They tend to be grouped around blood vessels.

Therapeutic agents
Iron salts. The use of solutions of ferric sulphate and ferric chloride in the treatment of dermatitis has been followed by a reddish-brown tattoo [3,4]. The pigmentation may disappear after a few months or may persist indefinitely [5].

Occupational contact with iron salts [6] produced red-brown punctate perifollicular pigmentation of the forearms in a man employed in pickling metal in hydrochloric acid.

Crystal violet (gentian violet; hexamethyl pararosaniline chloride). This has, exceptionally, given rise to a tattoo when applied to a wound of the face [7].

Decorative tattoos (Chapters 23 and 122)
History and prevalence. From ancient times, the practice of tattooing has developed along more or less parallel lines in most cultures. Tattoos have traditionally been based on aesthetic considerations, i.e. to accentuate beauty, or as a permanent adornment in a more sociological or cultural context to make a statement. Occasionally, when used in a sociocultural context, tattoos serve to accentuate aggression or ugliness in order to make the wearer more intimidating. Tattoos with words or a name as a symbol of dedication or devotion have always been popular. Tattoos have also been used for more sinister motives. Tattoos were used as a means of identification by the Nazis in the Second World War for members of concentration and labour camps as well as for members of the SS. Formerly associated with religious ceremonies, fertility and marriage rites, tattooing in contemporary westernised civilisations thus fulfils a number of diverse functions and in so doing it survives and flourishes.

Contemporary life finds tattooing more popular than ever [8], even among the elite [9]. Tattoos are no longer the exclusive preserve of street gangs, prisoners and members of the armed forces [8,9].

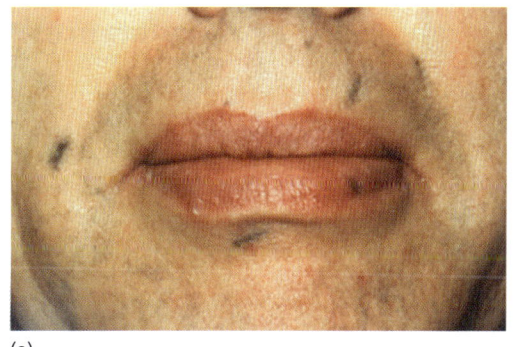

(a)

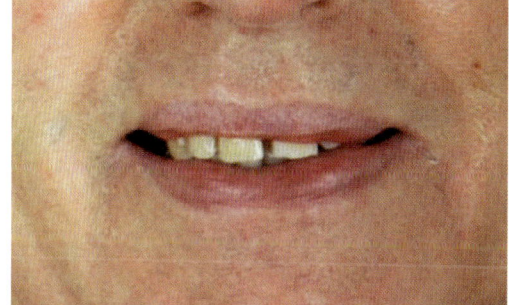

(b)

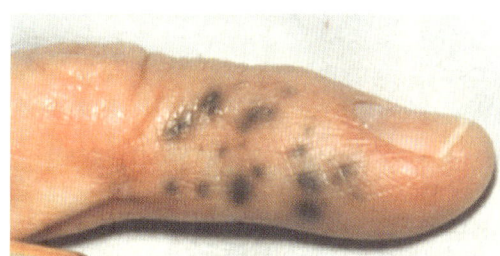

(c)

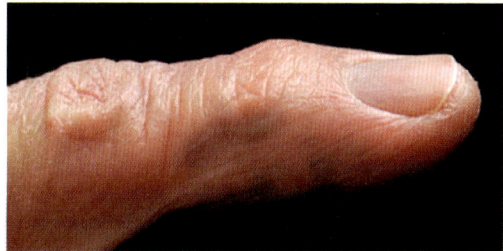

(d)

Figure 86.61 (a–d) Traumatic tattoo: accidental tattoo following explosion during school chemistry experiment; excellent response to Nd:YAG laser.

Tattooing is viewed by many as an acceptable fashion accessory like any other, and is increasingly popular in western societies with the young and with women, as well as the more traditional male stereotypes [8,9]. Tattooing and body piercing are now so common that health care workers are advised to maintain a non-judgemental attitude to tattoos [8], even in the face of the unexpected [10]. The decision to have a tattoo may be taken when an individual is in no position to make such a lifelong commitment, for example when intoxicated, under peer pressure or when mentally unwell [11,12]. Tattoos may also be a manifestation of deliberate self-harm [11,12].

Another contemporary trend is the use of temporary black henna 'tattoos' [13,14]. These are not true tattoos but represent application of a black dye to produce a tattoo-like appearance that lasts for a few days. Unfortunately, a high concentration of the well-known contact sensitiser *para*-phenylenediamine is usually present in these 'tattoos', which results in a risk of contact allergy [13,14].

Techniques and materials. The professional tattooist uses an electric needle to introduce particles of pigment into the dermis (Chapter 23). The amateur, often a child, pricks particles of soot or Indian ink into skin with any pointed object. The pigments commonly employed include the following:
- Blue-black (carbon).
- Red (cinnabar and vegetable dyes).
- Light blue (cobaltous aluminate).
- Green (chromic oxide or chromium sesquioxide).
- Yellow (cadmium sulphide).
- Brown (ochre, iron oxides).

Complications of tattoos. Infection, allergy to tattoo pigments (Figure 86.62) and koebnerisation of other disorders, particularly sarcoidosis, to tattoos represent the most common complications of tattoos. A sarcoidal granuloma in a tattoo may be the presenting manifestation of generalised sarcoidosis [15]. Foreign-body

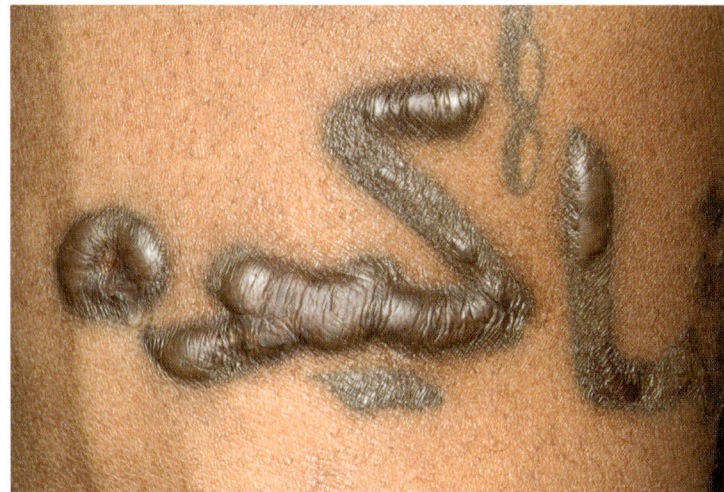

Figure 86.63 Keloid reaction to decorative tattoo: flattened areas have responded to the injection of triamcinolone.

granulomas of sarcoid type are, however, extremely unusual after decorative tattoos, but have been reported in ochre tattoos, which have a high silica content [16]. Tattooing may also be complicated by keloids (Figure 86.63). Complications of tattoos are discussed in further detail in Chapter 122.

Removal of tattoos. Although most people who choose to have tattoos are satisfied with them, there are many who wish to have them removed [17]. In a recent study of 154 attendees with tattoos at a sexual health clinic in Denmark, 21 (13.6%) expressed regret about one or more of their tattoos [18]. Fortunately, the technology for removing them has improved greatly in recent years. Small tattoos may be amenable to removal by simple surgical techniques. Lasers are also widely used for tattoo removal [19]. Their use is discussed in detail in Chapter 23.

Key references

The full list of references can be found in the online version at https://www.wiley.com/rooksdermatology10e

Skin pigmentation and the melanocyte
The colour of the skin
1 Abdel-Malek Z, Kadekaro AL. Human pigmentation: its regulation by ultraviolet light and by endocrine, paracrine, and autocrine factors. In: Nordlund JJ, Boissy RE, Hearing VJ et al., eds. *The Pigmentary System*, 2nd edn. Oxford: Blackwell Publishing, 2006:410–20.

The melanocyte
4 Brenner M, Hearing VJ. The protective role of melanin against UV damage in human skin. *Photochem Photobiol* 2008;84:539–49.

Biochemistry of melanogenesis
1 Hearing VJ. Determination of melanin synthetic pathways. *J Invest Dermatol* 2011;131:E8–11.
2 Rees JL. The genetics of human pigmentation disorders. *J Invest Dermatol* 2011;131:E12–13.
3 Hearing VJ. Invited editorial: unraveling the melanocytes. *Am J Hum Genet* 1993;52:1–7.

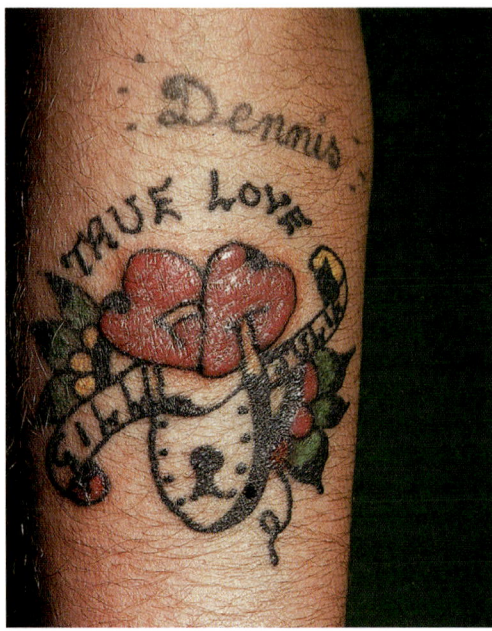

Figure 86.62 Lichenoid reaction in the red areas of a tattoo.

Constitutive pigmentation, human pigmentation and the response to sun exposure

5 Fitzpatrick TB. The validity and practicality of sun-reaction skin types I through VI. *Arch Dermatol* 1988;124:869–71.

Acquired hypermelanosis
Facial melanoses

Melasma

16 Gupta AK, Gover MD, Nouri K, Taylor S. The treatment of melasma: a review of clinical trials. *J Am Acad Dermatol* 2006;55:1048–65.

23 Picardo M, Carrera M. New and experimental treatments of cloasma and other hypermelanoses. *Dermatol Clin* 2007;25:353–62.

Photocontact facial melanosis

7 Pérez-Bernal A, Moñoz-Pérez MA, Camacho F. Management of facial hyperpigmentation. *Am J Clin Dermatol* 2000;1:261–8.

Poikiloderma of Civatte

2 Pérez-Bernal A, Moñoz-Pérez MA, Camacho F. Management of facial hyperpigmentation. *Am J Clin Dermatol* 2000;1:261–8.

Hypermelanosis in other systemic disorders

Neoplastic diseases

1 Wright TS. Cutaneous manifestations of malignancy. *Curr Opin Pediatr* 2011;23:407–11.

3 Sebaratnam DF, Venugopal SS, Frew JW et al. Diffuse melanosis cutis: a systematic review of the literature. *J Am Acad Dermatol* 2013;68:482–8.

6 Bell HK, Poston GJ, Vora J, Wilson NJ. Cutaneous manifestations of the malignant carcinoid syndrome. *Br J Dermatol* 2005;152:71.

Hypermelanosis of drug origin

Drug-induced hyperpigmentation

1 Dereure O. Drug-induced skin pigmentation. Epidemiology, diagnosis and treatment. *Am J Clin Dermatol* 2001;2:253–62.

2 Lerner EA, Sober AJ. Chemical and pharmacologic agents that cause hyperpigmentation or hypopigmentation of the skin. *Dermatol Clin* 1988;6:327–37.

Tetracyclines

1 Dereure O. Drug-induced skin pigmentation. Epidemiology, diagnosis and treatment. *Am J Clin Dermatol* 2001;2:253–62.

Ashy dermatosis and erythema dyschromicum perstans

1 Zaynoun S, Rubeiz N, Kibbi A-G. Ashy dermatoses: a critical review of the literature and a proposed simplified clinical classification. *Int J Dermatol* 2008;47:542–4.

Treatment of hypermelanosis

1 Picardo M, Carrera M. New and experimental treatments of cloasma and other hypermelanoses. *Dermatol Clin* 2007;25:353 62.

3 Cestari TF, Dantas LP, Boza JC. Acquired hyperpigmentations. *An Bras Dermatol* 2014;89:11–25.

Acquired hypomelanosis
Vitiligo

1 Bologna J, Pawelek JM. Biology of hypopigmentation. *J Am Acad Dermatol* 1988;19:217–55.

2 Ezzedine K, Lim HW, Suzuki T et al. Revised classification/nomenclature of vitiligo and related issues: the Vitiligo Global Issues Consensus Conference. *Pigment Cell Melanoma Res* 2012;25:E1–13.

11 van Geel N, Speeckaert R, Taieb A et al. Koebner's phenomenon in vitiligo: European position paper. *Pigment Cell Melanoma Res* 2011;24:564–73.

12 Richmond JM, Frisoli ML, Harris JE. Innate immune mechanisms in vitiligo: danger from within. *Curr Opin Immunol* 2013;25:676–82.

33 van Geel N, Mollet I, Brochez L et al. New insights in segmental vitiligo: case report and review of theories. *Br J Dermatol* 2012;166:240–6.

36 van Geel N, Speeckaert M, Chevolet I et al. Hypomelanoses in children. *J Cutan Aesthet Surg* 2013;6:65–72.

39 Whitton ME, Pinart M, Batchelor J et al. Interventions for vitiligo. *Cochrane Database Syst Rev* 2015;Issue 2:CD003263.

40 Taieb A, Alomar A, Böhm M et al. Guidelines for the management of vitiligo: the European Dermatology Forum consensus. *Br J Dermatol* 2013;168:5–19.

Chemical depigmentation

2 Lerner EA, Sober AJ. Chemical and pharmacologic agents that cause hyperpigmentation or hypopigmentation of the skin. *Dermatol Clin* 1988;6:327–37.

Non-melanin pigmentation
Endogenous non-melanin pigmentation

Cutaneous haemosiderosis

1 Jeghers H. Pigmentation of the skin. *N Engl J Med* 1944;231:88–100.

2 Kim D, Kang WH. Role of dermal melanocytes in cutaneous pigmentation of stasis dermatitis: a histopathological study of 20 cases. *J Korean Med Sci* 2002;17:648–54.

3 Caggiati A, Rosi C, Franceschini M, Innocenzi D. The nature of skin pigmentations in chronic venous insufficiency: a preliminary report. *Eur J Vasc Endovasc Surg* 2008;35:111–18.

5 Satoh T, Yokozeki H, Nishioka K. Chronic pigmented purpura associated with odontogenic infection. *J Am Acad Dermatol* 2002;46:942–4.

Jaundice and bronze baby syndrome

5 Kar S, Mohankar A, Krishnan A. Bronze baby syndrome. *Indian Pediatr* 2013;8:624.

6 Maisels MJ, McDonagh AD. Phototherapy for neonatal jaundice. *N Engl J Med* 2008;358:920–8.

Carotenoderma

6 Jen M, Yan AC. Syndromes associated with nutritional deficiency and excess. *Clin Dermatol* 2010;28:669–85.

Ochronosis

1 Lubics A, Schneider I, Sebok B, Havass Z. Extensive bluish gray skin pigmentation and severe arthropathy. Endogenous ochronosis (alkaptonuria). *Arch Dermatol* 2000;136:548–52.

2 Martins VM, Sousa AR, Portela N de C et al. Exogenous ochronosis: case report and literature review. *An Bras Dermatol* 2012;87:633–6.

3 Turgay E, Canat D, Gurel MS et al. Endogenous ochronosis. *Clin Exp Dermatol* 2009;34:865–8.

5 Jain A, Pai SB, Shenoi SD. Exogenous ochronosis. *Indian J Dermatol Venereol Leprol* 2013;79:522–3.

Exogenous pigmentation

Metals

Argyria

1 Pariser RJ. Generalized argyria. *Arch Dermatol* 1978;114:373–7.

2 Bleehen SS, Gould DJ, Harrington CI et al. Occupational argyria: light and electron microscopic studies and X-ray microanalysis. *Br J Dermatol* 1981;104:19 26.

4 Marshall JP, II, Schneider RP. Systemic argyria secondary to topical silver nitrate. *Arch Dermatol* 1977;113:1077–9.

6 Park SW, Shin HT, Lee KT, Lee DY. Medical concern for colloidal silver supplementation: argyria of the nail and face. *Ann Dermatol* 2013;25:111–12.

Arsenic

2 Majumdar KK, Guha Mazumder DN. Effect of drinking arsenic-contaminated water in children. *Indian J Public Health* 2012;56:223–6.

Bismuth

1 Dummett CO. Oral mucosal discolorations related to pharmacotherapeutics. *J Oral Ther* 1964;1:106–10.

2 Lueth HC, Sutton DC, McMullen CJ et al. Generalized discoloration of skin resembling argyria following prolonged oral use of bismuth. *Arch Intern Med* 1936;57:1115–24.

Chrysiasis

1 Smith RW, Leppard B, Barnett NL *et al*. Chrysiasis revisited: a clinical and pathological study. *Br J Dermatol* 1995;133:671–8.
2 Leonard PA, Moatamed F, Ward JR *et al*. Chrysiasis: the role of sun exposure in dermal hyperpigmentation secondary to gold therapy. *J Rheumatol* 1986;13:58–64.

Mercury

2 Kennedy C, Molland EA, Henderson WJ, Whiteley AM. Mercury pigmentation from industrial exposure. *Br J Dermatol* 1977;96:367–74.
4 Burge KM, Winkelmann RK. Mercury pigmentation. *Arch Dermatol* 1970;102:51–61.

CHAPTER 87

Acquired Disorders of Hair

Matthew J. Harries[1], *Susan Holmes*[2], *Amy McMichael*[3] *and Andrew G. Messenger*[4]

[1] University of Manchester, MAHSC and NIHR Manchester Biomedical Research Centre, Salford Royal Hospital, Northern Care Alliance NHS Foundation Trust, Salford, Greater Manchester, UK
[2] Alan Lyell Centre for Dermatology, Glasgow Royal Infirmary, Glasgow, UK
[3] Wake Forest Baptist Medical Center, Winston-Salem, NC, USA
[4] University of Sheffield, Sheffield, UK

Rook's Textbook of Dermatology, Tenth Edition. Edited by Christopher Griffiths, Jonathan Barker, Tanya Bleiker, Walayat Hussain and Rosalind Simpson.
© 2024 John Wiley & Sons Ltd. Published 2024 by John Wiley & Sons Ltd.

Introduction

The hair follicle (HF) is one of the defining features of mammals, instrumental for their ongoing survival and reproductive success. For animals, hair is vital for protection and camouflage, whereas in humans it serves a crucial role in society for social identity, personal style and sexual attractiveness. Therefore, it is unsurprising that hair loss, or excessive hair growth, can have a profound impact on someone's emotional well-being. However, hair growth changes may also be an important sign of a serious underlying medical condition or nutritional deficiency. Thus, the key to managing any hair disorder is accurate diagnosis and awareness of evidence-based treatments, while also supporting the sometimes marked psychological sequelae that may accompany these conditions.

Hair biology

Mammals probably evolved from Therapsid reptiles during the Late Triassic period over 200 million years ago. The earliest direct evidence of hair in mammals comes from fossilised casts and impressions in coprolites and pellets from the Late Palaeocene beds of Inner Mongolia [1]. Hairs from at least four extinct mammalian taxa have been identified, notably the multituberculate *Lambdopsalis bulla*, all showing striking preservation of the cuticular scale pattern. The three surviving mammalian groups – monotremes, marsupials and placental mammals – all possess hair, indicating its presence prior to the divergence of therian mammals from monotremes, which probably took place between 170 and 230 million years ago [2,3]. The multituberculate lineage extends back into the Triassic, suggesting that hair is a very ancient and possibly defining feature of mammals.

Compared with scale-covered animals, hair represents a more versatile integument. Ongoing regeneration and replacement of the coat, as opposed to intermittent shedding of skin (e.g. in reptiles), avoid exposing the creature to episodes of heat loss, thereby providing a survival advantage [4]. Further, hair may even serve a rudimentary excretory role by sequestering toxic material within the hair shaft, allowing complete elimination by hair shedding [5].

Whatever its origin, warm-blooded mammals owe much of their evolutionary success to the properties of the hairy pelage as a heat insulator. Paradoxically, the movement of humans from the ancestral forest home to a more open, hunter-gatherer existence is linked with a reversion to relative nudity and an ability to keep cool. Moreover, hair serves other purposes: in particular, it is concerned with sexual and social communication by constructing adornments such as the mane of the lion or the beard of the human male or assisting in the dispersal of scents secreted by complexes of sebaceous or apocrine glands.

For these evolutionary reasons, HFs are not all under identical control mechanisms. To match the animal coat to seasonal changes in ambient temperature or environmental background requires moulting and replacement of the hairs. The process appears to involve an inherent follicular rhythm, modified by circulating hormones such as melatonin, prolactin, androgens or thyroxine, whose secretion is geared to environmental cues through the pineal gland, hypothalamus and pituitary.

The control of sexual hair growth must be differentiated from that of the moult cycle. The development of pubic, axillary and other body hair is delayed until puberty because it is dependent upon androgens in both sexes. In all mammals including humans (apart from possibly merino sheep and the poodle dog), HFs show intermittent activity. Thus, each hair grows to a maximum length, is retained for a time without further growth and is eventually shed and replaced.

Types of hair

Different types of hair may be produced by different kinds of follicles, and the type of hair produced in a follicle can change with age or under the influence of hormones. Animals characteristically have both an overcoat of stiff guard hairs and an undercoat of fine hairs [6]. Many species also have large vibrissae or sinus hairs, which are sensory and are produced from special follicles containing erectile tissue, but there are no such strictly comparable follicles in humans. In humans, a prenatal coat of fine, soft, unmedullated and usually unpigmented hair, known as lanugo, is normally shed *in utero* in the eighth to ninth month of gestation. Postnatal hair may be divided at the extreme into two kinds: vellus, which is soft, unmedullated, occasionally pigmented and seldom more than 2 cm long; and terminal hair, which is longer, coarser and often medullated and pigmented. However, there is a range of intermediate kinds. Before puberty, terminal hair is normally limited to the scalp, eyebrows and eyelashes. After puberty, secondary sexual 'terminal' hair is developed from vellus hair in response to androgens.

Development and distribution of hair follicles

The process of *de novo* HF formation in developing embryonic skin is called morphogenesis. Recently reclassified [7], morphogenesis involves 10 stages driven by various critical signals (including wingless (Wnts), fibroblast growth factor 20 (FGF-20), sonic hedgehog (Shh) and bone morphogenic proteins (BMPs)) that drive each stage. Briefly, dermal signals induce the overlying epidermal cells

Table 87.1 Hair follicle density in human fetal and adult skin. In adults, hair follicle density is highest on the head and is much lower on the trunk and limbs. At 24 weeks' gestational age hair follicle density is similar on the forehead and thigh skin. There is a pronounced reduction in thigh hair follicle density by adult life but only a small fall on the forehead.

Skin area	Fetal skin (follicles/cm²)				Adult (follicles/cm²)	
	24 weeks		Full term			
	Mean	± SE	Mean	± SE	Mean	± SE
Cheek					830	40
Forehead	1060		1060	110	765	20
Scalp					350	50
Forearm					95	15
Thigh	1010	250	480	40	55	5
Lower leg					45	10
Abdomen					70	15
Chest					75	25

Adapted from Szabo 1967 [8].
SE, standard error.

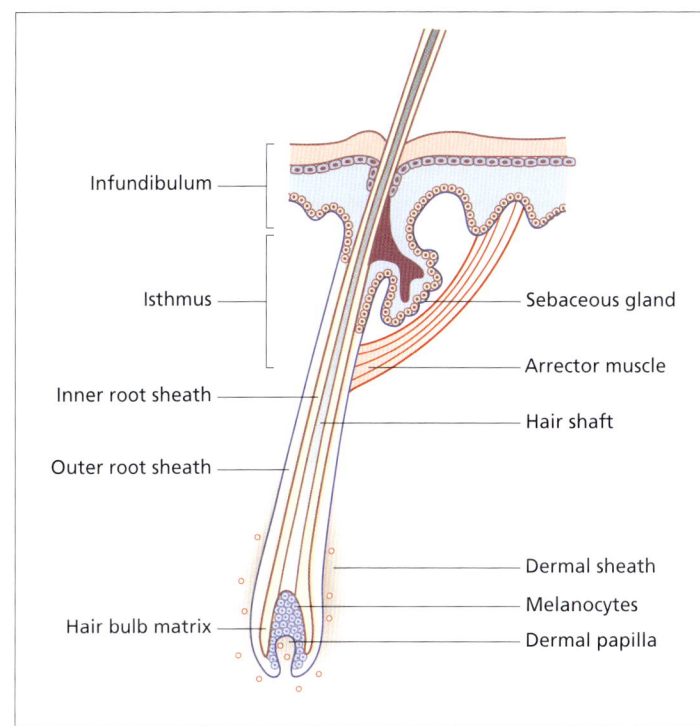

Figure 87.1 Diagram of an anagen hair follicle.

to thicken to form an area called the placode. Underlying the placode, a dermal condensate of mesenchymal cells develops. Over time the placode thickens, the dermal condensate becomes more defined and the epidermis starts to invaginate into the dermis producing the germ. This proximal extension continues with the column of cells next forming a rudimentary hair peg, enveloping the mesenchymal component, before eventually producing a fully formed HF [7].

Human HFs appear first in the regions of the eyebrows, upper lip and chin at about 9 weeks of embryonic development, and in other regions in the fourth month. Hair over most of the scalp passes through a complete cycle and is shed *in utero*, so follicles in these regions have re-entered anagen by the time of birth. In the occipital scalp, telogen is delayed until after birth giving rise to a patch of hair loss in this region in the neonatal period. A fuller account of embryonic development is given in Chapter 2.

In humans, the full complement of HFs is probably established by the time of birth. Follicle density is highest in the fetus, when it may be similar across the skin surface. With growth there is a progressive reduction in follicle density, which continues until adult life, as skin surface area increases (Table 87.1). This occurs to a greater degree over the trunk and limbs than over the head so that the reduction in follicle density is less marked on the head than elsewhere [8]. The highest hair follicle densities, in the region of 800/cm², are found on the forehead and cheeks, with rather lower values for the visible vellus hairs on the forehead in young adults of both sexes, and on the cheeks in women (400–450/cm²) [9]. Lower hair densities of 50–100/cm² are found on the chest and back in both sexes [9,10], and approximately 50/cm² on the thigh and leg [8]. Scalp hair density shows a normal distribution in the population with a wide range [11]. There is also racial variation in scalp hair density: published values for average scalp hair density in white people vary between 250 and 320 hairs/cm² [11–14]; whereas average hair densities in Africans (187/cm²) [15], African Americans (171/cm²) [16] and Koreans (128/cm²) [17] are lower than values seen in white people.

Anatomy of the hair follicle

The HF is a tube-like structure, continuous with the epidermis at its upper end, which produces the hair fibre (Figure 87.1). Follicles are sloped within the dermis and can extend into subcutaneous tissue. An oblique muscle, the arrector pili, runs from a point in the papillary dermis close to the dermal–epidermal junction to the mid-region of the follicle wall. Above the muscle, one or more sebaceous glands, and in some regions of the body apocrine glands, open into the follicle.

The hair fibre, inner root sheath (IRS) and outer root sheath (ORS) are all derived from highly proliferative epithelial cells in the hair bulb at the proximal part of the HF. The HF also has a specialised mesenchymal component, which includes the dermal (or connective tissue) sheath surrounding the follicle, and the dermal papilla, which invaginates the hair bulb.

The HF is conventionally divided into two regions: the upper 'permanent' part, consisting of the infundibulum and isthmus, and the lower 'cycling' part, comprising the hair bulb and suprabulbar region. The upper follicle is a relatively constant structure, whereas the lower follicle undergoes repeated episodes of regression and regeneration during the hair cycle. On the scalp, and some other regions of the skin, HFs are arranged in groups of three or more follicles known as follicular units (Figure 87.2). Several follicles within a follicular unit may coalesce so that hairs emerge through a common infundibulum.

Infundibulum

The infundibulum extends from the skin surface, where it merges with the epidermis, to the opening of the sebaceous duct at the junction with the isthmus. Infundibular epithelium differentiates in a similar manner to epidermis, producing a granular layer and stratum corneum, which desquamates into the follicular lumen [18].

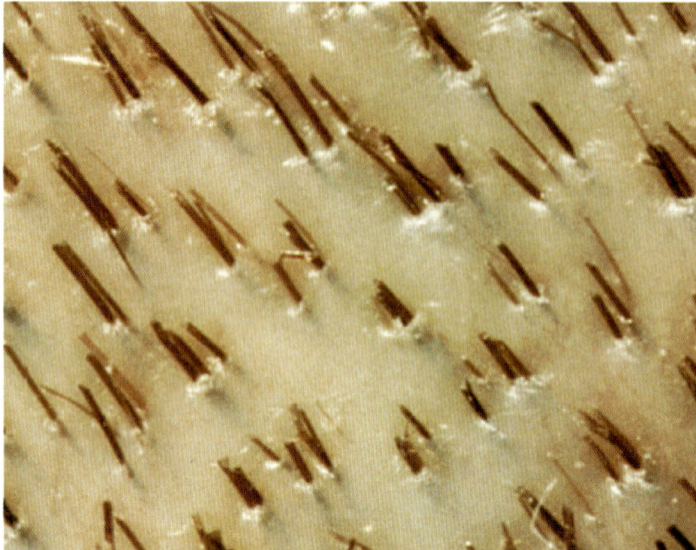

Figure 87.2 Grouping of hairs in follicular units on the human scalp. In some groups, multiple hairs emerge from a single follicular opening.

Isthmus and bulge region

The isthmus extends from the opening of the sebaceous gland duct to the proximal point of insertion of the arrector pili muscle. It consists of a multilayered ORS that is continuous with the infundibulum but differs in its structure. The innermost cells undergo abrupt keratinisation without formation of a granular cell layer, a pattern of differentiation known as trichilemmal keratinisation. The keratinised IRS, which lies within the ORS, disintegrates at or about the level of the sebaceous duct. The arrector pili muscle loops around the follicle in the manner of a sling [19]. Each follicular unit is supplied by a single arrector pili muscle, which splits to encircle each follicle within the follicular unit [20].

HF stem cells reside in the lower part of the isthmus, in an area called the bulge, at the insertion of the arrector pili muscle [21]. During embryogenesis, and in adult follicles in other species, this region shows a distinctive thickening (hence the name), although in humans a clearly defined bulge is often not seen. Therefore, the bulge really represents a biological concept, not a physical protuberance. However, distinctive protrusions in the ORS, termed follicular trochanter, are recognised anatomical markers sometimes seen in this region [22].

Epithelial HF stem cells (eHFSCs) show distinctive biochemical properties; they are slow cycling, label-retaining cells that proliferate only during the onset of anagen. Daughter cells, known as transient amplifying cells, input into the ORS of the lower part of the HF migrating downwards. On entering the hair bulb matrix, they proliferate and undergo terminal differentiation to form the hair shaft and IRS [23]. The progeny of eHFSCs may also migrate distally to form the sebaceous gland and, under certain circumstances such as wound healing, can repopulate the epidermis.

HF stem cells can be identified by various immunohistochemical markers, with positive staining for keratin 15, keratin 19 and CD200, but negative staining for connexin 43, currently the best way to identify eHFSCs in humans [24]. Interestingly, CD34, a key bulge marker in mice HFs, is not a stem cell marker in humans. Laser capture microdissection and gene expression profiling in both

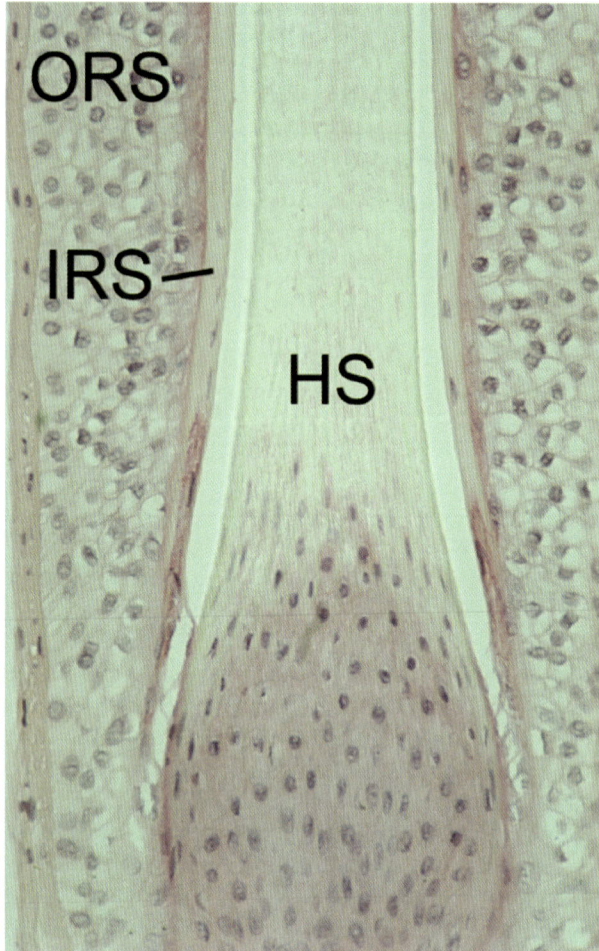

Figure 87.3 Longitudinal section through the suprabulbar region of an anagen follicle showing the keratogenous region of the hair shaft (HS). The inner root sheath (IRS) is keratinised at this level. ORS, outer root sheath.

mouse and human HFs have identified various gene signatures that characterise the stem cell niche, with functions that support the quiescent nature of this region [21,25,26]. Further, the HF stem cell compartment appears to signal with other skin sources, including lymphatics, blood vessels, neurons and local immunocytes, controlling quiescence, activation and cycling of the HF (reviewed in [27]).

Suprabulbar region

The suprabulbar region of the follicle, below the isthmus and above the hair bulb, is composed of three layers (from outermost to innermost): the ORS, IRS and hair shaft (Figure 87.3). The ORS is a multilayered epithelium enclosing the IRS which, at this level, is a fully keratinised structure. Cells of the hair shaft, at the centre of the follicle, undergo terminal differentiation within the keratogenous zone in the middle part of the suprabulbar region. Keratinisation of the IRS precedes that of the hair shaft, suggesting that the IRS has a role in 'moulding' the shape of the hair fibre.

Hair bulb

In large terminal follicles, the deepest part of the follicle, the hair bulb, is situated in the subcutaneous fat (Figure 87.4). The hair bulb is invaginated at its base by the dermal papilla, which is connected

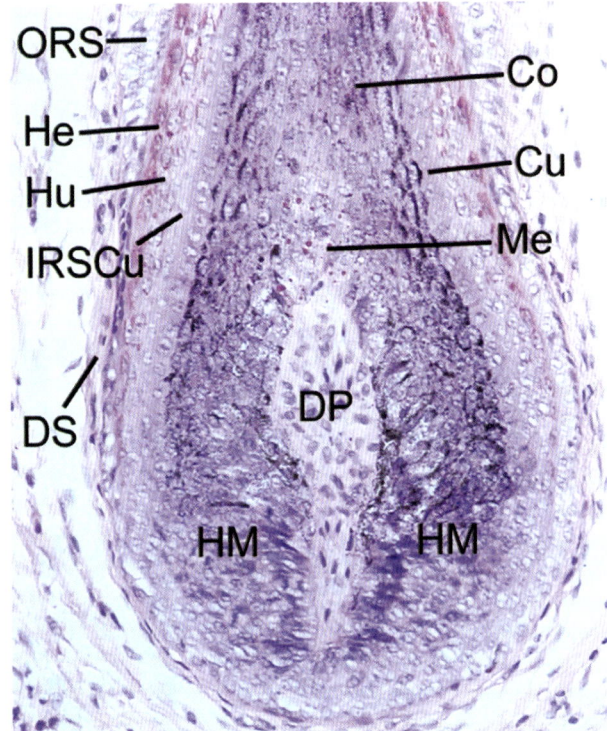

Figure 87.4 Anagen hair bulb. Co, hair cortex; Cu, hair cuticle; DP, dermal papilla; DS, dermal sheath; He, Henle layer; HM, hair matrix; Hu, Huxley layer; IRSCu, inner root sheath cuticle; Me, melanocyte; ORS, outer root sheath.

to the perifollicular dermal sheath by a narrow stalk. The hair shaft and IRS are derived from epithelial cells surrounding the dermal papilla, in a region known as the hair bulb matrix or germinative epithelium. Proliferating hair matrix cells are located below the Auber line, identified as a perpendicular line drawn through the widest part of the dermal papilla [28]. These cells have a high mitotic rate, with a rate of cell turnover similar to bone marrow. Daughter cells migrate in an upwards direction and differentiate in a highly ordered fashion to form the concentric layers of the IRS and the hair shaft. The IRS derives from cells in the lower, more lateral part of the matrix, whereas the hair shaft is formed from the upper, centrally situated cells. In pigmented HFs, highly pigmented melanocytes are situated among cells destined to form the hair cortex. The ORS surrounds the IRS.

Dermal papilla

In anagen follicles, the dermal papilla is a flask-shaped structure that invaginates the base of the HF. It is made up of specialised fibroblast-like cells embedded in an extracellular matrix rich in basement-membrane proteins and proteoglycans, and in large follicles the dermal papilla often contains a loop of capillary blood vessels. It is connected to the dermal sheath surrounding the follicle by a narrow stalk. Both the dermal papilla and the dermal sheath are derived from a condensation of mesenchymal cells, which appears at an early stage in follicular embryogenesis. Tissue recombinant studies have shown that the dermal papilla plays an essential part in the induction and maintenance of follicular epithelial differentiation [29–33]. It is responsible for determining the follicle type, so that cultured dermal papilla cells derived from rat vibrissae follicles

induce the formation of a vibrissa-like follicle when implanted into ear skin [30]. The volume of the dermal papilla may also be responsible for controlling the size of the HF and hair fibre [34,35]. This is of relevance to androgen-dependent changes in human hair growth as the dermal papilla is probably the primary target of androgen action in the HF.

Dermal sheath

A collagenous layer known as the dermal sheath (within the connective tissue sheath in humans) envelops the lower part of the HF. Like dermal papilla cells, fibroblasts of the dermal sheath are specialised. In particular, the dermal sheath cup cells located at the bottom of the hair bulb are contiguous but morphologically and molecularly distinct from the dermal papilla, containing a stem cell population. In experimental circumstances, these cells can reconstitute the dermal papilla and induce the formation of new HFs in adult human skin [36]. As we move distally along the HF, above the level of the arrector pili muscle insertion, the dermal sheath becomes less distinct, both structurally and functionally, as it merges with the interfollicular dermis.

Recently, α-smooth muscle actin has been identified as a dermal sheath marker, indicating these HF-lining cells are smooth muscle of fibroblastic origin. Further, in mice it has been shown that contraction of the dermal sheath is vital for relocating the dermal papilla into the correct position during catagen by focusing forces to pull the dermal papilla upwards [37].

Inner root sheath

The IRS consists of three layers (from outermost to innermost): the Henle layer, Huxley layer and IRS cuticle. IRS cells accumulate filaments approximately 7 nm thick and, in contrast with the hair cortex, amorphous trichohyalin granules appear in the cytoplasm. As the cells move up the follicle towards the surface, the filaments become more abundant, and the number and size of the granules increase. Each of the three layers of the IRS undergoes abrupt keratinisation. This occurs at different levels in each layer, although the patterns of change are identical. In the hardened cytoplasm, however, only filaments can be seen. The changes occur first in the outermost Henle layer, then in the innermost cuticle and lastly in the Huxley layer, which is situated between them. Cells of the IRS cuticle become flattened and overlap, with their free edges pointing downwards to interdigitate with the upwards-pointing cells of the hair shaft cuticle, thus anchoring the hair shaft within the HF. The IRS hardens before the presumptive hair within it, and it is consequently thought to control the definitive shape of the hair shaft.

Outer root sheath

The ORS forms the most peripheral layer of HF epithelium, enclosing the IRS. At the lower tip of the hair bulb, it consists of a single layer of cuboidal cells, becoming multilayered in the region of the upper hair bulb. The cytoplasm of ORS cells is rich in glycogen, giving a clear appearance with routine histological stains. In some follicles, particularly large beard follicles, there is a distinct single-cell layer interposed between the outer and inner root sheaths, known as the companion layer [38]. Companion layer cells are flattened along the axis of the follicle and are relatively devoid of glycogen. They show numerous intercellular connections to the IRS and are thought to migrate distally along with the IRS to be lost in the isthmus region. The direction of movement of ORS cells is unclear but they may migrate downwards towards the hair bulb, the companion layer forming the plane of slippage between the inner and outer root sheaths. The ORS of the suprabulbar region merges imperceptibly with the isthmus where the innermost cells undergo tricholemmal keratinisation.

Hair fibres

Cuticle

The hair cuticle is formed initially as a single-cell layer, but the cells become progressively imbricated (tile-like) as they move peripherally. The cells become flattened, first in a direction at right angles to the plane of the follicle, and then becoming progressively angulated so that the outer edges of the cells point in an upwards direction. The flattened cells overlap, their free edges directed towards the tip and interlocking with the cuticle of the surrounding IRS. In the fully formed hair shaft, the cuticle consists of 5–10 overlapping cell layers, reminiscent of roof tiles, each 350–450 nm thick (Figure 87.5). Viewed with electron microscopy the cuticle is composed of three layers: the A layer, outer exocuticle and inner endocuticle (Figure 87.6).

The cuticle has important protective properties, acting as a barrier to physical and chemical insults, and maintaining the integrity of the hair shaft. Wear and tear (e.g. from cosmetic procedures) leads to gradual degradation of the cuticle (called 'weathering'), with breaking and lifting of the free margins of the cuticular cells. Eventually this process may lead to exposure of the cortex and fracture of the hair shaft (see 'Abnormalities of the hair shaft' later in this chapter).

Cortex

Cells destined to form the cortex gradually become more fusiform in shape as they migrate upwards from the hair bulb. They develop a dense filamentous cytoskeleton in the upper hair bulb to become fully hyalinised in the suprabulbar region (the keratogenous zone) setting the hair fibre shape (Figure 87.7). The hard α-keratin intermediate filaments (α-KIF) are the major structural component of the mammalian hair cortex. The molecule in α-KIF is an obligate heteropolymer containing a type I and type II polypeptide chain [39–41], in which right-handed α-helices coil round one another in a left-handed manner to form a rod-like dimeric structure (a 'coiled coil') (Figure 87.8). The 8 nm keratin filaments (microfibrils) are formed from multiple α-KIF molecules, on average 16 molecules or 32 chains in cross-section [42]. Keratin filaments are cross-linked to cell-membrane complexes (keratin-associated proteins), which form a matrix between the filaments. More than 100 hair keratin-associated proteins have been found in various species. They are classified into three major families: high sulphur, ultrahigh sulphur and high glycine–tyrosine proteins [43]. In some species, notably sheep, the cortex can be divided into two regions: the orthocortex and paracortex, which differ in the arrangement of KIFs and the proportion of keratin-associated proteins. In humans, the hair cortex appears to contain mixtures of KIF arrangements within each cell [44].

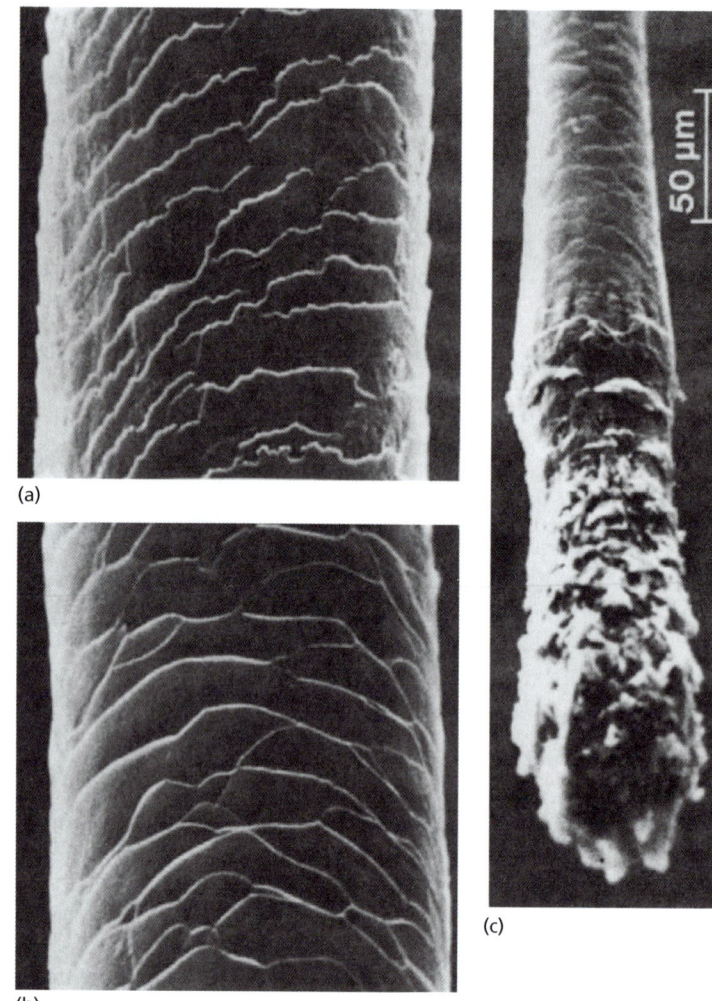

(a)

(b)

(c)

Figure 87.5 (a) Surface view of weathered cuticular scales in the distal portion of the hair shaft. (b) Surface view of undamaged cuticular scales in the proximal part of the hair shaft. (c) Low-power view of the proximal end of a hair shaft. Courtesy of Dr D. Jackson, University of Sheffield, Sheffield, UK.

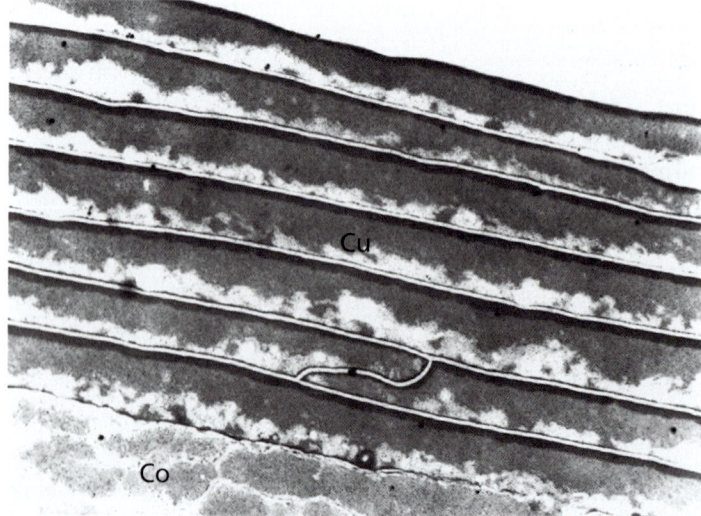

Figure 87.6 Cross-section through hair shaft showing cuticle layers (Cu) surrounding the central cortex (Co). Transmission electron micrograph, silver methenamine stain.

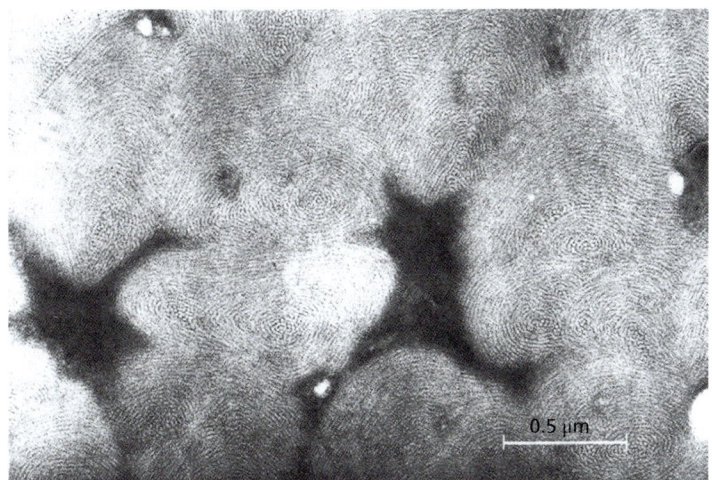

Figure 87.7 Cross-section of transformed cortical cells of human hair. The relatively translucent filaments, set in a more dense sulphur-rich matrix, appear as concentric lamellae (macrofibrils), giving a characteristic fingerprint pattern.

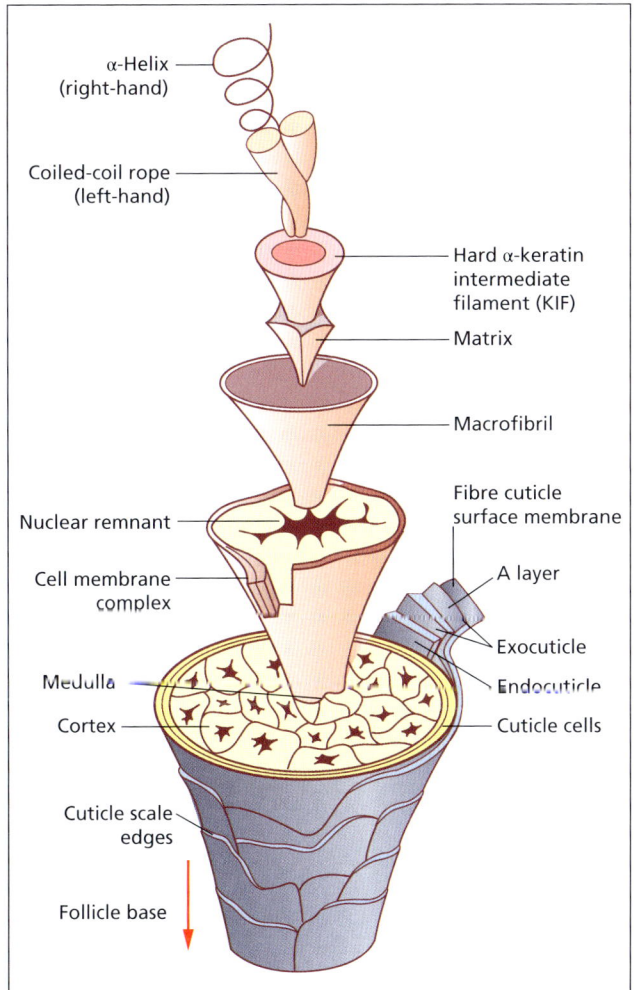

Figure 87.8 Exploded view of the major structural components comprising a human hair fibre. Pigment granules that are normally dispersed throughout the cortex are not included. Reproduced from Jones 2001 [44] with permission of Elsevier.

Medulla

The medulla is a variable structure in human hairs, where it may be continuous, discontinuous or absent. Large-diameter hairs are more likely to contain a medulla, although the relationship between hair diameter and medullation is not clear-cut.

Hair shape

There is significant variation in the degree of hair curl seen in human populations that does not always correlate with skin type or ethnicity. Hair curl is classified into eight types [45,46]. A recent genome-wide association study (GWAS) and meta-analysis identifies 14 single nucleotide polymorphisms (SNPs) from different genes that 'significantly and independently contribute to hair shape variation' [47]. Curly hair is produced by curled HFs and the hair shaft is often elliptical or D-shaped in cross-section. It is thought that asymmetrical cell proliferation forming the IRS and ORS, along with IRS hardening, contributes to hair curl development (reviewed in [48]).

Hair follicle innervation

A plexus of longitudinally aligned sensory nerve fibres surrounds the isthmus region. Small nerve fibres may also be arranged in a circular fashion outside the longitudinal fibres. Several different types of nerve endings are found around human HFs, including free nerve endings, pilo-Ruffini nerve endings and Merkel nerve endings. In other species, lamellated nerve endings are found in richly innervated sinus hair follicles (e.g. vibrissae follicles), which have specialised sensory function. The HF is densely innervated, particularly around the bulge region. In mice, nerve signals maintain a subpopulation of eHFSCs [49], and certain immune-inhibitory neuropeptides (e.g. calcitonin gene-related peptide (cGRP), vasoactive intestinal peptide (VIP)) support HF immune privilege (see 'Hair immune system' later in this chapter). Psychoemotional stress and neurogenic inflammation can inhibit hair growth via release of pro-inflammatory neuropeptides, such as substance P, that threaten HF immune privilege, induce catagen onset and trigger mast cell degranulation [50–52].

Hair cycle

Hair follicles undergo a repetitive sequence of growth and rest known as the hair cycle (Figure 87.9). The timing of the phases of the hair cycle and its overall duration vary between species, between follicles in different regions of the skin in the same species and, in some animals, between different follicle types, such as guard hairs and under-hairs in the same region of the skin.

The period of active hair growth is known as *anagen*, with the duration of this phase responsible for determining the final length of the hair. In most HFs in most animals, anagen is relatively brief, lasting a few weeks at most, with most hair remaining in telogen. This is probably because short periods of anagen growth are a more energy-efficient way of maintaining hair coverage compared with continuous growth. However, in some HFs, such as those on the human scalp, horse's tail, lion's mane and wool follicles in merino sheep, anagen may continue for several years, so that very long hairs are produced. Under normal circumstances, 80–90% of HFs on the human scalp are in anagen at any one time.

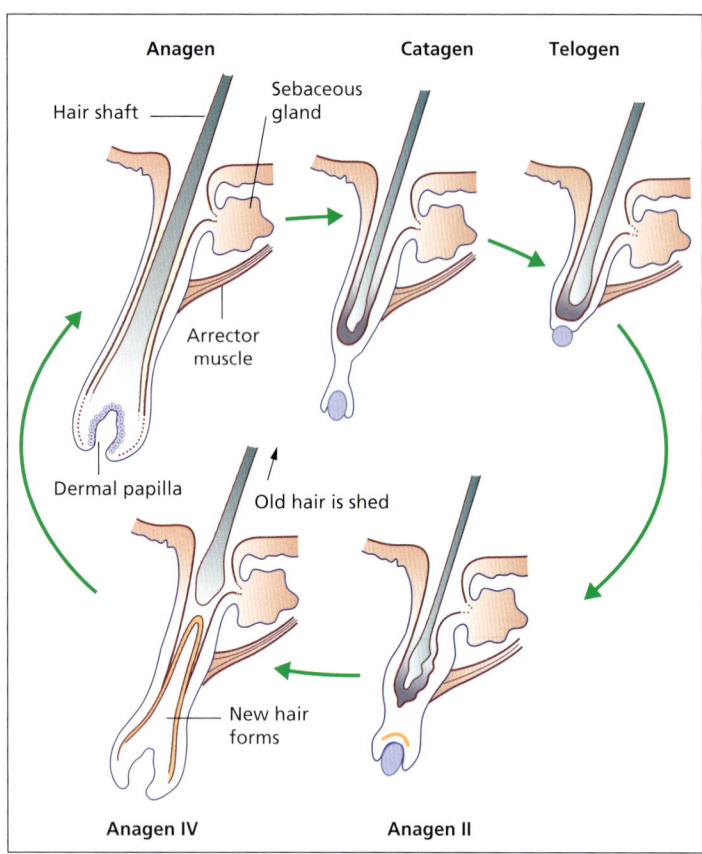

Figure 87.9 The hair cycle. Reproduced from Olsen 1994 [121] with permission of McGraw-Hill.

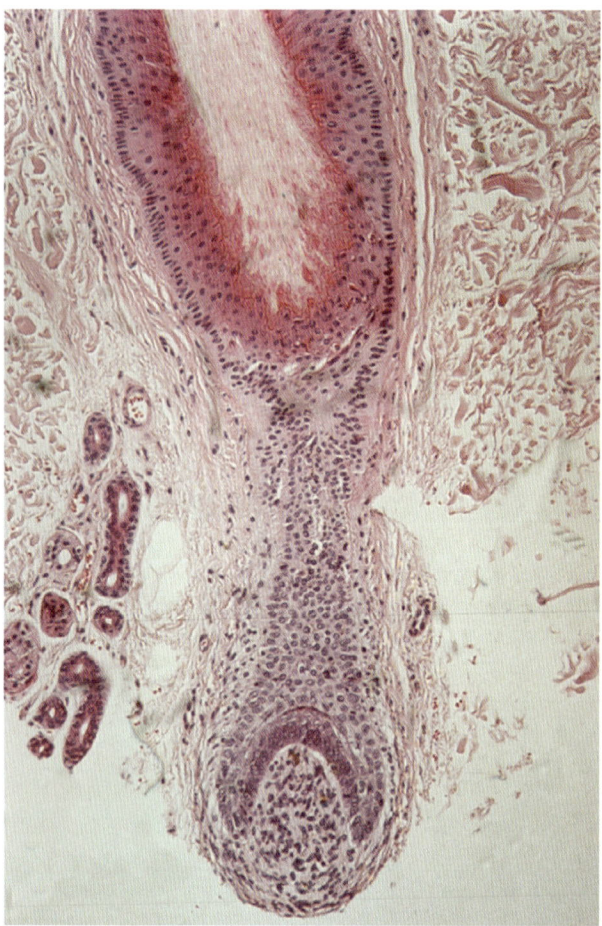

Figure 87.10 Scalp hair follicle in the anagen 2 stage of development. The club hair from the previous cycle is still present within the follicle. Courtesy of Dr A. J. G. McDonagh, Royal Hallamshire Hospital, Sheffield, UK.

The entry of a resting telogen HF back into anagen is heralded by the onset of mitotic activity in an epithelial cell population (called the secondary hair germ) that sits just above the regressed dermal papilla and beneath the club hair root at the proximal part of the permanent follicle. The secondary hair germ contains a subpopulation of epithelial progenitor cells identified by EpCAM/Bur-EP4 staining, but negative for keratin 15 and keratin 19 [24]. In most follicle types (vibrissae follicles are an exception), the lower part of the follicle elongates downwards along a preformed dermal tract (the stele). The developing hair bulb partly envelops the dermal papilla, and epithelial cells start to differentiate to form the IRS and the hair shaft (Figure 87.10). The dermal papilla expands from a tightly packed ball of cells into a flask-shaped structure where the cells become separated by an extracellular matrix rich in proteoglycans and basement membrane proteins. A network of capillary blood vessels develops around the lengthening follicle, extending into the dermal papilla in larger follicles. In the fully developed anagen follicle, epithelial cells in the hair bulb undergo vigorous proliferative activity. Their progeny move distally and differentiate in an ordered fashion to form the layers of the IRS and the hair shaft.

At the end of anagen, epithelial cell division declines and ceases, and the follicle enters an involution phase known as *catagen*. During catagen, the proximal end of the hair shaft keratinises to form a club-shaped structure and the lower part of the follicle involutes by apoptosis (Figure 87.11). The basement membrane surrounding the follicle becomes thickened and corrugated to form the 'glassy membrane'. The base of the follicle, together with its dermal papilla,

moves upwards, eventually to lie just below the level of the arrector insertion. Dermal sheath contraction appears important in successfully completing this stage [37].

The period between the completion of follicular regression and the onset of the next anagen phase is termed *telogen*. The club hair lies within an epithelial sac to which it is attached by tricholemmal keratin. In mice, telogen follicles are unable to respond to anagen-inducing signals immediately following catagen (termed 'refractory' telogen). This is thought to prevent excess regeneration. After approximately 1 month these HFs become 'permissive' and can now respond to anagen induction [4].

The club hair is eventually shed through an active process termed *exogen* [53]. In many species, follicles re-enter anagen prior to shedding of the club hair so that the old hair is not shed until the follicle is well into its next growth phase. This may also be seen in human follicles, although it is unusual for a club hair to be retained much beyond the mid-stage of anagen development. In the human scalp, HFs may remain empty, in a state of latency, known as *kenogen*, for a prolonged period after the club hair is shed [54].

Accurate recognition of different hair cycle stages is vital for experimental study in both *in vivo* animal models and *ex vivo* HF organ culture, with detailed morphological depiction of hair cycle substages described [55,56].

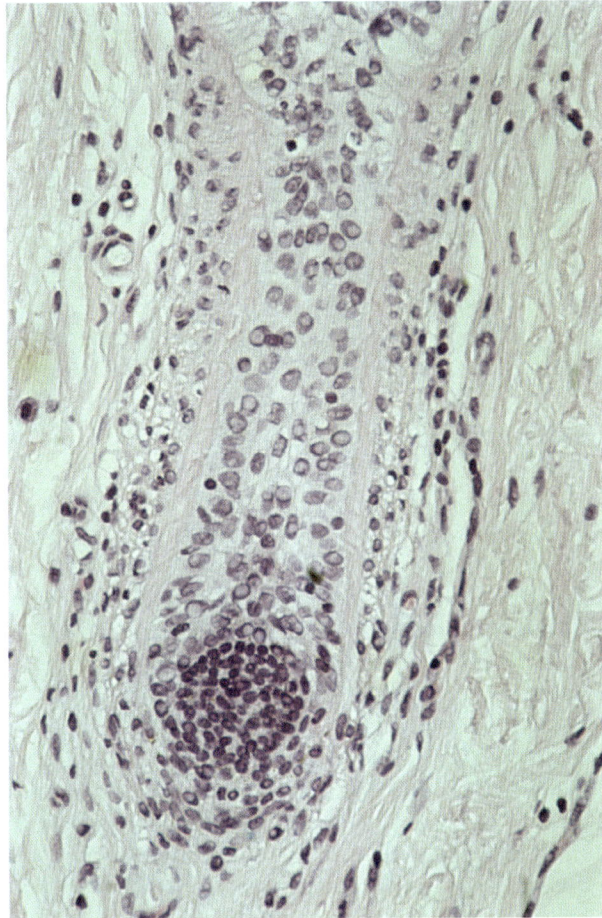

Figure 87.11 Human hair follicle in mid-catagen. There is a prominent glassy membrane surrounding the regressing epithelial column. The dermal papilla has rounded and condensed. Courtesy of McGraw-Hill.

Control of the hair cycle

Hair cycling is controlled primarily within individual HFs, but this intrinsic behaviour may be modulated by both local and systemic factors. In most newborn mammals, including humans, hair cycles are coordinated in a wave-like fashion (moult waves) that cross regions of the skin in the neonatal period. Moult waves are regulated within the skin and are accompanied by changes in other skin structures, such as epidermal and dermal thickness. In many mammals, living in their natural environment in temperate and higher latitudes, moult waves continue into adult life and occur on a seasonal basis. This allows adaptation of the thickness of the coat, and sometimes its colour, to different climatic conditions in summer and winter (Figure 87.12).

Seasonal moulting is regulated by the endocrine system under the influence of environmental signals. The most important of these is change in day length (the photoperiod). The production of melatonin by the pineal gland, which transduces visual signals, and prolactin by the pituitary play a key role in orchestrating endocrine control of seasonal hair growth [57–60]. Vestiges of seasonal variation in hair growth are present in humans [61], although the magnitude is seldom sufficient to be noticeable (see 'Telogen effluvium' later in this chapter).

Although local and systemic factors modulate the hair cycle in some species, in adult humans and some other mammals hair

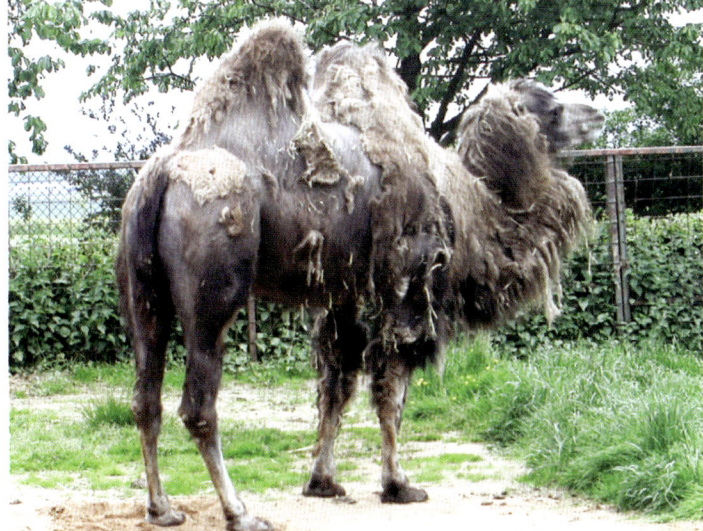

Figure 87.12 Bactrian camel in a spring moult.

cycling is asynchronous. HFs in different regions of the skin may also cycle differently. In humans, for example, the duration of anagen on the scalp may last several years, whereas on the eyebrows anagen is very brief. Even in animals showing seasonal hair growth, hair cycles in different follicle types in the same skin region are not necessarily in phase. When scalp hair follicles are transplanted into other regions of the skin they retain the cyclical behaviour of the donor site, indicating that cycle control is determined within the follicle or its immediate tissue environment. Interactions between two key cell populations in the hair follicle (i.e. the eHFSC in the bulge region and mesenchymal cells in the dermal papilla and dermal sheath) are thought to underlie intrinsic control of hair cycling, with a large number of molecules implicated in this process [62]. Fluctuations in the inhibitory influence of BMPs and the stimulatory Wnt/β-catenin pathway appear to play a key role in regulating stem cell activity during hair cycling. A wide array of other signalling molecules with hair growth stimulatory (e.g. follistatin, transforming growth factor β_2 (TGF-β_2), FGF-7, FGF-10) and inhibitory (e.g. Dkk1, FGF-18, 17β-oestradiol) influences have also been implicated but, such is their complexity, a comprehensive model of hair cycle control has yet to be achieved [63].

Hair growth
Rate of hair growth

The rate of hair growth varies from species to species, and within one species from region to region, as well as with sex and age. Published rates of scalp hair growth in humans vary between 0.3 and 0.5 mm per day, slightly faster in adult women than men but greater in prepubertal boys than girls. Male beard growth has been recorded at 0.27–0.38 mm/day. Vellus hair growth is much slower: 0.03 mm/day on the forehead in one study [10]. Interestingly, grey hair grows faster than pigmented hairs.

Androgens and hair growth

Androgens influence hair growth in several ways. Firstly, they participate in the endocrine control of moulting in animals that show seasonal hair growth. Secondly, in some mammals, androgens stimulate the growth of HFs in certain regions of the skin following sexual maturity. Thirdly, in humans and some other primates, androgens are necessary for the development of balding on the scalp.

Androgen-stimulated hair growth

The growth of obvious facial, trunk and extremity hair in the male, and of pubic and axillary hair in both sexes, is dependent on androgens. The development of such hair at puberty is, in broad terms and at least initially, in parallel with the rise in levels of androgen from testicular, adrenocortical and ovarian sources, which occurs in both sexes and is somewhat steeper in males. That testosterone from the interstitial cells of the testis is responsible for the growth of beard and body hair in male adolescence and that testicular activity is itself initiated by gonadotrophic hormones of the pituitary is unquestioned. However, the findings that growth hormone-deficient boys and girls are less than normally responsive to androgens, and that growth hormone is necessary as a synergistic factor to allow testosterone to be fully effective with respect to hair growth [64], as well as protein anabolism and growth promotion, suggest that pituitary hormones also have a more direct role. Direct evidence of the role of testicular androgen is that castration reduces growth of the human beard, whereas testosterone stimulates beard development in eunuchs and elderly men. The role of androgen is further demonstrated in the treatment of hirsute women with the antiandrogen cyproterone acetate [65,66], which is shown to reduce the definitive length, rate of growth, diameter and medullation of examined thigh hairs [65].

At puberty, terminal hairs gradually replace vellus hairs, starting in the pubic regions. In both sexes the first pubic hair is sparse, long, downy, slightly pigmented and almost straight. It later becomes darker, coarser, more curled and extends in area to form an inverse triangle. A British study showed that boys had the first recognisable pubic hair at an average age of 13.4 years, and the full adult 'male' pattern at 15.2 years, approximately 3.5 years after the start of pubertal development of the genitalia [67]. The corresponding mean ages for girls were considerably earlier, namely 11.7 years and 13.5 years [68]. In approximately 80% of men and 10% of women, the pubic hair continues spreading until the mid-twenties or later; there is no absolute distinction between male and female patterns, only one of degree.

Axillary hair first appears approximately 2 years after the start of pubic hair growth. The amount, as measured by the weight of the fully grown mass, continues to increase until the late twenties in males as well as in females, although in women it is less at any age. The mean amounts grown per day increase from late puberty until the mid-twenties and thereafter decrease steadily.

Facial hair in boys first appears at about the same time as the axillary hair, starting at the corners of the upper lip, and spreading medially to complete the moustache and then the cheeks and beard. Terminal hair development is continued in regular sequence on the legs, thighs, forearms, abdomen, buttocks, back, arms and shoulders [69]. The extent of terminal hair tends to increase throughout the years of sexual maturity, but most patterns occur over a wide age range. The adult pattern is not achieved until the fourth decade, when the androgen levels are already somewhat lower than in early adult life. Moreover, aural hairs do not appear until late

middle age, and a study of coarse sternal hair in men showed that the hairs continue to increase in length and number from puberty to the fifth or sixth decade.

There is considerable racial variability in androgen-dependent hair growth. The growth of facial and body hair is greater in European men than in Chinese men and there is also variation within these broad racial categories – southern European men tend to be hairier than men from northern Europe [70].

Androgenetic alopecia

See the section 'Androgenetic alopecia and pattern hair loss' later in this chapter.

Androgen synthesis and metabolism

Testosterone is the major circulating androgen, but in most body sites apart from the axillae and pubic region, the effect of testosterone on hair growth is mediated by its more potent metabolite 5α-dihydrotestosterone (DHT). The conversion of testosterone to DHT is catalysed by the enzyme 5α-reductase. There are three isoforms of 5α-reductase, which are encoded by different genes [71,72]. Type 1 5α-reductase is widely distributed in the skin, but expression of the type 2 isoform is restricted to androgen target tissues such as the prostate and epididymis. Evidence from studies in men with a genetic deficiency of 5α-reductase type 2, and from the response of androgenetic alopecia and female hirsutism to finasteride, an inhibitor of 5α-reductase type 2, indicates that this isoform plays the key role in regulating androgen-dependent hair growth. The type 3 isoform is widely expressed but it is not yet known whether it regulates androgen responses in the skin [73].

Androgen receptor

The tissue effects of androgens are mediated through binding to the intracellular androgen receptor. The androgen receptor is a nuclear hormone receptor [74], and like other members of the nuclear hormone receptor superfamily it acts as a gene transcription factor following ligand binding. Mutations in the androgen receptor gene are responsible for the androgen insensitivity syndrome [75]. Individuals with the complete form of the syndrome, in which there is failure of functional androgen receptor expression, have intra-abdominal testes but female external genitalia, breast development and psychosocial development. After puberty, circulating testosterone is in the normal or elevated male range, but pubic and axillary hair fail to develop and there is no beard growth and no balding. Polymorphisms in the *AR* gene may facilitate receptor activation, predisposing to androgen-related conditions [76].

Mechanism of androgen action on the hair follicle

The specificity of the response of HFs to androgens is determined within the skin. HFs in occipital skin, a site that shows little or no response to androgens, retain their site-specific behaviour (including size and curl) when transplanted into balding areas on the frontal scalp [77]. Conversely, HFs from a balding scalp continue to regress when transplanted into skin of the forearm [36]. The success of micrografting techniques, in which individual follicles are transplanted, shows that androgen responsiveness is determined at the level of the follicle or its immediate tissue environment. Three lines of evidence suggest that the dermal papilla is the primary target of androgen action in the hair follicle:

1 Androgen receptor expression in the lower part of the follicle is restricted to dermal papilla cells [78,79].
2 The size of the hair follicle is probably determined by the volume of the dermal papilla [34,80].
3 Dermal papillae express 5α-reductase type 2 whereas hair follicle epithelium expresses only 5α-reductase type 1 [81].

Androgens may act on hair growth by altering the number of cells in the dermal papilla and its extracellular matrix [80]. Cells cultured from dermal papillae of human beard HFs also release growth factors in response to androgens that stimulate the proliferation of keratinocytes [79,82], and the pattern of androgen metabolism by cultured and intact dermal papilla cells is consistent with that expected from their site of origin [83,84]. There is one report that dermal papilla cells grown from balding scalp follicles secrete TGF-β in the presence of testosterone [85]. TGF-β is a growth factor known to inhibit hair growth [86]. Hence the variable response of hair growth to androgens may reflect site-dependent differences in the types of growth factors produced by the dermal papilla.

Hair immune system

Hair follicles are a potential portal of entry for microbes into the body. Thus, the HF has evolved a robust hair immune system, comprising both innate and adaptive elements, which are predominantly located around the infundibulum and distal follicle to respond to pathogenic threats [18,87]. Further, antimicrobial peptides are part of an evolutionary conserved innate anti-infective mechanism that can be induced in response to the presence of certain microbial species (see the section on the HF microbiome).

Hair follicle immune privilege

Immune privilege describes a set of mechanisms in defined tissue compartments that shield (auto)-antigens generated in that area from immune surveillance. This process is seen in various tissue sites, including the eye, brain, testes and maternofetal unit, and is thought to protect these vulnerable structures from excessive immune responses. The proximal HF (from bulb to bulge) has also been shown to be an immune privilege site [88–90]. The reason is unclear, but it may represent an evolutionary advantage to prevent autoimmune hair loss (e.g. a real threat to survival should this occur in a polar bear).

Immune privilege is relative and dynamic. Various components all contribute to the immune privilege state, including (i) *restricted immune cell recruitment and trafficking* (e.g. lack of lymphatics); (ii) *reduced antigen presentation* (e.g. downregulation of major histocompatibility complex (MHC) class I and II expression); (iii) *active immunosuppression* (e.g. local production immunosuppressant α-melanocyte-stimulating hormone (α-MSH), TGF-β and interleukin 10 (IL10); expression of 'no danger' signals CD200; downregulation of danger signals MHC class 1 polypeptide-related sequence A (MICA) and UL16 binding protein 3 (ULBP3)); and (iv) *promotion of peripheral tolerance* [90,91]. Immune privilege can be collapsed experimentally with the pro-inflammatory cytokine interferon γ (IFN-γ) and neuropeptide substance P, but re-established using the various local immunosuppressants listed above [92]. Collapse of

HF immune privilege appears central to the pathogenesis of both alopecia areata and lichen planopilaris [91,93].

Hair follicle microbiome

The HF is a moist, less acidic and ultraviolet (UV) protected skin site conducive for microbial survival. The HF microbiome varies between skin sites, sexes and racial groups. Various commensal bacteria (e.g. *Cutibacterium* spp., *Staphylococcus* spp.), fungi (e.g. *Malassasia* spp.), viruses and mites (e.g. *Demodex*) make up the normal HF microbiome. These resident organisms, further controlled by antimicrobial peptides and immune tolerance mechanisms, probably maintain the HF homeostasis. However, increasingly it is recognised that microbiome dysbiosis is important in the development of multiple diseases, and so better understanding as to how the microbiome influences immune responses, and the link between skin, diet and gut health on immune functioning, will be a clear focus of future research [94–96].

Neuroendocrinology of the hair follicle

The HF is a unique miniorgan responsive to signals from the internal and external environment, with perhaps these mechanisms representing evolutionary conserved processes for responding to seasonal changes in climate. The HF not only contains various hormone receptors but is also a site of hormone synthesis [97,98].

Hypothalamic–pituitary–adrenal axis

Stress response is controlled centrally by the hypothalamic–pituitary–adrenal (HPA) axis, with the hypothalamus secreting corticotrophin-releasing hormone (CRH) that stimulates adrenocorticotrophic hormone (ACTH) from the pituitary, and then cortisol from the adrenal glands. Surprisingly, within defined HF regions CRH is transcribed and the CRH receptor expressed (cf. the hypothalamus). Exposed HFs upregulate pro-opiomelanocortin transcription, increasing ACTH and α-MSH (cf. the pituitary), and express ACTH receptors generating interfollicular cortisol (cf. the adrenals). Further, external cortisol suppresses CRH in HFs via a feedback loop [98,99]. The functional significance of these local stress responses is currently unclear, but all components of the HPA axis negatively impact hair growth, with CRH and ACTH also promoting mast cell degranulation.

Hypothalamic–pituitary–thyroid axis

Thyroid hormones directly impact HF biology by prolonging anagen and upregulating keratin 15. Both thyrotrophic-releasing hormone (TRH) and thyroid-stimulating hormone (TSH) receptors are expressed within the follicular unit, but in defined locations, so the presence of a functioning peripheral HPT axis is still unclear [98].

Prolactin

High circulating prolactin suppresses gonadotrophin-releasing hormone from the hypothalamus, which reduces luteinising hormone/follicle-stimulating hormone secretion, resulting in amenorrhoea (in women) and impotence (in men), along with galactorrhoea. Prolactin and prolactin receptor are expressed in the HF and appear important for HF functioning. Interestingly, prolactin effects are both sex and scalp location dependent, with anagen prolongation seen in human female frontotemporal HF, whereas catagen is triggered in male occipital HF; in mice prolactin inhibits hair growth [100,101].

Hair pigmentation

Hair colour is one of the most striking of mammalian characteristics. In humans, hair colour is determined by melanin incorporated into the hair shaft, with the relative proportions of eumelanin (black-brown) and phaeomelanin (yellow-red), and the number and degree of melanisation of melanosomes, important in determining the final phenotype. Other structural factors, such as hair fibre diameter, medullation and cuticle integrity, may also affect its visual perception [102–104].

Biology of hair pigmentation

Hair melanin is formed by melanocytes situated in the hair bulb epithelium around the upper half of the dermal papilla among cells destined to form the hair cortex (called the hair follicle pigmentary unit (HFPU)) [105]. The pathway of melanogenesis is described in Chapter 142. Ultrastructurally, hair bulb melanocytes appear more melanogenic than epidermal melanocytes and their population density is much greater than in the epidermis. In humans, hair bulb melanocytes donate melanosomes almost exclusively to cells undergoing early differentiation to form the hair cortex (Figure 87.13). Therefore, there is a close spatial and functional relationship between hair bulb melanocytes and the cells that act as pigment receptors (i.e. cortical keratinocytes). No pigment is transferred to presumptive cuticular and IRS cells, although pigment granules have been detected in the cuticle of human nostril hair and in the coats of many animals.

Melanocytes are also present in the basal layer of the infundibulum and ORS where they are unpigmented but identifiable by their expression of the melanocyte marker NK1beteb. A population of melanocyte stem cells (melanoblasts) are located in the bulge region [106]. Like eHFSCs these are undifferentiated, slow cycling and undergo proliferation only during early anagen, remaining quiescent through the rest of the hair cycle. Melanocyte stem cells are non-pigmented, do not express the marker gp100 and have no, or very few, dendrites. TGF-β signalling from surrounding epithelial stem cells appears vital for maintaining melanocyte stem cell quiescence [107]. Depletion of melanocyte stem cells ultimately leads to permanent hair greying [105]. There is also a subpopulation of immature amelanotic melanocytes in the proximal and lateral matrix that may function as an alternative non-bulge melanocyte stem cell pool.

Melanogenic activity in the hair follicle is intricately linked to the hair cycle. In early anagen, melanocyte stem cells are activated, and their progeny differentiate and populate the developing hair bulb. They congregate in the upper part of the anagen hair bulb forming the HFPU. Melanogenesis begins well after epithelial proliferation has started and coincides with the onset of morphological evidence of cortical differentiation. Tyrosinase activity becomes apparent in anagen 3 and pigment transfer to cortical epithelium begins in anagen 4 stage of development [108]. In pigmented hair follicles, intense melanogenesis continues throughout the

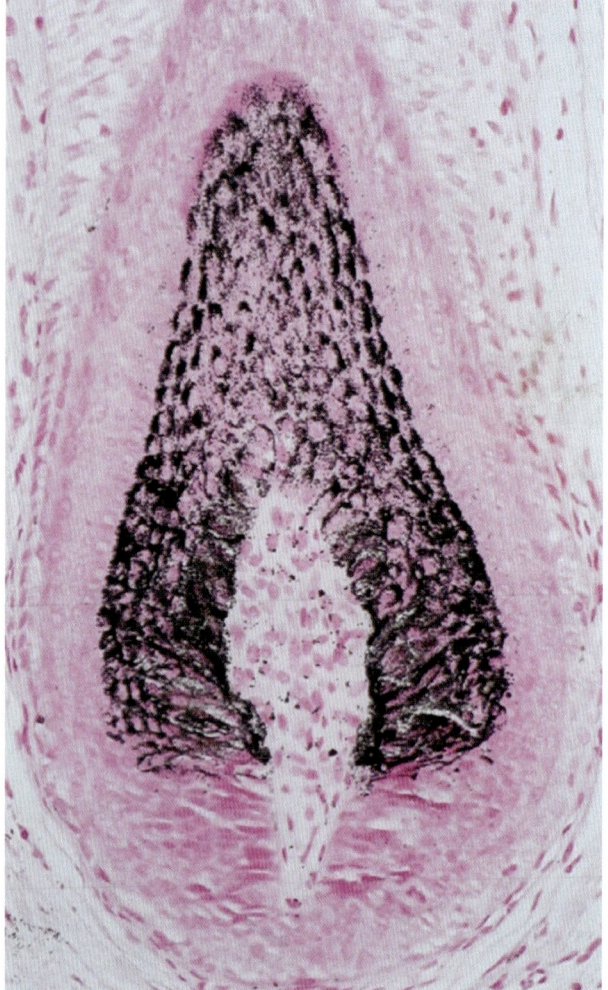

Figure 87.13 Human anagen follicle showing pigment donation to the hair cortex. There is pigment incontinence in the dermal papilla. Masson–Fontana stain.

remainder of anagen (anagen 5 and 6) and then ceases with the onset of catagen. The close anatomical and functional association of hair bulb melanocytes with cells to which pigment is donated, cells destined to form the hair cortex, suggests that interaction between these two cell types has a key role in regulating pigmentary activity. In catagen, the HFPU undergoes apoptosis, with some proximal melanocytes in the matrix also repopulating the secondary hair germ [105,109,110].

There are multiple regulators of HFPU pigmentation. Positive regulators include α-MSH, thyroid hormones, TRH, CRH and β-endorphin; negative regulators include BMAL1 (brain and muscle ARNT-like 1), cortisol and PER1 (period circadian regulator 1) (reviewed in [105]).

Melanogenesis releases reactive oxygen species (ROS), although these are controlled by various antioxidants (including catalase, methionine sulfoxide reductase A and B, Bcl-2, nuclear factor erythroid 2-related factor 2, tyrosinase-related protein 2 and eumelanin itself) that can scavenge ROS. Highest ROS levels are seen in the precortical zone, just distal to the matrix, in an area termed the 'ring of fire'. In this area ROS are thought crucial for hair shaft formation and keratinocyte differentiation [111]. Collapse of the HFPU antioxidant system, excessive hydrogen peroxide levels and accumulation of senescent melanocytes are all thought to underlie hair greying.

Variation in human hair colour

Variations in human hair colour occur most commonly in European populations. Non-European hair is predominantly dark brown to black in colour although pockets of lighter shades do exist in some parts of the world. Hair colour, along with skin and eye colour, is determined by multiple genes, classified as SHEP genes by MIM (227220). These include *OCA2*, *MC1R* and *TYRP*. Polymorphisms in the *OCA2* gene are associated with blond and brown hair in Icelanders [112], and blond hair in a Melanesian population is associated with variation in the *TYRP1* gene [113]. The current catalogue of genes affecting human hair colour is undoubtedly far from complete – over 100 genes involved in regulating murine hair pigmentation have been documented. Recently, a GWAS and meta-analysis identified 123 autosomal and one X-linked loci associated with hair colour in humans, confirming the polygenic nature of these complex phenotypes [114]. It is unclear why hairs darken in many children around puberty, but this change may be due to hair diameter increase with age.

Experimental techniques

Various experimental techniques have been used to understand HF biology. Some of the most used methods are summarised here.

Hair follicle organ culture

A technique first described by Philpott *et al.* allows ongoing human HF growth *ex vivo* [115]. It is predominantly used to test drugs and substances that can accelerate or delay the switch from anagen to catagen. Therefore, this technique is a useful model for both alopecia and hirsutism research. The disadvantage is that the whole hair cycle cannot be explored with this method, and so study of anagen induction is not possible. Established culture protocols and catalogues of catagen inhibitory and promoting agents are available as benchmarks [116].

Mouse models

Mouse models are the most widely used techniques for studying basic HF biology. A key advantage is that the murine hair growth is synchronised allowing study of the complete hair cycle. Further, various genetic mutants, and potential for genetic manipulation, allow detailed exploration of specific mechanisms through phenotype observation or gene knock-down [117]. Murine hair cycle stages are well defined [118]. However, findings in mice do not always directly correlate with human HF biology, with different stem cell markers, variable responses to hormone stimulation, shorter synchronised hair cycle stages and increased skin permeability all differing between human and mouse skin.

Recently a humanised mouse model has been developed using human skin xenografted onto SCID mice [119]. This technique is the only preclinical model allowing study of the whole human HF cycle, but the technique is expensive and specialised, so is often used in conjunction with other complementary techniques [120].

How to approach assessment and management of patients with hair loss

Introduction

It is well recognised that alopecia has a significant impact on patients' self-esteem and emotional and psychological well-being. Studies examining health-related quality of life scores demonstrate that alopecia patients have scores comparable with those of patients with psoriasis or atopic dermatitis [1,2]. The degree of patient distress is often not proportional to objective clinical assessment of alopecia severity [3] and many patients with mild, minimal or clinically imperceptible hair loss harbour fears that they will lose all their hair. Further, many alopecia patients feel that their problems have been trivialised, dismissed or ignored by medical professionals [2] and some become angry and frustrated. Therefore, it is important to treat patients' concerns seriously, and the use of quality of life measures in the out-patient clinic can provide an invaluable insight into the psychological impact of alopecia on the individual. Alopecia is often chronic, thus establishing a good rapport with patients is crucial. Clear explanation of the diagnosis and prognosis is important, as is the use of high-quality up-to-date patient information, in leaflet form or online. Patient support groups and alopecia charities can often provide support for patients and their families and it is helpful to signpost these at an early stage. Advice on cosmetic camouflage is also an important part of patient management. As the diagnosis of alopecia can be challenging, expert second opinion may be sought. In many countries, there are regional, national and international networks of clinicians with a special interest in hair disorders who can review and advise on complex cases.

History

A detailed history is as important to making the correct diagnosis as clinical examination. There are several key questions that help with establishing the diagnosis. Disease onset and duration are important; conditions such as alopecia areata and acute telogen effluvium (TE) are characterised by rapid onset and often extensive loss, and patients tend to present quickly. Female pattern hair loss (FPHL) and most scarring alopecias have an ill-defined onset and patients become gradually aware of hair loss over months and years. Whether hair loss is patchy or diffuse should be established: acute TE and FPHL cause diffuse hair thinning and scarring alopecias and alopecia areata tend to present with patchy hair loss. The area of scalp affected may provide a clue to diagnosis. Thinning on the top of the scalp is typically due to (male or female) patterned hair loss. Hairline involvement is characteristic of frontal fibrosing alopecia (FFA) and ophiasis-pattern alopecia areata. Involvement of the vertex, with extension onto the frontal scalp, is typical of folliculitis decalvans (FD) and pseudopelade of Brocq (PB). Dissecting cellulitis (DC) and acne keloidalis nuchae (AKN) typically affect the occipital scalp and nape of the neck.

The quantity of hair shedding is also useful to establish. This may be difficult for patients to estimate and the use of a shedding score can be helpful [4]. Significant hair shedding characterises severe alopecia areata and acute and chronic TE. The presence of symptoms should also be established. Many patients with alopecia have no or minimal symptoms. Patterned hair loss and alopecia areata are typically asymptomatic. Itch is a feature of lichen planopilaris (LPP) and chronic discoid lupus erythematosus (CDLE) but less so FFA. Pain, crusting and pustules are features of FD and DC. Scalp burning or dysaesthesia (trichodynia) can occur as a primary phenomenon or in association with alopecia (of any type). Hair breakage occurs with traction alopecia and some hair shaft disorders. Textural hair changes may occur with patterned hair loss or acquired hair shaft disorders (e.g. trichorrhexis nodosa), it may be due to medication (e.g. systemic retinoids) and occasionally occurs on hair regrowth following severe loss (e.g. anagen effluvium due to chemotherapy). Hair loss away from the scalp should also be assessed. Patients will usually report loss of facial hair such as eyebrows, lashes and the male beard, but gradual loss of hair from limbs is rarely recognised, especially by females.

Previous medical and dermatological history may provide useful information to support a diagnosis. Atopy is commonly found in association with alopecia areata. Severe acne (congolobata) or hidradenitis suppurativa may be present with DC. A history of mucocutaneous lichen planus may be found with LPP but is much less common with FFA. Sudden severe hair shedding (suggesting TE) should prompt enquiry regarding significant illness, operations, weight loss, new medications or severe stress in the previous 2–3 months. Relevant family history should be established, particularly if a genodermatosis (e.g. monilethrix) is suspected. With alopecia areata, an affected first-degree relative increases the risk of the disease 10-fold. Autoimmune disease (particularly thyroid) is also common with alopecia areata.

Examination

Establishing a standard method of scalp examination will help to avoid missing relevant pathology. It is important to examine the entire scalp and not just the area(s) indicated by the patient. Good lighting, an illuminated magnifier and dermatoscope are essential tools. An initial global visual assessment is useful – is there obvious hair thinning? Is it localised? Assessment of hair density can be achieved by performing a series of partings around the scalp and observing how easily the underlying scalp can be seen. This will also allow identification of any patches of loss. The entire hairline should also be examined. Close inspection of the scalp is required to identify diagnostic patterns of inflammation. The typical trichoscopic features of alopecias are now well described [5] and trichoscopy is a mandatory part of a complete examination (Figure 87.14). However, it is important to remember that not all scalp inflammation will be relevant to hair loss. Conditions such as seborrhoeic dermatitis and scalp psoriasis are common but are rarely the cause of significant alopecia. However, scalp inflammation may contribute to symptoms and may reduce efficacy of topical treatments such as minoxidil.

Various methods of pulling hair (gently) can aid diagnosis. Easy removal of short, broken (exclamation mark) hairs is characteristic of alopecia areata, whereas with trichotillomania, pulling similarly short, fractured hairs will not remove them. Easy removal of

any anagen hairs, such as around the margins of an active patch of scarring alopecia, is always abnormal. Active hair shedding can be assessed by a hair pull. A group of around 50 hairs are gripped near the scalp and constant gentle traction applied, pulling away from the scalp. This needs to be done at multiple sites over the scalp. Extraction of several telogen hairs at each pull is to be expected; however, in conditions such as TE, large numbers of telogen hairs can easily be removed. It should be noted that the pull test may be affected by how recently the hair has been washed or brushed, and a normal pull test does not exclude a diagnosis of TE.

The face (eyebrows, lashes, male beard) and body should also be examined for evidence of alopecia. This is seen commonly with alopecia areata and FFA but much less commonly with LPP. Loss of vellus facial hairs occurs frequently with FFA but is rarely noted by patients. Excessive body hair in females can be a sign of androgen excess and this may be relevant to patterned hair loss in women. Associated skin disease may be present and the skin, mouth and nails should be examined as appropriate.

An algorithmic approach to aid diagnosis is presented (Figure 87.15).

Investigations

It is helpful to confirm that there are no significant underlying medical conditions that might contribute to alopecia such as anaemia or thyroid dysfunction; routine bloods including full blood count (FBC), ferritin and thyroid function tests should be considered. If CDLE is suspected, antnuclear antibodies (ANA) should also be checked. Most females with pattern hair loss do not have evidence of androgen excess; however, an androgen screen should be considered in certain circumstances such as females in their teens and early 20s, if there are associated menstrual irregularities, the presence of other androgen-related disorders (acne, hirsutism, virilism) or severe hair loss and Hamilton–Norwood pattern hair loss. When pustules are present, swabs should be taken for bacterial culture and sensitivity. Scale and hairs should be sent for microscopy and mycological culture where appropriate. Tinea capitis is particularly common in children, and in adults it can masquerade as inflammatory scarring alopecias such as DC.

Trichograms (forcible extraction of 50–60 hairs) are now rarely performed. Examining the numbers of anagen, catagen and telogen hairs from a small area of scalp rarely yields useful diagnostic information. The phototrichogram [6] is a non-invasive method of accurately assessing hair growth but is generally a research tool. One or two 1 cm^2 representative areas of scalp are shaved or clipped as short as possible and an image taken; 2 or 3 days later, a further image is taken. Anagen hairs will be seen to grow, whereas telogen hairs remain the same length. This allows assessment of the anagen : telogen ratios. With appropriate software, hair density and hair shaft diameters can easily be calculated.

Light microscopy of hair is required for the investigation of possible hair shaft disorders, although many hair shaft disorders can be observed by trichoscopy [7]. In these conditions not all hairs will be affected and therefore a sufficiently representative sample (at least 50 hairs) is required. Hairs should be cut close to the scalp,

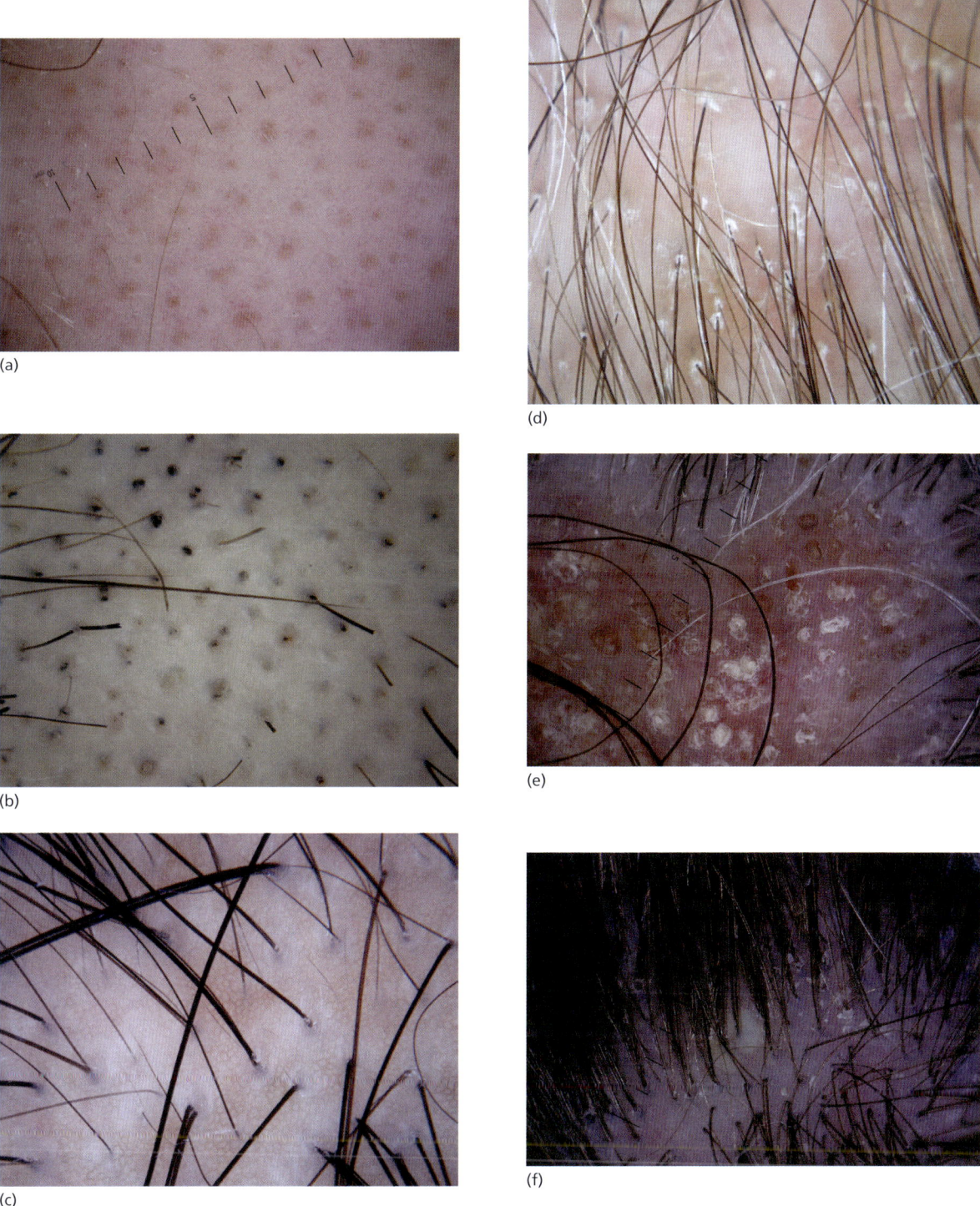

Figure 87.14 Trichoscopic images. (a) Yellow dots in alopecia areata. (b) Black dots and broken hairs in alopecia areata. (c) Variation in hair fibre diameter in female pattern hair loss. (d) Follicular hyperkeratosis in lichen planopilaris. (e) Follicular plugging in discoid lupus erythematosus. (f) Tufting and pustule in folliculitis decalvans.

not plucked, unless loose anagen syndrome is suspected in which case a small number of hairs should be plucked for examination of the roots. Trichoscopy can be used to identify abnormal hairs to improve sampling. For light microscopy, hairs should be spread out on a microscope slide (bone pathology slides are larger than standard slides and are ideal for this purpose) and a coverslip placed on top. Mounting medium is usually not required. In some hair disorders, the abnormalities are only seen using polarising filters (e.g. tiger tail pattern in trichothiodystrophy). Certain hair shaft disorders (e.g. pili trianguli et canaliculi) are best seen using

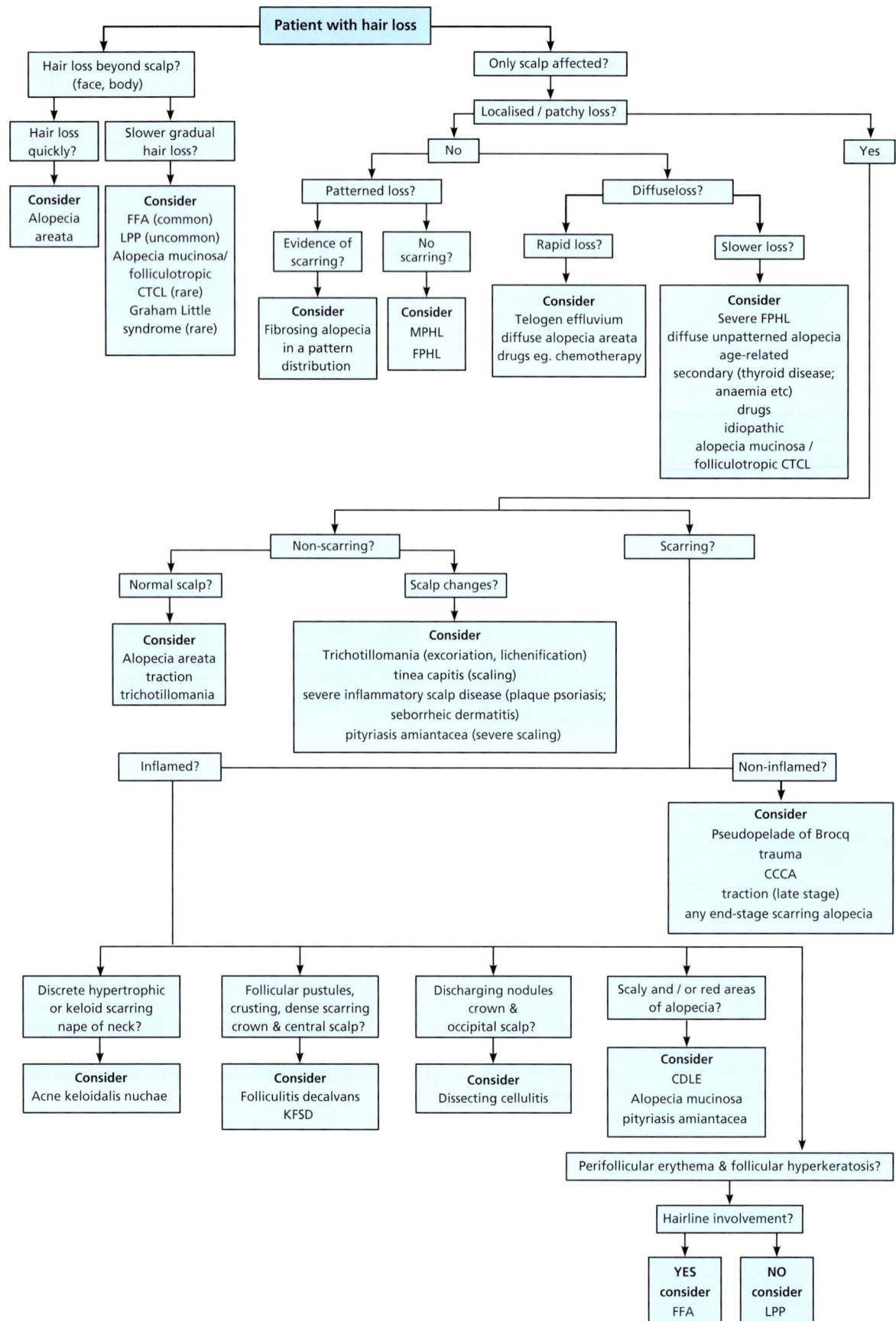

Figure 87.15 Diagnostic guide to assist hair loss evaluation. CCCA, central centrifugal cicatricial alopecia; CDLE, chronic discoid lupus erythematosus; CTCL, cutaneous T-cell lymphoma; FFA, frontal fibrosing alopecia; FPHL, female pattern hair loss; KFSD, keratosis follicularis spinulosa decalvans; LPP, lichen planopilaris; MPHL, male pattern hair loss; TTM, trichotillomania.

scanning electron microscopy although this is not available in most pathology departments. While light microscopy can be performed in the out-patient clinic, expert opinion is often required, and advice can be sought through regional or national networks of specialist hair societies. If sending hair samples, at least 50 hairs should be carefully folded within a piece of white A4 paper.

Histology can be useful in the evaluation of hair disease [8]. It will distinguish between non-scarring and scarring alopecia and differentiate between primary lymphocytic and neutrophilic cicatricial alopecias. It can also be useful in identifying the presence of follicular miniaturisation in patients with increased hair shedding but without clinical reduction in hair density, such as when attempting to distinguish between early FPHL and TE. Diffuse hair loss due to unsuspected alopecia areata or lupus erythematosus may also be identified on scalp biopsy, as will rare causes of alopecia such as sarcoidosis, secondary syphilis, cutaneous lymphoma and scalp metastases.

The choice of biopsy site and biopsy technique are crucial to obtaining a useful pathology report. For scarring alopecias, the selection of the biopsy site depends on what information is needed. A biopsy from the centre of a patch of hair loss will confirm the presence of scarring but will not generally provide useful information on causality. This is best obtained by sampling the active edge of a patch of loss. Active areas of alopecia may show signs of follicular inflammation and/or hyperkeratosis, features which can best be appreciated by trichoscopy. Similarly, a biopsy from the edge of a patch of alopecia areata where broken (exclamation mark) hairs are present is more likely to show the classic peribulbar inflammatory infiltrate, whereas a sample from the centre of a patch may not show diagnostic features. In patterned hair loss, it can be useful to sample the affected area and a control area (vertex and occiput) for comparison purposes.

Recommended practice is to take two 4 mm punch biopsies [8]. Biopsies should be orientated in the direction of hair growth in order to include as many intact follicles as possible and should extend into the subcutaneous fat (Figure 87.16). In scarring alopecia, one biopsy is usually sectioned longitudinally (vertically) and the second transversely (horizontally) (Figure 87.17). In non-scarring conditions, it may be more useful for both biopsies to be sectioned horizontally (Figure 87.18). A transversely sectioned 4 mm scalp biopsy may allow up to 30–40 hair follicles to be examined. Sections can be cut at different levels from the bulb to the isthmus and infundibulum. The opinion of a dermatopathologist experienced in hair pathology should be sought if there is uncertainty.

Alopecia monitoring and assessment

Accurate methods of assessing and monitoring alopecia are essential to evaluating disease progression and treatment efficacy. However, most currently used methods are at best suboptimal. Photographs are the most used means of monitoring alopecia. However, there are pitfalls which can lead to misinterpretation. Ideally, the help of an experienced photographer should be enlisted in order that lighting, background and head position are standardised. The use of stereotactic devices can assist with the latter. For assessment of hair density (e.g. central frontal scalp and vertex in patterned hair loss), the hair should be parted centrally and smoothed (but not held) down and the head tipped forward. To demonstrate patches

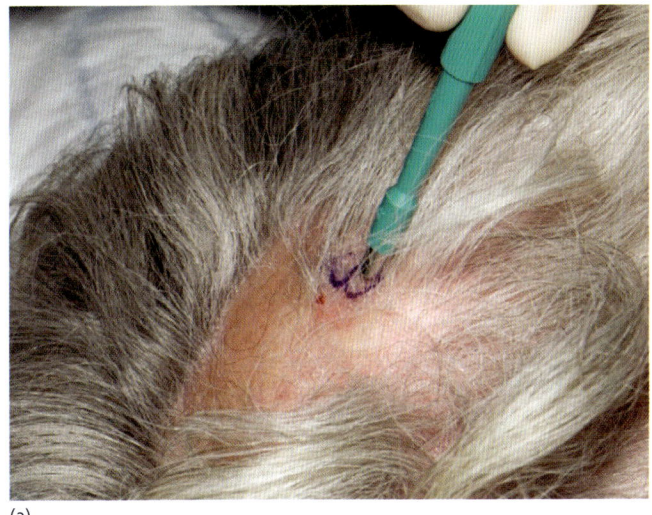

(a)

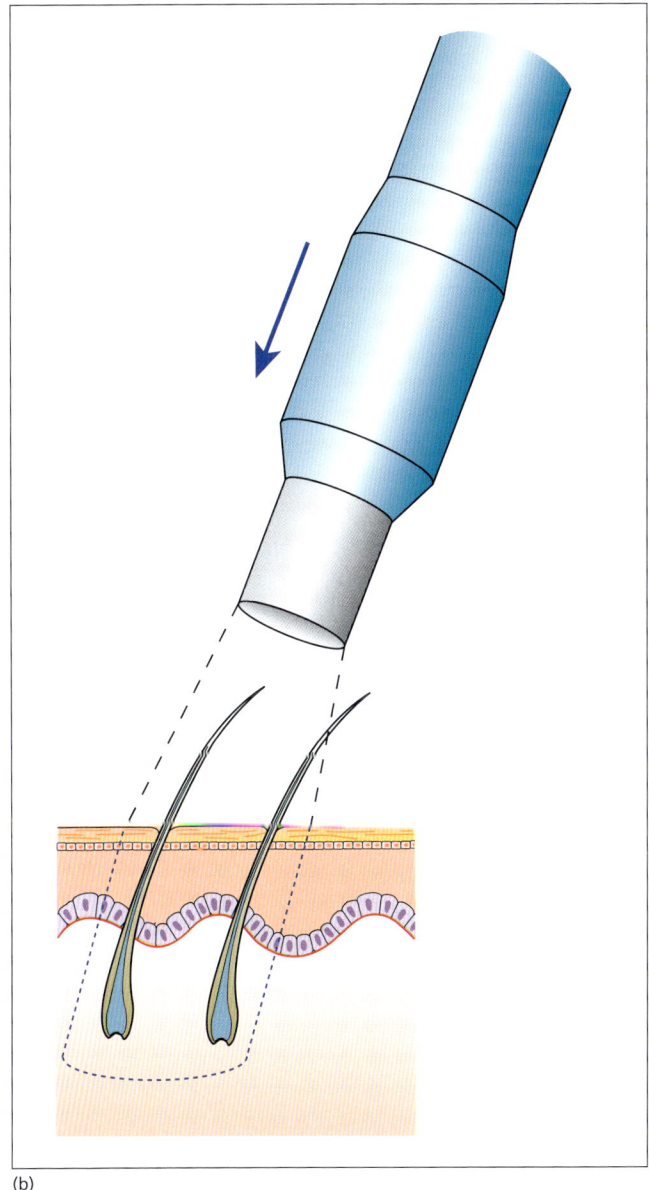

(b)

Figure 87.16 (a, b) Orientation of the punch biopsy in the direction of hair growth.

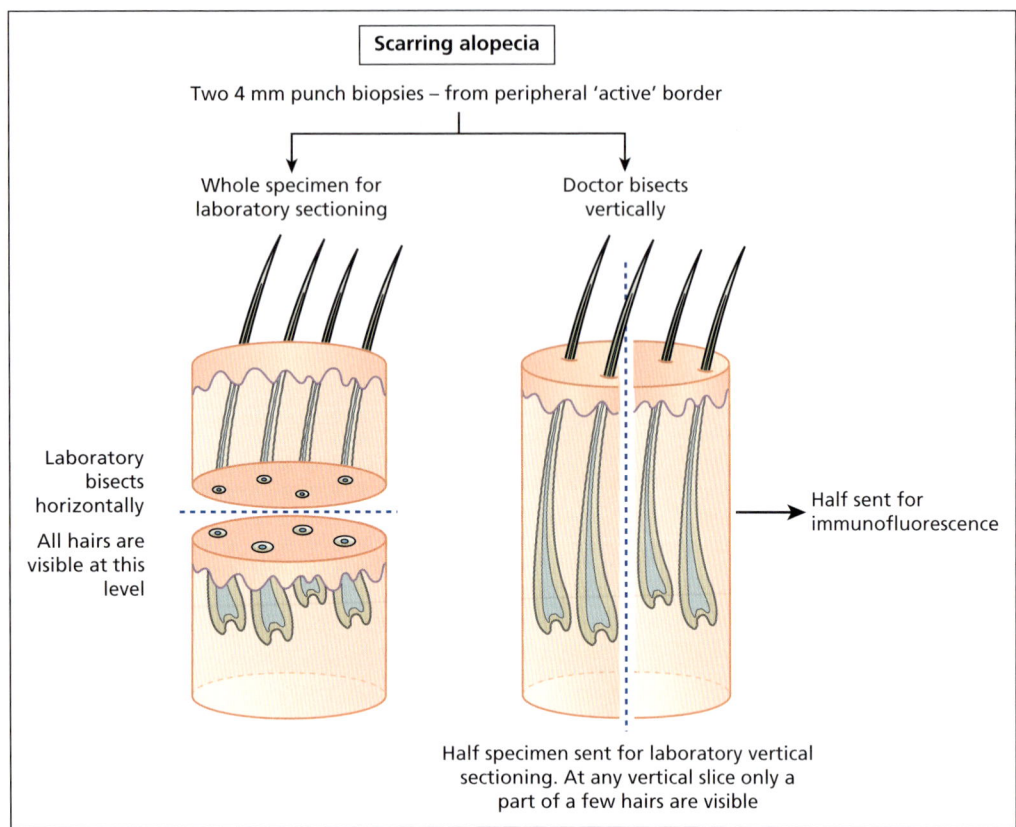

Scarring alopecia

Two 4 mm punch biopsies – from peripheral 'active' border

Whole specimen for laboratory sectioning

Doctor bisects vertically

Laboratory bisects horizontally

All hairs are visible at this level

Half sent for immunofluorescence

Half specimen sent for laboratory vertical sectioning. At any vertical slice only a part of a few hairs are visible

Figure 87.17 Biopsy – scarring alopecia protocol.

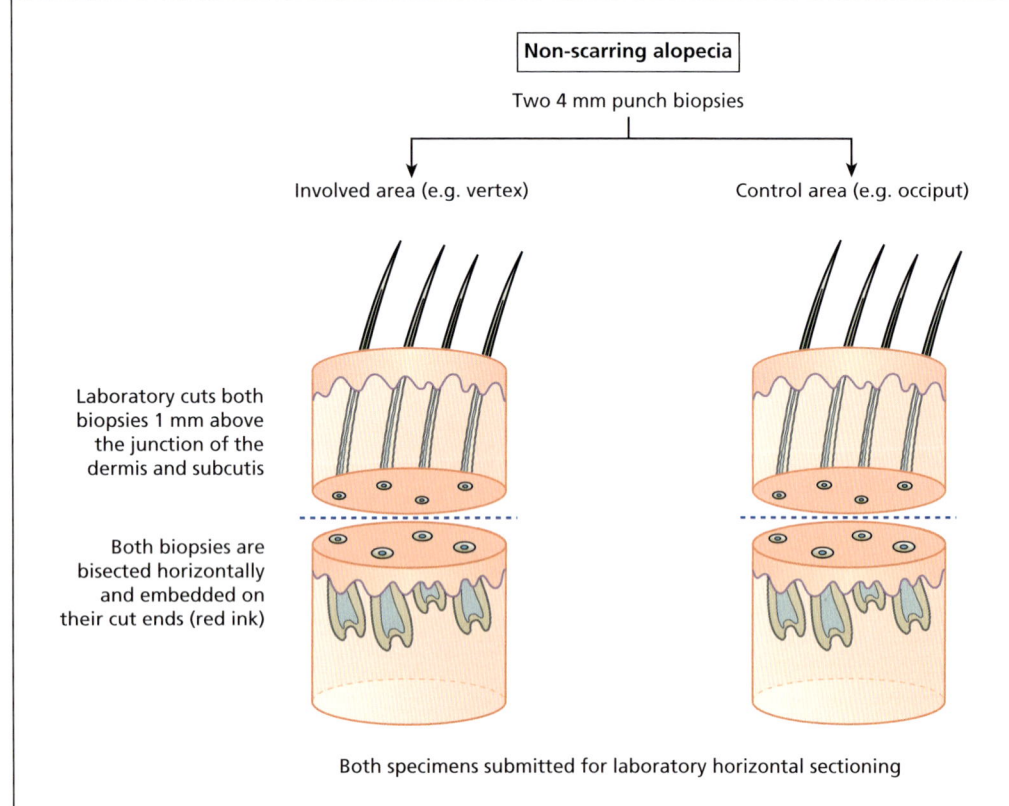

Non-scarring alopecia

Two 4 mm punch biopsies

Involved area (e.g. vertex)

Control area (e.g. occiput)

Laboratory cuts both biopsies 1 mm above the junction of the dermis and subcutis

Both biopsies are bisected horizontally and embedded on their cut ends (red ink)

Both specimens submitted for laboratory horizontal sectioning

Figure 87.18 Biopsy – non-scarring alopecia protocol.

of alopecia, surrounding hair should be brushed away from patches such that the entire patch can be seen. The use of photographic scales and inclusion of anatomical landmarks in images is also helpful. When there are multiple patches of alopecia throughout the scalp, accurate photographic assessment is challenging. One method that can be employed is taking serial images of a sequence of partings made several centimetres apart across the affected area of scalp, each time sweeping hair away to entirely expose patches. Imaging of the hairline is generally easier as hair can more easily be swept up to expose the hairline. Sometimes hair bands are used to evenly pull hair back, but care should be taken to avoid producing kinks of hair that protrude forward over the true hairline.

Taking measurements of alopecia can be a useful strategy in disease monitoring. Patches of alopecia can be measured in a variety of ways; however, these can be difficult to accurately reproduce. Drawing outlines of patches on clear plastic templates can be useful. In FFA, there are a variety of measurement techniques employed (e.g. measuring from fixed anatomical points to the new hairline; measuring from the original to new hairline) but again, there are issues of accuracy and reproducibility. There are also several scoring systems that have been devised to categorise alopecia severity. These include [4,9–21]:

- Severity of alopecia tool (SALT) and AA investigator global assessment for alopecia areata.
- Ludwig, Sinclair and female pattern hair loss severity index (FPHL-SI) scores for FPHL.
- Hamilton and Norwood scores for male pattern hair loss.
- Frontal fibrosing alopecia severity index (FFASI) and frontal fibrosing alopecia severity score (FFASS) for FFA.
- Lichen planopilaris activity index (LPPAI) for LPP.
- Central scalp alopecia photographic scale for central centrifugal cicatricial alopecia (CCCA).
- Marginal traction alopecia severity (M-TAS) score) for traction alopecia.
- Cutaneous lupus erythematosus disease area and severity index (CLASI) for chronic discoid lupus erythematosus.
- Sinclair hair shedding scale for TE/pattern hair loss.

Cosmesis

As treatment of alopecia is often difficult, camouflage is an important part of management. There is an extensive range of camouflage options for patients with alopecia and it is usually helpful to discuss these at an early stage – see the cosmetics section later in this chapter.

Resources

Further information

Institute of Medical Illustrators, hair loss photography standards: https://www.imi .org.uk/resources/professional-resources/national-guidelines/.

Patient resources

Alopecia UK: www.alopecia.org.uk.
British Association of Dermatologists: www.bad.org.uk/for-the-public/patient-information-leaflets.
National Alopecia Areata Foundation: www.naaf.org.
Scarring Alopecia Foundation: https://scarringalopecia.org/.
(All last accessed May 2023.)

HAIR LOSS PRESENTATIONS

ALOPECIA AREATA

Alopecia areata

Introduction and general description

Alopecia areata is a common, chronic, inflammatory disease that causes non-scarring hair loss. The severity ranges from small patches of hair loss, which usually recover spontaneously, to complete alopecia where the prognosis for hair regrowth is poor. The nails may also be affected. Current evidence indicates that alopecia areata is caused by a T-cell-mediated autoimmune mechanism occurring in genetically predisposed individuals. Environmental factors may be responsible for triggering the disease.

The first description of alopecia areata is generally attributed to the Roman physician Celsus (about 25 BC to AD 50) although treatments for a type of hair loss resembling alopecia areata were advocated in a 3500-year-old Egyptian papyrus [1]. Under the heading 'areae' Celsus described two types of hair loss; the first, known as 'alopecia', ' … spreads no certain form. It is found in the hair of the head, and in the beard.' The second type, called 'ophiasis', ' … begins at the hinder part of the head … it creeps with two heads to the ears … ' [2]. The term alopecia areata was first used by Sauvages in 1763 (cited by Hebra and Kaposi [3]). In the English literature Robert Willan described alopecia areata under the title 'porrigo decalvans', illustrated in Thomas Bateman's 1819 atlas (Figure 87.19). The first detailed account in more recent times was by Hebra and Kaposi [3] – many aspects of their description of the clinical features, the natural history and the response to treatment could appear in a modern textbook. Early ideas about the aetiology were numerous and included infectious, metabolic, vascular, neuropathic and trophoneurotic theories. The current view, that alopecia areata is an autoimmune disease, was first suggested by Rothman in a discussion of a paper presented by Van Scott [4], although an association with thyroid disease and vitiligo had been recognised from the early years of the 20th century [5].

Epidemiology
Incidence and prevalence
In a Mayo Clinic population study of alopecia areata from Olmsted County, Minnesota, USA between 1975 and 1989, the overall

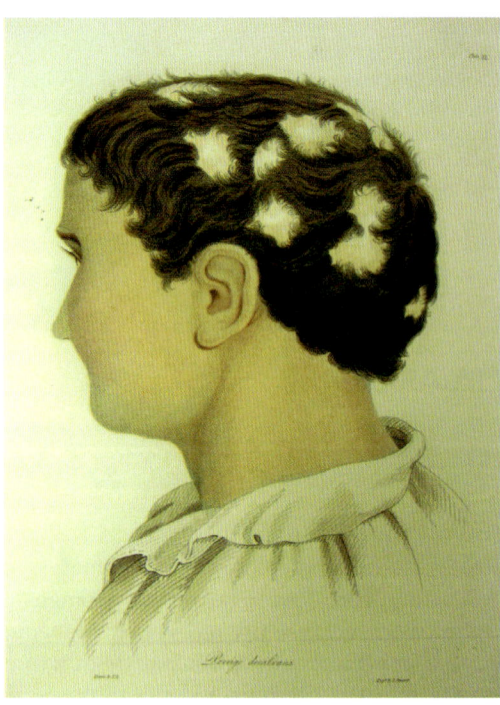

Figure 87.19 'Porrigo decalvans' (alopecia areata). Plate XL from Thomas Bateman's atlas *Practical Synopsis of Cutaneous Diseases*, 1819.

incidence rate was 0.20 per 1000 person-years with a projected lifetime risk of 1.7% [6]. A slightly higher incidence of 0.21 per 1000 person-years and lifetime risk of 2.1% was reported in an extension of the original study between 1990 and 2009 [7]. In a much larger population study in UK primary care, comprising over 4 million people, the incidence of alopecia areata was 0.26 per 1000 person-years between 2009 and 2018 [8].

Age
The onset of alopecia areata may occur at any age. However, in most affected individuals the first episode occurs before the age of 40 years, with the peak age of onset between 25 and 29 [8].

Sex
In the US population study, the frequency of alopecia areata was similar in both sexes [7]. In the UK study, the incidence was slightly, though significantly, greater in females [8].

Ethnicity
As far as is known, alopecia areata occurs in all ethnic groups but there may be interethnic variations in its frequency. In a study from the USA, self-reported alopecia areata was more common in female nurses of black and Hispanic ethnicity than in white nurses [9]. An increased frequency of alopecia areata in people of non-white ethnicity was also found in the UK study. The effect was particularly pronounced in those of Asian ethnicity where the incidence was threefold greater than in white people [8].

Associated diseases
Autoimmune disease. Numerous studies have shown an increased risk of other autoimmune diseases in patients with alopecia areata [10]. There is variation between studies in the level of risk for individual diseases, but the overall theme is constant. In the largest study of its type, incorporating 4334 patients with alopecia areata and over 700 000 controls, Chu and colleagues reported significant associations with vitiligo, thyroid disease, lupus erythematosus, psoriasis and rheumatoid arthritis [11]. The frequency of type 1 diabetes is not increased in patients with alopecia areata, but diabetes is more common than expected in their relatives, suggesting a protective effect of the diabetes genotype [12,13]. An association with coeliac disease has been suggested from some small case series [14] but does not feature in larger population studies [11]. Although improvement in alopecia in coeliacs taking a gluten-free diet has been reported, the numbers are too small to confidently exclude spontaneous remission [14].

Atopic disease. Atopic disease, especially atopic dermatitis, is more common than expected in alopecia areata, and is associated with early onset and more severe forms of hair loss [10,11,15,16]. Atopic dermatitis in a Korean population was significantly more common in patients with early-onset alopecia areata, whereas thyroid disease was the most common in late-onset disease [17].

Down syndrome. In two studies on institutionalised people with Down syndrome alopecia areata was diagnosed in 60 out of 1000 (6%) cases in the first study [18] and in 19 out of 214 (8.9%) in the second study [19]. These frequencies are well in excess of that expected in the population at large. Other autoimmune diseases are also common in Down syndrome.

Autoimmune polyendocrinopathy syndrome type 1 (APS-1). APS-1 is a genetic disease due to mutations in the autoimmune regulator gene (AIRE) at chromosome 21q22. AIRE protein is expressed in the thymus and is involved in the deletion of self-recognising T cells. The cardinal features of APS-1 are Addison disease, hypoparathyroidism and chronic mucocutaneous candidiasis, but other autoimmune diseases are also common and alopecia areata occurs in about 50% of cases [20].

Quality of life and mental health disorders. Impairment in quality of life in people suffering from alopecia areata has been reported by many studies [21,22]. Adverse effects on mental health, vitality, social functioning and emotions are common themes [23]. Time off work and unemployment are also more common than in the population at large [24]. Women appear more likely to suffer reduced quality of life than men but the evidence for a contribution of other factors, such as disease duration and severity of hair loss, is conflicting. It is important to recognise the serious impact that alopecia areata can have on quality of life. On the other hand, not all patients with alopecia areata experience a reduction in quality of life due to their disease – it was found to be 57% in one study [25].

Bullying is a common problem in children with alopecia areata. In one study, 23% of children across all age groups had experienced bullying, and additional psychological impact, including impairment of social and home life, was also common [26].

The prevalence of psychiatric disorders, particularly depression and anxiety, is greater in patients with alopecia areata than in the general population [27–29]. The association appears to be bidirectional. Thus, those with alopecia areata are at increased risk of subsequently developing depression and a history of depression is itself a risk factor for developing alopecia areata [24,30]. An association between depression and circulating levels of the pro-inflammatory cytokines IL-17E and IL-22 has been reported in patients with alopecia areata [31].

Pathophysiology
Pathology

Anagen follicles at the margins of expanding patches of alopecia areata characteristically show a perifollicular and intrafollicular inflammatory cell infiltrate, concentrated in and around the hair bulb (Figure 87.20). The inflammatory infiltrate is composed mainly of activated T lymphocytes, with a preponderance of CD4 cells, and an admixture of macrophages, Langerhans cells and cells expressing natural killer (NK) cell markers [32–34]. In contrast to the inflammatory scarring alopecias, little or none of the inflammatory infiltrate is seen around the isthmus of the HF, the site of HF stem cells. This may explain why follicles are not destroyed in alopecia areata. Lymphocytic infiltration of the dermal papilla and bulbar epithelium may be accompanied by increased expression of MHC class I and II antigens and of intercellular adhesion molecule 1 (ICAM-1) [35–37]. Normal numbers of follicles are found in established bald patches and in alopecia universalis. Both anagen and telogen follicles are found in these sites, with a higher proportion in telogen than in a normal scalp. Follicles are smaller than normal and anagen follicles do not develop beyond the anagen 3/4 stage [38]. The inflammatory infiltrate tends to be less pronounced than in early lesions and is associated mainly with anagen follicles.

Alopecia areata causes a disturbance in the normal dynamics of the hair cycle. Anagen follicles are precipitated into telogen. This may occur as a centrifugal wave, reminiscent of a moult wave [39]. Follicles can re-enter anagen but, while the disease is active, are unable to progress beyond the anagen 3/4 stage [38]. It has been suggested that follicles then return prematurely to telogen and that truncated cycles continue until disease activity wanes (Figure 87.21) [40].

Cells of several different types and differentiation pathways are found in the hair bulb, but which of these is the primary focus of the pathology is unknown. Epithelial cells in the hair bulb matrix undergoing early cortical differentiation may show vacuolar degeneration [41,42] and are also the predominant cell type showing

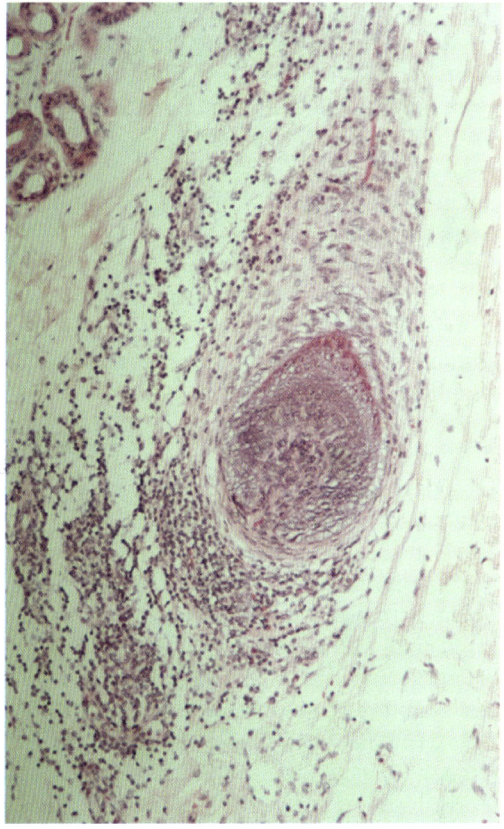

Figure 87.20 Lymphocytic inflammatory infiltrate surrounding an anagen hair bulb in alopecia areata.

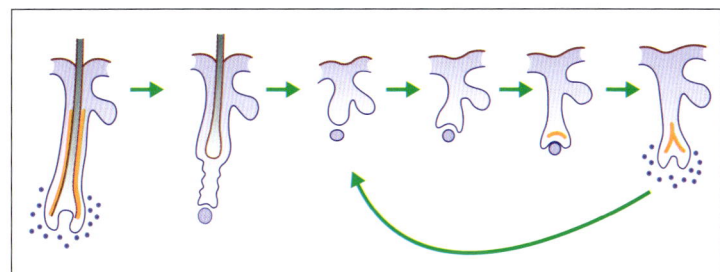

Figure 87.21 Proposed pathodynamic changes in alopecia areata. An inflammatory attack on anagen follicles precipitates follicles into telogen. Follicles re-enter anagen but development is halted in anagen stage 3–4 and follicles return to telogen prematurely.

aberrant MHC expression. The pigmentary features of alopecia areata have also raised the possibility that alopecia areata is primarily a disease of hair bulb melanocytes. The interruption of anagen in established alopecia areata occurs at the 3/4 stage of development when hair cortex differentiation and melanisation first become apparent in the normal hair cycle [43].

Pathobiology

Alopecia areata as an autoimmune disease. Since it was first proposed by Stephen Rothman in 1958 following a paper presented by Eugene Van Scott [4] the idea that alopecia areata is an autoimmune disease has been widely accepted [44,45]. The evidence can be summarised as follows:

- There is an increased frequency of other autoimmune diseases in patients with alopecia areata.
- There is an increased frequency of organ-specific autoantibodies in patients with alopecia areata. Serum antibodies to HF tissue also occur with increased frequency in alopecia areata although these antibodies appear not to bind to HFs *in vivo* and their pathogenetic significance is not known.
- The pathology is characterised by the infiltration of hair bulbs by activated T lymphocytes.
- In animal models of alopecia areata, depletion of CD4+ and CD8+ T cells results in hair regrowth [46].
- Hair regrows in human alopecic skin when transplanted onto immunodeficient mice [47].
- T cells isolated from the scalps of patients with alopecia areata and cultured with HF homogenates induced both hair loss and the pathological findings of alopecia areata when injected into autologous scalp grafted onto immunodeficient mice, indicating the HF lesion is mediated by T cells [48]. Passive transfer of patient serum in the same model fails to induce hair loss [49].
- Alopecia areata shares genetic associations with several autoimmune diseases, particularly with genes of the MHC.

The identity of the putative autoantigen(s) is not known. The pathology suggests the target for an immune-mediated assault is a product of differentiation in the anagen hair bulb. The pigmentary features of alopecia areata have implicated epitopes associated with melanogenic pathways on hair bulb melanocytes and cortex keratinocytes. One study has identified epitopes derived from trichohyalin and tyrosinase-related protein 2 as possible candidates [50].

Immune privilege. Like some other tissues, such as the anterior chamber of the eye, the brain and the testis, the HF is thought to be an immunologically privileged site that is relatively shielded from immune surveillance [51]. HF immune privilege is maintained by several mechanisms including extremely low or absent expression of class I and II MHC molecules by cells in the lower part of the follicle, the local secretion of immune-inhibitory substances and the action of other cells such as Treg lymphocytes [52]. The breakdown of HF immune privilege is believed to be a key event in the pathogenesis of alopecia areata, leading to invasion of the HF by NK cells and CD8+ cells. These cells release pro-inflammatory cytokines, including IFN-γ, that results in a release of IL-15 and IL-15Rα by follicular keratinocytes and promotes and sustains CD8+ T-cell autoreactivity.

Is alopecia areata a reaction pattern? Although it is conventionally regarded as a CD8+-driven disease, there is growing evidence that other IFN-γ-releasing cells such as NK cells and 'unconventional' T cells may trigger the collapse of follicular immune privilege in an autoantigen-independent manner [53]. Using a humanised mouse model Gilhar and colleagues showed that peripheral blood mononuclear cells derived from healthy donors, and enriched for NKG2D+/CD56+ cells, induced hair loss with typical alopecia areata pathology when injected into normal human skin transplanted onto immunocompromised mice [54]. This and other observations led to the proposal that alopecia areata is best viewed as a stereotypical reaction by anagen HFs to IFN-γ-mediated immunological damage leading to the collapse of follicular immune privilege [53].

Th2 activity in alopecia areata. Although most research has focused on Th1 pathways in the pathogenesis in alopecia areata there is increasing evidence for Th2 activation as well [55,56]. This is in keeping with the well-recognised association of alopecia areata with atopy and the observation that allergy may play a part in triggering the disease in some patients [57].

Genetics

The importance of genetic factors in alopecia areata is apparent from the high frequency of a positive family history [58]. In most reports this ranges from 10% to 20% of cases, but mild cases can be overlooked or concealed, and the true figure may be greater. A family history of alopecia areata is more common in those with disease onset before the age of 30 years [59]. The lifetime risk of alopecia areata in the children of a proband is around 6% [60,61]. There are several reports of alopecia areata in twins [62–64]. Two studies found a concordance rate of 55% and 42% for alopecia among monozygotic twins with 0% and 10% concordance, respectively, among the dizygotic pairs [65,66].

Case–control studies have identified associations between alopecia areata and a variety of genes involved in regulating immune and inflammatory responses [67]. The strongest associations to date have been with genes of the MHC, particularly the class II alleles HLA-DQB1*0301 and HLA-DRB1*1104 [68,69]. GWAS have confirmed the strong association with human leukocyte antigen DR (HLA-DR) and identified several other genomic regions associated with alopecia areata [**70**]. These include genes controlling activation and proliferation of T-regulatory lymphocytes and some genes expressed in the HF. There is a strong association with genes within the *ULBP* cluster coding for activating ligands of the NKG2D receptor, supporting a role for NK and certain CD8+ T cells in the pathogenesis of the disease. Some of the risk loci identified for alopecia areata are shared by other immune-mediated diseases including Graves disease, inflammatory bowel disease, coeliac disease, vitiligo, rheumatoid arthritis, systemic lupus erythematosus and psoriasis.

Environmental factors

The idea that alopecia areata is triggered by infection, either directly or as a consequence of a remote 'focus of infection', has a long history. It was predominant until well into the 20th century and sporadic reports connecting alopecia areata with infective agents continue to appear.

The 'external' factor most frequently implicated in triggering alopecia areata is emotional stress or a traumatic life event. In older, uncontrolled case series, the published frequencies of a stressful event preceding the onset of alopecia areata vary widely, between 4% and 85%, to the extent that no firm conclusion can be drawn. More recent controlled studies have also given conflicting results, with some studies finding a significant relationship between stressful events and the onset of hair loss, and others not [71].

The association between atopic disease and alopecia areata is well established but our understanding of its pathobiological significance is limited. Li and colleagues have suggested that dust mite allergy has a role in early-onset alopecia areata [72] and seasonal relapse of alopecia areata following allergic rhinitis has also been reported [73].

Several cross-sectional studies have reported an increased frequency of vitamin D deficiency in alopecia areata compared with unaffected controls. Vitamin D may have immunomodulatory functions and low levels of vitamin D have been reported in other autoimmune diseases [74]. However, one large prospective study found no association between the incidence of alopecia areata and predicted vitamin D levels, suggesting that deficiency may be a consequence rather than a cause [75]. No trials of oral vitamin D supplementation have yet been reported.

Deficiencies of other micronutrients that have been linked to alopecia areata include zinc, iron and folate. However, the studies are small, and the results are conflicting to the extent that no firm conclusion as to their significance can be drawn [76].

Despite the uncertain nature of some of the evidence it is entirely possible that environmental factors are responsible for triggering alopecia areata in some patients. If so, it seems likely that a diversity of factors can operate in this way.

Clinical features

The characteristic initial lesion of alopecia areata is a circumscribed, hairless, smooth patch. The skin within the bald patch appears normal or slightly reddened (Figure 87.22a). Short, easily extractable broken hairs, known as exclamation mark hairs, are often seen at the margins of the bald patches during active phases of the disease (Figure 87.22a, b). A strongly positive hair pull test around the margins of a bald patch is an indicator of actively progressing disease. A hair pull test may also be positive at scalp sites away from areas of obvious hair loss. The subsequent progress is unpredictable; the initial patch may regrow hair within a few months, or further patches may appear after varying intervals. A succession of discrete patches may coalesce to give large areas of hair loss. In some cases, this progresses to total loss of scalp hair (alopecia totalis) or loss of all hair on the body (alopecia universalis). The initial hair loss is occasionally diffuse without the development of discrete bald areas. Regrowth is often at first fine and non-pigmented, but usually the hairs gradually resume their normal calibre and colour. Regrowth in one region of the scalp may occur while the alopecia is extending in others.

The scalp is the first affected site in most cases, but any hair-bearing skin can be affected. In dark-haired men, patches in the beard are conspicuous and are often the first to be noticed (Figure 87.22c). The eyebrows and eyelashes are lost in many cases of alopecia areata and may be the only sites affected. The extension of alopecia along the back of the scalp is known as ophiasis (Figure 87.22d).

Trichoscopy can be helpful in confirming a diagnosis of alopecia areata. In a review of the published literature the reported features and their frequencies were yellow dots (6–100% of patients), short

vellus hairs (34–100%), black dots (also known as cadaverised hairs, 0–84%), broken hairs (0–71%) and exclamation mark hairs (12–71%) (Figure 87.14a, b) [77]. None is specific for alopecia areata, and their significance needs to be interpreted in the context of the gross clinical features. Yellow dots, which are due to follicular infundibula filled with keratinous material, predominate in chronic disease although they may also be seen in the acute stage. Black dots are a feature of actively progressing disease.

In patients with grey hair, where there is a mixture of pigmented and non-pigmented hair, alopecia areata may preferentially affect pigmented hair so that non-pigmented or white hair is spared. This may result in a dramatic change in hair colour if the alopecia progresses rapidly and is probably the explanation for historical accounts of people 'going white overnight'. Sparing of white hair is a relative phenomenon and white hairs, although less susceptible to the disease, are not immune. During the regrowth phase hairs may be non- or hypopigmented but hair pigmentation usually recovers completely (Figure 87.23). In cases where regrowing hairs remain non-pigmented, the possibility of concurrent vitiligo should be considered.

Alopecia areata may also involve the nails. Published frequencies vary widely, ranging from 7% to 66% [78], possibly reflecting differences in case mix as nail disease is more common in the context of severe hair loss. Alopecia areata typically causes fine, stippled pitting of the nails (Figure 87.24). Some cases show less well-defined roughening of the nail plate (trachyonychia) or a non-specific atrophic dystrophy. Less common features include red spotting of the lunula and longitudinal splitting of the nail plate. For some patients, severe nail dystrophy is the most troublesome aspect of the disease if it interferes with manual activities.

Clinical variants

Diffuse alopecia areata. Alopecia areata occasionally presents in a diffuse fashion rather than forming well-defined patches of hair loss. The onset is typically acute with a large increase in hair shedding and a diffuse, although not necessarily uniform, reduction in hair density. Hair may be lost from other sites such as the eyebrows and limbs. A pull test is usually strongly positive. Dermoscopy shows features of alopecia areata including yellow dots, exclamation mark hairs and cadaverised hairs. The term *acute diffuse and total alopecia* has been used to describe a form of rapidly progressive diffuse alopecia areata that affects young adult women, that usually recovers spontaneously within 6 months and has a good prognosis. Most cases have been reported from East Asian countries [79–81]. The histology shows typical features of alopecia areata including peribulbar inflammation.

Alopecia areata incognita. This entity was first described by Rebora in 1987 [82]. Most cases are adult women who present with a rapid onset of increased hair shedding resembling acute TE. There is no rarefaction of scalp hair unless the shedding persists and only a small proportion of cases (1–2%) develop small patches of hair loss. Only scalp hair is affected. A pull test is strongly positive showing telogen roots; dystrophic forms are rare. Histology shows follicular miniaturisation and an increase in telogen follicles [83]. Subtle peribulbar lymphocytic inflammation is seen in a small proportion of cases. The status of alopecia areata incognita is uncertain;

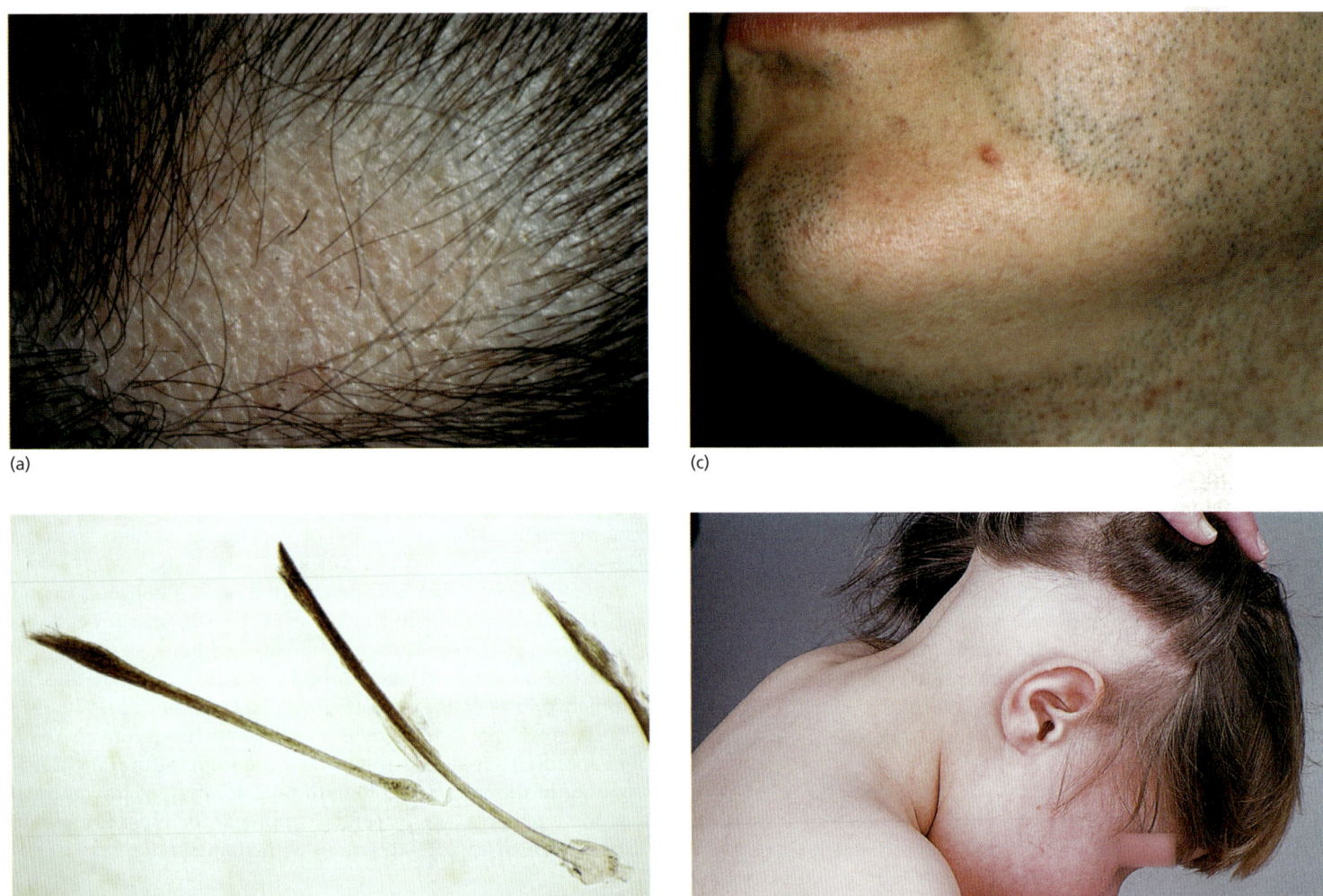

Figure 87.22 Alopecia areata. (a) Patch of alopecia areata showing broken exclamation mark hairs towards the margins. (b) Close-up of exclamation mark hairs. (c) Alopecia areata affecting the beard. (d) The ophiasis pattern of alopecia areata.

in particular, whether it truly represents a form of alopecia areata. Yellow dots are a consistent feature on trichoscopy but yellow dots may also be seen in other conditions, including FPHL [84].

Differential diagnosis

In children the main sources of difficulty are tinea capitis and trichotillomania. Tinea capitis should always be considered in children presenting with patchy hair loss. There is usually evidence of scalp inflammation, but this may be limited to mild scaling. The hair loss in trichotillomania may be asymmetrical or occur in artificial shapes. Broken hairs are usually present across the areas of hair loss, giving a bristly texture and, unlike exclamation mark hairs, are firmly anchored in the scalp. In most cases the true diagnosis will become evident with time; a biopsy is useful when doubt remains. Occasionally, the early stages of scarring alopecia can resemble alopecia areata. The diffuse form of alopecia areata is perhaps the most difficult to identify. A history of previous episodes of hair loss, nail dystrophy and the usually rapid progression may provide clues, but other causes of diffuse hair loss may need to be excluded. Pattern hair loss and TE are the main differential but lack the broken hairs, black dots and exclamation mark hairs seen on trichoscopy

of alopecia areata. Secondary syphilis and lupus erythematosus can cause both patchy and diffuse hair loss.

The development of alopecia totalis/universalis in infancy should always raise the possibility of a genetic atrichia due to mutations in the *HR* (human hairless) gene or *VDR* (vitamin D receptor) gene.

Classification of severity

Alopecia areata is conventionally classified as patchy, alopecia totalis and alopecia universalis. In addition to these simple criteria a more detailed classification should include the disease duration and, regarding patchy alopecia, the extent of the hair loss. A description of the pattern should include the presence of ophiasis, the involvement of sites on the trunk and limbs and the presence of nail disease. Several scoring systems have been devised of which the severity of alopecia tool (SALT) is the most widely used and is readily applicable to clinical practice (Figure 87.25) [85]. The impact of alopecia areata on patient quality of life can be assessed using a variety of instruments, both disease-specific and non-specific. The dermatology life quality instrument (DLQI) is straightforward, and most dermatologists are familiar with its use, although other more disease-specific methods have been devised [86,87].

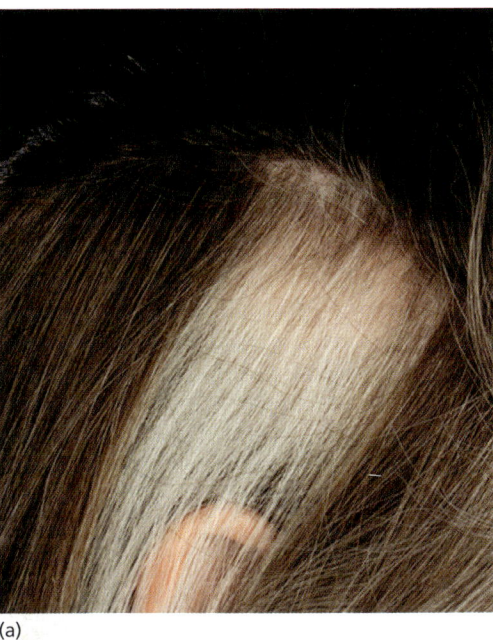

(a)

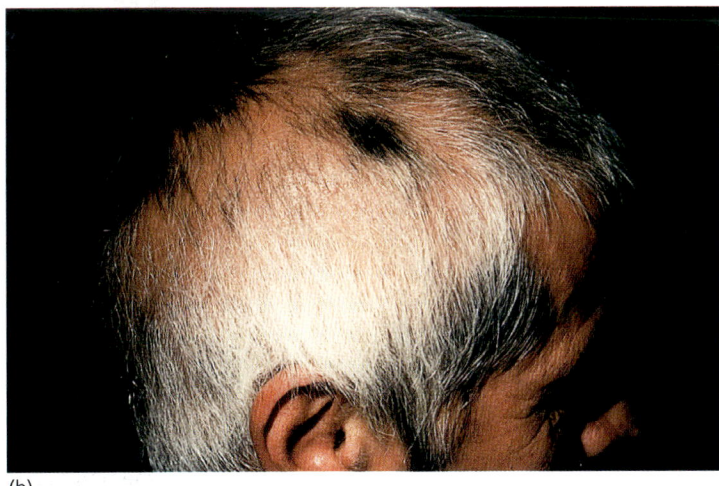

(b)

Figure 87.23 (a) Sparing of white hairs in a patch of alopecia areata. (b) Regrowth of hypopigmented hair in alopecia areata.

Disease course and prognosis

Alopecia areata does not destroy hair follicles, and the potential for regrowth of hair is retained for many years and is possibly lifelong. In some patients, patches of hair loss occur at infrequent intervals interspersed with long periods of normal hair growth. In others, alopecia areata is more persistent, so that new patches of hair loss continue to develop at the same time as regrowth occurs elsewhere. In a relatively small proportion of patients, hair loss progresses to involve all of the scalp (alopecia totalis) or the entire skin surface (alopecia universalis); in these cases, spontaneous recovery is the exception rather than the rule.

Data from secondary and tertiary referral centres indicate that 34–50% of patients will recover within 1 year, although almost all will experience more than one episode of the disease, and 14–25% progress to alopecia totalis or alopecia universalis, from which full recovery is unusual (less than 10%) [88–90]. A study from Japan

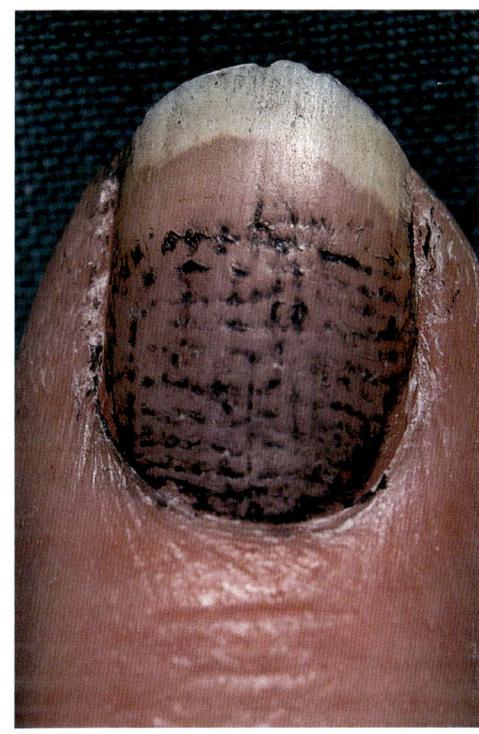

Figure 87.24 An organised pattern of pitting present on all fingernails 8 months prior to the onset of alopecia areata. The pits are highlighted with mascara.

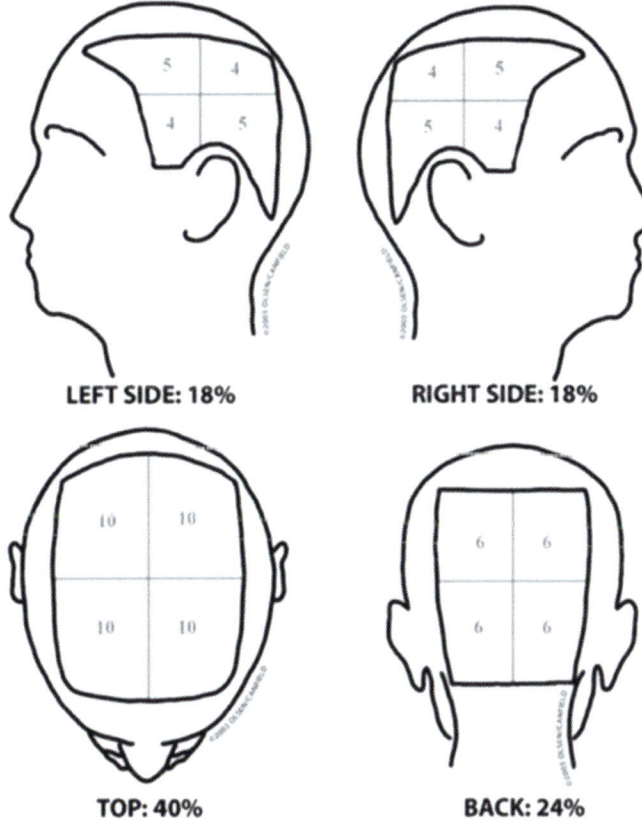

LEFT SIDE: 18%   **RIGHT SIDE: 18%**

TOP: 40%   **BACK: 24%**

Figure 87.25 Severity of alopecia tool (SALT) score. This is used to assess the extent of hair loss in alopecia areata by estimating percentage scalp hair loss. Adapted from Olsen *et al.* 2004 [51].

PART 8: SPECIFIC CUTANEOUS STRUCTURES

reported that spontaneous remission within 1 year occurred in 80% of patients with a small number of circumscribed patches of hair loss [15]. The prognosis is less favourable when onset occurs during childhood [90,91] and in ophiasis [91].

Investigations

In most cases alopecia areata can be diagnosed clinically and investigations are usually not needed. If there is diagnostic uncertainty a biopsy may be necessary, although the histological features may be subtle and require a pathologist experienced in the interpretation of hair pathology. Situations where a biopsy can be helpful include diffuse alopecia and possible early scarring alopecia. In selected cases other diagnostic tests may include:

- Fungal culture.
- Serology for lupus erythematosus.
- Vitamin D serology.
- Full blood count and iron studies.
- Syphilis serology.

Unless relevant symptoms and signs are present it is debatable whether routine 'one-off' screening for other autoimmune diseases is appropriate as the risk is small and lifelong, but screening for thyroid disease is often recommended.

Management

General principles of management

Several treatments can induce hair growth in alopecia areata, but none has been shown to alter the course of the disease. Few treatments have been subjected to randomised controlled trials and there are limited published data on long-term outcomes. These difficulties mean that counselling of the patient and, where relevant, of their family is of paramount importance. This should include discussion of the nature of the disease and its natural history, the treatments available and their chances of success. Assessment of the psychosocial impact of the disease is an important part of the consultation. Some patients have great difficulty coping with alopecia areata and require considerable support. Sources of support may include the physician, specialist nurses, other patients, formal patient support groups and, in some circumstances, professional counselling services. In helping patients to cope with their hair loss, normalising relationships with health care providers, significant others and peers has been cited as pivotal to positive adjustment [92].

Most patients presenting to clinicians want to receive treatment although, after counselling, some will prefer to leave their alopecia untreated. In those with limited patchy hair loss of short duration there is a high rate of spontaneous remission. The prognosis in long-standing and/or extensive alopecia is less favourable. However, all treatments have a significant failure rate in this group and some patients prefer not to be treated, other than by cosmetic measures, such as wearing a wig, if appropriate.

Management strategies

Limited patchy alopecia areata. A potent topical steroid (e.g. clobetasol), delivered in cream or foam formulation, may hasten recovery of hair growth in mild degrees of alopecia areata [93,94]. Treatment should be continued for at least 3 months. Folliculitis is an occasional complication, and skin atrophy can occur with prolonged use. With simple non-occluded application, topical steroids are ineffective in alopecia totalis/universalis. One study reported sustained hair regrowth in 5 of 28 patients with alopecia totalis/universalis when clobetasol ointment was used under plastic film occlusion [95]. Folliculitis was a common complication and, in some patients, was severe.

Intralesional steroid is generally the most effective local treatment in limited patchy alopecia areata, although the formal evidence base is of low quality [96]. One study reported complete regrowth in 63% of patients at 4 months [97] and, in a second, 82% showed more than 50% regrowth at 12 weeks [98]. A depot steroid is administered by fine-needle injection into the upper subcutis or using a needleless device. Triamcinolone acetonide 5–10 mg/mL is the most widely used agent [99] although a small study comparing different steroid concentrations found that 2.5 mg/mL was as effective as higher concentrations [100]. Multiple injections are usually needed. There is no set upper dose, but most practitioners limit the total dose of triamcinolone to 20 mg. Local atrophy is a common side effect, but this recovers within a few months. Intralesional steroid will not prevent the development of alopecia at other sites and is not suitable for patients with rapidly progressive alopecia or alopecia totalis/universalis [99]. Intralesional steroid may also be used to treat alopecia of the eyebrows and beard; lower concentrations (2.5–5 mg/mL) are advisable in these sites in view of the risk of atrophy.

The use of dithranol (anthralin) to induce an irritant dermatitis was first proposed in 1979. Early studies failed to show a consistent response. However, recent case series using more aggressive treatment regimens have suggested that dithranol can promote worthwhile regrowth in some patients [101,102]. Limiting factors include coping with a sore scalp, discoloration of the hair and staining of fabrics.

Topical minoxidil has been widely used but the evidence for efficacy is poor [**103**].

Extensive and rapidly progressive alopecia areata. The place of systemic steroids in treating alopecia areata is controversial, except for a general acceptance that a worthwhile response in alopecia totalis/universalis is very unlikely. Clinical experience provides some support for the use of relatively short courses of systemic steroids in managing exacerbations or rapidly progressive alopecia areata. Long-term treatment with systemic corticosteroids will produce some regrowth of hair in some patients with chronic patchy disease but the benefits are generally outweighed by the risks. Several protocols have been published, including daily oral dosing and various high-dose pulsed oral and intravenous regimens, but it is unclear whether any is more effective or safer than any other [104–108].

Extensive patchy alopecia or alopecia totalis/universalis. Since its introduction in the early 1980s, contact immunotherapy has been the most effective and best-documented treatment for extensive alopecia areata. Although the cost of contact immunotherapy in terms of materials is relatively low, the high costs associated with specialist clinical staff administering the treatment and patient travel, and its non-licensed status, have limited its widespread use and, in some countries, its use has been largely replaced by Janus kinase (JAK) inhibitors.

The patient is sensitised to a potent skin allergen by application to a small area on the scalp and the same allergen is then applied to the scalp, usually at weekly intervals, in a concentration sufficient to induce a mild contact dermatitis. The allergens that have been used in the treatment of alopecia areata include dinitrochlorobenzene, squaric acid dibutylester and diphenylcyclopropenone (DPCP). Most centres now use DPCP [109,110].

In an analysis of 45 published studies comprising 2227 patients, albeit most of low quality, 56% of those with patchy alopecia and 29% of those with alopecia totalis/universalis had major hair regrowth with contact immunotherapy [111]. Adverse prognostic features included SALT scores greater than 50, atopic disease, nail involvement and disease duration greater than 1 year. Almost half of all patients relapsed following treatment; the relapse rate was lower in those receiving maintenance treatment (38%) than in those not receiving maintenance (49%). Although its nature precludes blinded controlled trials, the validity of contact immunotherapy is supported by studies showing ipsilateral hair regrowth when only one half of the scalp is treated.

Most practitioners discontinue treatment after 6 months if no response is obtained, although one study from Canada reported better results with more prolonged treatment [112]. Two case report series of contact immunotherapy in children with alopecia areata reported response rates of 33% [113] and 32% [114]. A third study found a similar short-term response in children with severe alopecia areata, but less than 10% experienced sustained benefit [115].

Most patients will develop occipital and/or cervical lymphadenopathy during contact immunotherapy. This is usually temporary but may persist throughout the treatment period. Severe dermatitis is the most common adverse event, but the risk can be minimised by careful titration of the concentration. Uncommon adverse effects include urticaria and vitiligo. Cosmetically disabling pigmentary complications, both hyper- and hypopigmentation (including vitiligo), may occur if contact immunotherapy is used in patients with pigmented skin. Contact immunotherapy has been in use for over 30 years and no long-term side effects have been reported. Sensitisation of health professionals involved in delivering contact immunotherapy (doctors, nurses, pharmacy technicians) is a significant problem and they must take care to avoid skin contact with the allergen. The mode of action of contact immunotherapy is unknown.

Some clinicians use systemic immunosuppressive drugs (ciclosporin, azathioprine, methotrexate) in severe alopecia areata, either stand-alone or as steroid-sparing agents. A systematic review of case series concluded that ciclosporin is more effective, and the relapse rate is lower, when used in combination with systemic steroids [116], but it is less clear whether ciclosporin is effective when used alone [117]. Positive results have been reported for azathioprine in a few small case series [118] but there are no controlled studies. Methotrexate has probably been the most widely used drug in this category, first reported in 2006 [119]. Several case series have since been published. A critical review concluded there was insufficient evidence to say whether methotrexate is useful for maintaining regrowth in extensive alopecia areata, although there was some evidence to suggest that hair regrowth may be induced by methotrexate when used in combination with systemic corticosteroids [120]. Nevertheless, methotrexate is a relatively safe drug, most dermatologists are experienced in its use and, despite the rather weak evidence base, it is worthy of consideration in certain cases.

Janus kinase inhibitors. Many cytokines activate immune cells via the JAK/STAT signalling pathway. Drugs that inhibit JAK prevent the development of hair loss, and reverse it, in a mouse model of alopecia areata [121]. The oral administration of the JAK inhibitors ruxolitinib [121] and tofacitinib [122] also promotes hair regrowth in patients with alopecia areata. Two phase III randomised controlled trials of baricitinib, an inhibitor of JAK1 and JAK2, in 1200 patients with severe alopecia areata (SALT score ≥50) were published in 2022 [123]. At 36 weeks 36–39% of those taking baricitinib 4 mg daily achieved 80% scalp coverage (SALT score ≤20) and 23% had complete or near-complete regrowth (SALT score ≤10). Positive results have also been reported for other investigational JAK inhibitors in phase II trials [124,125]. In 2022 baricitinib was authorised for the treatment of severe alopecia areata in the USA. JAK inhibitors are immunosuppressive but reported side effects (in alopecia areata) appear minor, with upper respiratory infections the most common complaint. Preliminary evidence indicates that continued treatment is needed to maintain the response in most patients and some uncertainty remains over long-term safety, which will need to be monitored carefully.

Other treatments. *Platelet-rich plasma* (PRP): in a randomised controlled trial in limited patchy alopecia areata, PRP was more effective than intralesional corticosteroid at stimulating hair regrowth and produced more lasting remissions [126]. A small number of subsequent studies have supported the idea that PRP is at least as effective as intralesional corticosteroid in limited patchy disease [127]. One case series found that that PRP did not produce sustained benefit in severe (>50%) alopecia areata [128].

Phototherapy: the use of various forms of phototherapy in alopecia areata has a long history. These have included UVB, UVA, photochemotherapy (psoralen and UVA (PUVA)) and photodynamic therapy (PDT). UVB and PDT do not work. The evidence for PUVA is slightly stronger but there are no controlled trials [129]. Both topical psoralens with local UVA to the scalp and systemic psoralens with whole body irradiation have been used but continued treatment is usually needed to maintain any response, leading to unacceptably high cumulative doses of UVA.

Laser therapy: several small, controlled trials and case series in patchy alopecia areata have reported hair regrowth following treatment with a 308 nm excimer laser [129]. Overall, about 50% of patches appear to respond. However, there is little or no published information on relapse rates and the treatment regimens are arduous (e.g. twice weekly for 12 weeks).

Children with alopecia areata. Alopecia areata presents a particular therapeutic challenge in children as the treatment options are more limited, compounded by the often severe nature of the disease in this age group. Intralesional injections are rarely tolerated by young children and there is a reluctance to use systemic drugs such as corticosteroids or immunosuppressives. Possible options include topical corticosteroids, topical minoxidil and anthralin, but these are unlikely to help in extensive alopecia areata. Very young children are often oblivious of their hair loss, and it is the parents who are more likely to need support, but older children may struggle to cope – teasing and bullying at school are common problems. Patient support groups or charities aimed at helping those with visible skin disorders can provide invaluable advice for patients and their families; occasionally input from a paediatric clinical psychologist is needed.

Nail disease. Published data on the treatment of nail disease are limited to case reports and small case series. Improvement has been reported from intralesional steroid although the disease eventually relapses. There are several reports of a good response to treatment with oral tofacitinib even when there is little or no hair growth response. Nail disease may remit spontaneously in children [130].

Non-medical treatments. Women with extensive alopecia will usually benefit from wearing a wig [131], hairpiece or bandana. A few brave patients prefer not to conceal their lack of hair. Men tend to shave their heads although some opt for a wig. The use of semipermanent tattooing can be helpful to disguise loss of eyebrows.

Resources

Patient resources
Alopecia UK: http://www.alopeciaonline.org.uk.
British Association of Dermatologists, patient information: https://www.bad.org.uk/pils/alopecia-areata/.
National Alopecia Areata Foundation: http://www.naaf.org.
(All last accessed May 2023.)

OTHER NON-SCARRING, PATCHY OR DIFFUSE ALOPECIAS

The following diagnoses may also be confused with alopecia areata.

Temporal triangular alopecia

Synonyms and inclusions
• Congenital triangular alopecia

Introduction and general description

Temporal triangular alopecia (TTA) was first described by Sabouraud in 1905 as 'alopecia triangulaire congenitale de la temp' [1]. Although infrequently described in the literature, TTA is likely more common than originally thought, being underreported, overlooked or misdiagnosed [2].

Pathophysiology

It is a congenital defect, most likely representing a mosaic disease with para-dominant inheritance [3]. Associations with other congenital conditions, including Down syndrome and phakomatosis pigmentovascularis, are described [3,4].

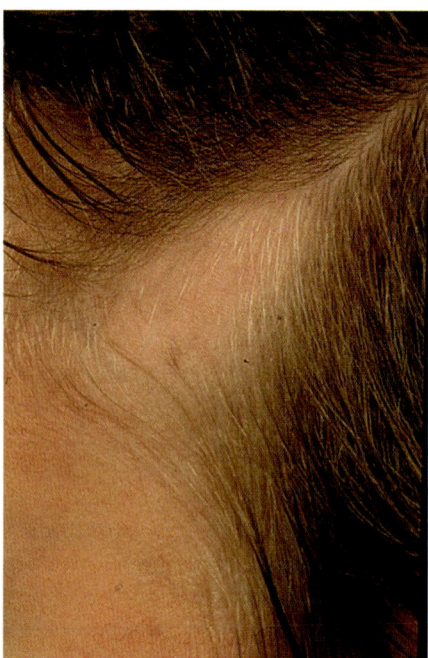

Figure 87.26 Triangular alopecia.

Clinical features

Temporal triangular alopecia usually presents at around 3–6 years of age and is often not noticed at birth [2,4–6]. Typically, the alopecia patches are triangular (with the triangle base orientated towards the anterior hairline), oval or lancet-shaped and may be unilateral (>80% of cases) or bilateral (Figure 87.26). The patch itself contains fine vellus hairs only, although completely bald areas and 'islands' of retained terminal hairs are recognised [7]. The patches are asymptomatic and remain unchanged in shape and size over time. Diagnostic criteria are described [8].

Differential diagnosis

The main differential diagnosis is alopecia areata. In TTA, yellow dots, exclamation mark hairs and broken hairs are not present.

Investigations

Skin biopsy is usually not required. Histology shows normal vellus hairs and hair density, but no terminal hairs [9].

Management

Topical minoxidil may stimulate growth, but ongoing treatment is needed to maintain a response [10]. Triangular alopecia can be treated surgically, either by simple excision or by hair transplantation.

Atrichia with papular lesions

Synonyms and inclusions
• Papular atrichia
Classification links
• MIM: 209500

Introduction and general description

Atrichia with papular lesions (APL) is a rare genetic disorder causing complete hair loss that may be misdiagnosed as alopecia universalis [11].

Pathophysiology

This is an autosomal recessive condition caused by mutations in the *HR* gene on chromosome 8p21 [12]. The *HR* gene encodes a zinc finger transcription factor protein that results in a dysregulated hair cycle, immature HF structures and keratin-filled follicular cysts. The first hair cycle is normal, after which signalling between the dermal papilla and bulge becomes perturbed, resulting in catagen follicles unable to re-enter anagen [13].

Clinical features

Most children with APL are born with a full head of hair. However, within a few months all the hair is shed and not replaced, resulting in complete and irreversible alopecia indistinguishable from alopecia universalis. Papular lesions typically develop later in childhood but can sometimes regress, leaving pitted scars [11,12]. Diagnostic criteria are described (Box 87.1) [12].

Box 87.1 Diagnostic criteria for atrichia with papular lesions

Major criteria (four of five required for diagnosis)
- Permanent and complete absence of scalp hairs by the first few months of life
- Few to widespread, smooth, whitish or milia-like papules on the face, scalp, arms, elbows, thighs or knees from infancy or childhood
- Replacement of mature hair follicle structures by follicular cysts filled with cornified material on scalp histology
- Mutation(s) in the *HH* gene through genetic testing
- Clinical and/or molecular exclusion of vitamin D-dependent rickets

Minor criteria (supplementary criteria)
- Family history of consanguinity
- Absence of secondary axillary, pubic or body hair growth and/or sparse eyebrows and eyelashes
- Normal growth and development (including normal bones, teeth, nails and sweating)
- Lack of response to any treatment modality

From Yip *et al.* 2008 [12].

Differential diagnosis

The alopecia of APL is indistinguishable from the hair loss seen in alopecia universalis and vitamin D-dependent rickets (see later in this chapter).

Investigations

Genetic testing for *HR* gene mutations is the gold standard for diagnosis. Characteristic histological features can also help secure the diagnosis [14]. Histology demonstrates replacement of the proximal two-thirds of remaining HFs with vertically orientated epithelial structures, follicular remnants and variable-sized keratin-filled cysts [13].

Management

There is no treatment for APL.

Vitamin D-dependent rickets type 2a

Definition, nomenclature and classification

Vitamin D-dependent rickets type 2a (VDDRIIa) is a rare hereditary condition caused by target-organ resistance to vitamin D resulting in bone changes, developmental delay and hair loss.

Synonyms and inclusions
- Vitamin D-resistant rickets

Classification links
- MIM: 277440

Pathophysiology

This is caused by mutations in the *VDR* gene on chromosome 12q12-q14. The *VDR* gene is expressed in multiple target tissues, including bones, kidneys and HFs. Phenotypic expression is variable and dependent on the specific *VDR* mutation and residual receptor activity [15].

Clinical features

Hair growth is usually normal at birth, but alopecia develops within the first 2 years in about two-thirds of cases. Complete alopecia is an early feature in VDDRIIa and is indistinguishable from APL or alopecia universalis. Importantly, papular lesions may also be seen in VDDRIIa. Bone pain and bone deformity (e.g. leg bowing when the child becomes ambulatory), muscle weakness, hypotonia, recurrent infections and growth retardation develop if left untreated [16].

Differential diagnosis

The alopecia of VDDRIIa is indistinguishable from the hair loss seen in alopecia universalis and APL (see earlier in this chapter).

Investigations

Typical biochemical changes include hypocalcaemia, hypophosphataemia, raised alkaline phosphatase and secondary hyperparathyroidism. Scalp biopsy shows thinned and hypoplastic HFs with no inflammation.

Management

High-dose oral or intravenous calcium is required to correct bone and mineral abnormalities; there are no effective treatments for the alopecia.

Anterolateral lower leg alopecia

Synonyms and inclusions
- Peroneal alopecia

Introduction and general description

Anterolateral alopecia is a non-scarring alopecia of the lower legs, first described in 1920. It is commonly seen in middle-aged and older men and has an estimated prevalence of up to 35% [17], yet it is rarely described in the literature [18].

Pathophysiology

The cause is unclear, but friction from clothing and leg crossing is suggested. Certainly, convincing cases of frictional alopecia from socks are described with clear demarcation of hair loss in areas covered by tight garments [19]. Other proposed associations include male pattern hair loss, hypothyroidism and peripheral vascular disease [17,18].

Clinical features

Anterolateral alopecia presents as symmetrical, circumscribed, smooth patches of alopecia affecting the anterolateral lower leg (in the distribution of the peroneal nerve), and sometimes spreading to the thighs.

Differential diagnosis

The main differential diagnosis is alopecia areata. Typical clinical and dermoscopy features and history of regrowth can usually differentiate this condition, although skin biopsy may be considered if diagnosis is unclear.

Investigations

Skin biopsy shows lack of HFs only [20].

Management

No treatment has been shown to regrow hairs in this condition. Reduction of friction and exclusion of associated conditions are recommended. Patient education and reassurance are usually all that is required.

Other circumscribed (congenital) alopecias

Circumscribed alopecia of congenital origin usually presents little difficulty if a reliable history is available.

Sebaceous naevus (organoid naevus). Sebaceous naevus usually presents in childhood as a hairless patch on the scalp, often in a linear configuration. The affected skin may have a yellowish hue and thickened rugged surface. See Chapter 73.

Aplasia cutis. Aplasia cutis is a heterogeneous group of conditions characterised by the localised absence of a portion of skin at birth. It most commonly presents as a single patch on the scalp vertex, but lesions may be multiple and other parts of the skin may be involved. At birth, the affected skin may be superficially or deeply ulcerated or may have healed leaving an atrophic scar. Aplasia cutis is usually an isolated defect, but it can be associated with a variety of malformation syndromes.

Sutural alopecia. Multiple patches of hair loss overlying the cranial sutures are a feature of the Hallermann–Streiff syndrome, in which dysmorphic facies, skeletal anomalies, microphthalmia, congenital cataract and hypodontia are also found. See Chapter 66.

Medical traumatic hair loss

There are instances where medical intervention may result in scalp trauma and be implicated in scarring alopecia. Scalp electrodes, infusions or forceps delivery in the neonate can result in trauma [21]. Marks from such interventions need to be distinguished from aplasia cutis, which can sometimes be the underlying diagnosis [22].

Interventions in adulthood, directly through scalp and brain surgery or indirectly through local embolisation procedures, can result in scarring. Adler *et al.* described a case in which ischaemic necrosis of the occipital scalp occurred following embolisation and surgery for a large convexity meningioma [23].

Pressure-induced alopecia

Synonyms and inclusions
• Postoperative alopecia

Introduction and general description

Pressure-induced alopecia was first described by Abel and Lewis in eight women undergoing gynaecological surgery [24]. Any cause of prolonged immobility or scalp pressure effects (e.g. tight headbands or facemask straps) may result in this condition.

Pathophysiology

Pressure-induced alopecia is due to localised pressure-induced ischaemic injury and hypoxia to the scalp tissue and HFs.

Clinical features

Circumscribed areas of hair loss develop at pressure points of the scalp, with the occiput being the commonest site affected [25,26]. Localised swelling and tenderness may initially be seen, associated with exudation, crusting and ulceration; however, hair loss may be the only presenting feature. Usually the alopecia is temporary, generally regrowing within 4 months. Sometimes permanent alopecia may result, particularly with longer surgery durations [26]. Dermoscopy may reveal redness along with black dots, broken hairs and thin residual hairs reminiscent of changes seen in alopecia areata, but the absence of yellow dots and tapered hairs helps to differentiate these conditions [27–29].

Investigations

Early histological changes include thrombosis, hair bulb necrosis and variable inflammation. In areas of alopecia virtually all hairs are in the catagen/telogen phase. Trichomalacia, pigment casts and increased apoptosis are prominent [30,31]. Scarring alopecia may be present in longstanding cases.

Management

The key to management is prevention. Longer procedures, patient positioning (e.g. Trendelenburg position) and patient factors are risks for alopecia development. Pressure-reliving cushioning [32,33] and frequent repositioning are recommended [26]. The role of topical corticosteroids in the acute inflammatory phase and topical minoxidil as adjunctive treatment is still to be determined.

Traction alopecia

Introduction and general description

First described in Greenlandic women in 1907 [34], traction alopecia is brought about by hairstyles that impose sustained pulling on the hair roots. Various cultural or religious hairstyle practices predispose to traction alopecia development and it is particularly common in women with afro-textured hair. A population study from South Africa reported an incidence of traction alopecia in 17.1% of schoolgirls and 31.7% of adult women [35,36].

Pathophysiology

Traction alopecia occurs due to sustained mechanical damage to the HF, predominantly affecting terminal hairs. It is regarded as a 'biphasic' alopecia, completely reversible if identified early, but can become permanent if the traction is sustained. Certain hair types, particularly highly curled hair, are more susceptible to traction due to increased tension forces within the HF [37].

Clinical features

The alopecia pattern reflects the hairstyle used, with hair loss occurring in the areas of maximal tension. The most common pattern seen is patchy alopecia at the temporal regions, in front and above the ears, due to tight ponytails. However, hair loss can involve any part of the scalp depending on the style. Hair loss between cornrows or braids (Figure 87.27), occipital alopecia due to chignon or bun styles, marginal loss due to hair twisting in Sikh males (Figure 87.28) [38] and tight scarf styles can all result in hair loss [39]. Problems typically start in childhood, where they may initially be reversible if identified early [40].

Patches of traction alopecia typically show reduced hair density, preferential loss of terminal hairs with preservation of vellus hairs,

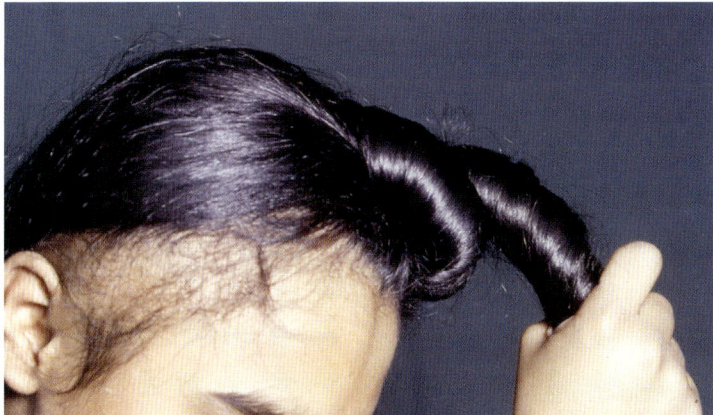

Figure 87.28 Traction alopecia in a Sikh boy.

and a fringe of retained terminal hairs (fringe sign) at the furthest point away from the tension. Features that suggest ongoing significant traction include visible 'tenting' of the skin, folliculitis and the presence of hair casts at the alopecia margins. Trichoscopic features include broken hairs, vellus hairs and hair casts; fibrotic white dots and loss of follicular ostia suggest chronic traction with scarring. Tulip hairs and the Flambeau sign are also described [41].

Khumalo *et al.* found that traction alopecia was significantly more likely in those who had previously experienced painful braids or papules at the base of the braids [42]. However, a history of traction is not always apparent as 'excessive tension' is subjective and difficult to quantify. Scalp symptoms (e.g. pain, stinging, crusting) and skin tenting suggest high-risk hairstyles for traction development.

Clinical variants

Various grooming practices, including night-time techniques used for hairstyle maintenance [43], may increase the risk of traction alopecia. High-risk styles are shown in Box 87.2 [44].

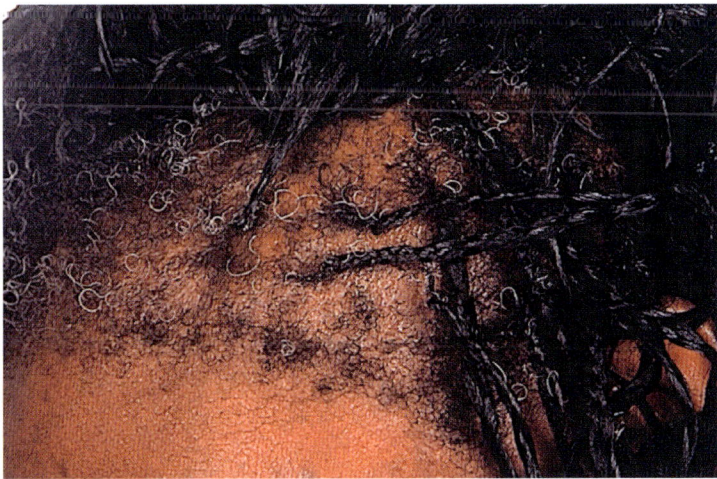

Figure 87.27 Traction alopecia from braiding.

Box 87.2 Risk categories for different hairstyles

High risk
- Frequent use of tight buns or ponytails
- Application of weaves and/or braids to relaxed hair
- Hair extensions applied to relaxed hair
- Tight braids, cornrows or dreadlocks
- Any hairstyle causing pain, stinging, crusting, tenting or pimples

Moderate risk
- Looser of braids, cornrows or dreadlocks
- Weaves and/or braids applied to natural hair
- Hair extensions applied to natural hair
- Wigs worn with cotton or nylon wig cap
- Permanent waving

Low risk
- Loose hanging ponytails or buns
- Wigs worn with satin wig caps
- Natural/unprocessed hair

From Haskin and Aguh 2016 [44].

Cicatricial marginal alopecia is a name given to a pattern of marginal hair loss, reminiscent of alopecia areata, without a good history of significant traction [45]. Clinical features and histopathology suggest this condition is best regarded as an end-stage variant of chronic traction alopecia.

Differential diagnosis

Frontotemporal recession of androgenetic alopecia and patchy or ophiasis alopecia areata may occasionally mimic traction alopecia. FFA can present with frontal hairline recession and a 'pseudofringe' [46].

Investigations

Histological features in early traction include an increased proportion of telogen hairs and trichomalacia. Late traction is characterised by follicular drop-out with preservation of sebaceous glands and deeper fibrous tracts. Follicular plugging, pigment casts, ORS tears and perifollicular haemorrhage may also be seen [37,47].

Management

Photography and the marginal traction alopecia severity score can be used to monitor severity and treatment response [48].

Treatment depends on the disease stage. The best approach is prevention; educational programmes targeting at-risk populations are advocated to raise awareness of the problem [49]. The patient, or parents of affected children, needs to be educated to adopt hairstyles that do not pull the hair tight and to change styles frequently. In early stages traction alopecia is reversible. If it is inflamed, potent topical or intralesional corticosteroid, as well as topical or oral antibiotics, can be helpful. Topical (or oral) minoxidil is frequently used to stimulate hair regrowth [47]. Once traction alopecia is established and follicles have been lost, the hair loss becomes permanent. In this situation, hair transplantation and scalp reduction surgery are the only options.

Trichotillomania

Synonyms and inclusions

• Hair pulling disorder

Introduction and general description

Trichotillomania (TTM) was first described by Hallopeau in 1889 and originates from the Greek words 'thrix' (hair), 'tillein' (to pull) and 'mania' (madness) [50]. TTM is a behavioural disorder characterised by compulsive hair pulling that presents with an often bizarre pattern of hair loss with no clear biological explanation. Compulsive hair rubbing (trichoteiromania) [51], biting hair (trichodaganomania) and hair cutting (trichotemnomania) [52] fall into the same general category. The lifetime prevalence of TTM is estimated as 1–3% [53].

TTM occurs in two main forms:

1 In infants and young children, it is usually a habit akin to thumb sucking and nail biting. It seems slightly more common in boys and usually resolves spontaneously or with minimal treatment.

Parents who have not noticed hair-pulling behaviour in their offspring may deny the diagnosis.

2 In older age groups (adolescents and adults), TTM is seen predominantly in females, and evidence of some form of psychological or behavioural stress is often apparent. Coexisting major depression and anxiety are common and are associated with more severe TTM symptoms. Feelings of shame frequently lead to social avoidance and withdrawal [54–56].

Pathophysiology

The American Psychiatric Association classifies TTM as an obsessive–compulsive spectrum disorder in the fifth edition of the *Diagnostic and Statistical Manual of Mental Disorders* (DSM-5) (Box 87.3) [56]. In DSM-5, TTM is grouped with obsessive–compulsive disorders, body dysmorphic disorder, nail biting disorder, skin picking disorder, tic disorders and eating disorders, as these all have an overlapping genetic predisposition, clinical features and treatment responses [54,56].

Box 87.3 DSM-5 diagnostic criteria for trichotillomania

• Recurrent pulling out of one's hair, resulting in hair loss
• Repeated attempts to decrease or stop hair pulling
• The hair pulling causes clinically significant distress or impairment in social, occupational or other important areas of functioning
• The hair pulling or hair loss is not attributable to another medical condition (e.g. a dermatological condition)
• The hair pulling is not better explained by the symptoms of another mental disorder (e.g. attempts to improve a perceived defect or flaw in appearance in body dysmorphic disorder)

From American Psychiatric Association 2013 [56].

Clinical features

In young children, the hair pulling tic develops gradually and unconsciously. Hair is plucked most frequently from one frontoparietal region. This results in a patch of hair loss, often in a bizarre or angular pattern, in which the hairs are twisted and broken at various distances from the clinically normal scalp.

Older patients present with an area of scalp on which the hair has been reduced to coarse stubble. The plucked area may be asymmetrical and sometimes quite extensive, covering the entire scalp but typically sparing the scalp margins (Figure 87.29). It is unusual for hair to be lost completely within the affected area (in contrast with alopecia areata) and the remaining hairs are short, broken and attached to the scalp. The scalp skin appears normal. Over time the extent of hair loss can vary, and hair growth may recover temporarily. There appear to be two main types of TTM: 'automatic' where people may not be fully aware they are pulling and 'focused' where specific hairs are identified and removed due to them being perceived as 'not right' or 'out of place' [55,57,58].

Specific features

Hair in sites other than the scalp can also be affected, such as eyelashes, eyebrows and beard. Exceptionally, the patient may pluck hair also, or only, from other regions of the body, such as the mons

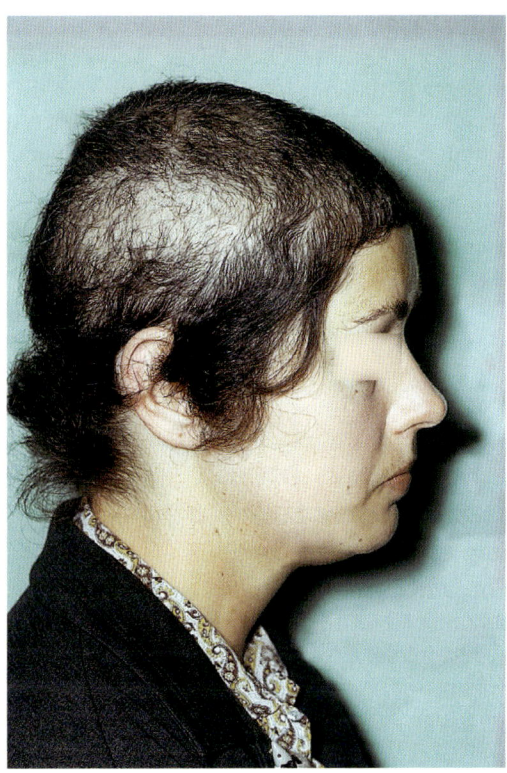

Figure 87.29 Trichotillomania showing a characteristic 'tonsure' pattern with the scalp margin hair spared.

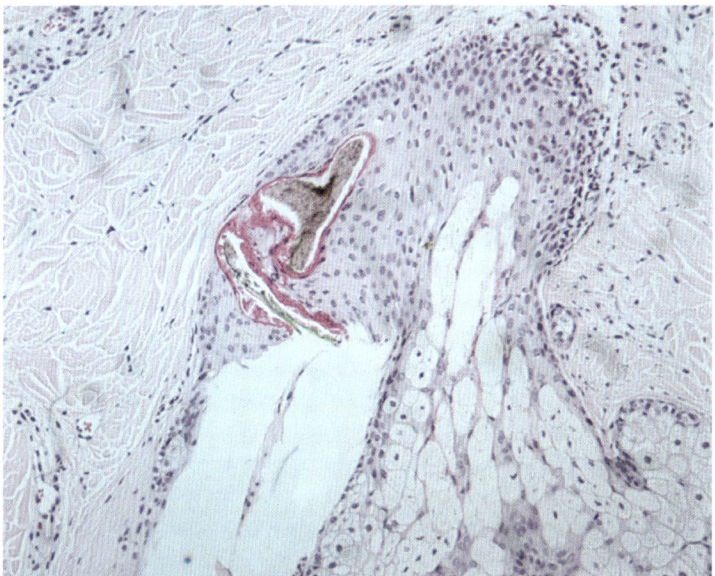

Figure 87.30 Histology of trichotillomania showing fragmentation of the hair shaft.

pubis and perianal region. Repetitive rituals, such as eating or biting hair, after pulling are common. A hairball (trichobezoar) is a rare complication of TTM and may present with abdominal pain, vomiting or bowel obstruction requiring surgical intervention [59].

Differential diagnosis
The minor form in young children can be confused with ringworm or alopecia areata. Alopecia areata may be difficult to exclude with certainty at the first examination, but the course of the condition usually establishes the correct diagnosis. Unlike alopecia areata, it is unusual for hair to be lost completely in TTM and, in contrast with exclamation mark hairs, the broken hairs of TTM are firmly anchored in the scalp. Where doubt remains a skin biopsy will usually establish the correct diagnosis. However, there are reports of the coexistence of alopecia areata and TTM [60]. In rare cases, genetic disorders characterised by increased hair fragility may resemble TTM and should be excluded by hair microscopy.

Investigations
Hair shaft microscopy may identify hairs of different length in an affected area. These may be broken (where trauma has snapped the shaft) or tapered regrowing hairs (where trauma is in the form of plucking). The scalp itself is usually clinically normal except in the instances where the trauma is rubbing or scratching. In these instances, there are often scalp symptoms and the problem may present primarily as a scalp dermatosis – even if it is wholly artefactual. Rubbing can also lead to hair breakage or interfere with the normal anagen cycle without specifically altering the hair shaft.

Several trichoscopy features are described in TTM including broken hairs of differing lengths, black dots, longitudinal split hairs,

irregular coiled hairs, 'hair powder' (residue of totally damaged hair shaft), 'flame hairs' (semitransparent hair residue that is wavy and cone shaped), 'tulip hair' (short hairs with darker tulip-shaped ends) and the 'V sign' (two hairs from one ostia of the same length). Importantly, many of these features may also be seen in alopecia areata, although yellow dots are uncommon in TTM and may help differentiate these conditions [61].

Scalp histology varies according to the severity and duration of the hair plucking, displaying many features also seen in traction alopecia. Increased catagen/telogen numbers and numerous empty canals are the most consistent findings. Some follicles may be severely damaged, showing follicular plugging, clefts in the hair matrix, separation of the follicular epithelium from the surrounding connective tissue sheath, intraepithelial and perifollicular haemorrhage, and intrafollicular pigment casts (Figure 87.30). Injured follicles may form only soft twisted hairs (trichomalacia) [62].

Management
The establishment of a relationship between the physician and the patient, or with the parents of an affected child, is an important step in the management of TTM. A confident diagnosis is essential, but this is not always easy and may require observation over time and sometimes a scalp biopsy.

The habit tic in young children is often self-limiting, but distraction techniques (e.g. furry toys) and sometimes input from a paediatric psychologist may be needed. TTM in adolescents and adults is a different proposition, and can be intractable [63]. Patients with insight should be referred to a psychiatrist or clinical psychologist.

A systematic review and meta-analysis of published studies found cognitive–behavioural therapy with habit reversal training superior to drug treatment and showed the largest benefit in controlling TTM symptoms [64]. Habit reversal training focuses on three main areas: (i) awareness training (to help identify pulling behaviours and triggers); (ii) response training (to develop alternative behaviours to prevent pulling when the urge is there); and (iii) social support (to build support networks and adherence) [65].

Pharmacological therapy may be preferred if cognitive–behavioural therapy and habit reversal training are unsuccessful, if the patient has other co-morbid psychiatric conditions or if they lack insight into the condition. Clomipramine, olanzapine and the glutaminergic agent *N*-acetylcysteine have demonstrated significant benefit over placebo in randomised controlled trials. Importantly, there was no convincing benefit from treatment with selective serotonin reuptake inhibitors [64,66–68]. Electronic awareness devices to alert to pulling behaviour are being developed [69].

Some patients are helped by contact with fellow sufferers, and there are several patient support groups and websites devoted to TTM. Patients who fail to admit the self-inflicted nature of the hair loss present difficulties as they are unlikely to accept psychiatric referral and, as with dermatitis artefacta, a confrontational approach will probably be unsuccessful. Management should be aimed at helping the patient recognise the cause for themselves. This can be a long and slow process requiring skill and empathy on the part of the physician.

Resources

Patient resources

National Health Service (NHS), patient information: https://www.nhs.uk/mental-health/conditions/trichotillomania/.
Trichotillomania Support: https://www.trichotillomania.co.uk/.
(Both last accessed May 2023.)

Psoriatic alopecia

Introduction and general description

Three main types of psoriatic alopecia are described: (i) alopecia localised to psoriatic plaques; (ii) generalised TE associated with erythrodermic/generalised pustular psoriasis; and (iii) scarring psoriatic alopecia (rare) [70]. Interestingly, increased hair growth in psoriasis plaques is also described [71].

Pathophysiology

Perturbed cytokine regulation of sebaceous gland gene signatures and sebaceous gland atrophy in psoriatic alopecia suggest that sebaceous gland dysfunction may underlie this presentation [72]. The cause of scarring psoriasis is less clear; potential causes include coincidence (with psoriasis just coexisting with a separate underlying scarring alopecia process) [73], psoriatic inflammation causing direct HF destruction or a genetic psoriasis variant that predisposes to more severe scalp involvement and scarring [74]. Scratching behaviour and secondary infection may also be a factor.

Clinical features

Hair loss in psoriatic alopecia is usually confined to the psoriasis plaques, with reduced hair density in these areas, which generally regrow when the plaques resolve [75]. However, rare cases of scarring psoriatic alopecia are described, usually in longstanding cases with more severe scalp involvement [74,76]. Here, patchy scarring alopecia with associated psorisiform skin changes is seen.

Investigations

The histopathology features of psoriatic alopecia include typical psoriasis changes in the interfollicular epidermis, reduction in size and number of sebaceous glands, increased catagen and telogen hairs, follicular miniaturisation, variable perifollicular inflammation and infundibular dilatation [75]. In scarring psoriatic alopecia HF fibrosis, follicular infundibular inflammation and overlying psoriasis changes are seen.

Management

Treatment regimens for scalp psoriasis should be followed (Chapter 35).

Tumour necrosis factor inhibitor-associated alopecia

Introduction and general description

The introduction of antitumour necrosis factor (anti-TNF) biological therapy has resulted in a recognition that paradoxical immune reactions, such as psoriasis, vitiligo and patchy alopecia, may develop in people previously unaffected with these conditions when treated with these agents [77]. TNF-inhibitor alopecia typically shows both psorisiform and alopecia areata features; TNF-inhibitor-induced LPP has also been reported [78]. Reassuringly, a recent large population study using the Korean National Insurance database found no significant increased risk for alopecia areata development with anti-TNF therapy in >11 000 cases and matched controls [79].

Pathophysiology

Tumour necrosis factor α regulates the maturation of plasmacytoid dendritic cells that secrete the pro-inflammatory cytokine IFN-α. Thus, TNF inhibition can result in increased plasmacytoid dendritic cell numbers, paradoxically increasing IFN-α expression, which drives the psoriasiform skin changes and hair loss seen. Genetic variations in the TNF pathway may explain why some people develop this complication.

Clinical features

Patchy alopecia with variable surface psorisiform skin changes is characteristic. Proposed diagnostic criteria include (i) recent initiation of anti-TNF treatment; (ii) no prior history of psoriasis (or flare of psoriasis) after starting the anti-TNF treatment; (iii) alopecic plaque(s) on the scalp; and (iv) red scaly patches and/or pustular lesions on the scalp and elsewhere on the body [80]. Typically, this complication appears more common in female patients and those with rheumatoid arthritis or Crohn disease.

Investigations

Histological features are like those of psoriatic alopecia; however, the presence of eosinophils, plasma cells and alopecia areata-like peribulbar lymphocytic inflammation suggests TNF-inhibitor-associated psoriatic alopecia [81].

Management

The type and severity of the adverse skin reaction, and alternative treatment options, should determine the management of this side effect. Treatment with topical anti-inflammatory therapy, methotrexate or ciclosporin may allow ongoing anti-TNF therapy. If the reaction is severe consider stopping the anti-TNF agent and choosing an alternative likely to address the presentation (but note that switching to an alternative anti-TNF generally does not help). Interestingly, for TNF-inhibitor-associated alopecia areata there was no clear difference in alopecia resolution between those who continued or discontinued their anti-TNF therapy [82].

Dupilumab and alopecia areata

Introduction and general description
Dupilumab is a biological agent recently licensed to treat atopic eczema. Reports of both regrowth of coexisting alopecia areata and new-onset alopecia areata-like patchy areas during treatment are described [83].

Pathophysiology
Dupilumab is an anti-IL-4/IL-13 biologic agent that downregulates Th2 cytokine pathways, important in atopic dermatitis pathogenesis. As alopecia areata also has both Th1 and Th2 components, dupilumab may improve hair growth by reducing IL-4-induced inflammatory mediators (e.g. mast cells) and reduce Th2 impact on regulatory T cells (Tregs), allowing hair to regrow [83,84]. In those developing new-onset alopecia areata lesions, the reduced Th2 signals may promote a Th1/Th17 imbalance, predisposing to alopecia areata-like lesion development [84,85].

Clinical features
Regrowth of existing alopecia areata was seen more frequently in women and those with longstanding eczema and multiple associated atopic conditions. Those who developed hair loss during dupilumab treatment were predominantly male with fewer associated atopic co-morbidities. The clinical presentation in these patients was typical alopecia areata patches, or an alopecia areata-like pattern with scalp redness and scaling [84,85].

Management
Dupilumab-induced alopecia areata may be reversible with standard therapy without requiring treatment discontinuation [86].

INFECTIONS AND HAIR LOSS

Tinea capitis

See Chapter 32.

Infestations

See Chapter 34.

Syphilis

Syphilis is a sexually transmitted infection caused by the bacterium *Treponema pallidum*, whose clinical manifestations are variable and often imitate other diseases [1]. Alopecia occurs in approximately 2.9–7% of cases of secondary syphilis and may be the presenting feature [2–4]. The hair loss typically has a moth-eaten appearance, but may be diffuse, mimicking TE [5]. Other features of secondary syphilis are also usually present, including rash (typically involving the palms and soles), malaise, fever, lymph node enlargement and hepatomegaly, although hair loss may be the only sign of infection [4]. Trichoscopy reveals reduced hair density, yellow dots, broken hairs and increased vellus hairs; pigtail and zig-zag hairs are also recognised [6].

Histological features include an increase in catagen and telogen forms, and a peribulbar lymphocytic infiltrate, similar to the changes seen in alopecia areata, although the absence of eosinophils and presence of plasma cells help differentiate syphilis from alopecia areata [5]. The serpiginous nodulo-squamous syphilide of tertiary syphilis may affect the scalp, and syphilitic gumma are a cause of scarring alopecia. See Chapter 29.

Human immunodeficiency virus infection

A variety of alterations in hair growth have been described in patients with human immunodeficiency virus (HIV) infection. Potential triggers include chronic HIV-1 infection itself, secondary infections (e.g. tinea capitis; syphilis), nutritional deficiencies and drugs. Diffuse hair loss is common and associated with lower CD4 counts, potentially representing a clinical marker of disease progression [7,8]. Sudden hair greying [9] and straightening of the hair (independent of nutritional status) in HIV-infected black patients are described [10].

Antiretroviral-induced alopecia is well recognised, with protease inhibitors (particularly indinavir), followed by the nucleoside reverse transcriptase inhibitors (especially lamivudine), being the main culprits. Median time to onset of hair loss was 2.5 months, which resolved by changing the treatment regimen [11].

Several reports associate the onset of alopecia areata in patients with new HIV infection [12–14], although remission of chronic alopecia universalis following HIV diagnosis has also been observed [15].

There are several reports of hypertrichosis of the eyelashes (trichomegaly) in HIV infection [16,17]. The cause of this striking and unusual feature is not known. It is usually associated with advanced disease and has been noted to regress with antiretroviral treatment. Various forms of folliculitis are seen in HIV infection, including acneform eruptions, staphylococcal folliculitis and eosinophilic pustular folliculitis [18]. See Chapter 31.

Herpes infections

Shingles is a common dermatomal blistering rash due to reactivation of the varicella-zoster virus (VZV) in dorsal root nerve ganglia. Herpes-infected cells are frequently identified in HFs, predominantly affecting the bulge and infundibulum – areas with a rich nerve supply [19]. Scalp involvement in VZV may include a dermatomal VZV folliculitis, alopecia areata-like lesions or rarely scarring alopecia [20]. An association between alopecia areata and VZV is reported, with stress, immune dysfunction and HF immune privilege collapse potentially contributing to the observed increased risk [21]. See Chapter 25.

Leprosy

Leprosy is due to an infection with *Mycobacterium leprae* that affects peripheral nerves, usually in areas of the skin with relatively lower temperatures. Clinical manifestations depend on both the number of bacilli present and the host immune response. Although loss of eyebrow and body hair may occur in lepromatous leprosy, the scalp is viewed as relatively immune to infection, probably due to the higher skin temperature in this area [22]. When scalp involvement does occur, hair loss is generally mild. See Chapter 28.

Trichodysplasia spinulosa

Trichodysplasia spinulosa is a rare disease caused by the trichodysplasia-associated polyomavirus (TSPyV) [23,24]. It is reported mainly in patients receiving immunosuppressive drugs, particularly following solid-organ transplantation [25,26], but is also described in HIV infection and lupus erythematosus. Recent evidence suggests that trichodysplasia spinulosa is due to a primary infection with TSPyV, and not virus reactivation [27].

It presents as small, skin-coloured, follicular papules with central keratin spines (spicules) and alopecia [25]. These occur most commonly on the nose and central face, although other sites elsewhere on the skin may also be involved; eyebrow hair loss is common (Figure 87.31).

The histopathology is distinctive, showing a dilated HF, keratin plugging and absent hair shaft with aberrant keratinisation of the IRS containing viral inclusions positive for polyomavirus

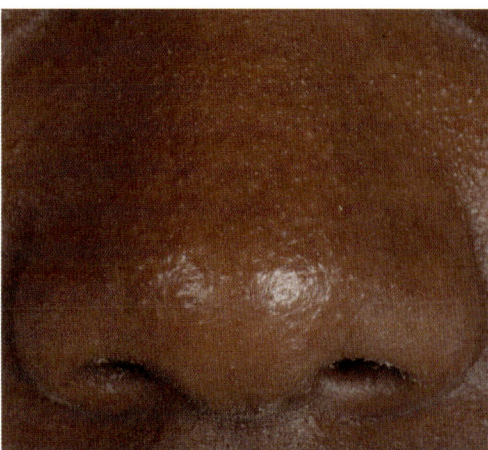

Figure 87.31 Trichodysplasia spinulosa.

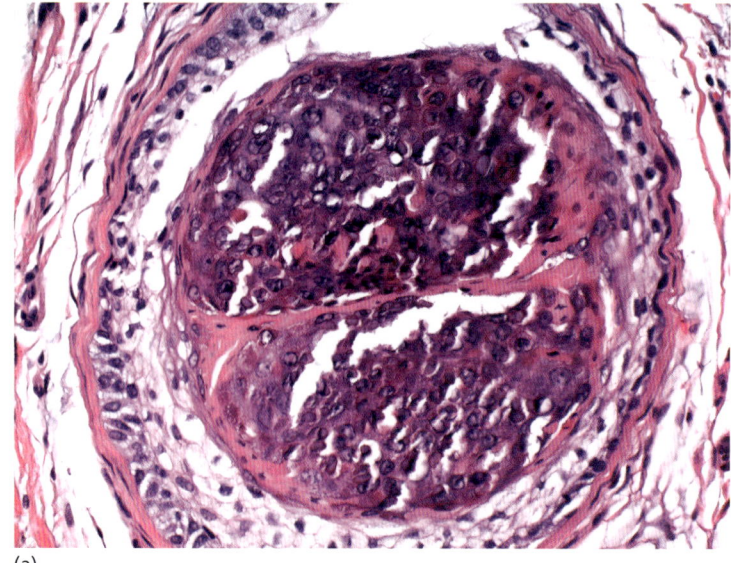

(a)

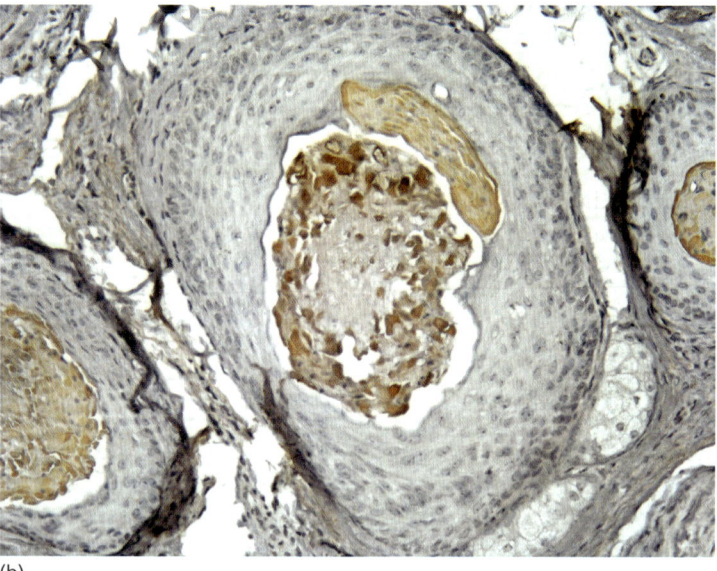

(b)

Figure 87.32 Trichodysplasia spinulosa histopathology. (a) Aberrant keratinisation of the inner root sheath. (b) Positive immunohistochemical staining for polyomavirus in the inner root sheath. Courtesy of Dr Misha Rosenbach and Dr Karolyn A. Wanat.

on immunohistochemistry (Figure 87.32) [24,27–29]. Diagnosis confirmation is by TSPyV polymerase chain reaction [25].

Treatments with reported success include reduction in immunosuppression, 3% topical cidofovir, systemic valganciclovir, physical extraction of spicules and oral leflunomide [25,30].

SCARRING ALOPECIAS

Introduction and general description

Cicatricial or scarring alopecia describes hair loss that occurs as a result of permanent damage to HFs and in which significant hair regrowth is not expected. The term scarring can be considered to describe several pathognomonic features; namely, permanent loss of HF stem cells within the bulge region of the follicle; permanent loss of HFs and their replacement by fibrous stellae; and the absence

Table 87.2 The North American Hair Research Society classification of primary cicatricial alopecias [1].

Inflammatory infiltrate	Diagnosis
Lymphocytic	Chronic cutaneous lupus erythematosus
	Lichen planopilaris (LPP):
	Classic lichen planopilaris
	Frontal fibrosing alopecia
	Graham–Little syndrome
	Classic pseudopelade (of Brocq)
	Central centrifugal cicatricial alopecia
	Alopecia mucinosa
	Keratosis follicularis spinulosa decalvans
Neutrophilic	Folliculitis decalvans
	Dissecting cellulitis/folliculitis
Mixed	Folliculitis (acne) keloidalis (nuchae)
	Folliculitis (acne) necrotica
	Erosive pustular dermatosis
Non-specific/end-stage	

of follicular openings on the scalp surface and a textural change of affected areas of the scalp. Scarring alopecias can be genetic or acquired. Acquired scarring alopecias occur as a result either of a primary disorder of the HF (Table 87.2) or secondary to other skin conditions or trauma that result in follicle destruction. Any hair-bearing skin can be affected by alopecia although most disorders primarily affect the scalp. In contrast to non-scarring alopecias, scarring alopecias are more often associated with symptoms including itch, burning, discomfort, scaling and crusting. The course of scarring alopecias tends to be chronic and treatment is focused on suppression of disease activity to minimise the extent of permanent hair loss. The focus of this section is the acquired primary cicatricial alopecias (PCAs). The generally accepted classification of PCA was devised by the North American Hair Research Society (NAHRS) and is based on the predominant inflammatory infiltrate observed histologically [1].

Epidemiology

Little is known about the prevalence of PCA within the population; however, scarring alopecias occur much less frequently than non-scarring disorders. Previous estimates from specialist hair clinics had shown that between 3.2% and 7.3% of patients with hair loss had a scarring alopecia, with LPP being the most common [2,3]. A 2012 survey of UK dermatologists found PCA to represent around 0.7% of all new dermatology referrals, with general dermatologists seeing an average of 9.6 new PCA cases annually [4]. A recent global point prevalence survey of specialist hair clinics in Europe, North and South America, South Africa and Australia showed that 26.8% of patients had a scarring alopecia. FFA was the commonest scarring condition, comprising 10.8% of all patients seen and 40% of all scarring alopecias [5]. As FFA was first described in 1994 [6] and remained uncommon during the 1990s, this represents a significant rise in incidence.

Pathophysiology

Scarring alopecias are characterised by the permanent loss of eHFSCs from the bulge area within the isthmus of the HF, located close to the insertion of the arrector pili muscle. In PCAs, inflammation at this level of the follicle leads to irreversible loss of stem cells and the inability of the follicle to regenerate during the normal hair cycle, leading to permanent hair loss [7]. The human HF bulge area has been established as a site of relative immune privilege [8], similar to the hair bulb, anterior eye chamber and brain. Within the HF bulge, both MHC class Ia and II are downregulated and there is strong upregulation of the 'no danger' signal CD200. There is also upregulation of so-called HF immune guardians including TGF-β, indoleamine-2,3-dioxygenase, α-MSH and macrophage migration inhibitory factor [9]. Thus, this immune-inhibitory milieu protects eHFSCs from immune-mediated injury.

Understanding of the pathogenesis of PCAs is based on the model of the lymphocytic alopecia LPP [10]. IFN-γ is a key mediator in the pathobiology of many autoimmune disorders and is established as playing a pivotal role in the development of LPP, inducing HF bulge immune privilege collapse and the subsequent immune-mediated keratin 15+ eHFSC destruction and pathological epithelial-to-mesenchymal transition (EMT) [11,12]. Key markers of bulge immune privilege maintenance (CD200, TGF-β_2) are downregulated, while indicators of immune privilege collapse (MHC class I and class II, β2 microglobulin) are upregulated in lesional HFs. IFN-γ-inducible CXCR3-binding chemokines CXCL9–11 are prominently upregulated in lesional bulge cells, and cytotoxic CD8+ T cells and CD123+ IFN-secreting plasmacytoid dendritic cells are increased around affected HFs [13]. Reduced peroxisome proliferator-activated receptor (PPAR)-γ signalling in eHFSCs has been implicated as an early event in LPP pathogenesis [14].

The sequence of events in non-lichenoid primary scarring alopecias (folliculitis decalvans, dissecting cellulitis, etc.) is less well understood. However, destruction of eHFSCs by an inflammatory infiltrate around the HF bulge is the common factor in all PCA pathogenesis. Reports of familial cases of PCA suggest a genetic predisposition and genetic studies have identified candidate genes in FFA [15] and central centrifugal cicatricial alopecia (CCCA) [16,17]. Environmental factors such as infection and trauma may play a role as potential triggers of PCA in genetically susceptible individuals. *Staphylococcus aureus* has long been suspected to play a role in FD [18]. The identification of HF biofilms [19] and an abnormal subepidermal microbiota in FD [20] tends to support a possible role for a microbial trigger. In AKN, skin trauma is one of the factors postulated to trigger the condition [21].

Clinical features

Visible loss of follicular ostia (openings) is the clinical feature common to all scarring alopecias. This is best assessed using an illuminated magnifier such as a dermatoscope. Some degree of scalp textural change such as atrophy or sclerosis may also be noted. Textural changes may be subtle, such as in early FFA, or more marked, as is usually seen with established FD. Although distinctive patterns of inflammation characterise the different PCAs, inflammation may be entirely absent on the scalp surface. In some conditions such as CDLE, scalp dyspigmentation is common, particularly in darker skin types. Symptoms such as itch, pain and dysaesthesia occur more frequently in scarring alopecias than in non-scarring conditions.

Investigations

A clear history of the duration and course of the alopecia is important, as is noting the presence of symptoms such as itch, burning, pain, scaling and crusting. The area of scalp affected will often give a clue to the diagnosis: FFA affects the hairline, FD typically starts around the crown area and AKN localises to the nape of the neck. It is essential to enquire about hair loss at other sites (e.g. eyebrows, limbs) and skin disease elsewhere, including the mouth, nails and genitals. Associated medical conditions such as autoimmune disorders may be relevant and should be noted. Genetic susceptibility to acquired scarring alopecias is described increasingly and family history is of relevance. Finally, hair care and styling practices can have profound effects on hair and scalp, and it is important to record these.

A careful examination of the whole scalp should be undertaken using an illuminated magnifying lamp and a dermatoscope. The extent and distribution of alopecia should be assessed and inflammatory features such as perifollicular redness, follicular hyperkeratosis, scaling, crusting and pustules noted. The absence of follicular openings is best assessed by trichoscopy. A hair pull test at the margins of alopecia patches can help assess disease activity, and easy extraction of any anagen hairs is always pathological. In some conditions such as FFA, hair loss extending beyond the scalp is characteristic and assessment should be made of eyebrows, eyelashes, vellus facial and limb hair. Any skin disease (including the mouth and nails) should be examined.

Although scarring alopecia due to fungal infection is rare in adults, tinea capitis may mimic conditions such as FD [22] and appropriate samples should be taken for mycology. Any pustules should be swabbed for bacterial culture. Although scalp biopsy is often recommended in all cases of scarring alopecia, in practice, if the diagnosis is certain, it may not be necessary. However, when the diagnosis is unclear or it is uncertain clinically whether alopecia is scarring, histological assessment is required. High-quality photographic images are essential in monitoring alopecia and baseline images should be arranged. Taking measurements of frontal hairline recession in FFA and recording dimensions of alopecia patches can also be useful in disease monitoring, as can the use of severity scores which have been developed for several scarring alopecias (FFA, LPP, CCCA and CDLE) [23–27].

Management

The treatment of all scarring alopecias is challenging and it must be made clear to patients that improvement, in terms of significant hair regrowth, is usually not possible. Instead, the aim of treatment is to minimise, and ideally prevent, further hair loss and to reduce symptoms by suppressing inflammation. There are no generally accepted standard therapeutic approaches or guidelines for the management of scarring alopecias. Reports of treatments in the literature are often of small numbers of patients in case series, retrospective reviews or single case reports. There are few controlled trials. Topical minoxidil and, increasingly, low-dose oral minoxidil [28] are often used as an adjunct to anti-inflammatory treatments to maintain or enhance hair density on unaffected scalp, particularly if there is concomitant pattern hair loss. Cosmetic camouflage measures should be discussed at an early stage as these can be of significant benefit to patients' self-confidence. Surgical intervention is sometimes considered in the management of scarring alopecias. For example, chronic stable areas of alopecia may be suitable for scalp reduction surgery, with or without scalp expansion

techniques. Hair transplantation may be considered for some scarring alopecias, although the procedure is generally less successful than for non-scarring alopecias, and the opinion of an experienced hair restoration surgeon is essential.

PRIMARY LYMPHOCYTIC CICATRICIAL ALOPECIAS

Follicular lichen planus

Several variants of follicular lichen planus have been described. Typically, all show the classic clinical features of perifollicular redness, follicular hyperkeratosis and loss of follicular ostia. Histologically, follicular lichen planus is characterised by vacuolar interface change with a moderately dense, perifollicular lichenoid lymphocytic infiltrate around the bulge at the level of the infundibulum and isthmus.

Lichen planopilaris

Introduction and general description

Lichen planopilaris is an uncommon inflammatory scarring alopecia. The typical clinical appearance is of patchy scarring hair loss affecting any area of the scalp. Affected HFs surrounding patches of alopecia typically show perifollicular redness and follicular hyperkeratosis. LPP was previously considered to be the commonest scarring alopecia seen in specialist hair clinics; however, a recent study suggests that FFA, a clinical variant of LPP, is now the commonest scarring alopecia seen in this setting (10.8% versus 7.6% for LPP) [5].

Epidemiology

More women than men are affected, although estimates vary considerably from 2 : 1 and 3 : 1 to 13 : 1 female : male [29–31]. Mean age of onset is generally estimated to be early to mid-fifties [32], although a minority of patients may present in their twenties and thirties [33]. Symptoms of itch, pain and burning are frequent, occurring in around 60% of cases [29]. Loss of facial or body hair is uncommon, occurring in only 1–2.7% [29]. Mucocutaneous lichen planus is found in association with LPP, with reported frequencies varying between 2% and 50% of cases [29,33–35]. Associated autoimmune disorders, most commonly thyroid disease, are seen in around 30% [31,36]. An association with androgen excess/polycystic ovarian syndrome (PCOS) has been reported in women with LPP [36].

Pathophysiology

Lichen planopilaris is the prototypical model of a primary lymphocytic cicatricial alopecia [10]. Disease pathobiology is characterised by a Th1-mediated IFN-γ driven inflammation centred on the bulge area of the HF, leading to loss of keratin 15-positive eHFSCs due to immune privilege collapse and pathological EMT [37]. Cytotoxic CD8+ T cells and CD123+ IFN-secreting plasmacytoid dendritic cells are upregulated along with IFN-γ-inducible CXCR3-binding chemokines CXCL9–11. This results in HF immune privilege collapse, with upregulation of MHC class I and II and β_2-microglobulin, and loss of K15+ CD200+ eHFSCs through

EMT, whereby eHFSCs assume a fibroblast-like morphology. EMT is characterised by reduced expression of the epithelial marker E-cadherin and increased expression of mesenchymal markers such as vimentin and smooth muscle actin, along with snail family transcription factors. These changes result in permanent loss of eHFSCs, impacting the follicle's capacity to regenerate and cycle and ultimately resulting in permanent HF destruction, fibrosis and scarring [13]. The initial events leading to targeted HF bulge inflammation are unclear. However, defective or insufficient PPAR-γ signalling has been implicated. PPAR-γ is a nuclear hormone receptor that regulates gene transcription and is prominently expressed in the human pilosebaceous unit where it is involved in control of lipogenesis and inflammatory gene expression. In LPP it has been demonstrated that expression of PPAR-γ in both affected and unaffected scalp is significantly decreased, resulting in pro-inflammatory lipid production, infiltration of inflammatory cells and destruction of the pilosebaceous unit. Further, targeted deletion of PPAR-γ in mouse follicular stem cells results in a phenotype resembling a scarring alopecia. These studies suggest that PPAR-γ signalling is essential for normal healthy pilosebaceous units [14]. However, the typically patchy phenotype of LPP cannot be explained by reduced PPAR-γ signalling alone, since levels of expression were similarly reduced in both lesional and non-lesional scalps of affected individuals, suggesting additional pathogenic factors must be involved.

There is evidence of a possible role for xenobiotic metabolism of an environmental trigger in LPP pathogenesis. Microarray data from biopsies of unaffected and affected LPP scalps identified aryl hydrocarbon receptor (AhR) signalling as a significant toxicity pathway activated in LPP. Environmental toxins such as dioxin or dioxin-like compounds are known to inhibit the expression of PPAR-γ and exert their biological effects via the AhR [14]. PPAR-γ stimulation also plays a role in the normal function of mitochondria in human HFs, upregulating mitochondrial transcription factor A (TFAM), which is critical for mitochondrial DNA transcription and genome replication. Ultrastructural analysis of the bulge region of LPP scalp biopsies revealed significant abnormalities of mitochondria in both lesional and non-lesional HFs, with TFAM immunoreactivity significantly lower in lesional HFs. When immune privilege collapse was induced in healthy cultured HFs, a significant decrease in TFAM expression was observed in the bulge area. Taken together, these observations suggest a functionally important role for PPAR-γ in eHFSC mitochondrial dysfunction in LPP [38].

Analysis of the inflammatory infiltrate in LPP has revealed the involvement of cells of the innate immune system. An increased number of IL-17A/IL-23-producing IL-23R+ mast cells has been demonstrated, suggesting HF infiltration by mast cells may play a role in the pathogenesis of LPP via the IL-23/IL-17 axis [39]. The finding of increased perifollicular mast cells was confirmed in a second study, with increased degranulated mast cells also observed [40]. Further, increased numbers of IFN-producing CD123+ plasmacytoid dendritic cells have been identified around LPP HFs, as have CD68+ macrophages, the latter particularly prominent within partially destroyed HFs, supporting their function as scavenging phagocytes. Analysis of macrophage polarisation revealed increased numbers of M2 (wound healing CD163+, IL-4 secreting) macrophages in LPP when compared with FFA [40]. Interestingly, increased expression of the Treg marker FOXP3 was also identified

in LPP. Tregs produce TGF-β, an immune privilege guardian, which also acts to drive fibrosis [40].

Clinical features

Lichen planopilaris typically causes discrete patches of scarring alopecia anywhere over the scalp. The patches vary in size and several clinical patterns are recognised. Multiple small patches can result in a 'confetti' or reticular pattern which is easiest to appreciate when hair is cut short (Figure 87.33). Usually, several or multiple patches of alopecia are evident. Within areas of alopecia, the scalp appears pale and mildly atrophic but not red. The classic features of LPP, namely perifollicular redness and follicular hyperkeratosis, are characteristically seen affecting hairs surrounding the alopecia (Figure 87.34); however, in some cases, the typical inflammatory pattern is not present, and this can lead to diagnostic difficulty. In darker skin types, focal postinflammatory dyspigmentation may be present, representing resolving perifollicular lichenoid inflammation. Symptoms are common in LPP, with pruritus, burning and discomfort frequently described. Localised symptoms may correlate with focal disease activity and their presence can be used to direct topical or intralesional treatment. Although classic LPP can affect HFs extending beyond the scalp, this occurs much less frequently than with FFA. Loss of eyebrows, eyelashes or vellus facial hair is

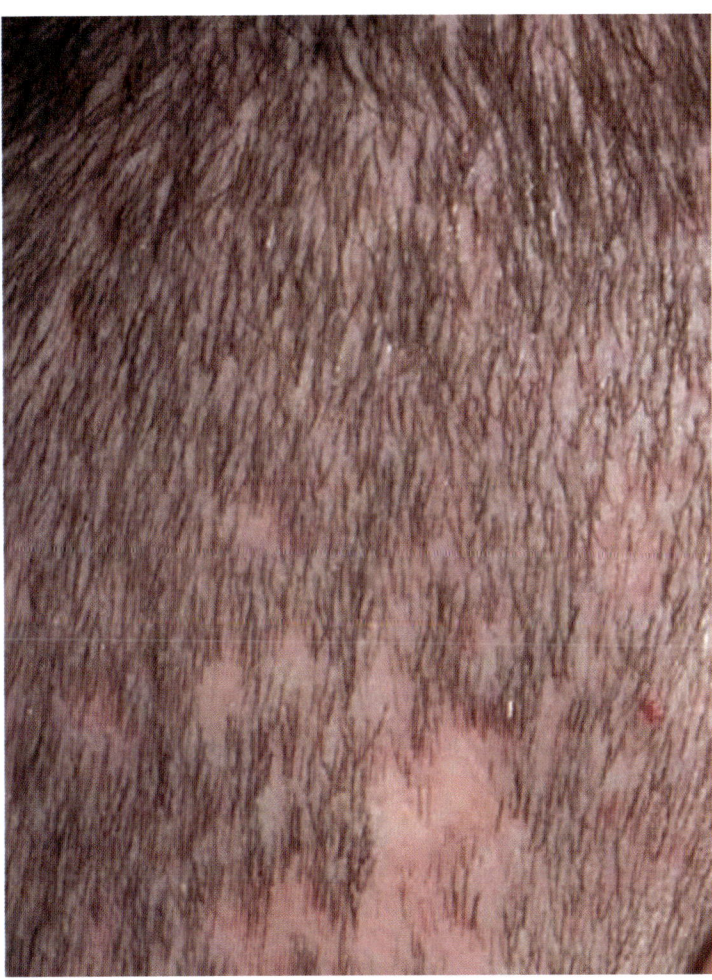

Figure 87.33 Lichen planopilaris showing multiple small patches of scarring alopecia, best appreciated when the hair is cut short.

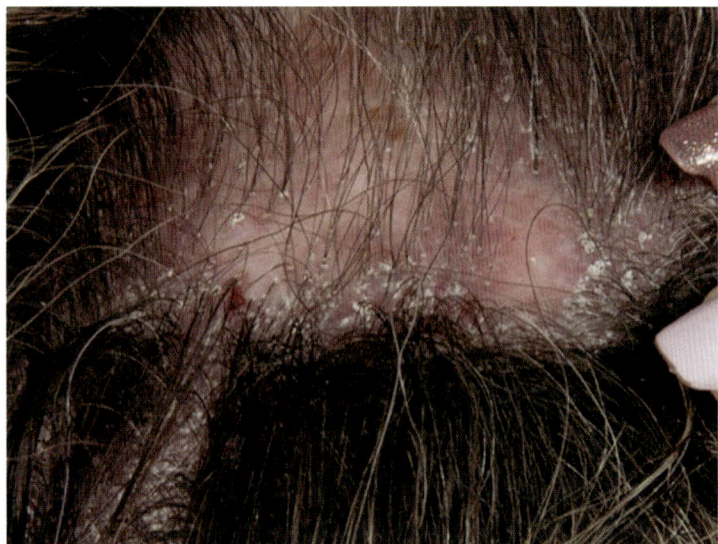

Figure 87.34 Lichen planopilaris showing central scarring alopecia with prominent perifollicular hyperkeratosis at the edge of the patch.

rarely reported with classic LPP but is a common feature of FFA. Loss of limb and torso hair is reported in 1–2.7% of LPP cases [29]. Lichen planus affecting the skin, mucosal sites (oro-pharyngeal, genital) or nails may occur. Reported estimates vary considerably between 2% and 50% of cases. More recent reviews of LPP report associated lichen planus in 2–21% of cases [29,33,35]. Trichoscopy of LPP reveals an absence of follicular openings, scarred white patches, follicular hyperkeratosis, perifollicular redness and blue-grey dots [41].

Differential diagnosis
When the typical features of LPP are present the diagnosis may be straightforward. However, when clinical inflammation is lacking, diagnosis is more challenging. Non-inflammatory LPP may initially be misdiagnosed as alopecia areata: when inactive, the typical features of alopecia areata (exclamation mark hairs, cadaver hairs) can be entirely absent and the affected scalp may be slightly depressed. Close inspection for follicular openings should be undertaken and if there is uncertainty, a biopsy to assess for scarring should be performed. In FFA, a minority of patients also have classic LPP affecting the scalp. A lack of hairline involvement, sparing of limb and facial hair (eyebrows, lashes and vellus hairs), tends to suggest classic LPP rather than FFA/LPP. PB can be indistinguishable from non-inflammatory LPP and there has been much debate as to whether these conditions represent the same entity [42].

Investigations
Histology is usually required to confirm a clinical suspicion of LPP. Biopsies should ideally be taken from actively inflamed hair-bearing skin at the edge of an area of alopecia, and trichoscopy can aid identification of suitable biopsy sites. Histology of early lesions shows vacuolar interface change with a moderately dense perifollicular lichenoid lymphocytic cell infiltrate at the level of the infundibulum and isthmus (Figure 87.35). Occasionally, the interfollicular epidermis may have an associated lichenoid infiltrate. End-stage LPP will show loss of elastic fibres in a superficial, dermal, wedge-shaped scar and loss of sebaceous glands. Direct

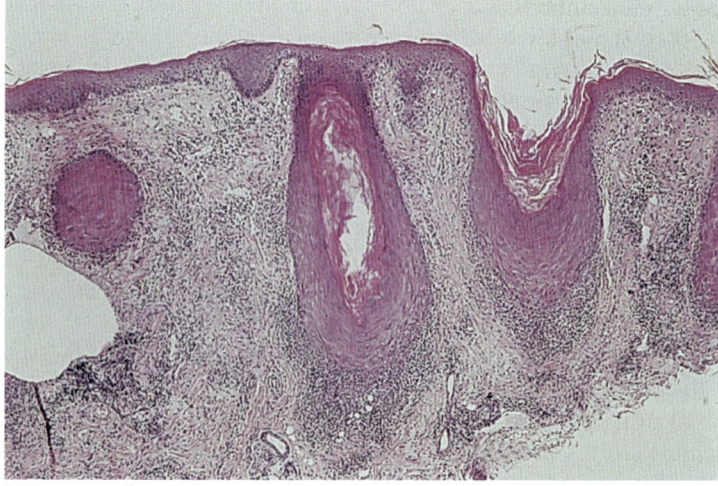

(a)

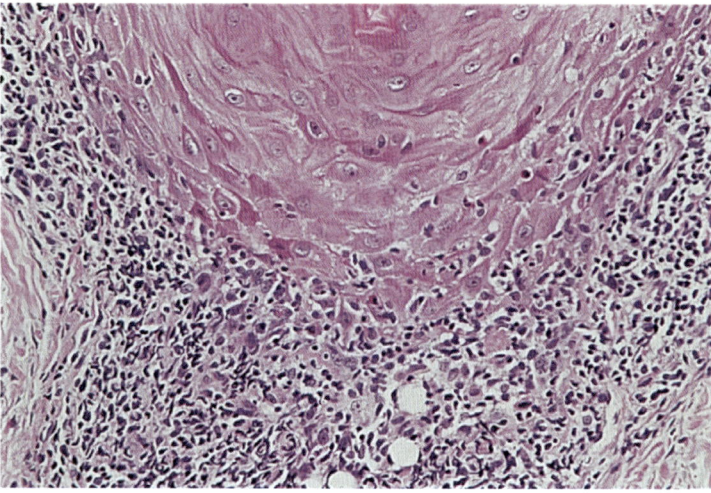

(b)

Figure 87.35 Lichen planopilaris. (a) Low-power photomicrograph showing follicular plugging and a periappendageal inflammatory infiltrate. (b) Base of the hair follicle showing hydropic degeneration of the basal layer and a lichenoid mononuclear cell infiltrate.

immunofluorescence highlights the presence of colloid bodies in the peri-infundibular/isthmic area staining with immunoglobulin M (IgM) [43].

Management
Serial photography can be useful in disease monitoring, as can measurements of larger areas of alopecia. A disease activity score has been developed (lichen planopilaris activity index or LPPAI) which scores symptoms, signs, disease activity and spreading [25]. Very potent topical steroid scalp applications should be prescribed in all cases and can provide symptomatic relief. Systemic treatment is usually required in all but the mildest of cases [44]. However, there are no evidence-based treatment guidelines. Hydroxychloroquine is the most frequently prescribed first option [45]. Methotrexate, mycophenolate mofetil and ciclosporin are considered second line options [25,46,47]. Systemic steroids are rarely used long term but short courses can be of value in rapidly progressive disease. Pioglitazone, a PPAR-γ agonist, has been tried with varying success [48,49]. Other treatments reported to be of benefit include

tetracycline antibiotics [50], oral retinoids [51], platelet-rich plasma (PRP) [52] and low-level light [53]. Given the similarities in pathobiology between LPP and alopecia areata, JAK inhibitors have also been tried in a small number of patients with benefit [54,55]. The prognosis for LPP is variable. Hair loss can remain minimal in some patients while for others there may be almost complete scalp hair loss.

Frontal fibrosing alopecia

Introduction and general description

Frontal fibrosing alopecia was first described in the early 1990s [6] and is generally agreed to be a clinical variant of LPP. However, in addition to having a distinct clinical phenotype, there are differences between FFA and LPP with regards to epidemiology, demographics and disease associations.

Epidemiology

Frontal fibrosing alopecia is now reported as the commonest scarring alopecia, comprising 10.8% of all alopecia patients seen and 40% of all scarring alopecias [5]. Initially described affecting postmenopausal women, this group remains the most affected (female : male 19 : 1), although increasing numbers of men and premenopausal women are reported [56]. Average age at diagnosis ranges between late fifties and 60 years, although several studies have shown that affected males appear to develop the condition earlier (median age 44–45 years) [5,56]. Although it has been reported in all ethnic groups, it is reported most frequently in white women (Fitzpatrick skin type II/III). Associated autoimmune disease is reported more commonly than in the general population, particularly thyroid disease, occurring in around a third of cases [56]. Reports of small numbers of familial cases have suggested a genetic predisposition. However, the increased incidence observed globally over the last 25 years has led to speculation regarding possible environmental trigger factors.

Pathophysiology

Genetic susceptibility has been confirmed by a GWAS involving 1016 UK and Spanish women and 4145 controls. Four genomic loci were identified including within the HLA region 6p21.1, where the class I allele HLA-B*07:02 has been implicated in conferring a fivefold increase in risk of FFA. A missense variant in CYP1B1 (also known as xenobiotic mono-oxygenase/aryl hydrocarbon hydroxylase), an enzyme involved in cellular xenobiotic metabolism and oxidative metabolism of oestrogens, was identified at 2p22.2. Supporting a role for T-cell dysfunction in FFA pathobiology was the finding of a likely causal allele at 8q24.22 within intron 1 of the ST3GAL1 gene encoding galactoside sialyltransferase, an enzyme linked to T-cell activation and homeostasis [15].

The pathobiology of FFA has been considered to be similar to that of LPP, namely a Th1-mediated IFN-γ-driven inflammation centred on the bulge area of the HF leading to immune privilege collapse and EMT and permanent destruction of eHFSCs [13]. Two recent studies have undertaken detailed immune profiling of FFA [40,57]. Both have shown increased CD8+ cytotoxic T cells, dendritic cells, FoxP3+ Tregs and mast cells. In addition, reverse transcription polymerase chain reaction analysis in one study demonstrated significant upregulation of Th1 pathways (IFN-γ, CXCL9 and 10), JAK signalling (STAT1, JAK3) and fibrosis-related markers such as vimentin (a marker of EMT). Although significant downregulation of K15+ CD200+ eHFSCs was demonstrated, there was not a complete loss of stem cell signalling. Intriguingly, one study demonstrated that while CD68+ macrophages are increased in both FFA and LPP, differences in macrophage polarisation were noted between the conditions, with M2 (wound healing type) polarisation in LPP. Taken together, these observations provide an insight into disease pathobiology that offers the prospect of novel disease-specific targeted therapy.

The striking rise in incidence over the past 25 years has led to debate regarding possible causes. Any possible trigger(s) for FFA must be biologically plausible and explicable in terms of the emergence and rapid rise in incidence since the mid-1990s. Associations have been demonstrated with use of sunscreens [58,59], however causality remains to be proven [60,61]. The finding of a missense variant in CYP1B1, an enzyme involved in oestrogen metabolism, implicates a possible role for exogenous hormones [15]. Increased rates of positive patch tests to allergens including fragrances (linalool, balsalm of Peru) have been reported in FFA [58,62] but the significance of these findings is unclear [63]. Low levels of androgens have been reported in women with FFA, in contrast to LPP where an association with androgen excess/PCOS has been documented [36]. However, another study showed that hormonal status in female patients with FFA was mainly normal [56]. A potential relationship between age-related decline in dehydroepiandrosterone (DHEA) activity, PPAR activity and FFA has been highlighted. DHEA is an immunomodulatory hormone essential for PPAR function. PPAR is a negative regulator of TGF-β_1-induced fibrosis and reduced PPAR-γ signalling has been implicated in the pathogenesis of LPP. Loss of PPAR function due to declining DHEA levels may result in impaired control of fibrosis by PPAR [64]. However, normal age-related decline in hormone levels alone would not explain the increase in FFA cases observed in recent years.

Clinical features

Frontal fibrosing alopecia is characterised by a band-like recession of the frontal hairline. The typical features of follicular LP, namely perifollicular redness and follicular hyperkeratosis, can be seen in most cases (Figure 87.36), although sometimes these features may be absent. Recession of the hairline results in a pale, rather atrophic band of alopecia over the frontal scalp which can be striking when contrasted with a sun-damaged forehead. Residual 'lonely' hairs are seen frequently. Any area of the hairline may be affected, with the temporal hairline the most frequently involved area after the frontal hairline. Here, hair thinning can be seen before hairline recession occurs. Occipital hairline recession is reported in 26–31% [56,65]. A minority of FFA patients (around 15%) also have classic LPP elsewhere on the scalp [56,65]. Scalp symptoms such as pruritus and dysaesthesia occur in a minority (79% no or mild pruritus [56]) and are less common than with LPP. Non-inflammatory loss of eyebrows is characteristic of FFA and is reported in 82–90.6% of cases [56,65] and may precede hairline loss [66]. Eyelash loss occurs less frequently (44.5%) [65]. Loss of vellus facial hairs is common but often unrecognised. This feature may help differentiate early FFA from early FPHL. Flesh-coloured

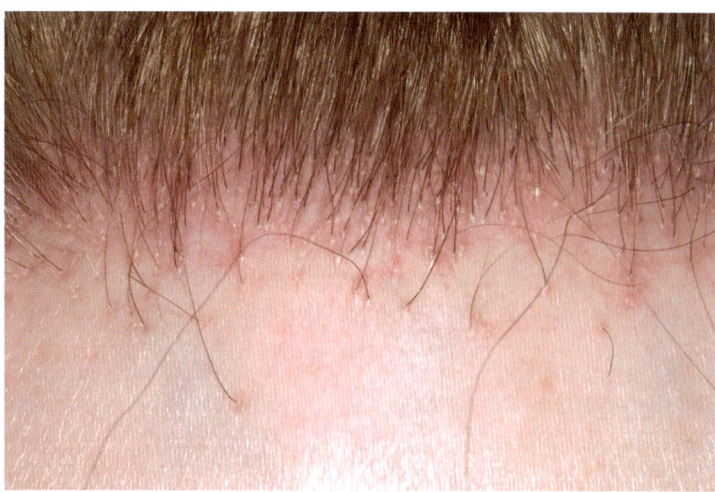

Figure 87.36 Frontal fibrosing alopecia showing perifollicular redness and scale involving the frontal hairline. A loss of follicular ostia and lonely hairs are also seen.

facial papules are seen around the temples in up to 40% of women and may be commoner in premenopausal Hispanic/Latino women and men [67]. Yellowish facial papules may also be seen affecting the temples, cheeks and lateral chin and appear to be due to prominent sebaceous glands on a background of poor connective tissue support. Follicular/glabellar red dots [68] and reticulate and diffuse rosacea-like redness may be seen on facial and extrafacial skin [67]. Dyspigmentation is common in darker skin types and overlaps with lichen planus pigmentosus [69,70]. Depression of frontal veins appears to be a unique finding associated with FFA, although the role of topical steroids in the aetiology of this feature is uncertain [71]. Non-inflammatory loss of limb hair is also common (45–77%) [56,65,72], although rarely complained of by women, and may predate scalp and facial hair loss [66]. In men, loss of the beard hair (55%) [56] and sideburns [73] is seen frequently and loss of limb hair is more easily appreciated. Associated mucocutaneous lichen planus is uncommon, reported in 9.5% of cases [65]. Trichoscopic features of FFA are indistinguishable from those of LPP and include the absence of follicular openings, scarred white patches, follicular hyperkeratosis, perifollicular redness and blue-grey dots [41].

Differential diagnosis

When the typical inflammatory features of FFA are absent, ophiasis-pattern alopecia areata should be excluded. In the early stages of FFA, if inflammatory features are not prominent at the frontal hairline, Hamilton–Norwood pattern hair loss should be excluded. The loss of vellus hairs on the forehead favours a diagnosis of FFA. Traction alopecia commonly occurs at the frontal and temporal hairline and exclusion relies on a good history of hair-styling practices. The fringe sign (retained hairs at the original hairline) is typical of traction alopecia; however, a pseudo-fringe sign can also be seen with FFA [74]. The gradual progressive loss of facial and body hair tends to support a diagnosis of FFA. In a reported 40% of cases, thinning and loss of eyebrows may precede hairline change and isolated eyebrow loss should prompt consideration of a diagnosis of FFA [75].

Investigations

A diagnosis of FFA can usually be made clinically. However, if there is diagnostic doubt, scalp biopsy should be undertaken. Histologically, the features are those of LPP – namely, vacuolar interface change with a moderately dense perifollicular lichenoid lymphocytic cell infiltrate at the level of the infundibulum and isthmus, concentric perifollicular fibrosis, reduced HF density and loss of sebaceous glands in end-stage disease [43]. Histopathology of non-scalp sites (eyebrow and limb) shows similar features [72]. A series of 21 eyebrow biopsies showed preservation of sebaceous glands in 38%, which the authors proposed may account for the observation of eyebrow regrowth seen in some cases of FFA [76]. Interestingly, biopsies from clinically normal scalp skin in patients with FFA/LPP showed lymphocytic perifollicular inflammation around the isthmus/infundibulum areas (65%) and perifollicular fibrosis (15%), suggesting more generalised scalp involvement than is evident clinically [77]. Histology of facial papules has shown features similar to scalp biopsies, with perifollicular lichenoid infiltrate around vellus follicles [78]. However, other studies of facial papules have shown prominent sebaceous lobules associated with an abnormal elastic framework [79].

Management

Assessment and monitoring of FFA can be challenging. The condition tends to progress slowly, and progression may occur only focally. The presence or absence of inflammatory signs (perifollicular redness, follicular hyperkeratosis) is often a poor guide to disease activity [80]. Serial photography can be useful in disease monitoring, as can hairline measurements. In addition, several severity scores have been developed [23,24,81]. Assessments of treatment efficacy need to be undertaken over an appropriate timeframe as the condition generally progresses slowly. Potent or very potent topical steroids are frequently prescribed for the affected hairline [56]. As these are often prescribed for prolonged periods, the frequency of application may require to be modified to minimise skin atrophy, which is also a feature of the condition [82]. The frequent use of topical steroids can lead to telangiectasia which may be misinterpreted as persisting perifollicular redness [83]. Topical tacrolimus and pimecrolimus are steroid alternatives, although ointment preparations are of limited usefulness on the scalp. They can also be applied to the eyebrow area. Intralesional steroids can be used to treat the entire hairline and are also useful where disease is focally active. A range of systemic treatments have been tried but there are no clinical trials or evidence-based guidelines to inform practice. Tetracycline antibiotics and hydroxychloroquine are relatively safe first treatment choices. Thereafter, options include retinoids (isotretinoin, acitretin, alitretinoin) [84], immunomodulators (methotrexate, mycophenolate mofetil, ciclosporin) and the PPAR-γ agonist pioglitazone. The 5α reductase inhibitors finasteride and dutasteride are also widely prescribed. Isotretinoin is reported to be of value in the treatment of facial papules [85] and dyspigmentation [86]. Given the similarities between the inflammatory profiles of FFA and alopecia areata, JAKI has been tried in small numbers of patients and further evaluation of these drugs in this condition is merited [54,55]. The prognosis for FFA is variable. Some patients develop extraordinarily little hairline recession even on no treatment, while others may experience hairline recession to the crown. Complete hair loss from FFA has not been reported.

Fibrosing alopecia in a pattern distribution

Introduction and general description
Fibrosing alopecia in a pattern distribution (FAPD) was first described in 2000 [87] and is a progressive cicatricial alopecia characterised by scarring hair loss on the central frontal scalp in the distribution of typical male (Hamilton–Norwood) or female (Ludwig) pattern hair loss. The condition is considered a composite of patterned hair loss and LPP, showing clinical and histological features of both.

Epidemiology
In a recent review of alopecias seen at specialist hair clinics, FAPD represented 1.8% of all alopecias (6.8% of all scarring alopecias) and most cases were postmenopausal females (89% female, median age 59 years) [5]. A Chilean study found FAPD affecting 0.64% ($n = 13$, 70% female) of all cases of alopecia seen over a 4-year period [88]. Familial cases are rarely reported. Anti-Ro antibodies have been identified in a small number of cases [89].

Pathogenesis
The pathobiology of FAPD is uncertain. It is classified as a variant of LPP; however, it has been suggested that in immunogenetically susceptible patients, it may represent a lichenoid reaction triggered by an unknown antigenic stimulus on HFs during miniaturisation [87].

Clinical features
Clinically, the typical features of follicular lichen planus are present, namely perifollicular redness, follicular hyperkeratosis and loss of follicular openings. In addition, affected follicles show features of patterned hair loss including anisotrichosis (variable hair diameter) and an increased proportion of follicular openings with single hairs. Unlike classic LPP, hair thinning is diffuse and symmetrical, not patchy. Symptoms including scalp dysaesthesia and itch occur in around a third of cases. Other reported clinical features include facial papules, reticulate red dots over the anterior chest and, rarely, involvement of eyebrows (reviewed in [90]).

Differential diagnosis
It is likely that FAPD is underrecognised and misdiagnosed. Where the diagnosis is considered, the main differential diagnosis to take into account is patterned alopecia with concurrent seborrhoeic dermatitis [90].

Investigations
As FAPD is rare, histopathological correlation is generally required. The histological features are those of both LPP and patterned hair loss; namely, HF miniaturisation and vacuolar interface change around the isthmus and infundibulum, with loss of HFs and replacement with fibrous tracts [90].

Management
There is little evidence to guide treatment of this condition. Documented management strategies are directed at the management of patterned hair loss (topical minoxidil, anti-androgens, e.g. finasteride) and anti-inflammatory drugs (potent topical steroids, hydroxychloroquine) [90].

Graham-Little–Piccardi–Lassueur syndrome

Introduction and general description
Graham-Little–Piccardi–Lassueur syndrome (GLPLS) is a rarely reported cicatricial alopecia described as a variant of LPP, occurring more frequently in women.

Epidemiology
In a recent survey of specialist hair clinics, only one case of GLPLS was reported (0.03% of 3133 diagnoses of alopecia) [5]. It is not clear whether it is a distinct entity or represents disseminated LPP of the scalp, flexures, torso and limbs.

Clinical features
The diagnosis of GLPLS is suggested by a patchy scarring alopecia, non-scarring hair loss of the axillae and pubic skin and keratosis pilaris-like hyperkeratotic papules on the torso and limbs.

Differential diagnosis
Disseminated LPP may be indistinguishable from GLPLS.

Investigations
Biopsies of affected HFs show a lichenoid folliculitis identical to LPP [43].

Management
Treatments reported in a small number of cases are like those used in the management of LPP and include topical and intralesional steroids, hydroxychloroquine, doxycycline and ciclosporin.

Chronic discoid lupus erythematosus

Introduction and general description
Chronic discoid lupus erythematosus is a chronic scarring photosensitive dermatosis, which is part of the disease spectrum of lupus erythematosus. See Chapter 51.

Epidemiology
It is the most common form of cutaneous lupus seen in dermatological practice and scalp involvement is frequent. In a recent point prevalence survey of specialist hair clinics, CDLE represented 1.9% of all alopecia diagnoses. It was more common in females (88% female; female : male 7 : 1) and those of African descent and represented 7.1% of scarring alopecias [5]. However, many cases of CDLE are managed in a general dermatology setting rather than a specialist hair clinic and it is likely that CDLE represents a greater proportion of the total burden of cicatricial alopecias.

Pathophysiology
The pathogenesis of cutaneous lupus is covered in detail in Chapter 51. Briefly, both genetic susceptibility and environmental

triggers (primarily UV light) play a role in disease pathogenesis. Several major and non-major histocompatibility complex genetic polymorphisms have been identified. Most of these genetic variants are associated with mechanisms attributed to disease pathogenesis, including pathways involved in IFN and vitamin D regulation, and UV light exposure [91]. DNA from UV-induced apoptotic keratinocytes and neutrophils activates the innate immune system via Toll-like receptors on plasmacytoid dendritic cells, upregulating type 1 IFN expression. Inflammatory mediators including IFN-γ, CXCL9 and CXCL10 drive continued recruitment of inflammatory cells [92]. Release of IFN-γ by Th1 cells initiates activation of the JAK/STAT pathway, suggesting a possible role for JAK inhibitors in treatment [93].

Clinical features

It typically presents as one or more discoid red scaly patches on the scalp with scarring hair loss (Figure 87.37). In the early stages, the affected areas may be diffusely red and as the disease progresses, pale depressed areas of atrophic scarring alopecia appear centrally. There is often marked hyperkeratosis, and follicular plugging (carpet-tack scale) is a characteristic feature of CDLE (see Figure 87.14e). Redness and hyperkeratosis do not localise to HFs as is typical with LPP, and when the condition is active, inflammatory activity is most pronounced centrally within the area of scarring hair loss. Lesions are typically pruritic when active. In darker skinned individuals, marked dyspigmentation may occur. Trichoscopy shows an absence of follicular openings and scarred white patches, identical to those seen in LPP. Prominent features in CDLE include follicular keratotic plugs, follicular red dots and telangiectasia. Blue-grey dots represent follicular pigment incontinence [41].

Differential diagnosis

When the typical inflammatory features of CDLE are present clinically and histologically, diagnosis is usually straightforward. In the absence of active inflammation, other scarring alopecias such as LPP and PB should be excluded.

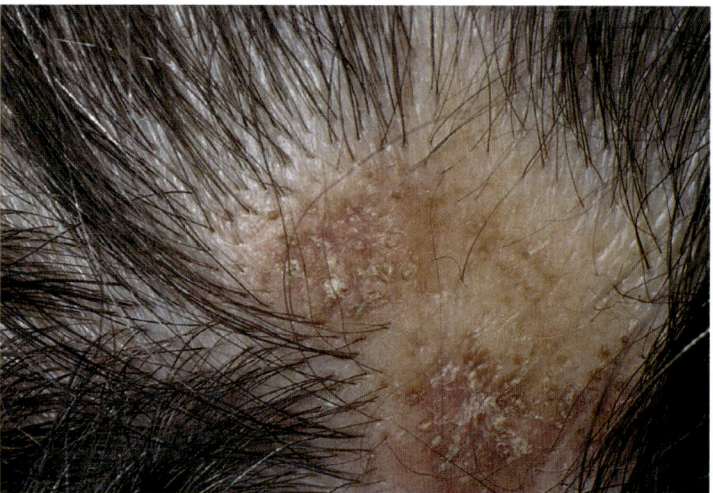

Figure 87.37 Discoid lupus erythematosus showing scarring alopecia with scalp redness and follicular plugging.

Investigations

Skin biopsy is generally performed to confirm a diagnosis of CDLE, and the histological features are usually unequivocal. The finding of CDLE on the scalp should prompt careful examination of the skin elsewhere, especially sun-exposed sites such as the face and neck. ANA ± extractable nuclear antigen (ENA), anti-dsDNA, FBC, biochemical profile, erythrocyte sedimentation rate (ESR) and urinalysis should be undertaken along with a careful history and assessment for systemic symptoms of lupus. Histopathological features include follicular hyperkeratosis and a vacuolar interface folliculitis at the level of the infundibulum. The interfollicular epidermis may also show vacuolar interface change. Superficial and deep perivascular and periappendageal lymphoid and plasma cell infiltrate are typical (Figure 87.38). Late stages are characterised by concentric lamellar perifollicular fibroplasia and by basement membrane zone thickening (highlighted by periodic acid–Schiff). Suprabasal dyskeratosis, pigmentary incontinence and dermal mucin may also be seen. Direct immunofluorescence will confirm the diagnosis with granular deposits of IgG and C3 along the epidermal and follicular basement membrane zone (Figure 87.39) [43].

Management

Very potent topical steroids are first line management for CDLE and can be useful for symptomatic relief. Intralesional steroids can be useful in focally stubborn disease. In many cases, systemic treatment is required, and hydroxychloroquine is the most effective treatment option in most cases (although efficacy is reduced by smoking). Second line options include methotrexate, mycophenolate mofetil and azathioprine. Newer agents such as biologics (rituximab, belimumab) may be used in the context of severe extensive cutaneous disease unresponsive to second line agents [94].

Pseudopelade of Brocq

Introduction and general description

Pseudopelade of Brocq is a rare, chronic, patchy scarring alopecia first described in 1888. It is classified as a primary lymphocytic alopecia under the NAHRS classification of PCAs [1]. However, it is a somewhat controversial entity as there are no specific diagnostic patterns of inflammation clinically or histologically. Given this absence of specific clinical and histological features, there has been uncertainty as to whether PB is a specific disease entity or represents the end stage of other cicatricial alopecias such as LPP or CDLE. PB diagnostic criteria were proposed by Braun-Falco and include typical clinical features (irregularly defined and confluent patches of atrophic alopecia; female > male; prolonged slowly progressive course, which may remit spontaneously) and histological findings (scarring/fibrotic streamers; reduced or absent sebaceous glands; normal epidermis; absence of inflammation and follicular plugging; negative immunofluorescence) [95]. A histological study reviewing biopsies of PB cases diagnosed using the Braun-Falco criteria found that around two-thirds of cases showed histological features of either LPP or CDLE [96]. More recently, a comparison of gene expression profiles in scalp biopsies taken from untreated active cases of LPP and PB diagnosed clinically suggested that these two

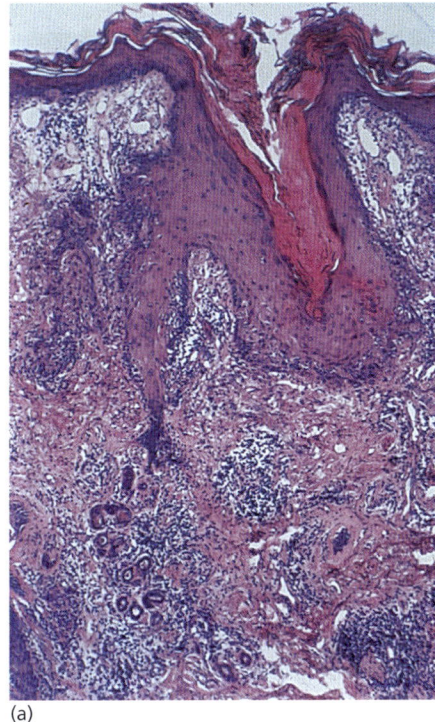

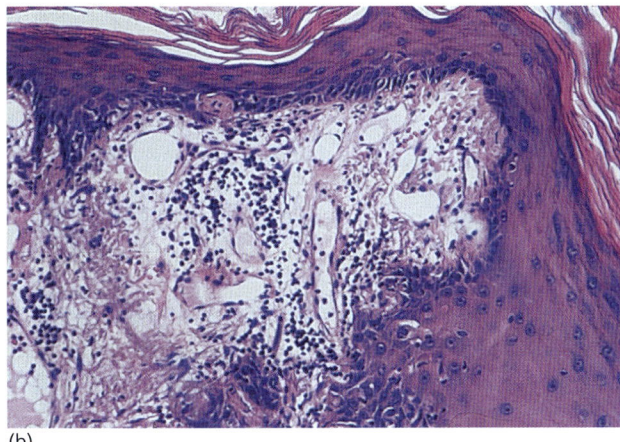

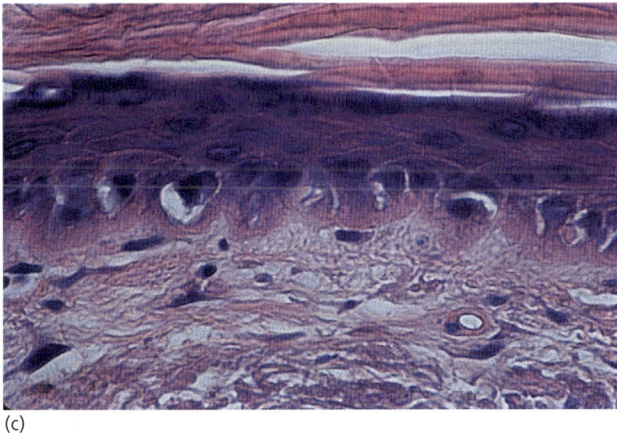

Figure 87.38 Discoid lupus erythematosus. (a) Low-power photomicrograph showing follicular plugging and superficial and deep perivascular and periappendageal lymphocytic infiltrate. (b) High-power photomicrograph showing hydropic degeneration of the basal layer and the mononuclear cell infiltrate. (c) Higher-power photomicrograph showing hydropic degeneration of the basal layer. Courtesy of Dr G. Mason, Melbourne, Australia.

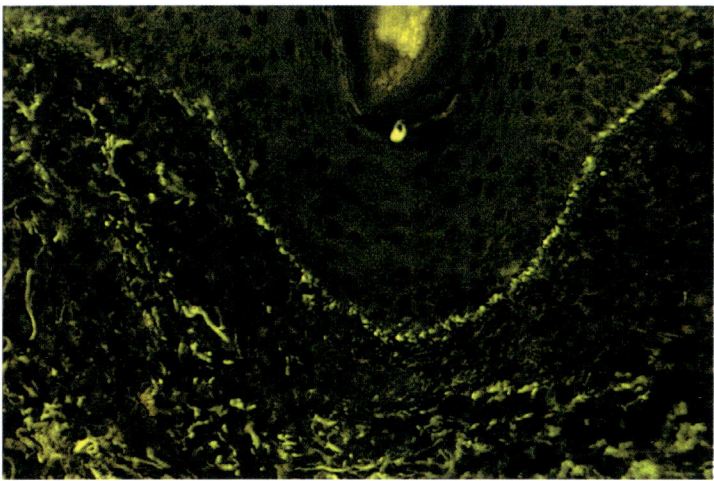

Figure 87.39 Positive linear immunofluorescence to IgG: the lupus band test. Courtesy of Dr G. Mason, Melbourne, Australia.

conditions are distinct and unrelated. Of 504 genes differentially expressed between LPP and PB with statistical significance, 479 genes were upregulated and 25 downregulated in LPP as compared with PB. Only 35 genes were similarly expressed in both LPP and PB compared with normal scalp [42].

Epidemiology

In a review of alopecias seen at specialist hair clinics, only one case of PB was reported (0.03% of 3133 diagnoses of alopecia) [5]. It is predominantly described in white females aged 30–50 years.

Pathophysiology

The pathogenesis of PB is unknown.

Clinical features

The characteristic features of PB are small, discrete, depressed, pale ovoid patches of scarring alopecia, usually starting around the vertex, and extending over the central and parietal scalp (Figure 87.40). Classically, the patches are described as 'footprints in the snow'. There is no inflammation evident clinically either within or surrounding the patches and the patches are soft and non-indurated. Over time, the areas of alopecia may coalesce into larger irregular areas of hair loss. The condition generally progresses slowly.

Differential diagnosis

The appearance of asymptomatic non-inflammatory patches of scalp hair loss may prompt a diagnosis of alopecia areata and a scalp biopsy should be performed to identify whether scarring is present. It may be difficult to confidently distinguish between PB and the end stage of other scarring alopecias such as CDLE or LPP. CDLE may be excluded based on history (itch, redness, scaling, photosensitive rashes, etc.) and typical histological features. LPP can be diagnosed if a lichenoid folliculitis (perifollicular redness, follicular hyperkeratosis) is identified on careful examination of the scalp and typical histological features are present. A history of mucocutaneous lichen planus would tend to support a diagnosis of LPP.

PART 8: SPECIFIC CUTANEOUS STRUCTURES

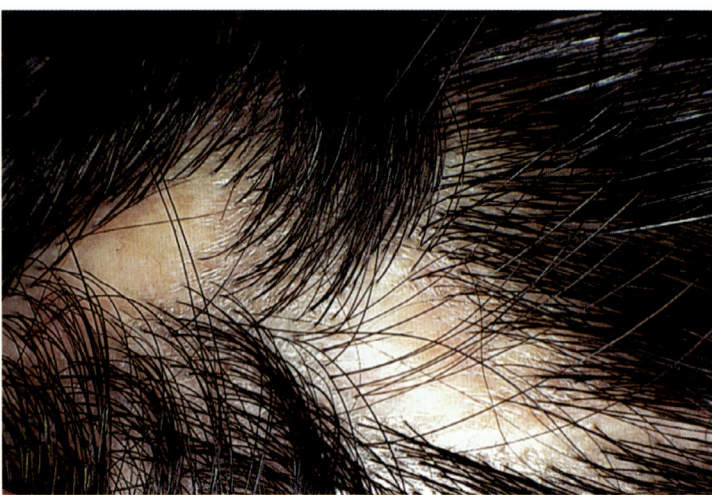

Figure 87.40 Pseudopelade of Brocq.

Investigations

Pseudopelade of Brocq is a diagnosis of exclusion so scalp biopsy is generally recommended. Histopathology shows non-specific features of an end-stage scarring alopecia, with concentric perifollicular lamellar fibrosis, loss of sebaceous glands, loss of follicular units with follicular scars and a minimal residual inflammatory cell infiltrate [43].

Management

The literature on treatment of PB is limited and options which have been tried are generally those used in the management of LPP; namely, very potent or intralesional steroids, hydroxychloroquine, oral steroids and mycophenolate mofetil [97].

Central centrifugal cicatricial alopecia

Synonyms and inclusions
- Follicular degeneration syndrome
- Hot-comb alopecia

Introduction and general description

Central centrifugal cicatricial alopecia is a chronic, progressive, scarring alopecia affecting the vertex and central scalp.

Epidemiology

It occurs almost exclusively in black women of African ancestry, in whom it is the most common cause of scarring hair loss [98]. Severe disease has been estimated to affect 2.7–5.6% of black women [99,100]. In a recent global survey of alopecia patients seen at specialist hair clinics, CCCA represented 1% of all alopecia diagnoses and 3.6% of all cicatricial alopecia. Cases were almost exclusively female (97%), with median age 46 years (range 27–72 years). CCCA represented 2.8% of all alopecia diagnoses in North America and 6% of all African cases [5].

Pathophysiology

The condition is likely to have a multifactorial aetiology. Reports of familial cases suggest a genetic predisposition [101]. A recent study identified several missense mutations in the *PADI3* gene in around 25% of CCCA cases [16]. *PADI3* encodes peptidyl arginine deiminase type III, an enzyme that post-translationally modifies proteins essential to hair shaft formation and shaping. The mutations were predicted to be pathogenic, causing protein misfolding. *PADI3* is one of three genes, mutations of which have been found in association with cheveux incoiffables (uncombable hair syndrome) in which characteristic hair shaft abnormalities (pili trianguli et canaliculi) are present [102]. Increased hair breakage has been identified as an early sign of CCCA [103] and hair shaft abnormalities reminiscent of pili trianguli et canaliculi (longitudinal grooving of the hair shaft and triangular cross-sectional shape) have been reported in a case of CCCA [104]. The risk of certain fibroproliferative disorders such as keloid scarring is increased in people of African descent and fibroproliferative genes (platelet derived growth factor (PDGF) gene, collagen (COL) I and III genes, matrix metallopeptidase (MMP) 1, 2, 7 and 9 genes) have been shown to be upregulated in the affected scalp of individuals with CCCA. A potential role for antifibrotic therapies in the treatment of CCCA has been proposed [17]. Women with CCCA have also been shown to have a nearly fivefold increased risk of uterine leiomyomas (fibroids) [105]. The precise role of hair-styling practices in triggering the condition is uncertain, however practices that induce significant hair traction (braiding, weaves) have been associated with more severe disease [101].

Clinical features

In the earliest stages of the condition, increased hair breakage around the vertex and central scalp may be reported. Reduction in hair density over the vertex and central scalp results in a slowly progressive centrifugal expansion of an area of scarring alopecia. The area of alopecia and surrounding scalp generally appear non-inflammatory, and the affected scalp is soft and non-indurated. The condition may be asymptomatic, although some patients experience burning, pruritus, pain, redness and scaling. On trichoscopy, reduced hair density and variable hair shaft diameter are evident. A preserved honeycomb pigment network with irregularly distributed pinpoint white dots can be seen, as well as irregular white patches due to follicular scarring. Grey-white peripilar halos are typical of CCCA. Broken hairs and black dots may sometimes be noted [41].

Differential diagnosis

In the early stages of CCCA, FPHL should be excluded, with anisotrichosis, single HFs and the presence of follicular ostia favouring the latter. Other scarring disorders such as LPP and CDLE may be excluded based on history, clinical features and histology. However, in the inactive phase, confident exclusion of these conditions may be difficult.

Investigations

Where diagnosis is uncertain, scalp biopsy should be performed. Histopathology is that of a typical scarring alopecia with perifollicular concentric fibrosis, mild perifollicular and perivascular lymphoid cell infiltrate, destruction of the follicular epithelium, naked hair shafts in giant cells and follicular drop-out. The most distinctive finding is below the isthmus and is characterised by premature desquamation of the IRS and eccentric thinning of the follicular epithelium [43]. Premature desquamation of the IRS can be found in inflamed follicles in other conditions such as LPP; however, in CCCA premature desquamation of the IRS may be observed in otherwise normal, unaffected HFs, suggesting that it is a characteristic feature of the condition [106]. Characterisation of the inflammatory infiltrate has demonstrated a CD4-predominant T-cell infiltrate with increased Langerhans cells extending into the lower hair follicle [107].

Management

A grading system for CCCA [26] allows staging and monitoring of disease progression. Serial photography ± measurements of the area of alopecia may also be helpful. Reducing trauma to hair and avoiding hair-styling practices that cause hair traction are generally recommended. Treatment of any associated scalp conditions such as seborrhoeic dermatitis can be managed with regular use of a medicated shampoo. Topical steroids can be used for symptom relief or if there is inflammation clinically. Intralesional steroids can be tried for focally resistant symptoms or inflammation. Systemic anti-inflammatory agents may be tried empirically, even in the absence of inflammation clinically. Tetracycline antibiotics and hydroxychloroquine are the most frequently used systemic agents, with mycophenolate mofetil, ciclosporin and short courses of oral steroids also reported [108]. Topical and low-dose oral minoxidil may be used empirically. PRP therapy and topical metformin have also been used [109,110]. Prognosis is generally considered to be poor.

Alopecia mucinosa

Introduction and general description

Alopecia mucinosa (AM) is a rare cause of scalp hair loss which may be non-scarring or, rarely, scarring. The term was first used by Pinkus in 1957 to describe hair loss in association with follicular mucin accumulation histologically [111]. The term alopecia mucinosa is sometimes used interchangeably with follicular mucinosis; however follicular mucinosis should be considered a histological tissue reaction pattern which can occur as a primary phenomenon (as in AM) or secondary to a wide range of skin conditions (e.g. spongiotic dermatitis, lichenoid eruptions, melanocytic naevi, CDLE, polymorphic light eruption, arthropod bites and skin malignancies) [112,113].

Pathophysiology

The pathogenesis of AM is uncertain.

Clinical features

Alopecia mucinosa presents as one or several red scaly patches associated with hair loss. Plaques may be tumid and indurated, with prominent follicular openings. On the head and neck, the scalp and eyebrows are predominantly affected but any area of hair-bearing skin may be involved. Lesions found on the limbs often lack redness and scaling and a well-defined patch of hair loss may be the only clinical feature. Pruritus is the commonest symptom.

As some cases of AM are associated with folliculotropic mycosis fungoides (MF)/cutaneous T-cell lymphoma (CTCL), there has been much debate as to whether idiopathic AM running a benign course and lymphoma-associated follicular mucinosis represent a clinicopathological continuum or are two distinct entities [114]. Cases of AM that tend to run a benign course usually occur in children and young adults with no associated underlying conditions. The extent of disease may be limited to the head and neck or develop more widely on the limbs and torso. Limited disease tends to have a better prognosis and may resolve spontaneously, whereas extensive disease tends to run a more chronic course [115]. While AM associated with MF/CTCL generally occurs in older adults, a case of AM in association with folliculotropic MF has been reported in a child [116]. Confirmation of the diagnosis can be challenging and long-term follow-up is essential, maintaining a high index of suspicion and repeating biopsies when indicated [114].

Differential diagnosis

On the scalp, CDLE may appear similar to AM and should be excluded histologically. Scalp disorders such as seborrhoeic dermatitis and psoriasis are not generally associated with significant focal hair loss. On the face, CDLE and chronic localised dermatitis should be excluded. Alopecia areata, FFA and LPP should be considered in the differential diagnosis of patchy alopecia on the torso and limbs.

Investigations

Histological assessment is mandatory for any case of suspected AM and investigations should include mucin stains, immunohistochemistry and T-cell gene rearrangement studies. There is currently no single diagnostic test that can provide certainty as regards malignant potential, and assessment of histological, molecular and clinical features is required [114]. The key histological feature is mucinous degeneration of the ORS and sebaceous glands usually associated with a perifollicular lymphocytic infiltrate.

Management

As AM is rare most reported treatments are based on small numbers of patients. Potent topical steroids are considered first line treatment. Topical calcineurin inhibitors (tacrolimus, pimecrolimus) have also been reported as being helpful [117,118], as has topical bexarotene gel in a case of idiopathic (non-lymphoma-associated) AM [119]. Phototherapy may be of value in widespread AM. PDT has also been reported as beneficial [120]. Systemic treatments reported to be of benefit include oral tetracyclines [121], hydroxychloroquine [122], retinoids, dapsone and indomethacin. Long-term follow-up is required, and biopsies should be repeated if clinical features change.

PART 8: SPECIFIC CUTANEOUS STRUCTURES

Keratosis follicularis spinulosa decalvans

Introduction and general description

Keratosis follicularis spinulosa decalvans (KFSD) is a rare genodermatosis characterised by widespread keratosis pilaris-like lesions on the face, torso and limbs associated with development of a scarring alopecia. It is classified as a distinct variant of keratosis pilaris atrophicans. A loss of eyebrows is commonly seen and there may also be loss of eyelashes. Other cutaneous features include facial redness, woolly hair [123] and palmoplantar keratoderma [124]. Reported extracutaneous features include photophobia, keratitis, blepharitis and enamel hypoplasia.

Epidemiology

Most cases of KFSD occur in males who develop a more severe phenotype than affected females, and the condition demonstrates an X-linked pattern of inheritance, although autosomal dominant mode of transmission and sporadic cases are reported. KFSD has been reported in association with AKN [125].

Pathophysiology

Genetics

Mutations have been identified in the *MBTPS2* (membrane-bound transcription factor peptidase, site 2) gene (MIM: 300294) located on chromosome Xp22.1 [126–128]. *MBTPS2* encodes a membrane-embedded zinc metalloprotease known as site 2 protease (S2P), essential for the cleavage of the sterol regulatory element-binding proteins (SREBPs) that function as downstream transcription factors. S2P also functions as a putative endoplasmic reticulum stress sensor through regulation of the unfolded protein response. Defects in these pathways are thought to impair cholesterol and other lipid biochemical pathways in the skin, leading to changes in epidermal differentiation. Mutations in *MBTPS2* also underlie ichthyosis follicularis, alopecia and photophobia (IFAP) syndrome (MIM: 308205), which presents with clinical features similar to KFSD [126].

Investigations

Keratosis follicularis spinulosa decalvans is underrecognised, and diagnosis is often delayed. Diagnosis is based on typical clinical features (early-onset extensive keratosis pilaris, followed by scarring alopecia and loss of eyebrows) in association with other typical disease features (particularly ocular disorders). Scrapings should be taken to exclude tinea capitis and any pustules should be swabbed for bacterial culture. Although the histological features are not diagnostic, scalp biopsy is advised. Established lesions show a perifollicular lymphohistiocytic infiltrate, follicular hyperkeratosis, fibrosis and destruction of the HF. Genetic assessment and counselling are advised, and ophthalmology assessment required.

Clinical features

It usually begins in early childhood with keratosis pilaris on the face, progressing to the torso and limbs. Cicatricial alopecia of the scalp, eyebrows and eyelashes develops during later childhood and early adolescence. The affected scalp is inflamed, with follicular hyperkeratosis, scarring and hair tufting. Pustules from secondary bacterial infections are common. Clinically, the scalp changes appear similar to FD.

Differential diagnosis

The differential diagnosis of keratosis pilaris-like lesions associated with follicular atrophy includes atrophoderma vermiculata and keratosis pilaris rubra atrophicans faciei (ulerythema ophryogenes). IFAP syndrome presents with similar, although generally milder, clinical features and the associated alopecia is non-scarring. In adults, FD is the main clinical differential diagnosis.

Management

Effective treatment of KFSD is challenging. When inflammation is present, potent topical steroids are first line therapy. Intralesional steroids may be helpful for focally stubborn inflammation. Systemic treatments which have been tried include retinoids [125,129], tetracycline antibiotics [125] and dapsone [130]. Several cases of successful response to laser hair removal have reported [131].

PRIMARY NEUTROPHILIC CICATRICIAL ALOPECIAS

Folliculitis decalvans

Synonyms and inclusions
- Tufted folliculitis

Introduction and general description

Folliculitis decalvans is an uncommon, chronic, inflammatory scarring alopecia arising on the vertex of the scalp. The condition tends to slowly expand centrifugally over the scalp, resulting in solitary or multiple patches of densely scarred alopecia. The affected scalp is often intensely inflamed, and painful pustules and crusting can be seen affecting involved HFs.

Epidemiology

A recent survey of specialist alopecia clinics found that FD represented 2.8% of all alopecia diagnoses. It was commoner in men (male : female 2 : 1), in whom it accounted for 6.8% of all alopecia. The median age at onset was 40 years [5]. Familial cases have been reported [132,133], as has occurrence limited to punch grafts after hair restoration surgery [134].

Pathophysiology

The pathogenesis of FD has been much debated; however, recent research suggests chronic HF dysbiosis and supports a role for a microbial trigger. *Staphylococcus aureus* has long been suspected to play a role, given the ubiquity with which it can be isolated from pustules and the response (albeit often transient) to antistaphyloccocal antibiotics [18,19]. However, factors such as the absence of significant *S. aureus* infections elsewhere on FD patients' skin, the lack of demonstrable immune dysfunction in FD patients and the lack of association between FD and immunosuppression argued against it being a simple infective process in susceptible individuals [18]. The identification of microbial biofilms in the infra-infundibular region of the HF in both FD and normal controls suggested that commensal bacterial biofilms are ubiquitous in normal HFs and that in FD they may undergo a pathogenic shift [19]. It was subsequently demonstrated that when *S. aureus* is present on lesional FD skin, it also colonises non-lesional and subepidermal skin in 80% of cases and is the only bacterial species present in more than two-thirds of the FD cases. In contrast, the subepidermal microbiota of the normal scalp is composed almost exclusively of *Cutibacterium acnes* and coagulase negative staphylococci. Antibiotic treatment leads to clinical improvement and the clearance of *S. aureus* in superficial (non-lesional and lesional) and subepidermal skin in almost all FD patients. However, clearance of *S. aureus* is accompanied by an incomplete return of the normal superficial and subepidermal microbiota, suggesting a persistent defect of the epidermal barrier. It is postulated that FD may occur when there is a breach of the normal epidermal barrier whereby an opportunistic bacterium such as *S. aureus* invades the subepidermal HF and colonises non-lesional scalp. Antibiotic treatment results in clinical improvement and clears pathogenic bacteria but does not restore a normal follicular microbiota, resulting in chronic follicular dysbiosis which, coupled with a subepidermal reservoir of pathogenic bacteria, causes chronic reinfection [20]. The restoration of normal HF microbiota may offer a novel therapeutic approach in FD [20].

The presence of a neutrophilic inflammatory infiltrate in FD suggests a role for the innate immune response. An immunohistochemical investigation of the expression of markers associated with the activation of innate immune signals (inflammasomes (NALP1 and NALP3), IL-1β, IL-8 and type I IFN) demonstrated significantly increased NALP1, NALP3 and IL-1β expression in FD HFs compared with controls and LPP. There was no difference found in inflammatory marker levels for both active and inactive FD, suggesting that in inactive FD there is a persistent inflammatory stimulus, supporting a possible role for bacterial biofilms [135].

Clinical features

Folliculitis decalvans typically starts on the vertex of the scalp as a painful folliculitis. As the condition progresses, it slowly expands, particularly over the central scalp, resulting in solitary or multiple patches of sclerotic alopecia. Pustules, often crusting, are seen affecting HFs at the margins of the patches of alopecia. Hair tufting (tufted folliculitis or polytrichia) of six or more hairs is a prominent feature of the condition (Figure 87.41). The scalp surrounding the patches of scarring alopecia can be intensely inflamed and, in some cases, most of the scalp may be inflamed. Perifollicular hyperkeratosis and scalp scaling are also frequent features. Involvement of other body sites is rare but is reported affecting the face and beard area [132,136]. Trichoscopy highlights pustules, crusting, scaling and tufting. Coiled dilated capillaries are also typical [41].

Differential diagnosis

While the presence of pustules, crusting, hair tufting and dense scarring around the vertex of the scalp is highly suggestive of FD, redness and follicular hyperkeratosis affecting the surrounding scalp can be suggestive of LPP, and in some cases these two conditions may coexist [137,138]. Fungal infection should be excluded. FD can occur in association with AKN [139]. Drug-induced eruptions

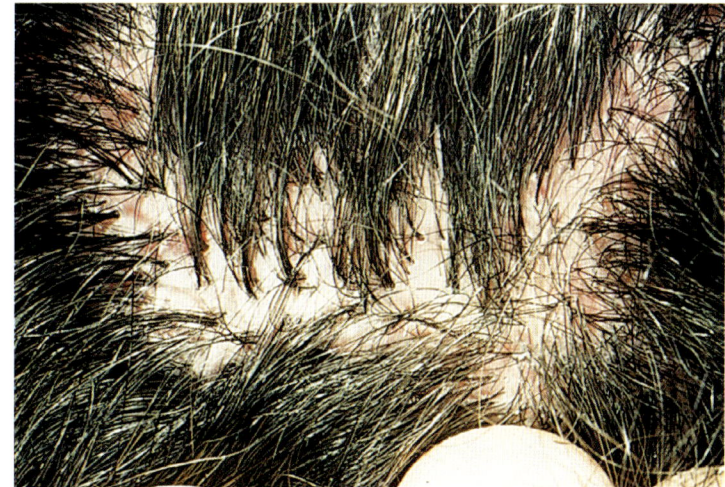

Figure 87.41 Tufted folliculitis.

suggestive of FD have been reported with ixekizumab and erlotinib [140,141].

Investigations

Samples for bacteriological culture and sensitivity should be taken from any active pustules. Scale should be sent for mycological examination as cases of tinea capitis mimicking FD are reported [22]. Biopsy from an area of active disease should be considered if the diagnosis is uncertain. Histology of early lesions shows features characteristic of an acute, dense, dermal perifollicular neutrophilic infiltrate. As the follicle ruptures, an intrafollicular and perifollicular infiltrate of neutrophils, lymphocytes, histiocytes and plasma cells is seen. Perifollicular fibrosis with fibrous tracts replacing the HFs, follicular tufting and interstitial dermal fibrosis are all features observed in late stages [43]. Interfollicular epidermal hyperplasia has been identified as a prominent feature in FD [142] and in cases of neutrophil-poor FD, where distinction from LPP may be challenging, a significant difference in the average interfollicular epidermal thickness between FD and LPP has been demonstrated [143].

Management

Management of FD largely relies on systemic antimicrobials [144]. Prolonged courses of oral ± topical tetracycline antibiotics are often used first line and can be effective in controlling inflammation in many cases [132,133]. A 10-week course of rifampicin and clindamycin (or doxycycline/ciprofloxacin/clarithromycin) appears to be an effective treatment option in active disease [18,132,133]. Fusidic acid in combination with other antimicrobials or oral zinc is also reported to be of benefit [145,146]. Isotretinoin has been reported to be an effective treatment in several retrospective studies [147,148]. There are also reports of benefit from dapsone [148]. Systemic PDT has been shown to be of benefit in one case of recalcitrant disease [149], although reports of the efficacy of topical PDT are more variable. Anti-inflammatory drugs such as adalimumab [150], infliximab [151], apremilast, tofacitinib [152] and ciclosporin [153] have been reported to be of benefit in a small number of cases. In recalcitrant disease, hair removal by neodymium:yttrium-aluminium-garnet (Nd:YAG) laser treatment may be a useful strategy [154]. In addition to systemic agents, potent topical steroids can be of benefit in symptom relief. The regular use of an antiseptic shampoo, such as those containing benzalkonium chloride, should be considered, given both the likely role of pathogenic bacteria and the risk of antimicrobial resistance as a result of long-term antibiotic use [155].

Dissecting cellulitis

Synoyms and inclusions

- Perifolliculitis capitis abscedens et suffodiens
- Hoffmann disease

Introduction and general description

Dissecting cellulitis is an uncommon primary neutrophilic cicatricial alopecia of uncertain aetiology. It is part of the 'follicular occlusion tetrad' along with hidradenitis suppurativa (HS), acne conglobata (AC) and pilonidal sinus.

Epidemiology

Estimates of the frequency with which DC is found in association with other follicular occlusion disorders vary (HS: 0–23.8%; AC: 14–29%; HS and AC: 3.9–4.7%) [156–159]. It is significantly more common in men (85–98% males) [158,159] and was thought to be commoner in males of African descent. However, in a European study, 85% of cases were white skinned [159]. The average age at onset is between 26 and 32 years [158,159]. Familial cases, including monozygotic twins, are reported [160]. In a recent survey of specialist hair clinics, DC represented 0.9% of all alopecia diagnoses, 2.7% of all alopecia diagnoses in males and 3.4% of all scarring alopecias [5]. However, some cases of DC may be managed in a general dermatology setting rather than in a specialist hair clinic, therefore these figures may underrepresent the true prevalence.

Pathophysiology

The relationship between DC, HS and AC suggests a possible common pathobiology. In HS, a genetic predisposition and lifestyle factors (e.g. obesity, which may induce cutaneous microtrauma) lead to microbiome alteration, subclinical inflammation around HFs and follicular hyperkeratosis, resulting in HF occlusion, stasis and dilatation and excessive growth of anaerobic bacteria. Subsequent HF rupture initiates an innate immune response. The innate immune system relies on recognition of conserved structures on pathogens, termed pathogen-associated molecular patterns (PAMPs) and/or tissue damage-associated molecular patterns (DAMPs), by pattern recognition receptors (PRRs, e.g. Toll-like receptors) on macrophages and dendritic cells. On PAMP/DAMP recognition, PRRs trigger activation of inflammasome component NLRP3 leading to release of IL-1β and TNF-α, further amplifying local immune responses [161]. Whether similar disease mechanisms are responsible for DC is not clear. There are several reports of the condition apparently being triggered by the use of anabolic steroids [159,162] and occurring after IFN-β1a treatment [163] and scalp trauma [158].

Clinical features

Dissecting cellulitis presents as painful, deep, fluctuant nodules and abscesses predominantly around the vertex and occipital scalp. The lesions appear similar to those seen in AC. Interconnecting sinuses often result in a purulent discharge and crusting and secondary infection are common. Hair is lost from affected nodules and may become permanent in severe or untreated disease. When extensive, coalescing lesions may result in a rather cerebriform appearance of the scalp. On trichoscopy of areas of alopecia overlying inflamed nodules, yellow dots and broken hairs (black dots) may be seen on a background of diffuse scalp redness and dilated blood vessels [41].

Differential diagnosis

Tinea capitis should be excluded, particularly in adolescents. Other scarring alopecias including FD and AKN should also be excluded.

Investigations

Samples for bacteriological culture and sensitivity should be taken from any discharge. Scale and hair should be sent for mycological examination as cases of tinea capitis mimicking DC are reported, particularly in adolescents [164–166]. Generally, diagnosis is made on clinical grounds, but if there is diagnostic uncertainty or failure to respond to treatment, incisional biopsy should be performed. Histology of the affected scalp demonstrates a dense, deep dermal and subcutaneous predominantly neutrophilic infiltrate, with follicular rupture and abscess formation. Formation of sinus tracts lined by squamous epithelium with surrounding dense fibrosis is characteristic [43].

Management

A moderate response to oral tetracycline antibiotics is reported; however, relapse on stopping is common [158]. Oral isotretinoin seems to be accepted as the most effective treatment [157]. Dosages range from 0.25 to 1.0 mg/kg/day, with some studies using standard doses of 30, 40 or 80 mg/day. Significant benefit may sometimes be achieved by around 3 months of treatment but slow responses and relapse on discontinuation are common; therefore, prolonged courses at a low dose may be required. There may also be a role for maintenance therapy [157]. In severe disease, anti-TNF therapies (adalimumab, infliximab) are reported to be of benefit, although not in all cases [157]. Other reported treatments for which there appears to be limited evidence of benefit include oral zinc, dapsone and PDT [167,168]. In severe extensive refractory disease, radical surgical resection and reconstruction with skin grafting have been reported to be of benefit [169].

MIXED INFLAMMATORY INFILTRATE

Acne keloidalis nuchae

Synonyms and inclusions

- Folliculitis keloidalis nuchae

Introduction and general description

Acne keloidalis nuchae is a chronic scarring folliculitis affecting the nape and occipital scalp. Despite the name, it is unrelated to acne vulgaris.

Epidemiology

It is seen most frequently in men of African descent but is reported in white and other ethnic groups. It rarely occurs in females although several recent studies [5,170] report a male : female ratio of 7 : 1. Estimated prevalence in African male populations is 0.7–10.5%, and it is 0.5–13.6% in African American males [21]. In a 2017 survey of specialist hair clinics, AKN represented 0.5% of all alopecia diagnoses and 1.8% of all alopecias in men (median age 32 years). AKN in the South African cohort represented 9% of all alopecia diagnoses [5]. It is rare before puberty and it is unusual to develop it after the age of 55 years.

Pathophysiology

The pathogenesis of AKN is uncertain although several factors have been implicated [21]. As the condition predominantly affects men between puberty and 55 years, a role for androgens has been suggested. However, the areas affected tend to be those spared by androgenetic alopecia. The role of skin trauma/irritation/occlusion in the aetiology of AKN remains uncertain, although symptoms are reported to worsen following cutting or shaving hair [21]. Chronic friction from collars, caps and helmets has also been implicated. The shape and curl of African hair have been postulated to play a role, as occurs with pseudofolliculitis barbae [21]. AKN is reported to be seen in association with FD in 21% of cases, with lesions of both conditions seen adjacent on the occipital scalp in 67%, prompting suggestions that both diseases may share similar pathogenic mechanisms [139]. A suspected association between AKN and the metabolic syndrome [170] has been confirmed in a population study involving 2677 AKN cases and 13 190 controls. Obesity demonstrated the strongest association with AKN, followed by type 2 diabetes and hypertension [171]. A similar population study identified an association with HS [172].

Clinical features

Firm follicular papules are typically seen on the nape of the neck and lower occipital scalp and hairline. Inflammation and pustules are often present, and symptoms include pruritus, pain and bleeding. Secondary infection with *Staphylococcus aureus* is common. Chronic inflammation results in scarring and permanent hair loss, with loss of follicular ostia and hair tufting. In some individuals, larger plaques of scarring or keloid develop.

Differential diagnosis

Conditions such as FD can coexist with AKN and may be found adjacent on the occipital scalp. DC should be excluded clinically.

Investigations

The clinical features of AKN are usually diagnostic and biopsy is often not required. Samples for bacteriological culture and sensitivity should be taken from any active pustules. If there is diagnostic doubt, biopsy can be performed; however, the histopathology of AKN depends on the duration and activity of the area biopsied and findings are not pathognomonic. Early in the disease there is follicular dilatation with neutrophils and follicular rupture with perifollicular abscesses. Late lesions show perifollicular granulomas around naked hair shafts mixed with a lymphoplasmacellular infiltrate, and hypertrophic scarring with broad eosinophilic hyalinised keloidal collagen bundles and loss of sebaceous glands [43].

Management

Given the possible aetiological role for trauma and irritation, it is essential that those affected are counselled to avoid practices that may aggravate the condition, such as closely shaving the hair, wearing tightly fitting caps or helmets and tight collars. Potent topical steroids (possibly with antiseptics or topical antibiotics such as clindamycin if mild secondary infection is present) are the first line management choice. Systemic antibiotics are often required for more marked secondary infection and inflammation and oral tetracyclines are the drugs of choice. Intralesional steroids can be useful for hypertrophic lesions. Laser epilation can be effective, especially in those with small papular lesions [173]. Severe disease such as the presence of extensive keloid scarring can prove challenging and surgical excision that includes the posterior hairline may be required [174].

Overlap/coincident alopecias

It is common to find features of more than one type of alopecia when examining a scalp. Male and female pattern hair loss are the most frequently seen alongside other disorders. Alopecia areata is common and when present with other types of alopecia can cause diagnostic confusion such as is reported with cases of FFA [175,176]. The presence of more than one type of scarring alopecia is not rare, occurring most frequently in FFA, where classic LPP is seen in a minority of cases (around 15%) [56,65]. AKN and FD are also seen in association in up to 21% of cases [139].

NON-SPECIFIC CICATRICIAL ALOPECIA

In some cases of scarring alopecia, the clinical and histological features are non-diagnostic. This is particularly true when alopecia is no longer active (end stage). In cases where the extent of alopecia is stable, no medical treatment is required. If hair loss is extensive and the alopecia is stable, surgical resection can be considered. If the area(s) of alopecia continues to extend, treatments may be trialled empirically. Very potent topical steroids can be tried first line and may be of benefit if there are symptoms such as pruritus; however, they are rarely sufficient to halt progress of a scarring alopecia. Intralesional steroids may be worth trying on localised areas of disease extension. If hair loss is more extensive and continues to progress, it may be useful to seek expert review. Systemic therapy can also be considered. The treatments of choice tend to be those used in the management of lichenoid alopecias, such as hydroxychloroquine, methotrexate, ciclosporin or mycophenolate mofetil.

Table 87.3 Secondary cicatricial alopecias

	Disease	Cross reference
Traumatic	Radiodermatitis	'Chemotherapy-induced alopecia' section
	Physical trauma	
	Postoperative (e.g. flap necrosis)	
	Burns	
	Dermatitis artefacta	
	Traction alopecia	'Traction alopecia' section
Sclerosing disorders	Morphoea (including en coup de sabre)	
	Scleroderma	
	Lichen sclerosus	
	Sclerodermoid porphyria cutanea tarda	
	Chronic graft-versus-host disease	
	Facial hemiatrophy (Parry–Romberg syndrome)	
Granulomatous	Sarcoidosis	
	Necrobiosis lipoidica	
Inflammatory	Psoriatic alopecia	'Psoriatic alopecia' section
	Immunobullous (e.g. Brunsting–Perry pemphigoid, cicatricial pemphigoid)	
	Temporal/giant cell arteritis	
	Lupus profundus	
	Chronic graft-versus-host disease	
	Dermatomyositis (rarely)	
Infectious:		
Bacterial	Folliculitis/carbuncle/furuncle	
Fungal	Kerion	
	Favus	
	Tinea capitis (rarely scarring)	
Viral	Varicella/shingles	'Infections and hair loss' section
	HIV	'Infections and hair loss' section
Protozoal	Leishmaniasis	
Treponemal	Syphilis	'Infections and hair loss' section
Mycobacterial	Tuberculosis	
Neoplastic:		
Benign	Cylindroma	
	Other adnexal tumours	
Malignant, primary	Basal cell carcinoma, squamous cell carcinoma, melanoma, angiosarcoma	
	Cutaneous T-cell lymphoma	
Malignant, secondary	Renal, breast, lung and gastrointestinal tumours	
'alopecia neoplastica'	Lymphoma, leukaemia	
Developmental defects and hereditary disorders	Aplasia cutis	'Aplasia cutis' section (under 'Other circumscribed (congenital) alopecias)
	Epidermal naevi	
	Hair follicle hamartomas	
	Incontinentia pigmenti	
	Focal dermal hypoplasia of Goltz	
	Porokeratosis of Mibelli	
	Ichthyosis	
	Epidermolysis bullosa	
	Polyostotic fibrous dysplasia	
	Conradi–Hünermann syndrome (chondrodysplasia punctata)	

SECONDARY CICATRICIAL ALOPECIAS

Secondary cicatricial alopecias (Table 87.3) result from skin conditions or trauma that cause non-targeted HF destruction. There are a wide range of possible causes, which fall into the broad categories of trauma, infection, inflammatory disorders and neoplasia. If there are no diagnostic clinical features to suggest a primary scarring alopecia, then a secondary cause should be sought. A careful history and complete skin and scalp examination are required, and biopsy is generally necessary. Many of the causes of secondary alopecias are rare but some may be encountered more frequently than others. En coup de sabre largely occurs in children and adolescents, more commonly in females. It presents as a linear depressed band of hair loss and atrophic skin changes affecting the frontal scalp and forehead. Imaging of the skull and brain is required as associated central nervous system abnormalities may occur. Alopecia due to malignancy should be considered, particularly in older patients with a new solitary patch of alopecia. Hair loss within skin cancers (e.g. squamous cell carcinomas) is seen commonly; however, some scalp malignancies present as an area of alopecia without a clinically obvious tumour and diagnostic biopsy is required. Rarely, scarring alopecia may be a manifestation of chronic graft-versus-host disease, clinically resembling LPP [177,178].

HAIR LOSS ASSOCIATED WITH INCREASED HAIR FALL

Telogen effluvium

Synonyms and inclusions
• Telogen defluvium

Introduction and general description

Telogen effluvium describes an increase in the proportion of telogen hairs due to changes in the hair cycle, resulting in increased hair shedding and reduced hair density. First coined by Kligman in 1961 [1], TE described a non-specific reaction pattern of the HF to a triggering insult. Thus, the observation of increased telogen hair shedding does not infer a cause. To establish the cause a careful history is required to identify known triggers, biochemical investigation to exclude endocrine, nutritional or autoimmune aetiologies and, in persistent cases, histology to determine if there is evidence of the earliest stages of androgenetic alopecia.

Pathophysiology

In infancy, hairs have a synchronised hair cycle resulting in multiple HFs all growing, involuting and then shedding at the same time, producing a so-called moult wave moving front to back across the scalp. These moult waves are also frequently seen in animals, and often persist throughout the lifetime of the creature. However, in humans, hair cycle synchronisation is lost in early childhood, superseded by individual follicles growing and cycling independent from one another. Therefore, normally small numbers of hairs across the scalp are constantly lost and replaced each day, often going unnoticed by the person [2].

The normal daily turnover of hair is not well defined, but frequently cited as up to 100 hairs lost per day. Various estimations of hair shedding have been extrapolated from white patients using mean percentage telogen counts derived from trichogram or scalp biopsy studies combined with estimated total scalp hair numbers and duration of different hair cycle phases. Using scalp plucked hair values, an average of 86% hairs are in anagen, 1% in catagen and 13% in telogen, whereas data from horizontal scalp biopsies put these figures at 93% in anagen and 7% in telogen [3]. Accordingly, based on scalp biopsy results, if the average number of scalp hairs is 100 000, then 7000 hairs should be in telogen at any one time. As the approximate duration of telogen is 100 days, 70 hairs should be shed each day.

As mentioned, most people are unaware of this level of daily hair shedding. The threshold amount of shed hair that is normally noticed is poorly defined, but it is likely that when people are concerned they are losing hair, they look harder and find more. Thus, introspection might very well heighten one's powers of detection [4], enhanced by other factors such as longer hair length and certain environments (e.g. flooring or lighting).

Headington [5] described five functional types of TE, based on different phases of the follicular cycle:

1 *Immediate anagen release* occurs when anagen follicles are prematurely forced to enter telogen, resulting in increased hair shedding approximately 3 months later when the telogen phase is complete. This is the commonest mechanism recognised, and is caused by various triggering factors including physiological stress and medications. When the triggering event is removed or resolves, a normal hair cycle resumes and excessive hair fall stops.

2 *Delayed anagen release* occurs when the anagen duration is abnormally prolonged, resulting in a reduced proportion of hairs in the telogen phase. When this anagen-prolonging driver subsides the hair cycle rebalances, with a higher proportion of anagen hairs transitioning into telogen at the same time, resulting in shedding 3 months later. This mechanism is thought to underlie postpartum TE and hair loss following cessation of the combined contraceptive pill.

3 *Short anagen syndrome* is caused by shortening of the duration of anagen so that proportionately more hairs enter telogen each day. These patients have an inability to grow their hair past a certain length and can suffer persistent telogen hair shedding. It is estimated that every 50% reduction in anagen duration will result in doubling of the numbers of telogen hairs. Shortening of anagen duration is also a key component in androgenetic alopecia associated with hair miniaturisation. Thus, increased shedding commonly precedes visible balding of the scalp in this condition.

4 *Immediate telogen release* results from premature exogen (teloptosis) and may also be associated with a shortening of telogen duration. However, exogen does not necessarily initiate the onset of the next anagen phase, so telogen follicles may remain empty for many weeks before the next anagen starts. These empty telogen follicles are called kenogen. Drugs such as minoxidil can precipitate exogen, and this explains the temporary increase in hair shedding commonly noticed 4–6 weeks after commencement of minoxidil therapy for hair loss. Other external factors, such as retinoid therapy and excessive UV exposure, can also promote exogen, whereas endogenous triggers include scalp inflammation from seborrhoeic dermatitis. Modulation of proteolytic activity appears central in controlling exogen [6].

5 *Delayed telogen release* occurs when anagen restarts after a prolonged telogen phase. This mechanism is seen in animals with synchronous hair cycles to control their winter and summer coats. It may occur seasonally in some humans.

Although the need for a new classification has been questioned [7], Rebora has proposed an alternative classification of telogen hair loss to simplify the definitions [8]:

1 *Premature teloptosis*, which is analogous to Headington's immediate telogen release.

2 *Collective teloptosis*. This definition combines Headington's delayed anagen release and delayed telogen release groups. It occurs in situations where the hair cycle has become synchronised.

3 *Premature entry into telogen phase*, which is analogous to Headington's immediate anagen release. The amount of hair loss is dependent on the severity of the triggering insult, and the phase in the hair cycle when this occurred.

An additional type of TE is also described by the same authors, which they call 'autoimmune (or inflammatory) TE'. Here, excessive telogen shedding is associated with marked trichodynia, strong autoimmune associations (e.g. high thyroid peroxidase antibodies) and response to topical corticosteroids [9]. The relationship of this condition with diffuse alopecia areata requires further clarification.

Various biological factors may contribute to the hair cycle changes seen in TE, including oxidative stress [10], mast cell degranulation and neurogenic inflammation [11] and exposure to catagen-inducing pro-inflammatory cytokines [12].

Clinical features

Acute TE is an acute-onset scalp hair loss that typically occurs 3 months after a triggering event such as a febrile illness (e.g. SARS-CoV-2), surgical trauma, sudden starvation or hemorrhage (Table 87.4; Figures 87.42, 87.43 and 87.44) [1,4,5]. The functional mechanism for this acute shedding is immediate anagen release. The patient may be particularly aware of increased loss on the brush or comb, or during shampooing. The daily loss ranges from under 100 to over 1000 hairs. If the lower rates of shedding are continued for only a short period there may be no obvious baldness, but if shedding occurs at higher rates, diffuse reduction in hair density is produced (Figure 87.45). Acute TE does not produce total baldness.

Unless the trigger is repeated, spontaneous regrowth occurs within 3–6 months. The proportion of follicles affected, and hence the severity of the subsequent alopecia, depends partly on the duration and severity of the precipitating cause and partly on unexplained individual variations in susceptibility. In approximately a third of cases of acute TE no trigger can be identified. Acute TE is commonly attributed to emotional stress, but the evidence for this is weak. Significant emotional stress, proposed by J. Shapiro as the 'three Bs' (break-up, bankruptcy and bereavement), may induce hair loss in some people. However, the normal stresses of everyday life appear insufficient to induce significant hair fall.

Chronic diffuse telogen hair loss refers to telogen hair shedding persisting for longer than 6 months. It can be a result of an idiopathic change in hair cycle dynamics (primary chronic TE; see later in this chapter) or be secondary to a variety of causes. Before a potential trigger can be accepted as a true cause of chronic TE, the relationship between the causative factor and the hair loss must fit chronologically. The hair loss should reverse when the causative factor is corrected and the hair shedding resume when the trigger is reintroduced. Other known causes of shedding, in particular androgenetic alopecia, also require exclusion.

Clinical assessment should include a careful history for potential triggers, including review of all medication. Patients frequently bring evidence of the amount of hair lost daily (the so-called bag sign, Figure 87.46) which can be a clue to diagnosis. Examination should record the extent of hair loss, assess the degree of shedding and exclude other conditions (particularly androgenetic alopecia and alopecia areata) that may present with increased hair fall. Trichoscopy shows short regrowing hairs in TE, with no variability in hair shaft diameter.

Trichodynia is the term given to unpleasant scalp symptoms, including paraesthesia, pain, burning or itch, associated with hair

Table 87.4 Causes of telogen effluvium.

Causes and references	Examples
Acute illness [1]	Febrile illness (>39°C)
	Major surgery
	Trauma
	Haemorrhage
Chronic illness [36,62–65]	Hypo- or hyperthyroidism (Figure 87.42)
	Malignancy
	Lymphoproliferative disorders
	Chronic infections (e.g. HIV, syphilis, TB)
	Chronic renal or liver disease
	Connective tissue diseases (e.g. SLE, dermatomyositis) (Figure 87.43)
Hormonal changes	Telogen gravidarum
	Changing or discontinuing the oral contraceptive pill
Medications [29]	Oral retinoids
	'Anti-medications':
	Antihypertensives (e.g. β-blockers)
	Anticoagulants
	NSAIDs
	Antidepressants
	Antiarrhythmic
	Antithyroid drugs
	Immunisations, plus many more
Severe emotional stress	Break-up
	Bankruptcy
	Bereavement
Malnutrition [66–69]	'Crash' dieting/starvation
	Low protein intake
	Chronic nutritional deficiency (e.g. iron, zinc, vitamin B_{12} and vitamin D) (Figure 87.44)
Heavy metal poisoning [70]	Arsenic
	Thallium
Physiological	Seasonal hair moult (spring and autumn)
	Neonatal hair loss
Inflammatory scalp disorders	Seborrhoeic eczema
	Psoriasis
Early androgenetic alopecia	

Adapted from Chien Yen *et al.* 2021 [32] and Cunningham *et al.* 2012 [61].
HIV, human immunodeficiency virus; NSAIDs, non-steroidal anti-inflammatory drugs; SLE, systemic lupus erythematosus; TB, tuberculosis.

loss. Trichodynia is seen more frequently in TE compared with androgenetic alopecia and controls and was positively associated with higher depression scores [13–15]. Trichodynia may be focal or diffuse, may be correlated with scalp telangectasia and is more common in women [7,16]. A clear association with abnormal laboratory readings has not been made, although possible association with low vitamin B_{12} levels has been reported [14,17]. The proposed pathogenesis of trichodynia is neurogenic inflammation and mast cell degranulation with the neuropeptide substance P playing a central role [16].

Objectively assessing hair shedding can be challenging. The following techniques are described:

1 *The hair pull test.* This is regarded as abnormal if >10% pulled hairs are removed. However, a recent study of 182 people suggests the normal value of removed hair is consistently lower than this, and so the normal value should be changed to two hairs or fewer per pull [18]. In TE hairs can be removed throughout the scalp, whereas in androgenetic alopecia hairs are predominantly removed from the vertex. Unfortunately, the hair pull test

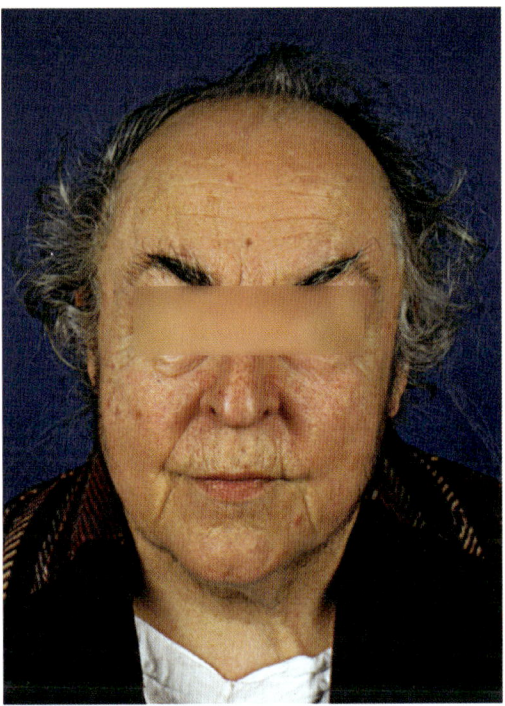

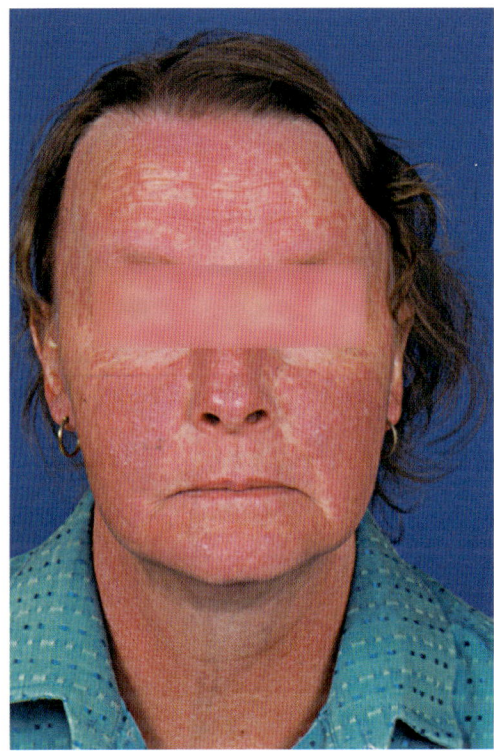

Figure 87.43 Hair loss and photosensitivity caused by systemic lupus erythematosus.

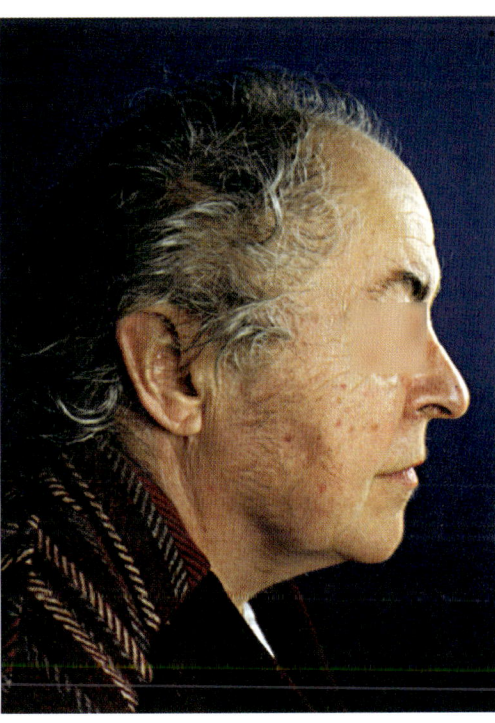

Figure 87.42 Diffuse alopecia in association with hypothyroidism.

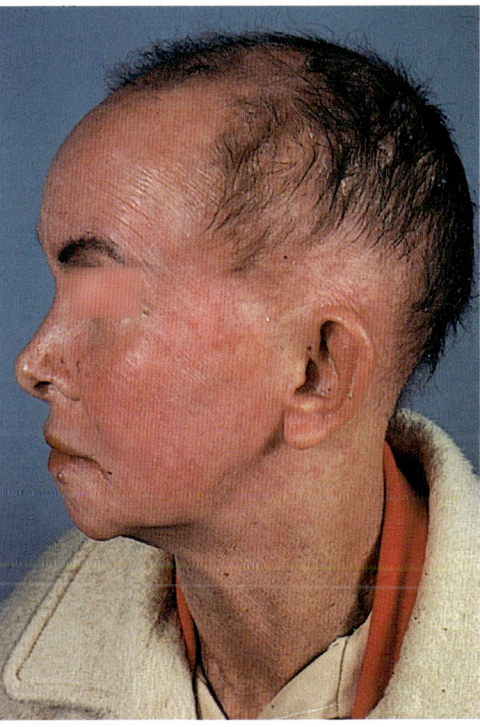

Figure 87.44 Acquired zinc deficiency resulting from prolonged parenteral feeding and inadequate zinc supplementation.

PART 8: SPECIFIC CUTANEOUS STRUCTURES

is notoriously difficult to interpret, with significant interobserver variation. Further, the pull test can be difficult to assess in cases where the hair is short or the curl pattern is tight. In acute TE the hair pull test is usually strongly positive for telogen hairs at the vertex and the scalp margins; however, a negative hair pull test does not exclude the diagnosis.

2 *Trichogram/hair microscopy* (Figure 87.47). Analysis of a hair pluck sample usually shows >25% telogen hairs in acute TE [1]. Microscopy will reveal predominantly typical clubbed telogen hairs, although 'atypical' telogen hairs (e.g. with a tail and/or remnent root sheath) are more prominent [19,20]. Suprabulbar shaft thinning may also be seen in acute TE, suggesting that triggers for TE may impact on anagen before telogen is eventually triggered [21].

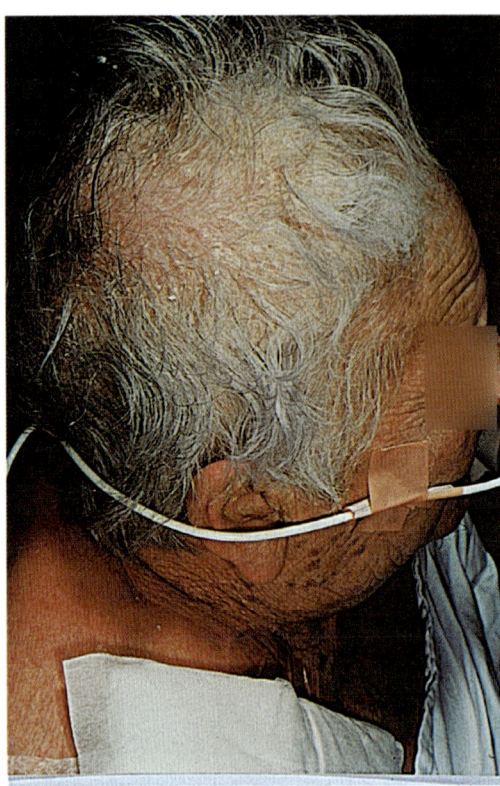

Figure 87.45 Acute telogen effluvium.

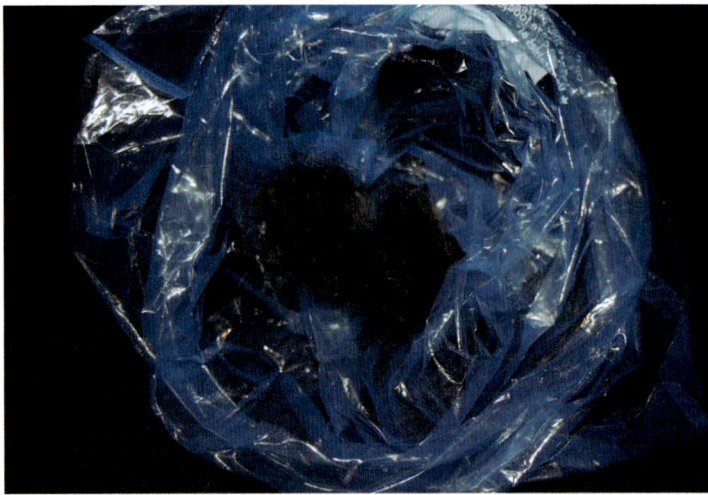

Figure 87.46 The 'bag sign' demonstrating increased hair shedding.

3 *Phototrichogram.* Due to practical issues, this technique is more suitable for research.

4 *Sixty-second hair count.* This involves shampooing daily for 3 days, and on the fourth day the hair is combed over a sheet or towel for 60 s; these hairs are collected and counted. Hair counts should be recorded on three consecutive days [22].

5 *Modified wash test (MWT).* Briefly, this requires abstinence from hair washing for 5 days before the hair is shampooed and shed hairs are collected in gauze over the plughole. All hairs are then counted and divided into <3 cm (vellus) and >3 cm (terminal) hairs. The following interpretation has been proposed: 'Patients with <100 hairs and ≥10% vellus hairs are diagnosed as having androgenetic alopecia; those with ≥100 hairs and <10% vellus hairs as having TE; those with ≥100 hairs and ≥10% vellus hairs as having androgenetic alopecia + TE; and those with <100 hairs and <10% vellus hairs as being normal or having TE in remission' [23,24].

6 *Visual hair shedding scales.* The original visual scale was presented by Sinclair with straight blond hair grouped and photographed in bundles of various sizes. Groups of 10, 50, 100, 200, 400 and 750 hairs were presented, and the patient asked to estimate loss on both wash and non-wash days. Losses of 400 and 750 hairs were regarded as abnormal (Figure 87.48) [25]. Subsequent attempts to reproduce this scale using short, medium and long curly hair types have been reported [26].

7 *Scalp biopsy* (see 'Investigations' later in the TE section).

Clinical variants

Drug-induced telogen effluvium. Drug-induced TE usually starts 6–12 weeks after instigation of treatment and is progressive while the drug is continued [27,28]. The commonest mechanism for premature catagen onset is immediate telogen release, although stopping drugs that promote anagen (e.g. combined oral contraceptive pill/minoxidil) or medications that trigger exogen (e.g. retinoids) may also result in increased telogen shedding. Further, some medication may indirectly precipitate shedding through exacerbation of androgenetic alopecia [29].

The diagnosis of drug-induced telogen hair loss is made by demonstrating a compatible chronology of drug exposure and the onset of the hair loss, and exclusion of the other causes of alopecia. If a particular drug is suspected, testing involves stopping it for at least 3 months. Regrowth following discontinuation and recurrence on re-exposure to the drug support the conclusion that the drug caused the alopecia. Many drugs are associated with TE [29].

Postpartum telogen effluvium. Postpartum TE (syn. telogen gravidarum) refers to the telogen hair loss seen 2–3 months after childbirth [31]. It is thought that raised oestrogen levels prolong anagen and synchronise the hair cycle, resulting in a higher proportion of anagen hairs during pregnancy that are then lost when the hormone levels subside. Telogen gravidarum is most common after the first pregnancy and occurs in around 20% of women [32,33]. Stress of delivery and autoimmune sequelae (e.g. postpartum thyroiditis) have also been proposed as contributory to this phenomenon [32,33].

Seasonal hair shedding. A northern hemisphere study ($n = 823$) investigated seasonal change in hair growth using trichogram assessment [34]. It found the maximum peak telogen hair levels were in summer (July), with a second smaller peak in spring (April) and the lowest telogen levels in winter. This suggests that there is seasonal variation in human hair growth. Although most people do not recognise seasonal changes in their hair, coexisting hair conditions (e.g. androgenetic alopecia) may exacerbate appreciation of this phenomenon. Seasonal shedding may be an evolutionary throwback allowing thicker hair growth in winter, thought to be controlled by the altered photoperiod influencing neuroendocrine signalling and UV intensity precipitating premature exogen [9,34].

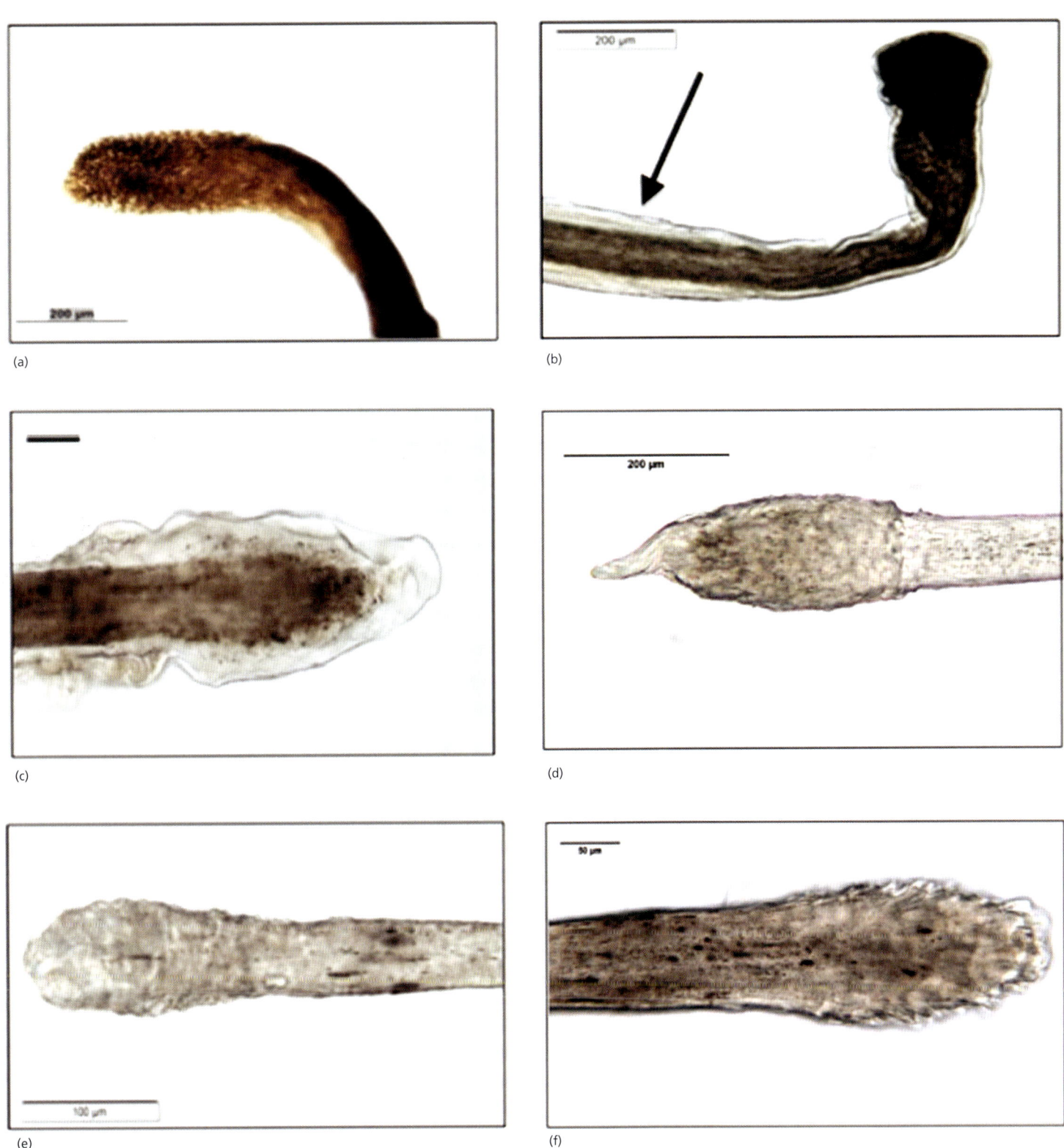

Figure 87.47 Hair root appearances using light microscopy. (a) Anagen with elongated root. (b) Anagen with follicular tissue. (c) Catagen with root end rounding and follicular tissue attached. (d) Late catagen transitioning to telogen. The presence of a follicular tag indicates it has not completed the transition. (e) Telogen with a bulbous root end and no follicular tissue. (f) Telogen with bulbous root end, pigment and ovoid bodies. Courtesy of Forensic Science and Wildlife Matters Pty Ltd. Reproduced from Koch *et al.* 2020 [71] with permission of John Wiley & Sons.

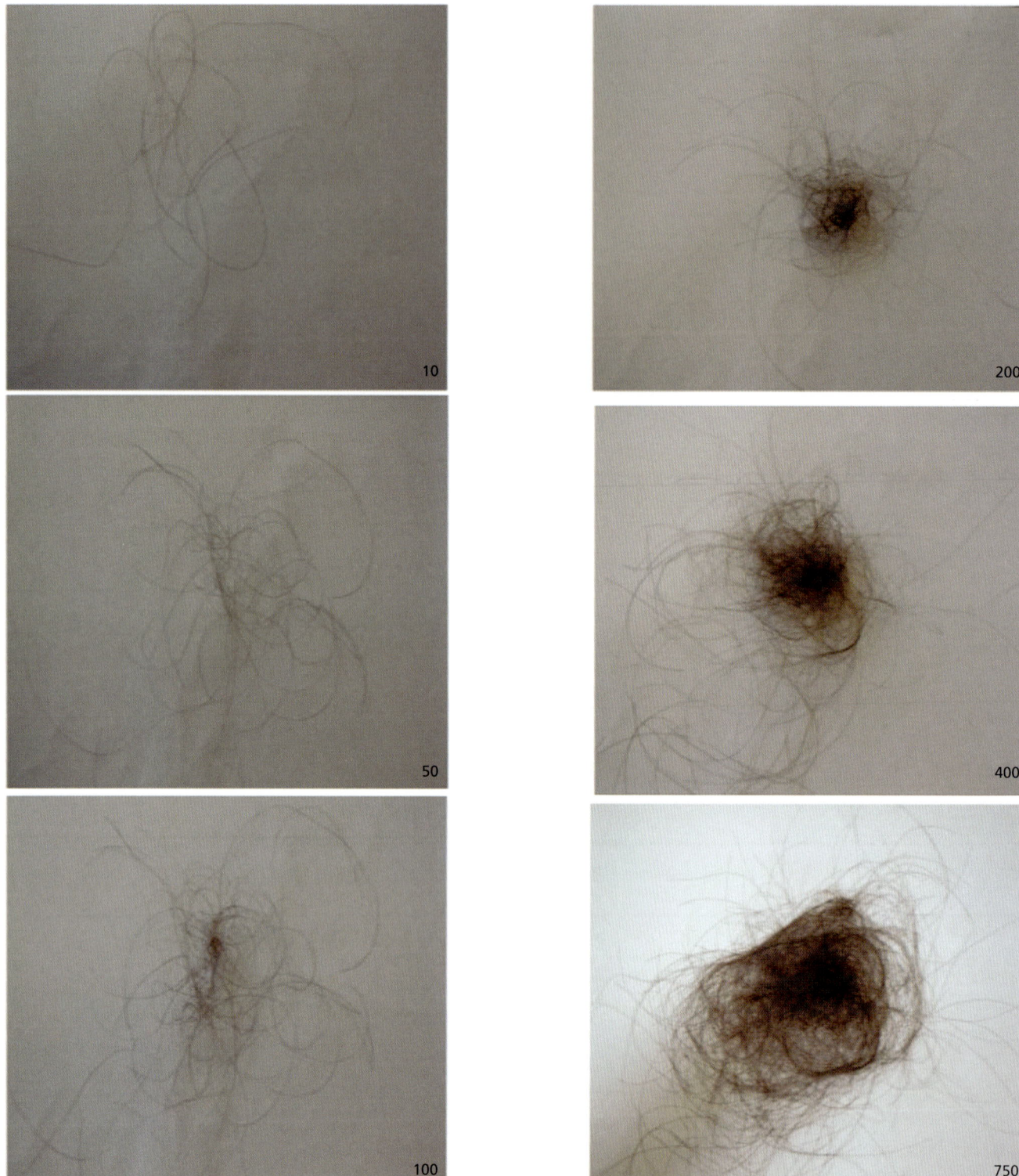

Figure 87.48 The Sinclair hair shedding scale. Reproduced from Sinclair 2015 [25] with permission of Oxford University Press.

Cronkhite–Canada syndrome. Cronkhite–Canada syndrome is a rare idiopathic disease characterised by gastrointestinal polyposis, diarrhoea, protein-losing enteropathy and weight loss; diffuse hair loss is also seen. Limited histological data indicate that the hair pathology is non-inflammatory and that anagen–telogen conversion is the early event [35], with follicular miniaturisation also reported [36]. Recently, hair features more reminiscent of alopecia areata are described [37,38].

Differential diagnosis

Shedding in the early stages of androgenetic alopecia can be diffuse and episodic and can mimic TE. Alopecia areata incognita results in diffuse hair thinning and increased shedding (see 'Alopecia areata' earlier in this chapter). The hair 'colour transition sign' can help differentiate TE from alopecia areata incognita [39]. However, scalp biopsy may be required to confirm the diagnosis of TE and exclude these conditions.

Investigations

Blood tests should be considered in those presenting with increased hair fall without a clear cause (Box 87.4). This is to identify reversible underlying drivers for the hair loss. Certain conditions are clearly associated with TE, including thyroid dysfunction, iron deficiency anaemia, renal or liver failure and acrodermatitis enteropathica. However, the role of isolated blood test changes without frank deficiency, and what values are required for optimal hair growth, is more complex and controversial [40].

Box 87.4 Screening blood tests for telogen effluvium

- Full blood count
- Ferritin/iron studies/erythrocyte sedimentation rate
- Thyroid function tests
- Renal and liver function tests
- Calcium/vitamin D
- Zinc
- Vitamin B_{12} and folate
- ± Connective tissue disease screen
- ± Syphilis serology
- ± Hormone profile

From Cunningham *et al.* 2012 [61].

Ferritin

Ferritin is a sensitive marker of body iron stores. The direct role of iron on the HF is unclear, but it appears to regulate various HF genes and may influence nuclear factor κB-controlled gene expression [41]. A mouse model of iron deficiency anaemia shows that hair regrows with iron replacement [42]. However, in humans evidence linking iron deficiency without anaemia, TE and hair regrowth with treatment is weak and often conflicting. Most studies are retrospective case–control comparisons of ferritin levels between TE and other groups. Lower ferritin levels in TE are reported by some [43–47] but not others [48–50] – and summarised in [41]. Interestingly, a series of studies by Rushton *et al.* [51–53] demonstrated increased ferritin levels and reduced shedding in chronic TE patients treated with iron and L-lysine (1000–1500 mg daily). L-lysine and vitamin C may help improve absorption of iron and zinc.

There are some practical issues that need to be considered when appraising these studies [51]:

- What is iron deficiency? Laboratory normal ranges for ferritin are derived from a large population of people, many of whom will be iron deficient, thereby falsely reducing the value. This is high- lighted by the observation that 39% of women have ferritin levels below the lowest value in men, despite no biological reason for differing iron requirements.
- How do ferritin levels correlate with iron stores? Ferritin is an excellent marker of iron stores. However, a ferritin >70 μg/L is

needed to achieve a 99% confidence limit for iron staining in bone marrow. Thus, despite ferritin levels lying within the 'normal range' the body iron stores may still be inadequate.
- Does anything influence ferritin levels? Ferritin is an acute phase reactant so inflammation may falsely elevate ferritin levels. There- fore, it is recommended to also check an inflammatory marker (e.g. ESR <10 mm/h) to be confident the value is accurate.

The conflicting studies mentioned use various cut-off values for ferritin, and many have prescreened their patients prior to analysis, making interpretation more challenging. Considering these arguments, at present it seems sensible to recommend that in people with low/normal ferritin levels and increased hair shed- ding, the aim should be to maintain their ferritin levels >70 μg/L with iron-rich foods and supplementation. Investigations for iron deficiency should also be considered based on local protocols.

Zinc

Zinc is a cofactor to many enzymes, playing a vital role in skin homeostasis. Acrodermatitis enteropathica and acquired zinc defi- ciency brought about by longstanding parenteral nutrition can lead to a severe TE (Figure 87.44). However, it is unclear if isolated low zinc levels found on routine blood biochemistry screening for TE are relevant. Again, the evidence is poor, but some studies highlight an association between low levels and increased hair shedding [46,54]. Zinc supplementation and improved absorption (e.g. with L-lysine) can be considered in those with low zinc levels.

Other

Low vitamin B_{12} [17], biotin deficiency [55,56] and low vitamin D [45,47,57] have also been associated with telogen hair loss.

Scalp biopsy using horizontal sectioning may be needed to con- firm the diagnosis of TE and to exclude other conditions that may present with increased hair fall, particularly androgenetic alopecia and diffuse areata alopecia. In TE there are normal follicular units and a normal terminal to vellus hair ratio, but an increased percent- age of telogen hair.

Management

When an obvious explanation exists for acute TE, expectant man- agement and observation are appropriate. Shedding can be expected to cease within 3–6 months but full recovery may take a further 6 months to be seen. Any underlying cause should be addressed. Some recommend topical steroids, particularly if trichodynia is present [9,16], but this approach risks steroid side effects. Topical and oral minoxidil may have a role in chronic TE, but not acute TE [58]. Other novel therapies recently reported include an olfactory receptor (OR2ATA) topical solution [59] and a topically applied arrector pili muscle constrictor that increases the force required to remove hairs during washing and brushing [60].

Primary chronic telogen effluvium

Introduction and general description

Primary chronic TE is an idiopathic and sometimes self-limiting condition that predominantly affects middle-aged women. The trigger for shedding is obscure, the problem is often only noticed by the individual and the process continues for over 6 months. However, importantly, hair density is maintained despite the protracted course.

Pathophysiology

Primary chronic TE appears to result from a reduction in the variance of anagen (i.e. resulting in a narrower spread of anagen duration values), which contrasts with the shortening of anagen seen in androgenetic alopecia [1]. The reason for this change in variance is unclear, but hypotheses include age-related effects or fluctuations in oestrogen levels in the perimenopausal period, influencing central and peripheral clock gene functions [2]. Chronic TE has also been associated with *VDR* gene polymorphisms [3] and heavy metal exposure [4]. The female squirrel monkey is a potential animal model for chronic TE [5].

Clinical features

This condition is almost exclusively described in women in their fourth to sixth decades, although there is one report in a long-haired man [6], potentially highlighting hair length as a factor in presentation. Typically, sudden-onset increased hair shedding occurs and persists for at least 6 months, often on a background of high hair density and ability to grow very long hair when younger (Figure 87.49) [7]. There is no associated visible widening of the central parting line, although mild temporal recession is sometimes seen. Trichoscopy is normal and there is no miniaturisation of HFs on scalp biopsy [8,9]. Trichodynia may accompany chronic TE.

Differential diagnosis

Chronic TE must be distinguished clinically from FPHL as women with early androgenetic alopecia may present with periods of increased hair shedding without a discernible pattern to the loss [10]. Psychogenic pseudo-effluvium is a type of body dysmorphic disorder where a person is preoccupied with concerns of hair loss without objective evidence of alopecia. Underlying mental health problems and introspection likely drive this presentation.

Investigations

The diagnosis of chronic TE is made by the exclusion of other causes of diffuse telogen hair loss. Careful history and examination may suggest the diagnosis, but scalp biopsy is often required to differentiate it from early androgenetic alopecia. Interestingly, Whiting proposed that scalp biopsy in chronic TE is also therapeutic, providing reassurance that hair levels are maintained despite the persistent hair fall seen [8,9].

Scalp histology on horizontal sectioning shows features similar to controls, where the terminal to vellus ratio is maintained (9T : 1V) but showing a slightly higher telogen rate (89% anagen and 11% telogen hairs) [8,9]. Multiple biopsies may improve diagnostic accuracy but these are only required to exclude androgenetic alopecia in those with relatively normal hair densities (Sinclair midline hair density grade 1 or 2), as higher grades (Sinclair 3–5) are strongly correlated with androgenetic alopecia on biopsy, allowing the diagnosis of androgenetic alopecia on clinical features alone [10,11]. Despite the assertion that chronic TE is a self-limiting process that does not evolve into androgenetic alopecia, its natural history remains poorly characterised with only one published longitudinal study [12].

Management

Clear explanation of the condition is important. No treatment is necessary as, while the hair continues to shed, it is replaced, and this condition does not lead to baldness. Antiandrogens have little effect on chronic TE. Topical and oral minoxidil can reduce hair shedding and may also improve trichodynia [13,14].

Androgenetic alopecia and pattern hair loss

Introduction and general description

The term androgenetic alopecia (AGA) has long been used to describe a common form of patterned hair loss on the scalp, in which there is a gradual decline in the production of hair that may eventually lead to balding. AGA is also known as male balding or male pattern hair loss (MPHL), and in the great majority of men is a genetically determined trait that requires androgens and age for its phenotypic expression. A similar type of hair loss affects women and has also been termed AGA but – although androgen-dependent scalp hair loss undoubtedly occurs in women – in the majority the roles of androgens and genetics are less conclusive than in men. Although the follicular changes appear similar in both sexes, the predominant patterns of hair loss differ between men and women and there is an increasing preference to use the non-aetiological term 'female pattern hair loss' in women rather than AGA, although this terminology also has its limitations as AGA may occur in a 'female' pattern in some men and in a 'male' pattern in some women.

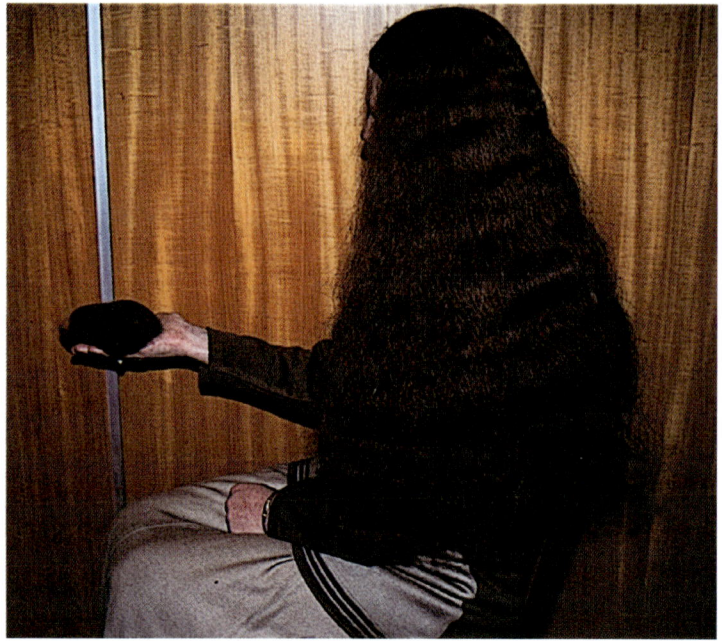

Figure 87.49 Idiopathic chronic telogen effluvium.

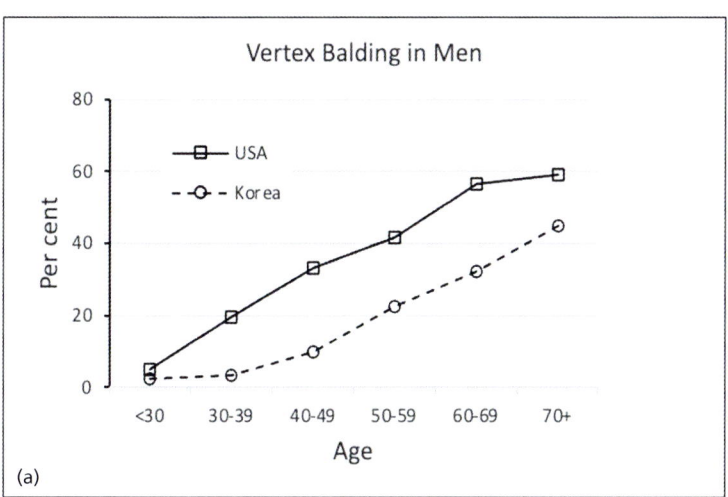
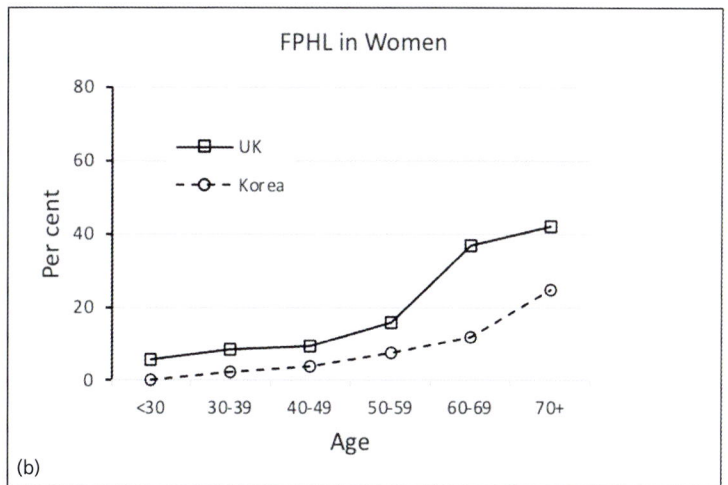

Figure 87.50 (a) Frequency of vertex balding (Norwood–Hamilton IIIv–VII) in Norwood's study in white US men [2] and the study by Paik *et al*. in Korean men [8]. The Korean data also include men with a female pattern of hair loss (FPHL). (b) Frequency of FPHL in the study by Birch *et al*. in white UK women [10] and in the study by Paik *et al*. in Korean women [8].

Epidemiology
Male pattern hair loss
Almost all white men develop some recession of the frontal hairline at the temples during their teens [1]. Deep frontal recession and/or vertex balding may also start shortly after puberty, although in most men the onset is later. Hair loss progresses to a bald scalp in 50–60% of men by the age of 70 years [1–4]. A small proportion of men (15–20%) do not show balding, apart from postpubertal temporal recession, even in old age. Balding is less common in Asian men although there is quite a wide variation in published frequencies (Figure 87.50a). Two studies from Thailand and Singapore found prevalence rates not far short of those in white European men [5,6]. A Japanese study reported that male balding starts approximately one decade later in Japanese men than in white men and that the prevalence is about 30% lower in each decade group [7]. In Korean men, the frequency is also 20–40% lower than in white men in the 40–70-year age group, although the difference becomes less pronounced with advancing age [8], and a large study in Chinese men reported that 41.4% of men aged over 70 had AGA [9]. Preservation of the frontal hairline was a common feature in the series reported from Korea: 11.1% of Korean men showed a 'female' pattern of hair loss, although this was less common (3.7%) in the Chinese study.

Female pattern hair loss
The frequency and severity of pattern hair loss are lower in women than in men, but it still affects a sizeable proportion of the population (Figure 87.50b). Two studies in white women in the UK and USA reported prevalence rates of 3–6% in women aged under 30 years, increasing to 29–42% in women aged 70 and over [10,11]. A higher prevalence was reported in a multiracial Brazilian population (Fitzpatrick skin types I–VI) of 350 women between the ages of 20 and 75 years [12]. Here, almost 10% of women aged 20–29, increasing to 70% in women aged 65–75, were reported to have FPHL, and there was no difference in prevalence between white and darker skinned women. These significantly higher rates likely reflect the diagnostic criteria used, with a high proportion of early FPHL (Sinclair grade 2) identified by trichoscopy. As in

Asian men, pattern hair loss is less common and appears to start later in life in Asian women, although nearly 25% of Korean women over 70 years of age show evidence of hair loss [8]. There are no published data on the prevalence in African women, although clinical experience suggests that its frequency is similar to that in other racial groups.

Pathophysiology
Aetiology
Male androgenetic alopecia.
Endocrine factors. Male balding is an androgen-dependent trait. The American anatomist James Hamilton observed that men castrated before puberty do not go bald unless treated with testosterone [13]. Testosterone is the major circulating androgen in men. However, DHT, the 5α-reduced metabolite of testosterone, is primarily responsible for driving hair loss. The conversion of testosterone to DHT is catalysed by the enzyme 5α-reductase. There are three isoforms of 5α-reductase (SRD5A1, -A2, -A3) which are encoded by different genes [14]. Types 1 and 3 5α-reductase are widely distributed, but expression of the type 2 isoform is limited to certain androgen target tissues such as the prostate, the epididymis and HFs in certain regions of the skin [14,15].

The role of DHT in hair growth was first recognised through observations in men with a genetic deficiency of type 2 5α-reductase (type II pseudohermaphroditism, pseudovaginal perineoscrotal hypospadias) [16]. The external genitalia are ambiguous at birth but enlarge and masculinise at puberty, together with deepening of the voice and typical male musculoskeletal development. Serum testosterone is at normal male levels, but DHT levels remain low. There is growth of pubic and axillary hair but elsewhere body hair and beard growth are absent or scanty and these individuals do not develop balding. These observations were extended by the demonstration that treatment with a 5α-reductase inhibitor prevented the development of balding [17] or increased scalp hair growth [18] in macaques, a primate that develops androgen-dependent hair loss. Confirmation of the role of DHT in human hair growth came from the results of clinical trials showing that finasteride, an inhibitor of type 2 5α-reductase, prevents or slows progression of

PART 8: SPECIFIC CUTANEOUS STRUCTURES

balding in most men and stimulates some recovery of hair growth in about two-thirds [19]. This latter finding also shows that, contrary to Hamilton's conclusions from his observations in eunuchs, male balding is partially reversible.

Studies where circulating androgen levels were measured in balding men have yielded mixed results. In some, total testosterone and DHT levels have not differed from non-balding controls [20–22] although elevated levels have been reported in case series of early-onset balding from Korea and India [23,24]. Some studies, although not all, have found raised free testosterone levels [22,25], and an increased DHT : testosterone ratio has also been reported [26]. Two studies have reported increased hair growth on the arms in balding men [20,22]. Some men with early-onset balding show a hormonal profile that resembles that seen in women with PCOS, leading to the proposal that this presentation represents the male equivalent of PCOS [27].

The essential role for androgens in the aetiology of male balding is incontrovertible. Nevertheless, other factors are clearly involved as not all men develop balding despite most having similar androgen levels to those that do. Information from human GWAS, from hair growth research in other species and from studies using cultured human HFs has implicated several other hormones in the pathogenesis of balding, including prolactin, melatonin (both of which play a key role in seasonal moulting), parathyroid hormone and insulin-like growth factor [28].

Prostaglandins. Prostaglandins have been implicated in the pathogenesis of male balding. Garza *et al.* showed elevated levels of prostaglandin D2 synthase mRNA and protein in bald compared with haired scalp in men [29]. The product of its activity, prostaglandin D2 (PGD2), was also elevated in the bald scalps and inhibited hair growth in explanted human follicles and when applied topically to mice. K14-Ptgs2 transgenic mice, which show elevated PGD2 in the skin, developed alopecia and miniaturisation of HFs. Further experiments in transgenic mice and cultured HFs indicated that the inhibitory effect of PGD2 on hair growth was via the GPR44 receptor.

Heritable factors. Twin studies demonstrate that the predisposition to male balding is very largely inherited [30,31]. Published concordance rates for monozygotic twins are around 80–90%, with consistently lower rates in dizygotic twins. Several studies have shown there is a high frequency of balding in the fathers of bald men. For example, Ellis and colleagues reported that 32 of 54 bald men (59.3%) had fathers with a greater degree of baldness, whereas only 1 of 65 sons of 50 non-bald controls had type III baldness or greater [32]. In a study involving 572 men aged 16–91 years, the risk of balding in young men with a balding father was significantly greater than in those with a non-bald father (odds ratio (OR) 5.5; 95% confidence interval (CI) 1.26–23.99). The risk fell with increasing subject age to approach unity in elderly men [3]. The opposite trend was seen in non-bald men where the risk of non-balding in men with a non-bald father increased with age (OR 3.2; 95%CI 1.82–5.58 in subjects aged 70 and over).

Like other common traits, the predisposition to male balding is highly polygenic and the number of genetic loci linked to it is now over 600 [33]. The first to be reported was an association

with the gene for the androgen receptor (AR) on the X chromosome [34]. Later studies have shown the strongest association is with a genomic region located between AR and the gene for the ectodysplasin A2 receptor (EDA2R). The association with the AR/EDA2R locus has been confirmed in several GWAS [28], which have also identified many other loci linked to AGA throughout the genome. A meta-analysis of eight GWAS identified 63 loci associated with AGA which, together, explained about 39% of the phenotypic variance [35]. Six loci were located on the X chromosome and 57 were autosomal. A larger GWAS using DNA from over 70 000 men identified 71 loci associated with male pattern baldness that explained about 38% of the risk [36]. The authors calculated a SNP-based heritability (h^2_{SNP}) of 94%, similar to the value derived from twin studies, indicating the risk for male balding is almost entirely genetic with little environmental contribution. The results of these studies have highlighted several plausible candidate genes (SRD5A2, FGF5, IRF4, DKK2) and pathways (androgen metabolism and signalling, melatonin signalling, adipogenesis, Wnt signalling) that may participate in the pathophysiological features of male AGA. These studies have also shown that male balding is not an isolated trait; at a genetic level it shares substantial overlap with other human traits and diseases, such as height, lifespan, risk of cancer and neurodegenerative disorders, that may have evolutionary implications.

Female pattern hair loss. Less is known about the aetiology of FPHL than male balding and there is a body of thought that it represents a multifactorial trait rather than a single entity.

Endocrine factors. The role of androgens in FPHL is less clear than it is in male balding. Scalp hair loss can undoubtedly be a feature of hyperandrogenism in women, although it is less common than hirsutism. Indeed, loss of hair was reported in women with androgen-secreting tumours prior to Hamilton's observations in men [37,38]. Cohort studies from the USA and China have reported pattern hair loss in 22% and 23%, respectively, in women with PCOS [39,40]. This compares with hirsutism in 70% and 58% of the same subjects. On the other hand, Azziz and colleagues reported hair loss in only 4% of over 800 women presenting with hyperandrogenism (75% had hirsutism) [41], a figure not dissimilar from the population frequency. There are isolated case reports of FPHL occurring in the absence of androgens [42], in complete androgen insensitivity syndrome [43] and in severe hypoandrogenism due to 17α-hydroxylase deficiency [44].

Several investigators have noted that, on average, women with hair loss are more likely to have elevated androgen levels or show an increased frequency of other features of androgen excess than women without hair loss. Futterweit and colleagues studied 109 women with hair loss and reported that 38.5% showed clinical or biochemical evidence of androgen excess [45]. In a series of 187 women with hair loss, Vexiau *et al.* reported abnormal hormonal profiles, mostly of minor degree, in 67% of women with hair loss alone and in 84% of women who were also hirsute [46]. In a series of 89 women presenting to a trichology clinic with hair loss, 67% showed ultrasound evidence of polycystic ovaries compared with 27% in a control group of 73 women, and 21% were significantly hirsute compared with 4% of controls [47]. However, other investigators have failed to find evidence of raised androgen levels in women with FPHL [48] and in all studies there is a variable proportion of women with hair loss who do not show clinical or biochemical signs of androgen excess.

Antiandrogens are widely used to treat FPHL but the quality of evidence for efficacy is poor [**49**]. A randomised controlled trial of finasteride 1 mg daily in postmenopausal women with FPHL failed to show any benefit after a year of treatment [50], although improvement has been reported in uncontrolled case series using higher doses of finasteride [51]. A 1-year trial comparing topical minoxidil with cyproterone acetate (CPA) reported improvement in the minoxidil group but overall deterioration in those receiving CPA [52]. Subgroup analysis did show a small improvement in women with menstrual irregularities taking CPA, possibly suggesting that antiandrogen treatment may work in women with hyperandrogenism.

Paradoxically, a questionnaire study in women receiving testosterone implants for symptoms of androgen deficiency reported improvement in scalp hair growth although almost all developed hirsutism [53]. Androgen levels in women decline progressively from early in the fourth decade [54] and this parallels the decline in hair density and hair diameter in the female population that occurs with advancing age [10]. It was suggested that testosterone may have an anabolic effect on hair growth that is distinct from a virilising effect via the 5α-reductase pathway.

A role for other endocrine factors in FPHL is also uncertain. Thyroid deficiency is often linked to hair loss, but it has been the subject of little research. There is some evidence that hypothyroidism may cause an increase in hair shedding, which can be reversed by thyroid replacement [55]. One study on diffuse hair thinning in hypothyroid women found features near identical to those of FPHL [56], but whether this was improved by thyroid replacement was not reported. Indirect evidence for a protective effect of oestrogens on human hair growth comes from the increasing prevalence of FPHL following the menopause, the prolongation of anagen during pregnancy [57] and reports of hair loss in women taking tamoxifen or aromatase inhibitors for the treatment of breast cancer [58]. One study found lower oestrogen : androgen ratios in premenopausal women with FPHL compared with a control group, suggesting a protective effect of oestrogen on hair loss, although the number of subjects was quite small [59]. On the other hand, there is no clear effect of oestrogen supplements on human hair growth, and several studies have shown an inhibitory effect of oestrogens on hair growth in other species [60].

Iron and vitamin D. The place of low iron stores in the aetiology of FPHL is controversial. Both lower [61,62] and similar [63] serum ferritin levels compared with control groups have been reported in women with FPHL. There are no controlled trials that have tested the hair growth response to iron supplementation in women with FPHL. One study reported a response to antiandrogen therapy in women with serum ferritin levels above 40 μg/L, but not in those with serum ferritins below this level [64].

Reduced vitamin D levels have been reported in women with FPHL compared with control subjects [65,66] but there are no published studies to show a hair growth response to vitamin D supplementation.

Heritable factors. Published models based on family histories have generally assumed that FPHL is the same entity as male balding, has a similar aetiology and shares a similar genetic predisposition. In 1916, Osborn proposed that balding is due to a single gene with balding (B) and non-balding (b) alleles [67]. Men homozygous for B (BB) or heterozygous (Bb) would develop balding but only BB women would bald, and she presented family histories to support this hypothesis. In support of Osborn's idea, Smith and Wells found that first-degree male relatives of women with hair loss showed an increased frequency of balding compared with the male relatives of non-balding women [68], although they did posit the idea of a multifactorial aetiology. Küster and Happle argued that the predisposition to balding is a polygenic trait in which clinical expression represents a threshold effect determined by androgens [69]. We now know that male balding is indeed polygenic, but the case remains unproven in women, partly because the relevant studies have not yet been done.

Somewhat surprisingly, a twin study in women found a strong heritable component to hair greying and to frontotemporal recession in women but none to diffuse thinning over the top of the scalp [70]. All the subjects were aged 59 years and over, and clinical experience does suggest there is a familial component to FPHL in young women. Nevertheless, the study was performed in similarly aged subjects, and drawn from the same population as the Danish study that showed strong heritability in male AGA [31].

Molecular genetic studies have been limited to case–control studies and, to date, there are no GWAS in FPHL. Two independent studies in women have suggested a weak association with the oestrogen receptor gene *ESR2* [71,72]. A German/UK study in women with FPHL analysed 12 gene loci that are associated with male AGA. There was a weak association with the *AR/EDA2R* locus in the UK cohort with early-onset hair loss, but not in the German sample, and there was no association with the other 11 loci in either group [60].

These findings suggest there is some commonality between early-onset FPHL and male balding but otherwise imply there are significant differences in aetiology.

Pathology

The follicular changes in pattern hair loss are similar in men and women. In essence, there is a gradual decline in the production of hair by affected HFs which eventually become smaller, a process referred to as miniaturisation, and may eventually be deleted.

Hair cycle dynamics. Pattern hair loss is characterised by a reduction in the duration of anagen in terminal follicles; thus, where anagen may have previously lasted several years, it is now only a matter of a few months or weeks. The time to exogen in telogen follicles is unchanged at 2–3 months but the duration of kenogen is lengthened, although not to the same degree as the shortening of anagen. Prolongation of kenogen increases the number of 'empty' follicles, further contributing to the balding process. These changes have been clearly demonstrated by longitudinal studies in both men and women [73,74].

Hair follicle miniaturisation. Ultimately, HFs shrink in size to produce smaller and thinner hair fibres, a process known as miniaturisation. Miniaturised follicles are often referred to as vellus follicles although they differ from vellus follicles in other sites that have not previous passed through a period of terminal growth, such as those on the cheeks of a child. The cross-sectional area of individual hair shafts remains constant throughout fully developed anagen indicating that the HF, and its dermal papilla, remains the same size through each individual anagen stage of the cycle. Thus, miniaturisation occurs between rather than within cycles. Follicular miniaturisation has traditionally been thought to occur in a stepwise fashion over several cycles. There have been suggestions that it occurs rapidly, possibly in the space of a single hair cycle [10,75], although this idea has been disputed [76]. A histopathological study in FPHL showed a progressive reduction in total follicle counts with increasing severity of hair loss in the subjects, suggesting that miniaturisation may not be the end point of the process and that follicles are eventually deleted [77]. Whiting's study also showed a lower total follicle count in biopsies from balding men than non-balding controls [78]. Both studies were cross-sectional in nature but there is also evidence from longitudinal phototrichogram studies that miniaturised hairs eventually disappear [79].

Follicular miniaturisation leaves behind stelae as dermal remnants of the full-sized follicle. These stelae, also known as fibrous tracts or streamers, extend from the subcutaneous tissue up the old follicular tract to the miniaturised hair and mark the former position of the original terminal follicle. Arao–Perkins bodies may be seen with elastic stains within the follicular stelae. An Arao–Perkins body begins as a small cluster of elastic fibres in the neck of the dermal papilla. These clump in catagen and remain situated at the lowest point of origin of the follicular stelae. With the progressive shortening of anagen hair seen in AGA, multiple elastic clumps may be found in stelae, like the rungs of a ladder [80].

Hairs on the scalp exist in groups known as follicular units. Hairs within follicular units may share a common infundibulum, emerging from a single pore. The diffuse hair loss pattern seen in FPHL is due to a reduction in the number of terminal hairs per follicular unit rather than miniaturisation of entire follicular units [81]. Baldness occurs only when all the hairs within the follicular units are miniaturised and is a relatively early event in men and a late event in women. Therefore, FPHL is generally less severe than male balding, occurs later and presents with diffuse thinning rather than a bald spot. This diffuse thinning that precedes baldness is also observed in men with early AGA and can be readily identified on close examination of the scalp.

Inflammation. Some degree of perifollicular inflammation is common in pattern hair loss although it is also common in the normal scalp. Whiting reported the presence of inflammation in 70% of biopsies from male AGA patients and in 40% of biopsies from non-balding controls. Mild inflammation was seen in about one-third of cases of male AGA and in a similar proportion of controls. In contrast, a moderate lymphohistiocytic inflammation is found in another one-third of cases of male AGA, but in only 10% of controls [78]. The infiltrate is composed mainly of lymphocytes and histiocytes; occasional esosinophils, mast cells and neutrophils

may also be seen. The infiltrate occurs mainly around the upper part of follicles and may be associated with perifollicular fibrosis. Perifollicular inflammation may also be seen in FPHL [77,82]. A role for inflammation in the pathogenesis of pattern hair loss was proposed by Jaworsky and colleagues [83], but whether this is the case is not yet established and treatment with anti-inflammatory agents or immunosuppressive drugs is not conspicuously associated with its reversal.

Arrector degeneration. In a study of eight scalp biopsies from patients with pattern hair loss, degeneration of the arrector pili muscle and replacement by fat tissue were observed [84]. The precise mechanism remains unclear, but the authors speculated that degeneration of the arrector pili muscle might be related to depletion of follicular stem or progenitor cells. The authors did not state whether samples were from men or women.

Histopathology

The key elements of the histology of pattern hair loss in both sexes are a reduction in the number of terminal HFs, an increase in miniaturised HFs with associated angiofibrotic streamers, a variable increase in the proportion of telogen and catagen hairs and a mild or moderate perifollicular lymphohistiocytic infiltrate, with or without concentric layers of perifollicular collagen deposition (Figure 87.51) [77,78,85,86].

Most of these changes are best seen on horizontally sectioned scalp biopsies. Miniaturised follicles can be identified by their small size – Whiting proposed that the diameter of the vellus hair is less than the thickness of its IRS – and the presence of an angiofibrotic streamer beneath the follicle that extends into the subcutis. There is a change in the ratio of terminal to vellus hairs from $\geq 7 : 1$ to $\leq 2 : 1$ in both male AGA [78] and FPHL [86].

As the balding scalp loses its protective covering of hair, solar degenerative changes may be seen.

Clinical features
Male pattern hair loss
In most men, balding is patterned, the two major components being frontotemporal recession and loss of hair over the vertex. Hairs become shorter and may, although not always, become finer in calibre. Ultimately this may lead to complete hair loss except at the lateral and posterior margins of the scalp where hair is retained. In elderly men, hair may also be lost in these parts of the scalp. A small proportion of men show a diffuse pattern of hair loss over the crown and frontal scalp with retention of the frontal hair line, similar to female pattern hair loss. Hamilton classified male balding into several stages [1] and the revision of his classification by Norwood is still widely used (Figure 87.52) [2]. Although the grades are imprecise measures of the continuum of hair patterns that are seen in adult men, they are useful as diagnostic aids and in the classification of extent of hair loss for record-keeping or clinical research.

Diffuse unpatterned alopecia is an uncommon form of miniaturising hair loss seen in some men. It is characterised by a diffuse global reduction in scalp hair density that affects the sides and back of the scalp as well as the top and frontal regions [87]. Involvement of the potential donor site means that this type of hair loss is not suitable for hair transplant surgery.

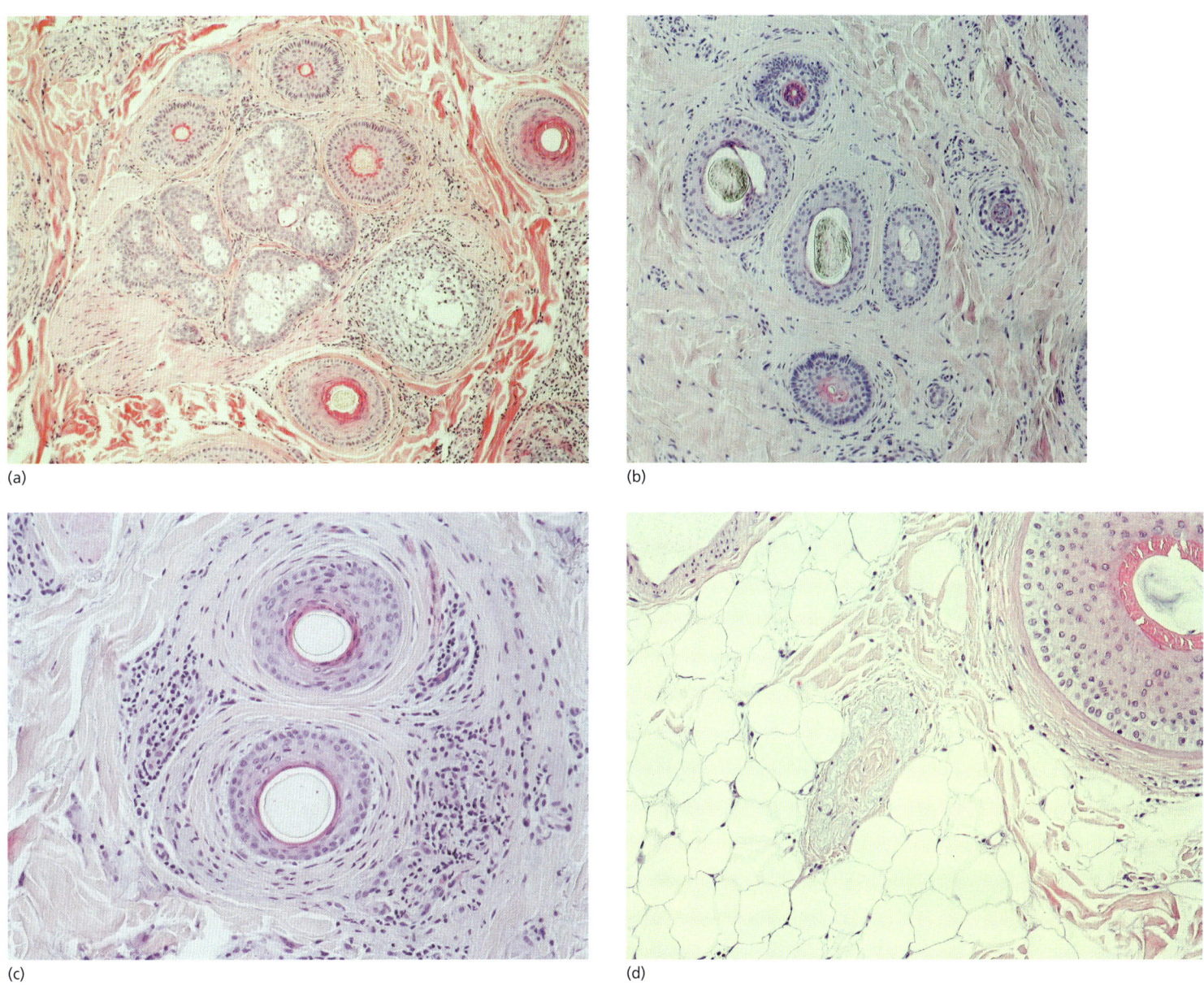

(a) (b) (c) (d)

Figure 87.51 Histopathology of female pattern hair loss. (a) Increase in telogen forms – three of five follicles in a follicular unit are in telogen. (b) Follicular miniaturisation – three of five follicles in a follicular unit are miniaturised. (c) 'Onion-skin' perifollicular fibrosis and mild inflammation at the infundibular level. (d) Fibrous tract adjacent to the terminal follicle.

PART 8: SPECIFIC CUTANEOUS STRUCTURES

Female pattern hair loss

Most women with FPHL present with a history of gradual thinning of scalp hair, often over a period of several years. The hair loss can start at any age from puberty onwards. There is sometimes a history of excessive hair shedding and/or of loss of hair volume, which may pre-date a clinically obvious reduction in hair density. Examination of the scalp shows a widening of the central parting with a diffuse reduction in hair density mainly affecting the frontal scalp and mid-scalp regions [88]. In some women the hair loss is accentuated over the frontal scalp giving rise to the 'Christmas-tree pattern' described by Olsen [89]. The frontal hairline is typically retained although many women develop a minor degree of postpubertal recession at the temples (equivalent to a Hamilton–Norwood II frontal hairline), whether or not they have diffuse hair loss. Some women have more pronounced temporal recession although this usually manifests as thinning rather than the complete loss of

temporal hair seen in men. Some women show a more global reduction in hair density that, unlike male AGA, involves the parietal and occipital regions.

FPHL was first classified by Ludwig into three grades of severity (Figure 87.53) [88]. A later classification introduced by Sinclair comprises five grades, with grade 1 representing normal hair density and grade 5 the most severe hair loss [90]. Sinclair grading is more sensitive and has largely replaced the Ludwig scale (Figure 87.54).

The hair pull test is usually used to assess a hair cycle disturbance, such as TE, and may be normal in pattern hair loss. However, an increase in easily extracted telogen hairs may be found in active pattern hair loss.

Trichoscopy can be helpful in the early stages of FPHL, revealing differing hair density between the mid-frontal and occipital scalp. Over the occipital scalp it is common to see two or three terminal hairs of equal fibre diameter emerging from a single ostium.

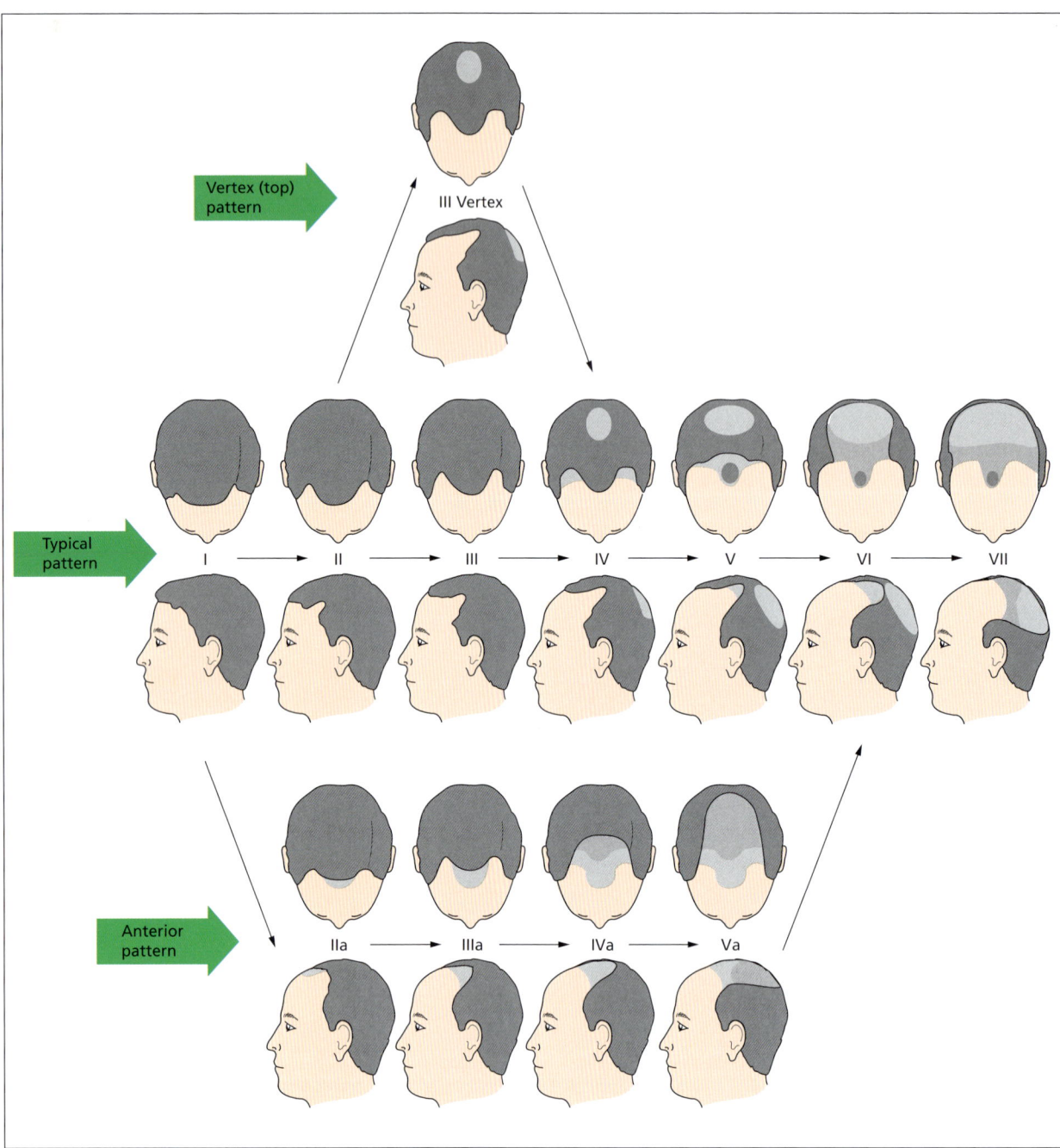

Figure 87.52 Hamilton–Norwood scale for grading male pattern hair loss. Reproduced from Norwood 1975 [2] with permission of Wolters Kluwer Health.

In comparison, the number of terminal hairs per ostium is reduced to one or sometimes two over the mid-frontal scalp. Early FPHL is also characterised by an increase in the variability of hair diameters known as hair diameter diversity [91]. Bhamla and colleagues reported that 75% of women complaining of hair thinning, but with no widening of the central parting and who showed features of FPHL on biopsy, had more than 20% hair diameter diversity on trichoscopy compared with 32% of non-hair loss controls showing the same trichoscopic features [92]. They concluded that trichoscopy is 75% sensitive and 62% specific in diagnosing early FPHL and that low hair diameter diversity is more reliable in ruling the diagnosis out than is high hair diameter diversity at ruling it in. In advanced

hair loss, trichoscopy is valuable in demonstrating the non-scarring nature of the process.

Androgenetic alopecia in children and adolescents

There is little discussion in the literature of pattern hair loss in children and adolescents (<18 years). Reports of prepubertal AGA are rare, with the youngest reported case being in a 6-year-old [93]. Both prepubertal girls and boys usually present with a 'female' pattern of hair loss, characterised by widening of the central hair part, with frontal accentuation ('Christmas-tree pattern') being common [93,94]. In adolescents, the 'female' pattern is also seen more commonly in both sexes, although most males will show the typical male

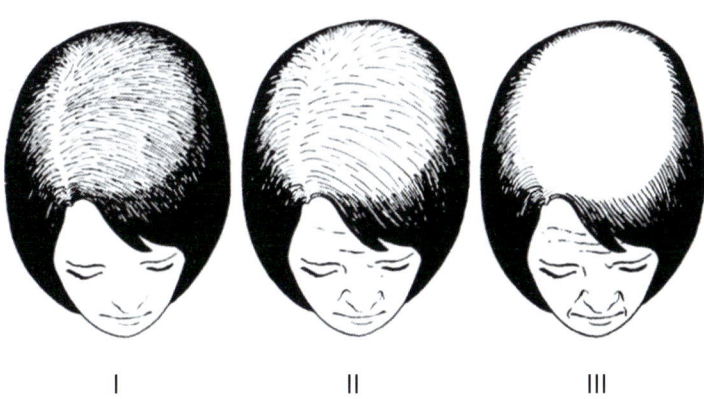

Figure 87.53 Ludwig scale for grading female pattern hair loss. Reproduced from Ludwig 1977 [88] with permission of Oxford University Press.

pattern of hair loss. Seborrhoeic dermatitis and acne are prominent in the group, with signs of hyperandrogenism important in identifying teenage girls presenting in this way [95]. Alternative causes of hair loss should be considered and an endocrine assessment to exclude causes of hyperandrogenism/precocious puberty is recommended [96].

A strong family history of AGA is consistently reported in children presenting with pattern hair loss, with usually one and sometimes both parents being affected [93,94]. There are no licensed treatments for AGA in children, but topical minoxidil is the most common agent used, although theoretical increased systemic absorption or accidental oral ingestion of topical minoxidil is a risk in this group. There are also odd reports of finasteride (in adolescent boys) and antiandrogens (in adolescent girls) being used successfully.

Why pattern hair loss develops before puberty is unclear. In the series of children reported by Tosti *et al.*, all participants showed postadrenarche blood DHEA-S levels but had no clinical signs of puberty [94]. Adrenarche typically starts 2 years before puberty, and certain factors such as obesity are associated with an earlier onset. Also, there has been a general trend towards adrenarche and puberty developing at a younger age. Thus, it is possible that increased adrenal androgen levels in adrenarche are sufficient to trigger pattern hair loss in genetically susceptible children. Alternatively, as discussed earlier for FPHL pathogenesis, it is possible the hair loss seen in this cohort is not primarily driven by androgen

Senescent alopecia

The concept of androgen-independent hair loss in older age groups, both men and women, was first promoted by Kligman [97]. He described the typical presentation as a diffuse thinning process in people over the age of 50 years with no family history of balding. On histology, those with senescent alopecia showed a modest increase in telogen follicles compared with non-balding subjects and a reduction in the size of follicles, but not to the extent of being classified as miniaturised. Inflammation was uncommon compared with male AGA. Later, Whiting disputed these findings on histological grounds, maintaining that most hair loss in the elderly is androgen dependent [98]. However, his data included a large cohort with diffuse hair loss and normal terminal : vellus ratios. In support of senescent alopecia as an entity separate from AGA, Karnik and colleagues showed differences in gene expression profiles in scalp

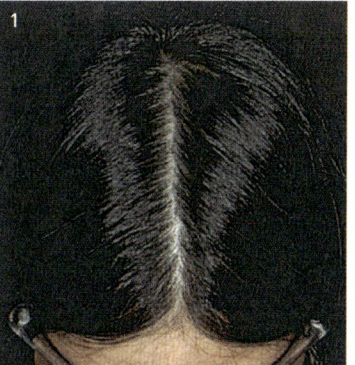
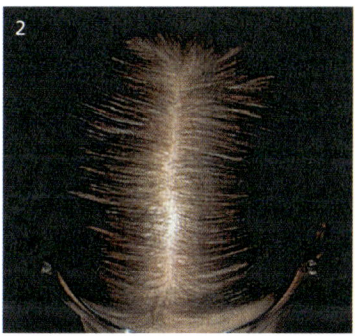
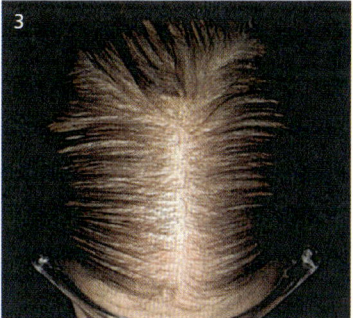
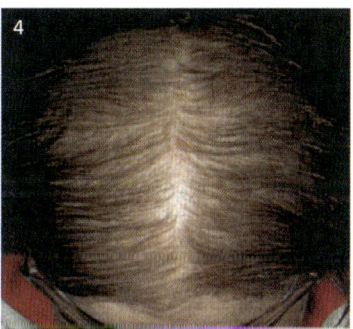
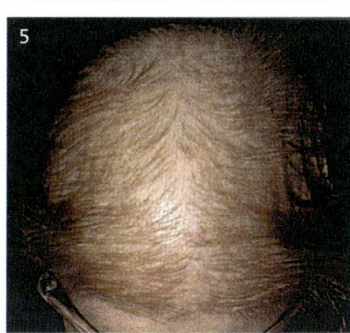

Figure 87.54 Sinclair scale for grading female-pattern hair loss. Women with grade 1 present with increased hair shedding and loss of hair volume but no reduction in hair density. Reproduced from [90].

PART 8: SPECIFIC CUTANEOUS STRUCTURES

biopsies from age-matched men with diffuse hair loss with onset after the age of 50 years and men with early-onset male AGA [99].

Differential diagnosis

The diagnosis of androgenetic alopecia in men rarely causes difficulties. In cases presenting with general thinning other causes of diffuse hair loss should be considered, particularly when the hair loss progresses quickly. The differential diagnosis of early FPHL includes chronic TE [86] and FAPD [100].

In women with skin of colour, the differential diagnosis must include CCCA. Women with chronic TE present with chronic diffuse hair shedding without noticeable widening of the central parting. They may describe a loss in volume of the ponytail of up to one-third, and there is commonly mild bitemporal recession. Scalp biopsies of women who present in this fashion reveal pattern hair loss in approximately 60% of cases and chronic TE in 40% [90]. In women with CCCA, there is a localised thinning over the vertex scalp, a loss of follicular openings and usually a more localised area of loss than is typically seen in FPHL.

Other potential differential diagnoses, albeit rare, include diffuse alopecia areata and systemic lupus erythematosus.

Complications and co-morbidities

Several studies have reported an increased risk of coronary heart disease in men with vertex balding but not frontal balding (mean relative risk (RR) 1.18–1.44) [101]. The risk increases with earlier onset and severity of hair loss.

A possible association between male AGA and prostate cancer has also been studied extensively, with mixed results. Two meta-analyses have concluded there is an increased risk of prostate cancer in men with vertex balding, but not with other balding patterns (mean RR 1.18–1.24) [102,103].

An increased frequency of metabolic syndrome in balding men has been reported in some studies [104,105] but this was not found in a large study from Korea [106].

An increased prevalence of metabolic syndrome has also been reported in women with FPHL [104,106,107]. In the Korean study, the frequency correlated with the severity of hair loss [106]. Birch and colleagues found that in women with FPHL, those with hirsutism had raised body mass index levels compared with control subjects, whereas the non-hirsute cohort did not, suggesting that normo-androgenic women with FPHL are less likely to develop features of metabolic syndrome [108].

Investigations

Investigations are usually unnecessary in men unless there is diagnostic uncertainty.

In women, the diagnosis of FPHL is mainly clinical and requires a careful history and examination. A key issue is whether hair loss is due to hyperandrogenism. The presence of a male pattern of hair loss, especially vertex balding, should always raise this possibility, although a female pattern is probably a more common manifestation. Other features of hyperandrogenism should be sought, including hirsutism, acne, menstrual disturbance, subfertility and acanthosis nigricans. How far to investigate women with evidence of hyperandrogenism depends on a variety of factors, such as the time course of the complaint, the age of the patient and the presence of associated features, and is usually best done by an endocrinologist. The most important cause, albeit rare, is an androgen-secreting ovarian or adrenal tumour; virilisation typically progresses rapidly in these patients. In the absence of clinical evidence of hyperandrogenism, extensive metabolic and endocrinological work-up is not routinely necessary. A multidisciplinary taskforce established by the Androgen Excess and PCOS Society recommended the following blood investigations in FPHL [109]:

- Serum total and free testosterone.
- Blood iron studies.
- Thyroid profile.
- Vitamin D.
- Serum zinc.
- Prolactin.

A scalp biopsy is seldom needed but it may be useful to distinguish between early FPHL and chronic TE in women with excessive shedding and minimum reduction in hair density. If FAPD is suspected a biopsy is needed to demonstrate scarring.

Management

Male balding is a biologically normal process. Under normal circumstances it has no adverse effect on physical well-being apart from increasing the risk of chronic photodamage to unprotected scalp skin. Under exceptional conditions a full head of hair may also contribute to thermoregulation – the French military surgeon Dominique-Jean Larrey observed that the bald men (and men without fur hats) were the first to die during the Russian campaign in the winter of 1812 [110]. Yet balding still has a powerful effect on the human psyche, to the extent that few men would choose to go bald were the choice available. Many men accept loss of their hair and prefer to let nature take its course. However, for some men balding is important enough for them to seek treatment and, for a few, concerns about hair loss reach the level of a body dysmorphic disorder. Men in the latter group are important to recognise, as treatment aimed at addressing the perceived hair problem is unlikely to be successful. Several studies have shown that male balding has an adverse effect on quality of life (although this is almost inevitable in those seeking professional advice) [111]. Nevertheless, balding is often seen as a trivial issue (mainly by non-sufferers), which may make men reluctant to approach their physician as they perceive, rightly or wrongly, that they will not receive a sympathetic response.

In most women FPHL is also a physiological trait. In contrast to the prevailing attitude to male balding, however, society generally regards it as abnormal for women to lose their hair. Consequently, the adverse effect of balding on quality of life tends be more severe in women than in men. As a group, women seeking medical advice for their hair loss experience more negative body image feelings, greater social anxiety, poorer self-esteem and lower psychosocial well-being than control subjects with non-visible skin disease, as well as dissatisfaction with their hair. In quality of life studies, individual responses were more related to self-perception of hair loss than to objective or clinical ratings, and those women most distressed by hair loss were more poorly adjusted and had a greater investment in their appearance [112,113]. The physician needs to be alert and sensitive to these issues and needs counselling and psychotherapeutic skills that go beyond merely prescribing treatment.

Counselling should include an explanation of the nature of the condition and its natural history. For those interested in preventing further progression or improving their hair status the treatment options, together with a realistic explanation of what can be achieved by treatment, will also need to be discussed. For those with a body dysmorphic disorder, involvement of a clinical psychologist or psychiatrist should be explored. Hair loss is an emotive issue and sufferers are vulnerable to exploitation by the unscrupulous. Patients should be advised against parting with large sums of money on unproven and valueless remedies.

Cosmetic approaches and camouflage

In women, a good hair stylist can help to disguise the appearance of thinning hair. In men, the 'comb-over' has fallen out of favour, to be largely replaced by the shaven-head approach.

Camouflage is the simplest, easiest and cheapest way of dealing with mild pattern hair loss. Balding becomes most noticeable when the scalp can be seen through the hair. Camouflage treatments involve either adding small fibres held in place electrostatically or dyeing the scalp the same colour as the hair to create the illusion of thicker hair. Several brands are available, each in a range of colours. Scalp tattooing is a more permanent approach and good practitioners can achieve impressive results.

A prosthesis is needed to cover extensive hair loss. These come in a range of forms and prices, from relatively cheap acrylic fibre wigs to expensive bespoke human hair appliances that are woven into existing hair. Because interwoven wigs lift as the hair beneath grows, they require periodic adjustment. Advice on wigs is available from alopecia patient support groups in the UK, USA and Australia.

Medical treatment

Treatment options for male AGA and FPHL are outlined here. See also the summary in 'Common treatments for hair disorders' later in this chapter for further information on these different options.

Treatment in male patients. At present two medical treatments, minoxidil and finasteride, are licensed for the treatment of male balding. Both drugs will stimulate some regrowth of hair in some men but are perhaps better regarded as preventative treatments. It follows that the earlier treatment is started, the more hair is retained [114]. Neither drug will regrow hair on completely bald scalps and continued treatment is necessary to maintain the response.

Minoxidil. Minoxidil is licensed for the treatment of male AGA as a 2% topical solution, 5% topical solution and 5% foam, each as a twice daily application. Clinical trials using various end points including hair counts, hair weight and global photography have confirmed improvement in male balding with the use of minoxidil lotion [115,116]. The mean increase in target area hair counts is about 8% with 2% minoxidil lotion and 10–12% with the 5% formulation. When assessed by global photography, nearly 60% of men show improvement with 5% minoxidil lotion and 40% with 2% lotion, compared with 23% with placebo. The response to minoxidil in terms of increased hair counts and hair weight is rapid and peaks by 16 weeks, although the cosmetic response may take longer to

become apparent. Trials that continued for up to 5 years suggested the improvement is sustained above baseline providing treatment is maintained [117]. Any positive effect on hair growth is lost within 4–6 months of stopping treatment. The rapid response of hair growth to minoxidil suggests that the drug promotes entry into anagen of terminal follicles in the kenogen stage of the hair cycle. This has been confirmed by phototrichogram studies, which also show some prolongation of anagen by minoxidil. Minoxidil does not reverse follicular miniaturisation [117].

Adverse effects of minoxidil are mainly dermatological. Constituents of the vehicle occasionally cause scalp irritation, more commonly with the 5% formulation. Allergic reactions to minoxidil or propylene glycol (a component of the vehicle) are rare but necessitate stopping treatment.

Finasteride. Finasteride 1 mg daily is licensed as a prescription-only drug for the treatment of male AGA. Taken orally it reduces DHT levels in serum and in the scalp by up to 70% [119]. Large, long-term, placebo-controlled studies using hair count and global photographic technology show that finasteride prevents or slows the progression of male balding in most men and about two-thirds experience some improvement [19]. The improvement peaks at around 12 months. A study using hair weighing to measure the response showed that men taking finasteride had maintained the improvement after nearly 4 years on the drug, whereas those on placebo continued to lose hair [120].

The response to finasteride is slower than to minoxidil, with the increase in hair counts taking up to 12 months to maximise. The effect is largely down to prolongation of anagen and, as with minoxidil, there is little evidence that miniaturisation is reversed [79].

Most men experience no adverse effects from finasteride. Clinical trials have shown a small increase in sexual dysfunction which resolved when the drug was discontinued. However, some men complain of persistent side effects after finasteride is stopped including sexual difficulties and depression (see 'Post-finasteride syndrome' later in this chapter).

Dutasteride. This drug inhibits both type 1 and type 2 5α-reductase and suppresses serum and scalp DHT to a greater degree than finasteride. Clinical trials have confirmed its efficacy in treating male AGA [121,122]. A meta-analysis of the results of dutasteride and finasteride clinical trials found a significantly greater degree of hair growth with dutasteride than finasteride [123]. The side effect profile is similar to that of finasteride. Dutasteride is licensed in many countries for treating benign prostatic hypertrophy; at present, it is licensed for male balding only in Japan and South Korea.

Treatment in female patients. Some women are content to be reassured that their hair loss is not a manifestation of a serious disease and that it is very unlikely that they will go bald. For those who are keen to be treated, there are two medical options – minoxidil and antiandrogens. In both cases it should be stressed that treatment will, at best, produce only a modest increase in hair density and that it is not possible to fully reverse hair loss. Furthermore, in those who respond, treatment must be continued to maintain the response. As in men, surgery is the only method capable of restoring the appearance in the presence of severe hair loss.

Topical minoxidil. Minoxidil 2% topical solution twice daily, and minoxidil 5% foam once daily, are licensed for the treatment of FPHL in most countries. Clinical trials in the early 1990s using hair counts as a primary end point reported a mean increase in hair growth of 15–33% in the minoxidil-treated groups compared with 9–14% in the vehicle control groups [124–126]. One small study using hair weight as the end point found an increase of 42.5% in hair weights in the minoxidil group compared with 1.9% in the controls [126]. In the investigator and subject assessments, minoxidil was superior to the vehicle but about 40% of subjects appeared not to respond to minoxidil [124,126]. A later trial comparing 5% and 2% minoxidil lotion found increases of 18% and 14%, respectively, in mean non-vellus hair counts after 48 weeks' treatment, compared with a 7% increase in the placebo group [128]. As in men, the increase in hair counts following treatment with minoxidil lotion is noticeable within 8 weeks and has peaked by 16 weeks.

Topical minoxidil is a safe treatment. Some patients complain that it leaves unsightly deposits on the hair. Occasionally, it causes scalp irritation which may be severe enough to cause a temporary increase in hair shedding and patients should be warned about this. Hypertrichosis on the face is occasionally a problem and has been reported particularly when higher concentrations of minoxidil are used [129]. This resolves if treatment is stopped. Occasionally, patients notice an increase in hair shedding 2–8 weeks after starting treatment. This is self-limiting and patients should be forewarned not to stop treatment if this happens.

The gains from treatment with topical minoxidil are modest and it is helpful to have an objective measure, such as serial standardised clinical photographs, to convince the patient (and the physician) of the response. Perhaps the major gain is halting or slowing the progression of hair loss, but this only becomes apparent on long-term follow-up and is not easy for the patient to detect.

Oral minoxidil. In recent years, oral minoxidil has come into favour as a treatment for hair loss, although it was tried (unsuccessfully) in alopecia areata in the 1980s [130]. In 2018, Sinclair reported the outcome of a small pilot study using oral minoxidil with spironolactone in women with FPHL, suggesting efficacy and safety [131]. Since that time, many investigators have evaluated the use of oral minoxidil in doses ranging from 0.5 to 5.0 mg in patients with various forms of alopecia including FPHL and male AGA. A randomised controlled trial comparing oral minoxidil 1 mg daily with minoxidil topical solution 5% once daily in the treatment of FPHL showed the two treatments had similar efficacy [132]. A large multicentre study of 1404 patients showed safety, with the most common treatment side effect being hypertrichosis, leading to drug withdrawal in 14 patients. The most common systemic side effects included lightheadedness (1.7%), fluid retention (1.3%), tachycardia (0.9%), headache (0.4%), periorbital oedema (0.3%) and insomnia (0.2%), leading to drug discontinuation in 29 patients (1.2%). No life-threatening adverse effects were observed [133].

Antiandrogens. The antiandrogens cyproterone acetate, spironolactone, flutamide and bicalutamide have all been used to treat FPHL, as has the 5α-reductase inhibitor finasteride, although none is licensed for this purpose and there is little clinical trial evidence of efficacy for any of them [**49**].

In a randomised controlled trial in 66 women with female AGA cyproterone acetate was compared with minoxidil lotion 2% [52]. After 12 months of treatment non-vellus hair density increased significantly in the minoxidil-treated group but fell in the cyproterone acetate group. However, subgroup analysis showed a small improvement in hair density in women with menstrual irregularities receiving cyproterone acetate. This study suggests that antiandrogens may be beneficial in women with evidence of androgen excess but not in those without.

Spironolactone is a competitive inhibitor of aldosterone receptors. It also blocks androgen receptors and increases metabolic clearance of testosterone. It has been widely used to treat FPHL as well as hirsutism. There are no controlled trials of its use in FPHL. In an open uncontrolled case series of 80 women treated for 1 year with spironolactone (200 mg daily) or cyproterone acetate, 35 women (44%) showed improvement in hair growth as assessed by standardised photography [134].

Flutamide is a pure androgen receptor blocker. A randomised trial from Italy compared flutamide 250 mg daily with cyproterone acetate and finasteride in the treatment of 48 hyperandrogenic women with AGA. Those treated with flutamide showed a modest improvement in hair growth whereas those treated with cyproterone acetate or finasteride did not [135]. The study appears not to have been blinded and the method of assessment, using Ludwig grading, was relatively crude. Some clinicians now use bicalutamide, an alternative non-steroidal androgen receptor blocker, that appears safer than flutamide [136,137].

In a large randomised controlled trial in postmenopausal women with FPHL finasteride 1 mg daily proved ineffective in preventing hair loss [50]. However, improvement has been reported in several uncontrolled cases series [138–140]. For example, in one study 62% of women taking finasteride 2.5 mg daily showed some improvement as assessed by global photography [139]. A meta-analysis of nine published studies concluded that finasteride does not increase hair density in FPHL but it may improve the clinical evaluation of hair loss, and that higher doses (2.5–5 mg daily) are more effective [51].

Antiandrogen treatment is not without problems. As with minoxidil, treatment must be continued to maintain a response and women taking antiandrogens should not become pregnant because of the risks of feminising a male fetus. Dose-related side effects of cyproterone acetate, including weight gain, fatigue, loss of libido, mastodynia, nausea, headaches and depression, are common. There is a significant risk of hepatotoxicity with flutamide, and cyproterone acetate is also potentially hepatotoxic in high doses. Spironolactone may cause breast soreness and menstrual irregularities but is probably the safest option. Finasteride is well-tolerated and is worth considering in postmenopausal and infertile women.

Iron. The idea that body iron stores, usually measured as serum ferritin, are important in hair growth is controversial and, as yet, unsubstantiated in a randomised controlled clinical trial. In an open trial of cyclical treatment with cyproterone acetate in women with serum ferritin levels above and below 40 µg/L (10 subjects in each group), hair densities increased by about 15% in the high ferritin group after 1 year of treatment but were unchanged in the low ferritin group [64]. In the absence of more conclusive data, it seems reasonable to check serum ferritin levels and advise dietary supplementation with iron in those with a level below 40 μg/L. Patients should be advised that iron treatment alone will not halt or reverse hair loss but it may improve the response to specific treatments.

Treatment in transgender patients. Transgender patients who present with pattern hair loss can require manipulation of oral and topical medications that may differ from typical prescribing patterns. For transgender women, hair loss can be particularly distressing, since the loss can serve as sign of the unwanted male phenotype. Often, oestradiol and spironolactone are used to maintain the female phenotype, and titration of these medications can help to promote hair growth in those experiencing pattern hair loss [141]. In transgender men, pattern hair loss can worsen after masculinising hormone therapy; 5a-reductase inhibitors can be helpful in their treatment [142]. The typical treatments described here, such as topical or oral minoxidil, may also be used in this population as well as surgical restoration [143].

Other treatments.
Surgery. See 'Surgery' later in this chapter.

Platelet-rich plasma. Several studies report increased hair density in patients with male AGA treated with PRP [144], although the efficacy of PRP in women is less clear [145]. A recent meta-analysis of seven randomised controlled trials identified significant increased hair density for PRP treatment compared with placebo. The pooled mean improvement in hair density was 30 hairs/cm^2 but with a wide confidence interval, and considerable heterogeneity and potential bias in the studies evaluated [146]. The optimal treatment regimen for PRP in pattern hair loss is not known, but most studies support monthly treatment for the first 3 months followed by maintenance treatment as an effective approach [144]. Interestingly, efficacy of PRP treatment has now been demonstrated in a preclinical humanised AGA mouse model [147].

Low-level laser light therapy. A systematic review and network meta-analysis ranked low-level laser light therapy as the most effective non-surgical interventions for pattern hair loss when compared with finasteride, dutasteride, topical minoxidil, PRP and placebo, although the quality of evidence of was rated as low or very low [148]. Combining low-level laser light therapy with minoxidil appears more effective than monotherapy based on improvements in global photography and hair density assessments [149].

Summary

Whether or not one regards pattern hair loss as a medical condition worthy of treatment [150], there is little doubt that it can have a significant adverse effect on quality of life. The emotive aspect of hair loss means that it is not necessarily a trivial issue for the sufferer and, consequently, managing the patient with AGA can be difficult and time consuming for the physician (the same is true of other hair loss disorders). Nevertheless, it can be rewarding to manage patients with pattern hair loss and, despite their limitations, current treatments can be of significant benefit providing the patient is fully aware of what can be achieved.

HAIR LOSS ASSOCIATED WITH CANCER TREATMENT

Chemotherapy-induced alopecia

Introduction and general description

Alopecia is a common and often distressing complication of systemic chemotherapy, occurring in up to 65% of regimens [1]. Chemotherapy-induced alopecia (CIA) is a particularly feared complication of cancer therapy, with 47% rating it as the most traumatic aspect of treatment, and 8% rejecting chemotherapy because of this side effect [2]. The risk of CIA depends on several factors including the specific agent and treatment protocol used (Table 87.5), whether combination therapy is required and the route of administration [3]. Further, patient factors such as performance status, nutrition, age and presence of pre-existing hair disorders also contribute to the ultimate degree of hair loss experienced [4].

Classification of alopecia severity in oncology clinical trials typically uses the Common Terminology Criteria for Adverse Events system (CTCAE v5.0) [5], with grade 0 (no hair loss), grade 1 (<50% hair loss not obvious from a distance, not requiring a wig or hair piece) and grade 2 (>50% hair loss readily apparent to others, requiring a wig or hair piece) categories available. However, these criteria are broad and do not supply good phenotypic description or identification of the type of alopecia induced [4].

Pathophysiology

The hair matrix in the anagen hair bulb is very metabolically active and is particularly vulnerable to chemotherapy agents, causing rapid and profound cessation of hair growth soon after administration. Importantly, slow-cycling stem cells in the HF bulge are relatively resistant to chemotherapy, allowing hairs to regenerate after treatment is completed.

Table 87.5 Drugs causing chemotherapy alopecia

Agents that usually cause hair loss	Agents that sometimes cause hair loss	Agents that uncommonly cause hair loss
Cyclophosphamide	Amsacrine	Capecitabine
Daunorubicin	Bleomycin	Carboplatin
Docetaxel	Busulphan	Carmustine
Doxorubicin	Cytarabine	Cisplatin
Epirubicin	5-Fluorouracil	Fludarabine
Etoposide	Gemcitabine	6-Marcaptopurine
Ifosfamide	Lomustine	Methotrexate
Irinotecan	Melphalan	Mitomycin C
Paclitaxel	Thiotepa	Mitroxantrone
Topotecan	Vinblastine	Procarbazine
Vindesine	Vincristine	Raltritrexate
Vinorelbine		Streptozotocin

Reproduced from Trueb 2010 [3].

The mechanism of HF damage and recovery in chemotherapy has been studied in a murine model using cyclophosphamide administration [6]. Two types of follicular dystrophy were identified:

1 Dystrophic anagen occurs at lower chemotherapy doses. Here less severe HF damage occurs, so the hair initially recovers in the same anagen phase (termed primary recovery) before eventually progressing through catagen/telogen to a new anagen hair cycle (secondary recovery).

2 Dystrophic telogen occurs with a more severe HF insult. Hairs skip the primary recovery phase, progressing directly to catagen/telogen before secondary recovery occurs. Thus, dystrophic telogen is a shorter pathway to complete regrowth.

In humans, CIA causes a prominent anagen effluvium but also increased telogen rates are identified on serial trichograms, suggesting that the HF response is determined by its stage in the hair cycle at the time of the insult. It is thought that this observed TE response occurs in late-stage anagen HF [7].

Clinical features

Hair shedding typically occurs within 1–3 weeks and is complete within 1–2 months after the initiation of chemotherapy. Hair loss is rapid, diffuse and extensive, associated with significant hair shedding. Trichoscopy reveals multiple black dots and broken hairs. In the remaining hairs a Pohl–Pinkus constriction may be seen due to temporary cessation of hair growth (analogous to Beau lines in the nails) [8]. Hair loss is most marked in areas of increased friction [1]. In most cases hair loss is temporary and recovers fully within a period of months following cessation of the causative insult [7]. Changes in hair colour and shape (curly/straight) are described with hair regrowth [1].

Investigations

Specific investigations are not usually required.

Management

The focus of CIA management has traditionally centred around psychological preparation and cosmetic support, with the provision of wigs during the treatment period.

Various methods have been employed to prevent the development of CIA. The most widely used is scalp cooling using ice packs or custom-designed cooling caps. The rationale for treatment is that cooling causes vasoconstriction, reduces uptake of the chemotherapy drug into cells and supresses metabolic activity, thereby limiting the effects of chemotherapy on the HF [9–11]. The results are variable but there is good evidence for efficacy in some patients. However, cold caps require additional treatment time, can be uncomfortable, may not be available in all centres and are contraindicated in certain haematological malignancies. Concern that scalp cooling increases the risk of scalp metastases in solid tumours is probably unfounded [12,13]. Topical minoxidil is not effective at preventing CIA.

Certain treatments may limit the impact of CIA by promoting hair regrowth. One small trial suggested that topical minoxidil can hasten recovery from chemotherapy alopecia [14].

The psychological impact of CIA should not be overlooked [15,16]. Hair loss has been shown to have a profound impact on body image and self-esteem, acting as a constant reminder of someone's illness.

Sex-specific responses are seen, with impact on beauty, femininity and sexuality particularly affecting women, and feelings of appearing less macho, child-like and vulnerable specifically affecting men. Interestingly, some view CIA positively as the hair loss demonstrates the treatment is working.

Loss of eyebrows and eyelashes is common and can have a significant cosmetic and functional impact on the patient. Topical bimatoprost 0.03% liquid applied to the upper eyelid margin has been shown to rapidly restore eyelashes post-chemotherapy, improving eyelash length, thickness and pigmentation [17–19].

Persistent chemotherapy-induced alopecia

Introduction and general description

Although CIA is usually reversible, persistent CIA (pCIA) (syn. permanent CIA) may be seen. It is particularly associated with conditioning regimens for bone marrow transplantation and taxane-based regimens for breast cancer, with higher doses appearing to increase the risk of persistent hair loss [1,20]. A recent UK survey identified self-reported hair loss persisting more than 6 months after treatment in 23.3% of breast cancer patients receiving docetaxel and 10.1% paclitaxel (P <0.01) [21].

Pathophysiology

The pathophysiology of pCIA remains unclear but is likely to result from associated HF stem cell damage inhibiting regeneration and ongoing hair cycling [1,22]. Whether an occult pre-existing hair loss process is unmasked by the CIA is yet to be determined. A reduced function mutation in the *ABCB1* gene, which encodes the p-glycoprotein efflux pump that removes drugs from cells, holds a genetic risk for pCIA development [23].

Clinical features

The definition of pCIA is 'absent or incomplete hair regrowth 6 months beyond the completion of chemotherapy'. Clinically, this manifests as either a non-scarring diffuse alopecia or hair loss that clinically and histologically resembles severe FPHL [1,22,24] (Figure 87.55). Trichoscopy shows variability of HS diameter, increased vellus hairs and predominantly single hairs per follicular ostia. Rarely pCIA may present as an inflammatory scarring alopecia.

Differential diagnosis

Other causes of diffuse hair loss should be excluded.

Investigations

Reversible causes of diffuse hair loss should be excluded (see 'Telogen effluvium' earlier in this chapter). A scalp biopsy with horizontal and vertical sectioning shows reduced hair density, decreased terminal to vellus ratio and end-stage fibrous streamers.

Management

The best approach to management is prevention, with scalp cooling dramatically reducing the risk of pCIA [1,20]. Although the

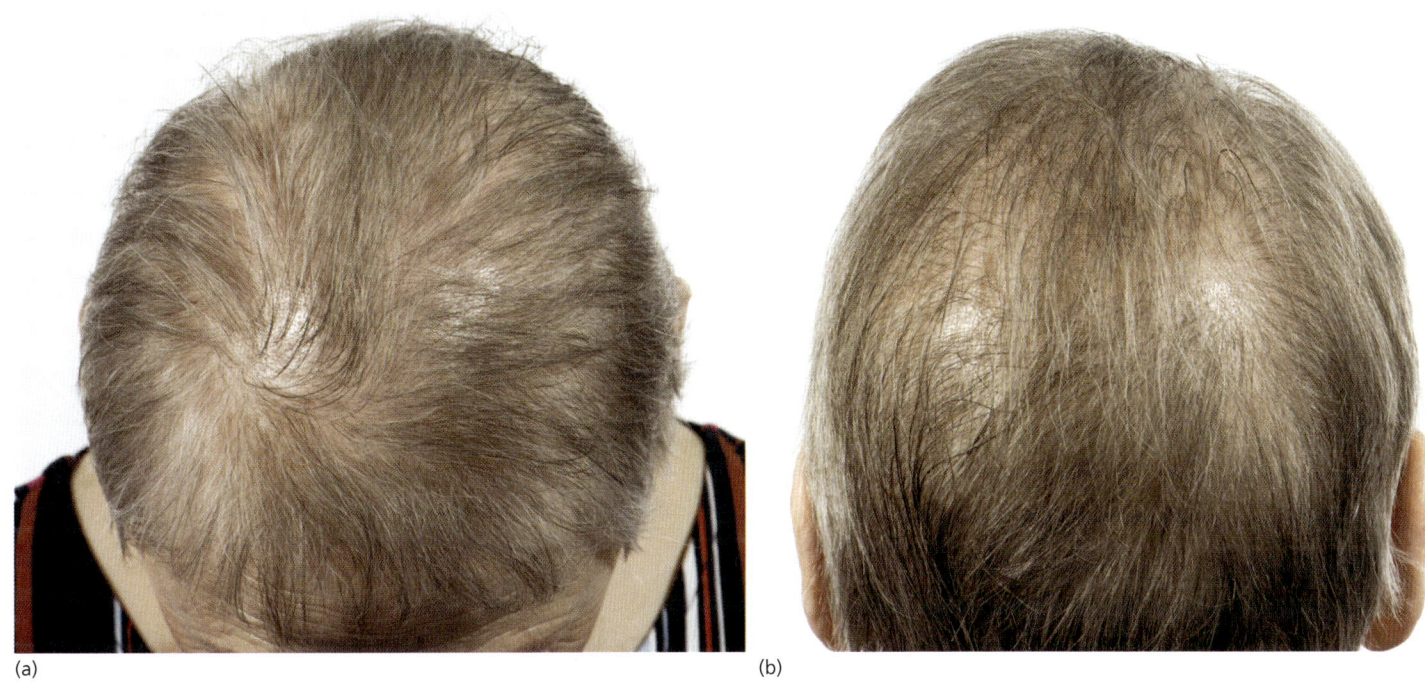

(a)   (b)

Figure 87.55 Persistent chemotherapy-induced alopecia on (a) the vertex and (b) the posterior scalp, showing diffuse non-scarring alopecia with a reduction in density predominantly over the vertex, reminiscent of female pattern hair loss.

evidence is limited, both topical and oral minoxidil can improve hair density [25]. Sometimes antiandrogen therapy (e.g. spironolactone/bicalutamide) may be tried, although caution is required in hormone-sensitive cancers and close liaison with the primary oncology team is recommended if this approach is considered.

Eyelash regrowth can be improved post-chemotherapy with topical bimatoprost even when starting treatment is delayed by up to 6 months [18].

Therapies for cancer that can cause hair loss
Endocrine therapies
Seventy per cent of breast cancers are hormone receptor positive. Antioestrogen therapies, such as oestrogen receptor modulators (e.g. tamoxifen), aromatase inhibitors (e.g. anastrazole, letrazole) and gonadotrophin-releasing hormone agonists (e.g. leuprolide), are frequently employed as suppressive therapy for 5–10 years after the initial treatment. Hormone therapy-induced alopecia (HTIA) was shown to occur in 4.4% of cases with a relative risk of 12.88 (95%CI 7.46–22.24; P <0.001) [26]. Clinically, HTIA presents as a diffuse alopecia mimicking FPHL. Onset is often slow, with a mean reported onset of 16.8 months. The loss of the anagen-promoting effects of oestrogen along with a relative switch in the hormonal profile towards an androgen dominant position may all contribute to this presentation [1,22].

Targeted oncology therapies
Targeted oncology therapies are revolutionising cancer treatment. Along with their powerful anticancer effects, a whole spectrum of cutaneous toxicities is now being recognised. Importantly, these novel side effects are providing insight into normal skin and HF homeostasis and can act as clinical biomarkers for treatment response in some situations. Thus, awareness of these nuances is important and highlights the need for a personalised and multidisciplinary approach when faced with these side effects.

Epidermal growth factor receptor inhibitors and mitogen-activated protein kinase inhibitors
Overexpression of the epidermal growth factor receptor (EGFR) is seen in various cancers, including lung and colon cancers. This has led to the development of inhibitors targeting EGFR, and the downstream mitogen-activated protein (MAP) kinase, in oncology treatment. Cutaneous reactions are common and occur in 75–90% of patients [27,28]. Typically, an itchy papular and pustular reaction develops over the face, chest and back within the first few weeks of treatment. Although acneform in appearance, the absence of comedones and distal follicular inflammation suggests this is better classified as a folliculitis [29]. Rarely, scarring alopecia reminiscent of folliculitis decalvans may be seen [30]. Trichomegaly (i.e. increased length and density of the eyelashes) is seen in up to 10% of cases [28,31].

Importantly, the presence of a rash appears to correlate with the drug's antitumour effect. Therefore, treatment should be continued where possible. Regular emollients and sun protection are recommended, but if symptoms are significant then topical corticosteroids, oral tetracycline antibiotics and sometimes isotretinoin may be required [28,31]. Patients with trichomegaly should regularly trim their eyelashes to prevent eye issues.

Tyrosine kinase inhibitors and hair pigmentation
Tyrosine kinase inhibitors block signal transduction within the cell, reducing proliferation and providing anticancer effects. However, they also frequently result in both skin and hair depigmentation, by influencing the modulatory effect of c-kit on tyrosinase activity and melanin synthesis. Interestingly, when treatment is paused,

pigmentation can return in the same hair fibre, leading to a striped appearance within the hairs [32].

Immune checkpoint inhibitors and autoimmune reactions

Immune checkpoint inhibitors are increasingly being used in oncology to harness the immune system to fight cancer development. However, immune-related toxic reactions affecting any organ may develop, with pneumonitis, endocrinopathies and colitis commonly being seen. Skin toxicities such as dermatitis, vitiligo/poliosis, alopecia areata and LPP are also described and may suggest a good therapeutic response [29]. The onset of these changes may be delayed, sometimes appearing many months after starting therapy [29,33–36].

Hedgehog pathway inhibitors

Abnormal activation of the hedgehog pathway is seen in >90% of basal cell carcinomas leading to the development of hedgehog pathway inhibitors (e.g. vismodegib, sonidegib) [37]. Adverse effects of these drugs are related to the important role of this pathway in normal homeostasis, including hair cycle control. Although these reactions are generally low grade, the long-term dosing required to suppress cancer development makes these side effects less tolerable as time passes. Diffuse alopecia affecting the scalp and body hair is common, seen in 46–66% of cases across all studies of vismodegib. Pretreatment assessment of associated hair loss conditions, nutrition and thyroid status is recommended to reduce the impact of alopecia development. Reported treatments include topical minoxidil, bimatoprost to the eyelashes/eyebrows and sometimes antiandrogen treatment. Cosmetic support is important. Dose adjustment may be required if side effects are severe [1,37].

Post-radiotherapy alopecia

Although HF stem cells are relatively chemotherapy resistant, they are more sensitive to ionising radiation. Therefore, radiotherapy treatment of head and neck cancers can frequently result in persistent alopecia [22]. Patterns of alopecia include localised areas of hair loss relating to the treatment field or a diffuse alopecia from whole brain irradiation; sometimes a radiation dermatitis may also be seen. Hair usually regrows 2–4 months after treatment, but persistent radiation-induced alopecia (defined as 'total loss or incomplete regrowth 6 months following completion of treatment') may be seen, particularly when higher doses are used or when combined with chemotherapy [1]. Treatment involves controlling any radiation dermatitis with topical steroids, stimulation of hair growth with minoxidil and cosmetic camouflage, with surgical correction sometimes suitable for localised patches.

ABNORMALITIES OF THE HAIR SHAFT

Structural defects of the hair shaft usually result from either an intrinsic fragility of the hair fibre (rendering it abnormally susceptible to damage by minor degrees of trauma), or when changes occur to an otherwise normal hair fibre because of excessive external damaging factors. If hair breaks close to the scalp (<4 cm), causes of intrinsic hair fragility should be sought.

Hair microscopy can be a useful part of the clinical assessment [1], providing clues to the diagnosis [2,3]. Increasingly, trichoscopy [4] and high-magnification video trichoscopy [5] are being used to preliminarily screen for scalp and hair shaft disorders, prior to hair sampling and formal microscopy (Figure 87.56). Measurement of hair amino acid composition is an additional means of quantifying hair shaft damage both in cosmetic weathering and in genetically damaged hair [6].

The technique chosen to sample hairs depends on the clinical situation. Generally, cut hair samples are preferred as hair plucking is usually poorly tolerated in children and the force required may instead break the hairs at the point of fragility, thereby missing the area of interest when the fibres are examined [7]. At least 50 hairs should be cut close to the scalp, wrapped in paper and labelled. These dry hair samples provide flexibility for future analysis, allowing dry microscopy or embedding in mounting media, as well as electron microscopy studies or amino acid analysis, if required.

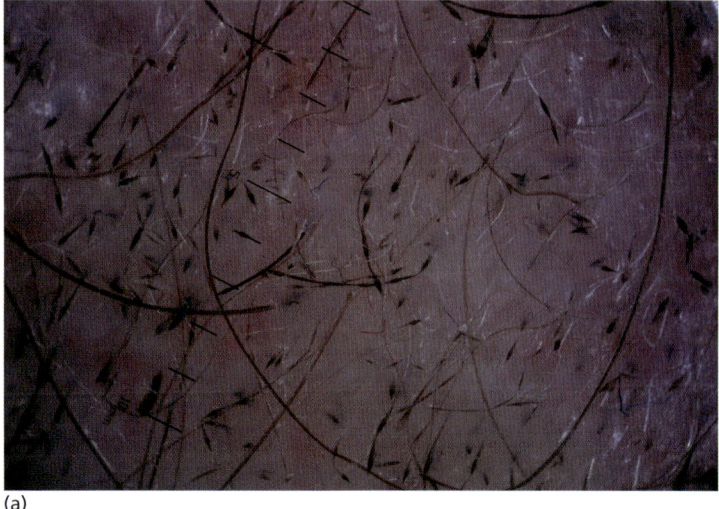
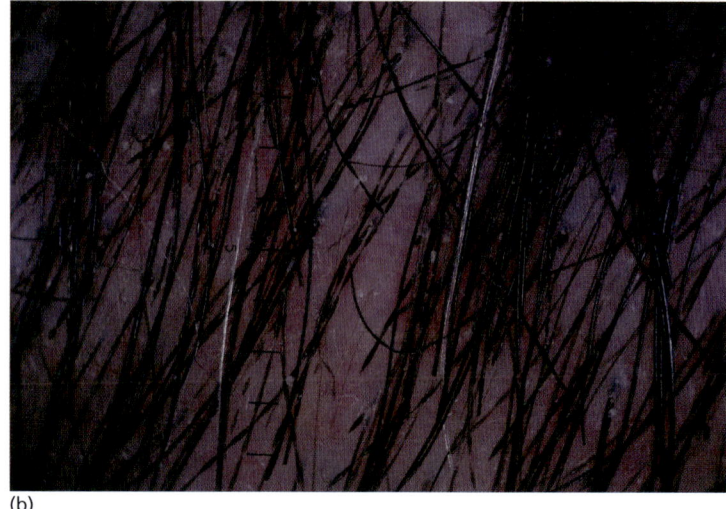

(a)   (b)

Figure 87.56 Trichoscopy as a real-time clinic-based tool for diagnosing hair shaft disorders. Typical beaded hair changes of monilethrix were seen in (a) a proband and (b) the proband's father.

Table 87.6 Fragile versus non-fragile hair shaft disorders.

Fragile disorders	Non-fragile disorders
Bubble hair	Pili annulati
Monilethrix	Pili bifurcate
Pili torti	Pili multigemini
Trichorrhexis invaginata	Uncombable hair syndrome
Trichorrhexis nodosa	Woolly hair
Trichothiodystrophy	

Hair shaft defects are usually divided into those with shaft fragility and those without (Table 87.6). Common descriptive hair shaft terminology is presented in Table 87.7.

STRUCTURAL DEFECTS WITH INCREASED HAIR FRAGILITY

Weathering of the hair shaft (including trichoptilosis)

Weathering describes the increasing cuticular damage ($\pm$ secondary cortical damage) acquired in all hair fibres as you move from the root to tip. Various external factors can increase hair damage, including excessive washing, brushing, UV radiation, swimming or chemical exposure. Therefore, longer hairs towards the tips are increasingly affected. Certain hair keratins appear more sensitive to oxidative damage from bleaching and chemical exposure [6].

Close to the scalp cuticle cells are tightly overlapped (likened to the tiles on a roof). As weathering develops the free edges of these cells start to lift and break up. Increased loss results in focal, then confluent, loss of the cuticle (Figure 87.57). Hair knotting and braids are a significant source of hair shaft trauma (Figure 87.58) [8]. Trichoptilosis is the term for 'split ends', appearing as whitish blurred ends to the hair fibre that are easily visible and mostly seen with other features of hair weathering [9].

Trichorrhexis nodosa

Introduction and general description

Trichorrhexis nodosa (TN) is the most severe form of weathering and is best regarded as a distinctive hair shaft response to injury [10,11]. Cuticle cells become disrupted, allowing the underlying cortical cells to splay out to form a node [8,12].

Pathophysiology

Trichorrhexis nodosa is due to focal cuticle loss on a background of hair weathering. Supporting this is the observation that TN can be induced in normal hairs under controlled laboratory stress [13].

Table 87.7 Terms used to define hair shaft pathology.

Term	Meaning	Associations
Bayonet hair	Slight kink in hair within 1–2 mm of tapered tip	Variant of normal
Brush end	When a trichorrhexis node breaks it leaves the proximal end looking like a chimney sweep's brush	See below
Bubble hair	Bubbles within the hair shaft	Arises due to extreme heat or singeing of hair; attributed to leaning over a fire, or hot hair treatments where thermostatic controls are faulty
Circle hairs	Circle and spiral hairs on the thigh and abdomen, usually trapped beneath the stratum corneum	Normal in more hirsute males; not the same as scurvy
Hair casts	Keratin cylinders moving freely on the proximal hair shaft and arising from the upper part of the internal root sheath	May be associated with scaling scalp conditions or hair styling where there is tension on the hair; sometimes referred to as 'pseudo-nits'
Nit	The egg case of a head louse adherent to the shaft	The egg case may be empty or still contain the louse nymph; only nits proximal on the shaft are likely to represent active infestation, which needs to be confirmed by identification of a live head louse
Pili torti	Twisting of hair through 180° within the long axis of the hair	Although this is a sign, it is sometimes used as a diagnosis; it is associated with the specific diagnosis of Menkes syndrome, but also presents as an isolated autosomal dominant condition
Pohl–Pinkus constriction	Zone of constriction within the hair shaft, possibly due to transient physiological compromise of hair growth; comparable with a Beau line	Period of ill health or cytotoxic medication, where not sufficient to precipitate telogen effluvium or anagen effluvium
Tapered hairs	The tip of a hair that has been generated de novo at the commencement of anagen will be tapered	Characteristic of hair that is regrowing after shedding or of hair with a short anagen phase, e.g. eyebrow
Tiger tail	Light and dark transverse stripes on a hair shaft when viewed with cross-polarisation, preferably in histological medium	Sulphur-deficient hair has a weakened cortex that loses its longitudinal rigidity and tends to become wavy; this alters light polarisation characteristics
Trichoclasis	A 'greenstick' fracture of the hair, where the cuticle is partly stripped in continuity with the fracture	Trauma and moderate fragility
Trichonodosis	Knots in hair	Usually a simple reef knot, seen where hair is rubbed or where the hair is markedly curly and predisposed to knotting; can contribute to fragility; most common in African hair
Trichoptilosis	Split ends – in continuity with the tip	Common outcome of cumulative brushing and chemical trauma
Trichorrhexis nodosa	Focal loss of cuticle revealing an area of exposed and splayed cortical fibres, forming a node	Marker of weathering and hair breakage. Seen in various hair fragility disorders
Trichoschisis	Clean transverse fracture across the hair	Typically associated with sulphur-deficient hair of trichothiodystrophy

PART 8: SPECIFIC CUTANEOUS STRUCTURES

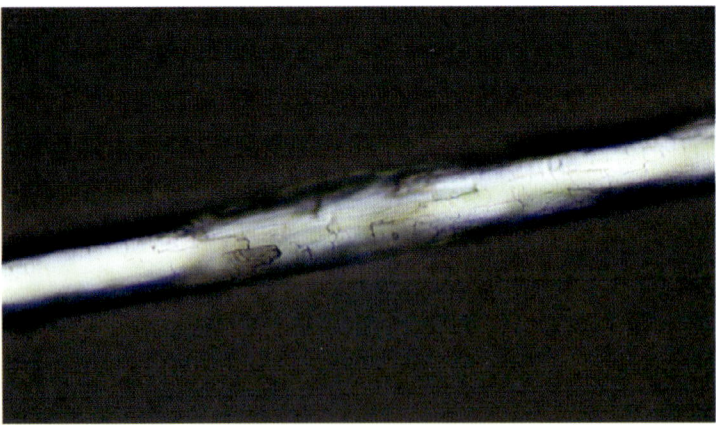

Figure 87.57 Focal loss of the cuticle in a weathered hair.

TN is particularly prominent in tightly curled African hair. However, this predisposition is shown to be predominantly due to mechanical factors causing trauma, as no intrinsic weakness or difference in cysteine-rich protein distribution has been identified in the hair of people of normal white, Asian and African heritage [14]. Hair amino acid analysis of TN-affected hairs shows a reduced cysteine level [15].

Clinical features

Trichorrhexis nodosa typically presents with dull, dry and brittle hair of variable length. Small grey-white nodules positioned irregularly along the shaft can be seen by eye, or with the aid of trichoscopy. Hair is fragile, demonstrated by performing the tug test, where hair breaks into small fragments when pulled firmly from each end.

The main clinical presentations of TN are:
- *Distal TN*. This occurs in all races and is more common in longer hair. It is often an incidental finding with a few whitish nodules near the ends of scattered hairs, although more extensive involvement can occur.
- *Proximal TN*. This is predominantly seen in women with African-textured hair. The scalp hair is short and brittle and demonstrates severe weathering on light microscopic examination (Figure 87.59). Other hair loss processes associated with traumatic hair care practices (e.g. traction alopecia, CCCA) may coexist.
- *Localised TN*. This can be seen in any pruritic dermatosis due to scratching (e.g. lichen simplex of the pubic area).
- *Congenital TN*. An isolated defect with autosomal dominant inheritance, termed 'trichorrhexis congenita', is described [16]. However, when TN presents in childhood other congenital hair fragility conditions should be excluded, particularly argininosuccinic aciduria. TN has also been associated with hypothyroidism, as well as zinc, iron and biotin deficiency [17–20].
- *Argininosuccinic aciduria* (MIM: 207900). TN is a feature of this rare metabolic defect [21]. Urine and serum amino acids should be analysed in children presenting with TN and hair fragility (Chapter 79).

Investigations

Trichorrhexis nodosa has a characteristic appearance on light or electron microscopy (Figure 87.60). At the nodes, the cuticle splits revealing the underlying splayed cortical fibres. This appearance is often likened to two paint brushes pushed together. These nodes are fragile, so breakage through the node is common, resulting in a 'brush end' appearance. Careful assessment for other diagnostic hair shaft abnormalities should be sought, which may reveal the underlying cause of the hair fragility.

Thyroid function, ferritin/iron studies and zinc levels should be checked [19]. Serum and urine amino acids should be requested in childhood presentations.

Differential diagnosis

Trichorrhexis nodosa is usually easily differentiated from pediculosis, hair casts, exogenous material, superficial mycoses and bubble hair with light microscopy.

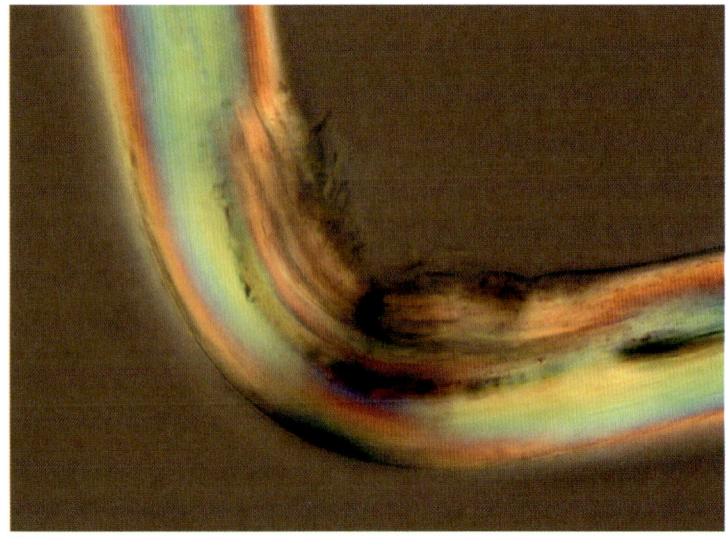

(a)   (b)

Figure 87.58 (a) Knotting of single and multiple hairs contribute to hair shaft trauma. (b) Braiding damages the hair shaft cuticle.

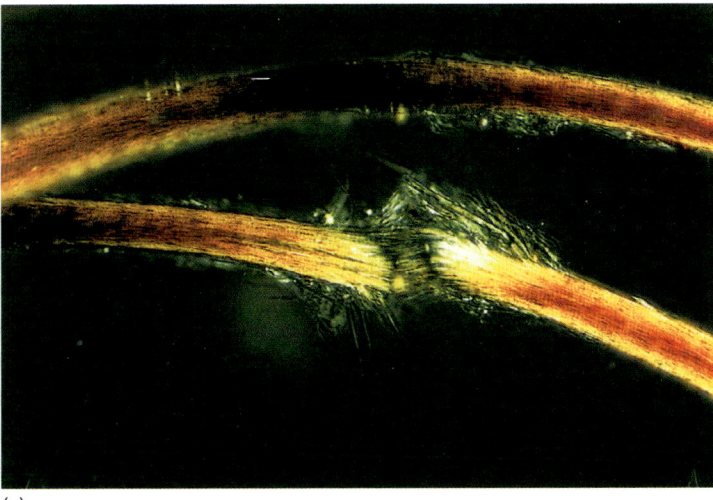

(a)

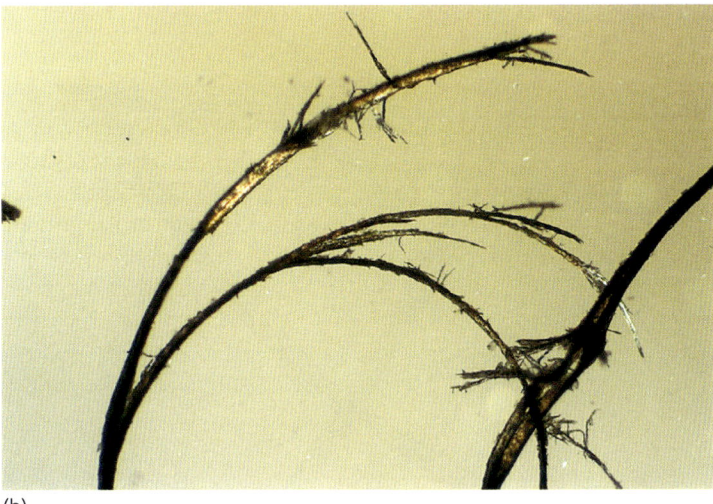

(b)

Figure 87.59 Trichorrhexis nodosa. (a) Polarised light examination demonstrating splayed cortical fibres radiating from the transverse fracture in a trichorrhexis node. (b) Proximal trichorrhexis nodosa nodes and dramatic split ends (trichoptilosis) visible in the hair from an Afro-Caribbean woman.

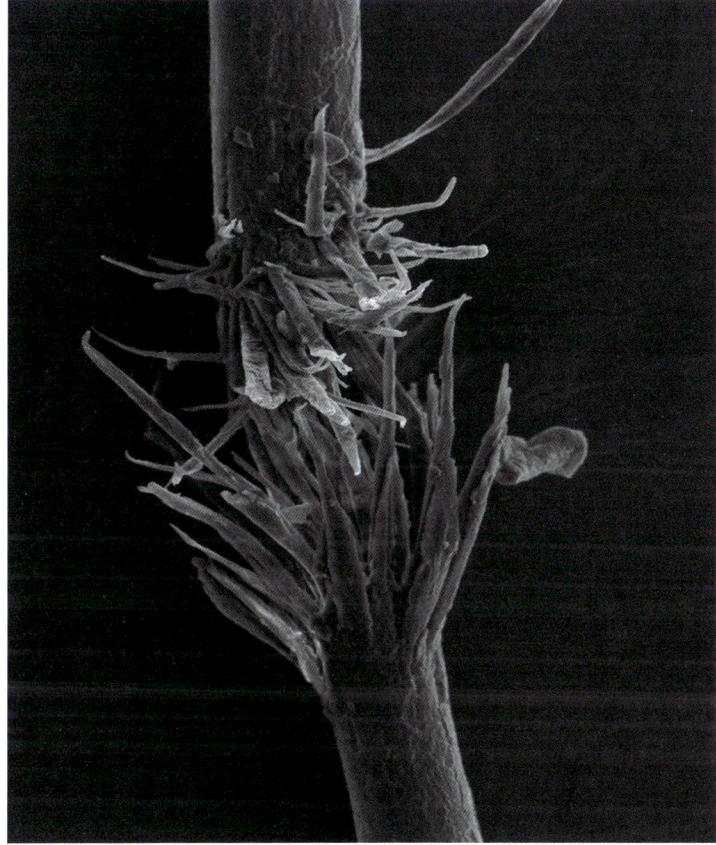

Figure 87.60 Scanning electron microscopy of trichorrhexis nodosa showing focal loss of the cuticle with splaying of the underlying cortical fibres. Courtesy of Dr Colin Malone.

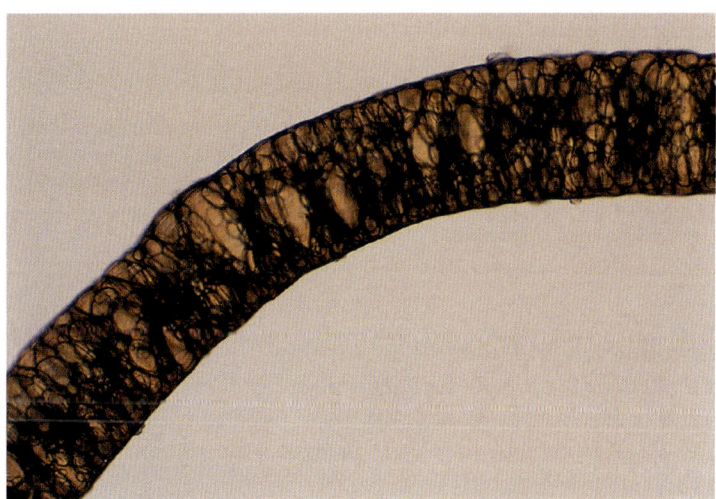

Figure 87.61 Appearance of normal scalp hair after exposure to a naked flame. Bubbles form within the cortex.

Management

The key to treating TN is minimisation of traumatic hair care practices. Frequency of shampooing will vary from person to person but should be sufficient to prevent excess build-up of hair products and oiliness. Mild shampoos and wash-out conditioners, as well as leave-in water-based conditioners, followed by thicker occlusive oil-based products (e.g. coconut oil) are advised to retain moisture and prevent further damage [22]. Nutritional deficiencies should be addressed [23,24]. Empirical biotin supplementation (e.g. 2.5–5 mg per day) may be considered.

Bubble hair

Introduction and general description

The characteristic appearance of bubble hair was first described by Brown *et al.* [25]. Bubble hair is caused by excessive heat, typically due to a faulty hairdryer or tongs at high temperature causing focal damage (Figure 87.61) [26].

Pathophysiology

Bubble hair can be intentionally created on any hairs using a naked flame or conducted heat. Although damp hair has been suggested as a contributory factor, it is not a requirement [27,28]. Light and electron microscopy assessment has demonstrated that the bubbles are gas-filled rather than containing fluid [26,29], with the high heat appearing to induce rapid gas expansion (i.e. vaporisation of water) within the hair shaft, resulting in loss of cortical cells and bubble formation [27].

Clinical features

Typically bubble hair is found in healthy young women who complain of focal hair breakage and hair textural change, associated with regular use of heated styling appliances. The hair breakage pattern relates to the styling technique used.

Differential diagnosis

Hair bubbles are also described in thallium toxicity, pili annulati and Favus infection.

Investigations

Although not always easily demonstrated by trichoscopy (as transmission of light through the defect is needed to demonstrate the bubbles) [4], bubble hairs may sometimes be identified in this way [30]. Light microscopy is usually required to confirm the diagnosis, and is made easier using a fluid slide-mounting medium to reduce reflection at the hair surface. Bubbles may be separate or adjacent and can be a single large cavity or have a 'Swiss cheese-like' appearance. The bubbles expand the hair shaft and predispose to breakage.

Management

Any appliances with hot components should be serviced or replaced. Affected hair can be trimmed to cut out the affected areas; subsequent hair will be normal.

Monilethrix

Synonyms and inclusions
• Beaded hair

Introduction and general description

Monilethrix is a fragile hair shaft disorder derived from the Latin 'monile' (necklace) and the Greek 'thrix' (hair), as a descriptive name for the characteristic hair shaft changes seen on light microscopy (Chapter 66) [31].

Clinical features

Monilethrix shows considerable variation in age of onset, severity, course and expression within a family. The hair shaft is beaded and breaks easily, particularly at sites of friction. Broken hair may be accompanied by follicular keratosis, most commonly on the nape and occiput (Figure 87.62).

The typical hair shaft changes can usually be readily identified on both trichoscopy and light microscopy (see Figure 87.56). Regularly spaced elliptical nodes (0.7–1 mm apart) are separated by narrower

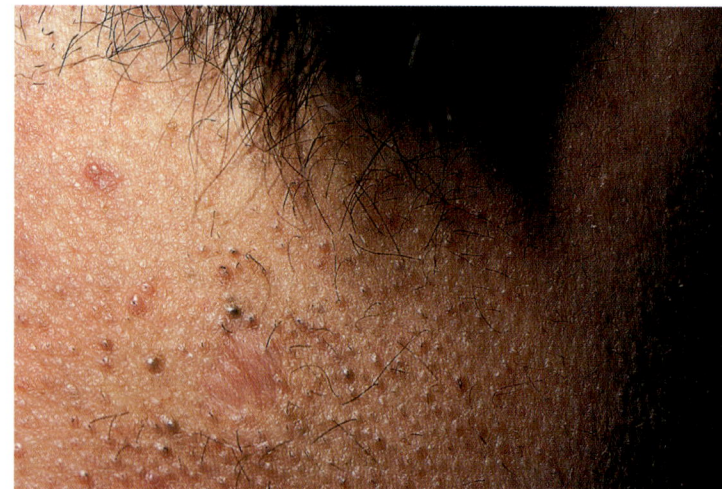

Figure 87.62 Monilethrix on the nape of the neck showing follicular keratoses and short, broken hairs.

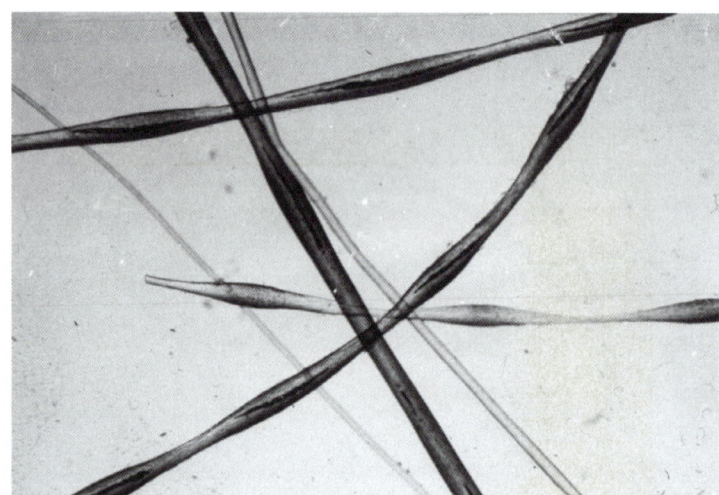

Figure 87.63 Monilethrix with swollen (node) and narrow (internode) fluctuations in the hair bore.

internodes, resembling a necklace (Figure 87.63). Breakages are typically seen at the internode sites of affected hair, although phenotypically normal hairs within an affected individual are also fragile.

Pili torti

Introduction and general description

The term pili torti is derived from the latin 'pili' (hair) and 'torti' (twisted). Hairs are flattened and at irregular intervals are completely rotated through 180° around their long axis (Figure 87.64). Hairs are fragile with the shape making them more vulnerable to the effects of weathering; TN may be seen at the sites of the twists [32]. Pili torti is a clinical sign and not a diagnosis, being seen in wide array of congenital and acquired defects (e.g. scarring alopecias).

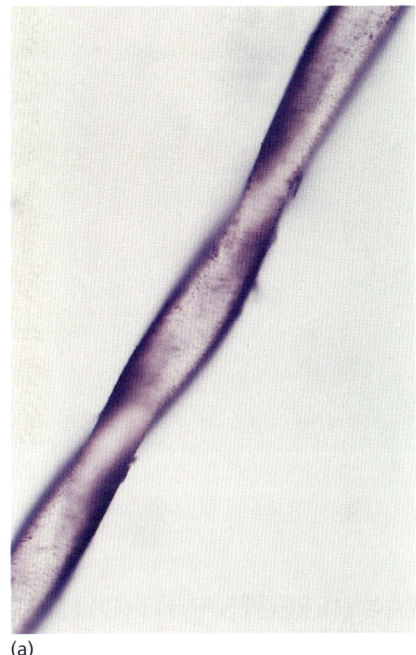

(a)

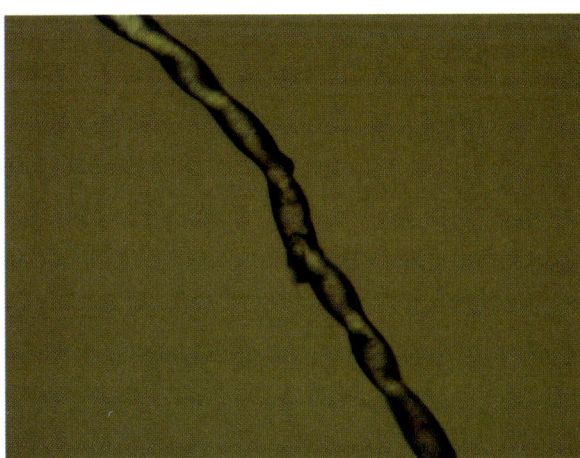

(b)

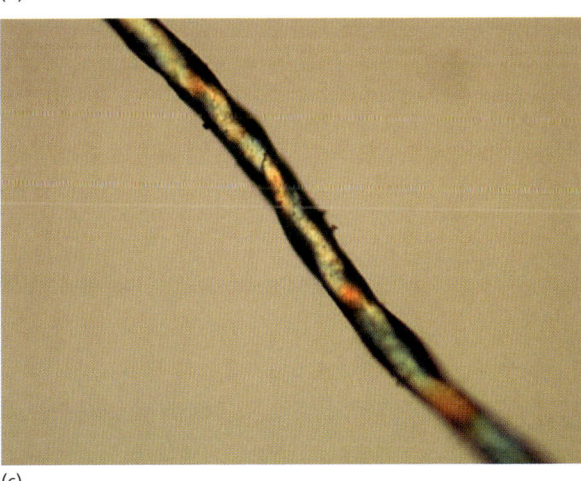

(c)

Figure 87.64 Pili torti. (a) Light micrograph showing 180° twists. (b) A hair from a 6-month-old boy with Menkes syndrome. (c) A hair from a 27-year-old woman with no personal or family history of associated disorders.

Clinical features

There is a wide variation from case to case in the fragility of the hair, and hence in the clinical severity. Affected hairs are brittle and may break off, particularly in areas subject to trauma, such as the occiput. Affected hairs have a spangled appearance in reflected light. Non-scalp areas (e.g. eyebrows/eyelashes) may also be affected. There are several syndromes in which twisted hair is a feature (Chapter 66).

Investigations

Rotations of the hair shaft run in groups of three to five twists before the shaft normalises [33]. Screening *in vivo* for abnormal hairs or where to sample scalp hair can be done with trichoscopy. However, sometimes the hair is so sparse as to be difficult to sample and is best assessed with light microscopy. Scanning electron microscopy has made it clear that twisted hairs occur in many different forms, and that not all twisted hairs are pili torti.

If pili torti is identified, a syndromic cause should be excluded. Assessment of hearing loss, serum copper/ceruloplasmin levels and/or nutritional deficiencies should be done depending on the clinical presentation (Chapter 66).

Netherton syndrome

Classification links
- MIM: 256500

Introduction and general description

Netherton syndrome is characterised by a triad of congenital ichthyosis, typical hair shaft abnormality and atopic diathesis (Chapter 63).

Clinical features

The hair in Netherton syndrome is short, dry, lustreless and fragile. The eyebrows and eyelashes are sparse or absent. The pathognomonic hair abnormality is trichorrhexis invaginata (syn. bamboo hair) that occurs due to a temporary arrest of longitudinal hair growth resulting in focal impaction of the proximal hair into the distal shaft with overgrowth of the proximal cuticle, producing a 'ball in cup' appearance. Intermittent nodes of trichorrhexis invaginata are seen along the hair shaft, giving a bamboo appearance to the hair, and these are the focus of hair breakage (Figure 87.65) [34].

When Netherton syndrome is suspected careful screening of hairs should be performed. Unfortunately, the diagnostic hair changes of trichorrhexis invaginata can vary over time and location. Therefore, it is important that samples of at least 100 hairs are carefully examined by light microscopy on several occasions before a definite negative is asserted. Alternatively, finding a single trichorrhexis invaginata node in a single hair is a conclusive positive. Trichoscopy is increasingly being employed to screen individuals suspected of having Netherton syndrome [35,36], with light microscopy (± electron microscopy) being used to confirm the diagnosis when affected hairs are identified.

Consider sampling eyebrows hairs as this is shown to increase the likelihood of successful diagnosis [35,37].

PART 8: SPECIFIC CUTANEOUS STRUCTURES

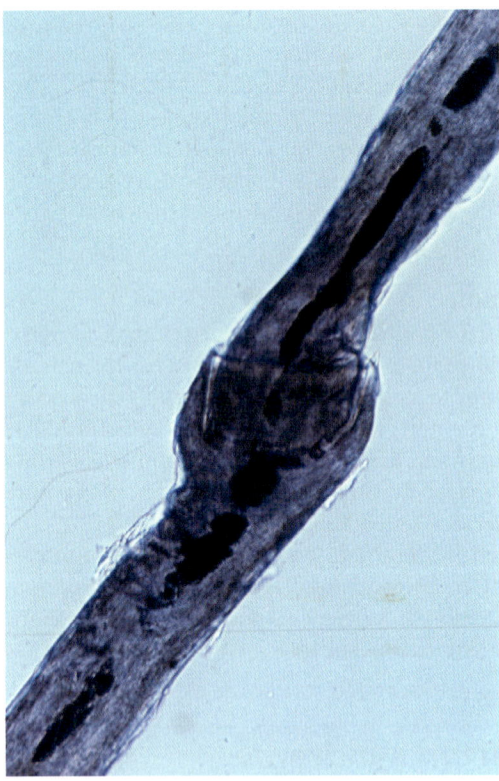

Figure 87.65 Trichorrhexis invaginata in Netherton syndrome.

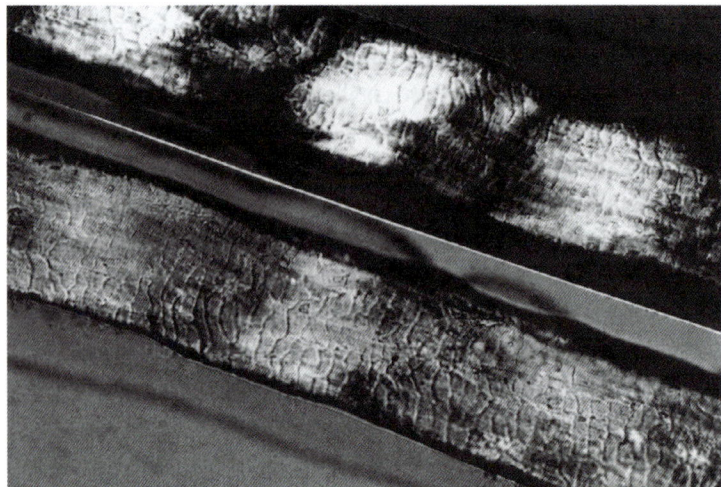

Figure 87.66 Trichothiodystrophy showing alternating bright and dark zones under a polarising microscope. Courtesy of D. Van Neste, Brussels.

Trichothiodystrophy

Introduction and general description

The term trichothiodystrophy (TTD) was coined to describe brittle hair with abnormally low sulphur content, derived from the Greek 'tricho' (hair), 'thio' (sulphur) and 'dystrophy' (faulty nourishment) [38]. The term covers a range of phenotypes, with low-sulphur fragile hair representing the central defining criterion [39,40]. TTD can be classified according to the constellation of features that accompany the hair changes (Chapter 66).

Clinical features

The hair in TTD is sparse, short and brittle, but the degree of alopecia varies considerably. A pathway to diagnosis by Cheng *et al.* proposes that TTD should be considered in anyone presenting with abnormal hair and/or a neuroectodermal syndrome [41]. Hair samples should be taken for light and polarised light microscopy, followed by hair amino acid quantification.

On light microscopy the hairs are flattened and can be twisted into various shapes – rather like a ribbon or shoelace. Weathering is often marked, with a loss of cuticle cells being prominent. A clean transverse break in the hair shaft (trichoschisis), TN and trichoptylosis may also be seen. Using crossed polarising filters, the hairs show alternating bright and dark zones likened to the appearance of a tiger tail. This appearance is formed due to loss of rigidity within the hair fibre, resulting in the longitudinal organisation of cortical fibres being thrown into a sine wave pattern. Usually >50% of hairs are affected in this way (Figure 87.66).

STRUCTURAL DEFECTS WITHOUT INCREASED HAIR FRAGILITY

Pili annulati

Synonyms and inclusions
- Ringed hair

Introduction and general description

Pili annulati is characterised by alternate light and dark bands along the length of the hair fibre resulting in an unusual, spangled appearance to the hair [1,2].

Clinical features

Pili annulati is often diagnosed coincidentally due to recognition of the unusual shiny, spangled appearance of the hair. The light bands identified by eye represent the air-filled cavities that are more easily seen in lighter hair colours. Trichoscopy is not reliable in pili annulati because the perception is based largely on light transmission through the hair and not reflection [4].

The diagnosis of pili annulati is readily established on microscopy of affected hairs, particularly when mounting medium is used [42]. The bright appearance of the abnormal bands in reflected light is caused by air spaces in the cortex (Figure 87.67), but when hairs are examined with transmitted light microscopy the abnormal bands appear dark due to light scattering.

Woolly hair

Introduction and general description

Woolly hair describes tightly coiled hair occurring over all or part of the scalp. In those of African origin, woolly hair is normal. Identifying woolly hair in non-African individuals is important as

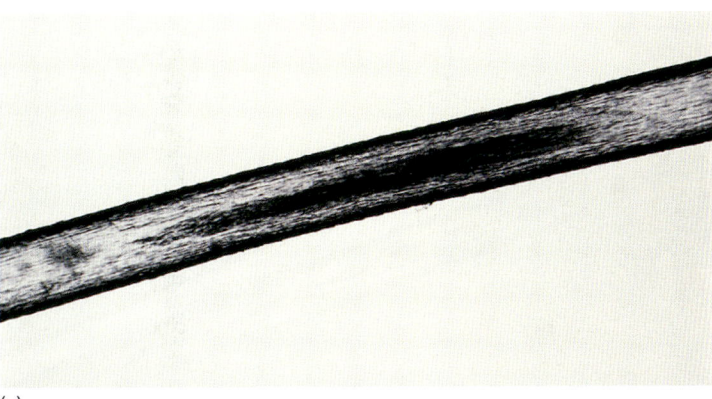

(a)

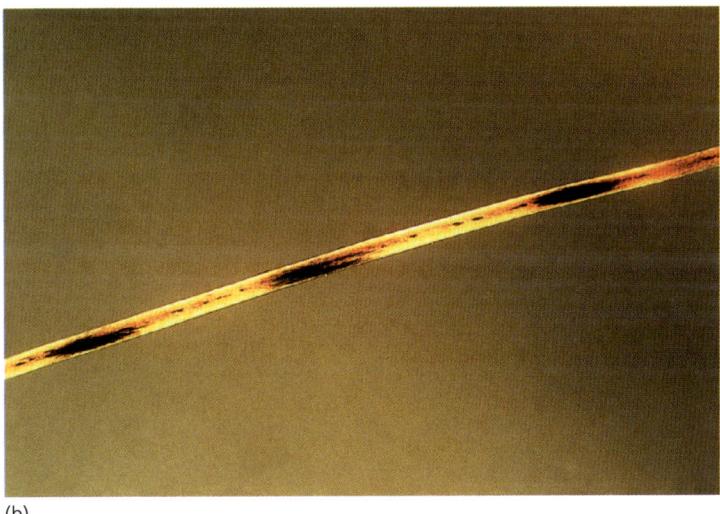

(b)

Figure 87.67 Pili annulati. (a) Hair shaft by transmitted light showing an abnormal dark band (central part) caused by multiple cortical air spaces. This corresponds to a bright region as seen by reflected light. (b) The abnormality is intermittent, causing a beaded or ringed appearance.

various inherited disorders may present with this phenotype, some of which have serious associated underling health implications.

Pathophysiology
Various distinct genetic defects have been identified that can all manifest with a woolly hair phenotype, highlighting the complex control of hair growth and curl development. Disorders of desmosomes, keratins and lipid mediators may all present with woolly hair [43].

Clinical features
Hair is tight coiled, with knots and fractures common. Trichoscopy shows kinking, flattening and twisting, with the appearance of some hairs likened to a 'crawling snake' [44].

Specific questions should be considered during assessment [43,45], including:
- Are the hair changes generalised or localised?
- Is it syndromic or non-syndromic?
- If non-syndromic, is it autosomal dominant or autosomal recessive inheritance?

Careful examination of the hands and feet, additional investigations, including genetic testing, and examination of other family

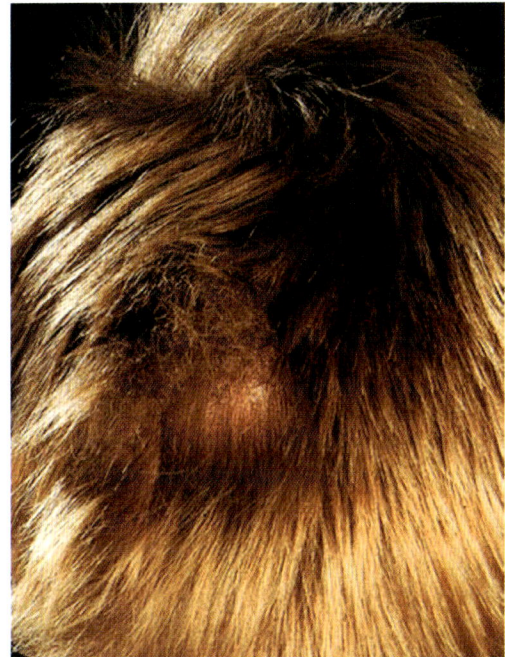

Figure 87.68 Woolly hair naevus.

members can help answer these questions. There will be a range of 'woolliness' in the same family.

Clinical variants
Generalised woolly hair (non-syndromic). Autosomal dominant woolly hair (ADWH)/hypotrichosis [43] or autosomal recessive woolly hair (ARWH)/hypotrichosis [43,46].

Generalised woolly hair (syndromic). Woolly hair and palmoplantar keratoderma (PPK). Naxos disease and Carvajal syndrome are characterised by woolly hair, striate PPK and systemic features including cardiomyopathy. These features are important to identify as the hair and skin phenotype appears early in life, with cardiac features only developing later in childhood and adolescence. Thus, early identification and prompt referral to cardiology are vital due to the risk of sudden death in these patients [47].

Localised woolly hair. Woolly hair naevus (Figure 87.68) [43,48–52].

Acquired progressive kinking of the hair. This is typically seen in young men and is strongly associated with rapid AGA development [53,54]; it is also known as whisker hair. A change in hair shape and texture at the frontotemporal and vertex regions is seen, associated with increased shedding and a positive family history for AGA [54]. Biopsy shows a reduced terminal : vellus ratio. The mechanism is unclear but may result from irregular proliferation within the HF bulb during hair miniaturisation.

Acquired woolly hair. This may also be caused by drugs such as valproate and retinoids [55,56].

Investigations
Hair microscopy in all the woolly hair disorders reveals non-specific features that are consistent with a woolly, stiff hair phenotype. For

localised woolly hair, additional investigations are usually not necessary. For generalised woolly hair, features of syndromic woolly hair should be sought. Cardiac investigation (electrocardiogram/echocardiography) may be indicated, and genetics referral should be considered in all generalised cases.

Uncombable hair syndrome

Synonyms and inclusions
- Pili triangulati et canaliculi
- Cheveux incoiffables
- Spun glass hair

Classification links
- MIM: 191480

Introduction and general description

The hairs of uncombable hair syndrome typically show a triangular or kidney-shaped cross-section causing them to be rigid and to stand up, resulting in a distinctive clinical presentation.

Clinical features

The hair is normal in quantity and sometimes also in length, but the wild, disorderly appearance totally resists all efforts to control it with a brush or comb [57]. The hair is often a silvery blond colour. The eyebrows and eyelashes are normal.

With light microscopy the three-dimensional aspect of the shaft changes can be difficult to establish. Polarised light microscopy may help, but scanning electron microscopy is the gold standard for identifying the typical changes [58]. The hairs are triangular or kidney-shaped in cross-section and longitudinal grooving is identified (Figure 87.69). Recently, techniques to identify the hairs in cross-section using epoxy resin [59] or frozen sectioning [60] have been described. Samples should show >50% abnormal hairs to make the diagnosis (Figure 87.70) [58,61].

Loose anagen syndrome

Introduction and general description

This condition features anagen hairs that are loosely anchored and easily pulled from the scalp [62–65].

Clinical features

Typically, loose anagen syndrome is seen in fair-haired children, aged 2–9 years and mostly girls [66]. The hair is slightly unruly, of uneven length and patchy in quality, with a history of not growing properly and never needing cutting. Hair is usually easily and painlessly plucked from the scalp. Diagnosis is suggested when 3–10 anagen hairs are easily removed using the hair pull test [65,67,68], although caution is required as the numbers of hairs removed can vary over time, so a single negative hair pull does not exclude the diagnosis [69]. Diagnosis can be confirmed by trichogram and requires at least 70% of hairs to be loose anagen hairs [65,66,68].

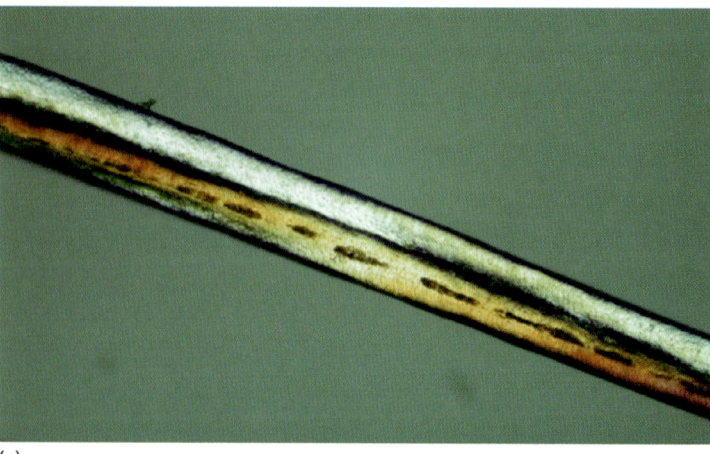

(a)

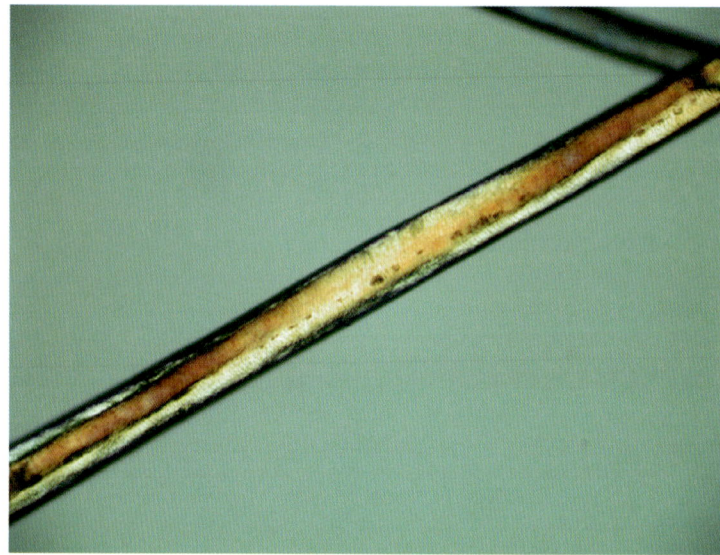

(b)

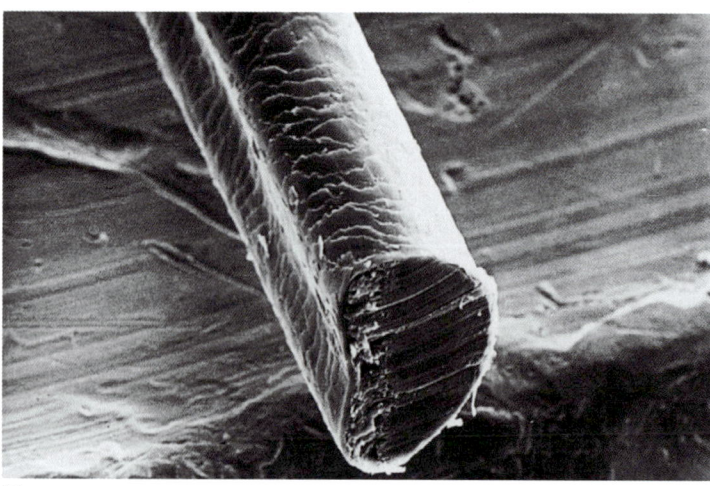

(c)

Figure 87.69 Uncombable hair syndrome. (a) The triangular cross-section of the hair contributes to its stiffness. (b) Light microscopy revealing grooving when using partially crossed polarising filters. (c) Scanning electron micrograph showing a triangular cross-section and canalicular depression or gutter along one side.

Figure 87.70 Hair fibres in uncombable hair syndrome showing a typical triangular shape in cross-section. Here hair fibres were embedded, sectioned horizontally, stained and viewed by microscopy.

Microscopy of loose anagen hairs shows ruffling of the cuticle adjacent to the anagen bulb, giving the appearance of a 'floppy sock' (Figure 87.71), along with the absence of an attached root sheath (helping to differentiate these hairs from normal plucked anagen hairs).

Differential diagnosis
Olsen *et al.* showed that 61% of normal children under 10 years have some degree of loose anagen hairs on hair pull, although the numbers of hairs removed were small (one or two loose anagen hairs per pull) compared with significantly higher numbers seen in loose anagen syndrome. This may reflect immature anchoring and higher anagen levels in this younger age group [67].

Short anagen syndrome

Introduction and general description
Short anagen syndrome is frequently confused with loose anagen syndrome (perhaps due to the similar name) but has distinct clinical features [70].

Pathophysiology
This condition is usually sporadic, resulting in poor hair growth due to a short anagen phase. As duration of anagen is the main determinant of hair length, hairs do not grow past a certain length in this condition and proportionately more hairs are in the telogen phase at any one time. It likely results from genetic and hormonal influence on anagen duration that are age and sex dependent. Shorter anagen durations of 4–10 months contrast with normal anagen durations of 2–6 years.

Clinical features
Typically, short anagen syndrome presents in early childhood (2–4 years) when shorter hair growth becomes apparent compared with the child's peers. It is mainly reported in white people with fine blond hair. The hair length is short, often <6 cm in length, and is described as 'not growing' or 'never needing cutting' [71]. The hair density may be low, with episodes of hair shedding, and a positive pull test is sometimes seen. However, the hair is of normal quality with no fragility or unruliness observed [70].

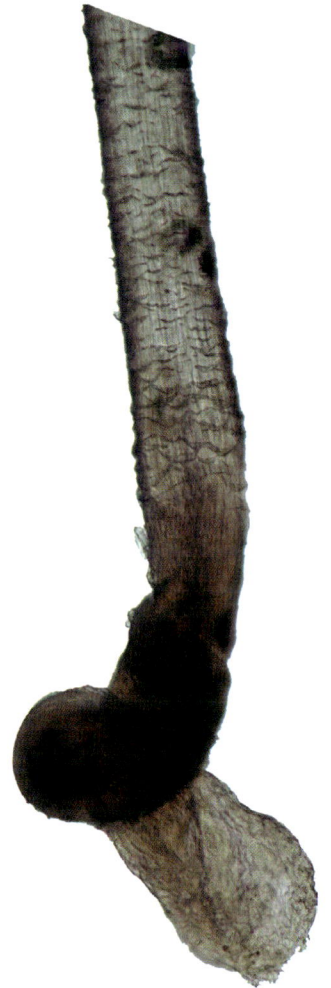

Figure 87.71 Plucked anagen hair in the loose anagen syndrome showing a vestigial root sheath and a ruffled cuticle.

Investigations
Hair microscopy should be performed to exclude other hair shaft abnormalities. Pointed tapered tips are seen on all hairs, showing that the shorter length is due to shorter hair growth and not cutting or breakage. Trichogram or scalp biopsy assessment is usually not necessary but may show an increased percentage of telogen hairs.

Management
Some improvement with age (especially during puberty) may be seen. Treatments to prolong anagen may be used, including topical or oral minoxidil. Low-level light therapy and PRP conceivably may help [71]; ciclosporin has also been used [72].

Trichostasis spinulosa

Introduction and general description
This is probably a normal, age-related phenomenon – which is easily overlooked – in which successive telogen hairs are retained in predominantly sebaceous follicles [73].

Pathophysiology

The cause of entrapment of vellus hairs within a hyperkeratotic infundibulum is unclear. A congenital dysplasia or abnormal angulation of the HF may predispose to entrapment of vellus hairs. External factors, such as dust or oils, may contribute. Follicles contain *Malassezia* yeasts and *Cutibacterium acnes*, but their role in pathogenesis is uncertain [74].

Clinical features

Usually an incidental finding, trichostasis spinulosa is reported at all adult ages, although it appears to be more common in the elderly. The lesions, which closely resemble comedones, occur predominantly on the nose, forehead and cheeks, but the trunk, interscapular area and limbs may also be affected [74,75].

Lesions are comedo-like with horny plugs and a retention of vellus hairs may be seen [76]. The classic variant affecting the face in elderly people is usually asymptomatic, whereas a pruritic variant occurring in younger people affecting the trunk and limbs is described [75,77]. The number of follicles affected varies greatly. Dermoscopy identifies tufts of multiple, slightly pigmented vellus hairs emerging from a dilated follicular ostium, with variable degrees of hyperkeratosis seen. Trichostasis spinulosa has been reported in association with the use of topical minoxidil and topical steroids, and in the clinical setting of chronic renal failure [78–80].

Differential diagnosis

The condition must be differentiated from the 'multiple hairs' of pili multigemini. Dilated pores, comedonal acne, Favre–Racouchot syndrome and keratosis pilaris should also be considered.

Investigations

On histology, affected follicles contain up to 50 vellus hairs embedded in a keratinous plug. Standard skin surface biopsy uses cyanoacrylate glue on a glass slide applied to the skin for surface sampling and identifies multiple vellus hair bundles in funnel-shaped structures [81].

Management

Keratolytic preparations are often disappointing. The most effective treatment is topical retinoic acid, which should be used as in the treatment of acne [82]. Depilatory wax, specialised cleaning pads and a variety of laser treatments have also been advocated [83].

Pili multigemini

Synonyms and inclusions
• Pili bifurcate

Introduction and general description

The term pili multigemini describes an uncommon developmental defect of HFs that fuse, resulting in multiple hairs from a composite follicular structure emerging through a single pilosebaceous canal [84,85].

Pathophysiology

Pili multigenini is due to a developmental defect of the HF. Two to 10 hairs develop with separate papilla, matrix and IRS, but sharing the same ORS.

Clinical features

Pili multigemini may occur anywhere on the body, but is typically found on the face, and especially along the jawline [84,85]. Isolated, thicker than average hairs are seen that may be flattened, oval or triangular. Their discovery is often a matter of chance, but the patient may complain of recurrent inflammatory nodules that leave scars. Dermoscopy reveals bundles of pigmented hairs of similar thickness emerging from one ostium, often surrounded by a peripilar cast. Numerous follicles showing this defect have been seen in a patient with cleido-cranial dysostosis, and a naevoid pattern on the back has also been described [86].

Differential diagnosis

This is different from compound or tufted follicles, where separate follicular bulbs generate hairs that fuse in the infundibular region and can emerge from a single opening.

Investigations

Microscopy of plucked hairs shows a typical 'bundle of sticks' appearance. Within the follicular canal, contiguous hairs may adhere, bifurcate and then re-adhere [87].

EXCESSIVE HAIR GROWTH

Growth of hair on the body may be considered excessive if it is increased compared with what would be considered normal for an individual of the same age, sex and race [1]. Hypertrichosis can involve any area of hair-bearing skin and affects both males and females. Hirsutism refers specifically to an increase in terminal pigmented hairs in an adult male (androgen-dependent) pattern in females.

Hypertrichosis

Hypertrichosis may be a generalised or localised phenomenon. Disorders resulting in hypertrichosis may be congenital or acquired. There are several mechanisms by which hypertrichosis is thought to occur [1]: (i) switching hairs from vellus to terminal (although the mechanism of vellus to terminal transition is poorly understood); (ii) changes to the HF growth cycle resulting in increased anagen duration and fewer telogen hairs (producing longer hairs and less shedding) thereby increasing hair density; or (iii) higher numbers of HFs than normal present at a particular body site.

The terminology relating to congenital hypertrichosis can be confusing and disorders are best described in terms of the specific genetic abnormality (if known), inheritance trait (autosomal dominant (AD), recessive (AR) or X-linked) and any associated abnormalities.

Congenital generalised hypertrichosis

Congenital generalised hypertrichosis (CGH) is rare. There are a small number of disorders in which generalised hypertrichosis is the main clinical feature. Inheritance may be AD, AR (MIM: 135400) or X-linked (MIM: 307150). Associated features may or may not be present, with gingival hyperplasia being the commonest association. The hair type may be specified as either lanugo or terminal. In cases of AD-CGH, copy number variations on chromosome 17 (17q24.2-q24.3) have been identified [2–4]. Recently, the overlapping genetic region for AD-CGH has been narrowed to two genes: *ABCA5* and *MAP2K6* [4]. *ABCA5* is a member of the superfamily of adenosine triphosphate (ATP) binding cassette transporters located at the lysosomal membrane and involved in efflux of lysosomal cholesterols. Loss of function in *ABCA5* may lead to the accumulation of endolysosomal cholesterol, defective lysosomes and impaired cellular cholesterol homeostasis, impacting normal HF biology [4]. In AR-CGH, a single base pair substitution in *ABCA5* has been identified [5]. A case report of isolated generalised hypertrichosis has been found in association with a duplication at 17q11.2. The duplicated region contained approximately 30 genes including *FOXN1*, a transcription factor involved with the differentiation of epithelial cells and regulation of keratinocytes, especially hair keratins [6].

X-linked CGH affects males more severely and, in different kindreds, has been associated with dental anomalies, deafness, scoliosis and spina bifida [7–9]. The condition has been mapped to chromosome Xq24-q27.1 and several studies have identified interchromosomal insertions at an extragenic palindrome site at Xq27.1 [9,10]. In one study, a gene surrounding the insertion, *FGF13* (fibroblast growth factor 13), was found to have significantly reduced mRNA levels. Immunofluorescence staining revealed a striking decrease in FGF13 throughout the ORS of affected HFs [10].

Cantu syndrome (MIM: 239850) is an AD syndrome characterised by congenital hypertrichosis, osteochondrodysplasia, characteristic facial anomalies and cardiomegaly [11]. The condition results from a gain-of-function mutation of the *ABCC9* gene that encodes SUR2, a subunit of ATP-mediated potassium channels [12–14]. Similarities between Cantu syndrome and the effects of the drug minoxidil were first noted in 2006 [12,15]. SUR2B is expressed on HF dermal papilla cells and is the pharmacological target of minoxidil [16–18].

Congenital hypertrichosis lanuginosa. Congenital hypertrichosis lanuginosa (syn. hypertrichosis universalis) (MIM: 145700) is an extremely rare disorder in which fetal lanugo hair is not shed *in utero*. To date, no genetic abnormality has been identified but the condition is inherited as an AD trait [19,20]. In reported cases, long, pale, silky lanugo hairs cover the entire body surface except the mucosae, palms and soles (Figure 87.72) [20,21]. Abnormal dentition is found in some cases [19–21]. Hypertrichosis may persist but improvement during infancy is reported [21].

Congenital hypertrichosis (Ambras type). There has been debate regarding the use of the term Ambras type congenital hypertrichosis (syn. hypertrichosis universalis congenita Ambras type) (MIM: 145701) [22,23]. It is recognised that cases described as Ambras-type hypertrichosis are associated with rearrangements of chromosome 8. Cytogenetic analysis of several cases of Ambras-type

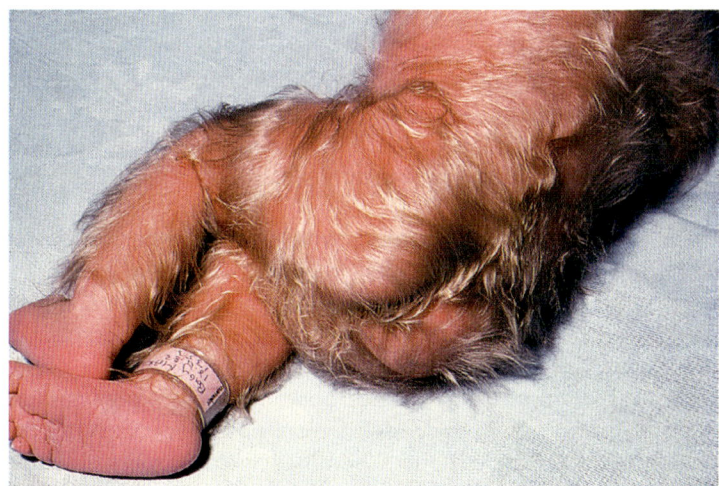

Figure 87.72 Congenital hypertrichosis lanuginosa. Courtesy of Dr Partridge, Leamington, UK.

hypertrichosis have identified breakpoints in the 8q22-8q24 region [24]. An 11.5 Mb candidate interval on chromosome 8q has been identified based on these breakpoints. *TRPS1*, a gene within this interval, was deleted in one patient with an 8q23 chromosomal rearrangement, and its expression was significantly downregulated in another patient with an inversion breakpoint 7.3 Mb downstream of *TRPS1*. These results suggest a position effect that downregulates *TRPS1* expression as the probable cause of hypertrichosis [24]. *TRPS1* is a transcription factor expressed in the nuclei of mesenchyme-derived dermal papilla cells and human HF epithelial cells [25]. Clinically, cases of congenital hypertrichosis with C8q breakpoints have widespread, long, fine, vellus-type hair, with accentuation of hair growth on the shoulders, ears and face; abnormal facial features are also described [24].

Other congenital disorders in which hypertrichosis is an important feature are described in Chapter 66. CGH may also arise in association with neonatal hypothyroidism [26] and non-genetic disorders such as fetal alcohol syndrome.

Congenital localised hypertrichosis

Congenital localised hypertrichosis may occur as a primary phenomenon or, more commonly, in association with other congenital conditions, naevi and hamartomas. Sometimes, such as with Becker naevus, increased hair is not evident in infancy, but develops later in childhood or adolescence. In some cases, focal hypertrichosis may be an indicator of significant underlying pathology, such as with spinal dysraphism.

Primary (naevoid) congenital hypertrichosis. Naevoid hypertrichosis (reviewed by Gupta *et al.* [27]) is a localised growth of terminal hair present at birth or shortly thereafter. It occurs in the absence of other abnormalities and can occur anywhere on hair-bearing skin. Patches are typically solitary; however, multiple patches have been described, some associated with a degree of lipoatrophy [28]. Multiple patches of hypertrichosis may be seen in association with other congenital cutaneous disorders such as hypomelanosis of Ito [29], and congenital syndromes such as Happle–Tinschert syndrome [30]. Several well-recognised patterns of localised hypertrichosis include hypertrichosis cubiti (MIM: 139600): 'hairy elbows', reviewed in [31]; anterior cervical hypertrichosis (MIM: 600457), reviewed in [32]; and hypertrichosis of the ears (syn. hypertrichosis pinnae auris) (MIM: 139500, 425500) [33].

Local hypertrichosis associated with other congenital naevi/hamartomas.

Hypertrichosis is frequently seen in association with congenital melanocytic naevi, although hairs may not become apparent until puberty. Hypertrichosis may also occur in association with neurofibromas, particularly plexiform lesions. Becker naevus occurs predominantly in males. Localised hyperpigmentation appears during childhood/adolescence, with hypertrichosis first evident after puberty due to the influence of androgens. Smooth muscle hamartomas, which can appear similar to Becker naevi, are often associated with hypertrichosis [34,35].

Localised hypertrichosis associated with spinal dysraphism.

Congenital focal hypertrichosis overlying the spine may be an indicator of spinal dysraphism (congenital abnormalities where defective closure of the neural tube is associated with abnormalities of the vertebral column, e.g. spina bifida). Approximately 50% of cases of spinal dysraphism have associated cutaneous abnormalities, with focal hypertrichosis one of the commoner cutaneous findings [36]. Localised lumbo-sacral hypertrichosis (syn. faun tail naevus) is a V-shaped patch of hair overlying the lumbo-sacral spine most associated with tethered cord and diastematomyelia (split spinal cord) (Figure 87.73) [36–38]. The appearance of the hairs is variable [39], and has also been reported overlying the upper thoracic spine in association with tethered cord [40]. Focal hypertrichosis may also be seen in association with cranial dysraphism, where it may overlie defects or encircle them. The hair collar sign is a ring of dark coarse hair surrounding exophytic scalp lesions such as encephaloceles and meningoceles [39].

Acquired hypertrichosis

Acquired hypertrichosis is usually classified as being either generalised or localised; however, these categories are not strictly defined and in some reported cases arguably either term could be applied. Some causes of hypertrichosis are reported to cause both localised and more generalised hair growth, such as the use of topical minoxidil or cetuximab, juvenile dermatomyositis and porphyria cutanea tarda.

Generalised acquired hypertrichosis.

The development of extensive hypertrichosis in an adult can be a cutaneous manifestation of internal malignancy and requires prompt investigation. More frequently, generalised hypertrichosis occurs as a side effect of systemic medication, but may also occur in association with several systemic conditions.

Malignancy-associated generalised hypertrichosis.

Malignancy-associated hypertrichosis lanuginosa (syn. 'malignant down', acquired hypertrichosis lanuginosa, paraneoplastic hypertrichosis lanuginose) is a rare paraneoplastic condition in which long, fine,

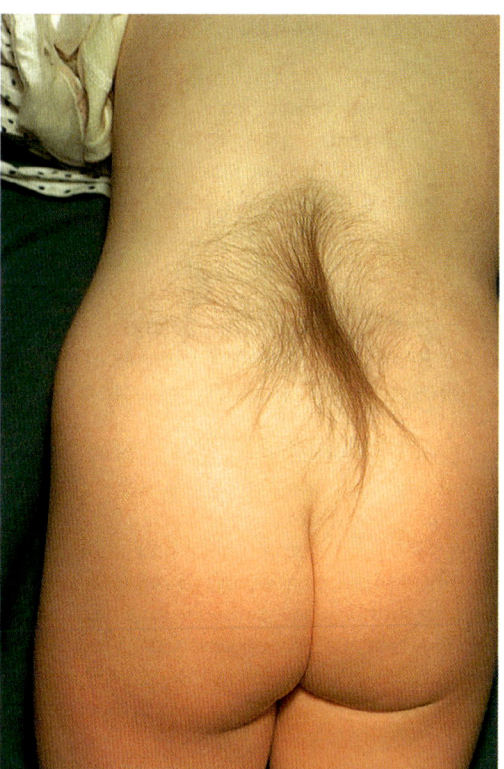

Figure 87.73 Lumbo-sacral hypertrichosis ('faun tail'), here associated with diastematomyelia.

lanugo-type hairs develop over the face and body in association with an underlying malignancy (reviewed in [41]). The condition is reported to occur most frequently in the fifth to eighth decades and is reported in women more frequently than men [41,42]. The condition is generally seen in association with advanced or metastatic cancer [41,42], although occurrence with early-stage breast cancer is reported [43]. The onset of hypertrichosis may precede tumour diagnosis by several years [42]. Striking downy hair growth starts on the face (particularly the eyebrows, forehead, cheeks, ears and nose) and progresses cephalocaudally, with sparing of the palms, soles and genital skin [42]. In women, colo-rectal cancer is the most observed associated malignancy, followed by lung and breast cancer. In men, lung cancer is the most frequent association, followed by colo-rectal cancer [41,42]. A wide range of internal malignancies have also been reported in association, including chronic lymphocytic leukaemia and extraskeletal Ewing sarcoma [44,45]. Hair growth tends to mirror the underlying cancer, regressing with successful treatment and recurring with cancer recurrence. A role for tumour-related growth factors and growth factor receptor ligands is speculated [41].

Non-malignancy-associated generalised hypertrichosis.

Drug-induced hypertrichosis. Hypertrichosis is a well-recognised side effect of several medications including minoxidil (oral and topical [46–50]), phenytoin, psoralens, ciclosporin and prednisolone. Generalised hypertrichosis in children is reported with inhaled corticosteroids [51]. Antihypertensives other than minoxidil may induce hypertrichosis, including diazoxide [52,53], verapamil [54], perindopril and amlodipine [55]. There are a number

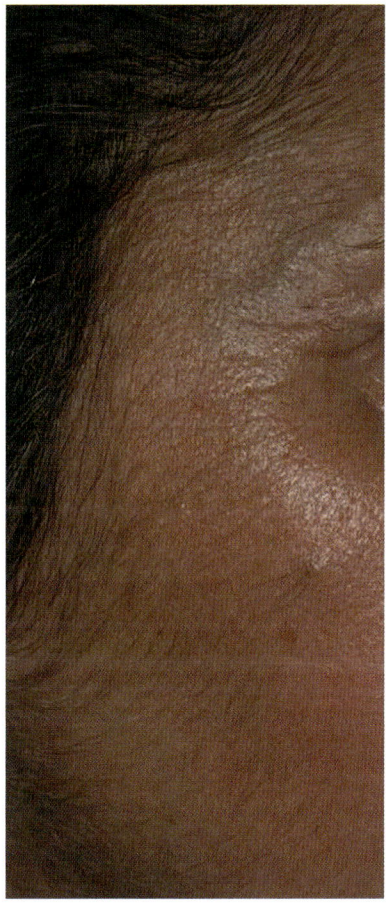

Figure 87.74 Facial hypertrichosis in porphyria cutanea tarda.

Table 87.8 Causes of localised acquired hypertrichosis

Cause	Examples and references
Medication	Topical minoxidil
	Topical intralesional corticosteroids
	Topical tacrolimus [68,69]
	Prostaglandin analogues (eyelash trichomegaly, facial hypertrichosis) [70,71]
	Infliximab [72]
	Dupilumab (injection sites) [73]
	Panitumumab (eyelash trichomegaly, ear hypertrichosis) [74,75]
	Erlotinib (eyelash trichomegaly, facial hypertrichosis) [76–78]
	Interferon α (eyelash trichomegaly) [79], interferon β (injection sites) [80]
	Cetuximab (face, scalp, eyelashes, eyebrows) [81,82]
Inflammatory and metabolic	Porphyria cutanea tarda (facial hypertrichosis)
	Pretibial myxoedema
	Juvenile dermatomyositis (infrapatellar) [83]
	Panniculitis [84,85]
Physical	Laser epilation (paradoxical hypertrichosis) [86]
	Chronic rubbing/skin trauma [87]
Infection	HIV (eyelash trichomegaly, eyebrows, ears) [88,89]
Miscellaneous	Vaccination sites [90]
	Sclerotherapy [91,92]
	Henna tattoos [93]
	Plaster casts/healing fracture [94]

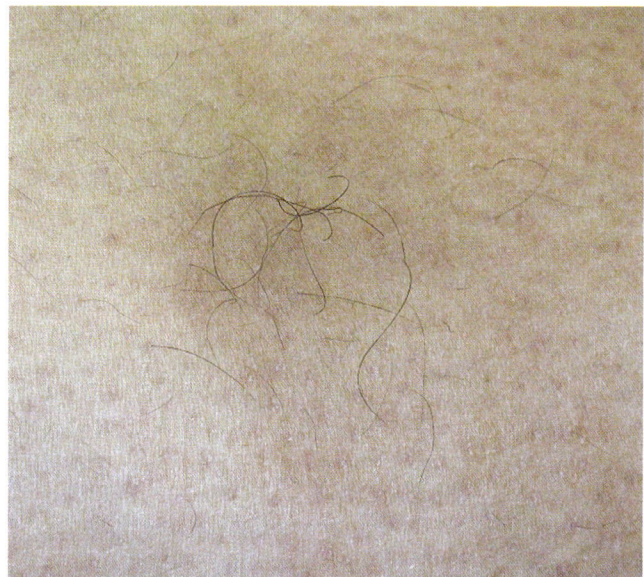

Figure 87.75 Localised hypertrichosis at the site of underlying panniculitis.

of reports of hypertrichosis occurring with biologic agents including secukinumab [56,57], ixekizumab [57], interferon-α [58] and cetuximab [59].

Hypertrichosis in association with medical disorders. Generalised hypertrichosis is reported to be a feature of several medical conditions including:
- Endocrine and metabolic disorders (juvenile hypothyroidism [60,61], Cushing disease, porphyria cutanea tarda (Figure 87.74) [62].
- Connective tissue disease (juvenile dermatomyositis) [63,64].
- Nutritional disorders (malnutrition, anorexia nervosa) [65,66].
- Haematological disorders (POEMS syndrome (polyneuropathy, organomegaly, endocrinopathy, monoclonal protein and skin changes)) [67].

Localised acquired hypertrichosis. Many causes of localised hypertrichosis are reported (Table 87.8), with medications constituting one of the most frequent associations. Eyelash trichomegaly is reported with several biologic treatments. Inflammatory disorders and physical causes (e.g. panniculitis (Figure 87.75)) are other well-recognised associations.

Hirsutism

Introduction and general description
Hirsutism is defined as excessive male pattern androgen-dependent terminal hair growth on the face and body of women. It is estimated to affect 5–10% of women of reproductive age worldwide and prevalence varies with age and ethnicity [1–4]. Most women with hirsutism (≥80%) will have an underlying disorder causing androgen excess [5]. However, the severity of hirsutism correlates poorly with androgen levels [3,6,7]. Hirsutism is frequently an emotional and financial burden for women, significantly impacting quality

of life [1,8]. While there are strict clinical definitions of hirsutism (usually assessed using the Ferriman–Gallwey scoring system [9]), it has been recommended that treatment be guided largely by patient distress experienced due to excessive unwanted hair growth [8].

Age, ethnicity and genetic factors influence the extent of female facial and body hair, and these factors are relevant to the epidemiology of hirsutism. Androgen levels tend to decrease with age [10]; thus, hirsutism tends to be more prevalent in younger women [11]. Hirsutism also varies with ethnicity, with significantly higher hirsutism scores seen in Mediterranean, Hispanic and Middle Eastern women compared with East Asian women (reviewed in [1]). A US population study examining hirsutism in black and white women of reproductive age found no statistically significant difference in abnormal hirsutism scores between the two groups (4.3% black women versus 5.4% white women) [12]. Hirsutism is a feature of several clinical disorders, most commonly polycystic ovarian syndrome (PCOS), but in a minority of cases it is idiopathic.

Pathophysiology

Pigmented terminal facial or body hair in a male pattern is controlled by androgens, and excessive hair growth occurs either due to increased androgen levels (hyperandrogenaemia) or, less commonly, increased HF sensitivity to normal levels of androgens. Hirsutism is an important clinical marker of underlying hyperandrogenism and is the most common clinical manifestation of hyperandrogenaemia in women [13].

Normal female androgen physiology [6,14]

In women, androgens are produced both by the adrenal glands and the ovaries. Adrenal androgen production (adrenarche) begins several years before the onset of puberty under the influence of ACTH. The major adrenal androgens are dehydroepiandrosterone sulphate, DHEA and androstenedione. Ovarian androgen secretion begins at puberty, stimulated by luteinising hormone. Ovarian tissues also secrete DHEA, androstenedione and testosterone. Testosterone is secreted by both the adrenals and ovaries; however, around 50% of testosterone is derived from the peripheral conversion of androstenedione in the skin and other extrasplanchnic sites. Circulating testosterone is bound avidly to sex hormone-binding globulin (SHBG), with around 20–25% loosely bound to albumin. Only around 1% of circulating testosterone is unbound; thus, levels of binding proteins such as SHBG are important modulators of androgen activity. DHT, the most potent androgen, is a product primarily of peripheral tissue conversion of testosterone via the activity of 5α-reductase. Only DHT and free (unbound) testosterone can bind to and activate androgen receptors. DHT has a fivefold greater affinity for the androgen receptor than testosterone.

Androgen excess

Excessive androgen levels are found in ≥80% of hirsutism cases and elevated androgens may be of ovarian or adrenal origin. Hirsutism without hyperandrogenaemia, and in which there are no other signs or symptoms indicative of a hyperandrogenic endocrine disorder and menses are regular, is described as idiopathic hirsutism [1,6]. It is unclear whether idiopathic hirsutism is due to altered androgen activity within the HF, increased HF sensitivity to androgens or abnormal local androgen concentrations [1,6,7,15]. DHT is the

primary androgen implicated in the transition of vellus hairs to terminal hairs in hirsutism. Activation of androgen receptors in HF dermal papilla cells promotes expression of genes that increase HF size, hair diameter and anagen duration [6].

A possible role for the androgen receptor in the pathogenesis of hirsutism has been considered. A variable number tandem repeat polymorphism consisting of CAG repeats is embedded in the *AR* gene [16]. These trinucleotide repeats have been found to be polymorphic among humans and the transcriptional activity of the *AR* gene is inversely correlated with the number of CAG repeats [17]. The normal CAG repeat number varies from 11 to 36, with an average of 20–23 repeats [17]. In one recent study of Turkish women with disorders of androgen excess and idiopathic hirsutism, short (<17) CAG repeats were found to be associated with both PCOS and idiopathic hirsutism [18]. Another study examined *AR* CAG repeats in healthy Jewish women of different ethnicities. For the group, there was a significant negative correlation between the number of CAG repeats in the *AR* gene and hirsutism scores, with longer CAG repeats associated with lower levels of hirsutism. Further, differences in the prevalence of hirsutism between the two ethnic groups correlated with CAG repeat length [19].

A study in 60 women with hirsutism and/or acne found that 8.3% of women had heterozygotic *CYP21A2* mutations. *CYP21A2* encodes for 21-hydroxylase, the enzyme most associated with non-classic (late-onset) congenital adrenal hyperplasia, an uncommon cause of hirsutism. The mutation rate in women with hirsutism was significantly higher than in the general population, although there was no significant difference in hormone levels between heterozygous carriers and subjects with normal *CYP21A2* genes [20].

Clinical features

The assessment of women presenting with a history suggestive of hirsutism should begin with a complete history and physical examination. Relevant factors in the clinical history include the patient's age and age at onset of hirsutism; menstrual history and pregnancies; medications; family history of endocrine disease; and history of hair removal. Clinical examination for other signs of hyperandrogenism and other endocrine disorders should also be undertaken [6].

The modified Ferriman–Gallwey score (mFGS) is the standard method of clinical evaluation of hirsutism (Table 87.9) [21,22]. Nine defined body areas (including upper lip, chin, anterior chest, back and proximal limbs) are assigned a score from 0 (no hair)

Table 87.9 Modified Ferriman–Gallwey score of hirsutism. Each site is assessed on a scale of 0 (no terminal hair growth) to 4 (extensive growth of terminal hair). A score of 8 or more is conventionally regarded as indicating significant hirsutism.

Area	Score
Moustache	0–4
Beard	0–4
Chest	0–4
Abdomen	0–4
Suprapubic, extending to umbilicus	0–4
Upper arms	0–4
Thighs	0–4
Upper back	0–4
Lower back	0–4
Total	*X/36*

to 4 (frankly virile) and these scores are added to give a total hirsutism score [1,21,22]. An mFGS above the 95th percentile for the female population of reproductive age is considered to constitute a diagnosis of hirsutism [1,3,22]. Epidemiological studies highlight variations in female body hair according to ethnicity: modified FGSs that define hirsutism in women of reproductive age in the USA and UK are values ≥8; for Mediterranean, Hispanic and Middle Eastern women values are ≥9–10; for South American women values are ≥6; and for East Asian women values are between ≥2 and ≥7, depending on ethnic group (reviewed in [1]).

Hirsutism is present when there is excessive terminal pigmented facial and/or body hair in a male distribution. Affected areas are most commonly the upper lip, chin and neck, anterior chest, lower abdomen and thighs [9]. Hirsutism should be distinguished from hypertrichosis, which is characterised by a generalised non-androgen-dependent increase in hair growth. When women are examined for signs of hirsutism, hair will often have been removed for cosmetic purposes. However, close inspection may reveal short cut and/or ingrowing hairs because of shaving, plucking or waxing. An accurate assessment of the mFGS may not be possible in women who have been treated by laser epilation or electrolysis. Other cutaneous signs of hyperandrogenism that may be present include seborrhoea, acne vulgaris and patterned hair loss. Other signs of androgen excess (virilisation) include clitoromegaly, deepening of the voice, increased muscle mass and male body habitus. Several endocrine disorders may be associated with hirsutism and signs such as acanthosis nigricans and cushingoid facies are important to recognise [23].

Investigations

Most women presenting with hirsutism (≥80%) will have biochemical hyperandrogenism. Given that the severity of hirsutism correlates poorly with androgen levels, all women with an abnormal hirsutism score should have biochemical assessment of circulating androgen levels. A short history of increasing hirsutism, particularly in association with other features such as virilism or signs of Cushing syndrome, indicates that prompt assessment is required. The most useful initial investigation is measurement of testosterone. An elevated result should be confirmed on a second sample, preferably using tandem mass spectrometry. Increasingly, the androgen profile is measured using tandem mass spectroscopy and an initial androgen screen might include total testosterone, androstenedione (predominantly an ovarian androgen) and 17-hydroxyprogesterone (to screen for non-classic congenital adrenal hyperplasia). Significant abnormalities of androgen biochemistry require further investigation and patients should be referred to the appropriate specialty, usually gynaecology or endocrinology. Further investigations may include extended androgen biochemical analyses, exclusion of other endocrine disorders (e.g. Cushing syndrome: urinary cortisol, dexamethasone suppression test), ultrasound evaluation of the ovaries (for suspected PCOS) and computed tomography/magnetic resonance imaging of the ovaries or adrenals (for suspected tumours).

Management

The two main aspects of management of hirsutism are treatment of excessive facial and body hair (cosmesis) and management of any underlying disorders causing hyperandrogenism.

Physical methods of hair removal

Most women will be familiar with the many options for the physical removal of hair. Many are cheap and easily available (shaving, plucking, depilatory creams, waxing, bleaching, threading, sugaring), although these methods frequently have side effects including skin irritation and pseudofolliculitis. Electrolysis is probably performed less frequently with the advent of hair removal lasers. Laser photoepilation is generally considered to be the most effective means of hair removal [1] and the best outcomes are seen when treating dark hairs in light-skinned individuals. Nd:YAG laser treatment is generally recommended for women with darker skin types [1]. Photoepilation of non-pigmented hairs is difficult and it has been suggested that electrolysis may be useful in this situation [1]. Paradoxical hypertrichosis is an uncommon side effect of photoepilation which is said to occur with increased frequency in Mediterranean and Middle Eastern women [24].

Topical treatments

Eflornithine cream reduces the rate of hair growth by inhibiting the enzyme ornithine decarboxylase. Clinical trial evidence suggests a modest benefit in the treatment of facial hirsutism, with around one-third of women considered a clinical success on completion of a 6-month trial using eflornithine cream, with an approximately 25% improvement in hair mass and length. Treatment must be continued to maintain the response [25]. There is some evidence that combining eflornithine cream with laser epilation results in a more rapid and greater reduction in unwanted hair compared with laser treatment alone [26]. The use of eflornithine cream following intense pulsed light (IPL) therapy has shown some benefit in maintaining IPL-induced hair reduction [27]. Eflornithine cream should be avoided during pregnancy.

Systemic therapies

The recommended first line systemic treatment for women with hirsutism is the combined oral contraceptive pill (OCP). Evidence suggests that no one type carries a significant advantage over another in terms of efficacy [1,28]. It has been recommended that if the response to treatment is suboptimal after 6 months combined OCP treatment, then an antiandrogen preparation should be added. Spironolactone 100 mg OD and flutamide 250 mg BD have been shown to be effective in treating hirsutism; however, some authors recommend against the use of flutamide for this indication, in view of hepatotoxicity associated with the use of this drug [1]. Bicalutamide appears to have a better safety profile than flutamide, however at present there are few data regarding its usefulness in the management of hirsutism. One trial comparing an OCP plus bicalutamide versus OCP alone demonstrated that OCP plus bicalutamide is well tolerated and significantly more effective than OCP alone in treating severe hirsutism [29]. Differing conclusions have been reached regarding the role of finasteride in the treatment of hirsutism. A systematic review concluded that finasteride was significantly more effective than placebo in the treatment of hirsutism, and its effectiveness comparable with spironolactone and flutamide [1]. However, an earlier systematic review concluded that while finasteride reduced the modified FGS, the reductions were inconsistent across studies [28]. Neither flutamide nor finasteride is licensed for use in hirsutism in the UK, and neither is used routinely. Metformin does not appear to be an effective treatment for hirsutism [1,28].

DISORDERS ASSOCIATED WITH HIRSUTISM

Hirsutism is a clinical sign and may be indicative of a serious underlying medical condition. The most common disorder associated with hirsutism is PCOS, which accounts for 70–80% of hirsutism diagnoses [2,4]. Idiopathic hirsutism (normal androgen levels, regular menses) accounts for approximately 5–15% of cases [1,2–4], and non-classic (late-onset) congenital adrenal hyperplasia 1.6–4.3% of cases. Androgen-secreting tumours are rare, accounting for only 0.2% of hirsutism cases [2,4,5].

Polycystic ovarian syndrome

Polycystic ovarian syndrome (syn. polycystic ovary syndrome) is one of the most common endocrine disorders, affecting an estimated 5–10% of women of reproductive age (depending on the diagnostic criteria used) [6]. The disorder is characterised by hyperandrogenism, chronic anovulation and ultrasound evidence of polycystic ovaries. The 2003 Rotterdam criteria require two of three of the following clinical features to diagnose PCOS: oligo- or anovulation; biochemical or clinical signs of hyperandrogenism; and ultrasound evidence of polycystic ovaries. Other conditions causing anovulation and hyperandrogenism, such as congenital adrenal hyperplasia, Cushing syndrome and androgen-secreting tumours, need to be excluded [7].

PCOS is a complex, multifactorial, polygenic disorder. Candidate genes suggested by GWAS relate to gonadotropin action, ovarian follicle development and insulin action [8]. However, although the heritability of PCOS is approximately 70% [9], the proportion of heritability accounted for by GWAS is less than 10% [6]. Several aberrant hormonal pathways are involved in disease pathogenesis. The hypothalamus secretes gonadotropin-releasing hormone with increased pulse frequency. This stimulates the anterior pituitary to preferentially release luteinising hormone, which in turn stimulates ovarian theca cells to produce androstenedione. Increased androgen levels arrest ovarian follicular development and cause the cutaneous signs of hyperandrogenism which are a feature of the condition (acne, hirsutism, patterned hair loss). Insulin resistance and hyperinsulinaemia also play a central role in disease pathogenesis, although the aetiology of this is unclear. Like luteinising hormone, insulin also stimulates ovarian theca cells to produce androstenedione. Suppression of hepatic SHBG by insulin further increases androgen levels by increasing free testosterone [6,10]. HAIR-AN (hyperandrogenism, insulin resistance and acanthosis nigricans) is a specific subtype of PCOS associated with severe insulin resistance [5,11].

Women with PCOS are at increased risk of a wide range of associated disorders including type 2 diabetes, hepatic steatosis, metabolic syndrome, hypertension dyslipidaemia, subfertility, endometrial cancer and psychiatric disorders [6,10].

Cutaneous manifestations of PCOS related to hyperandrogenism are hirsutism, acne and patterned hair loss. Insulin resistance is

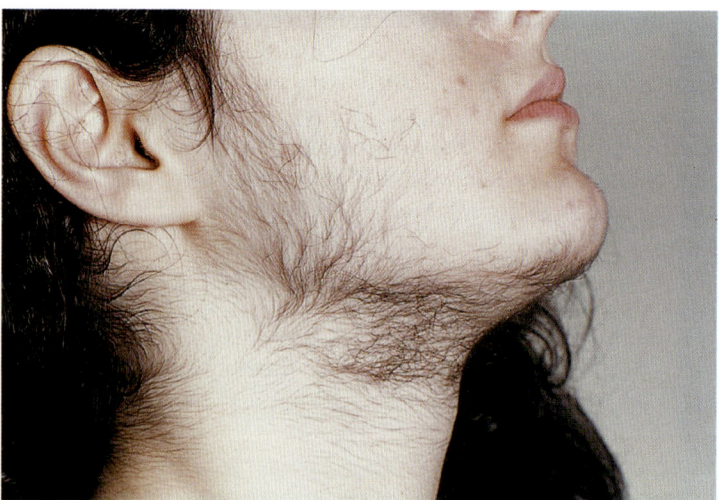

Figure 87.76 Facial hirsutism: in this case it was not associated with any systemic disease or detectable biochemical endocrine abnormality.

associated with acanthosis nigricans [10]. A study of the cutaneous features of PCOS demonstrated that over 90% of women had at least one typical skin feature. Hirsutism and acanthosis nigricans were found to be the best indicators of underlying PCOS, while acne and patterned hair loss were less reliable disease markers [12].

Ovarian hyperthecosis

Ovarian hyperthecosis is a non-neoplastic disorder usually seen in postmenopausal women and mimicks the clinical and metabolic features of PCOS. The aetiology is unknown; however, it is thought to be related to elevated postmenopausal gonadotropin levels. Women with ovarian hyperthecosis typically present with a long history of slowly progressive hyperandrogenism often resulting in virilisation. The hormonal profile is characterised by markedly increased serum testosterone levels (other androgens are normal), along with high gonadotropin levels. Severe insulin resistance and hyperinsulinaemia occur, resulting in central obesity and, in some cases, acanthosis nigricans [13].

Idiopathic hirsutism

Women with hirsutism but normal circulating androgens and normal ovulatory cycles and ovaries are described as having idiopathic hirsutism (Figure 87.76). Approximately 5–15% of all cases of hirsutism are idiopathic [3,4]. Idiopathic hyperandrogenism is defined as clinical hyperandrogenism in association with elevated androgen levels but with normal menstrual cycles and no identifiable ovarian abnormalities on ultrasound [4].

Congenital adrenal hyperplasia

Congenital adrenal hyperplasia comprises a group of rare autosomal recessive disorders due to enzyme deficiencies in steroid biosynthetic pathways. Non-classic (late-onset) congenital adrenal hyperplasia is an uncommon cause of hirsutism, occurring in approximately 5% of cases. The condition is usually due to 21-hydroxylase enzyme deficiency due to mutations in the *CYP21A2* gene. 21-Hydroxylase deficiency results in impaired conversion of 17-hydroxyprogesterone to other steroid hormones. Most females with non-classic congenital adrenal hyperplasia (80%) present between the ages of 10 and 40 years [14]. Some may remain asymptomatic with normal reproductive function [15]. However, most will present with symptoms of hyperandrogenism, clinically suggestive of PCOS [15]. Indeed, many (around 70%) will also have polycystic ovaries on ultrasound [4].

Endocrine disorders

Endocrinopathies such as Cushing syndrome, acromegaly, hyperprolactinaemia, thyroid disease and states of insulin resistance may be associated with hirsutism [1,2,13,16].

Androgen-secreting tumours

Androgen-secreting tumours are rare causes of hirsutism. The onset of symptoms is usually more rapid, and the clinical features may be more severe than with other causes of hirsutism. Virilism (clitoromegaly, deepening of the voice, increased muscle mass and male body habitus) is rare but more likely to be associated with androgen-secreting tumours [13,17]. In postmenopausal women, ovarian causes of virilisation are more common than adrenal ones. Adrenal androgen-secreting tumours tend to be diagnosed at a later stage when approximately 50% of cases are malignant [5].

Androgen-secreting ovarian tumours arise from the sex cord cells that surround oocytes, although some may originate from the stromal cells. These tumours are relatively rare and comprise 5–8% of all ovarian neoplasms. They may produce androgens and/or oestrogens. They are usually unilateral and have a low malignant potential [13]. They are subdivided further according to the cell of origin: Sertoli–Leydig cell tumours (androblastomas) (0.5%), granulosa cell tumours (2–3%; these usually produce oestrogens [18]), Sertoli cell tumours (0.1%) and hilus (Leydig) cell tumours (0.02%) [13,19].

Adrenocortical carcinoma is a rare malignancy arising from the adrenal cortex, with an annual worldwide incidence of 0.5–2 individuals per million population. In adults, the peak age of presentation is in the fourth or fifth decade. Around 60% will be sufficiently secretory to present with hormone excess. Hyperandrogenism is seen in 20–30% of affected females [20,21]. Cortisol secretion, or co-secretion of cortisol and androgens, is the most frequent pattern, with the latter highly suggestive of adrenocortical carcinoma. Patients present with a combination of virilisation and signs of hypercortisolism/Cushing syndrome [13,22]. Prognosis is generally poor with a median overall survival of approximately 4 years [20,21].

Exogenous androgens

Several drugs can result in hyperandrogenism and hirsutism including topical androgens, DHEA supplements, anabolic steroids and sodium valproate [1,13].

DISORDERS OF HAIR PIGMENTATION

HAIR GREYING (CANITIES)

The onset of hair greying is generally an unwelcome visible manifestation of the ageing process. However, many now 'embrace the grey' as a sign of life experience and maturity, while some younger women actively choose to colour their hair grey. Nonetheless, hair colouring products, including those to cover grey hair, are a multibillion-dollar market globally, suggesting greying hair remains a largely unwelcome occurrence.

The onset of hair greying tends to occur in white people by their mid-thirties, in Asians by their early forties and in those of African ancestry by their mid-forties [1]. An oft-quoted rule of thumb stated that 50% of the population aged 50 had at least 50% grey hairs [2]. However, these figures were obtained from a single ethnic population (fair-haired Australians) and additional variables have been demonstrated to be relevant in the epidemiology of hair greying [3]. A more recent study examined hair colour in healthy volunteers from a broad range of geographical and ethnic backgrounds. It was found that for those aged 45–65 years, the incidence of grey hair (defined as >5% grey hairs per hair sample) was 74%, with a mean intensity (percentage of greys) of 27%. At age 45 years, 57% already had grey hairs; however, mean intensity was low (approximately 15%). For those over 60 years, 91% had grey hair with a mean intensity of 40%. Men showed a higher incidence than women (78% M : 71% F), with greater grey intensity (29% M : 25% F). The occipital area appeared the least affected area irrespective of sex. In men, the temples showed a significantly higher incidence of greys. Both age at onset and rate of greying appeared to be linked to ethnic/geographical origin. The lowest incidences and intensities of grey hair were found in the darkest haired populations (Asian and African descent) and the highest were found in the lightest haired (white origin). Overall, a global range of 6–23% of people aged 50 years showed ≥50% grey hairs, varying with ethnic/geographical origin and natural hair colour [3]. Beard and moustache hair may grey before the onset of scalp greying, whereas eyebrows tend to grey later than scalp hair [1].

The visual impression of scalp hair greying is probably due to several factors including a reduced melanisation of pigmented hairs and the admixture of pigmented and white hairs on the scalp. Greying begins with a gradual decline in melanogenesis, including reduced tyrosinase activity, defective melanosome transfer and apoptosis of the hair follicle pigmentary unit (HFPU) melanocytes located in the anagen hair bulb [4]. Eventually, the bulge melanocyte stem cell pool becomes depleted leading to largely irreversible greying. Oxidative damage (due to intrafollicular ROS production

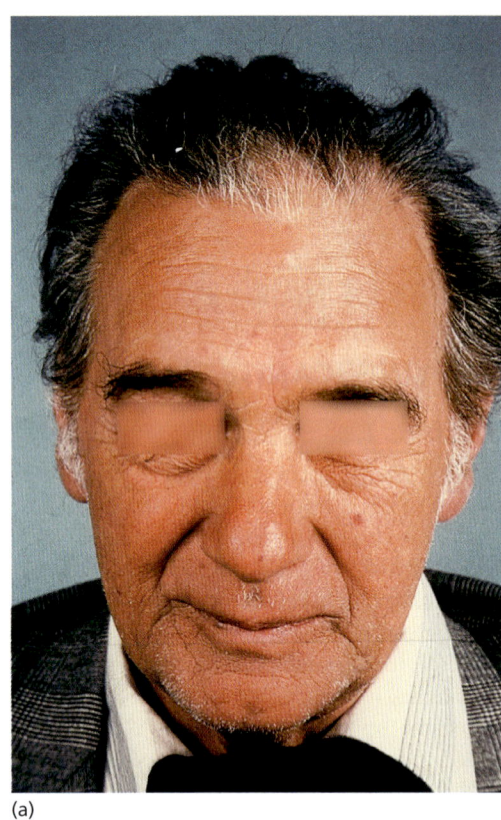

(a)

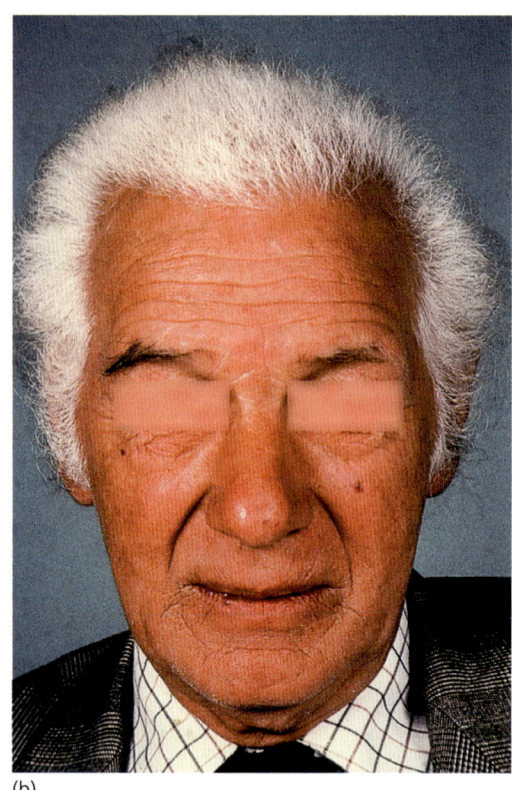

(b)

Figure 87.77 Rapid greying of the hair caused by alopecia areata. (a) A patient with slight greying of the hair, and (b) the same patient shown 1 week later. Courtesy of Dr D. Fenton, St Thomas' Hospital, London, UK.

and declining ROS scavenging and oxidative damage repair systems) is likely to be a crucial driver of the greying process, affecting HFPU melanocyte survival, melanocyte stem cell maintenance and melanogenesis [4]. While neuroendocrine factors such as α-MSH, ACTH and microphthalmia-associated transcription factor are well-known regulators of human HF melanocytes and melanogenesis, their role in greying is uncertain. A study in mice found that stress accelerated hair greying and that this effect was mediated via the sympathetic nervous system [5]. Two case reports of inhibition of human greying due to sympathectomy suggest this mechanism also operates in humans [6,7]. A recent study has demonstrated a clear link between stressful events and hair greying, with repigmentation occurring in some cases when the stress declined [8]. The role of genetics in hair greying remains poorly understood, but there are clear trends in greying onset within families and between populations, as well as greying occurring in association with genetic disorders, suggesting heritability [4]. A twin-controlled study in European females demonstrated that greying is highly heritable (90% heritability) [9]. By contrast, a study of a Latin American cohort demonstrated that hair greying had the lowest heritability of all traits studied, with greying-associated SNPs explaining only 6.7% of the observed phenotypic variation [10]. Further, the variation observed between pigmented and grey hairs on the same scalp indicates that factors additional to genetics are involved [4].

Rapid-onset 'overnight' greying of hair is a striking phenomenon of which there have been several notable historical cases including Sir Thomas More and Marie Antoinette, whose hair became grey over the night preceding their executions [11]. The probable mechanism is selective shedding of pigmented hairs in diffuse alopecia areata, with non-pigmented hairs being unaffected (Figure 87.77). In general, greying of the hair is progressive and permanent. However, repigmentation of previously depigmented hair has been reported in association with inflammatory alopecia (frontal fibrosing alopecia) [12], scalp melanoma [13–17], porphyria cutanea tarda [18], following herpes zoster infection [19] and hair transplantation [20], and due to medication including interferon, ribavirin, etretinate, thalidomide, lenalidomide, erlotinib, adalimumab, nivolumab, pembrolizumab and atezolizumab imatinib [4,21,22].

Premature greying

Hair greying is considered premature if it occurs before the age of 20 years in white people, 25 in Asians and 30 in those of African descent [1]. It may occur in association with autoimmune disease such as pernicious anaemia and hypothyroidism [23,24]. In a controlled study of 125 patients with pernicious anaemia, 11% had premature greying compared with 2% in the control group [25]. Premature greying also occurs in progeroid syndromes (rare premature ageing disorders caused by inherited defects in DNA repair pathways) such as Werner syndrome and Rothmund–Thomson syndrome. Associations with lifestyle factors such as smoking and obesity have also been suggested [26].

Poliosis

Poliosis is defined as the presence of a localised patch of white hair resulting from the absence or deficiency of melanin in a group of neighbouring follicles. Pigment absence can be congenital or acquired. In the former, it is brought about by physically or functionally abnormal melanocytes from birth, or abnormal migration during embryogenesis. Such migratory defects may be restricted to the skin, but there can be associated abnormalities in other organs such as the ear or eye, where melanocytes or related neural crest cells have an important role. Acquired forms of poliosis result from vitiligo or regrowth of non-pigmented hair following alopecia areata.

HEREDITARY DISORDERS OF HAIR PIGMENTATION

There are several hereditary pigmentary disorders that can affect hair colour. These include:
- Albinism (Chapter 68).
- Piebaldism (Chapter 68).
- Waardenburg syndrome (Chapter 68).
- Tuberous sclerosis (Chapter 78).
- 'Silver hair' syndromes (Griscelli, Elejalde and Chediak–Higashi syndromes) (Chapters 68 and 148).

ACQUIRED DISORDERS OF HAIR PIGMENTATION

In vitiligo, white patches of skin will often have white hairs within them. Scattered white hairs on the scalp may occur in children with vitiligo. In alopecia areata, regrowing hair is frequently white. This may persist although in most cases hair pigmentation recovers. Vogt–Koyanagi–Harada syndrome is a multisystem disorder characterised by ocular inflammation due to an aberrant T-cell-mediated autoimmune response directed against melanocytes [27]. The disease targets melanocyte-containing tissues in the uvea, skin, inner ear and leptomeninges, predominantly in genetically susceptible carriers of HLADRB1*04 haplotypes [28]. Viral infections and cutaneous trauma are reported as possible trigger factors [29]. Cutaneous pigmentary abnormalities are common, with poliosis (28–37%) reported in several large series of cases [30,31]. Alezzandrini syndrome presents similarly to Vogt–Koyanagi–Harada syndrome, but disease features (facial vitiligo, retinitis, hypoacusis and poliosis of the eyebrows and eyelashes) are unilateral [32,33]. Permanent loss of hair pigment may be induced by inflammatory processes that damage melanocytes (e.g. herpes zoster). X-irradiation often causes permanent hair loss, but less intense treatment leads to hypopigmented and, rarely, hyperpigmented hair.

Other causes of hair pigment changes
Drugs and chemicals
Some topical agents can temporarily change hair colour. Dithranol (anthralin) stains light-coloured or grey hair a purple/brown colour. Tar, as a topical preparation or from tobacco smoke, stains fair or white hair yellow, usually seen affecting frontal scalp hair in smokers, as well as the moustache in males [34]. Resorcin, formerly used extensively in treating skin disease, stains black or white hair a yellow-brown colour. Latanoprost (a prostaglandin analogue) and bimatoprost (a prostamide), used topically in the treatment of glaucoma, cause darkening of the iris and the eyelashes [35].

Several systemic agents are reported to cause changes in hair pigmentation. Chloroquine and hydroxychloroquine may occasionally cause hair depigmentation [36,37]. The tyrosine kinase inhibitor imatinib is reported to cause both hair repigmentation and depigmentation [37–40]. Other tyrosine kinase inhibitors (sunitinib, pazopanib dasatinib) have also been associated with hair depigmentation [37,41]. Several antiepileptics (valproic acid, phenytoin, phenobarbital) are reported to cause hair colour changes [37]. In addition to causing hypertrichosis, hair darkening is reported with ciclosporin [42]. Hair melanin may contribute to the excretion of heavy metals, chemicals and toxins from the body [1] as melanin avidly binds many inorganic elements, and hair colour changes are occasionally seen after exposure to certain substances. Exposure to high concentrates of copper in industry, or in tap or swimming pool water, may cause a green discoloration of hair, which is particularly visible in blond-haired subjects [43].

Nutritional deficiencies
Colour changes induced by nutritional deficiencies are rare. Tyrosinase is a copper-containing oxidase [44] essential to melanogenesis. In Menkes disease, an inherited defect in copper transport leads to low tissue copper levels [45], and low levels of both eumelanin and pheomelanin are reported in hair samples, with replacement therapy resulting in hair darkening [46]. Protein malnutrition, exemplified by kwashiorkor, is associated with generalised hypopigmentation of scalp hair, with dark hair initially turning reddish and evolving to a yellow/white-grey colour [47,48]. Intermittent protein malnutrition leads to the 'flag' sign of kwashiorkor (*signe de la bandera*), with alternating white (abnormal) and dark bands occurring along individual hairs [49]. Changes similar to those in kwashiorkor have been described after bowel resection such as the Whipple procedure [47] and in association with episodic malnutrition due to severe alcohol misuse [48,50].

Metabolic disorders
Metabolic disorders that may affect hair colour include:
- Phenylketonuria (Chapter 79).
- Homocystinuria (Chapter 79).
- Porphyria (Chapter 58).

Physical causes
The whiteness of hair seen when melanin is absent is an optical effect resulting from reflection and refraction of incident light from various interfaces where different refractive indexes meet. Thus, in general, non-pigmented hair with a broad medulla appears paler than non-medullated hair. Normal 'weathering' of hair along its length may lead to the terminal part appearing lighter than the rest because of a similar mechanism – the cortex and cuticle become disrupted and form numerous interfaces from internal reflection and refraction of light. This also applies in trichorrhexis nodosa, in

PART 8: SPECIFIC CUTANEOUS STRUCTURES

which patients often note a lightening in colour of the brittle hair, and in the white bands of pili annulati. Hairs on exposed parts may be bleached by sunlight.

Common treatments for hair disorders

The treatments outlined here have been successfully used in several hair loss conditions, either by directly targeting the underlying disease process or by augmenting hair growth in remaining hairs to allow better scalp coverage. For efficacy data of these agents in a specific disease, please see the appropriate treatment sections elsewhere in this chapter.

Topical minoxidil

Minoxidil was initially marketed as an oral antihypertensive agent. Serendipitous identification of increased scalp and body hair growth led to the development of topical minoxidil as a hair growth promotor, with the 2% strength lotion being licensed in 1988 in the UK and USA. Treatment is applied to the scalp one or twice a day.

Topical minoxidil is generally well tolerated. Side effects include local scalp irritation, facial hypertrichosis and headaches. Systemic absorption appears low, but dizziness and palpitations can sometimes occur. Patients should be warned about increased hair shedding in the first few weeks of treatment so that therapy is not stopped unnecessarily. This side effect settles after a few weeks, and probably heralds a successful treatment outcome. Minoxidil should be avoided during pregnancy and lactation. Minoxidil lotion contains propylene glycol to enhance solubility and HF penetration, but this can increase irritation. Minoxidil foam is propylene glycol-free and purportedly less irritating. Minoxidil should be used with caution on facial areas due to a higher risk of contact dermatitis and irritancy.

The biological effects of minoxidil include prolongation of anagen, as well as promoting new anagen growth by shortening the telogen phase and stimulating kenogen follicles to grow. If minoxidil is stopped the hair density will return to baseline within 6 months. Therefore, minoxidil treatment is generally regarded as a long-term treatment strategy [1].

The mode of action of minoxidil remains unclear, but includes (i) acting as a potent vasodilator, improving blood flow to the scalp; (ii) opening ATP-sensitive K channels that are important for cell cycle progression and cell proliferation; (iii) inducing vascular endothelial growth factor (VEGF) and hypoxia-inducible factor 1α stimulation to improve blood supply; and (iv) promoting prostaglandin synthesis (e.g. PGE2/PGE2R) which influences Wnt/β-catenin signalling in the dermal papilla [2].

Minoxidil is converted into its active metabolite minoxidil sulphate by the sulphotransferase enzyme (SULT1A1) in the follicle ORS. Importantly, this enzyme activity varies from person to person, explaining differences in the clinical response seen, with those expressing higher enzyme activity responding better than those with low levels [3]. Plucked hair sulphotransferase levels have been used experimentally to predict treatment response and inform dose selection. Importantly, aspirin/salicylate treatment can decrease sulphotransferase activity, reducing minoxidil efficacy [4].

Recently, direct application of the active ingredient minoxidil sulphate has gained popularity, although there are issues with the penetration and stability of this product.

Low-dose oral minoxidil

Oral minoxidil is increasingly being used at low doses (0.25–5 mg daily) to treat various hair loss conditions. It appears to be a convenient alternative to topical minoxidil that avoids the messy application and irritancy seen with topical therapy. These benefits have recently been highlighted as the '5 Cs of oral minoxidil': convenience, cosmesis, cost savings, co-therapy and compliance [5]. Others have added a 6th 'C' – complicated – suggesting that oral minoxidil can be an effective therapy when topical minoxidil has failed or not been tolerated [6].

Oral minoxidil is predominantly converted to minoxidil sulphate by liver and platelet sulphotransferase enzymes. Studies suggest that higher follicular accumulation may occur with the oral route, with lower SULT1A1 follicle bioactivation thresholds seen in oral compared with topical minoxidil administration [7].

The recommended starting dose for women is 0.5 mg daily, increasing every 3 months by 0.25 mg up to a maximum dose of 2.5 mg daily. For men, the starting dose is higher (as hypertrichosis is generally better tolerated in this group), beginning at 2.5 mg daily and increasing by 1.25 mg every 3 months to a maximum of 5 mg daily [8]. A similar dosing strategy that takes advantage of commercially available 2.5 mg minoxidil tablets (Loniten®, Pfizer) can be used instead, where 0.625, 1.25 and 2.5 mg dosing increments are achieved by quartering or halving the 2.5 mg tablets to obtain the required dose.

A major concern with oral minoxidil is treatment safety. However, growing experience suggests this therapy is well tolerated and side effects are predictable and dose related. A recent, large cohort study of 1404 patients found only 1.7% discontinued treatment due to side effects [9]. The main adverse events were body and facial hypertrichosis, low blood pressure symptoms (e.g. dizziness), fluid retention and tachycardia. Interestingly, reflex tachycardia occurs within the first day, blood pressure effects occur within the first week and hypertrichosis takes 3 months to manifest [9]. Routine laboratory monitoring is not generally recommended, and baseline electrocardiogram is not required at doses <5 mg/day if no significant cardiac or renal history is present [6,9]. The sublingual route of minoxidil administration is now also being explored [10].

Topical prostaglandins

Latanoprost and bimatoprost are prostaglandin F2α analogues that have been shown to stimulate eyelash growth following an observation of increased eyelash length, diameter and pigmentation with intraocular application during glaucoma treatment. Studies have since demonstrated enhanced eyelash growth effects with topical application of these agents to the upper eyelid margin in both idiopathic eyelash hypotrichosis and eyelash loss post-chemotherapy [11,12]. A cosmetic formulation of bimatoprost (Latisse®, Allergan) is now licensed by the Food and Drug Administration for eyelash hypotrichosis in the USA.

Bimatoprost 0.03% or latanoprost 0.005% ophthalmic solution can be applied to the upper eyelid margin (and eyebrows if necessary) each night using a cotton bud or brush applicator. Common side effects include irritation and hyperpigmentation of the skin. Caution is required to avoid application into the eyes as this may reduce intraocular pressure and can permanently discolour the iris. Prostaglandin F2α analogues work to promote anagen via vasodilatation and through being mitogenic [13].

Platelet-rich plasma

Platelet-rich plasma is an autologous preparation of platelets in concentrated plasma, generated by centrifugation of whole blood. PRP is commonly used in orthopaedic and dental practice, but its use has grown significantly in dermatology to improve wound healing, skin rejuvenation (the so-called 'vampire face-lift') and to promote hair growth [14]. Currently there are no standardised techniques for PRP isolation, although several commercially manufactured kits are now available, achieving platelet enrichment levels of 300–700%.

The patient's blood is taken, placed into the PRP kit and centrifuged. This separates the blood, revealing a platelet-rich layer that is drawn off before it is injected into the scalp skin. The procedure is uncomfortable, but side effects are generally only minor, including pain, swelling, bruising and headaches, with postoperative infections being exceedingly rare [14–16]. Currently, there is poor evidence to determine the optimal number of sessions or gap between sessions. However, efficacy appears to wane after >4 months following treatment, so many practitioners initially treat monthly for 3 months, followed by 3-monthly maintenance treatments.

The proposed mode of action is that activated platelets release various growth factors including VEGF, epidermal growth factor, insulin-like growth factor 1, FGF, PDGF and TGF-β that have been shown to exert hair growth-promoting properties, including decreased apoptosis, initiation of the Wnt/β-catenin pathway in the HF dermal papilla to stimulate proliferation, and increasing the vasculature and blood supply. Together they promote induction and prolongation of anagen, resulting in improved hair growth [14].

Microneedling

Microneedling, using electric pens or microrollers, causes controlled tissue injury and formation of microchannels in the skin. Optimal treatment protocols are yet to be determined, and it can be difficult to perform if the hair is long. Treatments are usually weekly to monthly and performed by rolling the device across the skin in different directions. The aim is to produce pinpoint bleeding and mild skin redness. Side effects include pain and localised infection.

The rationale for this approach is to trigger a wound healing response: releasing platelet-derived and epidermal growth factors, increasing VEGF and neovascularisation, with microchannels also potentially enhancing drug delivery through improved penetration into the skin [17].

Low-level laser light therapy

Low-level laser light therapy (LLLT) (also called cold laser or red laser) uses low-intensity red to infrared light (650–900 nm wavelength) to elicit a biological response in treated tissue called 'photobiomodulation' [18].

LLLT has been used in wound healing, nerve regeneration and pain reduction, but is increasingly being utilised in hair regeneration [18–20]. The mode of action is unknown but appears to incite photochemical reactions at a cellular level inducing transcription factors, activating various cell-signalling pathways, increasing mitochondrial energy production, promoting cell proliferation and reducing inflammation. In scalp therapy, LLLT promotes and prolongs anagen, manifesting as increased hair diameter and density [20].

Various devices are available including hoods, caps or combs, with the choice of device predominantly dependent on cost and lifestyle. A treatment duration of 15–30 minutes 3–4 times a week is recommended for mild to moderate hair loss as a longer-term treatment strategy. Side effects appear rare, but include scalp discomfort, urticaria, acne, skin dryness and risk of eye damage [18].

Autologous stem cell therapies

An area of great interest now is the use of adipose-derived stem cells for hair rejuvenation. Abdominal fat is removed under local anaesthetic, cleaned, degraded with enzymes and centrifuged, producing a stem-cell rich isolate. This isolate is then injected into the scalp under local anaesthetic. The treatment is expensive and unsubstantiated claims that this is a permanent solution should be viewed with caution until longer-term data are available [21]. The main side effects are bruising and oedema.

Hormone contraceptive pills

Combined oral contraceptive pills prevent pregnancy through the suppression of gonadotrophins and the inhibition of ovulation, whereas the progesterone-only pill (POP) works by increasing uterine mucus to prevent conception. The concern in various hormone-sensitive conditions, such as AGA and hirsutism, is that the different progestogens in the combined OCP or POP may exacerbate the already heightened androgenic susceptibility, thereby worsening the problem.

Some pills have reduced androgenic properties as the progestogen they contain does not oppose oestrogen induction of SHBG. This increased SHBG response reduces circulation of the active free hormone, resulting in a lower biological effect. Further, some progestogens have antiandrogen properties due to direct blockage of the androgen receptor. Although some pills may have more androgenic potential than others (i.e. a higher 'androgen index') it is probable that most combined OCPs have a net antiandrogen effect due to the oestrogen component (Table 87.10) [22,23].

Antiandrogens

Antiandrogens are frequently used off-licence to treat various hormone-dependent hair conditions such as AGA and hirsutism. Caution is required when used in premenopausal women as all agents have the potential to feminise a male fetus, so women should not become pregnant while taking them. Further, whether some of these agents increase the risk of breast or ovarian cancer is still unclear, so assessment of other cancer risk factors (e.g. family history) should be undertaken before prescribing.

Spironolactone

Spironolactone is a potassium-sparing diuretic and antihypertensive commonly used to treat oedema and ascites. It is also the most

PART 8: SPECIFIC CUTANEOUS STRUCTURES

Table 87.10 Combined oral contraceptive pill androgen index

Antiandrogen progestogens	Lower androgenic progestogens	Moderate to high androgenic progestogens
Dienogest (e.g. Qlaira®)	Drospirenone (e.g. Yasmin®)	Norethisterone (norethindrone) (e.g. Loestrin®, Brevinor®)
Cyproterone acetate (e.g. Dianette®)	Desogestrel (e.g. Gadarel®, Mercilon®, Marvelon®)	Levonorgestrel/norgestrel (e.g. Microgynon®, Levest®, Ovranette®, Rigevidon®)
Normogestrol (e.g. Zoely®)	Gestodene (e.g. Femodene®, Katya®, Millinette®)	
	Norgestimate (e.g. Cilest®)	

familiar and widely used antiandrogen in dermatology practice. Structurally related to aldosterone, spironolactone competitively binds to the androgen receptor on the HF, preventing androgen signalling as well as weakly inhibiting androgen biosynthesis.

Side effects are dose related and included menstrual irregularities, postmenopausal bleeding, breast tenderness and fatigue. The antialdosterone effect may result in an elevation of serum potassium and a slight reduction in blood pressure, although this is rarely significant in the absence of renal impairment. Therefore, regular assessment of renal function is generally not required in those <50 years with normal renal function [22,23]. A large cohort study involving almost 1.3 million women aged ≥55 years with a follow-up time of 8.4 million patient-years found no evidence of an increased incidence of breast cancer in those exposed to spironolactone [24].

Cyproterone acetate

Cyproterone acetate is a synthetic progestogen that blocks the androgen receptor, inhibits gonadotrophin secretion and suppresses activity of cutaneous 5α-reductase with longer-term use [25]. Various dosing regimens are proposed. In premenopausal women 50–100 mg/day for the first 10 days of each menstrual cycle is commonly used, whereas for postmenopausal women cyproterone acetate may be used continuously (e.g. 50 mg daily). The combination of cyproterone acetate and oral oestrogen therapy provides effective contraception and stabilises menstrual irregularities. Side effects are dose dependent and include weight gain, fatigue, loss of libido, breast tenderness, nausea, headaches and depression. Further, a strong dose effect has been reported between cyproterone acetate use and increased risk of intracranial meningioma, particularly affecting the middle skull base [26].

Flutamide and bicalutamide

Flutamide and bicalutamide are non-steroidal pure antiandrogens that act by inhibiting androgen binding. Flutamide has no antigonadotrophic effect (as binding to the central androgen receptor prevents negative feedback), so measurable serum androgen levels can go up with this treatment (note that bicalutamide does not cross the blood–brain barrier so this is not an issue). Rare, but potentially fatal, hepatotoxicity is seen with high-dose flutamide, limiting the use of this agent [27]. Recently bicalutamide has grown in popularity and appears to have a good safety profile [28,29], with doses of 25–50 mg daily generally being used. Regular monitoring of liver function is recommended throughout treatment.

5α-Reductase inhibitors

5α-Reductase inhibitors block the conversion of testosterone to DHT by potent and selective antagonism of the enzyme 5α-reductase. Although generally well tolerated, there is reasonable evidence that 5α-reductase inhibitors are associated with increased levels of depression, type 2 diabetes and gynaecomastia [30–33]. Suicide and erectile dysfunction are less clearly associated, with variable risks potentially dependent on age and treatment indication [34]. Recent data suggest that exposure to finasteride is not associated with increased breast cancer rates in men [35], although the risk in women is unknown.

Finasteride. Finasteride is a synthetic aza-steroid that inhibits 5α-reductase type 2. Finasteride 1 mg daily (Propecia®) is licensed to treat male pattern hair loss in adults. This oral dosage of 1 mg/day reduces scalp DHT by 64% and serum DHT by 68% [36]. Finasteride reduces serum prostate-specific antigen (PSA) levels by 50%; therefore, when PSA is checked the measured value should be doubled to correct for this finasteride effect. Finasteride has no effect on spermatogenesis or semen production [37], and no additional precautions are required to prevent exposure of finasteride in semen to female sexual partners.

Dutasteride. Dutasteride is a dual type 1 and 2 5α-reductase inhibitor. It produces a dose-dependent reduction in serum and scalp DHT levels with greater potency than finasteride. The usual dose of dutasteride is 0.5 mg daily, although lower-dose regimens (e.g. 0.5 mg weekly) have been advocated in some conditions [38]. Sexual side effects appear more common with dutasteride than finasteride, and are dose related. Because of the longer biological half-life, side effects may take many months to reverse.

Post-finasteride syndrome

Post-finasteride syndrome (PFS) is a collective term for an array of symptoms related to finasteride treatment that persist or develop despite cessation of therapy. Symptoms are broadly grouped into sexual side effects (e.g. loss of libido, erectile dysfunction, genital numbness, ejaculation problems), psychological complaints (e.g. suicidal thoughts, anxiety and depression, irritability, sleep problems), cognitive issues (e.g. poor concentration and memory, loss of confidence) and physical problems (e.g. muscle cramps, fatigue, gynaecomastia, dry skin) [39,40]. Accumulating postmarketing reports prompted changes to product labelling, and forums such as the Post-Finasteride Syndrome foundation (https://www.pfsfoundation.org; last accessed May 2023) have been set up to highlight this issue.

We know that 5α-reductase inhibitor therapy can have wide biological effects, including reduced synthesis of brain neurosteroids (important for mood, cognition and libido), and that impaired testosterone synthesis can increase oestrogen levels and reduce DHT effects on target tissue [40], although these revert to normal on stopping therapy. Therefore, it is currently unclear whether the spectrum of symptoms represented by the term PFS is truly related to previous finasteride therapy, as data in this area are generally of poor quality and are often uncontrolled and prone to bias [40,41]. Further, nocebo effects with finasteride are well documented [42]. Interestingly, studies of 5α-reductase inhibitor use in women only identify extremely low prevalence of side effects, with none persisting on stopping therapy, suggesting that at present PFS is solely a condition described in men [43].

Clinicians should be aware of PFS. It is recommended when initiating 5α-reductase inhibitor therapy to identify pre-existing depression or sexual dysfunction, as these patients may be at increased risk of developing persistent symptoms [44]. All patients should be counselled about the risk of sexual, physical or emotional side effects during treatment, and be warned that these side effects may persist in some people after stopping therapy. However, the cause of these ongoing symptoms, at present, remains unclear [40].

Surgery

Hair transplantation (or hair restoration) surgery has become a mainstream procedure for the treatment of male and female pattern hair loss, as well as some selected scarring alopecias [45]. The technique can not only restore hair on the scalp but can also be used to treat eyebrows and beard alopecia. The basic principle is redistribution of terminal hairs to cover affected areas. Generally, hair from the occipital scalp (termed the 'safe donor area') is used as these follicles are naturally resistant to hair miniaturisation in AGA. Hair is removed either by harvesting a strip of hair-bearing skin (strip technique) or by removing multiple individual follicular units (follicular unit extraction). Hairs are dissected into individual units and then transplanted into the area of alopecia. Up to 5000 follicular units may be transplanted in a single session. Hairs from transplanted follicles are usually shed following transplantation before new hairs appear after 3–4 months. It can take 6–12 months for the full results of a transplant to be seen. The advice of an experienced hair transplant surgeon is essential as some patients will not be suitable for this type of approach [46].

Patient selection is vital for a successful outcome. Important factors to consider include:

- Is there an adequate donor area? This is usually the safe donor area on the occipital scalp, but beard or body hair can sometimes be used (e.g. in scarring alopecia from burns) [47].
- How old is the patient? Surgery is not usually performed on people aged <25 years as it is difficult to predict hair loss progression at this age, and risks misplaced hairlines or an unnatural appearance years later as balding progresses.
- What sites are affected? Surgery for frontal hair loss is more effective than vertex balding, which tends to progress with time.
- Is the underlying process progressive? In pattern hair loss, the continuation of medical therapy is advised to preserve surviving native hairs. Unlike AGA where donor hairs are relatively resistant to hair miniaturisation (called 'donor dominance'), transplanted hair in PCA is not immune to the disease process, resulting in a progressive loss of the transplanted grafts over time [45,48].

Comparison of the advantages and disadvantages of strip versus follicular unit extraction is shown in Table 87.11 [49]. Complications

Table 87.11 Strip versus follicular unit extraction (FUE) hair transplantation

Strip method	FUE
Benefits	*Benefits*
Largest number of grafts per session	Less visible scarring (so able to maintain short hairstyles)
No head shaving	Used for beard/body donations
	Used in those not suitable for the strip method (e.g. poor scalp laxity)
	Allows harvesting of finer hairs (better for cosmetically sensitive areas, e.g. frontal hairline)
	Less pain and downtime post-procedure
Disadvantages	*Disadvantages*
Linear scar occipital scalp	Smaller number of grafts per session
Higher risk of postoperative wound issues	Higher graft transection rate
	Shaved donor area

of hair transplantation are as in any surgical procedure, including wound infection, bleeding and facial swelling. For both techniques, postoperative 'shock loss' (i.e. anagen effluvium) may occur post-procedure.

Small to medium-sized patches of stable permanent alopecia may be surgically excised, with or without scalp expanders or flap techniques.

Hair cosmetics and alopecia camouflage

For thousands of years, hair has been celebrated as the 'crowning glory' of human beauty and people have sought to enhance it by a variety of means [1]. Hair as a means of seduction is recorded in ancient Egyptian papyrus. The ancient Greeks and Romans considered hair to contain the essence of life and its presence represented power, with forced cutting seen as a means of emasculation or punishment. Therefore, throughout human history, beautiful hair has been considered highly prized and worthy of lavish attention [2].

The positive effects of attractive hair should not be underestimated, nor should the often profoundly negative effects of alopecia. Although washing and application of treatments to hair are not biologically necessary, most people consider hair care, at the very least, part of a normal cleansing regimen. More often, it is an essential component of enhancing personal appearance and well-being. There are now many different categories of hair products for every type of hair and cosmetic requirement, supporting a multibillion-pound cosmetic industry. As a result, commercial interests have driven many aspects of basic and clinical hair research.

Unfortunately, complete hair regrowth is not an achievable outcome for many patients with alopecia and therefore cosmetic camouflage is an important part of management. There are many camouflage options such that, in most cases, alopecia can be completely concealed, if this is what the patient wishes. Patient support groups and alopecia charities are often an excellent source of practical advice for patients (e.g. Alopecia UK: www.alopecia.org.uk; last accessed May 2023). In some instances, a change of colour or hairstyle can have significant positive cosmetic impact and the advice of an experienced hair stylist can be invaluable.

PART 8: SPECIFIC CUTANEOUS STRUCTURES

Shampoos

Shampoo is primarily a cleansing agent to remove excess sebum, sweat, environmental contaminants and styling products from a large surface area of hair (on average 4–8 m^2) [3–5]. The main active ingredient is a detergent, but many other components are necessary to ensure products not only cleanse hair but leave it pleasantly enhanced and conditioned. Patients with alopecia frequently ask how often they should wash their hair and the answer is generally as often as they need or wish to do so. Hair washing does not affect the course of alopecia, although any hairs at the end of the telogen phase of the hair cycle will be dislodged by the process, as they are with brushing and combing. However, as increased hair shedding is often most noticeable during hair washing, some patients assume that washing is the cause of the increased loss and as a result wash their hair less frequently. Delaying hair washing results in proportionately more telogen hairs being dislodged when the hair is washed, and patients can become locked in a distressing cycle of infrequent washing and apparently increased hair shedding.

Shampoo formulations

Shampoo is essentially an aqueous solution of detergent. Detergents are amphiphilic surfactants – that is, they possess both lipid (lipophilic) and water (hydrophilic) binding sites. Lipophilic sites bind to sebum while hydrophilic sites bind to water, allowing sebum to be rinsed away. There are five categories of shampoo detergents – anionic, cationic, amphoteric, non-ionic and natural surfactants (saponins) – and within each category there are several different chemical compounds. Each has differing cleansing and conditioning characteristics and modern shampoos often contain a combination of several different detergents. In addition to detergent, other typical components of shampoo include:

- Foaming agents: these create suds (not required for cleansing action but help spread shampoo over the hair).
- Conditioners: these are required to counteract the adverse effect of detergents on the hair shaft, particularly in shampoos for dry, damaged or coloured hair or those designed for daily use.
- Shampoo thickeners, opacifiers and pearlescents: a thick shampoo formulation is seen as more desirable and opacifiers add a pleasing pearly shine to the preparation.
- Stabilising agents: sequestering agents chelate calcium and magnesium ions prevent the formation of insoluble precipitates in hard water. Preservatives, pH buffers and UV filters may also be added.
- Perfume and colour: these are added to enhance product aesthetics.
- Active ingredients: these may have a medical purpose (e.g. tar, zinc pyrithione) or cosmetic benefits (e.g. panthenol, which enhances hair moisture content, or hydrolysed protein, which binds to damaged cortex).

There are many different types of shampoo, designed for different purposes (for dry hair, oily hair, daily use, etc.). Dry shampoos are becoming increasingly popular; they do not contain a detergent but rather a lipid-absorbing powder. Advantages include speed and ease of use, a reduced need for heat to dry/style and the addition of volume, texture and, in many preparations, colour.

Shampoo safety

Frequently used preparations such as shampoo must be non-toxic and must not irritate either the skin or eyes at concentrations used by the consumer. Shampoo formulations are extensively tested prior to marketing, particularly to assess eye irritancy. Skin irritation is not usually encountered from shampoos that have low eye irritancy potential. As detergents, all shampoos are potential irritants, but due to the short period of contact with skin during hair washing they rarely cause significant problems. However, allergic contact dermatitis may occur because of components such as fragrances and preservatives.

Conditioners

Dry hair appears dull, feels brittle, tends to tangle and is difficult to style [6–8]. It results from natural weathering and is worsened by the chemical agents (shampoo detergents, bleach, dyes, chemical relaxers) and excessive physical trauma (brushing, curling, heat application) that hair undergoes. Conditioners were introduced following the availability of shampoos with good detergent action, which remove excessive amounts of sebum from the hair shaft. Their purpose is to restore manageability, glossiness and softness normally provided by sebum. In addition, some constituents contribute to a reduction in static electricity, normalisation of hair pH, protection from UV radiation and possibly increased hair strength.

There are several constituents of hair conditioning products. Organic acids restore hair and scalp pH to a mildly acidic pH (around pH 5). Fatty compounds mimic the natural components of sebum and hair, and comprise fatty acids, alcohols and esters; natural triglycerides (e.g. almond, avocado, olive oils); waxes (e.g. beeswax, jojoba oil, lanolin); phospholipids (e.g. egg yolk, soya bean); and ceramides. Vitamins may be added, particularly D-pathenol, a precursor of vitamin B$_5$ and a normal constituent of hair, which has humectant properties and penetrates the hair shaft making it more manageable. Protein hydrolysates (e.g. from silk, collagen, keratins, gelatine and other proteins) bind to hair keratin, temporarily repairing damaged hair shafts and mildly improving hair strength. When hairs are coated with protein hydrolysates they have a temporary thickening effect, resulting in an improved cosmetic appearance. Cationic detergents (quaternaries or quaternary ammonium compounds) are effective in increasing adherence of the cuticular scales to the hair shaft, increasing the light-reflective properties of hair and improving shine and lustre. These positively charged compounds also neutralise static on negatively charged hairs, increasing manageability. Silicone derivatives spread over and coat hairs, adding shine, softness and manageability without making hair greasy. Cationic polymers (e.g. cationic polysaccharides, polyvinylpyrrolidones) form films over the hair shaft, temporarily filling hair shaft defects and thickening hairs to improve body, texture and shine. Their positive charge also neutralises static to improve manageability.

Conditioning products are available in a variety of forms and are widely used. They provide manageability and lustre to the hair and facilitate hair styling. Most commonly, short contact (instant) preparations are applied after shampooing and quickly rinsed off. They can also be combined with a shampoo in a 2-in-1 preparation. Deep conditioners are often thicker, more concentrated preparations which are applied to damp hair and left on for up to 30 minutes under a warm towel or cap. Some conditioners are designed to be leave-on, to assist hair styling, and these often contain film-forming cationic polymers such as polyvinylpyrrolidone. When hair is significantly prone to dryness or damage, conditioner may be used as a shampoo substitute ('co-washing'), much as a soap substitute is used for cleansing dry skin. The conditioner will mix with water to remove surface dirt and odour but will not subject the hair and scalp to the detergent effects of shampoo.

A recent trend is the use of products that are considered natural. This often includes oils or butters such as coconut, tea tree, argan, jojoba, shea butter and others. These products may impart shine to the hair shaft but may be comedogenic and cause scalp and facial irritation. There is little evidence that these kinds of products improve the overall strength of the hair shaft [9].

Temporary hair styling

Hair keratins are elastic, allowing hair to be stretched and shaped temporarily. Hair styling requires wet hair to be stretched and dried under tension (usually using a brush and hairdryer), resulting in a shaped style which holds when dry due to the formation of new ionic and hydrogen bonds [5,10]. The style will last only until the hair is washed again and factors such as atmospheric humidity can reduce the effect of styling. A wide range of products are available to prolong the hold of a hairstyle. These may be applied to wet hair before styling or to dry styled hair to maintain the shape. Products can have several physical properties (solidity, resistance, stickiness, hair-coating ability, hair finishing qualities) depending on the role for which the product is designed. For example, gels are intended to coat short hair, whereas foams are applied close to the scalp to add hold and volume at the root while leaving minimal residue on hair, and waxes are applied to only small areas of hair. The components of styling products include polymers to provide hold, polymer vehicles, thickeners for product texture, lubricants and conditioning agents for ease of styling and hair finishing, as well as perfumes, preservatives and colouring agents.

Permanent hair styling

Keratins in the hair cortex are linked by disulphide bonds that result in the physical and chemical stability of the keratin protein. To change the shape of a hair permanently, a proportion of these bonds must be broken and reformed. It should be noted that these processes expose hair to chemicals capable of causing severe damage not only to the hair but to the skin. Ideally, they should only be used by those experienced in their safe application.

Permanent waving ('perming') [7,10,11]

The process of permanent waving involves sections of hair being rolled onto curlers then a waving (reducing) lotion applied. The reducing agent (usually a thioglycolate) cleaves some of the disulphide bonds between keratin filaments, allowing hair reshaping. The pH of waving lotions is around pH 9 (achieved using alkalis such as ammonia), which allows the solution to penetrate the cuticle and reach the cortical keratin filaments. The hair's new shape is determined by the tightness of the curl around the curlers. This is then fixed by an (oxidising) neutralising solution, usually based on hydrogen peroxide, which reforms the disulphide bonds between keratin filaments.

Permanent straightening ('relaxing') [7,11–13]

Chemical straightening of hair (relaxing) is essentially identical to permanent waving except curly hair is permanently straightened. Disulphide bonds are cleaved using an alkaline reducing agent (relaxer) and the hair is mechanically straightened using a comb, to restructure the position of the disulphide bonds. The new bonds are then fixed using an oxidising agent. Generally, chemical relaxers are applied to new growth of the hair shaft near the scalp every 6–8 weeks. Relaxers can be lye or no-lye. Lye relaxers include sodium hydroxide and potassium hydroxide and are highly alkaline (pH 13–14). They can be subdivided into base (stronger, faster preparations that require a protective coating on the scalp) or no-base (weaker preparations that do not require scalp protection). No-lye relaxers are typically guanidine hydroxide (usually mixed with calcium hydroxide) or lithium hydroxide (no-mix). No-lye relaxers are less irritating but can leave mineral deposits on the hair, making it dry and brittle. More old-fashioned methods of hair straightening include hot combing (thermal straightening) whereby the hair is coated with petroleum jelly or liquid paraffin (which act as a heat-transferring agent), then a heated metal comb pulls the hair straight, causing the breakage and reforming of disulphide bonds. Chemical relaxing was previously very prevalent among African American women, with an estimated 80% using chemical relaxers 20 years ago. However, in the last decade, an increasing number are embracing a natural (chemically untreated) hairstyle.

Hair colouring

The desire to change one's hair colour is not a modern phenomenon. Records of the use of henna as a hair colouring date back to the ancient Egyptians and their contemporaries in India and Persia. The Romans used a variety of vegetable dyes to colour hair and eyebrows, and bleached blond hair was a particular Roman fashion [14]. Hair dyes can be classified as temporary, semipermanent and permanent. The penetration of dyes into the hair depends on molecular size and the aqueous swelling of the hair at the time of application of the dye; basicity of the dye is also important. The most successful dyes are relatively small molecules [15]. Given the widespread regular use of hair dyes by a significant proportion of the population (an estimated 50–80% of adult women and 10% of men >40 years old use hair dyes at some time in their life) [16,17], safety of preparations is paramount. The most common adverse effect of hair dye is allergic contact dermatitis, usually to *p*-phenylenediamine (PPD). An estimated 1.5% of the European population may be allergic to PPD, increasing to 4–6% of the patch-tested population in Europe and North America [18]. There have also been concerns that hair dyes may predispose to cancers. The International Agency for Research on Cancer classified occupational exposure to hair dyes as probably carcinogenic to humans, whereas personal use of hair dyes was not classifiable, as evidence from epidemiological studies has proved inconclusive [17]. A recent study of more than 100 000 US women found that those who had ever used permanent hair dyes had no significant increased risk of solid cancers, including bladder cancer, melanoma, hormone receptor-positive breast cancer and most of the major subclasses of haematopoietic cancer. However, basal cell carcinoma risk was slightly increased for users and higher cumulative hair dye exposure was positively associated with risk of hormone receptor-negative breast cancer and ovarian cancer. An increased risk of Hodgkin lymphoma was observed only for women with naturally dark hair, and a higher risk of basal cell carcinoma was observed for women with naturally light hair [17]. Genetic susceptibility from functional polymorphisms in genes such as those involved in arylamine activation or detoxification may modify the risk for individuals [16].

Excluding bleach, hair colourants can be classified as non-oxidation or oxidation dyes. Non-oxidation dyes include temporary colourants (effects last several days) and semipermanent (direct) colourants (fade slowly with shampooing). Plant-based (vegetable) dyes and metallic salts are non-oxidation dyes. Oxidation dyes provide permanent hair colouring and are generally aromatic ring derivatives belonging to three major chemical families: the diamines (includes PPD), aminophenols and phenols/naphthols [19].

Plant-based (vegetable) dyes [14]

Henna (also called red henna) has been used to colour hair and skin for thousands of years. It is derived from the dried crushed leaves of the shrub *Lawsonia inermis* which are mixed with water to form a paste that is applied to the hair. It produces a reddish brown colour in dark hair but turns white/blond hair orange. Red henna appears to be generally safe, with rare instances of contact allergy and type I hypersensitivity reactions [20]. However, children with glucose-6-phosphate dehydrogenase deficiency may develop life-threatening haemolysis after topical application of henna [20]. Black henna (a combination of red henna and PPD) is used for temporary tattoos and carries a risk of contact sensitisation [20]. Henna may be mixed with indigo powder (from the *Indigofera* plant genus) to give hair colours from chestnut to black. The flower heads of German or Roman chamomile contain a yellow dye (apigenin) that can tint hair. Crushed flower heads can be added to hot water to create a hair rinse or made into a paste to apply to hair. Other plant-based colourants can be derived from bark, wood, leaves and flowers (e.g. walnut shells), but are now rarely used.

Metallic dyes [14]

Regular application of dyes containing metallic salts (lead or silver) results in progressive hair colouring (darkening), particularly of grey hairs. Products are generally sold for at-home use by men. They tend to result in a dull leaden colour with a flat metallic appearance. They can damage the hair shaft and the colour cannot be removed.

Temporary colourants [14]

Temporary hair colourants can be considered as make-up for hair. Their effects last at most until the hair is washed. Dyes in this category include azo derivatives, triphenylmethane basic dyes (e.g. methyl violet), 'azine' derivatives (e.g. safranine) and indoamines/indophenols. Weak concentrations of semipermanent dyes such as anthraquinone derivatives may sometimes be used as temporary colourants. Preparations containing temporary colourants include shampoos, conditioners, rinses, mousses, coloured hair sprays and hair mascaras.

Semipermanent (direct) colourants [14]

Semipermanent dyes produce a change in hair colour that fades gradually with repeated shampooing. Colour should normally fade completely after 6 washes, but some dyes will persist for up to 12 washes. The dyes are intrinsically coloured small molecules that penetrate the hair cortex and are normally applied to natural non-bleached hair. They are used to add shades and tones to natural hair colour, and dye white hair a natural shade while minimising yellow discoloration. Semipermanent dyes include:

- 'Nitro' dyes (aromatic amines, aminophenols, nitrophenols).
- Solvent-assisted dyes (e.g. disperse dyes).
- Anion–cation complexes (e.g. azo acid dyes, anthroquinone acid dyes).
- Self-oxidising dyes (e.g. trihydroxybenzene derivatives).
- Cationic/basic dyes (e.g. basic red).
- Reactive dyes (e.g. dichlorotriazinyl group).

Permanent colourants [7,19]

Permanent hair colourants are the most used type of hair dye. The colour cannot be removed and new growth at the hair roots needs to be coloured approximately every 6 weeks. Permanent dyes can colour hair in an infinite variety of shades, including greys. The formulation of hair dye products to achieve reproducible, safe and permanent hair colour is a complex process. The most used agents are PPDs and aminophenols. These dyes are in fact colourless (primary) intermediates or bases. When oxidised by hydrogen peroxide, they produce small molecular compounds (quinone monoimine or quinone diimine) which can penetrate the hair cortex. Couplers (or modifiers) such as *m*-diamines, *m*-aminophenols or polyphenols then react with these products of oxidation to form permanent hair colourants. Permanent colouring is performed at an alkaline pH (pH 9–10) to allow penetration through the hair cuticle, and ammonia is commonly used as a pH adjusting agent. Permanent dye preparations also contain other agents including vehicles, surfactants, solvents, thickeners, antioxidants and metal chelating agents. A conditioner is often added to reduce hair damage.

The chemicals used in permanent hair dyeing are potentially hazardous. Hydrogen peroxide can cause structural damage to hair. Other components of hair dye preparations are potential irritants. The main concern is the potential for PPD (and to a lesser extent *p*-toluenediamine) to cause allergic contact dermatitis. In the UK, hairdressers are legally required to undertake patch tests for hair dye allergy prior to application, under Section 3 of the Health and Safety at Work Act (1974). All hair dyes in this group are sold to the public with instructions to carry out a standardised open patch test (allergy alert test) 48 hours before the product is used. The allergy alert test has been demonstrated to identify PPD allergy in >90% of allergic individuals [21]. Any redness, swelling or blistering implies allergy, and the product should not be used. If allergy to hair dye is confirmed, no PPD-containing dyes can be used and agents where cross-sensitisation is reported (e.g. sulphonamides, some local anaesthetics such as benzocaine and procaine) should also be avoided [18]. A negative patch test does not mean that subsequent allergy cannot occur but rather indicates that the subject is not allergic at the time of testing.

Hair bleaching [7,22]

Bleaching can be undertaken either to lighten hair colour or to prepare it to take up hair dyes. Hair lightening is achieved by oxidising melanin, and brown hair is easier to bleach than red hair. Bleaching can be highly damaging to the hair, causing dryness and fragility.

Bleaching solutions of hydrogen peroxide are usually 3%, 6% or 9% (10, 20 or 30 volume) and are mixed with ammonia to speed the reaction. The bleaching is terminated by shampooing with an acid pH product or acid rinse. The degree of bleaching will vary with contact time. Some degree of hair bleaching can occur with prolonged sun exposure.

Prosthetics

Wigs [23]

In most cases, NHS prescriptions for wigs can be issued by NHS dermatologists, but this is not true for every area of the UK [24]. Although there is a huge range of different wig styles available, there are essentially two types of wigs – synthetic or human hair ('real'). Each has its advantages and disadvantages, and careful thought should be given to the various pros and cons before obtaining a wig. Human hair wigs look natural and can be cut and styled. They are usually more expensive than synthetic wigs and last for around 1 year, with careful maintenance. Synthetic wigs are prestyled, easier to maintain and less expensive than real wigs, but are damaged by heat and have a shorter lifespan (3–6 months). Some wigs are designed specifically for complete hair loss (e.g. Supplex and Dermalite wigs). Vacuum wigs were also designed for complete hair loss; however, the remaining hair can be kept shaved to achieve the same result. Wig technology is constantly evolving, with newer types of wigs, include heat resistant synthetic wigs (which can be heat styled) and blended (real and synthetic hair) wigs, being developed. Patients are often concerned that wigs will fall off or be blown off by the wind. Therefore, it is best that wigs are fitted by a specialist wig salon. Most wigs have adjustable straps to ensure a close fit. Additional security can be obtained from the use of tapes, glues and clips. There are a variety of wig caps (bases) available (e.g. wefted, hand-tied, net, lace front; monofilament or silicone for suction wigs), each with different features. Full wigs are often not required when the area of alopecia is small and partial wigs may be more appropriate.

Hair systems (mesh integration/Intralace systems™)

Hair systems are essentially partial wigs that integrate the patient's own remaining hair and are fixed in place on the scalp. They are expensive and require regular maintenance. Although they can give an excellent cosmetic effect, they do not suit every individual.

Extensions and clip-ins

Hair extensions are extremely popular, adding length and increased volume to hairstyles. They are often of limited benefit to those with alopecia on the top of the scalp as they provide no scalp coverage in this area. Hair is added either by wefted panels or by individual attachment of multiple smaller groups of hairs. Attachment is achieved by a variety of methods including tapes, glues and beads, and this is usually done in a specialist salon, although clip-in extensions can be easily attached and removed by the person themselves.

Camouflage products

There is an extensive range of products that can be used to camouflage the scalp. Some are marketed specifically for use in alopecia (e.g. coloured fibres and sprays), while many others are intended for purposes such as coverage of grey roots or for use as dry shampoos. These can be remarkably helpful products for patients with small areas of alopecia or hair thinning. Make-up such as eyebrow pencils, eyeshadows, eyeliners and false lashes is helpful in camouflaging partial or complete loss of eyebrows and lashes.

Tattooing

Cosmetic tattooing (also called permanent make-up) can provide a more permanent solution to the loss of eyebrows and lashes, and the technique of microblading can produce the visual effect of eyebrow hairs. Tattoos often last 2–3 years but topping up the pigment every 18 months can optimise the appearance. Scalp tattooing or micropigmentation is a useful camouflage technique, particularly for men with short dark hair, and it can provide useful scalp coverage in women with thinning such as due to FPHL. The pigmentation does fade, and the procedure needs to be repeated every few years.

Acknowledgement

We would like to thank the previous authors (Dr Paul Farrant, Dr David de Berker and Professor Rodney Sinclair) for their contributions to this chapter and the images they supplied.

Key references

The full list of references can be found in the online version at https://www.wiley.com/rooksdermatology10e

Hair biology
105 O'Sullivan JDB, Nicu C, Picard M *et al.* The biology of human hair greying. *Biol Rev Camb Philos Soc* 2021;96:107–128.

Hair loss presentations
Alopecia areata
70 Petukhova L, Duvic M, Hordinsky M *et al.* Genome-wide association study in alopecia areata implicates both innate and adaptive immunity. *Nature* 2010;466:113–17.
103 Messenger AG, McKillop J, Farrant P, McDonagh AJ, Sladden M. British Association of Dermatologists' guidelines for the management of alopecia areata 2012. *Br J Dermatol* 2012;166:916–26.

Scarring alopecias
1 Olsen EA, Bergfeld WF, Cotsarelis G *et al.* Summary of North American Hair Research Society (NAHRS)-sponsored Workshop on Cicatricial Alopecia, Duke University Medical Center, February 10 and 11, 2001. *J Am Acad Dermatol* 2003;48:103–10.
13 Harries MJ, Jimenez F, Izeta A *et al.* Lichen planopilaris and frontal fibrosing alopecia as model epithelial stem cell diseases. *Trends Mol Med* 2018;24:435–48.

Hair loss associated with increased hair fall
Telogen effluvium
5 Headington JT. Telogen effluvium. New concepts and review. *Arch Dermatol* 1993;129:356–63.

Androgenetic alopecia and pattern hair loss
49 Van Zuuren EJ, Fedorowicz Z, Schoones J. Interventions for female pattern hair loss. *Cochrane Database Syst Rev* 2016;Issue 5:CD007628.

Hair loss associated with cancer treatment

1 Freites-Martinez A, Shapiro J, Goldfarb S *et al.* Hair disorders in patients with cancer. *J Am Acad Dermatol* 2019;80:1179–96.

Abnormalities of the hair shaft

1 Whiting DA, Dy LC. Office diagnosis of hair shaft defects. *Semin Cutan Med Surg* 2006;25:24–34.

Excessive hair growth
Hirsutism

1 Martin KA, Anderson RR, Chang RJ *et al.* Evaluation and treatment of hirsutism in premenopausal women: an Endocrine Society clinical practice guideline. *J Clin Endocrinol Metab* 2018;103:1233–57.

Disorders associated with hirsutism

1 Martin KA, Anderson RR, Chang RJ *et al.* Evaluation and treatment of hirsutism in premenopausal women: an Endocrine Society clinical practice guideline. *J Clin Endocrinol Metab* 2018;103:1233–57.

Disorders of hair pigmentation

4 O'Sullivan JDB, Nicu C, Picard M *et al.* The biology of human hair greying. *Biol Rev Camb Philos Soc* 2021;96:107–28.

CHAPTER 88

Acne

Alison M. Layton[1], Christos C. Zouboulis[2] and Heather Whitehouse[3]

[1]Skin Research Centre, Hull York Medical School, University of York, York; Department of Dermatology, Harrogate and District NHS Foundation Trust, Harrogate, UK
[2]Departments of Dermatology, Venereology, Allergology and Immunology, Staedtisches Klinikum Dessau, Brandenburg Medical School Theodor Fontane and Faculty of Health Sciences, Dessau, Germany
[3]The Leeds Centre for Dermatology, Leeds Teaching Hospitals NHS Trust, Leeds, UK

Acne vulgaris

Definition and nomenclature

Acne vulgaris is a chronic inflammatory disease of the pilosebaceous unit. The clinical lesions are closed and open comedones (Figure 88.1) and/or papules, pustules, nodules and cysts of varying degrees of inflammation and depth (Figure 88.2). The face, back and/or chest are the most frequently affected sites. Complications of acne include inflammatory macules, pigment changes (Figure 88.3), scarring (Figure 88.4) and psychological distress.

> **Synonyms and inclusions**
> - Acne (acne vulgaris)
> - Comedonal acne (acne comedonica)
> - Prepubertal acne
> - Nodulocystic acne (acne conglobata, conglobate acne)
> - Acne fulminans

Introduction and general description

Acne vulgaris is one of the most common skin diseases worldwide, affecting all ethnicities and races [1–5]. The highest prevalence of acne occurs in adolescence, affecting approximately 85% of young adults aged 12–25 years. A cross-sectional study in Brazil reported prevalence as high as 96%; the most prevalent form of acne was comedonal (61.1%), followed by mild (30.6%) and moderate (7.6%) papulopustular [6]. Prevalence rates vary globally, with lower rates of 4.6% in children aged 0–12 and 23.4% in adults with Fitzpatrick type V–VI skin in Angola [7].

The age of onset has changed over time, paralleling the earlier onset of puberty reported in recent years [2,3]. Acne commonly has a prolonged course, with acute or insidious relapse or recurrence over time, with persistent papulopustular acne reported in 68.3% of acne patients in a recent prospective observational study by Shah *et al.* [8].

Clinical presentation includes comedonal and/or inflammatory lesions extending over the face and/or trunk. Discomfort may be a significant manifestation of the inflammatory lesions. Seborrhoea is integral to acne and is evident in varying degrees. Higher sebum excretion is associated with more severe acne [9] and the degree of sebum correlates with more inflammatory lesions [10]. The combined impacts of acne frequently result in psychosocial morbidity. Successful treatment correlates with improvement of psychological factors in many cases [11]. Acne scarring is more likely if treatment is delayed (Figure 88.5) hence early treatment is advocated [12,13]. The burden of acne is significant [14]. Despite the lower prevalence with increasing age when compared with adolescence, the burden of acne remains high in adults [15] and data suggest prevalence is increasing globally [16]. It is unclear whether this increase is a result of higher prevalence of the western diet, earlier onset of puberty, genetic drift or other environmental factors [17].

Epidemiology

Age and sex

Once regarded as a transient disease of the teenage years, acne is now presenting earlier [17,18,19] and lasting longer [3,20]. It may develop *de novo* in adulthood. Earlier development of acne has been linked with earlier onset of puberty, which may also relate to diet/obesity and other lifestyle factors [21,22]; however, earlier recognition may also lead to earlier presentation. Acne most commonly presents between the ages of 10 and 13 years in both sexes. Large community-based surveys and detailed smaller-scale studies have shown that acne begins at a younger age in girls than boys, aligning with earlier puberty [23–25]. A number of studies have shown that adolescent acne is more common in males than females, but that conversely postadolescent acne is more common in females [6,26].

Comedonal acne can be detected in some children before any overt signs of puberty [27,28]. This is consistent with the pathophysiology of acne in which rising adrenal dehydroepiandrosterone (DHEAS)

PART 8: SPECIFIC CUTANEOUS STRUCTURES

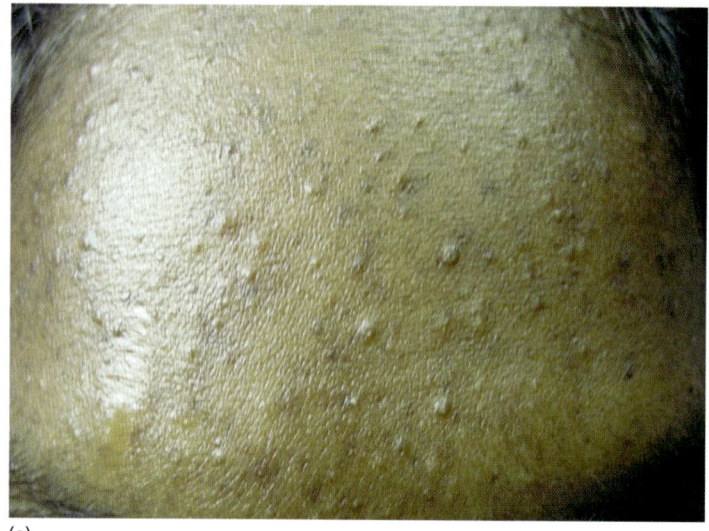

(a)

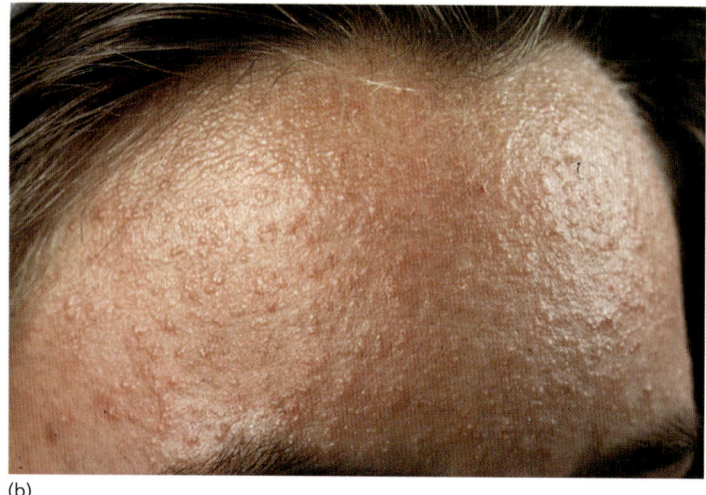

(b)

Figure 88.1 (a) Predominantly comedonal acne. (b) Comedonal acne. (a) Courtesy of Dr S. Chow, KL Skin Centre, Malaysia. (b) From Zouboulis 2014 [731] with permission from Springer Nature.

output is the trigger for sebum production by androgen-susceptible follicles in both girls and boys [28,29].

Early adrenarche in girls is a recognised risk factor for metabolic syndrome, polycystic ovary syndrome (PCOS) and insulin resistance [30]. The early development of comedonal acne in girls may be a predictor of more severe disease in later life.

Postadolescent acne, both persistent and late onset, is more common in women than in men [25,31,32]. This is supported by an observational study of patients of older than 25 years (both sexes) with acne, which found that 31.7% of patients had late-onset acne, of which 95% were female (Figure 88.6) [33]. A large multinational cross-sectional study found that 26% of women aged 31–40 years and 12% of women aged 41–50 years had clinical acne (range 7–22%) depending on ethnicity [34]. Data from a large-scale international study assessing the facial distribution of adult female acne surprisingly indicated that the acne distribution in almost 90% of cases is similar to that seen in adolescent acne, and the stereotype of adult female acne being due to hormonal disturbances

presenting as inflammatory acne localised only to the mandibular area was not found in the majority [35]. A personal or family history of acne in first-degree relatives, no previous pregnancies, having hirsutism, working as an office worker, reporting a higher level of psychological stress, a low consumption of vegetables or fruit and fish were all associated with female adult acne in a case–control study [36].

Peak prevalence occurred between the ages of 15 and 20 years in all ethnic groups. Although data for females were not reported separately, the lower prevalence of postadolescent acne 40 years ago is striking [14,27,28,37,38].

A historical review [23] identified a number of studies showing that males have more severe acne in late adolescence than females. Similar observations have also been reported in further studies [25,39–42]. A study looking at epidemiological modifiable and non-modifiable risk factors for acne severity and scarring found being male, being underweight and having current asthma were associated with higher grades of acne scarring. Consumption of cereals and milk for most or every day of the week reduces the risk of higher-grade acne scarring [43]. Tracking changes in the epidemiology of acne over time is problematic; however, data indicate that the age distribution of acne is widening (Figure 88.7) and this is happening in males and females, but more prominently in women over the age of 40 years [44].

Ethnicity

Acne is now considered to be among the 10 most common diseases worldwide [45]. Epidemiological studies demonstrate how challenging it is to unravel the effects of ethnicity and socioeconomic and cultural factors. However, ethnic variation in the prevalence of acne does appear to exist even when socioeconomic and cultural differences are accounted for. In the USA, where prevalence data are collected by the National Ambulatory Medical Care Survey (NAMCS), acne is the commonest or second most common reason for visits to dermatologists by all racial groups including Asian Pacific islanders [46].

The prevalence of acne appears to be lower and showing a slower rate of incline in developing versus developed countries (Figure 88.8) [17,47–49]. Many of these regions are racially diverse and heterogeneous in population, hence variance is most probably dependent on multiple factors rather than ethnicity alone.

A large systematic review of acne prevalence in mainland China found overall pooled prevalence rates were 39.2% (95% confidence interval (CI) 0.310–0.479). Interestingly, the authors found variation between the northern and southern regions of China, with the south (46.3%, 95%CI 0.374–0.555) having a higher prevalence of acne than the north (34.2%, 95%CI 0.242–0.458; $Z = 2.498$, $P = 0.012$). The authors suggested that this could be due to humidity, climate and dietary differences [50].

Acne is prevalent in all skin phototypes. Phototype has been reported as a risk factor for acne [51]. Phototype may impact on the type of acne lesion. A cross-sectional population-based study in Brazil using multivariate analysis reported that the morphology of acne lesions was different in adolescents with light or dark skin phototype [52]. Inflammatory lesions were noted more commonly in the light skin phototype and non-inflammatory ones in the dark phototype. Postinflammatory hyperpigmentation is more common

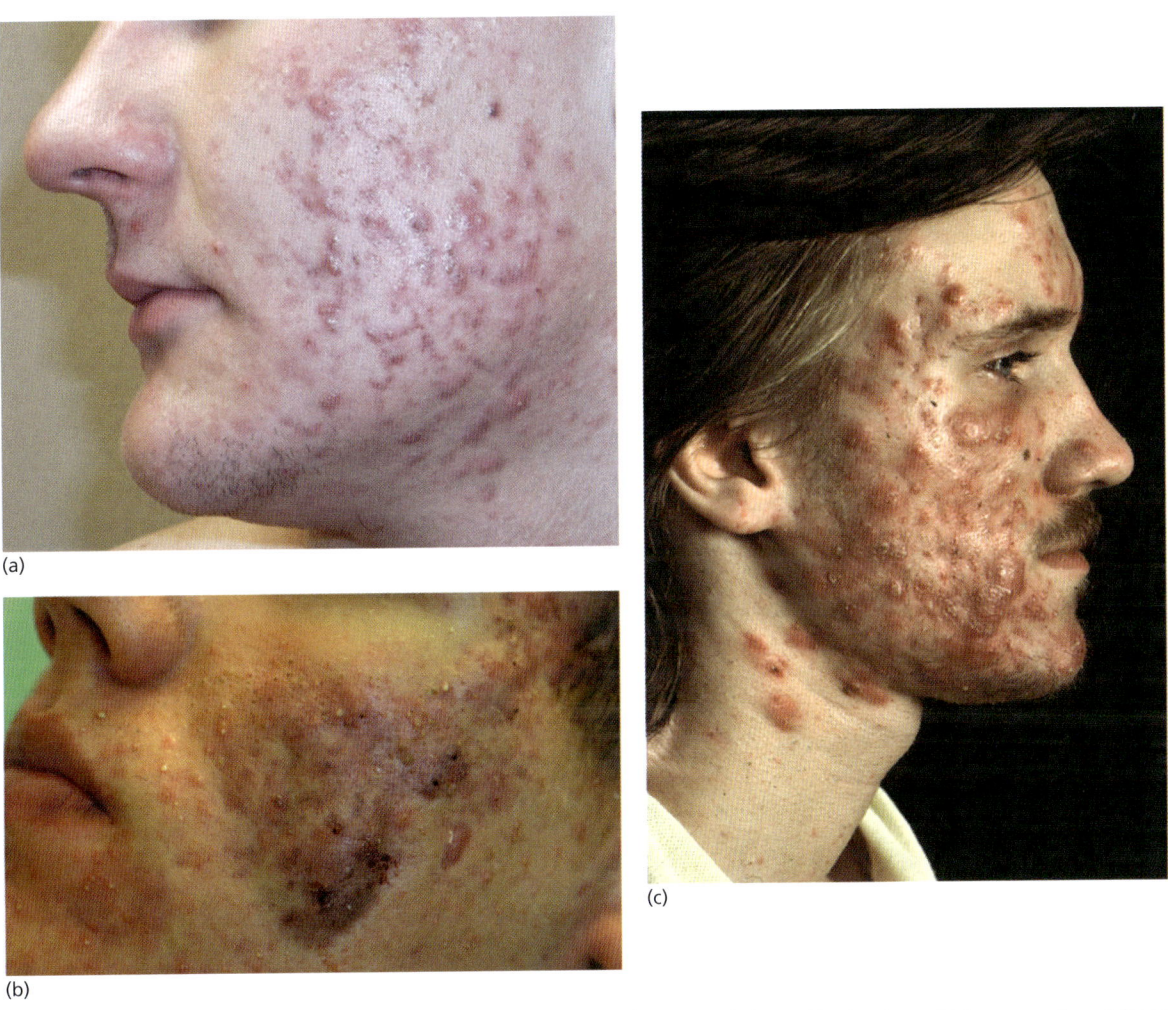

(a)

(b)

(c)

Figure 88.2 (a) Moderate to severe inflammatory acne including a mixture of comedonal and inflammatory lesions with seborrhoea. (b) Severe papulopustular acne. (c) Conglobate acne. (c) From Orfanos and Zouboulis 1998 [732] with permission from S. Karger AG, Basel.

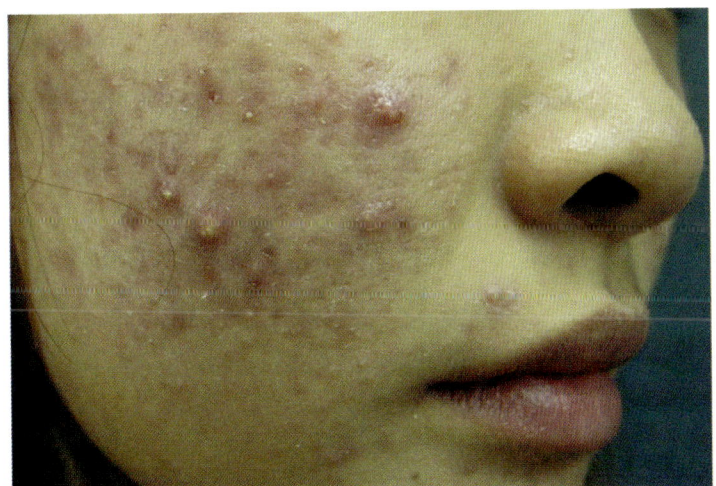

Figure 88.3 Postinflammatory macules and pigment changes interspersed with inflammatory acne. Courtesy of Dr S. Chow, KL Skin Centre, Malaysia.

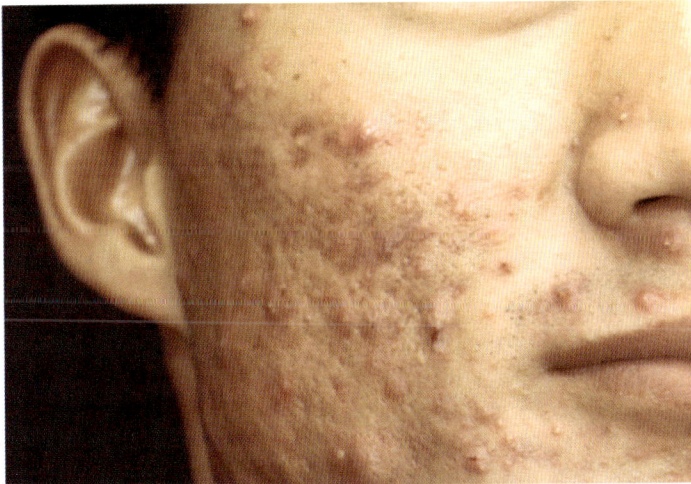

Figure 88.4 Active severe papulopustular acne with development of atrophic acne scars.

in darker phototypes and is a key concern for acne patients with skin of colour [53]. Cultural differences in skin and hair care practices should also be considered as a possible factor contributing to the variable incidence of acne among different ethnic populations. For example, within the black population cocoa butter, a highly comedogenic substance, is often used [54].

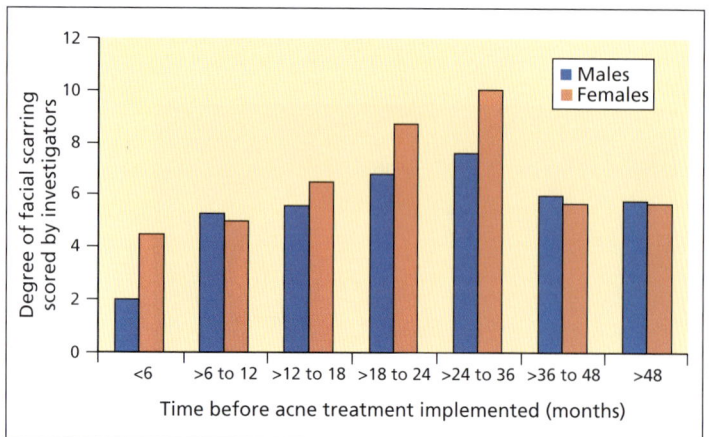

Figure 88.5 There is a correlation between acne scarring and duration of acne. Scarring is more likely to occur with delays in treatment. Adapted from Layton *et al.* 1994 [12] with permission from Wiley.

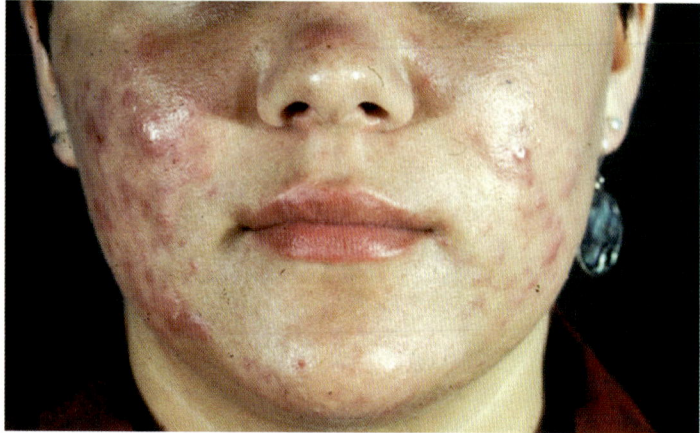

Figure 88.6 Acne tarda in a female patient. From Zouboulis and Piquero-Martin 2003 [733] with permission from S. Karger AG, Basel.

Associated diseases

Acne may be associated with a number of medical conditions in which there is a predisposition to inflammation or to be associated with an underlying metabolic disturbance involving androgenic steroids, insulin resistance and increased fibroblast growth factor receptor 2 (FGFR2) signalling. Table 88.1 summarises medical conditions that may predispose to or protect against acne and highlights the abnormalities associated with each condition that may influence the course of acne.

Most acne patients have no underlying endocrinological abnormalities although, as an androgen-mediated dermatosis, acne is often a symptom of diseases in which androgen metabolism is abnormal [55,56]. The term 'endocrine' acne should be reserved for cases associated with clear signs and symptoms of endocrine disturbance such as PCOS, late-onset congenital adrenogenital syndrome and Cushing disease. Of these, PCOS is by far the commonest endocrine disorder associated with acne. Female-to-male transgender patients receive masculinising doses of testosterone to induce virilisation and suppress menstruation. Elevated androgen levels in transgender men have been associated with an increased incidence of acne [57].

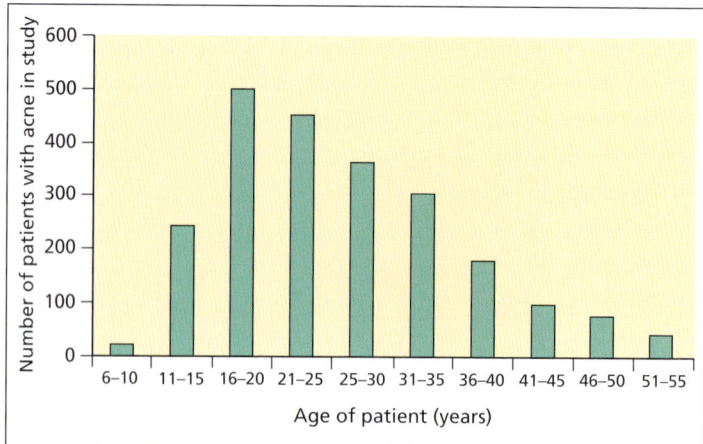

Figure 88.7 The age distribution of acne is widening in both sexes.

Polycystic ovary syndrome. PCOS is diagnosed according to the Rotterdam criteria [58] in which two of the following must be present:

- Overt symptoms of androgen excess (hirsutism, acne and/or alopecia).
- Ovulatory dysfunction (irregular or prolonged menstrual cycles).
- Polycystic ovaries.

In the USA, the alternative National Institutes for Health (NIH) criteria continue to be used (Table 88.2). Using the Rotterdam criteria, between 5% and 10% of adult women are classified as having the syndrome. PCOS almost certainly encompasses a spectrum of related ovarian endocrinopathies; subtypes are recognised (Table 88.3). Women with PCOS are frequently but not always overweight, have one or more raised serum androgen levels or a raised free androgen index and are insulin resistant, all of which predispose to acne. PCOS ovaries appear more sensitive to insulin than non-PCOS ovaries, resulting in excess androgen production. Hyperinsulinaemia is also associated with excess adrenal androgen synthesis. A systematic review of prevalence of acne among PCOS patients found pooled prevalence was 76% using the NIH definition and 36% by Rotterdam criteria with the highest prevalence of acne in PCOS patients reported in East Asia, being 3.5-fold higher than in non-PCOS counterparts [59].

Overall, acne is a common finding although there is one striking exception: adult Pacific Island women with PCOS have little or no acne [60], which is consistent with the absence of acne in the island population as a whole. PCOS is increasingly being diagnosed in adolescents [61] and has been linked to the obesity epidemic [62–64]. In teenagers, the onset of PCOS overlaps with the traditional acne-prone years, during which transient insulin resistance is common, making it difficult to attribute individual cases of acne to PCOS as opposed to normal puberty [65]. Most investigators have studied the prevalence of acne in women with PCOS and have shown a higher incidence [66–68] but others have examined the prevalence of PCOS or polycystic ovaries in female acne patients and demonstrated a higher prevalence of cystic ovaries in these patients [69,70].

Table 88.4 summarises studies providing data on the prevalence of acne among adult women with PCOS and demonstrates considerable variation [71–98].

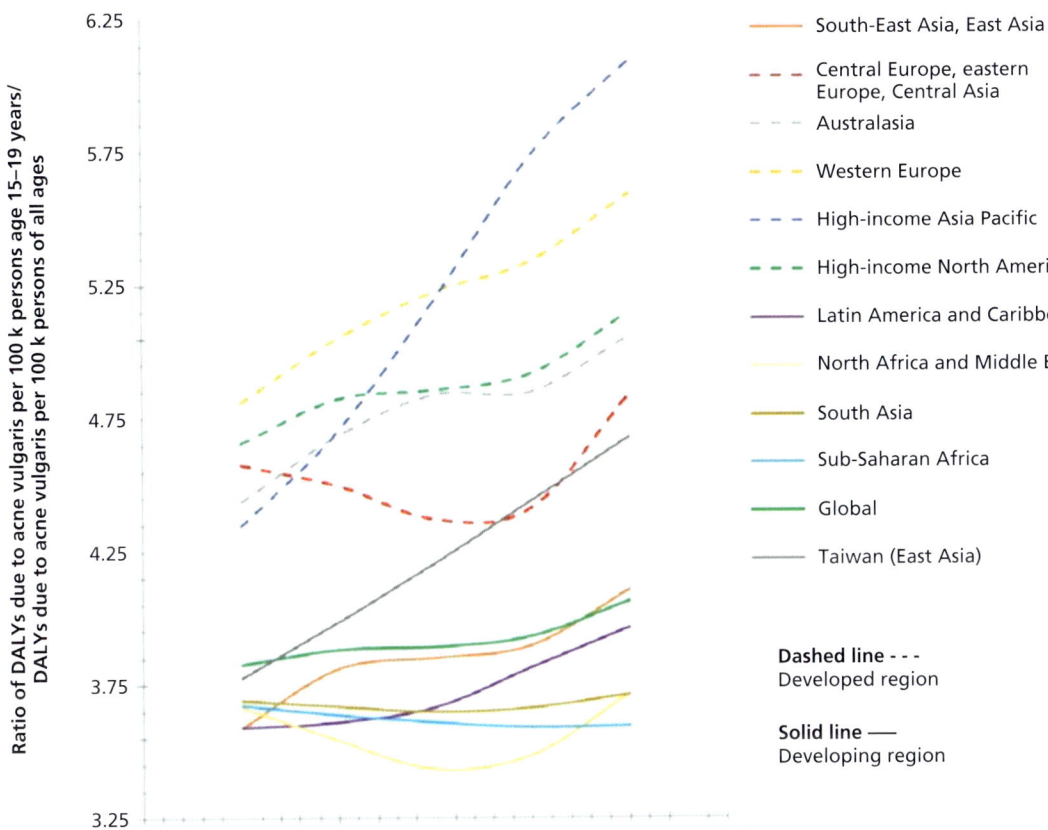

Figure 88.8 Acne vulgaris in late adolescence around the globe showing the proportional rate of disability-adjusted life years (DALYs) of 15–19-year-olds (both sexes) in a given region. Reproduced from Lynn *et al.* 2016 [**17**] with permission.

Adult women with PCOS often have other signs of peripheral hyperandrogenism including androgenic alopecia and hirsutism (Figure 88.9).

Late-onset congenital adrenal hyperplasia. Late-onset or non-classic congenital adrenal hyperplasia is a relatively common autosomal recessive disorder with an incidence reported as 1 : 500 to 1 : 1000 in white populations. Late-onset congenital adrenal hyperplasia arises due to mutations in the *CYP21A2* gene located at chromosome 6p21, which lead to 21-hydroxylase deficiency. 21-Hydroxylase is a key enzyme in the synthesis of mineralocorticoids and glucocorticoids (including cortisol) from progesterone and 17α-hydroxyprogesterone (17-OHP). In deficiency, intermediates proximal to the enzyme accumulate; elevated 17-OHP, progesterone and androstenedione concentrations are typically found (Figure 88.10). Raised serum 17-OHP, basally or following an adrenocorticotropic hormone (ACTH) stimulation test, is a diagnostic marker for late-onset congenital adrenal hyperplasia but is not 100% sensitive for carriers of mutations in *CYP21A2*. Table 88.5 outlines the clinical features; acne is not a consistent feature. Reported prevalence in women with androgen excess ranges from 0.6% to 9% [99]. Higher prevalences are seen in some Jewish, Mediterranean, Middle Eastern and Indian populations. The condition is most frequently diagnosed in late childhood or early adulthood but can present as precocious puberty. Severe, refractory or atypical forms of acne may represent late-onset congenital adrenal hyperplasia (Figure 88.11) [100–103]. If mild, it can go unnoticed until symptoms such as persistent acne, irregular menses or problems conceiving present. Late-onset congenital adrenal hyperplasia is a widely underdiagnosed disorder, particularly in males [104]. Box 88.1 outlines suggested assessment in males.

Box 88.1 Assessment of male patients with acne for congenital adrenal hyperplasia (CAH)

Medical history
- Acne/infertility

Physical examination
- Testicular examination

Biochemical investigations
- Basal level 17-hydroxyprogesterone (>6.1 nmol/L serves as a screening for non-classic adrenal hyperplasia)
- Adrenocorticotropic hormone stimulated plasma 17-hydroxyprogesterone (elevated basal levels or adrenocorticotropic hormone stimulated levels >260 ng/dL)
- Serum luteinising hormone, follicle-stimulating hormone
- Testosterone, dehydroepiandrosterone sulphate, androstenedione 21-desoxycortisol

Testicular ultrasound
Semen analysis

For the treatment of acne associated with late-onset congenital adrenal hyperplasia in male patients, oral glucocorticoids have been used. Systemic low-dose oral prednisolone (2.5–5 mg/day) or

Table 88.1 Medical conditions that may predispose to acne or in which acne prevalence is reduced.

Condition	Abnormalities associated with this condition and relevant to acne	Effect/comments
PCOS	Raised serum DHEAS, total and/or free testosterone and androstenedione, reduced SHBG. Also raised luteinising hormone, insulin, IGFBP-1 and IGF-1	Predisposes and/or worsens; effect on acne modified by BMI (or more correctly adiposity)
SAHA syndrome: subtype of PCOS	Serum androgens often but not always elevated. Subtypes can be characterised by which serum hormone levels are abnormal	Predisposes. According to Orfanos et al. [126], there are four types of SAHA: idiopathic, ovarian, adrenal and hyperprolactinaemic. Ovarian SAHA is associated with a more insulin-resistant profile
HAIR-AN syndrome: subtype of PCOS	Pronounced insulin resistance, with markedly raised serum insulin	Predisposes. May be a fifth subtype of SAHA syndrome. Insulin resistance is proportional to BMI. Onset is usually during puberty/adolescence
Premature adrenarche	Raised serum DHEA, DHEAS and androstenedione; often accompanied by insulin resistance	Much more common in girls than boys. Predisposes to earlier onset of acne and to PCOS. Rising insulin and IGF-1 appear to increase the adrenal sensitivity to ACTH, leading to overproduction of androgens
Premature puberty	Raised serum levels of gonadal androgens (highly variable depending on the cause)	Predisposes. Can be caused by premature adrenarche or tumours (of the pituitary or adrenal mainly)
Insulin resistance	Reduced IGF-1 and IGFBP-1	Predisposes
Hyperinsulinaemia	Raised serum insulin, IGF-1 and reduced IGFBP-3	Predisposes
Non-classic congenital adrenal hyperplasia associated with 21-hydroxylase deficiency (especially mild or heterozygous forms); more rarely 11β-hydroxylase or 3β-hydroxysteroid dehydrogenase deficiency	Elevated serum 17-OHP, progesterone, androstenedione, corticotrophin-releasing hormone and ACTH	Predisposes especially to early onset. May extend duration; reduces responsiveness to treatment
Apert syndrome	Associated with point mutations on *FGFR2*, which have been linked to acne	Predisposes to seborrhoea and an acne-like condition with involvement of the upper arms/forearms; responds to oral isotretinoin
Anorexia nervosa	Serum growth hormone raised, concomitantly IGF-1 is low	Predisposes
Turner syndrome	45,X. Rudimentary ovaries with reduced androgen synthesis leading to reduced serum levels of testosterone and androstenedione during puberty in affected girls	Only affects girls. Protects via reduced sebum production. Serum androgens are normal during adrenarche
Laron syndrome	Congenital deficiency of IGF-1	Protects
Mayer–Rokitansky–Küster–Hauser syndrome without *WNT4* mutation	Serum androgens are normal	?Protects. Lower prevalence of acne and PCOS but ovaries are intact
Mayer–Rokitansky–Küster–Hauser syndrome with *WNT4* mutation (may be a distinct condition)	Raised serum testosterone	Predisposes via inability to repress ovarian androgen synthesis
Cushing syndrome (iatrogenic and endogenous)	Elevated serum cortisol, ACTH and corticotrophin-releasing hormone	Predisposes. Can cause acne in pre-adrenarchal children
Ectopic ACTH syndrome	Elevated serum ACTH	Predisposes. Can cause acne in pre-adrenarchal children
PAPA syndrome	Mutations in *PSTPIP1*. IL-1β and circulating neutrophil granule enzyme levels in serum are raised. Impaired production of IL-10 and increased production of GM-CSF	Acne is one of three diagnostic features of this syndrome; pyogenic sterile arthritis and pyoderma gangrenosum are the others
PASH syndrome	?Raised IL-1β (systemically or locally) or aberrant regulation of the function of this cytokine	Acne is one of three diagnostic features, suppurative hidradenitis and pyoderma gangrenosum are the others
PASS syndrome	?Raised TNF-α (systemically or locally) or aberrant regulation of the function of this cytokine	As PASH but with axial spondyloarthritis
SAPHO syndrome	*Cutibacterium acnes* sometimes recovered from bone samples	Acne is one of five diagnostic features of this syndrome, synovitis, pustulosis, hyperostosis and osteitis are the others. Syndrome is more likely to be associated with *C. acnes* than acne *per se*
Adrenal and ovarian tumours	Elevated serum androgens exclusively or with other raised hormones	Predisposes
Male pseudohermaphroditism	17β-hydroxysteroid dehydrogenase type 3 deficiency, 5α-reductase type 2 deficiency	Normal pubertal development, normal levels of sebum and no altered risk of acne
Complete androgen insensitivity syndrome	Mutation in the androgen receptor	Protects. These patients produce no sebum and do not get acne
Exaggerated adrenarche	Specific elevation of adrenal hormones produced by the zona reticularis in adults; exaggerated DHEAS and androstenedione responses to ACTH stimulation test	Predisposes

ACTH, adrenocorticotrophic hormone; BMI, body mass index; DHEA, dihydroepiandrosterone; DHEAS, dehydroepiandrosterone; GM-CSF, granulocyte–macrophage colony-stimulating factor; HAIR-AN, hyperandrogenism, insulin resistance and acanthosis nigricans; IGF, insulin-derived growth factor; IGFBP, insulin-derived growth factor binding protein; IL, interleukin; 17-OHP, 17-hydroxyprogesterone; PAPA, pyogenic sterile arthritis, pyoderma gangrenosum and acne; PASH, pyoderma gangrenosum, acne and hidradenitis suppurativa; PASS, pyoderma gangrenosum, acne, seronegative spondyloarthritis; PCOS, polycystic ovary syndrome; SAHA, seborrhoea, acne, hirsutism and androgenetic alopecia; SAPHO, synovitis, acne, pustulosis, hyperostosis and osteitis; SHBG, sex hormone-binding globulin; TNF-α, tumour necrosis factor α.

Table 88.2 Criteria used to diagnose polycystic ovary syndrome.

Rotterdam diagnostic criteria – requires two of the following:	NIH diagnostic criteria – requires both the following:
1 Oligo- or anovulation	**1** Oligo- or anovulation
2 Clinical and/or biochemical signs of hyperandrogenism	**2** Clinical and/or biochemical signs of hyperandrogenism
3 Polycystic ovaries	**Plus:** exclusion of other aetiologies such as congenital adrenal hyperplasia, androgen-secreting tumours and Cushing syndrome
Plus: exclusion of other aetiologies such as hyperthyroidism, hypoprolactinaemia, congenital adrenal hyperplasia, androgen-secreting tumours and Cushing syndrome	

NIH, National Institutes for Health.

dexamethasone 0.25–0.75 mg/day) can be given, although the latter may have a higher risk of adrenal suppression [105].

Hypercortisolism. This describes signs and symptoms associated with prolonged exposure to inappropriately high levels of cortisol or in consequence of Cushing disease.

Cushing disease. Cushing disease refers to hypercortisolism secondary to excess production of ACTH from a corticopituitary adenoma. ACTH levels are often lower in Cushing syndrome. For primary hypercortisolism, see Box 88.2 which outlines the symptoms and signs associated with Cushing disease.

Box 88.2 Symptoms and signs associated with Cushing syndrome

C – central obesity, collagen fibre weakness, comedones (acne)
U – urinary free cortisol and glucose intolerance
S – striae, suppressed immunity
H – hypercortisolism, hypertension, hyperglycaemia, hypercholesterolaemia
I – iatrogenic (increased administration of corticosteroids)
N – non-iatrogenic (neoplasms)
G – glucose intolerance, growth retardation

Acromegaly. Acromegaly, which relates to excess growth hormone production, has been associated with the development of acne [106]. Growth hormone and excess insulin-like growth factor 1 (IGF-1) can stimulate sebaceous gland differentiation and androgen-induced sebaceous lipogenesis [107–109]. Affected subjects may notice increased sebum production [109] and in some cases acne is the only presenting symptom [106].

Synovitis, acne, pustulosis, hyperostosis and osteitis syndrome (SAPHO). This acronym, first described in 1987, represents a syndrome of pustular dermatoses together with aseptic osteoarticular lesions including synovitis, acne, pustulosis, hyperostosis and osteitis [110,111]. In the classic syndrome, patients present with sudden-onset haemorrhagic and ulcerative acne on the face and trunk, sterile pustular lesions on the palms and soles and pain especially affecting the anterior chest wall. In mild cases, the condition is underdiagnosed. Skin manifestations are commoner in adults than in children and severe acneform skin disease, including acne fulminans, acne conglobata and/or hidradenitis suppurativa (HS), is seen, predominantly in males. The disease may represent an immune reaction to an unspecified antigen. *Cutibacterium acnes*, previously called *Propionibacteria acnes*, has in some cases been isolated in osteitic bone lesions; the bony lesions fail to respond to antibiotics suggesting that they do not represent primary haematogenic spread [112]. Reports suggest that biphosphonates will improve bony lesions but they have no impact on the cutaneous manifestations [113,114]. Increased levels of tumour necrosis factor α (TNF-α) have been identified. In isolated cases, benefit has been noted following treatment with infliximab [115] and ustekinumab [116]. Opposing effects on skin and osteoarticular symptoms may occur with TNF-α antibodies (articular improvement/cutaneous deterioration) as well as with isotretinoin (cutaneous improvement/articular deterioration) [117,118].

HAIR-AN syndrome. This syndrome consists of hyperandrogenism (HA), insulin resistance (IR) and acanthosis nigricans (AN) [119]. Patients present with typical signs of hyperandrogenism, hyperseborrhoea, hirsutism, acne, menstrual irregularities and androgenetic alopecia. They may also show other features including deepening voice, clitoromegaly and increased muscle mass [120]. Other autoimmune or endocrine diseases may be associated with HAIR-AN, including Graves disease, Hashimoto thyroiditis, Cushing syndrome, Cohen syndrome, acromegaly, congenital

Table 88.3 Subtypes of polycystic ovary syndrome (PCOS).

	Type I classic PCOS	**Type II PCOS**	**Type III PCOS**	**Type IV PCOS**
Hyperandrogenism	Present	Present	Normal	Present
Menstruation	Oligomenorrhoea	Irregular	Irregular	Regular
Ovarian cysts	Present	No cysts	Present	Present
Cardiovascular risk	High – metabolic syndrome 3× higher in these patients Relatively higher BMI Insulin resistance Dyslipidaemia with increased small dense LDL and lipoprotein		Lowest cardiovascular risk may be similar to those with no signs of PCOS	Lower BMI Lesser degree of hyperandrogenism Mildest degree of metabolic syndrome versus other subtypes Still at higher risk of CVD than those without PCOS

BMI, body mass index; CVD, cardiovascular disease; LDL, low-density lipoprotein.

Table 88.4 Prevalence of acne among women with polycystic ovary syndrome (PCOS).

Number of women, nationality	Age range (years); mean ± SD	Prevalence of acne (%)	Notes	Reference
87 British (47 South Asians, 40 white skin)	Asian 26 ± 4; white skin 30.1 ± 5	66 Asian, 30 white skin		[71]
716 Mexican	27.7 ± 7.3	15	Very low figure – article does not say how acne was defined	[72]
316 American	Three groups: 26.3 ± 6.9; 27.3 ± 6.9; 30 ± 7.8	19	Very low prevalence of acne for American women with PCOS	[73]
German	28	50	Versus 33% for women without PCOS	[74]
273 Chinese	24.83 ± 5.31	45		[75]
295 Taiwanese	14–40; 26.7 ± 5.4	48	Compared with 18% for age-matched women without PCOS	[76]
32 Tanzanian	29.3 ± 4.5	41	Compared with 17.6 for 68 women without PCOS	[77]
103 American	13–20	33		[78]
70 American	11–22; 16.2	70		[79]
49 Indian	12–19	67		[80]
51 Indian	15–32 22.2 ± 5.4	55		[81]
42 Indian	17–31 22.4 ± 5.53	54		[82]
62 Saudi Arabian	29–43	39		[83]
115 Turkish	15–41	53	35% had seborrhoea	[84]
210 Iranian	17–18	27	Severe acne only	[85]
58 American	9–18	74	Five girls were premenarchal	[86]
318 Taiwanese	24.5 ± 5.0	39		[87]
74 Greek				[88]
365 Croatian	26.1 ± 5.9	50		[89]
136 Indian girls: 49 with PCOS,	18.8 ± 8.5 PCOS	33	Versus 14.9 in those without PCOS	[90]
87 without PCOS	19.8 ± 0.67 non-PCOS			[90]
100 Indian	20–38	13	Very low	[91]
133 Turkish	17–36	26 moderate or severe; 65 mild	Used Global Acne Grading System. Women with mild acne may be misclassified as no acne using a less stringent method	[92]
196 American	11–20; 15.7 ± 1.7	18 moderate or severe; 53 mild		[93]
10 Palestinian	18–24	80	Versus 37.2% in those without PCOS	[94]
149 American (121 white skin, 28 Asian)	28 ± 5.4 white skin; 29.6 ± 5.9 Asian	68 white skin versus 74 Asian	Difference not significant	[95]
40 Korean	Two groups: 24.7 ± 5.1; 25.7 ± 8.2	95	Seborrhoea in 45%	[96]
254 American	Two groups 28.8 ± 5.67 27.8 ± 6.10	61		[97]
59 Turkish	21.49 ± 4.18	46		[98]

adrenal hyperplasia and insulinoma [120–122]. The primary abnormality is hyperinsulinaemia, while elevated or upper limit levels of testosterone and androstenedione are frequent. The degree of excess insulin correlates directly to androgen levels [123]. The hyperinsulinaemia and hyperandrogenaemia stimulate epithelial proliferation and melanin accumulation resulting in the cutaneous changes seen. In some patients with HAIR-AN, a reduction in insulin receptors has been demonstrated and/or mutations in the receptor gene [124]. The binding of insulin to IGF receptors and insulin receptors on keratinocytes and fibroblasts leads to epidermal thickness which is thought to induce the changes seen in acanthosis nigricans [120,125].

SAHA (seborrhoea, acne, hirsutism and androgenetic alopecia) syndrome. In 1982, the association of seborrhoea and acne with hirsutism and/or androgenetic alopecia in females was defined as SAHA (Figure 88.12) [126]. The syndrome is classified into idiopathic, ovarian, adrenal and hyperprolactinaemic types. All four major clinical signs are only present in about 20% of cases, seborrhoea is a consistent finding and acne is evident in around 10% of cases [126].

PAPA (pyogenic sterile arthritis, pyoderma gangrenosum and acne) syndrome and PAPA spectrum disorders. PAPA, first described in 1997, represents a rare autosomal dominant autoinflammatory disease caused by mutations in the gene for proline/serine/threonine

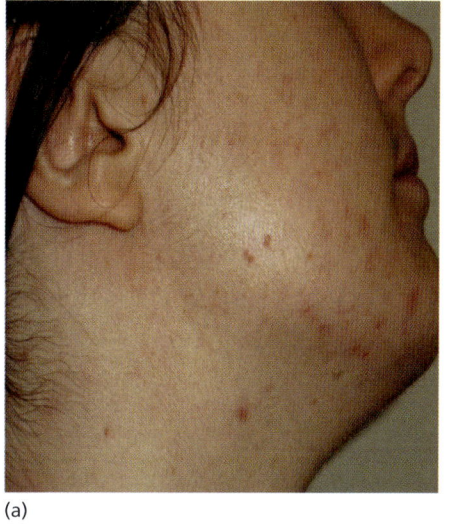
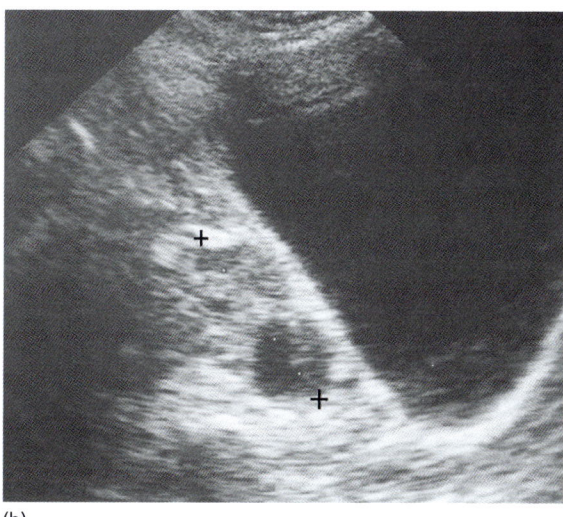

(a)   (b)

Figure 88.9 (a) Acne in an adult female with polycystic ovary syndrome associated with hirsutism and seborrhoea. (b) Ultrasound scan showing cysts (+) on the ovaries.

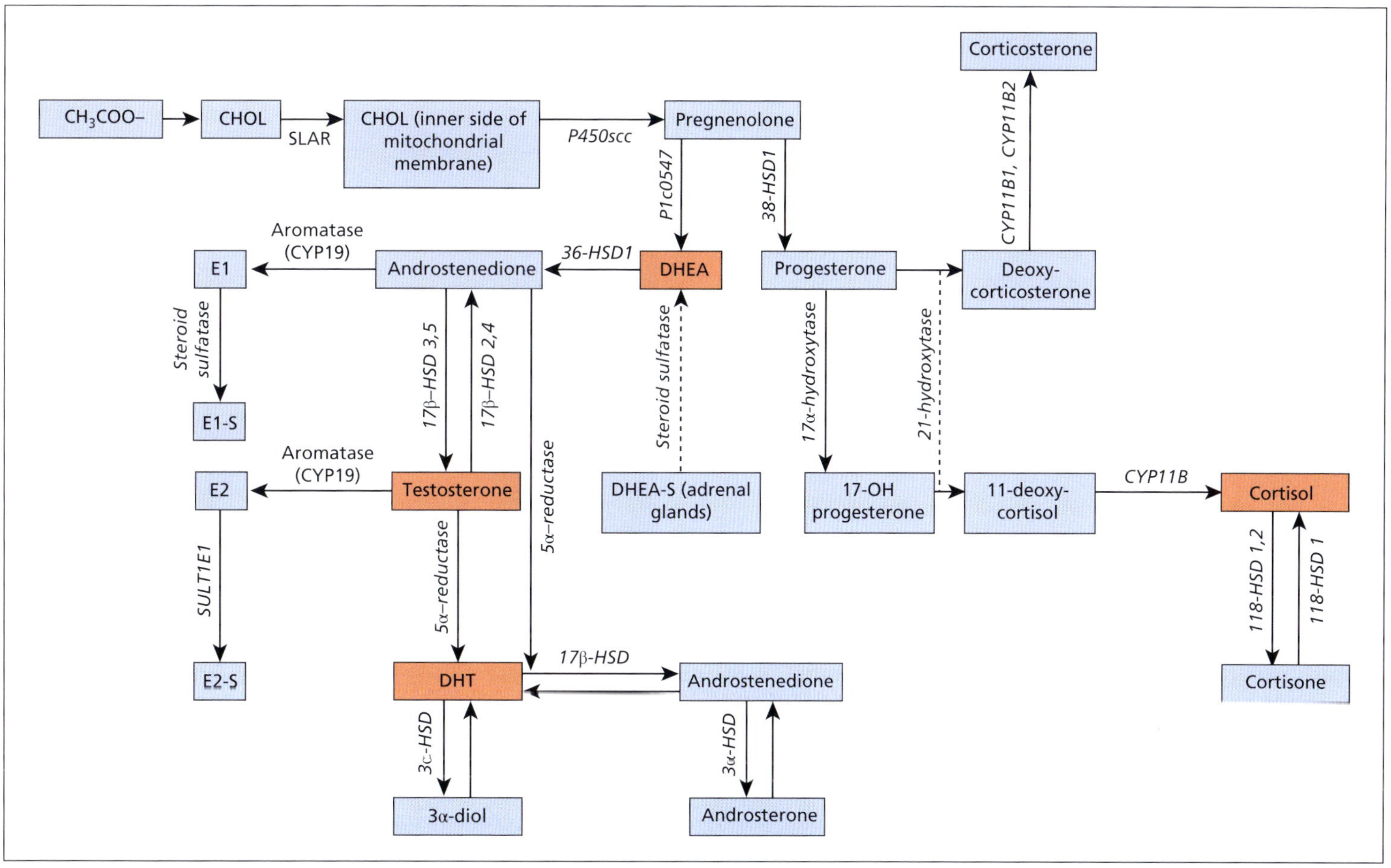

Figure 88.10 Schematic representation of the role of 21-hydroxylase in the adrenal steroid genesis pathway. CHOL, cholesterol; DHEA, dehydroepiandrosterone; DHEA-S, dehydroepiandrosterone sulphate; DHT, dihydrotesterone; 17-OH, 17-hydroxyprogesterone; SLAR, steroidogenic acute regulatory protein.

phosphatase interacting protein 1 (PSTPIP1; also known as CD2BP1). PSTPIP1 is a cytoskeleton-associated adaptor protein expressed predominantly in haematopoietic cells that modulates T-cell activation [127] and interleukin 1β (IL-1β) release [128].

Other syndromes similar to PAPA have been subsequently identified and can be unified under PAPA spectrum disorders (Table 88.6): PASH syndrome (pyoderma gangrenosum, acne and hidradenitis suppurativa (HS)), PASS (pyoderma gangrenosum, acne, seronegative spondyloarthritis, with or without HS), PAPASH (features of PASH with pyogenic arthritis), PsAPASH (PASH with psoriatic arthritis) and PAC (pyoderma gangrenosum, acne and ulcerative colitis). PAMI syndrome (PSTPIP1-associated

Table 88.5 Clinical features of 21-hydroxylase late-onset adrenal hyperplasia.

Adulthood	Childhood
Short stature	Tall stature
Hirsutism	Pseudoprecocious puberty
Acne	Cystic acne
Testicular enlargement in boys	Premature pubarche
Oligospermia	
Menstrual irregularities	
Infertility both sexes	

myeloid-related proteinaemia inflammatory syndrome) is a PAPA variant with haematological manifestations [129].

PAPA typically presents with recurrent sterile erosive arthritis in childhood occurring spontaneously after minor trauma, occasionally resulting in joint destruction. The joint problems tend to subside by puberty and there is a transition to cutaneous disease. Skin problems include pathergy, with abscesses developing at the sites of injections; severe nodulocystic acne appears in adolescence followed by recurrent sterile ulcers often diagnosed as pyoderma gangrenosum [130]. A review of PAPA spectrum disorders identified acne in 37 of the 49 identified cases with a phenotype of severe or more (nodulocystic, acne fulminans or severe but without the characteristics of the two previous phenotypes) in 83% of cases. The topography of the lesions was that of acne vulgaris (face, trunk), with four cases involving the scalp [129]. Pyoderma gangrenosum and acne may be present for several decades once present.

Systemic or locally administered glucocoticosteroids are usually helpful for the inflammatory symptoms. In most cases, systemic treatments are employed to treat clinical aspects other than the acne. These treatments include TNF-α blockade and IL-1 receptor antagonists such as anakinra or canakinumab which have been used successfully in case reports and have improved the acne lesions associated with PAPA syndrome [131–135].

Apert syndrome. Apert syndrome, also known as acrocephalosyndactyly, was first described in 1906 [136]. The prevalence is estimated at 15/1 000 000 births based on a population-based study [137]. Apert syndrome is characterised by craniosynostosis and early epiphyseal closure which results in deformities of the skull, hands and feet. The characteristic facial abnormalities are hypertelorism, a flattened occiput, proptosis due to shallow orbits, prognathism, a parrot-beaked nose and fused shortened digits. Severely delayed tooth eruption, shovel-shaped incisors and malocclusion of teeth occur. Abnormalities of the upper and lower respiratory tracts include a cleft soft palate and bifid uvula [138]. Moderate to severe acne, which generally presents early in puberty, is a characteristic feature of Apert syndrome [139–141]. The acne typically presents on the trunk and face but also extends to unusual sites such as the forearms and buttocks (Figure 88.13) [142].

Early epiphyseal closure is an androgen-mediated event. No difference in the androgen receptor expression has been demonstrated suggesting that the underlying problem in Apert syndrome relates to abnormal sensitivity to normal circulating levels of androgens [143–145]. Other cutaneous changes reported in Apert syndrome include seborrhoea, hyperhidrosis, nail dystrophy,

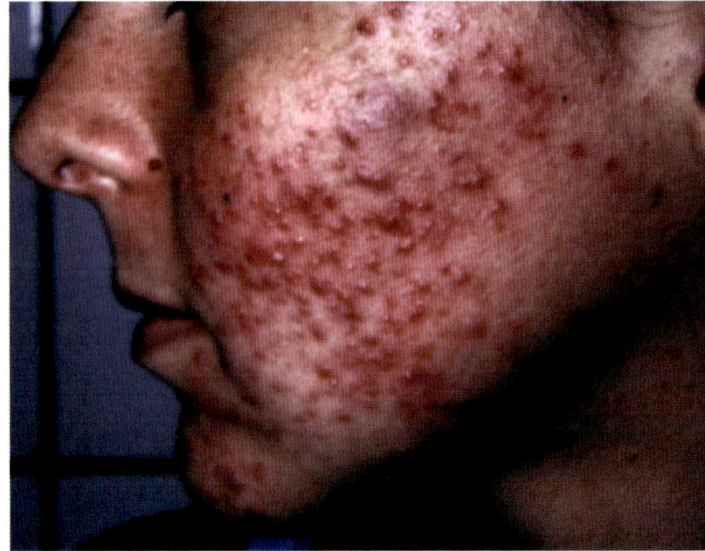

(a)

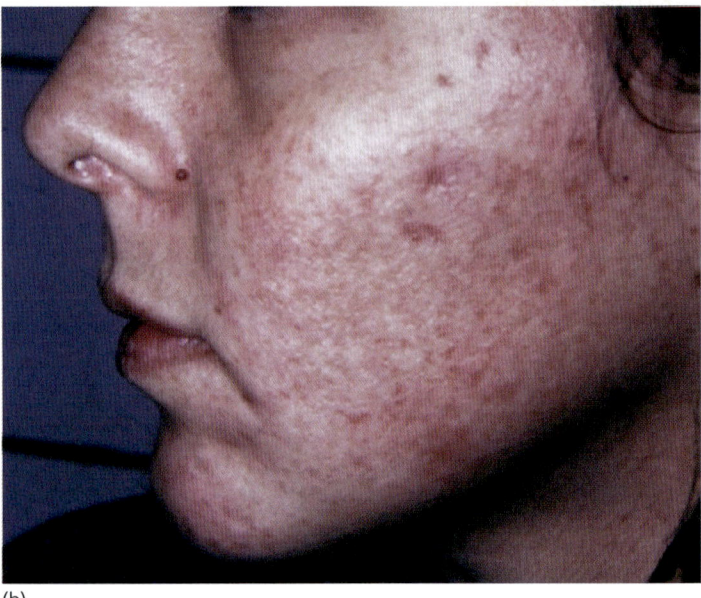

(b)

Figure 88.11 (a) Non-classic congenital adrenal hyperplasia in a 16-year-old with oligomenorrhoea pre-treatment. (b) Post-therapy with 2 mg oral prednisolone daily. Courtesy of Dr P. Troielli, School of Medicine, University of Buenos Aires, Argentina.

hyperkeratosis of the plantar surfaces and ocular and cutaneous hypopigmentation [146]. Apert syndrome may be inherited as autosomal dominant or may be due to a new mutation of paternal origin. Two specific heterozygous missense germ-line mutations of the *FGFR2* gene have been identified. The mutations of adjacent amino acid residues of *FGFR2*, either S252W or P253R, are localised in the linker region between D2- and D3-immunoglobulin-like regions of the *FGFR2* ligand-binding domain. Two major isoforms of *FGFR2* are formed. *FGFR2b* is exclusively expressed on epithelial cells, whereas *FGFR2c* is expressed only on dermal and mesenchymal cells. Both receptor isoforms and their specific ligands are involved in mesenchymal epithelial signalling leading to downstream effects of activated *FGFR2* signalling on follicular keratinocyte proliferation, sebaceous lipogenesis and inflammatory cytokine response [147]. The acne in Apert syndrome frequently

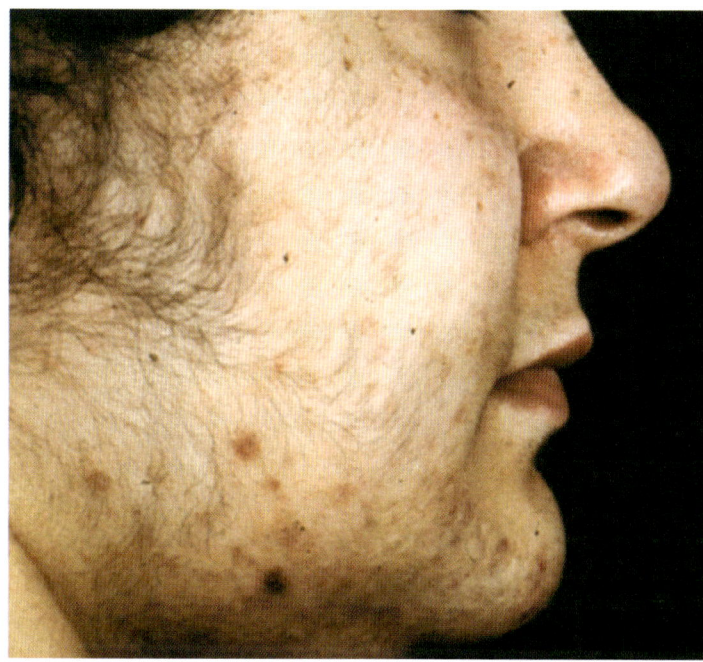

Figure 88.12 Seborrhoea, acne, hirsutism and/or androgenetic alopecia (SAHA) syndrome in a 22-year-old obese female with HAIR-AN. From Zouboulis and Dessinioti 2014 [734] with permission from Springer Nature.

requires oral isotretinoin [148,149]. Etretinate has also been effective in refractory cases [150].

Drug-induced acne. Some drugs may cause acneform reactions; these account for about 1% of all drug-induced skin eruptions. Drug-induced acne embraces monomorphic inflammatory lesions with an absence of comedones, often presenting acutely on sites not commonly affected by acne. The face and upper trunk are most frequently affected. The interval between the start of the implicated drug and the onset of the acneform eruption depends very much on the agent provoking the response. Several reviews provide lists of drugs associated with acne or acneform rashes [151,152]. Table 88.7 identifies drugs that have been implicated in acneform eruptions.

Corticosteroids. Corticosteroids may provoke an acneform reaction regardless of their route of administration (Figure 88.14)

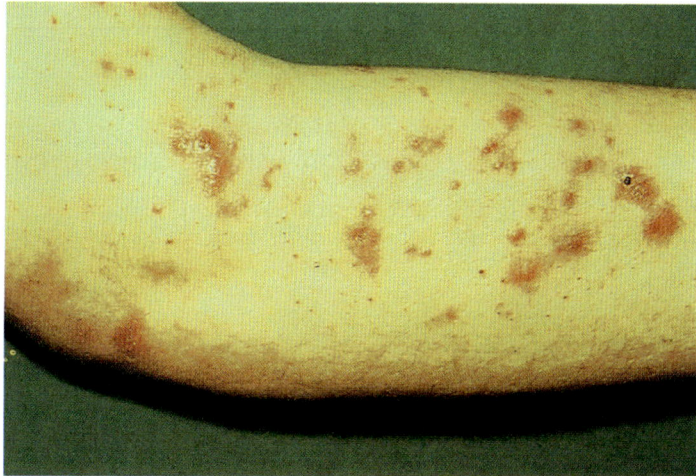

(a)

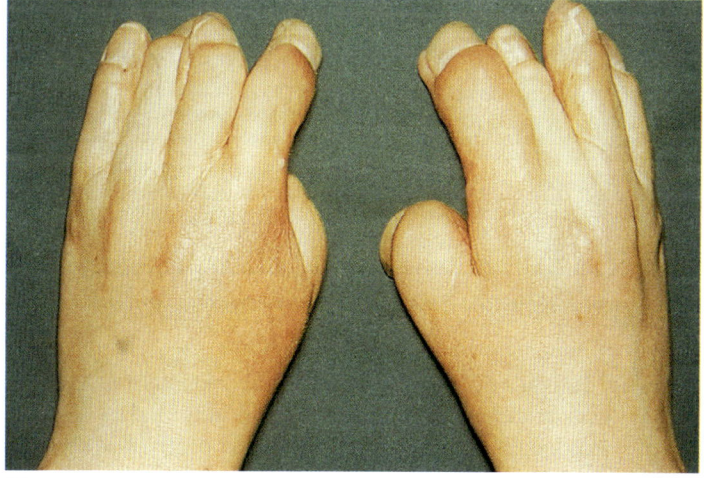

(b)

Figure 88.13 Apert syndrome. (a) The unusual extent of acne in a patient with Apert syndrome. (b) Typical appearance of the fingers of a patient with Apert syndrome.

[153–160]. The precise mechanism is uncertain. Steroid acne is usually more monomorphic than true acne vulgaris; however, both inflammatory and comedonal lesions may be present on the face, back and chest [160]. Abuse of androgenic anabolic steroids,

PART 8: SPECIFIC CUTANEOUS STRUCTURES

Table 88.6 Summary of PAPA spectrum disorders.

Syndrome (see text for name in full)	Involved gene or chromosomal alteration	Added features
PAPA	PSTPIP1	Pyogenic sterile arthritis, pyoderma gangrenosum and acne conglobata. Arthritis is the predominant feature, which is juvenile in onset and has a destructive course
PASH	PSTPIP1, NCSTN, MEFV, NOD2, NLRP3	Absence of pyogenic sterile arthritis distinguishes PASH syndrome from the PAPASH and PAPA syndromes
PASS	Unknown	Characterised by pyoderma gangrenosum, acne, hidradenitis suppurativa and spondylarthritis
PAPASH	PSTPIP1, IL1RN, MEFV	Similar to the PAPA syndrome with additional features of hidradenitis suppurativa
PsAPASH	Unknown	Pyoderma gangrenosum, acne, suppurative hidradenitis and psoriatic arthritis
PAC	PSTPIP1	Pyoderma gangrenosum, acne and ulcerative colitis
PAMI	PSTPIP1	Hypercalprotectinaemia and hyperzincaemia, raised serum myeloid-related protein plus hepatosplenomegaly, arthritis, pancytopenia and failure to thrive

IL1RN, interleukin 1 receptor antagonist; MEFV, Mediterranean fever; NCSTN, nicastrin; NLRP3, NOD-, LRR- and pyrin domain-containing protein 3; NOD2, nucleotide-binding oligomerisation domain-containing protein 2; PSTPIP1, proline/serine/threonine phosphatase interacting protein 1.

Table 88.7 Drug classes and types of medication that may exacerbate or cause acne.

Drug class or type	Examples
Corticosteroid:	
Topical	Betamethasone
Oral	Prednisolone
Inhaled	Budesonide
ACTH	ACTH, synthetic ACTH
Anabolic steroid/synthetic androgen	Danazol, nandrolone, stanozolol
Anticonvulsant	Carbamazepine, phenytoin, phenobarbitone, troxidone, gabapentin, topiramate
Antidepressant	Lithium, sertraline, vortioxetine
Other neuroleptic/antipsychotic	Pimozide, risperidone
Antitubercular	Isoniazid, pyrazinamide
Antineoplastic/EGFR antagonists	Dactinomycin, pentostatin, cetuximab
Antiviral	Ritonavir, ganciclovir
Calcium antagonist	Nilvadipine, nimodipine
Halogen	Sodium fluoride, potassium iodine
Human growth hormone	Genetically engineered human growth hormone
Vitamins	Vitamin B_{12}, possibly other B vitamins
Miscellaneous	Buserelin, cabergoline, ciclosporin, sirolimus, tacrolimus, clofazimine, dantrolene, disulfuram, famotidine, follitropin alfa, isosorbide mononitrate, medroxyprogesterone, mesalazine, quinine, ramipril, sulphur, thiouracil, thiourea

ACTH, adrenocorticotropic hormone; EGFR, epidermal growth factor receptor.

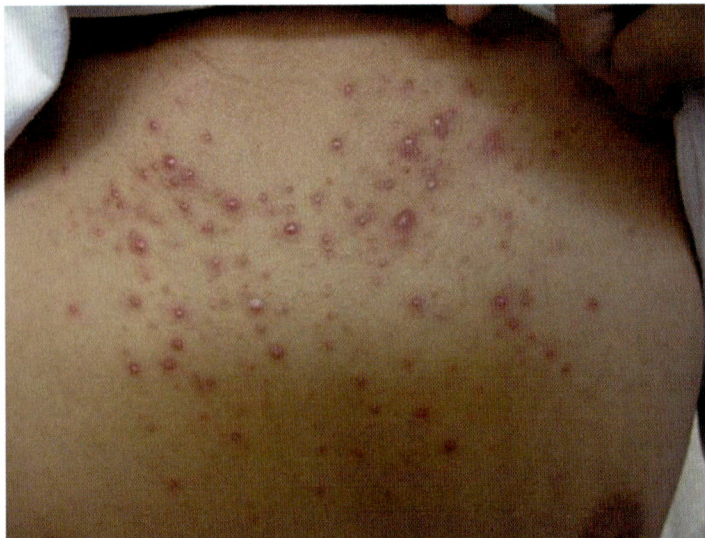

Figure 88.14 Monomorphic inflammatory papules and pustules associated with corticosteroid use. Courtesy of Dr S. Chow, KL Skin Centre, Malaysia.

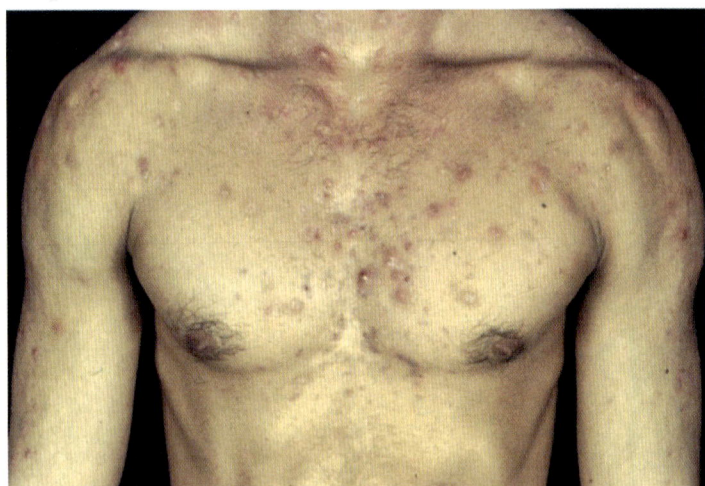

Figure 88.15 Severe acne vulgaris in a male body builder.

synthetic derivatives of testosterone and testosterone salts, can exacerbate acne vulgaris (Figure 88.15) and induce acne fulminans or acne conglobata [161]. Acne induction is partly due to androgen receptor binding leading to hypertrophy of the sebaceous glands with consequent increased sebum output and a concomitant increase in the population density of *Cutibacterium acnes*. However, not all androgenic anabolic steroids bind to the androgen receptor, suggesting that acne must be induced via other mechanisms [162,163]. Estimates suggest that as many as 43% of users have acne as a side effect [164].

Amino acid supplements. Branched-chain amino acids are becoming an increasingly popular exercise supplement, purported by the industry to help maintain and grow muscle mass, while reducing muscle fatigue. Leucine, an essential amino acid, is one of three branched-chain amino acids (the others are isolucine and valine) often found in protein supplements. Leucine stimulates mTORC1-SREBP signalling. Leucine is directly converted by sebocytes into fatty acids and sterols for sebaceous lipid synthesis and has been implicated in promoting acne [165,166].

Dehydroepiandrosterone A supplements. DHEA supplements are popular as they have been shown to increase lean body mass and decrease fat mass [167]. DHEA given in adrenal insufficiency reduces total cholesterol, improves well-being, sexual satisfaction and insulin sensitivity, and prevents loss of bone mineral density, making it hyped as an 'antiaging superhormone' whose benefits have been extrapolated to the general population [168]. However, side effects including hair loss and acne have been reported; this

is unsurprising given that DHEA is a major androgen ultimately responsible for the increased sebum production and recognised in acne pathogenesis.

Immunosuppressive drugs. Ciclosporin has been associated with induction of comedonal lesions 2–3 months after initiation of treatment and independent of dose. An acne-like eruption is seen as a consequence of immunosuppressive drugs used in transplant patients in up to 25% of cases [169]. The reaction may extend beyond the face and trunk, and a nodular component is common. Scalp folliculitis has been reported to occur within a few weeks of starting sirolimus [170]. Acne in this context can impact on quality of life (QoL) and may deter patients from taking their medication, particularly adolescent females [171]. Oral tacrolimus appears less likely to produce acneform reactions presumably due to the low accumulation in the skin. Localised acne has been reported in a patient using topical tacrolimus for vitiligo after 3 months of use [172]. Conventional acne therapies should be employed but if the acne

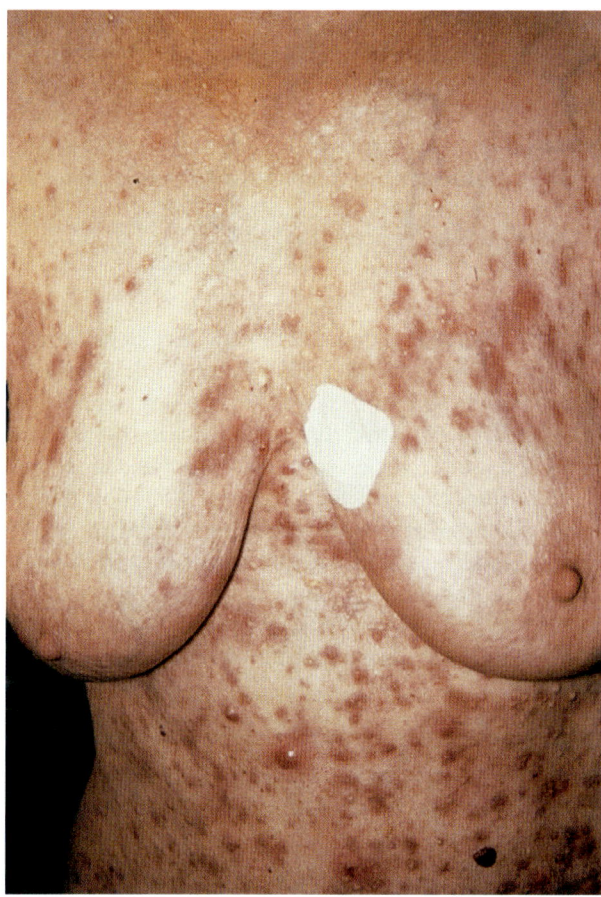

Figure 88.16 Lithium-induced acne which demonstrates an unusual location of the lesions beyond the seborrheic areas, a classical finding of drug-induced acneform rash. A monomorphic pattern is another common feature. Courtesy of Dr V. M. Yates, Royal Bolton Hospital, UK.

is severe and refractory, modification of the immunosuppressant therapy may be required.

Psychotropic drugs. Some psychoactive drugs including lithium (Figure 88.16), amineptine and vortioxetine can induce acne [173–178]. Lithium-induced acne frequently presents 2–3 months after starting therapy and severe forms such as acne conglobata have been described [176]. Male patients appear to be more susceptible to dermatological problems [177]. Lithium-induced acne is thought to occur through neutrophil chemotaxis and degranulation inducing an inflammatory cascade alongside a direct effect on follicular keratinocytes, leading to follicular plugging. Discontinuation of the lithium is recommended if possible. Tetracyclines can increase levels of lithium.

Most cases of amineptine-induced acne have involved adult females. Comedonal lesions are the most frequently seen lesions and inflammatory lesions are usually sparse. The mechanism has been postulated to be via selective decrease in the uptake of dopamine followed by an inhibitory effect of elevated dopamine on prolactin with subsequent increase in testosterone output [175]. Once 'acne' has been triggered, the drug should be withdrawn; response is variable and systemic therapy and physical treatment of the comedones may be required.

Progestins. Different progestins have varying androgenic effects (Box 88.3). The levonorgestrel-releasing intrauterine system, implants or mini-pills are all capable of exacerbating acne [179]. A recent review suggested that establishing the cause and effect is challenging and further research is required [180]. With the popularity of intrauterine progestogen contraceptives, often containing levonorgestrel, there is a delayed onset of acne.

Box 88.3 Relative androgenic effect of progestins in commonly used combined oral contraceptives and in implanted intrauterine contraceptives

Generic name	Androgenic effect
• Desogestrel	
• Norgestimate	
• Norethindrone	Increasing androgen effect
• Ethynodiol diacetate	
• Levonorgestrel	
• Norgestrel	
• Norethindrone	

Isoniazid. Slow inactivators of isoniazid may develop an acneform rash [181].

Antiepileptic drugs. Acne triggered by antiepileptic drugs has been reported but a study of hospitalised patients with severe epilepsy receiving different anticonvulsants, including phenytoin, showed no increased risk of acne compared with matched controls in the general population [182].

Iodides and bromides. Iodides and bromides commonly and rapidly cause follicular pustules [164,183]. Iodides may be found in non-prescription preparations for asthma, expectorants, kelp and teas. Sedatives and cold remedies often contain bromides. Chloracne (Figure 88.17) is a condition due to systemic poisoning most frequently found in occupational settings (see 'Occupational acne' later in this chapter). Dioxins are the most potent of these chemicals (Figure 88.18).

Vitamins B$_2$, B$_6$ and B$_{12}$. A monomorphic eruption consisting of small follicular inflammatory lesions on the forehead and chin, upper arms and trunk has been described with vitamin B$_{12}$ doses of 5–10 mg/day [184]. Women are almost exclusively affected and the onset of acne develops within the first 2 weeks post-injection. The acne-inducing dose of vitamin B$_6$ has not been established. A recent publication revealed that vitamin B$_{12}$ supplementation in *C. acnes* cultures promoted the production of porphyrins, which have been shown to induce inflammation in acne, providing a potential mechanism for this reaction [185]. Conventional acne therapies are usually unsuccessful but withdrawal of the drug results in resolution of the acneform rash within 10 days.

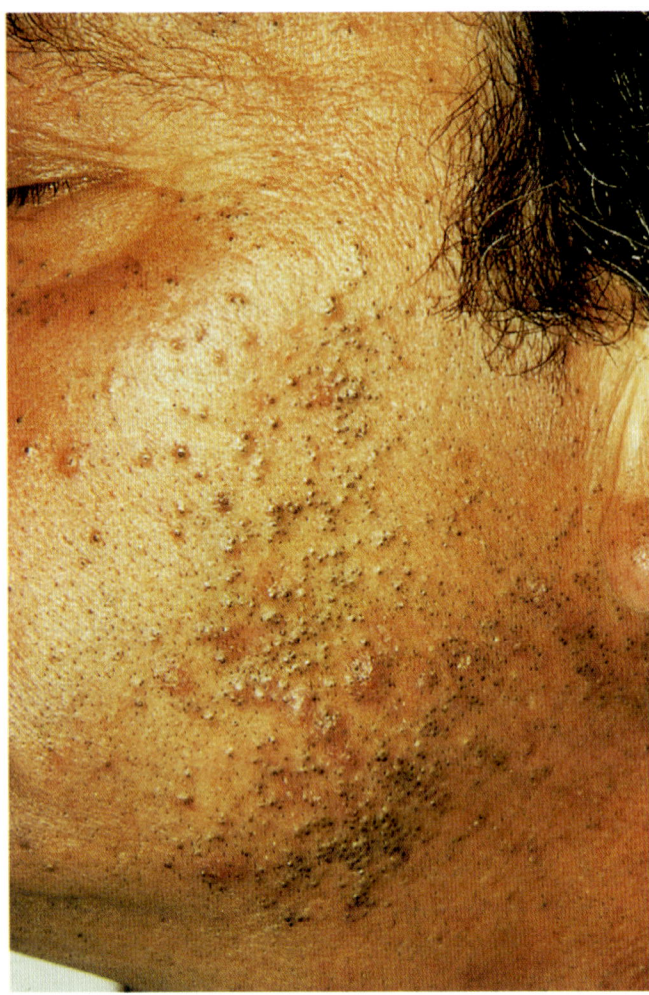

Figure 88.17 Chloracne showing multiple comedonal lesions on the face.

Epidermal growth factor receptor inhibitors. A follicular acneform eruption often within a few weeks of therapy has been reported in more than 50% of cancer patients treated with epidermal growth factor receptor inhibitors (Figure 88.19) [186,187]. The exact mechanism of how this occurs is not understood. Follicular papules and sterile pustules on the face and upper trunk occur and in severe cases the limbs may be affected. Comedones are not seen [188]. Histological examination of the lesions has found a superficial dermal inflammatory cell infiltrate surrounding a dilated follicular infundibulum. A direct correlation between efficacy to cancer therapy and severity of acneform reaction has been reported. Most reports suggest that topical acne therapies, oral tetracyclines and topical or oral corticosteroids are effective. Oral isotretinoin has also been used successfully [189].

Table 88.8 provides an aid for diagnosing acne associated with medications.

Pathophysiology

The classic concept is that acne results from the combination of increased sebaceous gland activity with seborrhoea, abnormal follicular differentiation with increased keratinisation, microbial hypercolonisation of the follicular canal and increased inflammation primarily through activation of the adaptive immune system. New research results have led to a modification of this classic explanation as more primary pathophysiological factors have been identified. Along with a genetic predisposition, other major factors include androgens, pro-inflammatory lipids such as ligands of sebocyte peroxisome proliferator-activated receptors (PPARs) and other inflammatory pathways. In addition, neuroendocrine regulatory mechanisms, diet and exogenous factors all may contribute to this multifactorial process [190–192,**193**].

Inflammation

Recently, there has been a debate as to whether hyperkeratinisation of the follicular duct precedes the influx of inflammatory cells or vice versa (Figure 88.20) [**193**]. Recent studies support the latter hypothesis by demonstrating that an increase in IL-1 activity occurs around uninvolved follicles and this triggers the activation of follicular keratinocytes and their hyperproliferation [**193**,**194**,195]. Expression profiling of acne-involved and uninvolved skin from acne patients and from subjects without acne via cDNA microarrays has provided a better insight into the aetiological factors giving rise to acne [196]. In inflammatory acne lesions, the majority of the upregulated genes are involved in inflammatory processes. These include matrix metalloproteinases, human β-defensin 4, IL-8 and granulysin. Nuclear factor κ B (NFκB), a transcription factor critical for upregulation of many pro-inflammatory cytokine genes, has been shown to be activated in acne lesions. NFκB-regulated cytokine mRNA levels of TNF-α, IL-1β, IL-8 and IL-10 are significantly upregulated in acne-involved skin compared with uninvolved normal adjacent skin [197]. Choi *et al.* showed that TNF-α induces lipogenesis in SZ95 sebocytes through the JNK and PI3K/Akt pathways [198]. IL-1β mRNA and the active processed form of IL-1β are abundant in inflammatory acne lesions [199].

Elevated expression of the chemokine IL-8 is able to attract inflammatory cells into the skin. Indeed, in early acne lesions (closed comedones), there is a marked increase in the presence of polymorphonuclear leukocytes as compared with the uninvolved skin, whereas lymphocytes are prominently visible in papules, pustules and nodules when compared to normal controls [197].

Kelhälä *et al.* illustrated the presence of IL-17A-positive T cells and the activation of Th17-related cytokines in acne lesions, indicating that the Th17 pathway is activated and may play a pivotal role in the disease process. However, additional studies are needed to assess the clinical relevance of IL-17 in acne [200]. Inflammation is further characterised by the action of active lipid mediators, such as leukotrienes, prostaglandins and 15-hydroxyeicosatetraenoic acids. These molecules are synthesised from arachidonic acid (AA) or linolenic acid by the enzymes lipoxygenase (LOX) and cyclo-oxygenase (COX), respectively. Both COX isozymes, COX-1 and COX-2, are expressed in human sebocytes *in vitro*, in particular COX-2 expression is selectively upregulated in acne-involved sebaceous glands *in vivo* [201]. Activation of the platelet-activating factor signalling pathway (1-*O*-alkyl-2-acetyl-*sn*-glycero-3-phosphocholine), which consists of a group of phosphocholines with various biological effects including modulation of keratinocyte function and skin inflammation, can regulate the expression of inflammatory mediators (e.g. COX-2 and prostaglandin E_2 (PGE_2)) as well as IL-8 in SZ95 sebocytes [202]. Transgenic keratin 5 promoter-driven overexpression of COX-2 in

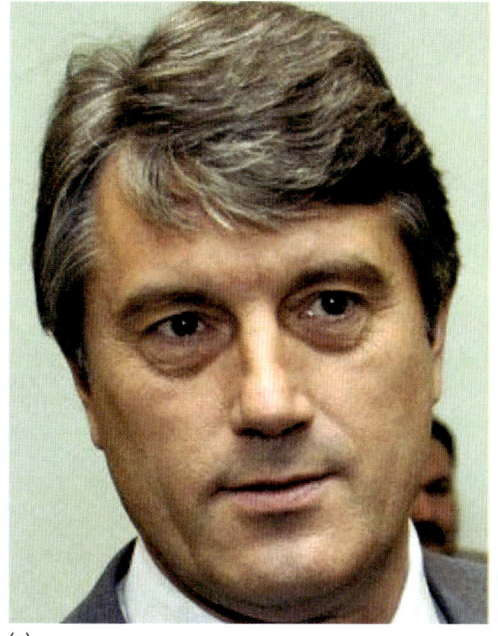 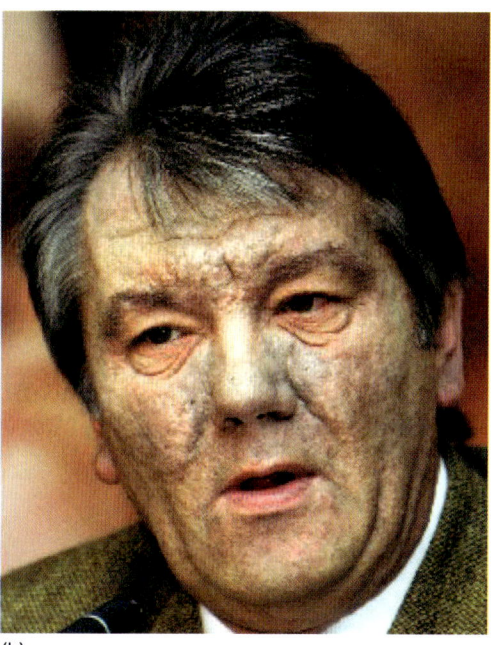

(a)   (b)

Figure 88.18 (a, b) Dioxin intoxication. Former president of Ukraine, Viktor Yushchenko, showing the effect of poisoning from 10 000 ppt tetrachlorodibenzodioxin (b). From BBC News; https://www.bbc.com/news/av/world-europe-43611547 (last accessed October 2023).

the basal compartment of the epidermis of the mouse and increased PGE_2 levels have been documented to cause sebaceous gland hyperplasia and overshooting sebum production. This points to a role of COX-2-mediated PGE_2 synthesis in this process [203].

Activation of PPAR-γ by UVB irradiation and the potent lipid-soluble oxidant *tert*-butylhydroperoxide induces COX-2 expression in SZ95 sebocytes. This finding indicates a PPAR-γ/COX-2-mediated pathway regulating sebocyte proliferation and/or lipogenesis [204].

Conversely, leukotrienes are potent pro-inflammatory mediators and neutrophil attractants produced from AA by 5-LOX. Human sebocytes express all the necessary enzymes for a functional leukotriene (LT) pathway. The enzymes 5-LOX and LTA_4 hydrolase are expressed in SZ95 sebocytes at the protein and mRNA levels. These enzymes are essential for the formation of LTB_4. However, 15-LOX shows a weak expression in SZ95 sebocytes, indicating that sebocytes do not play a significant role in the biosynthesis of the anti-inflammatory 15-HETE. Treatment of SZ95 sebocytes with AA stimulates 5-LOX expression and induces LTB_4 synthesis. In addition, AA induces the expression of the IL-6 and IL-8 cytokines. 5-LOX and LTA_4 hydrolase show a stronger expression in acne lesions than in normal skin and in uninvolved skin of acne patients. The involvement of 5-LOX in the pathogenesis of acne has led to new therapeutic strategies to deal with the disease, such as the 5-LOX inhibitor zileuton [205].

Neurophysiology

Human skin and in particular the human sebaceous gland has been shown to express functional receptors for neuropeptides (Figure 88.21) such as corticotropin-releasing hormone [206,207], the most proximal element of the HPA axis, melanocortins [195,208–211], β-endorphin, vasoactive intestinal polypeptide, neuropeptide Y and calcitonin gene-related peptide [212].

These receptors modulate the production of inflammatory cytokines, proliferation, differentiation, lipogenesis and androgen metabolism in human sebocytes [209–211,213]. Substance P, which can be elicited by stress, may promote the development of cytoplasmic organelles in sebaceous cells, stimulate sebaceous germinative cells and induce significant increases in the area of sebaceous glands. It also increases the size of individual sebaceous cells and the number of sebum vacuoles for each differentiated sebaceous cell, all of which suggests that substance P promotes both the proliferation and the differentiation of sebaceous gland cells. Facial skin from acne patients is characterised by rich innervation, by increased numbers of substance P-containing nerves and mast cells, and by strong expression of neutral endopeptidase (a potent neuropeptide-degrading enzyme) in sebaceous glands and E-selectin in venules around sebaceous glands, compared with normal skin [214,215]. These findings are attributed to local substance P activity. Recently, the ectopeptidases dipeptidyl peptidase IV (DP IV or CD26) and aminopeptidase N (APN or CD13), which have been shown to be involved in the degradation of several neuropeptides, especially substance P, have been found to be highly expressed in human sebocytes *in vivo* and *in vitro*. Further studies have shown unexpectedly that inhibitors of DP IV and APN can suppress proliferation and slightly decrease neutral lipids, but can also enhance terminal differentiation in SZ95 sebocytes. This suggests that ectopeptidases may be new targets to modulate certain sebocyte functions, and that ectopeptidase inhibitors may have potential therapeutic roles in acne pathogenesis [216].

Causative organisms

Propionibacterium acnes is a Gram-positive anaerobic rod commonly associated with acne vulgaris. In 2016, Scholz *et al.* [217] proposed a reclassification of the species within the genus *Propionibacterium* to the novel genus *Cutibacterium*. However, it is considered valid to continue to use the genus name *Propionibacterium* for the cutaneous

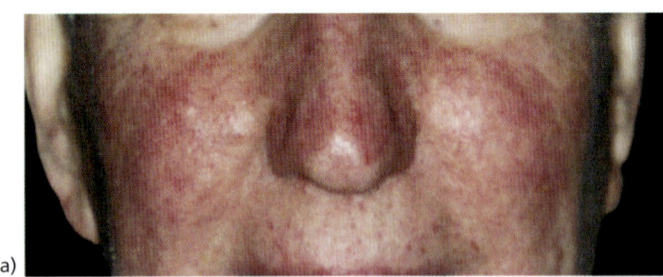

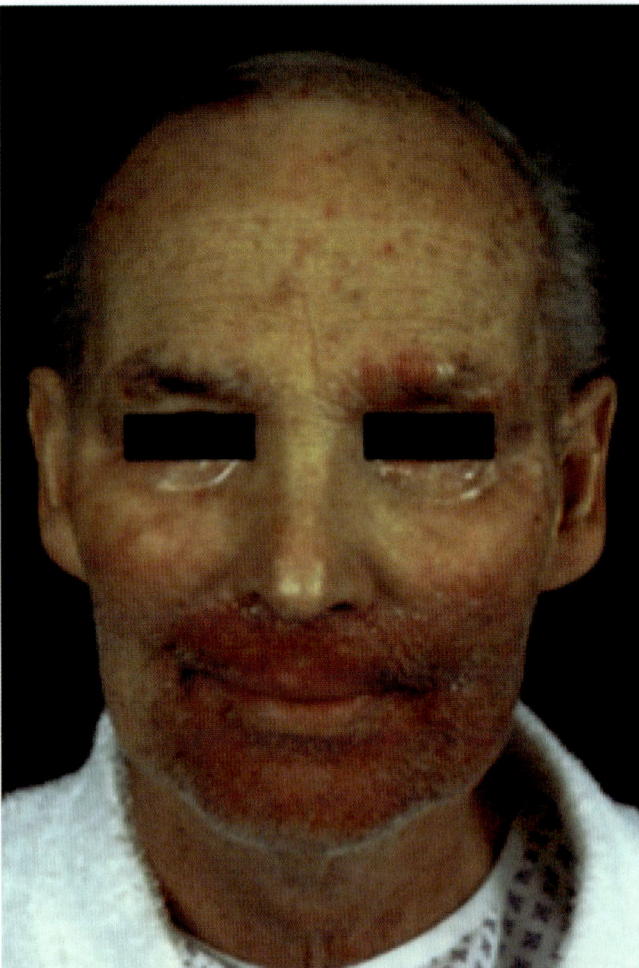

(a)

(b)

Figure 88.19 (a) Epidermal growth factor receptor (EGFR) inhibitor producing follicular acneform eruption on the face of a patient receiving treatment for colonic cancer. (b) Confluent perifollicular papules and pustules covered by yellowish crusts and prominent in the hairy regions of the scalp, the eyebrows and the beard under EGFR inhibitor treatment. (b) From Treudler and Zouboulis 2005 [309] with permission from S. Karger AG, Basel.

Table 88.8 Diagnosing drug-related acneform skin disease.

History	Secure a detailed history to include:
	• Onset of drug treatment
	• Dosage regimen
	• Duration of treatment
Exacerbating factors	Exclude triggers:
	• Hormonal therapy
	• Occupation
	• Cosmetics
	• Environmental factors
Temporal relationship of the treatment	Establish the relationship between:
	• The start of the drug and the clinical signs
	• Improvement on withdrawal of the drug

strain population structures were significantly different in the two cohorts. Certain strains were highly associated with acne, and other strains were enriched in healthy skin highlighting the importance of strain-level analysis of the human microbiome [219]. *P. acnes* strains modulate the expression of immune markers differently both at gene and at protein levels. *P. acnes* type III shows the highest pro-inflammatory potential by upregulating the expression of protease-activated receptor 2, TNF-α, matrix metalloproteinase 13 and tissue inhibitor of matrix metalloproteinases [220]. Treatment of cultured sebocytes with *P. acnes* and bacterial antigens (lipopolysaccharide (LPS)) significantly upregulates the expression of pro-inflammatory cytokines [221]. However, there is a difference in the cytokine production curve over time after treatment between *P. acnes* and LPS. While LPS stimulates CXCL8, TNF-α and IL-1α, *P. acnes* only stimulates CXCL8 and TNF-α; *P. acnes* has no effect on IL-1α. Furthermore, viable *P. acnes* – but not heat-killed organisms – can stimulate the release of cytokines such as IL-1β, granulocyte–macrophage colony-stimulating factor (GM-CSF) and IL-8 [222,223]. New reports suggest that *P. acnes* induces IL-17 expression in peripheral blood mononuclear cells and present evidence that IL-17+ cells are found in the perifollicular infiltrate of comedones, indicating that acne might be a T-helper type 17 (Th17) mediated disease [224]. In accordance with this, Kistowska *et al.* showed that, in addition to IL-17A, both Th1 and Th17 effector cytokines, transcription factors and chemokine receptors are strongly upregulated in acne lesions. *P. acnes* can promote mixed Th17/Th1 responses by inducing the concomitant secretion of IL-17A and interferon γ (IFN-γ) from specific CD4+ T cells *in vitro* [225]. *P. acnes* also triggers monocyte, macrophage and sebocyte NACHT, LRR and PYD domain-containing protein 3 (NLRP3) inflammasome activation [226].

Knocking down the expression of NLRP3 abolishes *P. acnes*-induced IL-1β production in sebocytes. The activation of the NLRP3 inflammasome by *P. acnes* is dependent on protease activity and reactive oxygen species generation [230]. Keratinocytes and sebocytes may act as immune cells capable of pathogen recognition and abnormal lipid presentation. Both cell types can be activated by *P. acnes* via Toll-like receptors (TLRs) and CD14 and CD1 molecules [231–233]. TLR2 is expressed in basal and infundibular keratinocytes and sebaceous glands, and its activation provokes the release of IL-1α from primary human keratinocytes *in vitro* [234].

group where needed to avoid confusion with earlier nomenclature which referred to corynebacterial acnes [218]. Many authors have now started to refer to *P. acnes* as *C. acnes* and this section uses them interchangeably according to the nomenclature used in the publication being discussed.

Fitz-Gibbon *et al.* compared the skin microbiome at the strain level and genome level of *P. acnes* (Figure 88.22) between 49 acne patients and 52 healthy individuals by sampling the pilosebaceous units on their noses [219]. Metagenomic analysis demonstrated that although the relative abundances of *P. acnes* were similar, the

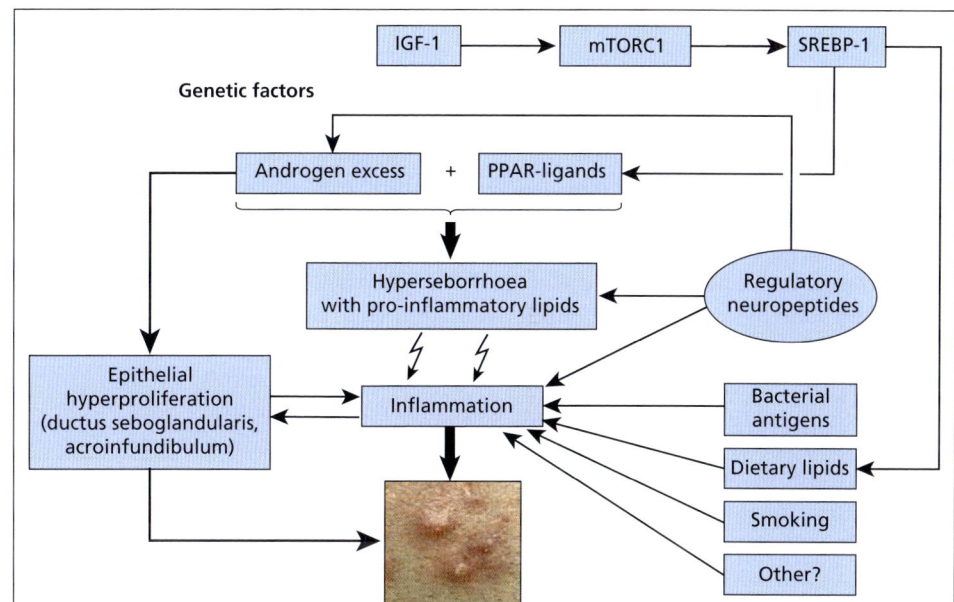

Figure 88.20 Inflammatory cascades involved in acne pathogenesis. IGF-1, insulin-like growth factor 1; mTORC1, mammalian target of rapamycin complex 1; PPAR, peroxisome proliferator-activated receptor; SREBP-1, sterol response element-binding protein 1. Adapted from Zouboulis *et al.* 2005 [2] with permission from John Wiley & Sons.

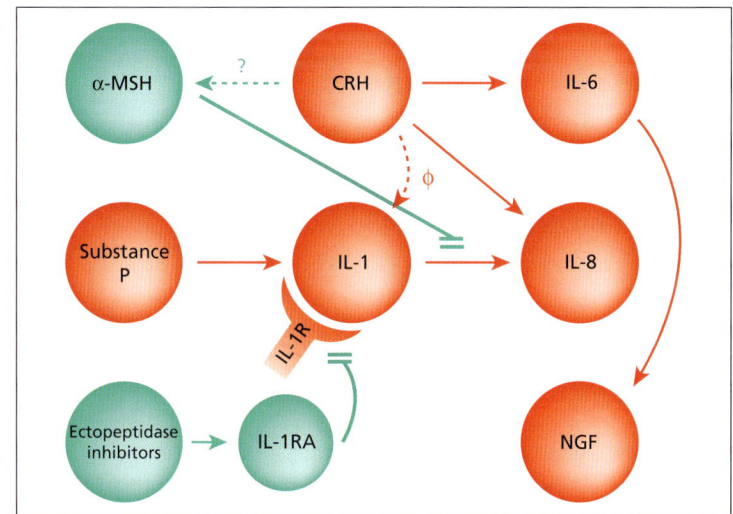

Figure 88.21 Neuropeptide–cytokine/chemokine signalling in human sebaceous glands and human sebocytes. Red: promoter of inflammation. Blue: inhibition of inflammation. α-MSH, α-melanocyte-stimulating hormone; CRH, corticotrophin-releasing hormone; IL, interleukin; II-1RA, II-1 receptor antagonist; NGF, neural growth factor; Ø, no influence; ?, unknown regulation in sebocytes; =, inhibition. From Zouboulis 2009 [735].

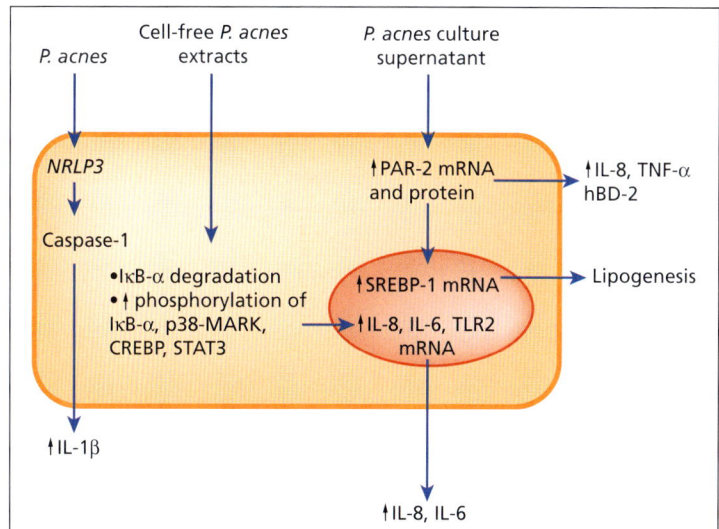

Figure 88.22 Effects of *Propionibacterium acnes* extracts on human sebocytes. CREBP, cAMP response element-binding protein; hBD-2, human β-defensin 2; IL, interleukin; p38-MAPK, p38 mitogen-activated protein kinase; PAR-2, protease-activated receptor 2; SREBP-1, sterol response element-binding protein 1; STAT3, signal transducer and activator of transcription 3; TLR2, Toll-like receptor 2; TNF, tumour necrosis factor. Courtesy of Lee *et al.* 2015 [227], Huang *et al.* 2015 [228] and Li *et al.* 2014 [229].

Bakry *et al.* documented statistically significant differences between acne-involved skin and normal skin and between acne-involved and non-involved skin regarding TLR2 expression intensity in pilosebaceous units and dermal inflammatory infiltrate [234]. Qin *et al.* showed that *P. acnes* induces robust IL-1β secretion in monocytes by triggering the activation of the NLRP3 inflammasome. *In vivo*, the encounter of *P. acnes* and macrophages in the perifollicular dermis could locally result in the release of substantial amounts of IL-1β and therefore exacerbate inflammation [235].

Human sebaceous glands may contribute to the skin immune defence by releasing antimicrobial peptides. For example, psoriasin, human β-defensins and cathelicidin are expressed in human pilosebaceous units, their expression is upregulated in acne lesions

[236,236a] and the levels are upregulated in the presence of *P. acnes* [222,237]. Each *P. acnes* strain has been shown to influence sebocyte viability and differentiation differently, which raises the possibility that certain *P. acnes* strains may be responsible for opportunistic infections worsening acne lesions [222,237,238].

A description of phylogenetically distinct *P. acnes* clusters has been already undertaken [238]. The monounsaturated fatty acids (MUFAs), mainly palmitoleic acid (C16:1) and oleic acid (C18:1) – both of which are bactericidal against Gram-positive organisms [239] – and stearoyl coenzyme A desaturase (SCD) 1, an enzyme responsible for the biosynthesis of MUFA, are also produced by the sebaceous glands [239]. The TLR-2 ligand macrophage-activating lipopeptide 2 stimulates both SCD and fatty acid desaturase 2 mRNA expression in SZ95 sebocytes [240]. Lauric acid (C12:0), one of the sebum free fatty acids (FFAs), has strong antimicrobial activity *in vitro* against skin bacteria, including *P. acnes*. Topical application or intradermal injection of lauric acid *in vivo* shows remarkable therapeutic effectiveness against *P. acnes*-induced inflammation and a significant reduction in the number of bacteria. Furthermore, lauric acid, palmitic acid (16:0) and oleic acid (C18:1, *cis*-9), which are the typical FFAs found in human sebum, enhanced the human β-defensin 2 expression and antimicrobial activity of human sebocytes against *P. acnes* [241]. This indicates that sebum FFAs are involved in the disinfecting activity of the human skin both through their direct antimicrobial characteristics and by inducing the expression of antimicrobial peptides in human sebocytes to enhance their innate immune defence ability [241].

Genetics

Twin studies show that inherited factors influence the acne phenotype in monozygotic and to a lesser extent dizygotic twins [243]. An Australian twin study estimated heritability at 0.85 (95%CI 0.82–0.87) [244]. Large cohort studies show that the risk of acne in a first-degree relative of someone who has had acne is approximately four to five times higher than in relatives of unaffected individuals [245,246]. A similar odds ratio has been found for the risk of adult (persistent or late-onset) acne in first-degree relatives of patients with acne aged 25 years or over [247].

A number of other studies have found adolescent and adult acne to be present in first- and second-degree relatives of acne patients at higher rates than in relatives of people without acne [248,249].

Heritability or susceptibility to adolescent acne seems to be more strongly linked to the maternal than to the paternal line and risk increases as more family members are affected [249–251]. Studies in different settings have confirmed that acne occurs earlier in patients with a positive family history and may affect clinical presentation and treatment outcomes [251].

There are a number of heritable traits that might predispose to acne (Table 88.9). Walton *et al.* [250] found greater concordance between sebum excretion rates (SERs) in monozygotic than dizygotic twins. Bataille *et al.* reported that 81% (95%CI 73–87%) of the variance of the disease in a twin study was attributable to additive genetic effects. The remaining 19% was attributed to unique (i.e. unshared) environmental factors. Of the potential risk factors tested in 400 acne twins and 2414 unaffected twins, only apolipoprotein A1 serum levels were significantly lower in acne twins even after adjusting for age and weight [251]. Genome-wide association studies in patients with severe acne continue to identify a growing number of loci that contribute to disease risk, and severity with variance of loci among different ethnic populations has been noted [252–254]. Functional characterisation of the genes at these loci implicates genes that impact on hair follicle development and maintenance and wound healing. A recent meta-analysis identified 29 new acne susceptibility loci, providing the potential to explore new therapeutic modalities [255].

Table 88.9 Heritable traits that may predispose to acne.

Factor	Effect
Sebum excretion rate (SER)	High SER predisposes – numerous genetic loci affecting sebaceous gland size and lipogenesis have been identified
Sebum composition	Poorly understood and may also be modulated by diet
Innate and acquired immune responses	Poorly understood – a number of candidate genes have been identified
Sex	Adolescent acne begins earlier in girls but tends to be more severe in males; being female is a risk factor for postadolescent acne
Ethnicity	Poorly understood; acne may be uncommon in all racial groups that have not adopted a western/urban lifestyle

Table 88.10 Lifestyle and environmental factors that may predispose to acne.

Factor	Strength of evidence
Diet	Moderate for glycaemic index and milk/milk products, low for other foodstuffs
Body mass index	Low
Smoking	High for comedonal acne in mature women with a history of chronic smoking; otherwise low
Alcohol consumption	Low
Psychological stress	Low
Cosmetics	Low
Prescription medicines	High for some drugs, low for others
Anabolic and androgenic steroids	High
Seasonal factors	High
Sunlight	Low
Lack of sleep/insomnia	Low

Environmental factors

A plethora of lifestyle and environmental factors that predispose to acne or modulate its course have been reported although data are frequently contradictory (Table 88.10). Confounding factors are multiple and frequently not controlled for. Systematic reviews have pooled data to summarise the factors that significantly modify the risk of presenting with acne [256].

The impact of diet continues to stimulate most debate and there has been a surge in studies focused on this. In most countries, it is rare to find families of any racial background with no acne. In contrast, acne is absent in some ethnic groups living in remote communities, for example the Kitavan Islanders of Papua New Guinea and the Aché hunter-gatherers of Paraguay do not suffer from acne in their native communities. Canadian Inuit only began to develop acne and other diseases of western civilisation following the urbanisation of their communities [257,258]. Leading epidemiologists have speculated that this is attributable to diet rather than race. Diet in these communities is characterised by local production and constancy, as well as a low consumption of milk, meat and processed carbohydrates. Academic interest has focused on milk, dairy produce and high glycaemic index (GI) foods as potential triggers for acne.

Diet. Many acne sufferers believe that diet modulates their skin condition [259–262] and unhealthy foods in particular are considered to make acne worse [263–265]. Some cross-sectional studies appear to support this [262,265,266] whereas others have found no link between diet and acne on multivariate analysis [25,52]. Like many other western diseases, acne is now also being linked to the obesity epidemic and to the rising prevalence of insulin resistance and hyperinsulinaemia [267]. A 2021 review by Baldwin and Tan summarises the most pivotal studies looking at the effect of diet on acne [**268**].

There has been a paucity of randomised controlled trials (RCTs) examining the link between diet and acne due to numerous possible confounding variables. Several investigators have used case–control, prospective cohort or cross-sectional studies to examine the link between current diet and acne and have adjusted odds ratios to take account of potential confounders. Table 88.11 excludes studies prior to 1990 that do not meet current quality standards. Trends and inconsistencies have begun to emerge. This demonstrates that several studies have shown a link between a high glycaemic load (GL) diet and acne while others have found no association [269–296].

More recent studies have focused on examining the mechanism by which diet may impact on acne. High GI/GL diet is thought to increase mTORC1 signal production. In acne, mTORC1 mediates sebaceous gland hyperproliferation, lipid synthesis and hyperplasia of keratinocytes [297–299].

IGF-1 has also been implicated [300]. Investigations of serum markers have been conducted in several studies examining the effects of a low GI diet but findings are contradictory [271,273, 274,280]. Dairy is a common constituent of western diets, and milk consumption has been reported to increase ILGF-1 [301]. Three studies from the same group consistently found that milk intake increased the risk of acne. However, it is unclear whether the risk is the same for whole and skimmed milk [302]. Other studies have also shown increased milk consumption in people with acne without testing for a causal link (Table 88.11). A meta-analysis of observational studies looking at the effect of milk consumption on acne found a significant increase of acne incidence in milk drinkers and that moderate to severe acne was linked to milk consumption, but that mild acne showed no association [302]. This was also demonstrated in a systematic review of all dairy products, which reported an association with yoghurt consumption, but borderline association for cheese [303].

A case–control study argued that a large number of foodstuffs such as red meat and chicken do not have any GI value as they do not have any carbohydrate value, hence the insulin index should be evaluated instead. When they looked at 202 acne patients against matched controls (sex and body mass index (BMI)) using logistic regression analysis they showed ≥3 servings of cola, instant coffee with powdered milk, feta cheese, and ≥1 serving of peanuts consumption were significantly higher in patients with acne [304]. A positive correlation was found between the global acne grading system (GAGS) score and cola consumption. The insulin index value is higher than the GI of cola, milk, feta and peanuts and the authors suggested it is the raised insulin index rather than the GI

that is the likely cause for the association of milk with acne [304]. Any definite link with dairy products such as yoghurt, cheese and chocolate remains unproven.

Non-food components are rarely considered in studies examining the impact of diet. Modern foodstuffs contain many ingredients, and a lot of these are biologically active. Reduced level of zinc, calcium and vitamin A have been demonstrated in acne patients compared with controls [305,306].

While many foods are considered acne-genic, others are under scrutiny because they may protect against acne. To date, most interest has been in healthy diets (e.g. Mediterranean, Paleolithic) and fish/fish oils/polyunsaturated fatty acids [236,266,285,307,308]. In a small randomised dietary intervention study, Ω-3 fatty acid and γ-linoleic acid supplementation were independently shown to reduce acne severity and the amount of IL-8 around acne lesions [310]. The skin and gut microbiota and probiotics are an increasing area of interest for their therapeutic potential [311–318].

A prospective, randomised, open-label trial comparing oral minocycline with and without a probiotic supplement showed significant improvement and fewer *Candida* infections in the probiotic group compared with the minocycline alone group [319]. Another study on 36 acne patients showed that consuming a fermented dairy drink containing *Lactobacillus* improved acne within 12 weeks [320]. Further investigation into the use of probiotics in clinical practice is necessary to support these early findings.

Body mass index. Numerous studies have examined the relationship between acne and BMI, especially in adult women as acne and obesity coexist as symptoms of PCOS (Table 88.12) [321–341]. Taken together, studies to date suggest the risk of having acne and the severity appear to increase with age-adjusted BMI in adolescents. Paradoxically, acne may be less prevalent in overweight women with postadolescent acne [341].

25-Hydroxy vitamin D_3. At a molecular level vitamin D has been demonstrated to reduce serum inflammatory biomarker expression and inhibit C. *acnes*-induced Th-17 differentiation and increase antimicrobial peptide production in sebocytes [342]. The clinical impact of 25-hydroxy vitamin D on acne has been examined by a number of studies showing an association between deficiency and acne prevalence, but no difference in acne severity [343–346].

Smoking. The weight of evidence suggests smoking has little, if any, effect on the prevalence or severity of acne in teenagers and young adults. Some studies have found acne is more common in postadolescent smokers [347]. Mature women who are persistent smokers seem to be susceptible to a particular type of acne, characterised by numerous comedones and macrocomedones [347]. In a large cross-sectional study, people without acne were more likely than those with acne to use tobacco, whereby smoking tobacco reduced the probability of acne by approximately 30% [348]. Maternal cigarette smoking has been found to be associated with earlier onset of acne but not of puberty in their sons [349].

PART 8: SPECIFIC CUTANEOUS STRUCTURES

Table 88.11 Key findings from pivotal studies on acne and diet.

Type of study and reference	Main findings	Strength of evidence and reason	Reference
Two arm investigator-blind RCT comparing low GI and normal diet over 12 weeks	Low GI diet significantly reduced acne severity, fasting insulin, DHEAS and FAI, and increased SHBG and IGFBP-1	**Low.** Low GI and normal diet differed in several other respects. Changes could be partly associated with weight loss in low GI group	[269]
RCT (subset of 2007)	No change in the amount of sebum produced on low GI diet. Ratio of saturated fatty acids to mono-unsaturated fatty acids increased significantly in low GI group and correlated with decrease in total lesion count	Strong evidence that diet affects sebum composition but not (in this case) sebum output. Cannot attribute change to GI though	[270]
Case–control study in young adults with and without acne	Significantly lower IGF-1 and markedly raised IGFBP-3 in acne patients but no difference in GI or GL. No insulin resistance associated with acne	**Low.** Dietary information unreliable; GI estimated by questionnaire. Calculation of GI and GL flawed by exclusion of numerous CHO-containing foods	[271]
Seven-day controlled feeding trial comparing high and low GI diet in 12 males with acne	Fasting insulin and HOMA-IR index significantly reduced in low GI group. FAI markedly increased in high GI group. IGFBP-1 and IGFBP-3 rose in low GI group compared with baseline	Some preliminary evidence from this study that the low GL diet improved insulin sensitivity but small sample size and males only	[272]
Case–control study in 47 355 US nurses	Milk (but not chocolate or chips) especially skimmed milk intake associated with severe acne. Positive correlations also found for total and supplemental vitamin D	**Low.** Acne status (except severe – verified by physician) and milk consumption during adolescence based on recall. Associations of acne and dietary components were weak. All grades less than severe acne included in control group	[273]
Prospective cohort studies in 6094 girls and 4273 boys aged 9–15 years in USA	Found greater milk consumption was associated with acne in girls and boys. No association with vitamin D	**Low.** Annual questionnaire study in which acne and diet were self-assessed. In girls, association was for all types of milk, in boys for skimmed milk only. Adjusted odds ratios all 1.2 or less	[274,275]
Cross-sectional study in 1002 Iranian students	Regular consumption of sweets, nuts, chocolates and oily foods was associated with increased acne severity	**Low.** Incomplete dietary information collected but acne was clinically assessed	[275a]
Cross-sectional study in 18- and 19-year-olds in Oslo, Sweden	No association of acne with consumption of sugary soft drinks or fatty fish. In males, significant associations were found with chocolate/sweets and crisps. In females, the only dietary association was with low intake of raw vegetables	**Low.** Acne self-reported and prevalence lower than expected in both sexes. Dietary associations differed between the sexes. In adjusted models, only the link with raw vegetables remained	[276]
Case–control study in 1245 Koreans (783 with acne)	Consumption of vegetable and fish significantly lower in those with acne. Consumption of selected meats, junk food, nuts, fizzy drinks and high GL foods higher in the acne group. Irregular dietary patterns also more prevalent in the acne group. Serum IGF-1 raised in subgroup who thought their acne was aggravated by food	**Moderate.** Acne was clinically assessed	[262]
Comparison of high and low GI diets over 8 weeks in adolescent males	Acne improved slightly on both diets – no significant difference between the groups. IGFBP-1 fell significantly on the low GI diet versus the high GI diet. IGF-1, IGFBP-3, SHBG, DHEAS and HOMA-IR unchanged	**Low.** Not random allocation. Underpowered. Findings inconsistent with those of Smith *et al*. Other dietary components more balanced in this study. Can infer from discussion there was no weight loss on low GI diet	[276a]
Case–control study in Italians aged 10–24 years	Cases drank significantly more milk (whole and skimmed) and ate less fish than controls	**Moderate.** Control group included mild acne. Acne was physician assessed from photos. Major foods (e.g. cereals, rice, yoghurt) omitted from questionnaire	[277]
Case–control study in Malaysians aged 18–30 years	GL and consumption of milk and ice cream significantly higher in cases than controls. BMI same in both groups. No difference in consumption of chocolate, nuts or yoghurt. Adjusted odds ratios for GL lost significance except for GL >175, for which the risk of acne was increased 25-fold	**Moderate.** Diet assessed from 3-day food diaries	[278]
Investigator-blind RCT comparing low glycaemic load diet and a calorie-adjusted control diet over 10 weeks	Low GL diet reduced global acne severity, inflamed and non-inflamed lesion counts at 10 weeks; inflamed lesion count also reduced at week 5. Although significant, reductions were modest. Reduced sebaceous gland size and less IL-8 observed in skin of the low GI group	**Moderate.** Small sample size ($n = 32$). No change in BMI in either group	[279]

(continued)

Table 88.11 (*continued*)

Type of study and reference	Main findings	Strength of evidence and reason	Reference
Case–control study in Italian adolescents investigating the effect of a Mediterranean diet on acne	Adherence to a Mediterranean diet, characterised by high intake of vegetables, fruit, nuts, cereals, fish and olive oil and low intake of dairy products and meat, was significantly less in group with acne. Score of ≥6 is protective	**Moderate.** Examined patterns of consumption over a long period. Collected data on intake of specific food items but did not report these. Adherence to the diet was categorised as low (score 0–2), moderate (3–6) or high (7–9)	[280]
Cross-sectional study in 248 young adults aged 18–25 years in the USA	Participants with moderate to severe acne reported significantly greater dietary GI, added sugar, total sugar, number of milk servings per day, saturated fat and transfatty acids, and fewer servings of fish per day compared with those with no or mild acne	**Moderate.** Used a validated food frequency questionnaire. Acne self-assessed against given set of criteria	[265]
Pilot open study in 10 US males who consumed increasing amounts of 100% chocolate bars	Total number of acne lesions increased on day 4 and day 7. Good correlation between the amount of chocolate consumed and the number of lesions	**Low.** Open study. Risk of expectation bias	[281]
Double-blind, placebo-controlled RCT in 13 US males aged 18–35 years with minimal acne comparing a single exposure to increasing amounts of unsweetened 100% cocoa versus hydrolysed gelatin	Significant exacerbation of acne (total lesions and comedones) noted on day 4 and day 7 post consumption of cocoa. Inflamed lesions increased on day 4 only. Low correlation with dose of cocoa consumed	**Low.** Only two subjects studied per dose. Data for all doses combined to generate means	[282]
Cross-sectional study in 10 521 people age 15–24 years from Belgium, Czech and Slovak Republics, France, Italy, Poland and Spain	Chocolate, but not pasta or sweets, consumption was independently associated with acne in multivariate analysis	**Moderate.** Large sample size, but acne self-reported using a new unvalidated online questionnaire	[283]
Parallel randomised controlled design to compare the effect of a low GI and GL diet to usual diet on biochemical factors after 2 weeks	GF-1 concentrations decreased significantly among participants randomised to a low GI and GL diet between pre- and postintervention time points. No differences in changes in glucose, insulin or IGFBP-3 concentrations or insulin resistance between treatment groups	**Moderate.** RCT design. No weight loss in low GI group. No assessment made on acne severity	[284]
Cross-sectional study of young, non-obese people with acne and healthy controls	GI and GL levels were significantly higher ($P = 0.022$ and $P = 0.001$, respectively) and serum adiponectin levels were significantly lower ($P = 0.015$) in patients with acne than in the controls	**Low.** Cross-sectional design, small sample size $n = 50$. Acne not assessed	[285]
Cross-sectional study of 24 452 participants in the French NutriNet-Santé study	Fatty and sugary products, sugary beverages and milk were associated with current acne in adults after adjusting for confounders	**Moderate.** Large sample size and 24-hour dietary record more accurate than frequency questionnaire. Unclear whether the association of chocolate and confectionery consumption with acne was due to the high GI of these foods or whether having acne causes an increased intake of chocolate and sweets	[286]
Cohort study of 2489 15–16-year-olds with 3 years' follow-up	High intakes (≥2 glasses per day) of full-fat dairy products were associated with moderate to severe acne. No significant associations were found between acne and intake of semiskimmed or skimmed dairy products, and not with moderate intakes of any fat variety of dairy products	**Moderate.** Potential for recall bias. Dairy product consumption and acne severity were self-reported	[287]
Case–control study ($n = 3826$ and 759 controls)	Positive correlation with chocolate, bread, green tea, milk, white sugar, ripe banana, ice cream, apple, orange and red meat consumption. Statistically significant relationship for acne severity and dietary factors such as chocolate, dairy and sunflower seed consumption	**Moderate.** Only included patients with mild/moderate to severe acne. Data collected by consecutive interviews	[288]
Cross-sectional study of 2201 18-year-old males	Daily consumption of whole milk or yoghurt was found to be associated with inflammatory acne in crude analysis; the association with milk was not detected and that with yoghurt was low in multivariate analysis	**Low.** Acne graded by assessor and females not included	[52]

(*continued*)

Table 88.11 (*continued*)

Type of study and reference	Main findings	Strength of evidence and reason	Reference
Case–control study (*n* = 40 and 20 controls)	Significantly higher serum IGF-1 level found in patients with acne compared with controls and cytoplasmic expression of FoxO1 was significantly greater in the acne group. High GL diet was significantly associated with higher serum levels of IGF-1	**Moderate.** A diet questionnaire was administered by a blinded physician (nutritionist). Randomised blood samples were taken. Physcian assessed acne severity, but sample size was small	[289]
Case–control study of 40 females and 40 matched controls in Iran	Serum MDA levels were significantly higher (*P* = 0.01) and HDL-C levels were significantly lower (*P* = 0.02) in acne patients compared with healthy controls. No difference in 25-hydroxy vitamin D, adiponectin, TAC, triglycerides, total cholesterol and LDL-C levels. A higher fibre intake was shown to be a protective factor (OR = 0.87, *P* = 0.04)	**Low.** Small sample size. 24-hour dietary recall used to collect data. Matched for nutrient intake, age, weight, height and BMI. However, significantly higher family history of acne in first-degree relatives in cases than controls	[290]
RCT of 84 patients with grades 1, 2 and 3 acne randomised to receive a low GL diet and no dietary intervention, respectively. Acne lesions (face) were scored and graded at baseline and 4, 8 and 12 weeks	Both groups showed significant reduction in acne counts at 12 weeks (*P* = 0.931) with no statistically significant difference between the groups	**Moderate.** RCT design, but low GL group lost weight with statistically significant difference in BMI between the groups as a confounder	[291]
Case–control study of 57 patients with acne and 57 age-, sex- and ethnicity-matched controls aged >14 years. The comprehensive acne severity scale (CASS) was used to categorise patients' demographics, family history, smoking habits and dietary intake. Data were collected using a self-administered questionnaire	Milk consumption was significantly higher in patients (63.2%, *n* = 36) versus controls (43.9%, *n* = 25) (OR = 2.19, *P* <0.05). In addition, chocolate consumption was also significantly higher in patients (43.9%, *n* = 25) versus controls (24.6%, *n* = 14) (OR = 2.4, *P* <0.05). No significant association was found with the intakes of sweets, potatoes, chips, nuts, yoghurt, ice cream or carbonated drinks	**Low.** Small study, cross-sectional design	[292]
Case-control study of 200 acne patients with 200 age- and sex-matched controls	Patients with acne consumed significantly higher daily amounts of sodium chloride compared with controls (*P* <0.001). A negative correlation between the amount of NaCl in the diet of patients with acne and the age of onset of acne lesions was detected (*r* = −0.216, *P* = 0.031). However, neither salty nor spicy food correlated with duration or severity of the disease	**Moderate.** Relatively small sample size. Authors suggest studying and comparing different populations could be of interest due to different rates of sodium excretion	[293]
Case–control study of 53 patients with acne vulgaris aged between 13 and 44 years and 53 controls with no significant difference in age, BMI and body fat percentage	Statistically significant increased intake of cheese in the acne group. No significant association was found with the intakes of milk, yoghurt, ice cream, kefir, carbohydrate, fat and protein. Acne severity increased as carbohydrate consumption increased in the acne group. Acne severity was not affected by milk and dairy products, protein or fat consumption	**Moderate.** Small study but acne severity was calculated according to the global acne grading system (GAGS). Potential for bias as acne scores and food consumptions of the patients were evaluated by the researchers	[294]
Cross-sectional study of 8226 students who underwent health examinations and a questionnaire survey inquiring about the intake of soft drinks	Frequent intake (≥7 times per week) of carbonated sodas (aOR 1.61, 95%CI 0.96–2.72), sweetened tea drinks (aOR 2.52, 95%CI 1.43–4.43) and fruit-flavored drinks (aOR 1.90, 95%CI 1.18–3.07) was associated with moderate to severe acne after adjustments for confounders. Sugar intake ≥100 g/day was significantly associated with moderate to severe acne (aOR 3.12, 95%CI 1.80–5.41)	**Moderate.** Skin examination by dermatologist	[295]
RCT of 50 patients aged 15–30 years with acne. Controls had no sunflower seeds; the intervention group consumed 25 g sunflower-containing food daily for 7 days	Primary outcome of interest was 10% increase/decrease in the baseline acne severity index (ASI), sustained to the end of the follow-up period on day 14. The ASI increased in the sunflower group from 62 at baseline to 86.8 after 2 weeks (*P* <0.001) and did not change in the control group. The GAGS score did not significantly change in either of the groups	**Moderate.** Small sample size. Convenience sampling and short-term investigation	[296]

aOR, adjusted odds ratio; BMI, body mass index; CHO, carbohydrate; CI, confidence interval; DHEAS, dehydroepinandrosterone; FAI, free androgen index; GF, growth factor; GI, glycaemic index; GL, glycaemic load; HDL-C, high-density lipoprotein cholesterol; HOMA-IR, insulin resistance; IGF, insulin-like growth factor; IGFBP, insulin growth factor-binding protein; IL, interleukin; LDL-C, low-density lipoprotein cholesterol; MDA, malondialdehyde; OR, odds ratio; RCT, randomised controlled trial; SHBG, sex hormone binding globulin; TAC, total antioxidant capacity.

Table 88.12 Studies that have examined the relationship between body mass index (BMI) and acne.

Reduced risk of acne and reference	Increased risk of acne	No change in risk or severity of acne	Study population	Reference
Reduced risk of moderate to severe disease in subjects aged 10–24 years who are underweight (BMI <18.5); trend stronger in males than females		Risk not increased in subjects of either sex who were overweight (BMI >23)	Dermatology out-patients in Italy	[277]
Reduced risk of acne (any grade) in children aged 6–11 years with low BMI	Increased risk in children of both sexes who were overweight		Schoolchildren in Taiwan	[321]
Trend for reduced risk with low BMI (both sexes combined data)	Increased risk in children aged 9–16 years who were overweight. No separate analysis by sex		Schoolchildren in Ghana	[322]
	Increased acne prevalence in children aged 7–19 years who were overweight. No separate analysis by sex		Lithuanian schoolchildren	[323]
	Increased risk in girls aged 18 or 19 years who were overweight or obese	No effect of BMI on risk of acne in boys aged 18 or 19 years	Final-year schoolchildren in Norway	[324]
	Men with acne had higher mean BMI than age-matched controls		Italian males with and without acne	[325]
		No difference in BMI between subjects aged 18–30 years with acne versus age- and sex-matched controls	Acne patients in tertiary care and students or staff of local university in Malaysia	[280]
Women with acne were more likely to be overweight or obese than controls. There was a positive correlation between BMI and acne severity			Turkish women with acne	[326]
Obese women had a lower prevalence of acne than non-obese women			Taiwanese women of reproductive age	[327]
Lower prevalence of acne in overweight/obese (BMI >25) versus non-obese women with PCOS			Female out-patients with PCOS in Taiwan	[327]
Adult women with PCOS but no acne had higher mean BMI than those with PCOS and acne)			Female out-patients attending reproductive endocrinology clinic in Taiwan	[86]
Lower prevalence of acne in obese versus non-obese women with PCOS			Female out-patients with PCOS in Croatia	[328]
Reduced acne severity in women with PCOS who were overweight or obese (BMI ≥27)			Female out-patients with PCOS in Turkish hospital	[329]
	Acne strongly associated with obesity in women with PCOS		Female out-patients with PCOS in Saudi Arabia	[330] [331]
	Acne more common in overweight than normal-weight women with PCOS			
		Prevalence of acne similar in normal (63%) and overweight (73%) girls with PCOS	Female adolescent out-patients with PCOS in the USA	[94]
Trend for less acne with lower BMI (<23, NS)			Indian women with PCOS	[332]
Trend for less acne with increase in BMI (NS)			Indian women with PCOS	[332]
Less acne with higher BMI in both adolescent and postadolescent groups (P <0.001)			Turkish pre- and postadolescent males and females with acne	[334]

(continued)

Table 88.12 (continued)

PART 8: SPECIFIC CUTANEOUS STRUCTURES

Reduced risk of acne and reference	Increased risk of acne	No change in risk or severity of acne	Study population	Reference
	Obese/overweight adolescents were more likely to have acne compared with adolescents with normal weight in univariable and multivariable analysis		School children in Kuwait	[335]
	Prevalence of respondents with BMI >30 was 38%; significant association (P = 0.005) between occurrence of acne and high BMI		484 residents of Hail City, Saudi Arabia	[336]
	Overweight or obese students (BMI ≥25) had a higher prevalence of acne (age- and sex-adjusted OR = 2.7; 95%CI 1.81–3.92) than normal or underweight students (BMI <25)		Elementary school children aged 7–12 years; 693 children enrolled	[19]
		Prevalence of acne did not differ significantly between teenagers with different BMIs. However, overweight or obese teenagers suffered from inflammatory acne more often compared with underweight, slim or normal-weight teenagers (P = 0.03)	143 consecutive acne patients aged between 12 and 18 years who attended a single school in Poland	[337]
	Prevalence of acne was 81.7% among adolescents with BMI >25, 61.1% in those with BMI 18.5–24.99 and 42.0% among adolescents with BMI <18.5 (P <0.001) but BMI was not significantly associated with severity of acne (P = 0.830)		1079 students aged 9–20 years in four co-educational schools in Nigeria	[338]
Lowest odds of acne in severely obese participants (males: aOR 0.53, 95%CI 0.42–0.64; females: aOR 0.5, 95%CI 0.37–0.62)			Data on 600 404 youths during compulsory military service	[339]
	Positive association of obesity with acne with a more pronounced effect in women (OR 14.526, 95%CI 2.961–71.272, P <0.001) than in men (OR 3.528, 95%CI 1.553–8.014, P = 0.002). Obesity was associated with truncal acne (OR 4.480, 95%CI 2.182–9.196, P <0.001)		Chinese Han population aged 10–25 years attending out-patient departments; 364 patients with acne and 295 controls	[340]
BMI negatively associated with number of acne lesions in Taiwanese women with moderate to severe postadolescent acne			Taiwanese women with moderate to severe postadolescent acne	[341]

aOR, adjusted odds ratio; CI, confidence interval; NS, not significant; OR, odds ratio; PCOS, polycystic ovary syndrome.

Table 88.13 Proportion of women experiencing a premenstrual flare of acne vulgaris.

Nationality and reference	Number studied	Age range (or mean age) in years	Percent with premenstrual flare	References
American	100	–	72	[352]
American	400	12–52	44	[353]
French	3305	25–40	78	[354]
Saudi-Arabian	200	Mean age 14.8	9.8	[355]
Jordanian	83	13–34	98	[356]
Indian	137	13–45	57.7	[357]
			35.5	[358]
Korean	–	Mean age 24	60.1	[359]
French	591	10–25	55	[360]
Korean	756	10–56	61.3	[361]
Indian	230	Over 25	11.7	[362]
Thai	392	18–41	>50	[363]

Alcohol. No conclusions can be drawn about alcohol as a risk factor for acne at any age. Two cross-sectional studies [25] suggest that alcohol consumption and acne are related whereas another found no association between acne and drinking alcohol [256]. No link between acne and alcohol consumption was found in the Glasgow Alumni Cohort Study [350].

Menstrual cycle. It is documented that about 70% of women complain of a flare of acne 2–7 days before the onset of menstruation when progestogen levels are rising [25,28,351–354]. This appears to affect all ethnic groups but perhaps not equally (Table 88.13) [352–363].

Stress and sleep deprivation. A number of small studies have examined the impact of acne and stress and found changes in stress scores significantly correlate with frequency of acne or changes in acne severity when confounding variables are adjusted for [36,189,363,364]. Some investigators have found that acne sufferers report stress as an aggravator [356,361,364,365,366–370] or have shown that stress is a risk factor for more severe acne [189,243,371]. One study looked at the consequence of acne and found the presence of acne is highly associated with stress (odds ratio (OR) 1.975, 95%CI 1.588–2.457, P <0.0001), fatigue upon waking, sleep disorders and reduced sexual activity, demonstrating the adverse effect acne can have on QoL [372]. Stronger evidence of the link between acne and stress comes from data on the role of elements of the hypothalamopituitary–adrenal (HPA) axis on sebaceous gland function [373,374]. Substance P, a neuropeptide which is a stress mediator that can stimulate sebaceous precursor cells, showed a positive, significant correlation with stress scales in acne patients in a small case–control study. The sample size and predominantly female participants were a limitation and more evidence is needed to assess the correlation between stress scales, serum substance P level and severity of acne [375]. Another study has shown acne patients presented with a higher average substance P level than the controls, but no statistically significant correlation was observed for acne severity [376]. Weak evidence is available to show that sleep deprivation or insomnia is associated with both adolescent and postadolescent acne [377].

Preliminary studies have looked at stress management as a treatment for acne. A pilot non-blinded, randomised study of 30 female patients with the intervention arm receiving normal care plus a novel cognitive-based stress management intervention called Pythagorean self-awareness intervention (PSAI) reported statistically significant improvements in clinical grade of acne, perceived stress and negative affect [378,379].

Cosmetics

Acne cosmetica. This represents an acne variant associated with chronic use of cosmetics containing potentially comedogenic substances. Cited agents include lanolin, petrolatum, certain vegetable oils, butylstearate, lauryl alcohol and oleic acid. Skin bleaching agents containing steroids can cause or exacerbate acne in women with skin of colour [380,381]. Of note, some women believe cosmetics worsen acne and others overzealously use skin care products leading to exacerbations of otherwise mild acne. Ingredients may be less important than how the preparations are used. The use of cosmetics has been shown to be significant in some studies [24,382], but not in others [383].

Pomade acne. Pomades are greasy preparations used to defrizz curly hair. They can trigger comedonal acne (Figure 88.23) [384]. Restriction of the pomades and treatment with topical retinoids achieve resolution.

Detergent acne. This uncommon form of acne develops in patients who wash many times each day in the mistaken hope of improving their existing acne. Trauma and the alkaline nature of soap are likely to be involved in the mechanism. Inflammatory lesions are most noticeable [385]. Several bacteriostatic soaps contain weak acne-genic compounds, such as hexachlorophene.

Ultraviolet radiation. The assumed beneficial effect of ultraviolet (UV) radiation was questioned when 139 people in Munich were asked what happened to their acne during the summer months [386]. One-third said it improved, one-third said it worsened and one-third said it stayed the same. A number of studies have shown seasonal variation with fewer patients seeking treatment in the summer months [387–389]. Others have shown no impact of UV

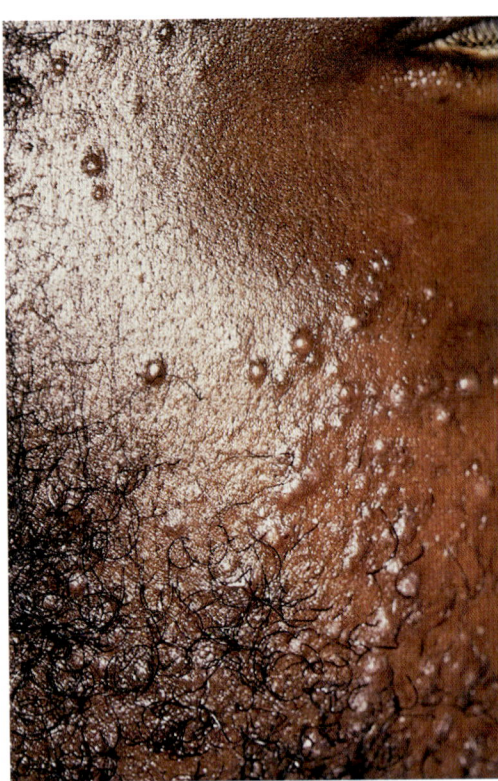

Figure 88.23 Pomade acne, characterised by multiple closed comedones and some papules on the forehead and temples. Note that pustules are rare.

radiation on disease, with most of the subjects participating in the study (64%) reporting that sun exposure had no significant impact on the disease [390]. Workers in a hot humid environment may be susceptible, for example troops in the Second World War suffered badly when posted to South-East Asia [391]. Hence, high temperatures and humidity may negate any beneficial effects of sunlight. An acne variant, acne aestivalis or Mallorcan acne, has been reported in patients exposed to sunshine on vacation. Small follicular papules appear, especially on the upper trunk, during or after a holiday in a hot humid environment. A small number of patients receiving psoralen and UVA (PUVA) treatment have been reported to develop a perioral dermatitis and/or an acneform eruption on the face [392,393]. Squalene monohydroperoxide is formed from squalene exposed to UVA and this compound appears to be responsible for comedogenicity [394]. UV radiation exposure has also been shown to alter the content of both pro- and anti-inflammatory cytokines in comedones *in vivo* [395]. Thus, evidence would support the fact that UV radiation may promote acne on sun-exposed skin in susceptible individuals not using adequate photoprotection.

Pregnancy. Among 415 Scottish women, 57.5% thought their acne improved during pregnancy and just 5.4% reported a deterioration [396]. In comparison, 75% of women thought their acne improved after giving birth and only 12% said it worsened. In South Korea [397], 28.4% of 756 women experienced a worsening of acne during pregnancy, whereas 10% observed an improvement.

Birth weight. A large study conducted among Turkish schoolgirls found that acne was more common among those with a birth weight at term of less than 2500 g [398]. Low birth weight has also been linked to acne associated with an increased risk of insulin resistance and other features of PCOS [399,400].

Miscellaneous factors. Lifestyle factors that have been proposed to modulate the risk of acne but for which there is virtually no evidence are hygiene/frequency of washing, touching the skin, mood, pollution, physical activity, use of recreational drugs, drinking water and sex.

Summary. While the effects of some dietary components are becoming clearer, there is not enough evidence to inform treatment guidelines and most acne guidelines support adoption of a healthy balanced diet with appropriate intake of water. It is not certain that being overweight predisposes to acne or that drinking alcohol has any effect. In some women with PCOS, being overweight seems to reduce the risk of acne. The relationship between smoking and acne appears complex; a variant of acne in adult women appears to be linked to habitual smoking over a long period while smoking might be protective in the early stages of inflammatory acne. It is virtually impossible to disentangle the impact of ethnicity and cultural factors, although it looks like a range of lifestyle factors including what we put on our skin, the medicines/supplements we take and the recreational activities we pursue may all play a part. While many people are convinced psychological stress makes their acne worse, the scientific evidence currently available is weak. The best advice to give patients who believe a lifestyle factor exacerbates their acne is almost certainly to avoid it for a while and keep a diary of how their skin reacts over a minimum period of several weeks. The exception is diet for which the best advice currently would be to eat healthily with everything in moderation and nothing in excess. There is reasonably good evidence that the presence of acne before puberty is a prognostic factor for more severe disease.

Clinical features
History
Acne is predominantly a chronic disease of adolescence lasting on average 7 years. However, acne may present in children as young as 6 years depending on the onset of adrenarche and adults may develop acne *de novo* or as a continuum of their adolescent problems. Despite a better understanding of acne pathogenesis over the last decade reasons for these age differences remain unclear.

Presentation
Acne is a polymorphic inflammatory disease of the skin that occurs most commonly on the face (in 99% of cases) (Figure 88.24) and to a lesser extent on the back (60%) (Figure 88.25) and chest (15%). The reasons for this varied distribution and extent are not clear. Seborrhoea along with scarring and persistent macular redness and/or pigment changes are common features (Figure 88.26). These may all contribute to a significant physical and psychosocial impact.

The clinical picture can vary from very mild comedonal acne, with or without sparse inflammatory lesions, to aggressive fulminant disease with associated systemic upset. Comedonal lesions are the earliest lesions to develop in younger patients and embrace both open (blackheads) and closed (whiteheads) comedones. Open comedones frequently appear in a mid-facial distribution

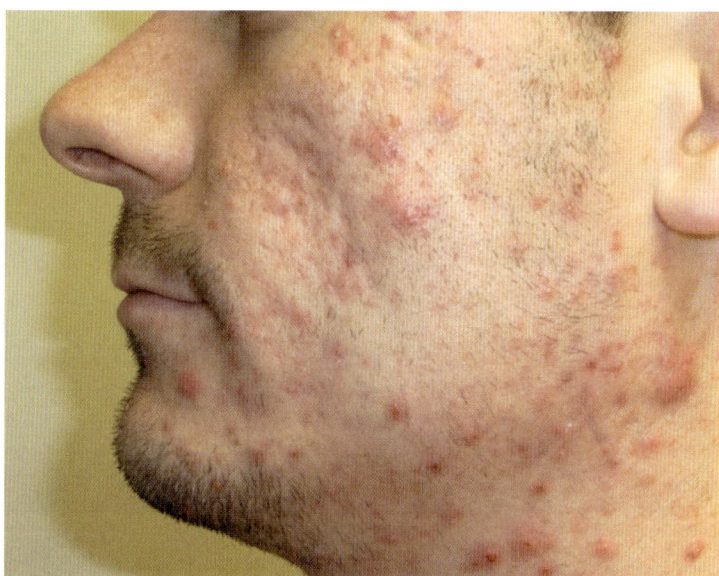

Figure 88.24 Moderate to severe inflammatory acne on the face.

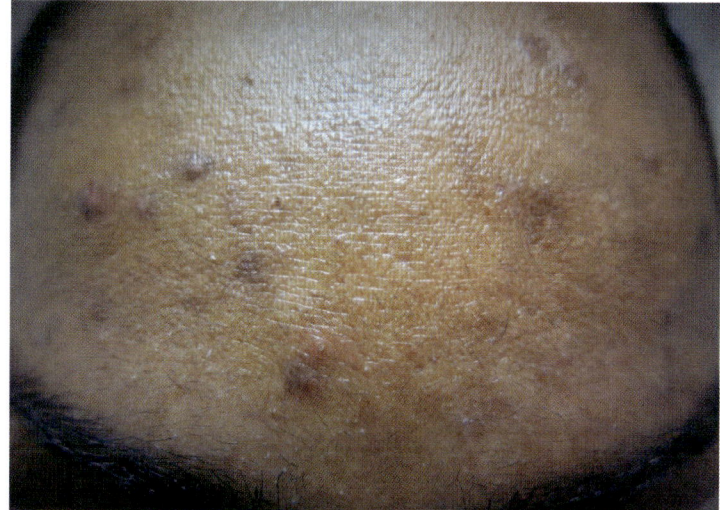

Figure 88.26 Persistent redness and pigment changes on the forehead. Courtesy of Dr J. Del Rosso, Las Vegas Skin and Cancer Clinic, Las Vegas, Nevada, USA.

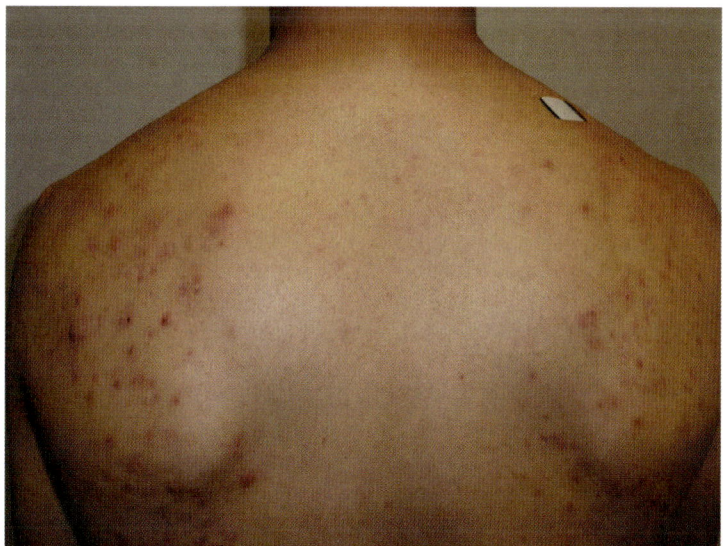

Figure 88.25 Acne on the back showing sparing of the central back and a Sebutape® used to assess skin surface sebum levels.

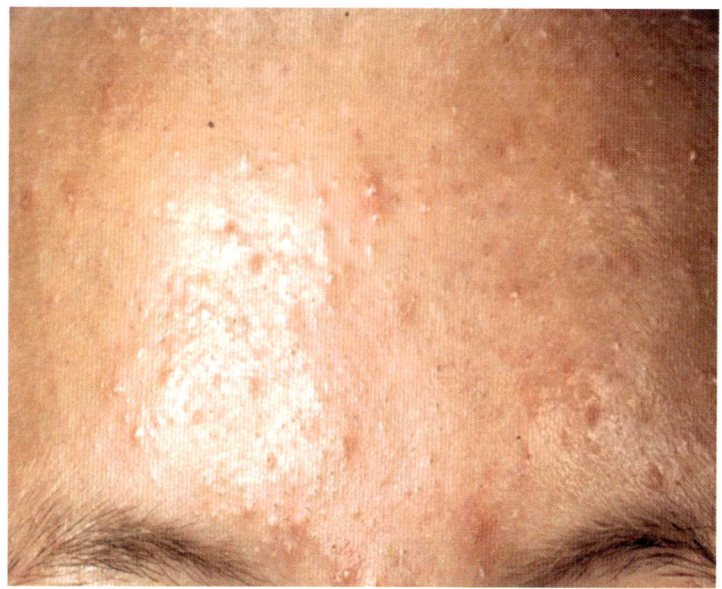

Figure 88.27 Comedonal acne with mid-facial distribution. This distribution is associated with poor prognosis.

PART 8: SPECIFIC CUTANEOUS STRUCTURES

(Figure 88.27), and when evident early they indicate poor prognosis [18]. Closed comedones are generally 1 mm in diameter, skin coloured and have no visible follicular opening. If greater than 1 mm they are described as macrocomedones. These lesions are often inconspicuous and require adequate lighting and stretching of the skin to be seen. Most patients have a mixture of lesions.

Several subtle subtypes of comedones have been described:
- 'Sandpaper' comedones consist of multiple, very small whiteheads, frequently distributed on the forehead (Figure 88.28), which produce a roughened, gritty feel to the skin.
- Macrocomedones (Figure 88.29) are large whiteheads greater than 1 mm in diameter. Both macrocomedones and sandpaper comedones respond poorly to conventional topical treatments.
- 'Submarine' comedones (Figure 88.30) are large comedonal structures greater than 0.5 cm in diameter and occur more deeply in the

skin; they are frequently associated with recurrent inflammatory nodular lesions.

Inflammatory lesions arise from the microcomedo and can remain superficial or deep in nature. Lesions embrace papules and pustules (5 mm or less in diameter) and can be extensively distributed on the face and/or trunk (Figure 88.31); deep-seated pustules and nodules (>5 mm) may also occur (Figure 88.32). Sinus tracts may develop between nodules and/or deep pustules leading to inevitable scarring (Figure 88.33). These lesions are frequently very tender, chronic and more resistant to treatment.

Itching is a rare symptom of acne and possibly relates to the release of histamine-like compounds from *C. acnes* which is implicated in disease pathogenesis.

Secondary lesions may occur as a result of acne. These include inflammatory macules which represent regressing lesions that may

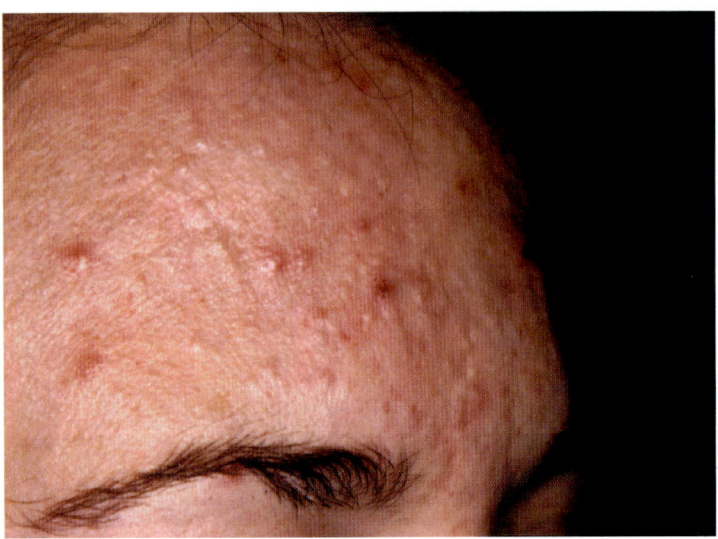

Figure 88.28 Sandpaper comedones on the forehead.

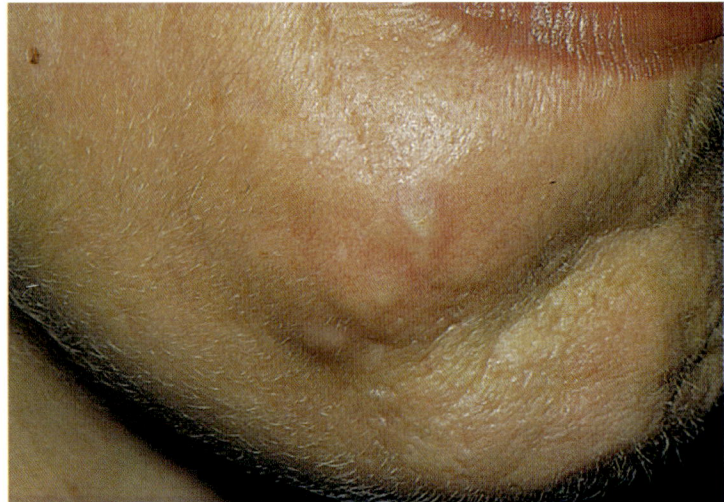

Figure 88.30 Submarine comedones. This patient required stretching of the skin in order for them to be seen.

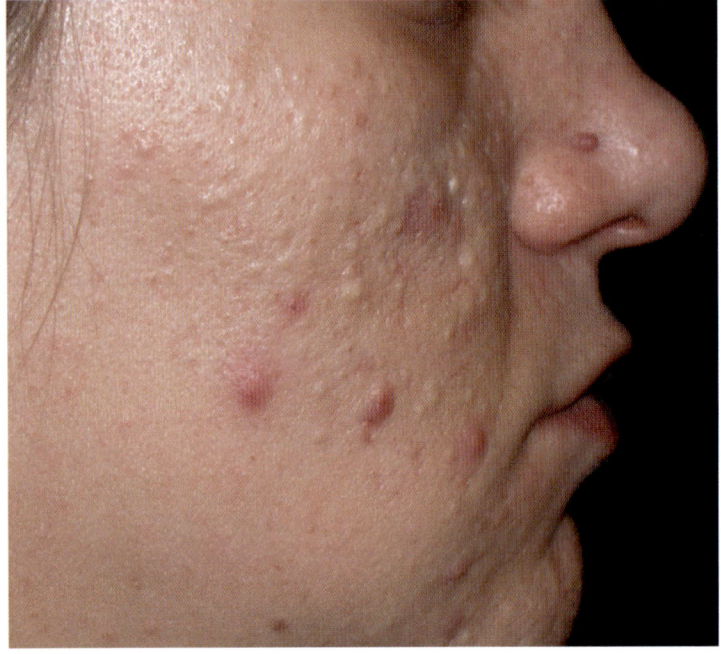

Figure 88.29 Multiple macrocomedones interspersed with some inflammatory lesions on the cheeks of a female patient with acne. Courtesy of Professor M. Jackson, University of Louisville, Kentucky, USA.

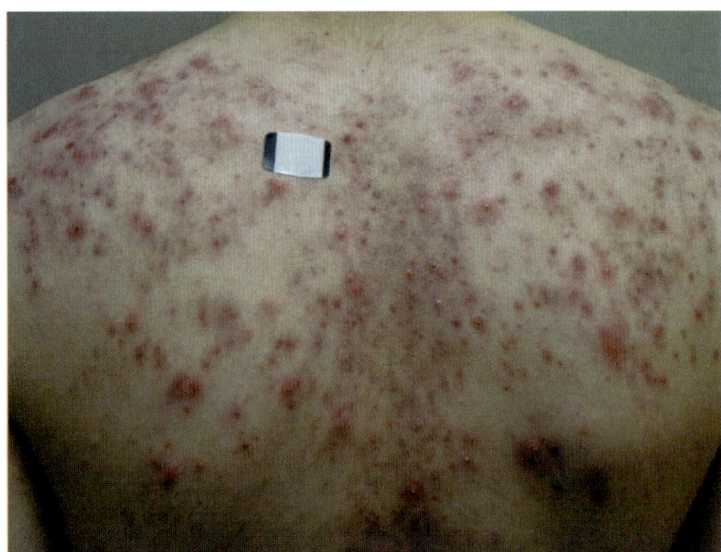

Figure 88.31 Severe acne of the back with many inflammatory papules and pustules and a Sebutape®.

persist for many weeks and contribute markedly to the general inflammatory appearance seen in acne (Figure 88.34). Scarring is also a common consequence of acne and can present as atrophic scarring (Figure 88.35) due to loss of tissue or, conversely, excessive tissue can arise in hypertrophic and keloid scarring (Figure 88.36).

Clinical variants
A number of variants of acne are recognised as follows:
- Severe forms (see 'Acne fulminans' and 'Acne conglobata' later in this chapter).
- Drug-induced acne (see 'Pathophysiology' earlier in this chapter).
- Cosmetic acne (see 'Pathophysiology' earlier in this chapter).
- Occupational acne (see 'Occupational acne' later in this chapter).

- Acne associated with psychological problems:
  - Acné excoriée.
  - Body dysmorphic disorder (BDD).
  - Eating disorders.
- Granulomatous acne.
- Acne mechanica.

Acne associated with psychological problems
Acné excoriée (synonyms: excoriated acne, picker's acne). Acné excoriée is seen predominantly in adolescent girls (Figure 88.37) although the incidence is increasing in mature females and is frequently associated with stress. Acné excoriée is regarded as a self-inflicted skin condition in which the sufferer compulsively picks real or imagined acne lesions predominantly on the face. A personality or psychological problem often underlies the condition

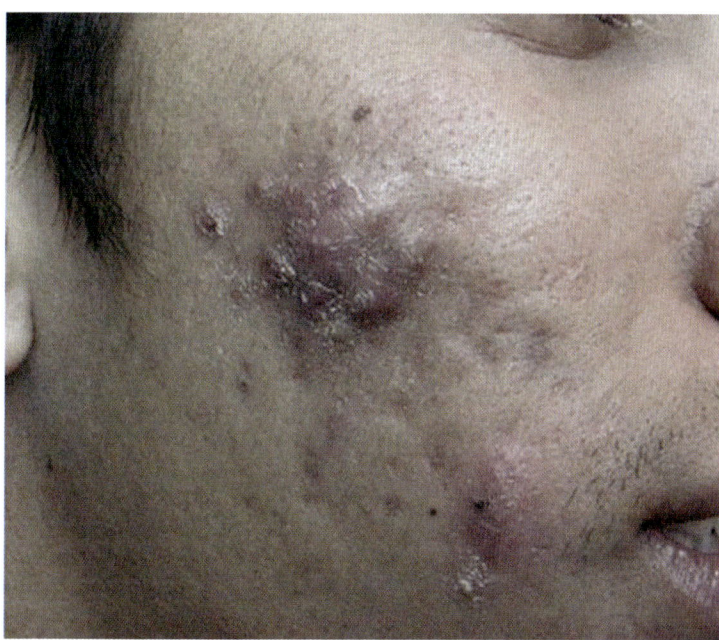

Figure 88.32 Nodular acne of the right cheek with scars. Courtesy of Dr S. Chow, KL Skin Centre, Malaysia.

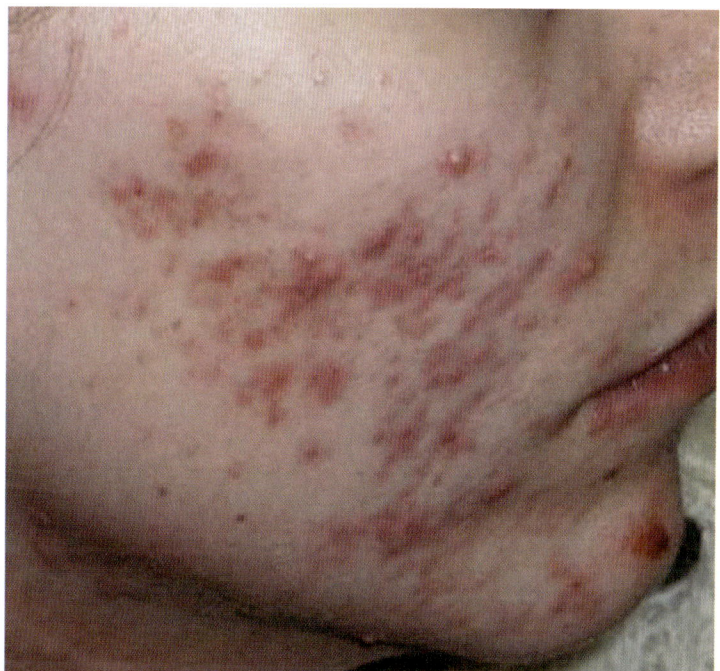

Figure 88.34 Inflammatory macules contribute to the redness seen in acne.

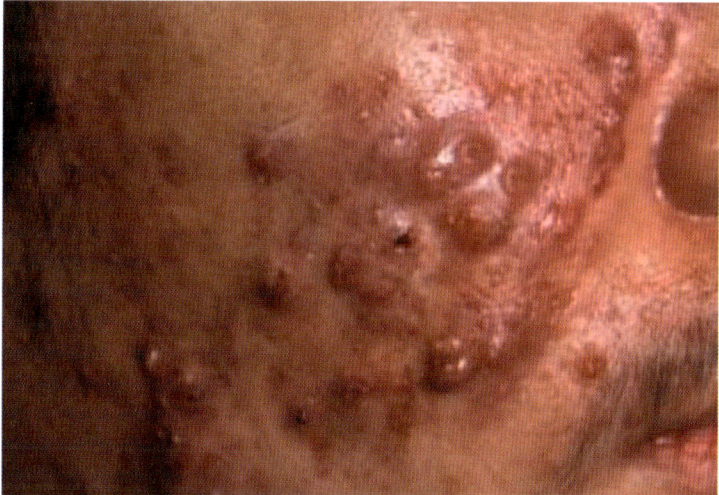

Figure 88.33 Nodular/conglobate acne with sinus tracts. Courtesy of Dr C. L. Goh, National Skin Centre, Singapore.

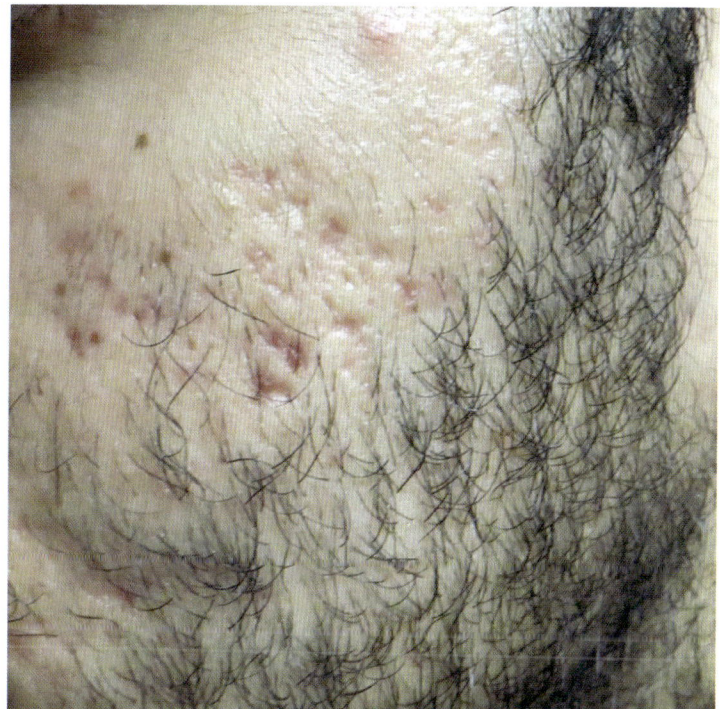

Figure 88.35 Atrophic scarring with associated inflammatory change. Courtesy of J. Del Rosso Las Vegas Skin & Cancer Clinic, Las Vegas, Nevada, USA.

including obsessive compulsive disorder and bodily focused anxiety. BDD may be associated and contribute to the pathophysiology [401,402]. Evidence of linear erosions is suggestive of self-mutilation and underlying psychiatric disease should be suspected [403]. An atopic background may be evident. A contact dermatitis should be considered and excluded [404]. The persistent trauma frequently results in significant scarring.

Treatment is challenging; acne should be treated but topical treatments have a tendency to irritate. Some patients with acné excoriée may just need to break the habit of picking while others may have a compulsive skin picking disorder which may require psychological therapy or psychotropic drug treatments [405]. Hypnosis and cognitive behavioural therapy using habit reversal techniques may be effective [406,407]. Selective serotonin reuptake inhibitors including fluoxetine, paroxetine, sertraline and fluvoxamine are treatments of choice and are frequently employed alongside psychotherapy. Treatment for facial scarring and ulceration resulting from acné excoriée has been improved using the 585 nm pulsed dye laser along with cognitive psychotherapy [408].

PART 8: SPECIFIC CUTANEOUS STRUCTURES

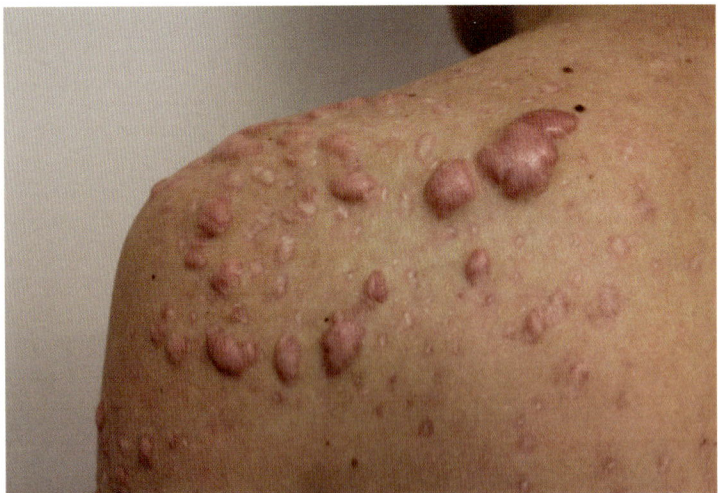

Figure 88.36 Acne keloidalis.

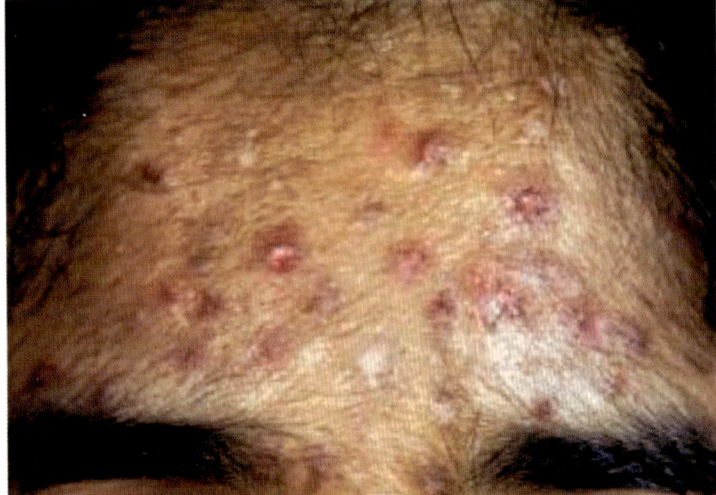

Figure 88.37 Acné excoriée on the forehead of a young female. Courtesy of Dr C. L. Goh, National Skin Centre, Singapore.

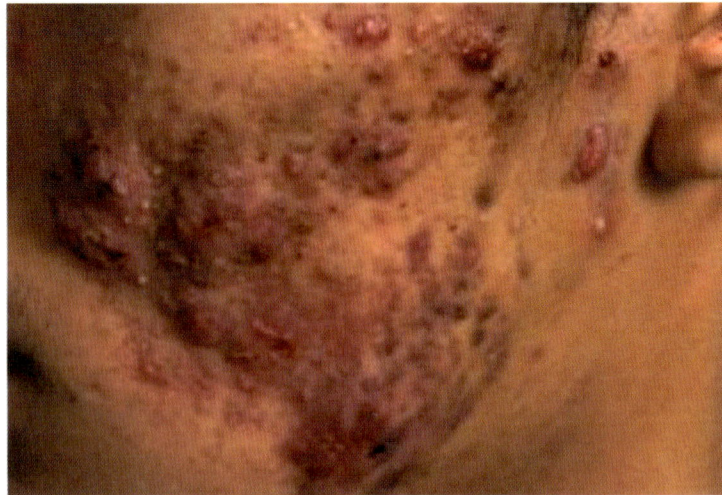

Figure 88.38 Granulomatous acne of the face. Courtesy of Dr C. L. Goh, National Skin Centre, Singapore.

Body dysmorphic disorder and acne. A small number of patients with BDD have acne as their prime symptom [409]. The perceived acne is out of proportion to physical signs. Patients require significant support; they are often depressed or have obsessional compulsive behaviours or anxiety. A significant risk of suicide has been reported [410]. Patients with BDD require dermatological and psychiatric management as many have global mental disorders. It has been suggested in the literature that some patients with BDD as the only behavioural symptom may gain relief by treating their mild acne aggressively. Off-licence use of oral isotretinoin has been described in this context but 'relapse', either real or perceived, is common and therefore this does not necessarily provide a solution to the problem [411] (Chapter 84).

Acne and eating disorders. Acne has been reported in anorexia nervosa. Acne itself may be a predisposing factor for anorexia in vulnerable teenage groups who adopt a diet in an attempt to control their acne [412]. Serum growth hormone has been shown to be raised in anorexia nervosa and concomitantly IGF-1 is low.

Granulomatous acne. The precise mechanism producing localised granulomatous acne is not known. The clinical picture is usually that of deep, well-demarcated lesion(s), especially on the cheeks (Figure 88.38). Response to therapy is slow and often unsatisfactory; antibiotics and isotretinoin are of limited benefit, and oral steroids are often required.

Mechanical acne (synonym: acne mechanica). This term describes acne that occurs at the site of repeated mechanical trauma and/or frictional obstruction of the pilosebaceous outlet resulting in comedo formation [413,414]. Examples include 'fiddler's neck', which may occur on the neck of violin players, and is characterised by well-defined plaques with the presence of comedones, lichenification and pigmentation. Headbands, tight bra straps, suspenders and collars as well as turtleneck sweaters may cause localised acne in the frictional sites [415]. This has also been reported in amputees [416]. Treatment should include elimination of the causative force(s) as well as management of comedonal and inflammatory lesions.

Differential diagnosis
A number of conditions may be considered in the differential diagnosis of acne vulgaris.

Milia. Closed comedones may be confused with milia. Milia represent intraepidermal keratin cysts predominantly infraorbital in distribution (Figure 88.39).

Syringomas. Syringomas are non-inflammatory papules that occur primarily around the eyelids and upper cheeks. They are seen more frequently in Japanese women. Histology demonstrates a dense fibrous stroma with dilated cystic spaces that have small comma-like tails resembling tadpoles (Chapter 137).

Fibrofolliculomas. Fibrofolliculomas are 2–4 mm dome-shaped papules seen most commonly on the face (Figure 88.40), neck and upper trunk. They are characteristically seen in Birt–Hogg–Dube

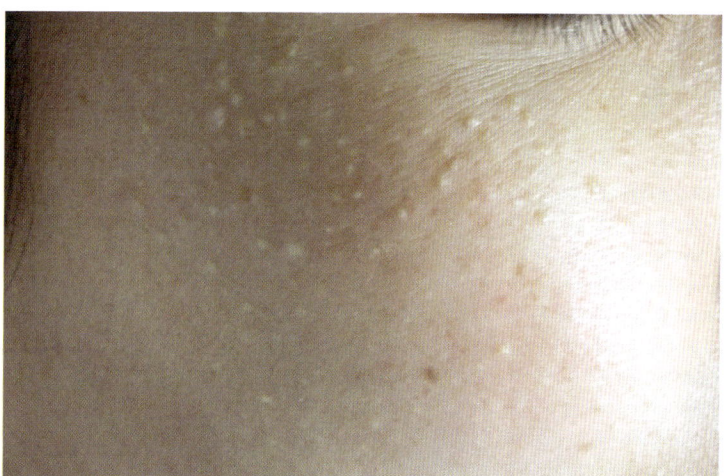

Figure 88.39 Multiple milia on the upper cheek. Courtesy of Dr J. Del Rosso, Las Vegas Skin and Cancer Clinic, Las Vegas, Nevada, USA.

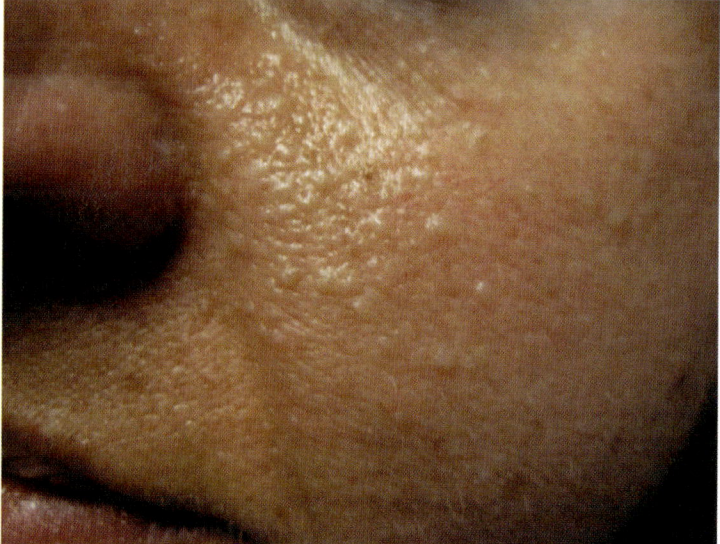

Figure 88.40 Fibrofolliculomas: Birt–Hogg–Dube syndrome. Courtesy of Dr J. Del Rosso, Las Vegas Skin & Cancer Clinic, Las Vegas, Nevada, USA.

(BHD) syndrome. This is a rare autosomal dominant inherited condition characterised by the development of benign tumours on the face and upper body including fibrofolliculomas, trichodiscomas and acrochordon. People with this syndrome are at increased risk of colon or kidney cancer as well as spontaneous pneumothorax due to pulmonary cysts. BHD syndrome is due to mutation in the *BHD* gene on chromosome 17p12-q11.2 encoding folliculin. If positive for the gene, patients with BHD syndrome should undergo renal ultrasound and/or abdominal computed tomography/magnetic resonance imaging, chest X-ray and colonoscopy to determine any associated malignancies (Chapter 137).

Ectopic sebaceous glands (synonym: Fordyce spots). These are heterotopic sebaceous glands that can occur around the vermilion border of the lips or within the oral mucosa (Chapter 91). They are commonly multiple, and appear as symmetrical discrete yellow papules [417]. They are present in 25% of the population over the age of 35 years and are usually asymptomatic but can be disfiguring. Oral isotretinoin has been used with some success for extensive lesions [418]. Carbon dioxide ablative laser therapy has also been used with good effect [419]. Lesions may occur on the penile shaft and may become inflamed and a cause for concern. The areolar of the breast is another site occasionally affected [420].

Pilosebaceous naevoid disorders. Some of these disorders are only tenuously linked with the pilosebaceous system.

Acneform naevi. Symmetrical areas of normal skin set in the midst of severe acne on the back [421] or acne localised to one side of the back have been described. Reduced sebum excretion and surface bacteria have been demonstrated in the normal-looking areas.

Comedo naevus (synonyms: naevus comedonicus, naevus follicularis, naevus unilateralis comedonicus). This uncommon naevus is usually a developmental defect of the hair follicles [422–426]. The associated sebaceous glands may be normal, hypoplastic or hyperplastic. Lesions usually occur on the scalp, face and trunk, and occasionally at unusual sites such as the genitalia. The individual lesions consist of keratin-filled pits, often grouped or linear in arrangement (Figure 88.41). Occasionally, inflammatory acne lesions may be found. Although usually present at birth, they often become more prominent at puberty. *FGFR2* mutations have been identified in a comedonal naevus but not in the adjacent normal skin [427]. The somatic heterozygous Ser252Trp-FGFR2 mutation has been confirmed within the affected skin lesions of a male patient presenting with a unilateral acneform naevus [428]; association with epidermolytic hyperkeratosis has also been reported [429]. Treatment is usually of only limited success. Topical retinoids and 12% aqueous ammonium lactate solution have been reported to be of benefit. Gentle cautery may help less severe cases [430].

Familial comedones. This uncommon genetic disorder presents with single comedonal lesions, but later the face may become extensively involved with gouped comedones and cysts; scarring may ensue. New lesions may continue into middle age.

Sebaceous naevus (synonym: naevus sebaceus of Jadassohn). This is an organoid naevus consisting of a mixture of relatively normal-looking epidermis, dermis, sweat and sebaceous glands. It usually presents on the scalp as an area of alopecia [431,432]. At puberty, the sebaceous glands enlarge and the epidermis becomes verrucous. Co-occurrence with aplasia cutis has been reported. Trichoepithelioma and eccrine syringoadenoma have been noted in sebaceous naevus [433]. An unusual haematopoietic proliferation at birth that spontaneously resolved at 4 months has been documented [434]. Excision is usually recommended because of the potential to develop a squamous or basal cell carcinoma with a lifetime risk reported between 5% and 22% [435].

Favre–Racouchot syndrome (synonymous with senile comedones and solar comedones). Multiple open and closed comedones occur on periorbital and malar areas of elderly people in the context of chronic sun exposure (Figure 88.42) (Chapter 94). UV radiation

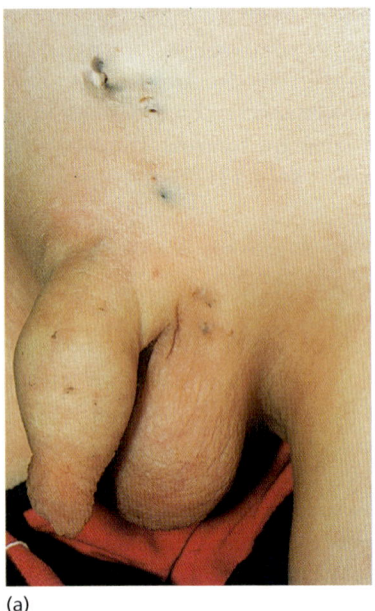

(a)

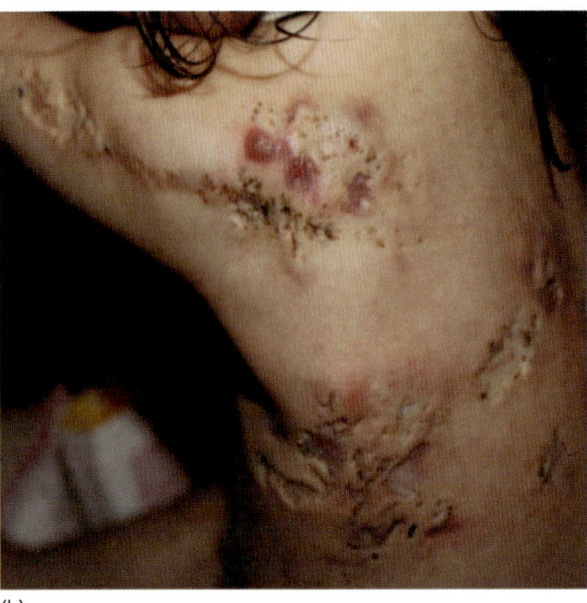

(b)

Figure 88.41 (a) A patient with comedo naevus (naevus comedonicus) predominantly consisting of blackheads on the lower abdomen. (b) Multilocular naevus comedonicus. (b) From Chiriac *et al*. 2016 [736] with permission from the University of California.

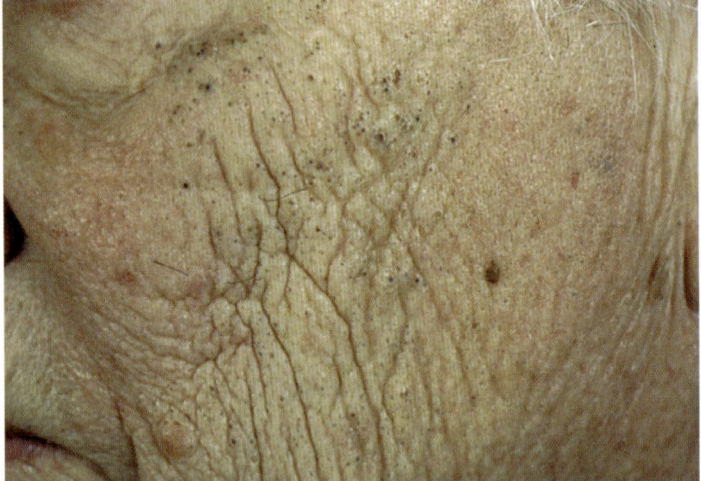

Figure 88.42 Favre–Racouchot syndrome (senile comedones). From Zouboulis *et al*. 2019 [737] with permission from Elsevier.

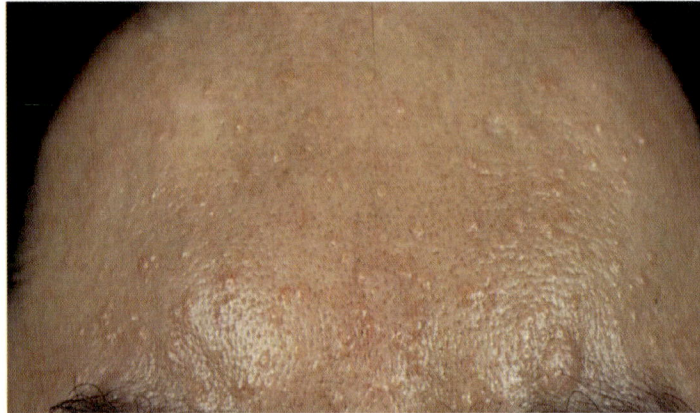

Figure 88.43 Sebaceous gland hyperplasia on the forehead. From Zouboulis and Boschnakow 2001 [738] with permission from Oxford University Press.

results in solar damage to the supporting dermis, causing the pilosebaceous duct to become distended with impacted corneocytes. Occasionally, lesions are unilateral. Histology demonstrates increased elastic tissue with thickened and tortuous fibres in the upper and mid dermis [436]. Similar change may be seen in pseudoxanthoma elasticum or post radiotherapy. A comedo extractor will remove lesions but they frequently recur. Topical retinoids and electrocautery may be of benefit.

Sebaceous gland hyperplasia, adenoma and carcinoma. Sebaceous gland hyperplasia represents a benign proliferation of the sebaceous gland producing yellow/pink lesions 1–3 mm in diameter on the face (Figure 88.43) (Chapter 91). They may also present on the light-exposed skin of renal transplant patients receiving ciclosporin [437]. Treatment is rarely requested but gentle cautery, cryotherapy, trichloroacetic acid, carbon dioxide and

pulsed dye lasers may help [438,439]. Lesions are occasionally diffuse, producing a yellowish hue to the skin. Oral isotretinoin used off-licence has benefited some cases [440]. Co-cyprindiol (Dianette® and Estelle-35®), with or without additional oral cyproterone acetate, will also produce regression of sebaceous hyperplasia in some females. Photodynamic therapy using aminolaevulinic acid has also been shown to be successful in reducing sebaceous hyperplasia [441].

Adenoma sebaceum (synonym: angiofibromas)**.** Adenoma sebaceum are small, translucent, waxy-looking papules symmetrically distributed over the central face. Multiple lesions are associated with tuberous sclerosis. Histology of the lesions demonstrates dermal fibrosis and vascular proliferation and dilatation.

Sebaceous gland tumours. These are uncommon but may be associated with internal malignancy and systemic disease.

Sebaceous adenoma. This is a benign tumour composed of incompletely differentiated sebaceous cells. It occurs in both sexes, predominantly in the elderly on the face or scalp [442]. The waxy pink/yellow tumours are usually 10 mm or less in size and may form ulcerative plaques. Excision is recommended but they are radiosensitive. Rarely, sebaceous gland adenomas can be associated with multiple visceral carcinomas, which present relatively early (45 years). This association is referred to as the Muir–Torré syndrome (MTS) (Chapter 137). MTS is a rare genodermatosis defined clinically by the occurrence of a sebaceous neoplasm (adenoma, epithelioma or carcinoma) and at least one internal malignancy in the absence of other predisposing factors. Most patients present with sebaceous adenomas but cystic sebaceous neoplasms have been reported as specific markers of MTS. Gastrointestinal and genito-urinary malignancies are the most commonly reported with colo-rectal cancers presenting at or proximal to the splenic flexure contrary to most sporadic colo-rectal cancers [443,444]. MTS is most frequently found as a variant of the autosomal dominant hereditary disorder non-polyposis colo-rectal cancer (HNPCC) [445], with tumours demonstrating microsatellite instability and germline mutations in the DNA mismatch repair genes Muts homologue *MSH2* and *MLH1*. However, the distribution of gene mutations in patients with MTS is slightly different from that seen in all patients with HNPCC and some cases of MTS arise spontaneously [446]. Clinicians should consider a diagnosis of MTS in patients presenting with sebaceous neoplasms, and immunohistochemical examination of tumours for MSH2 and MLH1 protein can be used as a screening test for MTS. The neoplasms of MTS tend to follow a more indolent course than the sporadic cases, which can be quite aggressive. Careful follow-up and active treatment are required for both familial and sporadic cases. Evidence suggests that patients with MTS and HNPCC should undergo colonoscopy every 1–2 years from the age of 25 years or at an age 10 years younger than the family member who originally presented with the disease. Others recommend annual history, physical examination, including thorough review of the skin, and urinalysis as well as endometrial sampling and transvaginal ultrasound for females.

Sebaceous carcinoma. This is a rare malignant tumour arising from the sebaceous glands (Chapter 137). It is commoner in men over the age of 40 years and presents as a firm, solitary, yellow-orange lesion usually on the face and scalp. It can ulcerate (Figure 88.44). Sebaceous carcinomas have a well-recognised association with MTS. The tumour grows slowly, but those arising in the eyelid (from the Meibomian glands) are more likely to metastasise [447]. Treatment is by excision or radiotherapy [448]. A tumour diameter of 10 mm or greater and/or tumours classified as T4 on the T classification of the tumour/node/metastasis staging system are linked to a poor prognosis [449].

Sebaceous (epidermoid) cysts and steatocystoma multiplex. The classic 'sebaceous' cyst is an epidermal structure; strictly, it should be referred to as an epidermoid cyst (Chapter 133). However, true sebaceous cysts occur as so-called steatocystoma multiplex (SM), a naevoid condition that histologically shows a mixture of a keratinising epithelium and sebaceous lobules attached to the epidermis by a thin epidermal strand [450,451]. A clinical and histological study examined 64 sporadic cases with an average age of onset of 26 years. They confirmed the presence of multiple,

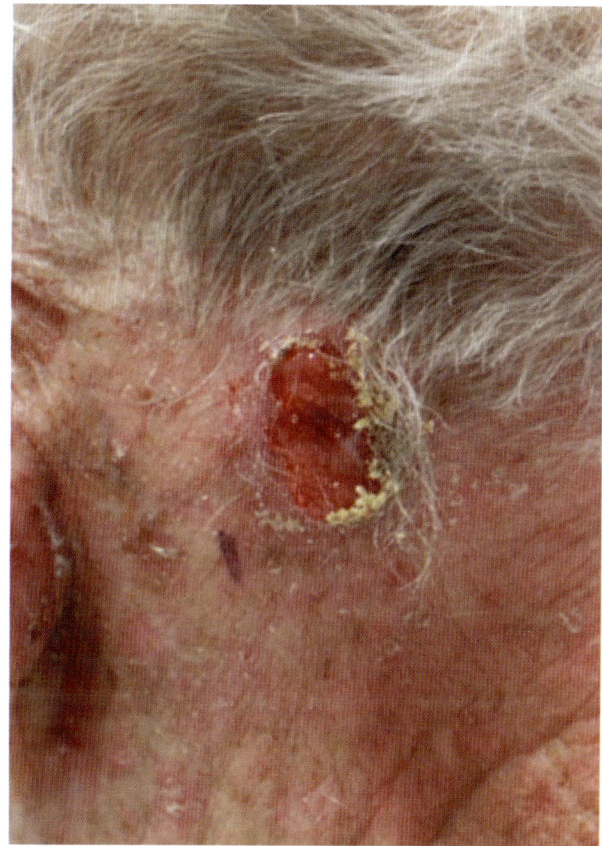

Figure 88.44 Sebaceous carcinoma.

smooth, yellow dermal swellings varying from a few millimetres to 20 mm in size distributed on the arms, chest, neck and axillae and appearing and/or enlarging at puberty (Figure 88.45). When extensive these can produce SM suppurativa, which mimics acne conglobata. SM shares many clinical features and may show overlapping histopathological features with eruptive vellus hair cysts (EVHCs). In a case series, all exhibited eosinophilia and lack of granular layer, and 17–42% displayed vellus hair, hair follicles, keratin and smooth muscle components within the cavity, in the wall or adjacent to it. The results of this study suggest that SM is a hamartomatous condition and that SM and EVHCs are variants that originate in the pilosebaceous duct [452]. SM is rare and is occasionally associated with type 2 pachyonychia congenita (PC-2 or Jackson–Lawler syndrome), in which natal teeth are also a feature [453–456]. Histologically, the cysts in PC-2 may be true steatocysts, EVHCs or keratinous cysts, even in the same family or in an individual [457–461].

To date, mutations in the Ia domain of keratin 17 (K17) have been found in all cases [456,459,460]. In some families with clinically and histologically typical SM, mutations in the *K17* gene are also found [460]. Close inspection demonstrates that some members have nail changes which are usually but not always milder than those of PC. Familial SM has also been associated with natal teeth in the absence of nail dystrophy [460] and it seems likely that these cases are also due to keratin gene mutations. However, in a case of SM/EVHC and in another of EVHC, mutations in *K17* were not found along the Ia domain [461]; this would suggest that SM is genetically heterogeneous.

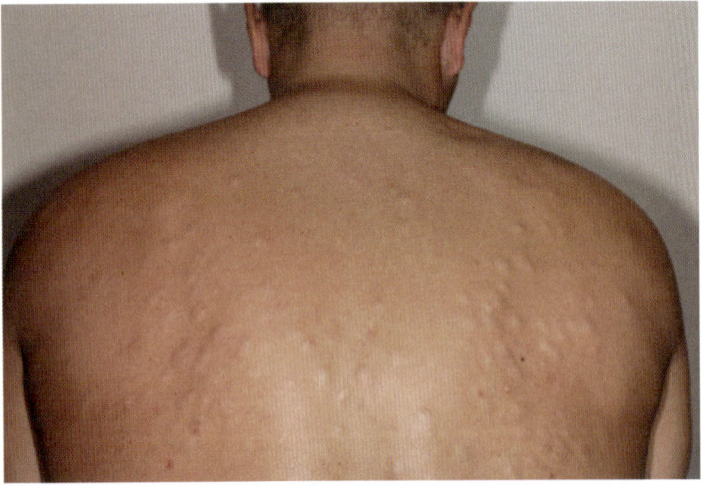

(a)

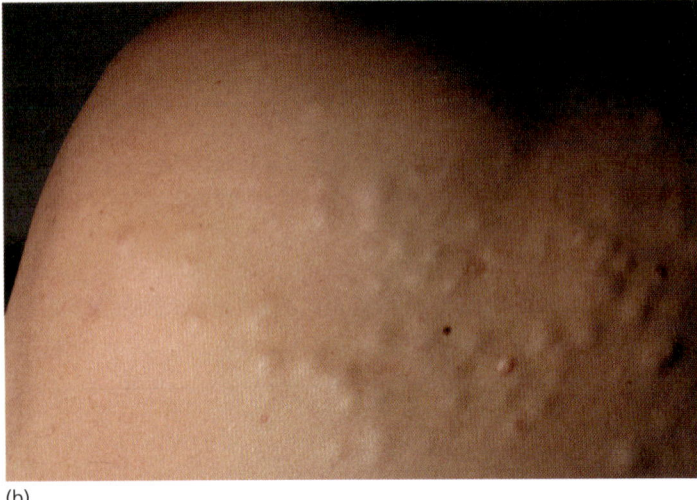

(b)

Figure 88.45 (a) Steatocystoma multiplex of the back. (b) Steatocystoma close-up of multiple cystic lesions. Courtesy of Dr N. Veien, the Dermatology Clinic, Aalborg, Denmark.

Treatment is challenging [450]; excision of the larger cysts is possible but total removal of all cysts is impractical. Successful treatment employing a vein hook to locally extract cysts has been reported [462]. One study also utilised the carbon dioxide laser with some improvement [463]. Topical therapy is of limited benefit. Systemic antibiotics may reduce inflammation and/or suppuration and oral isotretinoin reduces inflammation but does not affect the primary disease process.

Granulomatous rosacea (synonyms: lupus miliaris disseminatus faciei, acne agminata). Other diseases that may produce diagnostic difficulties include granulomatous rosacea (Figure 88.46) (Chapter 89).

Keratosis pilaris. Occasionally, inflammatory keratosis pilaris may masquerade as acne. Keratosis pilaris is most commonly seen on the proximal extremities (Figure 88.47), and is characterised by follicular keratotic papules in hair-bearing areas which may or may not be associated with redness (Chapter 85). It has a familial tendency

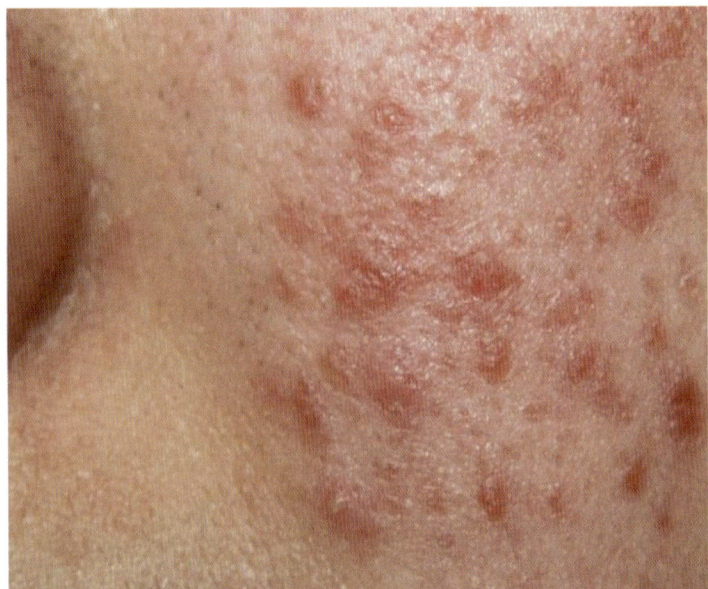

Figure 88.46 Granulomatous rosacea synonymous with acne agminata seen on the cheek.

and is reported in the context of genetic syndromes such as chromosome 18p depletion in which there may be prominent and extensive keratosis pilaris [464–466]. One study suggested that the presence of moderate to severe keratosis pilaris on the arms is associated with a lower prevalence of acne vulgaris and lower severity of facial lesions in adolescents and young adults [467].

Rosacea. Rosacea may be mistaken for inflammatory acne. Rosacea usually occurs in an older age group of patients (30–50 years of age), and lacks comedones or scarring and rarely affects the trunk (Figure 88.48). The presence of facial flushing and specific triggers, including heat, spicy food or alcohol, is more in keeping with a diagnosis of rosacea. Rosacea patients may also have ocular involvement. Some patients have features of both diseases [468] and clinical acne may evolve into more typical rosacea later in life (Chapter 89).

Pyoderma faciale. Synonymous with rosacea fulminans (Chapter 89), pyoderma faciale usually presents very acutely on the face in adult females (Figure 88.49). The lesions are deeply inflamed. Nodules, cysts and occasionally sinus tracts may form. Histology demonstrates a mixed inflammatory infiltrate in the upper and mid dermis with extravasation of red blood cells and haemosiderin deposition.

Perioral dermatitis. In perioral dermatitis the papules and pustules present on a red and/or scaling base localised symmetrically around the mouth with a clear zone around the vermillion border. Lesions frequently itch in perioral dermatitis and no comedones are evident (Figure 88.50) (Chapter 89).

Folliculitis. Gram-negative folliculitis due to Gram-negative organisms can occur as a complication of long-term oral or, less frequently, topical antibiotic therapy used to treat acne [469–471]. It has also been reported in human immunodeficiency virus (HIV)-positive

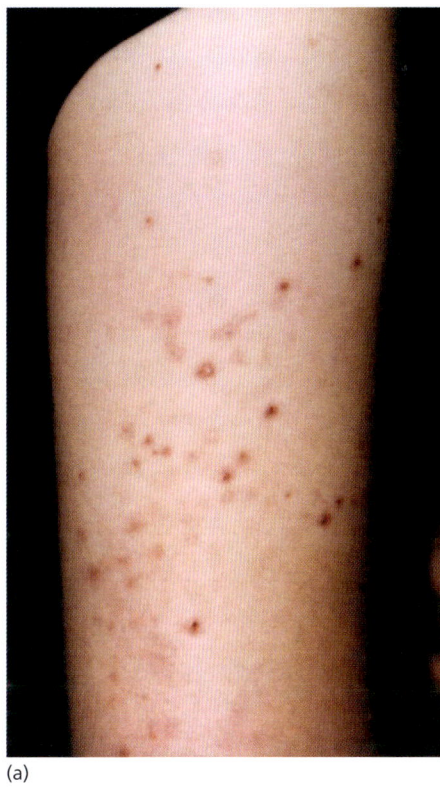

(a)

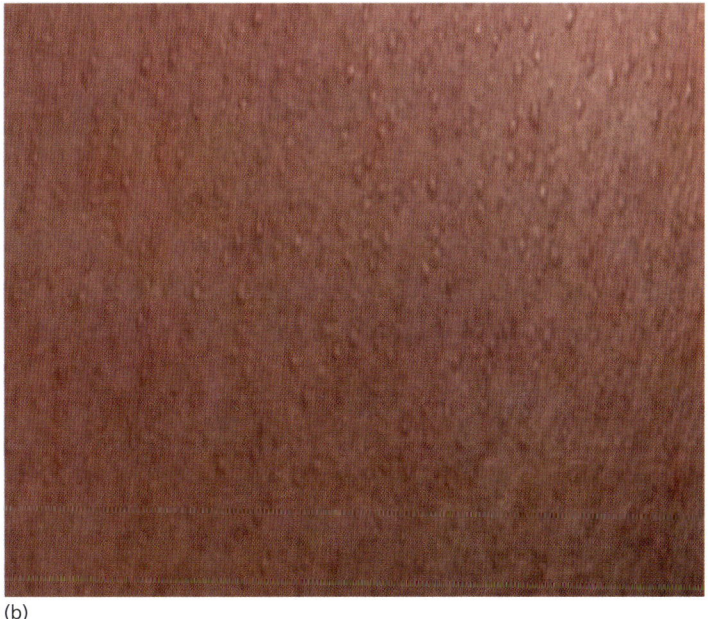

(b)

Figure 88.47 (a) Keratosis pilaris of the upper arms associated with some inflammation and excoriation. (b) A close-up view of keratosis pilaris. (b) From Liakou *et al.* 2014 [739] with permission from John Wiley & Sons.

patients and after hot tub immersion. Clinical features include a sudden eruption of multiple, small, follicular pustules or occasionally nodular lesions, most frequently localised around the perioral or perinasal skin (Figure 88.51). This results from overgrowth of Gram-negative organisms including *Klebsiella*, *Escherichia coli*, *Serratia marescens*, *Proteus mirabilis* and *Pseudomonas aeruginosa*. These organisms replace the Gram-positive flora of the facial skin

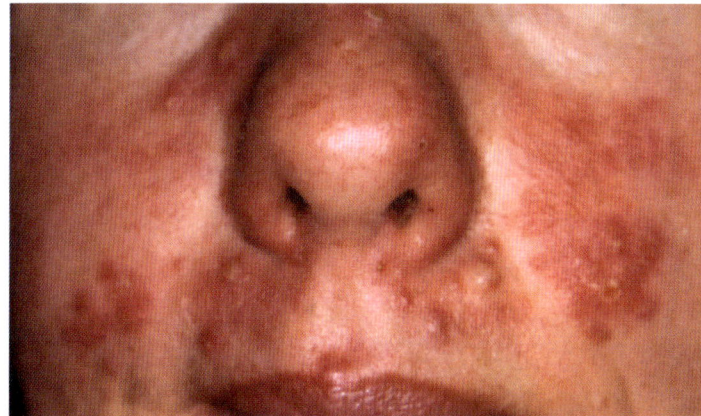

Figure 88.48 Rosacea on the mid-face with periorbital sparing.

and mucous membranes. The current antibiotic should be discontinued, replacing it with either ampicillin (250 mg four times a day) or trimethoprim (400–600 mg/day). However, response may be slow and relapse is common. Isotretinoin has been used very effectively off-licence for Gram-negative folliculitis and results in lower relapse rates than antibiotics [472–474].

***Malassezia* folliculitis** (synonym: pityrosporum folliculitis). *Malassezia* folliculitis is due to proliferation of the yeast within the hair follicles. It presents most frequently on the upper trunk as a monomorphic acne-like eruption with many papules or pustules which may itch (Figure 88.52). Topical or oral antifungal agents are generally helpful. In some cases oral isotretinoin to reduce the seborrhoea is beneficial [475,476].

Scalp folliculitis (synonyms: acne necrotica miliaris, proprionibacteria folliculitis). Scalp folliculitis is an inflammatory disorder of the hair follicles characterised by small itchy pustules on the scalp often around the hairline, resulting from an inflammatory reaction to microorganisms including bacteria (*C. acnes*, *Staphylococcus aureus*), yeasts (*Malassezia* spp.) and mites (*Demodex folliculorum*) (Chapter 91). Patients receiving oral isotretinoin may develop scalp folliculitis due to *S. aureus* infection, which responds well to oral flucloxacillin. A persistent scalp folliculitis has been recorded in patients with cyclical neutropenia [477].

Folliculitis keloidalis (synonyms: acne cheloidalis nuchae, acne keloidalis). Folliculitis keloidalis represents an unusual chronic form of folliculitis affecting the nape of the neck (Figure 88.53) and is associated with cicatricial alopecia (Chapter 91). Folliculitis keloidalis is more common in black males. The lesions present as small, itchy, raised papules within or close to hair-bearing areas of the occiput; secondary infection with *S. aureus* can ensue. The chronic process results in hairless scarring. Tufted hairs may be present representing multiple hair shafts emerging from single follicular openings. The cause is unknown but proposals include trauma following close shaving and ingrowing hairs which irritate the wall of the hair follicle; an association with obesity and the metabolic syndrome has been noted. Treatment is challenging and includes avoiding friction from clothes and close haircuts,

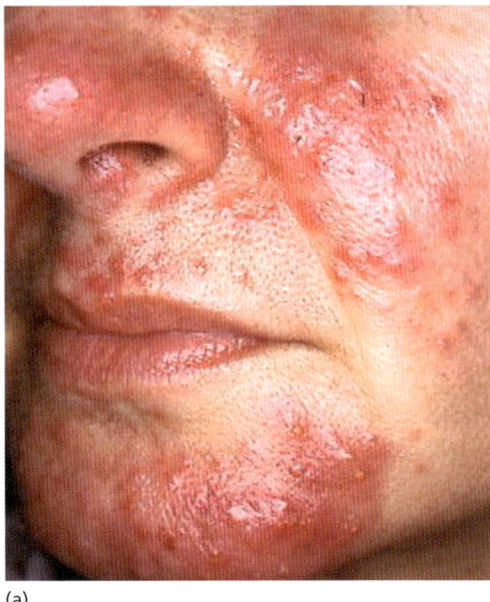

(a)

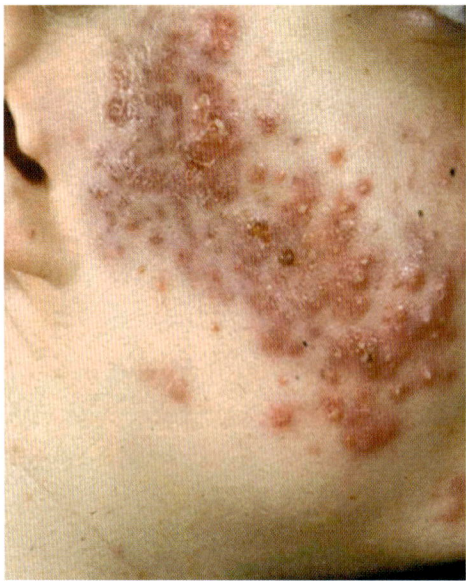

(b)

Figure 88.49 (a, b) Pyoderma faciale. (b) From Massa *et al.* 2017 [740] with permission from S. Karger AG, Basel.

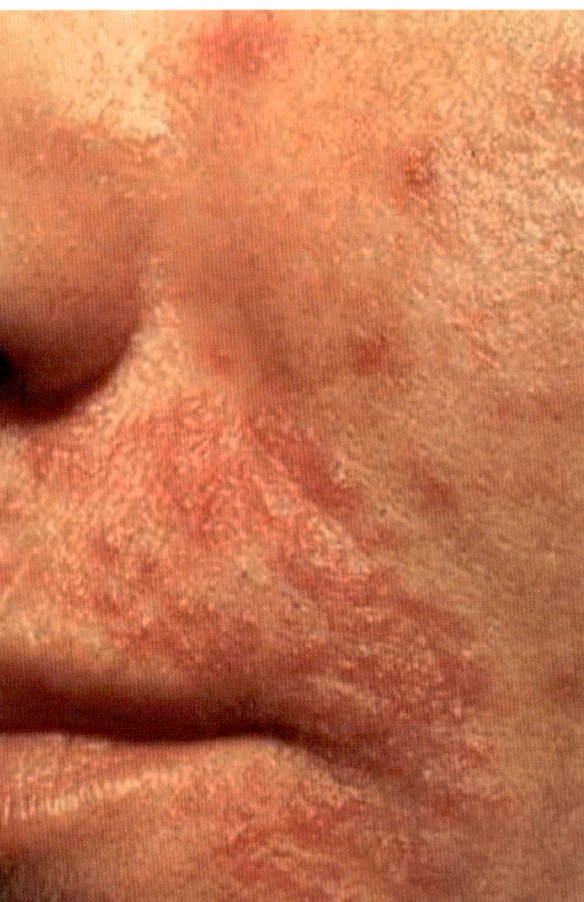

Figure 88.50 Perioral dermatitis demonstrating small papules on a red base.

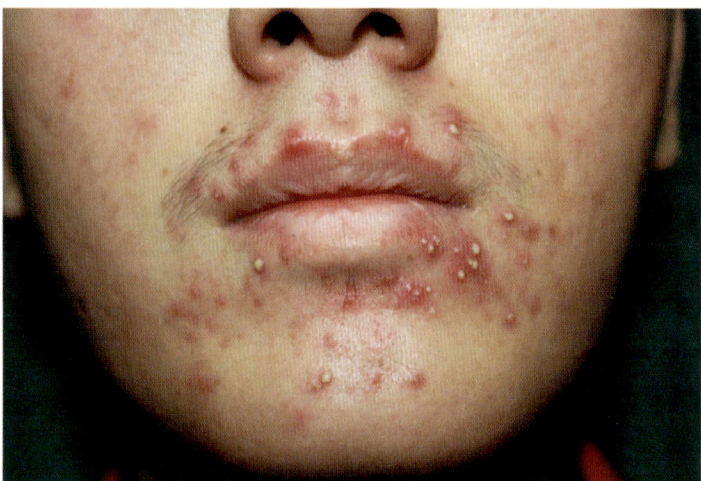

Figure 88.51 Gram-negative folliculitis after long-term antibiotic use showing multiple pustules. Courtesy of Dr S. Chow, KL Skin Centre, Malaysia.

significant scarring has occurred. Surgery, laser vaporisation [478] or excision has been used to remove large nodules and plaques. Systemic isotretinoin has also been used off-licence with some success, as has radiotherapy [479].

Folliculitis decalvans (synonym: tufted folliculitis). Folliculitis decalvans is a chronic disorder of the hair-bearing areas on the scalp that leads to scarring, alopecia and atrophy [480–482] (Chapter 87). Areas of tufted folliculitis have been identified in cases of folliculitis decalvans and the histological features include hyperkeratosis, follicular plugging and perifollicular inflammation. The aetiology is unknown and treatment is difficult. It has been suggested that folliculitis decalvans may be the result of an abnormal host response to toxins from *S. aureus*. If *S. aureus* is identified, systemic antibiotics are required; oral clindamycin or rifampicin may help by offering better tissue penetration. One case report suggests added benefit by also using topical mupirocin [483]. An isolated

antimicrobial washes, topical steroids for small papules and intralesional steroids for large papules and nodules. Oral tetracyclines as anti-inflammatories or clindamycin and rifampicin have been used successfully. Laser and hair removal have also been shown to be of benefit. Optimum results occur if treatment is started early before

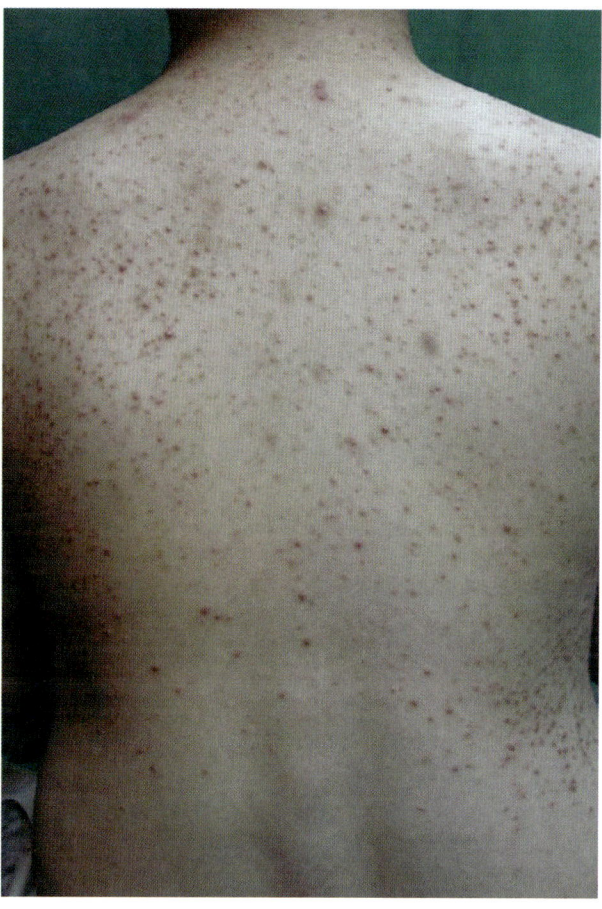

Figure 88.52 Pityrosporum folliculitis in an immunocompromised male. Courtesy of Dr S. Chow, KL Skin Centre, Malaysia.

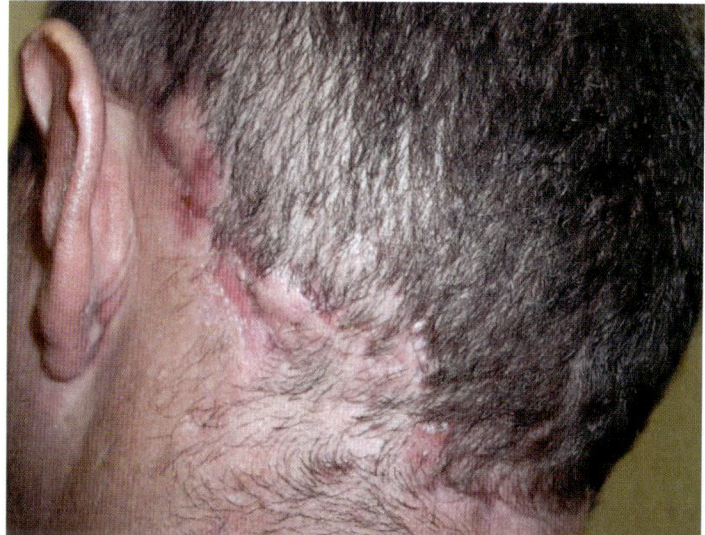

Figure 88.53 Folliculitis keloidalis affecting the nape of the neck and hairline resulting in cicatricial alopecia.

case report advocates the use of oral clindamycin in combination with oral isotretinoin and steroids [484]. Topical fusidic acid and oral zinc have also been used with some success in one series [485]. Radiotherapy and treatment with dapsone have been reported in isolated cases [486,487].

Dissecting cellulitis of the scalp (synonym: perifolliculitis capitis abscedens et suffodiens). This condition is predominantly seen in black males in their second to fourth decades. It is an uncommon, chronic, suppurative disorder of the scalp of unknown aetiology [488–494] (Chapter 105). Together with acne conglobata, HS and pilonidal cysts it is a component of the 'follicular occlusion tetrad'. Patients present with multiple, tender, inflammatory nodules and abscesses most commonly on the vertex and occiput of the scalp. Lesions frequently coalesce into sinus tracts. Scarring alopecia frequently results from the chronic suppurative changes. Follicular hyperkeratosis appears to be the primary feature in pathogenesis but secondary bacterial infection frequently occurs. Histology demonstrates a neutrophilic perifolliculitis with follicular destruction, granulomas and fibrosis. Lesions characteristically last for many years and are cosmetically disfiguring, painful and malodorous. It has been reported to occur with marginal keratitis [488] and squamous cell carcinoma may result in chronic cases [492]. Three cases of keratitis, ichthyosis and deafness (KID syndrome) have been reported in association with the follicular occlusion

triad [493]. Response to therapy is poor. Options include high-dose systemic antibiotics used for acne (minocycline 100 mg twice daily or trimethoprim 300 mg twice daily). Success with oral zinc sulphate 135 mg three times a day [489] and topical isotretinoin [490] has been reported. Oral isotretinoin is advocated as the most effective treatment [491]. Other treatment options include potent topical, intralesional and systemic steroids and widespread surgical excision with skin grafting [492]. One case of dissecting cellulitis associated with KID syndrome responded well to alitretinoin [494].

Hidradenitis suppurativa. HS is described in more detail in Chapter 90. It may be associated with severe nodular/conglobate acne. There is often a family history and the onset is usually in late adolescence; the disease prevalence gradually decreases with increasing age [495–497]. HS is a chronic disease that affects the axillae, breasts, genital and perianal areas (Figure 88.54), and may sometimes spread extensively onto the buttocks and lower back. There is clinical evidence of open comedones (often polyporous), deep nodules, large abscesses, sinus tracts and scarring. The inflammatory lesions are frequently deep seated, exudative, painful and malodorous, resulting in significant compromise of daily activities and a high degree of morbidity [496]. It is primarily a disorder of follicular occlusion. Aetiological factors such as obesity, smoking and local irritation (e.g. from excessive sitting) may be relevant aggravating factors.

Miscellaneous causes of papular facial rashes. Papular facial rashes may be mistaken for acne. Rarely, dermatitis herpetiformis may present as a vesicular pustular facial eruption, but it is usually very itchy, unlike acne. Linear immunoglobulin A (IgA) disease can also rarely present as a papular facial rash without comedones. Biopsy, including immunofluorescence studies, is essential to confirm the diagnosis. Facial lesions in micropapular sarcoid (Chapter 96) are relatively monomorphic papules, often skin coloured or with a brownish appearance, but if inflamed may be mistaken for inflammatory acne lesions [498–500]. A dental sinus

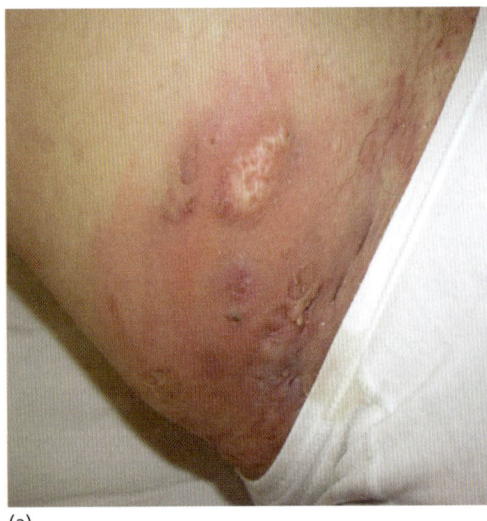

(a)

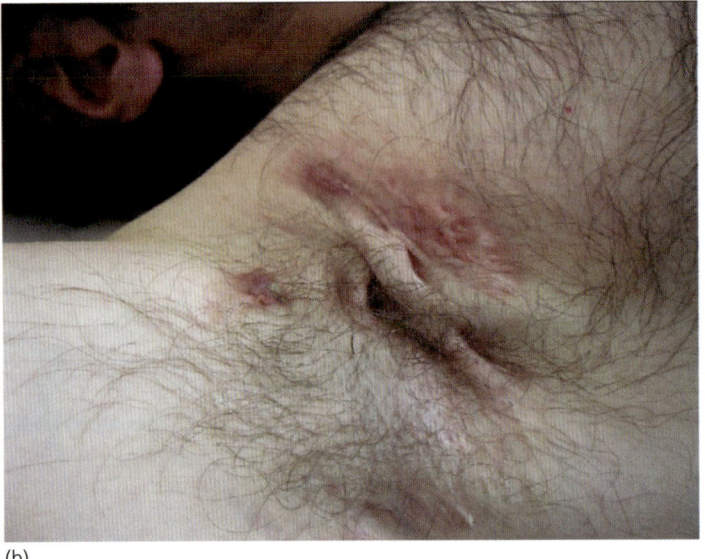

(b)

Figure 88.54 (a) Hidradenitis suppurativa of the groin showing inflammation, comedonal lesions and cribriform scarring. (b) Hidradenitis suppurativa of the right axilla. Courtesy of Professor V. Bettolli, University of Ferrara, Ferrara, Italy.

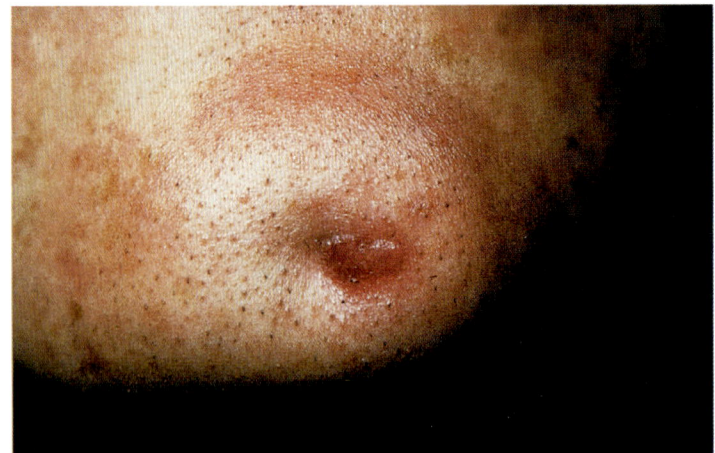

Figure 88.55 Dental sinus confused with persistent facial acne nodule.

can be confused with a persistent facial acne nodule (Figure 88.55). Epidermoid cysts may become inflamed and be mistaken for acne nodules. The severe papulopustular eruption associated with zinc deficiency can be mistaken for marked acne, and several cases have been reported after prolonged intravenous feeding without zinc supplementation [501].

Mimics of acne scarring. Scarring due to hydroa vacciniforme (Chapter 126), ulerythema ophryogenes (Chapter 87), folliculitis keloidalis (Chapter 91), varioliform atrophy and porphyria cutanea tarda (Chapter 58) can all masquerade as acne scarring. Acne necrotica varioliformis (necrotising lymphocytic folliculitis; Chapter 91) is associated with itching and smallpox-like scars, particularly around the scalp margin [502]. It can be mistaken for severe acné excoriée. Response to isotretinoin has been reported to be excellent [503].

Classification of severity

Accurately assessing outcome measures in acne is notoriously challenging. Many different approaches have been adopted but few are validated, challenging the interpretation of results from clinical trials [504]. In clinical practice, the severity of acne is assessed visually according to the extent of the disease and number and type of lesions and is frequently described as mild, moderate or severe. The clinical assessments of lesions utilised as a measure of outcome can be divided into grading or counting. The evaluation can be further divided into (i) overall or 'global' assessment; (ii) separate evaluations of individual lesions; and (iii) evaluation according to the predominant lesion type. Mechanisms to assess acne lesions using multimodal imaging are being evaluated [505] and patient-reported outcomes are now considered an important part of assessment, as are poor prognostic risk factors [506].

The Acne Core Outcome Research Network has identified through a Delphi consensus seven core domains that require measurement when assessing acne, and work is progressing to identify the best tools to measure the agreed domains [**507**].

The comprehensive acne severity system (CASS) was developed by application of a pre-existing six-category facial investigator global assessment scale ranging from clear through to very severe grading (Table 88.14) to include the chest and back [508]. This has been validated and provides a global system that includes a restricted number of categories to allow for a practical and comprehensive approach when assessing treatment outcomes.

Lesion counts are essential for clinical trials as this offers a reliability not evident in global systems; however, counting remains impractical for use in the day-to-day clinic. It is now widely recognised that there are other important factors and outcome measures that should be considered when assessing the severity and impact of acne as well as the effect of therapy. These include the extent and sites of involvement, the degree of seborrhoea, the patient's demographic and family history, evidence of sequelae such as scarring and pigmentation, patient satisfaction with treatment, their adherence to a therapeutic regimen, the speed of action of treatment, tolerability and adverse effects of therapy and impact on QoL.

The use of QoL measures captures the impact of acne and treatment on the patient's life and helps to identify those vulnerable

Table 88.14 The comprehensive acne severity system (CASS).

Grade	Description	Face	Back	Chest
Clear	No lesions to barely noticeable ones. Very few scattered comedones and papules			
Almost clear	Hardly visible from 2.5 m away. A few scattered comedones, a few small papules and very few pustules			
Mild	Easily recognisable, less than half the affected area involved. Many comedones, papules and pustules			
Moderate	More than half the affected area involved. Numerous comedones, papules and pustules			
Severe	Entire area affected. Covered with comedones, papules and pustules and a few nodules and cysts			
Very severe	Highly inflammatory acne covering the affected area, with nodules and cysts present			

to psychological complications. Adopting a QoL measure as an integral part of acne management is recommended.

Several simple questionnaires including combinations of generic and dermatology-specific questionnaires are available (Box 88.4). Generic tools allow comparison between different diseases whereas the disease-specific questionnaires assess the impact of the acne and allow comparison of acne response to treatment over time.

Box 88.4 Measurements available to assess the impact of acne on quality of life

Generic measures
- Euro-QoL (EQ-5D)
- SF-36

General health questionnaire (GHQ)
- UK sickness impact profile (UK SIP)
- Preference-based measures of utility

Dermatology-specific measures
- Dermatology life quality index (DLQI)
- Skindex
- Dermatology quality of life scales (DQOLS)
- Dermatology-specific quality of life instrument (DSQL)
- Children's dermatology life quality index (CDLQI)

Acne-specific quality of life instruments
- Acne/Cardiff acne disability index (CADI)
- Acne-specific quality of life questionnaire (Acne-QoL)
- Acne quality of life scale
- Acne quality of life index (Acne-QOLI)
- Assessments of the psychological and social effects of acne (APSEA)
- CompAQ
- Acne-Q

Acne also affects functional abilities. Patients are prone to embarrassment and social withdrawal, depression, anxiety and anger. The combined use of QoL and psychosocial questionnaires (see 'Complications and co-morbidities' later in this chapter) is essential to adequately understand just how severely the disease is affecting a patient, and can aid in assessing the efficacy of therapy. Acne scarring and pigment should also be included in the assessment of acne severity. Scars and pigment can produce significant disfigurement and psychosocial impairment in their own right. The difficulty in the evaluation of scars and pigment is manifold and there is currently no one simple clinically reproducible tool for evaluating the extent or volume deficiency of acne scars or the extent of pigmentary change.

Complications and co-morbidities

The main complications from acne relate to psychosocial and physical scarring. Persistent redness or pigment changes may occur, and rarely solid facial oedema and osteoma cutis have been reported. Pyogenic granulomas may occur in severe disease or result from treatment with isotretinoin. Seborrhoea may be a significant issue in some patients.

Psychosocial effects of acne. There have been many studies over the years investigating the specific psychological effects produced by acne using different measures. A recent comprehensive systematic review examining the impacts of acne identified more than 408 studies with 138 questionnaires that have been used [50].

Impact on QoL and perception. Studies have shown that many acne patients experience shame (70%), embarrassment and anxiety (63%), lack of confidence (67%), impaired social contact (57%) as well as problems with unemployment [510,511]. Severe acne may be related to increased anger and anxiety [512]. When compared with other serious organic diseases, acne patients describe levels of social, psychological and emotional problems as great as those reported with chronic disabling diseases such as asthma, epilepsy, back pain, arthritis and diabetes (Table 88.15) [513]. Research has confirmed that physically attractive strangers attribute more positive qualities such as friendliness, intelligence and higher social skill levels to each other, compared with physically unattractive strangers [514]. Studies assessing independent reactions to photographs of patients with acne, acne scarring and pigment change versus no acne, acne scarring or pigment change have identified that those suffering disease are perceived more negatively [515,516].

Anxiety, depression and suicide. Clinical depression has been demonstrated in acne patients and this does not necessarily correlate with the clinical severity of disease. Suicide in acne patients has been reported in the literature [517] and the depressed acne patient should be assessed for suicide risk. Acne patients compared with other skin patients using a depression test inventory may have depression levels reaching those identified from patients hospitalised with psoriasis [518]. Higher anxiety using the state-trait anxiety inventory (STAI) has also been identified in acne patients versus controls [519].

Acne scarring. This is a common consequence of acne and may occur, albeit mild in most instances, in up to 90% of patients as a result of acne lesions [520]. The duration of inflammation relates to scar production hence a delay in appropriate management is more

Table 88.15 The impact of acne on quality of life (QoL) compared with other medical conditions using the QoL SF-36.

	Social functioning	Role fulfilment for emotional reasons	Mental health	Energy and vitality
Acne	**11.1**	**7.4**	**13.4**	**7.0**
Asthma	5.9	6.3	4.2	6.0
Diabetes	8.7	9.5	5.9	9.1
Back pain	8.9	6.9	4.1	8.5
Epilepsy	7.4	5.3	3.4	5.9

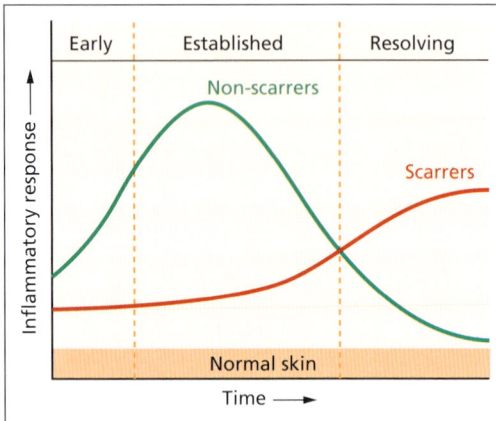

Figure 88.56 Immune responses vary between scarring and non-scarring acne patients.

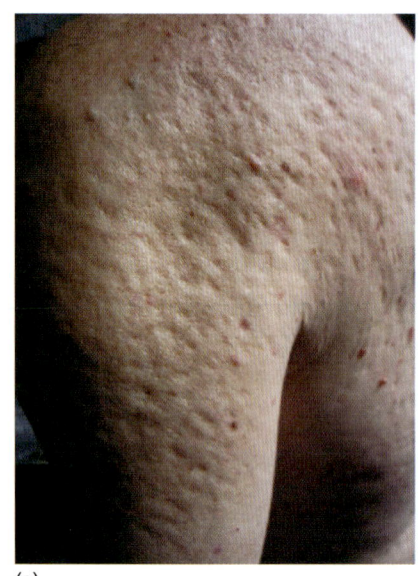

(a)

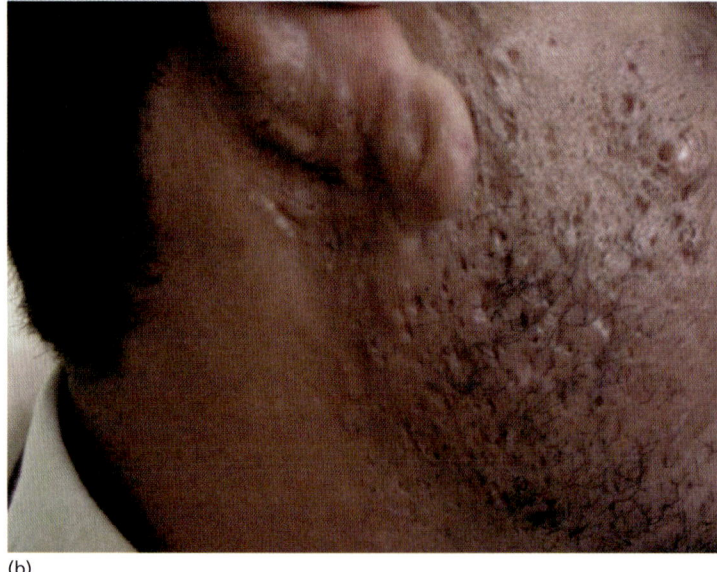

(b)

Figure 88.57 (a) Severe scarring of the arms and back showing soft distensible scars as a result of acne. (b) Fibrotic atrophic acne scars of the face. (a) Courtesy of Dr S. Chow, KL Skin Centre, Malaysia.

likely to result in significant scarring [521,522]. A cell-mediated immune response has been found to be involved in the inflammatory events in acne. Holland *et al.* [523] investigated the differences in cell-mediated immune responses in developing and resolving inflamed lesions between those acne patients who were prone to scarring and those with the same degree of inflammatory acne not prone to scarring. Clear differences in the cellular infiltrate were identified. In acne patients not prone to scarring, the time course was typical of a type IV delayed hypersensitivity response, and effective resolution occurred by both non-specific/innate and adaptive immune mechanisms. In lesions from acne patients who were prone to scarring, a predominantly adaptive immune response was present, which was persistent and upregulated in resolving lesions (Figure 88.56). A further more recent study also reported [524]. This suggested that effective management of inflammation during the development and resolution stages of acne may help to control scarring. Scars may show increased collagen (hypertrophic scars and keloids) or be associated with loss of collagen (i.e. atrophic scars). Keloids by definition extend beyond the extent of original inflammation and are most prevalent on the trunk. Hypertrophic scars in contrast to keloids do not extend beyond the extent of the original inflammation.

Limited morphological classification of scarring has been described and to date there is poor consensus and clinical assessment of scars demonstrates significant variation between assessors [525]. A tool to assess atrophic scars has been developed called FASET [526]. However, the lack of an accepted standardised objective quantification or qualitative scoring to estimate the global scar severity makes comparisons of treatments for scarring challenging. Atrophic scars are frequently multiple, they may be soft and

distensible or fibrotic (Figure 88.57). They often retain a vascular hue for many months before becoming less conspicuous. Perifollicular elastolysis is commonly found on the trunk and consists of multiple follicular atrophic-looking lesions, sometimes seen without evidence of acne [527]. Calcification is a rare complication of scarring

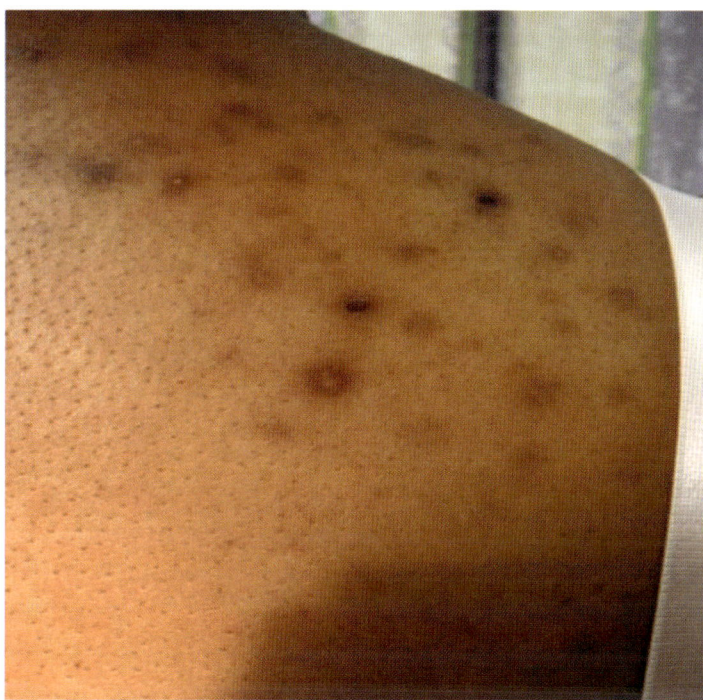

Figure 88.58 Acne-induced hyperpigmentation in Fitzpatrick type IV skin.

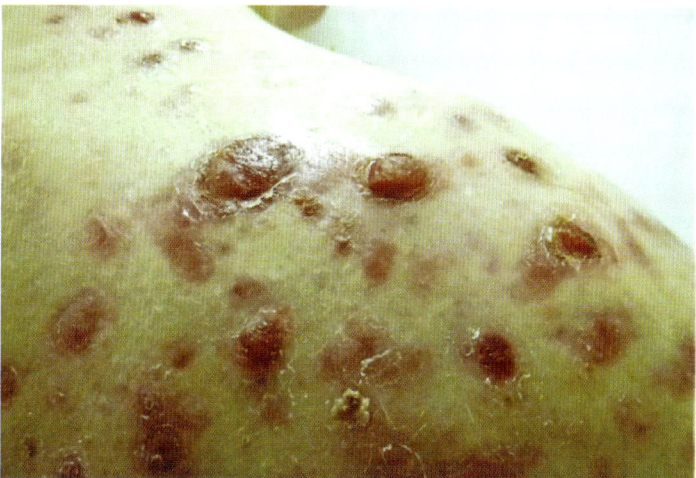

Figure 88.59 Pyogenic granulomas in severe acne.

[528,529]. Persistent hyperpigmentation, seen most frequently in pigmented skin (Figure 88.58), and persistent macular redness are both common and cosmetically disfiguring. The pigmentary change can take many months to resolve or may persist. A recent study conducted by the Asian Acne Board demonstrated many patients had evidence of acne-induced pigment change for 5 years or longer [530].

Solid facial oedema (Morbihan disease). This is a rare and disfiguring complication of acne [531] that has been reported in twins [532]. It is also reported as a consequence of rosacea (Chapter 89) [533] and in Melkersson–Rosenthal syndrome. Thickened, woody, facial oedema leads to significant distortion of the midline face and cheeks due to soft-tissue swelling most likely due to pre-existing hypoplastic lymphatics. The disorder is frequently progressive, and the associated acne must be treated aggressively to prevent permanent swelling. Successful treatment with oral isotretinoin alone or in combination with clofazamine or ketotifen has been reported [534–536]. Short or intermittent courses of oral steroids may also help the inflammatory component.

Osteoma cutis. This represents focal ossifications in the subcutaneous and dermal tissue. This uncommon complication of acne is described more commonly in women with longstanding inflammatory acne and usually needs no treatment [537–539]. The calcification presents as small 2–4 mm persistent papules which are firm to the touch. Histology confirms calcified trabecular bone formation surrounded by a perivascular proliferation, often with increased fibrous tissue formation. Treatment modalities are limited. Topical tretinoin may promote transepidermal elimination of osteomas in small superficial lesions [540,541]. Surgical ablative

therapy is most effective; techniques reported include combined dermabrasion and punch biopsy, scalpel incisions and curettage, extirpation of the small bone fragments after microdissection and laser therapies. The erbium:yttrium-aluminium-garnet (Er:YAG) laser is said to be associated with minimal thermal injury with better cosmetic results than the carbon dioxide laser [542–546].

Pyogenic granulomas in acne. Pyogenic granulomas are occasionally seen on the trunk [547,548] in patients with very severe acne (Figure 88.59). They can also rarely (<1 : 10 000) be precipitated during treatment with oral isotretinoin and may be a feature of acne fulminans. Lesions may respond to clobetasol propionate cream applied topically twice daily and carefully to the lesions over a 2–3-week period.

Seborrhoea. Excessive sebum production may impact on QoL and can persist after the acne has regressed [549]. Underlying systemic causes such as acromegaly or parkinsonism should be considered. Justification for the use of systemic isotretinoin or antiandrogen therapy in females should be considered carefully as their use in this context is outside the recognised product licence.

Disease course and prognosis

Although acne may be considered as a 'rite of passage' during the teenage years, a significant number of people suffer acne for many years. According to World Health Organization criteria, acne can be defined as a chronic disease [550]. Predisposing factors for developing acne are discussed elsewhere; certain factors link to severity of acne and risk of relapse (Table 88.16) [551].

Investigations

Investigations may be required as part of monitoring or to exclude an underlying endrocrinopathy. Box 88.5 summarises the signs and symptoms that may indicate an underlying endocrinopathy. Table 88.17 outlines hormonal investigations required to identify an endocrine problem. Although not routinely done, quantifying sebum excretion may support the selection of therapy as people with a higher sebum production respond less well to antibiotics [9] and there is a correlation between high sebum and acne severity [10].

PART 8: SPECIFIC CUTANEOUS STRUCTURES

Table 88.16 Summary of factors associated with acne severity and relapse.

Specific factor	Impact
Positive family history	Linked to
	Earlier occurrence of acne
	Increased retentional lesions
	Increased relapses
Early onset	Infantile acne shown to link to:
	Resurgence of acne in teenage years
	More severe acne in teenage years
	More frequent relapse in teenage
	Mid-facial years comedonal lesions in prepuberty
	linked to more severe disease
	Earlier onset of acne relative to menarche related to
	more severe disease
Duration of acne	Prolonged duration of disease associated with
	reduced efficacy
	A family history of acne >25 years associated with
	more adult acne in relatives
Seborrhoea	High sebum production correlates with more severe
	acne
	High sebum production relates to reduced response
	to systemic antibiotics
Extent, location and nature of lesions	Truncal acne associated with reduced efficacy to systemic therapy when compared with acne on the face

Table 88.17 Hormonal investigations required to identify endocrine problems.

Suspected clinical diagnosis	Hormonal evaluation
PCOS	Luteinising hormone
	FSH
PCOS	Total free testosterone
PCOS	Prolactin
CAH	DHEAS
CAH	17-hydroxyprogesterone
CAH	ACTH stimulation test
NCAH	TSH
Ovarian tumour	Free testosterone
Adrenal tumour	DHEAS

ACTH, adrenocorticotropic hormone; CAH, congenital adrenal hyperplasia; DHEAS, dehydroepiandrosterone; FSH, follicle-stimulating hormone; NCAH, non-classic congenital adrenal hyperplasia; PCOS, polycystic ovary syndrome; TSH, thyroid-stimulating hormone.

Assessment of sebum in the clinic can easily be performed using a microporous hydrophobic polymer film (i.e. Sebufix® or Sebutape®). The Sebutape measures the active follicle distribution but cannot measure the amount of sebum directly. After cleaning the skin with an alcohol wipe the tape is applied to the skin. The Sebufix shows the distribution of sebum with the aid of a UV light camera and calculates the sebum secretion area from the area evaluated [552]. Figure 88.60a shows Sebutape on the forehead of a patient and comparison of two Sebutapes demonstrating the difference between patients with and without acne (Figure 88.60b, c). Gravimetric assessments of sebum can also quantify the sebum output but these are labour intensive and not viable for use in the clinic.

Box 88.5 Signs and symptoms that may indicate an underlying endocrinopathy suggesting the need for investigation

Signs of hyperandrogenism alongside acne
- Seborrhoea
- Hirsutism
- Androgenic alopecia
- Cushingoid features
- Increased libido
- Deepening of voice
- Clitoromegaly
- Acanthosis nigricans

Acne reported to be
- Therapy-resistant acne
- Rapidly relapsing
- Very severe
- Marked seborrhoea
- Sudden onset particularly in the context of other signs of hyperandrogenism

Investigating for antibiotic-resistant strains of *C. acnes* may be of interest as there is a correlation between the presence of these strains and poor clinical response to antibiotics in some cases. Other investigations that should be considered in acne management relate to the treatment prescribed (see under specific treatments for acne).

Management

A medical assessment should include a personal and family history, a record of present and previous therapies including response, a careful physical examination and a psychosocial review.

General principles of management

The aims of acne management are summarised in Box 88.6. Patients should be reassured that effective treatments are available but should be informed that response is slow and resolution is directly linked to good adherence. Whereas therapy is largely determined by the severity and extent of the disease, it should be tempered by other factors such as duration, response to previous treatments, predisposition and evidence of scarring, persistent redness and pigmentation, as well as patient preference, lifestyle and treatment cost [553,554]. There are no standardised acne grading systems, but it is often categorised as mild, moderate or severe in guidelines and treatment recommendations. This is useful in helping treatment selection, but is dependent on a subjective assessment by the clinician [553]. Identifying the number of lesions as a means of providing a measure of moderate to severe disease as indicated in the 2021 National Institute for Health and Care Excellence (NICE) acne vulgaris guideline provides an objective assessment [555]. However, lesion counts alone do not accurately convey subjective aspects of acne, such as variations in lesion size and visibility. More generic definitions of acne severity have been adopted by the European evidence-based S3 acne guideline (Table 88.18) [556] and other treatment algorithms such as the Global Alliance algorithm, developed with the implicit aim of improving outcomes in acne (Table 88.19) [553]. These guidelines all provide treatment recommendations.

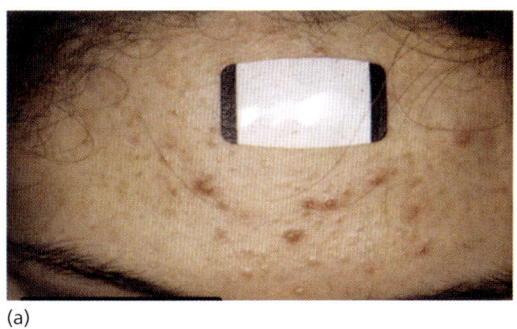 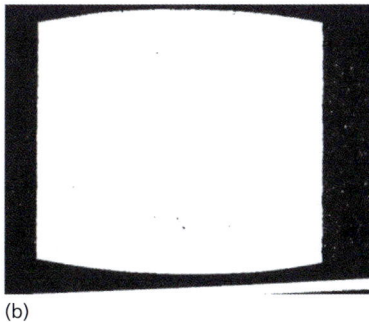 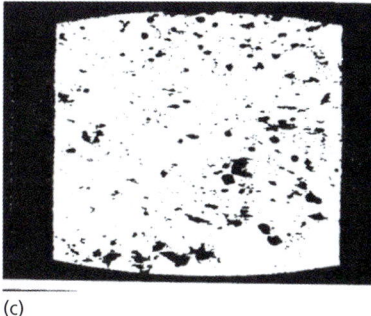

(a)   (b)   (c)

Figure 88.60 Sebutape® analysis. Comparison of two Sebutapes demonstrating the difference between patients with and without acne. (a) Sebutape assessment of sebum. (b) Acne patient with very few secreting follicles. (c) Acne patient with high sebum production, actively secreting follicles and heterogeneity.

Table 88.18 Defining the severity of acne according to lesion type and extent.

Type of acne	Description of clinical lesions
Comedonal acne	Non-inflamed lesions embracing both open (blackheads) and closed (whiteheads) comedones
	Comedones arise from the microcomedo seen at a histological level early in the course of the disease development
Mild acne	Mixed but fairly localised inflamed and non-inflamed lesions. Superficial inflammatory lesions usually <5 mm diameter
Mild to moderate papulopustular acne	More extensive papulopustular lesions frequently in association with comedonal lesions
Severe acne	Many inflammatory papulopustular lesions, frequently deep seated and may evolve into nodules and deep pustules. Small nodules are defined as firm inflammatory lesions >5 mm; large nodules are >1 cm
	At least 35 inflammatory lesions or three or more nodules
	Large nodules extend over large areas and frequently result in painful lesions, exudative sinus tracts and disfiguring tissue destruction and scarring
	Acne conglobata includes multiple grouped comedones, interspersed with papules, tender inflammatory nodules of varying sizes, some of which are suppurative and coalesce to form sinus tracts. Extensive scarring is a frequent outcome

---

Box 88.6 Aims of acne management

- Alleviate symptoms
- Clear existing lesions
- Limit disease activity by preventing new lesions forming as well as scars developing
- Avoid negative impact on quality of life

Adolescents' knowledge and beliefs about acne, help-seeking behaviour and treatment preferences have been studied [557] – highlighting patient and parent education is key in optimising treatment outcomes, including treatment adherence which has been shown to be low in acne [558,559].

Management in patients with skin of colour
Patient perceptions, preferences and decisions on treatment vary across different cultural beliefs and should hence be taken into consideration when deciding on treatment, and acne can be problematic in skin of colour (Figure 88.61). A study exploring the impact of racial differences in acne management found white people were more likely than East Asians and South Asians to see a health care professional about their acne, while East Asians used the Internet more frequently as a source of information about causes of acne and treatments compared with all other groups ($P = 0.04$). Race was not statistically significant as a predictor for willingness to pay [560].

Treatment options for patients with Fitzpatrick skin types III–VI are predominantly the same as for all acne patients, but with some notable additional considerations. Hyperpigmentation and atrophic scars are more common in skin types III–VI with acne-induced pigment being a primary driver in why patients seek treatment [561]. Treatment should therefore focus on targeting pigment and avoid regimens that may exacerbate existing pigmentary change. Patient education confirming the potential persistence or slow improvement of pigment is key, as is the need for early effective treatment of acne to limit inflammation and prevent pigment formation. Regular use of photoprotection and need to avoid excoriating lesions should also be recommended. A number of topical treatments have been shown to improve pigmentation including topical retinoids and azaleic acid, although few studies specifically look at pigment in darker skin types. A notable study by Kircik reported that azelaic acid gel 15% twice daily improved both mild to moderate acne and pigment in 20 adults with Fitzpatrick skin type V and VI, and by week 16 at study conclusion pigment was cleared in 31% of subjects [562]. Similarly, at least a one-grade improvement in pigment severity was found in 75% of patients with Fitzpatrick skin type V or VI with moderate facial acne treated with clindamycin phosphate 1.2%/benzoyl peroxide 3.75% gel (CL-BP 3.75%) once daily for 16 weeks [561].

Physical therapies such as chemical peels and lasers have been used to treat acne-induced pigment, but conversely they can exacerbate hyperpigmentation and therefore should be used with care in skin types III–VI. Microneedling has been suggested as being more advantageous than laser as it does not carry the potential risk of thermal activation of melanocytes and it does not target specific chemopores [563]. Fabbrocini *et al.* investigated the use of microneedling for acne scars and directly compared the outcomes in Fitzpatrick skin types I–VI. There was improvement of acne scars in all groups, adverse effects were comparable between skin types and no dyspigmentation was reported in darker skin types [564]. However, hyperpigmentation was reported at 16% in patients

Table 88.19 Treatment options and improving outcomes in acne. (a) Global Alliance algorithm. (b) National Institute for Health and Care Excellence (NICE) recommended treatment options.

(a)	Mild		Moderate		Severe
	Comedonal	**Papular/pustular**	**Papular/pustular**	**Nodular[a]**	**Nodular/conglobate**
First choice	Topical retinoid	Topical retinoid + topical antimicrobial	Oral antibiotic + topical retinoid ± BPO	Oral antibiotic + topical retinoid ± BPO	Oral isotretinoin[b]
Alternatives[c]	Alt. topical retinoid Or Azelaic acid[d] Or Salicylic acid	Alt. topical antimicrobial + alt. topical retinoid Or Azelaic acid[d]	Alt. oral antibiotic + alt. topical retinoid ± BPO	Oral isotretinoin Or Alt. oral antibiotic + alt. topical retinoid ± BPO/azelaic acid[d]	High-dose oral antibiotic + topical retinoid + BPO
Alternatives for females	See first choice	See first choice	Oral antiandrogen + topical retinoid/azelaic acid[d] ± topical antimicrobial	Oral antiandrogen + topical retinoid ± oral antibiotic ± alt. antimicrobial	High-dose oral antiandrogen + topical retinoid ± alt. topical antimicrobial
Maintenance therapy	Topical retinoid	Topical retinoid ± BPO			

(b)	**Mild to moderate**	**Moderate to severe**	**Severe**
Treatment recommendations	Fixed combination of topical adapalene + topical BPO[e] Or Fixed combination of topical tretinoin + topical clindamycin[e] Or Fixed combination of topical benzoyl peroxide + topical clindamycin[e]	Fixed combination of topical adapalene + topical BPO OD[e] Or Fixed combination of topical tretinoin + topical clindamycin OD[e] Plus either oral lymecycline or oral doxycycline taken OD[f] Or Topical azelaic acid applied BD, plus either oral lymecycline or oral doxycycline taken OD[f] In females with PCOS, consider adding ethinylestradiol with cyproterone acetate (co-cyprindiol) or alt. combined oral contraceptive pill to their treatment Consider photodynamic therapy in those 18 years and over if other treatments are ineffective, not tolerated or contraindicated	Treatments as for moderate–severe, but also consider oral isotretinoin[g] if aged ≥12 years and acne is resistant to adequate courses of standard therapy with systemic antibiotics and topical therapy or acne is at risk of permanent scarring Consider treating severe inflammatory cysts with intralesional injection of triamcinolone acetonide
Maintenance therapy	Topical retinoid ± BPO or if one component of the combination is contraindicated, consider topical monotherapy with adapalene, azelaic acid or benzoyl peroxide		

Adapted from Gollnick *et al.* 2003 [741] and NICE 2021 [**555**].
[a] With small nodules (>0.5–1 cm).
[b] Second course in case of relapse.
[c] Consider physical removal of comedones.
[d] There was no consensus on this alternative recommendation; however, in some countries, azelaic acid prescribing is appropriate practice.
[e] Consider topical benzoyl peroxide monotherapy as an alternative treatment to the options in Table 88.19a if these treatments are contraindicated, or the person wishes to avoid using a topical retinoid or an antibiotic (topical or oral).
[f] If cannot tolerate or have contraindications to oral lymecycline or doxycycline, consider replacing with trimethoprim or an oral macrolide (e.g. erythromycin).
[g] If an acne flare occurs after starting oral isotretinoin, consider adding a course of oral prednisolone *and* consider adding oral prednisolone at commencement of isotretinoin for patients with acne fulminans to prevent an acute flare.
Alt., alternative; BD, twice daily; BPO, benzoyl peroxide; OD, once daily.

with skin types III–IV treated with microneedling for acne scars in another study, hence patients should be warned about the potential risk [565].

First line therapy for mild, moderate and severe acne

Indications for topical therapy include mild acne, moderate to severe acne in conjunction with systemic treatment and as potential maintenance therapy. When considering management it is important to steer clear of monotherapy with either a topical or oral antibiotic due to the increased potential for antimicrobial resistance. Recently there has been some focus on strong topical therapies for their potential oral antibiotic-sparing role in treating moderate to severe facial acne. Stein Gold *et al.* reported that for severe acne (grade 3 on the European Union scale or grade 4 on the US Food

and Drug Administration (FDA) scale) fixed combination adapalene/benzoyl peroxide (BPO) 0.3% showed significantly greater efficacy in achieving success (clear or almost clear or a three-grade improvement) and reductions in lesion counts compared with vehicle [565]. However, systemic antibiotics alongside topical treatment is advocated for more moderate to severe disease, especially when the acne extends to sites other than the face. Topical and systemic combinations and oral isotretinoin should be considered earlier in patients demonstrating poor prognostic factors who have not responded to combined treatment regimens and are at risk of permanent scarring as outlined in Table 88.16 [566]. Figures 88.62, 88.63 and 88.65 outline first, second and third line management based on evidence and expert opinion according to lesion type and severity.

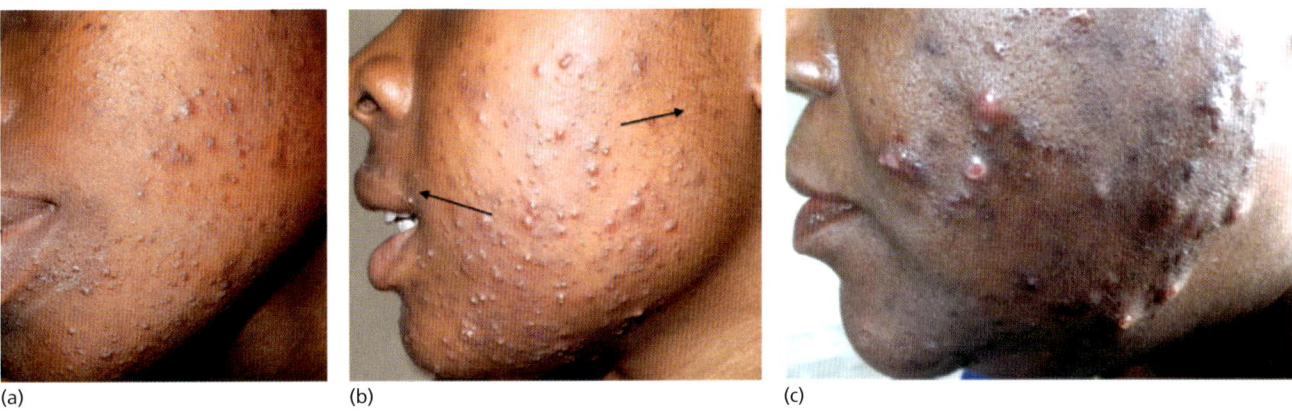

Figure 88.61 Acne in patients with skin of colour. (a) Comedonal acne with closed and open comedones. (b) Minor hirsutism (arrows), a sign of hyperandrogenism in female patients with darker skin. (c) Active acne nodulocystica with keloid development in darker skin. From Zouboulis *et al.* 2018 [742] with permission from Springer Nature.

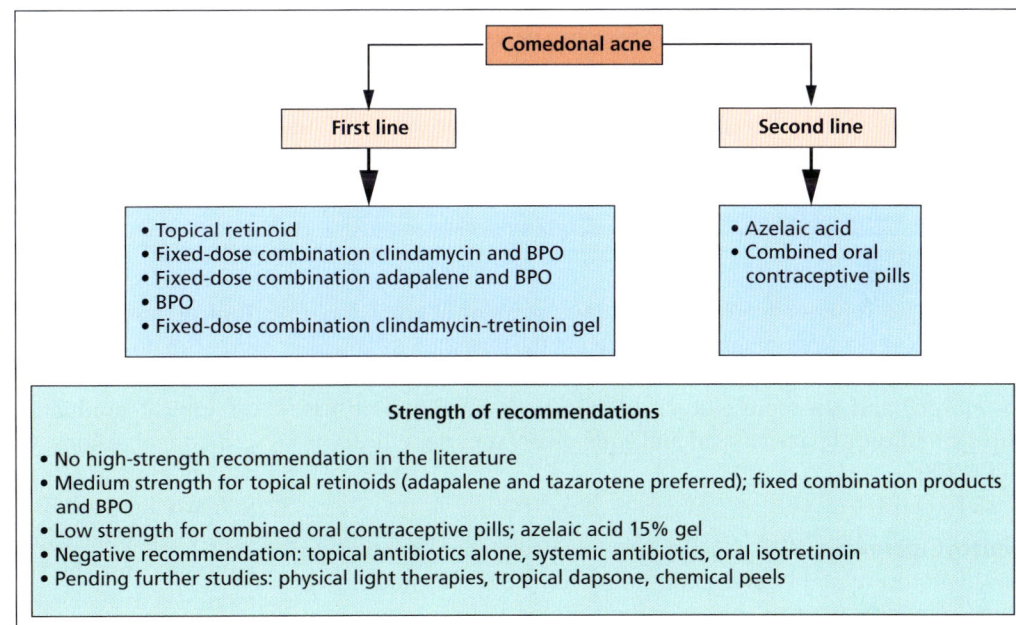

Figure 88.62 Treatment algorithm for comedonal acne. BPO, benzoyl peroxide.

Topical therapy should be applied to all areas of affected skin as the histology of normal-looking skin from an acne-prone site demonstrates microcomedones as the precursors of all clinical lesions. Topical retinoids target microcomedones and are frequently considered in an acne regimen as a means of preventing progression of the microcomedo to active visible lesions. To enhance treatment success, a combination of agents should be employed to impact multiple aetiological factors. Combination products are more convenient for patients to use and aid adherence [**555,556**].

Management of comedonal acne

There are a paucity of clinical trials addressing comedonal disease as it rarely exists as a single entity. Figure 88.62 summarises the treatment for comedonal lesions.

Topical retinoids. Topical retinoids are recommended for comedonal acne [565]. All-*trans* retinoic acid (tretinoin, vitamin A acid) is available in 0.01% up to 0.05% concentrations as either a gel or a cream. Newer formulations, microsponge and polymer

formulations are reportedly less irritant than original formulations [567]. Isotretinoin 0.05% gel is a second-generation retinoid. The third-generation retinoid, adapalene 0.1% cream or gel, has significant and rapid anti-inflammatory action and has a greater benefit/risk ratio than tretinoin. In the USA and a few other countries, the fourth-generation retinoid tazarotene is available for acne on prescription [568,569]. Retinoids reduce abnormal growth and the development of keratinocytes within the pilosebaceous duct. The reversal of hypercornification within the follicular canal as well as the induction of the follicular epithelium helps to 'unplug' the follicle [570]. This also inhibits the development of the microcomedo and non-inflamed lesions, resulting in less anaerobic conditions with fewer *C. acnes*, making the microenvironment less favourable for the development of inflammation. In addition, some of the novel retinoids reduce rupture of the comedones into the surrounding skin which results in less inflammation [571–573].

In vitro, adapalene and tretinoin downregulate TLR2 expression and function, which in turn influences the production of pro-inflammatory cytokines [574–577]. Topical retinoids have been

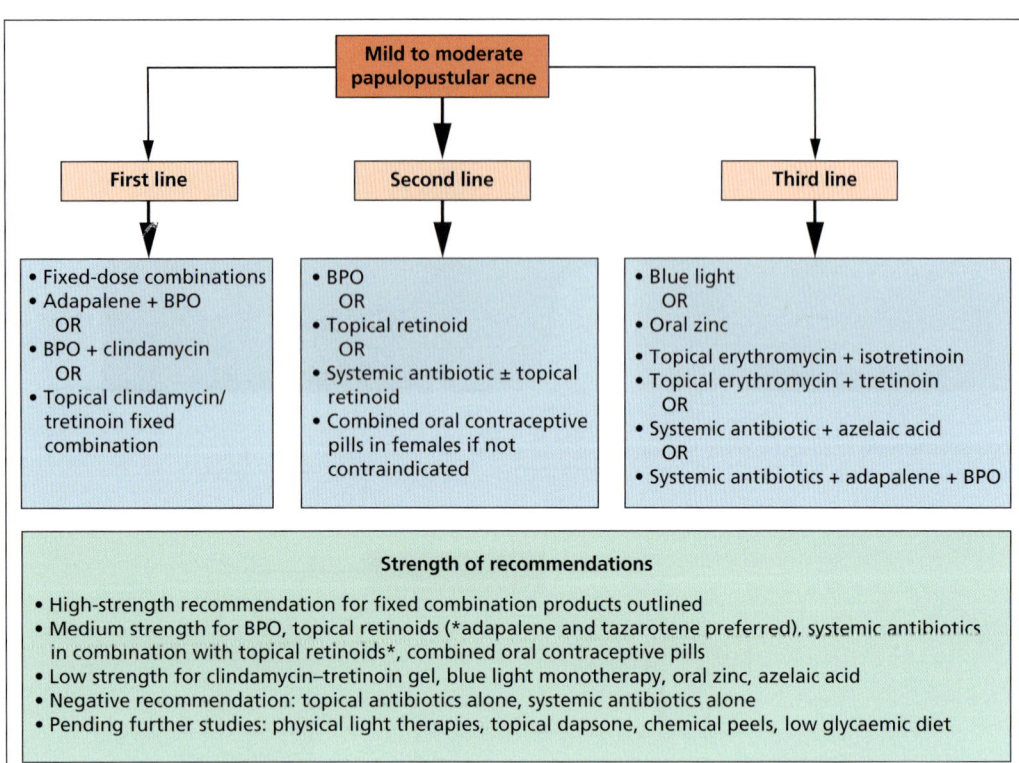

Figure 88.63 Treatment algorithm for mild to moderate papulopustular acne. BPO, benzoyl peroxide.

shown to be superior to placebo for the treatment of comedones and when used as monotherapy in reducing the formation of micro-comedones. Adapalene and tazarotene have the strongest evidence for efficacy and are more efficacious than tretinoin. Tretinoin has superior efficacy to azelaic acid and equivalent/superior efficacy to BPO [578].

Benzoyl peroxide. BPO is currently available in a number of different formulations and concentrations (2.5%, 5% and 10%), some of which are available over the counter. BPO is a powerful antimicrobial [579,580] and rapidly destroys both surface and ductal *C. acnes* and yeasts [581,582]. The lipophilic nature of BPO allows it to penetrate the pilosebaceous duct. Once applied to the skin it decomposes in the sebaceous follicles to release free oxygen radicals with potent bactericidal and anti-inflammatory activity [581,583]. BPO has some comedolytic activity and has been shown in RCTs to reduce the number of non-inflamed lesions by decreasing fol-licular hyperkeratosis [583]. Like other topical agents it does not impact on sebum production. There is no evidence to support a dose–response effect of BPO but potential adverse effects, including irritancy and bleaching, are increased with the 10% concentration [584]. Allergic contact dermatitis has been reported with BPO but is rare with other topical agents [585]. BPO bleaches clothes and hair and the patient must be informed of these inconvenient side effects.

Current evidence suggests that BPO as monotherapy or add-on treatment may be more effective than placebo or no treatment for improving acne, and there may be little to no difference between BPO and either adapalene or clindamycin. This efficacy evi-dence is based on participant self-assessment; trials of BPO versus erythromycin or salicylic acid did not report this outcome [586].

Topical antibiotics. Topical clindamycin has been shown to be superior to placebo when compared with vehicle for comedones but inferior to tretinoin. BPO has been shown to be superior to all topical antibiotics when used as monotherapy for treating comedonal lesions. Azithromycin 2% gel was at least as effective as clindamycin 1% gel in the treatment of mild to moderate acne vulgaris in an RCT and may have the added benefit of reduced *C. acnes* resistance [587]. Topical antibiotics as monotherapy are not advocated for the treatment of comedones as there are superior therapies available and when used alone they have the potential to drive selection of antibiotic-resistant bacteria. A novel topical antibiotic 4% minocycline foam has recently been approved by the US FDA. It is suggested that this can very effectively penetrate the pilosebaceous follicle and reach concentrations that preclude bacterial resistance emerging [588].

Fixed combination therapy. Fixed combination clindamycin/BPO is equivalent to BPO alone and superior to clindamycin alone for the treatment of comedonal acne. Fixed-dose adapalene/BPO is superior or equivalent to BPO and adapalene alone for the treatment of comedones. Both fixed combination products adapa-lene/BPO and clindamycin/BPO have similar efficacy and receive a medium-strength recommendation for comedonal acne [589]. A fixed combination clindamycin/tretinoin recently introduced has shown superior efficacy to its component monotherapies with respect to comedonal acne and favourable improvements in QoL and treatment tolerability in an observational study [590].

Topical dapsone. There are insufficient data to recommend topical dapsone for comedonal acne. One study analysing two RCTs using topical dapsone in acne reported an 8% improvement in comedones after 12 weeks [591]; however, this is unlikely to be of clinical significance. A study comparing efficacy in teenage and adult females of dapsone 5% gel showed statistically significant reduction in comedonal lesions in the older female group [592].

Azelaic acid. Azelaic acid reduces comedones by normalising the disturbed terminal differentiation of keratinocytes in the follicle infundibulum [593], and 20% azelaic acid cream has shown superiority to placebo in the treatment of comedonal acne. In one study, 20% azelaic acid cream had similar activity to 0.05% topical isotretinoin with approximately 80% reduction in comedonal lesion counts at 6 months [594]. However, based on available data this was given a low-level recommendation for comedonal disease in the European S3 guidelines [556].

Management of mild to moderate papulopustular acne

Topical therapy. Contrary to popular belief, studies have demonstrated that topical acne treatments can be as efficacious as oral antibiotics [556]. Tazarotene has shown good efficacy versus vehicle in moderate to severe acne [595,596]. No single topical agent is able to impact on the main aetiological factors implicated in acne pathogenesis and no topical agents have a significant sebosuppressive effect. Recent evidence-based guidelines have advocated combination regimens in order to target as many aetiological factors as possible (Figure 88.63).

Topical retinoids. All topical retinoids assessed in the European S3 guidelines [556] were found to be superior to placebo or vehicle in the treatment of papulopustular acne. The efficacy of adapalene was found to be equivalent to BPO and tretinoin for the treatment of inflammatory lesions [597]. Tazarotene has been noted to be superior to vehicle for inflammatory lesions and superior to or equivalent to adapalene and tretinoin for the treatment of inflammatory lesions and superior in reducing postinflammatory hyperpigmentation [598]. A medium-strength recommendation for topical retinoids in the treatment of mild to moderate papulopustular acne is suggested. A systematic review of retinoids found the differences in efficacy of topical retinoids appears minor, but adapalene had a superior tolerability profile [599]. The novel topical retinoids are less irritant than some of the older established retinoids such as tretinoin and less likely to produce an early treatment flare; and the newer formulations of tretinoin (microsponge or polymer based) are said to be less irritating than the early formulations [599]. Trifarotene, a new-generation retinoid with selective retinoic acid receptor γ agonist action, showed overall success. Both investigator and global assessment (IGA and PGA, respectively) success was 57.9% at week 52 in the same patient in a long-term safety and efficacy study [600]. Retinoids are associated with teratogenicity but significant absorption of topical retinoids has not been demonstrated [601,602].

Benzoyl peroxide. BPO is more efficacious than vehicle in the treatment of papulopustular acne. It is equivalent to adapalene and conflicting evidence exists regarding its equivalence to tretinoin for the treatment of inflammatory lesions [556]. BPO receives a medium-strength recommendation for mild to moderate papulopustular acne. Certain antibiotic/BPO combinations are less irritating than BPO alone, possibly explained by the anti-inflammatory action of the antibiotic.

Topical antibiotics. Topical antibiotics demonstrate superior efficacy compared with placebo in the management of inflammatory acne. However, their use as monotherapy in acne is not advocated due to the risk of emerging bacterial resistance, so they have received a negative recommendation as monotherapy in the management of acne [556]. A detailed analysis of 144 clinical trials of topical antimicrobial therapy rejected over 50% of the studies because of poor trial design [603]. Adequate conclusions could not be drawn from the remaining data because of the different protocols, but BPO emerged as a successful treatment and appeared similar in effectiveness to topical erythromycin and clindamycin.

Fixed-dose combination topical therapy. Fixed-dose clindamycin/BPO is more efficacious than BPO alone for papulopustular acne. Both clindamycin/BPO and adapalene/BPO are superior to adapalene monotherapy and have been shown to be equivalent in efficacy for the treatment of papulopustular acne [556,604]. These agents have received a high strength of recommendation for mild to moderate papulopustular acne. Fixed-dose clindamycin/tretinoin gel is efficacious for inflammatory acne and superior to vehicle, topical 1.2% clindamycin and topical tretinoin 0.025% alone. As clindamycin resistance has not been assessed in studies conducted for longer than 12 weeks, fixed-dose clindamycin/tretinoin gel is currently given a moderate-strength recommendation for mild to moderate papulopustular acne and is not currently advocated for longer than 12 weeks' use. Fixed-combination 0.3% adapalene/BPO has been shown to be effective in moderate to severe facial acne and in a split face study demonstrates potential for less scarring and reduction in scarring over time [605].

Topical dapsone. Topical dapsone 5% gel has been shown in two placebo-controlled trials to improve acne severity more than vehicle [606,607]. This is not deemed clinically significant against criteria used in the European S3 guidelines and there are no comparative studies against other active agents to assess the potential benefit of this novel preparation. A pilot study ($N = 20$) evaluated monotherapy using once-daily topical application of dapsone 7.5% gel for moderate to severe truncal acne. By the end of the study (week 16), the percentage of subjects achieving a two-grade improvement in IGA rating and the percentage of subjects graded as clear or almost clear were 55% and 45%, respectively. Caution must be used if combining topical dapsone with BPO, as a temporary yellow discoloration of the skin has been reported [608].

Azelaic acid. Azelaic acid (1:2-heptanedicarboxylic acid) is available as a 20% cream for acne. It is not sebosuppressive but has been reported to reduce the numbers and function of *C. acnes* [609,610]. A number of RCTs have compared azelaic acid with placebo, vehicle, BPO, tretinoin and 2% erythromycin. In mild to moderate papulopustular acne, the studies suggest that 20% azelaic acid has equivalent efficacy to 5% BPO, 0.05% tretinoin, adapalene and 2% topical erythromycin at 5–6 months but inferior efficacy to systemic tetracycline. The European S3 guideline gives azelaic acid a moderate-strength recommendation for mild to moderate papulopustular acne [556].

PART 8: SPECIFIC CUTANEOUS STRUCTURES

General side effects of topical treatments. The most common side effect of topical acne products is a primary irritant dermatitis which often subsides with time and can be managed by reducing the frequency of application, using emollients and, if severe, short-term application of a type I potency topical corticosteroid.

Systemic therapy. Systemic therapy is generally advocated when there is a significant inflammatory component and/or the acne is extensive rendering topical applications impractical. Systemic therapy for the treatment of mild papulopustular acne includes antibiotics, hormonal options, zinc, oral isotretinoin and/or steroids for unresponsive disease. Other drugs such as dapsone, clofazimine and vitamin A acid (10–20 mg/day) are occasionally used but evidence to support their effectiveness is limited.

Systemic antibiotics. Oral antibiotics are the most widely prescribed agents in acne and are indicated for severe acne, moderate facial acne not responding to topical therapies and/or extensive truncal acne. Response to systemic antibiotics varies. Young males with marked seborrhoea and truncal acne respond less well than females with purely facial acne.

Cyclines (tetracycline, oxytetracycline, doxycycline, lymecycline, minocycline, sarecycline) are the antibiotics of choice; however, there is insufficient evidence to support one agent or dose. They are contraindicated in pregnancy and children younger than 8 years as they can affect cartilage and bone growth, and cause yellow discoloration of the teeth [611]. The second-generation cyclines may aid adherence and of these lymecycline and doxycycline should be used in preference to minocycline [556]. Sarecycline is a tetracycline-derived narrow-spectrum oral antibiotic, specifically designed for acne, approved by the US FDA in 2018 for the treatment of inflammatory lesions of non-nodular moderate to severe acne in patients 9 years of age and older [612,613]. Spontaneous mutation rates of bacteria (*C. acnes*, *Staphylococcus aureus* and *S. epidermidis*) cultured in the presence of sarecycline are very low, showing reduced likelihood of bacterial resistance. This favourable characteristic is attributed to structural modifications that overcome tetracycline resistance mechanisms, changing bacterial ribosome binding [614]. Unlike the broad spectrum tetracyclines, sarecycline is minimally active against Gram-negative bacilli and normal microflora. This specificity translates to a reduction in off-target antibacterial effects, making it an attractive choice over others in its class [615]. In phase III trials sarecycline demonstrated therapeutic effect on both facial and truncal inflammatory acne. It also showed significant improvement in comedonal lesions compared with placebo.

Due to reports of potential serious adverse effects, minocycline is not recommended as first line therapy. Adverse effects with minocycline include drug hypersensitivity syndrome (DHS) occurring within 3 months of treatment initiation, characterised by fever, malaise, arthralgia and a diffuse exanthematous skin eruption. Systemic involvement may include pulmonary eosinophilia and hepatitis. Early recognition and withdrawal of the agent is essential, and repeat exposure may result in a recurrence of DHS within a few days [616]. A lupus-like reaction has also been reported occurring after 6–48 months of treatment. Patients are usually female and present with fever, malaise and polyarthralgia. A cutaneous rash is not always evident but urticaria, vasculitis and non-specific redness have all been reported. Some patients have concomitant liver disease, which may occur in the absence of joint symptoms. Serology for lupus is evident with a positive antinuclear antibody (ANA), along with positive perinuclear antineutrophilic cytoplasmic antibodies (pANCA) and raised C-reactive protein. Severely deranged hepatic enzymes and rarely liver damage requiring liver transplantation have also been reported [617]. Positive antihistone antibodies are rarely identified. The lupus-like reaction is reversible if the drug is withdrawn but abnormal serology may persist. Minocycline should be avoided in patients with a personal or family history of systemic lupus erythematosus. Before embarking on long-term minocycline it is advisable to check hepatic function and ANA at baseline and to repeat hepatic function, ANA and pANCA every 3–6 months.

A large RCT conducted in UK community practice demonstrated that oral minocycline and oral tetracycline were of similar efficacy to each other and comparable in terms of efficacy to topical BPO [618]. This study, which compared five antimicrobial regimens for mild to moderate facial acne in the community, suggested that maximum improvement was reached at 6 weeks with both oral antibiotics and topical BPO [618].

The prescribing of *macrolides* (erythromycin, clindamycin, azithromycin) for acne has increasingly fallen out of favour due to the emergence of antibiotic-resistant strains of *C. acnes* and although limited there is evidence showing tetracycline to be equivalent or superior in efficacy to erythromycin [619]. The antibiotic resistance profile of microbial strains isolated from Korean acne patients showed higher proportions of *C. acnes* isolates were resistant to clindamycin (30%) and erythromycin (26.7%) than to azithromycin (6.7%) and doxycycline (6.7%) [620]. A meta-analysis of RCTs comparing pulsed azithromycin with doxycycline showed similar efficacy, but more favourable pharmacokinetics and side effect profile for azithromycin [621]. If antibiotic therapy is required in pregnancy, oral erythromycin is thought to be safe although there are no data available evaluating chronic use over prolonged periods in pregnancy. A recent review of this published by the Medicines and Healthcare products Regulatory Agency (MHRA) found more evidence for erythromycin use in pregnancy, compared with azithromycin or clindamycin (>24 000 first-trimester exposures) [622]. Only 2 of the 11 studies suggested an increased risk of major congenital or cardiovascular malformations. However, the quality of the observational data was low and they concluded that the available evidence was insufficient to confirm the presence of small increased risks of major congenital malformations or cardiovascular malformations following first-trimester exposure to erythromycin, or an increased risk of miscarriage following exposure to clarithromycin or azithromycin in early pregnancy. Hence the MHRA caution that macrolide antibiotics should only be used during pregnancy if clinically needed and the benefit of treatment is expected to outweigh any possible risk [622]. The safest therapies in pregnancy are therefore topical BPO and/or topical erythromycin [623]. Erythromycin remains the preferred option in children (aged 8–12 years depending on national licences) as tetracylines are contraindicated due to potential musculoskeletal problems and discoloration of permanent teeth.

Table 88.20 Systemic antibiotics in the treatment of acne vulgaris: dosage and adverse effects.

Antibiotic	Dosage	Adverse effects
Oxytetracycline	500 mg BD, 30 min before food and not with milk; makes adherence to medication problematic for some	Common: gastrointestinal upset, vaginal candidaisis Rare: onycholysis, photosensitivity, benign intracranial hypertension, Sweet syndrome
Lymecycline (not available in the USA)	408 mg daily	As oxytetracycline but tolerated better
Doxycycline	100–200 mg OD	As oxytetracycline Photosensitivity (dose dependent)
Minocycline	100 mg OD	Rare but serious: headaches and dizziness associated with benign intracranial hypertension, pigmentary changes, autoimmune hepatitis/lupus erythematosus-like syndrome
Sarecycline (US FDA approved)	<54 kg: 60 mg OD 55–84 kg: 100 mg OD 85–136 kg: 150 mg OD	As oxytetracycline but better tolerated
Erythromycin	500 mg BD	Common: gastrointestinal upset, nausea, diarrhoea
Azithromycin	250 mg three times a week	Generally well tolerated, mild gastrointestinal effects Rare: Stevens–Johnson syndrome, hypersensitivity reactions, blood dyscrasias, small absolute increased risk of arrhythmias
Trimethoprim	200–300 mg BD	Common: gastrointestinal upset, maculopapular rash

Clindamycin is highly lipophilic and very effective in acne but adverse effects, including diarrhoea seen in 5–20% of cases, and potential pseudomembranous colitis from overgrowth of *Clostridium difficile* has discouraged use [624,625].

Trimethoprim may also be helpful in acne management at a dose of 400–600 mg/day [626,627] but has lower evidence of efficacy compared with tetracycline [628]. Adverse effects with trimethoprim include haematological reactions such as agranulocytosis, thrombocytopenia and pancytopenia. The risk of these developing is linked to higher dose regimens and those with folic acid deficiency and/or megaloblastic haematopoiesis [626,629]. It is advisable to take a baseline full blood count prior to starting any extended courses of trimethoprim and to repeat this monthly while the patients remain on treatment. DHS has been rarely been reported with trimethoprim [630].

Despite reports of efficacy in acne, the use of azithromycin, trimethoprim and other antibiotics including cephalosporins and fluoroquinolones should be discouraged as they are commonly used to treat a variety of systemic infections [624]. Exceptions to this rule may include short-term use for extremely refractory disease and/or evidence of Gram-negative folliculitis where other agents are not acceptable and in cases where tetracyclines are contraindicated.

Table 88.20 outlines dosage regimens for systemic antibiotics recommended for the treatment of acne and considers potential adverse effects.

Interactions of antibiotics with oral contraceptives. There is concern that combined oral contraceptive (COC) efficacy may be impaired when used alongside antibiotics based on the hypothesis that broad spectrum antibiotics reduce bacterial flora in the gut and thus may interfere with oestrogen absorption. However, pharmacokinetic studies have demonstrated that serum levels of oestrogen are unaffected by tetracycline and doxycycline. The failure rate of COCs when used with tetracycline resulting in pregnancy is reported as 1.2–1.4 pregnancies per 100 woman-years of oral contraceptive use, which is no greater than background failure rate

of COCs. The only antibiotic that has been shown to reduce COC efficacy is rifampicin [631–634].

General side effects of oral antibiotics. All oral antibiotics for acne can produce mild adverse effects (Table 88.20). Several studies have confirmed that the use of antibiotics for acne drives bacterial resistance [635,636]. The presence of antibiotic-resistant *C. acnes* may correlate with poor clinical response to antibiotics [637]. A study characterising patients carrying clindamycin-resistant *C. acnes* found clindamycin-resistant strains were frequently isolated from patients with older median age (≥24 years) and moderate to severe acne [638]. The concentration of ductal antibiotics varies considerably and may fall below the minimal inhibitory concentration for *C. acnes*. A low drug concentration in tissues will encourage the acquisition of antibiotic-resistant *C. acnes* [639]. Poor adherence to therapy will potentially reduce drug availability, and a high sebum excretion is likely to dilute an effective drug concentration [640].

A number of publications have proposed how antibiotics should be administered to achieve optimal therapeutic response while avoiding antibiotic resistance and have produced antibiotic prescribing policies (Table 88.21) [556]. Recent NICE guidelines suggest oral antibiotics should not be prescribed for longer than 12 months except in exceptional circumstances [555]. Suggestions to reduce exposure to antibiotics include (i) restricting the duration of antibiotics; (ii) the use of combination regimens from the onset of therapy to expedite response and reduce duration of antibiotic courses; (iii) the utilisation of BPO either to reduce the emergence of or to treat antibiotic-resistant strains of *C. acnes*; (iv) the avoidance of using chemically dissimilar antibiotics; and (v) regular switching of antibiotics. Table 88.22 summarises possible factors that might indicate the presence of antibiotic-resistant *C. acnes*. Resistance is not the only reason for poor response to treatment (Table 88.23).

Hormonal therapy

Clascoterone. Clascoterone, a first-in-class topical androgen receptor inhibitor, has been approved by the FDA in a twice-daily

Table 88.21 Antibiotic prescribing policies.

Strategy to avoid propionibacterial resistance emerging	Comments
Avoid inappropriate use of topical and systemic antibiotics	Use oral antibiotics for 3 months in the first instance and only continue if clinical improvement continues
If extending the duration of oral antibiotics, utilise combination therapy	Combine with an agent that reduces the likelihood of promoting antibiotic propionibacterial resistance, e.g. benzoyl peroxide
If repeated courses of antibiotics are required and the initial clinical response was favourable, reuse the same drug	This will avoid multiple resistant strains emerging
Avoid prescribing different oral and topical antibiotics concomitantly	This will avoid multiple resistant strains emerging
Consider using topical retinoids and non-antibiotic antimicrobials wherever possible	These do not promote resistant isolates and when used with antibiotics may achieve more rapid efficacy and so reduce the duration of the antibiotic course
Topical benzoyl peroxide (BPO) can be used for 7 days between antibiotic courses	BPO is fully active against sensitive and resistant strains of *Cutibacterium acnes* and able to eradicate resistant isolates
Remember to check medical adherence	Poor adherence to antibiotic therapies promotes resistance

Table 88.22 Reasons to suspect poor response relates to resistance to antibiotic therapies.

Reason to suspect possible antibiotic-resistant *Cutibacterium acnes*	Comments
Failure to respond to antibiotic therapy	Confirm good adherence to therapy
Deterioration in acne despite continuing antibiotic therapy	Patients often confirm initial good results
History of poor adherence	Thought to lend itself to resistance emerging
Multiple courses of oral and topical antibiotics	Particularly when used as monotherapy

Table 88.23 Reasons to suspect poor response to treatment.

Reason for poor response to therapy	Comments
Need for improved education of doctor or patient	Understanding of how to use therapies is mandatory for successful treatment
Poor adherence to therapy	Steadily diminishing adherence may lead to relapse
Presence of relevant antibiotic resistant *Cutibacterium acnes* in patient complying to therapy	Colonisation with resistant isolates from the start results in poor response; subsequent colonisation leads to relapse
Development of Gram-negative folliculitis	See section on differential diagnosis earlier in chapter
Incorrect diagnosis	See section on differential diagnosis earlier in chapter
Presence of macrocomedones prior to starting isotretinoin	Can result in significant flare of acne
Refractory subtypes of acne	See individual sections
Intolerance to or side effects of treatment	See treatment section
Inadequate dose of antibiotics	Patients of high body weight or marked seborrhoea may require a higher dose

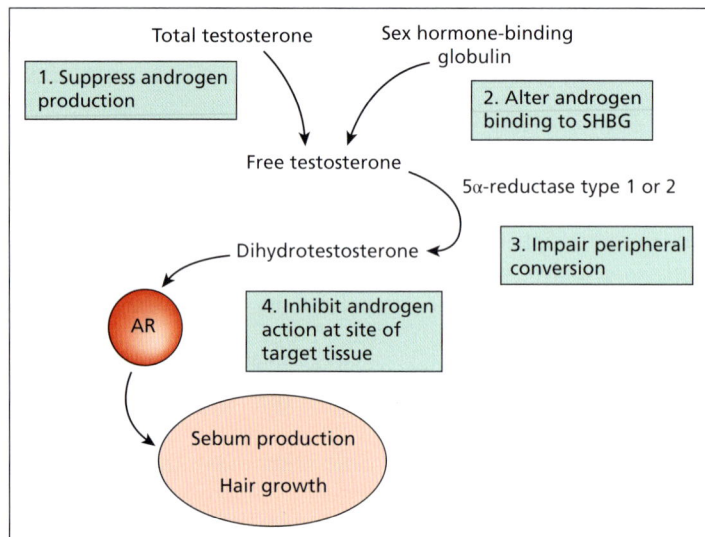

Figure 88.64 Potential mechanism of action(s) using antiandrogens in the management of acne. AR, androgen receptor; SHBG, sex hormone-binding globulin.

most common local skin reaction [641]. Unlike systemic antiandrogens, it can be used in males as well as females and so presents an attractive prescribing option for clinicians.

Systemic hormone preparations are available for acne in female patients. Current guidance advocated their use in adult females with acne who also require a contraceptive and/or have need for menstrual control. They may offer an alternative as part of a combination regimen when oral isotretinoin is inappropriate or not available.

Topical therapy and systemic antibiotics can be prescribed in conjunction with hormonal regimens and this will enhance efficacy. Potential hormonal treatments for acne include inhibitors of androgen production by the ovary (oral contraceptives) or adrenal gland (low-dose corticosteroids), androgen receptor blockers and antiandrogens that block the effect of androgens on the sebaceous gland. Figure 88.64 outlines the mechanisms of action [642,643].

Oestrogens and progestins. COCs generally contain oestrogen (most commonly ethinyl oestradiol) and a progestin. Oestrogens increase the synthesis of sex hormone-binding globulin (SHBG) leading to increased binding of testosterone and reduced levels

application, 1% cream formulation to treat acne in patients aged 12 years and over [641]. Phase II and III trials have demonstrated a statistically significant reduction in inflammatory and non-inflammatory lesions with clascoterone use and a favourable safety profile for up to 9 months of use, with redness being the

of free circulating testosterone. Hence all oral contraceptives potentially improve acne. In addition, oral contraceptives suppress ovulation by inhibiting the production of ovarian androgens which results in reduced serum androgens and lower sebum production. Progestins in COCs include estranes and gonanes, which are derivatives of 19-nortestosterone, cyproterone acetate (CPA) and drosperinone. The third-generation progestins (gestodene, desogestrel, norgestimate) are less selective for the androgen and more selective for the progesterone receptor. Drosperinone is a novel progestin derived from 17α-spironolactone and has antiandrogenic activity, making it potentially helpful in acne. Yasmin® contains drospirenone 3 mg combined with ethinyl oestradiol 30 μg and Yaz® contains the same dose of drospirenone with 20 μg of ethinyl oestradiol. Box 88.3 outlines the androgenic effect of progestins in COCs.

A Cochrane systematic review determining the effectiveness of COCs for the treatment of facial acne compared with placebo or other active therapies confirmed that COCs reduced acne lesion counts, severity grades and self-assessed acne compared with placebo [643a]. Limited data suggested that chlormadinone or CPA achieved better efficacy than levonogestrel, and a COC containing CPA may produce better outcomes than one containing desogestrel. Limited data were available comparing COCs with other therapies [643a]. A cohort study showed that the continued use of ethinylestradiol 20 μg/dienogest 2 mg COC reduced inflammatory and non-inflammatory acne lesions in 94% of women between 18 and 30 years of age over a 12-month period; 23% of women had a 100% reduction in acne lesions at the 12-month follow-up [642].

Androgen receptor blockers. Androgen receptor blockers suppress sebum and so offer potential for the treatment of acne. The antiandrogen CPA is licensed for acne in most European countries, but not in the USA, and directly inhibits the androgen receptor. Co-cyprindiol (Dianette and Estelle-35) is an oral contraceptive that ameliorates acne. It is as effective as oral tetracycline 1 g/day given over a 6-month period, although slower in action [643]. CPA 2 mg with ethinyl oestradiol (35 μg) has a greater risk of deep venous thrombosis embolism than first- and second-generation COCs [644]. As a result the current recommendation is that once the acne is under control, co-cyprindiol formulations should be replaced by a COC containing a lower dose of oestrogen. In summary, based on low-grade evidence and expert opinion, COCs may be helpful in the treatment of adult female acne in the context of those also requiring a hormonal therapy, being mindful of the fact there are associated risks which need to be explained to patients and that these agents are not necessarily licensed for acne.

Spironolactone in acne management. Spironolactone is reported in the literature as an effective treatment for acne. It is usually prescribed at a dose of 50–100 mg daily with meals, but many women with sporadic outbreaks do well with doses as low as 25 mg daily [645]. Although spironolactone is used in this context with clinical success there is a paucity of studies to confirm evidence of its effectiveness due to very small sample populations studied and poor trial design [646]. A hybrid systematic review emphasised this as it found that all trials were at a 'high risk' of bias with low quality of evidence. Only one crossover trial demonstrated

statistical superiority of a 200 mg daily dose versus inflamed lesions compared with placebo [647]. Barbieri *et al.* have now shown similar clinical effectiveness to oral tetracyclines as the odds ratio for being prescribed a different systemic agent within 1 year was 1.07 (95% CI 0.99–1.16) for those prescribed spironolactone when compared with oral tetracycline-class antibiotics in a retrospective cohort [648]. The main side effects are menstrual irregularity, breast tenderness, occasional fluid retention and, rarely, melasma. The frequency of menstrual irregularity can be significantly reduced by concomitant use of a COC. Pregnancy should be avoided due to potential abnormalities to the male fetus and serum. There is a theoretical risk of hyperkalaemia as spironolactone is a potassium-sparing diuretic, however data from the systematic review just mentioned supported the recommendation that routine monitoring is not required in this patient population [647]. A study has just recently been completed and preliminary results support the efficacy of spironolactone in adult women [649].

All hormonal regimens should be combined with appropriate topical therapies.

Comparative effectiveness of hormonal treatment with other approaches. There are few good studies comparing hormonal approaches to antibiotics and isotretinoin. Isotretinoin has been shown to be more effective than co-cyprindiol for acne patients [650]. One systematic review assessed mean weighted effects across different reported variables. Isotretinoin scored 85 ± 10% improvement compared with baseline, whereas tetracyclines and hormonal treatments were less effective, scoring 54 ± 3%, and CPA plus ethinyl oestradiol showed 65 ± 4% improvement compared with baseline levels [651].

Oral isotretinoin. Systemic isotretinoin is considered the most potent and effective therapy for acne. There are few studies comparing efficacy of isotretinoin with other treatments. A combination of high-dose doxycycline (200 mg daily) plus BPO/adapalene has been shown to be non-inferior to oral isotretinoin in the treatment of severe nodular acne [652], but oral isotretinoin has been shown to be superior to tetracycline plus adapalene in an earlier study [653]. Conventional doses of isotretinoin aiming for 1 mg/kg/day are extremely efficacious in most cases of acne. Due to the adverse side effect profile, national and international guidelines recommend that isotretinoin should be reserved for those with severe disease, defined as nodulocystic acne, acne conglobata or acne at risk of permanent scarring that has failed to respond to adequate courses of previous treatment. Some studies examining isotretinoin dose regimens found that lower doses of 0.25 mg/kg/day or 20 mg on alternate days were as efficacious as higher doses in the management of papulopustular disease [654,655]. However, there are no well-designed studies that are adequately powered to be clear if low- versus high-dose oral isotretinoin results in similar efficacy, with lower adverse effects and equal long-term remission. See the section on the use of oral isotretinoin in severe disease.

Oral zinc. Two double-blind studies showed a significant benefit for treatment of inflammatory lesions, particularly with zinc gluconate (200 mg/day). Comparison with minocycline 100 mg/day demonstrated that the antibiotic improved acne by 63% in contrast to 32%

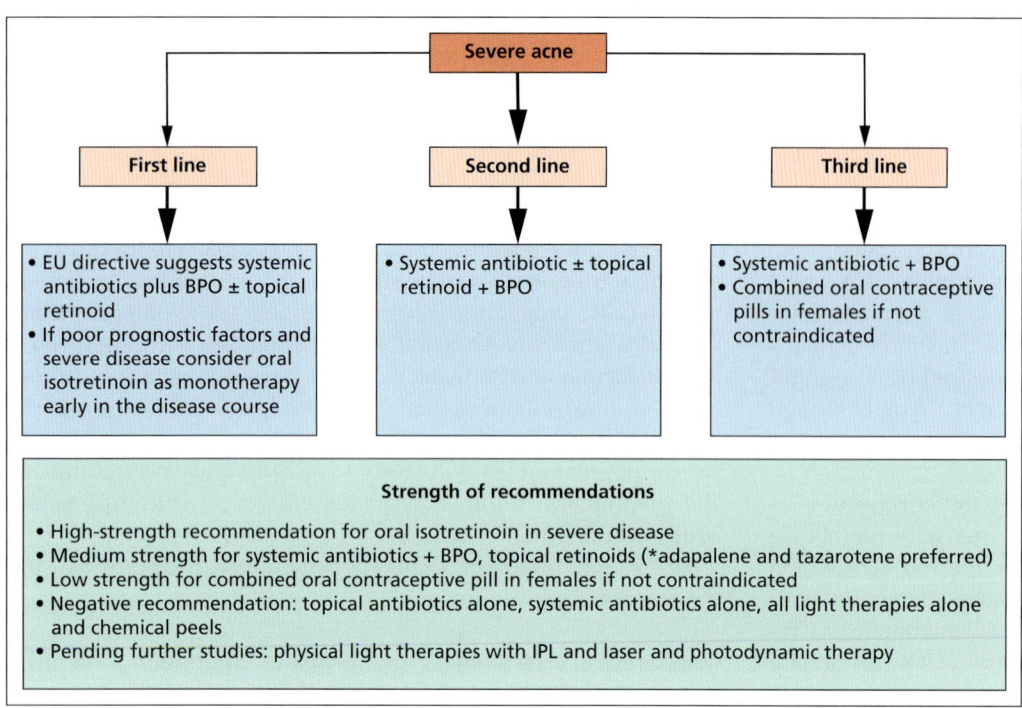

Figure 88.65 Treatment algorithm for severe acne. BPO, benzoyl peroxide; IPL, intense pulsed light.

with 30 mg/day of elemental zinc after 3 months; no placebo was included in the study [656]. The S3 European guidelines give zinc a low-level strength of recommendation for mild to moderate papulopustualar acne [556].

Management of severe acne

Clinical evidence for the treatment of severe acne is limited. Figure 88.65 outlines a suggested algorithm for the treatment of severe acne. Oral isotretinoin is regarded as the treatment of choice for severe acne that has failed to respond to conventional therapy. However, if this is contraindicated or not acceptable, topical adapalene or fixed-dose BPO/adapalene may be used in combination with systemic antibiotics, with the best evidence in support of doxycycline.

Systemic antibiotics. A combination of systemic antibiotic combined with BPO with or without adapalene has been given a medium-strength recommendation for severe acne [556]. Given the concerns about antibiotic resistance, monotherapy with systemic antibiotics is not recommended.

Hormonal therapy. Evidence for the use of hormonal therapy in severe acne is lacking. In the UK, ethinyloestradiol/CPA is officially indicated for the treatment of severe acne unresponsive to systemic antibiotics and other available treatments.

Oral isotretinoin. Oral isotretinoin (13-*cis*-retinoic acid) is a synthetic vitamin A analogue which was first approved by the US FDA in 1982 for the treatment of severe recalcitrant acne. Isotretinoin remains the most clinically effective acne therapy, producing long-term remission and significant improvement in many patients. It is licensed for the treatment of severe acne that has failed to respond to conventional antibiotic therapies. National

and international guidelines recommend isotretinoin should be reserved for those with severe disease defined as nodulocystic acne, acne conglobata or acne at risk of permanent scarring that has failed to respond to adequate courses of previous treatment [555,556]. Most patients who receive oral isotretinoin will be free of acne after 4–8 months of treatment depending on the dose used. Clinical experience suggests that the long-term cure rate may be lower than initially thought. There is evidence to suggest that younger patients relapse more frequently than older ones. Over the years, isotretinoin has been used to treat many different and difficult cases of acne with varying degrees of success, as outlined in Table 88.24.

The European Directive (ED) on prescribing of isotretinoin was introduced to ensure that generic prescribing was harmonised throughout the European Union and to minimise the risk of adverse effects including pregnancy [657]. Table 88.25 summarises the recommendations, which include monitoring of laboratory parameters to include primarily fasting lipids, and liver function tests at baseline, 1 month after starting therapy and if stable 12-weekly thereafter [657]. There has been much debate as to whether liver function tests and blood lipids should be monitored during therapy [658]. Elevated levels unrelated to any clinical significance are common and rapidly return to pre-treatment levels after therapy has been discontinued [659,660]. Some authors only advocate repeat testing post-baseline in at-risk groups such as those with diabetes and patients with known familial hypertriglyceridaemia [659]. However, as there is no good evidence on when to taper dosage regimens or to discontinue therapy in the context of abnormal results, and the absence of a laboratory abnormality does not preclude an adverse clinical outome [660], it would currently seem prudent to follow the ED and to interpret results aligned to the individual on treatment.

Reductions in haematological parameters including thrombocytopenia and neutropenia have been reported while taking oral isotretinoin for acne but a large population-based study showed

Table 88.24 Relative success of isotretinoin in various acne and other clinical conditions.

Diagnosis	Excellent response	Moderate response	Limited response
Severe acne	×	–	–
Moderate acne[a]	×	–	–
Mild acne[a]	×	–	–
Acne fulminans[a,b]	×	–	–
Rosacea	×	–	–
Rosacea fulminans[a,b]	×	–	–
Acne conglobata	–	–	×
Gram-negative folliculitis	–	×	–
Solid facial oedema	–	–	×
Hidradenitis suppurativa	–	–	×
Vasculitic acne	–	–	×
Dissecting scalp cellulitis	–	–	×
Steatocystoma multiplex	–	–	×
Seborrhoea	–	×	–
Fordyce disease	–	×	–
Chemoprophylaxis of skin cancer:	–	×	–
Basal cell naevus syndrome			
Xeroderma pigmentosum			
Eruptive keratoacanthomas			

[a] Especially if associated with scarring and/or psychological problems.
[b] Also needs pre-isotretinoin therapy with oral steroids.

Table 88.25 Recommendations from the European Directive on isotretinoin prescribing.

	Pre-directive	Post-directive
Dosage	0.5–1.0 mg/kg/day	Start 0.5 mg/kg/day
Indications for use	Isotretinoin recommended as first line therapy for severe acne (nodular and conglobata) as well as acne not responding to 3 months' systemic antibiotics in combination with topical therapy	New recommendations suggest isotretinoin should only be used in severe acne (nodular and conglobata) that has or is not responding to appropriate antibiotics and topical therapy; the inference of this being that it should now not be used at all as first line therapy
Age	Previously no age limit	Not indicated in children <12 years
Monitoring	Liver enzymes and lipids should be checked before treatment and 1 month after the maximum dosage has been used	Baseline investigations as before but at 1 month and 3-monthly throughout the course of treatment

very few haematological abnormalities during treatment [660]. There are no explicit recommendations for the assessment of haematological parameters but the American Academy of Dermatology advises full blood counts alongside triglycerides, cholesterol and transaminases.

Regulatory authorities in each country have approved a pregnancy prevention programme (PPP). This programme includes advice on education, therapy management and control of the distribution of oral isotretinoin:

- *Education* – both patients and prescribers must be fully aware of teratogenicity. The patient should acknowledge the problem by signing a consent form and should accept detailed counselling by the clinician prior to and during treatment.
- *Therapy management* includes medically supervised pregnancy testing before, during and 5 weeks after a course of therapy and provides advice on contraception.
- *Distribution control of isotretinoin* suggests that only 30 days of oral isotretinoin can be supplied at one time to a female patient and the prescription will only be valid for 7 days.

The scope of the PPP suggests that it should include all females of child-bearing potential. Clinicians can exercise clinical judgement if they establish that the patient is not currently sexually active, but it is mandatory that clinicians check carefully at each 4-week follow-up visit and record as well as act on any change in circumstance.

Pregnancy testing is recommended pre- and 5 weeks post-therapy. It has been suggested that the initial test can be done up to 2 weeks prior to the start of treatment provided contraception is used in those who require it. In addition, monthly pregnancy testing is recommended throughout the treatment period. The treatment should ideally start on day 3 of the menstrual cycle. The programme suggests that where possible patients should agree to at least one, and preferably two, complementary methods of effective contraception, including a barrier method, before therapy is initiated.

Dispensing restrictions do not apply to males as the process is aimed at ensuring that females do not receive extended periods of treatment without pregnancy tests being performed. The responsibility for the assessment of pregnancy tests and the administration of further prescriptions lies with the clinician. Clinical problems relating to the implementation of this approach include difficulties in females with irregular menses, potential lack of continuity of treatment due to potential unavailability of patient and/or health care workers as well as forgotten tests. Given the potential side effects of oral contraceptives, it may not always be appropriate to insist on all patients using specific contraceptives, especially those not sexually active.

The USA has a robust prevention programme called iPLEDGE. This has very recently been reviewed and revised (see Resources). The key changes are as follows:

1 The requirement for prescribers to document monthly patient counselling in patients who cannot become pregnant will change only at enrolment. Pending implementation, this could eliminate need for monthly visits for persons of non-childbearing potential.

2 The waiting period requirement (also referred to as the 19-day lockout) for patients if they do not obtain isotretinoin within the first 7 day prescription window will be lifted such that if a window period is missed, a repeat pregnancy test can be secured and if negative there is no need to wait a month.

3 Prescribers can adopt the option of using home pregnancy testing for their patients during and after isotretinoin treatment. This allows for continued flexibility at least for follow-up visits.

4 The requirement that pregnancy tests must be performed in a specially certified (i.e. Clinical Laboratory Improvement

PART 8: SPECIFIC CUTANEOUS STRUCTURES

Amendments) laboratory has been removed. This will make it easier to do pregnancy tests in a clinic setting without needing to send the patient to a laboratory.

In the UK, the MHRA has recently conducted a robust review of oral isotretinoin and as a result introduced new safety measures to strengthen the safe use of this medication. The new measures include additional oversight of the initiation of treatment for patients under 18 years of age and through improved assessment and monitoring of mental health and sexual function issues. The Isotretinoin Expert Working Group of the Commission on Human Medicines has also made recommendations to strengthen the safety of isotretinoin treatment. Recommendations include new warnings, the need for consistent monitoring requirements for psychiatric side effects, the introduction of new monitoring requirements for sexual side effects and additional oversight of the initiation of treatment for patients younger than 18 years. The MHRA has also introduced a new rule that treatment with isotretinoin for patients under 18 must be approved by two prescribers.

Current guidance recommends starting oral isotretinoin at 0.5 mg/kg/day and to titrate the dose as tolerated up to 1 mg/kg/day. The half-life is 22 h and the bioavailability is 25%. Absorption of isotretinoin is markedly affected by the presence of fat and pharmacokinetic studies show that absorption can be doubled by taking isotretinoin with or after a meal compared with the fasting state [661,662]. It is therefore advisable to take the capsules with fatty food at the same time of day. However, the amount of fat required is high and it is unlikely that patients ingest enough fat to optimise absorption. A novel lipid formulation is now available in some countries, the bioavailability of which is not fat dependent [663].

To date, the duration of therapy varies according to the dose administered over the course of the treatment period. Many acne guidelines suggest that post-therapy relapse is minimised by treatment courses that amount to a total of least 120–150 mg/kg. However, there is not an *a priori* pharmacokinetic reason to support the concept of accumulation of drug or a cumulative dose effect and recent publications suggest that the dose should be tailored to the tolerability of the drug as well as the clinical response, and have demonstrated that the cumulative doses previously recommended may not be necessary in all patients [664]. The duration of therapy should be adjusted to give at least 90% clearance of acne based upon initial clinical acne grade scoring techniques followed by 4–8 weeks of consolidation.

Demographic factors, such as age, sex and duration of acne, may all govern the rate of response and relapse. Males with extensive truncal acne, more severe acne and/or suffering from acne for less than 7 years fail to respond as well as, and relapse more quickly than, female patients with predominantly facial acne of a less severe grade.

A number of studies have been published using different dosing regimens of isotretinoin [556]. However, none is controlled for dietary fat intake and confounding factors that may influence relapse. There appears to be a small cohort of patients who benefit from long-term low-dose isotretinoin. However, it is not clear whether this approach will result in long-term adverse effects and it is important to clarify with the patient that although nothing untoward has been reported to date, this approach lies outside recommended guidelines and the current product licence.

The physical and psychological severity of acne will play a role in the decision whether to prescribe isotretinoin. Some patients may require repeat courses of therapy. There are no reports of cumulative toxicity from using repeat courses and tachyphylaxis has not been noted.

Although the ED suggests isotretinoin should not be used in patients under 12 years of age, there are reports in the literature of up to 0.5 mg/kg/day being used successfully in a number of neonates or juveniles with acne who have not responded to all appropriate topical or oral therapies [665,**666**,667]. Evidence-based paediatric guidelines suggest oral isotretinoin should be considered for paediatric patients with acne if there are sufficient clinical indications [**666**] (see section on prepubertal acne later in this chapter). Apert syndrome is a rare disorder associated with a hyperresponse of the epiphyses and sebaceous glands to androgens, which results in premature epiphyseal fusion and acne (see section on Apert syndrome earlier in this chapter). These patients frequently respond well to oral isotretinoin [668].

Side effects of isotretinoin. Isotretinoin has many side effects but most are predictable and rarely interfere with patient management. Tables 88.26–88.28 and 88.29 outline the potential and reported side effects and relative risk of occurrence. The common mucocutaneous side effects are dose dependent and are managed by modification of the dose and/or regular use of emollients or false tears. Occasionally, retinoid dermatitis (Figure 88.66), a severe retinoid cheilitis (Figure 88.67) or conjunctivitis complicated by secondary *Staphylococcus aureus* (Figure 88.68) may occur. These patients may need treatment with an intermediate-strength corticosteroid ointment combined with an antiseptic or oral antistaphylococcal therapy such as flucloxacillin and/or topical mupirocin 2% ointment [669]. Teratogenicity is well recognised and regarded as one of the most serious potential adverse effects of isotretinoin [670]. Fifty per cent of pregnancies spontaneously abort, and of the remainder

Table 88.26 Adverse effects of isotretinoin: very common.

Type of disorder	Very common side effects
Blood and lymphatic system	Anaemia
	Increased red blood cell sedimentation rate
	Thrombocytopenia
	Thrombocytosis
Eye	Blepharitis
	Conjunctivitis
	Dry eyes
	Eye irritation
Hepatobiliary	Increased transaminase
Skin and mucosal tissues	Cheilitis
	Dermatitis
	Dry skin
	Localised exfoliation
	Pruritus
	Redness
	Skin fragility
Musculoskeletal and connective tissue	Arthralgia
	Myalgia
	Back pain
Investigation	Increased triglycerides
	Decreased high-density lipoprotein

Table 88.27 Adverse effects of isotretinoin: common.

Type of disorder	Common side effects
Blood and lymphatic system	Neutropenia
Nervous system	Headache
Respiratory, thoracic and mediastinal	Epistaxis
	Nasal dryness
	Nasopharyngitis
Investigation	Increased blood cholesterol
	Increased blood glucose
	Haematuria
	Proteinuria

Table 88.28 Adverse effects of isotretinoin: rare.

Type of disorder	Rare side effects
Immune system	Allergic skin reaction
	Anaphylactic reactions
	Hypersensitivity
Psychiatric	Depression
	Aggravated depression
	Aggressive tendencies
	Anxiety
	Mood alterations
Skin and subcutaneous tissues	Alopecia

about half of the infants are born with cardiovascular or skeletal deformities.

The question whether neuropsychiatric problems result from oral isotretinoin remains a controversial issue. Disentangling the individual impacts of acne, adolescence and medication is challenging. Acne commonly affects adolescents at a time of significant transition, and mood changes and depression are common and may occur independently of acne. The past decade has seen an increase in mental health problems in young people. A recent millennium study confirmed that three-quarters of the people affected with psychological distress, self-harm and/or suicide first experienced their mental illness before the age of 20 years. High levels of severe mental health difficulties were reported in this study, with 24% of females experiencing high levels of depressive symptoms by 14 years of age. By 17 years self-harm in the preceding 12 months was reported in 28.2% and by the same age females demonstrated a lifetime risk of suicide of 10.6% [671].

Acne is known to have a negative psychosocial impact on patients and can result in anxiety and depression [672]. A cross-sectional questionnaire in Norway found suicidal ideation and suicide attempts are approximately twice as common in acne sufferers [673].

A systematic review and meta-analysis conducted to assess whether isotretinoin treatment for acne was associated with risk of depression found no evidence to support an association between isotretinoin and depression after pooling data from 31 prospective studies published from inception to 2016 [674]. Many of these studies demonstrated that oral isotretinoin ameliorated any negative psychosocial issues.

A large national US population study of acne patients over a 14-year period from 2004 to 2017 assessed the differential effects of antiacne treatments on depressive and distress symptoms over the

Table 88.29 Adverse effects of isotretinoin: very rare.

Type of disorder	Very rare side effects
Infection	Gram-positive (mucocutaneous) bacterial infection
Blood and lymphatic system	Lymphadenopathy
Metabolism	Diabetes
	Hyperuricaemia
Psychiatric	Abnormal behaviour
	Psychotic disorder
	Suicidal ideation
	Suicide attempt
	Suicide
Nervous system	Benign intracranial hypertension
	Convulsions
	Drowsiness
	Dizziness
Sexual dysfunction	Reduced libido
	Erectile dysfunction
Eye	Blurred vision
	Cataract
	Colour blindness
	Contact lens intolerance
	Corneal opacity
	Decreased night vision
	Keratitis
	Papilloedema
	Photophobia
	Visual disturbances
Ear	Impaired hearing
Vascular	Vasculitis (i.e. granulomatosis with polyangiitis, allergic vasculitis)
Gastrointestinal	Colitis
	Ileitis
	Dry throat
	Gastrointestinal haemorrhage
	Haemorrhagic diarrhoea
	Inflammatory bowel disease
	Nausea
	Pancreatitis
Hepatobiliary	Hepatitis
Skin and subcutaneous tissues	Acne fulminans
	Aggravated acne (acne flare)
	Redness (facial)
	Exanthema
	Hair disorders
	Hirsutism
	Nail dystrophy
	Paronychia
	Photosensitivity reaction
	Pyogenic granuloma
	Skin hyperpigmentation
	Increased swelling
Musculoskeletal and connective tissue	Arthritis
	Calcinosis (calcification of ligaments and tendons)
	Premature epiphyseal fusion
	Exostosis
	Hyperostosis
	Osteopenia
	Tendonitis
Renal and urinary	Glomerulonephritis
General	Increased formation of granulation tissue
	Malaise
Investigation	Increased creatine phosphokinase

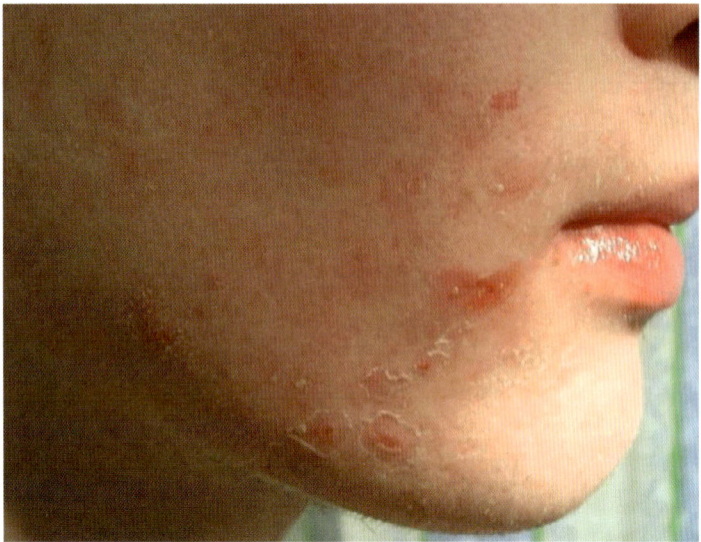

Figure 88.66 Retinoid dermatitis as a result of oral retinoids.

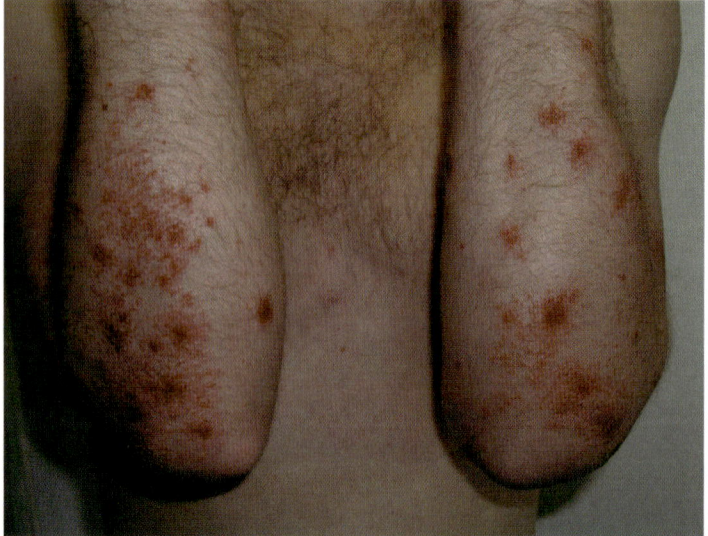

Figure 88.68 *Staphylococcus aureus* colonising discoid eczema induced by oral retinoids.

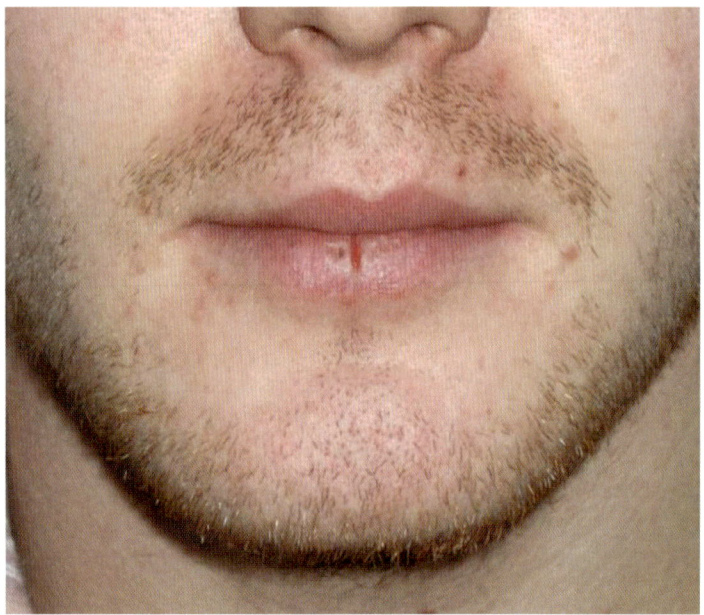

Figure 88.67 Cheilitis and fissure of the lower lip induced by oral retinoids.

course of treatment using validated questionnaires. After adjusting for sociodemographic characteristics, patients on oral isotretinoin had significantly fewer depressive symptoms than patients on oral antibiotics (isotretinoin 0.280 versus oral antibiotics 0.656), which was significant (P <0.01). Patients on isotretinoin also had less psychological distress than patients on oral antibiotics (isotretinoin 2.494 versus oral antibiotics 3.433, $P = 0.043$). The authors concluded that the negative psychological state of acne patients is likely attributable to having acne itself rather than potential iatrogenic effects of systemic treatments [675]. More recent population studies examining psychiatric disorders, mental health issues and/or suicide have reported similar findings including lower rates of suicide in patients treated with oral isotretinoin when compared with the normal population and no triggers for suicide [676–678]. Droitcourt *et al*. also demonstrated that predisposing risk factors correlated

with suicide attempts, highlighting the need to screen carefully for risk factors prior to commencing oral isotretinoin [677].

A review of all the psychiatric adverse effects for patients on oral isotretinoin, reported to the FDA in 1997–2017, identified over 17 800 such events in total with depressive disorders, emotional lability and anxiety disorders being reported most frequently. However, the authors suggested the reporting did not confirm causality. Eating disorders were reported more commonly in females as a possible confounder and acne itself was recognised as a contributing factor. The authors reported that the rate of completed suicide in those receiving oral isotretinoin was significantly lower than in the general population [679].

As plausible mechanisms of action have been proposed that implicate oral isotretinoin as a potential cause of an unpredictable idiosyncratic reaction leading to significant neurospychiatric morbidity [680], and given the high incidence of mental health problems in the population being treated, current guidance supports clear discussion with patients concerning all potential adverse effects and advocates involvement of their family and friends whenever possible. A direct enquiry to elicit any mental health problems should be undertaken at review. Validated tools used to screen for depression and mood change are now recommended following MHRA review in 2023. Provision of appropriate psychological support should also be considered.

Significant systemic effects are uncommon; headaches may uncommonly be an early feature of benign intracranial hypertension and arthralgia is seen most frequently in those patients participating in regular and heavy exercise. Tetracyclines, including doxycycline and minocycline, must not be prescribed with isotretinoin, as both drugs may produce benign intracranial hypertension [681].

An acute flare of acne early in a course of isotretinoin is a recognised problem in about 6% of cases and is clinically significant in half of these [682]. The physician should inform patients accordingly and provide rapid access if this occurs as these flares can be aggressive, producing physical and psychological sequelae. If the acne is very inflammatory, a lower dose of isotretinoin alongside

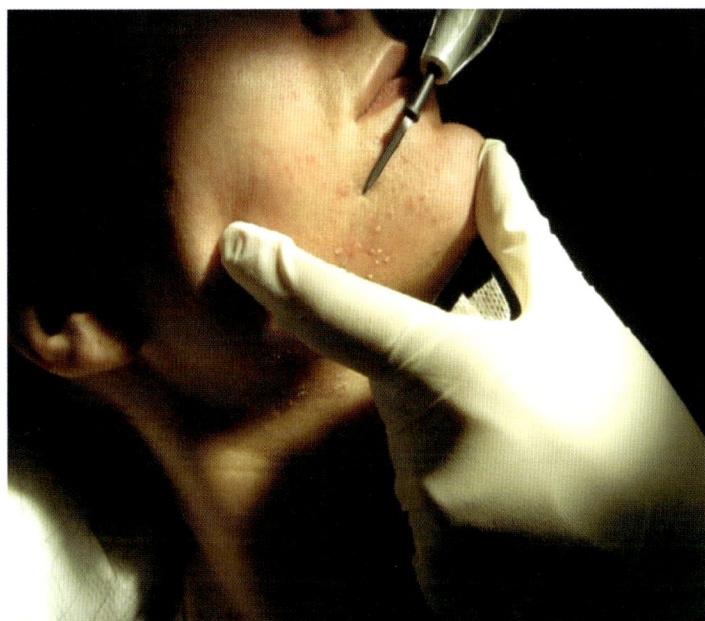

Figure 88.69 Hyfrecation of macrocomedones.

oral corticosteroids may be required (e.g. 0.5–1.0 mg/kg/day for 2–3 weeks). Predisposing risk factors for a flare include the presence of macrocomedones and nodules. If macrocomedones are present, light cautery or hyfrecation should be done prior to starting the isotretinoin. A local anaesthetic cream should be applied to the lesions beneath an occlusive dressing prior to starting the isotretinoin (Figure 88.69) [683]. If a severe flare occurs, 0.5–1.0 mg/kg/day oral prednisolone is needed over a period of 2–3 weeks followed by a tapering of dose over the following 6 weeks. The isotretinoin should either be stopped or reduced. If stopped, the drug can be slowly reintroduced at a dose of 0.25 mg/kg/day, and then increased or decreased as response dictates.

Reduced efficacy has been noted when isotretinoin is taken with heavy alcohol intake [684]. Isotretinoin is metabolised by cytochrome P450 enzymes, inducible by ethanol and inhibited by some drugs, for example ketoconazole. Hence, increased drug levels of isotretinoin may occur if combined with imidazole fungistatics. If salicylic acid and acidic drugs with a high affinity for albumin are present in the blood in high therapeutic concentrations, they may displace isotretinoin from protein-binding sites, resulting in an increase in the unbound concentration of the drug. Carbamazepine plasma levels decrease when concurrent isotretinoin is taken, hence careful monitoring should be considered in people with epilepsy on carbamazepine if requiring isotretinoin. Vitamin supplements containing vitamin A should be avoided alongside isotretinoin, as additive toxic effects could ensue.

Other therapies for acne

Topical therapies. The efficacy of other topical treatments has not been established by controlled studies, but dermacosmetics are increasingly used by patients as adjunct treatments [685–687]. Therefore, it has become important for dermatologists to understand dermocosmetics to effectively and appropriately advise patients on their use.

Topical zinc. A study comparing erythromycin (2% w/v) with zinc acetate (1.2% w/v) as 'topical gel' and erythromycin (2% w/v) gel alone for treating mild to moderate inflammatory acne vulgaris found that while both were effective in reducing acne there was no statistically significant difference between the two groups [688].

Topical nicotinamide. Topical nicotinamide 4% has anti-inflammatory actions and does not induce *C. acnes* resistance [689]. Double-blind studies have shown it to be better than vehicle alone against inflamed lesions, although the improvement with placebo was also considerable (32–76%) [690]. A comparison of 4% nicotinamide gel demonstrated it to be similar in efficiency to 1% clindamycin gel [691]. Comparable efficacy was also seen for 4% niacinamide + 1% gallic acid + 1% lauric acid compared with 5% BPO and 5% BPO + 3% erythromycin in a retrospective review [692].

Salicylic acid. Salicylic acid 2% has been shown to be more effective in reducing comedonal and inflammatory acne lesions than alcoholic vehicle at 12 weeks in an RCT [693,694]. A fixed-dose combination therapy with hydrogen peroxide (4%), salicylic acid (0.5%) and D-panthenol (4%) gel, plus daily SPF50 protection, was shown in mild to moderate acne vulgaris to improve global severity scale and to have good tolerability. This was in a small retrospective review, and no control group was used in the study [695].

Sulphur. A longstanding antiacne therapy, which may be both comedogenic and comedolytic [696,697], sulphur is unpopular because of its smell, and is rarely used.

Corticosteroids. A few topical preparations contain weak corticosteroids but proof of their efficacy is lacking. Potent steroids such as clobetasol propionate applied twice a day for 5 days can dramatically reduce the inflammation in an active inflammatory nodule [698].

Oral therapies
Oral vitamin C. A small case–control study comparing doxycycline (100 mg) capsules OD after a meal in combination with vitamin C (500 mg) chewable tablets OD, versus doxycycline 100 mg monotherapy, showed immunologically doxycycline plus vitamin C was more effective in reducing serum levels of IL-8, IL-1β, IFN-γ, TNF-α and TLR2 in comparison with doxycycline alone [699]. The authors proposed vitamin C as a potential adjunct to treating inflammatory conditions such as acne and rosacea. Further methodologically robust studies looking at the clinical benefits of oral vitamin C are needed.

Metformin. As discussed earlier, IGF-1 and activation of mTORC1 have been established in the pathogenesis of acne. Metformin, through the inhibition of mTORC1, has been investigated for its therapeutic potential. A randomised, open-label study evaluated the efficacy and safety of metformin as an adjunct for moderate to severe facial acne in 84 patients who received either oral tetracycline 250 mg BD and topical benzoyl peroxide 2.5% with or without metformin 850 mg daily. Results showed statistically significant higher success rates in the metformin group, but improvements in the Cardiff acne disability index score and lesion counts did not reach significance [700]. Further RCTs to evaluate the role of metformin are needed.

Complementary therapies. Herbal remedies have been used for centuries to treat skin ailments. Herbal extracts are being increasingly adopted by the cosmeceutical industry for topical treatments for a number of dermatological disorders, including acne. They are popular with consumers as they are seen as non-medicinal and have assumed safety. Data have been published on the potential value of traditional 'herbal' medicines [701,702]. Fisk *et al.* reported high-quality evidence, defined as randomised clinical trials receiving ≥3 points on the Jadad scale, that suggested that tea tree oil (TTO), seaweed extract, Kampo formulations, Ayurvedic formulations, rose extract, basil extract, epigallocatechin gallate (the main polyphenol in green tea) and green tea extract are promising therapies for acne [702]. However, they also caution that most of these botanicals have been studied in only one or two small clinical trials with methodological flaws, a sentiment echoed by other reviewers.

A systematic review of RCTs examining TTO in dermatological conditions, including acne, showed there were some promising data suggesting that TTO might be effective for acne and further investigation was advocated [703]. An RCT that compared the purported antioxidant active ingredient in milk thistle, silymarin, with doxycycline and doxycycline plus silymarin showed improvement in all groups with acne. The synergistic use of silymarin with doxycycline showed a favourable, but not statistically significant, improvement in GAGS score or acne severity index over doxycycline alone [704]. In addition, the following have been evaluated for their use in acne: green tea, cedar (*Ziziphus spina-christi*) [705], *Rhodomyrtus tomentosa* (Myrtaceae) leaf extract [706], myrtle [707] and cheongsangbangpoong-tang [708]. Bakuchiol has shown some effect on acne-induced hyperpigmentation in skin of colour [709].

Further validation for the safety and efficacy of all these therapies is required. A review article of complementary therapy trials compared 31 trials and found inconsistent effects in terms of whether acupuncture, herbal medicine or wet-cupping therapy was superior to controls in increasing remission or reducing skin lesions [710].

Devices and physical modalities for treating active acne. There are a variety of specially shaped tools available for blackhead macrocomedo removal (Figure 88.70). Light cautery or hyfrecation has been shown to help patients with multiple macrocomedones; these are usually whiteheads but occasionally blackheads (up to 1.5 mm diameter), and chloracne can be improved [711,712]. A topical anaesthetic preparation is applied beneath an occlusive dressing. The cautery or hyfrecation should be set as low as possible to produce little or no pain. The aim is to produce very low-grade thermal damage. The treatment of each lesion takes seconds and is associated with very little scarring or postinflammatory pigmentation. This therapy is more effective than topical tretinoin for macrocomedones [713].

Visible light. In a split face trial of 49 patients examining the efficacy of chromophore gel-assisted blue light, the group with a baseline IGA grade of 3 (moderate) demonstrated a success rate of 81.8% and 90.0% at weeks 6 and 12 and those with a grade of 4 (severe) demonstrated a success rate of 100% at both weeks [714]. The rate

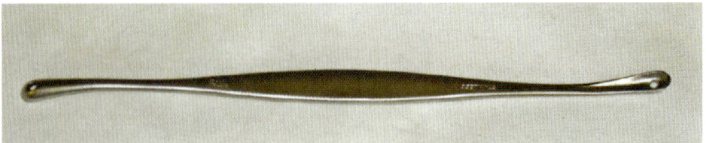

Figure 88.70 Comedo extractor.

of return to baseline in severity at 24 weeks was 15.5%, indicating a long duration of effect. However, efficacy was not compared with conventional acne treatments. A 2019 systematic review of blue light included 14 RCTs that investigated blue light with any intervention other than light (including placebo; topical agents such as retinoids, benzoyl peroxide or antibiotics; or oral antibiotics or isotretinoin). This review concluded that methodological and reporting failings of the trials (small sample size, limited duration, detection and reporting bias) limited the conclusions that can be drawn about the effect of blue light therapy. All reported improvements in the intervention group compared with the comparator, although the number of people and proportion of benefit varied [715]. Blue light has been given a low-strength recommendation in the management of mild to moderate papulopustular acne.

Lasers and photodynamic therapy. There has been increased interest in the use of lasers and light-based devices for acne over the last few years. Light therapy destroys propionibacteria by targeting porphyrins produced by these bacteria. These regimens also suppress a range of pro-inflammatory cytokines. A significant number of RCTs embracing light of diverse wavelengths have been conducted, but results from these studies have been contradictory. A Cochrane systematic review of light therapies concluded many of the studies included small numbers, short follow-up periods and had adopted non-standardised regimens [716]. The studies have also not compared these therapies with conventional treatments used for acne, hence making it challenging to draw firm conclusions to guide decisions in practice, especially considering the cost of light-based treatments [716].

Liu *et al.* compared photodynamic therapy (PDT), intense pulsed light (IPL) and blue-red light-emitting diode (LED) phototherapy in the treatment of 150 Chinese patients with moderate to severe facial acne. They found PDT was the fastest acting treatment as it required the least number of treatments to achieve >90% clearance (mean number of sessions required was 3 ± 1.52 PDT, 6 ± 2.15 IPL and 9 ± 3.34 LED) [717]. The 2021 UK NICE guidelines for the management of acne have reviewed the evidence base for physical therapies and have provided a 'consider' recommendation for PDT, which had the largest evidence base among physical therapies, as an alternative option for people with moderate to severe acne aged 18 years and over, if other treatments are ineffective, not tolerated or contraindicated [**555**]. They also made a research recommendation that further trials are needed. No robust studies are available to support the use of lasers or photodynamic therapy for comedonal acne. The most commonly reported adverse events associated with PDT treatment are pain, burning/itching sensation of the skin, redness and oedema. There is no widely accepted protocol for treating inflammatory acne patients with PDT. Increased incubation times suggest improved outcomes but increased short-term side effects

[718,719]. Newer preparations, such as 5% aminolevulinic acid in thermosetting gel, have been developed, which could allow for a more convenient application without occlusion [720]. One study comparing conventional PDT with daylight PDT found similar efficacy but a statistically significant lower visual analogue scale (VAS) pain score in the daylight PDT group (1.8 ± 0.2 versus 5.8 ± 0.3, $P < 0.05$) [721].

Chemical peels. Chemical peels are believed to promote desquamation, which reduces corneocyte cohesion and keratinocyte plugging, so enabling the extrusion of inflammatory contents. Peeling agents include α-hydroxy acids (glycolic acid), salicylic acid and trichloroacetic acid. Guidelines and evidence for their use have been considered in a Japanese review [722]. A further review of the efficacy of a variety of chemical peels for acne showed an average reduction in comedones by 35%; however, published studies are limited by sample size and design [723]. Peels with 30% azeliac acid reduced acne lesions and normalised the activity of the sebaceous glands in one study, although the sample size was small [724]. A number of studies have compared chemical peels with other physical therapies with mixed results [725,726]. Evidence for the use of chemical peels in the treatment of acne is therefore lacking but they are relatively safe and inexpensive and many dermatologists worldwide use light chemical peels with the aim of helping to remove comedones as well as superficial scarring and hyperpigmentation.

Novel treatments. Novel drug delivery strategies are a point of interest for researchers as they offer the potential for enhancing dermal delivery of the active antiacne drug and increasing effectiveness while concomitantly reducing side effects. Strategies include niosomes, liposome, emulsomes, transferosomes, microemulsion, nanoemulsion and nanolipid carriers [727].

New drugs are also under investigation for their suitability to treat acne. There is a phase II RCT investigating the use of once-weekly, high-dose oral finasteride (23.5 or 33.5 mg) compared with placebo for the treatment of severe nodulocystic acne in males. To date, no results have been published [728].

Novel physical therapies are under investigation too. Photothermal therapy using gold nanoparticles showed significant reductions in acne lesions after the use of gold photothermal therapy (papules $P = 0.001$; pustules $P < 0.001$; comedones $p = 0.001$) and patients showed an average 50% improvement on PGA in a 12-patient trial [729]. The findings aligned with a 2019 open-label pilot study by Fuchs et al. [730].

A single-centre pilot study on nine self-selected male and female patients with atrophic acne scars used a twice-daily application of synthetic epidermal growth factor (EGF) to scarred areas over 12 weeks. Patients showed improvement mesures by IGA and self-assessment measures. Further larger trials for the effect of topical EGF on acne scars are needed.

Resources

Further information
Eichenfield LF, Krakowski AC, Piggott C et al. American Acne and Rosacea Society. Evidence-based recommendations for the diagnosis and treatment of pediatric acne. *Pediatrics* 2013;131(Suppl. 3):S163–86.

Medicines and Healthcare Products Regulatory Agency. *Treatment with isotretinoin for patients under 18 must be approved by two prescribers, under new MHRA rules.* MHRA, 2023. https://www.gov.uk/government/news/treatment-with-isotretinoin-for-patients-under-18-must-be-approved-by-two-prescribers-under-new-mhra-rules (last accessed December 2023).

Nast A, Dréno B, Bettoli V et al. European evidence-based (S3) guideline for the treatment of acne – update 2016 – short version. *J Eur Acad Dermatol Venereol* 2016;30:1261–8.

National Institute for Health and Care Excellence (NCIE). *Acne Vulgaris: Management. NG198.* London: NICE, 2021 (last updated 2023). https://www.nice.org.uk/guidance/ng198 (last accessed June 2023).

Thiboutot DM, Dréno B, Abanmi A et al. Practical management of acne for clinicians: an international consensus from the Global Alliance to Improve Outcomes in Acne. *J Am Acad Dermatol* 2018;78(Suppl. 1):S1–23.e1.

US Food and Drug Administration. *iPLEDGE Risk Evaluation and Mitigation Strategy (REMS).* FDA, 2023. https://www.fda.gov/drugs/postmarket-drug-safety-information-patients-and-providers/ipledge-risk-evaluation-and-mitigation-strategy-rems (last accessed December 2023).

Patient resources
British Association of Dermatologists patient information leaflets: http://www.bad.org.uk/for-the-public/patient-information-leaflets.
Talk Health: http://www.talkhealthpartnership.com/.
(Both last accessed June 2023.)

Acne fulminans

Definition and nomenclature
Acne fulminans is a rare and severe, destructive form of acne presenting primarily in adolescent males. It most frequently affects the trunk but can affect the face and presents acutely in association with systemic symptoms.

> **Synonyms and inclusions**
> - Acne fulminans
> - Acne maligna
> - Sine fulminans

Introduction and general description
Acne fulminans was first described in 1959 as acne conglobata with septicaemia [1]. The disease was later distinguished from acne conglobata by Plewig and Kligman in 1975 [2]; they emphasised the characteristic features of sudden onset and severity of systemic upset as distinct features. It is a rare form of acne and the incidence appears to be diminishing, possibly due to more effective and earlier use of treatments [3]. A subset of patients with no systemic symptoms but with severe acne comparable to that seen in acne fulminans has been described as 'sine fulminans' [4].

Epidemiology
Age and sex
Acne fulminans is predominantly seen in young white males aged between 13 and 22 years [5], although there have been rare cases reported in females [6].

Ethnicity
There are globally reported cases of this condition, but its incidence seems to be declining. However, the frequency and severity of acne

fulminans are notably greater in patients of northern European descent compared with those of East Asian origin [7].

Associated diseases

Acne fulminans has been found in association with SAPHO syndrome (see section earlier in this chapter). This suggests that systemic inflammatory cytokinaemia might be responsible. This proposal is supported by the fact that infliximab has been used to treat acne fulminans associated with SAPHO syndrome [8].

Acne fulminans has also been reported at the onset of Crohn disease but the significance of this association remains unclear [9]. There is just one case report of acne fulminans and ulcerative colitis in a 19-year-old Japanese male patient, suggesting any association is very rare [10]. In a further single case report, a male with a leukaemoid reaction also developed posterior scleritis of his eyes and a pyoderma–gangrenosum eruption on the legs suggesting an autoimmune mechanism [11].

PAPA syndrome and acne fulminans. PAPA syndrome was described in 1997; it affects mainly the skin and joints, and the acne may present as acne fulminans or conglobata. The susceptibility gene is the CD2-binding protein 1 (*CD2BP1*) gene. The CD2BP1 protein interacts with pyrin and a mutation in the protein may increase its ability to bind to pyrin, then reducing the inhibitory effect of the IL-1β pathway and innate immunity, resulting in autoinflammatory reactions [12].

Pathophysiology

The pathophysiology of acne fulminans remains unclear. Infection, genetic predisposition and immunological causes have all been suggested. One theory suggests acne fulminans is an autoimmune complex disease; in favour of this is the rapid response to systemic steroids, increased levels of γ-globulins and decrease in complement levels seen in a number of patients. Immune complexes are found predominantly in patients with musculoskeletal problems. The association with autoinflammatory disorders described has led to the hypothesis that abnormal innate immunity, such as in the IL-1 pathway, may be involved in the pathogenesis of acne fulminans.

Predisposing factors

Acne fulminans is seen most frequently in young males and there is some evidence to suggest that elevated blood levels of testosterone may play a role [13]. The increase in physiological levels of testosterone in males at puberty may explain this predisposition. There are reports of patients developing acne fulminans after receiving high-dose testosterone for the treatments of excessively tall stature, Klinefelter syndrome and Marfan syndrome [14–17]. One case of acne fulminans has also been reported in a young man with androgen excess as a result of late-onset congenital adrenal hyperplasia [18].

A number of case reports have cited anabolic-androgenic steroids as a trigger for acne fulminans [3,19–21]. As derivatives of the hormone testosterone, anabolic steroids lead to hypertrophy of the sebaceous glands, increased sebum production and as a result of this an increased density of *C. acnes* [22].

Paradoxically, another predisposing factor is the use of isotretinoin. In some patients, mild cystic acne rapidly evolves with ulcerative and necrotic lesions. In these patients, the dose of isotretinoin is usually 0.5–1.0 mg/kg/day and the treatment had been administered for an average of 3 weeks (range 1–7 weeks) before deterioration occurred [3]. Kellet *et al.* reported circulating immune complexes in two cases with a flare of acne fulminans apparently triggered by isotretinoin [23].

Causative organisms

The presence in some patients of microscopic haematuria, erythema nodosum, increased response to *C. acnes* antigen on skin tests and depressed response to intradermal purified protein derivatives is in favour of an abnormal immunological response. Skin tests with *C. acnes* demonstrate a very extensive, immediate or delayed reaction, the immunohistology of which reveals a type III or type IV hypersensitivity reaction [24]. Isotretinoin can cause a significant flare of acne fulminans in some patients. Hypotheses to explain this suggest that the isotretinoin-induced fragility of the pilosebaceous duct epithelium allows significant exposure of C. *acnes* antigens and/or *C. acnes* chemoattractants to the immune system. An exaggerated response to intradermal injection of *C. acnes* suspended in saline has been demonstrated in a case of acne fulminans and erythema nodosum suggesting *C. acnes* may act as an antigen in this context [23]. Another theory is that genetically determined changes in neutrophil activity/hyperreactivity to chemoattractants may result in reduced phagocytosis of *C. acnes*. Authors have suggested that C. *acnes* destruction results in increased neutrophil chemotaxis, which may be responsible for the isotretinoin flares seen when patients start treatment. It has been suggested that patients who develop very severe flares of acne after starting isotretinoin may have an exaggeration of this response [25].

A retrospective observational study examined *C. acnes* phylotype distribution in patients with acne fulminans. The predominant phylotype was IA1 in 60% of patients, corresponding to the predominant phylotype in acne vulgaris, which supports the hypothesis that acute inflammation associated with acne fulminans is related to an abnormal cutaneous innate immunity activation rather than specific subtypes of *C. acnes* [26].

Genetics

Hereditary factors may play a role [27–29] as acne fulminans has been reported in identical monozygotic twins who presented at the same age with identical clinical presentation. Two siblings presenting with acne fulminans were noted to have identical human leukocyte antigen (HLA) phenotypes. A genetic predisposition associated with the *HLA-Cw6* gene has been described. A genetically determined change in neutrophil activity has also been proposed as a determinant.

Environmental factors

Infection as a trigger for acne fulminans has been reported. One case report indicated an association 2 weeks after a measles infection, implying that the virus may trigger a transient release of inflammatory cytokines, resulting in acne fulminans in a predisposed individual [30]. An acne fulminans-like picture has been reported in association with Epstein–Barr virus infection [31].

Clinical features

History

Most patients with acne fulminans describe mild to moderate acne for 0.5–5 years (mean 2 years) before a sudden onset of febrile, ulcerative, necrotic acne lesions alongside arthralgia, fever and various systemic inflammatory signs and symptoms [3]. Patients typically fail to respond to antibacterial therapy.

Presentation

Acne fulminans always presents as a severe cutaneous inflammatory process with varying systemic signs and symptoms. Patients present with numerous, inflammatory, tender and ulcerative nodules covered with haemorrhagic crusts (Figures 88.71 and 88.72). These are predominantly distributed on the upper chest, back and

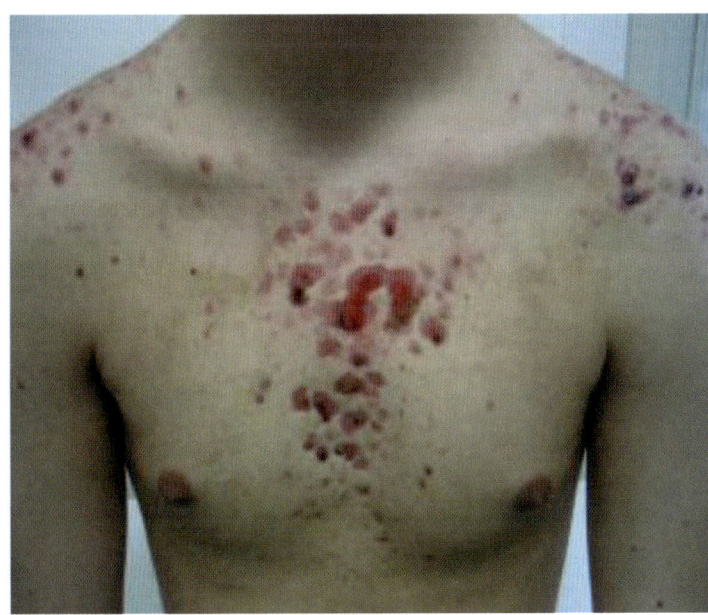

Figure 88.71 Acne fulminans in a young male.

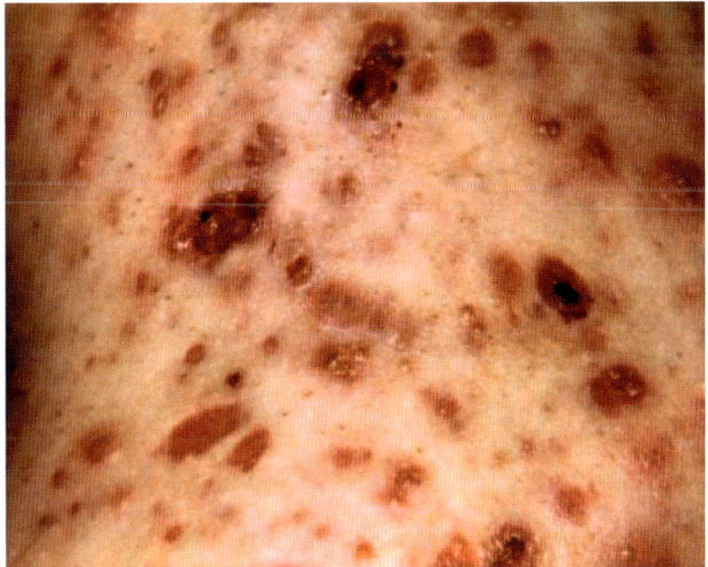

Figure 88.72 Erosive crusting lesions on the back of a young male with acne fulminans.

Table 88.30 The main features of acne fulminans.

Feature	Comments
Gender	Male gender dominant
Age	13–22 years
Pathogenesis	Unclear
Onset	Acute and sudden
Localisation	Upper chest and back, shoulders, face
Clinical picture	Ulcerative lesions covered with haemorrhagic crusts healing with scarring
Laboratory findings	Leukocytosis, increased erythrocyte sedimentation rate, anaemia, proteinuria, microscopic haematuria
Response to conventional antibiotic therapy	Poor
Treatments of choice	Systemic corticosteroids combined with isotretinoin

shoulders and pyogenic granulomatous-like lesions may be present. The face may also be involved and the lesions undergo rapid degeneration resulting in ulcerations filled with necrotic debris. Comedonal lesions are rare [3,32].

Systemic signs and symptoms are present in the majority of patients and include malaise, arthralgia, joint swellings, polyarthritis, myalgia, fever, anorexia and weight loss. A marked leukocytosis which may be leukaemoid is frequent; patients may also demonstrate anaemia (Table 88.30).

Painful splenomegaly [33], erythema nodosum [34] and bone pain due to aseptic osteolysis [35,36] have also been reported. Bone involvement is common [37]: in a series of 24 patients, 48% had lytic bone lesions on X-ray and 67% showed increased radiolabel uptake; 25% showed destructive lesions resembling osteomyelitis [37,38]. The sites of predilection for bone lesions include the anterior chest, particularly the clavicles and sternum, but osteolytic lesions have also been reported in the ankles, hips and humerus. Sacroiliitis has also been described.

Clinical variants

Acne fulminans may occur in the context of SAPHO syndrome and is considered by some as a spectrum of this autoinflammatory disorder [39,40].

Differential diagnosis

The main differential diagnosis is severe acne conglobata (see later in this chapter). The latter is seen in both men and women and has a more insidious onset, whereas acne fulminans is generally very acute and rarely seen in females. Patients present with acne conglobata at an older average age and the condition has a protracted and more chronic course than acne fulminans with few or fewer systemic symptoms. Comedonal lesions are generally much more florid in acne conglobata (Table 88.31).

Complications and co-morbidities

Radiographic changes such as hyperostosis and sclerosis may persist but the symptoms and signs associated with any bony changes typically resolve with treatment. Mild musculoskeletal discomfort has been reported as a persistent symptom following

Table 88.31 Differential diagnosis of acne fulminans and acne conglobata.

Feature	Acne fulminans	Acne conglobata
Gender	Male	Male
Age	Adolescence (13–16 years)	20–25 years
Onset	Sudden	Slow
Location	Face, neck, chest and back	Trunk and upper limbs, facial lesions are rare
Clinical features	Haemorrhagic ulcerations	Nodules, inflammatory cysts, grouped comedones
Systemic symptoms	Very common	None

the acute episode. The most common complication is significant and disfiguring scarring.

Course and prognosis

The prognosis for patients treated effectively with corticosteroids and isotretinoin is extremely good. Recurrent acne fulminans is very rare. Relapse may occur as corticosteroid therapy is reduced but the risk reduces over time and is unusual after a year.

Investigations

There are no consistent laboratory abnormalities in acne fulminans. Bacterial cultures from blood, joint fluid and skin are generally sterile. There is one report describing a patient with acne fulminans and a lytic bone lesion from which *C. acnes* was cultured [41]. This contrasts with another report in which a patient had osteomyelitis and acne fulminans but cultures from bone were negative for *C. acnes*, although red fluorescence in the affected bone characteristic of *C. acnes* was noted [42]. Abnormal laboratory findings may include an increased erythrocyte sedimentation rate, elevated C-reactive protein and thrombocytosis, together with a normochromic and normocytic anaemia. Characteristically, a leukocytosis is found sometimes with an associated leukaemoid reaction. There are a couple of reports in the literature in which 0.5–1.5% myeloblasts, promyelocytes and myelocytes were found in the peripheral blood [7,43]. Elevated liver enzymes and microscopic haematuria, proteinuria and other kidney abnormalities may be identified. Circulating immune complexes have been identified in some patients with acne fulminans and erythema nodosum [34,42]. Bone involvement is common and approximately 50% of patients have lytic bone lesions demonstrated by radiographs and 70% show increased uptake

using technetium scintigraphy. Destructive lesions resembling osteomyelitis are demonstrated on radiographs in 25% of patients [44]. When present, bone biopsies have been performed to rule out malignancy; the histology usually reveals reactive changes only but a neutrophilic infiltrate with mononuclear cells and granulation tissue can mimic osteomyelitis. Patients with osteolytic lesions may have elevated serum alkaline phosphatase [45].

Management

The acute myalgia, arthralgia and fever can be treated with oral salicylates or non-steroidal anti-inflammatory drugs and graduated physical exercise. Crusts should be removed by soaking the skin with emollient oil and this should be followed by the use of a potent steroid/antimicrobial cream for 2–3 weeks.

First line

Oral prednisolone therapy should be commenced first line (0.5–1.0 mg/kg/day) and decreased slowly over 2–3 months. Low-dose oral isotretinoin (0.25–0.5 mg/kg/day) should be cautiously introduced either after 3–4 weeks of systemic steroid therapy or can be considered in parallel with the corticosteroids and then gradually increased as tolerated and according to clinical response. A prospective case series of 26 patients given isotretinoin 0.5 mg/kg/day and prednisolone 30 mg/day concomitantly with the prednisolone being tapered after the first month showed resolution of systemic signs in 100% of patients and a >50% skin lesion improvement in 17 patients (65%) (Figure 88.73) [46]. It is advisable to use oral isotretinoin with caution as paradoxically it has been reported to induce acne fulminans in some patients [47–49].

Alternative therapies

Clofazimine 200 mg three times a week has been shown to improve acne fulminans [50]. Pulsed intravenous corticosteroids administered alongside isotretinoin have been used to control the disease in a 16-year-old male with good effect [51]. Isotretinoin in combination with dapsone has been used successfully to treat acne fulminans associated with erythema nodosum [52]. Combining systemic steroids with azathioprine or ciclosporin has been shown to avoid relapses on withdrawal of steroids [53–55].

In cases of acne fulminans which appear in the context of autoinflammatory disease, the effective use of biologics has been described in some cases but others have noted improvement in the musculoskeletal symptoms without much impact or in some cases a deterioration in the cutaneous problems. Table 88.32 outlines the systemic treatment options reported in the literature.

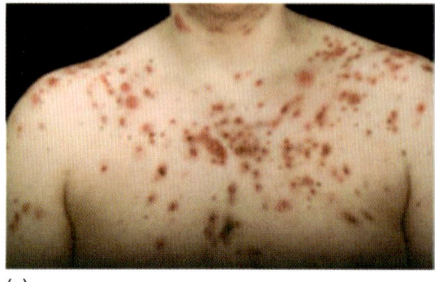
(a)

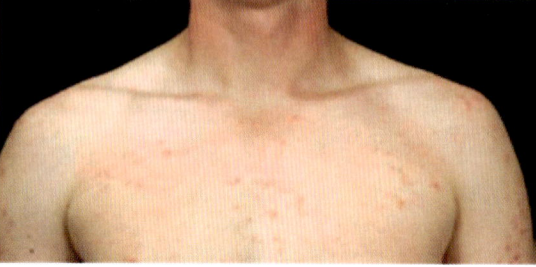
(b)

Figure 88.73 Young male with acne fulminans before (a) and 1 month after (b) treatment with isotretinoin 0.5 mg/kg body weight/day and prednisopone 30 mg/day. From Massa *et al.* 2017 [46] with permission from S. Karger AG, Basel.

Table 88.32 Systemic treatments used for acne fulminans.

Treatment recommendation	Duration/outcome/number of cases	Reference
0.5–1 mg/kg/day prednisolone for 4–6 weeks reducing thereafter	Assessment of 25 cases treated over 25 years	[2,3,46,56]
Commence oral isotretinoin week 4 at 0.5 mg/kg/day and gradually increase until clearance	Continued isotretinoin until clear	
Low-dose/cautious introduction of oral isotretinoin 4 weeks post start of systemic steroids at doses ranging from 0.2 to 0.5 mg/kg/day	Repeat isotretinoin may be required in many cases	
Systemic steroids plus 0.5–1 mg/kg/day isotretinoin	3–5 months, resolution	
Systemic steroids plus azathioprine	Poor response to steroid resolution after addition of azathioprine over months	[57]
Isotretinoin in combination with dapsone	No steroids required, one case report	[52]
Systemic steroids plus ciclosporin A (5 mg/kg/day)	Addition of ciclosporin avoided relapse on withdrawal of steroids. Case report in a patient developing acne fulminans in the context of the autoinflammatory disorder PAPA syndrome	[58]
Systemic steroids plus dapsone 50–150 mg daily	Dapsone is an alternative to isotretinoin if not available. Case report	[59]
Pulsed systemic steroids followed by isotretinoin	Case report	[51]
Isotretinoin 30 mg/day	Ciclosporin discontinued at 4 months as lesions resolved	[60]
Followed by ciclosporin 5 mg/kg in place of prednisolone	Isotretinoin 100 mg/kg given over 4 months	
Clofazimine (200 mg three times a week) has been shown to improve acne fulminans	Case report	[50]
Acne fulminans with sacroiliitis successfully treated with methotrexate and isotretinoin 0.25 mg/kg per day and prednisone 0.5 mg/kg per day. Initial clinical response was adequate, with a marked improvement in articular and cutaneous symptoms, but attempts to taper corticosteroids caused cutaneous and articular relapses. Complete response, treatment with methotrexate (15 mg weekly) and folic acid supplementation was added	Case report	[61]
Acne fulminans with SAPHO syndrome treated with infliximab	Case report	[62]

PAPA, pyogenic sterile arthritis, pyoderma gangrenosum and acne; SAPHO, synovitis, acne, pustulosis, hyperostosis and osteitis.

Acne conglobata

Definition
Acne conglobata represents a rare and severe form of acne characterised by multiple and extensive inflammatory papules, tender nodules and abscesses which commonly coalesce to form malodorous draining sinus tracts. Multiple polyporous, grouped comedones are typical and extensive disfiguring hypertrophic and atrophic scars are also common features [1,2].

Introduction and general description
Acne conglobata has a chronic and persistent course – it may occur in the context of existing papulopustular acne or may present as a recrudescence of acne that has been in abeyance for many years. Lesions typically occur on the trunk and upper limbs but frequently extend to the buttocks. In contrast to acne fulminans, systemic features are generally not a feature. The malodorous, discharging sinus tracts and significant scarring frequently result in psychological impairment [2].

Epidemiology
Incidence and prevalence
Acne conglobata is a rare disease.

Age and sex
Acne conglobata usually presents in the second to third decade and may persist into the forties and fifties. Males are more frequently affected than females.

Ethnicity
There are no studies to indicate that acne conglobata is seen more frequently in different ethnic groups [3].

Associated diseases
Acne conglobata may occur in the context of a number of inflammatory disorders.

Hidradenitis suppuritiva. A significant association has been found between HS and acne conglobata, demonstrated by a meta-analysis which demonstrated that patients with HS were associated with a 3.4 higher odds of having acne vulgaris/conglobata compared with control cases [4]. In these cases the HS may involve the perineal and gluteal regions extensively [5]. HS and folliculitis decalvans have also been described in association with acne conglobata [3,6], as have pilonidal cysts.

Arthritis. The association of acne conglobata and arthritis is rare but has been reported in a number of case reports [7–9]. Spondyloarthritis associated with acne conglobata, HS and dissecting folliculitis of the scalp is also recognised [10].

Pyoderma gangrenosum. Acne conglobata has been described in association with pyoderma gangrenosum [11].

A number of autoinflammatory syndromes cite acne conglobata as a possible clinical presentation within the context of the syndrome; these are described in more detail in Chapter 49.

SAPHO syndrome. This represents synovitis, acne conglobata, pustulosis, hyperostosis and osteitis [12–14].

PAPA syndrome. This is severe acne conglobata with sterile pyogenic arthritis and pyoderma gangrenosum, and has been reported as part of a related group of inflammatory disorders including psoriasis, uveitis and inflammatory bowel disease [15].

PASH syndrome. PAPA syndrome is also related to the triad of pyoderma gangrenosum, acne conglobata and suppurative hidradenitis known as PASH syndrome [16].

PASS syndrome. A new linkage designated PASS syndrome has also been described; this includes pyoderma gangrenosum, acne conglobata, suppurative hidradenitis and seronegative spondyloarthritis [17].

Pathophysiology
The primary cause of acne conglobata remains unknown.

Predisposing factors
Acne conglobata, like acne fulminans, can be triggered by testosterone and may be induced by anabolic steroid abuse and can occasionally occur after withdrawal of testosterone [18]. Although rare, patients should be advised of this risk. Acne conglobata may also occur in the context of an androgen-secreting tumour and has been described following ingestion of thyroid medications and halogens or exposure to aromatic hydrocarbons (see 'Occupational acne' later in this chapter). More recently, it has been reported following initiation of adalimumab, despite this drug's success in treating severe cystic acne [19]. The exact mechanism of this is unknown, but some authors suggest a paradoxical reaction, similar to the occurrence of anti-TNF-α-induced psoriasis [20].

Histopathology
Draining sinuses are characteristic of acne conglobata. Histologically, they consist of elaborate, epithelialised galleries connected to the skin surface at multiple points. The draining sinus contains corneocytes, hairs, bacteria, serum, inflammatory cells and epithelioid granulomas [21].

Causative organisms
It has been postulated that *C. acnes* may be implicated in acne conglobata but to date no causative organisms have been clearly implicated in the pathophysiology of acne conglobata. Gram-positive bacteria are often found secondarily infecting active lesions. *Mycobacterium chelonae* infection has been described as a mimic of acne conglobata in an immunocompetent host [22].

Genetics
Familial cases have been reported with linkage to chromosome 15q24-26 in the region of the IL-16 and *CRABPI* genes [23]. Chromosomal defects in the XYY karyotype of Klinefelter syndrome are believed to protect from severe acne; however, there is one case report in the literature with the unusual combination of Klinefelter syndrome and acne conglobata [24]. PAPA syndrome has been mapped onto the long arm of chromosome 15 and it has been suggested that the distinct clinical entities seen in PAPA may share the same genetic aetiology [23]. Novel mutations in the nicastrin (NCSTN) transcription regulator in HS and acne conglobata have

been identified. NCSTN is a γ-secretase protease, part of the Notch signalling pathway [25]. Notch is responsible for cell fate during differentiation of the epidermis and hair and is associated with cyst formation [4].

The association with specific HLA phenotypes has been studied but antigen frequencies in one cohort of 65 patients with acne conglobata were found to be normal. A further group of patients with both HS and acne conglobata were studied: four of six patients had cross-reacting antigens and all had HLA-DRw4 [26]. PAPA was originally reported in a three-generation kindred with autosomal dominant transmission [23].

Environmental factors
Exposure to halogenated aromatic hydrocarbons or ingestion of halogens should be considered (see 'Occupational acne' later in this chapter).

Clinical features
History
Acne conglobata may develop in the setting of acne vulgaris that has been quiescent for a number of years but frequently the onset is insidious with a chronic and unremitting course. It is more common in males. Active inflammatory lesions may persist for many years and typically continue until the fourth decade of life. The healing of lesions is slow and associated with significant discomfort and disfiguring scarring (Figure 88.74). Patients typically fail to respond to antibacterial therapy.

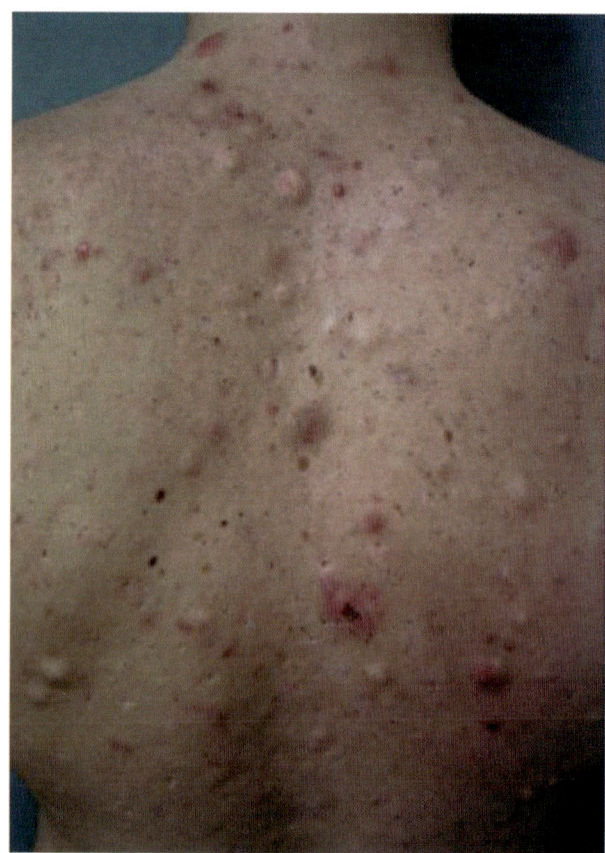

Figure 88.74 Acne conglobata of the back with multiple inflammatory lesions, grouped comedones, cysts and scarring.

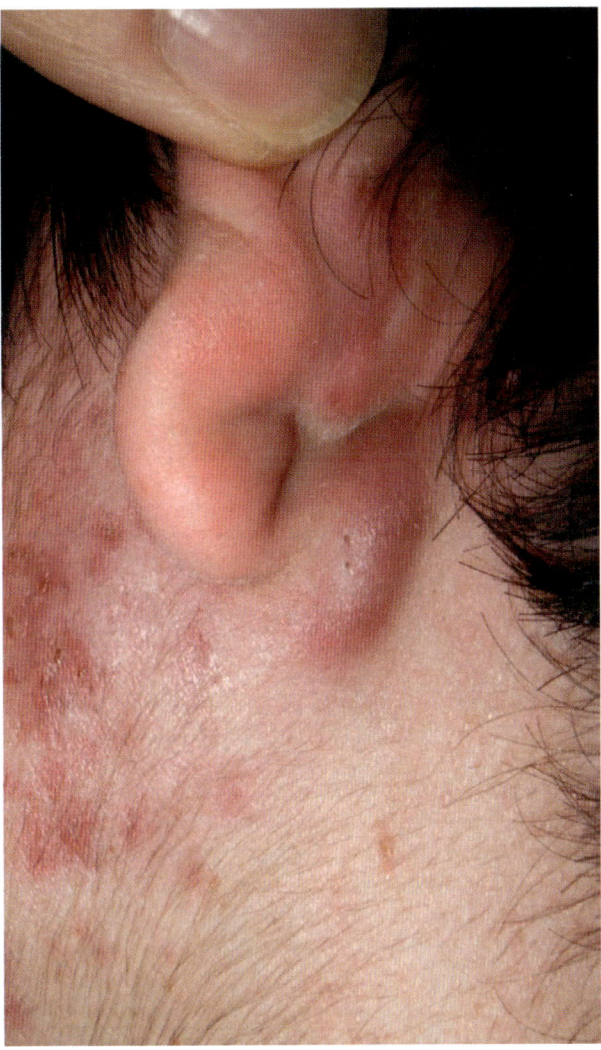

Figure 88.75 Patients with acne conglobata present with grouped comedones and deep-seated inflammatory lesions.

Table 88.33 The main features of acne conglobata.

Features	Comments
Sex	Males affected more frequently than females
Age	18–30 years
Pathogenesis	Unclear
Onset	May be an insidious onset with a chronic course on the background of previous acne or an acute deterioration of existing inflammatory acne
Localisation	Face, trunk and limbs extending to the buttocks
Clinical picture	Deep-seated inflammatory lesions, abscesses and cysts, causing interconnecting sinus tracts
	Polyporous grouped comedones and significant scarring
Laboratory findings	Gram-positive bacteria producing secondary infection
Response to conventional antibiotic therapy	Poor
Treatments of choice	Oral isotretinoin alongside systemic corticosteroids to reduce inflammation
	Systemic antibiotics to treat secondary infection and reduce inflammation
Other treatments described in the literature	Infliximab, etanercept and adalimumab
	Dapsone, ciclosporin or colchicine plus isotretinoin
	Carbon dioxide laser and external beam therapy, photodynamic therapy and some surgical procedures

Presentation

Patients with acne conglobata present with multiple comedones often in groups (Figure 88.75) and demonstrate highly inflammatory papules, pustules, tender nodules, interconnecting abscesses and draining sinus tracts (Table 88.33). The nodules characteristically increase in size and deep ulcers may develop beneath the nodules which interconnect and produce draining sinus tracts (Figure 88.76). Hypertrophic and atrophic scars are frequently present.

Clinical variants

As outlined earlier, acne conglobata may either be part of a number of collective inflammatory conditions or present as a distinct clinical entity.

Differential diagnosis

The main differentials are severe inflammatory acne or acne fulminans. The latter has an acute onset and is rarely seen in females. Patients present with acne conglobata at an older average age and the condition has a protracted and more chronic course than acne fulminans with fewer systemic symptoms (see Table 88.31).

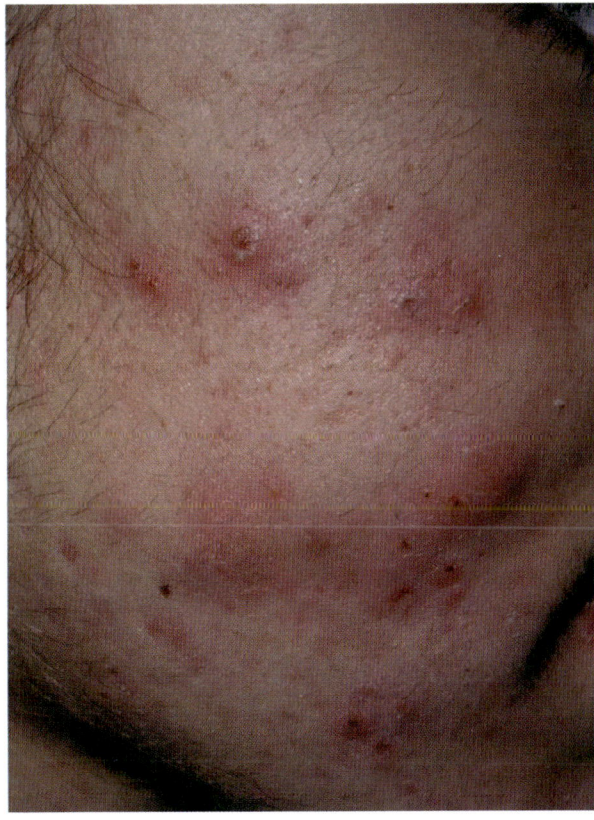

Figure 88.76 Patient with acne conglobata presenting with abscesses and cysts, causing interconnecting sinus tracts.

PART 8: SPECIFIC CUTANEOUS STRUCTURES

Table 88.34 Treatment options for acne conglobata.

Number of cases	Treatment employed	Duration/outcome of treatment
–	Oral isotretinoin (0.5–1 mg/kg/day) for 4–6 months. With or without systemic steroids	Reduction in some inflammatory lesions and better control of disease but not clearance in many
1 patient	Etanercept	Successful treatment
64-year-old male	Infliximab 3 mg/kg on weeks 0, 2 and 6. Alternate months thereafter. Isotretinoin 0.8 mg/kg/day used in conjunction with infliximab – failed to control the acne conglobata prior to infliximab	Reduction of lesions at week 6 No new lesions after week 6 Isotretinoin tapered off Control maintained with infliximab
–	Infliximab infusion	Successful treatment of acne with infliximab
–	Vaporisation of covering cyst wall with CO_2 laser, and topical tretinoin	Clinical improvement with laser, maintained with tretinoin
–	Isotretinoin and dapsone	Successful treatment achieved
53-year-old male	8 treatments of modern beam radiation over 2 weeks localised to the bilateral mandible cheeks	3 weeks post radiation reduced cyst size, absent drainage, reduced pain and improved self-esteem
1 male	Infliximab infusion	All dermatologocal and rheumatological manifestations reported to regress with infliximab. Previously failed on etanercept
–	Interleukin 1-β blockade	
18-year-old male	Adalimumab 80 mg loading dose followed by 40 mg twice monthly	Marked decrease in size and degree of inflammation of nodular lesions by 4 weeks; at 12 weeks full resolution of nodular lesions. At 12 months on treatment sustained efficacy
42-year-old male	Etanercept 25 mg twice a week and isotretinoin 20 mg weekly for 3 months. Etanercept then tapered to once a week for 1 month then alternate weeks for 2 months and isotretinoin reduced to 10 mg daily	Reduction in lesions and activity of the disease

Comedonal lesions are generally much more florid in acne conglobata and present in a characteristic grouped manner. Severe acne vulgaris, occupational acne and drug-induced acne should be considered in the differential diagnosis.

Classification of severity

Acne conglobata always presents as a severe cutaneous inflammatory process with significant scarring resulting in disfigurement in most cases. Psychosocial sequelae as a result of the disease process and resultant scarring are very common [27].

Disease course and prognosis

The disease course is insidious and chronic. It leads to significant psychosocial morbidity as a result of extensive scarring and discomfort and malodour associated with the inflammatory lesions.

Complications and co-morbidities

The most common complication is extensive and disfiguring scarring. Psychosocial impairment including anxiety and depression is frequent. Renal amyloidosis has been reported with acne conglobata [28]. Malignancy has also been reported in chronic scars attributed to acne conglobata [29].

Investigations

No consistent laboratory abnormalities are identified in acne conglobata. Bacterial cultures from the skin are generally sterile but in some cases lesions are secondarily infected with Gram-positive bacteria. In cases where there is malodour, assessing cultures and treating with appropriate antibiotics may be helpful. An IgA gammopathy has been observed in a patient with pyoderma and acne conglobata [30].

Management

Therapy is challenging. Treatment should aim to reduce the morbidity associated with discomfort and malodour with the use of appropriate analgesia alongside antiseptic washes and, if necessary, antibiotics. Treatment should also aim to prevent complications by reducing inflammation associated with resultant scarring [27].

Large nodules may be aspirated and injection with intralesional triamcinolone or cryotherapy may be beneficial [31]. More extensive surgical excision of interconnecting nodules and laying open of sinus tracts my also prove helpful [32]. There are reports of benefit with laser therapy and modern external beam radiation [33,34]. There are very few clinical trials assessing treatment in this refractory condition but one small study examining photodynamic therapy using 5% aminolaevulinic acid and red light demonstrated some advantage to control therapy [35]. A combination of medical and surgical approaches may be required to manage this refractory condition.

Biologic therapies have been demonstrated to be effective treatments for acne conglobata presenting in isolation or as part of the SAPHO syndrome [35–41]. However, larger-scale RCT studies are still lacking and would help better determine the efficacy of anti-TNFs in treating acne conglobata.

First line

Oral isotretinoin (0.5–1 mg/kg/day) for 4–6 months is the treatment of choice. Isotretinoin may need to be combined with oral antibiotics such as erythromycin or trimethoprim. Concomitant use of systemic steroids such as prednisolone 1 mg/kg/day for 2–4 weeks may also provide benefit to control the inflammatory component of the disease at its initial onset and intermittently during acute exacerbations. Surgery may be required to lay open abscesses and sinus tracts. Resultant scarring may be improved with the fractional laser after surgical intervention [27].

Second line

Tetracycline antibiotics are frequently prescribed to reduce the inflammation but are notoriously ineffective.

Alternative therapies

Alternative options for the management of acne conglobata include long-term high-dose antibiotics, dapsone with isotretinoin [42], ciclosporin and/or colchicine in conjunction with topical retinoids and antimicrobial therapy [43]. One case report has demonstrated the benefit of carbon dioxide laser in combination with tretinoin to open up cysts and to prevent the emergence of new lesions [33]. Potential treatments for acne conglobata as reported in the literature are outlined in Table 88.34.

Occupational acne

Definition and nomenclature

Occupational acne is a group of disorders characterised by the formation of acne-like lesions in patients not previously prone to acne after exposure to occupational agents, in most cases chemical compounds.

Synonyms and inclusions
- Chemically induced acne
- Chloracne

Introduction and general description

Environmental pollution can result in an acneform dermatosis imitating acne, which was first described in 1887 by Von Bettman and later by Herxheimer in 1899 [1]. Herxheimer suggested that the disorder was caused by chlorine exposure and hence called it 'chloracne' based on the similarity of its clinical features with acne vulgaris. Occupational acne can be induced by diverse environmental agents and can, therefore, be classified as acne venenata/acne cosmetica, tropical acne/hydration acne, oil acne/pomade acne, detergens acne, coal-tar acne and chloracne (Table 88.35) [2–4].

Chloracne is caused by certain polyhalogenated organic (aromatic) compounds containing naphthalenes, biphenyls and phenols (herbicides and herbicide intermediates) and is considered to be one of the most sensitive indicators of systemic poisoning by these compounds (Box 88.7) [1].

Box 88.7 Chloracne-inducing chemicals

Polyhalogenated naphthalenes[a]
- Polychloronaphthalenes
- Polybromonaphthalenes[b,c]

Polyhalogenated biphenyls
- Polychlorobiphenyls (PCBs)
- Polybromobiphenyls
- Polychalogenated dibenzofurans[a]
  - Polychlorodibenzofurans, especially tri-, tetra-, penta- and hexachlorodibenzofuran
  - Polybromodibenzofurans, especially tetrabromodibenzofuran

Contaminants of polychlorophenol compounds
Especially herbicides (2,4,5-trichlorophenol and pentachlorophenol) and herbicide intermediates (2,4,5-trichlorophenol)
- 2,3,7,8-tetrachlorodibenzo-p-doxin (TCDD)
- Hexachlorodibenzo-p-dioxin
- Tetrachlorodibenzofuran

Contaminants of 3,4-dichloroaniline and related herbicides
- 3,4,3',4'-tetrachoroazoxybenzene (TCAOB)
- 3,4,3',4'-tetrachoroazobenzene (TCAB)

Other
- Dihydrotrifluoromythylphenylbenzothiopyrazolone
- 1,2,3,4-tetrachlorobenzene (experimental)
- Dichlobenil (herbicide, clinical)
- Crude trichloronezene (DDT)[c]

[a]May occur as contaminants in some PCBs.
[b]May occur as contaminants in some PBBs.
[c]Not confirmed as chloracnegens.

Dioxins, a large family of halogenated aromatic hydrocarbons, are the most potent environmental chloracnegen. The most potent environmental chloracnegen of this group is 2,3,7,8-tetrachlorodibenzo-p-dioxin (TCDD) [5]. The chloracnegens are structurally similar, containing two benzene rings with halogen atoms occupying at least three of the lateral ring positions (75 isomers).

Epidemiology

Most cases of chloracne have resulted from occupational and non-occupational exposures. Non-occupational chloracne mainly resulted from contaminated industrial wastes and contaminated

PART 8: SPECIFIC CUTANEOUS STRUCTURES

Table 88.35 Differential diagnosis of occupational and environmental acne.

	Aetiology	Location	Lesions
Acne venenata/acne cosmetica	Cosmetics	Face	Closed comedones
Tropical acne/hydration acne	Heat/humidity	Back, neck, buttocks, proximal extremities	Nodules, cysts
Oil acne/pomade acne	Oil	Arms, thighs, buttocks	Red papules, pustules
Detergens acne	Alkalic soaps, detergents	Hands, face	Red papules, pustules
Coal-tar acne	Tar/pitch	Exposed facial areas, especially malar	Open comedones
Chloracne	Polyhalogenated organic (aromatic) compounds	Malar, retroauricular, mandibular	Comedones, straw-coloured cysts (0.1–1 cm)

Adapted from McDonnell and Taylor 2000 [16] © Springer.

Table 88.36 Large-scale single dioxin accidents in the latter half of the 20th century.

Year of outbreak	Country/city (reference)	Number of registered victims	Pollutants	Occurrence	Long-term follow-up of chloracne prevalence (survey year)
1953	Germany/Ludwigshafen [7]	248	TCP/TCDD	Leakage of byproducts of TCP production from a chemical reactor	10.1% (1989)
1963	Netherlands/Amsterdam [8]	145	TCDD	Explosion of a factory producing crop-protection agents	48.9% (1983)
1976	Italy/Seveso [9]	193[a]	TCP/TCDD	Explosion of a TCP reactor	1 of 193 (1989)

Adaptd from Ju *et al.* 2012 [3] © Elsevier.
[a] 193 detected cases with chloracne (170 younger than 15 years of age).
TCDD, 2,3,7,8-tetrachlorodibenzo-*p*-dioxin; TCP, trichlorophenol.

Table 88.37 Massive intoxication through ingestion of contaminated oils in the latter half of the 20th century.

Year of outbreak	Country/city (reference)	Number of registered victims	Pollutants	Occurrence	Long-term follow-up of chloracne prevalence (survey year)
1968	Japan/Kyushu (Fukuoka, Nagasaki) [10]	1684	PCB/PCDF	Contamination of PCB in rice bran oil	7.8% (1993)
1979	Taiwan/Changhua, Taichung [11]	2061	PCB	Contamination of PCB in rice bran oil	17% (1993)

Adapted from Ju *et al.* 2012 [3] © Elsevier.
PCB, polychlorinated biphenyls; PCDD, polychlorinated dibenzofurans.

food products. The identification of dioxin as an elicitor of occupational acne was made with the cooperation of the dermatologists Schulz and Kimmig with the chemist Sorge in Hamburg, Germany, who investigated patients with atypical acne in a chemical plant [6].

Since then, there have been several large accidents caused by occupational exposures or food contaminations. After the Second World War, several episodes of large-scale dioxin poisoning were reported after industrial work explosions, each with more than 100 victims (Table 88.36) [7–9].

Massive intoxication has so far happened twice through ingestion of contaminated oils: 'Yusho' in Japan in 1968 and 'Yu-Cheng' in Taiwan in 1979; both terms meaning 'oil syndrome' (Table 88.37) [10,11]. The real prevalence of chloracne among Vietnamese civilians and American soldiers caused by Agent Orange (containing phenoxyl herbicide contaminated with dioxins) during the Vietnam War (1962–71) is unknown [12]. The most recent sensational case report of a chloracne incident was the TCDD poisoning of Viktor Yushchenko, a former president of Ukraine, in late December 2004 (see Figure 88.18) [13].

Due to their extensive long-term developmental and neurological toxicity, hormonal and immunological disruption as well as cancer promotion, the production of polychlorinated biphenyls has been prohibited by the Stockholm Treaty on Persistent Organic Pollutants made effective from 2004.

Clinical features

Chloracne can be diagnosed by the history of exposure to chloracnegens, characteristic clinical manifestations such as acutely emerging comedones, papules, nodules and cysts (see Figure 88.17) followed by scars and specifically the detection of high serum concentration of chloracne. A history of exposure to chloracnegens,

Table 88.38 Differential signs of chloracne versus acne vulgaris.

Clinical signs	Chloracne	Acne vulgaris
Usual age	Any	Adolescent
Comedones	Many (essential sign)	Present
Inflammatory papules and cysts	Uncommon	Common
Straw-coloured cysts	Pathognomonic	Rare
Temporal comedones	Diagnostic	Rare
Retroauricular involvement	Common	Uncommon
Nose involvement	Often spared	Involved
Associated systemic findings	Common	Rare

Adapted from McDonnell and Taylor 2000 [16] © Springer.

progressively emerging comedones, papules, nodules and cysts followed by scars, skin xerosis and decreased sebogenesis, and high serum concentration of chloracnegens, differentiate chloracne from acne vulgaris (Table 88.38).

Investigations

As the assessment of chloracnegens in serum can only be carried out in specialised laboratories and the serum titres of dioxins are usually within the normal range, histopathological changes also offer important clues in the diagnosis of chloracne [14] as follows:
- Epidermal hyperplasia.
- Follicular hyperplasia – replacement by keratinising epidermal cells.
- Sebaceous glands disappear and are replaced by keratinising epidermal cells.
- Sebaceous gland involution after a complete loss of structure. The remaining sebocytes appear normal. Sebaceous gland involution is due to cessation of sebocyte replenishment.

Management

The aim of treatment is to lower or to eliminate the accumulated dioxins in the body at the very beginning of intoxication, for example by using dioxin-chelating substances such as synthetic dietary fat substitutes. The problem of dioxin contamination and its potential health hazards should be taken seriously during the current wave of industrial globalisation. Management is as follows:

- Olestra potato chips (Pringles® fat-free potato chips, 10 g olestra/ 28 g potato chips) over 38 days, using five different dosing regimens (from 15 to 66 g olestra daily) lasting 7 days each [15].
- Topical tretinoin over 1 year.

Prepubertal acne

Definition and nomenclature

Acne before the onset of puberty is uncommon. Descriptive terms used for acne in preadolescent children are generally based on age and include neonatal, infantile, mid-childhood and prepubertal or preadolescent acne. A recent classification of acne in children based on expert consensus included five subtypes according to age: neonatal, infantile, mid-childhood, preadolescent and adolescent. However, the distinction between preadolescence and adolescence by age can be challenging; the term prepubertal acne has been adopted for use in this text.

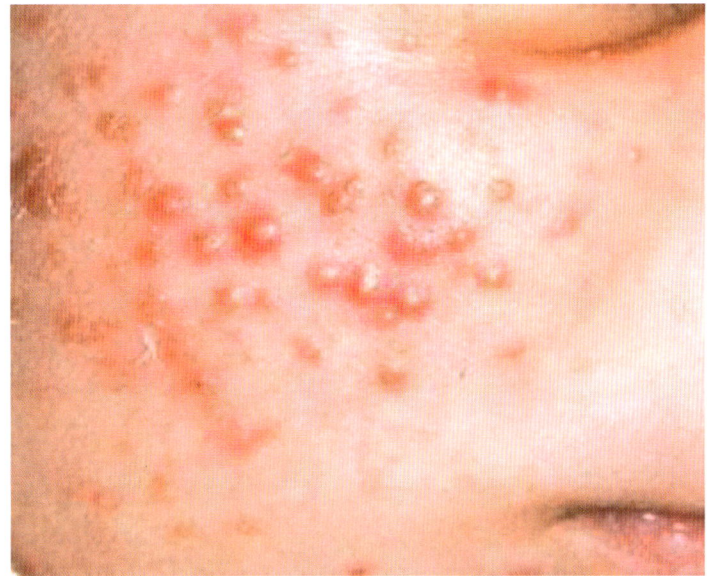

Figure 88.77 Neonatal cephalic pustulosis. From Firooz et al. 2019 [61].

Synonyms and inclusions

- Neonatal acne
- Infantile acne
- Mid-childhood acne

Introduction and general description

Prepubertal acne includes a number of clinical presentations and may be misdiagnosed. The definition by age does not necessarily identify children who are at risk of treatable forms of virilisation and a focused history and examination should be adopted to ensure that underlying hormonal abnormalities and adrenal or gonadal tumours are identified. A broad range of treatment options are available but some medications used in the management of adult acne are contraindicated in children [1].

Epidemiology

Incidence and prevalence

Neonatal acne is defined as the presence of even a small number of comedones and may affect up to 20% of neonates; however, this may reflect an overestimate as papulopustular conditions may masquerade as neonatal acne [2,3]. The most well recognised is neonatal cephalic pustulosis, an acneform eruption thought to be caused by *Malassezia* (Figure 88.77) [4].

Infantile acne is less common than neonatal acne and mid-childhood acne is very rare [1,5,6].

Prepubertal acne is defined as acne that commences before the onset of puberty. Acne has been reported in 60–71.3% of premenarchal females [7]. A mid-facial comedonal distribution is associated with poor prognosis (Figure 88.78) [8,9]. A 2021 retrospective anal-

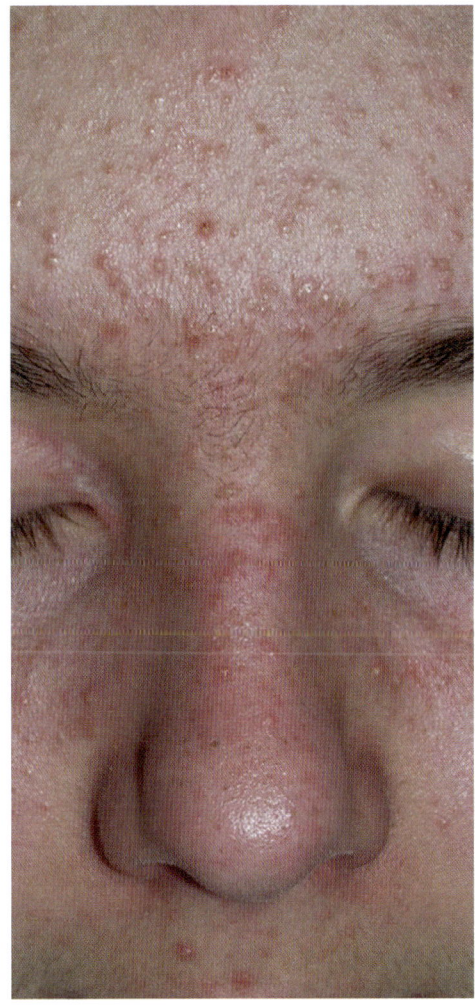

Figure 88.78 Mid-facial comedones are associated with poor prognosis.

Table 88.39 Prepubertal acne defined according to age.

Acne description	Age of onset
Neonatal	Birth to up to 8 weeks
Infantile	8 weeks up to 1 year
Mid-childhood	1–7 years
Preadolescent	7 years up to 12 years or menarche in girls
Adolescent	12 years up to 19 years or after menarche in girls

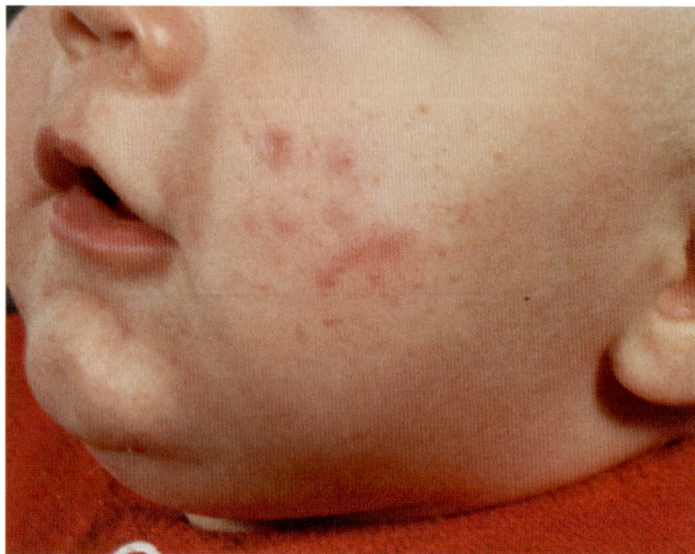

Figure 88.79 Infantile acne on the cheek. Courtesy of Dr J. Ravenscroft, Queens Medical Centre, Nottingham, UK.

ysis of 683 patients aged 7–12 years found a female preponderance (75%) and a high predominance of phylotype IA1 of *C. acnes* [10].

Age and sex
Based on recent consensus data [11], prepubertal acne can be defined as acne according to age as outlined in Table 88.39.

A neonate is defined as a newborn up to the equivalent of 8 weeks of age. Neonatal acne presents at birth through to the equivalent age of 8 weeks and is seen more frequently in boys (5 : 1) [11–14].

Infantile acne typically presents between 3 and 12 months but may occur as late as 16 months (Figure 88.79) [11,12,14–16]. It shows a male predominance.

Mid-childhood acne occurs from age 1 to 7 years [11].

Prepubertal acne presents before true puberty. Adrenarche represents maturation of the adrenal glands with adrenal production and increase in the zona reticularis and the acquisition of enzymes that facilitate synthesis of androgens from cholesterol. Adrenarche occurs at the age of 6–7 years in females and 7–8 years in boys. Prepubertal acne may occur from age 7 to 11 years [11]. However, depending on the age of puberty this will vary. Girls may present with acne as young as 8 years of age.

Ethnicity
There are no good studies comparing ethnicity in prepubertal acne but slight variation in the onset of puberty may influence the age of

onset. The mean age of puberty in white girls is 10.2 years compared with 9.6 years in African Americans [17].

Associated diseases
Prepubertal acne may be associated with underlying endocrinopathies and virilising tumours. SAPHO syndrome has been reported in childhood. Chronic cutaneous lesions were identified in 80% of children with SAPHO at follow-up visits at the University Children's Hospitals in Bern and Zurich, and of 260 cases reported in the literature 25% had inflammatory skin problems with 6% of these presenting with severe acne [18]. There are other medical conditions in which acne is either absent or very mild. This includes Turner syndrome [19]. There appears to be a reduction of peripheral androgen production in these patients and the use of conventional hormonal replacement therapy that further decreases testosterone and dihydrotestosterone may explain the absence of moderate to severe acne in Turner syndrome.

Pathophysiology
The underlying pathogenesis of neonatal acne is not clearly understood but is thought to relate to hyperactivity of the sebaceous glands stimulated by neonatal androgens from the testes in boys and adrenals in girls and boys [20]. Maternal androgens are thought to be transferred transplacentally and the hyperactive neonatal adrenal glands in both sexes result in an increased production of DHEA and the sulphated form DHEAS. During the neonatal period and for approximately 1 year afterwards, the adrenals secrete androgens. This restarts in mid-childhood, around 7 years of age, at which time the zona reticularis produces androgens again.

From birth through 6–12 months, there are pubertal levels of luteinising hormone; in boys, this results in additional testosterone production as a result of the high levels of luteinising hormone stimulating the testes. This may explain the increased incidence of neonatal acne in boys. Increased sebum production in the first few months returns to normal at about 6 months [21].

The aetiology of infantile acne also remains poorly understood. Similar to neonatal acne, it may be associated with increased levels of androgens produced by adrenal glands in both sexes and by the testes in boys. DHEA from the adrenal glands stimulates sebum production up to 1 year of age or until the DHEA levels drop at about 6–12 months [21].

During adrenarche, the secretion of androgens DHEA and DHEAS by the adrenal gland starts to increase, resulting in androgen-mediated sebum production. DHEAS levels have been reported to be significantly higher in prepubertal girls with acne when compared with controls [7]. Gonadal secretions of androgens are very low at this stage. The development of mid-facial comedonal acne is considered a predictor of acne severity [8,9].

Acute onset, persistent or severe acne, particularly in the presence of virilisation between 1 and 7 years of age, should always raise the possibility of an underlying endocrinopathy. Infantile acne has been reported as an initial sign of an adrenocortical tumour in a 23-month-old boy with accelerated growth and signs of virilisation [22]. In females, ovarian androgen excess is most commonly related to PCOS but rarely may be a consequence of benign or malignant ovarian tumours [23]. In boys, recalcitrant or severe acne may be a presenting sign of NCCAH [24].

Predisposing factors
See section on acne vulgaris earlier in this chapter.

Causative organisms
Cutibacterium acnes is implicated in the pathophysiology of acne (see section on acne vulgaris earlier in this chapter). The onset of sebum production triggers the expansion of *C. acnes* and this occurs earlier in children who develop acne than in those who do not [25].

In the case of neonatal cephalic pustulosis, a relationship has been suggested between the clinical presentation and *Malasezzia furfur*, *M. sympodialis* and other species [26,27].

Genetics
See section on acne vulgaris earlier in this chapter.

Environmental factors
Certain medications may be implicated in prepubertal acne as identified in the section on drug-induced acne earlier in this chapter. Maternal ingestion of phenytoin has been implicated [28]. Exposure to certain substances including greasy emollients, hair gels and occlusive topical agents as well as aromatic hydrocarbons and halogenides may be a trigger.

Clinical features
Presentation
Neonatal acne presents at or shortly after birth with red papulopustular lesions commonly distributed on the cheeks, chin and forehead (Figure 88.80). Occasionally, these extend to the neck, scalp and upper trunk.

Infantile acne presents later than neonatal acne. The central cheeks are frequently affected with a combination of inflamed

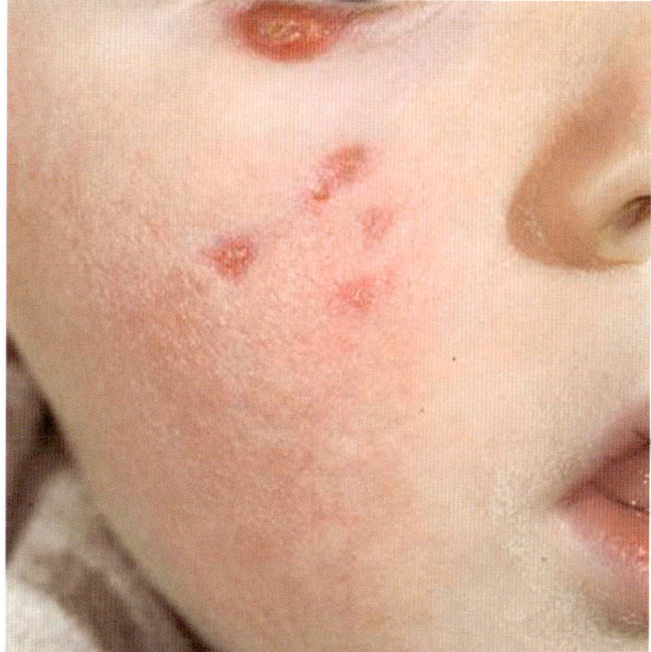

Figure 88.81 Infantile acne may involve cystic lesions and scarring. Courtesy of Dr J. Ravenscroft, Queens Medical Centre, University of Nottingham, UK.

papules and pustules with open and closed comedones. The presentation is usually more widespread than neonatal acne. A study of 29 patients with infantile/juvenile acne seen in a specialist centre over a period of 25 years demonstrated the median age of onset was 9 months; the disease was mild in 24%, moderate in 62% and severe in 14% [29]. In 59%, the acne was predominantly inflammatory. Five patients (17%) were left with scarring. Acne conglobata can present in infants, resulting in severe inflammatory cystic lesions, sinus tract formation and significant scarring (Figure 88.81) [30].

Acne developing during mid-childhood should always raise the suspicion of androgen excess.

Acne in prepubertal children usually presents with comedonal lesions with or without some inflammatory papules. Lesions are frequently located in a mid-facial distribution and may precede any other signs of maturation [7]. Mid-facial comedonal acne (see Figure 88.78) can be the first sign of pubertal maturation in females, preceding areolar development, pubic hair and the menarche. The development of acne in childhood along with premature adrenarche may be an initial sign of PCOS or metabolic syndrome [31,32]. Follow-up and anticipatory guidance are indicated in these children.

Clinical variants
Neonatal cephalic pustulosis has been considered by some as synonymous with neonatal acne but others consider it a separate entity as there are more inflammatory papules, significant pustules and a lack of comedonal lesions.

Acne conglobata is a severe variant of acne that can present in infants resulting in severe inflammatory cystic lesions, sinus tract formation and significant scarring [30].

Differential diagnosis
The differential diagnoses for neonatal acne are outlined in Box 88.8.

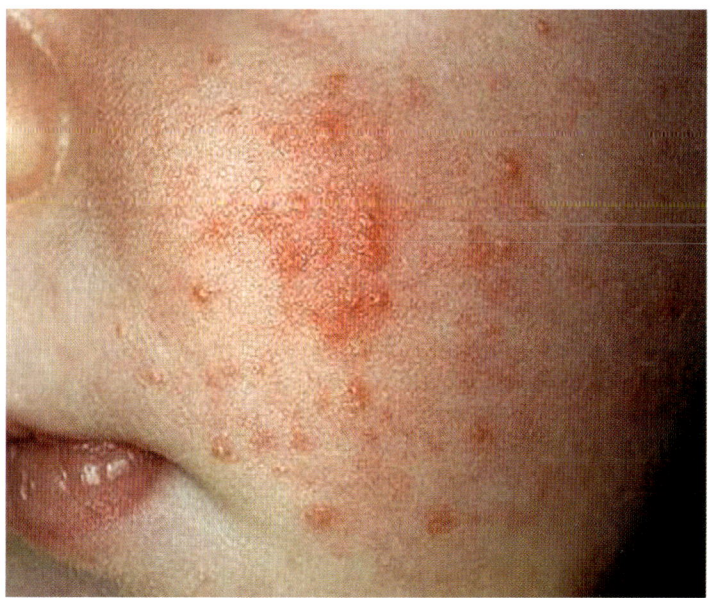

Figure 88.80 Neonatal acne presenting in the first few weeks of life.

Box 88.8 Differential diagnoses of acne in the neonate

Infections
- Bacterial
- *Staphylococcus aureus* (bullous impetigo)
- *Streptococcus* (β-haemolytic group B)
- *Pseudomonas aeruginosa*
- *Haemophilus influenzae*
- *Listeria monocytogenes*
- Fungal
- Candidiasis
- Pityrosporum folliculitis
- Viral:
  - Herpes simplex
  - Varicella-zoster
  - Cytomegalovirus
- Parasitic:
  - Scabies
- Non-infectious:
  - Erythema toxicum neonatorum
  - Infantile acropustulosis
  - Transient neonatal pustular melanosis

Other
- Milia
- Sebaceous gland hyperplasia
- Pustular miliariasis
- Eosinophilic pustular folliculitis of infancy
- Acneform eruptions
- Acne venenata infantum
- Acneform drug eruptions (steroids, lithium, hydantoin)
- Chloracne

Neonatal cephalic pustulosis was first described in 1991 and is historically referred to as neonatal acne [33,34]. It usually presents in the first 3 weeks of life (see Figure 88.80), and prevalence varies between 10% and 66% of newborns in the literature. It is characterised by red papular/pustular lesions especially on the cheeks but also on the chin, eyelids, neck and upper chest. Comedonal lesions are not usually seen. It has been postulated that neonatal cephalic pustulosis develops in association with *Malassezia sympodialis* and *M. globosa*; however, the exact aetiological role of *Malassezia* is uncertain as the organism is part of the normal flora of neonatal skin, and up to 38% of cases had negative smears in one study [35]. Another explanation is that neonatal cephalic pustulosis relates to an overgrowth of lipophilic yeasts at birth that results in an inflammatory reaction leading to monomorphic papules and pustules in predisposed neonates with more sebum production.

Treatment is usually not required for neonatal cephalic pustulosis as it is a self-limiting disorder which usually heals without scarring in 1–3 months. If the condition does persist beyond this time and/or is widespread and unsightly, topical ketoconazole cream expedites recovery [36].

The differential diagnoses of infantile acne include neonatal acne, acne venenata infantum, chloracne and hyperandrogenism.

The differential diagnoses of mid-childhood acne include keratosis pilaris and milia alongside endocrinopathies and conditions relating to hyperandrogenism.

The differential diagnoses of prepubertal acne include childhood granulomatous periorifacial dermatitis, lupus miliaris disseminatus faciei and childhood granulomatous rosacea alongside endocrinopathies and disorders associated with androgen excess.

Classification of severity

There is no recognised or validated grading system for prepubertal acne. Severity is assessed as mild, moderate or severe and the persistence or appearance of scarring should be considered as a less favourable prognostic factor.

Complications and co-morbidities

Acne scarring can result from acne lesions as in adult acne. In one study examining cases of infantile acne, secondary scarring affected 17% of the cases [29]. Acne conglobata is rarely seen in infants but the incidence of scarring is high in these patients [37,38]. Patients with infantile acne may develop a resurgence of their acne as teenagers and the likelihood of developing acne in adolescence is greater in these patients than in their peers [39].

Infantile acne is very rarely associated with other clinical features of androgen excess such as hirsutism or premature closure of the epiphyses; very occasionally, there may be transient or more persistent high plasma levels of testosterone, luteinising hormone and follicle-stimulating hormone.

Disease course and prognosis

Neonatal acne usually settles spontaneously and leaves little scarring. Infantile acne has a more persistent and variable course than neonatal acne and although most cases resolve by 5 years of age others may persist until puberty. Scarring from the deep-seated inflammatory lesions may ensue. Patients with infantile acne may develop a resurgence of their acne as teenagers and parents should be advised accordingly [39].

Predictive factors for severity and persistence include a high number of comedones, mid-facial distribution, early development of comedones, and high levels of DHEAS and free and total testosterone and earlier menarche in females.

Investigations

A focused history and examination for signs of accelerated growth, precocious puberty and hirsutism or other signs of hyperandrogenism should be employed. It is important to consider underlying endocrinopathies and investigate accordingly with the support of a paediatric endocrinologist (Box 88.9). One study has indicated that there is a relatively low risk of true endocrinopathy in preadolescent children in the context of no other symptoms or signs of androgen excess [36].

Box 88.9 Examination and investigations that should be considered to rule out an endocrinopathy in prepubertal acne

History and examination
- Age of menarche in girls
- Tanner stage
- Telarche (palpable breast tissue below the areolae in girls, testicular enlargement in boys)
- Pubarche (presence of pubic hair)
- Growth chart
- Height, weight, body mass index
- Bone age (left hand and wrist X-ray for those with high growth parameters)

Endocrine work-up
- Free and total testosterone
- Dehydroepiandrosterone, luteinising hormone, follicle-stimulating hormone
- Prolactin
- 17-hydroxyprogesterone (to rule out congenital adrenal hyperplasia)

Table 88.40 Algorithm of therapeutic options for neonatal, infantile, mid-childhood and prepubertal acne.

Acne category	Treatment options
Neonatal	Gentle cleansers, oil-free emollients
	If marked pustules, use topical azole cream
Infantile and prepubertal	***First line***
	Benzoyl peroxide (BPO) or topical retinoid (if primarily comedonal)
	Fixed combination products for mixed lesions from 12 years with the exception of 0.1% adapalene/2.5% BPO which is indicated from 9 years
	Second line (for more severe disease)
	Oral erythromycin (oral trimethoprim if allergic to macrolides) combined with BPO to avoid emergence of antibiotic-resistant *C. acnes* ± topical retinoid
	Third line
	Severe recalcitrant scarring acne, exclude underlying hyperandrogenism
	Consider oral isotretinoin
Mid-childhood	Exclude underlying pathology and treat as infantile and prepubertal

Management

General principles of management

The principles of treating acne in children involve adopting simple regimens that target the clinical lesions and pathophysiological factors implicated in acne while avoiding adverse effects. Most acne therapies are approved for children of 12 years and older. The exceptions include erythromycin which is approved for children 8 years and older by the FDA, adapalene/BPO gel approved for patients 9 years and older and tretinoin approved for patients 10 years and older. Apart from tetracycline antibiotics that should not be prescribed below 12 years of age in the UK because of the risk of damage to developing bones and permanent discoloration of dentition, most acne treatments are not contraindicated in younger children. However, regulations do vary by country regarding tetracycline use, with some evidence that adult teeth are fully formed by 8 years of age [40]. It is important to ensure parents are fully informed if medications are prescribed off-licence [41].

For mild disease, topical therapies such as topical retinoids and/or topical antimicrobials are recommended. For moderate disease, a topical retinoid and/or BPO combined with a systemic antibiotic such as erythromycin (as ethyl succinate, 125 mg TDS) should be adopted. Systemic trimethoprim has also been used (up to 100 mg BD) [40]. If prescribing an antibiotic, topical BPO should be used alongside the agent to reduce the likelihood of bacterial resistance emerging in resident *C. acnes*. The literature also reports the use of other antibiotic agents such as amoxicillin [42], cephalexin [43] and azithromycin, although concerns about antimicrobial resistance with azithromycin limit its use (see acne vulgaris management section earlier in this chapter). Infantile acne may take several months to resolve – the more inflammatory the disease, the longer the duration.

Isotretinoin is rarely needed, and only for severe non-responding cases. Successful treatment with isotretinoin has been reported in the literature using doses of 0.36–2 mg/kg/day for 4–6 months in children younger than 5 years [40]. Topical retinoids may provide maintenance following successful therapy [44].

In most cases of neonatal acne, daily cleansing is all that is needed; however, if more extensive, topical agents aimed at treating comedonal and/or apparent inflammatory lesions should be employed.

First line

In neonatal acne, if lesions are causing concern or are moderate to severe in nature an approach as outlined in Table 88.40 should be adopted for acne pre-adrenarche.

Second line

If oral antibiotics are required for more moderate to severe disease, erythromycin is the treatment of choice [40]. Of note, oral tetracycline is contraindicated in children of less than 8 years of age in the USA and 12 years in Europe as it can cause damage to developing dentition and bones.

Third line

Clinicians face a dilemma when a patient presents with severe recalcitrant acne that is causing scarring and cosmetic sequelae, where treatment with oral isotretinoin could be beneficial. Currently, oral isotretinoin is approved by the FDA and European Commission for the treatment of nodulocystic recalcitrant acne in children over 12 years of age.

There are reports in the literature confirming the safe and successful use of oral isotretinoin in patients ranging from 5 to 20 months of age. All patients had recalcitrant scarring acne that had failed to respond to topical and oral medications usually used for acne. The ideal dose of isotretinoin is not defined, although published reports suggest a dose range from 0.2 to 2 mg/kg/day divided in doses with food or milk to maximise absorption (Table 88.41) [45–59].

Administering capsules can be challenging in children of this age. Isotretinoin is highly light sensitive and oxygen labile so splitting

Table 88.41 Dosage regimens used for isotretinoin in childhood acne [45–59].

Sex	Onset age of acne (months)	Isotretinoin dosage (mg/kg/day)	Duration (months)	Side effects
Female	18	0.5–1	5	Reduced hair growth, mood changes, high lactate dehydrogenase
Male	2 (comedones), 10 (cystic)	0.36–0.67	5	High serum glutamic-pyruvic transaminase and glutamic-oxaloacetic transaminase
Male	12	1	4	Mild eczema on neck
Male	6	0.5	4	None
Female	20	1 then 2 (+ prednisolone)	6 5	Transient umbilical granulation
Male	?	0.5	4	?
Female	20	0.5–0.6	7	None
Female	6	0.2–1.5	14	None
Female	7	0.5	5	None
Male	9	?	–	None
Male	6	?		None
Male	0	0.5	12	Transient perioral exanthema, diarrhoea 3 weeks
Male	4	0.5	4	None
Male	5	0.5–1	6	Slight lip desquamation

capsules may reduce potential efficacy if not conducted in dim light. Although mixing with food has been advocated this may affect the stability of the drug. Freezing the capsule to a solid constituency enables it to be divided into halves or quarters to deliver the desired dose. This prevents drug wastage, minimises degradation of the drug and masks any unacceptable taste. Given that the use of isotretinoin is an off-licence indication in this context, clinicians should ensure parents are well informed if using oral isotretinoin for acne in this age group.

Complementary therapies in the paediatric population have been reviewed by Gurnee *et al.* [60]. They note few studies have compared complementary therapies with commonly used acne therapies, such as topical antibiotics or oral antibiotics, and none has compared efficacy with topical retinoids.

Key references

The full list of references can be found in the online version at https://www.wiley.com/rooksdermatology10e

Acne vulgaris

13 Tan J, Kang S, Leyden J. Prevalence and risk factors of acne scarring among patients consulting dermatologists in the USA. *J Drugs Dermatol* 2017;16:97–102.

14 Layton AM, Thiboutot D, Tan J. Reviewing the global burden of acne: how could we improve care to reduce the burden? *Br J Dermatol* 2021;184:219–25.

17 Lynn DD, Umari T, Dunnick CA *et al.* The epidemiology of acne vulgaris in late adolescence. *Adolesc Health Med Ther* 2016;7:13–25.

29 Mourelatos K, Eady EA, Cunliffe WJ *et al.* Temporal changes in sebum excretion and propionibacterial colonization in preadolescent children with and without acne. *Br J Dermatol* 2007;156:22–31.

35 Dréno B, Thiboutot D, Layton AM *et al.* Large-scale international study enhances understanding of an emerging acne population: adult females. *J Eur Acad Dermatol Venereol* 2015;29:1096–106.

45 Hay RJ, Johns NE, Williams HC *et al.* The global burden of skin disease in 2010: an analysis of the prevalence and impact of skin conditions. *J Invest Dermatol* 2014;134:1527–34.

193 Zouboulis CC. Is acne vulgaris a genuine inflammatory disease? *Dermatology* 2001;203:277–9.

194 Jeremy AH, Holland DB, Roberts SG, Thomson KF, Cunliffe WJ. Inflammatory events are involved in acne lesion initiation. *J Invest Dermatol* 2003;121:20–7.

268 Baldwin H, Tan J. Effects of diet on acne and its response to treatment. *Am J Clin Dermatol* 2021;22:55–65. Erratum in: *Am J Clin Dermatol* 2021;22:67.

507 Layton AM, Eady EA, Thiboutot DM, Tan M, Members of the Acne Core Outcomes Research Network (ACORN) Outcomes Identification Group. Identifying what to measure in acne clinical trials: first steps towards development of a core outcome set. *J Invest Dermatol* 2017;137:1784–6.

521 Tan J, Kang S, Leyden J. Prevalence and risk factors of acne scarring among patients consulting dermatologists in the USA. *J Drugs Dermatol* 2017;16:97–102.

523 Holland DB, Jeremy AH, Roberts SG *et al.* Inflammation in acne scarring: a comparison of the responses in lesions from patients prone and not prone to scar. *Br J Dermatol* 2004;150:72–81.

553 Thiboutot DM, Dréno B, Abanmi A *et al.* Practical management of acne for clinicians: an international consensus from the Global Alliance to Improve Outcomes in Acne. *J Am Acad Dermatol* 2018;78(Suppl. 1):S1–23.e1.

554 Zaenglein AL, Pathy AL, Schlosser BJ *et al.* Guidelines of care for the management of acne vulgaris. *J Am Acad Dermatol* 2016;74:945–73.e33.

555 National Institute for Health and Care Excellence (NICE). *Acne Vulgaris: Management. NG198.* London: NICE, 2021 (last updated 2023). https://www.nice.org.uk/guidance/ng198 (last accessed June 2023).

556 Nast A, Dréno B, Bettoli V *et al.* European evidence-based (S3) guidelines for the treatment of acne. *J Eur Acad Dermatol Venereol* 2012;26(Suppl. 1):1–29.

647 Layton AM, Eady EA, Whitehouse H, Del Rosso JQ, Fedorowicz Z, van Zuuren EJ. Oral spironolactone for acne vulgaris in adult females: a hybrid systematic review. *Am J Clin Dermatol* 2017;18:169–91.

648 Barbieri JS, Choi JK, Mitra N, Margolis DJ. Frequency of treatment switching for spironolactone compared to oral tetracycline-class antibiotics for women with acne: a retrospective cohort study 2010-2016. *J Drugs Dermatol* 2018;17:632–8.

649 Renz S, Chinnery F, Stuart B *et al.* Spironolactone for adult female acne (SAFA): protocol for a double-blind, placebo-controlled, phase III randomised study of spironolactone as systemic therapy for acne in adult women. *BMJ Open* 2021;11:e053876.

666 Eichenfield LF, Krakowski AC, Piggot C *et al.* Evidence based recommendations for the diagnosis and treatment of pediatric acne. *Pediatrics* 2013;131(Suppl. 3):S163–86.

Prepubertal acne

44 National Institute for Health and Care Excellence (NCIE). *Acne Vulgaris: Management. NG198.* London: NICE, 2021 (last updated 2023). https://www.nice.org.uk/guidance/ng198 (last accessed June 2023).

CHAPTER 89

Rosacea

Esther J. van Zuuren[1], *Jerry Tan*[2], *Mireille M. D. van der Linden*[3] *and Martin Schaller*[4]

[1]Department of Dermatology, Leiden University Medical Centre, Leiden, the Netherlands
[2]Department of Medicine, Western University, Ontario, Canada
[3]Department of Dermatology, Amsterdam University Centre, Amsterdam, the Netherlands
[4]Department of Dermatology, Universitätsklinikum Tübingen, Tübingen, Germany

Rosacea

Definition, nomenclature and classification

Rosacea is a chronic inflammatory disease affecting the cheeks, chin, nose, forehead and frequently the eyes. It is often characterised by periods of remission and exacerbation [1–4]. Clinical features include transient erythema (flushing), persistent erythema, telangiectasias, inflammatory papules/pustules, phyma and ocular involvement [1–4]. Outdated synonyms or misnomers (such as 'acne rosacea', 'couperose', 'Kupferrose', 'facial erythrosis' and 'Rotfinne') may be confusing and should be avoided [5,6].

In 2002, the National Rosacea Society Expert Committee (NRSEC) proposed standard criteria for rosacea diagnosis and classification [7]. They deemed that any one of the following primary features in a centrofacial distribution would be sufficient for diagnosis: flushing, non-transient erythema, papules/pustules or telangiectasias. Secondary features such as burning/stinging, erythematous plaques, dry appearance, oedema, peripheral location, phymatous changes and ocular manifestations could present concomitantly with primary features or appear independently [2,7]. Furthermore, they established four subtypes and one variant based on clinical patterns: erythematotelangiectatic, papulopustular, phymatous, ocular and granulomatous (the variant), respectively [3,7]. This paradigm has subsequently dominated rosacea research, publications and patient management [2,3,8,9]. However, shortcomings have been increasingly recognised including inadequate consideration of features into those of greater or lesser predictive value in diagnosis, and conflation of multiple features into subtypes [1–4,8,9]. The latter ignores variability of patient presentation, negates evaluation of temporal sequence of feature development and forces assessment of multiple features within single subtypes [1,2]. To address these problems, rosacea diagnosis and classification are now based on presenting signs and symptoms: the phenotype approach [2,3]. Phenotype describes observable characteristics of an individual that can result from genetic and/or environmental factors [2,3]. In rosacea, this patient-centred approach is based on weighting of features relevant to diagnosis and removes the restrictions of subtyping [2,3,7].

Rosacea can be diagnosed by at least [2,3]:
• One diagnostic feature *or*
• Two major features (Table 89.1).
Minor or secondary features may appear with one or more diagnostic or major features, but are not diagnostic [2,3].

Whilst we have moved away from the term 'erythema' in favour of 'redness' in this edition of *Rook's Textbook of Dermatology*, where erythema is used in conjunction with referenced publications or diagnostic criteria, we have not changed it, as in this chapter.

Introduction and general description

'Rosacea' encompasses a spectrum of features involving the face and frequently involves the eyes [1]. These features usually appear between 30 and 50 years of age. While more frequently observed in those with fair skin, it is likely underdiagnosed in darker photo types [1,4]. The combination of bothersome symptoms (stinging, burning, pain and itching) and the ready visibility of facial features contribute to adverse impacts on quality of life, anxiety, depression and stigmatisation [10–12].

As the cutaneous features of rosacea are characteristic and pivotal to diagnosis and classification, they are further described to facilitate recognition and assist in standardisation. These are presented under the 'Clinical features' section later in this chapter [2,8].

Management should be tailored towards features most bothersome to the patient [9,13,14]. Beyond visible aspects, enquiry regarding cutaneous and ocular symptoms should be undertaken as the impact of these can be underestimated. As no single treatment can

PART 8: SPECIFIC CUTANEOUS STRUCTURES

Table 89.1 Diagnostic, major and minor features of rosacea [2].

Diagnostic features	Major features	Minor features

Persistent centrofacial erythema with periodic intensification by potential trigger factors
Phymatous changes
	Flushing/transient centrofacial erythema
	Inflammatory papules and pustules
	Telangiectasias (excluding alar involvement)
	Ocular manifestations:
	  Lid margin telangiectasias
	  Blepharitis
	  Keratitis/conjunctivitis/
	  sclerokeratitis
		Burning sensation of the skin
		Stinging sensation of the skin
		Oedema
		Dry sensation of the skin

address the entire spectrum of rosacea features, management may require a combination of options individualised to presenting signs and symptoms [13,14]. Management should include education on rosacea, counselling on general skin care and trigger avoidance. Individualised treatment options include topical, systemic and procedural options.

Epidemiology
Incidence and prevalence
There is a wide range of reported rosacea prevalence from less than 1% on the Faroe Islands to more than 20% in Estonia [15]. The proximity of these regions and similar population demographics suggest potential differences in case ascertainment or case definition. Using population-based survey methodology with a screening algorithm for rosacea and subsequent dermatologist verification provides a means to establish population prevalence in a more accurate, credible and standardised manner. A validated population screening survey and algorithm for rosacea detection [16] followed by dermatologist verification was used to determine prevalence in Russia and Germany [17]. This validated population survey methodology provided nationwide rosacea prevalence estimates of 5% and 12%, respectively [17]. This narrow range encompasses the 5.5% global prevalence estimate from a meta-analysis of 32 published studies [18]. No gender difference in rosacea was detected in this analysis. Prevalence studies of rosacea in darker skin phototypes are sparse. Centrofacial erythema as a diagnostic criterion in dark phototypes may confound case finding [8,19,20].

The incidence of rosacea was addressed in only one study, from the UK, and this estimated it to be 1.65 per 1000 person-years [21].

Age
Rosacea onset is typically in middle-aged adults (30–50 years old). Childhood cases of rosacea exist but there is a paucity of information [15]. In studies reporting age distributions, an equal distribution of rosacea among different age groups was observed, with highest prevalence at 45–60 years [15,18].

Sex
In contrast to prior observations that rosacea was more prevalent in women [1,3,17], a recent systematic review of population-based and dermatological out-patient surveys on the incidence and prevalence of rosacea demonstrated that genders were equally affected [18]. However, rhinophyma occurs more frequently in men, and often at a more advanced age [1,22,23]. This may be partially due to inadequacies in clinical detection at earlier stages of phyma where findings may be more subtle.

Ethnicity
Rosacea has been considered to predominantly affect fair haired, pale-skinned, sun-sensitive individuals with particular susceptibility in those of Celtic origin (sometimes referred to as the 'curse of the Celts') [1,20,24,25]. However, rosacea might be underdiagnosed in darker phototypes as erythema and telangiectasia are more difficult to discern [20,25,26]. There is a paucity of general population prevalence metrics in patients of colour. However, statistics for ambulatory care visits in the USA indicate that of all patients diagnosed with rosacea 2% were black, 2.3% Asian/Pacific Islander and 3.9% Hispanic/Latino [25].

Delayed diagnosis as well as misdiagnoses may contribute to greater morbidity and burden of the disease [17,20,25,26]. While signs and symptoms of rosacea are likely similar across phototypes, a high index of suspicion is required as centrofacial persistent erythema may be inapparent [20,25–27].

Associated diseases
Co-morbidities associated with rosacea include cardiovascular, gastrointestinal, neurological, autoimmune, psychiatric, endocrine/metabolic, rheumatological and other diseases [28–34]. However, causality has not been determined [28–32]. Confounding variables such as shared environmental or lifestyle factors, concomitant medications and selection bias may have influenced outcomes [28,29,31]. These associations have led to the hypotheses that rosacea is a cutaneous manifestation of a systemic inflammatory disease or that it shares common pathophysiological mechanisms as these co-morbidities [28,29,31]. Therefore, further controlled prospective studies are required to establish directionality and confirm these findings [29,31].

Pathophysiology
The spectrum of triggers and clinical features in rosacea implies involvement of multiple pathogenic pathways [35]. Current evidence supports contributions from innate, adaptive, inflammasome and neurogenic mechanisms. However, the biological features underlying individual susceptibility to initiation of these pathways in rosacea is unknown.

External triggers of rosacea may act differentially to activate these pathways. Innate immune activation may be elicited by bacteria (*Bacillus oleronius* and *Staphylococcus epidermidis*) [36], *Demodex* and their associated microbial proteases [37–39], and physical triggers such as heat and ultraviolet (UV) light. These initiating events upregulate proteinase-activated receptor 2 (PAR-2) and Toll-like receptor 2 (TLR-2) leading to cytokines, chemokines, proteases and angiogenic factors eliciting erythema, telangiectasia and inflammation [40]. The cathelicidin LL-37 is erythemogenic and angiogenic [41]. PAR-2 is upregulated in rosacea and mediates inflammation, pruritus and pain. Both TLR-2 and PAR-2 activate the NLRP3 inflammasome resulting in the release of interleukin

1β (IL-1β), tumour necrosis factor α (TNF-α) and prostaglandin E2, contributing to papules/pustules, pain and vasculopathy [42]. An adaptive immune Th1/Th17 profile in rosacea has been shown by immunohistochemical and transcriptome analysis across multiple rosacea cutaneous presentations [43].

Neurogenic pathways may be activated by physical factors (heat, exercise, UV light) and ingestants (spicy food, alcohol) via transient receptor potential (TRP) subfamilies [44]. The release of mediators such as substance P, pituitary adenylate-cyclase activating peptide, and calcitonin gene-related peptide can induce neurogenic inflammation and vasoreactivity.

Mechanisms underlying fibrosis in phyma may involve mast cells and their interaction with fibroblasts [45]. Dermal mast cells may have a primary role in inducing fibrosis by stimulating fibroblast chemotaxis via histamine and tryptase and may promote proliferation via vascular endothelial growth factor (VEGF) and basic fibroblast growth factor (FGF). Monocyte chemoattractant protein-1 (MCP-1) and matrix metalloprotease (MMP) from mast cells can also promote fibrosis [46].

Predisposing factors

Multiple predisposing factors for rosacea have been identified including early-onset signs, phototype, family history and external factors.

In childhood, a potential prognostic indicator for rosacea risk was the development of styes – conferring a 3.8 times greater prevalence than age-matched controls for subsequent adult rosacea [47].

In adults, rosacea risk was significantly higher with a positive family history of rosacea, previous smoking status and light phototypes I and II [48]. While light skin has been implicated as a predisposing factor in rosacea, large epidemiological studies on rosacea have primarily been performed in the USA and northern Europe using facial redness as a pivotal diagnostic criterion. However, as redness is not readily visible in darker phototypes, there may be an inherent survey population pre-bias and flawed case definition. Thus, use of this criterion in diagnosis may underestimate true prevalence in dark phototypes [18,21]. Patients with rosacea have a greater odds of a positive family history, implying genetic mechanisms either directly or indirectly [49], or shared environmental factors within a family [50].

Outdoor occupations, as a proxy for UV exposure, have been found in one study to be a higher risk for moderate and severe rosacea. However, that study did not predefine nor exclude those with heliodermatitis [48]. A Korean study found that the severity of erythematotelangiectatic rosacea correlated with extent of sun exposure rather than papules/pustules [51]. A higher risk of rosacea has been found to be associated with alcohol consumption >25 units per week [21,52]. Of alcoholic beverages, only white wine and liquor were found to be significantly associated with increased rosacea risk [52]. Alcohol consumption has also been significantly associated with severity of rhinophyma, especially in moderate to excessive drinkers [23].

Cigarette smoking and caffeine intake appear to reduce the risk of rosacea. The former is thought to result from the immunosuppressive and vasoconstrictive effects of cigarette smoking [53]. Conversely, the higher risk of rosacea among ex-smokers was attributed to withdrawal of these effects [48]. The association between caffeine

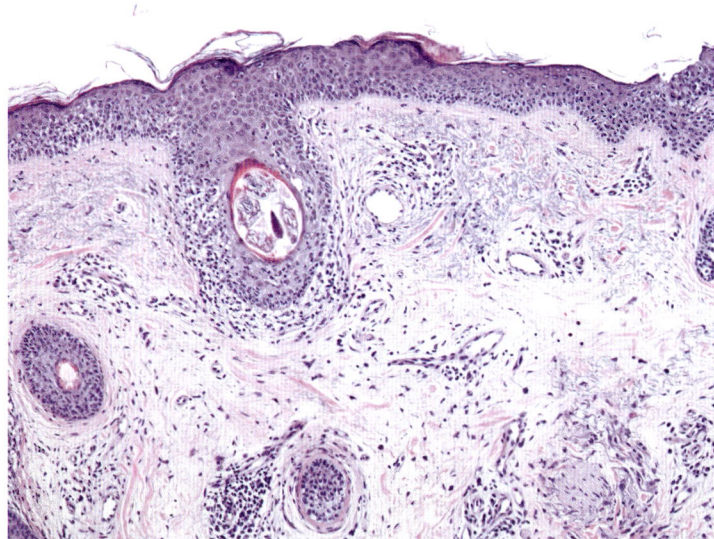

Figure 89.1 Biopsy demonstrating perifollicular lymphocytic inflammatory cell infiltrate with presence of *Demodex folliculorum* inside the follicle and enlarged lumina. Courtesy of Dr S. Forchhammer, Eberhard Karls University Tübingen, Tübingen, Germany.

intake and reduced risk of developing rosacea may also be due to immunosuppressive effects. Additional mechanisms include vasoconstrictive and antioxidant effects of caffeine and polyphenols in coffee [54].

Pathology

In a comprehensive histological study of cutaneous rosacea involving skin biopsies from 86 patients, primary histological features of rosacea were identified [55]. These included abnormalities of cutaneous vasculature, oedema and increased inflammatory cell infiltrates with lymphocytes, mast cells and macrophages. Furthermore, *Demodex* was typically found in the infundibular regions (Figure 89.1) [55]. In addition, standardised skin scrapings from involved skin showed higher *Demodex* densities [39,40].

In contrast to telangiectatic photoageing, histology in erythematous and telangiectatic rosacea showed more inflammation, less dermal collagen damage, less solar elastosis and increased mast cell degranulation [56]. In erythematous and telangiectatic presentations of rosacea, a characteristic feature was unusual telangiectasias with enlarged lumina, tortuous contours and intraluminal projections extending throughout the superficial and mid dermal regions. Also present was oedema presenting as a zone of lucency in superficial papillary and reticular dermis. Perivascular dermal inflammatory infiltrates comprised lymphocytes, histiocytes, plasma cells and mast cells [55]. Papules and pustules of rosacea were characterised by perifollicular infiltrates of plasma cells, neutrophils, mast cells and occasional eosinophils. Neutrophil collections were especially prominent at infundibular regions, often corresponding to the presence of *Demodex* [39,40,55,57].

Phyma was characterised by fibrosis and enlarged sebaceous lobules with normal glandular structure (Figure 89.2). Perifollicular inflammation composed primarily of lymphocytes, neutrophils and occasional small granulomas was ubiquitous but less prominent than in papules and pustules [55].

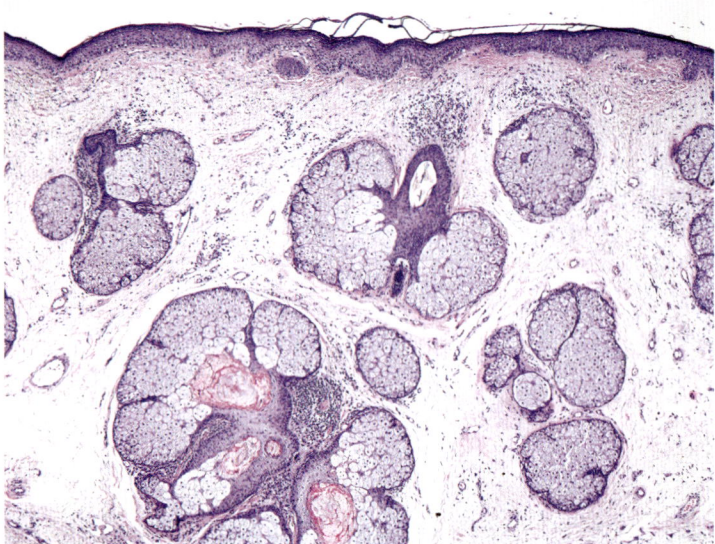

Figure 89.2 Biopsy showing increased density of sebum glands, enlarged and increased capillary vascular structures as well as lymphoplasma cellular inflammatory infiltrates. Courtesy of Dr S. Forchhammer, Eberhard Karls University Tübingen, Tübingen, Germany.

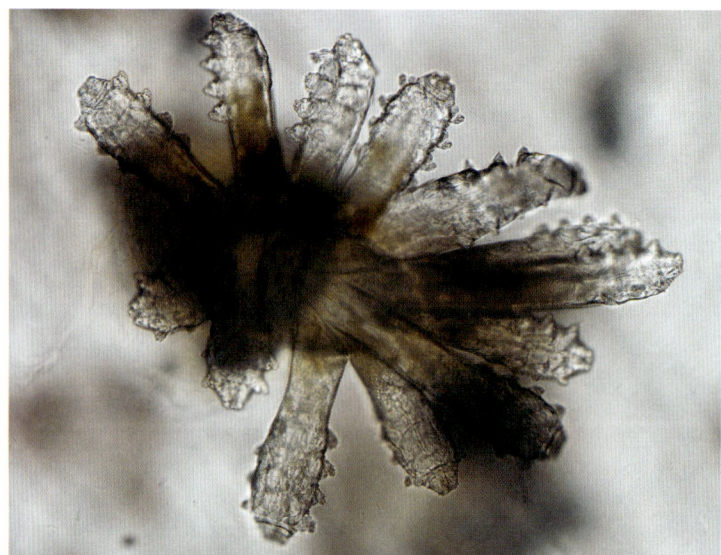

Figure 89.3 *Demodex folliculorum* mites showing their elongated worm-like posterior body (opistostoma) and four sets of short legs on the upper body (podostoma). The mouth parts (gnathostoma) are at the front of the podostoma. Magnification 100×.

In ocular rosacea, blepharitis, inspissation of glandular orifices, hordeola, chalazia and lid margin telangiectasias result from chronic inflammation and meibomian gland dysfunction. Histology of conjunctival epithelium in ocular rosacea showed inflammatory cell infiltrates of lymphocytes, phagocytes and macrophages, while the corneal stroma had dense chronic inflammatory infiltrates and occasional granulomas [58].

Causative organisms

The potential role of microorganisms in the pathogenesis of rosacea is supported by upregulation of pattern recognition receptors, e.g. TLR2, and antimicrobial peptides (cathelicidin) [59,60], and by the efficacy of antibiotics and ivermectin in the treatment of rosacea [61]. Recent reviews of microorganisms that might induce rosacea have identified several possible candidates including *Staphylococcus epidermidis*, *Chlamydophila pneumoniae* and the *Demodex*-associated bacteria *Bacillus oleronius*, *Bacillus cereus* [62] and *Corynebacterium kroppenstedtii* subsp. *demodicis* [63].

The biological significance and possible pathogenic potential of these bacteria remain unknown. In contrast, there is increasing evidence that *Demodex* mites (Figure 89.3) contribute to erythema, papules and pustules by inducing inflammation and vasodilatation not only in cutaneous but also in ocular rosacea. Two systematic reviews of case–control studies and meta-analysis have documented a significant association between the degree of *Demodex* infestation and the presence of rosacea [39,64]. While *Demodex* are normally present as a follicular commensal in humans, their pathogenic potential may relate to the size of the mite population [65]. Uncontrolled mite population growth might induce inflammatory reactivity resulting in erythema [66] and the typical papulopustular inflammatory lesions [65,67]. This is supported by studies showing that a high density of *Demodex* induced the release of inflammatory mediators by sebocytes, whereas lower numbers did not [57]. The immunomodulatory effect was also confirmed by a different *in vivo* approach, demonstrating downregulation of IL-8, LL-37, HBD3, TLR4 and TNF-α gene expression levels, together with significant reduction of the *Demodex* density in patients with moderate to severe rosacea, by topical ivermectin 1% [68].

Role of the microbiome. Beyond *Demodex folliculorum*, the role of the cutaneous microbiome in the pathogenesis of rosacea is otherwise unclear. For example, the Gram-negative bacterium *Bacillus oleronius* isolated from the gut of *Demodex* of one rosacea patient has been posited as a trigger to inflammation in rosacea [69]. However, this observation has not been repeated.

A case–control 16S ribosomal RNA sequencing study investigated the skin microbiota in patients with rosacea compared with controls. In erythematotelangiectatic rosacea, skin microbiota was depleted in multiple bacterial species (e.g. *Roseomonasis*), suggesting that certain strains may promote healthy skin. A relative abundance of *Corynebacterium kroppenstedtii* in rosacea was observed to be highest in affected skin, followed by unaffected skin in patients with rosacea. This suggests that *C. kroppenstedtii* levels must reach a certain population threshold before papulopustular rosacea features manifest [70].

Associations between rosacea and inflammatory gastrointestinal tract disorders have been reported, but the pathogenic mechanisms including the potential role of the gut microbiome remain unclear [34,71–74]. Observations of an increased prevalence of rosacea in SIBO (small intestinal bacterial overgrowth) patients and the effect of SIBO eradication with the non-absorbable antibiotic rifaximin, leading to enduring improvement of rosacea in almost all patients, imply a pathogenic role [75].

Genetics

A positive family history of rosacea in up to 50% of patients with rosacea suggests a strong familial inheritance [48]. Rosacea-associated genes have been identified in a genome-wide association study. These included single-nucleotide polymorphisms (SNPs) on chromosome 6 and three HLA alleles (HLA-DRB1, HLA-DQB1, HLA-DQA) [49].

A genetic cause for early-onset rosacea associated with *Demodex* has been described in several unrelated families, with a gain-of-function mutation in *STAT1* [76].

Environmental factors

Increased environmental temperature and dietary influences (ingesting hot liquids, spicy foods, large meals, alcohol, etc.) are often cited as potential exacerbating factors. A cohort-based twin study investigated genetic and environmental factors affecting rosacea and found that approximately half of the contribution could be accounted for by genetics and the other half by environment. Correlations between rosacea and UV radiation exposure, alcohol, smoking, skin cancer history, cardiac co-morbidity and age have been identified [50].

Clinical features

Rosacea usually presents with peak onset between 30 and 50 years and a spectrum of signs and symptoms. Each of these features can vary in degree of severity. Independent assessment of the severity of each feature will provide accuracy in assessment [2,3,19]. A 'rosacea tracker' including descriptions of the features and considerations for severity assessment has been developed for dermatologists, ophthalmologists and patients to monitor changes in disease features, as well as patient impact and response to treatment [8].

History and presentation

The multiplicity of clinical features of rosacea is reflected by the variety of clinical symptoms including flushing, itch, pain, stinging, burning and ocular irritation. In society, a red face has negative connotations including unhealthy lifestyle (sunburn, alcoholism), shame, anger or embarrassment. This has led to the use of foundations and camouflage make-up to conceal redness [5]. Along with persistent redness, the flushing, papules, pustules and/or phyma of rosacea can lead to embarrassment, anxiety, low self-esteem, lack of confidence, depression, social anxiety disorder, body dysmorphic disorder and stigmatisation [4,77–82]. As expected, rosacea has an adverse impact on quality of life (QOL) [83–88].

The impact of rosacea on QOL correlates with disease severity, however profound adverse impact can also be seen in those with lesser severities [10]. Persistent rosacea features with periodic flares were reported by most patients. The majority of patients modify their behaviours to avoid trigger factors such as sun exposure, alcohol, spicy food, high temperatures and exercise. Even a few flares per year could adversely impact QOL. Those with greater QOL impact spent more time on daily skin care and had higher rates of absenteeism from work or school.

In a survey of the general population evaluating digital photographs with and without facial erythema (redness) associated with rosacea, facial erythema was associated with being sick, tired and stressed and with being less relaxed, healthy and rested. Attributes conferred on images of facial erythema associated with rosacea were that the person shown was less trustworthy, successful and confident [78].

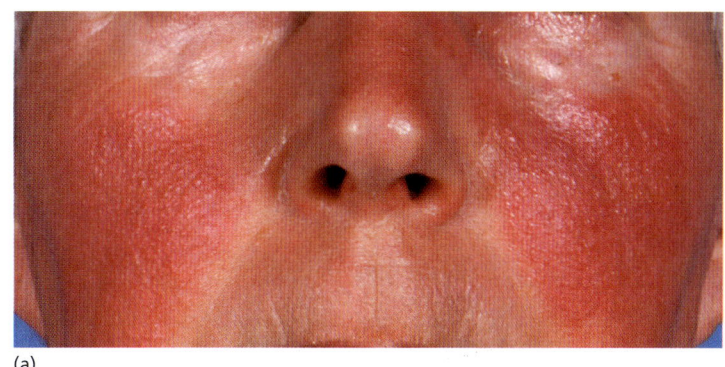

(a)

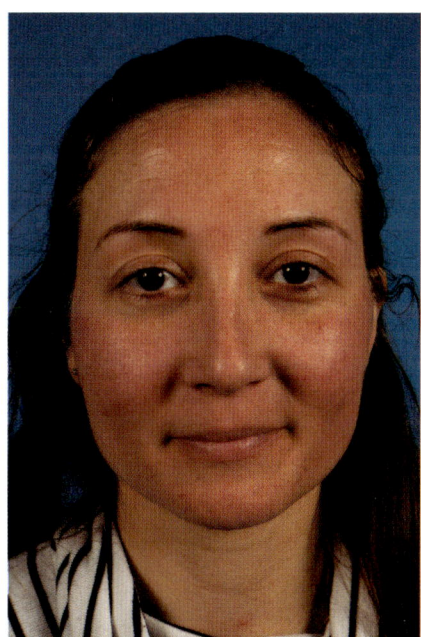

(b)

Figure 89.4 (a) Persistent erythema in the centrofacial area. (b) Subtle persistent erythema with few papules and some oedema.

Diagnostic features

Persistent erythema. Patients with persistent erythema usually complain of a gradual increase in facial redness which may intensify in response to triggers [2,3,8]. While the central face is the typical location (Figure 89.4a), the lateral cheeks, ears and sometimes lateral neck can also be affected. As erythema is often more difficult to recognise in darker skin, extra attention should be paid to the history, symptoms and signs at the central face (Figure 89.4b).

Phymatous rosacea. Phyma most often involves the nose, 'rhinophyma', but has also been described at chin (gnatophyma), ears (otophyma), forehead (metophyma) and eyelids (blepharophyma). Rhinophyma has been reported most frequently in white men, between the fifth and seventh decades. However, occurrence in Asian or African (American) men has also been reported [22]. In women phyma is very rare [89]. Rhinophyma may be preceded by inflammatory lesions and/or erythema or may appear *de novo*. Skin changes include thickening, an increase of prominent follicular openings and tortuous telangiectasias (Figure 89.5a). Inflammatory phyma is characterised by soft tissue prominence, erythema and

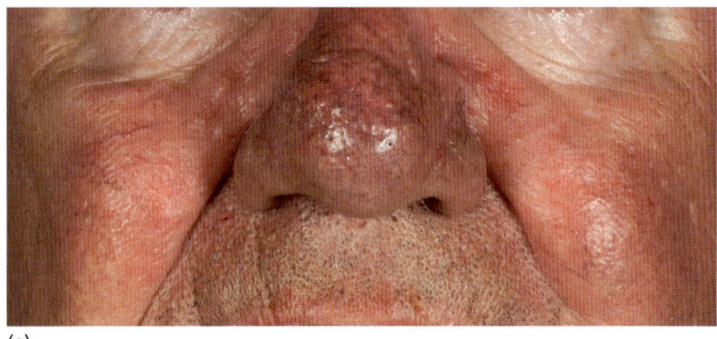

(a)

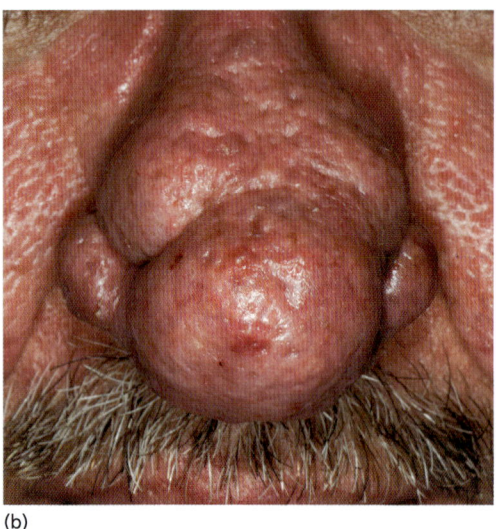

(b)

Figure 89.5 (a) Mild phymatous changes showing a peau d'orange appearance of the prominent nasal follicles. (b) Severe phymatous changes showing nasal distortion.

papules/pustules. Over time, phyma with soft tissue distortion and bulbous protuberances may lead to deformity (Figure 89.5b), complaints about oily skin and malodor with manipulation.

Major features

Transient erythema (flushing). Transient erythema or flushing is temporary centrofacial redness that may spread to the entire face, ears, neck and upper chest, and may include sensations of warmth, heat, burning and/or pain usually lasting at least 10 min [90]. Sweating is not an associated feature of flushing in rosacea. Due to its transitory nature, flushing may not be present during a consultation [2,3]. Therefore, physicians should enquire about and address possible triggers, which can differ between patients. In skin of colour, flushing might not be visibly apparent but may be described symptomatically as a transient warm or burning sensation of the face [3,20].

Papules and pustules. Patients with papules/pustules often have a history of 'spots, red bumps or pimples' that are located principally in the centrofacial area (Figure 89.6a). Their appearance is characterised by prominent lesional erythema. In severe cases, these coalesce into plaques. There may also be mild facial oedema, which is most noticeable if there are widespread inflammatory lesions. Individual lesions may be slightly tender. Pustules (Figure 89.6b) can accompany papules, with most being relatively superficial [3].

Papules often appear to be in different stages of evolution and untreated lesions wax and wane spontaneously over a course of weeks. Lesions that resolve typically heal without scarring but may leave persistent postinflammatory erythema and in darker skin postinflammatory hyperpigmentation (Figure 89.6c).

Telangiectasias. Telangiectasias in rosacea are superficial, visible, dilated blood vessels appearing as red arcuate lines at the central face (Figure 89.7). It can be difficult to distinguish telangiectasias due to rosacea from photodamage (see Differential diagnosis section later in this chapter). Telangiectasias contribute to facial redness and can become more prominent over time. Dermatoscopy may assist in detection of telangiectasias in darker phototypes [3,20].

Ocular rosacea. Up to three-quarters of patients with rosacea have ocular symptoms such as foreign body sensation, dryness, burning, itching, redness, photophobia, tearing and blurred vision [91–93]. These may develop concurrently or independently of cutaneous features [92,94]. A frequent ocular complaint is irritation or a 'gritty' sensation. Ocular features typically occur bilaterally, but there are cases of unilateral or sequential involvement [94]. Ocular manifestations are telangiectasias of the eyelid margin, crust and collarette scale formation around eye lashes (Figure 89.8), thickened lid margin, meibomian gland dysfunction (plugging), interpalpebral conjunctival injection and neovascularisation, spade-shaped infiltrates in the cornea, chalazia, scleritis and sclerokeratitis [3,95]. Minimum diagnostic criteria for ocular rosacea include either the combination of lid margin telangiectasias and interpalpebral injection, or scleral inflammation with corneal abnormalities [2]. Severity of ocular rosacea and clinical findings can be mild (mild blepharitis and lid margin telangiectasias), mild–moderate (blepharoconjunctivitis), moderate–severe (blepharokeratoconjunctivitis) or severe (sclerokeratitis or anterior uveitis) [2]. Other severe manifestations include corneal ulcers and loss of vision [91–93,95,96]. Ocular rosacea can range from nuisance to debilitating including loss of vision. Corneal ulcers and sudden vision loss mandate immediate ophthalmology referral.

However, most common are blepharoconjunctivitis with eyelid margin inflammation and meibomian gland dysfunction. The latter results in tear film dysfunction [94]. Symptoms and signs of ocular rosacea are not specific for the disorder (see Differential diagnosis). Ocular rosacea is insufficiently recognised in children and in individuals with skin of color [97]. In pediatric rosacea, ocular symptoms can be predominant and often precede cutaneous features [98,99]. A high level of suspicion is needed as ocular involvement in children can be severe.

Minor features. Burning and stinging are experienced by many patients with rosacea, especially in those with persistent and transient erythema. Their facial skin is sensitive and easily irritated with daily skincare products. Burning and stinging are often exacerbated by sunlight and wind exposure. A dry sensation with the skin feeling rough, tight, scaly and/or itchy is also commonly reported [3,8]. Although itch and pain are not considered typical of rosacea, they are frequently present and underestimated by physicians [10]. Facial oedema may be present especially when there are many

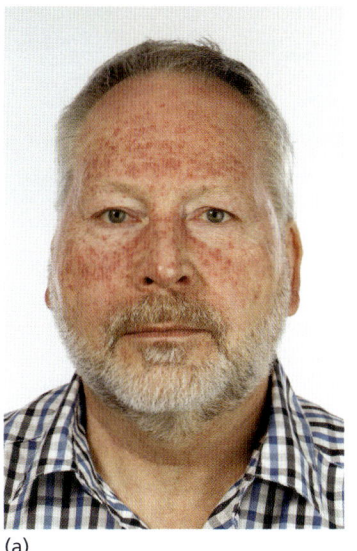
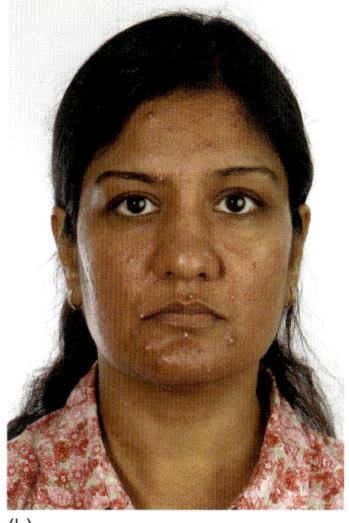
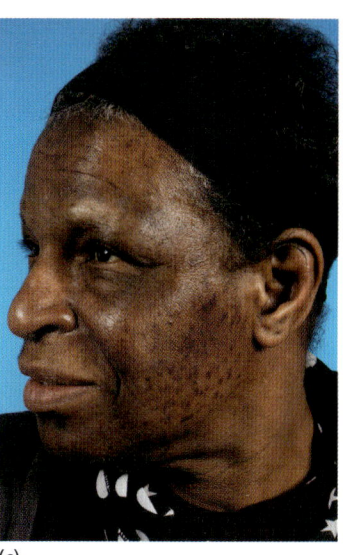

Figure 89.6 (a) Papules in the centrofacial area. (b) Pustules in the centrofacial area. (c) Postinflammatory hyperpigmentation.

(a) (b) (c)

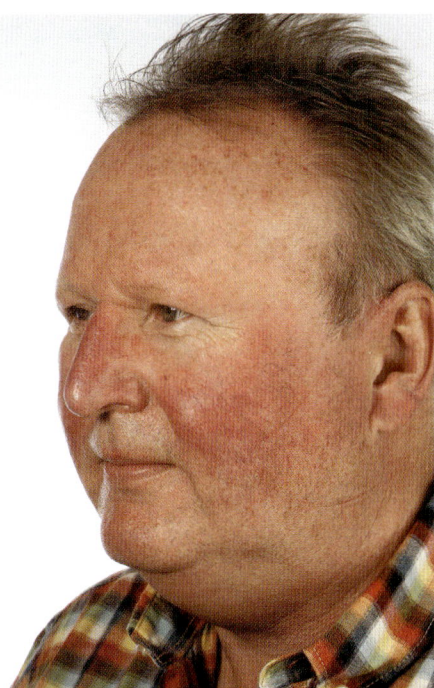

Figure 89.7 Prominent telangiectatic vessels centrofacial and on the lateral cheeks.

inflammatory lesions or may be due to prolonged erythema [3,8]. Oedema can be soft or firm and may vary in duration [8].

Clinical variants

Atypical distribution. Papules/pustules in rosacea may be asymmetrical or involve areas beyond typical centrofacial locations (periocular and postauricular) (Figure 89.9). Male patients with inflammatory papules/pustules and androgenetic alopecia frequently develop similar inflammatory lesions on their bald scalp.

Granulomatous rosacea. Granulomatous rosacea (GR) is uncommon and presents with persistent monomorphic, firm, yellow, red to brown papules or nodules around the mouth, eyes, cheeks and lateral sides of the face and neck (Figure 89.10) [100–102]. In severe

cases, scarring may occur [7,90]. Lesions may vary in size between individuals but are usually less variable in an individual. Extrafacial involvement has been reported involving ears, neck, axillae, shoulders, groins, thighs and knees [102]. Other features of rosacea such as flushing, telangiectasias and erythema may be present [90] with similar exacerbating factors [100]. Dermoscopy demonstrates diffuse or focal orange-cream structureless areas [103]. Large pandermal granulomas with or without caseation are characteristic for GR [55]. Lupus miliaris disseminatus faciei (LMDF) has been considered a variant of GR by some because of similarities in its histopathology and clinical picture but as a distinct entity by others (see section on LMDF later in this chapter). GR should be differentiated from sarcoidosis. Evaluations should involve clinical assessment, skin biopsy and laboratory testing [90,100,102,104]. Treatment is difficult, and there is no standard treatment although case reports suggest tetracyclines as initial treatment and isotretinoin for recalcitrant cases [102,105].

Differential diagnosis

The differential diagnoses vary according to clinical features at presentation (phenotypes).

Erythema. Centrofacial erythema with potential for episodic intensification is a diagnostic feature of rosacea on exclusion of differential diagnoses [3]. In rosacea, erythema which is *persistent and diffuse* (background erythema), without inflammatory lesions, must be distinguished from *lesional erythema*, which is related to the presence of inflammatory papules/pustules [106,107]. When both features are present, it can be extremely difficult to distinguish the contribution to erythema due to papules/pustules and persistent erythema.

Persistent, diffuse erythema (background erythema). Differential diagnoses of persistent, diffuse erythema (background erythema) include the following.

Heliodermatitis. Heliodermatitis (or photodamage) presents as persistent erythema together with telangiectasias due to chronic UV

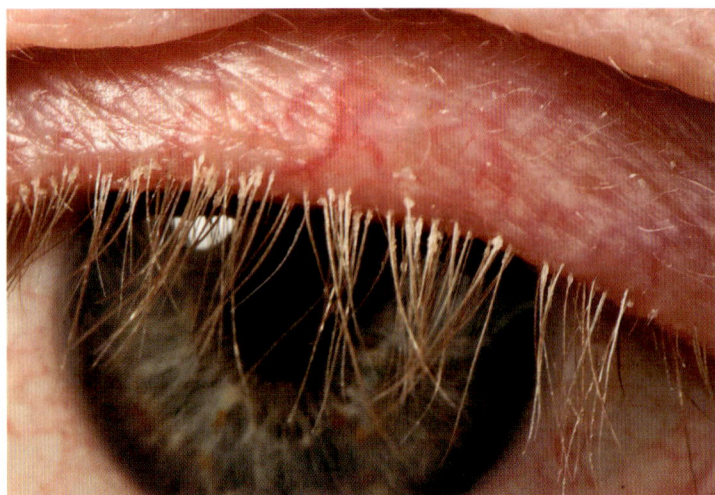

(a)

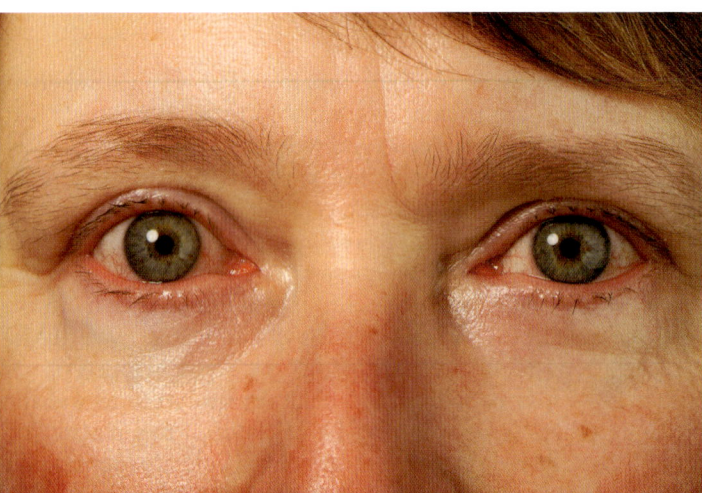

(b)

Figure 89.8 Ocular rosacea: (a) crust and collarette scale formation around the base of eye lashes; and (b) lid margin telangiectasias and conjunctival injection.

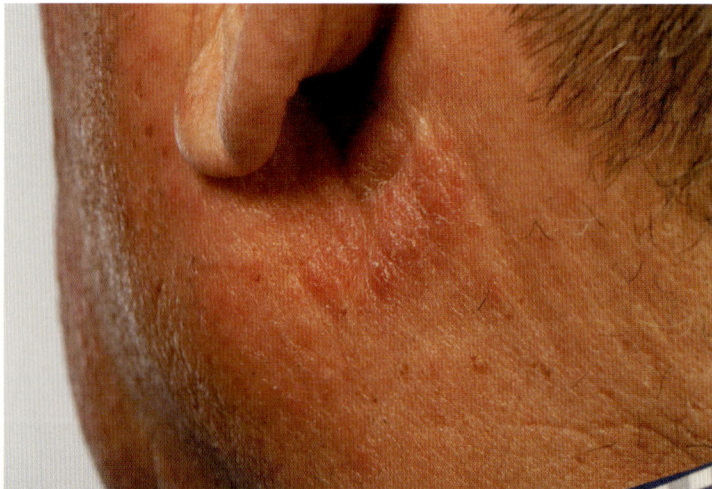

Figure 89.9 Grouped papules behind the ear of a patient with moderate rosacea with papules and pustules. This is a commonly overlooked location of inflammatory lesions.

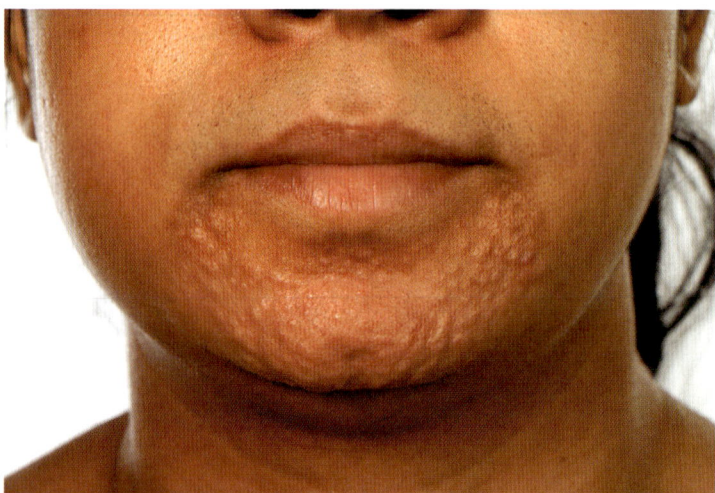

Figure 89.10 Granulomatous rosacea. There is a profuse eruption of small, firm, monomorphic, plum-red, dome-shaped papules on the chin. Histology showed multiple dermal granulomas.

exposure (Figure 89.11) [56,108,109]. In heliodermatitis, erythema often extends to the lateral face and neck and there is a history of outdoor activities, occupational or recreational [56,109].

Seborrheic dermatitis. This is a common dermatosis characterised by patchy scaly erythema at the perinasal, scalp, periauricular, glabella and eyebrow regions (Figure 89.12). It often coexists with rosacea but in contrast to rosacea tends to improve with sun exposure.

Facial contact dermatitis. This results in itchy erythema at sites of irritant or allergen application. This may involve the entire face if applications are panfacial. In facial aerocontact dermatitis, full facial involvement including the periocular regions without a zone of sparing, unlike rosacea, is a differentiating factor.

Systemic lupus erythematosus and (sub)acute cutaneous lupus erythematosus. These may present with photo-distributed erythema. In addition to evaluation of other clinical features, skin

biopsy and serological testing may be required for definitive diagnosis.

Dermatomyositis. This should be suspected with red-violet discoloration of the eyelids, red papulosquamous eruption of extensor regions of the extremities and torso, along with limb–girdle muscle soreness and weakness (Figure 89.13) [110].

Ulerythema ophryogenes. This is mostly seen in children and young adults presenting with facial erythema. The characteristic follicular keratosis in ulerythema ophryogenes enables differentiation from rosacea [111].

Transient erythema (flushing). Transient erythema or flushing is caused by increased cutaneous blood flow from temporary vasodilatation [112]. Common causes for flushing other than rosacea include benign cutaneous flushing, fever, hyperthermia and menopause. Uncommon, serious causes include carcinoid

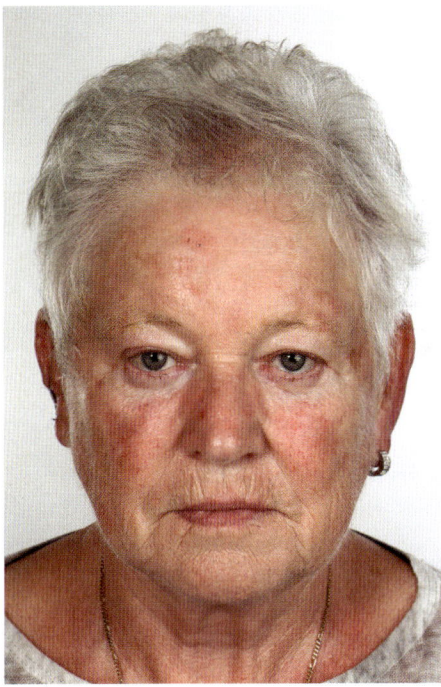

Figure 89.11 Telangiectasias on sun-exposed area.

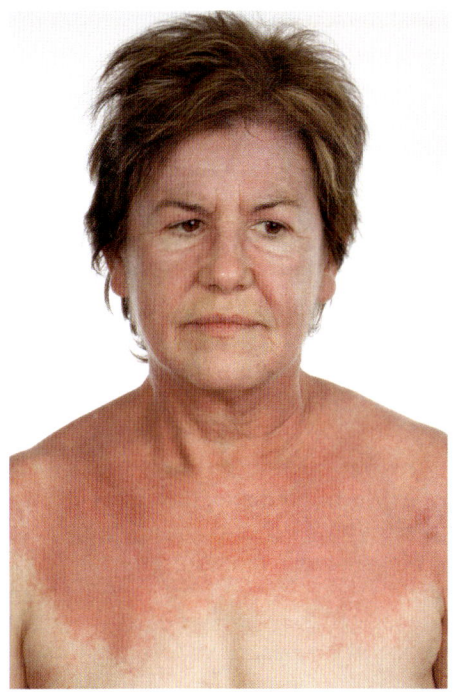

Figure 89.13 Photodistributed erythema reaching over the 'V' area of the anterior chest.

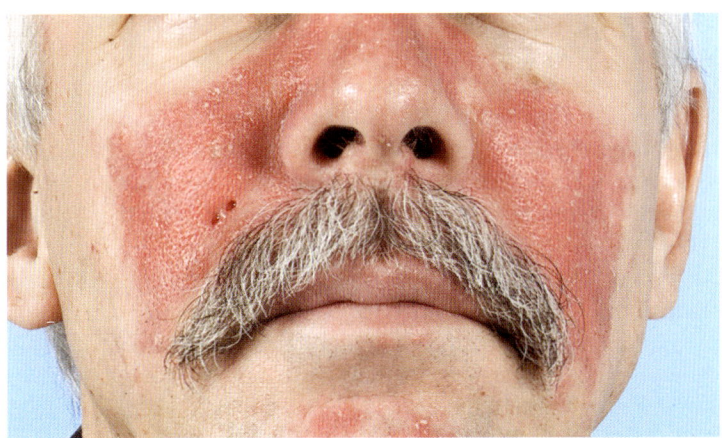

Figure 89.12 Perinasal seborrhoeic dermatitis with distinct erythematous patches and scaling, extending on the cheeks.

Table 89.2 Differential diagnoses of uncommon, serious causes of transient erythema (flushing).

Differential diagnosis	History, clinical picture, further investigations
Carcinoid syndrome	Weight loss, increased 5-hydroxyindole–acetic acid in urine
Mastocytosis	Hypotension, tachycardia, increased histamine and tryptase in plasma, increased mast cells in skin biopsy
Pheochromocytoma	Hypertension, palpitations, headache, sweating, catecholamine and (nor)metanephrine excess in urine/plasma
Other causes: Pancreatic neuroendocrine tumour Medullary thyroid cancer Endogenous Cushing syndrome Renal cell carcinoma Drugs	History, physical examination, specific laboratory tests, advanced imaging techniques

syndrome, pheochromocytoma, mastocytosis and rare malignancies [113,114]. Cardiac disease and drugs are also implicated such as vasodilators, calcium-channel blockers, nicotinic acid, opiates, ciclosporin, beta-blockers, angiotensin-converting enzyme inhibitors and alkylnitrites (recreational drugs) [113]. Further investigations may be appropriate based on history, associated signs and symptoms (Table 89.2).

Inflammatory lesions (papules/pustules) with or without erythema. Differential diagnoses of inflammatory lesions (papules/pustules) with or without redness include the following.

Acne vulgaris. This may be mistaken for papules/pustules of rosacea especially in late-onset acne. However, comedones, the hallmark lesions of acne, are present. Furthermore, sequelae of cysts

and scars are unique to acne, although the latter may be evident from prior acne. Rosacea papules/pustules and erythema mostly involve the central face while acne lesions extend to the lateral cheeks, jawline, temples, neck and torso [3,8]. Eye symptoms and flushing are not characteristic of acne [3]. Sun exposure may worsen rosacea, whilst ameliorating acne. These conditions can coexist.

Granulomatous rosacea. Granulomatous rosacea is discussed under 'Clinical variants' earlier in this chapter.

Periorificial facial dermatitis (PD). This includes perioral dermatitis and periorbital dermatitis. Monomorphic, small papulopustules or papulovesicles dominate the clinical picture. Both topical and inhaled corticosteroids increase the risk of this condition (see 'Facial dermatoses with an uncertain nosological relationship' later in this chapter).

Lupus miliaris disseminatus faciei (LMDF). This is an infrequent granulomatous inflammatory condition, with a distinct clinical presentation, mainly affecting the face of young male individuals. While self-limiting, it may persist for several years (see 'Facial dermatoses with an uncertain nosological relationship' later in this chapter).

Tinea faciei. This can present with erythema, papules and pustules and can be difficult to distinguish from atypical rosacea. The peripheral scaling, typical itch and expanding edges are suggestive. Confirmatory fungal skin scraping on microscopy and culture is diagnostic.

Jessners lymphocytic infiltrate. This is a rare condition that can present with papules, mostly asymptomatic, that can last for weeks or months before spontaneous resolution (Chapter 134).

Pityriasis folliculorum. This can result in rosacea-like skin eruptions with high-density *Demodex* mite infestation in the follicles. It can induce irritation and a burning sensation. Slight erythema and occasional papules and pustules might be seen. Digitate keratosis is typical due to follicular scaling. Dermoscopy, skin scrapings and/or biopsy are useful to identify *Demodex* infestation.

Rosacea-like dermatoses due to medication. These can occur with topical and systemic corticosteroids (see 'Facial dermatoses with an uncertain nosological relationship' later in this chapter). Furthermore, psychotropic medications, calcineurin blockers, hormones, aromatic anticonvulsants and drugs such as epidermal growth factor blockers (e.g. cetuximab), small-molecule tyrosine kinase inhibitors (e.g. erlotinib) and MEK (mitogen-activated extracellular signal-regulated kinase) inhibitors (e.g. trametinib) can induce acneiform lesions. Medication history and temporal association are valuable in making this diagnosis.

Phymatous rosacea. Differential diagnoses of phymatous rosacea include the following.

Sarcoidosis. In sarcoidosis (lupus pernio) affected tissue shows a dark red-violaceous enlargement with a firm, indurated consistency (Figure 89.14). In phyma associated with rosacea, large follicular openings are typical and the tissue is less indurated. Furthermore, phymatous tissue is mostly skin colored or slightly erythematous. Only the angiomatous form of rhinophyma shows dark red to purple coloration. In sarcoidosis, diascopy shows the typical 'apple-jelly' colour, characteristic of granulomatous skin lesions. Histological examination shows non-caseating granulomas with little surrounding inflammation. Additional investigations (increased level of serum angiotensin-converting enzyme, chest X-ray, pulmonary function tests) might be necessary.

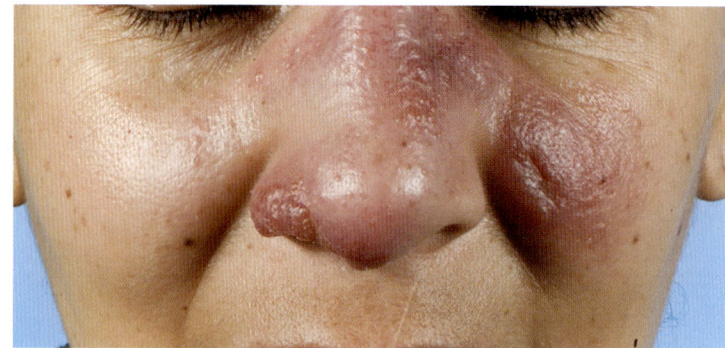

Figure 89.14 Lupus pernio. A skin biopsy showed the characteristic non-caseating granulomas of sarcoid.

Discoid lupus erythematosus. This is characterised by erythema, scaling, follicular plugging, absence of enlarged follicular openings and tendency to scarring. A skin biopsy including direct immunofluorescence should establish the diagnosis.

Solid facial lymphoedema (Morbihan disease). This mostly affects the central and upper aspect of the face and may resemble rhinophyma when it involves the nose. The clinical picture consists of persistent erythema and firm, non-pitting swelling (see 'Facial dermatoses with an uncertain nosological relationship' later in this chapter).

Lymphocytoma cutis. Lymphocytoma cutis or cutaneous pseudolymphoma is rare and considered to be a reactive lymphoproliferative process (Chapter 139). The combination of clinical signs, such as a solitary or several red or blue-red papules or plaques on the face and ears, in combination with histology can establish the diagnosis [115].

Neoplasms. Neoplasms such as keratinocyte carcinomas, lymphomas and angiosarcoma involving the nose can be confused with rhinophyma. Diagnosis is based on histology.

Granuloma faciale. This is a rare, benign, chronic dermatosis presenting with single or multiple facial and occasional extrafacial reddish-brown asymptomatic plaques [116] (Chapter 100). There are no strictly defined histopathological criteria but the presence of many eosinophils is characteristic.

Ocular rosacea. Other common inflammatory skin diseases such as seborrhoeic dermatitis, atopic dermatitis and psoriasis can also be accompanied with ocular involvement [117]. However, ocular findings suggestive of rosacea include lid margin telangiectasias and interpalpebral injection, or corneal abnormalities and scleral inflammation [2].

Complications and co-morbidities

The most frequent consequences of rosacea are psychosocial, including adverse impact on QOL, embarrassment, anxiety regarding flares, loss of self-confidence, social anxiety, depression and stigmatisation. In rosacea, common concomitant conditions include acne, seborrhoeic dermatitis and atopic dermatitis [118–121].

Table 89.3 Potential exacerbating factors and triggers [1,4,14,123].

Exposure	Food and drinks
Psychological stress (anger, anxiety, embarrassment)	Alcohol
	Coffee/tea
Climate (cold, heat, humidity, UV light, wind)	Dairy products
	Chocolate
Fever	Chili, curry, peppers, capsaicin
Exercise	Tomatoes
Hot flushes	Spinach
Microorganisms (*Demodex*,	Soya
Helicobacter pylori,	Vinegar
Staphylococcus epidermidis)	Citrus fruits
	Avocado
	Eggplant

Topical irritants	Drugs
Alcohol-containing facial cleansing products	Capsaicin
	Corticosteroids
Fragrance/aftershave	Doxorubicin
Facial cleansing wipes	Interferon
Menthol	Infliximab
Shaving foam	Niacin
Peeling products	Nifedipine
Waterproof cosmetics	Nitroglycerin
Soap	Prostaglandin E
	Rifampicin

Additionally, treatment for one condition (e.g. topical steroids for atopic or contact dermatitis) may aggravate rosacea.

Disease course and prognosis

Rosacea is a chronic disease with periodic remission of papules/pustules. Individual features may progressively worsen without treatment. Erythema can become more pronounced and may intensify with increasing telangiectasias. Crops of inflammatory lesions can occur during flares, but these dissipate with increasing age. The developmental sequence of signs and symptoms in rosacea may initiate with flushing (transient erythema) followed by persistent erythema and telangiectasias. Papules/pustules may then develop and phyma is of even later onset [122].

Rhinophyma can result in adverse QOL impact, facial disfigurement and, in severe cases, airway obstruction [22].

Ocular rosacea-like cutaneous rosacea is chronic with recurrent flares. Early and ongoing treatment provides for symptomatic improvement and ongoing care may reduce the risk of corneal complications [3,94,97].

Investigations

Investigations are not required for patients who present with the typical clinical features of rosacea. In atypical presentations or those with unusual symptoms, alternative diagnoses should be considered. There is no specific test that will establish the diagnosis of rosacea. Histology can be supportive but is not diagnostic.

Management

Management starts with educating patients and with helping them identify potential exacerbating factors and triggers [1,8,14,123].

In Table 89.3 potential exacerbating factors and triggers are summarised. Keeping a diary can assist patients with identifying triggers worsening their rosacea.

Although evidence is limited, clinical experience suggests that general skin care measures are important [1,8,14]. Impaired skin barrier function should be addressed with non-soap cleansers (e.g. synthetic detergents) and gentle moisturisers. As UV light can trigger erythema and flushing, sun protection with hats, sunglasses and sunblock is recommended (Box 89.1) [1,8,14]. The use of foundation and camouflage cosmetics can provide aesthetic improvement.

> ## Box 89.1 General measures and skin care guidance
>
> Identify and avoid triggers that aggravate the rosacea (such as cosmetics, environmental factors, exercise, foods or drinks and drugs)
>
> Advise patients to:
> - Avoid triggers whenever possible
> - Avoid direct sun exposure
> - Daily use of a sunscreen protecting against both UVA and UVB, minimum sun protection factor 30, preferably containing dimethicone, cyclomethicone or both to minimise irritation. Mineral sunscreens with zinc oxide and/or titanium dioxide tend to be better tolerated
> - Use soap-free facial skin cleansers, rinse off with lukewarm water and gently pat dry
> - Use a hydrating, non-irritating, non-occlusive moisturiser. Cosmetics with a green or yellow pigment can camouflage redness
> - Use a non-oily/greasy foundation and/or concealer if camouflaging redness is desired
>
> Advise patients to avoid:
> - Waterproof make-up, as removing is more difficult and can irritate the skin
> - Skin tonics, toner and astringents (i.e. products containing alcohol, menthol, lavender, peppermint, camphor, witch hazel or eucalyptus oil)
> - Cosmetics containing sodium lauryl sulphate, fragrance, fruit acids or glycolic acids
> - Rubbing, scrubbing and peeling of the skin (including facial sponges, scrub creams and washcloths)

First line

Initial management requires identifying the presenting features of rosacea, their clinical severity and patient impact. The burden of rosacea does not necessarily correlate with disease severity (see 'History and presentation' earlier in this chapter), therefore it is important to establish patient expectations, including their values and preferences. Treatment selection can then be based on evidence and the principles of shared decision making [10,14]. Multiple features can be treated simultaneously by combining treatments [8,13,14]. Achieving complete resolution of erythema and papules/pustules is associated with an improved QOL and an extended time to relapse [124]. Therefore, complete resolution may be an appropriate treatment goal, but more research is required for other rosacea features [8,14,124].

Ocular rosacea is discussed in a separate section.

PART 8: SPECIFIC CUTANEOUS STRUCTURES

Details regarding concentration, dosing regimen and treatment duration are discussed in the Treatment ladder at the end of this section.

Diagnostic features
Persistent erythema. Topical α-adrenergic agonists such as brimonidine or oxymetazoline hydrochloride can diminish the redness for up to 12 h [1,4,8,13,14]. However, not all patients benefit to a satisfactory extent and some may have worsening of erythema [125].

Phymatous rosacea. For mild inflamed phyma, topical retinoids [1,14] or ultra-low-dose isotretinoin may be considered [126,127].

Major features
Transient erythema (flushing). Although there is limited evidence for the efficacy of topical α-adrenergic agonists these can be considered [8,13,14]. The use of either topical brimonidine or oxymetazoline may result in less flaring and flushing.

Papules and pustules. The following topical products are available: ivermectin, metronidazole and azelaic acid [1,4,8,13,14]. Others that can be considered include sodium sulfacetamide 10% and sulphur 5% preparations, and more recently minocycline foam and encapsulated benzoyl peroxide [14,24]. Treatment should be continued for 8–12 weeks and followed by reassessment. Topical medications should be applied before a daily moisturiser or sunblock. Combining brimonidine with ivermectin results in a greater reduction of erythema and inflammatory lesions, supporting an additional effect of brimonidine to ivermectin cream [24,128]. Topical clindamycin is not effective for treating papules and pustules of rosacea [4].

Telangiectasia. Electrodessication can treat facial telangiectasias but risks scarring [1,8] and therefore has largely been replaced by intense pulsed light (IPL) therapy and vascular lasers, which are effective with lower scarring risks.

Second line
If there is intolerance, inadequate improvement, lack of access to first line treatment or higher levels of severity, second line options may be considered. These include systemic treatments or dermatological procedures [1,13,14].

Diagnostic features
Persistent erythema. Both IPL therapy as well as vascular laser therapy are widely used to treat erythema and telangiectasias. These are often effective in reducing telangiectasias and persistent erythema. However, the effect in diminishing erythema can sometimes be incomplete [1,4,8,13,14].

Phymatous rosacea. Clinically inflamed phyma may be treated with oral sub-antimicrobial doxycycline 40 mg modified release (MR) or doxycycline 100 mg [1,8,13,14,22]. Their presumed mechanism in rosacea is due to anti-inflammatory effects. Isotretinoin not only reduces inflammation, but also reduces the size of sebaceous glands, sebum production and oedema [22]. Low-dose isotretinoin

is recommended to prevent worsening ocular rosacea and may reduce phyma. However, isotretinoin is highly teratogenic and pregnancy prevention during treatment is imperative [1,14].

Major features
Transient erythema (flushing). Although there is limited evidence for the efficacy of α-adrenergic agonists or β-blockers in transient erythema, carvedilol, clonidine and propranolol can be considered [8,13,14]. Well-known adverse events include hypotension, bradycardia and dizziness [1]. Both IPL therapy and vascular laser can reduce the intensity of erythema during flushing.

Papules and pustules. Usually, topical treatment is continued with the initiation of systemic treatment. Doxycycline 40 mg MR once daily is the only systemic drug approved for inflammatory lesions of rosacea. The combination of doxycycline 40 mg with topical ivermectin enhances clinical improvement [129,130]. There is less robust evidence for systemic antibiotics other than doxycycline 40 mg MR. One study found doxycycline 100 mg daily to be as effective as doxycycline 40 mg MR with more adverse events (especially gastrointestinal) [4]. However, the experience of many dermatologists is that it is more effective than doxycycline 40 mg MR. Minocycline 100 mg daily may also be considered; however, rare but serious side effects of autoimmune hepatitis, drug-induced lupus erythematosus and hyperpigmentation (with prolonged use) have been reported [1,4]. If tetracyclines are not tolerated, azithromycin has been demonstrated to be effective for papules/pustules of rosacea [4].

Telangiectasia. Both IPL therapy and vascular lasers are effective in treating telangiectasias. Side effects consist mainly of transient pain and purpura. Less common are crusting, hyper- and hypopigmentation and scarring.

Third line
These treatments may be considered when first and second line treatments are inadequate, not tolerated or inaccessible or if severity at outset requires escalation in treatment.

Diagnostic features
Persistent erythema. Combining both topical α-adrenergic agonists and device treatments (IPL and vascular laser) may provide greater efficacy than either alone. Intradermal botulinum toxin injections have been shown to reduce facial erythema and flushing. However, these treatments require repetition every 3–6 months [131–134]. Localised bruising, transient pain and headache are the most frequently reported side effects.

Phymatous rosacea. Various ablative options are available to debulk phyma and remodel the affected area. Electrosurgery, scalpel sculpting and ablative laser therapy (e.g. carbon dioxide laser) can provide long-lasting, excellent results (Figure 89.15) [1,8,13,14,135].

Major features
Transient erythema (flushing). As for persistent erythema, botulinum toxin injections appeared to be effective and safe in several small studies for reducing flushing [131–134].

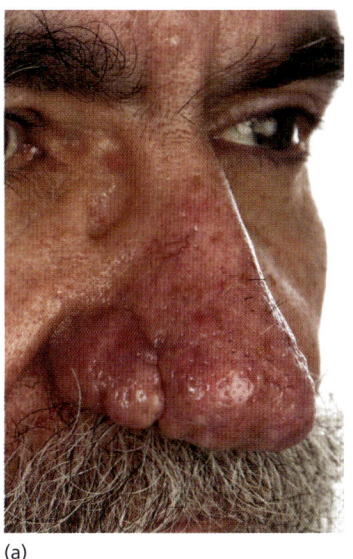 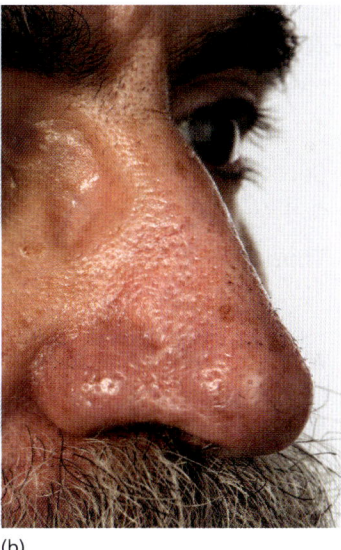

(a)   (b)

Figure 89.15 Rhinophyma before (a) and after (b) 4 months' treatment with scalpel excision.

Papules and pustules. Isotretinoin is effective for severe or refractory papules and pustules of rosacea [1,4,8,13,14]. To avoid worsening of ocular features by exacerbation of tear film dysfunction, isotretinoin should be used in the lowest effective dose.

Telangiectasia. Unresponsive telangiectasias or larger facial vessels may require sclerotherapy. This should be performed by an experienced injector with a thorough knowledge of vascular anatomy [136].

Maintenance treatment

Rosacea is a chronic condition and although remissions can be achieved, relapses are likely to occur. Therefore, ongoing attention to trigger avoidance and general skin care is advisable. Topical metronidazole, topical azelaic acid and topical ivermectin have been shown to maintain remission after clearance of papules/pustules of rosacea [1,4,13].

Ocular rosacea treatment

First line. Daily lid hygiene can be helpful for patients with early blepharitis and lid crusting [1,13,94,95,97,117]. Cleansing can be achieved by gentle application of diluted baby shampoo (add a few drops of baby shampoo in a shot glass with warm water) to the lid margins with a cotton applicator. Prior application of warm compresses may help liquefy the meibomian gland plugs to facilitate removal [94,95,97]. Artificial tears are helpful to address ocular dryness due to tear film dysfunction from reduced meibomian gland lipid excretion [137,138]. As saline does not replace the needed lipid component, eye drops containing hydroxypropyl-guar (HP-guar) four times a day are more effective and can restore the tear film and improve meibomian gland functionality [135,137,138].

Omega-3 supplementation improves dry eye symptoms as well as tear gland function [4,13,14,135].

Second line. In addition to lid hygiene, warm compresses, HP-guar-containing eye drops and omega-3 fatty acids, ciclosporin ophthalmic emulsion can reduce the signs and symptoms of ocular rosacea [1,4,13,14]. Other options to address bacteria and/or inflammation include topical fusidic acid, azithromycin, tacrolimus, ivermectin and metronidazole applied to the lid margins [1,4,14,94].

Third line. When the above are insufficient, or if ocular involvement is moderate to severe, systemic treatment should be considered and referral to an ocular specialist arranged [8,14,94,95]. Cutaneous rosacea should be taken into account when starting oral treatment to optimise treatment results for both cutaneous and ocular features. Both daily doxycycline 40 mg MR as well as doxycycline 100 mg have been shown to be effective in treating ocular rosacea [1,4,13,14,94,95,135]. Other options include azithromycin and minocycline [14,94]. Immediate referral to an ophthalmologist is warranted for corneal ulceration, sudden pain or visual decline and suspected ocular rosacea in children (see 'Management of paediatric rosacea') [1,13,14,94]. IPL and laser therapy have demonstrated beneficial effects on telangiectasias and meibomian gland dysfunction [14,95].

Treatment ladder for rosacea

Diagnostic features

Persistent erythema

First line
- General skin measures and avoidance of exacerbating factors and triggers
- Topical brimonidine 0.33% gel or oxymetazoline hydrochloride 1% cream once daily

Second line
- Intense pulsed light (IPL) or pulsed-dye laser (PDL) therapy, neodymium:yttrium-aluminium-garnet (Nd:YAG) laser or potassium-titanyl-phosphate (KTP) laser therapy

Third line
- Combined topical α-adrenergic agents and light/laser treatments
- Botulin toxin injections may be considered

Phymatous rosacea: inflamed phyma

First line
- General skin measures and avoidance of exacerbating factors and triggers
- Tretinoin 0.025% cream or 0.01% cream/gel once or twice daily for 8–12 weeks

- Isotretinoin 10 mg daily

Second line
- Doxycycline 40 mg MR, doxycycline 100 mg once daily for 2–4 months

Third line
- Low-dose isotretinoin 0.25–0.30 mg/kg/day for 3–6 months

Phymatous roseacea: non-inflamed phyma

First line
- General skin measures and avoidance of exacerbating factors and triggers

Second line
- Ablative surgery, electrosurgery or laser therapy to debulk and reshape (most frequently the nose)

Major features

Transient erythema (flushing)

First line
- General skin measures and avoidance of exacerbating factors and triggers
- Topical brimonidine 0.33% gel or oxymetazoline hydrochloride 1% cream once daily

Second line
- Carvedilol 6.25 mg 2–3 times a day, clonidine 50 μg twice daily or propranolol 20–40 mg 2–3 times a day
- IPL, vascular laser

Third line
- Botulin toxin injections may be considered

Papules and pustules

First line
- General skin measures and avoidance of exacerbating factors and triggers
- Topical ivermectin 1% cream once daily, metronidazole 0.75%/1% gel or cream twice daily or azelaic acid 15%/20% gel/cream/foam twice daily for 8–12 weeks
- Sodium sulfacetamide 10% and sulphur 5% twice daily, minocycline 1.5% foam once daily or encapsulated benzoyl peroxide 5% cream once daily for 8–12 weeks

Second line
- Doxycycline 40 mg MR once daily, doxycycline 100 mg once daily or minocycline 100 mg once daily for 2–4 months
- Azithromycin 500 mg three times/week for 4 weeks, then tapering to 250 mg three times/week for 4 weeks, and then 250 mg twice/week for 4 weeks

Third line
Isotretinoin 0.25 to 0.3 mg/kg/day for 3–4 months

Telangiectasia

First line
- Electrodessication, IPL or vascular lasers

Second line
- IPL, PDL, Nd:YAG or KTP laser therapy

Third line
- Sclerotherapy

Maintenance treatment

- Topical ivermectin 1% cream once daily, metronidazole 0.75%/1% gel or cream twice daily, azelaic acid 15%/20% gel/cream/foam twice daily for inflammatory lesions
- Topical brimonidine 0.33% gel or oxymetazoline hydrochloride 1% cream once daily for erythema
- Periodic treatment of erythema with IPL or vascular laser

Ocular rosacea

First line
- Lid hygiene
- Warm compresses and lid massage
- HP-guar-containing eye drops
- Omega-3 supplementation 360 mg eicosapentaenoic acid/240 mg docosahexaenoic acid twice daily for dry eye symptoms

Second line
- Ciclosporin 0.05% ophthalmic emulsion one drop twice daily
- Fusidic acid gel twice daily, azithromycin 1.0% ointment or 1.5% drops one drop twice daily, tacrolimus 0.03% twice daily, or ivermectin or metronidazole 0.75% gel twice daily applicated to the lid margins

Third line
- Doxycycline 40 mg MR once daily, doxycycline 100 mg once daily or minocycline 100 mg once daily for 12 weeks
- Azithromycin 500 mg 3 days a week for 3–4 weeks or azithromycin 500 mg for 1 day then 250 mg for a further 4 days
- IPL, PDL or Nd:YAG laser therapy

Management of paediatric rosacea

Rosacea appears uncommon in children and adolescents. The prevalence and incidence are unknown. The most common features are papules/pustules, while persistent erythema and telangiectasias occur less often (Figure 89.16). Ocular manifestations, which may be serious especially in girls, often predominate and precede cutaneous features in 50% of pediatric patients [99]. Flushing sometimes occurs, along with pruritus, burning and stinging [139]. Phyma does not occur in children.

Management of childhood rosacea includes identifying and avoiding triggers and UV protection with sunscreens [139–141].

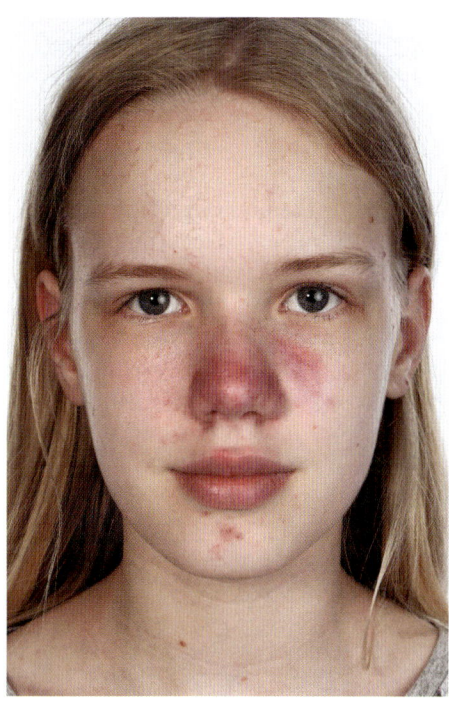

Figure 89.16 Pediatric rosacea showing papules and pustules in a young girl.

There is limited evidence for treatment. In several case reports and case studies, efficacy of topical and systemic treatment has been reported. Most treatments are not approved for children.

Treatment ladder for paediatric rosacea

First line

- Topical azelaic acid 15%/20% gel/cream twice daily, metronidazole 0.75%/1% gel or cream twice daily, permethrin 5% twice daily and ivermectin 1% cream once daily.

Second line

For more severe cases combinations of topical and systemic treatment are recommended for 8–12 weeks; prolonged treatment may be required [139–141]:

- Tetracycline 500 mg twice daily (tapering)*
- Minocycline 50–100 mg twice daily*
- Doxycycline 50–100 mg twice daily*
- Azithromycin 5–10 mg/kg once daily
- Erythromycin 30–50 mg/kg once daily
- Metronidazole 20–30 mg/kg once daily.
- Ivermectin single dose 200–250 µg/kg (children ≥15 kg)

For ocular involvement, ophthalmic consultation is recommended [95].

*Not for children younger than 8–9 years [144].

Management of rosacea in pregnant and lactating women

Few treatments are considered safe during pregnancy and lactation [1,142,143]. Well-controlled human studies of rosacea medications evaluating fetal and infant outcomes are not available. Accordingly, estimates of risk derive from animal or human pharmacokinetic studies (serum and breast milk levels in women). Benefit–risk ratio, patient preference as well as approval for this specific population by regulatory authorities such as the US Food and Drug Administration (FDA) and the European Medicines Agency (EMA) should be taken into account when making a treatment choice.

As both laser as well as IPL therapy can be painful and cause distress, treatment for erythema and telangiectasias can be postponed until postpartum. For papules and pustules the treatments in the treatment ladder can be considered [1,142,143].

Treatment ladder for rosacea in pregnant and lactating women

First line

- Metronidazole 0.75%/1% gel or cream twice daily
- Azelaic acid 15%/20% gel/cream/foam twice daily

Second line

- Azithromycin 500 mg three times/week for 4 weeks, then tapering to 250 mg three times/week for 4 weeks, and then 250 mg twice/week for 4 weeks

There is no evidence for the efficacy of clarithromycin nor erythromycin in rosacea [1,4]. Tetracyclines and isotretinoin are absolutely contraindicated in pregnancy.

Ocular rosacea

First line

- Lid hygiene and artificial tears
- Fusidic acid gel twice daily

Second line

- Ciclosporin 0.05% ophthalmic emulsion one drop twice daily

Resources

American Academy of Dermatology: https://www.aad.org/public.

British Association of Dermatology: www.bad.org.uk/.

European Academy of Dermatology and Venereology patient information leaflets: https://www.eadv.org/patient-corner/leaflets.

National Rosacea Society, USA: www.rosacea.org.

(All last accessed January 2022.)

FACIAL DERMATOSES WITH AN UNCERTAIN NOSOLOGICAL RELATIONSHIP TO ROSACEA

There are various facial dermatoses that share some features with rosacea but for which there is currently no consensus as to their nosological relationship with rosacea. These are described in this section.

PART 8: SPECIFIC CUTANEOUS STRUCTURES

Idiopathic facial aseptic granuloma

Synonyms and inclusions
• Pyodermite froide du visage

Idiopathic facial aseptic granuloma (IFAG), which only occurs in children, is characterised by one or more painless red or purple nodules, usually on the cheeks (Figure 89.17) [1]. Based on histopathology, which resembles granulomatous rosacea and because of frequent occurrence of chalazia, it is suggested that IFAG fits within the spectrum of childhood rosacea [2]. The condition typically resolves spontaneously or in response to antibiotic treatment [3].

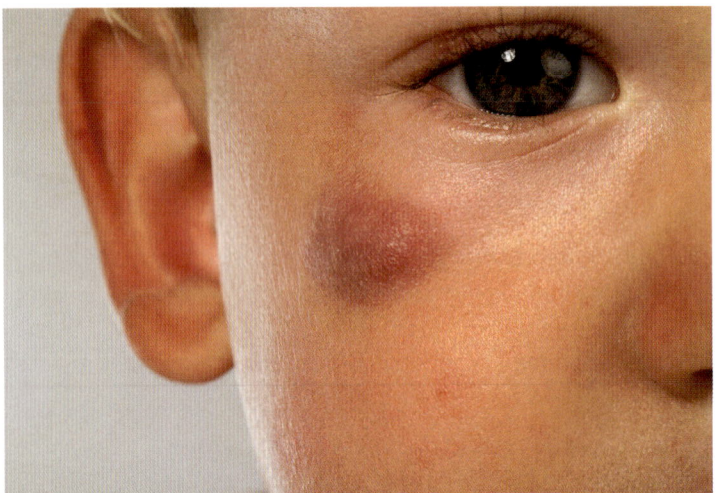

Figure 89.17 Idiopathic facial aseptic granuloma showing a well-defined plum-coloured nodule on the face.

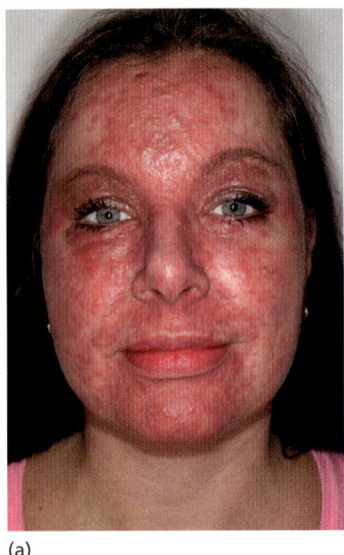
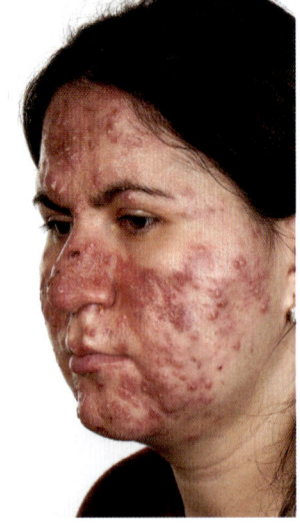

(a)   (b)

Figure 89.18 (a) Rosacea fulminans showing an abrupt onset of severe inflammation with extensive papules and to a lesser extent pustules in a young pregnant woman. (b) Rosacea fulminans showing marked erythema, inflammatory papules, pustules and nodules.

Rosacea fulminans

Rosacea fulminans, previously called pyoderma faciale, is a rare facial dermatosis characterised by sudden onset of marked erythema, inflammatory papules, pustules, nodules, cysts and indurated haemorrhagic plaques (Figure 89.18) [4]. Ocular involvement is reported [5–7] but extrafacial manifestations are rare [4]. The disease typically occurs in young women, the majority having a history of rosacea. Common identifiable triggers include pregnancy, emotional stress, medications and inflammatory bowel disease [4,7]. Histopathology is not specific but may exclude other disorders such as granulomatous rosacea [7]. Early treatment is recommended to prevent scarring [8]. The combination of oral isotretinoin and corticosteroids has been reported to be most successful. During pregnancy, a combination of oral antibiotics such as macrolides with oral corticosteroids or topical therapy is suggested, as oral antibiotic monotherapy may not be sufficient [4,5].

Solid facial lymphoedema

Synonyms and inclusions
• Morbihan disease

Introduction and general description

This is a rare condition of persistent, pronounced, mostly symmetrically distributed, firm, non-pitting oedema with erythema involving the upper two-thirds of the face (Figure 89.19) [9]. It may result in significant discomfort, visual impairment and cosmetic disfigurement [10]. The condition may occur spontaneously or develop in the context of rosacea [11]. Whilst most are reported in white middle-aged males, patients with skin of colour and younger individuals have been described [9]. It is a clinical diagnosis but other diagnoses such as thyroid disease, dermatomyositis, angioedema, systemic lupus erythematosus, Melkerson–Rosenthal syndrome and neoplastic disease (if presentation is asymmetrical) should be excluded [12,13].

Pathophysiology

The pathogenesis remains unclear. It has been postulated that chronic inflammation with inadequate lymphatic drainage and/or intralymphatic obstruction results in lymphoedema [14]. Histopathology shows features characteristics of rosacea but dilated lymphatic vessels, granulomas and clusters of mast cells are suggestive of the diagnosis [9,14].

Management

Prolonged treatment over at least 4–6 months with tetracycline-based antibiotics, isotretinoin and oral corticosteroids may be required. These may also be used in combination with antihistamines, intralesional triamcinolone injections and debulking surgery. Improvement is often only partial and transient [9,14]. Very good results have been recently published with long-term ultra-low-dose isotretinoin in combination with antihistamines [15].

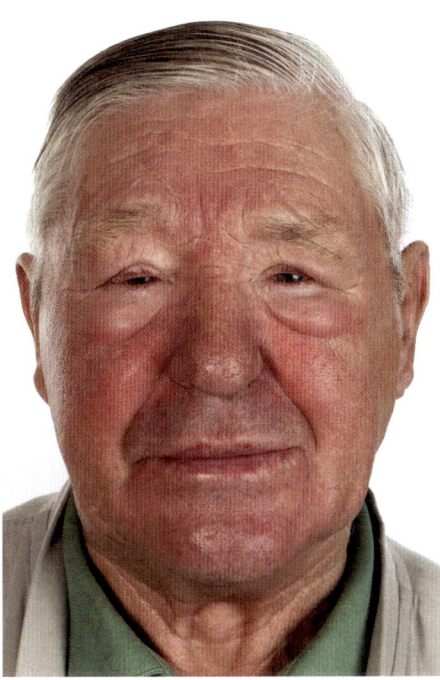

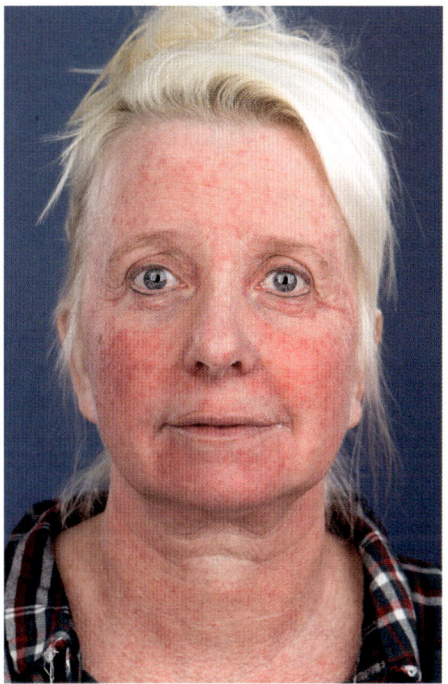

Figure 89.19 Solid facial lymphoedema is characterised by the presence of persistent, non-tender, firm, upper facial swelling. Note the creases under the eyes in this patient indicating the presence of this unusual type of facial erythema and swelling.

Figure 89.20 Corticosteroid-induced rosacea-like facial dermatosis.

Corticosteroid-induced rosacea-like facial dermatosis

Introduction and general description
Steroid-induced rosacea is caused by long-term application of mid- to high-potency topical steroids to the face. Women are most often affected, but children and men may develop the condition.

Pathophysiology
Various factors are involved in the pathogenesis of steroid-induced rosacea. Accumulation of multiple metabolites, such as nitric oxide, and alterations in the skin microbiome are implicated [16]. Withdrawal of the topical steroid is essential, either rapidly or gradually [17].

Clinical features
The clinical picture is initially characterised by fixed erythema and telangiectasias. Subsequently, atrophy and rosacea-like features may develop such as papules, pustules and scaling (Figure 89.20) [18]. These usually develop after 6 months or more, but have been observed at 2 months [19]. Symptoms include itching, burning, skin hypersensitivity and intense redness. Progressive increase in corticosteroid potency is undertaken to control symptoms and signs but withdrawals lead to exacerbation. This results in an escalating cycle of steroid abuse: temporary improvement followed by worsening, then escalation of steroid potency with improvement followed by worsening. The differential diagnoses include allergic corticosteroid-induced contact dermatitis, acne vulgaris, seborrhoeic dermatitis, systemic lupus erythematosus and dermatomyositis [20].

Management
Management comprises topical steroid withdrawal along with use of topical pimecrolimus, metronidazole or combinations thereof. The addition of oral antibiotics such as doxycycline, tetracycline or azithromycin for 4–8 weeks may augment resolution and reduce withdrawal flares [17,21]. Tacrolimus has also been recommended though tacrolimus-induced rosacea-like dermatitis has been reported [22]. It may take several weeks or even months before complete resolution is achieved.

Periorificial facial dermatitis

Synonyms and inclusions
- Perioral dermatitis
- Periorbital dermatitis

Introduction and general description
Periorificial facial dermatitis (PD) typically affects females 16–45 years of age but may occur also in children [23,24]. Childhood periorificial dermatitis should be differentiated from childhood *granulomatous* periorificial dermatitis (CGPD), a self-limited condition (see 'Childhood granulomatous periorificial dermatoses' later in this chapter).

Pathophysiology
Overuse of cosmetics, physical sunscreens and fluoridated toothpaste have been considered potential causative factors [25–27]. Other potential causes that may have a role include microbiological factors (*Candida albicans*, fusiform bacteria and *Demodex* mites) [28,29], weather conditions (UV light, wind, heat), hormonal factors

(oral contraceptives) and skin-barrier impairment [30,31]. Patients often possess an atopic diathesis [32].

The mechanism(s) through which these factors contribute to PD is unknown. Histopathology of PD resembles rosacea with non-specific inflammation, but with fewer signs of actinic damage [24,33].

Clinical features
History
In most cases of PD, there is a history of prolonged use of corticosteroids (topical, inhaled or ophthalmic). These corticosteroids can initially improve but subsequently perpetuate the condition. Furthermore, prior attempts at discontinuation of these preparations may have led to exacerbations [34,35].

Presentation
Small papules and pustules or vesicles on patchy erythema around the mouth, with a sparing zone around the lips, and in the melolabial folds, with a tendency to extend to the chin, cheeks and lateral parts of the face, are characteristic (Figure 89.21a, b) [32,36,37]. Lesions can also develop around the eyes and sometimes on the eyelids (Figure 89.21c) [38]. Symptoms include skin tightness, and sometimes moderate burning, pain and pruritus [32,36].

Differential diagnosis
Differential diagnoses of PD include rosacea (see 'Differential diagnosis' of rosacea, earlier in this chapter), granulomatous rosacea and CGPD.

Management
Management starts with discontinuation or tapering of topical corticosteroids and suspected skincare products [24,36,37]. Flares often occur in the first few weeks and patients need reassurance that discontinuation of the corticosteroid and offending cosmetics is necessary to achieve remission over time. Unless causative agents are used again, remission is usually complete and permanent [24]. Treatment depends on severity and adherence. Self-care regimens including daily cleansing with water and use of gentle moisturisers are suggested [37]. Topical medications like ivermectin, metronidazole, azelaic acid and pimecrolimus can be helpful. In contrast, topical tacrolimus may induce a rosaceiform dermatitis [24,36,39,40]. In more severe cases, oral tetracycline, doxycycline, minocycline or erythromycin can be considered [32,36].

Childhood granulomatous periorificial dermatoses

Synonyms and inclusions
• Facial Afro-Caribbean childhood eruption (FACE)

Introduction and general description
Childhood granulomatous periorificial dermatoses (CGPD) is considered a variant of PD, while others consider it a variant of

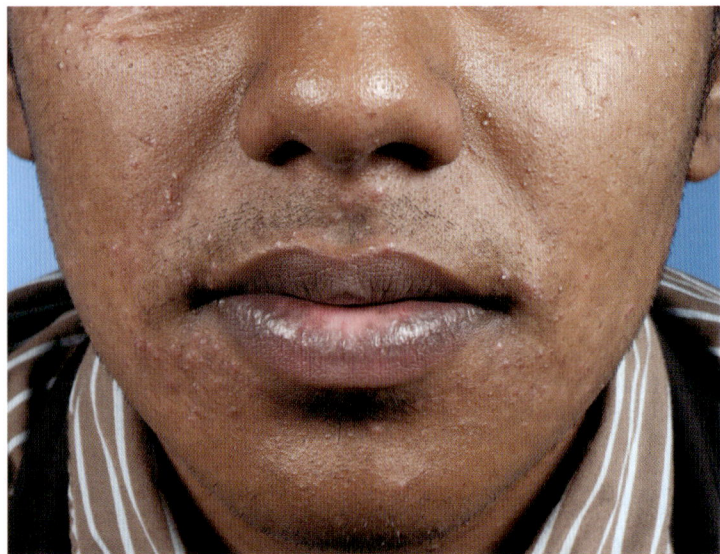
(a)

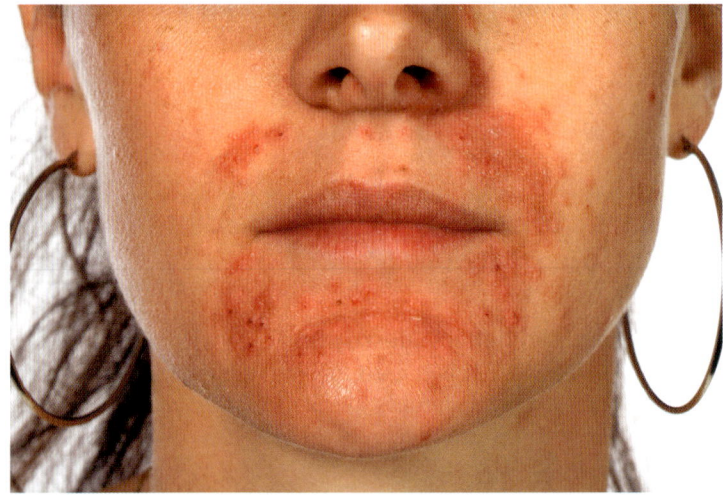
(b)

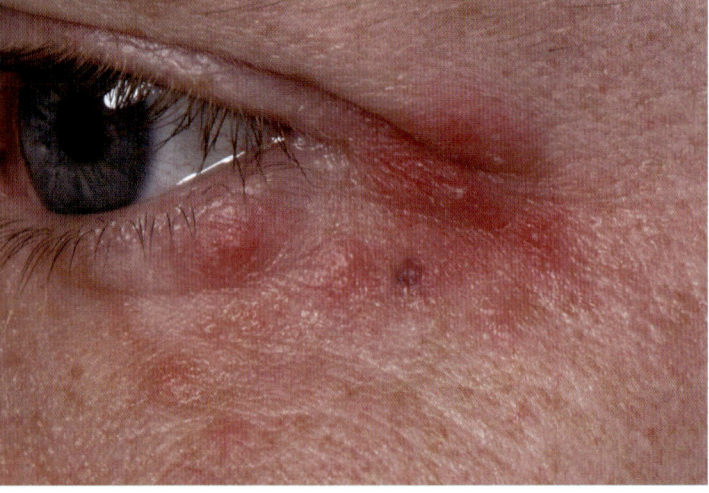
(c)

Figure 89.21 (a) Perioral dermatitis showing papules/pustules around the mouth. (b) Perioral dermatitis showing papules/pustules with spare zone around the lips and in the melolabial folds and on the chin. (c) Dermatitis periorbitalis.

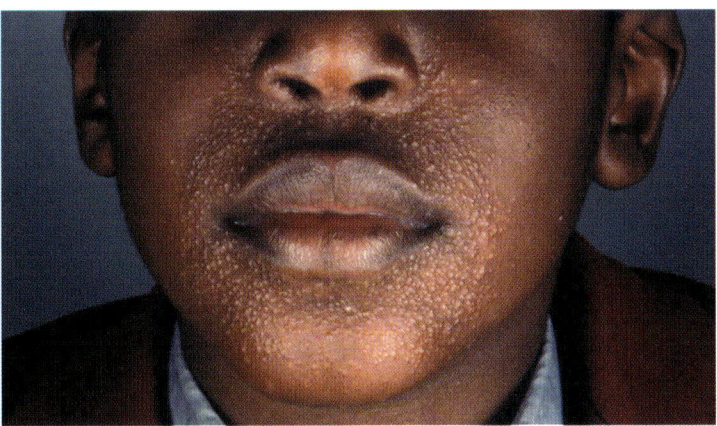

Figure 89.22 Childhood granulomatous periorificial dermatitis. Courtesy of Professor Hywel Williams, University of Nottingham, UK.

granulomatous rosacea [24,41,42]. CGPD generally occurs in prepubertal children of African descent although the condition has also been reported in children with light phototype [43].

Pathophysiology
Histologically, CGPD demonstrates non-caseating granulomatous infiltrates of lymphocytes, histiocytes and giant cells in the mid and upper dermis with perifollicular involvement [41,44]. The etiology and pathogenesis of CGPD are unknown [42].

Clinical features
Presentation
The clinical features are characterised by symmetrical distribution of monomorphic flesh-colored, pink and yellow-brown papules around the mouth, nose and eyes (Figure 89.22) [41]. Occasionally extrafacial involvement (ears, neck, trunk, upper limbs, genital area) along with blepharitis and conjunctivitis has been reported [45].

Management
The condition is self-limiting, and may result in some scarring [24,42]. Treatment with topical therapy including metronidazole, pimecrolimus, tacrolimus and erythromycin is effective in most cases.

Lupus miliaris disseminatus faciei

Synonyms and inclusions
- Acne agminate
- Lupoid rosacea
- Lewandowsky eruption

Introduction and general description
Lupus miliaris disseminatus faciei (LMDF), an uncommon granulomatous inflammatory dermatosis primarily affecting the face, has been considered a variant of GR by some and a distinct entity by others. There are differences in clinical presentation and age of onset [46,47], with LMDF usually presenting in young male adults and GR usually in middle age of both genders [46].

Pathophysiology
Histopathology shows large caseating and non-caseating granulomas with perifollicular inflammation of lymphocytes, histiocytes and multinucleated giant cells [46]. Although these histological features are similar to those of granulomatous rosacea, the latter is differentiated by the presence of *Demodex* and smaller non-caseating granulomas. The development of scars correlates with histological fibrosis in older lesions [48].

Clinical features
The dermatosis LMDF is characterised by multiple, yellow-brown, red dome-shaped papular and nodulocystic lesions at the medial and lateral face, often involving the eyelids, and extending onto the neck and chin [46]. Extrafacial involvement includes axillae, neck, groin and/or extremities [49]. Papular lesions appear like 'apple jelly' on diascopy [47]. LMDF is self-limiting, persisting for months to years, but may lead to scarring [48].

Differential diagnosis
Differential diagnoses include sarcoidosis, granulomatous rosacea and infectious granulomatous dermatoses. The latter, including cutaneous tuberculosis, should be considered in regions of high prevalence [46]. Compared with granulomatous rosacea, extrafacial involvement is not unusual in LMDF, but there are no features of rosacea such as flushing, background erythema and exacerbation caused by triggers of rosacea or ocular involvement [46]. Sarcoidosis should be considered in the presence of extracutaneous manifestations or systemic complaints. Histological characteristic features of sarcoidosis include non-caseating granulomatous infiltration. In view of the differential diagnoses, the following tests should be considered: skin biopsy with Ziehl–Neelsen staining for acid-fast bacilli, serology, chest X-ray, Mantoux test, deep fungal/mycobacterial cultures and polymerase chain reaction using organism-specific primers [46].

Management
Although self-limiting, early treatment of LMDF is recommended due to the risk of scarring [50]. LMDF has been reported to respond better to oral corticosteroids than to tetracycline-class antibiotics. Other options include oral prednisolone with dapsone (100 mg daily), oral dapsone with topical tacrolimus [50] and low-dose isotretinoin [51].

Key references

The full list of references can be found in the online version at https://www.wiley.com/rooksdermatology10e

Rosacea
1. Van Zuuren EJ. Rosacea. *New Eng J Med* 2017;377:1754–64.
2. Tan J, Almeida LM, Bewley A *et al.* Updating the diagnosis, classification and assessment of rosacea: recommendations from the global ROSacea COnsensus (ROSCO) panel. *Br J Dermatol* 2017;176:431–8.
3. Gallo RL, Granstein RD, Kang S *et al.* Standard classification and pathophysiology of rosacea: the 2017 update by the National Rosacea Society Expert Committee. *J Am Acad Dermatol* 2018;78:148–55.

PART 8: SPECIFIC
CUTANEOUS STRUCTURES

4 Van Zuuren EJ, Fedorowicz Z, Tan J *et al*. Interventions for rosacea based on the phenotype approach: an updated systematic review including GRADE assessments. *Br J Dermatol* 2019;181:65–79.

8 Schaller M, Almeida LMC, Bewley A *et al*. Recommendations for rosacea diagnosis, classification and management: update from the global ROSacea COnsensus 2019 panel. *Br J Dermatol* 2020;182:1269–76.

13 Schaller M, Almeida LM, Bewley A *et al*. Rosacea treatment update: recommendations from the global ROSacea COnsensus (ROSCO) panel. *Br J Dermatol* 2017;176:465–71.

14 Thiboutot D, Anderson R, Cook-Bolden F *et al*. Standard management options for rosacea: the 2019 update by the National Rosacea Society Expert Committee. *J Am Acad Dermatol* 2020;82:1501–10.

18 Gether L, Overgaard LK, Egeberg A, Thyssen JP. Incidence and prevalence of rosacea: a systematic review and meta-analysis. *Br J Dermatol* 2018;179:282–9.

40 Buddenkotte J, Steinhoff M. Recent advances in understanding and managing rosacea. *F1000Res* 2018;7:1885.

41 Yamasaki K, Gallo RL. Rosacea as a disease of cathelicidins and skin innate immunity. *Investig Dermatol Symp Proc* 2011;15:12–15.

CHAPTER 90

Hidradenitis Suppurativa

John R. Ingram[1], Hessel H. van der Zee[2] and Gregor B. E. Jemec[3]

[1] Division of Infection and Immunity, Cardiff University, Cardiff, UK
[2] Department of Dermatology, Erasmus Medical Center, Rotterdam, the Netherlands
[3] Department of Dermatology, Zealand University Hospital, Roskilde; Faculty of Health and Medical Sciences, University of Copenhagen, Copenhagen, Denmark

Hidradenitis suppurativa

Definition and nomenclature

Hidradenitis suppurativa (HS) is a chronic, inflammatory, follicular disease that usually presents at or after puberty. Painful, deep-seated inflamed skin lesions occur in apocrine gland-bearing areas, most commonly the axillary, inguinal and ano-genital regions. The disease is defined clinically, based on the San Francisco modification of the Dessau criteria [1]. All three of the criteria described in Box 90.1 must be met to confirm the diagnosis.

Box 90.1 Essential criteria for a diagnosis of hidradenitis suppurativa to be made

1 Typical lesions	Deep-seated painful nodules, abscesses, draining tunnels, bridged scars and paired or multiheaded open pseudocomedones	
2 Typical topography	Axillae, groin, perineal and perianal region, buttocks, infra- and intermammary folds	
3 Chronicity and recurrence of lesions	Recurrent flares of painful lesions over time in the same or differing skin sites (at least two flares in a 6-month period)	

Synonyms and inclusions

- Acne inversa
- Verneuil disease
- Velpeau disease

Introduction and general description

Velpeau was the first to describe the condition of recurrent, painful, inflammatory abscesses of the axillae and groin in 1839 [2]. Verneuil later coined the term hidradenitis suppurativa, a misnomer derived from the historical hypothesis that the disorder related to inflammation of the sweat glands [3]. Current evidence demonstrates that HS is a primary disorder of the hair follicle.

HS is a chronic, inflammatory, follicular disorder characterised by recurrent painful nodules, abscesses, draining skin tunnels and scarring. It localises to areas of apocrine gland-bearing skin, predominantly the axillae, groin and ano-genital sites. Disease staging, from mild to severe, is defined by the Hurley system, which helps to determine initial therapy [4]. Management is challenging and requires a combined medical and surgical approach, ideally in a multidisciplinary setting for severe disease. Complications of severe disease include contractures, anaemia, lymphoedema and squamous cell carcinoma [5]. The psychosocial and quality of life impact can be substantial [6], and even includes an increased risk of completed suicide [7].

Epidemiology

Incidence and prevalence

Prevalence figures vary 80-fold, from 0.05% using US insurance-based data [8] to 4% observed in young adults attending a sexually transmitted disease clinic [9]. Population- and symptoms-based studies in Europe, which also identified undiagnosed patients, demonstrated an estimated prevalence of 1–2% [10,11].

Annual incidence figures vary considerably as well, from 11.4 per 100 000 person-years using US insurance data [12] to 28.3 using UK population-based data [11]. Incidence rates are rising in some regions, probably because of increasing recognition of the condition [12].

Age

The average age of sufferers is 24.2 years (± 12 years) [13]. Diagnosis of HS is most often made in the third decade of life and, factoring in an average diagnostic delay of 7 years [14], this fits with the concept that HS typically presents at or after puberty. There is a sharp decline in onset after the fifth decade, and onset after menopause is uncommon. Prepubertal onset is rare.

PART 8: SPECIFIC CUTANEOUS STRUCTURES

Rook's Textbook of Dermatology, Tenth Edition. Edited by Christopher Griffiths, Jonathan Barker, Tanya Bleiker, Walayat Hussain and Rosalind Simpson.
© 2024 John Wiley & Sons Ltd. Published 2024 by John Wiley & Sons Ltd.

Sex

In Europe, women are more frequently affected than men, in a ratio of 3 : 1 [11]. The reported ratio is reversed in Asia, with a female : male ratio of 1 : 2 [15]. The topographical distribution of lesions can vary between sexes. Perianal and gluteal disease more commonly affects males; females are more likely to have genito-femoral and submammary lesions [16].

Ethnicity

From a systematic review of the scarce number of retrospective cohort and other studies reporting ethnicity data, HS prevalence rates are highest in African American populations (1.3%), followed by Caucasian populations (0.75%), and lowest in the Hispanic/Latino ethnic group [17]. Limited data from Africa imply prevalence rates comparable with those of white-skinned populations [18].

Associated diseases

Diseases associated with HS include disorders of the follicular occlusion tetrad, cardiovascular disease, systemic inflammatory disorders and mental health problems [5].

Follicular occlusion tetrad. Acne conglobata (Chapter 88), dissecting cellulitis of the scalp (Chapter 105) and pilonidal sinus (Chapter 111) can coexist with HS; together they comprise the 'follicular occlusion tetrad'. Typical acne vulgaris is more common and severe acne at atypical sites is more common in male patients with HS [11,13].

Cardiovascular disease. There is a strong association between HS and metabolic syndrome due to higher rates of obesity, insulin resistance, type 2 diabetes, dyslipidaemia and hypertension. The prevalence of metabolic syndrome in people with HS is 40% and a meta-analysis confirmed an odds ratio of 2.2 for metabolic syndrome in HS compared with controls [19,20]. Adding in higher rates of smoking in HS, it is not surprising that people with HS have a greater risk of cardiovascular (CV) disease, with an incidence rate of 1.6 for myocardial infarction and 1.3 for ischaemic stroke [21] compared with matched controls without HS. Risk of death from CV disease in HS is twice as high as in unselected controls and 1.6 times higher than in those with severe psoriasis. Higher rates of CV disease make up the largest proportion of increased all-cause mortality in HS, with mean life expectancy in HS being 61 years, compared with 71 years for those with psoriasis and 75 years in healthy controls [22].

Inflammatory disorders. A strong association exists between HS and Crohn disease (Chapter 95), which shares epidemiological, histological and therapeutic features with HS. In one study 17% of patients with Crohn disease were considered likely to have had coexistent HS [23]. There is also a link between HS and ulcerative colitis, however the association is weaker [24]. An inflammatory spondyloarthropathy of axial and appendicular joints, which is HLA-B27- and rheumatoid factor-negative, has been associated with HS [25].

Mental health. There are higher rates of depression and anxiety in HS which, at least in part, is probably due to HS being a painful, chronic condition that can be socially isolating [6,26]. There is a 2.4-fold higher rate of completed suicide in those with HS compared with controls [7].

Additional associations. Most case–control studies confirm a link between HS and polycystic ovary disease [27]. Rates of HS in people with Down syndrome are five times higher than controls [28]. There is also an association with obstructive sleep apnoea, which is probably secondary to obesity [29].

Syndromic HS. Rarely, HS can present as part of a syndrome of other inflammatory disorders including PASH (*p*yoderma gangrenosum, *a*cne conglobata and *s*uppurative *h*idradenitis) and PAPASH (*p*yogenic *a*rthritis, *p*yoderma gangrenosum, *a*cne and *s*uppurative *h*idradenitis) [25] (Chapters 45, 49 and 88).

Pathophysiology

Early studies implicated apocrine gland occlusion as a primary pathogenic event. However, histopathological observations have since demonstrated that follicular involvement is central to pathogenesis. The following sequence of events has been suggested: infundibular hyperkeratosis causing narrowing of the outlet, follicular dilatation/cyst formation, follicular rupture with subsequent inflammation, and skin tunnel formation by epidermal strands [30]. A perifollicular lymphocytic infiltrate found in healthy-looking perilesional skin suggests that subclinical inflammation precedes infundibular hyperkeratosis [31].

Predisposing factors

Obesity and smoking. Obesity and smoking are the two main environmental factors associated with HS. Obesity is implicated as a risk factor, with two-thirds of patients being either overweight or obese [32]. Obesity is associated with higher severity scores [32,33]. There are studies describing the beneficial effect on HS of weight loss, while bariatric surgery and weight loss reduce self-reported HS in the morbidly obese [34]. It has been hypothesised that increased pro-inflammatory cytokine release from visceral fat, physical occlusion and mechanical frictional stress at intertriginous skin sites may explain this association.

There is an increased prevalence of smoking among patients with HS compared with controls with an odds ratio of 4.3 for HS and current smoking [20]. The mechanism may be mediated by nicotinic acetylcholine receptors in the skin or could relate to smoking increasing follicular occlusion. A temporal or dose effect of smoking is not consistently demonstrated. It is not known if smoking cessation improves the course of disease.

Hormonal influences. Hormonal influences are supported by a female preponderance, observed perimenstrual disease flares and improvement in some cases during pregnancy [35]. Clinical signs of virilisation are, however, usually absent, circulating androgen levels are typically normal and no differences in androgen metabolism have been observed in large case series [36].

Autoinflammation. Alterations of both the innate and adaptive immune systems are thought to play a role in the disease pathogenesis. However, no major immune abnormalities have been found.

Some small studies reported aberrant immune functions including an enhanced production of free oxygen radicals by stimulated neutrophil granulocytes; an impaired secretion of tumour necrosis factor α (TNF-α) and interleukin 6 (IL-6) upon stimulation of monocytes by bacterial compounds; and a diminished proportion of natural killer cells in the blood [37]. However, another study found no abnormalities in granulocyte function or serum immunoglobulin levels [38]. Regarding the complement system, increased levels of the C3a and C5a components have been reported [39]. Fibroblastic stromal cells may also play a role in development and progression of HS [40].

Alterations in the skin (mRNA and/or protein levels) have been reported for IL-1β, CXCL-8/IL-8, IL-17/IL-17A, IL-32 and IL-36/IL-36α/IL-36β/IL-36γ [41–43]. Alterations in the serum (mRNA and/or protein levels) have been reported for IL-1β, IL-6, CXCL-8/IL-8, IL-10, IL-12p70 and IL-17/IL-17A [**44**,45].

The inflammatory IL-23/Th17 pathway seems to be activated, reflected by enhanced expression of IL-17A, IL-12 and IL-23 in HS skin [45,46].

Furthermore, keratinocytes isolated from non-lesional skin of patients with HS demonstrated a pro-inflammatory state with an enhanced production of the antimicrobial peptides human beta-defensin-2, psoriasin (S100A7) and calgranulin (S100A8). In addition, skin samples from HS lesions demonstrated increased expression of several Toll-like receptors [47–51].

Medications. There are cases reported of a paradoxical exacerbation or onset of disease following anti-TNF-α treatment of other chronic inflammatory diseases [52], probably due to immune disequilibrium, as well as lithium and sirolimus therapy [53,54].

Pathology

Histopathological changes vary with disease stage. Early changes, which precede clinically evident lesions, are characterised by a sparse lymphocytic infiltrate of the terminal follicular unit and sebaceous gland atrophy [55,56]. Follicular hyperplasia, perifollicular lymphocytic inflammatory infiltration, interfollicular psoriasiform hyperplasia and dilatation of the follicular lumen follow in developed lesions [30,55]. Cysts lined by stratified squamous epithelium containing lamellated keratin and free hair shafts appear [55]. During flares, abscess formation and ruptured follicular units are seen, associated with a dense, dermal, mixed inflammatory infiltrate including histiocytes and giant cells that extends to interfollicular apocrine and eccrine structures and deep into the subcutis. Skin tunnel formation and fibrosis follow [55].

Histopathological variations less frequently seen include isolated inflammation of the apocrine gland (apocrinitis in 5%), sebaceous gland necrosis, epithelioid granulomas and B-cell pseudofollicles [55,56].

Causative organisms

Hidradenitis suppurativa is currently regarded as a primary inflammatory disorder without a defined infectious trigger. The role of bacteria remains to be clarified. Microbiology from superficial and deep sampling often demonstrates negative culture or only normal skin flora, with multiple non-pathogenic bacterial species in the majority of cultures. The most common bacterial isolates are *Staphylococcus epidermidis* and *S. aureus*, followed by *Peptostreptococcus* species and *Cutibacterium acnes* [57–59]. Streptococcal antibodies are usually not found. Recent studies using S16 analysis suggest that a state of dysbiosis exists in all HS, with an overabundance of *Porphyromonas* and *Peptoniphilus* species in lesional skin, and relative lack of, for example, *Cutibacterium* compared with healthy controls [60].

Biofilm has also been suspected to play a role in HS. It is, however, absent from HS-prone healthy-looking skin, whereas a bacterial biofilm is present in healthy follicles in controls and more advanced HS [61]. Biofilm in early lesions is associated with a greater presence of regulatory T cells [62].

Genetics

Approximately one-third of patients have a family member with HS and inheritance is often consistent with an autosomal dominant pattern [63]. A twin study found that three-quarters of the susceptibility to HS came from shared genetics [64]. Loss-of-function mutations in the γ-secretase genes *Nicastrin*, *Presenilin-1* and *Presenilin enhancer-2* are found principally in Han Chinese HS patients but are rarely found in European cohorts [63,65], and there remains no genetic test for HS. Gamma-secretase regulates notch signalling, which plays a role in epidermal and terminal hair follicle differentiation, immune cell development and immune functions [63,65]. Deficient notch signalling in mice is associated with conversion of hair follicles to keratin-enriched epidermal cysts as a result of changes to the outer root sheath cells [65,66]. Phenotypic heterogeneity in HS complicates genotype–phenotype correlations [67].

Environmental factors

Mechanical irritation and shear forces are potential contributory factors, linked to flexural involvement. There is no evidence that poor hygiene, variation in routine depilatory techniques or use of antiperspirant is relevant to HS.

Clinical features

The diagnosis of HS is clinical and relies on the recognition of typical skin lesions in predominantly flexural sites, occurring in a chronic and recurrent manner (see Box 90.1)

History

Typical index lesions consist of painful subcutaneous nodules or abscesses that persist for a mean duration of 7–15 days. This is followed by spontaneous regression, partial regression (to form non-inflammatory, asymptomatic nodules) or progression to abscess formation with the rupture and release of purulent malodorous exudate which is frequently blood-stained. Typical sites are the axillae; the inguino-genital, perineal, perianal and gluteal areas; and infra- and intermammary skin.

Recurrence takes the form of acute intermittent or continuous disease, involving new skin sites or pre-existing non-inflammatory nodules. Acute intermittent flares consist of solitary or multiple lesions, which are localised or disseminated across regions. Periods of remission (characterised by normal skin or persistent

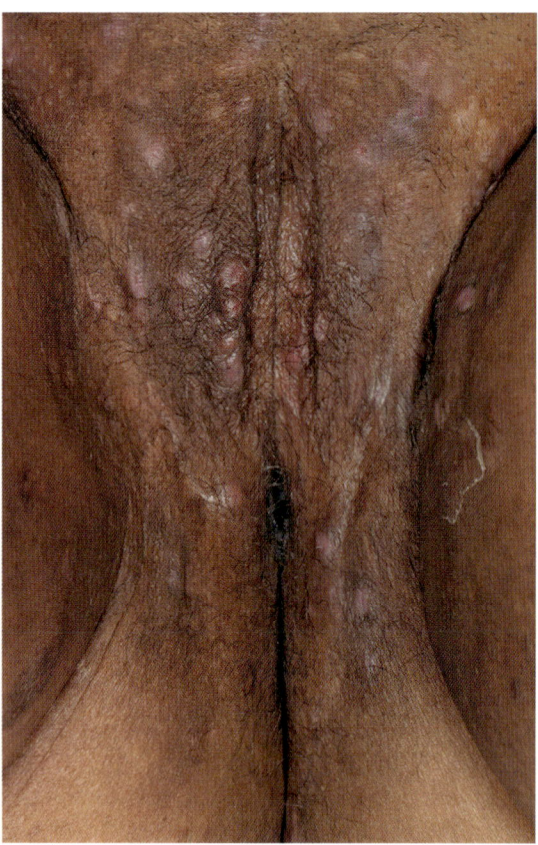

Figure 90.1 Multiple non-inflamed nodules in a patient with Hurley stage II disease of the genital area.

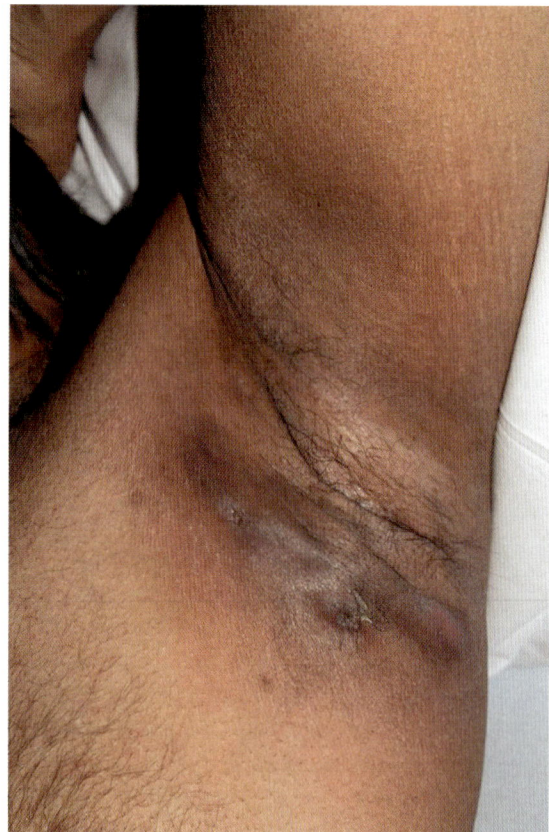

Figure 90.2 Classic axillary abscess as seen in hidradenitis suppurativa.

non-inflammatory nodules) may last for weeks to months. Continuous active disease can lead to the formation of coalescing nodules and skin tunnels forming an inflammatory plaque which may be associated with chronic, daily, purulent discharge and pain.

Presentation

Index lesions include inflamed and non-inflamed dermal and subcutaneous nodules (Figure 90.1), which may require palpation to identify; rounded (as opposed to 'pointing') abscesses (Figure 90.2); and draining or non-draining skin tunnels (Figures 90.3 and 90.4). The term 'tunnel' is preferred to 'sinus tract' to avoid confusion with fistulae. Scarring is typically bridged or 'rope-like', it can be hypertrophic or atrophic, producing depressions especially on the buttocks, and may be associated with contractures (Figure 90.5). Pseudo (secondary) comedones are often seen, typically paired, polyporous and grouped (Figure 90.6). Closed comedones are not seen.

Associated lesions include follicular papules and pustules, pyogenic granulomas at skin tunnel openings and indurated plaques. Epidermoid cysts are seen in some patients on external genitalia, the face and the thorax. Regional lymphadenopathy is not routinely seen, however regional dermatopathic lymphadenopathy can be associated with severe disease.

Lesions are typically localised to inverse (flexural) areas. The commonest sites are the axillae and inguinal and ano-genital regions, including the external genitalia and the perineal, perianal and gluteal skin (Figures 90.7–90.10). Sub- and intermammary skin can also be affected, as can, less commonly, retroauricular, preauricular

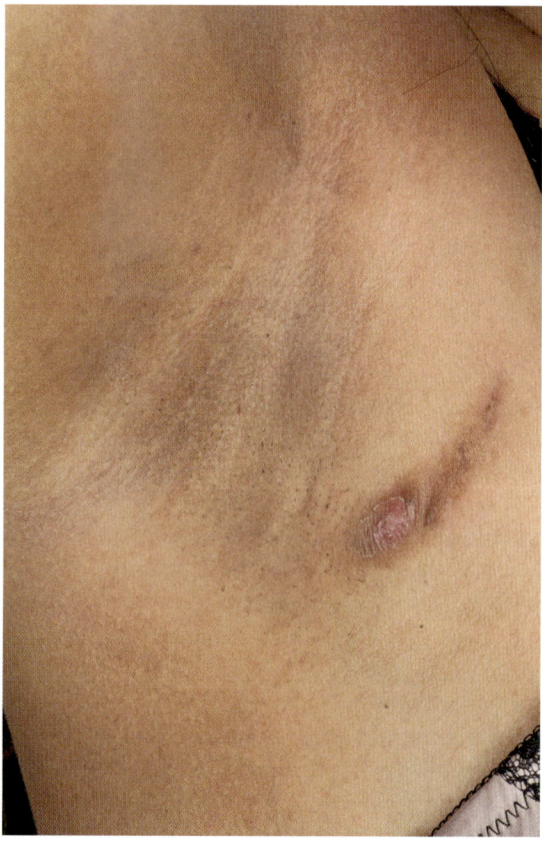

Figure 90.3 Non-draining tunnel, recognised by the palpable linear shape.

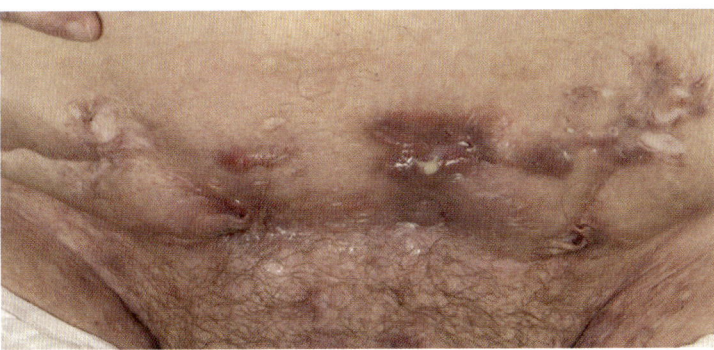

Figure 90.4 Multiple inflamed nodules and draining tunnels in active Hurley stage II disease of the mons pubis.

and occipital scalp locations (Figure 90.11). Truncal variants are also reported, for example in Han Chinese patients (Figure 90.12).

The clinical presentation varies with respect to the number of anatomical regions affected, the extent of the lesions and the types of lesions within a single region. The spectrum ranges from mild disease consisting of solitary nodules to severe disease comprising extensive inflamed confluent nodules, skin tunnels and scarring forming inflammatory plaques affecting an entire anatomical region.

Clinical variants

Hidradenitis suppurativa is a heterogeneous disorder. Epidemiological studies indicate that multiple phenotypic subtypes are likely to exist, grouped by topographical predilection and lesion subtype.

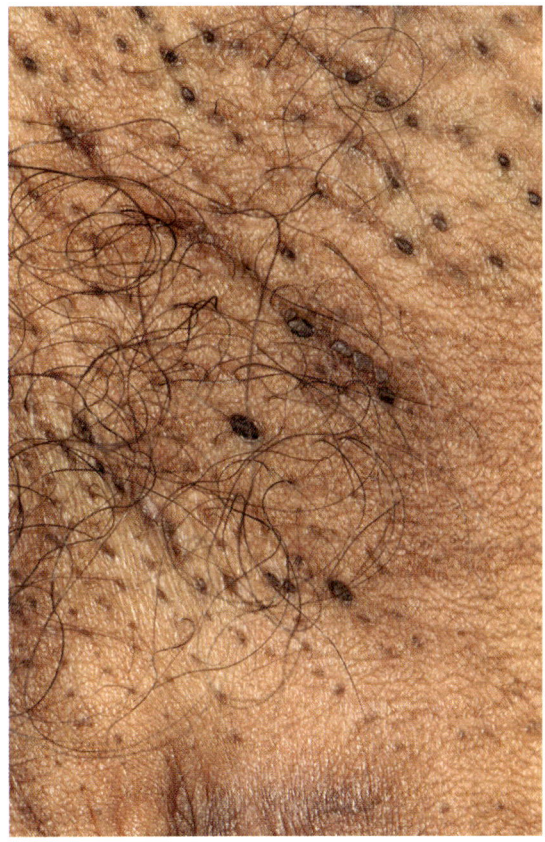

Figure 90.6 Tombstone comedones in the axilla.

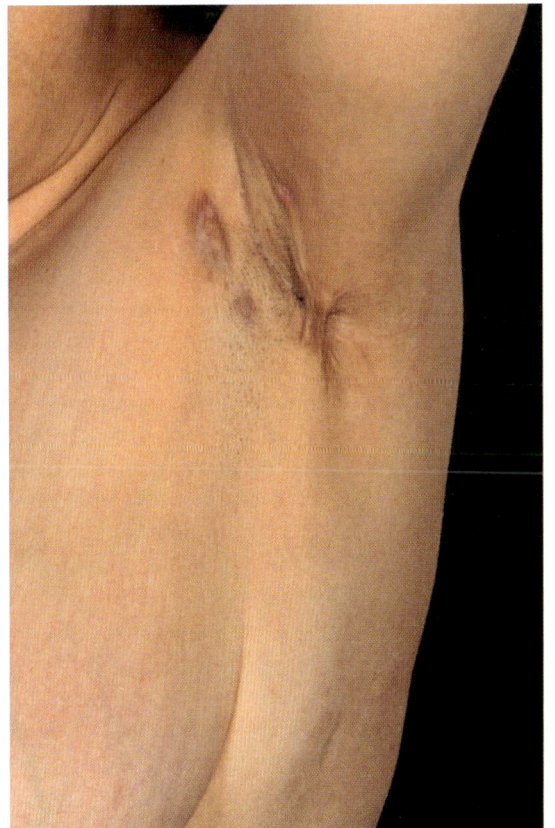

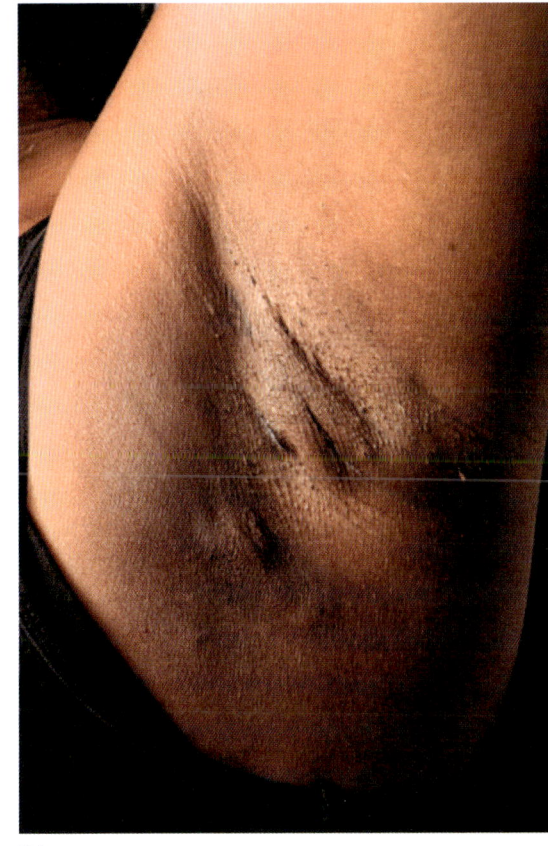

Figure 90.5 (a, b) Scars of rope-like bands formed by fibrotic tissue, most often seen in the axillae. (b) Copyright Cardiff & Vale University Health Board.

(a)

(b)

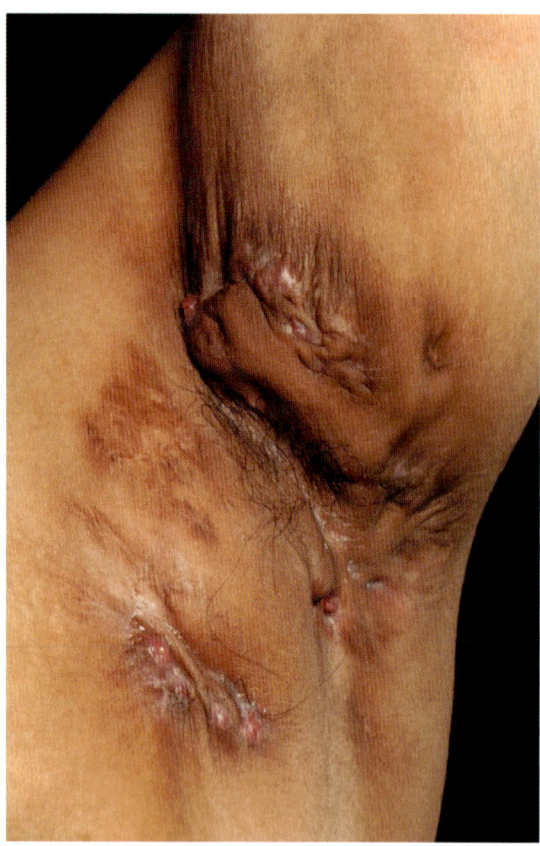

Figure 90.7 Multiple draining tunnels in the axilla, some with pyogenic granuloma-type lesions near their orifices. Copyright Cardiff & Vale University Health Board.

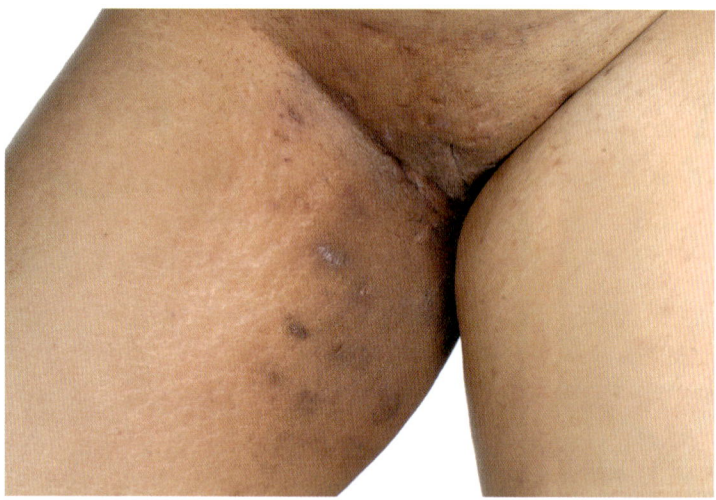

Figure 90.8 Follicular pattern involving the genito-femoral area showing non-active disease.

Several clinical variants have been suggested. However none is generally accepted yet [68].

Differential diagnosis
The differential diagnosis of HS includes several infectious and inflammatory skin conditions. Index lesions should be differentiated from abscesses, carbuncles or furunculosis associated with primary cutaneous bacterial infection (typically

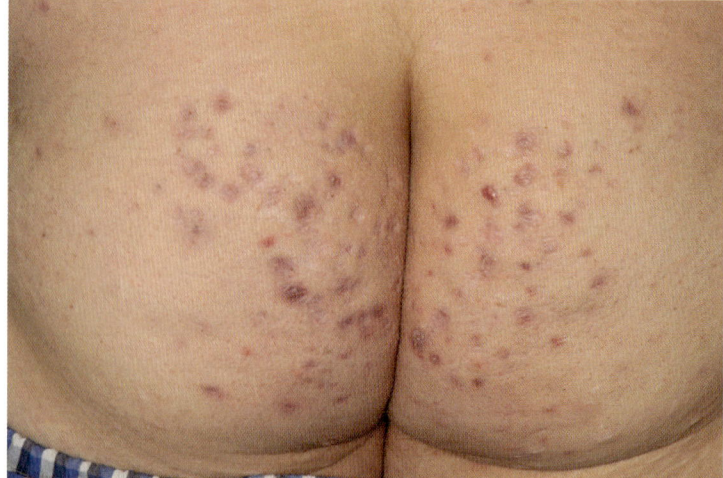

Figure 90.9 Follicular pattern involving the buttocks.

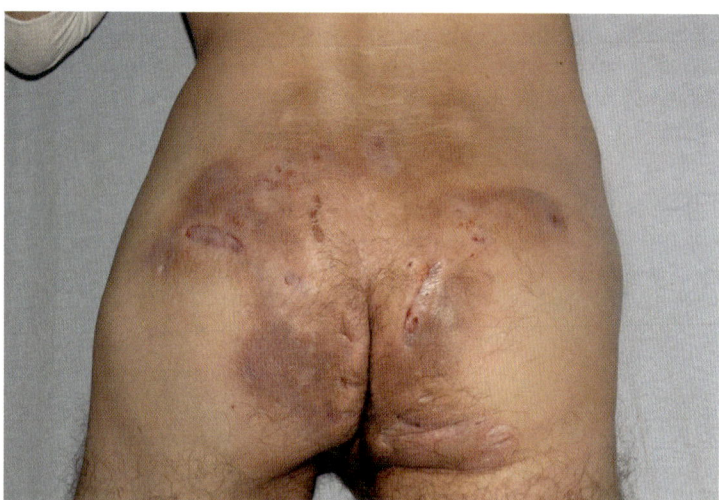

Figure 90.10 Nodules and sinus tracts involving the buttocks.

staphylococcal or streptococcal) or secondary infection of cystic structures (e.g. epidermoid cysts and Bartholin glands). Crohn disease can result in inflammatory abscesses and skin tunnels at ano-genital sites. However, in Crohn disease skin tunnels can involve the gastrointestinal tract, whereas in HS they do not. Of note, HS is associated with Crohn disease and so the two conditions may coexist. Rare infections, including tuberculosis, sporotrichosis, actinomycosis and lymphogranuloma venereum, can present with both abscesses and skin tunnels. Steatocystoma multiplex and neoplastic diseases such as Langerhans cell histiocytosis should also be considered in the differential diagnosis.

Classification of severity
The Hurley staging system refers to three stages based on the presence and extent of skin tunnels and scarring (Table 90.1) [4]. The system describes disease severity in a single affected region, rather than an overall stage across all affected regions. Baseline Hurley staging allows stratification of therapy but is not useful for assessing response to therapy.

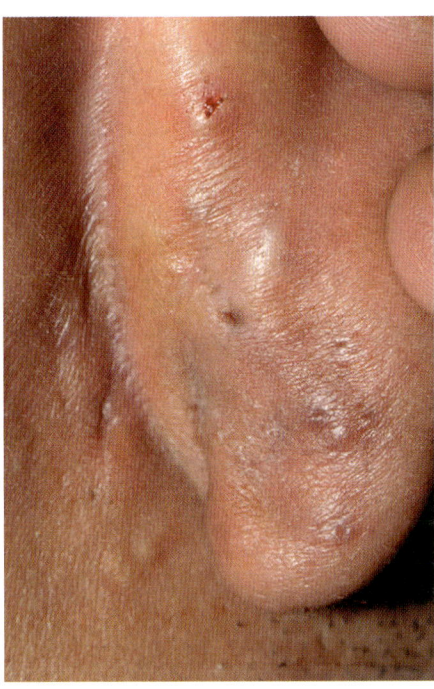

Figure 90.11 Ectopic disease with retroauricular involvement.

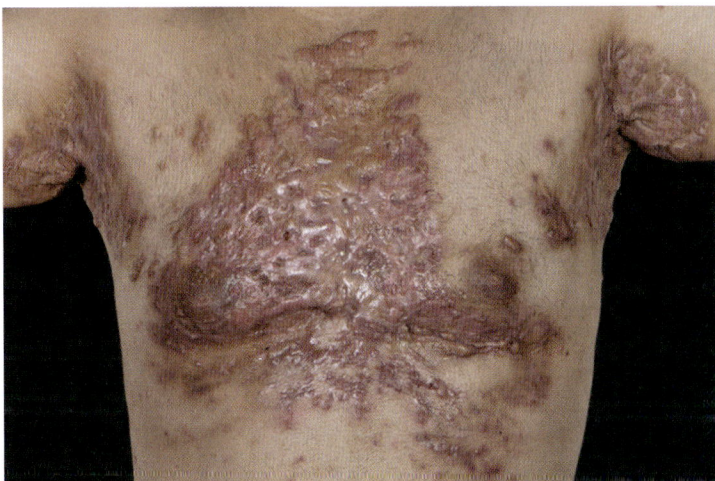

Figure 90.12 Ectopic plaque on the chest of a patient. Notice the classic involvement seen in the axillae.

Table 90.1 Definition of the three Hurley stages in hidradenitis suppurativa.

Stage	Features
I (Figure 90.13)	Recurrent inflammatory skin lesions without skin tunnels and scarring
II (Figure 90.14)	Recurrent inflammatory skin lesions with widely separated skin tunnels and scarring
III (Figure 90.15)	Multiple interconnected inflammatory lesions, skin tunnels and scarring diffusely involving an entire skin region

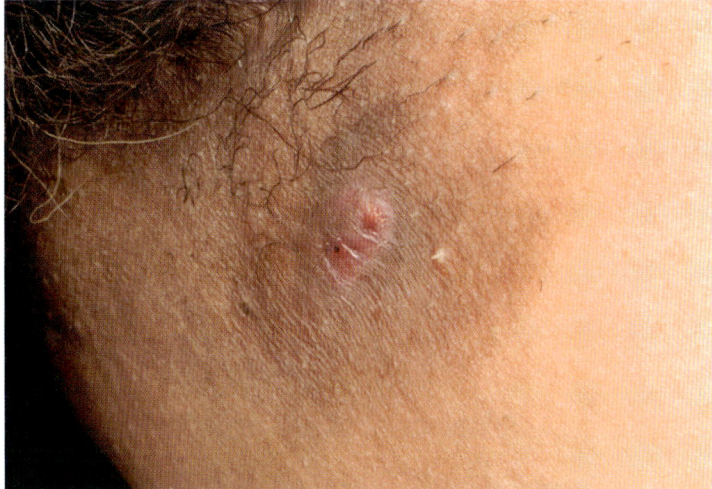

Figure 90.13 Hurley stage I disease of the genito-femoral area showing a solitary nodule. Notice the normal-looking surrounding skin and perilesional halo of discoloration indicating a recent episode of inflammation.

A number of instruments are used to measure HS disease severity dynamically in clinical practice. These include several different lesion count instruments, quality of life scales used in other areas of dermatology such as DLQI and Skindex, pain scores and flare frequency. An international HS core domains process (HISTORIC) is underway to reach consensus between HS patients and clinicians regarding what aspects of disease should be measured in all HS trials (domains) and how these domains should be measured (instruments). Six core domains have been identified: HS-specific quality of life, pain, physical signs, patient and physician global assessment, disease progression (flare frequency and time to recurrence) and symptoms (drainage and fatigue) [69].

Previously, most HS outcome scales were not validated in an HS setting [70]. The hidradenitis suppurativa clinical response (HiSCR) is a validated end point to determine treatment success, developed from the PIONEER trials of adalimumab for HS [71]. It is defined as a ≥50% reduction from baseline in the number of inflamed lesions (abscesses or inflamed nodules), without an increase in the number of abscesses or draining skin tunnels. Work continues to reach consensus on an instrument to dynamically measure changes in HS physical signs in trials, with candidates including IHS4 (International Hidradenitis Suppurativa Severity Score System) and HASI-R (Hidradenitis Suppurativa Area and Severity Index Revised) [72,73]. A HS-specific quality of life instrument, HiSQOL, is now available and validated [74]. Functional effects of pain are included within HiSQOL and the magnitude of pain can be measured using a numerical rating scale from 0 to 10.

Complications and co-morbidities

Superinfection can occur. Structural complications of longstanding disease include lymphatic obstruction leading to clinical lymphoedema. The ano-genital sites are most severely affected (Figure 90.16) and progression to scrotal elephantiasis can occur. Fistula formation to the gastrointestinal tract (anal canal and rectum), genito-urinary tract (urethra, bladder and vagina) and peritoneum is rarely described, and when seen should trigger

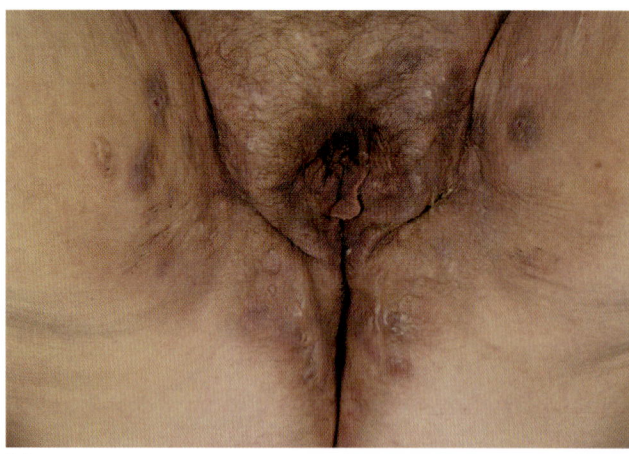

(a)

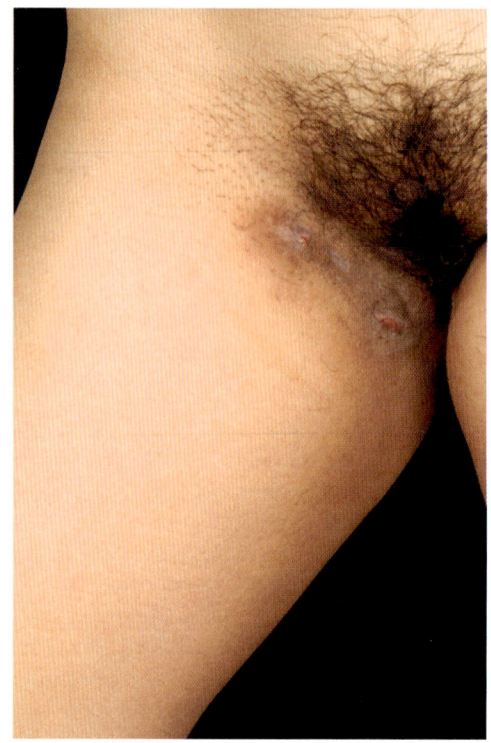

(b)

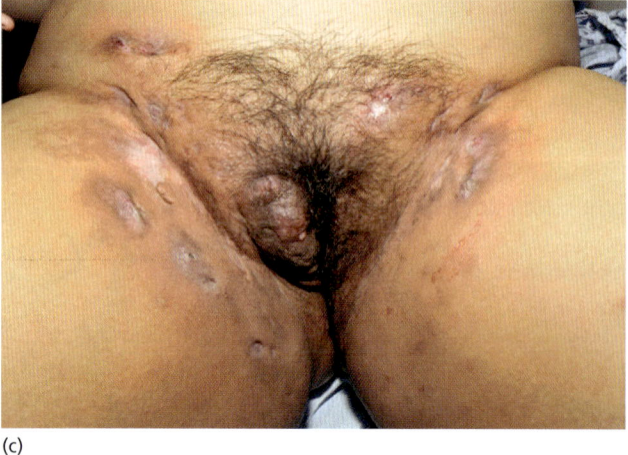

(c)

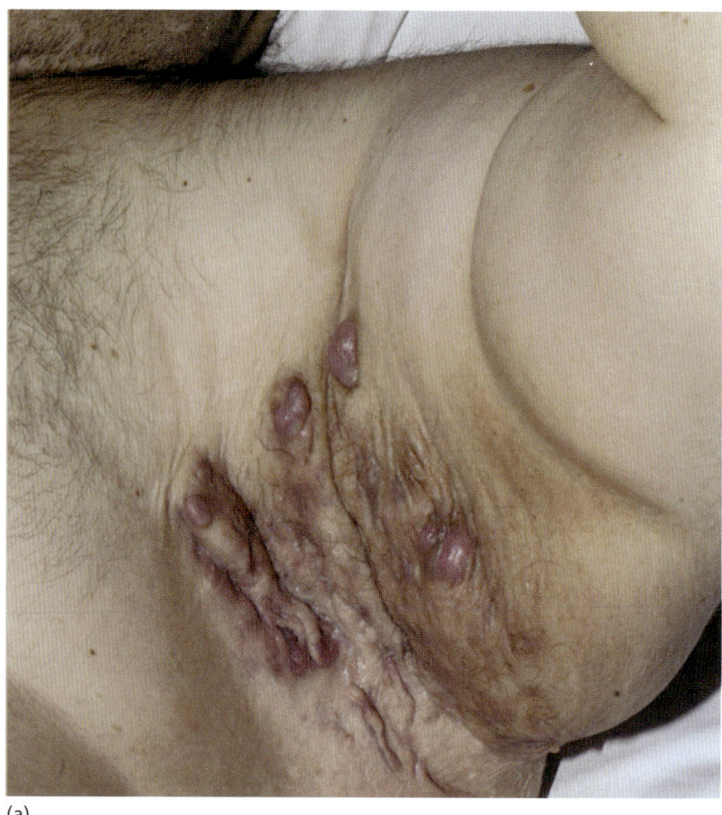

(a)

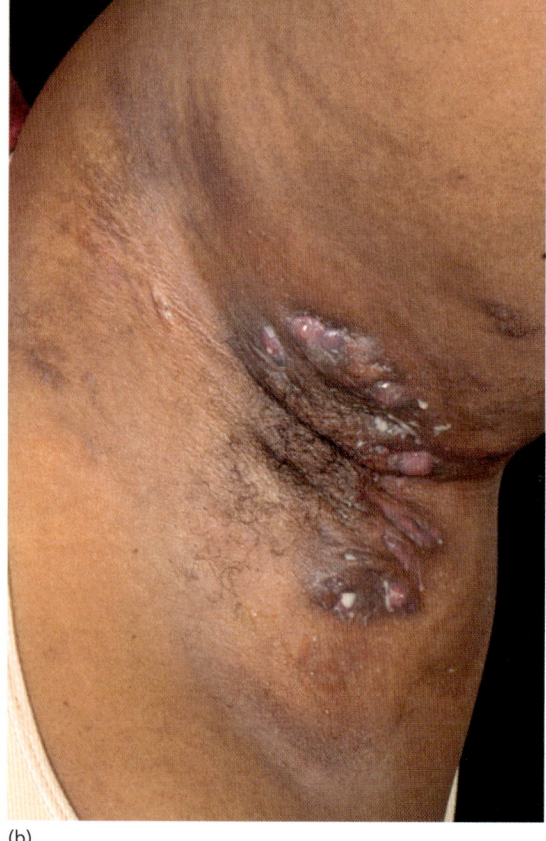

(b)

Figure 90.14 Hurley stage II disease of the genito-femoral area. (a) Hurley stage II is a broad category which may involve more severe disease as shown here. (b) Inactive, mild disease. (c) Active, multifocal disease. Notice the areas of normal-looking skin separating the lesions.

Figure 90.15 Hurley stage III disease. (a) Non-draining, confluent, chronic lesions involving the entire axilla. (b) Active draining lesions in the axilla.

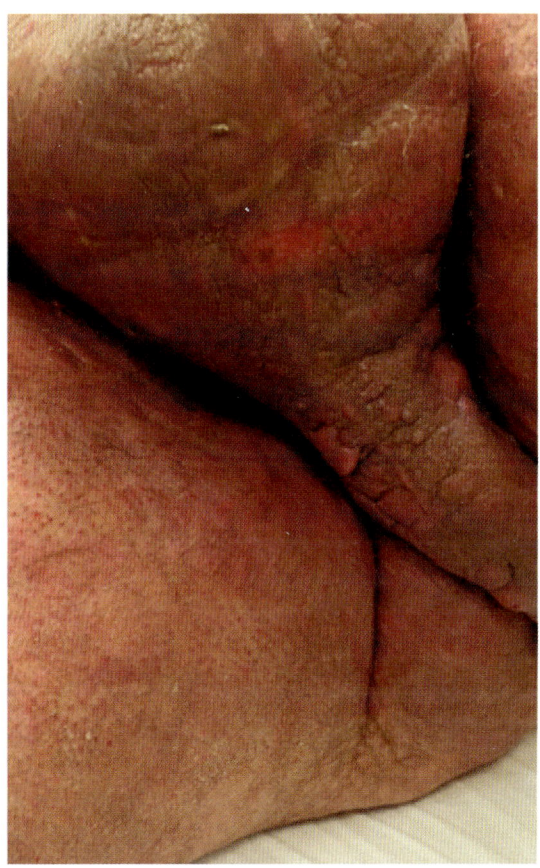

Figure 90.16 Scrotal lymphoedema secondary to chronic hidradenitis suppurativa affecting the region.

examination for Crohn disease. Cutaneous squamous cell carcinoma (SCC) can complicate chronic ano-genital disease, most commonly the perianal, perineal or buttock regions of male patients with longstanding inflammation, and carries a poor prognosis [75]. Other complications of chronic disease include anaemia (multifactorial), hypoalbuminaemia, hypergammaglobulinaemia and rarely amyloidosis and sacral bacterial osteomyelitis [76].

A profound impact on quality of life complicates disease at all stages of severity. Significant psychological, social and economic impact appears more commonly than in many other chronic inflammatory dermatoses [6]. As discussed in the section on associated diseases, depression is frequent and leads to a higher rate of completed suicide [7,26]. A higher incidence of CV risk factors leads to higher rates of CV disease [20,21].

Disease course and prognosis

Chronicity is the hallmark. The mean duration is 19 years [77]. Milder forms (Hurley stage I) are more frequent and reported to affect 45.5% of patients seen in secondary care, with moderate disease (Hurley stage II) affecting 41.5% and severe disease (Hurley stage III) 13% [13]. Both intermittent and continuous disease can be seen at each stage. Most patients do not progress beyond mild disease, however those who do progress tend to reach severe disease relatively rapidly, within 6 years after first symptoms [78]. In patients older than 50 years, the disease is less common, with increasing age suggesting that spontaneous remission may occur

over time. A long-term follow-up study has reported that remission occurs in approximately 40% of HS patients after a median follow-up period of 22 years [79].

Investigations

Microbiology (swabs, purulent exudate and tissue) and histopathology are occasionally indicated for refractory or atypical cases to exclude flare secondary to superinfection and to consider relevant differentials. Imaging (both ultrasound and magnetic resonance imaging) is helpful to define subclinical extension particularly in the perianal region, to check for complications of severe disease and to inform preoperative planning. Routine bloods in severe disease (Hurley stage III) may reveal anaemia (multifactorial), hypoalbuminaemia, polyclonal hypergammaglobulinaemia and elevated C-reactive protein. A screen for diabetes or impaired glucose tolerance should be considered, as well as a fasting lipid profile, to identify any associated CV risks.

Management

The treatment strategy should be individually based and take the following into account:

1 Systemic therapy is required when multiple skin regions are affected.
2 Surgical treatment should be considered for scarring HS, particularly where scars and skin tunnels are acting as foci for recurrent flares.
3 Integration of medical and surgical care, along with screening for co-morbidities and potential complications, is important to provide holistic care, ideally coordinated via a multidisciplinary team approach.
4 As a scarring condition in which increasing disease severity is associated with progressively greater impact on quality of life, management should aim to prevent disease progression.

A management flow chart for HS according to Hurley stage is shown in Figure 90.17.

Adjuvant treatment

Patients should be provided with an information leaflet and made aware of any local patient support groups. Body mass index should be calculated and a referral made to weight management services if necessary. Smoking cessation support should be offered where relevant. Loose-fitting clothes are recommended to minimise friction and patients with suppurative disease should be advised on how to obtain wound dressings [80]

Analgesics

Hidradenitis suppurativa is painful and patients should be offered appropriate analgesic therapy, including paracetamol and non-steroidal anti-inflammatory therapy, and, in selected cases, centrally acting analgesics are indicated [80]. However, chronic use of opioids should be avoided.

Topical and intralesional therapy

Topical clindamycin lotion 0.1% may be beneficial and appears to offer control of mild HS with more superficial lesions [81]. For single inflammatory nodules, intralesional triamcinolone (5–7 mg) often ameliorates symptoms rapidly; topical resorcinol 15% in a suitable

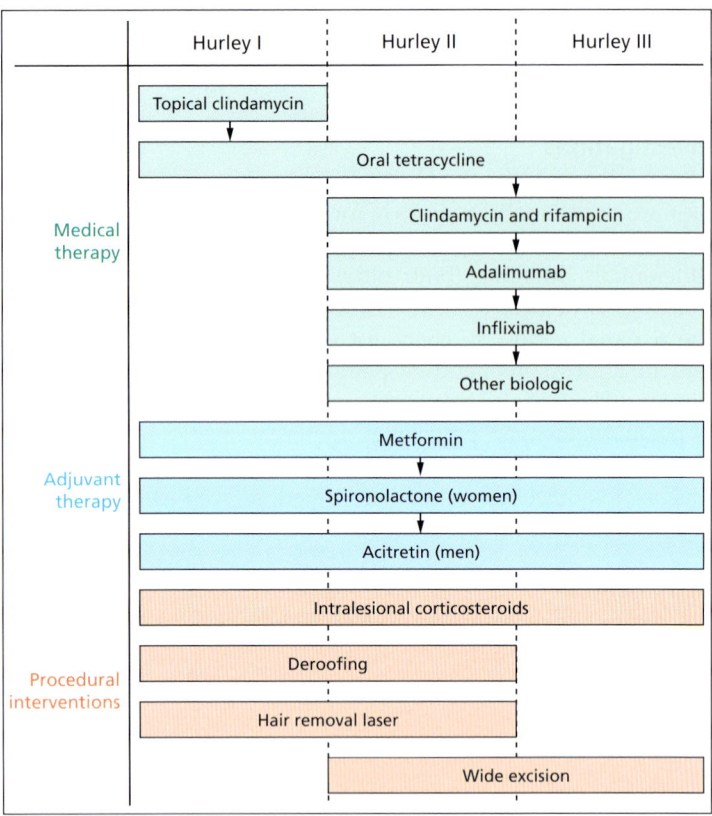

Figure 90.17 Management flow chart for the treatment of hidradenitis suppurativa (HS) according to Hurley stage. Arrows indicate the recommended sequence of interventions, however flexibility may be needed depending on patient preference, co-morbidities and the distribution of active HS lesions.

ointment may also be beneficial, however its use is limited by local availability. Potential benefits of antiseptics such as chlorhexidine washes or benzoyl peroxide remain unproven.

Systemic antibiotics

Oral tetracyclines are usually the initial oral therapy in mild to moderate disease. Double the standard acne dose may be required [80]. Initial treatment is for 12 weeks and longer-term treatment may be considered if they are effective at preventing HS flares. For more advanced cases, combined treatment with clindamycin 300 mg BD and rifampicin 300 mg BD given for 10–12 weeks should be considered. This regimen reduced disease severity by an average of 50% in retrospective case series data [82]. There are no formal studies of longer-term treatment, but responders may require repeated treatments for recurrences, and no additional safety issues with prolonged treatment have been identified [83]. Intravenous antibiotics may be necessary as rescue therapy for very severe suppurative disease unresponsive to oral antibiotic therapy. Intravenous ertapenem 1 g daily for 6 weeks provided substantial benefit in a case series of 30 patients [84].

Other oral therapies

Metformin and spironolactone are used in HS for their antiandrogen properties and case series evidence shows they have modest benefit either as concomitant therapy or monotherapy in some patients [85,86]. Metformin has an additional benefit in obese patients and/or those with impaired glucose tolerance, improving their metabolic profile and providing a degree of weight loss; it can also be used in pregnancy. Spironolactone treatment is restricted to women, at a dose of 75–100 mg daily. Finasteride is an alternative antiandrogen oral therapy in those who are intolerant to spironolactone [87]. Dapsone 50–100 mg daily can be helpful in mild to moderate HS, probably because of its antineutrophil action [88]. Short-term systemic prednisolone (0.5–1.0 mg/kg body weight) may be necessary for severe disease unresponsive to other therapies.

Retinoids

While isotretinoin is helpful for concomitant acne vulgaris, it is rarely effective in HS and its use for HS alone should be avoided. In contrast, case series evidence suggests that acitretin may be effective and in some cases offers long-term remission, however use is limited by avoidance in women of child-bearing potential [89].

Biologic agents

The anti-TNF-α therapy adalimumab is currently the only US Food and Drug Administration (FDA) and European Medicines Agency (EMA) approved treatment for HS. The results from three randomised controlled trials (RCTs) confirmed that adalimumab is effective when given at a dose of 40 mg weekly from week 4, after loading doses of 160 mg at week 0 and 80 mg at week 2 [90,**91**]. The HiSCR end point was achieved by approximately 50% of those on active treatment. In some cases it may be necessary to add in concomitant therapy, such as an oral tetracycline, for additional disease control.

An RCT of standard infliximab failed to reach its primary end point, but a *post hoc* analysis of the results indicated significant improvement in actively treated patients [92]. An RCT of etanercept for HS showed no benefit compared with placebo [93]. A small RCT in 20 HS patients showed benefit from MABp1, an anti-IL-1α biologic therapy [94]. Initial open studies investigating the anti-IL-17 therapy secukinumab and the anti-IL-23 therapy ustekinumab in HS have yielded promising findings and RCT results are now required [95,96].

Surgery

Several lesion-directed therapies can be considered for the management of HS. In general, the removal of larger areas of affected, or potentially affected, skin reduces the recurrence rates at the expense of longer healing times.

Incision and drainage. Classic incision and drainage are useful only for frank fluctuating abscesses. The inflamed nodules of HS are phlegmons rather than abscesses and therefore seldom contain drainable fluid and usually respond with additional scarring. Incisions carry a 100% recurrence rate and should only be used if manifest fluctuation is found [97].

Deroofing. Deroofing is a tissue-saving technique, whereby the 'roof' of a skin tunnel or static scar tissue is surgically removed either through electrosurgery (using a loop) or conventional surgery [98]. A blunt probe is inserted in tunnel openings discharging purulent exudate. If an opening cannot be identified, a small incision is made to introduce a probe into the lesions. The full extent of the lesion is explored systematically with the probe and the roof of the lesion surgically removed using the probe as a guide, leaving the partly epithelialised/granulating floor of the lesion exposed. The ensuing defect is left to heal by secondary intention.

Localised surgery. Single lesions can be surgically excised; this results in a lower recurrence rate than after incision and drainage [99]. Generally, complete surgical removal of the lesion is required, suggesting that wider excisions have a better result than more limited excision. Whether or not the defect should be closed is a matter of debate. Patients with few, clinically stable, non-inflamed lesions (nodules or skin tunnels) are most suitable for localised surgery.

Ablative lasers and electrosurgery. The removal of all involved tissue appears to be necessary for successful surgical treatment of HS. CO_2 laser evaporation provides a method whereby all visibly affected tissue can be vaporised using a scanner in a manner akin to macroscopic Mohs surgery, systematically evaporating abnormal tissue under visual guidance until healthy tissue is reached everywhere [100]. The technique offers radical treatment while still being tissue sparing. Postsurgical defects are usually left to heal by secondary intention. They normally heal sufficiently for resumption of work after 2–3 weeks, but it can take 8–10 weeks for the tissues to re-epithelialise fully.

Extensive surgery. In severe disease when entire sites are involved with multiple interconnecting skin tunnels, the only curative method is excision of the entire area involved. The margins of excision in case series range from 1 cm up to excision of all hair-bearing skin of the affected region. For extensive ano-genital disease, this may therefore require multidisciplinary collaboration with plastic surgery and, if a temporary colostomy is required, with colorectal surgery. Large defects are usually left to heal by secondary intention. Particular attention should, however, be paid to mobilisation of the affected areas in order to avoid the development of postoperative strictures, especially in the axillae. The defects can also be closed by split-skin grafts or flaps, for example in the axilla a thoracodorsal artery perforator flap may be used [101].

Non-ablative lasers/intense pulsed light

Hair removal using laser or light therapies appears to have a beneficial effect in HS. Studies have found significant improvement following monthly treatments with either neodymium:yttrium-aluminium-garnet (Nd:YAG) laser or intense pulsed light (IPL) [102,103].

Integrating biologic and surgical therapy

As both an inflammatory and scarring condition, moderate to severe HS may require a combination of biologic and surgical therapy. There may be a role for initial biologic therapy to delineate areas of scarring, allowing surgery to be more targeted. Experience suggests that biologic treatment should be continued during and after HS skin surgery to prevent a recurrence of inflammation delaying healing and to avoid postoperative relapse [104].

Screening for co-morbidities and complications

In partnership with primary care, dermatologists should be mindful of higher rates of depression, anxiety and CV disease in those with HS. Mental health problems can be detected by a screening questionnaire and blood pressure, HbA1c and/or an oral glucose tolerance test, and fasting lipid levels should be monitored.

Key references

The full list of references can be found in the online version at https://www.wiley.com/rooksdermatology10e

1 Zouboulis CC, Desai N, Emtestam L et al. European S1 guideline for the treatment of hidradenitis suppurativa/acne inversa. *J Eur Acad Dermatol Venereol* 2015;29:619–44.

5 Ingram JR. The epidemiology of hidradenitis suppurativa. *Br J Dermatol* 2020;183:990–8.

6 Matusiak Ł. Profound consequences of hidradenitis suppurativa: a review. *Br J Dermatol* 2020;183:e171–7.

7 Thorlacius L, Cohen AD, Gislason GH et al. Increased suicide risk in patients with hidradenitis suppurativa. *J Invest Dermatol* 2018;138:52–7.

44 Matusiak Ł, Szczęch J, Bieniek A et al. Increased interleukin (IL)-17 serum levels in patients with hidradenitis suppurativa: implications for treatment with anti-IL-17 agents. *J Am Acad Dermatol* 2017;76:670–5.

65 Pink AE, Simpson MA, Desai N et al. Gamma-secretase mutations in hidradenitis suppurativa: new insights into disease pathogenesis. *J Invest Dermatol* 2013;133:601–7.

69 Thorlacius L, Ingram JR, Villumsen B et al. A core domain set for hidradenitis suppurativa trial outcomes: an international Delphi process. *Br J Dermatol* 2018;179:642–50.

80 Ingram JR, Collier F, Brown D et al. British Association of Dermatologists guidelines for the management of hidradenitis suppurativa (acne inversa) 2018. *Br J Dermatol* 2019;180:1009–17.

91 Kimball AB, Okun MM, Williams DA et al. Two phase 3 trials of Adalimumab for hidradenitis suppurativa. *N Engl J Med* 2016;375:422–34.

98 Van der Zee HH, Prens EP, Boer J. Deroofing: a tissue-saving surgical technique for the treatment of mild to moderate hidradenitis suppurativa lesions. *J Am Acad Dermatol* 2010;63:475–80.

PART 8: SPECIFIC CUTANEOUS STRUCTURES

CHAPTER 91

Acquired Non-infective Disorders of the Pilosebaceous Unit

Kapil Bhargava[1,2], *Evangelos Christou*[2] *and Christos Tziotzios*[2]

[1] Barts and Royal London Hospitals, London, UK
[2] St John's Institute of Dermatology, Guy's and St Thomas' NHS Foundation Trust, London, UK

Introduction

The pilosebaceous unit consists of the hair shaft, hair follicle, sebaceous glands and the arrector pili muscles. These structures are under neural and hormonal influences, both local and systemic. In addition, the microbiome, immune system and environmental factors provide a dynamic homeostatic environment. Changes in these factors or in the physical structure of the pilosebaceous unit lead to many of the disorders observed.

Common pilosebaceous disorders, including acne and infective folliculitis, are covered in the preceding chapters. Acquired hair follicle disorders are discussed under superficial folliculitis in which the inflammation is restricted to the infundibular aspect of the follicle, and deep folliculitis where both the deeper follicle and the surrounding dermis are also involved. Sebaceous gland disorders are then discussed.

SUPERFICIAL FOLLICULITIS

Irritant folliculitis

Definition and nomenclature
Irritant folliculitis is a common self-limiting inflammatory disorder resulting from friction or the application of topical agents.

Introduction and general description
Irritant folliculitis often results from the occlusive or chafing effect of tight clothing, dressings and the application of topical medications, particularly ointments or other occlusive topical agents applied in a direction opposite to that of hair growth.

Epidemiology
Incidence and prevalence
The incidence is unknown as the condition is often self-limiting and patients rarely present to a physician.

Pathophysiology
Occlusion of the follicular ostia results in inflammation in the upper regions of the follicle.

Clinical features
Presentation
Follicular erythema and/or pustules occur at the site of contact or exposure to the irritant. Sites with terminal hair growth are more commonly affected

Complications and co-morbidities
A secondary bacterial folliculitis may result.

Management
The condition is self-limiting and removal of the causative agent results in improvement. Topical agents should be applied in the direction of hair growth where required.

PART 8: SPECIFIC CUTANEOUS STRUCTURES

Follicular eruptions due to systemic medications

Definition and nomenclature

Adverse cutaneous effects of systemic medications may present with follicular inflammation.

Synonyms and inclusions
- Acneiform drug eruption
- Drug-induced acne
- Drug-induced folliculitis

Introduction and general description

Follicular drug eruptions are a relatively uncommon type of adverse cutaneous reaction. However, they tend to occur more commonly with certain groups of medications. They are characterised by monomorphic morphology, with the absence of comedones, and arise following initiation of the culprit drug agent.

Epidemiology

Follicular drug eruptions are an uncommon presentation of a cutaneous drug eruption. However, they are well recognised with certain medications: more than 50% of patients taking epidermal growth factor receptor inhibitors (EGFRis), up to 50% of patients using anabolic androgenic steroids, up to 26.8% of women using etonogestrel implants, 15–25% of patients taking sirolimus and 16% of patients taking isoniazid [1].

Pathophysiology

The mechanisms of drug-induced follicular eruptions are related to individual classes of medications and include disturbance of follicular keratinocyte function, changes to sebaceous glands and modification of the microbiome.

EGFRis inhibit epidermal growth factor receptors in normal epidermal keratinocytes, including those in hair follicles. This causes keratinocyte apoptosis, and changes in cell growth and differentiation, which results in release of inflammatory chemokines causing follicular hyperkeratosis, plugging and microorganism growth in the upper follicular apparatus. Interestingly, sirolimus may induce acne because of direct inhibition of EGF activity through inhibition of the mTOR pathway [1,2].

Androgen and androgen-like induced effects on sebaceous glands (including sebocyte proliferation and lipid synthesis) are responsible for acneiform drug eruptions from steroids. Similarly, progestogens with high androgenic activity in hormonal contraceptives may produce adverse effects through a similar mechanism [1].

High-dose vitamin B12 supplementation is known to modulate the transcriptome of the skin microbiota, upregulating inflammatory porphyrins by *Propionibacterium acnes* [3].

Causative medications

A list of causative medications is given in Table 91.1.

Table 91.1 Medications that have an increased observation of follicular cutaneous drug eruptions. Reproduced from Du Thanh *et al.* 2011 [1] with permission from Springer Nature.

Hormones
Local and systemic corticosteroids
Corticotropin (ACTH)
Androgens and anabolic steroids
Hormonal contraceptives
Other hormones (thyroid-stimulating hormone, danazol)
Neuropsychotherapeutic drugs
Tricyclic antidepressants (amineptine, maprotiline, imipramine)
Lithium
Antiepileptic drugs
Aripiprazole
Selective serotonin reuptake inhibitors
Vitamins
Vitamins B_1, B_6, B_{12}
Cytostatic drugs
Dactinomycin (actinomycin D)
Azathioprine, thiourea, thiouracil
Immunomodulating molecules
Cyclosporine (ciclosporin)
Sirolimus
Others: topical tacrolimus, topical pimecrolimus
Antituberculosis drugs
Isoniazid
Rifampin (rifampicin)
Ethionamide
Halogens
Iodine
Bromine
Chlorine
Others: halothane gas, lithium
Miscellaneous
Dantrolene
Quinidine
Antiretroviral therapy
Targeted therapies
EGF inhibitors (cetuximab, panitumumab)
Multitargeted tyrosine kinase inhibitors (gefitinib, erlotinib, lapatinib sorafenib, sunitinib imatinib)
VEGF inhibitor: bevacizumab
Proteasome inhibitor: bortezomib
TNF-α inhibitors (lenalidomide infliximab)
Histone deacetylase inhibitor: vorinostat

EGF, epidermal growth factor; TNF-α, tumor necrosis factor α; VEGF, vascular endothelial growth factor.

Clinical features

Presentation

The eruption usually occurs within 2 weeks to 3 months of starting the medication, although it may appear many months after initiation of isoniazid, lithium or anticonvulsants. The age of onset may occur outside the characteristic age range for acne vulgaris.

The eruption is composed of monomorphic, follicular inflammatory papules and pustules, and comedones are usually *absent* in the inflammatory phase but may appear later (Figure 91.1). The distribution may extend beyond the seborrhoeic regions to include the arms, trunk and lower back.

Androgenic medications such as hormonal contraceptives may exacerbate pre-existing acne with characteristic lesions present including comedones. A sudden exacerbation in the severity of acne is a useful indicator in this situation.

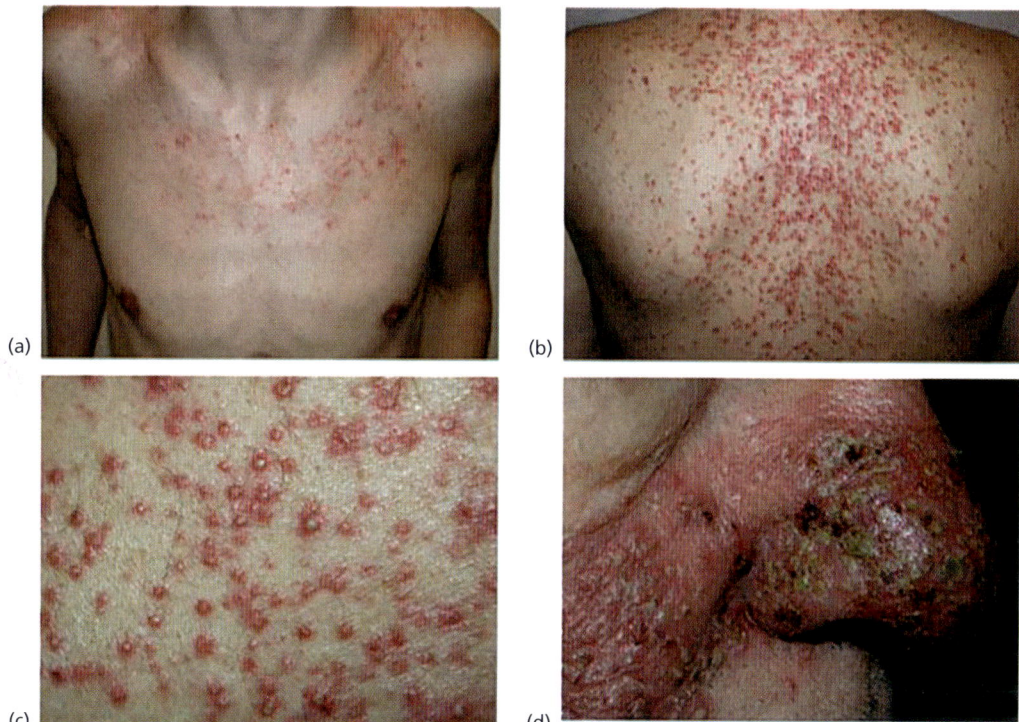

Figure 91.1 Acneiform eruption. (a) Papular lesions on the chest. (b) V-shaped papulopustular eruption on the back. (c) Close-up of follicular pustules. (d) Confluent pustules on the nose. Reproduced from Segaert *et al.* [4] with permission from Elsevier.

Differential diagnosis
Acne vulgaris and infective folliculitis.

Management
Withdrawal of the causative drug is likely to result in improvement over a few weeks. While good quality evidence is not available for the optimal treatment when the drug needs to be continued, the topical and oral treatments commonly used in acne are prescribed.

Topical therapies including benzoyl peroxide, clindamycin or erythromycin and retinoids may be helpful in patients with mild folliculitis. Systemic tetracycline antibiotics and oral isotretinoin can be beneficial in more severe folliculitis.

Randomised controlled trials in patients with EGFR-targeting agents show that oral doxycycline and minocycline are effective in reducing rash severity in primary prevention and treatment [4–7]. Lymecycline is often used in preference for its improved tolerability and is less photosensitising. Maintenance of the skin barrier through soap substitutes, regular moisturisation, avoidance of irritant products and use of sunscreen (when exposure cannot be avoided) are important adjunctive measures. Topical steroids may also be helpful. Epidermal growth factor ointment has been successfully trialled in one study to reduce EGFis-related skin toxicities [8].

Eosinophilic pustular folliculitis

Definition
Eosinophilic pustular folliculitis is an uncommon cutaneous reaction pattern characterised by infiltration of the pilosebaceous follicles by large numbers of eosinophils. Three different forms are recognised: classical, immunosuppression-associated and infantile.

Introduction and general description
Eosinophilic pustular folliculitis is an uncommon inflammatory cutaneous reaction pattern of poorly understood aetiology, which is characterised by infiltration of the pilosebaceous follicles by large numbers of eosinophils. The classical adult form, Ofuji disease, is predominantly facial and is reported principally from Japan [1,2]. Immunosuppression-associated eosinophilic pustular folliculitis is strongly associated with HIV infection and is more often extrafacial [3]. Infantile eosinophilic pustular folliculitis, which has also been termed infantile eosinophilic pustulosis, would seem to have little in common with the adult forms and is described separately later.

Epidemiology
Age
Classical and immunosuppression-associated pustular folliculitis typically occur in young adults, with the former demonstrating a peak between 30 and 40 years. In the paediatric population, patients aged 5–10 months are typically affected although neonates have been reported.

Sex
Male to female ratio 5 : 1.

Ethnicity
The majority of classical eosinophilic pustular folliculitis patients have been reported from Japan.

Pathophysiology

Predisposing factors

The cause of the immune dysregulation in eosinophilic pustular folliculitis is not understood. Immaturity or suppression of the immune system appears to be important, although this has not been demonstrated in the classical adult form. Many hypotheses, including hypersensitivity reactions to *Malassezia* spp., *Demodex* spp. or sebaceous gland-derived lipids, have been proposed [1]. Various chemotactic factors have been detected in the fluid of the pustules, which are sterile, and it has been suggested that they may serve to localise excessive circulating eosinophils [4]. Sebocytes may play a key role by inducing eosinophil chemotaxis around the pilosebaceous area through eotaxin-3 production upon prostaglandin D_2 (PGD_2) stimulation. There are several reports of the condition erupting during pregnancy [5–7]. Medications have been described as causal factors and more specifically carbamazepine, minocycline, allopurinol, indeloxazine hydrochloride and chemotherapy [8]. Additionally, it can occur in the background of a variety of haematological malignancies, such as Hodgkin and non-Hodgkin lymphoma, chronic lymphocytic leukaemia, acute and chronic myeloid leukaemias, acute lymphoblastic leukaemia, multiple myeloma, Waldenström macroglobulinaemia, Sézary syndrome, T-cell lymphomas and polycythemia rubra vera [9]. A case of facial eosinophilic pustular folliculitis has been described a few years following a nose and chin augmentation with subcutaneous silicone injections, while another has been reported to occur on a mastectomy surgical scar [10,11].

Pathology

The follicular inflammation is characterised by heavy infiltration of the outer root sheath and sebaceous gland by eosinophils accompanied by scattered mononuclear cells and neutrophils (Figure 91.2). This is best detected by serial horizontal sectioning of biopsies of fresh unexcoriated papules or pustules. Perifollicular and perivascular infiltration by eosinophils is also seen. In immunosuppression-associated eosinophilic pustular folliculitis, the inflammation may be more diffuse [3].

Mild to moderate peripheral blood eosinophilia is seen in up to 35% of patients [1,2,12] with classical type and in up to 50% with HIV-associated eosinophilic pustular folliculitis, which usually occurs when the CD4 count is less than 200 cells/mL [13].

Genetics

There is no known genetic predisposition.

Clinical features

Classical adult eosinophilic pustular folliculitis

This is a chronic relapsing disease in which crops of sterile follicular papules and pustules coalesce into inflammatory annular plaques with peripheral expansion and central clearing. It takes 7–10 days for the inflammation to subside before the cycle repeats itself a few weeks later [3]. The face is the commonest site of involvement (Figure 91.3): in a review of 91 Japanese cases, the face, trunk and extremities were involved in 88%, 40% and 26%, respectively [12]. Pustular inflammation of the palms and soles may be seen in up to a fifth of cases, even though follicles are not present in palmoplantar skin. This may cause diagnostic confusion with palmoplantar

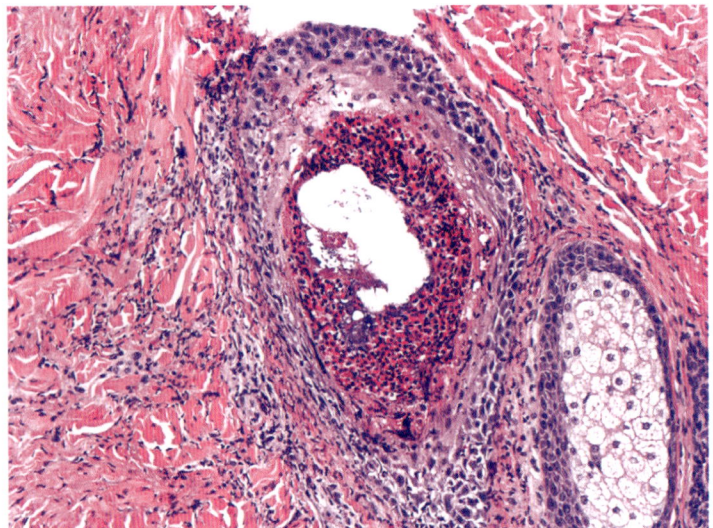

Figure 91.2 Histopathology of eosinophilic pustular folliculitis showing dense accumulation of eosinophils within the follicular canal. Courtesy of Professor Luis Requena.

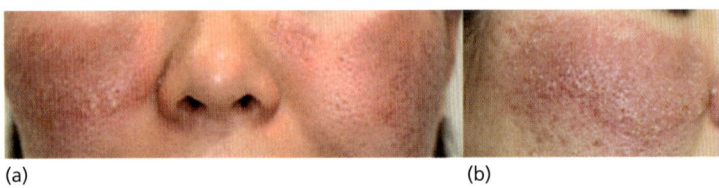

(a)   (b)

Figure 91.3 (a,b) Classical eosinophilic pustular folliculitis: well-defined, dark erythematous plaques with numerous pustules and crusts involving the cheeks. Reproduced from Ramdial *et al.* [5] with permission from Wolters Kluwer.

pustulosis [14]. The trunk and the upper outer arms are also frequently involved, and the legs and scalp occasionally. Widespread involvement has occurred [15].

The inflammatory plaques may reach 3–5 cm in diameter before subsiding to leave slight pigmentation. Lakes of pus and erosions are sometimes seen. Itch is frequent and may be severe but is not invariable. Patients are systemically well. The overall course is chronic with new crops of lesions repeatedly reappearing in affected areas, although a few cases have entered spontaneous remission. Eosinophilic folliculitis due to wearing protective gear in citizens volunteering for sanitation services during the Covid-19 pandemic has recently been described [16].

Immunosuppression-associated eosinophilic pustular folliculitis

This has been reported predominantly in association with HIV and AIDS, but also in the setting of bone marrow and stem cell transplantation [1,9,13,17,18] (Chapter 31). It differs in a number of respects from the classical form. It is not restricted to the Japanese and pruritus is typically much more intense. The pustular element is often not as prominent and clustering into plaques is not a characteristic feature [1]. Facial skin is less commonly involved. The clinical signs may be subtle, sometimes with just scattered follicular papules or excoriations (Figure 91.4), and multiple biopsies may be required to confirm the diagnosis.

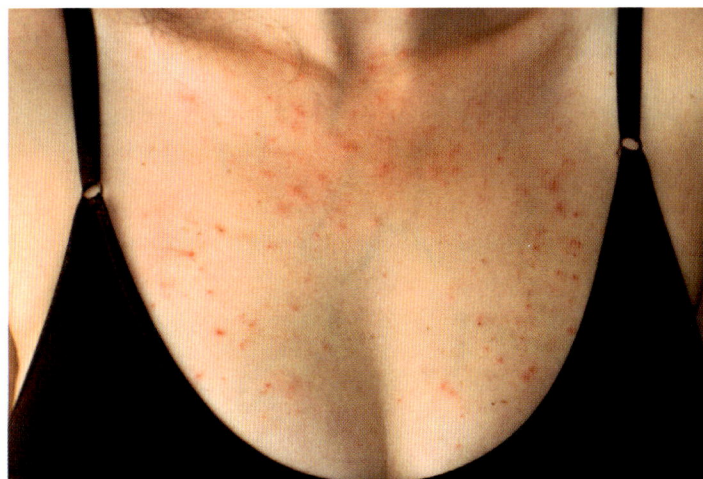

Figure 91.4 Immunodeficiency-associated eosinophilic pustular folliculitis in a 32-year-old woman with HIV infection: view of anterior chest. Courtesy of Professor Luis Requena.

Paradoxically, although eosinophilic pustular folliculitis may first develop after the CD4 count starts to rise with the introduction of highly active antiretroviral therapy (HAART), in which case it may be accompanied by the immune reconstitution inflammatory syndrome (IRIS), generally it improves with HAART, possibly through restoration of Th1 immune response [**19**].

Differential diagnosis

Folliculitis, follicular mucinosis, mycosis fungoides, dermatophyte infections, papular urticaria, acne, rosacea, lupus miliaris disseminatus faciei, palmoplantar pustulosis, subcorneal pustular dermatosis and drug-induced eosinophilic pustular folliculitis. As the clinical presentation is non-specific and differential diagnoses wide, biopsy of the lesions is recommended. For some cases the final diagnosis is made after careful interpretation of the clinical and histological findings, especially as the initial lesions of cutaneous T-cell lymphoma have the same histological characteristics [20].

Investigations

In the classical form a mild to moderate peripheral blood eosinophilia is present in about half of patients. In HIV disease the CD4 count is often <300 cells/mm^3. Infants may have an elevated serum IgE level.

Skin swabs for microscopy and culture will be useful in detecting infection and a biopsy with immunofluorescence and concurrent serum for desmoglein ELISA will be helpful to exclude pemphigus in vesicular presentations.

Management

A comprehensive review of the various treatments showed that no treatment is consistently effective, and treatment has to be tailored to the individual patient [17]. Systemic corticosteroids are usually but not always helpful; potent topical corticosteroids are sometimes of some value, while topical pimecrolimus and tacrolimus have also been advocated [21]. Oral non-steroidal anti-inflammatory drugs (NSAIDs) are widely used in Japan for the classical form: in a review of published Japanese cases, nearly 80% reportedly responded to indomethacin, possibly through interfering with the

PGD$_2$-induced chemotaxis of eosinophils [12,22]. The combination of low-dose oral indomethacin and topical tacrolimus was safe and effective in two cases, reducing the risk of NSAIDs side effects [8]. Dapsone is effective in some cases [22,23] and ultraviolet B (UVB) therapy was helpful in six HIV-associated cases [24], although maintenance treatment was required. Other reported therapeutic options with varied efficacy include topical permethrin, minocycline, isotretinoin, itraconazole, cetirizine, metronidazole and colchicine [12].

Treatment ladder

First line
- Topical pimecrolimus or tacrolimus
- Topical indomethacin
- Combination of low-dose topical indomethacin and topical tacrolimus
- Potent topical corticosteroids

Second line
- Oral indomethacin
- Narrow-band UVB phototherapy
- PUVA (psoralen plus ultraviolet A) phototherapy
- Dapsone
- Oral corticosteroids
- Oral antimicrobials (minocycline, itraconazole)
- Cetirizine
- Oral isotretinoin

Infantile eosinophilic pustular folliculitis

Definition and nomenclature

Infantile eosinophilic pustular folliculitis is an inflammatory pustular disorder of infants associated with cutaneous and peripheral blood eosinophilia.

Synonyms and inclusions
- Infancy-associated eosinophilic pustular folliculitis
- Infantile eosinophilic pustulosis

Introduction and general description

Infantile eosinophilic pustular folliculitis is an inflammatory pustular disorder of infants associated with cutaneous and peripheral blood eosinophilia. It was first reported in 1984 by Lucky *et al.* [**1**]. It is characterised by recurrent outbreaks of non-infective pustules containing eosinophils on the scalp of infants. In the majority of cases, the condition commences before the age of 6 months and remits by the age of 3 years. In two-thirds of cases, body areas other than the scalp are affected. The cause is unknown. It was originally considered and is still generally termed a folliculitis, but in a substantial number of cases no follicular involvement has been found [2,3].

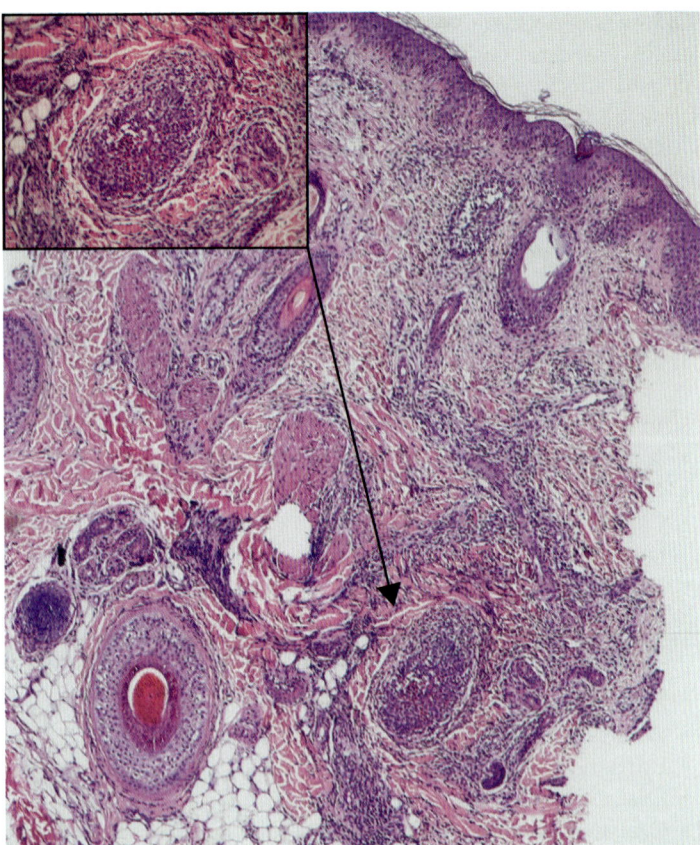

Figure 91.5 Infantile eosinophilic pustular folliculitis with dense infiltrate of eosinophils, spongiosis and microabscess formation within the follicle (inset). Reproduced from Alonso-Castro *et al.* [7] with permission from California Digital Library.

Epidemiology

Age
Average age at presentation is 6 months [4].

Sex
More common in boys, with a male to female ratio of 4:1.

Associated diseases
A case of HIV-associated infantile eosinophilic pustular folliculitis has been described in an infant [5]. It has also been associated with hyper-IgE syndrome and atopic disease [6].

Pathophysiology
Pathology
Tzanck smear shows an abundance of eosinophils. Biopsy shows an intense follicular polymorphonuclear and eosinophilic infiltrate (Figure 91.5), occasionally demonstrating flame figures [3]. Affected hair follicles were identified in only 63% of biopsies in a large case series [2], with eosinophils also affecting the perifollicular and periadnexal areas [3].

Causative organisms
Bacteriology is usually negative.

Genetics
It has been reported in brothers [3].

Clinical features
Presentation
It is characterised by recurrent crops of itchy sterile pustules, which recur over several months or years. The sterile pustules develop on the scalp predominantly (Figure 91.6), but lesions may occur at other sites such as face, trunk, palms, legs and soles. Children may develop axillary, inguinal or cervical lymphadenopathy [7]. Pustular lesions resolve spontaneously without scarring [8].

Differential diagnosis
Other neonatal and infantile pustular eruptions which should be considered in the differential diagnosis are shown in Table 91.2.

Disease course and prognosis
This is a self-limiting disease with frequent flares. Spontaneous resolution usually occurs from 4 months to 9 years of age, with up to 80% of cases resolving by 3 years of age [3].

Investigations
Tzanck smear, culture for bacteria and fungi, HIV test and IgE levels.

Management
Topical steroids are generally effective [4]. Because the condition is self-limiting, aggressive treatment is not recommended; however, oral indomethacin or dapsone can be helpful, particularly in recalcitrant or extensive disease [8,9]. Topical tacrolimus and antihistamines with anti-eosinophilic activity, such as cetirizine and cimetidine, can be effective alternative treatment options [3,10].

Treatment ladder

First line
- Expectancy
- Topical corticosteroids

Second line
- Antihistamines
- Topical tacrolimus

Third line
- Oral indomethacin
- Dapsone

Actinic folliculitis

Definition and nomenclature
Actinic folliculitis is a rare photodermatosis of unknown aetiology characterised by the development of pruritic monomorphic follicular papules and pustules appearing on photo-exposed sites several hours to days after sunlight exposure.

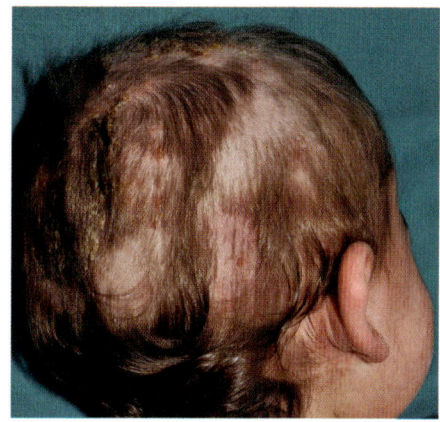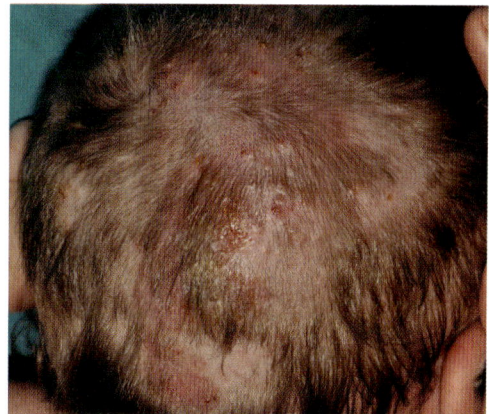

Figure 91.6 Sterile pustules in the scalp of a young boy with infantile eosinophilic pustular folliculitis. Courtesy of Dr Antonio Torrelo.

Table 91.2 Differential diagnosis of infantile eosinophilic pustular folliculitis.

Diagnosis	Incidence	Site	Lesions	Onset	Duration	Peripheral eosinophilia	Tzanck smear	Histology
Infantile eosinophilic pustular folliculitis	Rare	Scalp, trunk (± hands, feet)	Vesicles, pustules, crusts	Birth or later	Cyclical outbreaks for 3 months to 5 years	During outbreaks in some patients	Eosinophils	Eosinophilic spongiosis; subcorneal pustules; eosinophilic folliculitis
Erythema toxicum neonatorum	One-third of neonates	Face, trunk, limbs	Macules, vesicles, pustules	Birth–7 h	Resolves within 1 week	Up to 15%	Eosinophils	Eosinophilic folliculitis; subcorneal eosinophilic pustules
Transient neonatal pustular melanosis	4–5% of black infants; 0.1–0.3% of white infants	Neck, trunk, thighs, palms, soles	Vesicles, pustules, pigmented macules	Birth–2 h	Resolves within weeks	May occur	Neutrophils, occasional eosinophils	Neutrophilic intracorneal and subcorneal pustules
Infantile acropustulosis	Rare; mainly in black males	Hands, feet (± scalp, face, trunk)	Pruritic papules, vesicles, pustules	Neonatal period or later	Lesions last 7–10 days, crops recur for 2 months to years	May occur	Neutrophils, occasional eosinophils	Subcorneal pustules containing neutrophils; occasional eosinophils
Langerhans cell histiocytosis	Rare	Scalp, flexures	Papules, pustules, vesicles, crusts	Birth or later	Varies depending on systemic involvement	No	Histiocytes	Infiltrate of Langerhans cells; Birbeck granules on electron microscopy

Reproduced from Rahman *et al.* 2020 [3] with permission from John Wiley & Sons.

Synonyms and inclusions

- Actinic superficial folliculitis
- Acne aestivalis
- Mallorca acne

Introduction and general description

Actinic folliculitis is a rare photodermatosis of unknown aetiology characterised by the development of pruritic monomorphic follicular papules and pustules appearing on the face, neck, arms and/or upper trunk several hours to days after sunlight exposure. Photoprotection and abstinence from sun exposure normally lead to remission, with the lesions resolving within 10–14 days. Cultures for microorganisms are negative. Histologically, there is a superficial neutrophilic folliculitis with an admixture of lymphocytes [1].

Epidemiology
Age
Actinic folliculitis has been described in young to middle-aged adults of both sexes.

Sex
Males and females are equally affected.

Pathophysiology
Predisposing factors
Exposure to sunlight is a predisposing factor. Although the exact pathophysiological mechanisms are still not well understood, the reported seasonal variability and triggering of the lesions through window glass pinpoint a key role for ultraviolet A (UVA) [2] and provocation with iterative doses of broadband UVA has been shown [2]. UV radiation may induce occlusion of the follicular ostia through epidermal thickening and follicular infundibular thickening [3], although the aetiology is not confirmed.

Clinical features
Presentation
Monomorphic follicular papules and pustules erupt over the face, neck, upper arms, shoulders and/or upper chest following as little as a few hours to up to a week of sun exposure. In some patients it may appear in sunlight abroad, but not in the UK [2]. There may be a

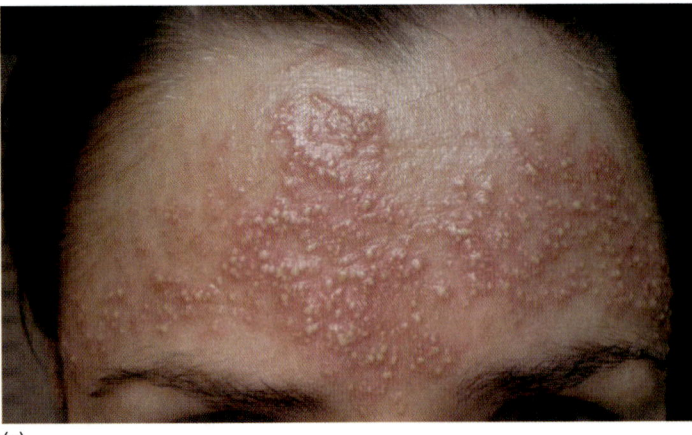

(a)

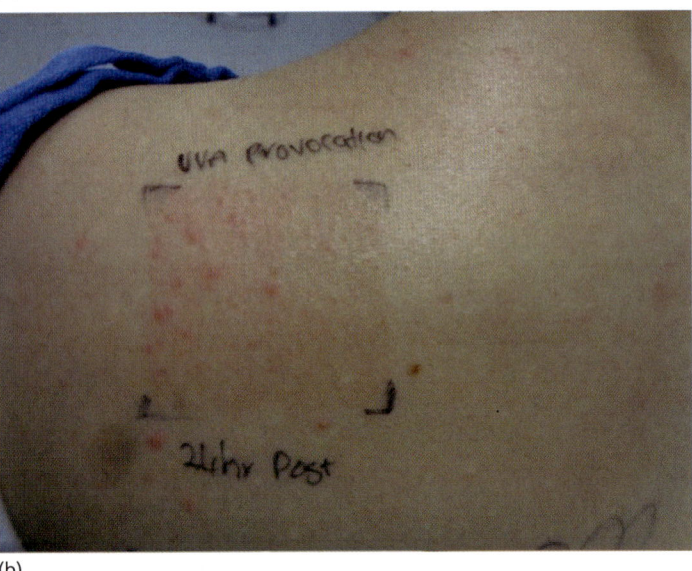

(b)

Figure 91.7 Follicular pustules on (a) the forehead and on (b) the left upper back 24 hours after irradiation with broadband UVA in a patient with actinic folliculitis. Reproduced from Butt *et al.* [2] with permission from John Wiley & Sons.

burning sensation or pruritus at the onset, resolving within 10 days [4,5]. Another report describes itchy pustules and papules on the lower face resolving within 4 days [6]. The mechanism is unknown.

Differential diagnosis

Polymorphic light eruption, miliaria, papulopustular rosacea, photoaggravated rosacea, photoaggravated acne vulgaris.

Disease course and prognosis

It may recur annually over many years and demonstrate seasonal variability, being most active at the beginning of the summer.

Investigations

Iterative broadband UVA provocation tests can be performed to support the diagnosis (Figure 91.7). Monochromator phototesting is usually normal, although a reduced minimal erythema dose (MED) has been observed [2].

Management

Photoprotection with behavioural modification, hats, clothing and high-factor sunscreen may be beneficial. Antibiotics, either oral or topical, are ineffective, but severe cases may respond to oral isotretinoin [6,7]. Topical retinoid application a few weeks in advance of the anticipated sun exposure could be an effective and well-tolerated alternative option. Narrowband ultraviolet-B (NB-UVB) phototherapy may provide useful and effective long-term desensitisation [2].

DEEP FOLLICULITIS

Pseudofolliculitis

Definition and nomenclature

Pseudofolliculitis is a chronic follicular and perifollicular inflammatory disorder due to foreign-body skin reaction to hair trapped beneath the skin surface.

Synonyms and inclusions

- Ingrown hairs
- Pili incarnati
- Pseudofolliculitis barbae
- Razor bumps
- Shave bumps

Introduction and general description

Pseudofolliculitis is a chronic follicular and perifollicular inflammatory disorder which occurs from penetration or retraction of the cut ends of hair into the skin following shaving or as the result of disturbed hair growth following plucking or waxing. Areas particularly affected are those most frequently shaved including the beard, pubic areas and lower legs.

Epidemiology
Incidence and prevalence

The exact prevalence is unknown. It is particularly common in men, but it can also affect females and generally those with curly hair. Pseudofolliculitis barbae occurs in 10–80% of adult black men, particularly those who shave closely on a regular basis [1].

Age
After puberty.

Sex
Males are more commonly affected than females.

Ethnicity
Men of African and Hispanic descent are particularly predisposed.

Pathophysiology
Predisposing factors

Pseudofolliculitis results either from the hair being cut too short,

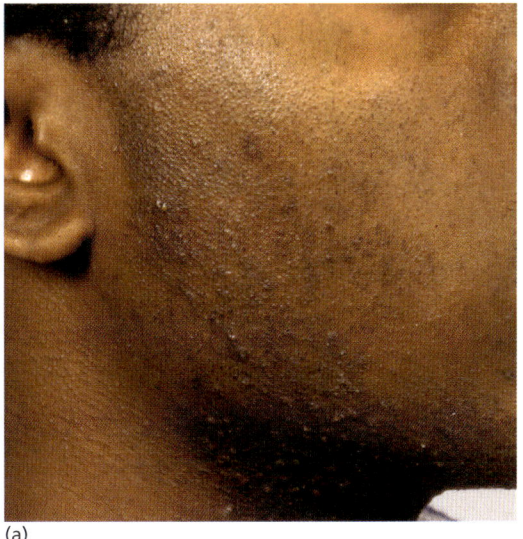
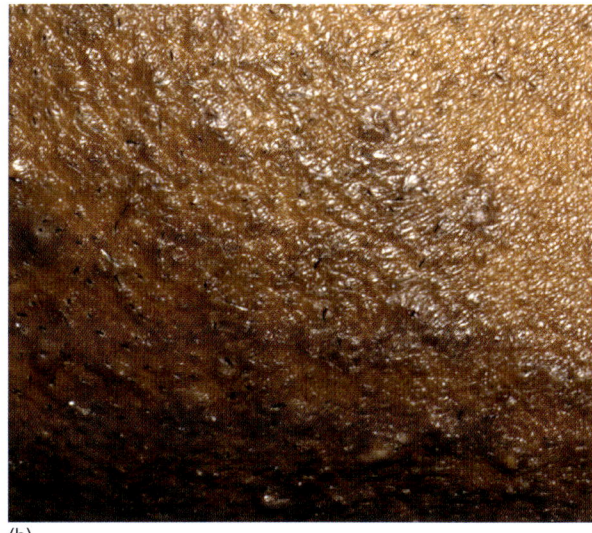

Figure 91.8 Pseudofolliculitis barbae showing typical distribution (a) and close-up view (b).

(a)   (b)

so that it may retract into the follicle and then directly penetrate the follicle wall, or from hair left to grow for a few days after being cut or shaved, such that the hairs curve backwards and penetrate adjacent skin [2,3]. Underlying genetic predisposition plays an important role in individuals who are genetically determined to have curly hair because they are more liable to both of these aberrations; the condition is very common and more severe in those with tightly coiled hair [3,4,**5**]. Skin folds or irregularities due to scarring may also allow ingrowth of straight hairs.

Shaving practices play an important contributory role to pseudofolliculitis, including daily shaving without pre- and post-shave care. Both plucking [6] and waxing [7] of hair, particularly on the limbs, commonly lead to pseudofolliculitis in females. Cut nasal hairs may act similarly [8]. Hyperandrogenism can be a contributing factor in females as it is associated with increased hair growth and the use of shaving or depilation for cosmetic reasons [9]. Pseudofolliculitis has also been reported as an adverse drug reaction to oral minoxidil [10].

Pathology
Penetration of aberrant cut ends of the hair into the follicle or surrounding tissue results in acute inflammation, microabscesses and foreign-body giant cell granuloma formation.

Causative organisms
Coagulase-negative staphylococci may sometimes be grown from the lesions. However, the condition is not primarily infective but rather a foreign-body inflammatory reaction.

Clinical features
Presentation
The condition typically manifests as multiple small firm papules and pustules on shaven skin. Any shaved surface in either sex may be affected, with the male beard area most commonly affected. The skin of the anterior and posterior neck and over the jaw is also commonly affected as well as the cheeks, chin, axilla, pubic area and legs (Figures 91.8 and 91.9). Papules may be large and may scar, with

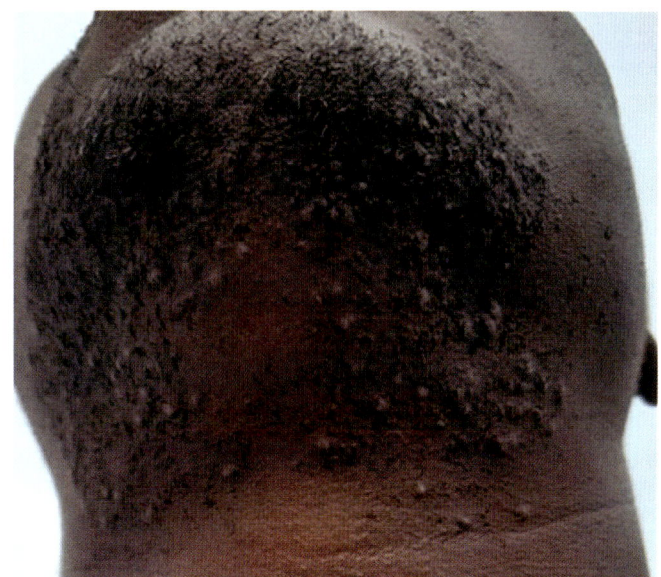

Figure 91.9 Pseudofolliculitis barbae affecting the chin and upper neck. Courtesy of Dr Ibrahima Traore.

keloid formation and hyperpigmentation possibly ensuing. It is generally possible to identify some penetrating hairs, but they may not be visible in all cases. Where there is clinical doubt, it is sometimes possible to extract a coiled hair using the tip of a sterile needle. The clinical appearance can lead to significant psychological distress.

The diagnosis is usually obvious based on the clinical findings. Dermoscopy aids diagnosis by demonstrating ingrown hairs, extrafollicular penetration, perifollicular and follicular papules and pustules. In cases where sites other than the beard area are affected, a history of shaving, plucking or waxing should help to clinch the diagnosis.

Differential diagnosis
Bacterial folliculitis including sycosis barbae and dermatophytosis, fungal infection, traumatic folliculitis, acne keloidalis nuchae and cutaneous sarcoidosis.

PART 8: SPECIFIC CUTANEOUS STRUCTURES

Complications and co-morbidities

Pseudofolliculitis, particularly of the beard area, can result in hypertrophic or keloid scarring. Postinflammatory hyperpigmentation is also a common complication.

Females with pseudofolliculitis are commonly affected by acne and disorders characterised by hyperadrogenism, such as polycystic ovarian syndrome (PCOS), hirsutism and infertility [9].

Disease course and prognosis

Pseudofolliculitis is a chronic condition with a relapsing and remitting course. Avoiding shaving can allow the skin to recover, otherwise intermittent treatment may be required. Permanent hair removal at high-risk sites may be appropriate in selected cases.

Management

Cessation of shaving/waxing for a minimum of 4–6 weeks will allow the inflammation to settle and the hairs to grow sufficiently long to prevent ingrowth. Resumption of shaving or waxing will often lead to relapse [3]. Therefore, alternative shaving and hair removal practices should be implemented. If clean shaving is required, shaving regularly, even daily, with light strokes and using a technologically advanced multiblade razor with pre-shave hair hydration and post-shave moisturisation has been shown not to cause exacerbations [11]. Lifting out re-entrant hairs with a needle can be helpful but tedious and brushing with an abrasive sponge or toothbrush to 'release' the hair is less effective but quicker. Plucking should be avoided. Hair removal with chemical depilatories or topical eflornithine hydrochloride cream may be helpful for some patients. Laser hair removal has been shown to be effective treatment by reducing the density and thickness of the hair and there is evidence that the combination of eflornithine cream and laser is better than laser depilation alone [12,13]. Some relief is possible with benzoyl peroxide, low-potency topical steroids and topical antimicrobial either alone or in combinations [1]. Topical retinoids and topical glycolic acid therapy have also be shown to be effective.

Treatment ladder

First line
- Stop shaving the affected area for 6 weeks and apply topical combination steroid/antibacterial cream

Second line
- Regular shaving, even daily, using a technologically advanced multiblade razor
- Perform pre-shave hair hydration and post-shave moisturisation
- Use chemical depilatories rather than physical hair removal

Third line
- Combination of eflornithine cream and laser hair removal in the affected area

---

Folliculitis keloidalis

Definition and nomenclature

Folliculitis keloidalis is a chronic scarring folliculitis involving principally the hair follicles of the nape of the neck and occipital scalp and leading to papules, plaques and hypertrophic scars.

Synonyms and inclusions
- Acne keloidalis nuchae
- Acne keloidalis
- Dermatitis papillaris capillitia
- Folliculitis keloidalis nuchae
- Folliculitis nuchae
- Keloidal folliculitis
- Sychosis nuchae

Introduction and general description

Folliculitis keloidalis is a chronic scarring folliculitis involving principally the hair follicles of the nape of the neck and occipital scalp and is considered to be a form of mixed primary cicatricial alopecia [1,2]. However, the term keloidalis is inaccurate as the condition is not associated with true keloids.

Epidemiology
Incidence and prevalence

Folliculitis keloidalis is a common disease, particularly in people of African, Afro-Caribbean and Hispanic descent [3]. A study from Nigeria reported that 9.4% of all patients attending a dermatology outpatient department had folliculitis keloidalis [4].

Age

Folliculitis keloidalis occurs in males after puberty and is most frequent between the ages of 14 and 25 years.

Sex

Males are most commonly affected, with an increased male to female ratio ranging from 7:1 to 20:1 [2,5].

Ethnicity

Most common in individuals of African, Afro-Caribbean and Hispanic descent [3].

Pathophysiology
Predisposing factors

This chronic inflammatory condition occurs mainly in males and therefore implies a possible pathogenetic role of sex hormones. Although friction from the collar is often incriminated, the evidence is unconvincing [6]. An association between frequent haircuts (at < two-weekly intervals) has been documented in older boys attending high school [7]. This finding and the observation of foreign-body granulomas surrounding fragments of hair have led to the suggestion that the process begins with penetration of cut hair into the skin as in pseudofolliculitis. However, no evidence of this was found on a detailed histological examination [8]. Moreover, it has been reported to occur secondary to several medications such

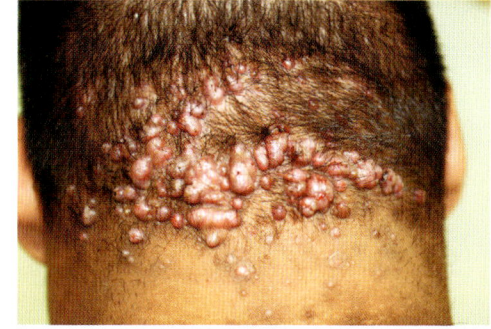
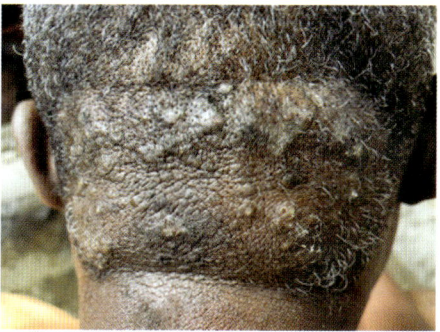

Figure 91.10 (a) Folliculitis keloidalis of the nape of the neck. Courtesy of Dr Ian Coulson. (b) Folliculitis keloidalis of the nape of the neck in a patient with skin of colour. Courtesy of Dr Ibrahima Traore.

(a)   (b)

as carbamazepine, diphenylhydantoin, cyclosporin, sirolimus and tacrolimus [5,9].

Pathology

The most frequent histopathological findings include follicular dilatation with neutrophils early in the disease course and chronic perifollicular inflammation with a lymphoplasmacellular cell infiltrate particularly affecting isthmus and lower infundibulum [1,10]. Disappearance of sebaceous glands, destroyed follicles, lamellar fibroplasia and acute inflammation around degenerating follicular components can also be found as well as perifollicular granulomas, abscesses and tufted hair folliculitis. Serial sections may show a foreign-body reaction to hair and follicular remnants. Furthermore, an increased number of interleukin (IL)-6 positive cells within the dermis of affected areas can be found, which suggests a possible pathogenetic role for IL-6 [10].

Causative organisms

Staphylococcus aureus and *Demodex* may be isolated from the skin, but it is uncertain whether these organisms can be implicated as primary pathogens [6,8].

Clinical features
Presentation

Follicular papules or pustules, often in irregularly linear groups, develop on the nape of the neck just below and within the hair line and on the occipital scalp (Figure 91.10). Less often and in more severe cases, they extend upwards into other areas of the scalp [5]. The early inflammatory stage may be inconspicuous and the patient may be unaware of the condition until hard keloidal papules develop at the sites of follicular inflammation. Also, the lesions may only be noticed following haircuts and it is assumed that the lesions occur due to an infection caused by the haircut instruments [10]. The papules may remain discrete or may fuse into horizontal bands, irregular plaques or tumorous masses [5]. In other cases, the inflammatory changes are persistent and troublesome, with undermined abscesses and discharging sinuses. The condition is chronic and new lesions may continue to form at intervals for years with signs of both active and chronic inflammation, which result in keloid-like scars and scarring alopecia [11]. Patients of African descent are prone to develop keloid-like masses and, less often, discrete papules and nodules compared with patients of different descent [3]. However, the condition is not associated with

an increased frequency of keloids elsewhere in the body because the prevalence of keloid formation in individuals with folliculitis keloidalis is similar to that in the general population [3].

Disease course and prognosis

The condition usually becomes chronic with episodic flares, leading to permanent scarring and cicatricial alopecia.

Co-morbidities

An increased frequency of acne, seborrheic dermatitis and pseudofolliculitis barbae as well as of folliculitis decalvans, dissecting cellulitis, hidradenitis suppurativa and the rare X-linked keratosis follicularis spinulosa decalvans has been reported [3,5,12]. Although there is no evidence to support a causal relationship between these conditions, a shared underlying predisposition cannot be excluded [3]. Moreover, patients may have hypothyroidism, acanthosis nigricans and features of metabolic syndrome such as diabetes mellitus, hypertension and dyslipidaemia [5].

Investigations

Skin swabs can be taken if bacterial infection is suspected.

Management

Bacterial infection should be treated if present and antiseptics may be used to prevent secondary infection. Close shaving of the hair on the nape of the neck and occipital scalp should be avoided. Intralesional steroids have been reported to be effective [13]. Potent topical corticosteroids may reduce scarring and inflammation and can be used either as monotherapy or in combination with topical antibiotics or retinoids [10]. Topical and oral antibiotics such as tetracyclines as well as oral isotretinoin have also been shown to be effective [13]. Treatment with a 1064 nm Nd:YAG laser or 810 nm diode laser has shown good therapeutic results [13,14]. The laser treatment causes miniaturisation of the hair shafts, which is thought to reduce subsequent inflammatory episodes. Additionally, NB-UVB phototherapy aids remission, possibly by reducing inflammation and regulating the expression of matrix metalloproteinases [13,15]. In those patients with extensive and refractory disease, surgery or cryosurgery with secondary intention healing as well as radiotherapy of the affected areas are effective alternatives [16].

Treatment ladder

First line
- Avoidance of close shaving of the hair on the nape of the neck and occipital scalp
- Topical antiseptics
- Intralesional steroids
- Topical steroids either as monotherapy or as combination with topical antibiotics or retinoids
- Topical and oral antibiotics such as tetracyclines
- Oral isotretinoin

Second line
- Laser-assisted hair removal
- NB-UVB phototherapy

Third line
- Surgery or cryosurgery with second intention healing
- Radiotherapy

Necrotising lymphocytic folliculitis of the scalp margin

Definition and nomenclature

Necrotising lymphocytic folliculitis is a rare and poorly understood chronic scarring follicular dermatosis characterised by necrotising inflammation of follicles close to the scalp margins and resulting in multiple small round varioliform scars [1]. It has historically been termed acne necrotica varioliformis but it is not considered as a variant of acne [2].

Synonyms and inclusions
- Acne frontalis
- Acne necrotica varioliformis
- Acne necrotica
- Acne pilaris
- Folliculitis necrotica

Introduction and general description

This uncommon condition is characterised by a necrotising folliculitis which appears in crops primarily along the frontal hairline and is a form of mixed primary cicatricial alopecia [3].

Epidemiology
Incidence and prevalence

It is a rare but underrecognised disorder. It affects individuals in their fourth and fifth decades [4].

Pathophysiology
Pathology

Early lesions are characterised by a dyskeratotic follicular epithelium with associated spongiosis. A prominent lymphocytic perifollicular and perivascular lymphocytic infiltrate is also seen as well as

subepidermal and perifollicular oedema [1]. As the lesions progress, more widespread necrosis appears involving the upper pilosebaceous unit, follicular epithelium, epidermis and dermis, and often containing fragments of hair. In later stages, the lesions are characterised by non-pathognomonic changes of perifollicular inflammation, making the diagnosis more challenging [5].

Causative organisms

Staphylococcus aureus, *Cutibacterium acnes*, *Malassesia spp*, *Demodex folliculorum* and *Herpes simplex* have been implicated but their role, if any, is uncertain [6].

Triggering factors

Aggravation in summer has been reported as well as its occurrence secondary to the use of phenylbutazone [1,6].

Clinical features
Presentation

Some patients experience mild pruritus but usually the disease onset is insidious, with the appearance of papules being most often in the frontal hairline, anterior scalp, nose, cheeks and the nape [4]. Some soreness may be associated with the evolving reddish-brown papules which gradually develop into pustules and umbilicate, developing focal areas of necrosis with crusting over the course of weeks, ultimately leaving depressed varioliform scars (Figure 91.11) [2].

Differential diagnosis

Potential differential diagnoses include papulonecrotic tuberculid, tertiary syphilis rosacea, repetitive excoriation, folliculitis decalvans, eczema herpeticum, dermatitis artefacta, pyogenic bacterial folliculitis, pityriasis lichenoides, molluscum contagiosum, nodular prurigo, bite and infestations, and drug reactions [5,7,8,**9**].

Disease course

It is characterised by spontaneous resolution or by chronicity with frequent recurrences and resistance to treatment [2,6].

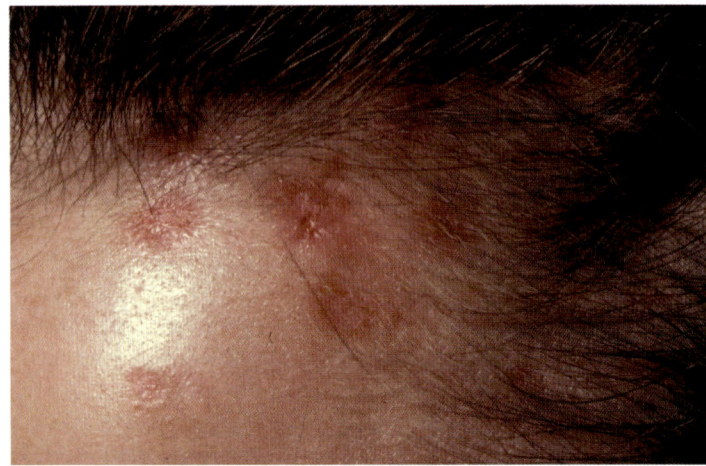

Figure 91.11 Varioliform scars at the scalp margin secondary to necrotising lymphocytic folliculitis.

Investigations
Careful culturing to establish whether *S. aureus* is present.

Management
Although strong evidence with regard to the treatment is lacking, the use of anti-staphylococcal antibiotics is recommended if *S. aureus* is found on culture. If this is not the case, oral tetracyclines or macrolides and antibacterial shampoos can effectively induce remission [5]. Topical, intralesional or systemic steroids, topical benzoyl peroxide and topical calcipotriol cream could also be of value, as well as oral isotretinoin in treatment-resistant patients, especially if *C. acnes* is found on culture [6].

Treatment ladder

First line
- Oral tetracyclines
- If *S. aureus* is found, antistaphylococcal therapy along with treatment of possible concomitant nasal carriage
- Antibacterial shampoos

Second line
- Oral isotretinoin
- Topical, intralesional or systemic steroids
- Topical benzoyl peroxide
- Topical calcipotriol cream

Chronic non-scarring folliculitis of the scalp

Definition and nomenclature
A non-scarring chronic superficial folliculitis of the scalp that is typically characterised by multiple minute, very itchy pustules distributed throughout the scalp.

Synonyms and inclusions
- Chronic scalp folliculitis
- Scalp folliculitis
- *Propionibacterium acnes* folliculitis of the scalp
- Acne necrotica miliaris

Introduction and general description
Chronic non-scarring folliculitis of the scalp is a relatively common but understudied chronic relapsing condition in which multiple minute itchy pustules form in the scalp. Maibach first recognised the condition in 1967 and since then several case series have been reported [1–3]. However, a confusing terminology has been used to describe it, either acne necrotica miliaris although no necrosis is seen; or *Propionibacterium acnes* folliculitis although *Cutibacterium acnes* (previously known as *Propionibacterium acnes*) does not have a pathogenetic role; or scalp folliculitis which is an umbrella term including chronic non-scarring scalp folliculitis, folliculitis decalvans, tufted folliculitis, acne keloidalis nuchae and dissecting cellulitis [1–3,4].

Epidemiology
Incidence and prevalence
Unknown but relatively common.

Age
Onset in third and fourth decades.

Sex
Male to female ratio 3:1.

Pathophysiology
Pathology
Neutrophilic folliculitis without necrosis and preserved sebaceous glands is typically seen. Immunochemistry may demonstrate increased IL-1β skin reactivity, induced possibly by macrophages [5].

Causative organisms
It has been supported to be an inflammatory condition within the group of neutrophilic dermatoses rather than being caused by an infective organism [4,5,6]. Several microbiological studies showed no pathogenetic role of an underlying microbial infection although a putative role of *C. acnes* and *S. aureus* had been suggested [4,5,6]. Moreover, the beneficial role of antimicrobial treatments is attributed to their anti-inflammatory effect [4,5,6].

Clinical features
Presentation
It is characterised by small papules and pustules associated with significant pruritis. Because of the itch, secondary excoriation and crusting are common (Figure 91.12).

Dermoscopy reveals pustules but no scarring, tufted hair or lack of follicular openings. It most commonly affects the occipital region but also the vertex, temporal and parietal regions, spreading to more than one region with disease progression [4].

Differential diagnosis
Acne vulgaris, folliculitis decalvans, tufted folliculitis, acne keloidalis nuchae, dissecting cellulitis, actinic folliculitis [4].

Disease course and prognosis
It is a recurring non-scarring folliculitis associated with frequent flares and temporary remissions [2].

Management
Low-dose tetracycline appears to be beneficial as well as the isotretinoin therapy and the combination of rifampin and clindamycin [2,4]. The use of topical steroids, clindamycin solution and benzoyl peroxide wash might be effective [4]. Moreover, discontinuation of treatment commonly leads to flares and often requiring long-term treatment to facilitate remission [4,5]. Additionally, the tumour necrosis factor inhibitor adalimumab has proven effective in

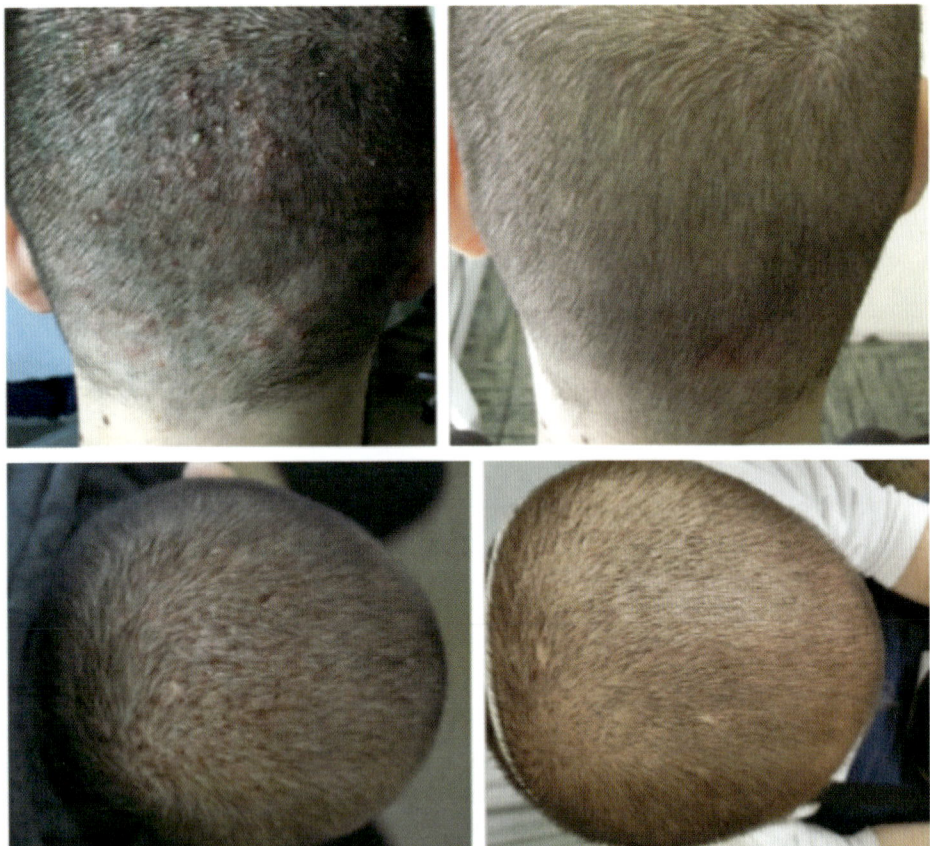

Figure 91.12 Chronic non-scarring scalp folliculitis before and after treatment with adalimumab. Reproduced from Soglia *et al.* [5] with permission from John Wiley & Sons.

a case report of a treatment-recalcitrant patient, further illustrating the possible pathogenetic role of the IL-1β and inflammasome [4,5].

Treatment ladder

First line
- Doxycycline

Second line
- Isotretinoin
- Combination of rimampin and clindamycin
- Topical steroids, clindamycin solution and benzoyl peroxide

Third line
- Adalimumab

Disseminate and recurrent infundibulofolliculitis

Definition
Disseminate and recurrent infundibulofolliculitis is a dermatosis of poorly understood aetiology affecting principally the chest, shoulders and upper arms of young black men. It manifests clinically as sheets of small monomorphic pruritic papules [1].

Synonyms and inclusions
- Hitch and Lund disease
- Infundibulofolliculitis of Hitch and Lund
- Disseminate and recurrent infundibular folliculitis

Epidemiology
Age
Begins in childhood or in adult life.

Sex
Mainly males.

Ethnicity
Mainly patients with dark skin.

Pathophysiology
Pathology
Histologically, it is characterised by disseminated inflammatory changes confined to the infundibular portion of multiple adjacent follicles and a mixed inflammatory infiltrate. Spongiosis and follicular exocytosis can be seen as well as follicular dilatation, fibrinoid

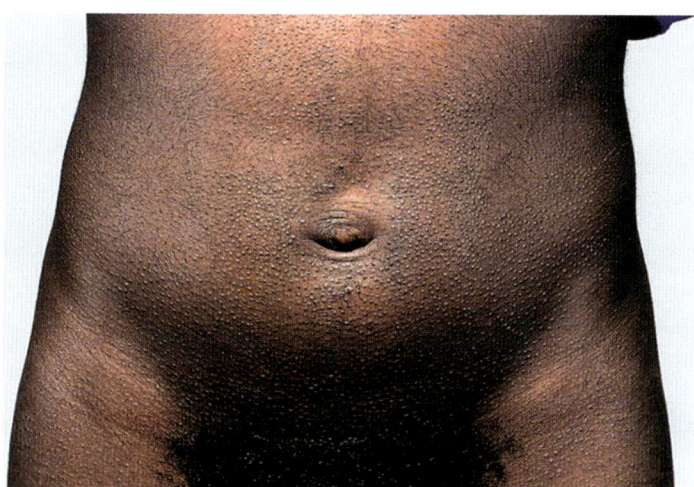

Figure 91.13 Disseminate and recurrent infundibulofolliculitis.

necrosis around the follicle, melanophages and transfollicular elimination of the follicular unit [2,3,4].

Causative organisms
No infective agent has been identified.

Genetics
Possible genetic predisposition is supported by two case reports, one of two affected siblings and another of a family with three affected members [2,5].

Clinical features
Presentation
A widespread eruption of small monomorphic follicular papules on the neck, chest, trunk and proximal extremities sparing the flexures (Figure 91.13). Less often the face, buttocks and lower extremities are affected [6]. Itch is often but not always present. Occasionally pustules develop.

Differential diagnosis
Bacterial and fungal folliculitis, pityrosporum folliculitis, keratosis pilaris, acneiform reactions, lichen spinulosus, lichen nitidus, follicular lichen planus, keratosis follicularis, alopecia mucinosa, follicular eczema and juxta-clavicular beaded lines [3,6,7].

Disease course
It tends to be persistent and as its name implies it may relapse periodically with spontaneous resolution [4].

Management
Although consensus about its treatment is lacking, high-dose vitamin A either as monotherapy or in combination with vitamin E [7] and oral isotretinoin [8] have each been proven to be beneficial. Topical corticosteroids [9], topical calcineurin inhibitors [8], PUVA and NB-UVB phototherapy [4,10] and oral doxycycline [2,4] have each been reported to be helpful in individual case reports.

Treatment ladder

First line
- Oral vitamin A either as monotherapy or in combination with vitamin E
- Oral isotretinoin

Second line
- Topical steroids
- Topical calcineurin inhibitors
- Oral doxycycline
- PUVA and NB-UVB

SEBACEOUS GLAND DISORDERS

Heterotopic sebaceous glands (Fordyce spots)

Definition and nomenclature
Fordyce spots are heterotopic sebaceous glands (i.e. not associated with hair follicles) which are located on mucosal surfaces or glabrous skin of the lips, oral mucosa or genitalia. Rarely, they have been reported in the eyes, palms, soles, tongue, salivary glands, larynx, thymus, oesophagus, gastroesophageal junction and uterus [1,2,3].

Synonyms and inclusions
- Fordyce granules
- Ectopic sebaceous glands

Introduction and general description
These common asymptomatic but readily visible skin and mucosal lesions easily attract the attention of both patients and physicians. Traditionally considered to be ectopic sebaceous glands, they should be considered as within the spectrum of normality.

Epidemiology
Incidence and prevalence
Fordyce spots on the lips and buccal mucosa are common from an early age and increase in prevalence with age. Fordyce spots were found in 1% of Swedish newborns [4]. The prevalence rises with age: oral or labial lesions were observed in 8% of a large cohort of preschool Brazilian children [5] and in 95% of a large cohort of adult Israeli Jews [6].

Sex
It remains unclear whether there is a sex predominance [1]. Vulval Fordyce spots are very common in women, with reported rates of 75–95% [7]. Fordyce spots on penile or scrotal skin were incidental findings in 9% of 400 Polish men who sought advice about other genital abnormalities [8].

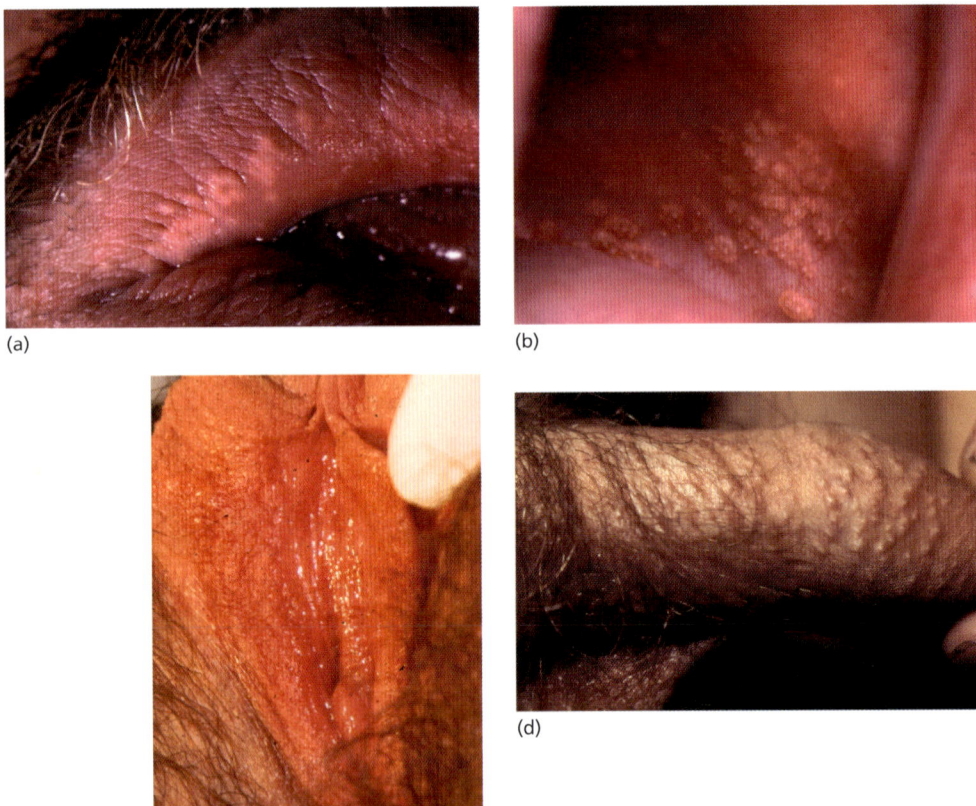

(a)   (b)   (c)   (d)

Figure 91.14 Fordyce spots on the vermilion of the upper lip (a), buccal mucosa (b), labia minora (c) and penis (d). (c) Courtesy of Dr Ekaterina Burova.

Pathophysiology
The aetiology remains unclear. The increased prevalence with age may point to hormonal changes. It has also been hypothesised that they may occur due to abnormal disposition during embryonic development [1].

Pathology
Fordyce spots are essentially sebaceous glands in which the duct is connected directly to the overlying epidermal or mucosal surface rather than into a hair follicle. They contain similar lipids to follicle-associated sebaceous glands [9,10].

Clinical features
Presentation
Fordyce spots manifest as multiple smooth, creamy white to yellow well-demarcated papules which may, however, coalesce into irregular plaques. They are usually 1–2 mm in diameter but may be larger and are slightly to moderately elevated above the skin or mucosal surface. They develop most commonly on the vermilion of the upper lip (Figure 91.14a), the buccal mucosa (91.14b) or the labia minora (Figure 91.14c). Advice is, however, most likely to be sought by adolescents or young men with prominent penile or scrotal involvement (Figure 91.14d).

Clinical variants
Heterotopic sebaceous glands may be located in the coronal sulcus of the penis to either side of the frenulum and in this location have been referred to as the glands of Tyson [11]. They are normal structures and require no treatment.

Sebaceous glands are found within the tubercles of Montgomery on the areola of the female breast. Typical Fordyce spots on the areolae have, however, been described in a man with coexistent labial and penile lesions [12].

Differential diagnosis
- Human papillomavirus infection
- Low-grade intraepithelial lesions
- Milia
- Molluscum contagiosum
- Post-herpetic changes

Investigations
In cases of doubt, a biopsy will provide the diagnosis.

Management
As the lesions are benign and asymptomatic, no treatment is necessary. However, if they cause significant distress for aesthetic reasons, local destruction may be performed with modalities including superficial cautery or electrodessication, topical trichloroacetic acid, carbon dioxide (CO_2) laser evaporation and micropunch excision therapy [1,13]. These may cause scarring dependent on the depth of injury. Systemic isotretinoin is an effective alternative, with a risk of recurrence upon discontinuation. Intralesional electrocoagulation with a proximally insulated single microneedle is a promising treatment option especially in cosmetically important areas such as the lip region [1,14].

Treatment ladder

First line
- Reassurance

Second line
- Local destruction with superficial cautery or electrodessication
- Topical trichloracetic acid

Third line
- Systemic isotretinoin
- Carbon dioxide laser evaporation
- Micropunch excision therapy
- Electrocoagulation

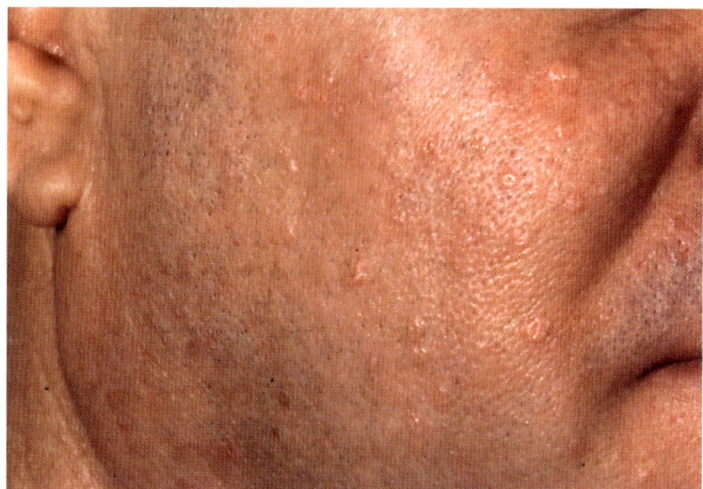

Figure 91.15 Sebaceous gland hyperplasia on the cheek of a 42-year-old man.

Sebaceous gland hyperplasia

Definition

Sebaceous gland hyperplasia presents as scattered, clinically obvious, flesh-coloured to yellowish papules resulting from hypertrophy of sebaceous glands.

Introduction and general description

Sebaceous gland hyperplasia is characterised by a benign proliferation of sebocytes within normal pilosebaceous units in hair-bearing skin (cf. Fordyce spots). It is most commonly seen in adults but may manifest in the neonatal period due to the passage of maternal androgens across the placenta.

Epidemiology
Incidence and prevalence

Sebaceous gland hyperplasia is a common disorder, affecting approximately 1% of the population [1]. Its prevalence in patients taking long-term immunosuppression is higher, ranging from 10% to 16% [1].

Age

Sebaceous hyperplasia is common in middle-aged or older adults [2]. It is uncommon in childhood and adolescence although neonates are often affected due to exposure to maternal androgens.

Pathophysiology
Associated diseases and predisposing factors

Immunosuppression with ciclosporin or tacrolimus in organ-transplant recipients may predispose to sebaceous hyperplasia [2–4]. It has been reported following use of systemic corticosteroids, dialysis and HAART in HIV patients [2,5]. It has also been associated with Muir-Torre syndrome, X-linked hypohidrotic ectodermal dysplasia syndrome and pachydermoperiostosis [5].

Pathology

The sebaceous glands are enlarged and surround and connect to a dilated central duct.

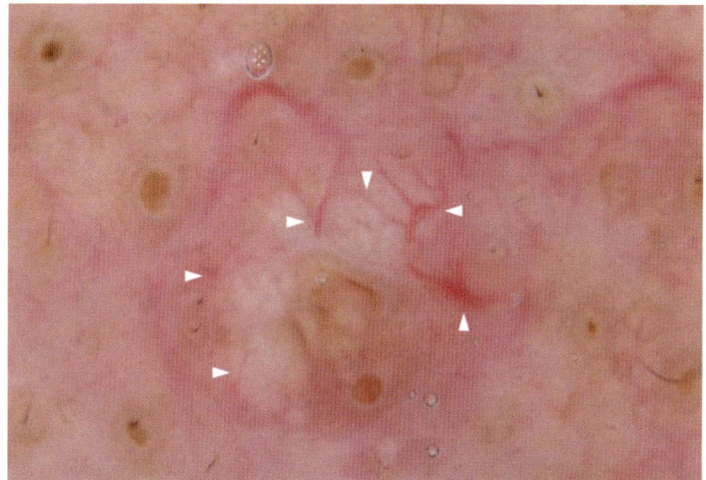

Figure 91.16 Crown vessels in a sebaceous hyperplasia. Crown vessels surrounding a white-yellow polylobular centre are a specific clue for sebaceous hyperplasia, while they sometimes mimic molluscum contagiosum (white arrowheads). Reproduced from Togawa 2017 [7] with permission from John Wiley & Sons.

Genetics

Familial cases presenting at a young age suggest the possibility of a genetic component [6].

Clinical features
Presentation

Sebaceous gland hyperplasia presents as individual asymptomatic flesh-coloured to yellow-pink papules measuring 1–3 mm in diameter, but may be larger (Figure 91.15). Closer inspection highlights that these are made up of smaller aggregated papules surrounding the follicular opening resulting in a umbilicated appearance with prominent blood vessels, easily seen with dermoscopy (Figure 91.16). These are distinct from the arborising pattern of vessels seen in basal cell carcinoma and may have 'crown vessels' that are specific for sebaceous gland hyperplasia [2].

A solitary nodule or multiple lesions may be present. They are most common on the forehead, temples and cheeks, but may occur on the oral mucosa, ear, carbuncle, upper trunk, vulva, areola and penile shaft. Their main clinical significance is that they may be mistaken for other disorders presenting with facial papules such as basal cell carcinoma.

Disease course and prognosis

Persistent but asymptomatic. However, in case of multiple lesions especially on the face, sebaceous gland hyperplasia can have an aesthetic and psychological impact.

Investigations

In cases of diagnostic doubt, biopsy will rule out neoplasm or other disorder (see Box 91.1 for differential diagnosis).

Box 91.1 Differential diagnosis of sebaceous gland hyperplasia

- Sebaceous adenoma (with associated Muir-Torre)
- Sebaceous carcinoma
- Heterotopic sebaceous glands (Fordyce spots)
- Basal cell carcinomas
- Trichepitheliomas and other adnexal tumours
- Fibrous papule of the face
- Granulomatous rosacea
- Milia
- Molluscum contagiosum
- Nevus sebaceous
- Sebaceous nevus
- Xanthoma

Management

Sebaceous hyperplasia is a benign asymptomatic disorder and no treatment is necessary. Where there is a cosmetic concern, physical treatments such as electrodessication, cryotherapy, trichloroacetic acid, shave or curettage or ablative laser (CO_2 or Er:YAG) may be used [8–11]. A 1720 nm laser is more specific for the sebaceous gland and improved outcomes over conventional methods have been described [12]. Optimal outcomes involve resolution of the lesions without scarring or dyspigmentation. Nanosecond pulsed electric field (nsPEF) technology has also been shown to be a safe and effective treatment option [1].

Oral isotretinoin is helpful. However, lesions recur on cessation of treatment. Anti-androgens, e.g. cyproterone acetate, in combination with a combined oral contraceptive preparation may induce regression of sebaceous hyperplasia in females [13]. Photodynamic therapy using aminolaevulinic acid or methylaminolaevulinate has also been shown to be useful for shrinking lesions of sebaceous hyperplasia and combination therapies may also be used.

Treatment ladder

First line
- Cosmetic camouflage

Second line
- Electrodessication

- Local destruction with lasers (CO_2, Er:YAG), cryotherapy and nanosecond pulsed electric field (nsPEF)
- Topical trichloracetic acid

Third line
- Systemic isotretinoin
- Cyproterone acetate combination with oral contraceptive preparation (COCP)
- Photodynamic therapy with or without lasers or other destructive modalities

---

Key references

The full list of references can be found in the online version at https://www.wiley.com/rooksdermatology10e

Follicular eruptions due to systemic medications
1 Du-Thanh A, Kluger N, Bensalleh H, Guillot B. Drug-induced acneiform eruption. *Am J Clin Dermatol* 2011;12:233–45.

Eosinophilic pustular folliculitis
19 Nervi SJ, Schwartz RA, Dmochowski M. Eosinophilic pustular folliculitis: a 40 year retrospect. *J Am Acad Dermatol* 2006;55:285–9.

Infantile eosinophilic pustular folliculitis
1 Lucky AW, Esterly NB, Heskel N *et al*. Eosinophilic pustular folliculitis in infancy. *Pediatr Dermatol* 1984;1:202–6.

Pseudofolliculitis
5 Nussbaum D, Friedman A. Pseudofolliculitis barbae: a review of current treatment options. *J Drugs Dermatol* 2019;18:246–50.

Folliculitis keloidalis
3 Umar S, Lee DJ, Lullo JJ. A retrospective cohort study and clinical classification system of acne keloidalis nuchae. *J Clin Aesthet Dermatol* 2021;14:E61–7.

Necrotising lymphocytic folliculitis of the scalp margin
9 Ross EK, Tan E, Shapiro J. Update on primary cicatricial alopecias. *J Am Acad Dermatol* 2005;53:1–37.

Chronic non-scarring folliculitis of the scalp
4 Romero-Maté A, Arias-Palomo D, Hernández-Núñez A, Córdoba-Guijarro S, Borbujo-Martínez J. Chronic nonscarring scalp folliculitis: retrospective case series study of 34 cases. *J Am Acad Dermatol* 2019;81:1023–4.

Disseminate and recurrent infundibulofolliculitis
4 Rekha S, Kumar V, Rao P, Kachhawa D. Disseminate and recurrent infundibulofolliculitis. *Indian J Dermatol* 2019;64:404–6.

Heterotopic sebaceous glands (Fordyce spots)
1 Lee JH, Lee JH, Kwon NH *et al*. Clinicopathologic manifestations of patients with Fordyce's spots. *Ann Dermatol* 2012;24:103–6.

Sebaceous gland hyperplasia
12 Simmons BJ, Griffith RD, Falto-Aizpurua LA, Bray FN, Nouri K; International League of Dermatological Societies; European Dermatology Forum. Light and laser therapies for the treatment of sebaceous gland hyperplasia a review of the literature. *J Eur Acad Dermatol Venereol.* 2015;29:2080–7.

CHAPTER 92

Disorders of the Sweat Glands

Ian H. Coulson[1] *and Niall J. E. Wilson*[2]

[1]Burnley General Teaching Hospital, East Lancashire NHS Trust IHC, Burnley, UK
[2]Liverpool University Hospitals NHS Foundation Trust, UK

Introduction

In this chapter the anatomy, physiology and diseases of the two types of sweat gland, eccrine and apocrine, are described. The clinical patterns, causes and associations of excessive sweating on the one hand and of reduced or absent sweating on the other are addressed in detail. Guidance is given on the management of hyperhidrosis and on the choice of appropriate therapy, including topical and systemic agents and surgery. The presentation and management of occlusive and inflammatory disorders of eccrine sweat glands is covered fully, as are the clinical features and management of abnormal sweat odour and colour and of apocrine miliaria. Brief reference is made to conditions associated with sweat gland inclusions; discussion of the latter and of neoplasms derived from sweat gland elements is to be found elsewhere in the book.

ECCRINE GLANDS

Anatomy and physiology of eccrine glands

Human eccrine sweat glands have two distinct functions [1,2,3,4]. They allow body cooling by evaporation and contribute in a major way to adaptation to a hot environment by humans. They also moisten the skin on the palms and soles at times of activity and thus improve their grip.

Eccrine sweat glands are distributed over the whole skin surface including the glans penis and foreskin, but not on the lips, external ear canal, clitoris or labia minora. The number varies greatly with site, from $620/cm^2$ on the soles, about $120/cm^2$ on the thighs to $60/cm^2$ on the back [5]. The total number on the body surface is between 2 and 5 million, and is similar in different ethnic groups. It has been calculated that the weight of the eccrine glands totals 100 g. The glands vary in size from person to person by a factor of five and this probably accounts for individual as well as regional differences in sweat rate (maximal individual gland secretion rates ranging from 2 to 20 nL/min/gland).

Embryologically, sweat glands are derived from a specialised downgrowth of the epidermis at about the third month of intrauterine life on the palms and soles and at about 5 months elsewhere; they resemble adult glands by 8 months. Sweat glands are morphologically normal at birth but may not function fully until about 2 years of age. No new eccrine glands develop after birth. Unlike the apocrine glands they have no developmental relationship with the pilosebaceous follicle, although some glands may eventually come to open into the follicular neck. The gland consists of a secretory coil in the lower dermis (Figure 92.1a) and subcutaneous tissue, and a duct leading through the dermis to the intraepidermal sweat duct unit (Figure 92.1b). Apoeccrine glands have features of both eccrine and apocrine glands but seem to be nearer to eccrine in function.

Rook's Textbook of Dermatology, Tenth Edition. Edited by Christopher Griffiths, Jonathan Barker, Tanya Bleiker, Walayat Hussain and Rosalind Simpson.
© 2024 John Wiley & Sons Ltd. Published 2024 by John Wiley & Sons Ltd.

PART 8: SPECIFIC CUTANEOUS STRUCTURES

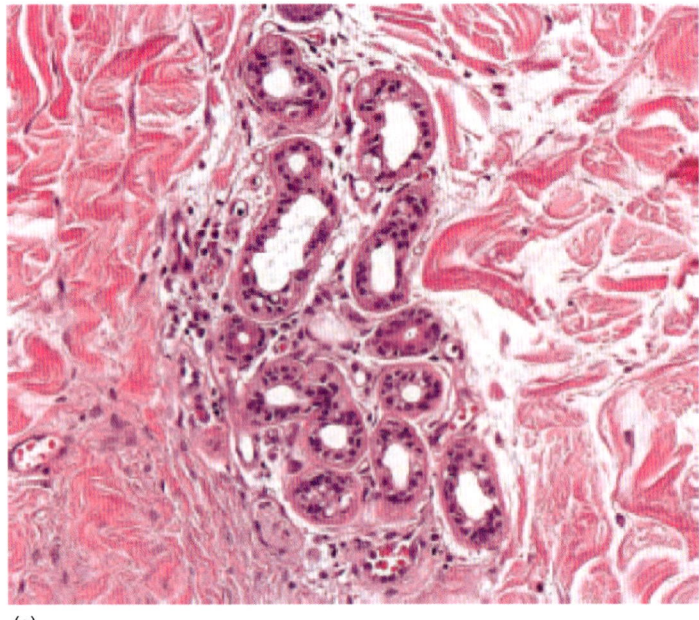

(a)

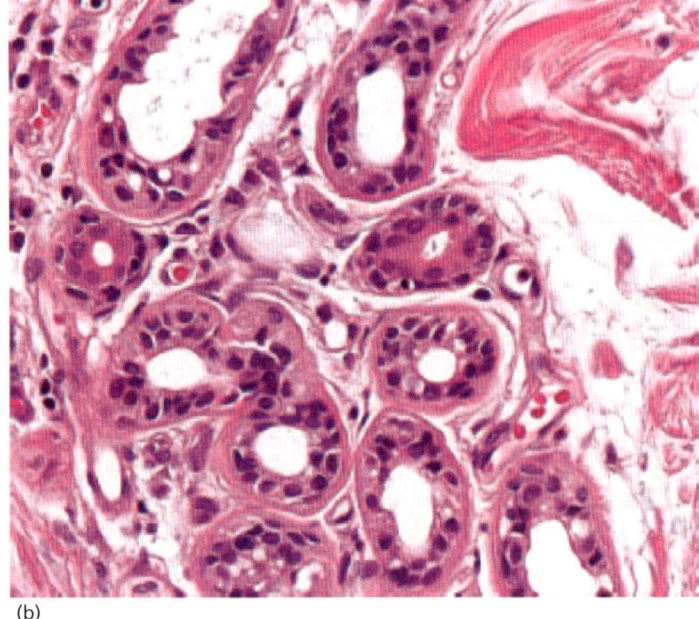

(b)

Figure 92.1 (a) A normal eccrine unit composed of secretory glands and ducts. Magnification 10× (H&E). (b) Closer view of eccrine glands showing the double layer of lining epithelial cells. Magnification 40× (H&E). Courtesy of Dr Arti Bakshi, Liverpool University Hospitals NHS Foundation Trust, UK.

They open onto the surface and produce a copious watery fluid. They may account for 10–45% of adult axillary glands [6].

The *secretory coil* contains three types of cell: large clear cells, which are the main secretory cells, small dark cells, which resemble mucus-secreting cells of other organs but whose function is not known, and myoepithelial cells [7]. The large and small cells of the secretory coil, unlike those of the duct, are attached to the basement membrane, although individual sections may at times suggest a double layer. Outside the basement membrane are the longitudinally arranged myoepithelial cells, whose function is probably to support the gland, but they may also help propel the sweat towards the surface. They respond to cholinergic stimuli. The function of the coil is to produce from plasma a watery isotonic secretion which can subsequently be modified by the duct. Ultrastructurally, the large clear cells are characterised by the presence of many mitochondria and by both intricate basal infoldings and intercellular canaliculi. *Para*-nitrophenyl phosphatase activity, which reflects catalytic activity of Na-K-ATPase, is evident in the basal infoldings but not the intercellular canaliculi, suggesting that the basal areas are the sites of active ion transport requisite for sweat secretion. The classic theory suggests that acetylcholine passively increases entry of sodium into the cell, and this is then pumped out by the sodium pump into the intercellular canaliculi rather than directly through the luminal margin. However, there are other theories [4]. Fluid secretion is believed to be mediated osmotically, but the mechanism by which water moves has long been obscure. The discovery of aquaporins (AQPs) may challenge this theory. AQPs are a group of intercellular membrane water channel proteins, which allow movement of large amounts of fluid. In animal models, sweat secretion in AQP5 null mice was markedly decreased [8]. AQP5 has been identified in the dark cells of human eccrine sweat glands but its role in human sweating is still not clear [9,10]. Many different monoclonal antibodies can be shown to react with different portions of the sweat glands, allowing distinction of the gland from other components of the skin [11].

The *duct* consists of two or more layers of relatively uniform cuboidal cells. About one-third of the coil has this histology, as well as the uncoiled part passing up to the epidermis. The basal cells are rich in mitochondria and their entire membranes are rich in Na-K-ATPase activity, suggesting sodium pumping occurs along the entire duct membrane, and performs an active part in modifying the secretion produced by the coil.

It has been suggested that sweat glands do not cool the skin only by evaporation of heat from the surface, but that they also act as heat pipes. According to this theory, evaporation of the fluid at the base of the duct allows water vapour to pass up the duct and condense nearer the surface, and thence return to the deeper parts by capillary action. Such systems are a very effective way of transferring heat quickly [12].

The *intraepidermal sweat unit* is lined by a layer of specialised cells that often may be distinguished only with difficulty from the surrounding epidermis. On the palms and soles, it has a well-developed coil structure that is not so apparent in other sites.

The techniques for studying the function of the eccrine sweat glands [12–14] include the following:
• Collection of sweat in bags or pads at rest, after exposure to heat, or after injection or iontophoresis of pilocarpine or other cholinergic agonists.
• Direct measurement of water loss.
• Microcannulation of the duct or coil [15].
• Measurement of electrical potentials and electrical resistance of the skin, which depends on both the sweat present on the epidermis and the column present within the duct [16,17].
• Visualisation of the individual sweat droplets. This may be achieved by direct microscopy, by *in vivo* staining, by forming plastic impressions [18] or by indicators that become coloured on contact with water, such as the starch/iodine technique [19],

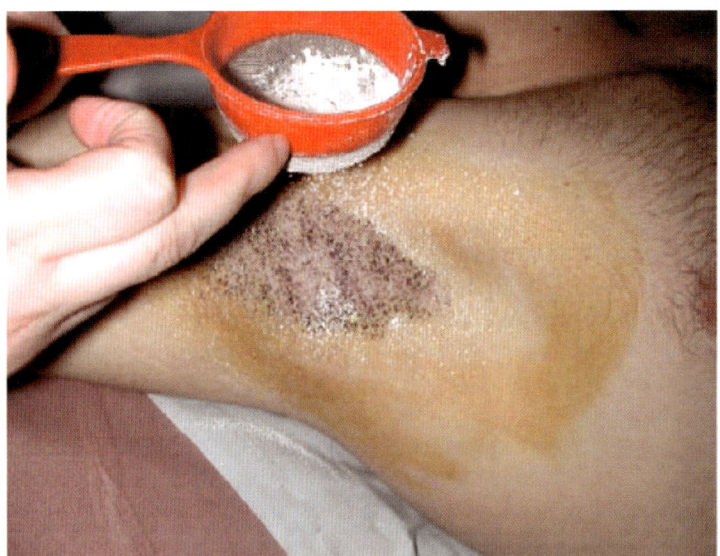

Figure 92.2 Identifying the extent of axillary hyperhidrosis – the skin has been cleaned with povidone iodine solution and then sprinkled with corn starch powder from a fine culinary sieve. The hyperhidrotic areas are blue-black.

bromophenol blue [13], quinizarin [20] and the food dye Edicol ponceau. The plastic or silicone impression techniques are probably the most reliable and can produce a permanent record. A simple modification of the starch/iodine test is to dry the skin, paint it with 2% iodine in alcohol, allow it to dry, and then press the skin against a good-quality paper. The starch in the paper reacts with iodine in the presence of water, so that each sweat droplet shows up as a minute dark spot. Alternatively, the starch may be suspended in castor oil (50 g in 100 mL) and painted onto the iodine-treated skin (Figure 92.2). Special dry starch/iodine powders can be dusted directly onto the skin [21].

- Isolated glands. It is possible to isolate single eccrine glands (and also hair follicles, sebaceous glands and apocrine sweat glands) by the relatively simple technique of shearing tissues with scissors [22,23]. This allows the physiology, biochemistry and tissue culture behaviour to be studied *in vitro*.

Control of eccrine sweating [1,2,3,4]

Eccrine gland secretion is influenced by a number of stimuli including thermal, osmotic, mental and gustatory factors, mediated by a complex of central and local control mechanisms. As a result, the quantity and composition of sweat is highly variable from minimal basal activity to a maximum of 3 L in 1 h.

Central control

Thermoregulatory sweating is primarily controlled in response to internal body temperature and secondarily influenced by skin temperature [24]. The effect of a rise in core temperature is nine times more efficient than the same rise in skin temperature in stimulating sweating. Central and peripheral changes in temperature influence the thermal receptors in the preoptic area and anterior hypothalamus. An increase in core temperature activates cooling mechanisms including sweating, panting and vasodilatation. Conversely, cooling promotes heat-preservation mechanisms such as vasoconstriction and shivering [25].

Although the precise neural pathway that mediates eccrine sweating in humans is still unclear, evidence from animal studies suggest that the efferent pathway from the hypothalamus includes the medulla, lateral horn of the spinal cord and sympathetic ganglia [26].

Osmotic factors also influence the rate of sweat production. Both hyperosmolality and hypovolaemia decrease sweat production, presumably in an attempt to prevent further loss of body fluid [27,28].

Centres and pathways controlling mental sweating are not fully known but areas within the frontal region of the brain have been identified. Functional magnetic resonance studies indicate that neural pathways for thermal and mental sweating are similar [29]. Mental stimuli enhance sweat production particularly from the palms and soles, potentially improving grip at times of stress.

Local control

From the sympathetic ganglia non-myelinated C fibres pass to eccrine sweat glands ending at many cholinergic terminals and a few adrenergic terminals [30]. Although stimulation of adrenergic nerves increases sweating this is much less marked than the response to cholinergic stimulation [31,32,33]. The relevant receptor is felt to be M3 muscarinic. The adrenergic nerve supply seems to play little part in the normal modulation of eccrine sweating in humans. In addition, vasoactive intestinal polypeptide, calcitonin gene-related peptide and nitric oxide may play some role in the control of eccrine sweating [24].

Other factors may modify the quantity and quality of sweat in the presence of an intact sympathetic nerve supply including hormones, circulatory changes and axon and spinal reflexes. Sweat coils contain androgen receptors [34], and androgens may be at least partly responsible for the increase in sweating around puberty and for the greater sweat activity in males.

The composition of sweat [4,33] varies greatly from person to person, time to time and site to site. It has a basic similarity to the plasma from which it is derived. The sweat duct is largely responsible for the modification in sweat constituent concentration that occurs, and this will therefore vary according to how rapidly the sweat is passing through the duct. The most important constituents are sodium, chloride, potassium, urea and lactate. Sweat is hypotonic and this is largely due to reabsorption of sodium in the duct. At increased sweat rates the sodium concentration rises, presumably because there is reduced time for ductal reabsorption. The normal sodium concentration is between 10 and 20 mmol/L at low sweat rates, and up to 100 mmol/L at high rates. Aldosterone can increase ductal sodium reabsorption and in Addison disease high sweat sodium can be demonstrated (70–80 mmol/L). Antidiuretic hormone may reduce sweat rates in humans, but it also induces local vasoconstriction.

An increase in sweat electrolytes occurs in cystic fibrosis and forms the basis of the sweat chloride test [35]. Mutations in the *CFTR* gene in cystic fibrosis result in abnormalities of chloride transport across epithelial cells on mucosal surfaces [36]. A raised level of chloride in sweat (above 60 mmol/L) is considered consistent with a diagnosis of cystic fibrosis although it is recommended that the test is repeated on two occasions [35].

Lactate is found in a concentration of 4–40 mmol/L, which greatly exceeds the concentration found in plasma. It is formed in the gland from glucose from the blood. It is interesting to speculate whether urea and lactate can act to moisturise the stratum corneum.

Glucose is present in small quantities only (usually 0–0.17 mmol/L, although levels up to 0.3 mmol/L may be found). High sweat glucose may be found in uncontrolled diabetes and this may create a favourable environment for skin infections. The pH is 4–6.8.

A variety of other substances may be found in sweat, including pharmacologically active substances and inhibitors, antigens, antibodies and drugs [4]. Some of these seem to be excreted and have no special function; others may have a definite function, for example a urokinase-type plasminogen activator may play a part in the digestion of glycoprotein plugs in sweat pores [37]. Active excretion or secretion of drugs such as griseofulvin and ketoconazole may contribute to their efficacy.

DISORDERS OF ECCRINE SWEAT GLANDS

Hyperhidrosis

Definition and nomenclature

Hyperhidrosis is defined as excessive production of sweat, that is, more than is required for thermoregulation [1]. It can be defined gravimetrically [2] as greater than 2 standard deviations above mean values of sweat secretion for a normal population in various sites (palmar 50 mg/min/m², plantar 50 mg/min/m², axillary 150 mg/min/m² and facial 50 mg/min/m²).

Synonyms and inclusions
- Excessive sweating

Introduction and general description

Hyperhidrosis can be a major inconvenience and embarrassment to sufferers, with a significant effect on quality of life. In theory, when there is overproduction of sweat it should be possible to determine whether this is due to abnormal sweat glands, pharmacologically active agents acting on the glands, abnormal stimulation of the sympathetic pathway between the hypothalamus and the nerve ending, or to overactivity of one of the three different 'centres' responsible for thermoregulatory, mental and gustatory sweating. Any difficult case should be approached from first principles in this way.

Most cases of hyperhidrosis can be classified as one of the following:
- Generalised.
- Focal – palmar, plantar, axillary, cranio-facial and inguinal.
- Localised naevoid.
- Compensatory.
- Hyperhidrosis with extensive anhidrosis (Ross syndrome).

Epidemiology

In a series of Polish medical students, 16% admitted to perceived hyperhidrosis. Fewer than half of these, however, were determined to have gravimetrically measured sweat secretion rates defined as greater than 2 standard deviations above the reference range for a

given site [2]. The incidence in the US population is estimated to be of the order of 4.8%. Generalised and focal naevoid hyperhidrosis are relatively rare. There is no sex or racial preponderance.

Generalised hyperhidrosis

Pathophysiology

There is marked physiological variation in thermoregulatory sweating from person to person in the absence of disease. An increase in the temperature of blood bathing the hypothalamus increases heat loss by sweating and vasodilatation. Some instability of the sweat regulating centre is caused by many febrile conditions, so that sweating may occur at times when there is no fever. This instability may persist for days, or even months, after the fever has subsided, and in some cases is such a prominent feature that the term 'sweating sickness' has been used [3]. Generalised sweating may occur in disorders of unknown aetiology that alter the setting of the thermoregulatory centre and may be associated with episodic hypothermia [1].

For a list of disorders associated with generalised hyperhidrosis see Box 92.1.

Box 92.1 Causes of generalised hyperhidrosis

- Febrile infective illnesses: tuberculosis, malaria, brucellosis, endocarditis, etc.
- Metabolic diseases: diabetes, hyperthyroidism, hyperpituitarism, hypoglycaemia, phaeochromocytoma
- Menopause
- Underlying solid malignancy and lymphoma
- Congestive heart failure
- Neurological disorders:
  - Brain disease:
    - Parkinson disease
    - episodic hypothermia with hyperhidrosis
    - generalised hyperhidrosis without hypothermia
  - Peripheral neuropathies:
    - familial dysautonomia (Riley–Day)
    - congenital autonomic dysfunction with universal pain loss
    - cold-induced sweating syndrome
- Drugs: fluoxetine
- Exercise-induced hyperhidrosis

Thermoregulatory sweating occurs during or after many infective processes, and may be the presenting manifestation of malaria, tuberculosis, brucellosis, lymphoma, subacute bacterial endocarditis, etc. Night sweats are often part of the clinical picture. A similar mechanism may account for the hyperhidrosis associated with alcohol intoxication or gout, and after vomiting. The mechanism of generalised hyperhidrosis that may be associated with diabetic autonomic neuropathy, hyperthyroidism, hyperpituitarism, hypoglycaemia, obesity, the menopause and malignant disease is unknown, although experiments in recently oophorectomised mice showed that the flushing and sweating of hot flushes could be antagonised by blocking calcitonin gene related peptide [3]. Increased sweating has been documented in some patients with Parkinson disease, but others have noted the combination of patchy anhidrosis and compensatory hyperhidrosis, suggesting autonomic dysfunction. Paroxysmal sweating, tachycardia and headaches strongly suggest a phaeochromocytoma. Hypertension is noted during attacks. Cases have been reported of patients who develop generalised sweating in a thermal pattern, but are induced by cold [4].

Hyperhidrosis is seen in association with peripheral neuropathies, as in familial dysautonomia, or Riley–Day syndrome, a recessively inherited disorder of Ashkenazi Jews comprising an absent axon reflex flare after histamine injection, pupillary meiosis, diminished tendon reflexes, diminished pain sensation and absent fungiform papillae of the tongue (Chapter 83). Excess sweating is thought to be due to sweat centre excitability. Congenital autonomic dysfunction with universal pain loss is similar, but individuals are not Ashkenazi Jews, have a complete absence of pain sensation with accidental self-mutilation, corneal opacities and episodic fever.

Generalised hyperhidrosis may be associated with brain lesions (diencephalic lesions, malformations of the corpus callosum, microgyria) and may be accompanied by episodic hypothermia. Exercise-induced hyperhidrosis can occur in athletes and can be severe; the highest sweat rate recorded in a man being in this condition (5.8 L/h) and contributes to rapid dehydration.

Drug-induced hyperhidrosis is an important consideration in any patient presenting with generalised symptoms and a careful drug history is mandatory. The main culprit drugs are listed in Box 92.2.

Box 92.2 Causes of drug-induced hyperhidrosis

- Selective serotonin reuptake inhibitors
- Tricyclic antidepressants
- Opioid analgesics
- ACE inhibitors
- Beta-blockers
- Calcium channel blockers
- Aromatase inhibitors
- Tamoxifen
- Isotretinoin
- Proton pump inhibitors
- Progestogen-containing contraceptives

In many cases of generalised hyperhidrosis of the thermal type, but with no obvious underlying disease, the aetiology remains unknown, even after extensive investigation.

Focal hyperhidrosis

Pathophysiology

Focal hyperhidrosis includes palmoplantar, axillary, inguinal and cranio-facial ('emotional') hyperhidrosis [5]. Emotional or mental activity increases sweating, especially on the palms, soles, axillae and, to a lesser extent, groin, face and scalp. It should be emphasised that mental activity devoid of any clear emotional content may provoke sweating. Thermal stimuli and physical effort increase this effect in many cases. Most cases of hyperhidrosis presenting to the dermatologist are of this type. Although mental or emotional factors are the usual trigger for this type of sweating, and in some patients deep-seated emotional disturbances may be found, in many there seems to be some facilitation of the nervous pathways causing physiological mental sweating.

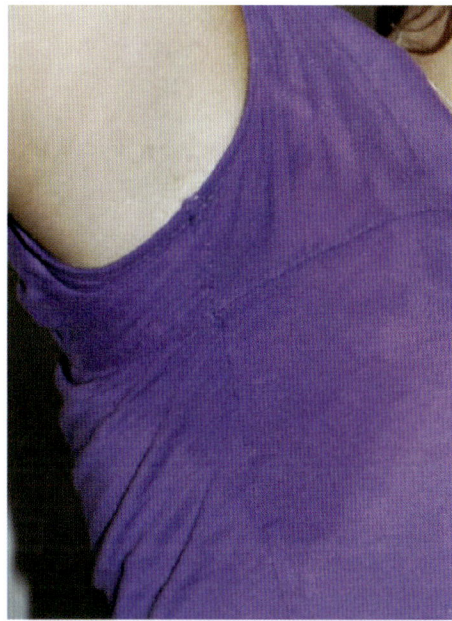

Figure 92.3 Axillary hyperhidrosis: patients often wear white or black garments as the wetness is not as visibly obvious as with coloured clothes.

Clinical features

Focal hyperhidrosis may be a significant disability and embarrassment, particularly if sweat drips from the hands onto the floor; rusting of metal objects may be an occupational problem, or clothing may be saturated. Patients with axillary hyperhidrosis often wear only black or white garments as these show the wetness less obviously than coloured clothes (Figure 92.3).

Hyperhidrosis may be associated with Raynaud phenomenon and reflex sympathetic dystrophy or may follow cold injury. Frequently there is a family history of excessive sweating.

Palmoplantar hyperhidrosis. Palmoplantar hyperhidrosis (Figure 92.4) occurs in both sexes, and commonly begins in childhood or around puberty. The sweating of the palms and soles may be either continuous or phasic [5]. When continuous, it is worse in the summer, and not so clearly precipitated by mental factors. When phasic, it is usually precipitated by minor emotional or mental activity and it is not markedly different in summer and winter. The hands may be cold and show a tendency to acrocyanosis. Hyperhidrosis may affect the hands, feet and axillae in any combination, but only a minority of patients with axillary hyperhidrosis also have involvement of the palms and soles. Troublesome hyperhidrosis of the feet occurs especially in young adult men. When this is associated with vasomotor changes, so that the sodden skin is also cold and cyanotic, the name 'symmetrical lividity' is sometimes applied. Palmoplantar hyperhidrosis is one component of various syndromes in which palmoplantar keratoderma occurs. It also occurs with the nail–patella syndrome (Chapter 67).

Axillary hyperhidrosis. This may be continuous, or more commonly phasic, and may or may not be aggravated by heat or mental activity. It is uncommon before puberty. Axillary sweating on undressing is very common. Axillary hyperhidrosis is due to overactivity of

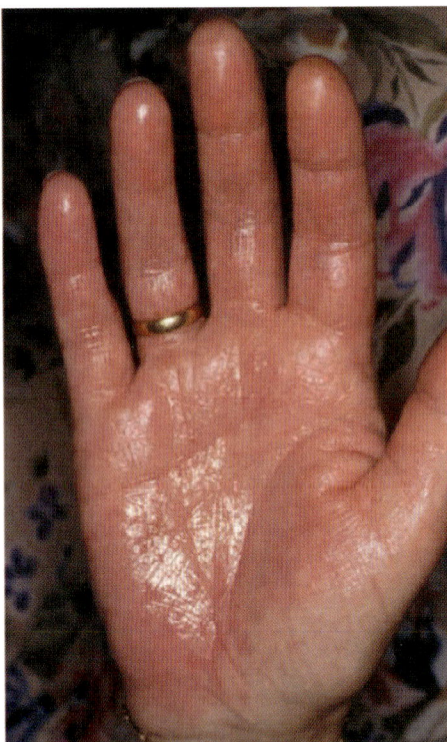

Figure 92.4 Palmar hyperhidrosis.

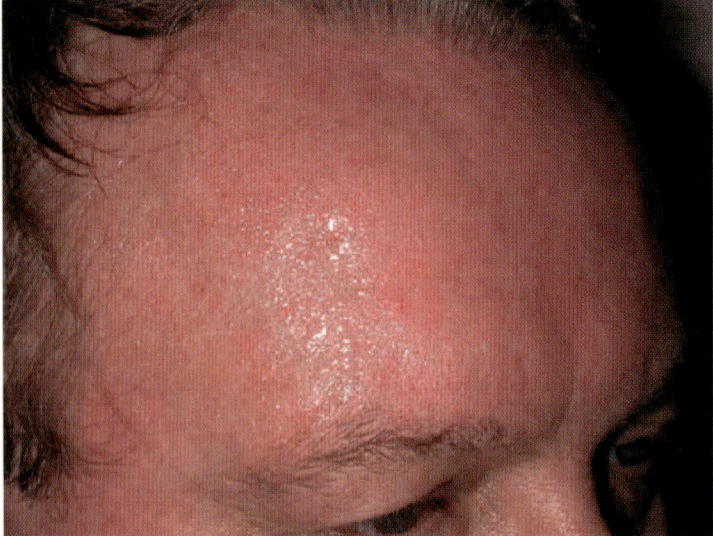

(a)

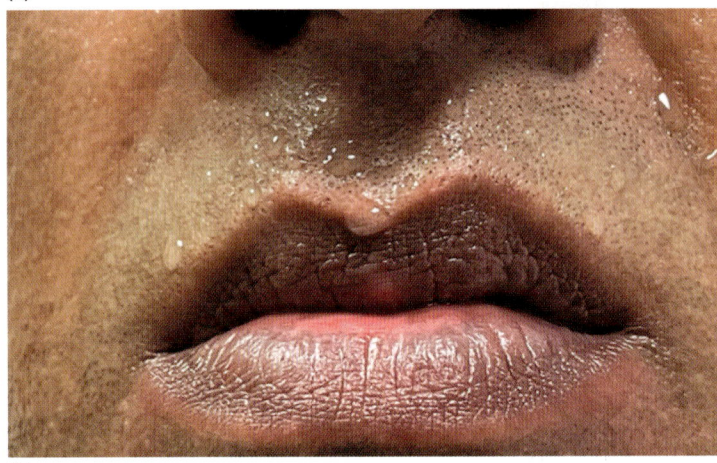

(b)

Figure 92.5 (a) Cranio-facial hyperhidrosis. It may be sufficiently profuse to drip off the face and wet the hair. (b) Cranio-facial hyperhidrosis – profuse facial sweating at rest in a cool room.

the eccrine glands, unlike axillary odour (bromhidrosis, see later in chapter), which is mainly apocrine in origin.

Cranio-facial hyperhidrosis. Cranio-facial hyperhidrosis (Figure 92.5) is often phasic, occurs in middle age and may be exacerbated by heat, exercise and eating but, unlike true gustatory hyperhidrosis, not exclusively so. It may be more persistent and usually presents at a later age than palmoplantar hyperhidrosis, and a postmenopausal variant is described [10]. The entire face and scalp may be affected; sweating sufficient to soak the hair is an additional embarrassment. Affected individuals may resort to wearing a towel around the neck to mop up excessive sweat.

Inguinal hyperhidrosis. The least common location for focal hyperhidrosis, bilateral disease (termed Hexsel hyperhidrosis) may be associated with focal axillary disease, is often familial, and saturation of the inguino-genital region may cause vulvitis [16].

Complications and co-morbidities

Palmoplantar hyperhidrosis predisposes to vesicular eczema (pompholyx) and allergic sensitisation to footwear constituents; control of sweating may thus reduce the risk of contact dermatitis to footwear materials. Maceration of the skin, particularly in the toe clefts, is common and may predispose to both dermatophyte and bacterial infection (see Chapters 26 and 32). Pitted keratolysis of the feet, due to infection with *Kytococcus sedentarius*, is strongly associated with hyperhidrosis (Figure 92.6).

Disease course and prognosis

Hyperhidrosis may persist for some years, but there is a tendency to spontaneous improvement of axillary and palmar hyperhidrosis after the age of 25 years.

Investigations

Thyroid function and gravimetric determination of sweat rate estimation are seldom helpful. Several severity tools for assessment of quality of life and effect of therapy are validated, such as the Hyperhidrosis Disease Severity Score (HDSS) and Hyperhidrosis Quality of Life Index (HidroQol).

Localised circumscribed and asymmetrical hyperhidrosis

Pathophysiology

The causes of localised hyperhidrosis are outlined in Box 92.3. Excessive sweating may be due to neurological lesions involving

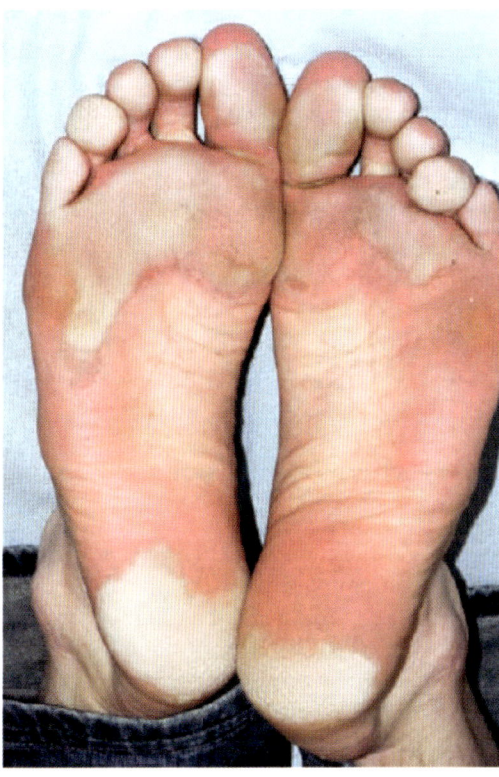

Figure 92.6 Plantar hyperhidrosis showing maceration of the plantar keratin and secondary pitted keratolysis due to infection with *Kytococcus sedentarius*.

Box 92.3 Causes of localised hyperhidrosis

- Spinal cord injury:
  - Hyperhidrosis associated with autonomic dysreflexia
  - Hyperhidrosis due to orthostatic hypotension
- Intrathoracic neoplasia
- Gustatory hyperhidrosis
- Frey syndrome
- Harlequin syndrome
- Granulosis rubra nasi
- Functional and true sweat gland naevi
- Sweating associated with local skin disorders:
  - Glomangioma
  - Blue rubber bleb naevi
  - Pachydermoperiostosis
  - Pretibial myxoedema
  - POEMS syndrome
  - Burning feet syndrome
- Compensatory: after sympathectomy, or with partial anhidrosis
- Idiopathic unilateral circumscribed hyperhidrosis

POEMS, polyneuropathy, organomegaly, endocrinopathy, M protein and skin changes.

---

any part of the sympathetic pathway from the brain to the nerve ending. It may be the presenting symptom, but it is quite exceptional for this to occur as an isolated phenomenon in the absence of other neurological symptoms or signs. Causative lesions may be within the central nervous system (cortex, basal ganglia or spinal cord), the sympathetic pathway and ganglia, or in the peripheral nerves [1,5,6,8,9,10,11,12–15]. It must be remembered that the distribution of the sympathetic nerves does not exactly correspond with sensory dermatomes. One sympathetic grey ramus may supply 10 or more sensory segments, and one white ramus extends over at least five. Asymmetrical sweating may also occur reflexively from visceral disturbances, adjacent to an area of anhidrosis or due to axon reflex stimulation, around a leg ulcer, for example, or around glomus tumours, blue rubber bleb naevi or a sudoriparous angioma.

Compensatory hyperhidrosis occurs in normal sweat glands when those elsewhere are not functioning because of neurological or skin disease, diabetes or after sympathectomy. It is also a component of Ross syndrome (see later).

Functional sweat gland naevi have been reported [14] but must be distinguished from sweat gland hypertrophy associated with local hyperhidrosis of some other aetiology. Areas of skin may be localised (Figure 92.7) [15], termed idiopathic circumscribed hyperhidrosis, or as extensive as one-half of the body [16] and may sweat continuously or, more commonly, with mental activity. They may represent functional naevi, where the eccrine glands show increased sensitivity to cholinergic neurotransmitters. In the absence of other

neurological symptoms or signs, they are seldom a manifestation of a progressive neurological lesion.

Cold-induced sweating syndrome

This rare condition presents in infancy with poor feeding and difficulty in suckling, followed in adulthood by paradoxically cold-induced hyperhidrosis and anhidrosis in heat [1]. There is an associated mild neuropathy, kyphoscoliosis, valgus deformity of the elbows, high arched palate and digital syndactyly. Inactivation of a cardiotropin-like cytokine, a second ligand for ciliary neurotrophic factor receptor, has been identified in this syndrome.

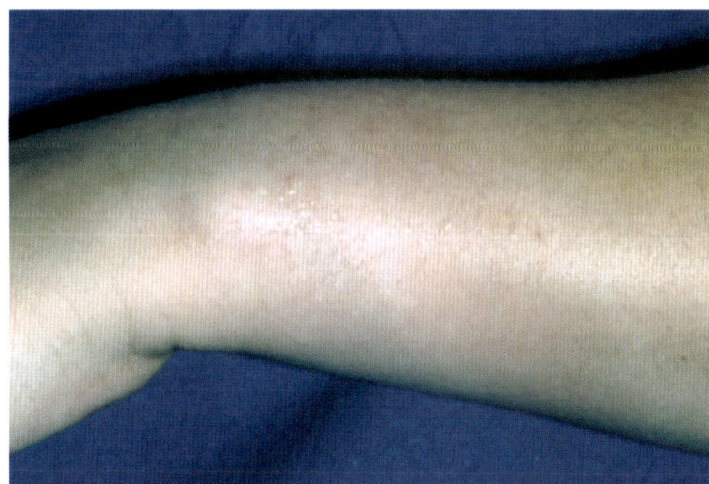

Figure 92.7 Circumscribed (naevoid) hyperhidrosis on the wrist. There is a solitary area of hyperhidrosis with normal sweating and neurology elsewhere on the rest of the skin.

Gustatory hyperhidrosis

Pathophysiology (Box 92.4)

Hyperhidrosis precipitated by eating specific foods can occur physiologically in many people [1]. Hot spicy foods are the most likely cause. The central connections of this reflex are not fully known.

Box 92.4 Classification of gustatory hyperhidrosis

- Idiopathic
- Central
- Postherpetic
- Postperipheral nerve injury:
  - Parotid surgery, injury and abscess
  - Auriculotemporal
  - Chorda tympani
  - Greater auricular
  - Cervical sympathectomy
- Peripheral autonomic neuropathy:
  - Diabetes

Gustatory hyperhidrosis also occurs in pathological conditions involving the autonomic nervous system. Localised areas of intense hyperhidrosis may occur on the face, and even on the knees [2]. These disorders are very rare, usually start in childhood and are not progressive. Their nature is little understood.

The commonest cause, however, is damage to the sympathetic nerves around the head and neck [3–5]. After such an injury, regeneration occurs not only from the proximal ends of the damaged sympathetic nerves, but also from damaged or undamaged parasympathetic nerves. In this way, abnormal connections are made. Thus, the reflex arcs that normally allow chewing or taste stimulation to cause parotid or gastric secretion may cause sweating in a localised zone corresponding to the area of skin in which the sympathetic innervation has been damaged. The commonest site is within the distribution of the auriculotemporal nerve, which may be injured by trauma, abscess or surgery in the parotid region (auriculotemporal or von Frey syndrome). Submental gustatory sweating follows injuries involving the chorda tympani, and sweating in the distribution of the greater auricular nerve commonly follows radical neck surgery [6]. Injury to fibres from the vagus may cause gustatory sweating localised to the upper arm after cervical sympathectomy.

Gustatory sweating may occur in diabetes as part of a widespread autonomic neuropathy [7]. It has also followed herpes zoster [8].

Clinical features

Gustatory sweating is not uncommon and occurs in 50–80% of patients subjected to operations on the parotid gland. Symptoms usually appear 4–7 months after the operation, and either persist indefinitely or wane after 3–5 years. The stimuli required to initiate the reflex vary, as does the severity. Sometimes chewing, without taste sensation, is the most important stimulus. In many cases it is merely a curiosity, but in others it can cause significant disability. As well as sweating there is usually vasodilatation, which in rare instances may occur by itself in the absence of visible sweating. For a classification and list of causes of gustatory hyperhidrosis see Box 92.4. Olfactory hyperhidrosis, in which the trigger stimulus is smell, has also been recorded [9].

Management

Treatment of severe cases may require surgical interruption of the parasympathetic pathway – for example, section of the glossopharyngeal nerve within the skull or tympanic neurectomy [4]. Excision of the auriculotemporal nerve is usually followed by recurrence. Topical therapy with aluminium chloride [10], topical glycopyrronium bromide [11] or botulinum toxin injections may be helpful [7].

Skin disorders where normal sweating can worsen the phenotype

In epidermolysis bullosa and pachyonychia congenita, normal sweating on the feet coupled with the skin fragility and friction from normal walking and weightbearing, may result in more blistering and hyperkeratosis. Studies have shown that reducing sweating with topical treatments and with botulinum toxin injections can reduce the incidence of blistering and pain [12]. Similarly, a placebo-controlled study in army cadets who have to run long distances as part of their training found that reducing sweating on the feet with a topical preparation of 15% aluminium chloride reduced the generation of friction blistering which could impede work performance [13].

Management of hyperhidrosis

Topical treatment

Topical anticholinergics. Atropine-like drugs may be absorbed sufficiently to produce a beneficial local effect without associated systemic side effects, but none of those at present available can be relied upon to do so [1]. Poldine methosulphate, 1–4% in alcohol, suppresses experimentally induced sweating, but unfortunately has not proved to be useful in clinical practice [2]. Topical 0.5% glycopyrronium bromide cream has been successfully used in gustatory hyperhidrosis in diabetics and at 0.5–2.0% for axillary hyperhidrosis [3]. A 2.0% aqueous solution has been used in scalp hyperhidrosis, and may be used to treat axillae. Recently, commercially available glycopyrrolate tosylate solution (2.4%) delivered on a wet wipe type towel has been introduced for axillary hyperhidrosis [4]. Other topical anticholinergic gels (sofpironium and oxybutynin) have shown suppression of axillary hyperhidrosis [5,6].

Eccrine duct-blocking agents. These drugs act by impeding the delivery of sweat to the skin surface. Formalin (40% aqueous solution of formaldehyde) 1% soaks have long been used for treatment of hyperhidrosis of the feet, but are unsuitable for the hands and axillae. Glutaraldehyde 10% in a buffered solution, pH 7.5, swabbed onto the feet three times weekly, has helped some patients [4], but stains the skin so that it is suitable only for the feet. There is a small risk of allergic sensitisation both to formaldehyde and to glutaraldehyde.

For axillary hyperhidrosis (as opposed to bromhidrosis), the most commonly used topical applications are aluminium or zirconium salts. Aluminium chloride, the first to be introduced, is in many ways the best, but may be irritant to the skin and damage clothes. Many other salts – for example, the chlorhydrates – are in use in cosmetic preparations [5]. Improved results can be achieved by applying 20% aluminium chloride in absolute ethanol at night after drying the axilla, with or without polythene occlusion. It should initially be applied nightly but may later be required only once every 1–4 weeks [6,7]. Commercial preparations are available. Mild irritation of the skin from such therapy may be helped by a weak topical corticosteroid and the use of a greasy emollient to protect the peri-axillary skin. The same treatment can also be tried on the hands and feet, or other localised areas of hyperhidrosis, but usually with rather less success. The mode of action of aluminium salts is uncertain, but they can be shown to affect both the duct and the secretory coil [8].

Iontophoresis. One of the more satisfactory methods of controlling hyperhidrosis of the hands and feet is by iontophoresis, using either tap water or anticholinergic drugs such as 0.05% glycopyrronium bromide solution [9–11,12]. The mode of action of tapwater iontophoresis is not known. In very soft water areas, adding sodium bicarbonate to the iontophoresis solution is reported to improve efficacy. Direct current is usually used, with each palm or sole being treated for 30 min with 20 mA, initially three times a week. Once euhidrosis is established, monthly maintenance treatment may be sufficient. Alternating current is less effective, but may usefully be combined with direct current (alternating current offset) to produce a safer, more comfortable treatment [13]. Once control has been achieved, a single treatment may prove effective for some weeks. Minor systemic side effects due to absorption of anticholinergic agents, such as dry mouth and eye symptoms, are not uncommon, and can be avoided if tap water alone is used. The authors' practice is to initiate thrice-weekly treatment on a hospital out-patient basis, and, if this is successful, a small battery-operated home unit can be purchased for maintenance therapy [14]. Less frequent treatment will then be required. When the sweating is controlled, the associated lividity, coolness and oedema improve. Similar treatment has also been used for the axilla, but is less often needed because topical applications or injections of botulinum toxin are more effective in this site. Devices have been designed to deliver iontophoresis to the chest and back affected by post-sympathectomy compensatory hyperhidrosis.

Botulinum toxin A injection. This compound produces prolonged blockade of neuronal acetylcholine release at the neuromuscular junction and in cholinergic autonomic neurons: it has been used to treat dystonic conditions for many years. In recent years, intradermal injection has been used to produce a marked reduction of sweating in hyperhidrotic areas associated with a variety of conditions [15,16–18]. Different preparations of botulinum A toxin have different activities, and dose schedules differ for each product;

0.1 mL of appropriately diluted botulinum toxin administered by high intradermal injection can be given to 1 cm^2 areas of skin appropriately anaesthetised – topical eutectic lignocaine/prilocaine is sufficient for axillary skin, but palms and soles may require regional nerve blockade, topical anaesthesia or application of ice. Each axilla usually requires 12 injections, hands 20 and each foot 24–36. A reduction in sweating is apparent within 48 h and the benefit will normally last for up to 8 months in axillary and 6 months in palmar and cranio-facial hyperhidrosis [19]. Reinjection seems to be effective, and to date resistance has not been seen in hyperhidrosis (although it eventually occurs in 5% of patients treated intramuscularly for dystonia). Botulinum toxin has been used for idiopathic circumscribed and gustatory hyperhidrosis including Frey syndrome, the hyperhidrotic areas in Ross syndrome, and frontal and cranio-facial hyperhidrosis and inguinal disease. A sight transient reduction of thenar and hypothenar muscle power is a minor problem after palmar injections [18]. The use of botulinum toxin on the forehead may produce short-lived frown reduction [19]. It is contraindicated in conditions affecting the neuromuscular junction and myasthenia.

Systemic drug treatment

Atropine-like drugs have been used to block the effect of acetylcholine on the sweat glands, but their side effects are often more troublesome than the hyperhidrosis itself. These include dryness of the mouth, constipation, urinary retention and disturbances of vision, due to paralysis of accommodation. More serious side effects, for example glaucoma, hyperthermia and convulsions, can occur. Atropine itself is seldom employed. Propantheline may be prescribed in doses of 15 mg three times daily, increasing, if tolerated, to as much as 150 mg daily [20], but overall the results are disappointing. Methantheline at a dose of 50 mg three times a day has recently been advocated [21]. The oral antimuscarinic agent oxybutynin, usually used to treat bladder instability, has been reported to be effective for generalised and focal hyperhidrosis. The dose is escalated from 2.5 mg daily to a maximum of 30 mg daily as tolerated, with an improvement in quality of life in 65% of those treated [22], although about 10% of those treated develop dryness of the mouth. Glycopyrrolate at a dose of up to 8 mg, in divided doses often gives useful sweat reduction without other marked anticholinergic effects [23]. Clonidine at a dose of 0.1 twice daily may be useful, but hypotension may limit its use. Ganglion-blocking drugs can inhibit sweating, but side effects from hypotension are usually too troublesome. Calcium-channel blockers, such as diltiazem, have helped some patients [24]. In cases with a pronounced emotional factor, sedative or tranquillising drugs are often useful, but psychiatric treatment may be necessary. Both clonazepam [25] and amitriptyline have helped isolated cases of unusual localised hyperhidrosis.

Surgical treatment

Sympathectomy. Sympathectomy, whether cervical, transaxillary or endoscopic, causes anhidrosis, if complete [26,27]. Sweating may return after a period of some years, due either to regeneration of sympathetic fibres or to fibres that do not pass through the sympathetic ganglia [28]. The former open approach has been largely replaced by an endoscopic procedure, which may be successful in treating palmar, axillary and cranio-facial hyperhidrosis. A pneumothorax is induced, and an operating endoscope inserted into the thorax via a small axillary incision, allowing visualisation of the sympathetic trunk. Interruption of the sympathetic fibres between the second and fourth thoracic ganglia can be achieved by surgical transection, radiofrequency ablation, phenol destruction, cautery, clamping or clipping [29]. The latter technique has the potential advantage of partial reversibility. Most surgeons treat both sides at a single session. Lumbar sympathectomy is occasionally justified for plantar hyperhidrosis.

With both the open and endoscopic approaches, satisfactory reduction of palmar hyperhidrosis is achieved in over 95% of cases; it is a little less successful for axillary hyperhidrosis. A recent consensus guideline [30] suggested that an international nomenclature should be adopted that refers to the rib levels (R) instead of the vertebral level at which the nerve is interrupted. It states that the highest success rates occur when interruption is performed at the top of R3 or the top of R4 for hyperhidrosis limited to the palms. R4 may offer a lower incidence of compensatory hyperhidrosis but moister hands. For hyperhidrosis involving the upper limbs and/or the axillae, interruptions at R4 and R5 are recommended. The top of R3 is best for cranio-facial hyperhidrosis.

In a series of 1731 patients who underwent endoscopic sympathectomy, the initial failure rate was 9%, and there was recurrence in 2%; overall, 98% of those treated were satisfied with the result. Compensatory hyperhidrosis occurred in 88% of patients and was severe in 27%. Only 2.5% of patients experienced regret for having the operation [31]. Large case series using endoscopic techniques in children show it to be an acceptable option, with a low recurrence rate [32].

Complications of sympathectomy include haemothorax, pneumothorax, chylothorax, nipple sensitivity and Horner syndrome. There are rare instances of transient or permanent bradycardia complicating the technique. Other disadvantages are that the palms or soles may become excessively dry, and irritant eczema after sympathectomy has been reported. In five patients who had undergone a clipping procedure and subsequently developed compensatory hyperhidrosis, removal of the clips resulted in a return of the palmar sweating and abolition of the compensatory hyperhidrosis [33]. It has been suggested that ablation at the level of the third thoracic ganglion does not produce this side effect. Management of post-sympathectomy compensatory hyperhidrosis is difficult; topical and oral anticholinergics are usually unhelpful. There has been recent interest in diffuse sympathectomy, where further ablation of R5 to R11 is undertaken, with resolution of excess sweating established in 80% of those treated. Abolition of severe facial blushing may be a desirable consequence and resolution of palmar eczema has been reported after endoscopic sympathectomy.

In general, only those patients with severe disability from hyperhidrosis of the hands or axillae warrant surgery, and in these selected cases the results can be very gratifying. Endoscopic sympathectomy has been used successfully in the treatment of severe cranio-facial hyperhidrosis [34]. Pedal sympathetic denervation requires lumbar sympathectomy; if more cranial lumbar ganglia are removed, ejaculatory impotence may occur. A selective retroperitoneal approach has recently been advocated that has no effect on sexual function in either men or women [35]. An endoscopic technique employing clips may also be employed with high patient satisfaction and minimal surgical morbidity.

Physical eccrine gland ablation. Minimally invasive techniques to ablate the eccrine sweat glands have been introduced in the last few years, and long-term efficacy is to be established. Microwave-delivering units causing selective thermolysis can result in prolonged and possibly permanent relief of axillary hyperhidrosis after one or two treatment sessions. Radiofrequency energy delivered to the upper dermis by microneedles results in thermal destruction of eccrine glands and reduction of hyperhidrosis after one or two treatments, although a side-to-side comparison with botulinum injection showed greater success with the latter therapy [36].

Excision of the axillary vault. Axillary hyperhidrosis may be greatly helped by local excision of the axillary vault [37,38]. Variations of this technique include subcutaneous curettage of the axillary skin [39], directly trimming the eccrine glands after reflection of the axillary skin using only a short incision [40], and tumescent liposuction of the axillae [41].

Treatment ladder for hyperhidrosis

First line
- Eccrine duct-blocking agents (aluminium chloride hexahydrate)
- Topical anticholinergics (glycopyrrolate)

Second line
- Iontophoresis with tap water or anticholinergics (hands, feet and axillae)
- Intradermal botulinum toxin (axillae, hands and face)
- Oral anticholinergics: propanthelene, methanthelene oxybutynin, glycopyrrolate
- Oral clonidine
- Oral β-blockers and anxiolytics
- Physical therapies – microwave or radiofrequency ablation

Third line
- Removal or ablation of eccrine glands (axillary)
- Sympathectomy (thoracic or lumbar)

Granulosis rubra nasi

Definition

Granulosis rubra nasi is a rare disorder characterised by hyperhidrosis of the nose and associated skin changes [1].

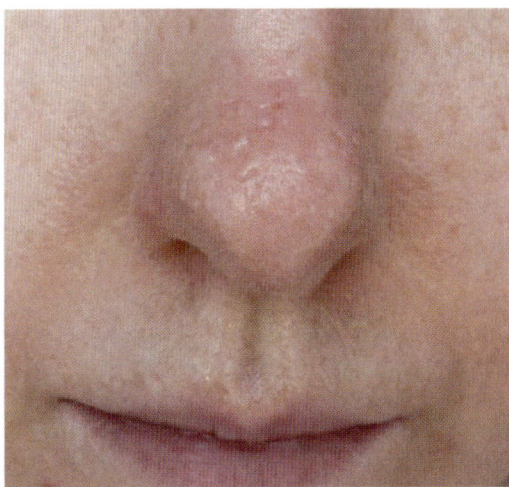

Figure 92.8 Granulosis rubra nasi in young adult female showing localised hyperhidrosis with beads of sweat on nose and philtrum together with multiple vesicles and mild erythema on dorsum of nose. Courtesy of Dr E.P. Burova, Bedford Hospital, UK.

Epidemiology and pathophysiology

The condition was first described by Jadassohn. The pathogenesis remains obscure but in some cases there is evidence of autosomal dominant transmission [2]. Symptoms develop from as early as 6 months but can occur at any age in childhood and occasionally in adults.

Clinical features

Initial presentation is with excess sweating localised over the tip of the nose. Droplets of sweat are usually visible. With time redness, papules, vesicles and telangiectasia may develop over the nose, cheeks and upper lips (Figure 92.8) [3]. In the vast majority of cases, resolution occurs around puberty, but persistent cases are recognised. Patients may also report peripheral acrocyanosis and palmoplantar hyperhidrosis. A single case has been described in association with phaeochromocytoma [4]. Skin biopsy demonstrates a chronic inflammatory cell infiltrate with dilatation of vascular spaces [3].

Investigations

These are not usually needed.

Management

Reassurance, given the natural history of the condition, is sufficient in most cases. Botulinum toxin has been reported as effective [5], and there are two case reports of response to topical tacrolimus [6].

Anhidrosis and hypohidrosis

Diminished sweat production may be partial (hypohidrosis) or complete (anhidrosis) [1]. Disturbance of any part of the physiological pathway of sweat production may decrease sweating. Causes may be broadly classified as being neurological (Box 92.5) or eccrine gland in origin (Box 92.6).

Box 92.5 Neurological causes of anhidrosis and hypohidrosis

- Organic brain lesions of hypothalamus, pons and medulla
- Spinal cord lesions:
  - Syringomyelia
  - Sympathectomy
- Congenital insensitivity to pain with anhidrosis
- Degenerative syndromes:
  - Shy–Drager syndrome
  - Ross syndrome
- Peripheral neuropathy:
  - Diabetes
  - Alcohol
  - Leprosy
- Autonomic neuropathy
- Drug-induced blockade of neurotransmission:
  - Ganglion-blocking agents
  - Anticholinergic agents
  - Calcium channel-blocking agents
  - α-adrenergic blockers

Box 92.6 Eccrine gland disorders producing anhidrosis and hypohidrosis

- Genetic disorders:
  - Bazex syndrome
  - Ectodermal dysplasia
  - Fabry disease
  - Incontinentia pigmenti
  - Naegeli–Franchetti–Jadassohn syndrome
- Atrophy or destruction of eccrine glands:
  - Scleroderma
  - Burns
  - Sjögren syndrome
  - Lymphoma
  - Acrodermatitis chronica atrophicans
- Obstruction of sweat ducts:
  - Miliaria
  - Eczema
  - Psoriasis
  - Lichen planus
  - Ichthyosis
  - Porokeratosis
- Drugs affecting eccrine gland function:
  - Topical aluminium salts
  - 5-Fluorouracil
  - Mepacrine
  - Topiramate
  - Checkpoint inhibitors
- Idiopathic:
  - Acquired idiopathic generalised anhidrosis

Impairment of sweat production interferes with the body's temperature control mechanisms. Symptoms include heat intolerance, fatigue, drowsiness and pyrexia. In severe cases death may result.

Examination of patients with hypo- and anhidrosis is often unremarkable. A novel bedside test demonstrating the reduced traction provided to a spoon stroked against the affected skin (the spoon test) may allow for its appreciation [2]. Autonomic function tests, in particular the quantitative sudomotor axon reflex test and the thermoregulatory sweat test (essentially a heat stress in a warmed room), may help delineate the distribution of anhidrosis and point towards a cause [3]. Skin biopsy is also helpful to identify eccrine sweat gland abnormalities.

Ross syndrome

This rare syndrome is characterised by a triad of segmental anhidrosis, tonic pupils (Figure 92.9a) and absent deep tendon reflexes [3]. It is a progressive degenerative disorder of sensory and autonomic nerves [4,5]. Accumulation of alpha synuclein has been demonstrated in cholinergic fibres [6]. Involvement of the cardiac sympathetic nerve supply has also been reported [7].

The main symptoms are those of heat intolerance and socially disabling compensatory hyperhidrosis (Figure 92.9b), which may be asymmetrical, patchy or unilateral. Hyperhidrosis arising in this situation has been successfully treated with iontophoresis and botulinum toxin [4,7].

Acquired idiopathic generalised anhidrosis

This term describes a heterogeneous group of very rare disorders characterised by progressive loss of sweating and heat intolerance [9]. Three subtypes have been proposed: idiopathic pure sudomotor failure, sudomotor neuropathy and sweat gland failure [10]. In a proportion of patients, lymphocytic infiltration of the eccrine glands is seen and the presence of such inflammation may explain the response to oral corticosteroids and ciclosporin observed in this condition [11]. Like some other autoimmune skin disorders, it has been seen in those receiving checkpoint inhibitors for melanoma. In some sufferers, optical coherence tomography has shown hyporefractile material below the stratum corneum, which was felt to be obliterating the eccrine duct. The majority of patients significantly improved with oral isotretinoin [12].

Miliaria

Definition and nomenclature

This is a common acute or subacute skin condition that arises due to the occlusion or disruption of eccrine sweat ducts in hot humid conditions, resulting in a leakage of sweat into the epidermis (miliaria crystallina and miliaria rubra) or dermis (miliaria profunda) [1–3].

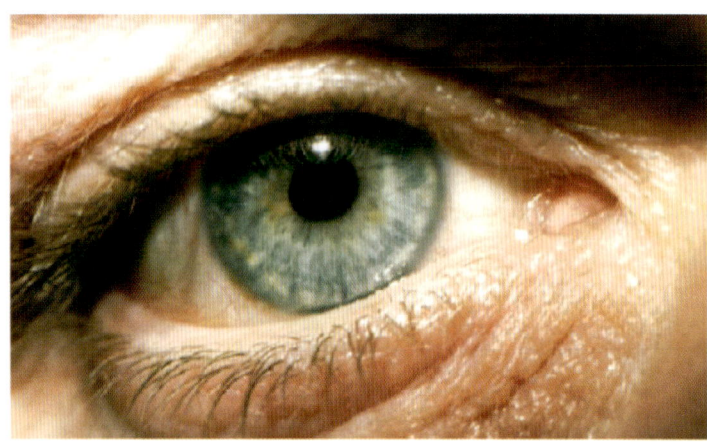

(a)

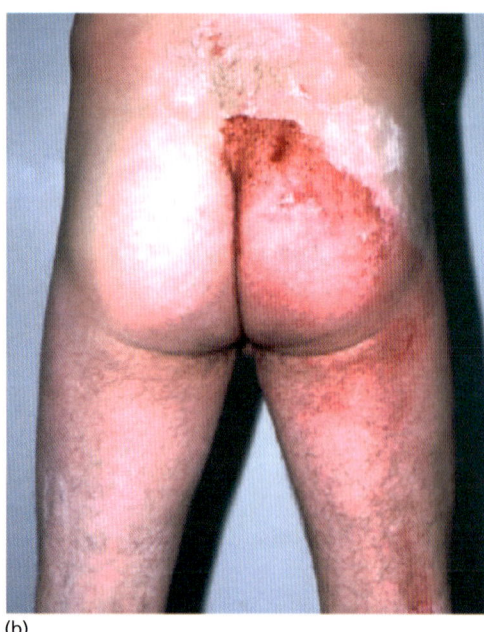

(b)

Figure 92.9 Ross syndrome. (a) The pupils are tonic, asymmetrical and irregular in outline. (b) Most of the skin is anhidrotic but the remaining areas of enervated eccrine glands demonstrate compensatory hyperhidrosis (demonstrated by Edicol ponceau powder, which turns red on hydration).

Synonyms and inclusions
- Prickly heat
- Miliaria crystallina
- Miliaria rubra
- Miliaria profunda

Introduction and general description

The three forms of miliaria – miliaria crystallina (sudamina), miliaria rubra (prickly heat) and miliaria profunda – occur as a result of either occlusion or disruption of the eccrine sweat ducts. They differ in clinical form due to the different levels at which occlusion occurs, although some authorities have suggested that disruption of the duct rather than occlusion is responsible [4]. In miliaria crystallina, the obstruction is very superficial, within the stratum corneum, and the vesicle is subcorneal, producing a vesicle containing clear fluid. In miliaria rubra, the later changes include keratinisation of the intraepidermal part of the sweat duct, with leakage and then formation of a vesicle around the duct. In miliaria profunda, there is rupture of the duct at the level of or below the dermal–epidermal junction.

Epidemiology

Miliaria crystallina occurs commonly in infants due to a delay in patency developing in the sweat ducts. In a large Japanese study, it was identified in 4.5% of babies, with a peak frequency at 1 week [5]. The incidence of miliaria rubra, and particularly miliaria profunda, is highest in hot, humid conditions, but it may occur in desert regions, affecting up to 30% of people exposed to these climatic conditions. It may begin within a few days of arrival in a tropical climate, but is maximal after 2–5 months. There is a striking variation in individual susceptibility. Infants are especially prone.

Miliaria rubra is common on the trunk in hospitalised patients who have to be nursed on their backs on bedding that has waterproof occlusive membranes below the sheets. It may also commonly be seen after occlusive therapy with polythene. Outbreaks on the legs in miners working in tropical climates have been reported [6].

Pathophysiology

Miliaria crystallina can easily be produced experimentally by minimal, non-specific epidermal injury and profuse sweating [7]. It has been identified by the use of tight fitting personal protective masks during the Covid-19 pandemic. It is often seen in febrile illnesses associated with profuse sweating. It occurs commonly in infants due to a delay in patency developing in the sweat ducts.

Miliaria rubra may be produced experimentally in susceptible subjects by epidermal injury [8]. It can be reproduced regularly by occlusion of the skin under polythene for 3–4 days, following which anhidrosis lasts for about 3 weeks. Prolonged exposure of the skin to sweat achieves the same effect. The first event may be an increase in the skin flora, perhaps with *Staphylococcus epidermidis* being responsible for producing an extracellular polysaccharide substance or slime that blocks the lumen of the sweat duct [1,9]. The parakeratotic plugs, which are a notable feature of the later stages of the disease, are not the primary cause of the obstruction, but arise in the repair process, and may further aggravate the obstruction. Leakage of sweat into the epidermis is responsible for the final production of the lesions, and for their further aggravation.

Miliaria profunda is due to more severe damage to the sweat ducts, and usually follows repeated attacks of miliaria rubra. It may be reproduced by experimental injury.

Rarely, miliaria may be associated with pseudohypoaldosteronism; high sweat sodium levels produce damage of the eccrine ducts, causing lesions similar to those seen in miliaria rubra. It can be precipitated by drugs (bethanechol, isotretinoin and doxorubicin).

Clinical features

Clinical features of the three types of miliaria are.

Miliaria crystallina. Clear, thin-walled vesicles, 1–2 mm in diameter without surrounding inflammation, are usually symptomless and develop in crops, mainly on the trunk. In persistent febrile illnesses, recurrent crops may occur. The vesicles soon rupture, and are followed by superficial, branny desquamation.

Miliaria rubra. Typical lesions develop on the body, especially in areas of friction with clothing, and in flexures. The lesions are uniformly minute red papules, which may be present in very large numbers (Figure 92.10). Characteristically, the lesions produce intense discomfort in the form of an unbearable pricking sensation. Relief is often instantaneous when the stimulus to sweating is

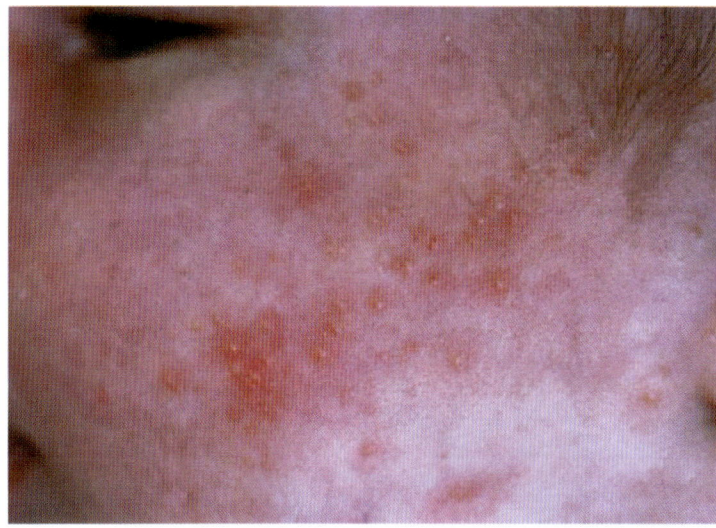

Figure 92.10 Miliaria rubra affecting the cheeks of an infant. Courtesy of Dr Richard Logan, Bridgend, UK.

abolished by a cool shower. In infants, lesions commonly appear on the occluded skin of the neck, groins and axillae, but also occur elsewhere. Patients often wrongly refer to polymorphic light eruption as 'prickly heat'; here the relationship of the rash to light, particularly on newly exposed sites, is usually straightforward.

Miliaria profunda. This nearly always follows repeated attacks of miliaria rubra and is uncommon except in the tropics. The lesions are easily missed. The affected skin is covered with pale, firm papules 1–3 mm across, especially on the body (Figure 92.11), but sometimes also on the limbs. There is no itching or discomfort from the lesions.

Disease course and prognosis

This depends mainly on environmental factors. If continued sweating occurs, recurrent episodes lasting a few days are usual, but discomfort may be continuous. However, after a few months some degree of acclimatisation occurs, and the disorder becomes less prevalent.

The most important complications of miliaria are secondary infection and disturbance of heat regulation. Secondary bacterial infection is common and sometimes serious. This may present as impetigo. In other cases, the pustules are more clearly related to sweat ducts, although in pustular miliaria factors other than bacterial infection are implicated [10]. Miliaria rubra in young infants may predispose to multiple superimposed staphylococcal abscesses [11]. In most cases of miliaria rubra the changes are reversible if further sweating is avoided, but permanent damage to the sweat duct may occur, especially after miliaria profunda.

Management

The only really effective prevention or treatment for miliaria is avoidance of further sweating. Even if this is achieved only for a few hours a day, as in an air-conditioned office or bedroom, considerable relief is experienced. For the very susceptible person,

PART 8: SPECIFIC CUTANEOUS STRUCTURES

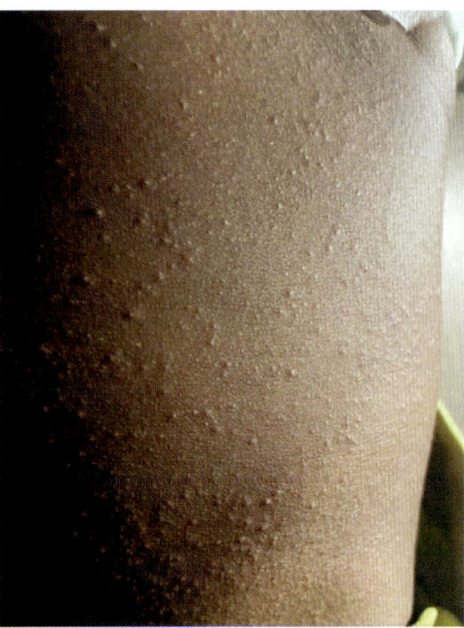

Figure 92.11 Milaria profunda in an African child. Courtesy of Dr Ibrahima Trauore, Guinea.

a move away from tropical climates may be essential. Avoidance of excessive clothing, friction from clothing, excessive use of soap and contact of the skin with irritants will reduce the incidence. The large number of treatments advocated for prickly heat is the best indication of their relative ineffectiveness if sweating is not reduced. In the absence of gross secondary sepsis, the effect of topical or systemic antibiotics or other antibacterial preparations on established miliaria is disappointing, but they may have some role in prophylaxis [1]. Oral ascorbic acid 500 mg twice daily was found to diminish the severity of miliaria, as was the degree of subsequent anhidrosis in experimentally induced disease [12]. Calamine lotion is probably as effective as anything for the relief of discomfort, but because of its drying effect, a bland emollient (e.g. oily cream or menthol in aqueous cream) may subsequently be required to prevent further epidermal damage. Isotretinoin was reported to help a recalcitrant case of miliaria profunda [13].

Treatment ladder for milaria

First line
- Control local environment (remove excess bedding, fans, air conditioning)
- Cool the skin (damp compresses, cool showers)
- Avoid tight or excessive clothing

Second line
- Menthol (e.g. 0.5% menthol in aqueous cream)
- Topical antibiotics if there is secondary infection
- Mild topical steroids

Third line
- Removal to cooler climate
- Prophylactic oral vitamin C

Neutrophilic eccrine hidradenitis

Definition and nomenclature
Neutrophilic eccrine hidradenitis refers to a rare clinical condition with non-specific features but characteristic acute inflammation of the eccrine sweat glands, seen on skin biopsy.

Synonyms and inclusions
- Chemotherapy-associated eccrine hidradenitis
- Idiopathic palmoplantar hidradenitis

Introduction and general description
Neutrophilic eccrine hidradenitis (NEH) may arise in a variety of very different clinical situations, producing an eruption with very distinct pathological features. It can be classified into the following types:
- Chemotherapy-induced NEH.
- Infectious NEH.
- Palmoplantar NEH.
- NEH with HIV infection.
- NEH with Behçet disease.

Epidemiology
This is a rare condition that may be considered a reaction pattern to a variety of stimuli [1,2,3]. Drug-induced NEH is primarily seen in patients receiving cytotoxic chemotherapy, while childhood NEH affects otherwise well children [4,5]. Attacks of childhood NEH are reported to be more frequent in the spring and summer. Disease-associated NEH and infectious NEH are both very rare.

Pathophysiology
The key pathological feature of NEH is necrosis of the eccrine epithelium in association with a dense neutrophilic infiltrate. In drug-induced NEH this is most commonly reported with the use of cytotoxic chemotherapeutic agents. Typical histological changes can be induced experimentally by the local injection of bleomycin into human skin, suggesting that the eccrine glands are subject to direct toxicity [6]. Other drugs reported in association with NEH include carbamazepine, tumour necrosis factor α antagonists, BRAF inhibitors and cetuximab [7,8,9].

Childhood NEH is not associated with underlying disease. However, it may follow physical exertion and exposure to damp footwear [10].

Infectious NEH is most frequently encountered in immune-suppressed individuals. Causative organisms implicated include *Serratia*, staphylococci, streptococci and *Nocardia* [11–13]. NEH has also been reported in HIV infection, Behçet disease and as a paraneoplastic phenomenon in both haematological and solid organ malignancies [12,13,14,15].

Clinical features
Drug-associated NEH typically occurs 8–10 days after starting chemotherapy. Painful red papules and plaques develop on the limbs, neck and face [2]. Facial redness and swelling may be severe

enough to mimic cellulitis [16]. The condition typically resolves within 2 weeks of treatment ending. Recurrence, however, may occur with subsequent courses of chemotherapy [17].

Childhood NEH has a particular predilection for the soles and less frequently the palms. Typically, tender plaques and nodules are seen. Attacks resolve spontaneously in 3 weeks but the condition may be recurrent [4,5,**18**].

Investigations

In drug-induced NEH, skin biopsy is diagnostic. Associated neutropenia is also common. Further investigations may be necessary to exclude sepsis. Investigation of childhood NEH is not usually necessary.

Management

In the majority of cases the condition resolves without any treatment. In adult NEH systemic corticosteroids, dapsone and colchicine have all been recommended [15,19]. Dapsone may also be helpful in preventing recurrent disease [20].

Eccrine syringosquamous metaplasia

Definition

Eccrine syringosquamous metaplasia is used to describe both histological change, seen within eccrine sweat glands, and also a distinct skin eruption associated with the use of chemotherapeutic agents [1].

Pathophysiology
Predisposing factors

Eccrine syringosquamous metaplasia is characterised by the transformation of cuboidal ductal epithelial cells into areas of squamous differentiation [2]. This process has been reported in a wide variety of different settings including pyoderma gangrenosum, panniculitis and infection [3,4]. It is considered a non-specific marker of eccrine duct damage and may be confused histologically with squamous cell carcinoma. Similar histological changes are seen in patients undergoing chemotherapy, presumably forming part of a spectrum of cytotoxic eccrine damage, which includes NEH [5].

Clinical features

In patients undergoing chemotherapy, eccrine syringosquamous metaplasia has been observed following the use of a range of drugs, most notably cytarabine and protein kinase inhibitors. The eruption develops during or shortly after chemotherapy and slowly resolves spontaneously. Widespread papulovesicular lesions, acral redness and an intertriginous eruption may all be seen.

Investigations
Skin biopsy is usually diagnostic.

Management
The condition resolves spontaneously but symptom control may be required.

Drugs and eccrine glands

A number of drugs are concentrated and secreted by eccrine glands. This may partially account both for their therapeutic effect and cutaneous toxicity. Drugs known to be secreted include sulfaguanidine, sulfadiazine, amphetamines, arsenicals, iodides, phenytoin, phenobarbitone, carbamazepine, griseofulvin, ketoconazole, fluconazole, ciprofloxacin, diamorphine, cocaine and nicotine [1]. Sweat testing may be used as an alternative to urine testing in the setting of substance abuse [2].

Disorders with sweat gland cellular inclusions

The accumulation of substances within eccrine secretory cells occurs in a number of metabolic conditions summarised in Table 92.1 [1–5].

APOCRINE GLANDS

Anatomy and physiology of apocrine glands

Apocrine sweat glands derive their name from the way their secretion appears (Greek apo- 'away' and krinein 'to separate'). On light microscopy, the secretions appear to be 'pinched off' by parts of the cytoplasm. They are epidermal appendages and develop as part of the pilosebaceous follicle in the fourth to fifth month of intrauterine life. In the embryo they are present over the entire skin surface, but most glands subsequently disappear, so that in the adult the characteristic distribution in the axillae, perianal region and areolae of the breasts is found [1–3,4]. So-called ectopic glands may be found elsewhere. The mammary glands and ceruminous glands in the external auditory meati are modified apocrine glands. Apocrine glands are poorly developed in childhood and begin to enlarge with the approach of puberty. The activity of the glands is androgen dependent, and the glands show marked testosterone 5α-reductase activity [5].

The glands are larger than eccrine glands, and in the dissected specimen are visible to the naked eye. They are situated in the subcutaneous tissue. Each consists of a tubule and a duct. The latter is often quite short and opens into the neck of the hair follicle above the

Table 92.1 Disorders with characteristic eccrine gland inclusion.

Microscopic changes	Disorder
Membrane-bound vacuoles in secretory cells	Mucopolysaccharidoses (Hurler, Hunter and Sanfillipo types)
Intracytoplasmic lipid inclusions	Sphingolipidoses
Secretory cell inclusions	Fabry disease, fucosidosis, Kanzaki disease, adrenoleukodystrophy and maltase deficiency
PAS-positive granules in outer duct cells	Lafora disease

PAS, periodic acid–Schiff stain.

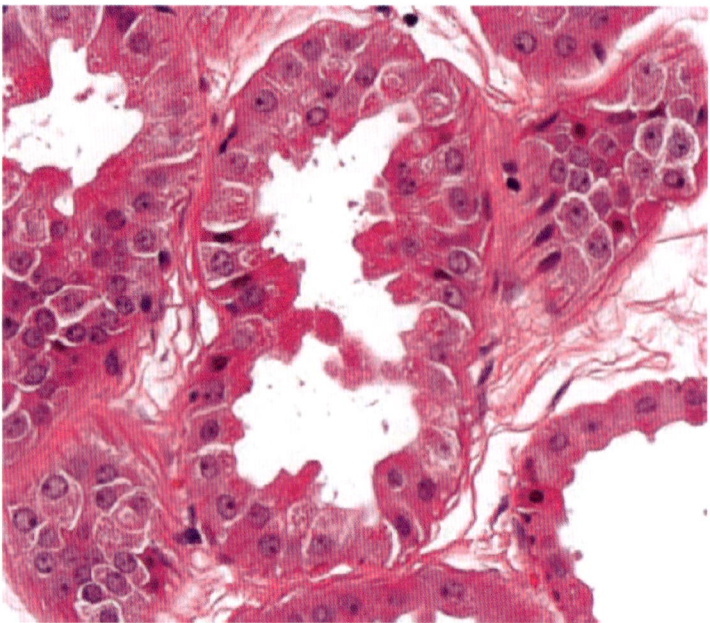

Figure 92.12 Normal apocrine glands lined by cells with abundant eosinophilic cytoplasm and decapitation secretions. Magnification 40× (H&E). Courtesy of Dr Arti Bakshi, Liverpool University Hospitals NHS Foundation Trust, UK.

sebaceous gland. Despite their embryological origin from the hair follicle, some apocrine glands eventually open on the surface of the skin. The secretory coil is a simple convoluted tube. It is lined by a single layer of columnar or cuboidal cells resting on a basement membrane. The free edge of the cells may show the appearance of apocrine secretion (Figure 92.12). Electron microscopy shows that this may be partly an artefact, but eccrine, apocrine and even holocrine secretion may all be found in places [3,6,7]. The apocrine duct closely resembles the eccrine duct and consists of a double layer of cuboidal cells. Outside the basement membrane of the gland and duct is a longitudinal layer of myoepithelial cells. Their function is to support the duct and to propel the secretion to the surface, and waves of peristalsis have been seen in them [8]. Where the duct opens into the neck of the hair follicle there is the equivalent of the acrosyringium of the eccrine duct, although it is less obvious [9]. Apocrine sweat glands have an adrenergic sympathetic supply but neural control appears to be unimportant [10].

Apocrine glands secrete small quantities of an oily fluid. This secretion is odourless on reaching the surface of the skin. Bacterial decomposition is responsible for the production of odiferous compounds. In particular, corynebacterial aminoacylase is responsible for the production of 3-methyl-2-hexenoic and 3-hydroxy-3-methylhexenoic acids [11]. Smaller quantities of odiferous sulphanylalkanols and steroids have also been identified [12,13]. The production of these metabolites is under the genetic control of the *ABCC11* gene, which encodes an ATP-driven efflux pump. Individuals homozygotic for a mutation in this gene produce much less odour. Mutation in this gene is predominant in South-East Asians, explaining racial variations in body odour [14].

There is evidence that products of apocrine sweat glands may act as human pheromones but the specific chemicals and pathways involved have not yet been elucidated [15].

DISORDERS OF APOCRINE SWEAT GLANDS

Abnormal sweat odour (bromhidrosis)

Definition and nomenclature
Human skin odour is largely due to the production of volatile chemicals by the actions of bacteria on secreted apocrine sweat.

> **Synonyms and inclusions**
> • Osmidrosis

Epidemiology
Human skin odour is largely determined by alteration or degradation of odourless substances secreted by apocrine glands by bacteria, especially *Corynebacterium* species, in the presence of hyperhidrosis [1]. Eccrine secretion is usually odourless but can contain odour-producing substances that are excreted in it, such as drugs, arsenic and garlic. Sebaceous secretion has some odour, as do the decomposition products of keratin, which can cause malodour in some hyperkeratinising disorders such as keratodermas and Darier disease. On occasion, malodour appreciated only by the patient may be a symptom of monosymptomatic delusion of malodour (olfactory reference disorder) which requires psychiatric intervention [2] (Chapter 84), or from an organic lesion of the central nervous system.

Incidence
There is marked individual and racial variation in body odour, and what is socially acceptable varies greatly with race and social upbringing.

Age
As apocrine secretion increases under androgen control, malodour usually develops at or after puberty. Cases of generalised bromhidrosis in children have been reported due to chronic retention of nasal foreign bodies, and as a result of precocious puberty.

Sex
Malodour is more evident in men, but men and women seek medical management with equal frequency [3].

Ethnicity
There is anecdotal evidence that axillary malodour is more prevalent in European and African individuals, and less so in East Asian, Chinese and Korean people.

Associated diseases
Recent studies have associated axillary malodour with wet-type ear wax, and this is the result of a single nucleotide polymorphism in the *ABCC11* gene [4]. This gene is responsible for the function of the apical efflux pump and the conjugation of some of the odour-producing thioalcohols. Dry ear wax individuals do not produce these substances.

Pathophysiology

In the axillae, high humidity due to eccrine sweating and sebaceous secretion results in a rich microflora, including bacteria of the genera *Staphylococcus*, *Micrococcus*, *Corynebacterium* and *Propionobacterium*. An increased axillary pH may facilitate the overgrowth of these bacteria. Late sudden onset of bromhidrosis has been associated with *Sphingomonas paucimobilis* infection of axillary skin, resolving with appropriate antibiotic therapy. Apocrine secretions are largely odourless, but biotransformation by bacteria, particularly corynebacteria, results in the liberation of short- and medium-chain volatile fatty acids (C2 to C10 branch length), 16-androstene steroids and thioalcohols, each of which may produce its own odour signature [1]. Studies have demonstrated histological differences between normal and bromhidrotic apocrine glands; in the bromhidrotics, the apocrine glands were larger and more numerous [5].

Clinical features

Presentation may be due to the patient being conscious of emitting odour, or as the result of comments from friends and relatives. Sniff testing may result in the appreciation of the character of the malodour, such as 'onion-like and beefy' or a 'lighter fruity' note.

Management

The treatment of axillary bromhidrosis includes the omission of foodstuffs such as garlic from the diet, frequent washing of the axillary regions and local antibacterial substances. There is no evidence that measures used to control axillary eccrine hyperhidrosis – for example, aluminium salts and anticholinergic drugs – have much effect on the apocrine glands, although excessive eccrine excretion may favour the spread of apocrine secretion and facilitate proliferation of the odour-producing microflora.

Deodorants are the mainstay of therapy as the fragrances disguise the undesired odour. A topical glycine-soya sterocomplex agent has shown encouraging improvement on both the intensity and quality of odour in patients with bromhidrosis [6]. A silver-zeolite powder has been shown to have strong antibacterial effects on axillary microflora and to diminish axillary malodour [7]. Botulinum toxin A has been used to treat axillary [8] and genital malodour [9] with good effect: the impact on eccrine sweating and rendering the area anhidrotic may prevent bacterial activity and thus have an effect on odour. There is some evidence that botulinum toxin reduces apocrine gland secretion and size. Surgical excision of axillary subcutaneous tissue by a variety of surgical techniques (axillary shave and subsection of subcutaneous glands, laser ablation, ultrasound ablation, intradermal alcohol injection, liposuction and hydrosurgical jet injection), which removes both eccrine and apocrine glands, has been performed with good effect in those dissatisfied with conservative measures [10,**11,12**]. Microwave devices used primarily for hyperhidrosis may also diminish bromhidrosis.

Treatment ladder for bromhidrosis

First line
- Regular washing
- Avoidance of odour-producing foodstuffs
- Deodorants

Second line
- Silver-zeolite powder
- Botulinum toxin

Third line
- Removal or ablation of apocrine glands

Trimethylaminuria

Definition and nomenclature

This disorder results from excessive amounts of the offensively smelling tertiary amine trimethylamine appearing in eccrine and apocrine sweat, breath and urine, and imparting an unpleasant rotting fish smell to sufferers [1].

Synonyms and inclusions
- Fish odour syndrome

Epidemiology

Incidence

The ability to N-oxidise trimethylamine into trimethylamine oxide (which has no odour) is distributed polymorphically, and sufferers are homozygous for an allele that determines this impaired reaction. One per cent of the population are heterozygous carriers of the allele.

Age

Most cases present in their late teens or early twenties.

Sex

The incidence does not vary by sex.

Pathophysiology

Affected individuals are unable to oxidise trimethylamine, which is produced by the intestinal bacterial degradation of choline and carnitine in food, to the odourless trimethylamine N-oxide. This can occur as a primary problem, as a result of a mutation in the flavin-containing mono-oxygenase3 (*FMO3*) gene [2]. Secondary trimethylaminuria can occur when there is an increased burden of trimethylamine and is seen when there is an increased production of it from its precursors by gut bacteria in conditions such as blind loop syndrome, uraemia and liver disease.

Clinical features

The unpleasant odour, which is often worse after eating seafood, during periods of stress or during menstruation, can be the source of much distress, rejection and resentment. Sufferers are sometimes unaware of their smell, which may be intermittent and may not be detected by physicians when consulted. Trimethylaminuria was found in 7% of a series of individuals who perceived themselves to be malodorous [3].

Investigations

The condition can be diagnosed by direct estimation of trimethylamine in the urine after a marine fish meal. Both affected individuals and heterozygous carriers have abnormally elevated excretion of trimethylamine after such an oral challenge.

Management

A diet low in carnitine and choline may help. Egg yolks, legumes, red meats, fish and beans should be avoided. Short courses of metronidazole or neomycin may temporarily reduce the bacteria that degrade the carnitine and choline in the gut. Charcoal and copper chlorophyllin have been shown to reduce urinary trimethylamine concentrations to normal levels in sufferers [4].

Treatment ladder for trimethylaminuria

First line
- Low carnitine diet

Second line
- Antibiotics (metronidazole and neomycin)
- Oral charcoal
- Oral copper chlorophyllin

Chromhidrosis

Definition

Chromhidrosis is the secretion of vividly coloured apocrine sweat [1,2]. It is most commonly a blue, yellow or green colour and is usually of apocrine origin, and seen in the axilla, areola of the nipple or face.

Pathophysiology

It results from the secretion of lipofuscins in apocrine sweat and may be associated with the secretion of coloured breast milk. The more oxidised lipofuscins appear deeper in colour; the lighter-coloured pigments may fluoresce.

Clinical features

Apocrine sweat may be tinged with a yellow, green or blue hue in up to 10% of the population. Only rarely does it occur to the striking degree that merits the term chromhidrosis. The diagnosis can be confirmed by finding lipofuscin pigment granules that may fluoresce on fluorescence microscopy in the apocrine secretory cells in affected skin. Affected individuals' clothes may also fluoresce on Wood's light illumination. The secretion of coloured sweat starts at puberty and persists until there is a gradual regression of apocrine function in old age. Coloured sweat may be discharged from the glands in response to exercise and emotional stimuli, and after manipulation of the skin. The axillae are the most frequently affected sites, although facial [3] and areolar [4] chromhidrosis are recorded.

Management

Treatment ladder for chromhidrosis

First line
- Topical capsaicin

Second line
- Intralesional botulinum toxin
- Topical capsaicin has satisfactorily reduced facial and nipple chromhidrosis
- Botulinum toxin has been used to successfully suppress facial chromhidrosis [5,6]

Pseudochromhidrosis

Pseudochromhidrosis is the secretion of clear sweat that changes to a coloured secretion after it exits the sweat duct. It may occur due to chromogenic or porphyrin-producing bacteria on the skin [7]. A case of facial red chromhidrosis in a child responded to erythromycin, the antibiotic eradicating a chromogenic bacterium, which was felt to be the cause of the abnormal colour [8].

Exogenous chromogens can affect eccrine sweat. Occupational and homeopathic medicinal exposure to copper salts has been reported to produce blue eccrine sweat; excessive consumption of a red food dye resulted in red sweat staining of underwear in one reported case [9].

Alkaptonuria (ochronosis) may result in dark perspiration.

Hematidrosis [1]

This is characterised by one or more episodes of spontaneous bloody sweat arising from non-traumatised skin (Figure 92.13). Microscopy shows normal erythrocytes within the eccrine sweat, distinguishing it from red chromhidrosis, although in many putative cases this has not been substantiated. In a review of 25 cases, most patients were adolescent women, with the face, eyes and ears being the sites affected. Stressful triggers were identified in many cases. Psychological support and beta blockers have been advocated; the condition resolves spontaneously.

Apocrine miliaria

Definition and nomenclature

Apocrine miliaria is a disorder of the apocrine glands comparable to prickly heat of the eccrine glands and caused by obliteration of the apocrine duct at the infundibulum [1]. It usually presents with an itchy papular eruption in the axillae, ano-genital area or on the areolae of the nipple.

Synonyms and inclusions
- Fox–Fordyce disease

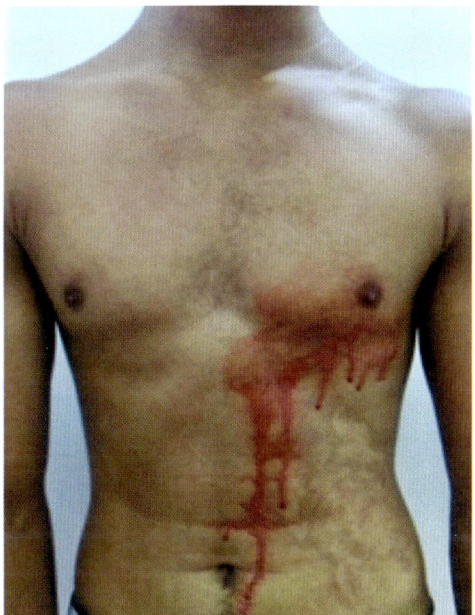

Figure 92.13 Hematidrosis on the chest. Courtesy of Dr Julio Salas, Guadalupe.

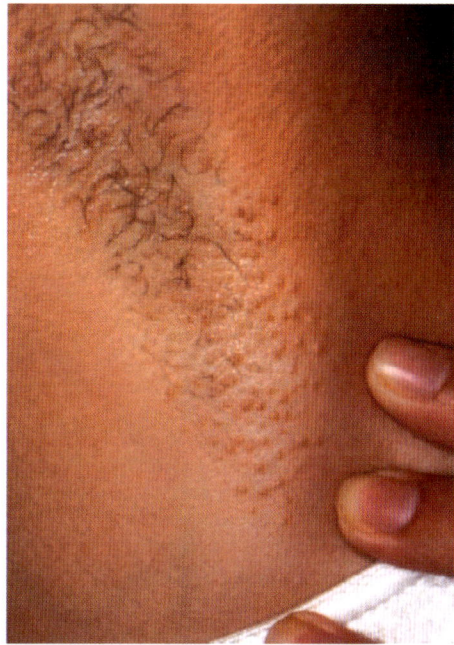

Figure 92.14 Axillary apocrine miliaria (Fox–Fordyce disease).

Epidemiology
Incidence and prevalence
It is uncommon.

Sex
It predominates in females. Familial twin and male cases are reported [2].

Pathophysiology
The condition occurs as a result of apocrine sweat duct occlusion by aggregates of epithelial cells of the apocrine or apoeccrine secretory cells [3]. The earliest pathological sign is a small vesicle in the apocrine duct. Later, the apocrine glands are seen to be enlarged, and as a consequence of repeated inflammatory events, perifollicular xanthomatosis with perifollicular foam cells expressing CD68 may develop [4].

Clinical features
The disease occurs mainly in women soon after puberty but can be postmenopausal [1]. It can occur in males or in children and has been reported in females with Turner syndrome and in identical twins. In recent years it has been reported after laser axillary hair epilation [5]. Itching, which may be intense, occurs in the axillae, and to a lesser extent in the ano-genital region and around the breasts. Objectively there may be little to see at first, but later skin-coloured or slightly pigmented, dome-shaped, follicular papules develop (Figure 92.14). Hair loss in the axillae usually ensues. The itching is often provoked by those emotional stimuli that normally cause apocrine secretion. The disease runs a very prolonged course and may persist until the menopause. Some remission may occur in pregnancy.

Differential diagnosis
It is usually easy to diagnose due to its distinctive clinical features.

Management
Response to treatment is unsatisfactory. Topical and intralesional steroids provide some benefit, but their use is limited by atrophy. It may respond to calcipotriol betamethasone or tacrolimus topically. Topical clindamycin is reported to have been of help [6]. Treatment with 4–6-weekly doses of ultraviolet radiation, sufficient to cause exfoliation, helps some patients [7]. Topical retinoic acid or adapalene may also be helpful, as may oral contraceptive agents and oral retinoids [8]. Other cases are sufficiently severe to require electrocautery [9], surgical excision of the affected skin or subcutaneous removal of the apocrine glands [10].

Treatment ladder for apocrine miliaria

First line
- Topical or intralesional steroids, calcipotriol with betamethasone
- Topical clindamycin lotion
- Topical retinoids

Second line
- Ultraviolet light
- Oral retinoids

Third line
- Surgery

PART 8: SPECIFIC CUTANEOUS STRUCTURES

Key references

The full list of references can be found in the online version at https://www.wiley.com/rooksdermatology10e

Eccrine glands
Anatomy and physiology of eccrine glands

1 Baker LB. Physiology of sweat gland function: the roles of sweating and sweat composition in human health. *Temperature (Austin)* 2019;6:211–59.

4 Sato K, Kang WH, Saga K *et al*. Biology of sweat glands and their disorders. *J Am Acad Dermatol* 1989;20:537–63, 713–26.

6 Sato K, Leidal R, Sato F. Morphology and development of an apoeccrine sweat gland in human axillae. *Am J Physiol* 1987;252:R166–80, 181–7.

24 Shibasaki M, Crandall CG. Mechanisms and controllers of eccrine sweating in humans. *Front Biosci (Schol Ed)* 2010;2:685–96.

26 Shibasaki M, Wilson TE, Crandall G. Neural control and mechanisms of eccrine sweating during heat stress and exercise. *J Appl Physiol* 2006;100:1692–701.

33 Wolf JE, Maibach HI. Palmar eccrine sweating – the role of adrenergic and cholinergic mediators. *Br J Dermatol* 1974;91:439–46.

Disorders of eccrine sweat glands
Hyperhidrosis

1 Sato K, Kang WH, Saga K, *et al*. Biology of sweat glands and their disorders. *J Am Acad Dermatol* 1989;20:537–63, 713–26.

2 Stefaniak TJ, Proczko M. Gravimetry in sweating assessment in primary hyperhidrosis and healthy individuals. *Clin Auton Res* 2013;23:197–200.

4 Hoorens I, Ongenae K. Primary focal hyperhidrosis: current treatment options and a step-by-step approach. *J Eur Acad Dermatol Venereol* 2012;26:1–8.

6 Chatterjee S, Ghosh K, Banerjee T. An intramedullary tumor presenting with hyperhidrosis. *Neurol India* 2004;52:39.

9 McCoy BP. Apical pulmonary adenocarcinoma with contralateral hyperhidrosis. *Arch Dermatol* 1981;117:659–61.

10 Eustace K, Wilson NJ. Postmenopausal craniofacial hyperhidrosis. *Clin Exp Dermatol* 2018; 43:180–2.

11 Moon MH, Hyun K, Park JK, Lee J. Surgical treatment of compensatory hyperhidrosis: retrospective observational study. *Medicine (Baltimore)* 2020;99:e22466.

Gustatory hyperhidrosis

1 Lee TS. Physiological gustation sweating in a warm climate. *J Physiol* 1954;124:528–42.

6 McGibbon BM, Paletta FX. Further concepts in gustatory sweating. *Plast Reconstr Surg* 1972;49:639–42.

Management of hyperhidrosis

1 McMillan FSK, Reller HH, Snyder FH. Antiperspirant action of topically applied anticholinergics. *J Invest Dermatol* 1964;43:363–7.

3 Mackenzie A, Burns C, Kavanagh G. Topical glycopyrrolate for axillary hyperhidrosis. *Br J Dermatol* 2013;169:483–4.

6 Anon. Aluminium chloride for hyperhidrosis. *Drug Ther Bull* 1981;19:101–2.

7 Shelley WB, Hurley HJ. Studies on topical antiperspirant control of axillary hyperhidrosis. *Acta Derm Venereol (Stockh)* 1975;95:241–60.

12 Stolman LP. Treatment of excessive sweating of the palms by iontophoresis. *Arch Dermatol* 1987;123:895–6.

15 Heckmann M, Ceballos-Baumann AO, Plewig G. Hyperhidrosis Study Group. Botulinum toxin A for axillary hyperhidrosis (excessive sweating). *N Engl J Med* 2001;344:488–93.

23 Cruddas L, Baker DM. Treatment of primary hyperhidrosis with oral anticholinergic medications: a systematic review. *J Eur Acad Dermatol Venereol* 2017;31:952–96.

24 James WD, Schoomaker EB, Rodman OG. Emotional eccrine sweating. *A heritable disorder. Arch Dermatol* 1987;123:925–9.

27 Drott C, Gothberg G, Claes G. Endoscopic transthoracic sympathectomy: an efficient and safe method for the treatment of hyperhidrosis. *J Am Acad Dermatol* 1995;33:78–81.

30 Cerfolio RJ, De Campos JR, Bryant AS *et al*. The Society of Thoracic Surgeons expert consensus for the surgical treatment of hyperhidrosis. *Ann Thorac Surg* 2011;91:1642–8.

39 Lawrence CM, Lonsdale Eccles AA. Selective sweat gland removal with minimal skin excision in the treatment of axillary hyperhidrosis: a retrospective clinical and histological review of 15 patients. *Br J Dermatol* 2006;155:115–18.

Anhidrosis and hypohidrosis

1 Shelley WB, Horvath PN, Pilsbury DM. *Anhidrosis. Medicine* 1950;29:194–224.

3 Ross AT. Progressive selective sudomotor denervation; a case with coexisting Adie's syndrome. *Neurology* 1958;8:809–17.

9 Chen YC, Wu CS, Chen GS *et al*. Identification of subgroups of acquired idiopathic generalized anhidrosis. *Neurologist* 2008;14:318–20.

11 Palm F, Löser C, Gronau W *et al*. Successful treatment of acquired idiopathic generalized anhidrosis. *Neurology* 2007;68:532–3.

Miliaria

1 Holzle E, Kligman AM. The pathogenesis of miliaria rubra. *Br J Dermatol* 1978;99:117–37.

2 Leithead CS, Lind AR. *Heat Stress and Heat Disorders*. London: Cassell, 1964.

3 Sargent F, Slutsky HL. The natural history of the eccrine miliarias. *N Engl J Med* 1957;256:401–8, 451.

4 Shuster S. Duct disruption, a new explanation of miliaria. *Acta Derm Venereol (Stockh)* 1997;77:1–3.

9 Mowad CM, McGinley KJ, Foglia A, Leyden JJ. A role of extracellular polysaccharide substance produced by *Staphylococcus epidermidis* in miliaria. *J Am Acad Dermatol* 1995;33:729–33.

Neutrophilic eccrine hidradenitis

2 Harris T, Fine JD, Berman RS *et al*. Neutrophilic eccrine hidradenitis. *Arch Dermatol* 1982;118:268.

9 Turan H, Kaya E, Gurlevik Z *et al*. Neutrophilic eccrine hidradenitis induced by cetuximab. *Cutan Ocul Toxicol* 2012;31:148–50.

14 Gómez Vázquez M, Peteiro C, Toribio J. Neutrophilic eccrine hidradenitis heralding the onset of chronic myelogenous leukaemia. *J Eur Acad Dermatol Venereol* 2003;17:328–30.

18 Simon M, Jr, Cremer H, von den Driesch P. Idiopathic recurrent palmoplantar hidradenitis in children. Report of 22 cases. *Arch Dermatol* 1998;134:76–9.

Apocrine glands
Anatomy and physiology of apocrine glands

1 Hurley HJ, Shelley WB. *The Human Apocrine Sweat Gland in Health and Disease*. Springfield, IL: Thomas, 1960.

2 Ebling FJG. Apocrine glands in health and disease. *Int J Dermatol* 1989;28:508–11.

3 Montagna W, Parakkal PF. *The Structure and Function of Skin*, 3rd edn. London: Academic Press, 1974.

5 Takayasu S, Wakimoto H, Itami S *et al*. Activity of testosterone 5μ-reductase in various tissues of human skin. *J Invest Dermatol* 1980;74:187–91.

7 Schaumburg-Lever G, Lever WF. Secretion from human apocrine glands. *J Invest Dermatol* 1975;64:38–41.

10 Robertshaw D. Neural and humoral control of apocrine glands. *J Invest Dermatol* 1974;63:160–7.

11 Natsch A, Gfeller H, Gygax P *et al*. A specific bacterial aminoacylase cleaves odorant precursors secreted in the human axilla. *J Biol Chem* 2003;278:5718–27.

12 Natsch A, Schmid J, Flachsmann F. Identification of odoriferous sulfanylalkanols in human axilla secretions and their formation through cleavage of cysteine precursors by a C-S lysase isolated from axilla bacteria. *Chem Biodiversity* 2004;1:1058–72.

13 Bird S, Gower DB. The validation and use of a radioimmunoassay for 5 alpha-androst-16-en-3-one in human axillary collections. *J Steroid Biochem* 1981;14:213–19.

14 Martin A, Saathoff M, Kuhn F *et al*. A functional ABCC11 allele is essential in the biochemical formation of human axillary odor. *J Invest Dermatol* 2010;130:529–40.

Disorders of apocrine sweat glands
Abnormal sweat odour (bromhidrosis)

1 James AG, Austin C, Cox D, Taylor D, Calvert R. Microbiological and biochemical origins of human axillary odour. *FEMS Microbiol Ecol* 2013;83:527–40.

3 Morioka D, Ohkubo F, Amikura Y. Clinical features of axillary osmidrosis: a retrospective chart review of 723 Japanese patients. *J Dermatol* 2013;40:384–8.

4 Nakano M, Miwa N, Hirano A, Yoshiura K, Niikawa N. A strong association of axillary osmidrosis with the wet earwax type determined by genotyping of the ABCC11 gene. *BMC Genet* 2009;4:42.

8 Wu CJ, Chang CK, Wang CY, Liao YS, Chen SG. Efficacy and safety of botulinum toxin A in axillary bromhidrosis and associated histological changes in sweat glands: a prospective randomized double-blind side-by-side comparison clinical study. *Dermatol Surg* 2019;45:1605–9.

11 Huang YH, Yang CH, Chen YH, Chen CH, Lee SH. Reduction in osmidrosis using a suction-assisted cartilage shaver improves the quality of life. *Dermatol Surg* 2010;36:1573–7.

12 Qian JG, Wang XJ. Effectiveness and complications of subdermal excision of apocrine glands in 206 cases with axillary osmidrosis. *J Plast Reconstr Aesthet Surg* 2010;63:1003–7.

Chromhidrosis

1 Shelley WB, Hurley HJ. Localized chromhidrosis: a survey. *Arch Dermatol Syphilol* 1954;69:449–71.

2 Hurley HJ, Shelley WB. *The Human Apocrine Sweat Gland in Health and Disease.* Springfield, IL: Thomas, 1960.

5 Wu JM, Mamelak AJ, Nussbaum R, McElgunn PS. Botulinum toxin A in the treatment of chromhidrosis. *Dermatol Surg* 2005;31:963–5.

7 Poh-Fitzpatrick MB. 'Red sweat.' *J Am Acad Dermatol* 1981;4:481–2.

Hematidrosis

1 Kluger N. Hematidrosis (bloody sweat): a review of the recent literature (1996-2016). *Acta Dermatovenerol Alp Pannonica Adriat* 2018;27:85–90.

Apocrine miliaria

1 Hurley HJ, Shelley WB. *The Human Apocrine Sweat Gland in Health and Disease.* Springfield, IL: Thomas, 1960.

3 Kamada A, Saga K, Jimbow K. Apoeccrine sweat duct obstruction as a cause for Fox-Fordyce disease. *J Am Acad Dermatol* 2003;48:453–5.

4 Bormate AB, Jr, Leboit PE, McCalmont TH. Perifollicular xanthomatosis as the hallmark of axillary Fox–Fordyce disease: an evaluation of histopathologic features of 7 cases. *Arch Dermatol* 2003;144:1020–4.

PART 8: SPECIFIC CUTANEOUS STRUCTURES

CHAPTER 93

Acquired Disorders of the Nails and Nail Unit

Marcel C. Pasch[1], Bertrand Richert[2] and Matilde Iorizzo[3]

[1] Radboud University Medical Center, Department of Dermatology, Nijmegen, The Netherlands
[2] Brugmann – St Pierre and Children's University Hospitals, Université Libre de Bruxelles, Brussels, Belgium
[3] Private Dermatology Practice, Bellinzona/Lugano, Switzerland

PART 8: SPECIFIC CUTANEOUS STRUCTURES

Rook's Textbook of Dermatology, Tenth Edition. Edited by Christopher Griffiths, Jonathan Barker, Tanya Bleiker, Walayat Hussain and Rosalind Simpson.
© 2024 John Wiley & Sons Ltd. Published 2024 by John Wiley & Sons Ltd.

ANATOMY AND BIOLOGY OF THE NAIL UNIT

Structure

Gross anatomy [1,2,3]

The components of the nail apparatus are shown in Figure 93.1. The nail plate (nail) is firmly attached to the nail bed. At the proximal side about one-quarter of the nail is covered by the proximal nail fold (or posterior nail fold). The proximal nail fold has two epithelial surfaces, ventral and dorsal; at the junction of the two, the cuticle projects distally onto the nail surface. A narrow margin of the sides of the nail is often occluded by the lateral nail folds. The lateral nail folds are in continuity with the skin on the lateral sides of the digit, and medially they are joined. When the nail plate is viewed from above, two distinct areas may be visible: the lunula proximally and the larger distal pink zone. The lunula is most prominent on the thumb and great toe and may be partly or completely concealed by the proximal nail fold in other digits. The reason for the white

colour of the lunula is not known [1,4]. The nail plate distal to the lunula usually appears pink, due to its translucency, which allows the redness of the vascular nail bed to be seen through it. On close examination, two further distal zones can often be identified: the distal yellowish-white margin and immediately proximal to this the onychodermal band [5]. Histologically, the onychodermal band is defined as the most distal attachment of cornified epithelium to the undersurface of the nail and has also been termed the nail isthmus [6]. As such, it is structurally significant for the adherence of the nail plate to the nail bed. Once breached, as in conditions such as psoriasis, separation of the nail bed from the nail plate can be progressive.

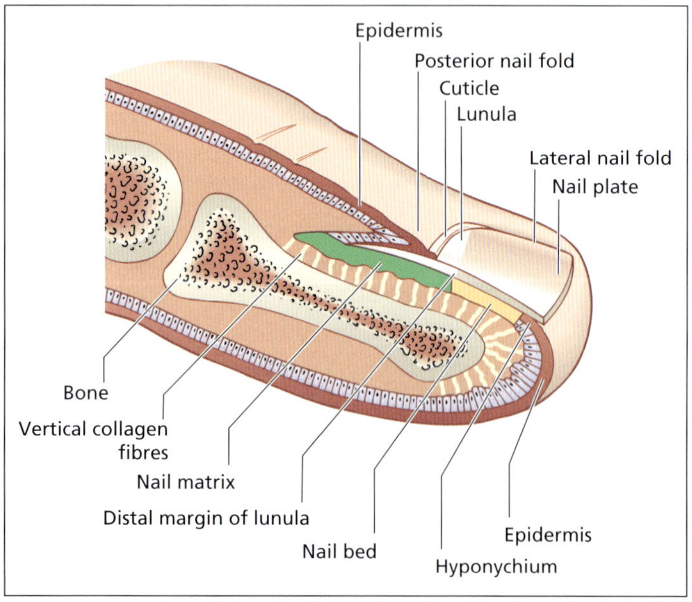

The definition of the nail matrix is controversial [7]. Mostly it is assumed that the nail is synthesised completely in the germinal nail matrix, which is situated under the proximal nail fold and its distal extension is visible as the lunula (half-moon lunule) [8] (green in Figure 93.1). The onychodermis below the nail matrix has been hypothesised to be the nail counterpart of the follicular dermal papilla [9]. For those who consider this region beneath the proximal nail to be the sole source of nail it is termed simply the matrix. The natural shape of the free margin of the nail is the same as the contour of the distal border of the lunula. While there is common acceptance that this localised region beneath the proximal nail produces the major part of the normal nail plate, there is some evidence that other epithelial and mesenchymal parts of the nail unit also play a role in the growth of the nail plate. Other epithelial parts are also sometimes attributed matrix status and can be subdivided into dorsal (the ventral aspect of the proximal nail fold), intermediate (germinal matrix or matrix) and ventral matrix sections (Figure 93.2). The ventral matrix section (nail bed) is also

Figure 93.1 Longitudinal section of a digit showing the components of the nail apparatus.

Labels (Figure 93.1): Epidermis; Posterior nail fold; Cuticle; Lunula; Lateral nail fold; Nail plate; Bone; Vertical collagen fibres; Nail matrix; Distal margin of lunula; Nail bed; Epidermis; Hyponychium

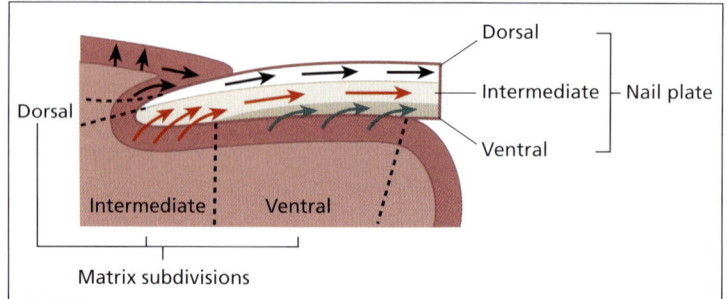

Figure 93.2 Direction of differentiation and cell movement within the nail apparatus.

Labels (Figure 93.2): Dorsal; Intermediate; Ventral; Nail plate; Dorsal; Intermediate; Ventral; Matrix subdivisions

termed the sterile matrix but its role in the production of the nail is unclear. Although it appears that the nail plate may thicken by 21% as it passes from the distal margin of the lunula to the end of the nail bed [10,11], this is not associated with an increase in cell numbers and may represent compaction of the nail from distal tip trauma rather than nail bed or nail plate production [12]. The situation may change in disease, where the nail bed changes its histological appearance to gain a granular layer [13] and may contribute a false nail of cornified epithelium to the undersurface of the nail [14].

In rheumatological literature it has become popular to consider the nail apparatus a musculoskeletal appendage [15]. A recent study showed that this assumption relies on an oversimplified anatomy and that the nail unit is an epidermal appendage with a specialised connection with the lateral periosteum [16].

Microscopic anatomy [17,18]

Nail folds

The proximal nail folds are similar in structure to the adjacent skin with sweat glands but devoid of pilosebaceous glands. There is a normal granular layer. From the distal area of the proximal nail folds, the cuticle adheres to the upper surface of the nail plate; it is composed of modified stratum corneum and serves as a seal to protect the structures at the base of the nail, particularly the germinal matrix, from environmental insults such as irritants, allergens and bacterial and fungal pathogens.

Nail matrix (intermediate matrix)

The nail matrix is composed of stratified squamous epithelium with long rete ridges. The basal compartment is broader than the same region in normal epithelium or in other parts of the nail unit, such as the nail bed [12]. There is no granular layer and cells differentiate into mature onychocytes with the expression of trichocyte 'hard' keratins alongside normal epithelial 'soft' keratins (see later) [17,19]. During this process of nail formation, cells become larger and paler and eventually the nucleus disintegrates. Occasionally, they may retain their nuclei until more distal in the nail plate. These retained nuclei are called *pertinax bodies*.

The nail matrix contains melanocytes, which can donate pigment to the onychocytes [20]. They are found in the basal and suprabasal layers and are most prominent in the distal matrix. In addition, the nail bed often contains melanocytes but they are sparse or absent with a mean of 0.43 per millimetre, and are restricted to the basal layer with thin cytoplasmic dendrites [21]. Melanocytes can occur in foci in normal nail beds, in which the melanocytic density can reach the level seen in the matrix. The presence of about seven melanocytes per millimetre of matrix basement membrane (range 4–14) can be considered a normal matrix melanocyte population [21,22], although higher numbers have also been reported [23]. Matrix melanocytes are distinguished from those elsewhere by their failure to produce melanin in normal circumstances in white people. This can change, with melanotic streaks presenting in local inflammatory, naevoid or neoplastic disease. In non-white people, brown streaks are common and are almost universal in Fitzpatrick phototyping scale V and VI by the age of 60 years.

Nail bed

The nail bed consists of epidermis with underlying connective tissue closely apposed to the periosteum of the distal phalanx. The nail bed epidermis is usually no more than two or three cells thick, although there may be tongues of epithelium that extend obliquely down. At the nail folds it becomes thicker and develops rete ridges. The transitional zone from living keratinocyte to dead ventral nail plate cell is abrupt, occurring in the space of one horizontal cell layer; in this regard it closely resembles the Henle layer of the internal root sheath of the epidermis [24]. Nail bed cells do not have any independent movement, and it is yet to be clearly demonstrated whether they are incorporated into an overlying nail plate as it grows distally [10,11,24]. The process of nail bed keratinisation has been likened to that seen in rat tail epidermis, possibly being affected by pressure changes [12]. The loss of the overlying nail results in the development of a granular layer, which is otherwise present only in disease states.

The nail bed dermis is sparse and without subcutaneous fat, although scattered dermal fat cells may be present. The collagenous adherence of the nail bed is firm and mainly orientated vertically, being directly attached to the phalangeal periosteum and the epidermal basal lamina. Within the connective tissue network lie blood vessels, lymphatics and a fine network of elastic fibres; at the distal margin, eccrine sweat ducts have been seen [2].

Nail plate

The nail plate is composed of three horizontal layers of compacted keratinised epithelial cells: a thin dorsal lamina, the thicker intermediate lamina and a ventral layer from the nail bed (Figure 93.2) [25]. This is apparent with silver stain and ultrasound but not always with normal light microscopy using routine stains, where the nail demonstrates a transition between flattened cells dorsally and thicker cells on the ventral aspect. It has been suggested that the ventral nail plate is only one or two cells thick [26] or may be a variable entity [27]. Electron microscopy shows squamous cells with tortuous interlocking plasma membranes [28,29]. At high magnification, the contents of each cell show a uniform fine granularity similar to the hair cuticle [4]. The nail plate gains thickness and density as it grows distally [30], although *in vivo* ultrasound suggests slight reduction in thickness distally [31].

The nail plate contains variable amounts of minerals and electrolytes, including sodium, potassium, nitrogen, calcium, iron, copper, zinc, magnesium, phosphorus and sulphur [32]. Mainly the dorsal and intermediate layers of the nail plate contain phospholipids, which contribute to its flexibility and water resistance. The contents of lipids and water in the nail plate is much lower than the stratum corneum: 0.1–1% lipids and 7–12% water in the nail plate, versus 10% lipids and 20–40% water in the stratum corneum [32].

Signalling pathways involved in nail formation

The primary nail field is the earliest discernible area and appears around the 10th week of gestation [32]. The nail plate grows from the 14th week of gestation and by the 17th week almost the entire nail bed area is covered. From then, nails continue growing till death. Many factors act upon nail growth and influence its appearance. A complex interaction through various signalling pathways between ectoderm and mesoderm are essential, which is coordinated by

Wnt signalling together with bone morphogenetic proteins (BMPs) [1,32]. Wnt signalling is crucial in both embryogenesis and adult nail maintenance. Genes influencing the presence or absence of malformation of nails have also been sought in connection with inherited abnormalities of the nail unit. Spondins are a family of proteins contributing to intracellular communication. When there are mutations in the *R-spondin* genes and others influencing the *Wnt/β catenin* signalling pathway, nail loss or reduction occurs [33–35]. This first became evident from mutations seen in the *R-spondin 4* gene in a family with an autosomal recessive pattern of anonychia [33]. Mice deficient to *R-spondin 2* have limb and phalangeal abnormalities and no nail unit [36]. *Frizzled-6* is a *Wnt* receptor gene. More subtle forms of nail dysplasia can be attributed to defects of *Frizzled-6* which, in common with *R-spondin 4*, enhances the *Wnt* signalling pathway and is found in inherited nail dysplasia [37]. In claw differentiation in *Frizzled-6* knock-out mice, it is associated with downregulation of hair keratins K86, K81, K34 and K31, and two epithelial keratins, K6a and K6b: all keratins with significance in nail formation and biology. Defects in other factors influencing the *Wnt* signalling pathway, including β catenin, have detrimental effects on nail formation [38]. Also, leucine-rich repeat-containing G protein-coupled receptor 5 and 6 (*Lgr5* and *Lgr6*) are part of the *Wnt* signalling pathway. In mice, *Lgr6* is assumed to be necessary for nail unit regeneration following loss [39]. Primary abnormalities in the *Wnt* signalling itself are also associated with inherited nail dysplasias such as Schöpf–Schulz–Passarge syndrome (*Wnt10a*) [40]. Mutations in other genes such as *LMX1B* are associated with multisystem disease such as nail–patella syndrome [41] which may have overlap with elements of *Wnt* signalling. Other relevant molecules include *histone deacetylase*, the serine/threonine protein kinase *Akt*, and the Forkhead box N1 transcription factor (*FOXN1*) [42].

Keratins [1]

Keratins belong to the family of intermediate filament proteins and represent 80% of nail mass, and their distribution and differentiation is pivotal. Keratin distribution in the nail and associated epithelium has been studied in adult, infant and embryonic digits [1,17,19,43]. Genome analysis demonstrated that humans possess 54 functional keratin genes [44]; 28 acidic type I keratins and 26 basic-to-neutral type II keratins. These keratins are subdivided into 'soft' epithelial keratins and 'hard' hair or trichocyte keratins. The nail plate contains approximately 10–20% soft keratins (keratin pairs K50/K58 and K48/K56) and 80–90% 'hard' keratins (K31 to K40 and K81 to K86) as they become incorporated into the nail plate [17,19]. K31 to K40 belong to the category of type I hard keratins, and K81 to K86 are type II hard keratins. Hard keratins are characteristic of hair and nail differentiation and keratins 31, 32, 34, 38, 81, 85 and 86 have all been demonstrated immunohistochemically in the nail matrix but not in the nail bed [1,17,19]. The higher sulphur content of amino acids (e.g. cysteine and methionine) in nail keratin results in disulphide bonds, which are responsible for their rugged physical qualities of the nail. This is matched by the resistance of hair keratins to dissolution in strong solvent. Proximally, the hair keratins do not extend onto the ventral aspect of the proximal nail fold (dorsal matrix) and distally their expression is limited to a margin taken as corresponding to the lunula. Their distribution appears to define a matrix consistent with the classic description of the germinal matrix (green in Figure 93.1).

Expression of soft 'epithelial' keratin pair K1/K10 is found in a suprabasal location in the matrix but is absent in the healthy nail bed [17]. Expression of K1 and K10 in the nail bed occurs in pathological situations in which cornification and terminal keratinocyte differentiation occurs together with development of a granular layer, such as in onychomycosis or psoriasis [17]. The nail bed contains keratins synthesised in normal basal layer epithelium, K5/ K14, which are also found in nail matrix. An antibody marking the epitope characteristically associated with keratin expressed in the basal layer is found throughout the thickness of the nail bed, but only basally in the matrix. Keratins 6, 16, 17 and 8 have all been found in different subungual locations and phases of nail matrix development with a variety of attributed functions [1]. K6/K16 is identified in the nail bed but not in the germinal matrix [19]. This is because proliferation is not a prominent feature. The nail bed has very low rates of proliferation [12,30], and it may be that K6/K16 more precisely illustrates a loss of differentiation, often associated with proliferation in skin but representing the resting state of nail bed epithelium. Nail bed expression of K6a, -6b, -16, and -17 has significance, because features of pachyonychia congenita develop in case of mutations in the genes for these keratins [45–51]. In this group of autosomal dominant disorders, there is thickening of the nail plate attributed to disease of the nail bed in variants of the disease attributed to abnormalities in each of these keratins [52,53]. Positive immunostaining for K8 and K20, specific for Merkel cells, has been noted in the nail matrix [54].

Nail immune system

The nail apparatus is constantly exposed to environmental threats. Effective immune responses are essential to prevent infection, but autoaggressive immunity and the loss of nail production has to be prevented. The nail immune system differs from the skin immune system, but shows similarities to the hair follicle immune system, including the establishment of an area of relative immune privilege [1]. This relative immune privilege may be essential to prevent autoimmunity and damage by inflammatory pathogens. Collapse of the nail immune privilege may be an underlying cause of nail lichen planus that may present with permanent loss of nails.

Compared with other regions of nail epithelium, human leukocyte antigen (HLA)-A/B/C expression is prominently downregulated on both keratinocytes and melanocytes of the nail matrix, whereas HLA-G(+) is upregulated here. Together with the expression of macrophage migration inhibitory factor in the nail matrix, this may serve to inhibit a natural killer cell attack on the major histocompatibility complex (MHC) class Ia-negative nail matrix. Langerhans cells are detectable in the matrix by CD1a staining [2] but their expression is reduced [1]. Also, the number of natural killer cells and mast cells, key players in the innate immunity, are reduced in number, while immunosuppressive mediators such as α-melanocyte stimulating hormone and transforming growth factor β1 have a prominent expression in the nail unit, contributing to the immune privilege [1,3]. Also, antimicrobial peptides (AMPs) have a broad spectrum of innate immune properties and their presence is increased in the nail unit [4,5]. They may contribute to the relative immune privilege of the nail matrix by playing a role in effective defence in the presence of continuous exposure of the nail to various microbiological agents. The nail unit has been shown to contain human cathelicidin LL-37, which can kill *Candida albicans* [4] and beta defensins hβD-2 and hβD-3 [5].

Blood and nerve supply

Blood supply [1]
There is a rich arterial blood supply to the nail bed and matrix derived from paired digital arteries, a large palmar and small dorsal digital artery on either side. The palmar arteries are supplied from the large superficial and deep palmar arcades [2]. The main supply passes into the pulp space of the distal phalanx before reaching the dorsum of the digit (Figure 93.3). Distally, the arteries are extremely tortuous and coiled, which allows them to be distorted without kinking to occlude supply. The superficial arcade lies just distal to the distal interphalangeal joint, and supplies the nail fold and extensor tendon, and has many branches to the germinal matrix. The nail fold capillary network has capillary loops which are more horizontal and visible than in the normal cutaneous plexus. There are two main subungual arterial arches (proximal and distal) supplying the nail bed and matrix, formed from anastomoses of the branches of the digital arteries. In the event of damage to the main supply in the pulp space, such as may occur with infection or scleroderma, there may be sufficient blood from the accessory vessels to permit normal growth of the nail. Venous drainage of the finger is by deep and superficial systems. The deep system corresponds to the arterial supply. The superficial system consists of a branching network of dorsal and palmar digital veins.

At a microvascular level, there are three patterns. Within the germinal matrix, vessels are longitudinal with helical twisting. The axis becomes more longitudinal in the nail bed without the tortuosity – a pattern that is also seen in the distal proximal nail fold. This orientation in the nail bed is reflected in the appearance of splinter haemorrhages. In the digit pulp, vessels follow the pattern of the dermatoglyphics [3].

There are many arteriovenous anastomoses beneath the nail – glomus bodies – which are concerned with heat regulation. These

neurovascular glomus bodies serve as regulators of capillary circulation and thus are important in maintaining acral circulation under cold conditions: arterioles constrict with cold but glomus bodies dilate [4]. The nail bed is richly supplied with glomus bodies which increase in number in a gradient towards the distal nail bed [5].

Nerve supply [1]
Paired digital nerves follow the course of the arterial blood supply. The periungual soft tissues are innervated by dorsal branches. The main branch of the digital nerve passes under the nail bed and innervates both nail bed and matrix [6]. There is often dual sensory innervation of the nail unit, which is relevant when applying ring block anaesthesia [7].

Nail growth and morphology

Clinicians experienced in observing the slow rate of growth of diseased or damaged nails are apt to view the nail apparatus as inert, although it is biochemically and kinetically active throughout life. In this respect, it differs from most hair follicles, which undergo periods of quiescence as part of the follicular cycle.

Cell kinetics
The kinetic activity of the matrix has been examined using many techniques, including immunohistochemistry, autoradiography, flow cytometry and direct measurement of matrix product (i.e. nail plate) by ultrasound, micrometre or histology.

A putative nail stem cell (SC) is assumed to reside within the nail matrix compartment and is responsible for maintenance of the cell population of nail plate forming onychocytes, but also may play a role in digit tip regeneration following amputation [1]. These relatively quiescent SCs with a high proliferative capacity have to be distinguished from their progeny, the transit amplifying cells (TACs), which also have a high proliferative capacity, but are fast cycling. The characterisation of the nail SC has been rather difficult and future studies may elucidate the issue. Candidate markers include PHLDA1 (Pleckstrin homology-like domain, family A, member 1), Gli1, Lgr6, keratins 14, 15, 17 and 19, CD29, CD34, and leucine-rich repeat-containing G protein-coupled receptor 6 (Lgr6) [2,3]. Highly proliferative K14+ and K17+ assumed SCs are localised to the proximal matrix. Expression and coexpression of keratin 15 and keratin 19 were detected suprabasal in the root of the nail by Korver [4] and on the ventral aspect of the proximal nail fold by others [2,5].

The TACs are situated in the broad basal compartment of proliferating cells in the matrix. TACs can be detected immunohistochemically with antibodies to proliferating cell nuclear antigen and Ki67/MIB1 (Figure 93.4) [6]. Ki67 expressing cells were detected in the dorsal matrix and, in particular, in the intermediate matrix but not in the nail bed [4], indicating no important contribution of the nail bed in the creation of the nail plate. The matrix is also the site of maximal inclusion of tritiated thymidine if injected into the peritoneum of squirrel monkeys and followed subsequently by autoradiography [7]. Although there was some inclusion of thymidine into the nail bed, Zaias and Alvarez [7] interpreted the findings as indicating that the nail bed had no role in the creation of the nail plate. Norton [8] drew a similar conclusion from work with

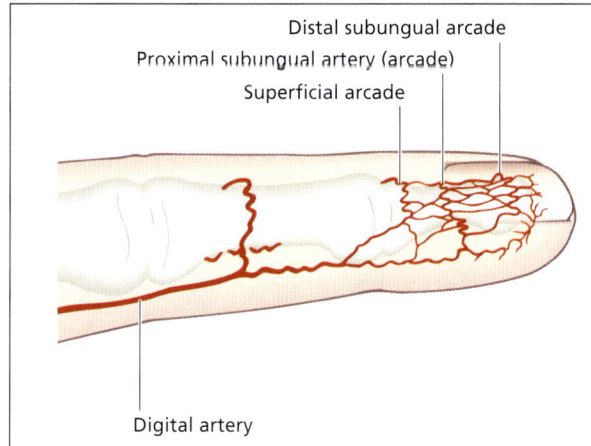

Figure 93.3 Arterial supply of the distal finger.

Distal subungual arcade
Proximal subungual artery (arcade)
Superficial arcade
Digital artery

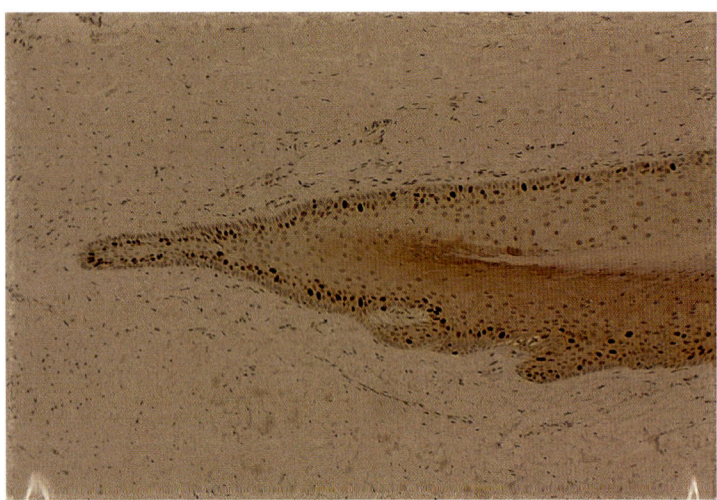

Figure 93.4 Proliferating epithelial cells of the matrix and ventral aspect of the proximal nail fold, staining with the antibody MIB-1.

Table 93.1 Physiological and environmental factors affecting the rate of nail growth.

Faster	Slower	Reference
Daytime	Night	
Pregnancy?	1st day of life	[19–21]
Right-hand nails/dominant hand	Left-hand nails /non-dominant	[22]
Youth, increasing age	Old age	[22]
Fingers	Toes	[23]
Summer	Winter or cold environment	[24–26]
Middle fingers	Thumb and little finger	[27,28]
Male gender	Female gender	[22,28]
Nail biting, friction		[29]

Table 93.2 Pathological factors and medication affecting the rate of nail growth.

Faster	Slower	Reference
Psoriasis	Finger immobilisation	[35–37]
Normal nails	Fever	[33,35]
Pitting	Beau lines	[35,38]
Onycholysis	Poor nutrition	[39,40]
Pityriasis rubra pilaris	Denervation	[27,29,41]
	Peripheral neuropathy	
Hyperthyroidism	Hypothyroidism	[27]
HIV	Yellow nail syndrome	[42,43]
Arteriovenous shunts	Congestive heart failure	[27]
	Onychomycosis	[44]
	Relapsing polychondritis	[45]
Levodopa	Methotrexate	[46,47]
Etretinate, rarely	Etretinate	[48]
Itraconazole	Azathioprine	[47,49]
Benoxaprofen	Targeted therapies and immunotherapies	[50,51]

live human subjects where labelled thymidine and glycine were injected locally to act as markers of proliferating and metabolically active keratinocytes, and both primarily labelled the matrix.

However, the earlier work of Lewis [9] suggested on histological grounds that the nail plate is a trilaminar structure originating from three separate matrix zones: the dorsal matrix (ventral aspect of proximal nail fold), intermediate matrix (germinal matrix) and ventral matrix (nail bed) (Figure 93.2). In support of this, Johnson *et al.* [10,11] demonstrated that 21% of the nail thickness is gained as it passes over the nail bed, implying that the nail bed is generating this fraction of the nail plate. De Berker *et al.* [6] noted that the increase in nail thickness did not coincide with corresponding increases of nail plate cells. This challenges the interpretation that nail thickens over the nail bed because of a contribution from underlying structures. An alternative explanation may be appropriate, such as compaction arising from repetitive distal trauma. Others have also debated this issue and, although the nail bed may have a significant contribution to make in disease [12], the evidence for its contribution at other times is conflicting.

Nail morphology

Why the nail grows flat, rather than as a heaped-up keratinous mass, has generated much thought and discussion [13–16]. It is reasonable to consider horizontal nail growth as being attributable to collaboration of several physical factors acting on the nail [17], including guiding restraint of the proximal nail fold [14], containment by the lateral nail fold, inductive influence of the underlying phalanx [18] and adherence to the nail bed [17]. In diseases such as psoriasis, the nail bed can lose its adherent properties, exhibiting onycholysis. In addition, there may be subungual hyperkeratosis. These combined factors make psoriasis the most common pathology in which up-growing nails are seen. Onychogryphosis is characterised by upward growth of thickened nail. In this condition, the nail may become bucket-shaped and the effect of the overlying proximal nail fold is lost.

The contour of the free edge of the nail is assumed to be attributable to the shape of the lunula. The free edge following the margin of lunula is visible in two situations with uneroded

or unmanicured outgrowth: at birth and with regrowth following avulsion. The nail bed may play a minor role in the shape of the free edge, because nail dystrophies following trauma of the nail bed give the edge a scalloped contour.

Linear nail growth [17,30–32]

Many studies were carried out on the linear growth of the nail plate in health and disease; these are listed in Tables 93.1 and 93.2 [17]. Most of these studies have been performed by observing the distal movement of a reference mark etched on the nail plate over a fixed period of time. Fingernails grow approximately 3 mm per month or 0.1 mm per day, and toenails at one-third of this rate. The height or weight of the individual makes no difference, nor do mild intercurrent illnesses, but severe systemic upsets disturb nail formation. Systemic upsets may result in reduced linear nail growth [33] and in transversal depressions upon the nail, known as Beau lines [34]. Also, local disease can influence linear nail growth and induce development of Beau lines.

NAIL SIGNS AND THEIR SIGNIFICANCE

A good knowledge of the anatomy and physiology of the nail apparatus is essential to make a correct diagnosis, because signs and symptoms caused by a disorder are strictly related to the affected anatomical area. Nail signs fall into categories of shape, attachment, surface and colour.

Abnormalities of shape

Clubbing

Synonyms and inclusions
- Hippocratic fingers
- Acropachy
- Watch glass nails

In clubbing, there is increased transverse and longitudinal nail curvature with hypertrophy of the soft-tissue components of the digit pulp. The nail can be 'rocked' and in causes associated with cardiopulmonary disease there may be local cyanosis.

There are three forms of geometric assessment that can be performed. *Lovibond's angle* is found at the junction between the nail plate and the proximal nail fold and is normally less than 160°. This is altered to over 180° in clubbing (Figure 93.5). *Curth's angle* at the distal interphalangeal joint is normally about 180°. This is diminished to less than 160° in clubbing (Figure 93.6). *Schamroth's window* is seen when the dorsal aspects of two fingers from opposite hands are opposed, revealing a window of light, bordered laterally by the Lovibond angles (Figure 93.7a). As this angle is obliterated in clubbing, the window closes (Figure 93.7b) [1]. Assessment of clubbing at the bedside shows poor agreement between examiners [2] in milder cases and there are problems in using firm morphometric analyses that do not lend themselves to routine clinical practice [3]. Ultrasound criteria for diagnosis can also be used and longitudinal images of the distal phalange can assist in the quantification of the profile and hyponychial angles [4].

Clubbing appears to be related more to increased blood flow through the vasodilated plexus of nail unit vasculature than to vessel hyperplasia, although MRI studies have also implicated

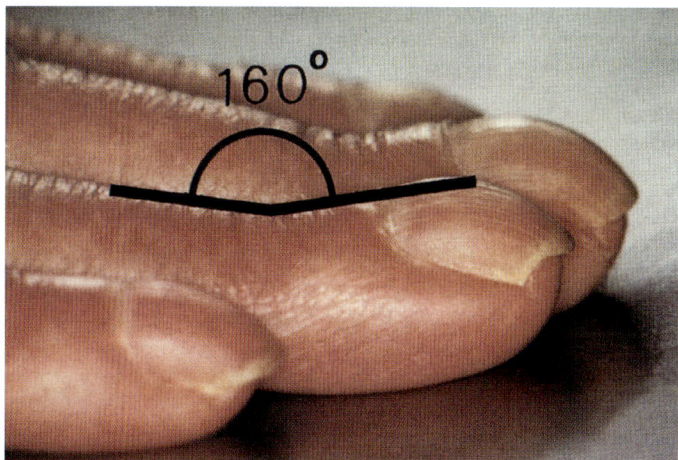

Figure 93.6 Clubbing: Curth's modified profile sign.

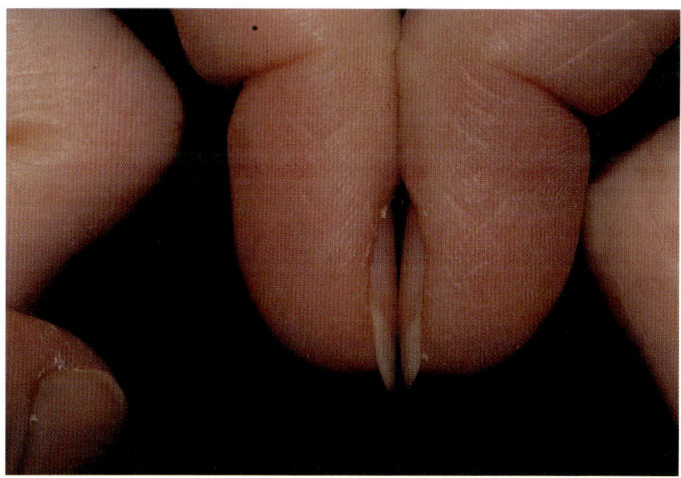

(a)

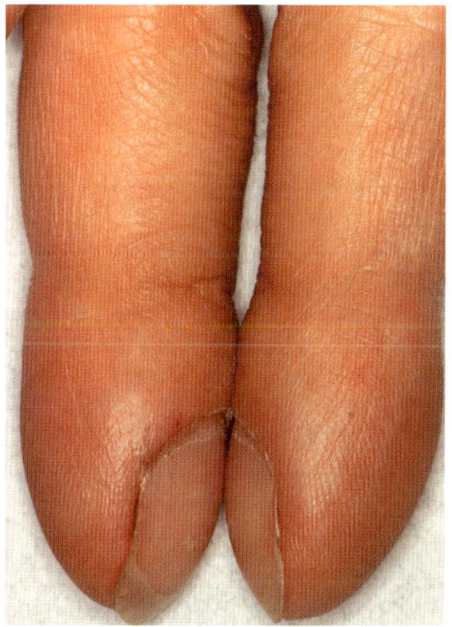

(b)

Figure 93.7 Schamroth's window is seen clearly as a window of light, bordered laterally by the Lovibond angles in this image of normal nails (a). Schamroth's window is obliterated in clubbing (b).

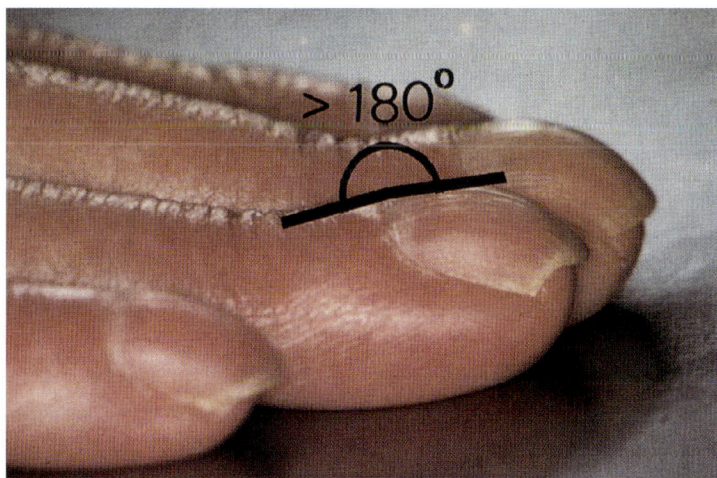

Figure 93.5 Clubbing: Lovibond's profile sign. The angle is normally less than 160° but exceeds 180° in clubbing.

Table 93.3 Causes of secondary nail clubbing.

Cause	Comment
Nasopharyngeal carcinoma	Clubbing can be an association with nasopharyngeal carcinoma in both children and adults
Asbestosis	Clubbing is found in about 40% of those with asbestosis
Thoracic carcinoma	Includes carcinoma of bronchus, pleura, lymphosarcoma, mediastinal lymphoma and metastatic disease in the lung arising outside the thorax (melanoma for example)
Mesothelioma	Clubbing is found in about 1/3 of those with mesothelioma and may in some instances be associated with the asbestosis which is a predisposing factor
Cystic fibrosis	This is acquired in adolescence or early adulthood. Clubbing can be used as a predictive factor for clinical progression of disease
Cryptogenic fibrosing alveolitis	Clubbing is an indicator of disease morbidity
Sarcoidosis	Clubbing can be a local manifestation of sarcoid within the distal digit or a feature of pulmonary involvement
Pulmonary arteriovenous malformation	Can be found associated with hereditary haemorrhagic telangiectasia
Cyanotic heart disease	Typically a patent ductus arteriosus or septal defect
Infective endocarditis	Clubbing can reverse when the infection is resolved
Hepatopulmonary syndrome	Associated with a shunt that gives rise to breathlessness and cyanosis
Carcinoma of the oesophagus	Usually associated with the pattern seen with hypertrophic osteoarthropathy
Inflammatory bowel disease	May be seen with hypertrophic osteoarthropathy
Laxative abuse	It is not clear whether clubbing resolves if laxative abuse stops
Liver disease	A range of liver diseases is implicated. When treatment is a liver transplant, the clubbing has been seen to reverse
Chronic parasitic infestation	Examples include dysentery caused by *Trichuris trichiura*
HIV	In one observational study, 37% of HIV patients had clubbing. The mean duration of the HIV was 4 years
Tuberculosis	Pulmonary tuberculosis is often associated with other diseases in turn associated with clubbing, such as HIV or coexisting lung disease
Thyroid disease	The distinction between thyroid acropachy, pachydermoperiostitis and clubbing is not always clear in reports
Lupus erythematosus	A rare association
POEMS syndrome	Found in 70% of patients with this rare syndrome of *polyneuropathy, organomegaly, endocrinopathy, monoclonal gammopathy and skin changes*
Hemiplegia	Typically associated with other soft-tissue changes in the hemiplegic hand
Subungual tumour	An isolated subungual tumour can create the shape of a clubbed digit, although the rocking of the proximal nail may be absent

hypervascularity [5]. Circulating vascular endothelial growth factor (VEGF) levels are elevated in patients with clubbing, producing nail bed angiogenesis. Altered vagal tone and microvascular infarcts have also been implicated [6,7]. Mutations in the *HPGD* [8] and *SLCO2A1* [9] genes have each been linked to pachydermoperiostosis (primary hypertrophic osteoarthropathy), of which clubbing is a component (primary clubbing): their gene products are involved in prostaglandin metabolism and prostaglandin transmembrane transport, respectively, suggesting that prostaglandins may be important. Other factors such as bradykinin and serotonin or reactive factors associated with hypoxia could have relevance [10].

The list of diseases associated with clubbing (Table 93.3) has a pattern where chronic inflammation of the bowel and lung are seen with or without precipitating infection. Some of these diseases can be clustered, with tuberculosis associated with underlying fibrotic lung disease or HIV, all of which are found to have independent associations. Vascular causes can be associated with central cyanotic ischaemia, as in heart disease, or local factors such as the unilateral soft-tissue changes of hemiplegia. Clubbing can be also a component of secondary hypertrophic osteoarthropathy where a subungual lymphocytic infiltrate and some associated fibrosis may create reactive bone changes and osteoarthropathy.

An isolated subungual tumour located within the mid-proximal zone of the subungual space can displace the nail unit upwards in a form similar to clubbing. However, some of the other features are typically lacking, such as the fluctuant quality of the proximal nail and nail fold [11,12]. This can be included in the category of pseudoclubbing which arises from local pathology such as osteolysis of the tip of the digit seen in systemic sclerosis.

A rare form of pseudoclubbing is represented by osteoid osteoma, a bone tumour that can occur in the distal phalanx, especially of the index finger. It is typically painful and responsible for thickening and enlargement of the nail plate. Increased sweating and tenderness could be observed in the digital pulp without any evident sign of inflammation. X-ray is diagnostic showing an area of rarefaction with surrounding sclerosis. MRI better defines the tumour that can be located in the medulla, cortex or subperiosteally. Surgery is not always able to restore the original shape of the finger that remains slightly bigger with macronychia.

Koilonychia

Synonyms and inclusions
- Spoon nails
- Petaloid nails

In koilonychia (Greek: *koilos*, hollow; *onyx*, nail), there is reverse curvature in the transverse and longitudinal axes giving a concave dorsal aspect to the nail (Figure 93.8). Fingers and toes may be affected, with signs most prominent in the thumb or great toe. The aetiologies are diverse but can be divided into hereditary, acquired and idiopathic causes. Pathogenesis is, however, poorly understood. It has been hypothesised that poor digital blood flow disrupts the subungual connective tissue, resulting in a relative depression of the distal matrix in comparison to the proximal matrix [1].

Koilonychia is common in infancy as a benign and idiopathic feature of the great toenail, although its persistence may be associated

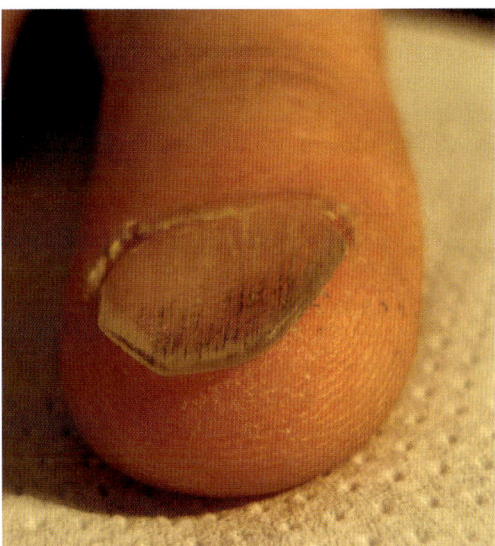

Figure 93.8 Koilonychia.

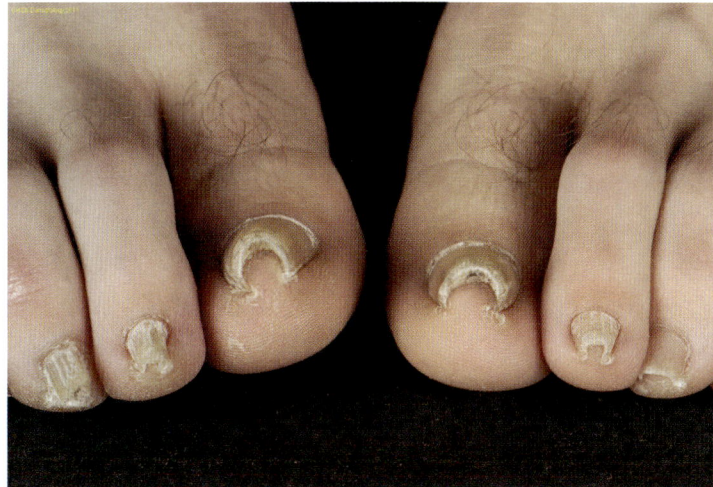

Figure 93.9 Pincer nails.

with a deficiency of cysteine-rich keratin [2] as in trichothiodystrophy. The most common systemic associations are with iron deficiency [3] and haemochromatosis, although the majority of adults with koilonychia demonstrate a familial pattern, which may be autosomal dominant [4]. In dermatoses such as psoriasis, lichen planus and dermatophyte infection, nail bed hyperkeratosis may push the nail up distally to produce a spoon-shaped nail. In mechanics, softening of the nail from contact with oil may be a factor [5] and, in hairdressers, permanent wave solutions may be causal [6].

Pincer nail

> **Synonyms and inclusions**
> - Trumpet nail
> - Arched nail

Pincer nails are characterised by transverse overcurvature of the nail plate that increases along the longitudinal axis of the nail towards the tip. At the tip of the digit the nail plate pinches the soft periungual tissues constricting, with pain, the underlying nail bed.

It presents in three patterns [1,2,3]. Probably the most common is in association with psoriasis, where the thumbs and big toes are the most likely to be affected, although the pattern is not as organised and symmetrical as that seen in the inherited version. In the latter, there is often a gradient of involvement, radiating from the thumbs and big toes outwards, which progresses with time (Figure 93.9). The third variant is the individual nail which develops a pincer deformity. In this instance, careful imaging and surgical exploration should be undertaken to exclude an isolated space-occupying lesion beneath the matrix [4–6]. An X-ray might be useful to evaluate a traction osteophyte on the dorsal side of the distal phalanx.

Treatment is usually done by surgery to relieve pain [7–9]. In the toes, it is usually best to perform a lateral ablation of the most embedded margin. This will sometimes lead to a shift of the nail such that the other side no longer embeds. If both sides require

ablation, the dimensions of the toenail may mean that it is better to ablate the entire matrix rather than to leave a central zone of nail. More complex procedures entail a Z plasty and a dermal flap but the cosmetic result is often worth the difficulty. When treating the thumbs or fingers, the chance of success with corrective surgery is higher, but the cosmetic and functional handicap of ablation may not be acceptable. Some surgeons advocate a combination of reconstruction and ablation [10]. Nail braces rarely produce long-term benefit, although promising outcomes have been reported [11].

Pachyonychia

Pachyonychia is characterised by thickening of the nail plate. Besides the congenital form (Jadassohn–Lewandowsky syndrome), this sign has been reported in psoriasis, pityriasis rubra pilaris, chronic eczema and onychomycosis. Pachyonychia is characterised by yellowish colour of the plate, increased transverse overcurvature with the free edge shaped as a horseshoe and extreme hardness. Fingernails are usually more severely affected than toenails. Histology shows a normal or moderately thickened plate but with a normal structure.

Anonychia/micronychia

Anonychia is the absence of the nail plate. Micronychia means a smaller nail plate [1]. Usually, the underlying phalanx is either absent or hypoplastic [2]. Both may be congenital, acquired or transient. An isolated congenital form of anonychia (Figure 93.10) is caused by a mutation in the *R-spondin4*, *Frizzled6* or *Wnt10a* genes (see Nail Biology), which play a part in *Wnt* signalling within the cell [3]. A variety of genetic syndromes are associated with anonychia or micronychia, but many of them involve other areas of the body thus facilitating the differential diagnosis (i.e. DOORS syndrome, COIF syndrome, Iso Kikuchi syndrome, ectodermal dysplasias).

Anonychia and micronychia at birth can be the result of alcohol and drugs (anticonvulsants, anticoagulants, morphine) taken by the mother during pregnancy. For this reason, when this abnormality occurs, it is advisable to check the mother's history before drawing conclusions concerning inheritance.

Acquired forms are due to scarring of the nail matrix. This can arise through burns, surgery or trauma, or be due to inflammatory

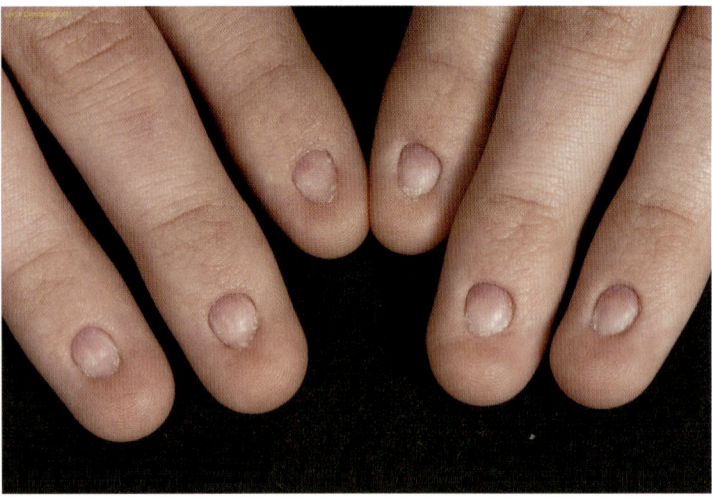

Figure 93.10 Congenital anonychia.

dermatoses such as lichen planus where the entire nail matrix is scarred and lost (onychoatrophy) [4]. Similar scarring can occur in variants of epidermolysis bullosa, with irreversible nail loss. Recently, anonychia has been described as a sign of cutaneous T cell lymphoma [5].

Brachyonychia (racquet nails)

In this condition the width of the nail plate (and the nail bed) is greater than the length. All digits or a single digit may be involved. It may occur as an isolated form or associated with a shortening of the terminal phalanx.

The 'racquet thumb' is usually inherited as an autosomal dominant trait and with a higher prevalence in females. The epiphyses of the terminal phalanx of the thumb are normally closing at the age of 13–14 years. In individuals with the hereditary form, the epiphyseal line is obliterated on the affected side at the age of 7–10 years.

Racquet nails have been reported in association with brachydactylia, multiple malignant Spiegler tumours, acroosteolysis and hyperparathyroidism.

Macronychia

The nails are larger than normal due to a larger nail bed and matrix. This may occur isolated or in association with megadactyly, as in von Recklinghausen disease. It has been associated also with Proteus syndrome, Maffucci syndrome and Klippel–Trenaunay–Weber syndrome. A hallmark of the Rubinstein–Taybi syndrome is the presence of broad thumbs and great toes. Macrodactyly most commonly manifests in the middle and index fingers.

Abnormalities of nail attachment

Nail shedding

Nails can be lost through different mechanisms:
1 Detachment of the nail plate from the proximal nail fold with the formation of a transverse whole thickness sulcus (*onychomadesis*). It is due to a severe insult producing complete arrest of nail matrix activity and it is considered a progression of a profound Beau line. This may reflect local or systemic disease and, in the latter, may result in temporary loss of all nails. Viral infections, severe metabolic stress, drugs and severe illness are usually the most common culprits [1–3]. When one or few nails are involved, local factors, such as trauma or paronychia might be the responsible agents [4].
2 Detachment from the nail bed (*onycholysis*) that generally starts distally due to disruption of the onychocorneal band and moves proximally. Proximal onycholysis is also possible. Local and generalised dermatoses may be responsible for this clinical sign [5,6].
3 An extreme case of detachment is represented by nail degloving, a postinflammatory avulsion of the nail's epithelial structures [7].
4 *Onychoptosis defluvium* or alopecia unguium describes a rare, familial, non-inflammatory type of nail shedding [8]. It may be periodic and associated with dental amelogenesis imperfecta.

Trauma is probably the most common cause of recurrent loss and may reflect the nature of the activity, such as football or some underlying abnormality of footwear or foot mechanics. It is often associated with subungual haemorrhages or hematoma [9]. Due to recurrent trauma and shedding, the nail may become thickened, and the nail bed may show irreversible alterations that prevent normal attachment of the plate to the nail bed.

Onycholysis

Onycholysis is the separation of the nail plate from the nail bed and can be graded according to severity [1]. It generally starts distally due to disruption of the onychocorneal band and moves proximally, but proximal onycholysis is also possible and it is usually a consequence of onychomadesis or tumours in the distal nail matrix. Onycholysis may be caused by traumatic, inflammatory or infective nail disorders, but also by drugs and nail bed tumours. Linking onycholysis to a specific cause is sometimes impossible (idiopathic onycholysis, see later).

The detached nail plate looks white (apparent leukonychia) due to the presence of air underneath. Green discoloration indicates the presence of *Pseudomonas* (Figure 93.22). Red discoloration is typical of drug-induced onycholysis or photo-onycholysis [2]. A yellowish colour is typical of onychomycosis. Dermoscopy is very useful to distinguish between traumatic onycholysis, psoriatic onycholysis and onycholysis due to onychomycosis (Figure 93.11) [3,4]. In traumatic onycholysis the line of detachment appears linear, regular and surrounded by a normally pale pink bed, without hyperkeratosis. The subungual space is usually whitish to yellow and splinter haemorrhages can be present due to traumas. In nail psoriasis, onycholysis is characterised by an erythematous and slightly dented border surrounding the distal edge of the detachment and by signs of nail bed inflammation (salmon patches/oily spots). In onychomycosis, white–yellow longitudinal striae/indentations (proximal progression of fungi) and fading colours are clearly recognisable.

Idiopathic onycholysis

Idiopathic onycholysis is typically seen in middle-aged women. Overzealous manicure, frequent wetting and cosmetic 'solvents' may be the cause but may not be always admitted by the patient. There may, however, be a minor traumatic element, as the condition occurs rather more often in persons who keep their nails abnormally long.

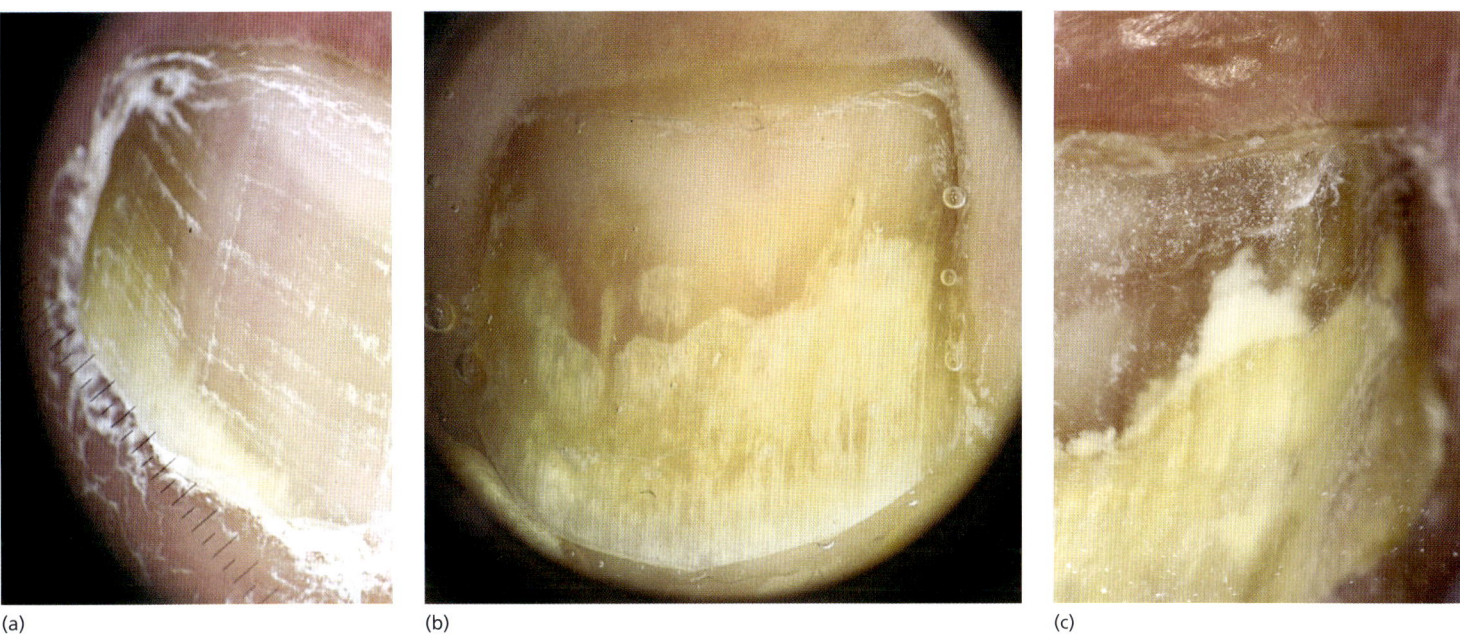

(a)   (b)   (c)

Figure 93.11 Dermoscopic differences in three types of onycholysis. (a) In post-traumatic onycholysis, the margin of the detachment is regular and most frequently localised at the lateral edge where the first toenail hits the second toenail. (b) In psoriatic onycholysis, the margin of the detachment is irregular and involves the whole free edge and may be surrounded by an erythematous border. (c) In the presence of onychomycosis, dermoscopy shows the ragged edge of the onycholytic area with the mycotic area in a proximal direction.

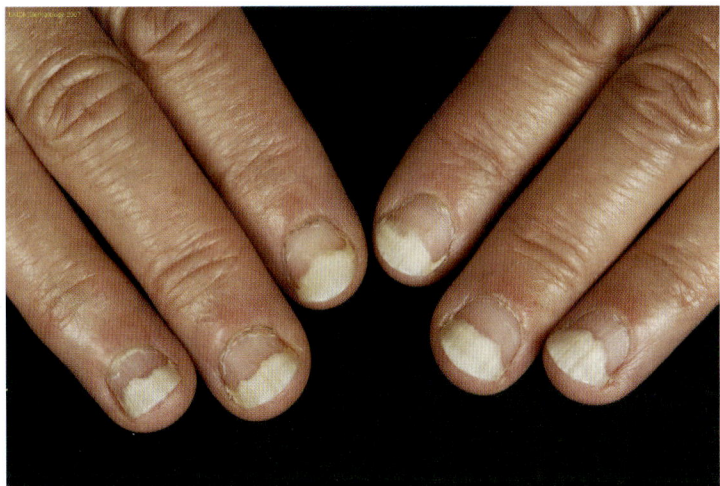

Figure 93.12 Onycholysis: idiopathic type.

The condition usually starts at the tip of one or more nails and extends to involve the distal third of the nail bed (Figure 93.12). Persistent manicure is attempted to remove the debris which accumulates within the onycholytic space and this can result in a crescentic margin of onycholysis matching the onychocorneal band and appearing similar in all involved digits. This clinical pattern is also known as *onycholysis semilunaris*. Pain occurs only if there is further extension as a result of trauma or if active infection supervenes. Fungi are usually secondary colonisers, and therefore treatment with antifungals does not improve the onycholysis. The longer the onycholysis lasts, the less likely is the nail to become reattached, due to keratinisation of the exposed nail bed [5].

The cornerstone of treatment is to minimise trauma to the affected digit and avoid water/irritant environments as much as possible

[6]. Try to clip away the onycholytic nail plate and repeat this procedure until the nail plate grows attached. The exposed nail bed should be carefully dried after each soaking. If clipping is not possible avoid aggressive cleaning under the nail plate because it promotes the spreading of the detachment.

Application of a topical antiseptic solution (twice a day) on the exposed nail bed is recommended to prevent infections. Others prefer a fixed combination of hydrocortisone cream with miconazole nitrate. Sodium hypochlorite 1% solution (Milton), 1 drop twice daily, or gentamicin eye drops, usually remove *Pseudomonas* when present.

Secondary onycholysis

There are many causes of onycholysis [7,8]. Psoriasis, fungal infection, contact dermatitis and trauma are among the most common. Thirty per cent of psoriatics with nail involvement will have onycholysis, with toenail involvement more common than fingernails. Onycholysis occurs in general medical conditions, including impaired peripheral circulation, hypothyroidism, hyperthyroidism, hyperhidrosis, yellow nail syndrome and shell nail syndrome [9,10]. Minor trauma is a common cause and many occupational cases are due to trauma. Immersion of the hands in soap and water may be considered traumatic, as well as the use of certain nail cosmetics. It has also been described after the application of 5% 5-fluorouracil to the fingertips for the therapeutic treatment of warts [11]. There is a condition of hereditary partial onycholysis associated with hard nails [12]. *Photo-onycholysis* (Figure 93.13) may occur during treatment with psoralens, demethylchlortetracycline and doxycycline [13,14], and rarely other antibiotics. This is sometimes associated with cutaneous photosensitivity. Drugs such as retinoids [15] and cancer chemotherapy can also be implicated, with taxanes eliciting nail changes in between 19% and 44% of patients, depending on the chemotherapy regimen [16]; cooling the hand with a specialised

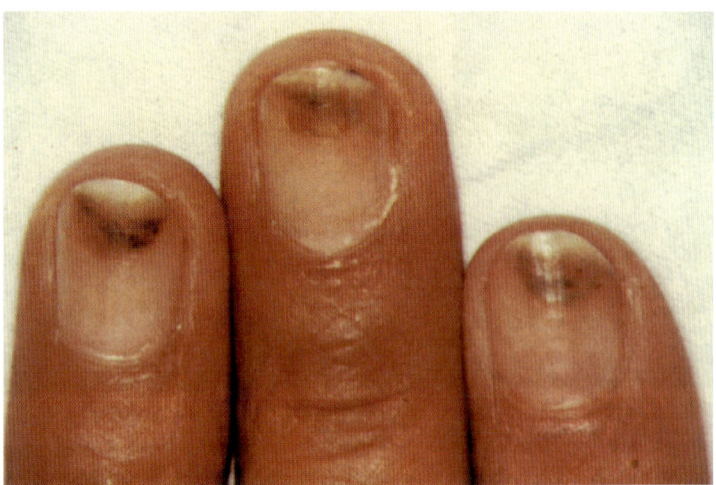

Figure 93.13 Photo-onycholysis with a uniform pattern of discoloured onycholysis in the midline.

glove has been demonstrated to help diminish or delay onset of these adverse effects [17].

Pterygium [1]

The term pterygium describes the winged appearance achieved when a central fibrotic band divides a nail proximally in two (Figure 93.14). However, the fibrotic tissue may not always grossly alter the nail and can extend from the lateral nail fold as well as the more typical proximal nail fold. A large pterygium may destroy the whole nail.

A trauma or inflammatory destructive process precedes pterygium formation. There is fusion between the nail fold and underlying nail bed and matrix. The fibrotic band then obstructs normal nail growth. Superficial abnormal vessels may be seen and there are no skin markings. It most typically develops in trauma or lichen planus and its variants, including idiopathic atrophy of the nail [2] and graft-versus-host disease [3]. It can also occur in leprosy, where it may represent scarring secondary to neuropathic damage and secondary purulent infection [4].

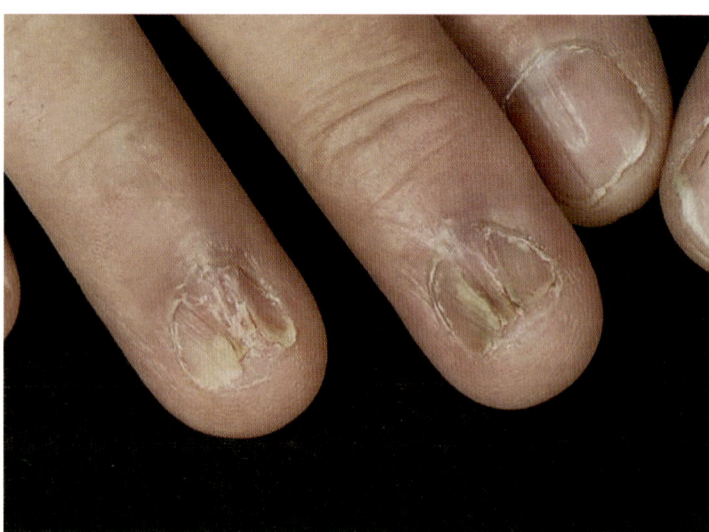

Figure 93.14 Nail pterygium due to lichen planus.

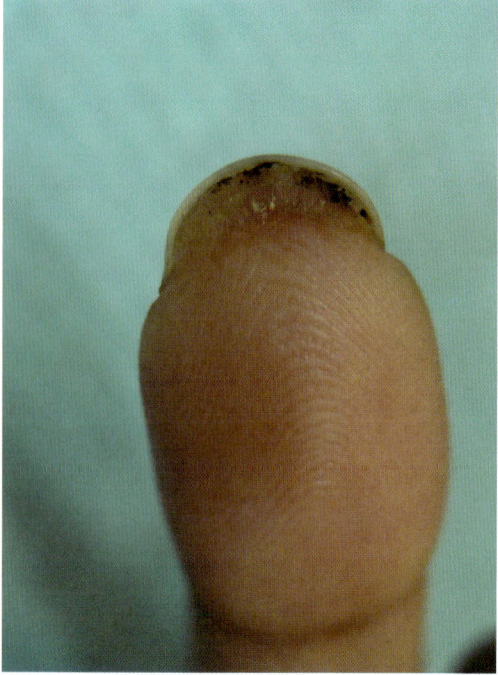

Figure 93.15 Ventral pterygium (post-traumatic).

Ventral pterygium

Ventral pterygium (Figure 93.15) or pterygium inversum unguis [1] occurs on the distal undersurface of the nail, with forward extension of the nail bed epithelium dislocating the hyponychium and obscuring the distal groove. The overlying nail may be normal, but adjacent soft tissues can be painful. Causes include trauma, systemic sclerosis [2], Raynaud phenomenon, lupus erythematosus, familial cases [3] and infections [4].

Reversible cases have been described in contact dermatitis due to nail cosmetics and are caused by temporary inflammation due to exposure to chemicals [5]. It is expected to improve completely after removing the exposure to the chemical culprit.

Changes in nail surface

Longitudinal grooves

Longitudinal grooves may run all or part of the length of the nail in the longitudinal axis and need to be distinguished from ridges which are part of the nail surface [1]. Grooves may be full or partial thickness.

The *median canaliform dystrophy of Heller* [2] is the most distinctive form (Figure 93.16) [3]. It has been seen in children under 10, but the literature is potentially misleading due to the confusion between midline transverse ridging of habit tic and true canaliform dystrophy [4]. The nail is split, usually in the midline, with a firtree-like appearance of ridges angled backwards. The thumbs are most commonly affected and the involvement may be symmetrical. The cuticle may be normal, as distinct from the cuticle in habit tic deformity ('washboard nails'). After a period of months or years the nails often return to normal, but relapse may occur [5] and a ridge may replace the original defect. Some patients give a definite history of trauma [1] and rarely the disorder can be attributed to oral retinoids [6].

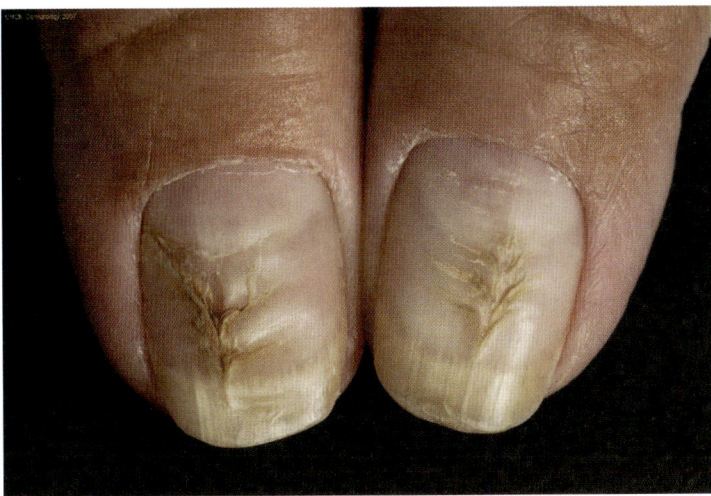

Figure 93.16 Median canaliform dystrophy of Heller.

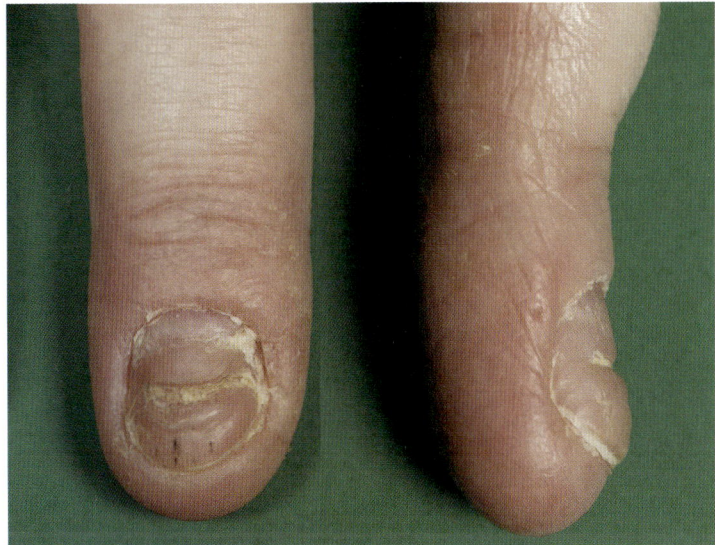

Figure 93.17 Beau lines present as transverse grooves in the nail matching the proximal margin of the nail matrix and lunula.

Although familial cases have been recorded, the majority of cases are sporadic and of unknown cause [7].

Tumours (e.g. viral warts, myxoid cysts, periungual fibromas) pressing on the matrix, or a proximal nail fold pterygium, may also produce a longitudinal groove.

Transverse grooves (Beau lines and onychomadesis) [1,2]

Transverse grooves may be full (*onychomadesis*) or partial (*Beau line*) thickness through the nail. When they are due to an endogenous cause, they have an arcuate margin matching the lunula. If exogenous, such as those due to manicure, the margin matches the proximal nail fold and the grooves may be multiple, as in washboard nails associated with a habit tic [3] or psoriasis. Transverse grooves may occur on isolated diseased digits (trauma, inflammation or neurological events) [4] or may be generalised, reflecting an acute systemic event such as a drug reaction [5], myocardial infarction, measles, mumps or pneumonia. *Beau line* arises through temporary interference with nail formation and become visible on the nail surface (Figure 93.17) some weeks after the precipitating event. The distance of the groove from the nail fold is related to the time since the onset of growth disturbance. The depth and width of the groove may be related to the severity and duration of disturbance, respectively. In many cases, grooves are seen on all 20 nails but are most prominent on the thumb and great toenail and are deeper in the midline of the nail. Full-thickness grooves can be associated with distal extension of the plane of separation of the nail plate, termed *onychomadesis*, leading to nail loss.

Nail pitting

Nail pitting presents as punctate erosions in the nail surface. Individual pits may be shallow or deep, with a regular or irregular outline [1–3]. The individual pits of psoriasis (Figure 93.63) are said to be less regular in form and in overall pattern than those of alopecia areata, but this is not always the case. When numerous, they appear randomly distributed upon the nail surface (psoriasis) or have a geometric pattern (alopecia areata). The latter may cause rippling or create a grid of pits. Mild pitting may also occur in association with different patterns of eczema but is usually more subtle or localised than psoriatic pitting. Extensive pitting combined with other surface irregularities results in the appearance of *trachyonychia*. An isolated large pit may produce a localised full-thickness defect in the nail plate termed *elkonyxis*, which is found in reactive arthritis, psoriasis and following trauma. Histologically, pits represent foci of parakeratosis in the proximal matrix, reflecting isolated nail malformation.

Trachyonychia

Trachyonychia presents as a rough surface affecting all of the nail plate and up to 20 nails. The former term '20-nail dystrophy' is not valid because several other nail diseases may affect 20 nails [1,2]. The nail plate surface is rough, sandpapered and opaque due to a severe inflammation in the proximal nail matrix. When the inflammation is milder and intermittent the result is the shiny variant. The original French term was 'sand-blasted nails', which evokes the main clinical feature of a grey, roughened surface (Figure 93.18). It is mainly associated with alopecia areata [3], psoriasis and lichen planus, but it can also be idiopathic. Histology shows spongiosis and a lymphocytic infiltrate [4] of the nail matrix. It may present at birth, as a self-limiting condition in childhood or as a more chronic problem in adulthood.

Onychoschizia (lamellar dystrophy)

Onychoschizia is also known as lamellar nail dystrophy and is characterised by transverse splitting into layers at or near the free edge (Figure 93.19) [1]. There is a subtle distinction between the static features, such as types of split, and the subjective experience of having brittle nails. Usually these characteristics coincide, although clinicians and patients may prefer to use one term over the other. Variants include splitting at the lateral margins alone and multiple crenelated splits at the free edge. It is seldom associated with any systemic disorder, although it has been reported with polycythaemia [2], HIV infection [3] and glucagonoma [4] and has been referred to as a 'syndrome' [5].

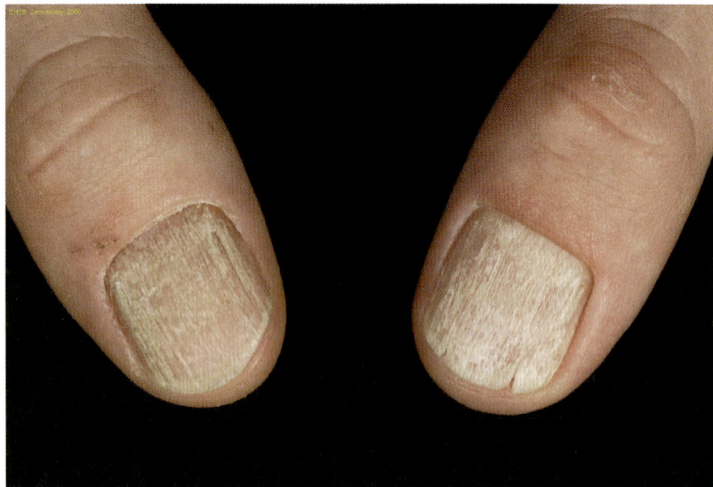

Figure 93.18 Trachyonychia: roughened surface.

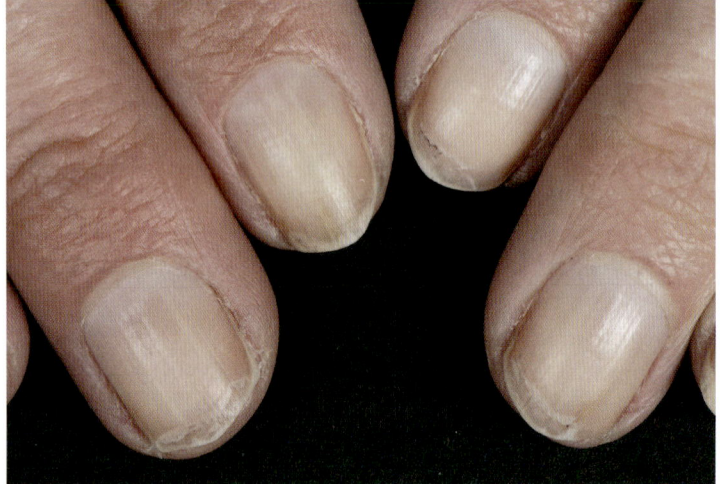

Figure 93.19 Onychoschizia (lamellar splitting).

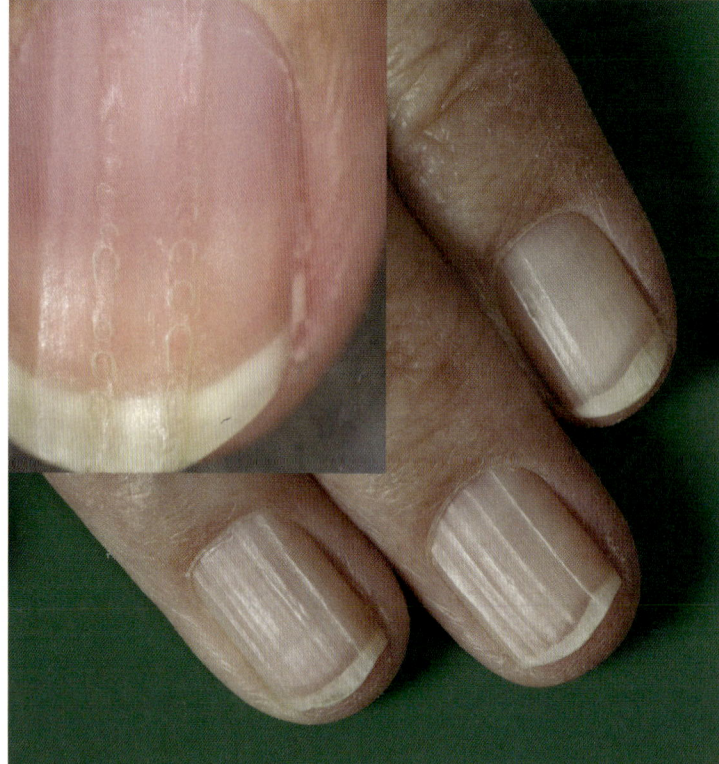

Figure 93.20 Longitudinal ridging of the nail. The inset shows beading. Both are physiological signs in the elderly.

Scanning electron microscopy illustrates the tendency of the lamellar structure of the nail to separate after repeated immersion in water [6], although case–control studies show that occupation is not a major determinant of the condition [7]. However, efforts at retaining hydration (gloves, emollient and base coat with nail varnish) may help reverse clinical changes. Biotin has been used as systemic therapy, but the evidence for its efficacy is weak [8–10].

Worn down nails

The affected nails present a triangular area of marked thinning that extend from the middle nail plate to the distal margin, which shows a wedge-shaped incision. A mild erythema of the nail bed surrounding the incision of the distal margin is also possible. They are usually caused by a frictional trauma and may be seen in severe chronic dermatitis. They have been described for the first time by Robert Baran who coined the term 'bidet nail' because he observed the abnormality in patients that frequently rubbed the fingernails against the glazed earthenware of the bidet because of an obsession about personal hygiene [1].

Beading and ridging

Beading and longitudinal ridging of the nails are common minor nail surface abnormalities which become more prominent with age (Figure 93.20). They are not an indication of disease.

Changes in nail colour

Alteration in nail colour may occur because of changes affecting the dorsal nail surface, the substance of the nail plate, or the undersurface of the nail or the nail bed.

Exogenous nail plate pigmentation

Exogenous pigment on the upper surface is easy to demonstrate by scraping the nail plate. If the proximal margin of the pigment is an arc matching the proximal nail fold, this is a further clue confirming an exogenous source. Nicotine is a typical pigment with the 'quitters' nail, which demonstrates the cessation of smoking and nicotine-free fingers for 2 months. Henna and spray tan are other common causes, but also colour coming off shoes (Figure 93.21). Fungal pigment (black, brown, orange) is also possible in the presence of superficial onychomycosis due to *Candida* sp. or moulds (*Aspergillus, Scytalidium*) [1]. In presence of onycholysis, the ventral surface of the nail plate can also become pigmented and the most common instance is the green colour seen from colonisation with *Pseudomonas aeruginosa* [2] (Figure 93.22).

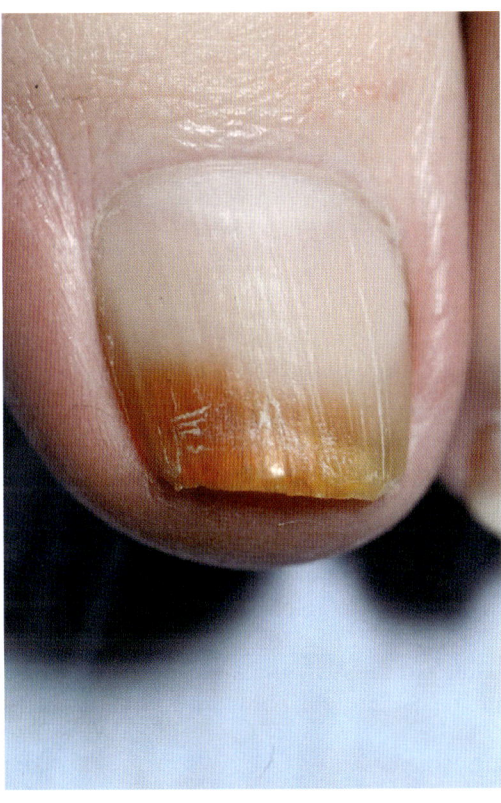

Figure 93.21 Orange pigmentation of onycholytic toenail due to orange dye from work-boots.

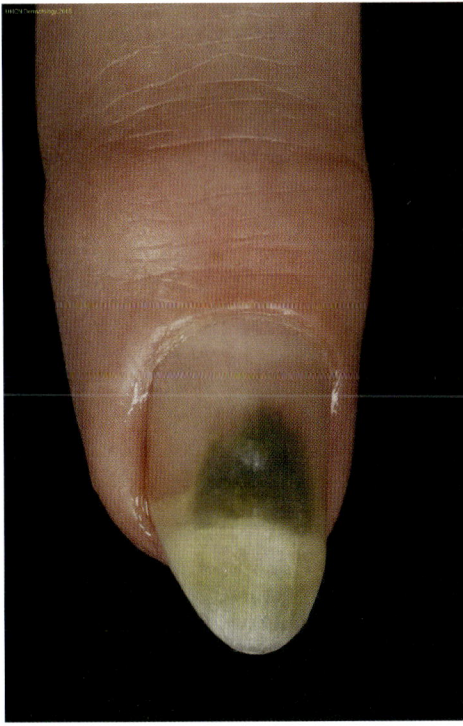

Figure 93.22 Green pigmentation of onycholytic fingernail due to *Pseudomonas*.

Melanonychia

Melanonychia describes the presence of melanin within the nail plate and can be due to melanocytic activation or to melanocytic hyperplasia, benign (lentigo, nevus) or malignant (melanoma) [3,4]. Nail matrix melanocytes are generally dormant, but in the distal matrix there is an active compartment. The nail bed hardly contains any melanocytes [5]. Activation of nail matrix melanocytes results in formation of pigment which is built into the onychocytes of the nail plate. Outgrowth of the nail results in a pigmented band, longitudinal melanonychia (Figure 93.55), starting from the cuticle or lunula and extending to the tip of the plate. Less often the pigmentation can involve the whole nail plate or presents as a transverse band.

When dealing with melanonychia it is always advisable firstly to consider possible causes of melanocytic activation, such as race, drugs, systemic diseases or inflammatory nail disorders (e.g. lichen planus, paronychia, onychotillomania, friction). In these cases, usually, several nails are affected. In cases of fungal infection [6] or nail tumours, a single digit can be affected by the pigmentation. A band caused by melanocytic hyperplasia can, however, be hidden within other bands of activation. This means that a careful evaluation of all bands is always advisable, and always with dermoscopy. The evaluation of nail melanic pigmentation is often difficult because the examined lesion shows melanin deposition and not the site of melanin production, i.e. the matrix or bed.

The evaluation of the free edge of the nail plate can provide useful information regarding the origin of the pigment. If the pigment is located in the upper portion of the free edge, the source is likely to be the proximal or dorsal portion of the matrix; if the pigment is found in the lower portion, it favours a more distal matrix location [7]. The origin of the pigment is very important because taking a biopsy from the distal matrix will result in a limited risk of permanent damage to the nail. Patients should be informed of this information before surgery.

At dermoscopy, a grey background with thin, regular and parallel lines suggests melanonychia due to nail matrix melanocyte activation. The presence of a brown background with longitudinal brown to black regular parallel lines often suggests a nevus. Brown background with longitudinal, brown to black lines with irregular colouration, spacing or thickness and parallelism disruption suggest melanoma but dermoscopy alone is insufficient to distinguish benign from malignant causes of melanonychia. Hutchinson sign (extension of the pigmentation to the periungual folds (Figure 93.23), is an important indicator of nail melanoma and can help the clinician in the diagnosis [8]. It should not be confused with the pseudo-Hutchinson sign that is represented by the pigment seen through the cuticle (Figure 93.24).

In children, nail melanoma is extremely rare [9,10], but the clinical and dermoscopic features of nail matrix nevi are frequently alarming and different from those observed in adults [11]. In children it is common to see pigmentation of the periungual tissues as well as a progressive enlargement and darkening of the band, without the presence of a melanoma. Thinning and splitting of the pigmented nail plate may also occur. In children, nail pigmentation may also spontaneously regress with age [12]. This phenomenon may be erroneously interpreted as a benign clinical sign. However, fading of the

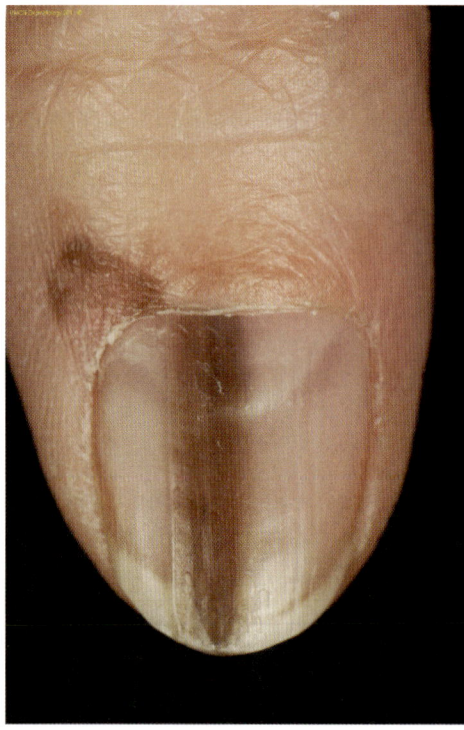

Figure 93.23 Hutchinson sign (extension of the pigmentation to the periungual skin) in a patient with melanoma of the nail unit.

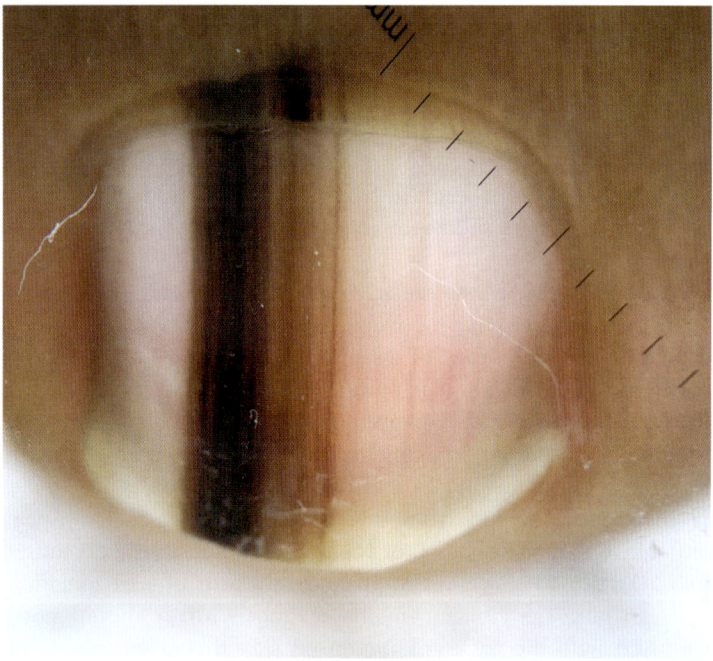

Figure 93.24 Pseudo-Hutchinson sign with hyperpigmentation that is seen through the cuticle.

pigmentation only indicates a decreased activity of the nevus cells and not a regression of the nevus itself.

Leukonychia

The term leukonychia means 'white nails' and it can be due to nail plate or nail bed abnormalities. The first one is named true leukonychia and the second one is named apparent leukonychia.

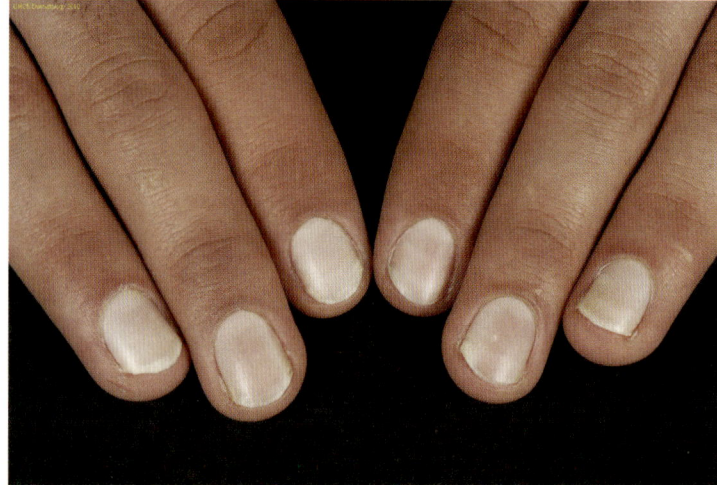

Figure 93.25 Total leukonychia.

True leukonychia is caused by parakeratotic cells within the ventral portion of the nail plate due to an abnormal keratinisation of the distal matrix. The white colour moves distally with nail growth and does not fade with pressure. Apparent leukonychia is due to abnormalities in the nail bed vascularisation. It does not move distally with the nail growth, but it fades with pressure.

True leukonychia
Total/subtotal leukonychia
In this rare condition, the nails are milky porcelain white. If the whole nail plate is affected, it is called total leukonychia (Figure 93.25). In subtotal leukonychia, the proximal two-thirds are white, becoming pink distally. This is attributed to a delay in keratin maturation, and the nail may still appear white at the distal overhang. It can be congenital, idiopathic or inherited as an isolated finding or part of a syndrome [1]. Different genes have been associated with leukonychia totalis/partialis: the most frequent is gene GJB2 located on chromosome 13 and encoding for connexin 26. Hearing loss is typically associated with leukonychia when this gene is involved.

Punctate leukonychia
It comprises white spots of 1–3 mm diameter attributed to minor matrix trauma (e.g. manicure) (Figure 93.26). It is seen in alopecia areata or psoriasis, but incidence is also very high in the normal population [2]. The pattern and number of spots may change as the nail grows. It is not related to calcium or iron content of the nail plate, as popularly believed.

Transverse leukonychia
It can reflect a systemic disorder, chemotherapy, arsenic/thallium poisoning (*Mees' lines*) [3], trauma [4] or systemic infection [5] affecting the matrix function. The 1–2 mm wide transverse band is in the arcuate form of the lunula and is analogous to a Beau line, with which it is occasionally found. Lines of transverse leukonychia have been described in mycotic nail infections in two situations: in the presence of proximal subungual onychomycosis where the fungus moves distally from the lunular area to the free edge and in the presence of recurrent infections in incompletely cured nails.

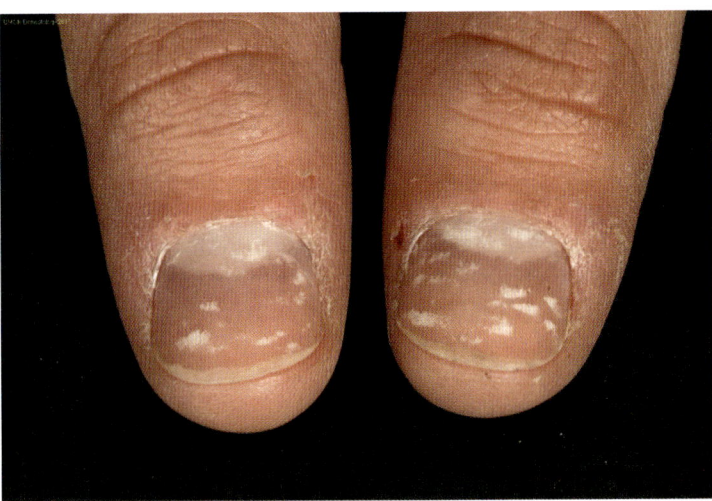

Figure 93.26 Punctate leukonychia.

Longitudinal leukonychia

It is a typical sign of Darier disease and typically associated with longitudinal erythronychia and distal splitting (*candy cane nails*). It can also be a sign of Hailey Hailey disease and nail matrix lichen planus.

Apparent leukonychia
Terry nail

It is a term used to describe nails which are white proximally and normal distally. All nails are uniformly involved and the lunula is invisible. It has been supposed that the erythematous distal crescent is a prominent onychodermal band. They have been attributed to cirrhosis, congestive cardiac failure or diabetes [1,2]. Nail bed biopsy reveals only mild changes of increased vascularity.

Half-and-half nails

It describes nails where there is a proximal white zone and a distal (20–60%) brownish sharp demarcation, the histology of which suggests an increase of vessel wall thickness and melanin deposition [3]. It has been stated that if the distal portion is less than 20% of the total nail length, we are facing Terry nails and not half and half nails. Half and half nails are seen in 9–50% of patients with chronic renal failure [4] and after chemotherapy (Figure 151.3). It is unclear whether Neapolitan nails, where there are bands of white, brown and red, is a version of half-and-half or Terry nails, or a feature of ageing.

Muehrcke paired white bands

White bands are parallel to the lunula in the nail bed, with pink between two white lines. They are commonly associated with hypoalbuminaemia, the correction of which by albumin infusion can reverse the sign. Bands are most commonly observed in the 2nd, 3rd and 4th fingernails.

Other nail bed changes

Vascular abnormalities can affect apparent nail colour as in blue nails from cyanosis and bright red nails from carbon monoxide poisoning. In addition to such generalised vascular changes there can be localised changes, as seen with nail bed tumours. The increased vascularity of a glomus tumour in comparison with the surrounding nail bed may be the sole method of determining its location. Subungual haemorrhages produce a variety of colour changes ranging from bright red to black. Splinter haemorrhages are longitudinally arranged and result from leakage of blood from nail bed capillaries and may be due to local trauma or to microemboli, classically but rarely from infective endocarditis. Subungual hyperkeratosis from dermatophyte infection or psoriasis may also change the apparent colour of the nail plate.

Colour changes due to drugs and chemicals

There are a number of colour changes which can be caused by drugs. An endogenous cause should be suspected when the colour change parallels the shape of the lunula. Yellowing of the nail is a rare occurrence of thiol compounds use, gold and *methotrexate*, or prolonged *tetracycline* therapy, which can also produce a pattern of dark distal photo-onycholysis [1,2]. Topical *5-fluorouracil* may also cause yellow nails: the whole nail is affected and returns to normal when the drug is discontinued [3]. A bluish colour is seen with *mepacrine* (quinacrine) [4]. *Hydroxyurea* has been reported to result in blue lunulae [5]. *Chloroquine* may produce blue–black pigmentation of the nail bed [6]. Other antimalarials may produce longitudinal or vertical bands of pigmentation on the nail bed or in the nail [7]. Hyperpigmentation due to increased melanin in the nail and nail bed has been noted in children after *doxorubicin* (adriamycin) [8]. However, in AIDS, longitudinal melanonychia may be seen in untreated cases [9,10] as well as in those receiving *zidovudine* [11]. Argyria may discolour the nails slate blue [12].

Yellow nail syndrome

The nails in yellow nail syndrome are yellow due to thickening, sometimes with a tinge of green possibly due to secondary infection with *Candida* or *Pseudomonas*. The lunula is obscured and there is increased transverse and longitudinal curvature of the nail plate with loss of cuticle (Figure 93.27). Occasionally, there is chronic paronychia with onycholysis and transverse ridging [1]. The condition usually presents in adults but may occur even at birth [2]. Familial forms have also been observed but never supported by genetic evidence [3]. Some of the clinical features may overlap with lichen planus [4], although the latter does not have the other systemic features normally seen in this syndrome.

The nail changes are often accompanied by lymphoedema [5] at one or more sites and by respiratory or nasal sinus disease. These conditions may appear sequentially making the diagnosis sometimes difficult. The nails grow at a greatly reduced rate: 0.1–0.25 mm/week for fingernails compared with the lowest normal rate of 0.5 mm/week. All 20 nails may be involved, although often a few are spared. Histologically, in the nail bed and matrix, dense fibrous tissue is found replacing subungual stroma, with numerous ectatic endothelium-lined vessels [6]. A foreign-body reaction has been noted [7]. It has been suggested that obstruction of lymphatics and defective lymphatic drainage by this dense stroma leads to the abnormal lymphatic function found in the affected digits in some [8] but not all [9] cases. Pathogenesis is, however, not fully understood.

The oedema is variable and may affect the legs, face or hands and occasionally it is universal. In some instances, the oedema

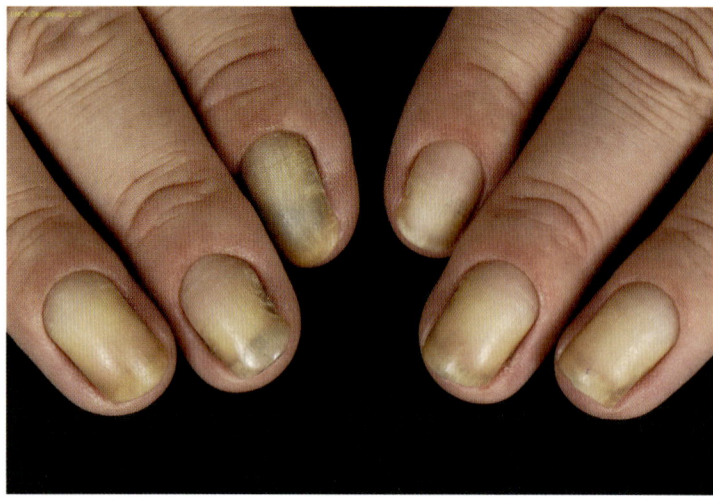

Figure 93.27 Yellow nail syndrome.

has been shown to be due to abnormalities of the lymphatics, either atresia or, in some cases, varicosity. Other cases have normal lymphatics, suggesting that a functional rather than an anatomical defect may be present, or that perhaps only the smallest lymph vessels are defective [10,11]. Although the nail changes may draw attention to the underlying lymphatic abnormality, they are found only in a minority of patients with congenital abnormality of the lymphatics. Recurrent pleural effusions have been noted [12,13]. Chronic bronchitis, bronchiectasis and pneumonias may also occur. The condition may be associated with an increased incidence of malignant neoplasms, but the hypothesis that yellow nail syndrome might be a paraneoplastic syndrome may be discharged [14,15]. Other associations include rheumatoid arthritis [16] and nephrotic syndrome [17].

In hypothyroidism and AIDS there may be yellow nails, but it is debatable whether these represent yellow nail syndrome or simply the discoloration of nail associated with retarded growth [18,19].

Nail features can fluctuate enormously over time. Attempted treatments include high dose vitamin E and the treatment of chronic infection at other sites [20–22]. There is debate as to whether itraconazole or fluconazole are of value as treatment. Itraconazole has been demonstrated to increase the rate of longitudinal growth, but an open trial in eight patients demonstrated that half gained no benefit with respect to nail changes [23]. It is reported that results are better when itraconazole or fluconazole are combined with high dose oral vitamin E (600–1000 IU once daily) [24]. Many authorities claim a resolution rate of about 50%, but it is not clear how much of this is part of the natural course [25].

Red lunulae

Erythema of all or part of the lunula may affect all digits, but it is usually most prominent in the thumb. Duration of the change will depend on the cause. When associated with cardiac failure, it may follow the course of management of the cardiac disease. When due to a subungual tumour such as a myxoid cyst or glomus tumour, it will remain until the tumour is removed. Inflammatory connective tissue causes may also result in a fluctuating course (lupus is a typical example). Erythema is less intense in the distal lunula, where it can merge with the nail bed or be demarcated by a pale line and can

be obliterated by pressure on the nail plate. The appearance can fade over a few days. Dotted red lunulae have been reported in psoriasis, lichen planus and alopecia areata [1–3].

Histopathological examination of red lunulae revealed an increased density of benign-appearing and mildly dilated vascular channels in the superficial papillary dermis of the nail matrix. These findings raise the possibility that systemic or local factors might be responsible for angiogenesis within the nail unit [4]. Recently, intraoperative dermoscopy confirmed these findings [5].

Longitudinal erythronychia (Figure 93.28)

A longitudinal red streak in the nail can have several causes [1,2]. All will have a corresponding band of thinned nail plate as part of the defect. The effect of this is a strip where vascularity in the underlying nail bed is seen more easily not only because the nail plate is thinner, but also because blood pools in the underlying nail bed capillaries as a result of reduced compression by the overlying nail plate. Splinter haemorrhages may lie longitudinally within the strip. The distal part of the thinned, and therefore vulnerable, strip is commonly split and onycholytic due to trauma from everyday activities. Such strips of thinned nail arise because of focally reduced proliferation within the distal matrix. This can be due directly to matrix pathology or may be secondary to focal pressure with secondary loss of function. The matrix pathology includes a spectrum of epidermal disorders. The most common are *lichen planus* and *Darier disease* [3]. Recently, it has also been described in a patient with *sarcoidosis* [4].

Pressure on the matrix may be exerted by any of the full range of dermal tumours as well as tumours of the bone and cartilage that arise from the distal phalanx.

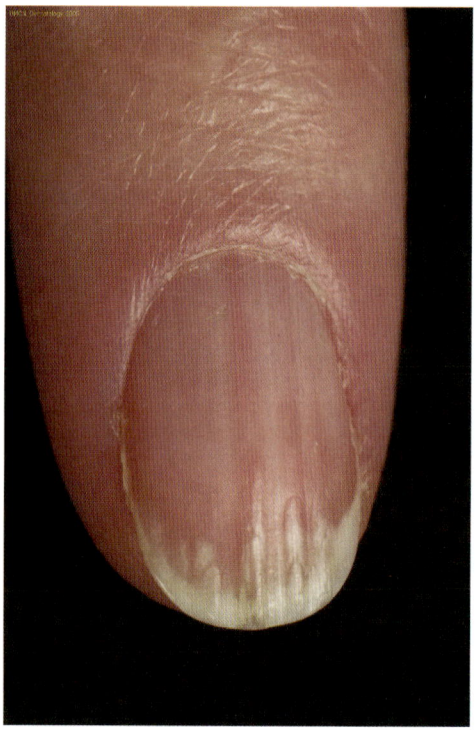

Figure 93.28 Longitudinal erythronychia in idiopathic polydactylous longitudinal erythronychia.

Baran and Perrin have coined the term 'onychopapilloma' to describe the isolated benign warty distal nail bed lesions found in association with longitudinal erythronychia for which no underlying cause can be identified [5]. Isolated longitudinal erythronychia needs careful assessment, however, as a similar clinical presentation can be due to conditions such as Bowen disease, squamous cell carcinoma [5,6] or basal cell carcinoma [7] of the matrix. Biopsy may be warranted if the erythronychia is observed to change or if the patient suffers any symptoms. Some patients seek medical evaluation because of pain in the associated distal digit.

Where no primary disease can be identified to explain erythronychia affecting multiple nails, the descriptive term 'idiopathic polydactylous erythronychia' has been proposed [8].

However, polydactylous longitudinal erythronychia usually coincides with a regional or systemic cause and biopsy is less often performed compared with the localised form [9,10].

TRAUMATIC NAIL DISORDERS

Nails may show signs of acute trauma, scars following acute trauma or consequences of chronic repetitive trauma.

Acute trauma

Acute trauma is classified with respect to severity, ranging from a small haematoma to digit amputation [1–3].

Subungual haematoma [1,2]
Subungual bleeding is a common sign. It may present as a feature of acute trauma, with pain due to the recent event in combination with pain arising from the pressure exerted by the subungual accumulation of blood. A haematoma arising within the matrix will be incorporated into the nail plate [3,4]. Where the haematoma is associated with acute trauma, there is usually pain and the diagnosis is obvious. However, with less extreme trauma, a haematoma may not develop immediately and may be painless. This is most common in the toes and may give rise to clinical uncertainty as to whether it represents early subungual melanoma. A history of traumatic sporting hobbies is useful, and signs of symmetrical nail trauma and inappropriate footwear all indicate trauma as the cause of the appearance. Dermoscopy will nearly always resolve the situation [5,6], but, if it does not, making a small punch in the surface of the nail may reveal old blood as the source of pigment. Malignancies can bleed and so confirmation of blood does not refute the possibility of a tumour; however, as an isolated finding in the absence of other clues, this test should be sufficient to obviate the need for surgical exploration. An alternative is to score a transverse groove in the nail at the proximal margin of the pigment and observe over a few weeks as the discoloration grows out. If pigment continues to spread proximal to the groove, surgical exploration is warranted.

The only treatment that can be offered is to relieve the pressure and if dealt with soon after the injury this can be done by puncturing the nail, for instance with a hot pointed implement, cautery, small drill or punch biopsy [7]. This procedure will relieve pain and may save the nail. The possibility of an underlying fracture must be considered for larger haematomas [1]. It is stated that if more than 50% of the visible nail is affected, the nail plate should be removed. However, a systematic review has shown that in the majority of cases, cosmetic outcome or complication rates are not better after nail plate avulsion than after trephination [1].

Nail bed laceration

The nail bed may be lacerated by incisions, avulsion or crush injuries. In simple lacerations there is displacement of the nail plate. Stellate lacerations and lacerations by crush injuries often involve fragmentation of the nail plate. Over 50% of all nail bed injuries have an associated distal phalanx fracture [1]. The management of nail bed lacerations is controversial and there is much debate about removal of the nail plate for repair of a nail bed laceration compared with simple trephining of even large subungual haematoma [2–7]. The success of nail bed repair diminishes with delay following injury, with recommended intervention within 2–3 days, but ideally sooner. Repair of stellate lacerations can have good outcomes while crush injuries have a poorer prognosis due to additional nail bed contusion.

The nail bed damage can be assessed by avulsion and then the nail can be replaced after any necessary nail bed repair has been performed using absorbable sutures or medical adhesive such as 2-octylcyanoacrylate (Dermabond) or n-butyl-2-cyanoacrylate (Histoacryl) [8]. After repair, the nail is used as a splint, also because the nail bed often is partially attached to the undersurface of the nail plate, and may grow back in position [9]; a small window for drainage of blood and exudate is made in the nail [10]. For bigger nail bed defects a split-thickness skin graft, split-thickness nail and full-thickness nail bed graft can be used; the latter two are preferred but may cause a donor site deformity [6]. The graft can be harvested either from uninjured areas of the involved finger or from other intact digits for larger defects. Distal tuft fractures and nondisplaced distal phalanx fractures are managed with nail bed repair and nail plate replacement. Displaced fractures or fractures proximal to the nail fold are treated with operative fixation of the bone. The nail plate should be removed to permit nail bed exploration for bone fragments and repair [2,6].

Delayed trauma

The most common kind of chronic deformities following an acute injury are onycholysis, ridged nail, split nail, nail horn, or reduction in the length of the nail bed with consequent overcurvature of the tip of the nail [1].

In cases of post-traumatic onycholysis or ridged deformity the application of a full thickness nail matrix graft harvested from the great toe could be applied after excision of the scar tissue [1]. Cure of a split nail deformity is difficult, with only a modest chance of success [2,3]. Sometimes, there is an associated pterygium. Treatment entails excision of the nail bed and matrix scar and, in the case of a pterygium, a split-skin graft or part of the nail plate may be placed on the ventral aspect of the proximal nail fold. This may help to prevent recurrence of the pterygium. Often wide undermining is necessary because the underlying bone and fragile nail bed and matrix limit the margins of the excision. It is important to keep the wounded aspects of nail bed or matrix separate from the overlying

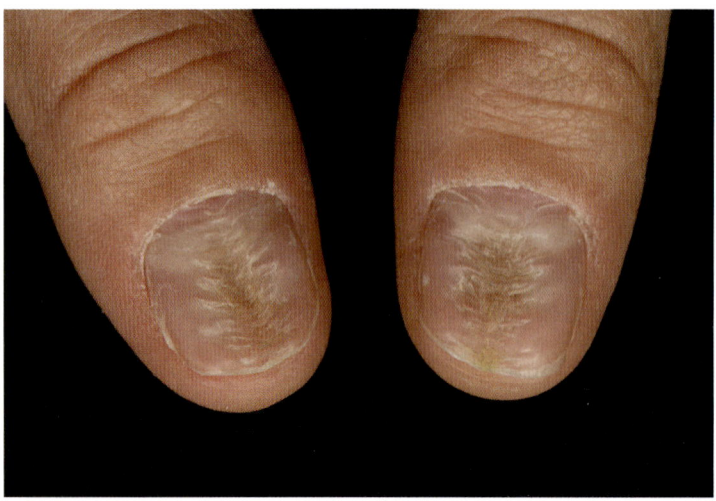

Figure 93.29 Transverse ridges resulting from habit tic.

nail fold after surgery. This is often best done by returning the nail plate because replacement with a silicone nail splint has a higher risk of development of nail deformities [4].

If treatment is required for a shortened distal phalanx with nail bed changes, there are several choices [1,5]: the entire nail can be phenolised or local flap to gain additional distal pulp can be performed; a V–Y advancement flap based on two neurovascular pedicles or a cross finger flap after sub-periosteal freeing of hooked nail bed followed by de-epithelialisation and split thickness sterile matrix grafting of the advancing edge of skin flap to lengthen the nail bed.

Chronic repetitive trauma

Chronic repetitive trauma may take several forms. Some have been considered in other sections detailing transverse ridges produced by a habit tic (Figure 93.29), the canaliform dystrophy of Heller (Figure 93.16) and chronic paronychia (Figures 93.59 and 93.60).

Nail biting and onychotillomania [1,2]

Synonyms and inclusions
- Onychophagia
- Nail picking
- Dermatitis artefacta of the nail

Classification links
- ICD-10: F98.8
- ICD-11: 6B25.Y

Onychophagia, defined as habitual nail biting, is a common problem in children and young adults. It is usually confined to the fingernails. Nail biters tend to bite all 10 fingers. The nail plate, periunguium and nail bed are all subject to nail biting. Onychotillomania can be defined as self-induced trauma of the nail unit, either by recurrent picking or pulling at elements of the nails, leading to nail dystrophy

or extraction of nails. Complications of nail biting and onychotillomania include damage to the nails, paronychia and secondary bacterial infections.

Epidemiology
Features of nail biting are found in up to 60% of children, 45% of adolescents and 10% of adults [3,4]. Onychotillomania affects 0.9% of the population [5]. Nail biting usually begins in childhood and adolescence; onychotillomania begins at a later age [5]. Biting is rarely seen in patients younger than 2–3 years old [1,4] and the median age of onset is 5 years old [4]. Onychotillomania may be allied to parasitophobia when the patient picks off pieces claiming that they contain parasites [6].

Pathophysiology
The aetiology of nail biting and onychotillomania is unknown, but genetic and environmental contributions are associated [1,2]. Both are variants of compulsion and may occur concurrently. Severe forms of onychophagia are classified under obsessive-compulsive and related disorders but the majority of moderate fingernail biters have no associated psychiatric disorder [4,5]. On the other hand, the majority of patients diagnosed with onychotillomania have psychiatric co-morbidities, specifically depression, anxiety disorders and obsessive–compulsive disorders [2]. Severe damage may be associated with genetic disorders with self-mutilation, such as Lesch–Nyhan syndrome and Smith–Magenis syndrome.

Clinical features
Nail signs in biting and onychotillomania show overlap. The nails in nail biting are typically short, with up to 50% of the nail bed exposed. The free edge may be even or ragged. Surface change may include splitting of the nail into layers or a sand-papered effect, and pterygium inversus (Figure 93.15). The nail may acquire a brown longitudinal streak [7–9] both in nail biting and onychotillomania and macrolunula may be present. A rough and irregular nail and nail fold may coincide with subungual splinter haemorrhages, and with nail fold haemorrhage and erosions. Nail fold erosions occur in cases where the nail folds are bitten in addition to, or as a substitute for, the nail (Figure 93.30). The most aggressive nail biting can produce subungual haemorrhage, strips of nail loss, with residual spurs or loss of the entire nail.

Self-induced trauma in onychotillomania can be inflicted by utensils or other nails, or with pushing back of the proximal nail fold as part of a habit tic. In more conscious forms of self-damage, sharp instruments are used to produce dermatitis artefacta of the nail unit, and the nail fold is commonly preserved [10]. The characteristic finding in onychotillomania is the habit tic deformity [2], a midline furrow along the length of the nail, with associated transverse ridges and depressions running up the midline of the nail, associated with loss of the cuticle (Figure 93.29). This is also known as wash-board nails. The central portion of the proximal nail fold is often red and slightly swollen in habit tic deformity, with focal detachment of the cuticle.

Differential diagnosis
Findings in nail biting are non-specific. The differential diagnosis includes acute and chronic paronychia, nail psoriasis, lichen planus,

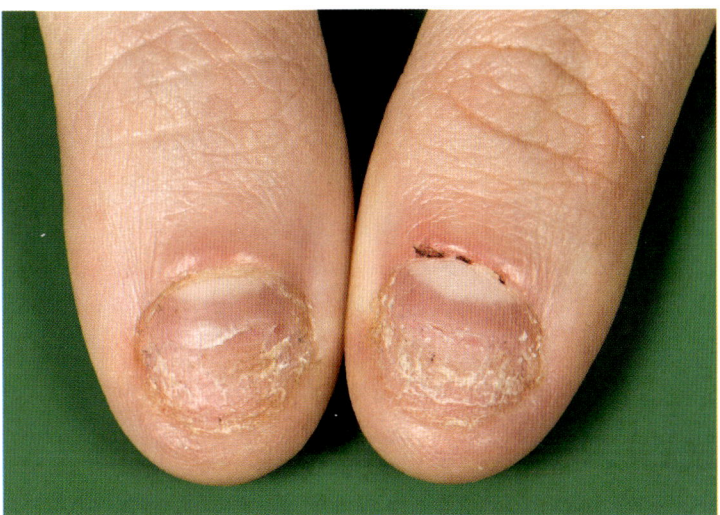

Figure 93.30 Nail biting can be extensive, with damage to the nail folds and nail plate causing subungual splinter haemorrhage.

trachyonychia, epidermolysis bullosa acquisita and onychomycosis [11]. Heller's median nail dystrophy is usually a separate entity but may occasionally overlap with onychotillomania in a subset of patients [11] and could be drug-induced (isotretinoin).

Complications and co-morbidities
Focal abnormalities, such as viral warts, are often a complication, whether as a cause or as a result of the Koebner effect after biting. Nail biting can also predispose to herpetic whitlow. Since nail biting can lead to transfer of MRSA to the oral cavity, the World Health Organization has strongly advised clean, short nails in health care workers. Dental problems can also arise due to nail embedded in gums or between teeth [12]. Trauma followed by secondary infection involving the matrix may make nail loss permanent or results in pterygium formation. Biting the nail folds can lead to bleeding and chronic paronychia with acute infective exacerbations. This in turn may lead to nail plate damage or ridging, nail fold scarring, or osteomyelitis of the terminal phalanx [13,14]. Irreversible shortening of the fingernails may develop as a result of chronic nail biting. A possible explanation for this is that if the distal nail bed is detached from the nail plate for a long time, the distal nail bed may become keratinised and disappears irreversibly, and this ultimately results in permanent shortening of the fingernails due to the shortened nail bed [15].

Investigations
The diagnosis of nail biting and onychotillomania is usually clinical. Subjects will sometimes deny nail biting and picking and attribute the appearance to a disease that stops nail growth. Transverse grooves scored proximally in the nail plate will confirm that the nail is growing by moving distally with time. In aggressive nail biting, the groove may be eroded from the surface. In onychotillomania, subjects often refuse to accept the causative relationship between their behaviour and the onychodystrophy.

Management
The nails usually return to normal after the behaviour is stopped for several months. Long-term nail dystrophy and melanonychia

may persist in those patients who have this behaviour for many years. There are two main approaches to treatment of the nail biting, namely, non-pharmacological and pharmacological. The non-pharmacological methods of treating onychophagia include punishment, aversive therapies (bitter tasting lacquer), competitive stimuli, as well as methods to try to 'unlearn' the habit, such as habit reversal [1], behavioural therapy [16] or a health promotion programme [17].

Treatment of onychotillomania is often unsuccessful and cure relies largely on the motivation of the patient. Where the patient acknowledges an element of self-damage, they may comply with the use of a dressing (Micropore) over the tip of the digit 24 h a day for 2–3 months. This needs to be replaced twice weekly to several times a day in some instances. In the first month, it may be helpful to combine the dressing with moderate potency topical steroid to suppress any inflammation. Ensure there is no infection prior to this. Local antiseptics and antimicrobial ointments may help settle the infection secondary to nail unit damage. Antiseptics or treatments with the most bitter taste are often prescribed in the belief that this will discourage biting. In severe forms of onychophagia and onychotillomania, behavioural therapy [16,18,19], oral N-acetylcysteine [16], clomipramine [20] and pimozide [21] may be beneficial and indicated in these cases. Antidepressants may be considered in cases with coexisting depression [2].

Damage from nail manicure instruments
Metal instruments, such as a nail file or scissors, wooden or plastic orange sticks, or nail whitener pencils may create acute or chronic injuries in the nail area. Onycholysis may result from using the sharp point for cleaning under the nail plate. Nails, however, are best cleaned with a nail brush and soap, because overzealous manicure and pushing back the cuticles, may result in leukonychia across several nails [1]. Cleaning around the nail with contaminated instruments may lead to acute or chronic paronychia. It is not advisable to cut or clip the nail plate, as this produces a shearing action that weakens the natural layered structure and promotes fracturing and splitting [2]. An emery board is preferred for shaping the fingernail by filing from the sides of the nail towards the centre.

Onychogryphosis and nail hypertrophy [1–3]

Synonyms and inclusions
- Onychauxis
- Ostler's nail
- Ram's horn nail

Classification links
- ICD-10: L60.2
- ICD-11: EE10.3

Introduction
Onychogryphosis and onychauxis are acquired dystrophies usually affecting the great toenail, which is thickened, yellow and, in case of onychogryphosis, twisted.

Epidemiology

Onychogryphosis most often is a disease of the elderly population in which a prevalence of 11–38% has been reported, mainly in people with long-standing poor personal care or neglect, in homeless persons, and in people with senile dementia [1]. Trauma, neglected onychomycosis, impairment of the peripheral circulation and biomechanical foot problems may, however, precipitate similar changes in middle age or earlier. There also are few reports of onychogryphosis inherited as an autosomal-dominant trait with onset within the first year of life, and as an autosomal recessive trait in Haim–Munk syndrome.

Traumatic causes may be major trauma to the nail, microtrauma caused by sport, improperly fitting footwear and anatomical anomalies (e.g. hallux valgus). At one time, onychogryphosis was known as ostler's nail, because some cases could be traced to injury caused by a horse trampling on the foot of the ostler. The injury, once sustained, is aggravated by improperly fitting footwear. As the nail becomes longer and thicker, damage from footwear becomes progressively more important.

Some cases of nail hypertrophy are intrinsic and this applies especially to toenails other than the nail of the great toe. The nail becomes thick and circular in cross section instead of flat, and thus comes to resemble a claw.

Clinical features

In the early stages onychogryphosis mimics nail hypertrophy, with the more classical features of onychogryphosis appearing later. In onychogryphosis, one or more nails become greatly thickened (Figure 93.31) and, with neglect, increase in length and becoming curved. It is often described as a 'ram's horn nail' or being 'oyster-like' in appearance, with an irregular surface marked by longitudinal and transverse striations, the latter of which are more frequent (Figure 93.32). The nails of the great toes are most often involved, but no toenail is exempt. In extreme cases, the free edge may press on or even re-enter the soft tissues of the foot. More common complications of onychogryphosis include ingrowing toenails, paronychia, secondary onychomycosis, and the inability to cut the toenail due to increasing hypertrophy of the nail plate [1].

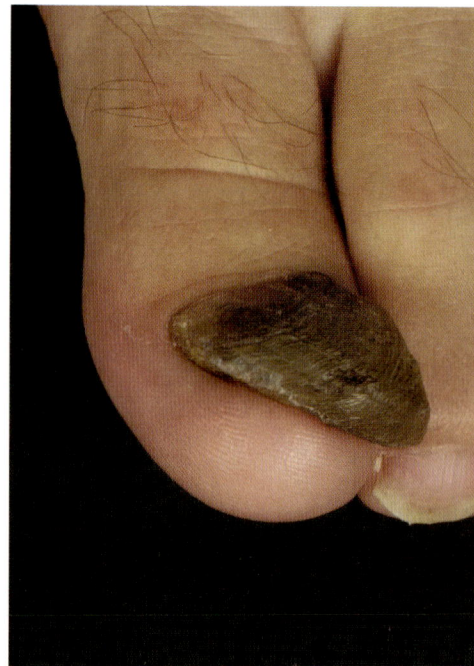

Figure 93.32 Typical onychogryphosis of a great toenail.

Differential diagnosis

Other causes of thickened nails include psoriasis, pityriasis rubra pilaris, Darier disease, fungal infections, retronychia, pachyonychia congenita, congenital ectodermal defects and congenital malalignment of the great toenails [4].

Management

Treatment is indicated in order to prevent complications and sometimes for aesthetic reasons. Footwear should always be reviewed to assess appropriate fit. The thickened nails are extremely hard and trimming is difficult. Treatment of onychogryphosis and nail hypertrophy may be either conservative or surgical [1]. Surgical treatment is recommended in those with good circulation (Figure 93.33). Options are a simple nail avulsion with or without any type of matricectomy, optionally with V-Y advancement flap [5]. Occasionally, one-half of the terminal phalanx is excised together with the nail fold (Syme method). Beware that onychogryphosis will recur after a simple nail avulsion. Conservative treatment is preferred in the elderly population and requires regular paring and trimming of the affected nails, usually by a podiatrist using nail clippers and a file or mechanical burr. Before nail trimming, cryotherapy on onychogryphotic nails with liquid nitrogen may make the nails very brittle and easy to trim within 1 second after cryotherapy [6].

Ingrowing toenail [1–4]

Synonyms and inclusions
• Onychocryptosis
• Unguius incarnatus
• Retronychia

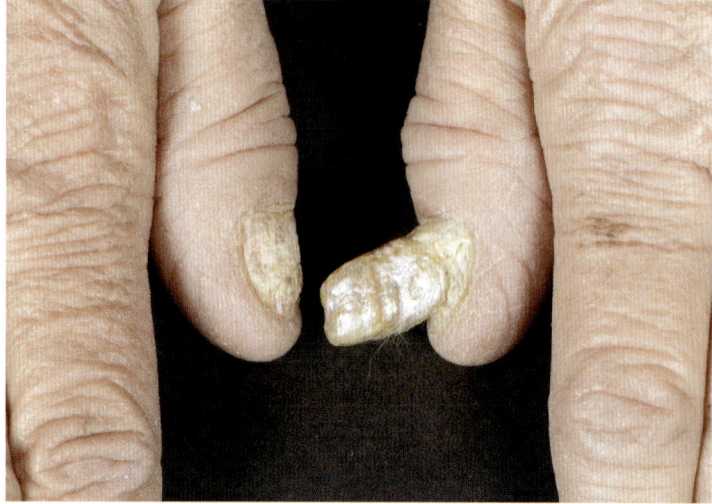

Figure 93.31 Onychogryphosis in nail psoriasis.

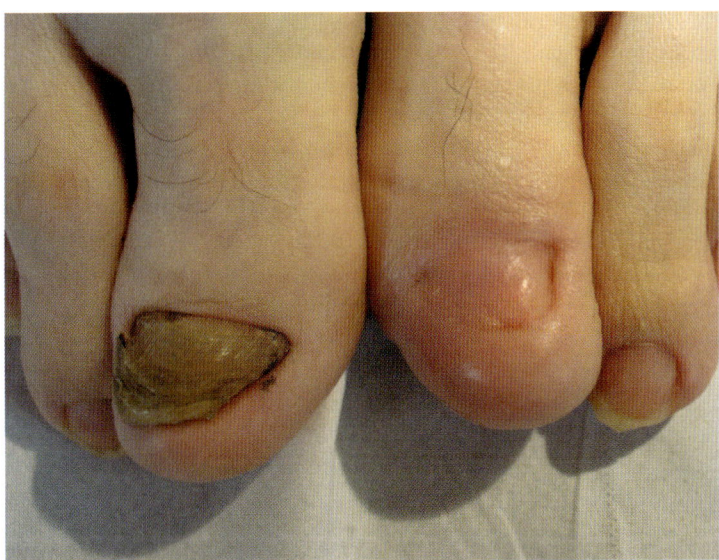

Figure 93.33 Onychogryphosis is often best treated with ablation of the nail matrix: right toe not operated, left toe 10 weeks after complete phenolisation.

Classification links
- ICD-10: L60.0
- ICD-11: EE13.1

Introduction

The nail can ingrow on any of its four margins, although lateral ingrowing is the most common pattern. The soft tissue at the side of the nail (lateral nail fold) is penetrated by the edge or spikes of the nail plate, resulting in pain, inflammation and, later, the formation of granulation tissue. Proximal ingrowing of the proximal nail plate is known as retronychia [5]. In all variants of ingrowing toenails, the big toes are involved in the majority of cases.

Epidemiology

An ingrowing toenail may present at any age, but most commonly it affects teenagers and adults in their 50s. Among teenagers, males are more often involved [1], while at an older age, females are more often affected [6]. An epidemiolocal study showed a 10-year overall incidence of 307.5/100 000 person-years [6].

Pathophysiology

Ingrowing toenails are caused by nail or nail spikes that penetrate the lateral nail folds leading to a painful inflammation and granulation tissue. The most common predisposing factor is the combination of ill-fitting footwear and improper nail trimming, in a half-circle instead of straight across. Other predisposing factors are bad foot hygiene, hyperhidrosis, trauma, the use of some medications and bone deformity, especially acquired hallux valgus, varus deformity and flat feet [1,6]. Also nail shape abnormalities, including pincer nails, congenital malalignment of the big toenails and thickening of the nail may lead to ingrowing nails.

In children, ingrowing is commonly distal rather than lateral and commonly occurs before shoes are worn. It is associated with crawling, 'pedalling' or the wearing of undersized jumpsuits [7].

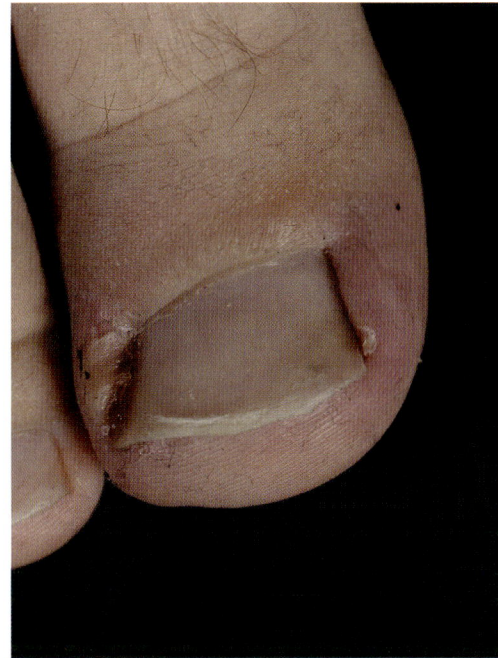

Figure 93.34 Ingrowing great toenail (stage 2).

Retronychia develops when the nail embeds in the proximal nail fold. This is provoked by disturbance of nail growth, usually through trauma. The result is dislodging of the nail upwards with a new nail growing beneath. The proximal aspect of the old nail then impacts on the ventral aspect of the proximal nail fold and this creates the same features of inflammation, ooze, swelling, redness and pain as seen when the lateral nail fold is affected.

Clinical features

Ingrowing toenail affects almost exclusively the toenails of the hallux and can affect one or both lateral nail edges. Involvement of the lateral toe edge occurs twice as often as the medial side [6,8]. Patients present with pain and redness. Physical examination shows signs of inflammation in the affected toe: pain, swelling, and erythema (stage 1). Stage 2 is characterised by more oedema and tenderness as well as drainage of seropurulent exudate and ulceration of the nail fold (Figure 93.34). This acute infection may develop towards a chronic infection with hypertrophic granulation tissue at the lateral nail fold (stage 3).

Excess nail fold granulation tissue can also be a feature of amelanotic melanoma [9] and is a rather frequently encountered reaction to medications such as retinoids (Figure 93.35), ciclosporin, antiretroviral drugs, methotrexate and conventional chemotherapy [10–16]. More recently, severe nail toxicities can be found after targeted therapies and immunotherapies, mainly with epidermal growth factor receptor inhibitors and selective pan-fibroblast growth factor receptor inhibitors 1–4, but also with mitogen-activated protein (MAP) kinase inhibitor and with mammalian Target of Rapamycin (mTOR) inhibitors [17].

Management

General measures focus on the elimination of predisposing factors. In particular, it is essential to insist that the patient wears sufficiently wide, high and pliable shoes to remove lateral pressure [18]. Nail

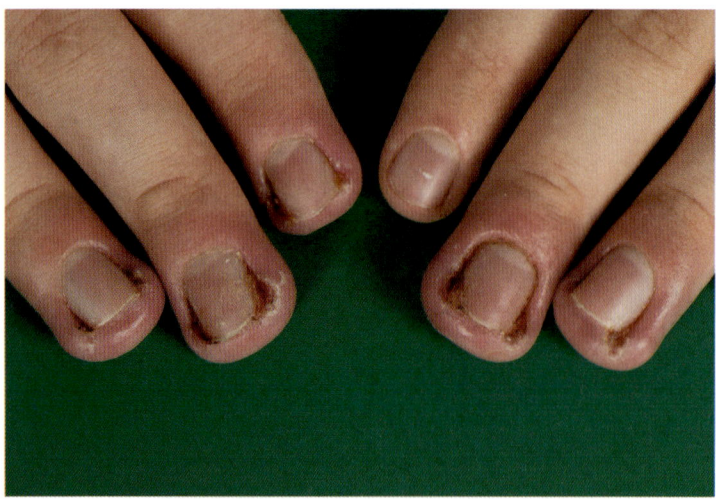

Figure 93.35 Ingrowing fingernails in patient on isotretinoin.

trimming habits in which the lateral edges are rounded off should be corrected; the nail must be allowed to grow until its edges are clear of the end of the toe before they are cut straight across. Other underlying factors also deserve attention, including hyperhidrosis, onychomycosis, bad foot hygiene, hyperhidrosis, trauma and bone deformity. Application of topical steroids to the granulation tissue may decrease inflammation [19]. They should, however, only be used after infection has been ruled out or is being actively managed. An appropriate systemic antibiotic should only be administered if the infection is more severe with local cellulitis [20]. When granulation tissue forms this should be destroyed by cauterisation with a silver nitrate stick.

Both conservative and surgical treatments are available for the treatment of ingrowing toenails. All treatments focus on restoration of a situation in which no nail or spikes grow into the nail fold. In general, conservative treatments can be applied in stages 1 and 2, while surgical treatment may be preferred in more refractory or disabling cases (stage 3). In paediatric ingrowing toenails, surgery is only occasionally required. In most instances, management is conservative with topical steroid and antiseptic preparations [21].

Many conservative techniques have been described [1]. Options to separate the ingrowing edge of the nail from the nail folds include insertion of material under or around the edge of the nail. Materials used are dental floss, cotton wisp or wedges of cotton wool. Taping the toe or applying plastic gutters between nail edge and nail fold are alternatives [22]. Conservative techniques can be supplemented with nail braces or with acrylic nail to build up a smooth surface able to push the nail fold away and relieve the ingrow [23].

If conservative measures fail or in the case of stage 3 ingrowing toenails, operative intervention will be necessary [3]. Removing the nail, or parts of the nail alone is likely to result in recurrence of ingrowing when the nail grows [24], and therefore should be combined with matricectomy. Chemical matricectomy is commonly performed using phenol (see Nail Surgery section) but also other denaturating agents can be employed, such as sodium hydroxide and trichloroacetic acid. Chemical matricectomy demonstrates a higher success rate and is less painful than surgical matricectomy [2]. Although surgical excision of the matrix can provide an excellent result, it is more than phenolisation dependent on

the skill of the practitioner. Nail fold resection without matricectomy, the Howard-Dubois and Vandenbos procedures, and the super-U technique are indicated when ingrowing nails are caused by hypertrophy of the nail folds [3,25,26]. Other techniques for treating ingrowing toenail have also been introduced, including electrocautery, radiofrequency ablation and carbon dioxide laser ablation [1]. Their exact position in treating ingrowing nails still needs to be established.

Retronychia is said to be self-limiting over a matter of several months as eventually the older nail is shed. Also taping has been presented as a treatment option in mild cases [4]. In most patients nail avulsion is the treatment of choice [27]. The replacement nail usually grows back without any problem [5] but to prevent distal ingrow of the nail after avulsion, an acrylic nail can be attached to the newly growing nail when it has reached one-third of its length.

TUMOURS UNDER OR ADJACENT TO THE NAIL

BENIGN TUMOURS

Lobular capillary haemangioma (pyogenic granuloma) of nail apparatus

Definition and nomenclature
Pyogenic granuloma (PG) is a common acquired benign vascular tumour frequently encountered at the nail apparatus (nail bed and folds).

Synonyms and inclusions
- Nail pyogenic granuloma
- Nail lobular capillary haemangiomas

Introduction and general description
Although lobular capillary haemangiomas (PGs) may occur at many different sites (Chapter 135), they have a particular predilection for the soft tissues around the nail.

Pathophysiology
Nail PGs are due to a range of causes that act through different pathogenetic mechanisms which are not yet clearly understood.

Predisposing factors
Nail PGs are secondary to four main causes as follows:
1 Trauma: local trauma is the most common cause of PGs involving the nail apparatus, friction from footwear [1], a range of self-induced disorders (onychotillomania, onychophagia and aggressive manicure) and accidental penetration of a foreign body may also promote the development of PGs [2].
2 Drugs: the main characteristic of drug-induced nail PGs is the involvement of multiple digits, both fingers and toes. Several drugs have been implicated including retinoids (systemic and

topical) [3,4,5–8], antiretroviral therapies (indinavir, lamivudine) [4,9,10], mitozanthrones [11], ciclosporin [12] and systemic 5-fluorouracil [13]. A number of new targeted therapies have become an increasingly important cause of PG. The antineoplastic therapies which are very commonly associated with multiple PGs are epidermal growth factor receptor (EGFR) inhibitors (cetuximab, gefitinib) [4,14], agents of the fluoropyrimidine family (capecitabine) [15–17] and agents of the taxan family (docetaxel, paclitaxel) [4,18,19]. Multiple eruptive PGs have also been reported in association with anti-CD20 antibody treatment for severe rheumatoid arthritis [20].

3 Peripheral nerve injury: different conditions, all having in common injury to the peripheral nerves, have been reported to be associated with nail changes and PGs of the proximal nail fold. Plaster cast immobilisation is one such condition, where poor application technique may result in peripheral nerve damage from mechanical compression [21]. Patients will often complain of paraesthesia and pain. A few days after cast removal, the nail plate detaches proximally from the bed (onychomadesis) and is associated with periungual swelling and PG formation under the proximal nail fold. Similar nail changes have been observed in reflex sympathetic dystrophy [22]. Periungual PGs have also been reported after Guillain–Barré syndrome [23], in patients with hemiplegia [24] and after multiple episodes of hypoxia [25].

4 PGs due to inflammatory systemic diseases: periungual PGs involving multiple fingernails and toenails have been reported in cutaneous sarcoidosis, psoriasis and seronegative spondyloarthritis [4].

Pathology
Histopathology shows the characteristic features of PG, irrespective of cause and location (Chapter 135). It should be differentiated from granulation tissue.

Clinical features
History
The patient's history usually identifies the cause of the PG.

Presentation
A PG starts as a minute red papule that rapidly grows to the size of a pea or even a cherry. It bleeds easily and the surface may become eroded by necrosis of the overlying epidermis. Partial epithelialisation may occur.

Clinical variants
PGs are commonly located at the proximal nail fold (Figure 93.36) but may develop distally in the hyponychium or on the nail bed. In the latter instance, which often results from prolonged frictional trauma, the PG is associated with onycholysis.

Differential diagnosis
When a PG is single, especially if it involves the nail bed, histological examination is necessary to rule out subungual exostosis, melanoma and squamous carcinoma.

Complications and co-morbidities
In some instances, PG may promote local infection.

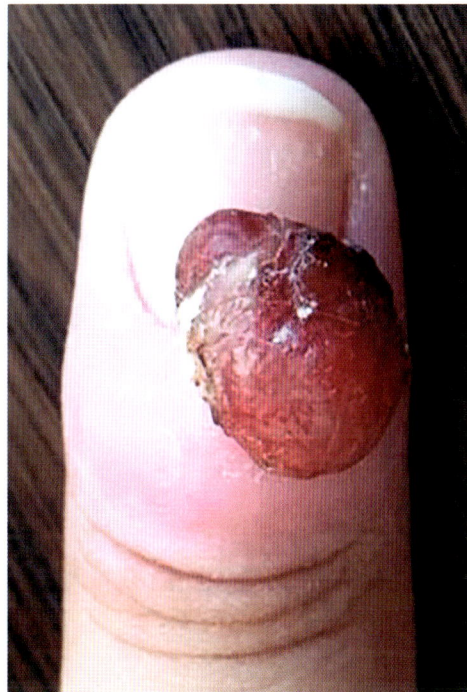

Figure 93.36 Pyogenic granuloma of the second left fingernail in a middle-aged woman – onset after improper cuticle removal.

Disease course and prognosis
If local trauma is suspected, the cause should be addressed (surgical removal of foreign body, stopping nail manipulation in onychotillomania, etc.). For drug-induced PGs, conservative treatment is recommended as they are likely to recur until the responsible drug is discontinued or replaced if necessary with a different agent. Topical beta-blockers may be of some help in nearly 2/3 of patients after one month [26]. PGs due to cast immobilisation usually heal with topical corticosteroids. PGs due to reflex sympathetic dystrophy or to systemic diseases are more difficult to treat and often need several cycles of topical therapy or surgical removal [4].

Investigations
X-rays will rule out a subungual exostosis. Histological examination should always be undertaken to rule out amelanotic melanoma or squamous cell carcinoma when faced with a single PG without a clear aetiology.

Treatment ladder

First line
- Potent corticosteroid cream (class I) under an occlusive dressing (best for drug-induced PGs) for up to 6 weeks

Second line
- Topical beta blockers (timolol)

Third line
- Curettage under local anaesthesia
- Remove cause (drug, plaster cast, etc.) if feasible

Glomus tumour

Definition and nomenclature

Glomus tumour, a benign tumour of the neuromyoarterial glomus, also known as glomus body or glomus apparatus (Chapter 135), is a common cause of severe pain under the nail [27,28].

Synonyms and inclusions
- Glomangioma

Epidemiology
Incidence and prevalence

This is an uncommon neoplasm which represents about 1–2% of all hand tumours [28].

Age

Glomus tumour occurs mainly in patients in their forties.

Sex

It affects predominantly women (up to 90% of cases) [28].

Pathophysiology

Glomus tumours arise principally in the pulp or nail bed or matrix of the distal phalanx, where the glomus bodies of Masson are numerous.

Pathology

A solid glomus tumour is composed of clusters of glomus cells surrounding capillaries. Glomus cells are uniform and round with pale eosinophilic cytoplasm, and a centrally located round nucleus. A basal lamina, highlighted by periodic acid–Schiff (PAS), surrounds each cell [29].

Presentation

Pain is the predominant symptom of a subungual glomus tumour. The pain may be pulsating, spontaneous or provoked by the slightest trauma. Variations in temperature, especially cold, may trigger pain radiating to the shoulder. Pain is sometimes described as worse at night. One case reports that even polishing the nail was unbearable [30].

Clinical variants

There are two main clinical presentations of subungual glomus tumour as follows:
- A small reddish or bluish spot (<1 cm) seen through the nail plate (Figure 93.37a).
- A longitudinal erythronychia with distal notching or overlying longitudinal fissure (Figure 93.37b).

Differential diagnosis

Differential diagnosis includes all causes of nail pain (Box 93.1). Exceptionally, glomus tumour might be totally painless.

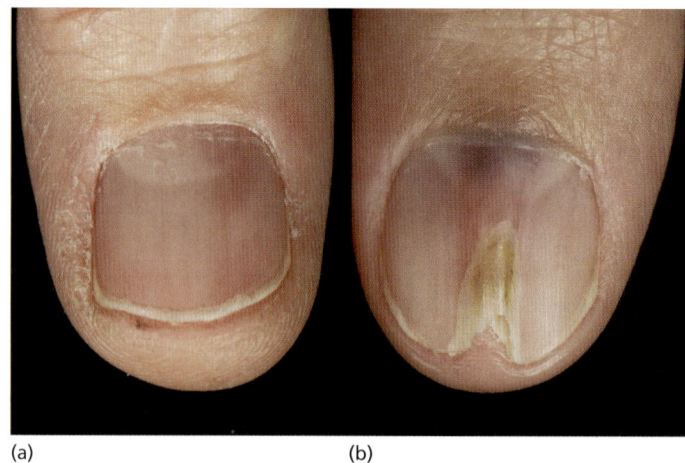

(a)   (b)

Figure 93.37 Painful glomus tumours. (a) Note the bluish hue under the nail bed and matrix. (b) A glomus tumour with longitudinal erythronychia and a distal fissure.

Box 93.1 Causes of nail pain

Tumours
- Glomus tumour
- Subungual keratoacanthoma
- Subungual exostosis
- Subungual horn
- Osteoid osteoma
- Enchondroma
- Intraosseous implantation cyst
- Metastasis

Inflammatory, infectious
- Bacterial paronychia
- Herpetic whitlow
- Osteomyelitis of terminal phalanx
- Onychomycosis

Inflammatory, non-infectious
- Ingrowing toenail
- Nail psoriasis
- Dermatomyositis

Vascular
- Frostbite
- Chilblains
- Acrosclerosis

Iatrogenic
- Taxanes
- Epidermal growth factor receptor inhibitors
- Retinoids
- Protease inhibitors

Complications and co-morbidities

Pressure of the glomus tumour on the underlying phalanx may induce bone erosion in 50% of cases [28,31].

Disease course and prognosis

Patients have been wrongly referred to psychiatrists due to misdiagnosed glomus tumour where no nail alteration was visible and no proper work-up performed.

Investigations

In most cases the clinical grounds suffice to establish the diagnosis [32]. Glomus tumour is the main indication for MRI of the nail unit [33]. It offers the highest sensitivity and best assessment of the extent of the tumour. The signal behaviour varies with the histological nature (vascular, cellular, myxoid) of the lesion [34]. MRI accurately determines the spatial location of the tumour, enabling a precise and radical surgical resection to be carried out [34,35]. Recurrent symptoms can usually be attributed to small synchronous satellite lesions [36]. New high-resolution ultrasound with colour Doppler flow imaging can obviously improve the diagnostic accuracy [37].

Management

Treatment consists of surgical removal of the tumour. Two approaches are possible: the direct approach after nail plate avulsion through the nail bed or the matrix followed by meticulous repair [38,39]; or the lateral approach on the volar aspect of the lateral nail fold. The latter gives a more restricted view of the tumour with a higher chance of incomplete excision compared with the transungual approach [40]. It should be recommended only for lesions that are proximal and deep seated [40,41].

Subungual exostosis

Definition

Subungual exostosis is an isolated slow-growing benign osteochondral outgrowth from the distal phalanx.

Most authors consider it to be a distinct clinicopathological entity [42], but some classify them with osteochondromas [43].

Epidemiology
Incidence and prevalence

Subungual exostosis is probably considerably underreported. The prevalence is unknown.

Age

Teenagers and young adults in their twenties are mostly affected [44–46].

Sex

The sex ratio varies from series to series but is most probably 1:1.

Pathophysiology

Subungual exostosis was previously thought to be a reactive process. It is now considered a true neoplasm harbouring a pathognomonic translocation t(X;6)(q22;q13-14) [47].

Predisposing factors

Trauma seems to be the most important aetiological factor [44].

Pathology

Histopathology shows a bony tumour with a hyaline cartilaginous cap [29].

Clinical features
History

The association of nail deformity and pain is highly suggestive, but pain is often not present.

Presentation

All large series ($n = 19$–45) have shown that the great toenail is affected in 75% of cases [44–46]. Subungual exostosis usually elevates the nail plate as it emerges from the hyponychium (Figure 93.38a) or from a lateral sulcus. In its early stages, the tumour may have a porcelain white hue with superficial telangiectasias and a collarette surrounding its base. As the tumour enlarges, it develops a thick hyperkeratotic surface. Onychoscopy may help in the diagnosis [48].

Clinical variants

Dorsal subungual exostoses may present as a nondescript erythematous patch seen through the nail plate, with or without onycholysis (Figure 93.38b,c).

Differential diagnosis

Differential diagnosis includes acral superficial fibromyxoma, verruca vulgaris, fibrokeratoma, PG, ingrowing toenail, squamous cell carcinoma, and amelanotic melanoma.

Complications and co-morbidities

Erosion and secondary infection of the nail bed may give rise to a subungual PG-like outgrowth [49] (Figure 93.39).

Investigations

Radiographic examination is the cornerstone in the diagnosis of subungual exostosis. Early lesions, mostly formed from cartilage, may not be visible.

Management

Treatment is resection of the outgrowth under full aseptic conditions [46].

Digital myxoid pseudocyst

Definition and nomenclature

Digital myxoid pseudocysts are the second most common benign tumours of the digits.

Synonyms and inclusions
- Digital myxoid cyst
- Digital mucoid cyst
- Ganglion cyst
- Digital synovial cyst

Epidemiology
Incidence and prevalence

The exact incidence and prevalence are not known.

PART 8: SPECIFIC CUTANEOUS STRUCTURES

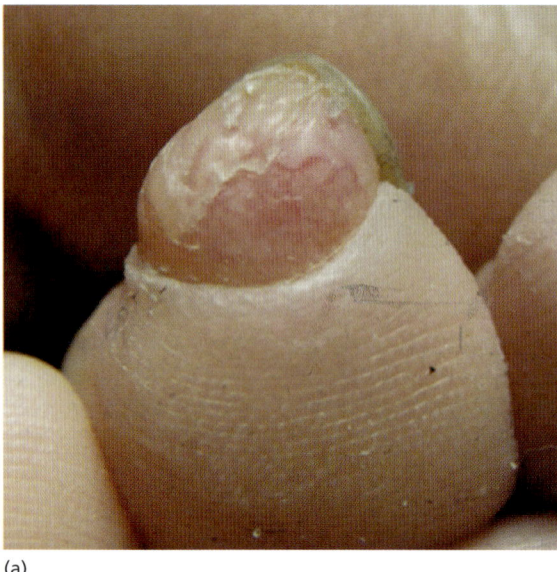 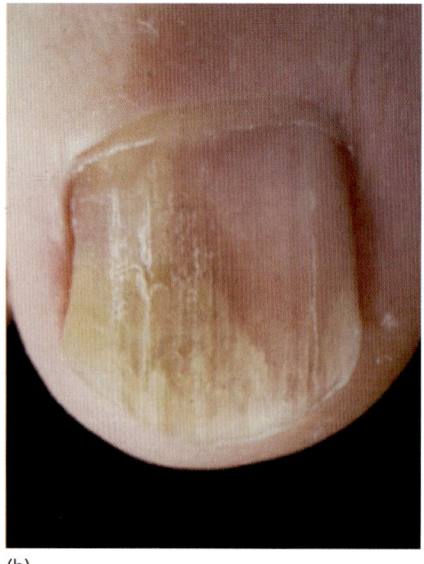 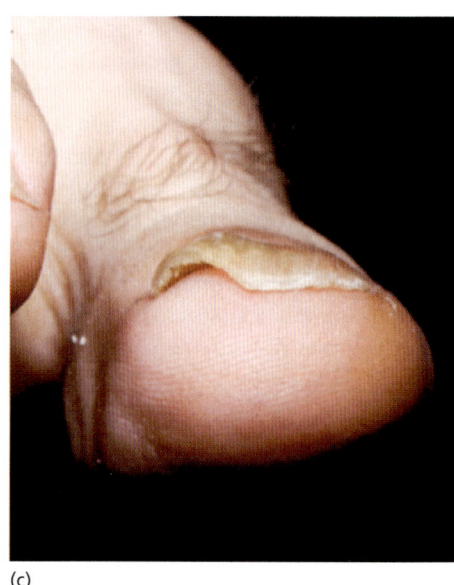

(a)   (b)   (c)

Figure 93.38 Subungual exostosis: exophytic growth of bone emerging from under the nail plate through collarette of skin (note the telangiectasias) (a); exostosis from the dorsal surface of the terminal phalanx presenting as painful onycholysis (b,c).

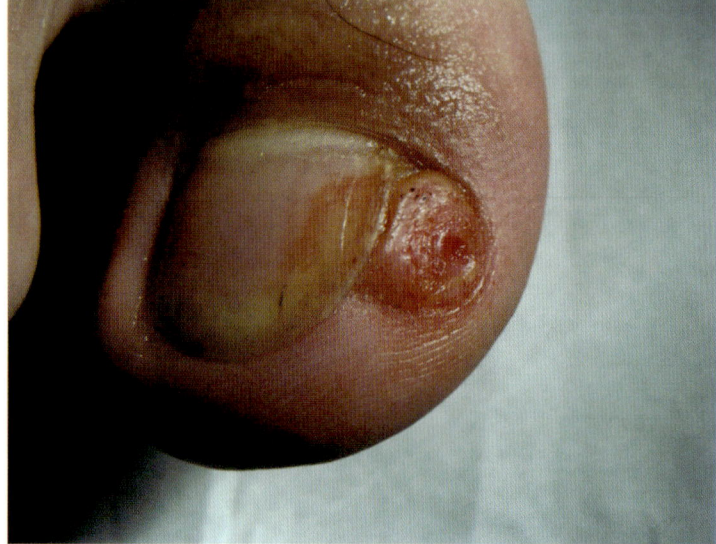

Figure 93.39 This lesion was mistaken for an ingrowing toenail. X-rays confirmed the presence of subungual exostosis.

Age
Over 50 years of age.

Sex
It is estimated that women are affected more than twice as often as men [50].

Associated diseases
Osteoarthritis.

Pathophysiology
It is now believed that digital myxoid pseudocysts result from leakage of synovial fluid through a breach in the joint capsule of the distal interphalangeal joint [51], as could be demonstrated in more than 85% of cases in a study using MRI [52].

Predisposing factors
The presence of osteophytes and reduction of the joint space from osteoarthritis or repetitive occupational trauma [53] promote leakage of joint fluid.

Pathology
Digital myxoid pseudocysts manifest as well-circumscribed but unencapsulated cyst-like dermal swellings, devoid of any lining. They consist of large mucin-filled spaces containing spindle-shaped and stellate fibroblasts without atypia [28].

Clinical features
Presentation
The clinical features depend upon their location in relation to the nail apparatus. De Berker *et al.* classified them into three subtypes [54,55] as follows:
- Type A: the most common presentation, the digital myxoid pseudocyst presents as a nodule between the distal interphalangeal joint and the proximal nail fold (Figure 93.40).
- Type B: the digital myxoid pseudocysts is in the proximal nail fold and presses on the underlying matrix resulting in a longitudinal groove in the nail plate (Figure 93.41a,b). The groove often varies in depth according to the fluctuating volume of the cyst (Figure 93.41c). A small keratotic tip protruding from under the proximal nail fold may also be observed.
- Type C: the digital myxoid pseudocyst exerts pressure from under the matrix, giving rise to a reddish or bluish lunula (Figure 93.42).

Differential diagnosis
Main differential diagnosis is fibrokeratoma in subtype B.

Disease course and prognosis
In most instances, digital myxoid pseudocysts are asymptomatic but unsightly and therefore may bother the patient. Increased pressure within the joint may be responsible for pain.

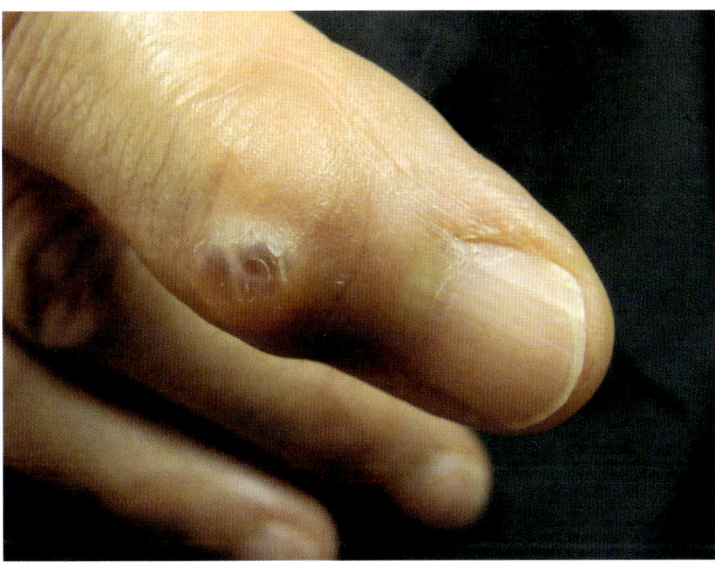

Figure 93.40 Digital myxoid pseudocyst type A.

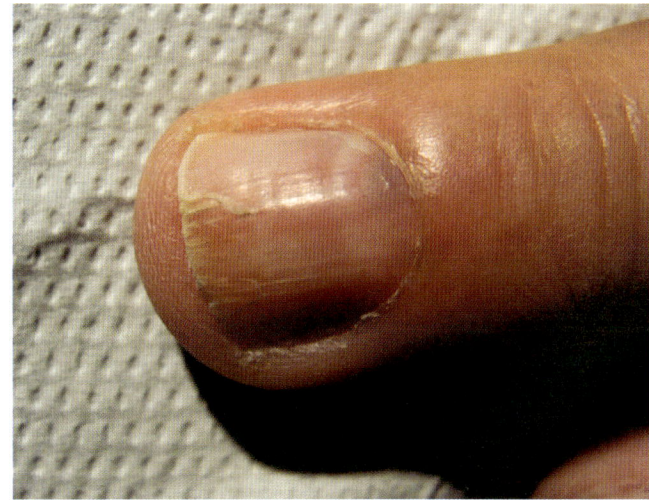

Figure 93.42 Digital myxoid pseudocyst type C. Note the red macule within the lunula.

Investigations

None are necessary except for type C, for which ultrasound or MRI may be needed. Transillumination may reveal the lesion.

Management

Numerous treatments have been recommended for this condition. Their aim is to obliterate the leakage from the joint, by inducing fibrosis around the capsule. The authors do not recommend the use of sclerosing agents as they may be responsible for local necrosis or unintentionally diffuse into the joint with subsequent limitation of mobility.

> **Treatment ladder**
>
> **First line**
> - Cryotherapy should be tempted at least twice for type A
> - Drainage followed by compression for several weeks for type B and C
>
> **Second line**
> - Methylene-blue guided surgery for ligature of the leak of joint fluid is a quick and effective technique as it provides a very highest success rate on the fingers (94%) [51]

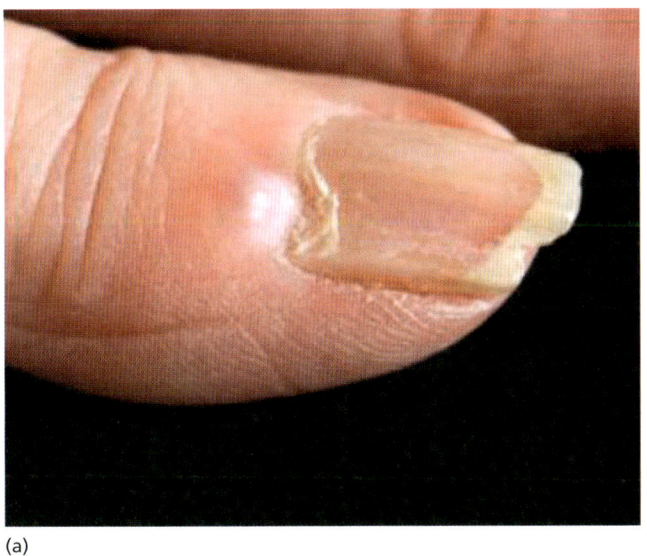
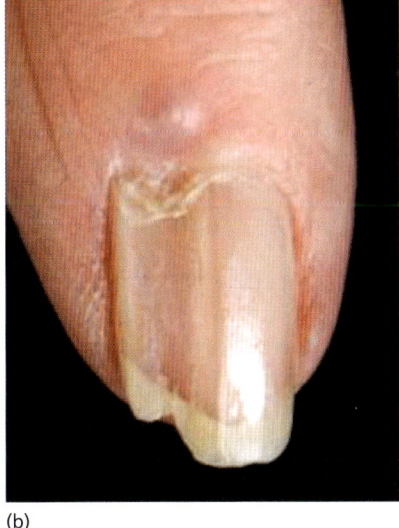
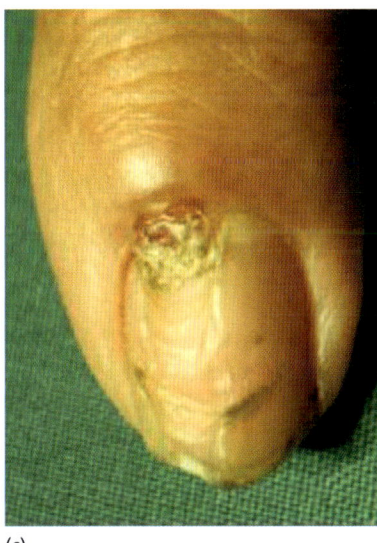

(a)   (b)   (c)

Figure 93.41 Digital myxoid pseudocyst type B. Note the longitudinal groove arising from underneath the proximal nail fold where the matrix is compressed by the overlying pseudocyst and extending to the free edge of the nail (a–c); any tumour compressing the matrix may give rise to a longitudinal gutter as shown in (a) and (b) but only a myxoid pseudocyst, which commonly fluctuates in size and therefore the pressure exerted on the matrix, may give rise to the irregular guttering as seen in (c).

PART 8: SPECIFIC CUTANEOUS STRUCTURES

Acquired ungual fibrokeratoma

Definition and nomenclature

Acquired ungual fibrokeratoma is a solitary benign asymptomatic nodule with a hyperkeratotic tip that forms in the periungual area or, rarely, within or under the nail plate.

Synonyms and inclusions
- Garlic clove fibroma
- Acquired periungual fibrokeratoma

Pathophysiology

Trauma is thought to be the major causative factor.

Pathology

Acquired ungual fibrokeratomas are pedunculated fibroepithelial lesions. The epidermis is hyperkeratotic and acanthotic, with thickened, often branching, rete ridges. The core of the lesions is composed of fibroblasts and dense collagen fibres. The vascular component is sometimes prominent [29]. No histological difference has been found between isolated acquired ungual fibrokeratomas and the Koenen tumours of tuberous sclerosis [56], although the latter has no prominent hyperkeratotic tip.

Clinical features
Presentation

Most of them emerge from under the proximal nail fold and lie in a longitudinal groove which extends to the free edge of the plate. Their size varies considerably from tiny (Figure 93.43) to prominent; they may sometimes be bifid.

Clinical variants

Rarely, an acquired ungual fibrokeratoma may originate from the matrix and grow into the nail plate (intraungual or dissecting fibrokeratoma) (Figure 93.44) to eventually emerge in the middle of the nail. Subungual fibrokeratomas arising from the nail bed are also rare.

Differential diagnosis

Fibroma, keloid, Koenen tumours, recurring digital fibrous tumour of childhood, cutaneous horn, exostosis, type C myxoid pseudocyst.

Investigations

Histology is mandatory as Bowen disease may present as a pseudofibrokeratoma [57,58]. When lesions are present on several digits, tuberous sclerosis should be ruled out. The lesions are then called Koenen tumours (Figure 93.45). They develop most commonly on the toes around puberty and their number increases with age.

Management

Surgical removal.

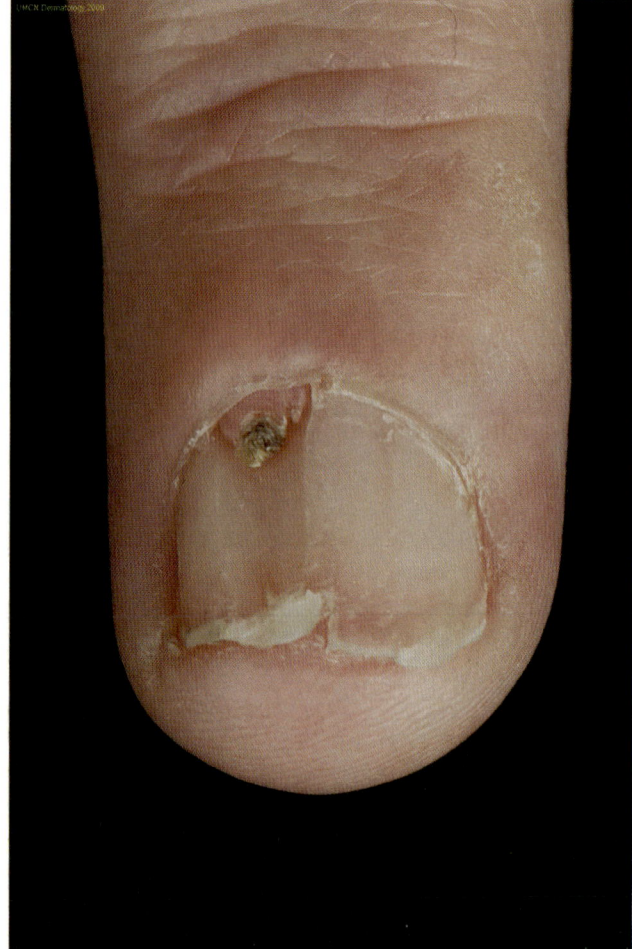

Figure 93.43 Supramatricial fibrokeratoma pressing onto the underlying matrix with subsequent longitudinal smooth groove.

Subungual keratoacanthoma

Definition

Subungual keratoacanthoma is a rare benign but rapidly growing and aggressive tumour that is usually situated in the most distal portion of the nail bed.

Epidemiology
Incidence and prevalence

Unknown.

Sex

Subungual keratoacanthoma occurs predominantly in males (75% of cases) [59].

Pathophysiology

The pathogenesis is not understood.

Predisposing factors

Trauma [59], oncogenic human papillomavirus [60] and, in one case of steel wool [61], have each been suggested as contributory factors.

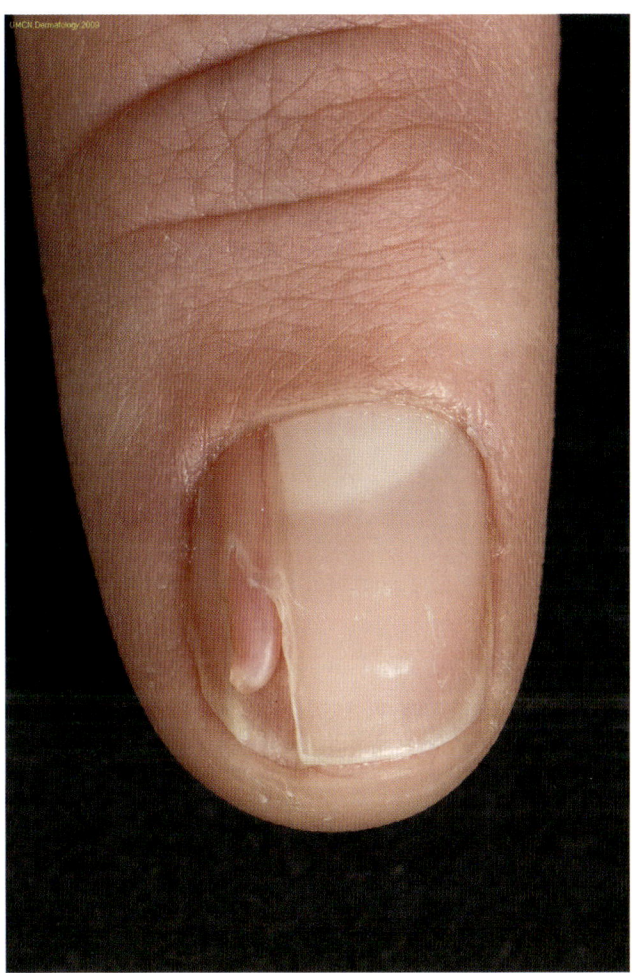

Figure 93.44 Intraungual (dissecting) fibrokeratoma. The lesion grows within the nail plate and emerges at its distal half.

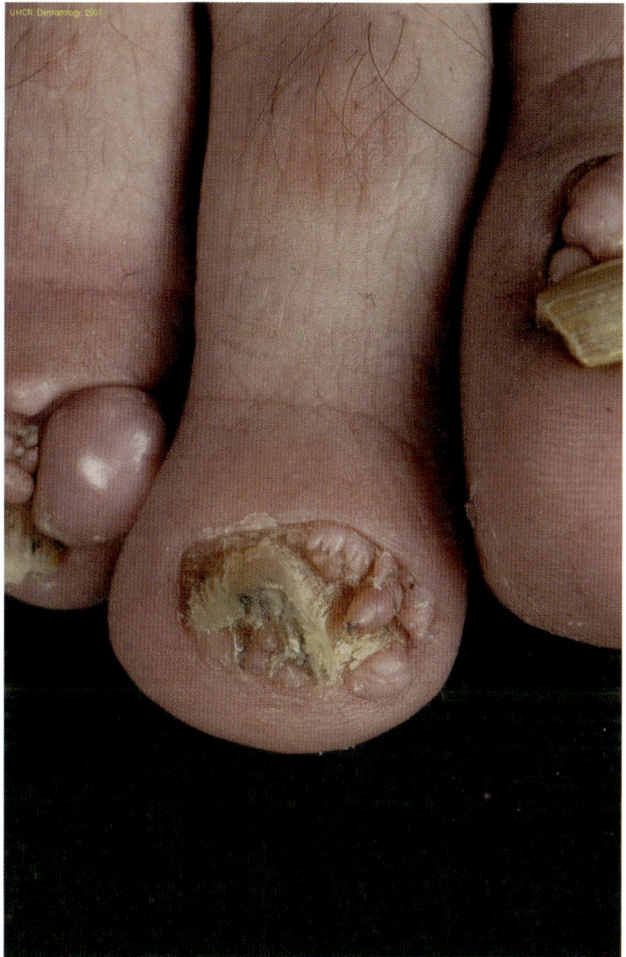

Figure 93.45 Multiple soft fibrokeratomas in tuberous sclerosis (Koenen tumours).

Genetics

In women, the development of multiple subungual keratoacanthomas may represent a late manifestation of incontinentia pigmenti. A mutation search of the *NEMO* gene should be performed.

Pathology

Microscopic examination shows a squamoproliferative lesion with a focal crateriform pattern and overlying hyperkeratosis with ortho- and parakeratosis. Lobules of squamous epithelium are often well differentiated, composed of large keratinocytes with copious 'glassy' eosinophilic cytoplasm. Dyskeratotic cells are numerous, but atypia and mitotic figures are rare. Tumour protein p53 and proliferation marker Ki-67 can help distinguish subungual keratoacanthomas from subungual squamous cell carcinomas [29].

Clinical features
History

Subungual keratoacanthomas are rapidly growing tumours (within weeks) which are always painful and are most often located on the distal part of the nail bed. They are most commonly located on the thumb but the index and middle fingers are also well-recognised sites [59].

Presentation

The tumour may start as a small and painful keratotic nodule just under the free edge of the nail, rapidly growing to 1–2 cm in diameter within 4–8 weeks. After clipping of the overlying nail plate, the typical gross appearance resembles that of keratoacanthoma at other sites as a dome-shaped nodule with a central crater plugged by keratinous material (Figure 93.46). The tumour may rapidly plunge deeper and erode the underlying bony phalanx.

Clinical variants

If located more proximally under the nail fold, subungual keratoacanthomas may present as a painful chronic paronychia [59,62].

Differential diagnosis

The three main differential diagnoses are: epidermoid implantation cyst, subungual wart and squamous cell carcinoma.

Complications and co-morbidities

Long-lasting lesions may lead to complete destruction of the distal bony phalanx.

Investigations

Standard X-rays consistently demonstrate a well-defined cup-shaped erosion of the underlying bone (Figure 93.47). The margins of the defect show no evidence of sclerosis or any sign of

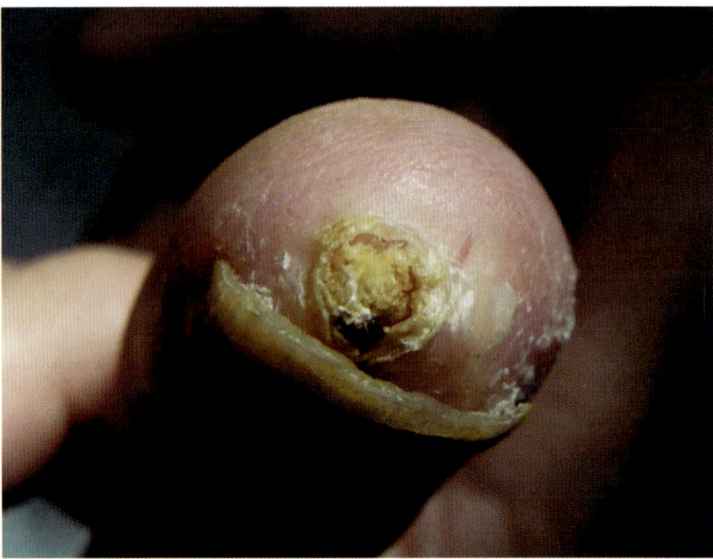

Figure 93.46 Subungual distal keratoacanthoma. Note the keratotic plug on the distal bed.

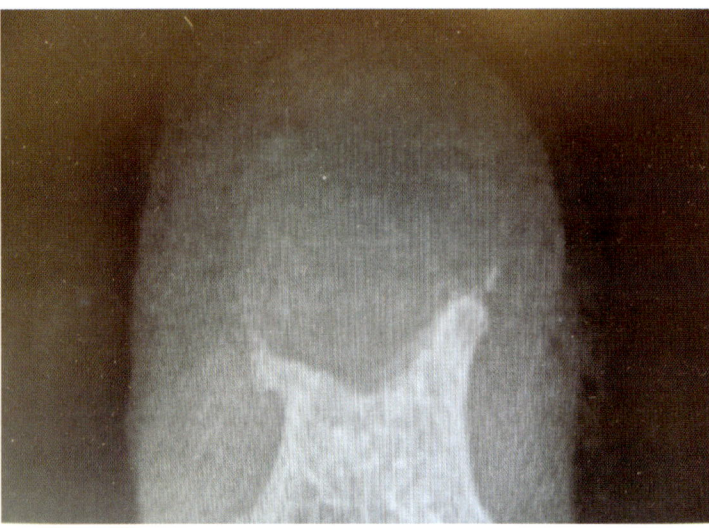

Figure 93.47 X-rays showing massive osteolysis of the distal bony phalanx associated with subungual keratoacanthoma.

periosteal reaction [63]. This lytic effect is attributed to the very rapid compression from the tumour rather than tumour invasion [64]. Long-term radiological follow-up data following subungual keratoacanthomas are sparse, but failure to reossify [64], partial repair of the bony defect [65] and spontaneous regression with full reossification [66] have all been reported.

Treatment ladder

First line
- Removal of the entire tumour with curettage of the cavity

Second line
- Amputation: only for multiple recurrences or massive bony destruction

---

Third line
- Acitretin 1 mg/kg/day may be attempted for multiple subungual keratoacanthoma associated with incontinentia pigmenti

---

Onychomatricoma

Definition and nomenclature
Onychomatricoma is a rare benign tumour of the matrix, with peculiar clinical and pathological features, first described in 1992 by Baran and Kint [67].

Synonyms and inclusions
- 'Onychoblastoma', 'unguioblastoma' and 'unguioblastic fibroma' are similar tumours of the nail matrix [68,69]

Epidemiology
Incidence and prevalence
Unknown.

Age
All published cases were adults in their 50s [70] except one in a child, in whom the diagnosis was purely clinical and without histopathological verification [71].

Ethnicity
The overwhelming majority of cases are reported in white people, and only exceptionally in non-Europeans [72].

Pathophysiology
The origin of the tumour remains obscure. It most probably stems from a disturbed differentiation of nail matrix cells. The tumour digitations are onychogenic and responsible for the thickening of the nail plate.

Pathology
Histopathology is unique. Two different zones may be observed as follows:

1 The distal zone is characterised by multiple 'glove finger' papillary projections covered by a matrix-type epithelium devoid of stratum granulosum that keratinises through an eosinophilic keratogenous zone.

2 The proximal zone is dome shaped in transverse sections and lined by a papillomatous matrix-type epithelium, with vertically oriented deep invaginations into the stroma. These invaginations surround optically empty cavities in a characteristic V-shaped configuration [28].

Clinical features
History
The condition is indolent and patients mostly seek medical advice for cosmetic purposes, when the tumour has been evolving for several years.

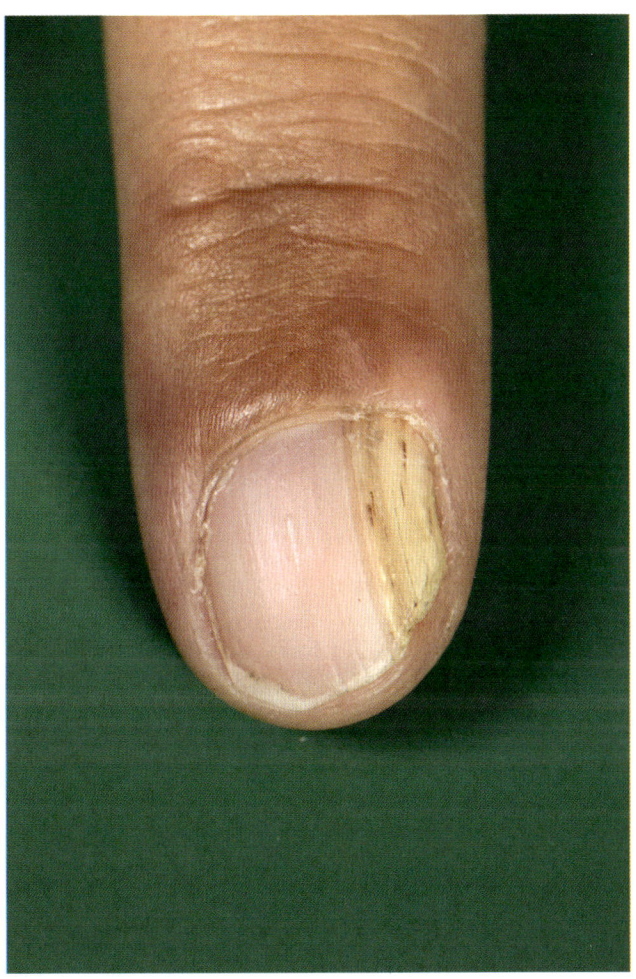

Figure 93.48 Onychomatricoma: note the very well-delimited longitudinal thickening of the plate.

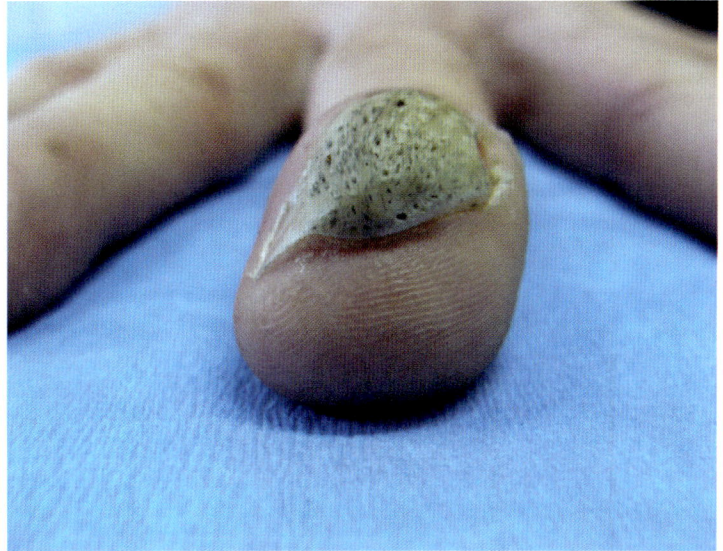

Figure 93.49 Onychomatricoma: 'woodworm' cavities in the nail plate are especially visible in this longstanding case (>40 years).

Presentation

Single fingers are most commonly affected (75%), mainly the middle finger [73]. Few reports mention involvement of the lesser toes [74] or exceptionally of several digits [75].

Several clinical signs are striking enough to either make the diagnosis or at least to arouse suspicion (Figure 93.48) as follows:

- Longitudinal xanthopachyonychia of various width, often sparing a part of normal pinkish nail.
- Transverse and longitudinal overcurvature of the affected portion of the nail.
- Longitudinal ridging, sometimes quite prominent on the surface of the nail.
- Splinter haemorrhages, mostly proximal but sometimes distal.
- Woodworm cavities at the free edge of the thickened nail plate (Figure 93.49).

Clinical variants

Some unusual clinical variants have been reported: giant form [76], association with dorsal pterygium [77,78] or associated with onychomycosis and longitudinal melanonychia [79]. Only rarely is the length of the digitations such that clipping of the free edge of the nail induces bleeding [80].

Differential diagnosis

Clinical presentation is characteristic but onychomycosis and Bowen disease [81] should be ruled out.

Disease course and prognosis

Excellent prognosis if skilled surgeons perform the surgery. Long lasting lesions may end in complete destruction of the nail plate.

Investigations

Dermoscopy confirms diagnosis in showing the woodworm perforations at the distal edge of the nail [82]. Recently, nail clipping of the diseased part of the nail has been shown to be a minimally invasive method to achieve the correct diagnosis of onychomatricoma [83]. MRI is typical and reveals a tumour emerging from the nail matrix [84]. Ultrasonography reflectance confocal microscopy and optical coherence tomography may be also helpful [85]. Nail avulsion is diagnostic as it exposes a villous tumour, reminiscent of a sea anemone, emerging from the matrix while the nail appears as a thickened funnel, storing filamentous digitations of matrix fitting into the holes of the proximal nail extremity (Figure 93.50).

Management

Surgical removal of the tumour is the only option. The tumour should only be tangentially excised from the underlying matrix [40].

Superficial acral fibromyxoma

Definition and nomenclature

Superficial acral fibromyxoma is a rare slow-growing soft-tissue tumour which has a predilection for the subungual and periungual regions of the fingers and toes in adults [86]. It is a distinct clinicopathological entity, recognised by Fetsch *et al.* in 2001 [87].

PART 8: SPECIFIC CUTANEOUS STRUCTURES

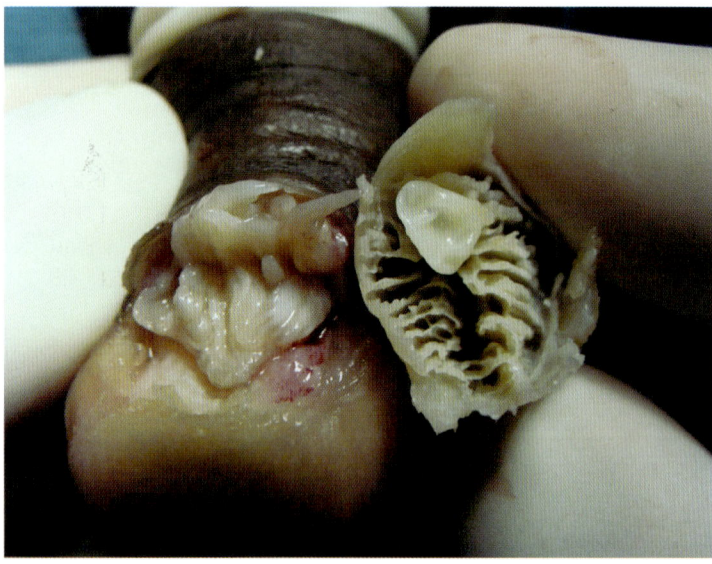

Figure 93.50 Onychomatricoma: showing the sea anemone-like matrix tumour and the cavities in the avulsed nail plate into which digitate projections from the tumour had infiltrated.

Synonyms and inclusions
- Digital fibromyxoma

Epidemiology

Incidence and prevalence
Unknown.

Age
Middle-aged adults.

Sex
Males are more commonly affected than women (male to female ratio: 1.6 : 1).

Pathology
It presents as a relatively well-circumscribed but unencapsulated dermal tumour composed of spindle-shaped cells integrated in a fibromyxoid matrix, sometimes invading the subcutis, often with accentuated vasculature and increased numbers of mast cells. Nuclear atypia is slight or absent and mitotic figures are infrequent. Immunohistochemically, more than 90% of cases are positive for CD34. CD99 and epithelial membrane antigen (EMA) are often focally positive [28,88].

Presentation
Superficial acral fibromyxoma is normally diagnosed on histology and its clinical presentation has not been well characterised. The tumour is located in the nail bed or nail folds. Some reports describe a dome-shaped, well-circumscribed, whitish to pink firm tumour, sometimes surrounded by a basal collarette, lifting up the plate (Figure 93.51) and covered with very thin fissured keratin; if located deep in the lateral nail fold, it presents as a swollen fold covered with normal skin. It may or may not be painful [89,90].

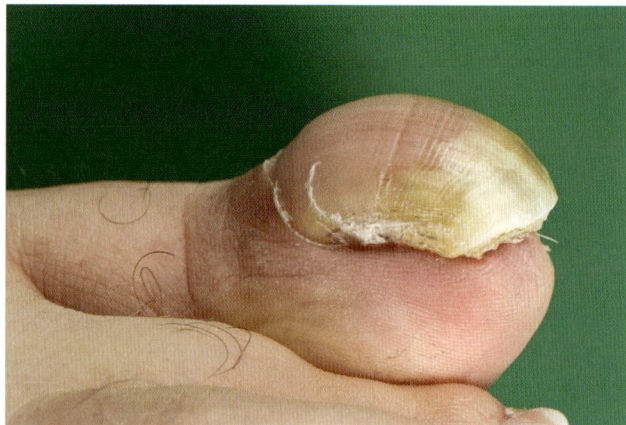

Figure 93.51 Superficial fibromyxoma of the nail bed elevating the nail plate.

Clinical variants
Exceptionally, superfical acral fibromyxoma may be located beneath the matrix [91].

Differential diagnosis
Subungual exostosis, lipoma, schwannoma and neurofibroma.

Complications and co-morbidities
Bony involvement occurs in one third of cases [91].

Disease course and prognosis
No metastases were observed in a large series of 124 cases with a mean follow-up of 35 months [92].

Investigations
Radiological imaging should be performed to rule out bony involvement.

Management
Complete surgical resection, as it has a propensity for local recurrence if incompletely excised [92].

Onychopapilloma

Definition and nomenclature
Onychopapilloma is a benign longitudinally orientated subungual tumour of unknown aetiology.

Synonyms and inclusions
- Multinucleate distal subungual keratosis [93]
- Nail-producing papilloma [94]

Epidemiology
It is usually seen in adults and rarely in adolescents, but exceptional cases have been reported in children [95].

Pathology

Onychopapilloma is characterised by: acanthosis and papillomatosis, mostly of the distal part of the nail bed; matrix metaplasia of the nail bed with an onychogenous zone; canaliform deformation of the ventral part of the nail plate; and a keratinous mass under the distal nail plate [28].

Clinical features

History

Patients seek medical advice either because of pain or because they catch the fissured free edge of the nail.

Presentation

Onychopapilloma usually presents as an isolated pink longitudinal nail streak (erythronychia) extending from the distal matrix to the free edge, from under which emerges a fine filiform subungual keratosis. It may be accompanied by distal onycholysis or a fissure [96]. Distal splinter haemorrhages are also common (Figure 93.52).

Clinical variants

Onychopapilloma may, albeit rarely, present as longitudinal melanonychia [97] or leukonychia [98].

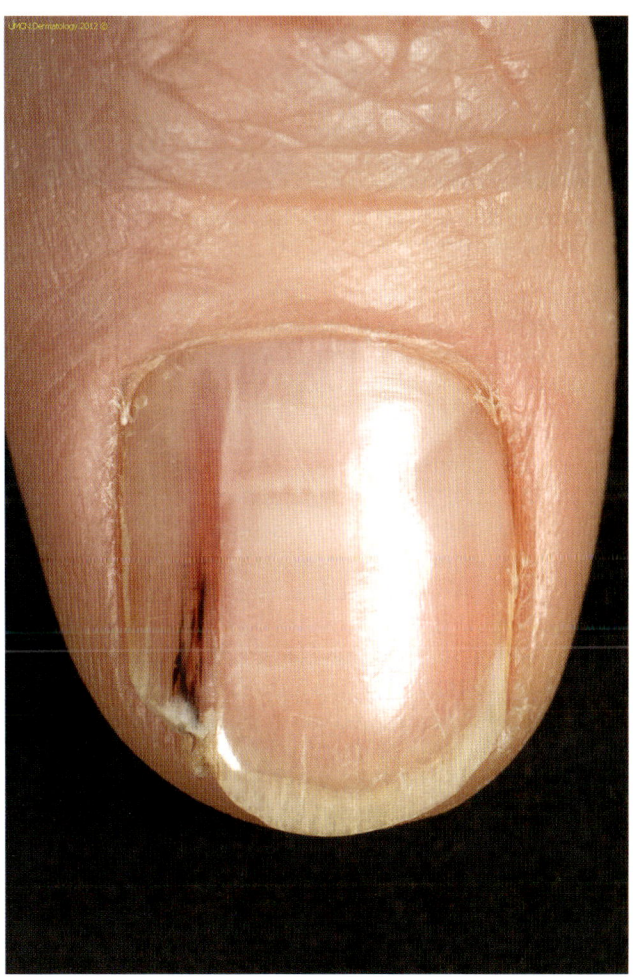

Figure 93.52 Onychopapilloma: note the longitudinal erythronychia starting in the distal matrix, the distal splinter haemorrhages and the onycholysis at its distal end.

Differential diagnosis

Bowen disease [99] and nail lichen planus [100] may present in rare instances as an onychopapilloma.

Management

The onychopapilloma is usually excised only if it bothers the patient or to rule out other tumours. Longitudinal excision with careful removal of the lesion from the inferior face of the nail plate and notching the distal matrix seems to be the most accurate surgical technique. In the pathology laboratory, longitudinal sections should be recommended. A recurrence rate of 20% is observed [95].

MALIGNANT TUMOURS

Squamous cell carcinoma

Definition

Squamous cell carcinoma is the most frequent malignant tumour of the nail apparatus, where presentation as *in situ* squamous cell carcinoma (Bowen disease) is more common than invasive squamous cell carcinoma [99].

Epidemiology

Age

The mean age at presentation is 60 years [99,101–103].

Sex

Three quarters of cases occur in males [99,102,103]. Some authors suggest that nail squamous cell carcinoma is a hidden high-risk HPV-associated reservoir and should be recognised as a sexually transmitted infection [104].

Pathophysiology

Predisposing factors

One third of patients with squamous cell carcinoma of the nail apparatus have a personal history of human papillomavirus-associated genital disease (genital warts, dysplasia or cancer of the cervix) or a similar history in a sexual partner. The average time between the onset of the genital disease and the appearance of the nail tumour is around 12 years [102]. It is estimated that genito-digital transmission of human papillomavirus is responsible for up to 60% of cases of squamous cell carcinoma of the nail apparatus (both *in situ* and invasive forms). Prolonged unprotected contact with chemical mutagens is another possible predisposing factor.

Causative organisms

Human papillomavirus, especially serotype 16, which is isolated in three quarters of cases [102], but also serotypes 2, 6, 11, 18, 26, 31, 34, 35, 56, 58 and 73 [105–108].

Environmental factors

Ionising radiation, arsenic, pesticides, paint/solvents, soluble oils, and stagnant water have been suggested as potential causative factors [109].

Pathology

The picture is identical to that of Bowen disease in other skin areas [110]. The most important feature to look for is the intact basement membrane defining the *in situ* form.

Clinical features

History

Patients are often not bothered by this indolent and painless condition and therefore tend to seek medical advice very late (mean delay 6 years) [99,111].

Presentation

The clinical presentation is protean, accounting for the delay in diagnosis. Bowen disease and invasive squamous cell carcinoma cannot be differentiated clinically. The largest published series identifies the right index and middle fingers as the most commonly affected. This finding is in agreement with the postulated genito-digital transmission of human papillomavirus [99]. The condition is usually solitary but, uncommonly, tumours may arise in more than one digit especially in immunocompromised patients [110,112–116]. The most common clinical findings are, in decreasing order of frequency, subungual hyperkeratosis (Figure 93.53), onycholysis (Figure 93.54), oozing and nail plate destruction. Oozing

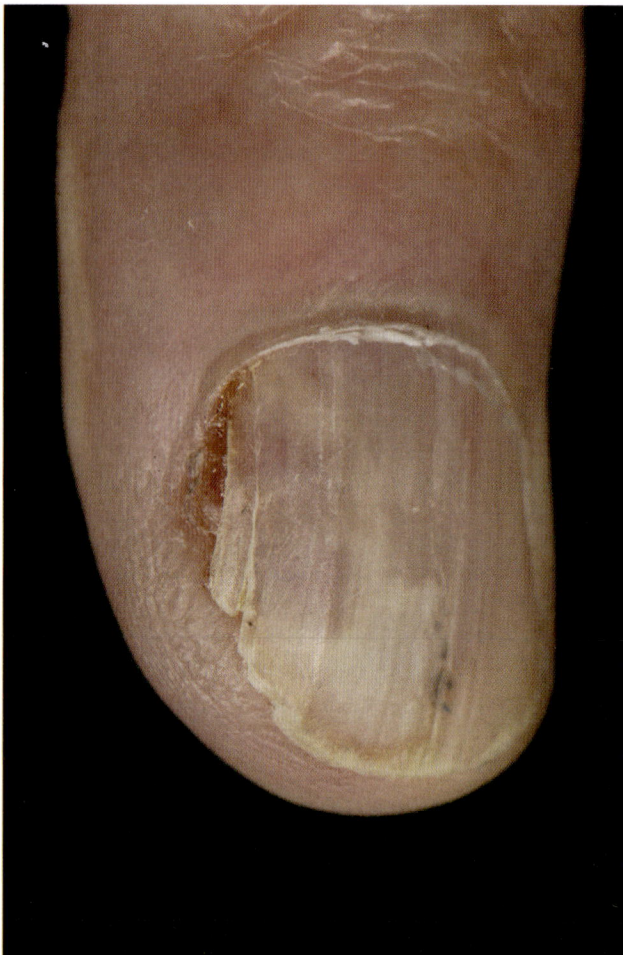

Figure 93.54 Onycholysis and oozing of the nail bed due to invasive squamous cell carcinoma secondary to Bowen disease.

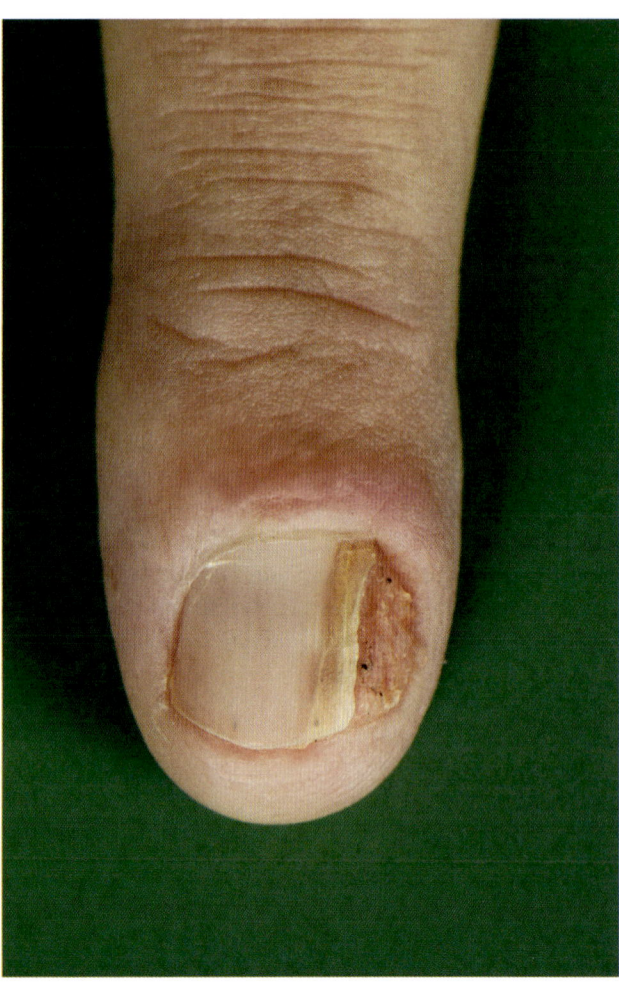

Figure 93.53 Bowen disease: warty lesion of the matrix and bed. The lesion was treated for several years as a wart.

is an important but underrecognised sign and is only occasionally reported in the literature [99,115].

Clinical variants

Squamous cell carcinoma may also present as longitudinal melanonychia [116], an onychopapilloma [95], a fibrokeratoma [56] or may simulate an onychomatricoma [81].

Verrucous carcinoma (carcinoma cuniculatum) of the nail apparatus is a rare low-grade variant of squamous cell carcinoma, characterised by a local aggressiveness but a low potential for metastasis. Very few cases have been reported in the literature [117–119]. It presents clinically as a slowly enlarging warty papillomatous plaque and, of reported cases, were most commonly located on the thumb, the hallux or the fifth toe.

Differential diagnosis

The main differential diagnosis is a wart [93].

Disease course and prognosis

Prognosis both of *in situ* and of invasive forms is excellent: metastases and deaths are extremely exceptional [103,106,111,112, 120–122].

Investigations

Radiological imaging should be performed to rule out bony involvement. It was detected in only 2% of cases in a large reported series [99] and up to 30% in another one [123] of squamous cell carcinoma of the nail unit.

Management

The goal of treatment is eradication of the tumour. However, even with sophisticated surgical techniques, recurrences are not uncommon, probably because human papillomavirus is difficult to eradicate [99]. HPV vaccination on the long term should make this condition progressively disappear.

Treatment ladder

First line
- Mohs surgery

Second line
- Conventional surgery with micrographic control of the margins on fixed tissue

Third line
- Imiquimod cream [124], 5-fluorouracil cream [125,126] with or without prior curettage, photodynamic therapy [127–131] and intra-arterial infusion with methotrexate [132]. None of these techniques allows histological control of tumour margins and they should therefore be considered as a treatment option only in special cases of histologically proven Bowen's disease

Fourth line
- Amputation is mandatory only when bone involvement occurs

Basal cell carcinoma

Definition

Basal cell carcinoma very rarely involves the nail apparatus: around 20 cases only have been reported in the literature.

Epidemiology

Age

The average age at diagnosis is 65 years.

Environmental factors

One basal cell carcinoma of the proximal nail fold was reported in a respiratory specialist using radioscopy for 30 years [133]. Another was reported in a worker dealing with azo dyes [134]. Nail polish has also been incriminated [135].

Pathology

The pathological features are identical to those observed on the skin (Chapter 139).

Clinical features

History

In the published cases, diagnosis was delayed by an average of about 10 years.

Presentation

The classical clinical features as observed on the skin are very rarely encountered, except on the periungual skin. There is no typical clinical presentation (see Differential diagnosis). Diagnosis was histological in all cases. The thumb is most frequently involved, followed by the hallux [136].

Clinical variants

Longitudinal melanonychia is a rare presentation [136,137].

Differential diagnosis

Chronic paronychia, PG, amelanotic melanoma, squamous cell carcinoma, bacterial or a mycotic infection and habit tic [138].

Investigations

Radiographic imaging to rule out bony involvement.

Management

Surgical removal.

Treatment ladder

First line
- Mohs surgery [139]

Second line
- Conventional excision

Third line
- Amputation if bone involvement

Melanoma

Definition

Melanoma (see also Chapter 142) of the nail apparatus is rare but associated with poor prognosis. Very early recognition and excision provides the best chance of survival.

Epidemiology

Incidence and prevalence

The prevalence ranges from 0.18% to 2.8% of all cutaneous melanomas [140]. The incidence has been estimated at 0.1/100 000/year [141].

Age

Average age of onset is between the sixth and seventh decade but can also be found at considerably younger ages. Melanoma of the nail apparatus is extremely exceptional in children, with only 13 reported cases to date (some being debatable) [142].

Ethnicity

The proportion of melanomas involving the nail apparatus is much higher in populations of African and East Asian ethnicity than in white people: about 25% of melanomas are located at the nail apparatus in Japanese and African Americans. However, the absolute incidence may well be similar in all racial groups [140].

Pathophysiology

Trauma is often mentioned as a potential causative factor, but no clear link can be established with certainty [143]. UV radiation is not responsible as the nail plate acts as a barrier to penetration of UV [144]; furthermore, the similar frequency of melanoma of the nail apparatus in dark- and fair-skinned peoples suggests that pigmentation is not protective [140]. New insights into the molecular pathogenesis of subungual nail melanoma reveal a high frequency of *KIT* and *NRAS* mutations in subungual melanoma, but a low incidence of *BRAF* mutations [145].

Pathology

Most cases are acral lentiginous melanoma. In melanoma of the nail apparatus, the histological subtype, the Clark's level, and the Breslow thickness are difficult to assess because of the peculiar nail anatomy [28]. Immunochemistry is particularly helpful for the diagnosis of early disease and for the determination of excision margins: HMB-45 is more sensitive than Mart-1 for detecting intraepithelial melanocytes and the latter is in turn more sensitive than S-100 protein. In invasive melanoma of the nail apparatus, however, S-100 protein is the most sensitive and was the only positive marker in cases of desmoplastic melanoma and in areas with chondroid differentiation [146].

Clinical features
History

Diagnosis is very often delayed and associated with poor prognosis. Patients do not suspect cancer at that site and by the time they consult the melanoma is already advanced with a thick Breslow thickness [147]. It has been shown that only one third of patients with longitudinal melanonychia seek medical advice [140].

Presentation

In three quarters of cases, melanoma of the nail apparatus starts in the matrix and presents as longitudinal melanonychia [148] (Figure 93.55). In the remainder, it arises from the nail bed and presents as a pigmented or amelanotic nodule, ulceration with bleeding, nail fold pigmentation, unexplained paronychia and/or partial destruction of the nail plate [149] (Figure 93.56).

Clinical variants

As many as 20–30% of melanomas of the nail apparatus are amelanotic [140]. Melanoma of the nail apparatus is even more treacherous when it manifests as isolated onychorrhexis [150] or as a fissure in the nail [151].

Hutchinson sign describes the presence of pigment on the proximal, lateral or distal nail fold. It represents the radial growth phase of subungual melanoma. Although this sign is highly suggestive of melanoma it is not pathognomonic.

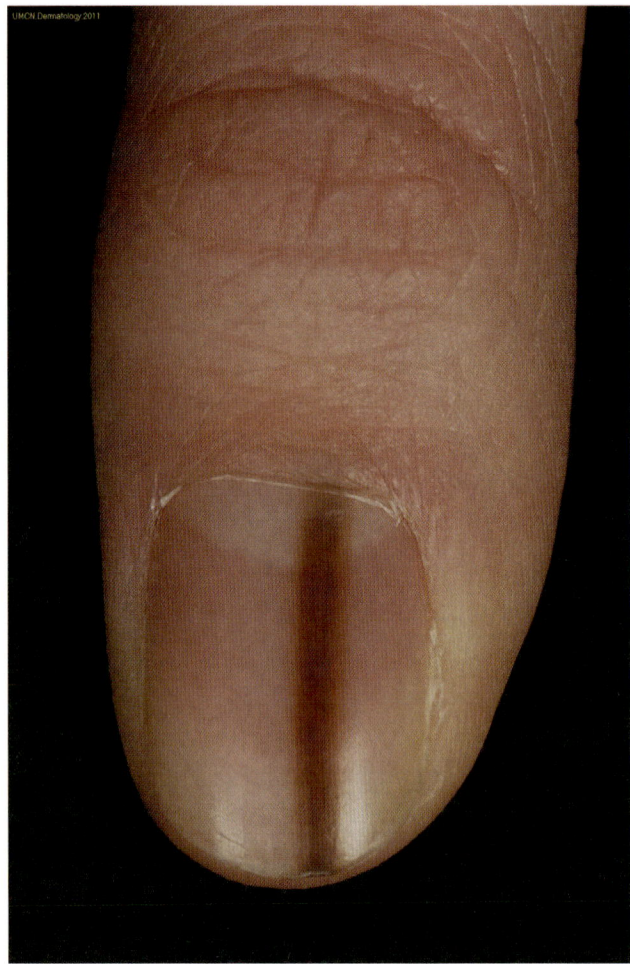

Figure 93.55 Narrow longitudinal melanonychia on a thumb. Dermoscopy showed loss of parallelism and the lesion was removed.

Differential diagnosis

All causes of longitudinal melanonychia and tumours of the nail bed (squamous cell carcinoma, PG, etc.).

Complications and co-morbidities

Metastasis.

Disease course and prognosis

Survival rate for *in situ* melanoma is reported as 100%. The 5-year survival rate was 88% for a Breslow thickness of less than 2.5 mm but only 40% for a thickness greater than 2.5 mm [152].

Investigations

The dermoscopic pattern is well established (brown background with brown to black lines which are unevenly pigmented, irregularly spaced, of variable thickness and with or without interruption of parallelism) but dermoscopy is not reliable enough to differentiate benign causes of melanonychia from melanoma [153–155]. A band occupying more than 40% of the width of the plate should be considered as suspicious [156]. Adult dermoscopic criteria should never be applied to children: a triangular sign as well as the presence of dots/globules, Hutchinson sign and an irregular pattern are very commonly found in benign pigmented nail lesions in children [157].

achieve deep excision margins, without amputation or removal of a layer of bone [165]. Many publications report that treatment of *in situ* melanoma of the nail apparatus by *en bloc* removal of the nail unit with 5–10 mm margins followed by a full-thickness skin graft results in excellent survival rates with optimal cosmetic and functional results [166–172]. Several meta-analysis confirmed that conservative surgery should be the treatment of choice for *in situ* or minimally invasive nail melanoma [173,174].

For thicker nail melanoma, as there is no evidence that aggressive amputation is associated with higher survival rates, amputation should be aimed at retaining the greatest function possible [163].

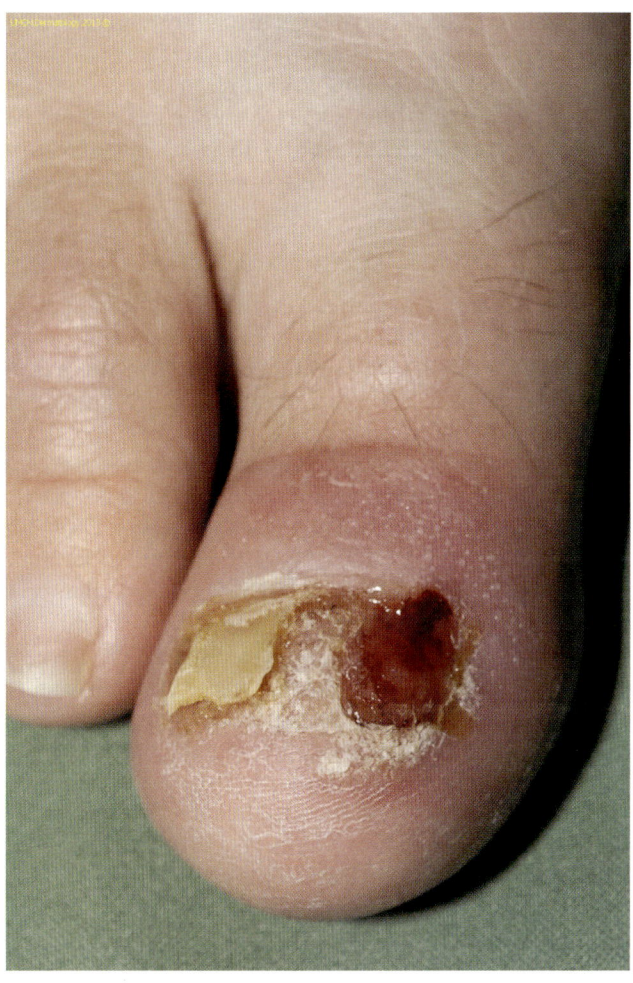

Figure 93.56 Friable granulation tissue under the plate of the great toenail. Pyogenic granuloma was suspected but histology revealed an amelanotic melanoma.

Some authors have performed matrix dermoscopy after nail avulsion and identified four dermoscopic patterns that showed high sensitivity and specificity [158]. The recent development of intraoperative reflection confocal microscopy examination of the nail matrix has enabled one-step surgical management [159].

Incisional biopsy is not recommended, as it does not allow complete histological examination of the pigmented lesion. Several excisional biopsy techniques are available [160,161]. Sentinel lymph node biopsy for melanomas of the nail apparatus greater than 1 mm in thickness is probably warranted but firm evidence of its benefit on survival is also lacking in this situation.

Management

Studies have demonstrated that amputation confers no survival advantage as long as the tumour is fully excised [140,162]. Only one study compared local excision with amputation in patients with melanoma of the nail apparatus. In this study of 62 patients with melanoma of the nail apparatus of mean thickness 1.68 mm, no significant differences in recurrence or survival rates were detected. Overall disease-free survival at 5 years was 92% [163].

Excision margins for melanoma of the nail apparatus remain controversial. Surgery poses a challenge because of the lack of surrounding soft tissue [164]. As the matrix is fixed to bone, it is difficult to

> ### Treatment ladder
>
> #### First line
> - *In situ* melanoma of the nail apparatus: en bloc removal of the nail unit with 5–10 mm margins
> - Invasive melanoma of the nail apparatus: amputation guided by a balance between tumour thickness and conservation of function

PERIONYCHIAL DISORDERS

Acute paronychia

Synonyms and inclusions
- Cellulitis of the finger/toe
- Perionychia

Classification links
- ICD-10: L03.0
- ICD-11: EE12.0

Introduction
This is one of the most common hand infections and it is characterised by acute inflammation, swelling and pain affecting the proximal and lateral nail folds. Abscesses can also occur.

Epidemiology
Fingernails are more commonly affected than toenails. The index finger and the thumb are those most commonly affected. These infections are three times more common in females than in males.

Pathophysiology
A minor trauma (mechanical or chemical) usually breaks down the cuticle, the physical barrier between the nail plate and the nail folds. This results in loss of the natural barrier against infectious organisms, allergens or irritants. Once infiltrated, infectious organisms cause an inflammatory reaction that impairs normal nail fold keratinisation and formation of a new cuticle, perpetuating the

cycle. In general, all traumatic work or activities can predispose to paronychia.

Staphylococcal infection, herpes and orf viruses, *Treponema pallidum* and some fungi can cause acute paronychia [1]. Some dermatological diseases like irritant and contact dermatitis, bullous disorders, psoriasis and pustular psoriasis, and systemic diseases like diabetes and immune/haematological abnormalities can predispose to paronychia.

In neutropenic patients with haematological or solid-organ malignancy, the most common causes of paronychia with cellulitis of the toe are *Fusarium* and, less frequently, *Aspergillus*. Moulds are, however, frequently responsible for acute paronychia with purulent discharge.

Artificial nails and gel polish have recently been identified as possible vehicles of bacteria due to their ability to harbour microorganisms inaccessible to routine hand hygiene practices and, for this reason, have to be included in the list of conditions predisposing to paronychia.

Acute paronychia also occurs frequently as an episode during the course of chronic paronychia, when other organisms may be involved including streptococci, *Pseudomonas aeruginosa*, coliform organisms and *Proteus vulgaris*. Bacterial paronychia may also present as a subacute infection [2].

Clinical features

Acute paronychia presents as a painful red swelling of the paronychial area (Figure 93.57). If the infection spreads to the nail bed, it may generate enough pressure to uplift the nail plate and damage the nail matrix: Beau lines and onychomadesis (nail shedding) may occur as a consequence. If left untreated, an infection of the paronychium may spread to the fingertip (felon), but also to the underlying bone (osteomyelitis). The degree of host immune competence is responsible for the severity of clinical manifestations.

Investigations

In many nail unit infections, the clinical presentation is non-specific and for this reason diagnostic tests are always advisable to guide treatment. Treatment should be targeted in order to avoid drug-resistance. Bacterial culture for pathogens is the standard test but consider checking for the presence of herpes simplex

virus. A Tzanck smear test or PCR usually give a fast response because non-bacterial and bacterial paronychia can be distinguished. Consider performing imaging or biopsy to exclude osteomyelitis or another underlying disorder in bacterial paronychia non-responding to treatment or with a high rate of recurrences. As trauma and terminal phalanx fractures can mimic acute paronychia, radiography is advised when the latter occurs after trauma [1].

Management

The key to successful management is early identification of the aetiology and initiation of the most appropriate treatment.

In the presence of a bacterial paronychia, if an abscess is present and it is superficial, it can easily be drained by incision with a pointed scalpel without anaesthesia. Sometimes a bullous pyoderma brings to light a narrow sinus. This may be a part of a 'collar-stud' abscess that may communicate with a deeper necrotic inoculation zone. This must be laid open and excised. Deeper lesions should be treated with penicillinase-resistant antibiotics initially. If there is no clear sign of response within 2 days, surgical intervention under local anaesthesia is required, particularly in children. The removal of the proximal third of the nail plate, cut transversally with nail-splitting scissors without initial incisional drainage, is advisable: this gives more rapid relief and more sustained drainage. In associated subungual infection, probing will determine the most painful area and provide an indication of where the nail plate should be cut away. Soaking the finger twice a day in an antiseptic solution such as chlorhexidine or 2–4% thymol in chloroform results in rapid healing. A topical combination of fusidic acid and betamethasone 17 valerate might be required. Systemic antibiotics are only for severe cases not responding to topical therapy, in the presence of osteomyelitis, or in frequent recurrences, as well as in populations at risk (diabetes, immunosuppression, peripheral vascular impairment, a prosthetic heart valve), but always according to sensitivities. A broad-spectrum antibiotic treatment such as amoxicillin/clavulanate or clindamycin is advisable when the antibiogram is not feasible [1,3].

Herpetic paronychia

Synonyms and inclusions
- Herpetic whitlow

Classification links
- ICD-10: L99.8
- ICD-11: 1F00.0Y

Introduction

This is an uncommon condition due to both herpes simplex virus, type 1 and type 2, which may cause nail unit infections if the virus is able to enter a disrupted epidermis in the nail region.

Epidemiology

Women and children are more frequently affected than adult men. Medical and dental personnel are particularly at risk. Fingernails,

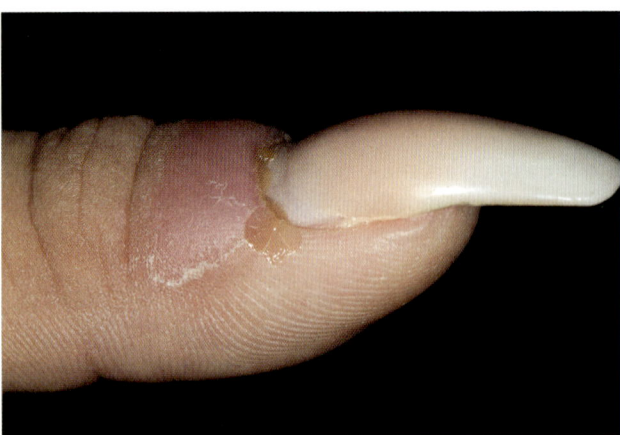
Figure 93.57 Acute bacterial paronychia of the finger.

especially the index finger, are more frequently affected than toenails.

Pathophysiology

It is due to primary inoculation of the virus from autogenous inoculation from another affected area (mouth/nose/genital area), exogenous inoculation from contact with a person actively shedding the virus, or due to virus that remained viable on surfaces.

Clinical features

Herpes simplex virus may affect the periungual skin of the terminal phalanx with the typical vesicles, but alternatively it may cause an acute and extremely painful paronychia often confused with bacterial paronychia [1]. After a prodromal period (up to 20 days, but <6 hours in recurrent infections) of local tenderness, erythema and swelling, clusters of small and tense vesicles appear around the perionychium. Clear at first, the blisters soon become purulent and may rupture and be replaced by crusts (Figure 93.58). The infection is usually very painful and takes about 3 weeks to resolve, with pain for half that time. More rarely the vesicles develop within the nail bed producing onycholysis. Lymphangitis sometimes occurs and may precede vesiculation.

Investigations

Diagnosis may be established by recovering the virus from a recent blister and by cytological examination of the blister floor (Tzanck

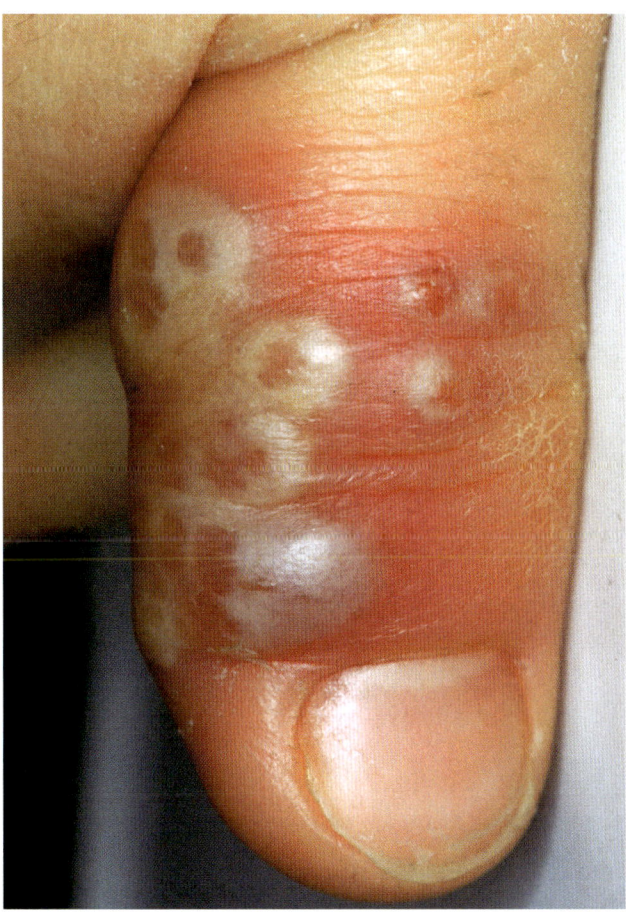

Figure 93.58 Herpetic paronychia. Courtesy of R. Baran, Cannes.

smear) [4]. This test is fast and cheap but cannot distinguish between type 1 and type 2, and herpes zoster virus. Differentiation is possible with PCR, culture and serologic testing. Among these three, culture is the gold standard, but PCR is faster and more sensitive. Serum analysis for herpes simplex virus antibodies is helpful to differentiate between type 1 or 2 and also helpful when the vesicles are localised to inaccessible areas such as the nail bed [4].

Management

Treatment probably does little to shorten the course of the disorder, but treatment with thymidine analogues, such as oral aciclovir, famciclovir and valaciclovir, may be useful if recurrences are frequent. Although widely used, topical aciclovir and topical famciclovir provide no relevant benefit in reducing the duration of symptoms. Moreover, the topical application will not reach the site of reactivation and does not influence the host immune response [1]. Numbness of the finger has been reported following infection, as well as persistent lymphoedema. Herpetic paronychia may cause complete destruction of the nail, bacterial superinfection and systemic spread that may cause meningitis.

Orf paronychia

Synonyms and inclusions
- Ecthyma contagiosum

Classification links
- ICD-10: B08.0
- ICD-11: 1E75

Introduction

Orf is a highly contagious zoonotic parapoxvirus infection that has been reported in subjects who have had a history of direct or indirect contact with sheep and goats. It is not uncommon among sheep farmers, shearers, slaughterhouse workers, butchers, vets and those who bottle-feed lambs.

Pathophysiology

Human lesions are caused by direct inoculation of infected material.

Clinical features

After a maculo-papular stage (early stage), the lesion acquires a reddish centre with an outer halo (target stage). In the acute phase it starts to weep and then it becomes dry (regenerative stage), crusty and then undergoes spontaneous resolution, with little or no residual scarring.

Investigations

Orf mainly is a clinical diagnosis, based on history of contact with animals. Biopsy is rarely indicated: keratinocytes that are infected with the virus have eosinophilic cytoplastic inclusion and irregularly shaped nuclei.

Management

The benign course justifies conservative management awaiting spontaneous resolution. Other approaches such as imiquimod, cidofovir, excision, cryotherapy and electrocautery have, however, been reported to be successful [5].

Syphilis on the finger

Classification links
- ICD-10: A51.2
- ICD-11: 1A61.2; 1A61.3; 1A62.22

Introduction

Syphilis on the perionychium may be due to occupational infection or sexual contact with the spirochete *Treponema pallidum*. Clinical pictures of the three stages are usually unspecific and additional diagnostic procedures are mandatory to make the diagnosis.

Epidemiology

The finger accounts for 5–14% of extragenital primary syphilitic chancres.

Pathophysiology

T. pallidum survives briefly outside of the body: this means that the transmission requires direct contact with the infectious lesion. *T. pallidum* rapidly penetrates intact mucous membranes or microscopic abrasions and, within a few hours, enters the lymphatics and blood to produce systemic infection. The clinical picture of primary syphilis is evident in 3 weeks at the site of inoculation. Even without treatment the primary lesion heals.

Secondary syphilis develops around 4–10 weeks later. Widespread mucocutaneous lesions are typical and involve the palms, the soles and oral mucosae. If left untreated, the infection evolves into latent and then tertiary stage.

Clinical features

Primary syphilis (chancre) may present as a deep horseshoe-shaped whitlow with diffuse induration of paronychial tissues and associated regional lymphadenopathy. Pain and tenderness of the fingertips with swelling and serous discharge may also be observed. Chancre in this region has usually a chronic course.

Secondary and tertiary syphilis may also involve the nail unit with secondary syphilis involving the nail matrix with various degrees of inflammation and nail plate dystrophies (fragility, splitting, lunular elkonyxis, Beau lines, onychomadesis, pigmentation, wedge thickness of the free edge) and tertiary syphilis involving the entire nail apparatus with granulomatous reaction, tissue necrosis and permanent nail loss [6].

Investigations

As stated, clinical pictures are not specific. Serological tests can be helpful. Biopsy typically reveals a plasma-cells infiltrate and endarteritis. Mononuclear leukocytic infiltrate, macrophages and lymphocytes are also typical. A more granulomatous reaction with palisaded macrophages is more typical of the tertiary stage. PCR is the gold standard of detection for all stages. The immune reaction is particularly high during the secondary stage.

Management

Penicillin is the drug of choice to treat syphilis. Doxycycline is the best alternative.

Chronic paronychia

Classification links
- ICD-11: EE13.2

Introduction

Chronic paronychia is an inflammatory dermatosis of the nail folds which causes retraction of the periungual tissues and loss of cuticle, with resultant secondary effects on the nail matrix, nail growth and soft-tissue attachments (Figure 93.59).

Epidemiology

Chronic paronychia is predominantly a disease of domestic and catering workers, bar staff and fishmongers. Handling of wet foods represents a particular hazard, as these often combine several

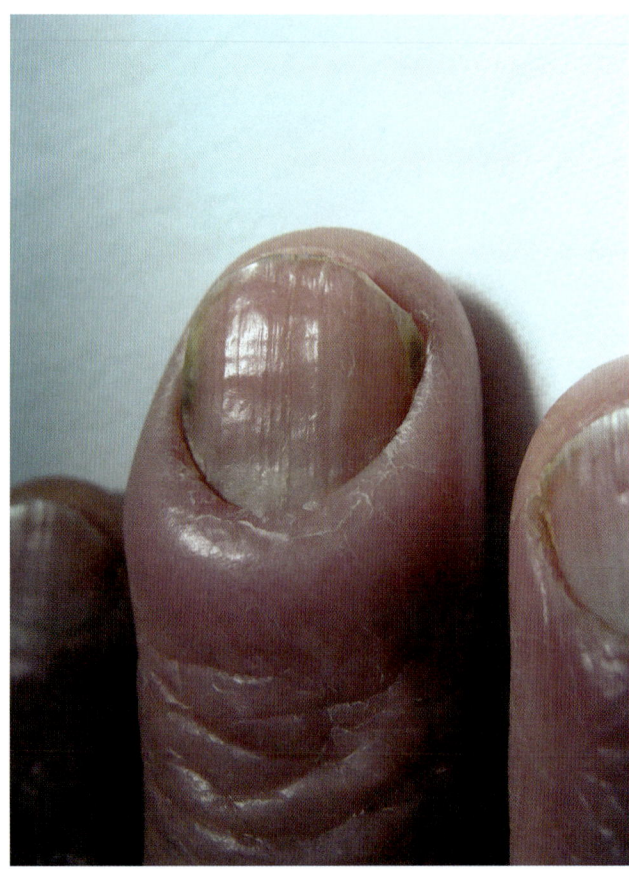

Figure 93.59 Chronic paronychia: paronychial swelling, loss of cuticle and dystrophic nail.

predisposing factors including wet working conditions, a cold environment and irritation from the food itself. The condition most frequently involves females. Any finger may be involved, but the first three fingers of the dominant hand are the most severely affected.

Pathophysiology

It can be the consequence of an acute paronychia, but depending on the major aetiological factor, chronic paronychia is generally classified into the following types: irritative reaction, contact allergy, food hypersensitivity, *Candida* hypersensitivity, true *Candida* paronychia. It is frequently seen with atopic eczema or psoriasis, where minor provocation can result in active disease [7].

Clinical features

The condition begins as a slight erythematous swelling of the paronychial tissues. It may be painless but, if tender, is much less so than in acute paronychia, except when pressed. The cuticle is lost. Inflammation adjacent to the nail matrix disturbs nail growth, resulting in irregular transverse ridges and other surface irregularities (Beau lines) which may be combined with discoloration. Concomitant darkening of the lateral edges of the nail plate may be due to the pigment of *Candida* spp. or *Neoscytalidium dimidiatum*, though it is sometimes associated with green staining of *Pseudomonas aeruginosa*. *Candida* paronychia can be observed in children who have oral candidiasis or a habit of thumb sucking.

In longstanding cases, the size of the nail may be reduced, and this reduction is exaggerated by the bolstering of the fold all around the nail. Most of the nail deformity is due to inflammation, which interferes with the formation of the nail, but a true *Candida* infection of the nail plate is occasionally seen, especially in patients with immunodeficiency.

Much of the chronic inflammation seen in this disorder probably arises from an irritant reaction to material sequestered beneath the proximal nail fold. The loss of the cuticle means that detergent and other solvents may gain access to this tight space, inducing or maintaining an inflammatory reaction. Acute exacerbations occur from time to time and are due to secondary bacterial infection (*Staphylococcus aureus* or *Staph. epidermidis*, *Proteus vulgaris*, *Escherichia coli*).

Investigations

Patch tests and food provocative tests can be performed when contact allergy needs to be excluded. Fungal/bacterial cultures are also other investigative options.

Management

Treatment mimics that of chronic hand eczema and is a combination of avoidance of precipitants, proper hand care and medication. Perhaps the most important part of the treatment, but the one most difficult to achieve, is keeping the hands dry. Patients involved in wet work should be advised to wear cotton gloves under rubber or plastic gloves and avoid manicure of the proximal nail fold. General hand care with emollients and protection from trauma and irritants is helpful. If these precautions are not followed, the condition is unlikely to settle whatever medical treatment is given.

A potent topical steroid may be used for short periods. Injections with triamcinolone acetonide in the nail fold (2.5–10 mg/mL

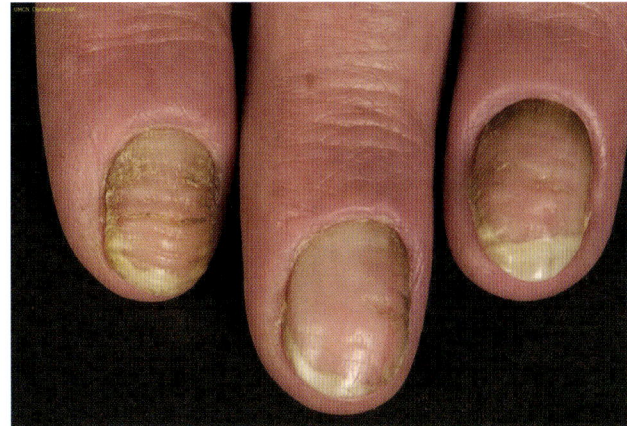

Figure 93.60 Chronic paronychia with a *Candida* superinfection causing brown discoloration.

monthly) are very useful. Topical imidazoles are usually sufficient to treat *Candida* and may provide modest activity against some bacteria. Systemic antifungals are useless because *Candida*, although often present (Figure 93.60), is not a primary pathogen [8]. Twice a day application of sodium hypochlorite solution is very effective against *Pseudomonas* superinfection. Chronic paronychia not responding to medical therapy should be treated surgically.

OTHER DISORDERS OF THE PERIONYCHIUM

Drug-induced paronychia

Paronychia may be caused by certain drugs such as retinoids, methotrexate, antiretrovirals and targeted therapies and can involve multiple digits [9–11]. Several nails are usually involved within 1 or 2 months after the drug intake. Loss of the nail plate can be associated. The pathogenesis is still unclear, but probably a toxic effect of the drug on nail epithelia or a pyogenic infection may be responsible for the clinical presentation. Paronychia resolves with drug interruption and is frequently followed by onychomadesis. Rechallenge is often positive.

It seems that paronychia due to anticancer treatments can be prevented with the application of topical beta blockers, both in adults and paediatric patients.

Hangnails

Hangnails are small portions of the horny epidermis that have split away from the lateral nail fold. They are often triangular in shape, with a hard pointed distal end and an adherent base (Figure 93.61). Hangnails are common in people who handle irritants or who work primarily with their hands. Inflammation is usually present causing pain, particularly if the hangnails are interfered with (onychotillomania). Attempts to remove them may be complicated by acute or chronic paronychia. In addition to classical hangnails, scaling of the nail folds with scattered small haemorrhages and focal erosions or

PART 8: SPECIFIC CUTANEOUS STRUCTURES

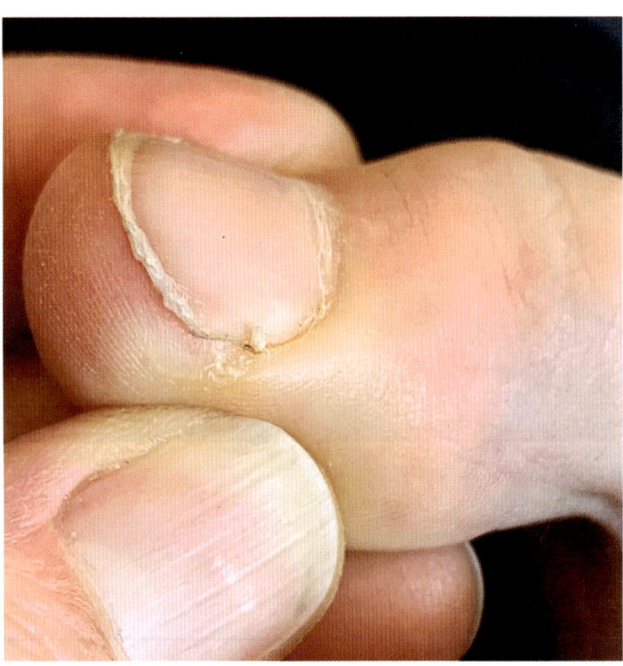

Figure 93.61 Hangnail.

necrosis may be observed, typically involving the toes. Hangnails should be snipped off using sharp-pointed scissors. Mupirocin or fusidic acid ointment may prevent or clear low-grade infection.

Painful dorsolateral fissures of the fingertip

This condition is not uncommon and occurs particularly in manual workers involved in wet work or in contact with irritants or solvents; it is also seen in patients receiving chemotherapy or targeted therapies where the fissures, often painful, are associated with xerosis and become infected [12]. Interestingly, the fissures are distal to and in line with the lateral nail groove (Figure 93.62). The discomfort experienced by the subjects may render many

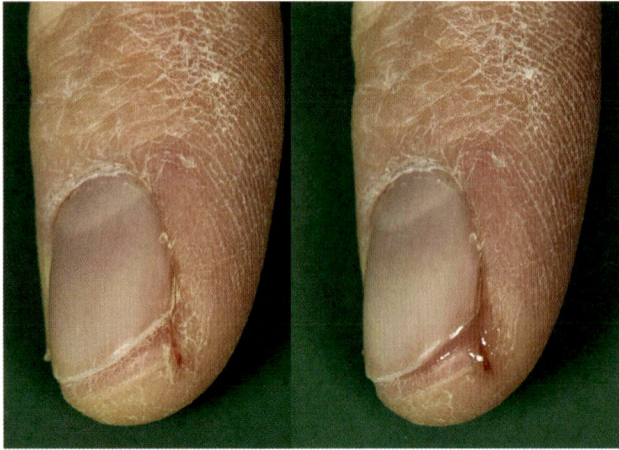

Figure 93.62 Painful dorsolateral fissure of the fingertip. At the right side: the same fissure after application of cyanoacrylate glue.

subtle tasks difficult and even impossible. There appears to be no anatomical basis for the site of fissure, although it could reflect some structural weakness distal to the lateral nail grooves. Application of cyanoacrylate glue in the fissure often results in an immediate relief of pain but contact allergies to skin adhesives such as cyanoacrylates have been reported.

DERMATOSES AFFECTING THE NAILS

There are a number of inherited and acquired conditions that cause nail changes. Here we describe the most common dermatoses that can have nail involvement. Please see specific chapters for description of nail changes that may occur in other conditions, e.g. Chapter 69, genetic blistering disorders for changes seen in epidermolysis bullosa.

Nail psoriasis

Synonyms and inclusions
- Psoriatic nail dystrophy
- Acrodermatitis continua of Hallopeau

Classification links
- ICD-10: L40.8
- ICD-11: EA 90.51

Introduction
About half of the patients who suffer from psoriasis also have changes affecting their nails. Psoriatic nail disease (see also Chapter 35) differs greatly in clinical appearance, severity and impact for individual patients. It is associated with significant pain and physical impairment as well as issues such as self-image and cosmetic concerns, difficulty with tasks involving manual dexterity, anxiety and/or depression, an increased number of missed workdays relative to patients without nail involvement and substantial impairments in quality of life.

Epidemiology
Psoriasis is probably the most common disorder affecting fingernails. Among plaque psoriasis patients, prevalence of nail psoriasis is over 50%, with an estimated lifetime incidence of 80–90% [1,2]. Nail psoriasis in the absence of cutaneous or joint disease is present in 5–10% of psoriatic patients [3]. Most frequently, both fingernails and toenails are involved [2]. De Jong et al. [4] reported that 93% of people with nail psoriasis considered it a significant cosmetic handicap, 58% found that it interfered with their job and 52% described pain as a symptom.

Nail psoriasis has the highest prevalence in patients between 35 and 64 years of age and is much rarer in children [5–7]. Psoriasis patients with psoriatic arthritis and genital psoriasis have an increased risk of developing nail psoriasis [8–10]. Psoriasis patients with nail involvement have a higher risk of developing psoriatic arthritis but most nail psoriasis patients will never develop psoriatic arthritis: the annual risk to develop psoriatic arthritis in psoriasis patients with nail involvement is 0.55–2.55% and in psoriasis patients without nail involvement this risk is 0.26–1.14% [11,12].

Pathophysiology

Environmental factors, genetic susceptibility, abnormal function of keratinocytes and immunological disturbances of the innate and acquired immune system are all postulated to play a role in the pathophysiology of psoriasis [13,14]. Nail unit psoriasis is a localised form of this inflammatory disease and the features represent a combination of local skin changes and secondary effects on nail plate growth.

Little is known about the role of environmental factors in the pathogenesis of nail psoriasis, while some data are available on genetic susceptibility: plaque psoriasis is positively correlated with HLA-Cw6; nail psoriasis patients are more frequently HLA-Cw6-negative, indicating a separate genotype [15,16]. Nail involvement appears to be also milder in HLA-Cw6-positive than in HLA-Cw6-negative psoriasis patients [16]. In Asian patients the Nail Psoriasis Severity Index (NAPSI) was significantly higher in HLA-B46–positive patients [17], and nail psoriasis was more frequent in HLA-A*02:07 carriers, HLA-B*46:01 carriers and HLA-C01*02 carriers, whereas C*6:02 carriers were less prone to have nail involvement [18]. Little is known about the role of the innate and adaptive immune system in nail psoriasis, but mast cells [19,20], antimicrobial peptides, including LL37, hβD-2 and hβD3 [21], and inflammatory mediators TNF-α, IL-6, IL-8 and NF-κB [20], may play a role.

Because of the close anatomical relationship between the soft-tissue attachments of the distal interphalangeal joint and the proximal element of the nail unit it has been assumed that enthesitis of the extensor tendon of the distal interphalangeal joint may play a role in the development of both nail psoriasis and of psoriatic arthritis [22,23]. However, the nail enthesitis theory is becoming obsolete because anatomical [24,25], ultrasound [26,27] and a prospective clinical study [28] indicated that enthesial thickening is not specific for nail psoriasis and instead represents non-specific inflammatory oedema of the whole involved area, including the enthesis.

Clinical features

The inflammatory reaction in nail psoriasis can be present in the nail folds, in the nail matrix and/or in the nail bed. Clinical manifestations differ according to which of these structures is involved. Nail fold psoriasis manifests with papulosquamous or pustular lesions or with paronychia as a result of psoriatic inflammation of the periungual region. Psoriasis of the nail matrix can cause pitting, leukonychia, red spots of the lunula, Beau lines, thickening and crumbling of the nail plate (Figures 93.63, 93.64 and 93.67). Psoriasis of the nail bed presents as oil-drop discoloration, splinter haemorrhages involving the distal third of the nail plate, subungual hyperkeratosis and/or onycholysis (Figures 93.64, 93.65 and 93.66).

Nail fold psoriasis

The epidermis of the dorsal surface of the proximal nail fold is much like its surrounding skin. Psoriasis here resembles psoriasis elsewhere on the skin or presents with signs of chronic paronychia with erythematous swelling of the proximal nail fold and loss of

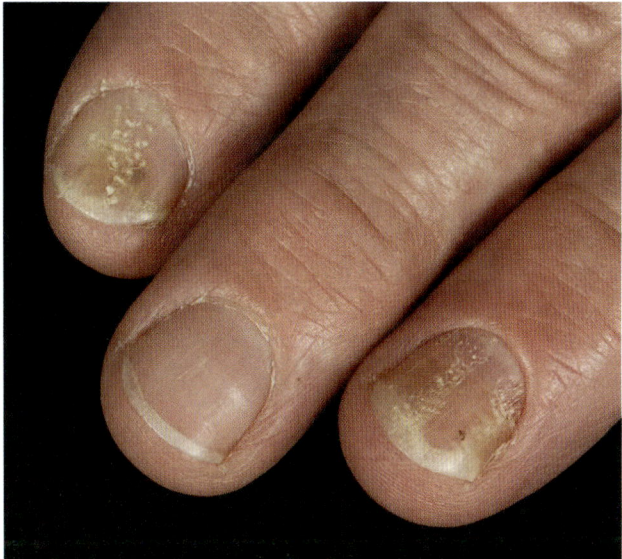

Figure 93.63 Psoriasis: pitting.

the cuticle. Periungual involvement may be dramatic and highly inflammatory with overflow of the inflammation to the underlying nail matrix. Loss of the nail may follow, with scaling of the nail bed or a deep transverse furrow. In milder cases the nail plate can become thickened or thin [29].

Nail fold psoriasis is commonly found in patients with psoriatic arthritis with nail involvement and is, like subungual hyperkeratosis, associated with the severity of both nail psoriasis and cutaneous psoriasis [30].

Nail matrix psoriasis

Red lunula. Red spotted lunulae (Figure 93.64) represent vasodilatation of the vessels beneath the nail. This may be induced by the psoriatic inflammatory reaction of the intermediate or ventral matrix.

Pitting. Pits more commonly affect fingers than toes (Figure 93.63 and 93.64). They represent punctate surface depressions arising from proximal matrix disease (Table 93.4). Psoriatic inflammation in the proximal matrix produces loose parakeratotic cells in the surface portion of the nail plate [31]. As the plate grows out, these cells are exposed to the environment and shed, resulting in the irregular punctate depression we know as a 'pit'. The pits typically are relatively large and deep. The distribution often is irregular but pitting also occurs in transverse/longitudinal rows. If the pits are widespread, shallow and small, the nail becomes dull and rough (trachyonychia). If pits are large and deep a punched-out hole in the nail plate (elkonyxis) may develop [32].

The matrix origin of pits means that they can be influenced by disease modification in the proximal nail fold and injection of triamcinolone into the nail fold alone suppresses this clinical feature [**33**].

Transverse depressions. Transverse depressions are, similar to pits, the consequence of psoriatic inflammation of the matrix. While pits are the result of focal parakeratosis, transverse grooves and ridges are the clinical reflection of a wider and compact area of psoriatic matrix disease. Serial transverse depressions or Beau lines may mimic 'wash-board nails' (Figure 93.64).

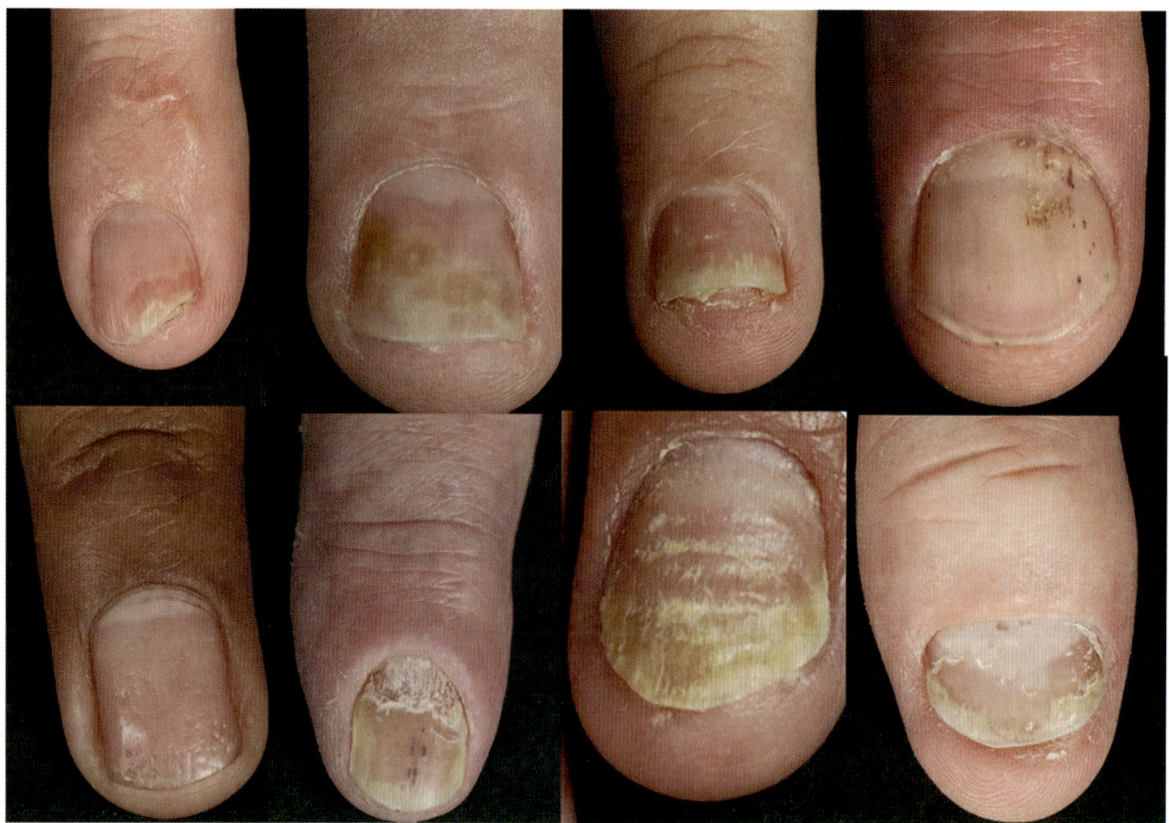

Figure 93.64 Psoriasis. Signs of nail psoriasis: Top: salmon patch, onycholysis, subungual hyperkeratosis splinter haemorrhage. Bottom: pitting, crumbling, Beau lines, red spots of the lunula.

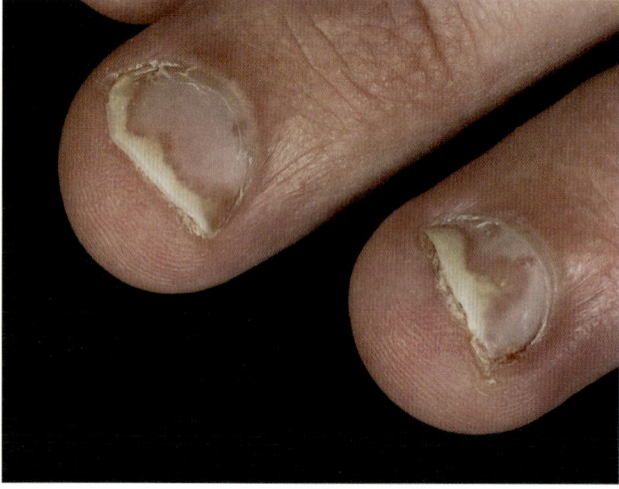

Figure 93.65 Psoriasis: distal onycholysis. Note also the salmon patch.

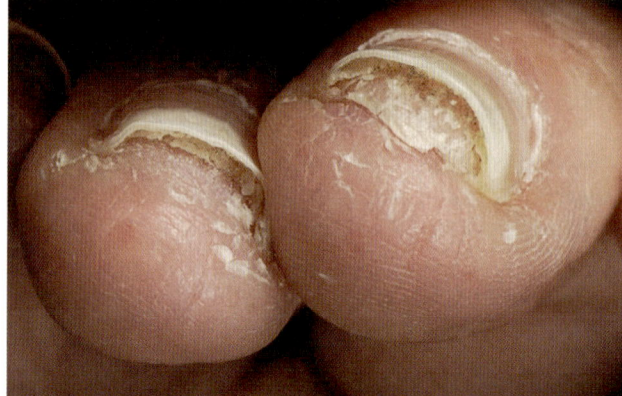

Figure 93.66 Psoriasis: subungual hyperkeratosis.

Onychomadesis and dystrophic crumbling of the nail plate. If psoriatic inflammation persists and involves the entire matrix the consequence can be twofold. A transverse groove can become complete and nail shedding (onychomadesis) occurs. When the whole matrix is affected the nail plate may also become off-white and crumbling (Figure 93.67).

Leukonychia. Inflammation of the mid- or distal matrix causes accumulation of trapped parakeratotic cells within the nail plate. This is recognisable as white spots *in* the nail plate (leukonychia). Leukonychia is rather non-specific for psoriasis and can also be found in many healthy people [34].

Nail plate thickening and discoloration. In cutaneous psoriasis epidermal hyperproliferation is responsible for the thickened plaques. Hyperproliferation of the nail matrix can cause thickened nail plates, which is a major factor in yellow discoloration of the psoriatic nail. Also, subungual hyperkeratosis may contribute to this appearance, which is particularly common in the toenails. The coincidence of onychomycosis and psoriasis is frequent in

Table 93.4 Relationship between clinical features and site of disease activity in psoriasis of the nail. From Zaias [31]

Clinical feature	Area of disease	Duration of disease
Changes in nail plate	***Matrix***	
Pits	Proximal matrix	Episodic: short
Transverse furrows	Proximal matrix; distal extension depends on depth of furrow	1–2 weeks
Crumbling nail plate	Entire matrix	Prolonged
Leukonychia with rough surface	Proximal matrix; leukonychia may involve distal matrix	Variable
Changes in nail bed and hyponychium	***Nail bed***	
Splinter haemorrhages	Nail bed dermal ridge haemorrhage	Short
Oily spot/onycholysis	Nail bed psoriasis	Prolonged
False nail following onychomadesis	Nail bed psoriasis	Prolonged
Subungual hyperkeratosis	Nail bed psoriasis	Prolonged
Yellow/green discoloration of nail bed	Secondary infection by yeasts or *Pseudomonas*	Prolonged

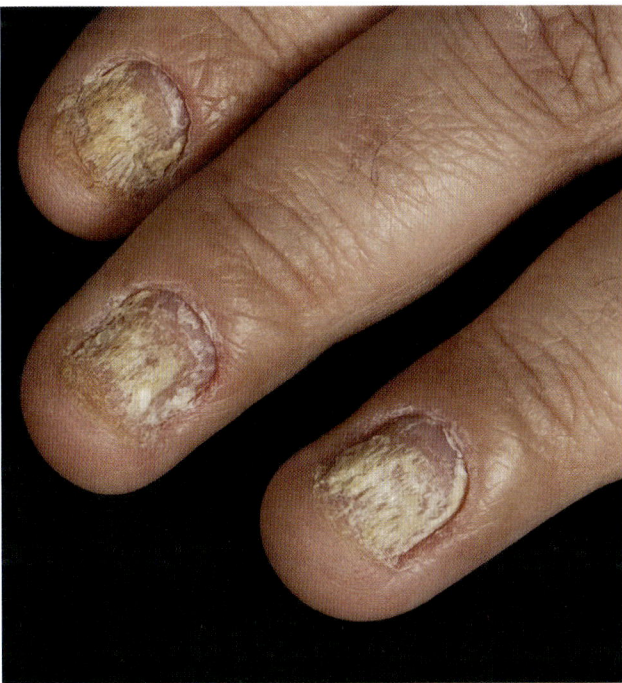

Figure 93.67 Nail crumbling in a psoriasis patient.

both toenails [35] and fingernails [36], and can modify the clinical appearances. *Candida* and *Pseudomonas* superinfections can result in brown or green discoloration.

Nail bed psoriasis

Oil dropping sign and onycholysis. Focal nail bed parakeratosis produces an 'oil spot' or 'salmon patch'. These patches of various size and variable duration can be observed through the nail plate. Extension to the free edge results in onycholysis, which typically has a reddish-brown proximal margin (Figure 93.64). Consequently, a clue to the diagnosis of psoriasis as the cause of

onycholysis is the characteristic salmon-coloured zone at the leading edge of onycholysis (Figure 93.65). Alternatively, onycholysis may commence at the distal edge, representing disruption of the onychocorneal band [37]. Once this band of firm attachment has been breached, the process is often progressive. Minor manicure, wet work and leverage from long nails exacerbate the problem.

Subungual hyperkeratosis. Subungual hyperkeratosis represents accumulation of keratinocytes in nail bed disease (Figures 93.64 and 93.66). The nail plate is raised off the nail bed due to the volume of the subungual cell material. Substantial apparent nail plate thickening may result: it is most marked distally and extends proximally. The colour of the hyperkeratosis can vary from yellow to white, but in psoriasis the subungual hyperkeratosis frequently has a less common silvery white colour. The fingertip may become very tender where there is gross thickening, as the nail plate attachment is greatly reduced and the nail can easily be caught and tug on the matrix attachment. Subungual hyperkeratosis is also a prominent feature of pityriasis rubra pilaris affecting the nails and is often associated with splinter haemorrhages [35,38].

Splinter haemorrhages. Capillary injury in the longitudinally oriented epidermal–dermal ridges manifests clinically as small linear haemorrhages, known as splinter haemorrhages. Splinter haemorrhages in psoriasis frequently occur under the distal third of the nail plate and are seen in the nail bed in up to 94% of nail psoriasis patients and in 37% of healthy controls [34]. Dermoscopy may facilitate the detection of splinter haemorrhages. Bleeding of the capillaries can be due to the increased capillary prominence and fragility in nail bed dermis in psoriasis and to the presence of dystrophy. Patients often consider the splinter haemorrhages as dirt and try to remove them, resulting in leverage and trauma, which results in more splinter haemorrhages and onycholyses.

Pustular variants of nail psoriasis

The nomenclature of sterile pustular conditions of the nail is confusing, perhaps because of the considerable overlap between acrodermatitis continua of Hallopeau, acropustulosis repens (Figure 93.68), palmoplantar pustulosis and acute generalised pustular psoriasis [39]. There is controversy regarding whether these conditions are separate entities or are on a continuum with pustular psoriasis. Acrodermatitis continua of Hallopeau [40] is the most frequent of these rare disorders and typically begins in one single finger or toe but involvement of multiple digits is common. It presents with paronychia and collections of sterile pustules around the nail fold and subungual. The nail may ultimately be shed and then the nail bed will present with scales and pustules. In severe acrodermatitis continua of Hallopeau the entire digits may be involved with resorptive osteolysis and loss of the tips of digits and nails [41,42]. Acrodermatitis continua of Hallopeau has a chronic relapsing course and is frequently refractory to many therapeutic modalities.

Differential diagnosis

The main differential diagnostic considerations are onychomycosis and lichen planus, and less commonly eczema or reactive arthritis (previously known as Reiter syndrome) where pitting may be

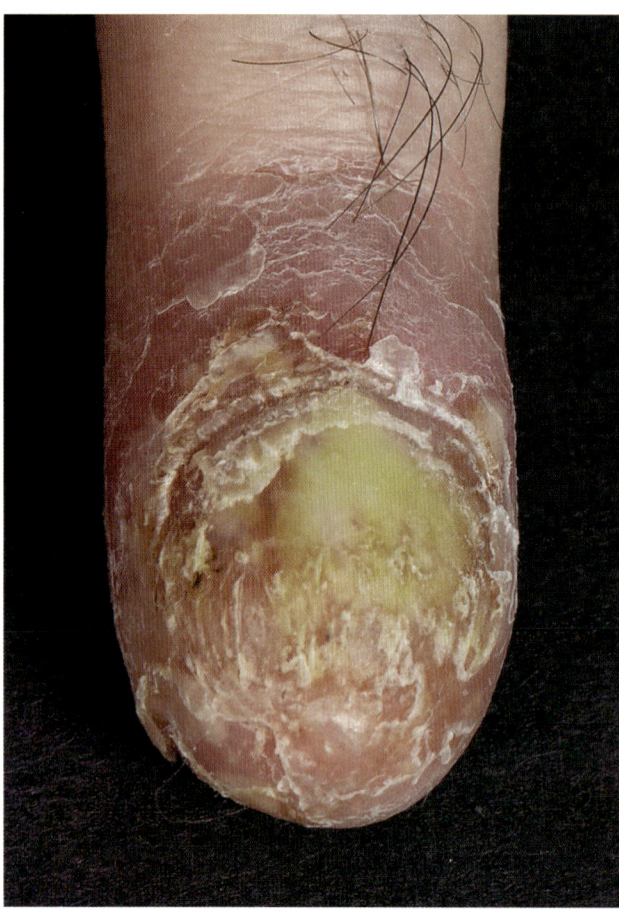

Figure 93.68 Acropustulosis: nail plate has been destroyed by intense pustular inflammation.

seen [43]. Onychomycosis more commonly affects the toenails, whereas the fingernails are more commonly involved in psoriasis. Furthermore, in psoriasis the nail surface alone is often affected, whereas in onychomycosis there are usually visible abnormalities within or beneath the nail plate. Onychomycosis of the fingernails tends to involve only one or a minority of digits, in contrast with psoriasis where multiple digits often are affected. Obviously, psoriatic skin changes or arthritis of the distal interphalangeal joint suggest a psoriatic cause of nail dystrophy.

Some forms of fingernail lichen planus are very difficult to distinguish from psoriasis. Both may result in roughened nails (trachyonychia) with subungual hyperkeratosis. If pits are prominent the diagnosis of psoriasis can be made, but if they are subtle and difficult to distinguish from other surface changes, they may be part of lichen planus. The nails in reactive arthritis and pityriasis rubra pilaris can also be difficult to differentiate from psoriasis [43,44] where distal subungual hyperkeratosis and splinter haemorrhages are common. Aggressive forms of atypical nail psoriasis presenting in later life may represent acrokeratosis paraneoplastica of Bazex (Chapter 148). The patient is usually male, with subungual hyperkeratosis and scaling of the periunguium, ears and nose associated with malignancies of the upper gastrointestinal or respiratory tract [45–47].

A variant of nail psoriasis presents with pain and soft-tissue swelling of the distal digit associated with psoriatic nail changes

and underlying bone erosion and periosteal reaction. This can develop in the absence of joint involvement and is called 'psoriatic onychopachydermoperiostitis' (POPP) [48,49].

Investigations

General accepted criteria for the diagnosis of nail psoriasis do not exist and the diagnosis is primarily based on clinical signs. A nail unit biopsy taken from the affected area of the nail unit may be considered gold standard, but also non-invasive techniques like dermoscopy [50] and ultrasound [51] have well-described features. The presence of structural damage of the nail plate and higher power Doppler signal are the main ultrasound findings supporting a diagnosis of psoriatic onychopathy. Other non-invasive imaging techniques, such as magnetic resonance image techniques [52] or optical coherence tomography [53], have also been introduced to facilitate the diagnosis of nail psoriasis.

Dermoscopy of the nail unit (onychoscopy) can be used to evaluate the nail plate surface, the free edge and the periungual tissues. The most common onychoscopic findings are dilated and tortuous capillaries in nail bed and hyponychium, present in 90% of patients [54,55]. Other onychoscopic features of nail matrix psoriasis are coarse pits/pitting, nail plate thickening, trachyonychia, transverse grooves, leukonychia and red spots in the lunula. The most common onychoscopic feature indicating nail bed involvement are splinter haemorrhages. Other nail bed features of nail psoriasis are salmon patches, onycholysis, dilated globule vessels, streaky capillaries, subungual hyperkeratosis and erythematous borders of an onycholytic area [56].

A nail unit biopsy can be used in case of doubt about the correct diagnosis. Histologically, psoriasis of the nail folds simulates psoriasis involving other cutaneous sites. Histopathological features of nail bed and matrix psoriasis are somewhat different from psoriasis elsewhere on the body [57]. The following histological features are characteristic for psoriasis of the nail bed and matrix: varying degrees of uniform hyperplasia, spongiosis, appearance of a granular layer, spongiform pustules and parakeratosis with neutrophils [58]. Unlike psoriasis elsewhere, nail bed and matrix histopathology reveals hypergranulosis in more than half of the cases. Conversely, the hyponychium, where a granular layer is normally present, no longer has one [59].

Biopsies taken from the nail bed are more helpful when subungual hyperkeratosis is present but areas of onycholysis generally do not produce useful histological information [60]. In a histological nail bed study, the feature found most frequently was hyperkeratosis with parakeratosis (78% of biopsies), followed by neutrophilic infiltration of nail bed epithelium (63%), hypergranulosis (58%), psoriasiform hyperplasia (53%), dilated capillaries (47%) and serum exudates in 43% of cases [61]. The use of nail clipping microscopy as a diagnostic tool for nail psoriasis has shown that the predominant histological features consistent with psoriasis are a thickened nail plate, subungual hyperkeratosis, neutrophils and parakeratosis [62–66].

Management [33,67–69]

Effective management of nail psoriasis is often complex, challenging and time-consuming. An optimal effect of any treatment may take up to 1 year. Numerous treatments have been described as treatments for nail psoriasis [67] but a successful therapeutic approach should include both general advice for all patients with nail psoriasis (Box 93.2) and an individualised choice from available pharmacological treatments. Onychomycosis, especially of the toenails, has been demonstrated to be more common in patients with psoriasis [36] and could koebnerise psoriatic nail disease. In case of onychomycosis, antifungal treatment should be prescribed along with nail psoriasis treatment [33].

Box 93.2 General advice for all patients with nail psoriasis. Reproduced from [33] with permission from Elsevier.

- Avoid biting, tearing and traumatising the nails; tangential filing; frequently applying and removing nail cosmetics; frequent water contact; artificial or gel nails; pulling, biting and cutting cuticles; wearing high heels or narrow toed shoes; and cutting toenails round at the edges
- Wear heavy duty cotton gloves for dry work and light cotton gloves underneath vinyl gloves for wet work
- Keep nails short in nail bed psoriasis
- Frequently use hydrating topical products on hands and nails
- An orthopaedist or podiatrist should be consulted for the fitting of proper shoes and shoe inserts if anatomical problems, such as bunions, improper foot strike, pronators or supinators, are present

---

Accepted treatment modalities include topical agents, intralesional injections, conventional systemic medications, small molecules and biologic agents. The role of non-pharmacological treatment options, including phototherapy, photodynamic therapy, radiotherapy and laser therapy is limited [67]. Topical treatments used to be the mainstay therapies in nail psoriasis. Gradually the focus in clinical research has shifted towards systemic treatment, in particular towards small molecules and biologics. However, it is reasonable to assume that in daily clinical practice many more patients with uncomplicated nail psoriasis are treated topically and intralesionally than with systemic therapies. High-potency corticosteroids with or without calcipotriol could be tried in mild nail bed or nail matrix psoriasis [70,71]. Intralesional therapy in nail disorders has several advantages above topical or systemic treatments [72]. It is able to treat unreachable parts of the nail unit as non-invasively as possible, avoids barriers to drug penetration resulting in effective levels of drugs at the site of action and may establish a tissue depot for a prolonged release of drugs. Locally injected steroids have a long history in the treatment of nail psoriasis and their efficacy is beyond dispute. Studies suggest that intralesional injection into the nail bed and matrix is particularly effective for alleviating lesions caused by psoriasis of the nail matrix, and also has moderate effects on nail bed signs. In addition to intralesional triamcinolone, intralesional treatment with methotrexate in nail bed or nail matrix is a potentially interesting therapy [73,74]. Systemic therapy with methotrexate is more frequently used in nail psoriasis than intralesional methotrexate. Systemic methotrexate can be used in both nail bed and nail matrix psoriasis and is rather effective but also slow acting. It may take up to 6 months before relevant clinical improvement can be noticed [75]. Acitretin is another systemic treatment which is

effective in nail psoriasis and as slow acting as methotrexate [76]. Ciclosporin might be somewhat faster and at least as powerful as methotrexate or acitretin [75] but its potential side-effects limit long-term treatment. It appears that the small molecule apremilast [77–82] and possibly also tofacitinib [83] are oral alternatives for conventional systemic therapies with methotrexate, ciclosporin or acitretin. Comparative studies are missing but efficacy and speed of onset with small molecules appears to be in the same range. Biologic therapies appear to act faster and might be more effective treatments for nail psoriasis [67] but comparative studies with conventional therapies and other biologics are sparse. Adalimimab is the only biologic which is FDA (but not EMA) approved for the treatment of nail psoriasis. This anti-TNF monoclonal antibody is an effective treatment for nail psoriasis [84,85] but probably not more effective than the other anti-TNFs – infliximab [86], etanercept [87], certoliziumab pegol [88], or golimumab [89]. Other groups of biologics used in psoriasis inhibit IL12, IL17 and/or IL23, and may be more powerful treatments for nail psoriasis than anti-TNF treatments, but it is too early to make a final judgement. Brodalimumab [90], guselkumab [91], ixekizumab [92], risankizumab [93], secukinumab [94] and ustekinumab [95] all can improve nails in psoriasis patients.

Concerning non-pharmacological treatment options it is possible that 595-nm pulsed dye laser or long-pulsed 1064-nm Nd:YAG laser treatment of nails has some beneficial effect in nail psoriasis. However, quality of life seems not to improve, nor is improvement noticed by a vast majority of treated patients [96]. A randomised study comparing laser treatment with sham laser treatment is therefore urgently needed to justify this painful treatment in patients with nail psoriasis. Also, UVB or PUVA phototherapy should not be advised in nail psoriasis patients because treatment results do not justify this intensive treatment [67]. Radiotherapy is rarely used in the daily clinical care of patients with nail psoriasis. Superficial radiotherapy, Grenz ray therapy, brachytherapy and electron beam therapy have been reported to have some efficacy [67,97] but cannot be advised because of too limited efficacy and safety concerns.

A summary of treatment recommendations of a consensus group of nail psoriasis experts can be found in Figure 93.69. In summary, in few-nail disease (≤3 nails involved) intralesional steroid injections were considered the treatment of choice in the case of matrix involvement only. The second-line treatment should be topical steroids, topical vitamin D analogues, topical vitamin D analogues in combination with topical steroids, topical retinoids, topical keratolytic agents (e.g. urea nail lacquer, salicylic acid), or topical 0.1% tacrolimus. Topical steroids alone or in combination with topical vitamin D analogues were suggested as first line treatment for nail psoriasis limited to the nail bed in few-nail disease. The steroids could be used under occlusion, both for matrix and bed disease, but occlusive treatment is recommended to not exceed 1 month due to possible local side effects. If both nail bed and nail matrix are involved in few-nail disease, the first line treatments of choice are intralesional steroid injections and/or topical steroids in combination with topical vitamin D analogues. Alternative treatments in these patients are topical vitamin D analogues, or topical steroids, or topical retinoids or topical 0.1% tacrolimus. If more than three nails are involved the treatment of choice largely should depend

PART 8: SPECIFIC CUTANEOUS STRUCTURES

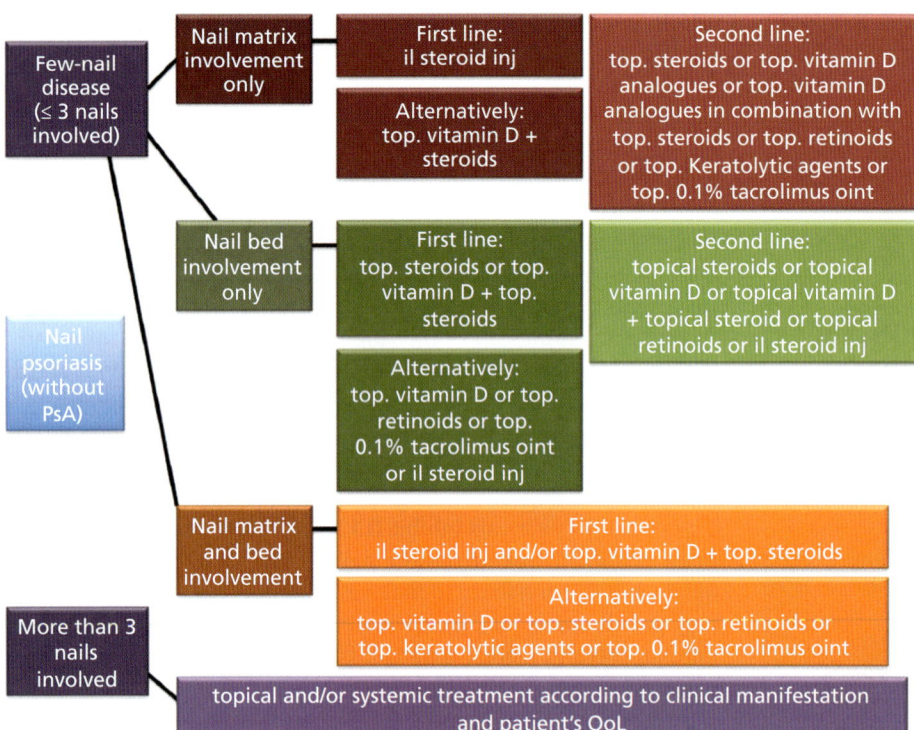

Figure 93.69 A summary of the treatment recommendations of a consensus group of nail psoriasis experts [**33**]. Clinical treatment algorithm for nail psoriasis according to the number of nails involved and the location of the psoriatic lesion. il, Intralesional; inj, injection; oint, ointment; PsA, psoriatic arthritis; QoL, quality of life; top., topical. Reproduced from [**33**] with permission from Elsevier.

PART 8: SPECIFIC CUTANEOUS STRUCTURES

on the discussion between the clinician and the patient in which the severity of nail involvement, the impact on quality of life and patient's preferences all are included. Both topical and systemic treatments are options in these patients. Acitretin, methotrexate, ciclosporin, small molecules and biologics may be employed for the systemic treatment of nail psoriasis. Acitretin should be initiated at 0.2–0.4 mg/kg for 6 months or until at least a moderate improvement is documented. Ciclosporin is only recommended for short-term treatment in doses of 3–5 mg/kg. Methotrexate can be employed in doses up to 15 mg/week and also as maintenance treatment. The nail expert group concluded that TNF-α inhibitors infliximab, etanercept, adalimumab and golimumab; IL-12/23 inhibitor ustekinumab; IL-17 inhibitors secukinumab and ixekizumab; phosphodiesterase 4 inhibitor apremilast; and Janus kinase (JAK) 1/3 inhibitor tofacitinib could be considered for systemic treatment of nail psoriasis. In patients treated for psoriatic arthritis or plaque psoriasis the pegylated TNF-α inhibitor certolizumab pegol and the IL-23 inhibitor guselkumab appear to have a positive effect on nail psoriasis [33]. Treatment with these agents results in rapid and significant improvement of nail psoriasis when used in patients with nail psoriasis and cutaneous disease, arthritis, or both.

Another consensus paper on treatment of nail psoriasis was developed by the Medical Board of the National Psoriasis Foundation and additionally defined scenarios for nail psoriasis patients with significant skin disease [98]: in patients with significant skin and nail disease, adalimumab, etanercept and ustekinumab were strongly recommended, and methotrexate, acitretin, infliximab and apremilast were recommended. Finally, for a patient with significant nail, skin and joint disease, adalimumab, etanercept, ustekinumab, infliximab, methotrexate, apremilast and golimumab were recommended.

Darier disease of the nails [1–3]

Synonyms and inclusions
- Dyskeratosis follicularis
- Darier–White disease

Classification links
- ICD-10: Q82.8
- ICD-11: EC20.2
- OMIM: 124200

Introduction
Nail involvement is common in Darier disease (see also Chapter 64) 92–96% of patients are reported to have acral changes of which nail changes are the most common [4,5].

Epidemiology
The estimated prevalence of Darier disease is 1:50 000.

Pathophysiology
Darier disease is an autosomal dominant inherited condition which is caused by mutations in the *ATP2A2* gene, encoding the sarco/endoplasmic reticulum Ca^{2+} adenosine triphosphatase isoform 2 (SERCA2), which plays a role in maintaining calcium homeostasis [6]. Since desmoplakin, a component of desmosomal adhesions, is calcium dependent, abnormal functioning of SERCA2 causes epidermal acantholysis and dyskeratosis, thus explaining the physical findings seen in Darier disease [7].

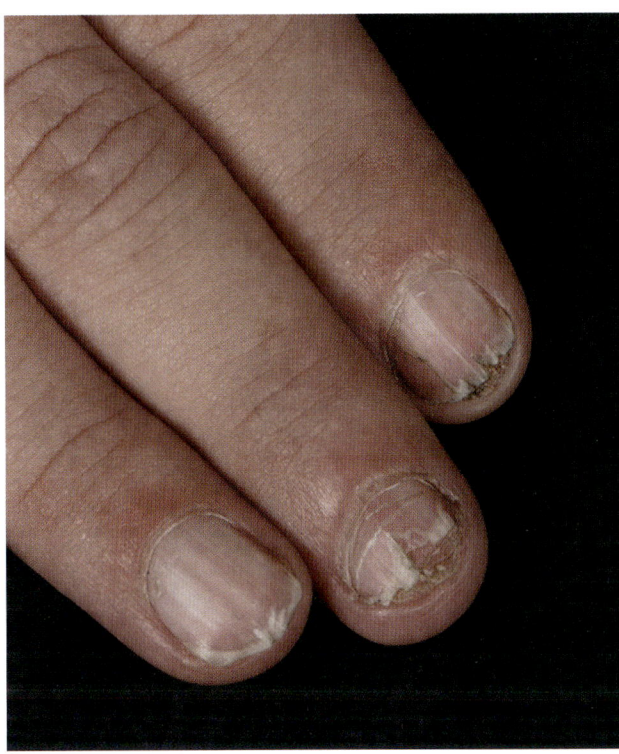

Figure 93.70 Darier disease: white and red longitudinal lines, distal notching and onycholysis.

Clinical features

Typically, Darier disease presents in early adult life with keratotic papules in a seborrheic distribution, palmar pits, white or flesh-coloured cobblestone papules on the oral mucosa and nail dystrophy [1]. Nail involvement is one of the typical expressions of Darier disease, and present in almost all patients [4,5]. Multiple nails with multiple red and white bands (longitudinal erythronychia together with longitudinal leukonychia) resembling 'candy-canes' are pathognomonic for Darier disease [1]. These red and white bands are essential for the diagnosis, but initially they can be very subtle. At the nail plate free margin the bands may have a fissure and a V-shaped notch, indicating the fragility of the streaks (Figure 93.70). In severe cases, the nails are almost lost by extension of the fragmentation process to involve the entire matrix. Subungual hyperkeratotic papules can be found in the hyponychium. Less specific nail findings include longitudinal ridging, total leukonychia, a rough nail surface, splinter haemorrhages and marked thickening of the nail plate [1,4,5,8].

The differential diagnosis includes conditions with polydactylous longitudinal erythronychia and/or leukonychia. Polydactylous longitudinal erythronychia can be idiopathic or seen in lichen planus, primary amyloidosis, graft-versus-host disease, acantholytic epidermolysis bullosa [1]. Hailey–Hailey nail disease presents with polydactylous longitudinal leukonychia [4,9].

A case of squamous cell carcinoma developing in a nail bed with chronic changes of Darier disease has been reported [10]. Pain or conspicuous uncharacteristic features in a nail apparatus affected by Darier disease may therefore be indications for biopsy.

Investigations

Histologically, matrix and nail bed changes resemble the acantholysis seen in involved skin, with the addition of multinucleate giant cells and epithelial hyperplasia in the nail bed [11]. These histological features make it possible to diagnose Darier disease when it is confined to the nail [12].

Eczematous nail dystrophy

Synonyms and inclusions
- Eczema
- Dermatitis

Classification links (as appropriate)
- ICD-10: L60.3
- ICD-11: EE13.5

Introduction

Eczema of the nail unit comprises nail changes induced by atopic dermatitis, nummular dermatitis, allergic contact dermatitis, irritant contact dermatitis and tylotic eczema. The inflammation may involve the nail folds, the nail matrix, the nail bed or the hyponychium, resulting in a wide range of potential clinical expressions.

Epidemiology

Almost all patients suffering from hand eczema have at least some nail involvement [1]. Prevalence of nail abnormalities in atopic dermatitis patients was reported to be 16% [2]. A combination of atopy and an exogenous irritant or allergic contact reaction is common. Selective exposure to allergens or strong irritants is as important as chronic low-grade irritation from milder irritants such as water and detergents seen in catering workers.

Pathophysiology

Nail changes in eczema may be seen in the context of eczema elsewhere, with hand eczema or as an isolated finding with periungual and subungual features. Endogenous and exogenous factors may contribute. Eczema in childhood is commonly due to atopic dermatitis, which can involve the hand and the periungual tissues. Nail signs are always associated with dermatitis of the dorsal or volar skin of the hand causing mild onycholysis, subungual hyperkeratosis, transversal ridges, pitting and melanonychia [3]. Finger sucking can also induce periungual eczema in children [4].

The most important allergens in contact dermatitis of the nail are toluene sulphonamide formaldehyde resin contained in nail lacquers and various types of (meth)acrylates contained in sculptured and artificial nails and preformed plastic tips [5–8], but also ethyl cyanoacrylate glue which is used to attach preformed nails [9,10]. Nail varnish allergy often induces dermatitis of the eyelids because of scratching [11] but another common expression of this is chronic hand eczema with cracked pulpitis, paronychia and nail dystrophy [12]. Other potential contact allergens may be applied topical drugs or emollients, or occupational exposure to (meth)acrylates,

Table 93.5 Differential diagnosis between four common nail disorders: fungal infections, psoriasis, chronic paronychia and dermatitis.

	Fungal infections	Psoriasis	Chronic paronychia	Dermatitis (all subtypes)
Colour	Often yellow or brown; part or whole of nail	May be normal or yellow or brown	Edge of nail often discoloured brown or black	May be normal
Onycholysis	Frequent	Frequent	Usually absent	Confined to tip or absent
Pitting	Infrequent	Often present and fine	Uncommon	Coarse pits frequent
Filaments or spores in potassium hydroxide preparations	Filaments, usually abundant	Up to 20% of psoriasis patients have an onychomycosis	May be spores in lateral edge of nail; filaments and spores in scrapings from nail fold	Absent
Cross-ridging	Absent	Uncommon	Frequent	Frequent
Other	Associated fungal infections elsewhere	Associated psoriasis elsewhere or family history of psoriasis	Predominantly women; wet work and cold hands cause predisposition	Recent history of dermatitis on hands

gasoline, paint removers and others [13]. Irritant contact dermatitis, inducing brittle nails, can also be the consequence of prolonged wearing of occlusive gloves [14]. Certain drugs, such as tetracyclines, capecitabine and 5-fluorouracil, can produce phototoxic dermatitis resulting in onycholysis that follows the shape of the proximal nail fold [13].

Clinical features (see also Pathophysiology)

Clinical expression of nail involvement in eczema reflects shiny smooth nails as a sign of persistent rubbing or nail signs secondary to involvement of components of the nail unit. Eczema on the proximal or lateral nail folds may result in redness and swelling with loss of the cuticle, resembling chronic paronychia. Loss of the cuticle may result in superinfection by bacteria or *Candida* species. Eczema of the proximal nail fold mostly induces involvement of the underlying nail matrix, resulting in abnormalities of the nail plate: the nail may become thickened, pitted, rough or discoloured [15] (Table 93.5). Beau lines are very common in eczema and represent variations in time and intensity of the inflammatory reaction.

In allergic and irritant contact eczema the nail bed and hyponychium also usually show signs, including splinter haemorrhages in an early phase, followed by onycholysis, subungual hyperkeratosis and paronychia in a later phase. Finally, erythema, scales and painful fissures may develop.

Associated hand dermatitis may show vesicles, scaling, erythema, cracks and swollen fingers, although the presence of vesicles will not always distinguish the condition from psoriasis, which should be sought at other sites.

Investigations

Patch testing may be indicated.

Management

General hand care is important, with the avoidance of soap, irritants, wet work and any identified cause. Protective gloves should be used, with copious emollient application. Cotton, transpiration absorbing gloves under protective gloves is advisable if gloves are worn for more than 15–20 minutes. Treatment of eczematous nail dystrophy mimics treatment of chronic paronychia and hand eczema, and includes moderate to high potency corticosteroids, calcineurin inhibitors and frequent application of an emollient. These topical drugs should be rubbed in around the nail folds. In the young, steroids may precipitate premature closure of the phalangeal epiphyses if too potent or used for too long. Osteomyelitis has also been reported in children using potent topical steroids in this area [16]. Antibiotics may be helpful in case of a bacterial superinfection.

Lichen planus of the nails and related conditions

Synonyms and inclusions
- Trachyonychia
- Idiopathic nail atrophy
- Lichen nitidus

Classification links
- ICD-10: L43.8
- ICD-11: EA91.5

Introduction

Nail lichen planus (NLP) is an uncommon inflammatory disorder that may present as an isolated variant or may be associated with mucosal or cutaneous lichen planus (see also Chapter 37). Lichen planus is assumed to be an autoimmune disease and nail involvement may lead to irreversible damage of the nail matrix resulting in pterygium formation. NLP is classified into three categories: typical NLP, twenty-nail dystrophy (or trachyonychia) and idiopathic nail atrophy [1].

Epidemiology

Nails are involved in 10–16% of cases of lichen planus of the skin, scalp or mucosa [2]. While overlap with mucosal lesions is not uncommon, most patients with NLP have no involvement of other body sites [3–6,7]. NLP has no propensity for race and can occur at any age, but the incidence peaks in the fifth and sixth decade of life [7–9]. Males may be involved slightly more often than females [7,10].

Clinical features

Fingernails are more commonly involved than toenails. Although the skin lesions in lichen planus may itch intensely, nail disease

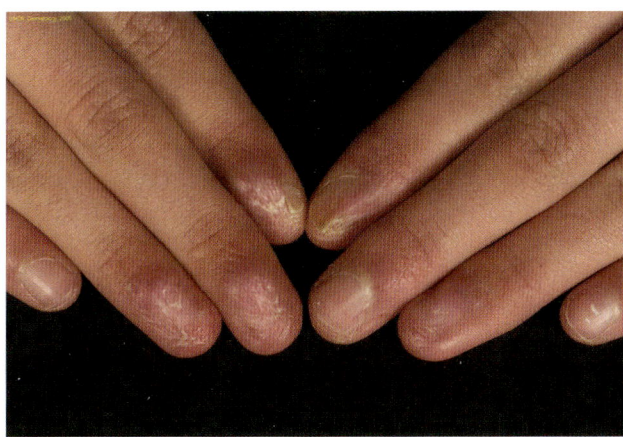

Figure 93.71 Severe onychatrophy from juvenile onset lichen planus of nails.

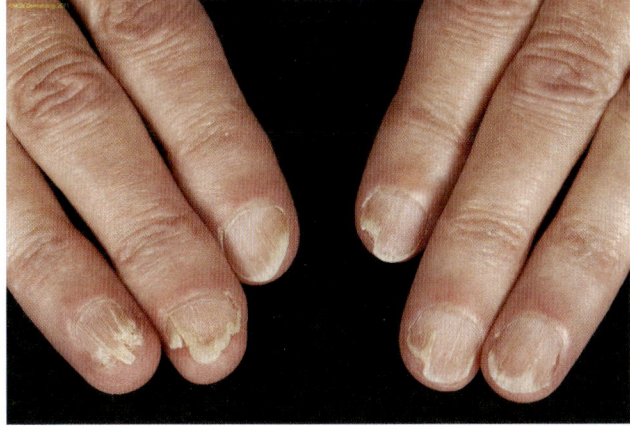

Figure 93.72 Typical lichen planus with trachyonychia, onychorrhexia and onycholysis.

is relatively asymptomatic except when nails are shed. Clinical features are determined by site and severity of the inflammation (Figures 93.71 and 93.72). The proximal nail fold, nail matrix and the nail bed can all be affected, but involvement of the matrix is most frequent [7]. Nail matrix involvement results in abnormalities of the nail plate, in particular in thinning, brittleness, longitudinal ridging, trachyonychia (surface roughening) and in distal splitting of the nail (onychorrhexia) (Figure 93.72) [7,9]. Also, longitudinal melanonychia [11], longitudinal erythronychia [12], leukonychia as a postinflammatory phenomenon, crumbling or fragmentation may be encountered as signs of nail matrix lichen planus. Thickening, with features resembling yellow nail syndrome, is a less common pattern of presentation [13]. When inflammation is intense and widespread within the nail apparatus, nails may be shed. Dorsal pterygium, the presence of a scarred midline band originating from the proximal nail fold, indicates late-stage matrix involvement. Dorsal pterygium is the consequence of a destructive local inflammation within the nail matrix resulting in fusion of the proximal nail fold with the nail bed. Proximal nail-fold involvement can be recognised as bluish discoloration or as pigmentation of the nail. Nail bed involvements manifests as onycholysis (Figure 93.73), subungual hyperkeratosis, nail bed atrophy or linear nail bed dyschromia [9,14].

Clinical variants

Trachyonychia (previously known as *twenty-nail dystrophy*) in which there is stippling of the nail plate (Figure 93.18), can be seen as a paediatric expression of NLP but is mostly considered idiopathic [15]. Contrary to typical NLP, longitudinal splitting and pterygium are absent. Trachyonychia may involve all 20 nails but may also affect as few as four or five. Trachyonychia is seen not only in NLP or idiopathic but may also occur in a range of autoimmune diseases [16], especially in alopecia areata [15,17], psoriasis, eczema and vitiligo [18], but also in sarcoidosis, primary biliary cirrhosis and possibly in pemphigus [15,19]. Even without treatment it has a reasonably good prognosis [15,18], in contrast to *idiopathic atrophy of the nails*, which may also occur in children. Idiopathic atrophy of the nails is the most severe variant of NLP, and is characterised by an acute onset and rapid course, culminating in diffuse, painless irreversible nail destruction in a few months [1]. If destructive lichen planus is not treated in childhood, there will be lifelong loss of nails. In the related disorder, *lichen nitidus*, nail involvement is associated with extensive cutaneous disease, but nail changes appear to be less severe than in lichen planus and are generally self-limiting [20,21]. Numerous pits giving a fine rippling effect have been reported [22]. Longitudinal ridging, beads and thickening may occur and the nails may become brittle. Clues to the diagnosis include the presence of subtle papules on the affected digit and swelling with hyperpigmentation of the nailfold [20].

Less common presentations of NLP include erosive lichen planus (Figure 93.73) and a bullous form with haemorrhagic lesions resulting in complete shedding of the nail plate with atrophy [23], splinter haemorrhages, koilonychia and yellow nail syndrome-like changes. Erosive lichen planus may affect the soles of the feet but may also involve the toenails. It is characterised by erosions of the nail bed, acute inflammation of nail folds and permanent anonychia (Figure 93.71) [24,25].

Lichen planus-like nail changes are seen in *graft-versus-host disease* [26–28] and in the *disseminated lichenoid papular dermatosis of AIDS*. There can be an overlap between lichen planus and *discoid lupus erythematosus*, both in the skin and nails. Coexistence of skin and nail *lichen sclerosus* has been reported [29]. *Lichen striatus* may extend down a limb to the nails [30]. Further differential diagnoses for the range of appearances of lichen planus in the nail unit include

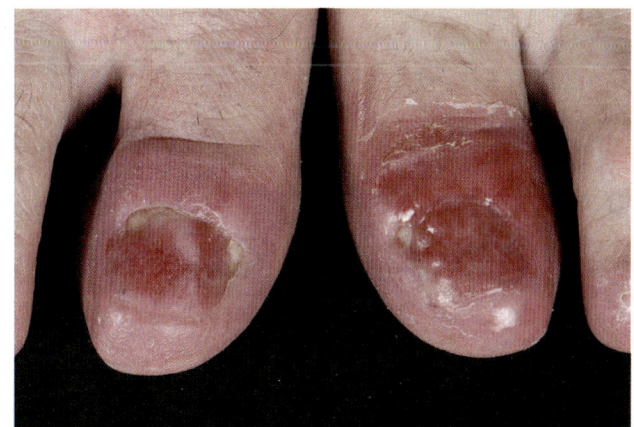

Figure 93.73 Erosive lichen planus.

PART 8: SPECIFIC CUTANEOUS STRUCTURES

Stevens–Johnson syndrome, infection, peripheral vascular disease, trauma and radiodermatitis. Scarring inherited abnormalities such as *dyskeratosis congenita*, *Schöpf–Schulz–Passarge syndrome*, *Darier disease* and variants of *epidermolysis bullosa* can also present with nail atrophy and scarring, with overlap with the appearance of lichen planus.

Investigations

In most cases the diagnosis of NLP is clinical. Dermoscopy can provide diagnostic information by highlighting the known clinical signs [14,31]. In questionable cases, obtaining a biopsy specimen is necessary, with the biopsy site selected according to the findings of the clinical examination. Histopathological studies reveal a band-like lymphocytic infiltrate of the nail matrix and /or nail bed dermis, sawtooth acanthosis, hypergranulosis and hyperkeratosis of the nail bed and nail matrix epithelium [7,10].

Management

The prognosis of NLP is variable. Typical NLP is slowly progressive and pterygium formation takes several months or may not occur. Some patients may have a more rapid worsening of nail signs or develop idiopathic atrophy of the nail variant.

Treating NLP is notoriously challenging, with high rates of failures, relapses and recurrences [7]. No randomised controlled trials have been completed for this condition [32], and treatment advice should therefore be regarded with some scepticism. The objective of treatment is to minimise irreversible scarring and nail damage but also to improve physical and cosmetic properties of the nail. Treatment needs to be commenced early and at sufficient potency to ensure that the disease does not progress while treatment is ongoing. Wait-and-see is not an advisable option because of the potentially destructive nature of NLP.

Topical corticosteroids have questionable effectiveness in NLP due to concerns of low drug penetration. Instead, intralesional and intramuscular triamcinolone acetonide should be considered first-line therapies [32]. Oral retinoids are second-line choices, and immunosuppressive agents may also be considered (Table 93.6). Considering the nail growth of 2–3 mm per month for fingernails, a minimum of 3–6 months is necessary to evaluate the results of any treatment. Growth of toenails is considerably slower, resulting in worse and slower treatment response.

In adults and children above the age of 14, triamcinolone acetonide can be injected intralesionally direct to the site of inflammation: the nail matrix or the nail bed. Injections in the nail bed are too painful without a digital block anaesthesia. Haematomas

and transient numbness of the distal digit are more frequent than serious side-effects. Triamcinolone acetonide should be injected in a concentration of 2.5, 5, or 10 mg/mL according to disease severity. This should be repeated every 4–5 weeks for a minimum of 4–6 months to appreciate the results. If improvements are seen, it is appropriate to continue until there is marked or complete improvement and then to taper for a few months. Intramuscular triamcinolone could be an alternative or adjunct to intralesional administration in case of severe disease, especially if more than three nails are affected. A dose of 0.5–1 mg/kg every month for at least 3–6 months is suitable for both children and adults, with dosages of 1 mg/kg/month advised during the active treatment phase. This low dose may appear rather homeopathic because 25–40 mg triamcinolone once a month is equivalent to 32–50 mg prednisone once a month which is only a fraction of the endogenous production of corticosteroids. However, this approach was advised by experts based on non-controlled retrospective studies [1,7,8]. If no clinical response after 6 months is achieved, a change of treatment should be considered. Oral retinoids are options. Acitretin 0.2–0.3 mg/kg/day [33] or alitretinoin 30 mg/day [34–36] can be tried for at least 6 months. Ciclosporin 3–5 mg/kg/day can be considered as monotherapy or as an adjunctive to steroid therapy in severe cases with poor response to steroids [37]. In refractory cases methotrexate [38], antimalarials [39] or etanercept [40] can be tried. Erosive lichen planus of the nail unit may benefit from oral corticosteroids [24] or eventually grafting the nail bed.

NAILS IN CHILDHOOD AND IN THE ELDERLY

Childhood

In early childhood, the nail plate may show physiological alteration [1–3]. The most frequent nail alteration in newborns is the incomplete development of the hallux nail, which is triangular, or sometimes trapezoidal or round-shaped. This may be the same as (apparent) congenital hypertrophy of the lateral folds of the hallux and regresses spontaneously within 1–3 months [2]. Nails in newborns can also be relatively thin and may show temporary koilonychia, onychoschizia or onycholysis [1]. Koilonychia is particularly prominent on the great toes. Neonatal fingernails often have an oval shape, are flat and the lunula may be absent [1]. Beau

Table 93.6 Systemic therapies in common dermatological diseases affecting the nail.

	Ciclosporin	Methotrexate	Systemic corticosteroids	Acitretin	Alitretinoin	Azathioprine	Biologicals
Psoriasis	++	++	−	+	−	−	++
Lichen planus	+	+	++	+	+	−	−
Eczema	++	+	+	−	+	+	+

Justification for all systemic treatments in nail disease may be based on the combined presentation of skin and nails. It is less common to prescribe on the basis of nail disease alone. Course duration can usually be limited to pulses of 3 months in a 9–12-month period, repeated if needed. Doses are as for the cutaneous disease.
++Good choice, with moderate evidence supporting its use.
+Reasonable choice, with case reports or small series supporting use.
−Little or no published evidence.

lines can be seen in up to 92% of normal infants between 4 and 14 weeks of age [4]. Transient light-brown or ochre pigmentation of the proximal nail fold can be found in young infants [5]. Normal surface markings of the nail can differ in children from those seen in adults. Toddlers may present with physiological punctuate leukonychia or pitting. A pattern in which the ridges are oblique and converge distally towards the centre is common up to the age of 3–7 years, and gradually diminishes with time [6]. This is also known as chevron nails or herringbone nails, and may reflect a gradual change in the pattern of matrix maturation [7]. Under the age of 5 years, nails are also prone to distal onychoschizia (lamellar splitting). This can be most prominent on sucked thumbs but is also seen on the toes. Sucking may also lead to paronychia, which can be a troublesome condition in childhood, with pain and nail dystrophy.

Diagnoses in older children frequently depend on the age category [8]. Infants in the 0 to <2 years old age category mainly exhibit congenital hypertrophy of the lateral nail folds and congenital malalignment of the great toenail. Fever-related Beau lines or onychomadesis are predominant in children in the 2 to <6 years old age group. Children in the 6 to <12 years old age group mostly present with trachyonychia and longitudinal melanonychia. Between 12 and 18 years old, trauma is the prevalent diagnosis. Other causes of nail abnormalities, including neoplastic, infectious, systemic, iatrogenic, and/or hereditary/syndromic (including ectodermal dysplasias) are rarer in these age categories. Among congenital and hereditary causes, the nail–patella syndrome, with its pathognomonic triangular lunula, should not be missed as recognition of the disease allows early diagnosis of relevant associated pathologies.

Congenital malalignment of the great toenail is characterised by lateral deviation of the nail plates, which are not parallel to the major axis of the distal phalanx. It is usually bilateral and presents in infancy or childhood [8–10]. The nails are discoloured, ranging from brownish-black to green-brown, and are sometimes shorter, curved, triangular and distally pointed in shape. These changes may subside within 5–10 years in over 50% of children [8,11]. Therefore, a conservative and expectant attitude, based on prevention and treatment of possible complications, is recommended. On the other hand, onycholysis, acute or chronic paronychia, and ingrowing nails may occur. Severe ingrowing toenails in congenital malalignment may be an indication for surgical intervention. If no spontaneous resolution occurs, the condition usually results in severe nail dystrophy and nail plate thickening, which may cause onychogryphosis. Surgical therapy may be considered in patients with severe or complicated forms. In adults it may be reasonable to begin with a conservative approach if the deformity is not psychologically distressing to the patient [12].

Ingrowing nails can cause pain and may present in different forms. At birth, there is often a degree of distal ingrowing, particularly in the great toe, as the nail has not surmounted the tip of the digit in its development [13]. In a more gross form, this may present as congenital hypertrophic lip of the hallux, where soft-tissue overgrowth may resemble fibrous tumours of the digit before it spontaneously disappears [14,15]. Painful distal embedding can lead to infection, but as long as the toenail is properly orientated with respect to the underlying phalanx, the condition usually subsides. In one series of seven children, two needed surgery due to painful persistence of the problem [14].

Trachyonychia or nail roughness is not a distinctive disease but only the clinical result of disorders that involve the nail matrix. It can be present at any age and can be associated with nail matrix localisation of an inflammatory dermatological disease, including alopecia areata, lichen planus, eczema or psoriasis. If no underlying cause can be distinguished it is known as (idiopathic) 20-nail dystrophy of childhood, which has a good prognosis.

Onychomycosis is relatively uncommon in children, with a prevalence of 0.3% [16] to 0.44% [17]. Although extremely rare, *Candida* onychomycosis can be found in neonates [18,19]. The presence of onychomycosis in a child mostly indicates an affected household contact. Both terbinafine and itraconazole are well studied in children with high cure rates of approximately 80% [20]. Both drugs are not licensed for use for treating onychomycosis in children in many countries, but are widely used. Despite the disappointing results of topical onychomycosis treatment, it is assumed that topical treatment may be somewhat more effective in the paediatric population.

Elderly [21–23]

Nail disorders are frequent among the elderly. Ageing causes obvious changes to the nail, some of which are inherently due to age, while others are due to other diseases/conditions which become more prevalent as we age, such as trauma, neoplasms, abnormal biomechanics, and, for example, the high rate of onychomycosis in diabetes, reduced immunity and impaired peripheral blood circulation. Changes in circulation, abnormal biomechanics and cumulative trauma affect the feet more than most other body sites [24]. Age-dependent alterations of the fingernails are mostly cosmetic, while alterations of toenails may cause pain, limit mobility and have profound impact, in particular among frail elderly.

Nail changes in the elderly that may be considered physiological are modifications in growth, contour, colour and consistency [21,25]. In adults, linear nail growth decreases by approximately 0.5–1.0% per year [24,26,27]. Contour changes seen in the elderly are flattening (platyonychia) or development of concave (koilonychia) or convex (clubbing) nails. Longitudinal ridges and a brittle free edge are also age-related phenomena which are present to some degree in most people after 50 years of age. Toenails may develop pincer nail deformity. The colour of the nails gradually will change towards white, yellow or grey, and may mimic Terry nails but without cirrhosis, uraemia or hypoalbuminemia. A modification in colour known as 'Neapolitan nail' is associated with ageing and may reflect an underlying disturbance of collagen: the nails have three different coloured zones: a white proximal part, a normal pink central part and an opaque free edge [28]. The appearance will become opaque and dull with decrease or disappearance of the lunula [29]. Fingernails tend to soften and weaken with age whereas toenails thicken (onychauxis or pachyonychia) and harden [30]. The softer fingernail often becomes fragile and prone to longitudinal fissuring and splitting into layers. The thick and hard toenails frequently have hyperkeratotic lesions and are difficult to cut.

For details of common traumatic abnormalities and changes due to inadequate pedicure or neglect, detailed texts should be consulted [21,31,32]. Nail problems in the elderly are often associated with more widespread mechanical changes of the foot, and it is often more important to focus treatment on maintaining mobility rather than the restoration of normal nails [33,34]. Repeated constraints between shoes and toes are mostly responsible for hyperkeratosis of the nail plate or of the nail bed. The big toenail and the fifth toenail are most often involved, because here friction is most prominent. A subungual clavus is extremely painful and can be seen under the big toenail, mostly in patients with a hallux erectus. In hammer toes, the contracted lesser toe induces hyperkeratosis of the hyponychium due to rubbing against the sole. Distal and lateral onycholysis of the big toenail is common in the elderly. It is caused by overlapping of the second toe on the first one, may be promoted by hallux valgus, or compression from ill-fitting footwear. Pincer nails may arise in patients with osteoarthritis of the distal interphalangeal joint. Also, the treatment of these disorders should focus on keeping the patient ambulant and reduction of pain. Podiatric care is more important than surgical intervention in most circumstances. Nail avulsion with partial or complete phenolisation of the nail matrix may be an option in specific cases. Nail dystrophy from neglected nail care may give rise to the development of onychogryphosis. The huge and abnormal-shaped nail may lead to injury of soft tissues of adjacent digits. Incorrect cutting may also lead to ingrowing toenails, which may have serious consequences in patients with vascular disease, diabetes or neuropathy.

Onychomycosis is one of the most common nail diseases of the elderly and is often combined with elements that will predispose to relapse after treatment, such as traumatic and other nail dystrophy, reduced peripheral circulation, slower growth of nails, suboptimal immune status, diabetes, reduced foot hygiene and increased exposure to disease-causing fungi [21]. The prevalence of onychomycosis is high (~40%) among individuals older than 60 years [35–38]. In patients older than 65 years fungal infections are the third most common dermatological complaint [39]. As in the younger population, dermatophytes are the most common causative agent [40]. There are concerns that drug interactions in this group, especially with azoles, might make systemic therapy a poor choice [41], but a patient in good health can be treated in the same manner as a young adult. In general, terbinafine is the drug of choice for dermatophyte onychomycosis, and adjunct debridement may improve the cure rates. In the elderly, cure rates of systemic treated onychomycosis might be similar or lower than in younger patients [42,43].

Some benign and malignant nail tumours have preference for the elderly. Nail tumours have been discussed in this chapter, but myxoid pseudocysts are the most common benign nail tumours in the elderly. Squamous cell carcinoma has a peak between the ages of 50 and 69 years [21], and mostly is a tumour of a fingernail. Clinically, it may be disguised for some time: it should be considered in all patients with a solitary, long-existing nail dystrophy. Melanoma of the nail unit often presents with longitudinal melanonychia and has a higher mortality rate than melanoma with the same Breslow thickness elsewhere on the skin. It has preference for the great toenail and thumb of elderly patients.

In older patients taking systemic medication, drug-induced nail disorders should be considered. In general, most or all nails (rather than a single nail) will be involved because of the systemic origin of drug-induced disorders. After withdrawal of a suspected drug, in most cases it will take months before this results in evident clinical improvement of the nails. Some frequent drug-induced nail disorders are melanonychia from hydroxyurea or cytostatics, digital necrosis, pincer nails or nail psoriasis from β-blockers, and onycholysis induced by the ACE-inhibitor captopril.

Nail changes in diabetic patients may be secondary to trauma, vasculopathy, infections and peripheral neuropathy. Diabetic microangiopathy in type I diabetes may present as periungual telangiectasias. Peripheral neuropathy or inadequate blood supply to the nail unit, caused by diabetes or other age-dependent factors, may influence both the function of the normal nail matrix and nail bed. Impairment of the matrix may result in the development of Beau lines, pitting, leukonychia punctata, or smooth yellow to yellowish green thickened or overcurved toenails. Nail bed involvement will present with apparent leukonychia or nail bed hyperkeratosis. Subungual hyperkeratosis makes the nails prone to onychomycosis. Other acral complications of diabetes mellitus include ulceration, gangrene and spontaneous development of bullae in patients with a diabetic foot. Bacterial and mycotic infections are common in type 2 diabetes patients. Severe bacterial infections make amputations unavoidable in some patients.

IMAGING OF THE NAIL

X-ray examination

Under normal circumstances, X-ray examination reveals little of the soft structures of the nail unit. It can, however, be useful in identifying a range of pathologies including bony outgrowths, bony resorption, calcification of soft tissues or radio-opaque foreign bodies.

Most isolated nail dystrophies should be X-rayed prior to surgical exploration. Benign space-occupying lesions may compress the underlying bone with corresponding upward convexity in the nail. Osteoid osteoma may be manifest through a characteristic nidus, although X-ray is not sufficient to rule out this pathology and may need to be supplemented with a bone scan or MRI. Chondroid tumours may be located externally to the bone but may be detected by X-ray as a lucency within the bone. Similarly, an X-ray may show evidence of bony invasion by locally invasive or metastatic malignancy.

Acquired acro-osteolysis, acronecrosis and distal phalangeal erosive lesions

Acro-osteolysis in adults is a predominantly bilateral lysis of the distal phalanges of the digits. Radiographs are poor at differentiating longitudinal from transverse acro-osteolysis [1]. Acquired varieties (Box 93.3) are by far the most frequent and usually secondary to a medical condition, trauma or toxins. Investigation of the cause is based more on clinical and laboratory data than on imaging. Idiopathic acro-osteolysis in adulthood may be sporadic or familial.

Occupational acro-osteolysis

Workers involved in the polymerisation of vinyl chloride have developed acro-osteolysis. The other features of this occupational condition are Raynaud phenomenon and scleroderma-like skin changes (Chapter 54). Exposure to vapours of synthetic materials

---

Box 93.3 Causes of acquired acro-osteolysis

- Vinyl chloride exposure
- Drugs (phenytoin, ergot)
- Snake or scorpion venom
- Connective tissue diseases
- Thermal injuries
- Biomechanical stress
- Neuropathic diseases
- Hyperparathyroidism

---

used in the production of other plastic products may occasionally produce similar abnormalities. The acro-osteolysis begins as small cortical erosions that enlarge to produce transverse defects in the terminal phalanges (Figure 93.74a). The isolated phalangeal tuft may then fragment and resorb. If exposure is eliminated, healing may occur with coalescence of phalangeal fragments resulting in pseudoclubbing, the thumb being more commonly affected than other digits.

Connective tissue diseases

Transverse acro-osteolysis is rarely associated with Raynaud phenomenon, rheumatoid vasculitis, psoriasis or scleroderma. When present, acro-osteolysis is almost certainly secondary to vascular compromise.

Bony erosions of the phalanges occur in 40–80% of patients with systemic sclerosis. Gradual resorption of the tuft leads to 'pencilling' of the phalanx and in some patients all of the distal phalanx may be destroyed. The presence of sclerodactyly and/or calcinosis cutis helps indicate the correct diagnosis. 'Whittling' or 'pencilling' of the tufts also occurs in psoriasis and can result in a peg-shaped phalanx (Figure 93.74b) [1]. In acronecrosis, the final stage of acro-osteolysis, the soft tissues in the fingertip telescope around the shortened tuft resulting in pseudoclubbing.

Thermal/biomechemical/neuropathic injuries

Thermal injuries (i.e. frostbite [2], electrical and chemical burns) can result in acronecrosis long after the initial insult and may be due to a combination of mechanical and vascular injury. Phalangeal microgeodic syndrome is an uncommon benign condition described by Maroteaux [3]. Clinical manifestations include swelling and redness of one or more phalanges of one or both hands. Radiological signs encompass multiple small osteolytic areas and sclerosis compatible with acro-osteolysis. A relation to cold exposure has been suggested since patients often present this during the colder months of the year [4]. Acro-osteolysis has been reported in young guitar players [5] probably related to persistent mechanical injury resulting in vascular compromise and avascular necrosis.

Hyperparathyroidism

In hyperparathyroidism and renal osteodystrophy, increased levels of parathyroid hormone produce excessive bone resorption and altered bone formation. The earliest radiological sign of this disease is cortical resorption of the phalangeal tuft [6].

Soft-tissue lesions
Intra-osseous epidermoid implantation cyst

This appears after a penetrating injury. Radiographic examination shows a well-defined cystic lucency in the distal phalanx. It occurs more commonly in the phalangeal tuft, rather than at its base.

Glomus tumour

Pressure on the bone may induce an extrinsic pressure erosion, smooth and concave in most cases [7], although occasionally, with a more 'punched-out' appearance [8].

Keratoacanthoma

Bony destruction of the distal phalanx is present in virtually all cases even shortly after clinical presentation. The destruction is characteristically well-defined, smooth, circular and limited to the tip of the phalanx. The margins of the radiological defect show no evidence of sclerosis or any sign of periosteal reaction [9]. This lytic effect may be attributed to the very rapid compression caused by the tumour rather than to tumour invasion itself. Some patients showed a partial or even complete re-ossification on a long-term follow-up.

Osseous neoplasms
Enchondroma

Enchondroma is a benign tumour arising from mature hyaline cartilage. It is a small well-defined cystic lucency in the phalanx, sometimes having scalloped margins or a sclerotic rim, and is most commonly located centrally in the bone. In the distal phalanx, the enchondroma is typically located at the base of the phalanx, abutting the articular surface.

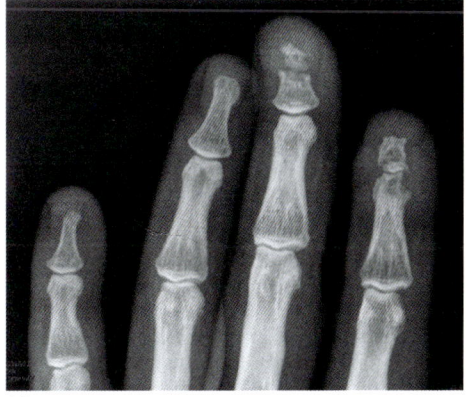
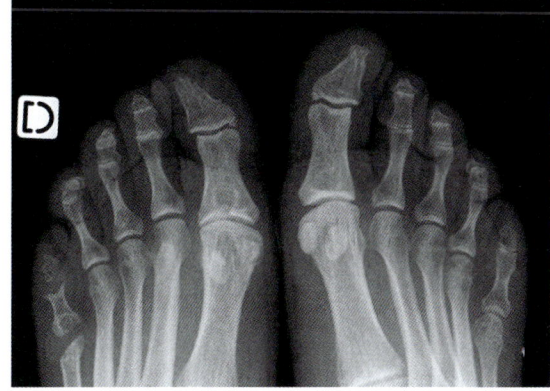

Figure 93.74 Transverse acro-osteolysis of the fingernail (a); acro-osteolysis of the toenail (b). Courtesy of J. L. Drapé.

(a)   (b)

Osteoid osteoma

Osteoid osteoma is a benign osteoblastic lesion consisting of a small oval or round mass, called a nidus, usually smaller than 1 cm. All those affecting the terminal phalanx have a similar appearance characterised by a sclerotic nidus with a radiolucent halo ('ring sequestrum') [10]. It is, however, better visualised on computed tomography.

Aneurysmal bone cysts and giant cell tumours

These tumours rarely occur in the distal phalanges. Both may have similar radiological features characterised by lytic expansive lesions involving the entire phalanx [11].

Haemangiomas

Haemangiomas may arise in the bone or soft tissue of the distal phalanx. When primary in the bone, they have a characteristic radiographic appearance of linear striations parallel to the shaft of the bone. Soft-tissue haemangiomas are more common and may manifest as local soft-tissue masses, localised bony overgrowth, phleboliths in the soft tissue and pressure erosion of the underlying bone.

Ultrasound imaging

Ideally, a hockey stick-shaped and variable-frequency probe that works with frequencies over 15 MHz should be used for the examination (Figure 93.75a). The machines are capable of detecting the blood flow of the nail bed in real time and three-dimensional reconstructions may also provide valuable information concerning tumour size, location, shape and internal characteristics (Figure 93.75b). Ultrasound can show submillimetre structures and discriminate tissue characteristics difficult to detect with CT or MRI units.

Ultrasound imaging is a powerful tool in daily practice in many nail conditions. It helps mainly to differentiate solid from cystic lesions and locate radio-opaque foreign bodies.

Ultrasound is playing an increasingly important role in the early diagnosis and monitoring of psoriatic arthritis. Both ultrasound and magnetic resonance imaging can be used to diagnose enthesitis and dactylitis due to psoriasis, especially in patients in whom symptoms may be difficult to discern [12].

Normal sonographic examination of a normal nail unit shows three main areas: the nail plate, the nail bed and the paronychial tissues. The dorsal and ventral plates present a bilaminar hyperechoic structure (two parallel lines) separated by a very thin hypoechoic layer (interplate space). Low-velocity arterial and venous vessels are usually detectable within the nail bed (colour Doppler with spectral curve analysis) (Figure 93.75c). The distal insertion of the lateral bands of the extensor tendon in the distal phalanx shows a fibrillar hyperechoic pattern, typical of tendinous structures. The bony margin of the distal phalanx shows a continuous hyperechoic line following the contour of the cortex of the bone that is only interrupted by the anechogenicity of the distal interphalangeal joint space, which contains fluid and cartilage (Figure 93.75d) [13].

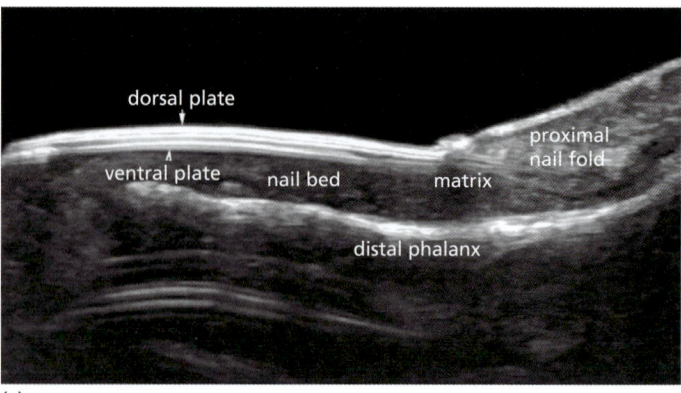

(a)

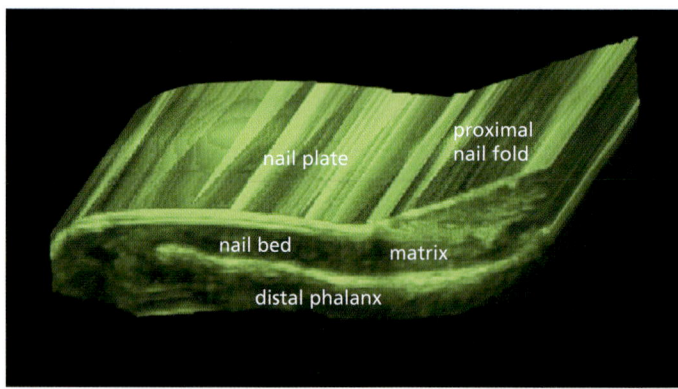

(b)

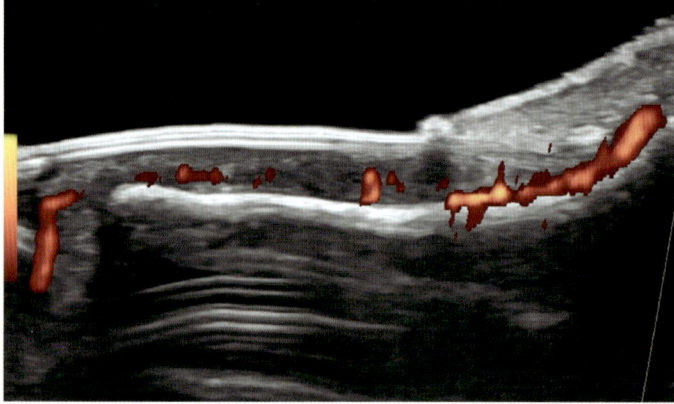

(c)

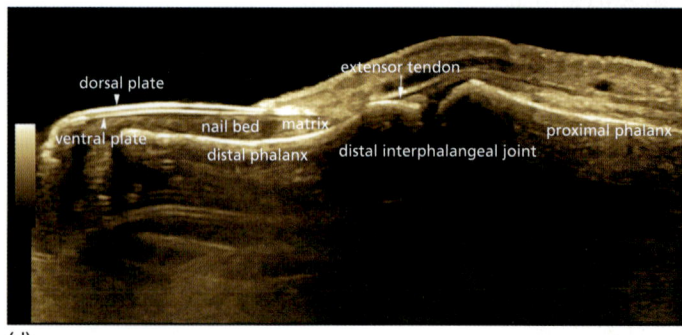

(d)

Figure 93.75 Ultrasound: grey scale ultrasound (longitudinal view) demonstrates the normal sonographic anatomy of the nail (a); 3D ultrasound reconstruction of the nail (longitudinal view) (b); power Doppler ultrasound (longitudinal view) shows the blood flow within the nail bed (c); extended field of view of the nail and periungual structures (longitudinal view) (d).

Optical coherence tomography

Optical coherence tomography (OCT) is an optical analogue of ultrasound, using infrared instead of acoustic waves [14]. The reflection of infrared light from the tissue is measured by interferometry and two-dimensional grey scale images are generated. Images reflecting the different layers may be either horizontal or vertical (similar to ultrasound). Functional aspects such as speckle variation and vascular flow may be included in some equipment. Three-dimensional images can be generated. OCT has a very high resolution (5–10 μm) but a very low penetrance (2 mm), thus limiting its use to very superficial tissues.

It has been claimed that OCT can differentiate morphological details and nail thickness better than high-resolution ultrasound and thus it has been advocated as an assessment tool for onychomycosis. One study showed that OCT may be a useful assistance tool to increase diagnostic sensitivity of nail scrapings – but cannot replace specific identification – as well as for monitoring treatment response in onychomycosis [15].

Furthermore, OCT imaging is consistent with both physical and ultrasound findings in patients with symptomatic psoriatic nail disease. Given that OCT can also measure nail plate thickness, OCT has the potential to provide more objective and informative quantitative data for use in outcome measures for interventional trials in psoriatic nail disease.

Reflectance confocal microscopy (RCM)

In RCM, a near-infrared light from a diode laser is focused on a microscopic skin target and is naturally reflected by the different cellular structures. The reflected light is then captured and recomposed into a two-dimensional grey scale image by computer software. RCM gives horizontal images of the analysed tissue. Penetration is around 200–300 μm and resolution is between 1.5 and 5 μm which is near histological resolution.

No stains are required for RCM imaging. Skin and nails are ideal locations for exploration by RCM. This mainly *in vivo* technique is only available in a few centres worldwide and has a very long learning curve.

Two main applications have interested dermatologists so far:

1 RCM and onychomycosis. Hongcharu *et al.* [16] first reported the possible application of *in vivo* RCM for the diagnosis of onychomycosis. A study on 58 patients demonstrated that RCM permitted a faster examination with the same accuracy as standard mycological tests (potassium hydroxide preparation and fungal culture) [17].

2 RCM and melanonychia. Intraoperative dermoscopy and RCM have recently been advocated for better visualisation of nail matrix pigmentation during exploratory nail surgery for melanonychia (Figure 93.76). In most cases, the RCM images obtained either *ex vivo/in vivo* revealed sufficiently atypical cytological and architectural features to indicate accurately the correct final diagnosis of melanoma with a good correlation with histopathology [18].

In skin and nails, RCM combines the advantages of dermoscopy (non-invasive examination of the whole area of interest without alteration of the epithelial surface) and histopathology (resolution at a cellular level). RCM enables melanocytes to be distinguished readily from adjacent structures and permits the visualisation of the architectural and cytological features of the melanocytic proliferation. *Ex vivo* examination can be used as a complementary technique if the data provided by *in vivo* examination are not diagnostically valid.

Computed tomography

This imaging technique is of very little value in the exploration of the nail unit except for osteoid osteoma where it shows a small lucent bone area within a focal hypertrophy of the phalangeal tuft.

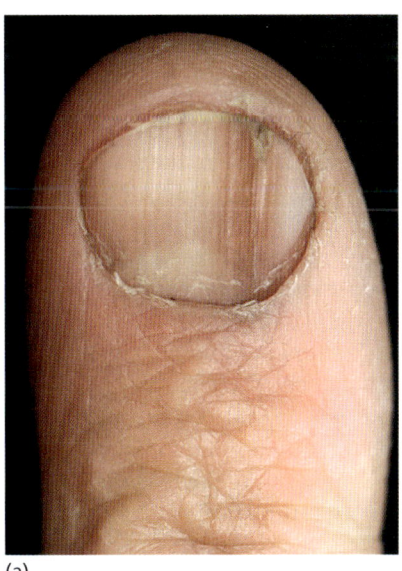
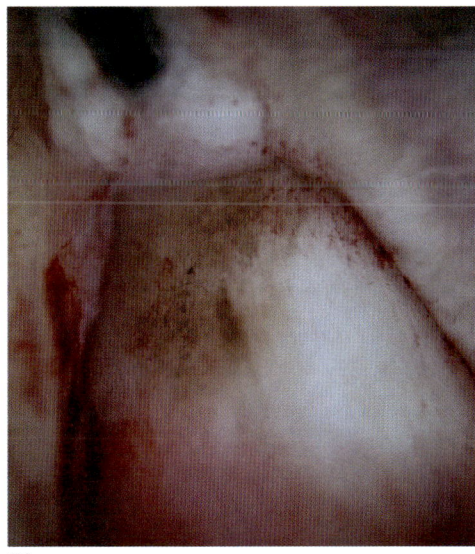
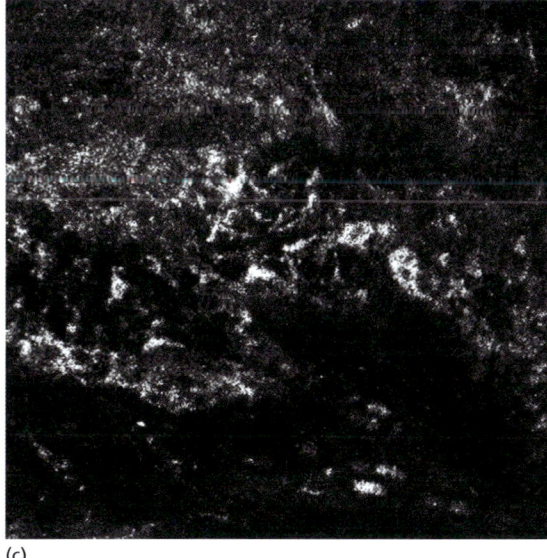

(a)   (b)   (c)

Figure 93.76 Nail melanoma: clinical presentation (a); dermoscopy (b) and *in vivo* reflectance confocal microscopy (c) of the nail matrix in the same patient. Courtesy of L. Thomas.

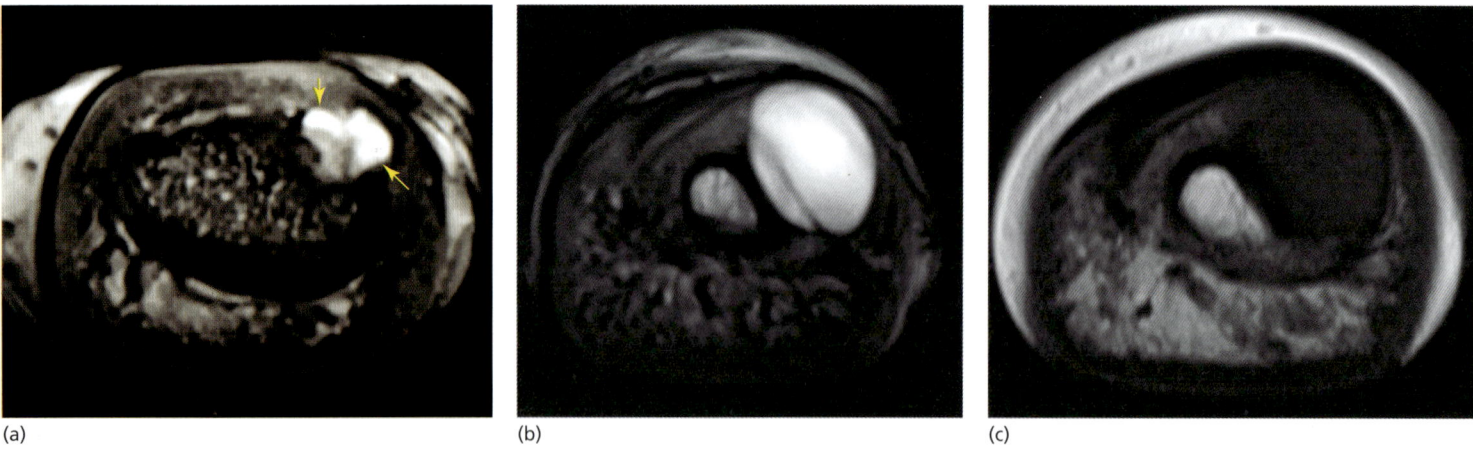

(a)   (b)   (c)

Figure 93.77 Axial T2-weighted image at the level of the distal interphalangeal joint (arrows): pedicle of the myxoid pseudocyst connected with the joint (arrows) (a). Axial T2 (b) and axial T1 (c) at the level of the nail cul-de-sac: lifting of the matrix and the root of the nail plate due to the cyst; bone scalloping of the dorsolateral aspect of the distal phalanx. Courtesy of J. L. Drapé.

Magnetic resonance imaging

Magnetic resonance imaging (MRI) is well known for its high contrast of soft tissue. At the nail unit, it is indicated when ultrasound findings are equivocal and will provide a more specific pattern of the tumours. Small surface coils dedicated to finger imaging are optimum and available with all 1.5 or 3 Tesla whole body MRI units [19]. MRI can detect tumours as little as 1 mm in diameter and defines their location and tissue characteristics, all of which facilitates surgical management. A T1-weighted sequence allows morphological evaluation of lesion contour and anatomical extent; a T2-weighted sequence defines tissue characterisation from signal intensity emitted by the tumour; gadolinium highlights the vascularisation of tumours and may improve definition of lesion contours. The signals obtained in the various sequences are characteristic and can distinguish the most common tumours encountered in the nail region [19].

MRI can be helpful for investigating a range of periungual neoplasms and cysts. It is the gold standard for assessing glomus tumours of the nail unit and is particularly useful for myxoid (synovial) cysts, where even normal soft tissues can be distinguished and an *in vivo* anatomical assessment made (Figure 93.77a–c and Figure 93.78). MRI can help identify the inflammatory changes of psoriatic arthritis [20], where it has consequences for the soft-tissue element of the nail unit resulting in abnormal nail growth and appearance.

Proximal nail fold capillaroscopy

Proximal nail fold capillaroscopy is a simple *in vivo* non-invasive and reliable technique used for evaluating superficial microvascular structures. The capillaroscope is composed of an optical microscope with a 50× to 200× magnification. A cold light source is used in order to avoid vasodilatation. It is of particular value for examining the microvasculature of the proximal nail fold, with its special arrangement of vascular loops parallel to the skin surface, which cannot be well visualised by the naked eye.

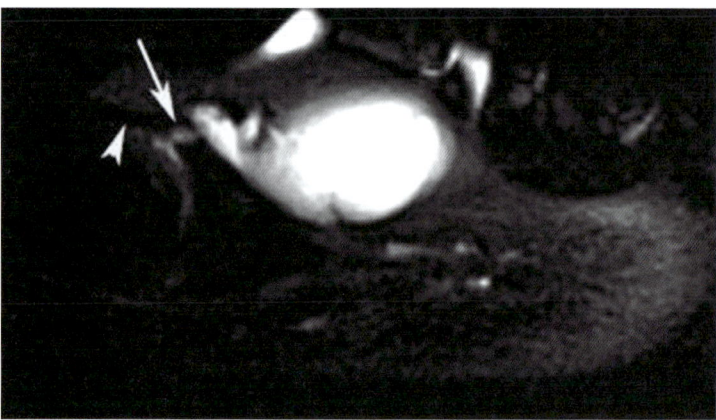

Figure 93.78 Sagittal section T2 fat saturated image: pedicle connecting with the joint (arrow) under the extensor tendon (arrow heads). Courtesy of J. L. Drapé.

Skin is 'prepared' with an ointment of cedar oil or liquid petrolatum in order to improve optical transmission. Second, third, fourth and fifth fingernails of both hands are examined consecutively. Some authors have suggested that a dermoscope (or an ophthalmoscope) can be used for capillaroscopic examination of the proximal nail fold. The lower magnification permits visualisation of megacapillaries but is insufficient to explore other components of the bloodstream in detail.

Useful information can be obtained by an overall examination of the microvascular structure of the proximal nail folds. Capillary loops physiologically have a hairpin shape and are arranged in two parallel longitudinal rows: usually 12–18 loops are found per millimetre (Figure 93.79a). Proximal to and arranged perpendicularly to them, the subpapillary veins can be visualised. It is important to recognise a number of different patterns of no pathological significance: these include a glomerular conformation and elongated and tortuous loops. Pathological changes include ramified vessels, elongated loops, megacapillaries, loss of the normal parallel arrangement of loops and microaneurysms. Under the highest magnification, blood flow can be directly observed: either a normal continuous flow or a pathological intermittent flow with

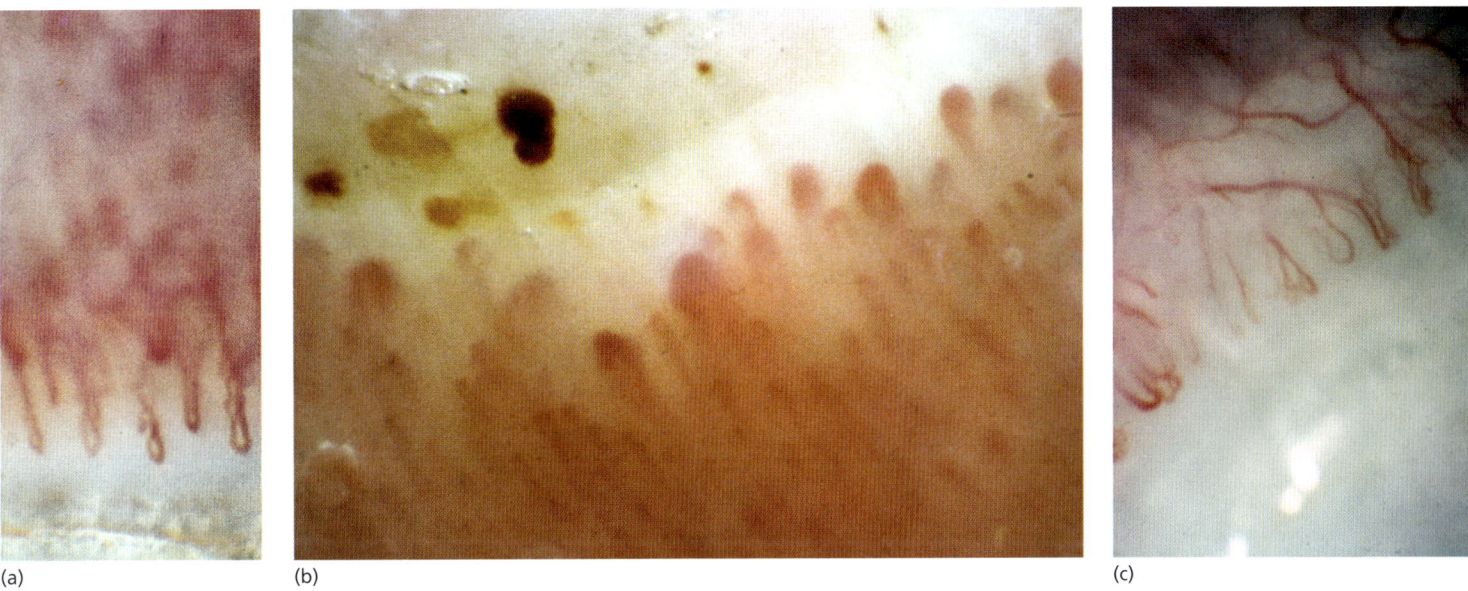

(a)   (b)   (c)

Figure 93.79 Normal nail fold capillaries (×60) (a); acrocyanosis showing dilatation of the nail fold capillaries, stasis and thrombosis of many vessels (b); rheumatoid arthritis showing rather elongated capillary loops (c).

irregular interruptions occurring over time. Vasomotor tone can be evaluated subjectively by detailed observation of a vascular field. It is overactive in idiopathic Raynaud phenomenon and decreased in acrocyanosis. In lupus erythematosus, rapid and marked changes in vasomotor tone can be observed within the same capillary loop. It should be noted that deep epidermal pigmentation may reduce the visibility of the capillary loops.

Examination of the background may also yield useful information. In lightly pigmented skin, the background colour is pinkish, but can be orange if there is venous stasis. A pericapillary halo can be observed in inflammatory conditions and in cases of vascular stasis. A 'hazy' appearance may be seen in systemic sclerosis. Haemorrhages are observed in cases of evolving microangiopathy: a 'pearl necklace' appearance differentiates these from trauma-induced haemorrhages where the appearance is blotchy [21].

Acrosyndromes
Raynaud phenomenon
Raynaud phenomenon may be either idiopathic, Raynaud disease, or associated with a connective tissue disease (Raynaud sign or symptom). The most important indication for capillaroscopy is in the differential diagnosis between these two situations with very different prognoses. In Raynaud disease capillaroscopy is normal. Rarely, efferent capillaries can be found to be somewhat enlarged and some subtle haemorrhages can be observed. During the vasoconstrictive phase, a whitish background and a reduction in the number of visible capillaries can be observed. The appearances in connective tissue disease are discussed below.

Acrocyanosis
Acrocyanosis is clinically characterised by a painless distal cyanosis often with hyperhidrosis and cold extremities. This disease is worsened by exposure to cold. Capillaroscopy shows a normal or slightly increased number of capillaries of slightly enlarged

diameter (especially in the efferent part of the loop). The loops are often tortuous over a cyanotic background. The blood flow is slowed and often has a granular appearance (Figure 93.79b).

Livedo
In livedo reticularis, capillaroscopy shows enlarged efferent loops intermixed with normal loops and the blood flow is slowed. In livedo racemosa ('broken livedo') microvasculitis can sometimes be detected.

Chilblains (perniosis)
In chilblains affecting the fingers, homogeneously dilated vascular loops are observed in association with normal loops.

Systemic autoimmune diseases
Rheumatoid arthritis
Signs of dermal vasculitis are observed with tortuous and ramified capillary loops (Figure 93.79c). In some cases, short parallel loops in a 'fish shoal'-like pattern are observed. Background is not hazy and the blood flow is granular and fast.

Dermatomyositis
The clinically visible telangiectasias of the cuticle correspond to megacapillaries as seen under the capillaroscope (Figure 93.80). However, in contrast with systemic sclerosis, there are no avascular areas.

Lupus erythematosus
In lupus erythematosus, observed abnormalities are morphological and rheological. Elongated loops, irregular enlargement of the afferent and/or efferent vessels, ramified and in some cases tortuous loops, and microaneurysms are the most common morphological changes (Figure 93.81a) [22].

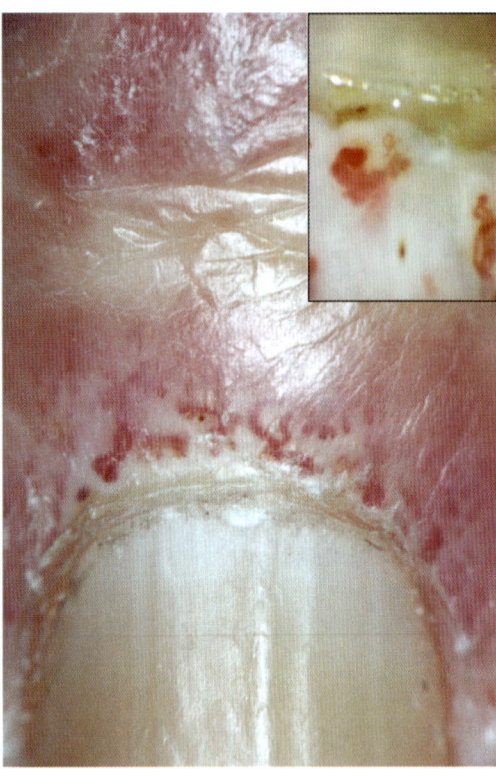

Figure 93.80 Dermatomyositis showing dilated nail folds capillaries and obstructed and thrombosed capillaries (×60) (inset).

Systemic sclerosis

Typical changes are observed in systemic sclerosis (Figure 93.81b) and nail fold video-capillaroscopy [23,24] is at present the most valuable tool for allowing an early diagnosis as follows:
- Rarefaction of the capillary loops with avascular areas.
- Megacapillaries of different size and shape often corresponding to the clinically visible telangiectasias of the cuticle.
- Granular blood flow.
- Few haemorrhages.

Four stages are usually recognised as follows:
- Stage I: appearance of a few 'open' loops, 'U-shaped' and a few slightly enlarged capillaries.
- Stage II: slight decrease in the number of capillary loops, a few megacapillaries among many normal loops, hazy background.
- Stage III: marked decrease in the number of capillary loops, many megacapillaries, atrophic capillary loops, very hazy background.
- Stage IV: many avascular areas, reduced number of megacapillaries, very hazy background.

Psoriasis

Cutaneous microcirculation is different in psoriatic patients and normal individuals.

Vascular changes have been reported in nail folds. For this reason, Ribeiro *et al.* [25] studied psoriatic nail fold video-capillaroscopy in 46 patients (mean age 50.5, median disease duration 10 years) and 50 healthy controls and found lower capillary density, increase of avascular areas and morphologically abnormal capillaries in psoriatic subjects. No association between changes in capillary density and duration, extent or severity of the disease was noted. However, the presence of avascular areas was more common in patients whose nails were affected by the disease (pitting or dystrophy).

Toxic diseases

Vinyl chloride poisoning produces sclerodactyly. Capillaroscopy shows megacapillaries without decreased vascular density or avascular areas. The background is not hazy.

NAIL SURGERY

Introduction and general description

Patients often fear nail surgery because of anticipated pain, both during anaesthesia and postoperatively. The potential for causing permanent postoperative nail dystrophy frightens the practitioner.

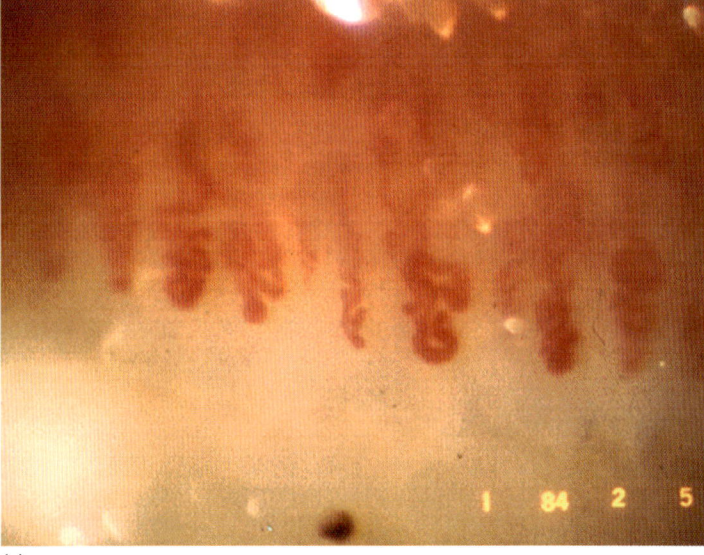

(a)

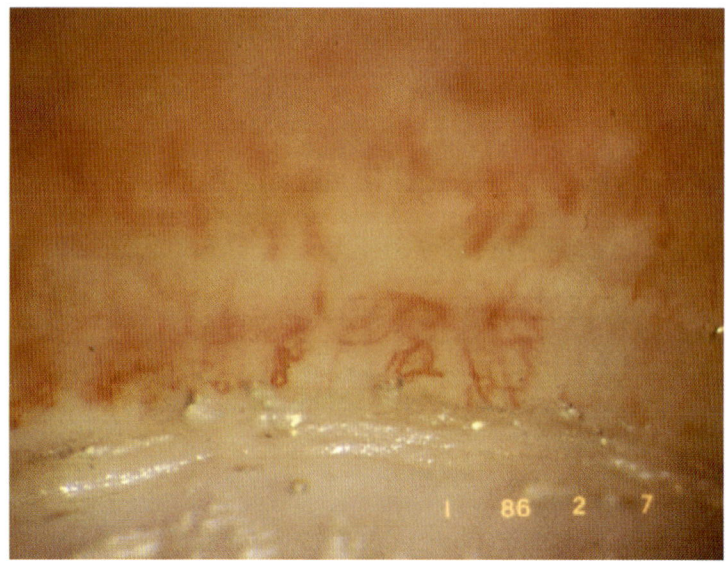

(b)

Figure 93.81 Lupus erythematosus (a) and systemic sclerosis (b). Courtesy of C. Mathys.

A good knowledge of anaesthetic techniques, nail anatomy and surgical procedures is a prerequisite for a successful nail surgery with almost no pain and minimal scarring. It is also mandatory to involve a dermatopathologist who is familiar with the histological idiosyncrasies of the nail unit.

Anaesthesia

Premedication

Premedication may be useful in anxious patients. Short action molecules should be preferred: hydroxyzine, diazepines, orally or sublingually, the latter acting more rapidly. The combination of hydroxyzine 25 mg the night before the operation with 0.5 mg lorazepam sublingually 1 h prior to surgery is very effective [1]. Midazolam is favoured by some surgeons as it has short-acting hypnotic, anxiolytic and retrograde amnesic properties [2]. The use of EMLA under an occlusive dressing prior to surgery will only alleviate the pain caused by needle insertion but not that due to injection of local anaesthetic and distension of tissues [3].

Equipment

Injections into the nail apparatus encounter high resistance and the use of a Luer lock syringe is mandatory. Using very thin needles (30 G) will decrease pain from puncture and limit the anaesthetic flow and rate of distension of the soft tissues. It is common for the physician to spend more time administering the anaesthesia than performing the surgical procedure.

Anaesthetics

Plain lidocaine 1% or 2% is the reference local anaesthetic. It acts for 60 min. As it is acid, pain during infusion may be reduced by prior alkalinisation [4]. Warming the anaesthetic to 37°C also reduces the pain associated with infusion [5].

Lidocaine with epinephrine (adrenaline) is safe in the digits [6–9] except in patients with vasospastic, thrombotic or severe medical conditions. However, the use of epinephrine is of little interest in nail surgery as, to achieve a bloodless field, a tourniquet must be placed at the base of the digit in almost all procedures. Bupivacaine 0.5% acts after 45 min for up to 480 min [10]. It may be added to lidocaine to lengthen the postoperative analgesia. An alternative is to inject 0.5 1 mL of bupivacaine immediately postoperatively into the lateral aspect of the digit: this will act as a 'volumetric' tourniquet and prevent further bleeding [11]. Ropivacaine has the same quick onset as lidocaine, provides better postoperative pain relief [12–14] and is less cardiotoxic than bupivacaine [15]. Pain at infiltration depends on concentration. For routine use, a 2 mg/mL concentration provides a very comfortable anaesthesia with full sensation restored by 7 h. Ropivacaine produces slight vasoconstriction at low dosages [16].

Procedures

The so-called 'ring block' is still very popular but it should no longer be recommended. Its main drawbacks are the 'late' anaesthetic effect, requiring up to 20 min to develop, and the potential hazard of compression and trauma to neurovascular bundles with subsequent postoperative oedema and prolonged pain [17].

The distal digital block is the technique of choice for many in nail surgery. The injection site is 1 cm proximal and lateral to the junction of the proximal nail fold and the lateral nail fold. The needle is pushed at a 45° angle directed distally, down to the bone. The branches of the dorsal nerve are anaesthetised by 0.5 mL of anaesthetic. The needle is then partially withdrawn and pushed down vertically skimming the lateral aspect of the phalanx towards the pulp where another 0.5 mL are deposited to block the branches of the palmar nerves. For complete anaesthesia, the procedure should be repeated on the opposite side. Anaesthesia takes effect immediately. (See Video 93.1 for a video of this procedure.)

Instrumentation

Basic nail surgery requires only very few specific instruments. The classic tray should include an elevator to detach the plate from its attachments (e.g. Freer or Locke elevator, or a dental spatula), a nail splitter, straight haemostat, fine iris or Gradle scissors, no. 15 surgical blade, fine-toothed Adson forceps, a fine-needle holder, 3/0 and 4/0 non-absorbable sutures.

Diagnostic surgery

Proximal nail fold biopsy

Two techniques are available for taking a biopsy in this area:
- When the indication is similar to a biopsy elsewhere on the skin, a punch biopsy (not over 3 mm) may be taken on the proximal nail fold, taking care that its distal margin is always preserved. The defect may be left for secondary intention healing.
- The shave biopsy technique is also very useful for this area. Haemostasis can be obtained with aluminium chloride solution.

Nail bed biopsy

Indications for nail bed biopsies are diseases of the nail bed presenting as onycholysis, subungual hyperkeratosis or tumour. In the absence of onycholysis, a partial or total nail avulsion (see later) should be performed to expose the area to be biopsied. As for skin, incisional biopsy is performed with a punch and excisional biopsy with a blade. The punch should be pushed down to the bone. No suture is required, as a defect up to 4 mm across will heal by secondary intention without dystrophy.

Elliptical biopsy of the nail bed is indicated to remove larger specimens (e.g. small tumours). The elliptical excision should always be orientated in a longitudinal axis. The nail bed is very fragile and tightly adherent to the bone so that reapproximation of the margins may be difficult. To overcome this, lateral undermining of the edges should be generous. Suturing may leave a gap that will heal by secondary intention.

Nail matrix biopsy

Matrix biopsies are most useful for longitudinal melanonychia. An accurate histological diagnosis requires examination of the entire pigmented lesion and therefore incisional biopsies are not recommended; only excisional biopsies should be performed. Dystrophic sequelae are unlikely if the pigment is confined to the distal matrix, as the latter synthesises the ventral part of the nail plate. The only consequence will be a nail plate thinned from below. Fortunately, in the majority of cases longitudinal melanonychia originates in the distal matrix [18]. If the pigment is located within or extends to the proximal matrix, a nail plate dystrophy is highly probable, as this part of the matrix generates the upper third of the nail plate.

Several techniques are available according to the width and shape of the band. Each of the following procedures starts identically in order to expose the whole nail matrix. Using an elevator, the proximal nail fold is detached from the nail plate; two lateral incisions at 45° enable it to be reflected. Then, a lateral avulsion ('sardine tin' avulsion) of the proximal third of the nail plate exposes the whole matrix and the most proximal part of the nail bed.

1 For a well-circumscribed round pigmented lesion of <3 mm in diameter located in the distal matrix, the punch biopsy technique is best [19]. A 3 mm punch encompassing the whole pigmented macule is pushed vertically into the matrix down to the bone (Figure 93.82a–d). The defect is left open and the nail plate is

laid back in place and sutured to the lateral nail fold. Punching through the nail plate at the origin of the longitudinal melanonychia before avulsing is very useful when dealing with lightly pigmented bands: the process of avulsion often detaches the superficial layers of the matrix epithelium and the origin of the band may then be difficult to identify. By performing a punch in this manner, the area to biopsy can be clearly seen once the nail plate has been avulsed [20].

2 If the source of pigment is orientated longitudinally, it should be excised using a longitudinal ellipse with minimal margins. The edges of the incision are widely undermined and reapproximated with 5/0 or 6/0 absorbable sutures (Figure 93.83a–d). The nail is laid back in place and sutured to the lateral nail fold. The proximal nail fold is returned to its anatomical position and the lateral incisions are sutured [20].

3 If the source of pigment is orientated horizontally, and for very extensive pigmentation (>6 mm in diameter), the tangential excision is recommended. A shallow incision is carried out around the pigmented zone. The scalpel is then held horizontally

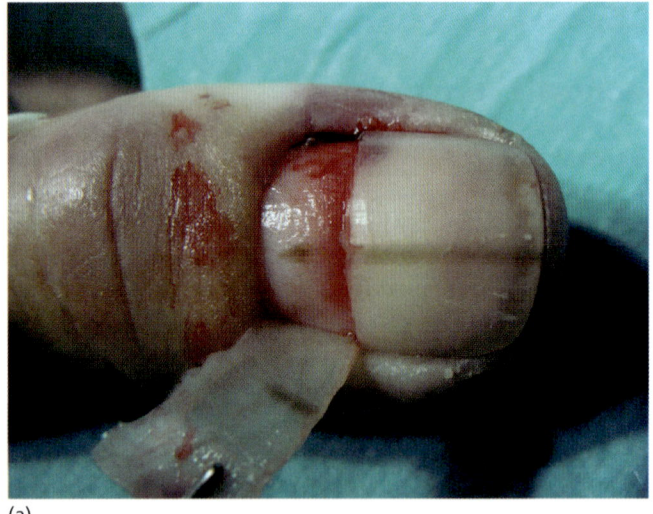

(a)

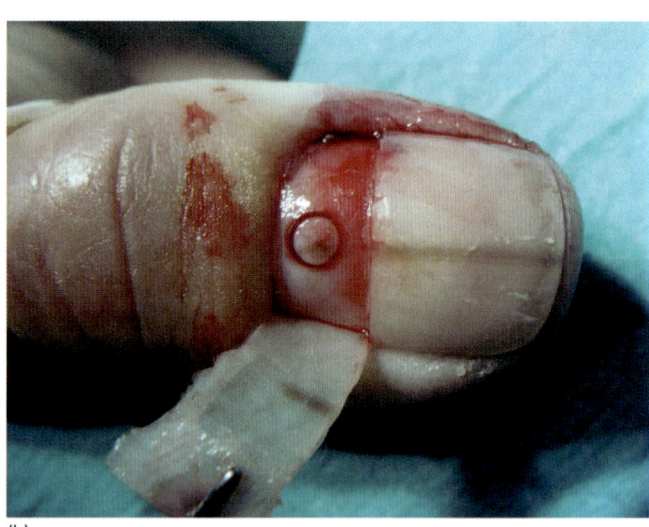

(b)

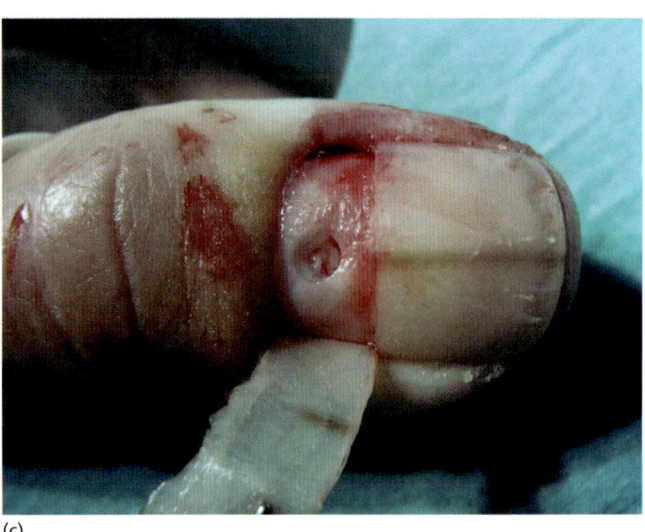

(c)

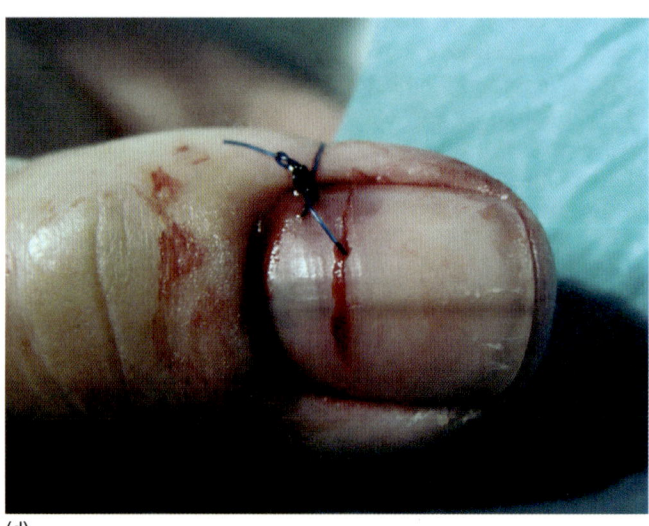

(d)

Figure 93.82 (a) Avulsion of the proximal third of the plate exposes the pigment area responsible for the longitudinal pigmentation. (b) A 3 mm punch is performed around the whole pigmented area. (c) The specimen is removed down to the bone. (d) The plate is put back in place and secured to the lateral fold.

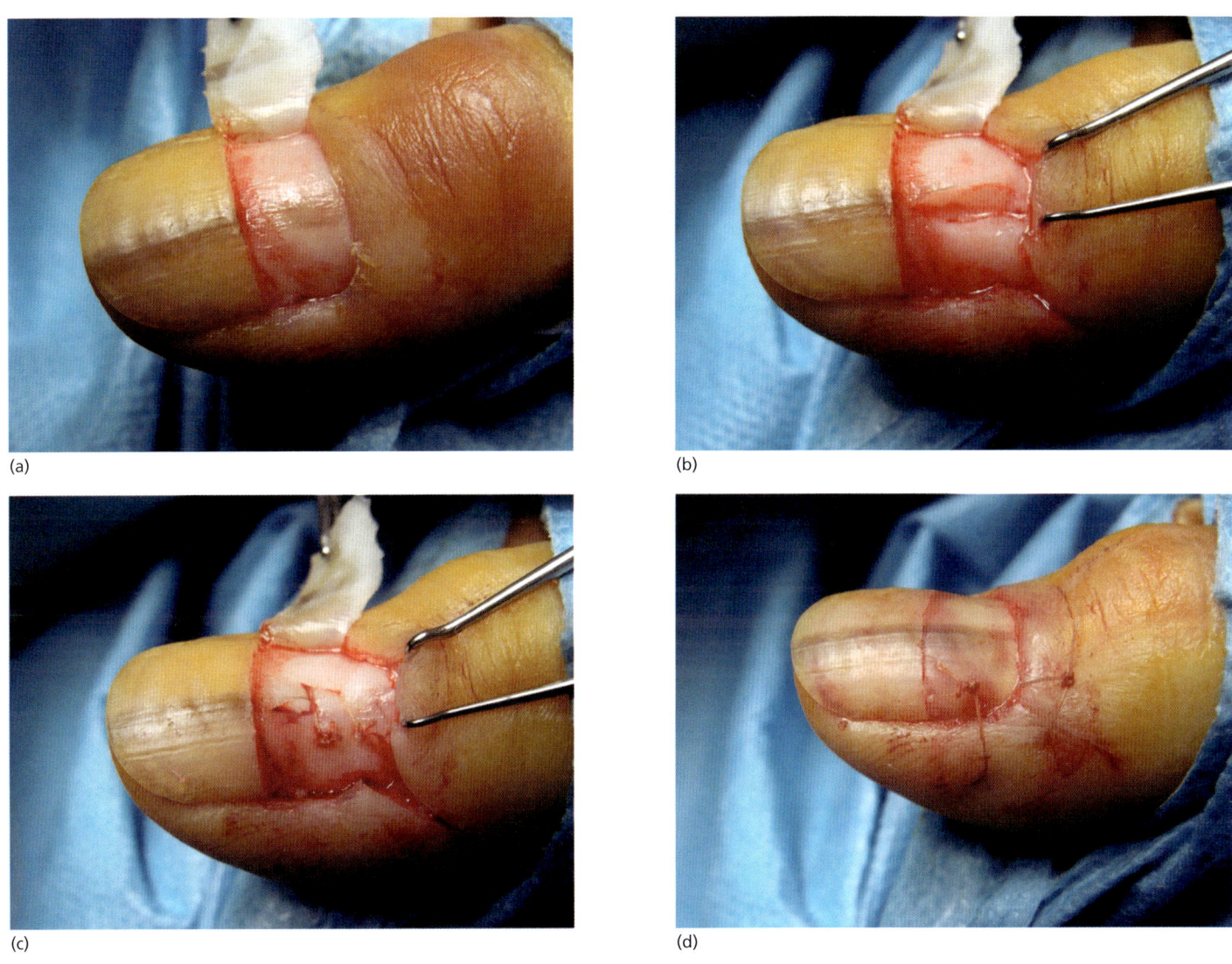

(a)   (b)

(c)   (d)

Figure 93.83 (a) Avulsion of the proximal third of the plate demonstrates that the pigment area responsible for the pigmentation extends longitudinally on the matrix. (b) The whole pigmented area is removed in a longitudinal elliptical excision. (c) After undermining the wedges, the defect is reapproximated with absorbable sutures. (d) The plate is put back in place and secured to the lateral nail fold.

and with sawing motions the lesion is removed from the deep dermis. It should not be thicker than 0.5 mm. The specimen is placed on filter paper and properly orientated for the pathologist. The avulsed nail is put back and secured to the lateral fold. This technique has proven sufficient to allow adequate diagnosis in all cases. Its main drawback is a recurrence of the pigmentation in about three quarters of cases [21]. This technique should be restricted to large pigmented bands that were formerly an indication for immediate total ablation of the nail unit (Figure 93.84a–d). This technique avoids mutilating surgery in cases where the pigment derives from a large benign lesion. If histopathology shows that the lesion is malignant, further surgery is required.

Biopsy of whole structures of nail apparatus

The lateral longitudinal biopsy permits study of all components of the nail unit: proximal nail fold, matrix, nail bed, nail plate and hyponychium. This is the most rewarding biopsy technique when dealing with a disease presenting as alterations of the nail plate

surface. This will narrow the nail permanently due to the partial amputation of the lateral horn of the matrix. In order to avoid any postoperative lateral deviation, the specimen should not exceed 3 mm in width [22]. The incision starts halfway between the cuticle and the crease of the distal interphalangeal joint and runs distally through the proximal nail fold, the nail plate and its bed to the hyponychium. At the junction of the lateral and proximal nail fold, the incision should follow a laterally curved direction extending halfway down the lateral aspect of the finger as far as the distal interphalangeal joint, in order to ensure removal of the lateral horn of the matrix. A second incision, starting from the distal extremity of the previous one, runs from the hyponychium into the lateral sulcus and joins the proximal end of the previous incision. The resulting sigmoid biopsy specimen (Figure 93.85) is then carefully detached from the bone with fine scissors. At the proximal end of the biopsy, care must be taken to include the matrix by avoiding lifting the scissors too soon and thus foreshortening the specimen. The defect is reapproximated with horizontal mattress sutures in order to recreate a lateral nail fold [23].

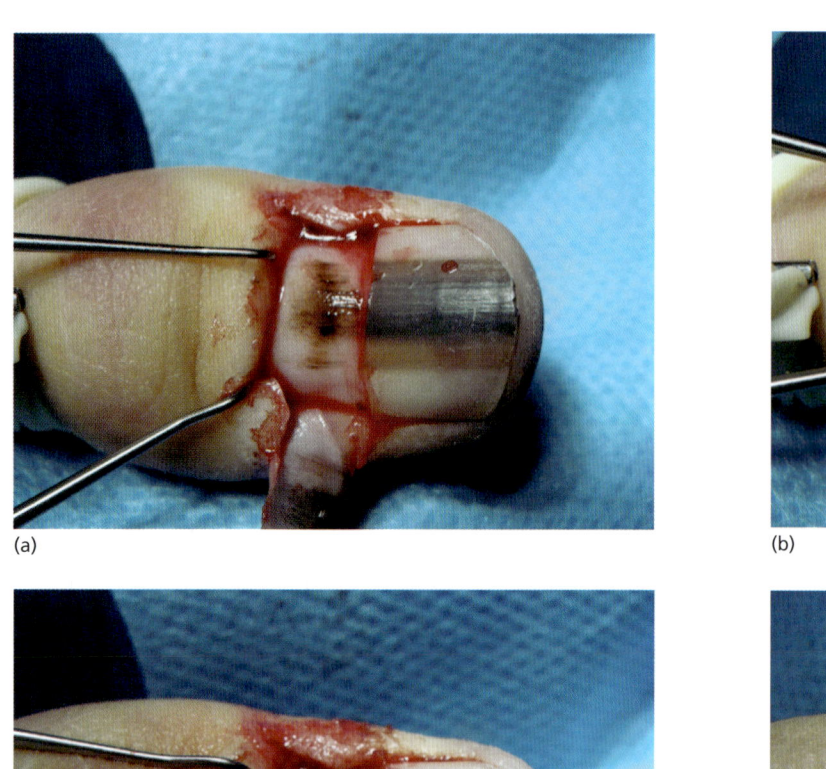

(a)

(b)

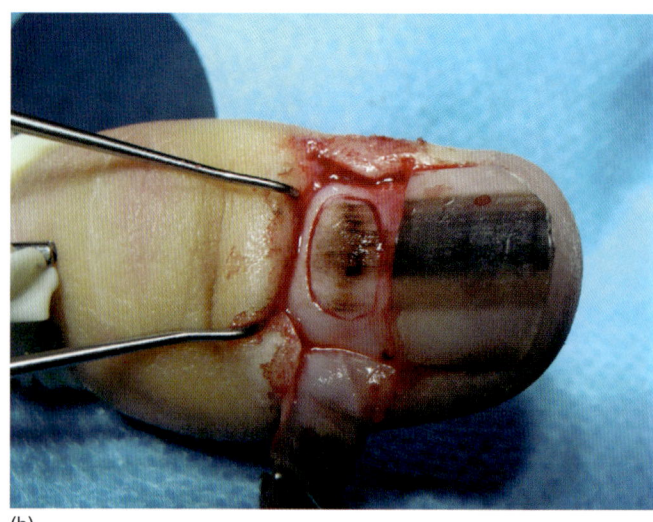

(c)

(d)

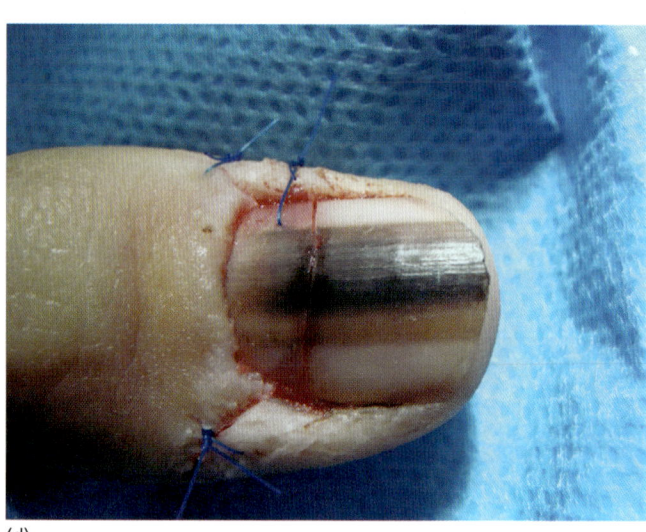

Figure 93.84 (a) Avulsion of the proximal third of the plate exposes the wide pigment area responsible for the longitudinal pigmentation. (b) An incision is carried out all around the whole pigmented area. (c) The specimen is tangentially removed as a whole. (d) The plate is put back in place and secured to the lateral nail fold.

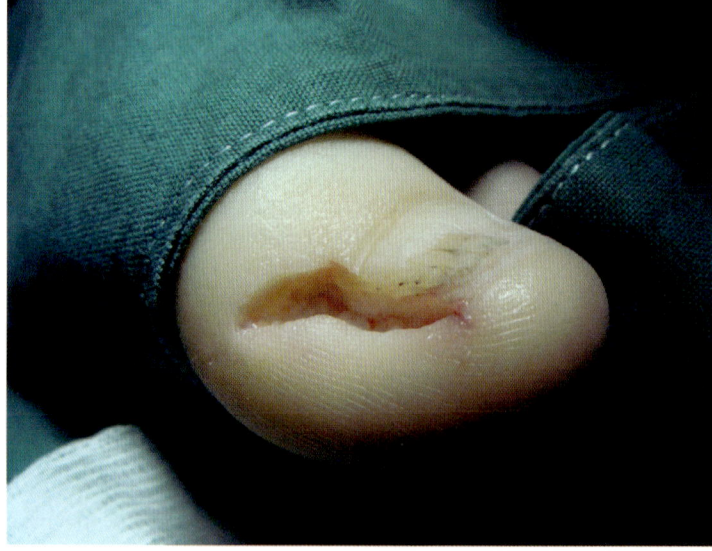

Figure 93.85 Lateral longitudinal biopsy. Note the sigmoid shape of the defect that can be easily closed.

Excisional surgery

Nail avulsion

Nail avulsion is a core procedure in nail surgery: it allows inspection of and access to a subungual lesion in the nail bed or matrix for biopsy or excision (Figure 93.86); it is an adjuvant treatment in onychomycosis as it reduces the fungal mass; it is part of the treatment of an acute paronychia and of ingrowing toenail. Total surgical removal should be discouraged: the distal nail bed may shrink and become distorted dorsally. In addition, the loss of counterpressure from the nail plate allows dorsal expansion of the distal pulp, promoting distal embedding. Partial nail avulsion should always be favoured. However, in some instances (e.g. prominent dystrophic total onychomycosis) total avulsion is unavoidable.

Total surgical nail avulsion

This may be carried out using either a distal or a proximal approach.

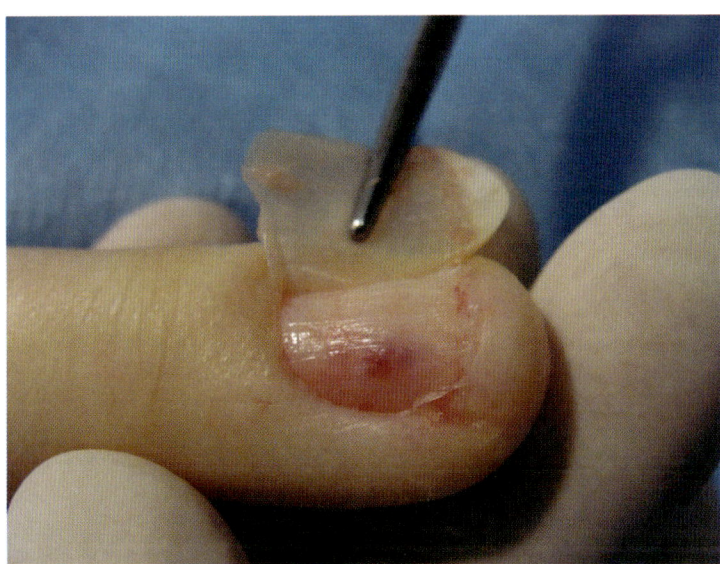

Figure 93.86 Lateral avulsion ('sardine tin' avulsion) allows exposure of the complete nail bed and excisional biopsy of the nail bed tumour.

Distal approach

An elevator is gently slid under the proximal nail fold in a back-and-forth motion from side to side, so avoiding injuring the fragile longitudinal nail bed ridges, until the proximal nail fold is freed from the nail plate. The elevator is then pushed under the nail plate from the distal free edge until the elevator gives way (meaning the elevator has reached the matrix area to which the nail plate is loosely attached). Caution must be taken to detach the lateral horns of the nail plate fully. A jaw of a sturdy haemostat is slid under the whole length of a lateral portion of the nail plate and grasped firmly. In an upward rotating motion, the nail plate is avulsed [24].

Proximal approach

The proximal approach is advised when the distal subungual area strongly adheres to the nail plate (e.g. thick hyperkeratosis) and it is then difficult to find a cleavage plane between the plate and the bed. The proximal nail fold is detached as described above. The elevator then reflects the proximal nail fold and is delicately inserted under the base of the nail plate where the adherence to the matrix is weak. The procedure is repeated along the whole width of the nail root. The avulsion progresses distally following the natural cleavage plane up to the hyponychium [24].

Partial surgical nail avulsion

The considerable advantage of this technique is that it leaves a large portion of normal nail plate that still exerts a pressure on the underlying soft tissues, reducing the risk of distal embedding. It is a must in the treatment of some types of onychomycosis (longitudinal streaks, lateral disease, dermatophytoma, onychomycosis due to moulds) [25] (Figure 93.87a,b). Partial nail avulsion is part of many surgical procedures: chemical cautery of a part of the matrix in ingrowing toenails, treatment of acute paronychia, surgical exploration of any nail bed or matrix tumour. It is performed in the same way as the distal approach method of total surgical nail avulsion but is restricted to a limited portion of the nail plate. For exposure of the matrix area, avulsion of the proximal third of the nail plate is best. It starts with two lateral incisions on the proximal nail fold at 45° enabling it to be reflected. A jaw of a nail splitter is inserted under the lateral border of the nail plate, approximately 5 mm distal to the lunula. The plate is cut horizontally to the other side. A haemostat grasps the lateral portion of the plate and lifts it up laterally, as for a sardine tin, exposing the whole matrix area (see Figures 93.82a, 93.83a and 93.84a). After surgery, the plate is laid back in place and sutured to the lateral fold.

Acute paronychia

Acute paronychia generates a lot of pain and prolonged pressure from the swollen paronychial soft tissues onto the matrix may impair the normal regrowth of the nail plate. Incision of the proximal nail fold is discouraged as it may result in a deformed eponychium. If the pus collection is located under the proximal

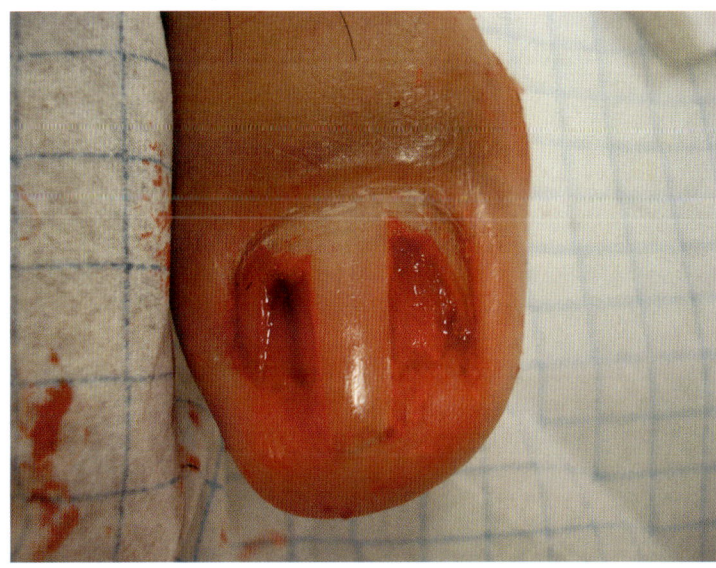

(a)   (b)

Figure 93.87 (a) Dermatophyte onychomycosis with longitudinal spikes. (b) After surgical removal of the yellow streaks.

PART 8: SPECIFIC CUTANEOUS STRUCTURES

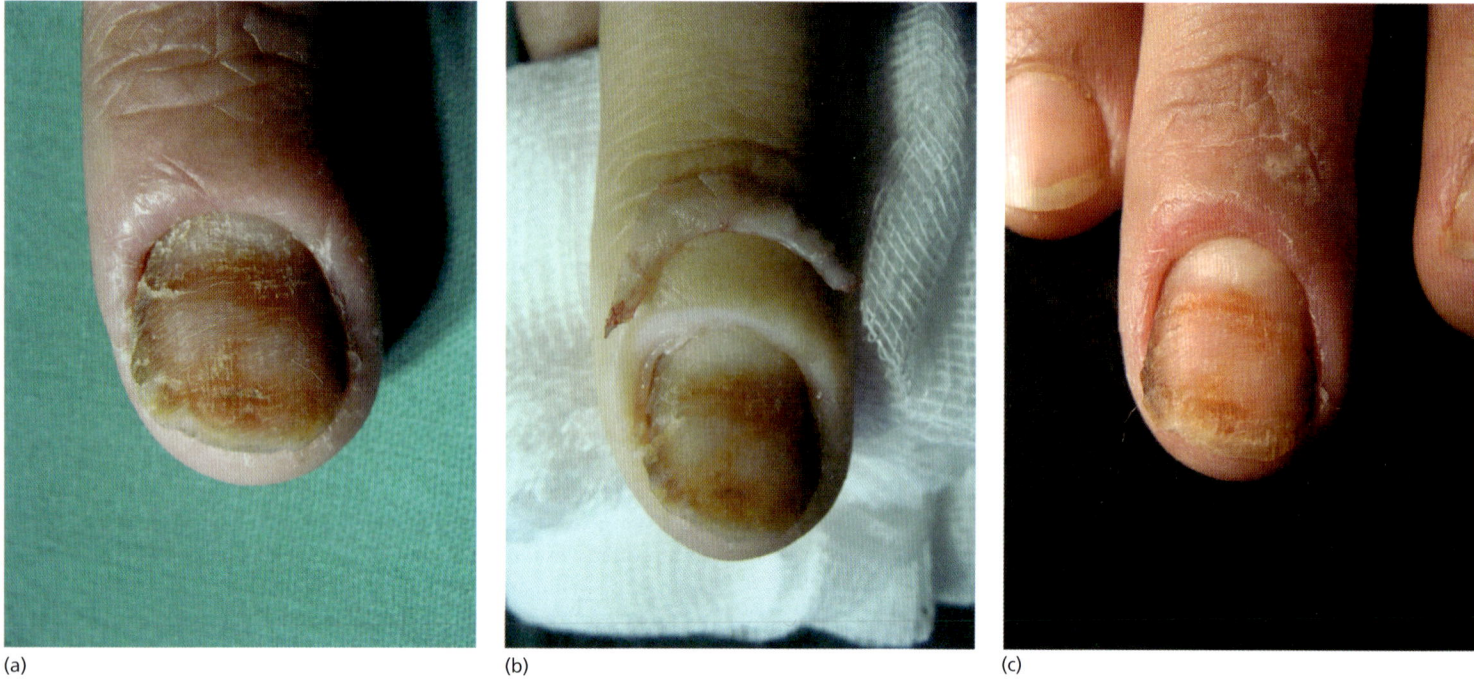

(a)   (b)   (c)

Figure 93.88 (a) Chronic paronychia resistant to topicals and steroid injections. (b) Crescent-shaped excision of a part of the proximal nail fold. (c) Complete re-epithelialisation at day 8. Note that the nail is now apparently longer.

PART 8: SPECIFIC CUTANEOUS STRUCTURES

nail fold, the best treatment is avulsion of the proximal third of the nail plate (see Partial nail avulsion earlier) to allow drainage of the pus. If the collection is in the lateral nail fold, avulsion of a lateral strip of nail plate should be carried out. Systemic antibiotics are prescribed empirically and adapted if necessary once culture results are known [26].

Chronic paronychia

Surgical treatment is indicated when medical treatment has failed. An elevator is inserted into the proximal nail groove under the proximal nail fold in order to protect the matrix and the extensor tendon. With a no. 15 surgical blade, a crescent-shaped excision of the proximal nail fold is performed: the incision should run from one side to the other, reaching its maximum width (5 mm) in the midline of the proximal nail fold. The incision should include the five most proximal millimetres of the lateral nail folds. The blade should be held obliquely at 45° down to the nail plate (Figure 93.88a,b). Complete healing by secondary intention will restore the proximal nail fold with its cuticle in less than 2 weeks (Figure 93.88c). However, the nail plate will appear a bit longer with a larger lunula [27,28]. This technique is also adequate for small very distal type B myxoid pseudocysts. An alternative procedure is the square flap technique where the proximal fold is elevated and its undersurface cleaned from the fibrotic tissue and put back in place and sutured. The downtime is very short and the main advantage is that the length of the ungual plate is maintained [29].

Fibrokeratoma resection

For a fibrokeratoma arising from the ventral surface of the proximal nail fold, reflection of the latter with two oblique incisions at 45°

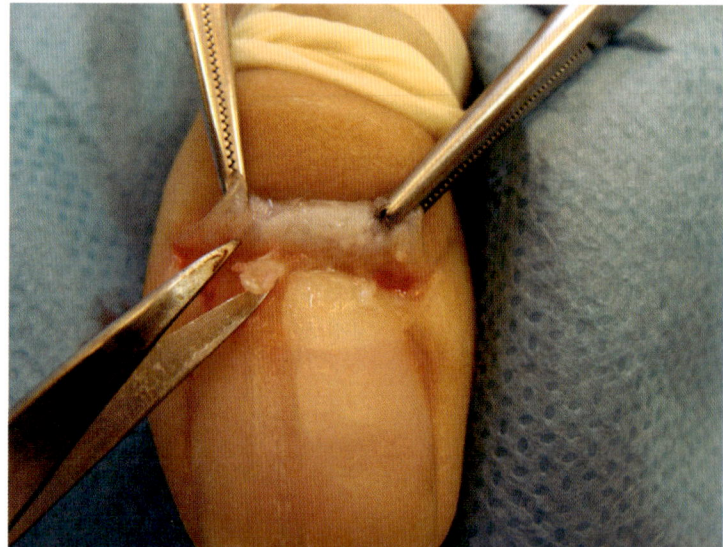

Figure 93.89 Two lateral incisions at 45° allow reflection of the proximal nail fold; visualisation of the tumour and its removal.

exposes the whole nail pocket (Figure 93.89). In most instances, the fibrokeratoma originates from the most proximal part of the ventral proximal nail fold. The tumour should be delicately dissected up to its base using fine iris scissors and then severed. Injuring the matrix is impossible as the nail plate is still in place. The proximal nail fold is then laid back and secured with 5/0 stitches or adhesive strips [30].

For a fibrokeratoma arising from the nail bed, a nail avulsion is required in order to expose the nail bed (Figure 93.90). The tumour is excised in the same manner as an elliptical biopsy of the bed

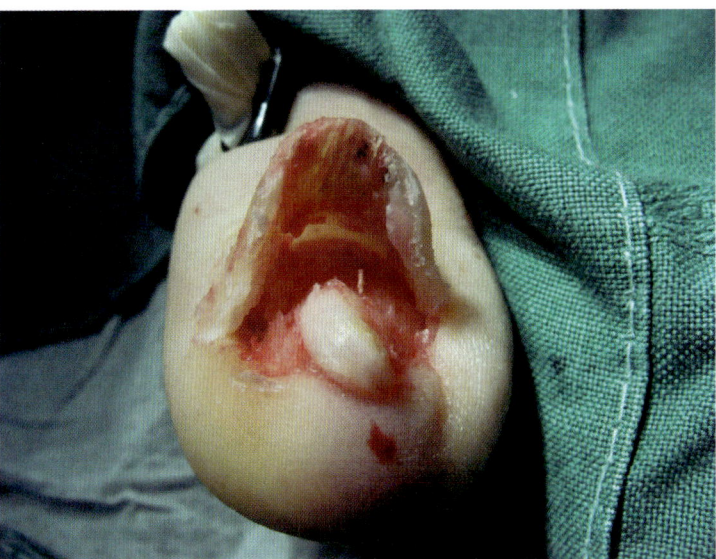

Figure 93.90 Trap door avulsion permits access to the nail bed tumour. The latter will be removed in a longitudinal excision.

(see Nail bed biopsy earlier). In both forms, incomplete resection leads to recurrence.

Chemical cautery for ingrowing toenails

The therapeutic aim of this procedure is a selective cautery of the lateral horns of the matrix to obtain a permanently narrowed nail plate that will solve the 'nail plate–lateral nail fold conflict' once and for all. This technique may be performed on both sides of pincer nails and suppresses immediately the 'pincer' effect of the lateral edge of the nail plate on the soft tissues. Chemical cautery with phenol is easy to learn and is very effective (<3% recurrence rate). It is the recommended procedure in several Cochrane reviews as it has a high success rate with low morbidity [31,32]. After a distal digital block, a 3–5 mm wide lateral strip of nail is avulsed up to its most proximal part. This partial nail avulsion exposes the lateral horns of the matrix at the proximal part of the cavity. Chemical cautery of the lateral horns of the matrix is carried out with a cotton-tipped applicator dipped into 88% phenol and then pushed into the cavity (Figure 93.91a–c). The applicator is left in place for 4 min [33]. To ensure the effect of the phenol, it is essential to work in a bloodless field using a tourniquet. Spillage of phenol onto the periungual tissues should be avoided as this causes unnecessary burns. For beginners, application of a greasy ointment onto the perionychium prior to cauterisation may protect the tissues. After the procedure, applying alcohol will not 'neutralise' the phenol but only dilute it [34]. Phenol induces coagulation of proteins from the matrix epithelium. Once coagulated, the epithelium becomes impermeable to any liquid. Release of the tourniquet will allow the blood proteins to inactivate any residual phenol. Patients have little postoperative pain as phenol has, apart from its caustic effect, important antiseptic and anaesthetic properties. The major drawback of this technique is the prolonged oozing from the phenolic burn. This may last up to 5 weeks. Daily home care (soakings and antiseptic ointment) are required until the wounds are completely dry. The ooze should not be mistaken for infection. As alternatives to phenol other caustics may be used such as 10% potassium hydroxide [35] and 100% trichloroacetic acid. Trichloroacetic acid achieves the same very high success rate as phenol but has no shorter oozing time [36].

Longitudinal melanonychia removal

See matrix biopsies.

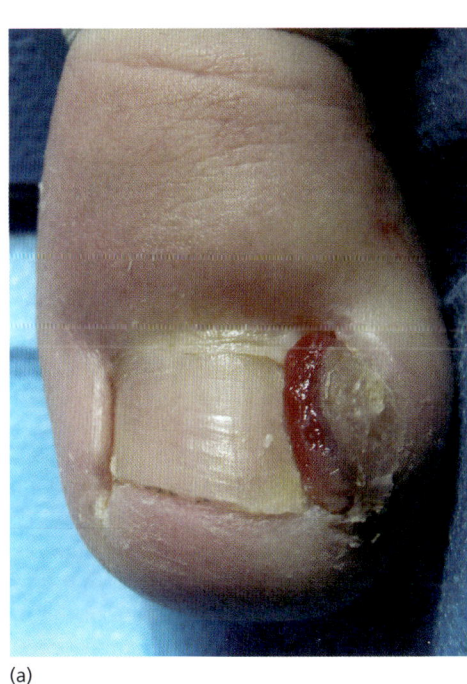
(a)

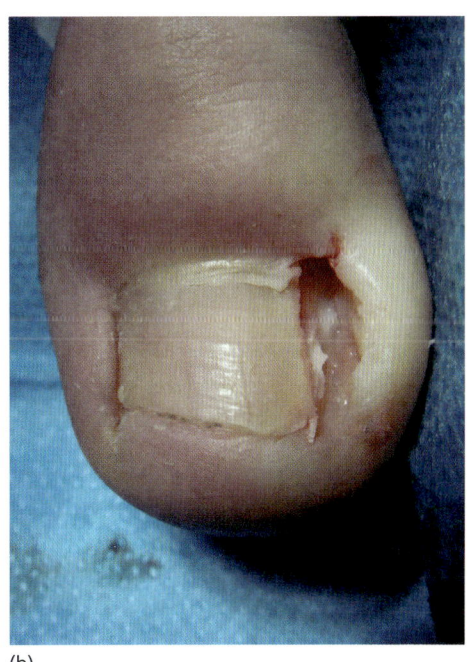
(b)

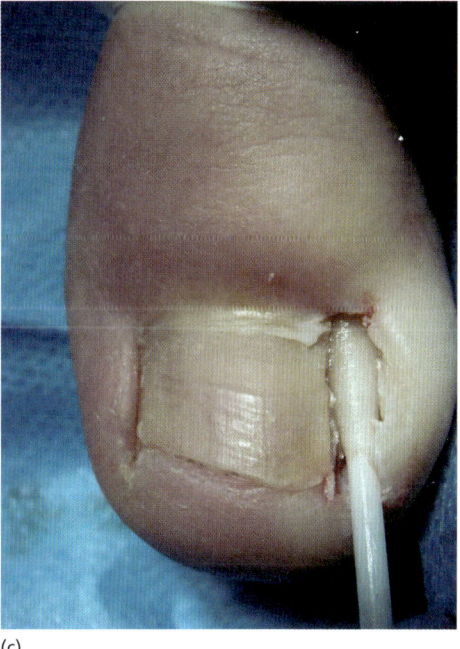
(c)

Figure 93.91 (a) Ingrowing toenail with pyogenic granuloma. (b) After curettage of the pyogenic granuloma, a lateral strip of nail is avulsed. (c) A cotton-tipped applicator, dipped into 88% phenol is pushed into the cavity. Note the bloodless surgical field.

PART 8: SPECIFIC CUTANEOUS STRUCTURES

Postoperative care

Dressings should include generous amounts of antiseptic ointment covered with petrolatum gauze to avoid adhesion to the wound and to facilitate removal of the dressing. Two to three fine mesh gauze squares and either tubular elastic net or elastic bandage complete it. A narrow bandage (4 cm) is a more flexible form of dressing which enables pressure to be applied more precisely over the wound. The dressing should provide no more than light compression in order not to compromise the blood flow. This bulky dressing will enable postoperative bleeding to be absorbed and will provide some protection against trauma. The limb should be kept elevated for 48 h to ease throbbing and facilitate healing. The patient should wear a sling if the surgery involves a finger, or keep the foot elevated for 2 days for toe surgery. This also means that the patient should not plan to drive home following surgery. Painkillers should be prescribed for 3 days. The dressing should be removed on day 2, if necessary, after soaking. Further care includes twice-daily dressings with antiseptic ointment covered by a plaster until complete healing has been achieved.

THE NAIL AND COSMETICS

Nail unit damage as a result of incorrect manicures is common. Nails should always be trimmed with as slight a curve as possible and with the corners left untouched to avoid ingrowing and paronychia. The free edge should be filed in only one direction with a cardboard file. The cuticles should be pushed proximally with an orange stick rather than a metallic cuticle pusher, which is less likely to cause injuries to the proximal nail fold. Cuticles must be left uncut to avoid Beau lines and paronychia.

Nail coatings represent an attractive nail enhancement. They may harden upon evaporation (nail varnish) or polymerise (sculptured nails, gels, preformed artificial nails) [1,2]. Although many of the products available on the market may be of great benefit to an individual user, unfortunately they may also be a source of significant adverse effects. Allergic contact dermatitis, for instance, continues to be one of the most important medical issues related to nail cosmetics, making it necessary for dermatologists to familiarise themselves with available products and their potential risks. Interestingly, some adverse reactions, such as distant allergic contact dermatitis, are more frequent with the use of nail polish than with the application of artificial nails. However, artificial nails have also been found to pose health risks directly to nails. Nail damage after the removal of nail polish (any kind) is also an issue. Recently, UVA lamps, which are used in nail salons to speed-dry manicures, have been considered as potential sources of skin cancer and skin ageing. They have been replaced with LED lamps, which also emit UV radiation, and can therefore be of equal risk. To play it safe, The Skin Cancer Foundation recommends applying a broad-spectrum (UVA/UVB) sunscreen to hands 20 minutes before manicuring or suggests wearing gloves during the procedure. Nail salons have also been investigated as potential sources of health hazards in relation to nail instruments and the store environment. Furthermore, an unsafe nail salon poses a risk not only to customers, but also the staff working there, who may suffer from long-term health consequences as a result of being exposed to the chemicals in nail products.

Coatings that harden upon evaporation

Nail varnish

The term 'nail lacquer' is sometimes used to include enamels, top coats and base coats, either as separate entities or combined in one product. Although chemically similar, they contain different ratios of the same constituents to lend different characteristics. The base coat is used to improve the adhesion or bonding of enamel to the nail. A top coat improves the depth and lustre of the enamel and increases its resistance to chipping and abrasion. Nail polishes consist of solids and solvent ingredients, the former representing about 30%, the latter 70% of the product. The ingredients can be divided into six principal groups (Box 93.4).

Box 93.4 Ingredients of nail polish

1 Cellulose film formers (e.g. nitrocellulose): provide gloss, body and gel structure
2 Resins (e.g. tosylamide formaldehyde resin; previously known as toluene sulphonamide formaldehyde resin): improve gloss and adhesion of the film
3 Plasticisers (e.g. camphor): give the film pliability, minimise shrinkage, and soften and plasticise the cellulose
4 Thixotropic suspending agents (e.g. bentonite) for non-settling and flow: keep pigments in suspension by preventing the particles from clogging together, so that they will disperse on shaking
5 Solvents and diluents: keep nitrocellulose, resin and plasticiser in the liquid state and control the application and drying time
6 Colour substances: these are either inorganic (iron oxides) or a variety of certified organic colours (such as D and C yellow aluminium lakes). 'Pearls' or 'frosts' are produced by bismuth oxychloride and titanium dioxide coated with mica and guanine (obtained from fish scales). 'Clears' contain a small tint

---

The base coat is formulated in a manner similar to standard lacquer, but it has a lower non-volatile content (less nitrocellulose) and lower viscosity, because a thinner film is desirable; it may also contain hydrolysed gelatine. In the top coat, the nitrocellulose content is increased and the resin reduced. A slight increase in plasticiser content improves the elasticity of the film. There is no pigment. The top coat often has an added sunscreen.

Reactions such as an allergic contact dermatitis to nail varnish frequently appear on any part of the body accessible to the nails, with paradoxically no signs in or around the nail apparatus [3–5]. The most commonly involved areas are the eyelids (Figure 93.92), the lower half of the face, the sides of the neck and the upper chest. Sometimes the use of nail polish on stockings to stop 'runs' or on nickel-plated costume jewellery to prevent nickel dermatitis may induce nail polish dermatitis on the legs or at the site of the metal contact. Connubial or transfer nail polish dermatitis may occur in the user's partner or other close contacts. Although any ingredient may account for distant allergic contact dermatitis, tosylamide formaldehyde resin is the most common culprit. After the nail

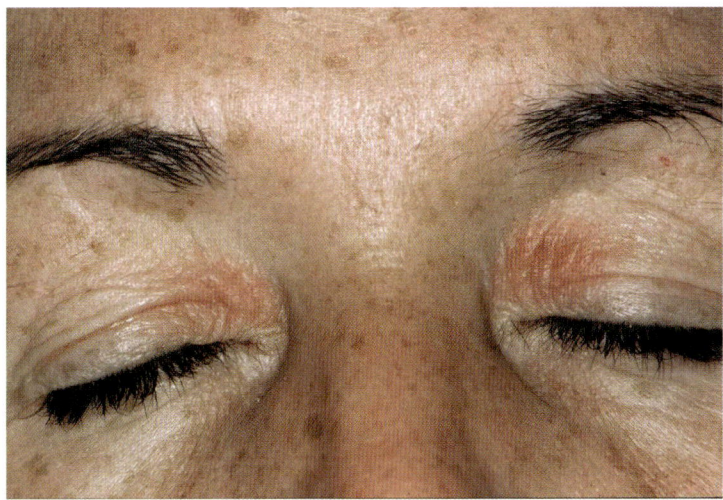

Figure 93.92 Allergy to nail varnish presenting as an eyelid dermatitis.

polish is removed, the dermatitis usually clears rapidly unless secondary infection or lichenification has occurred. Eluate from uncoated metal pellets present in some bottles to keep the varnish in a liquid state may cause nickel reactions and onycholysis.

Nail plate staining from the use of polish is most commonly yellow-orange in colour (Figure 93.93). It typically starts near the cuticle, extends to the nail tip and becomes progressively darker from base to tip. With time, the dyes penetrate the nail too deeply to be removed. Injury to the nail plate from nail lacquers is rare. However, 'granulation' of nail keratin (pseudoleukonychia), a superficial friability, can be observed in some instances where individuals leave nail lacquer on for many weeks or where there is poor formulation of the product. Onychoschizia and overall thinning are also a consequence.

For patch testing, several nail lacquers should be used and tested 'as is' using occlusive chambers (e.g. Finn Chambers® or IQ Ultra Chambers®); the lacquers should be allowed to dry for 15 min before application of the patches, because the solvents and diluents may cause false-positive reactions.

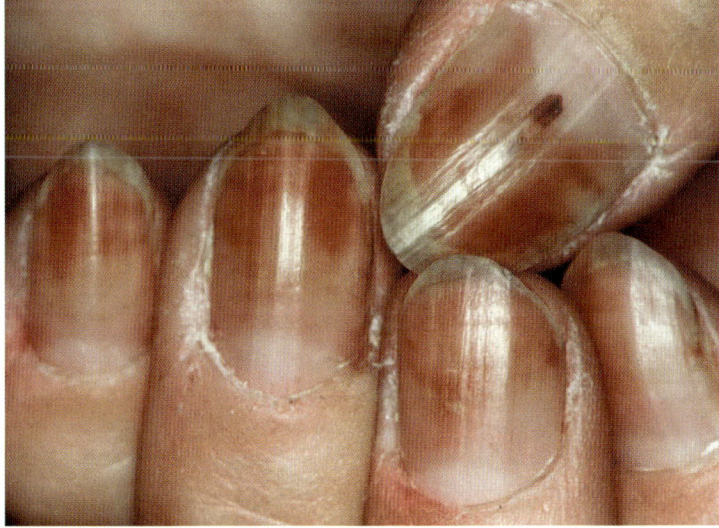

Figure 93.93 Staining of the nail plates from nail varnish.

The substances listed in Box 93.5 should be included in the test battery.

Various cosmetic companies now make varnishes that are formulated without the sensitising resin and are toluene free. The presence of nickel in any product can be detected using the dimethylglyoxime spot test, which is highly specific.

Box 93.5 Test battery for nail plate staining

- Tosylamide formaldehyde resin (10% in petrolatum)
- Nickel sulphate hexahydrate (2.5% in petrolatum)
- Glyceryl phthalate resin (polymer resin) (10% in petrolatum)
- Pearly material; guanine powder (as is)
- Formaldehyde (1% aqueous)
- Colophony (20% in petrolatum)
- Drometrizole trisiloxane (10% in petrolatum)
- Dyes: red 1, red 17, red 46, yellow 3 and orange 3

Nail polish removers. These are composed of various solvents such as acetone. Occasionally, nail polish removers cause trouble by excessive drying of the nail plate and may be responsible for some inflammation of the nail folds and onycholysis.

Coatings that polymerise

Sculptured nails

The nail is first thoroughly cleansed and painted with antiseptic and antifungal solutions. The nail is frequently dried with a diethyl ether-based nail dehydrating agent and sometimes 'primed' with methacrylic acid/solvent adhesion promoter which works like a double-sided adhesive tape, sticking to both the nail and to the acrylic.

Self-curing acrylic resins are obtained by blending a methyl, ethyl or isobutyl methacrylate monomer which comes in a liquid form and a polymethyl or ethyl methacrylate polymer, which is a powder. The monomer also contains a stabiliser such as hydroquinone and *N,n*-dimethyl-*p*-toluidine as an accelerator. The polymer contains benzoyl peroxide as a polymerisation initiator. Liquid monomer and powder polymer are mixed and the compound has to be moulded on the natural nail. Self-curing acrylic resins harden at room temperature. When hardened, the compound produces a prosthetic nail that is enlarged and elongated by repeated applications. The prosthesis can be filed and manicured to shape. As the plate grows out, further applications of acrylic can be made to maintain a regular contour.

Allergic reactions [6,7]

Allergic reactions due to sculptured nails may occur 2–4 months, or even as long as 16 months, after the first application. The first indication is an itch in the nail bed. Paronychia, which is usually present in allergic reactions, is associated with excruciating pain in the nail area, and sometimes with paraesthesia. The nail bed is dry and thickened, and there is usually onycholysis. The natural nail plate becomes thinner, splits and is sometimes discoloured. It takes several months for the nails to return to normal. Permanent nail loss is exceptional, as is intractable prolonged paraesthesia [8].

Allergic reactions frequently occur when the monomers are not completely polymerised. Home kits are especially at high risk due to the unprofessional procedure. Acrylates are also components of dentistry and orthopaedic material, and cross reactions are very frequently observed.

Irritant reactions

Irritant reactions to monomers occur. These manifest as a thickening of the nail bed's keratin layer, which can sometimes cause the entire nail bed to thicken with or without onycholysis. Nonetheless, the overwhelming majority of cases result from physical trauma or abuse.

Damage to the natural nail is not unusual after 2–4 months of wear of a sculptured nail. If it becomes yellow or crumbly, this means that the product was applied and maintained incorrectly. The patient should find a better-qualified nail technician. The problem may well not be the acrylic nail materials but rather the thinning of the nail due to excessive filing with heavy abrasives.

Primer (methacrylic acid) is a strong irritant, which may produce third-degree burns. It is hazardous if the cuticles are flooded or spills are not washed out immediately. Primer can permeate the plate and soak into the nail bed if the nails are too thin. Soap or baking soda dissolved in water are excellent neutralisers. If primer gets into the eye, it should be rinsed with water for at least 15 min and a Poisons Information Centre should be contacted.

Light-cured gels

Gel system products are a premixed variant of sculptured nails in a semi-liquid form, either acrylic based (14% of the market) or cyanoacrylate based (1% or less of the market). Their virtual lack of odour makes gels popular in full-service beauty salons. UV light-cured gels are the best known of the different gel technologies. These gels contain urethanes and (meth)acrylate compounds, a photoinitiator and cellulose, which necessitates anti-yellowing agents and a UV light unit. The proportion of resins to monomers determines the gel consistency. When the gel is exposed to light of an appropriate wavelength, polymerisation occurs, resulting in hardening of the gel. UV gels never involve catalysts and often do not require primers. Depending upon their composition, the gels can be used for different purposes as follows:

- Instead of the sculptured nail technique. However, they do not permit the formation of nails which are as long and resistant as those from the classical liquid–powder technique.
- Over preformed plastic tips: the nail surface is buffed. After disinfection, the preformed plastic tip is simply fixed with cyanoacrylate glue on the distal half of the nail.
- To protect a natural or varnished nail: this procedure is known as 'nail capping'.
- Capping with fabric (silk, linen or fibreglass fixed with cyanoacrylate glue) adds strength and is known as 'nail wrapping'.

The gel nails are useful in patients seeking treatment for cosmetically disfigured nails with the exception of psoriasis, where the risk of the Koebner phenomenon is high.

Gel enhancement products shrink by up to 20%, which may result in lifting and tip cracking. As an effect of excessive shrinkage, clients may comment that the enhancement feels tight on the nail bed. Other symptoms include throbbing or warmth below the nail plate. This may lead to tender and sore fingertips. Photobonded acrylate has been observed to cause nail reactions, sometimes with nail loss and paraesthesia. Hemmer *et al.* [9] have patch tested 'hypoallergenic' commercial products in patients wearing photobonded acrylic nails who had perionychial and subungual eczema. Triethyleneglycol dimethacrylate, hydroxy-functional methacrylates and (meth)-acrylated urethanes proved to be relevant allergens in photobonded nail preparations. Methacrylated epoxy resin sensitisation was not observed. The omission of irritant methacrylic acid in UV-curable gels does not reduce the high sensitising potential of new acrylates. Contrary to the manufacturers' declarations, all 'hypoallergenic' products continue to include functional acrylate monomers and therefore retain the potential for allergic sensitisation. Gels and acrylics, being chemically distinct entities, will not necessarily cross-react.

Unreacted UV gel in the dusts and filings may produce distant allergic reactions. Although sensitisation to butyl-hydroxytoluene is possible, gels usually contain acrylated oligomers and monomers. Acrylates are far more likely to cause sensitisation than methacrylates or stabilisers.

Finally, thick and ornately painted gel false nails that may be difficult to remove present a real challenge to pulse oximetry. It appears to be the polish more than the sculpted nail that interferes with the readings.

Gel polish

This is a manicure system applied in a salon by a nail technician. The application involves a base coat that is cured under a UVA/LED lamp, two layers of a proprietary nail varnish, and a top coat. During the curing process with a UVA/LED lamp, the manufacturer states that solvents evaporate and leave tiny 'tunnels' in the layer of varnish, connected by acetone-dissolvable polymers. Conventional UVA lamps have almost entirely been replaced by LED lamps, which are more expensive but faster and safer due to their narrower wavelength profile with less UV radiation. However, some gel nails still require UVA lamps for optimal polymerisation.

Preformed plastic nails

Preformed plastic nails are packaged in several shapes and sizes to conform to the normal nail plate configuration. Such nails are trimmed to fit the fingertip and are fixed with cyanoacrylate adhesive supplied with the kit. The usefulness of these prosthetic nails is limited by the need for some normal nail to be present for attachment. Normal physical and chemical insults to the nails cause the preformed plastic nails to loosen. If the preformed nails remain in place for more than 2–3 days, they may cause onycholysis and nail surface damage. Eczematous painful paronychia due to cyanoacrylate nail preparations may be observed after about 3 months. Dystrophy and discoloration of the nails may become apparent and last for several months. In some cases, distant contact dermatitis of the face and eyelids occurs. On patch testing, the patients react far more often to the adhesive than to the prosthetic nails (Figure 93.94). Suggested test substances are *p*-tertiary butylphenol resin (1% petrolatum); tricresyl ethyl phthalate (5% petrolatum); cyanoacrylates and other glues (5% in methylethylketone).

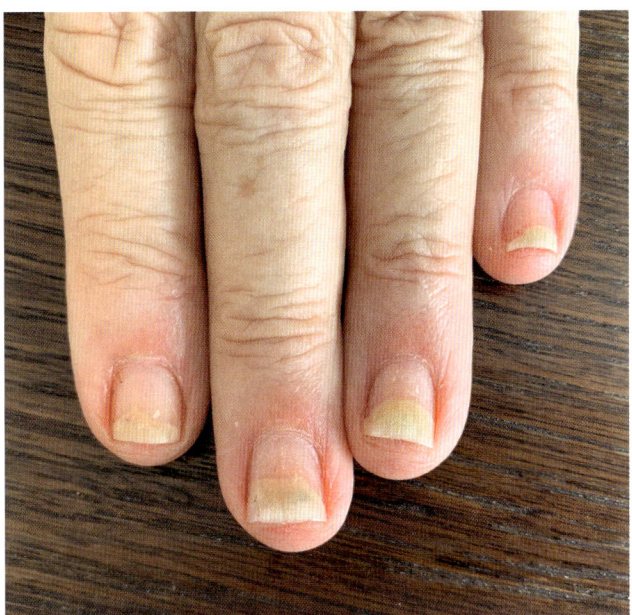

Figure 93.94 Complication of nail extensions: allergy to acrylate adhesive presenting as onycholysis.

Nail-mending kits

These include paper strips of a basic film-forming product to create a 'splint' for the partially fractured nail plate. The split is first bonded with cyanoacrylate glue, then the nail is painted with fibred clear nail polish. A piece of wrap fabric is cut and shaped to fit over the nail surface. This is then embedded in varnish of high solid content and several coats are applied.

Removal of nail coatings that polymerise

The most commonly used solvent for removal of self-curing acrylic is acetone. Warming the solvent with great care can cut product removal time in half. However, most gels are difficult to remove because they are highly cross-linked and resistant to many solvents. Therefore, if gel enhancements have to be removed, they should be slowly filed (not drilled) with a medium-grit file, leaving a very thin layer of product. They should then be soaked in warm product remover and, once softened, the remaining product may be scraped away with a wooden pusher stick.

Other nail cosmetics

Cuticle removers

These are lotions or gels containing approximately 0.4% sodium or potassium hydroxide. The lotion is left in place for 1–3 min and then washed off. Creams containing 1–5% lactic acid (pH 3–3.7) are also used.

Nail hardeners

There are two main groups of products that make nail-hardening claims.

Products in the first group provide a protective coating. The implied benefits come from the added strength and durability of the coating itself, rather than changes to the physical properties of the nail plate. Some consist of nail polish modified by the addition of extra ingredients including nylon fibres, acrylate resin and hydrolysed proteins: they function either as a base coat for nail polish or as a stand-alone treatment. Others applied as a base coat are essentially a modification of clear nail polish with different solvents and combinations of polyester, acrylic and polyamide resins designed to provide better adhesion of the coloured nail coating.

The second type of hardener chemically alters the structure of the nail. These products may contain up to 5% formaldehyde tissue fixative but are designed to be applied only to the free edge of the nail while the skin is shielded. Most products never exceed 3% formaldehyde and the more widely sold brands contain less than 1%. Higher concentrations of formaldehyde can adversely affect both the nail plate and the surrounding tissue. In some countries the use of formaldehyde in nail products is forbidden.

Nail changes due to hardeners may include pain, subungual haemorrhage and bluish discoloration of the nail. Formaldehyde nail hardeners have also been reported as causing onycholysis and both irritant and allergic contact dermatitis. Patch testing should be performed with formaldehyde (1 or 2% aqueous).

Silicone rubber nail prosthesis

For a wide variety of nail problems, ranging from deformed nail to complete loss of the terminal phalanx, a silicone rubber thimble-shaped finger-cover may be indicated. This prosthesis is easily fitted onto the finger stump, encasing the entire distal phalanx; it must be fine and flexible to maintain pulp sensitivity and have the same marking and colouring as the finger. The fixation is excellent and the nail form accepts nail varnish well. The most well-known are Pillet Hand Prostheses® (PHPs), which are available in the USA and some European countries. When there has been loss of tissue from the distal phalangeal pulp, a 'sub-mini' digital prosthesis is also available.

Nail buffing

Weekly buffing may be indicated for removing small particles of nail debris, thus enhancing the lustre and smoothness of the nail plate. Buffing creams, which contain waxes and finely ground pumice, and buffing powders are abrasive and should not be overused on thin nails.

Nail whitener

This is a pencil-like device with a white clay (kaolin) core used to deposit colour on the undersurface of the free edge of the nail.

Infection risks of artificial nails

Medical staff with artificial nails or nail extensions may put patients at risk through carriage of pathogens [10]. UK guidelines now require medical staff not to wear such embellishment. Nail varnish is also thought to be associated with bacterial carriage when it becomes chipped, although the evidence for this is weak. Infection through nail salons and the manicuring process is a further factor that adds to the risks for those with artificial nails. Manicure/pedicure instruments, if not properly sterilised, can also be responsible for infections, as can water that has been used for soaking hands and feet. Acute bacterial paronychia and warts are common complications after improper cuticle removal. *Pseudomonas* colonisation can also occur.

Conclusion

Nail beauty therapy is a flourishing and innovative industry with low overall risks of serious adverse events. In addition to enhancing normal nails, it can be very valuable for disguising unsightly nail conditions: it is not recommended for psoriatic nails as it may provoke the Koebner phenomenon. In general, acrylic-based manicures including gel polish can cause psoriasiform nail changes and pterygium inversum unguis [11,12]. Psoriasiform nail changes are usually due to acrylate sensitisation and pterygium inversum unguis has been linked to nail hardeners, acrylic nails and gel polish manicure. A typical form of traumatic onycholysis, the roller coaster onycholysis, is a typical consequence of improper cleaning of the subungual space with metal files. This is better identified at dermoscopy where haemorrhagic spots are detectable between the onycholytic area and the normal nail bed.

Video legend

Video for this chapter is available on the companion website (https://www.wiley.com/rooksdermatology10e).

Video 93.1 The distal digital block anaesthesia technique.

Key references

The full list of references can be found in the online version at https://www.wiley.com/rooksdermatology10e

Anatomy and biology of the nail unit
Structure
  1 De Berker D, Ruben BS, Baran R. Science of the nail apparatus. In: Baran R, de Berker DAR, Holzberg M, Piraccini BM, Richert B, Thomas L (eds) *Baran & Dawber's Diseases of the Nails and their Management*. Oxford: Wiley-Blackwell, 2019:1–58.

Nail signs and their significance
Abnormalities of shape
Pincer nail
  1 Baran R, Haneke E, Richert B. Pincer nails: definition and surgical treatment. *Dermatol Surg* 2001;27:261–6.

Changes in nail surface
Transverse grooves (Beau lines and onychomadesis)
  1 de Berker DAR. What is a Beau's line? *Int J Dermatol* 1994;33:545–6.

Trachyonychia
  3 Starace M, Alessandrini A, Bruni F, Piraccini BM. Trachyonychia: a retrospective study of 122 patients in a period of 30 years. *J Eur Acad Dermatol Venereol* 2020;34:880–4.

Changes in nail colour
Exogenous nail plate pigmentation/melanonychia
  3 Tosti A, Piraccini BM, de Farias DC. Dealing with melanonychia. *Semin Cutan Med Surg* 2009;28:49–54.

Yellow nail syndrome
  6 Vignes S, Baran R. Yellow nail syndrome: a review. *Orphanet J Rare Dis* 2017;12:42–52.

Longitudinal erythronychia
  1 de Berker D, Perrin C, Baran R. Localized longitudinal erythronychia: diagnostic significance and physical explanation. *Arch Dermatol* 2004;140:1253–7.

Dermatoses affecting the nails
Nail psoriasis
 33 Rigopoulos D, Baran R, Chiheb S *et al*. Recommendations for the definition, evaluation, and treatment of nail psoriasis in adult patients with no or mild skin psoriasis: a dermatologist and nail expert group consensus. *J Am Acad Dermatol* 2019;81:228–40.

Lichen planus of the nails and related conditions
  7 Goettmann S, Zaraa I, Moulonguet I. Nail lichen planus: epidemiological, clinical, pathological, therapeutic and prognosis study of 67 cases. *J Eur Acad Dermatol Venereol* 2012;26:1304–9.

Nail surgery
 28 Haneke E, Richert B, Di Chiacchio. Surgery of the proximal nail fold. In: Richert B, di Chiacchio N, Haneke E, eds. *Nail Surgery*. London: Informa, 2010:42–54.

CHAPTER 94

Acquired Disorders of Dermal Connective Tissue

Caoimhe M. R. Fahy and Christopher R. Lovell

Department of Dermatology, Royal United Hospital, Bath, UK

PART 8: SPECIFIC CUTANEOUS STRUCTURES

CHANGES IN DERMAL CONNECTIVE TISSUE DUE TO AGEING AND PHOTODAMAGE

Introduction and general description

Both intrinsic ageing and ultraviolet (UV) exposure result in alterations in dermal connective tissue that affect the appearance of the skin in old age [1–3,4]. The relative contributions of each vary in the individual from body site to body site and in the population at large according to environmental factors, particularly cumulative photodamage and cigarette smoking. The skin becomes increasingly thin and atrophic in elderly people. Changes in both the epidermis and the dermis result in age-related skin fragility characterised by translucent, lax and wrinkled skin with a tendency to easy bruising and stellate scars. The term 'dermatoporosis' has been coined to describe these changes [3]. The relative contribution of intrinsic ageing and environmental factors to the changes in

Rook's Textbook of Dermatology, Tenth Edition. Edited by Christopher Griffiths, Jonathan Barker, Tanya Bleiker, Walayat Hussain and Rosalind Simpson.
© 2024 John Wiley & Sons Ltd. Published 2024 by John Wiley & Sons Ltd.

dermal connective tissue, which manifest as skin ageing, determine the clinical appearance. Much of what is perceived as aged skin is due to photodamage with the development of actinic elastosis, lax skin and wrinkles. Recent research has helped to elucidate the pathomechanisms underlying these changes. There is reduced collagen biosynthesis and increased production of matrix metalloproteinases, which both inhibit collagen fibril synthesis and promote fragmentation of collagen fibrils, leading to a reduction in healthy collagen but accumulation of damaged collagen [5]. Studies using reflectance confocal microscopy highlighted features of photodamage that were also biopsy-proven including individual corneocytes, pleomorphism of keratinocytes, inflammatory cells in the dermis, increased vascularity and overall architectural disruption [4]. The topic is discussed in detail in Chapter 156. Some specific clinical manifestations associated with aged and photoaged skin are described later in this chapter.

Wrinkles

Definition and nomenclature

Wrinkles are a characteristic of ageing skin. They may be defined as creases or furrows in the skin surface.

Synonyms and inclusions
- Rhytides

Introduction and general description

Wrinkles are particularly prominent in hypertrophic skin photodamage [1] (Chapter 156). Facial wrinkles had a positive correlation with total standard erythema dose, adjusting for age, smoking and skin type, in a study that investigated various features of photodamage between Danish outdoor and indoor workers [2]. Cigarette smoking is also a potent independent cause of wrinkling. The so-called 'cigarette face' is characterised by pale, grey, wrinkled skin with rather gaunt features, so that heavy smokers can often be recognised from their facial appearance alone. Heavy smokers are five times more likely to be wrinkled than non-smokers of the same age, and cigarette smoking probably has at least as much effect on facial wrinkles as sun exposure [3].

Clinical features

Wrinkles are particularly prominent in hypertrophic skin photodamage (Chapter 156). Wrinkles can be classified into three morphological types [4].

1 Crinkles. This is a very fine wrinkling which occurs in aged skin, even in areas protected from sunlight. These fine wrinkles disappear when the skin is slightly stretched. They are caused by deterioration of elastin, especially the vertical subepidermal fine elastic fibres that keep the epidermis in tight apposition to the dermis [5,6]. Ultrastructural studies have shown that even in normal people the elastic fibres begin to deteriorate from the age of 30 years onwards, regardless of the amount of sun exposure, although sunlight undoubtedly increases the damage [7]. Crinkles are seen in a marked form in mid-dermal elastolysis.

2 Glyphic wrinkles. These creases are an accentuation of the normal skin markings. They occur on skin that has been prematurely aged by elastotic degeneration caused by sunlight, for example on the sides and back of the neck (see Actinic elastosis).

3 Linear furrows. These are long, straight or slightly curved grooves that are usually seen on the faces of elderly people. They include the horizontal frown lines along the forehead, the 'crow's feet' radiating from the lateral canthus of the eye and the creases from the nose to the corners of the mouth.

Actinic elastosis

Definition and nomenclature

Actinic elastosis is another component of hypertrophic skin photodamage. It is characterised clinically by yellowish discoloration and thickening of the skin (Figure 94.1), and histologically by a reduction in collagen and an accumulation of amorphous masses of degenerate elastic fibres in the papillary and upper reticular dermis (Figure 94.2) [1].

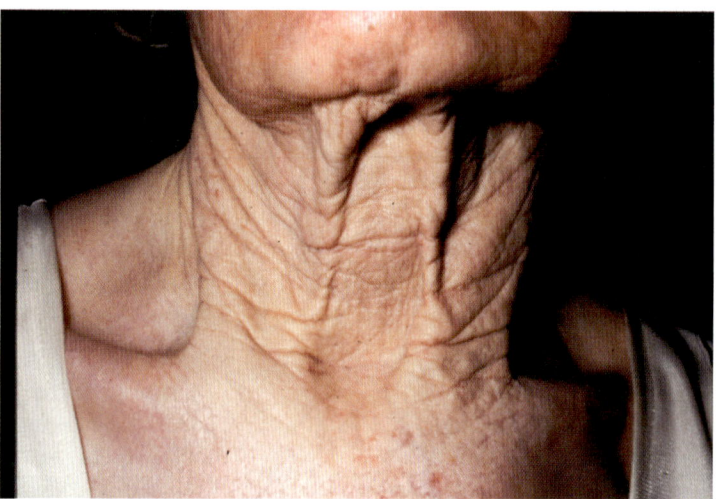

Figure 94.1 Actinic elastosis on the neck of an elderly female patient.

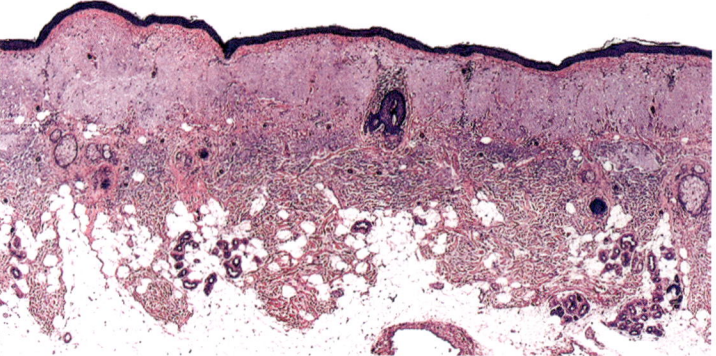

Figure 94.2 Actinic elastosis showing confluent masses of amorphous basophilic material in the papillary and upper reticular dermis with atrophy of the overlying epidermis.

Synonyms and inclusions
• Solar elastosis

Introduction and general description

Actinic elastosis usually results from prolonged exposure to sunlight [1], but it can also follow infrared irradiation [2].

Epidemiology

Incidence and prevalence

Actinic elastosis is related to the cumulative lifetime exposure to UV radiation rather than to episodes of intense UV exposure: it is more common in outdoor workers and in those living in sunny climates. There is, however, considerable variation in susceptibility between individuals.

Age

Actinic elastosis does not usually present until the fourth decade or later but cumulative sun exposure is more important than chronological age alone.

Ethnicity

Fair-skinned people are the worst affected, although actinic elastosis can occur in skin of colour [3].

Associated diseases

Severe actinic elastosis may occur in photosensitised skin, for example in porphyria cutanea tarda and erythropoietic protoporphyria (Figure 94.3) (Chapter 58).

Pathophysiology

Pathology

See Chapter 156.

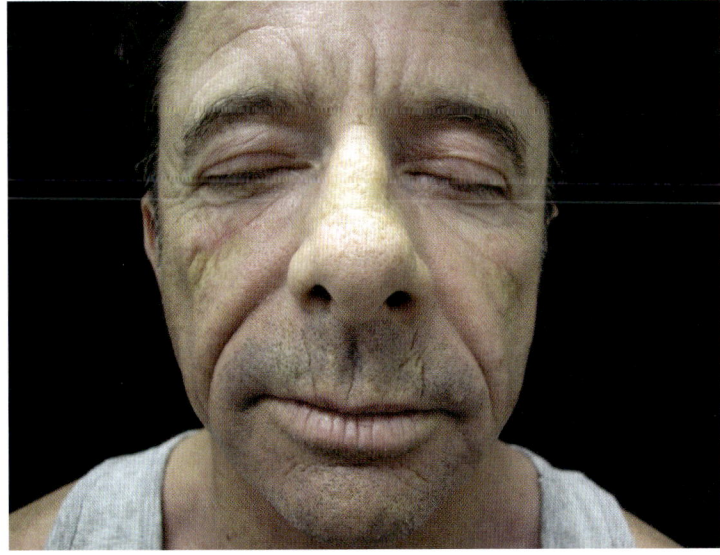

Figure 94.3 Patient with erythropoietic protoporphyria and actinic elastosis. Courtesy of Dedee Murrell.

Environmental factors

Cumulative UV exposure is the main exacerbating factor, although other factors such as infrared irradiation may play a part [2].

Clinical features

History

The characteristic changes develop gradually over the course of years.

Presentation

Actinic elastosis is part of hypertrophic photoageing [4]. The light-exposed areas are affected, particularly the forehead, bald scalp and the back of the neck. Mild degrees of elastosis may not be apparent until the skin is pinched up, when it may assume a wrinkled appearance. Elastosis is usually more advanced in the tissue than the clinical appearance would suggest.

The affected skin is diffusely thickened and yellowish (Figure 94.1) and on the neck it may be divided by well-defined furrows into an irregular rhomboidal pattern (cutis rhomboidalis nuchae). There may also be more sharply marginated, thickened plaques on the face or neck. These are usually, but not always, symmetrical. Recent studies suggest that elastotic skin in specific photo-exposed areas of skin may be protected from epithelial neoplasia [5].

Actinic elastosis may also be complicated by actinic granuloma (see later in this chapter).

Clinical variants

Actinic comedonal plaque. (Synonyms Favre–Racouchot syndrome, nodular actinic elastosis with cysts and comedones.) Actinic elastosis may form into confluent plaques studded with comedones. This is most commonly seen in the periorbital skin (Figure 94.4). It is usually symmetrical, but unilateral and circumscribed forms have been reported [6]. Rarely, a variant has been described with vesicular changes within zones of severe actinic elastosis [7]. Occasionally, similar plaques may form elsewhere than on facial skin, such as the forearm [8].

Elastotic nodules of the ear. In this variant of actinic elastosis, single or multiple firm papules occur on the anterior crus of the antihelix, usually in middle-aged or elderly males. Their significance is that they sometimes have a pearly edge, clinically suggesting basal cell carcinoma (BCC), but histology reveals large aggregates of amorphous elastotic material, sometimes with degradation of underlying cartilage [9–11]

Differential diagnosis

Plane xanthoma, pseudoxanthoma elasticum (PXE) and colloid milium may sometimes cause confusion, but the combination of the clinical and histological features is distinctive.

Classification of severity

Actinic elastosis is of cosmetic significance.

Disease course and prognosis

The process may be halted but not reversed by stringent photoprotection. Stopping smoking may be presumed to slow down progression [12].

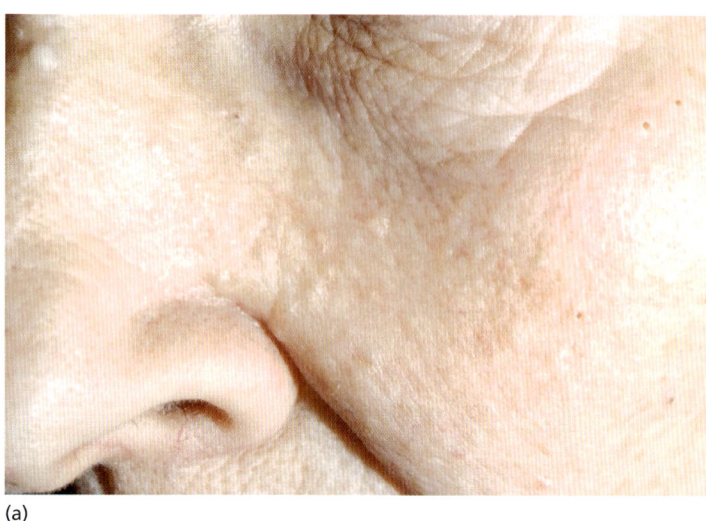
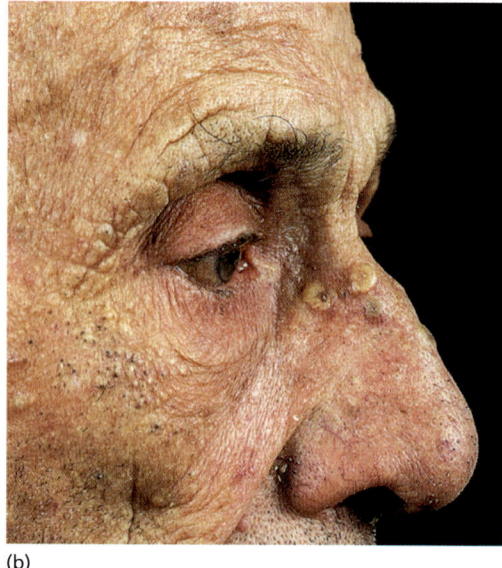

(a)   (b)

Figure 94.4 Nodular actinic elastosis with comedones and cysts (Favre–Racouchot syndrome): early stages in a 78-year-old woman (a) and advanced stage in an elderly man (b). (b) Courtesy of Professor R. Marks.

PART 8: SPECIFIC CUTANEOUS STRUCTURES

Investigations

Skin biopsy should be done if there is doubt about the diagnosis. Histological changes may be more florid than the clinical appearance.

Management (Chapter 156)

Sunscreens protect against the development of photodamage both in humans and animals [13]. In hairless mice exposed to UVB radiation, synthesis of subepidermal collagen has been demonstrated in animals protected with a sunscreen [14]. Topical application of α-hydroxy acids ('fruit acids', i.e. lactic, glycolic and citric acids), has been shown to lead to a modest improvement in photodamaged skin [15]. More impressive results have been obtained with topically applied tretinoin cream [16]. A double-blind study demonstrated a decrease in papillary dermal collagen type I in photodamaged skin, and subsequent treatment with 0.1% tretinoin cream for 10–12 months resulted in an 80% increase in dermal collagen [17]. Several studies have shown clinical and histological improvement after prolonged use [18]. Tretinoin may also repair skin changes due to intrinsic ageing [19]. Retinoids reduce matrix metalloproteinase 1 (MMP-1) expression *in vitro*, partially restoring levels of fibrillin 1 and collagens I and VII in the papillary dermis [20]. Similar results have been obtained in double-blind trials of topical isotretinoin [21] and tazarotene cream [22]. Antioxidants play a part in the prevention of photoageing [23] and may have a therapeutic role in established photodamage [24]. Non-ablative lasers, including the 1320 nm neodymium:yttrium-aluminium-garnet (Nd:YAG) and 1540 nm erbium (Er) glass lasers, are claimed to wound the upper dermis without epidermal damage [25]. Restoration of fibrillin I in the microfibrillar network of the papillary dermis may prove a useful 'biomarker' for the efficacy of topical products used in actinic elastosis [26,27].

Treatment ladder for actinic elastosis

First line
- Prevention by photoprotection

Second line
- Topical retinoids

Collagenous and elastotic marginal plaques of the hands

Synonyms and inclusions
- Digital papular calcific elastosis
- Keratoelastoidosis marginalis

Collagenous and elastotic marginal plaques of the hands is an acquired dermatosis affecting dermal connective tissue in which papules and plaques form on the dominant hand along the radial aspect of the index finger, the first web space and the ulnar aspect of the thumb (Figure 94.5a) [1,2]. Histologically, there is hyperkeratosis, with sawtoothing of the rete ridges. The dermal collagen fibres are thickened and arranged haphazardly; there are basophilic elastotic masses, often containing calcium, in the upper reticular dermis (Figure 94.5b) [3]. Cases are sporadic, unlike the clinically similar disorders acrokeratoelastoidosis and focal acral hyperkeratosis (see Acrokeratoelastoidosis later in this chapter) [4].

Chronic friction and photodamage have been proposed as aetiological factors; the condition has been reported in manual

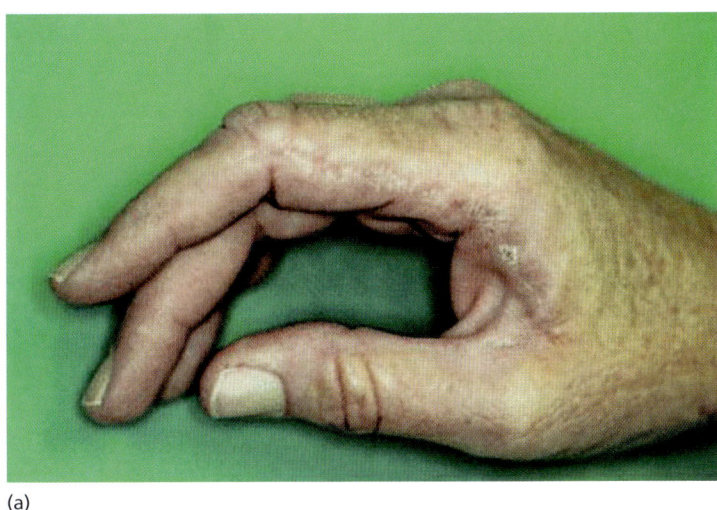
(a)

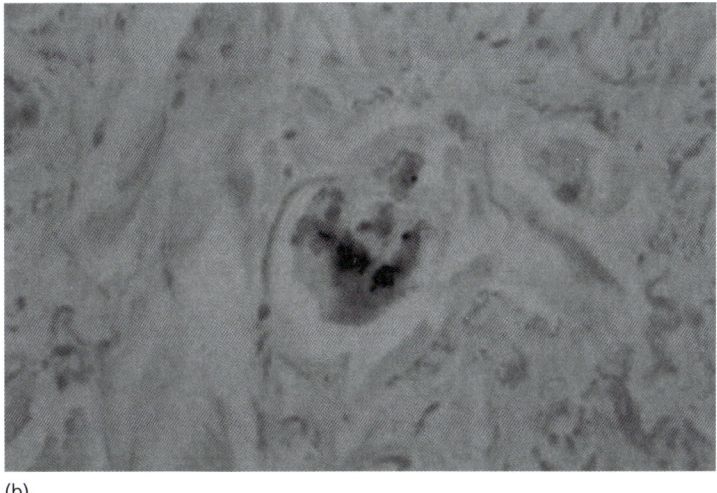
(b)

Figure 94.5 Collagenous and elastotic marginal plaques of the hands: linear plaque involving radial aspect of the right index finger of a 49-year-old woman from Queensland, Australia (a) and calcium deposits within collagen bundle (b). Reproduced from Mortimore and Conrad 2001 [7] with permission of John Wiley & Sons.

workers and from geographical areas with high solar irradiation. It is regarded as a variant of actinic elastosis [5] although actinic damage is not always observed clinically [6]; furthermore the papillary dermis is relatively spared by the elastotic process and the basophilic areas containing calcium differ from the changes normally seen in actinic elastosis [1].

Adult colloid milium and colloid degeneration of the skin

Definition and nomenclature
Colloid degeneration of the skin is a rare but probably underdiagnosed dermatosis that requires biopsy for definitive diagnosis [1]. It is defined histologically by the presence of colloid in dermal papillae and presents as yellowish, translucent papules, nodules or plaques on light-exposed skin. There are several clinical variants of which the commonest is adult colloid milium, which manifests as multiple milia-like papules on light-exposed skin, particularly on the face.

Synonyms and inclusions
- Colloid degeneration of the skin
- Colloid pseudomilium
- Nodular colloid degeneration
- Elastosis colloidalis conglomerata

Epidemiology
Incidence and prevalence
The condition is rare but usually affects fair-skinned, outdoor workers living in sunny climates [1,2].

Pathophysiology
The exact cause of adult colloid milium is uncertain but sunlight exposure is strongly implicated and actinic elastosis is usually

evident as well [3]. Occupational exposure to mineral oils has also been implicated [4,5]: an outbreak among refinery workers in the tropics was attributed to trauma and prolonged contact with photodynamic phenols in oxide fuel (gas oil) [4]. Cases have also been reported in association with ochronosis after the long-term application of strong hydroquinone bleaching creams [6].

Pathology
The earliest histological change is the appearance of colloid globules at the tips of the dermal papillae. Homogeneous fissured masses of amorphous colloid occupy the upper dermis, each surrounded by bands of collagen. There is characteristically a subepidermal uninvolved Grenz zone. The colloid is usually eosinophilic but may be basophilic. Within it, small blood vessels and the nuclei of fibroblasts are well preserved. In the larger, plaque-like lesions, the colloid change occurs diffusely throughout the dermis. The source of the colloid material is uncertain. It could be a protein synthesised by fibroblasts or it could be derived from degraded elastic fibres [2,7].

Environmental factors
Ultraviolet exposure can contribute to the deposition of colloid.

Clinical features
Presentation
Small dermal papules 1–5 mm in diameter, yellowish brown and sometimes translucent, develop slowly and more or less symmetrically in irregular groups in areas exposed to sunlight (Figures 94.6 and 94.7) [1]. They feel soft and may release their gelatinous contents when punctured. The most frequently involved sites are the face, especially around the orbits, the dorsa of the hands, the back and sides of the neck and the ears. There are usually other signs of actinic damage. The changes induced by prolonged light exposure are associated to varying degrees. Although colloid milium may become more severe and more extensive over the years, most cases reach their maximum development within 3 years and then remain unchanged.

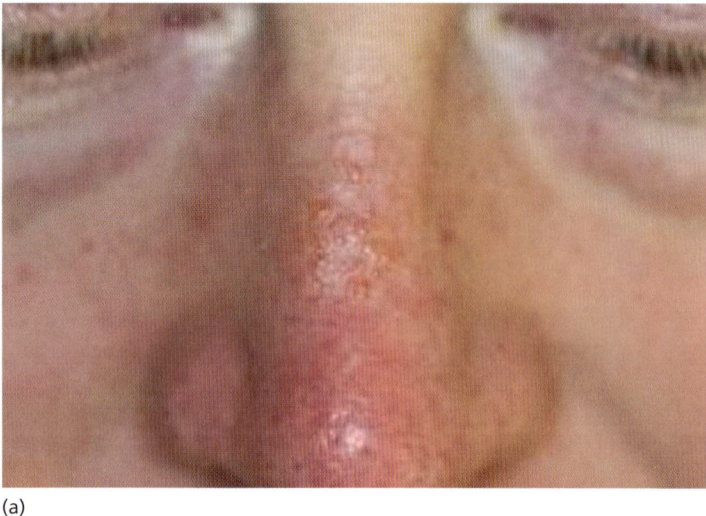

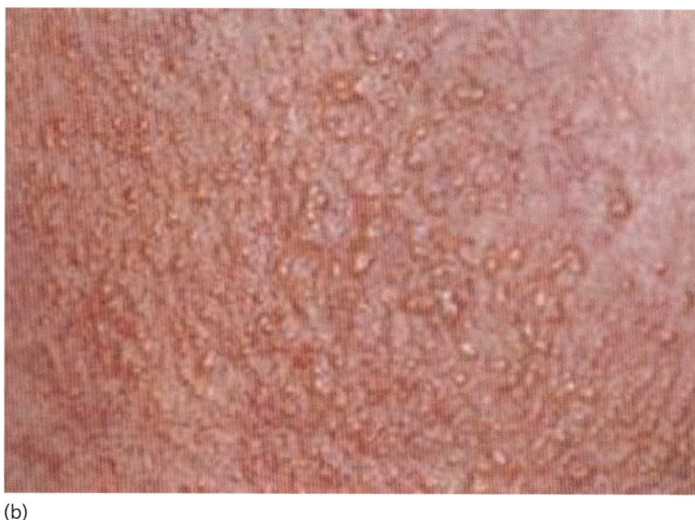

(a)   (b)

Figure 94.6 Adult colloid milium with multiple, tiny, yellowish translucent papules on the dorsum of the nose (a) with a close-up view of papules on the cheek (b). Reproduced from Mehregan and Hooten 2011 [1] with permission of John Wiley & Sons.

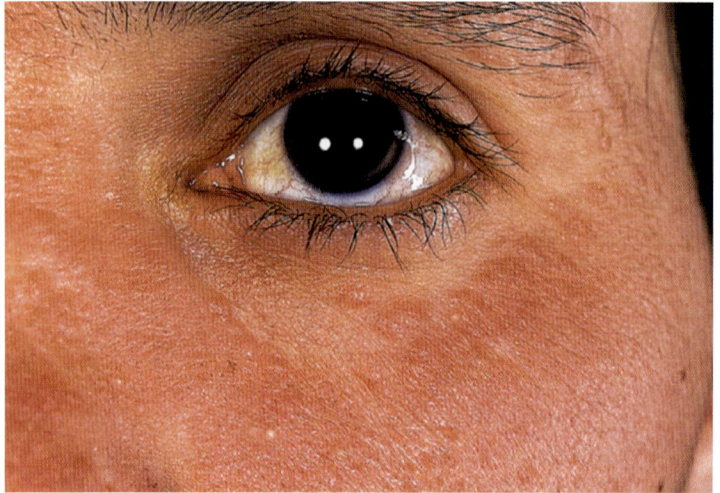

Figure 94.7 More advanced adult colloid milium manifesting as confluent plaques of the infraorbital region but with individual papules discernible at the margins.

Differential diagnosis

The differential diagnosis is presented in Table 94.1. The rare juvenile form manifests before puberty and is often familial [8,9]. It is thought to derive from degeneration of keratinocytes rather than elastic fibres [10].

Clinical variants

Nodular colloid degeneration usually presents as a single nodule up to 5 cm in diameter although multiple nodules may occur. It may be associated with myeloma [11] (Table 94.1).

Management

No completely satisfactory intervention has been found for this condition. Good results have been claimed for dermabrasion [12] and for the long-pulsed Er:YAG laser [13].

OTHER CAUSES OF CUTANEOUS ATROPHY

Introduction and general description

Atrophy of the skin is caused by a decrease in the dermal connective tissue. It is characterised by thinning and loss of elasticity. The skin usually appears smooth and finely wrinkled, and it feels soft and dry. Veins or other subcutaneous structures may be unduly conspicuous. There is often associated loss of hair follicles, and telangiectasia may also be present, due to the loss of connective tissue support of the capillaries. There may or may not be associated atrophy of the epidermis.

Atrophy of the skin occurs in varying degrees in several skin conditions, including naevi, and the underlying histological changes are also variable, because the several components of the connective tissue may be involved to a different degree. Atrophy that includes subcutaneous tissue or even deeper structures is referred to as panatrophy. Box 94.1 lists the main acquired disorders in which cutaneous atrophy is prominent.

Atrophy due to corticosteroids

Introduction and general description

Both systemic and topical glucocorticoid therapy can produce cutaneous atrophy by a dose-related pharmacological effect [1]. The effect is more severe with repeated use of the more potent steroids (as assessed by the vasoconstrictor assay test) but both fluorinated and non-fluorinated topical steroids can cause atrophy. The effect is most marked when potent steroids are applied topically under an occlusive dressing. The skin becomes thin, fragile and transparent, and striae and ulceration may develop (Figures 94.8, 94.9 and 94.10) [2].

Table 94.1 Differential diagnosis of colloid milium.

Deposition disorder	Clinical findings	Pathological characteristics	Staining pattern
Adult colloid milium	Multiple, symmetrical, yellow to flesh-coloured facial papules; associated with sun exposure	Homogeneous eosinophilic colloid masses in papillary dermis from degenerating elastic fibres, often with subepidermal Grenz zone	PAS + Congo red ± Cotton dye − Cytokeratin −
Juvenile colloid milium	Multiple, translucent, yellowish papules on cheeks, nose and perioral skin; onset before puberty; familial; associated with ligneous conjunctivitis	Secondary to UV-induced degeneration of keratinocytes	PAS + Congo red ± Cotton dye − Cytokeratin +
Nodular colloid degeneration	Flesh-coloured nodule on face, scalp or chest; usually solitary	May be associated with myeloma; lacks plasma cells	PAS + Congo red ± Cotton dye −
Acrokeratoelastoidosis of Costa	Multiple, tiny, skin-coloured umbilicated papules at the sides of hands and feet; familial; commonest in black skin	Fragmentation and degeneration of elastic fibres	Congo red − Cotton dye −
Collagenous and elastotic marginal plaques of the hands	Skin-coloured papules and plaques along radial border of index finger and ulnar border of thumb	Fragmentation and degeneration of elastic fibres	Congo red − Cotton dye −
Nodular amyloid	Single flesh-coloured nodule	Deposition of monoclonal immunoglobulin light-chain fragments from localised plasma cell infiltrate	Congo red + Cotton dye +

Adapted from Mehregan and Hooten 2011 [1].
PAS, periodic acid–Schiff; UV, ultraviolet.

Box 94.1 Selected acquired forms of cutaneous atrophy

- Generalised cutaneous thinning:
  - Ageing (see earlier in this chapter)
  - Rheumatoid disease (Chapter 155)
  - Glucocorticoids (exogenous or endogenous)
- Acquired poikiloderma
- Striae
- Atrophic scars:
  - Stellate pseudoscars
- Spontaneous atrophic scarring of the cheeks
- Acrodermatitis chronica atrophicans (Lyme borreliosis)
- Atrophodermas:
  - Follicular atrophoderma
  - Linear atrophoderma (Moulin)
  - Atrophoderma of Pasini and Pierini
- Paroxysmal haematoma of the finger (Achenbach syndrome)
- Panatrophy:
  - Local panatrophy
  - Facial hemiatrophy

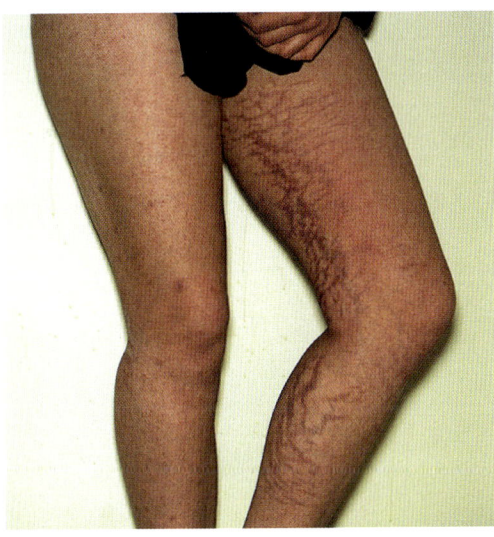

Figure 94.8 Striae of the legs due to long-term application of a potent topical steroid in a young woman with psoriasis.

Pathophysiology
Predisposing factors
Steroids are known to inhibit the formation of glycosaminoglycans. Hyaluronate and the major cell surface hyaluronate receptor CD44 are depleted in atrophic skin [4]. Topical corticosteroids rapidly suppress hyaluran synthase 2 in the dermis; this precedes alteration of dermal collagen [5]. The fibroblasts become shrunken, although their numbers do not decrease, but the number of mast cells is markedly reduced. Topical steroids also inhibit the activity of enzymes involved in collagen biosynthesis [6], and they have

Severe dermal atrophy can follow injection of intralesional steroids, such as triamcinolone acetonide (particularly if the higher concentration of 40 mg/mL is used, instead of the more usual 10 mg/mL, which is less likely to cause atrophy) (Figure 94.11). Inhaled corticosteroids also induce dermal thinning in adults and in children [3]. See Chapters 18 and 19, respectively, for more general discussions of topical and systemic corticosteroids.

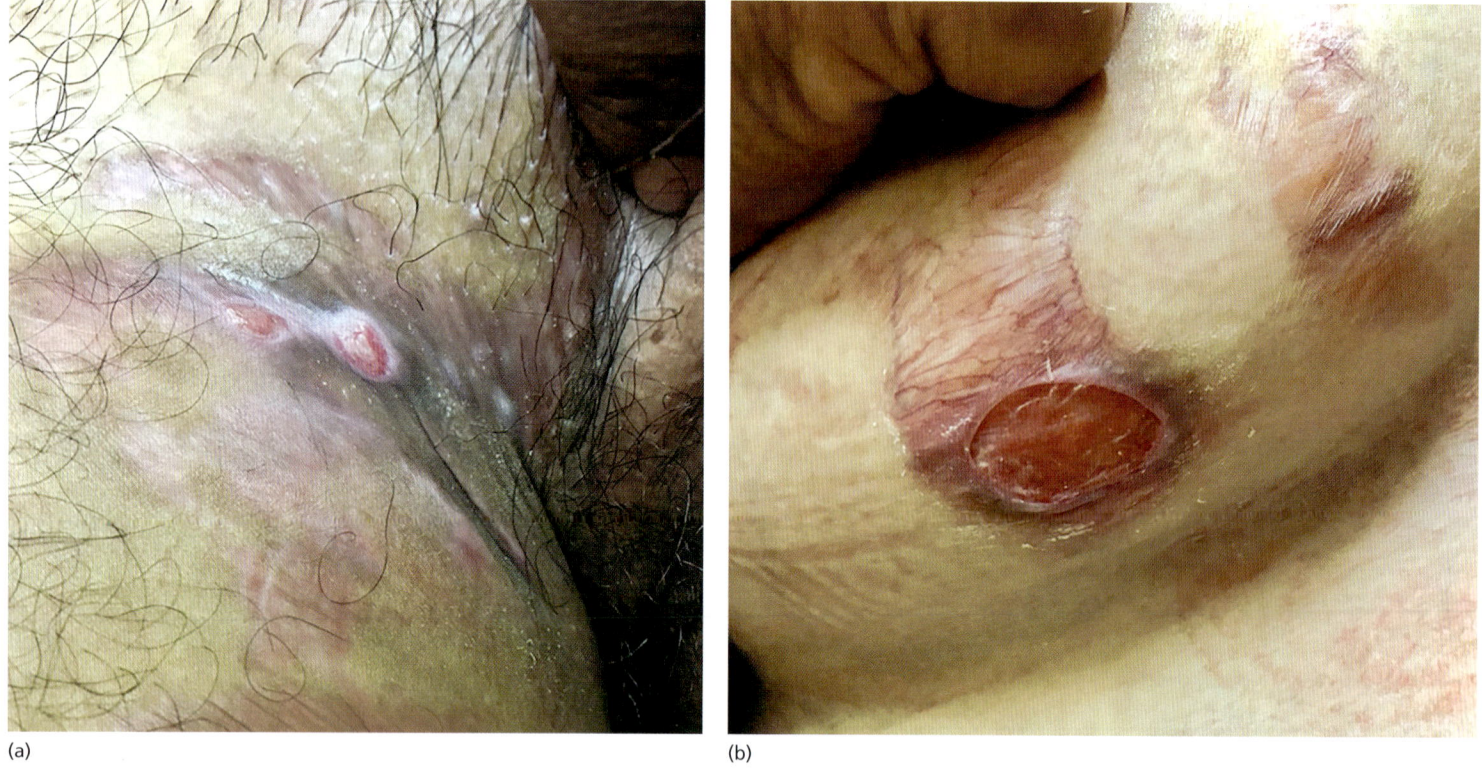

(a)

(b)

Figure 94.9 (a) Superficial ulceration over striae in the inguinal area. (b) Ulceration over atrophic stria with telangiectasia on the inferior breast surface. From Verma and Madke 2021 [2]/The Scientific Electronic Library Online (SciELO)/CC BY 4.0.

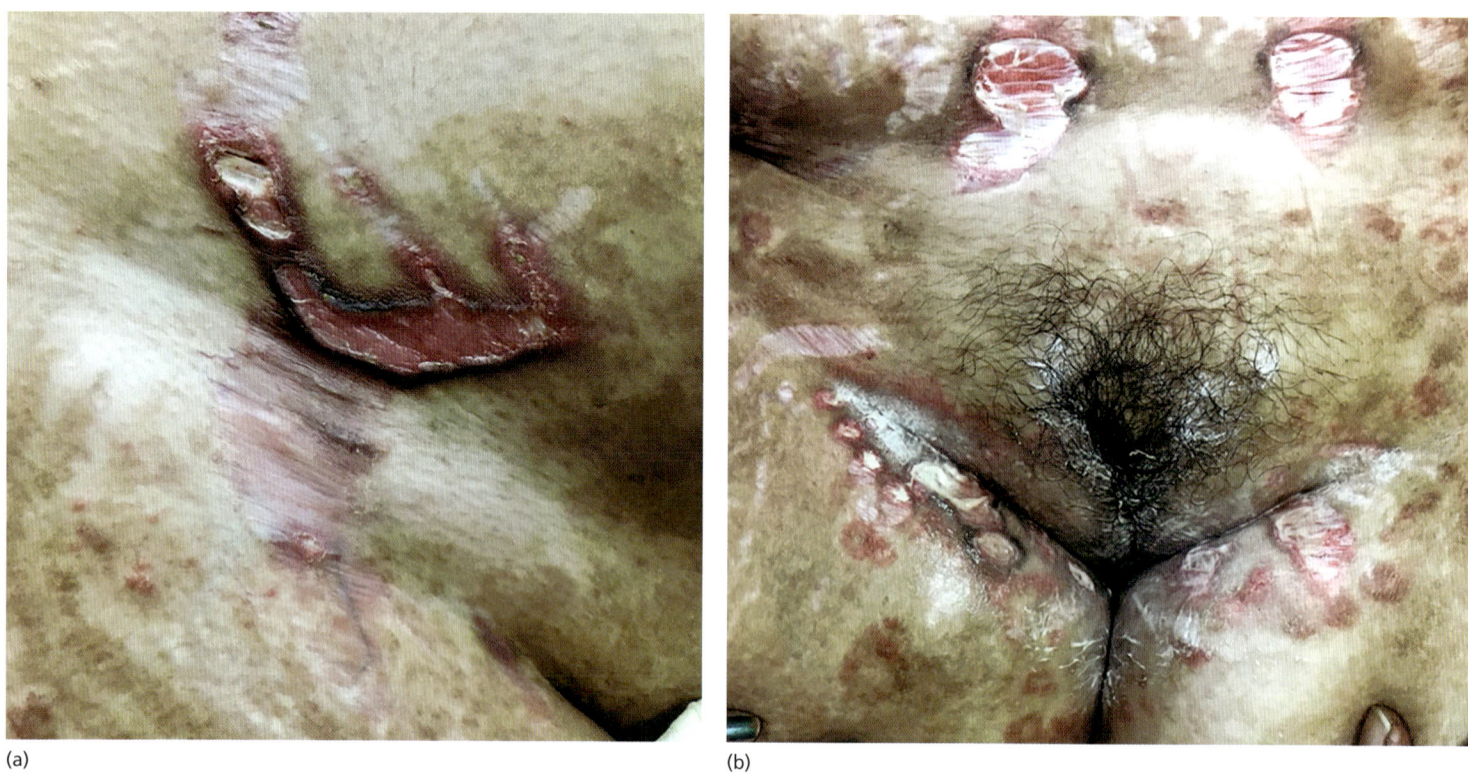

(a)

(b)

Figure 94.10 (a) Ulcerated striae on the abdomen. (b) Ulceration on the inguinal areas and lower abdomen. From Verma and Madke 2021 [2]/The Scientific Electronic Library Online (SciELO)/CC BY 4.0.

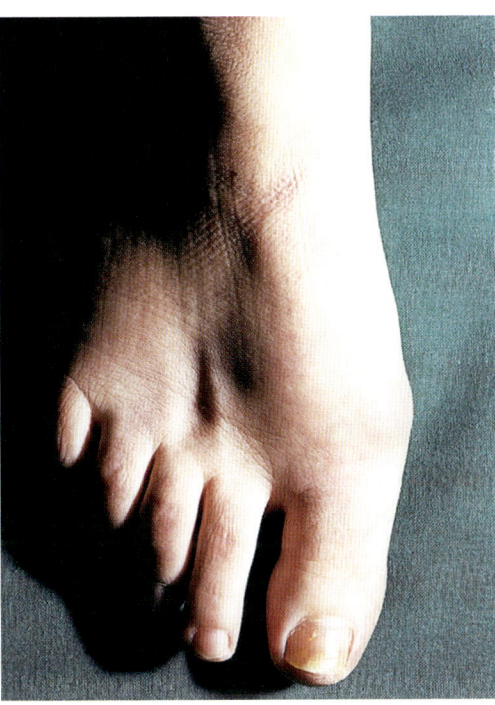

Figure 94.11 Localised atrophy due to injection of a steroid (triamcinolone 40 mg/mL) into the skin between the second and third metatarsals.

been shown to depress synthesis of types I and III collagen *in vivo* [7–9]. Type III collagen synthesis is preferentially reduced in fibroblast cultures [8]. Corticosteroids can also depress collagenase production and collagen breakdown [10], and the rate of collagen turnover is probably decreased. Even a weak steroid, such as hydrocortisone, can suppress the stimulatory effect of cyclic nucleotides on collagenase production. Studies of the effect of topical steroids on collagen and elastic fibres *in vivo* have given conflicting results [11–13]. Capillaroscopic studies have shown that steroid-induced vasoconstriction involves the superficial capillary network, and prolonged superficial ischaemia could also play a role in producing atrophy [6].

Pathology
The earliest histological change is marked thinning of the epidermis, with flattening of the rete ridges and decreased corneocyte size [1]. This is followed a few weeks later by thinning of the dermis, which can be measured by skinfold calipers, ultrasonography or a radiographic technique [14–16].

The epidermal thinning probably results from a reduction of mitotic activity in the germinal layer [17], but the mechanism by which dermal thinning is produced is uncertain.

Loss of dermal ground substance leads to a reorganisation of the dermal architecture. The spaces between the collagen and elastic fibres become smaller, so that the dermis becomes more compact but thinner [11].

Collagen microfibrils may form globular microfibrillar bodies, although the changes are not specific for steroid atrophy [18]. These ultrastructural changes can develop in the early stages before there is clinical or histological evidence of atrophy. Digestion of collagen fibrils in the endocytic vesicles of fibroblasts may be involved in the production of steroid-induced atrophy [10].

Environmental factors
Systemic, topical, intralesional or inhaled corticosteroids are implicated.

Clinical features
History
A careful history should be taken, including enquiry about the use of corticosteroid inhalers (Figure 94.12).

Presentation
The skin becomes thin and fragile with easy bruising. Changes are generalised in patients on systemic corticosteroids, although the changes are more marked at sites of photodamage and trauma. Thinning due to topical corticosteroids may be localised to the site(s) of application. Severe dermal atrophy can follow injection of intralesional steroids.

Differential diagnosis
Other causes of cutaneous atrophy should be considered.

Complications and co-morbidities
Corticosteroid-induced skin thinning leads to delayed wound healing and easy bruising, often after trivial trauma. Measurement of bone density is advisable in at-risk patients, although extensive skin thinning is not necessarily associated with steroid-induced osteopenia [8].

Investigations
Consider measuring blood glucose and bone density if systemic steroid toxicity is suspected.

Management
It has been suggested that local and oral vitamin C therapy might help restore the normal skin thickness [19]. Concurrent application of retinoic acid may partially prevent the epidermal atrophy due to steroids [2]. Intralesional saline injections can restore surface contour [21]. Hyaluronate fragments are reported to induce skin thickening in corticosteroid-induced atrophy [22]. There is a potential therapeutic role for antagonists of REDDI1 (regulated in development and DNA damage 1), a major driver of steroid-induced atrophy expressed on keratinocytes [23].

Prevention is clearly the best approach, including the use of steroid-sparing systemic drugs and topical agents such as calcineurin inhibitors to treat skin disease. In the future, more selective corticosteroid receptor agonists with potentially less atrophogenic effect may be developed [24].

Striae

Definition and nomenclature
Striae are visible linear scars that form in areas of dermal damage produced by stretching of the skin. They are histologically characterised by thinning of the overlying epidermis, with fine dermal collagen bundles arranged in straight lines parallel to the surface.

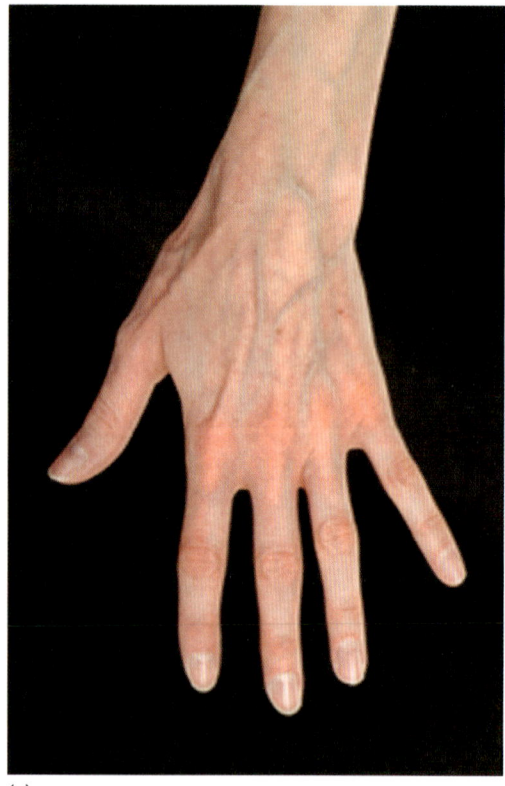

(a)

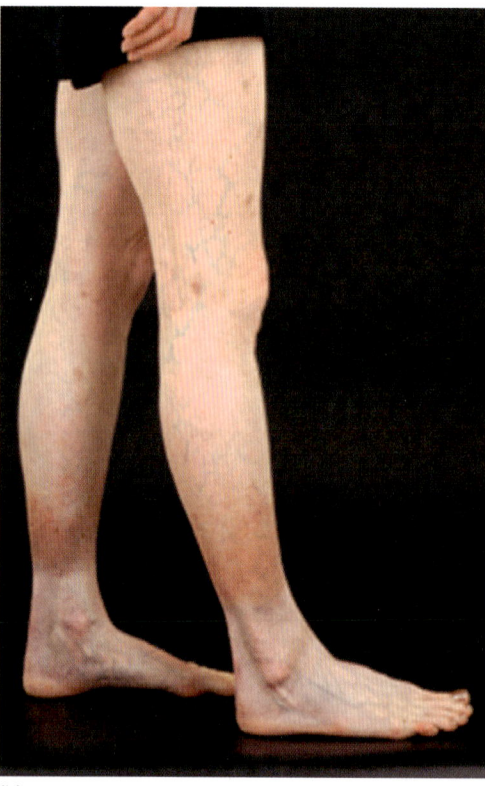

(b)

Figure 94.12 (a, b) Severe generalised cutaneous atrophy in a 29-year-old female as the result of using inhaled corticosteroids for asthma since the age of 7; (b) note haemosiderosis on the lower legs as a result of ready bruising of her atrophic skin.

Synonyms and inclusions
- Striae distensae
- Striae atrophicans
- Stretch marks

Introduction and general description

The factors that govern the development of striae are poorly understood. Many authors have suggested that striae develop following stress rupture of the connective tissue framework [1], but others disagree. It has been suggested that they develop more easily in skin that has a critical proportion of rigid cross-linked collagen, as occurs in early adult life [2]. They are common during adolescence [3], and they seem to be associated with rapid increase in size of a particular region. They are very common over the abdomen and breasts in pregnancy, and they may develop on the shoulders in young male weight-lifters when their muscle mass rapidly increases [4]. They are a feature of Cushing disease, and they may be induced by local or systemic corticosteroid therapy [2,5]. The effects of glucocorticoids on the dermal connective tissue are outlined earlier in this chapter. Together with other steroid-like effects, striae have been reported in human immunodeficiency virus (HIV) positive patients receiving the protease inhibitor indinavir [6].

Epidemiology

Incidence and prevalence

Striae are very common, and occur in most adult women, as they readily develop at puberty or during pregnancy.

Age

Adolescent striae may first develop soon after the appearance of pubic hair.

Sex

Abdominal striae gravidarum are extremely common in pregnancy. Striae are often associated with growth spurts in adolescent males (Figure 94.13).

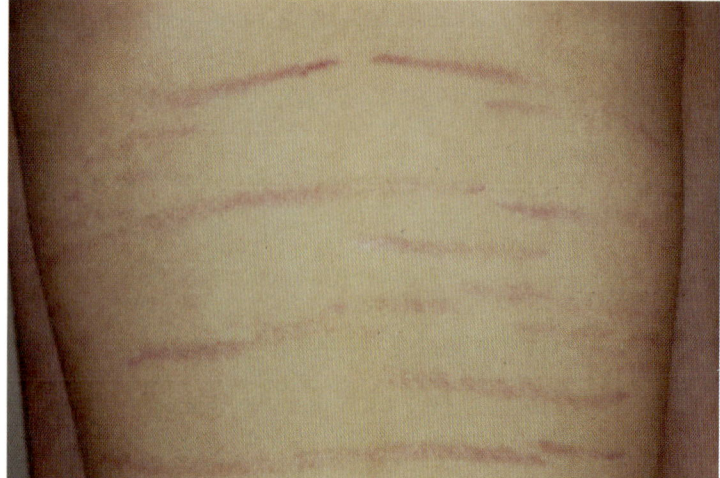

Figure 94.13 Pubertal growth striae across the back of an adolescent boy: note that these are normally all horizontally arranged right across the back (compare with Figure 94.14).

Associated diseases

Most striae occur in otherwise healthy individuals, although they are a feature of Cushing syndrome and Marfan syndrome.

Pathophysiology

Predisposing factors

Striae are associated with growth spurts, for instance body-building or pregnancy, but more rarely they may reflect structural abnormalities of connective tissue such as Marfan syndrome or the effect of glucocorticoids.

Pathology

In the early stages, inflammatory changes may be conspicuous; the dermis is oedematous and perivascular lymphocytic cuffing is present. In the later stages, the epidermis is thin with flattening of the dermal papillae [7,8]. The dermal collagen is layered in thin eosinophilic bundles, orientated in straight lines parallel to the surface in the direction of the presumed stress. Scanning electron microscopy shows amorphous sheet-like structures [9]. With Luna stain, the elastic fibres are numerous, close together, fine and straight, and in the same direction as the collagen bundles [10]. On scanning electron microscopy in collagen-free preparations there is an abundance of thin, curled and branched elastic fibres.

Genetics

The importance of genetic factors in determining the susceptibility of connective tissue is emphasised by their presence as one of the (minor) diagnostic criteria for Marfan syndrome [11] and congenital arachnodactyly, associated with mutations of the *fibrillin-1* and *fibrillin-2* genes, respectively. Striae may occur in the absence of other phenotypic features of Marfan syndrome [12], and their presence may be predictors for aortic dissection [13]. They are commonly absent during pregnancy in Ehlers–Danlos syndrome.

Recent genome-wide association analysis of apparently otherwise normal individuals with striae has revealed associations with genes affecting expression of matrix proteins such as collagen, elastin and fibronectin [14].

Clinical features

The commonest sites for obesity-related striae are the outer aspect of the thighs and the lumbosacral region in boys (Figure 94.14) and the thighs, buttocks and breasts in girls, but there is considerable variation, and other sites, including the outer aspect of the upper arm, are sometimes affected. Pseudoedematous striae have been described as a variant of striae seen in the groin and upper thighs of overweight individuals who use potent topical corticosteroids in the treatment of tinea cruris and corporis (Figure 94.15) [15]. Pubertal growth striae are concentrated symmetrically over, and on either side of, the spine (Figure 94.13).

Early lesions may be raised and irritable, but they soon become flat, smooth and livid red or bluish in colour. Their surface may be finely wrinkled. They are commonly irregularly linear, several centimetres long and 1–10 mm wide. After some years, they fade and become inconspicuous. They are then generally paler than the surrounding skin.

The striae in Cushing syndrome or those induced by steroid therapy may be larger and more widely distributed, and involve

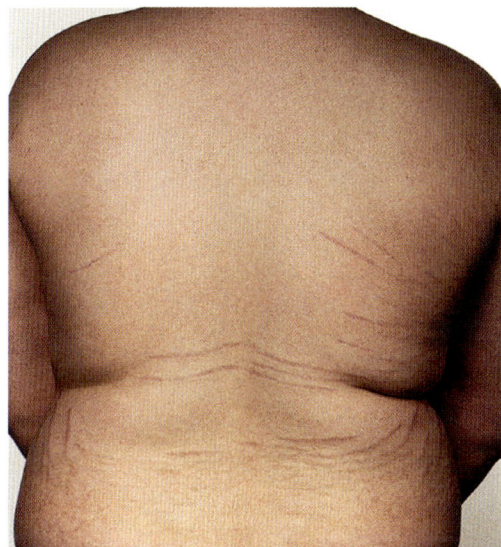

Figure 94.14 Striae due to obesity in a young man.

other regions, including sometimes the face. In pregnancy, the striae appear first and are most conspicuous on the abdominal wall, and later on the breasts, but may involve most or all of the pubertal sites [15]. The striae induced by topical corticosteroid therapy occur particularly in the flexures, but may appear in other sites if occlusive plastic films increase absorption (see Figure 94.8) [16,17].

Differential diagnosis

The diagnosis of striae is usually simple. The possibility of Cushing syndrome must be considered, although this is rarely the cause. Lay people may mistake adolescent growth striae for signs of physical abuse. In linear focal elastosis the lesions are yellow and palpable. Linear, often serpiginous, lesions, which tend to spare the back, are reported in patients with bartonellosis; there are generally associated urticated papules or plaques and the lesions respond rapidly to antibiotics [18].

Complications and co-morbidities

Usually, striae are no more than a cosmetic problem, but occasionally if extensive they may ulcerate or tear easily if traumatised.

Disease course and prognosis

Striae gravidarum generally improve after delivery and adolescent striae have an excellent prognosis. Even corticosteroid-induced striae may disappear or become less conspicuous when treatment is stopped.

Investigations

Exclude Cushing syndrome if suspected.

Management

In the case of common adolescent striae, the patient may be reassured that in time they will become less conspicuous. Numerous unproven remedies are available from cosmetic companies and there is no well-substantiated evidence that topical therapies prevent or accelerate healing of striae [19,20].

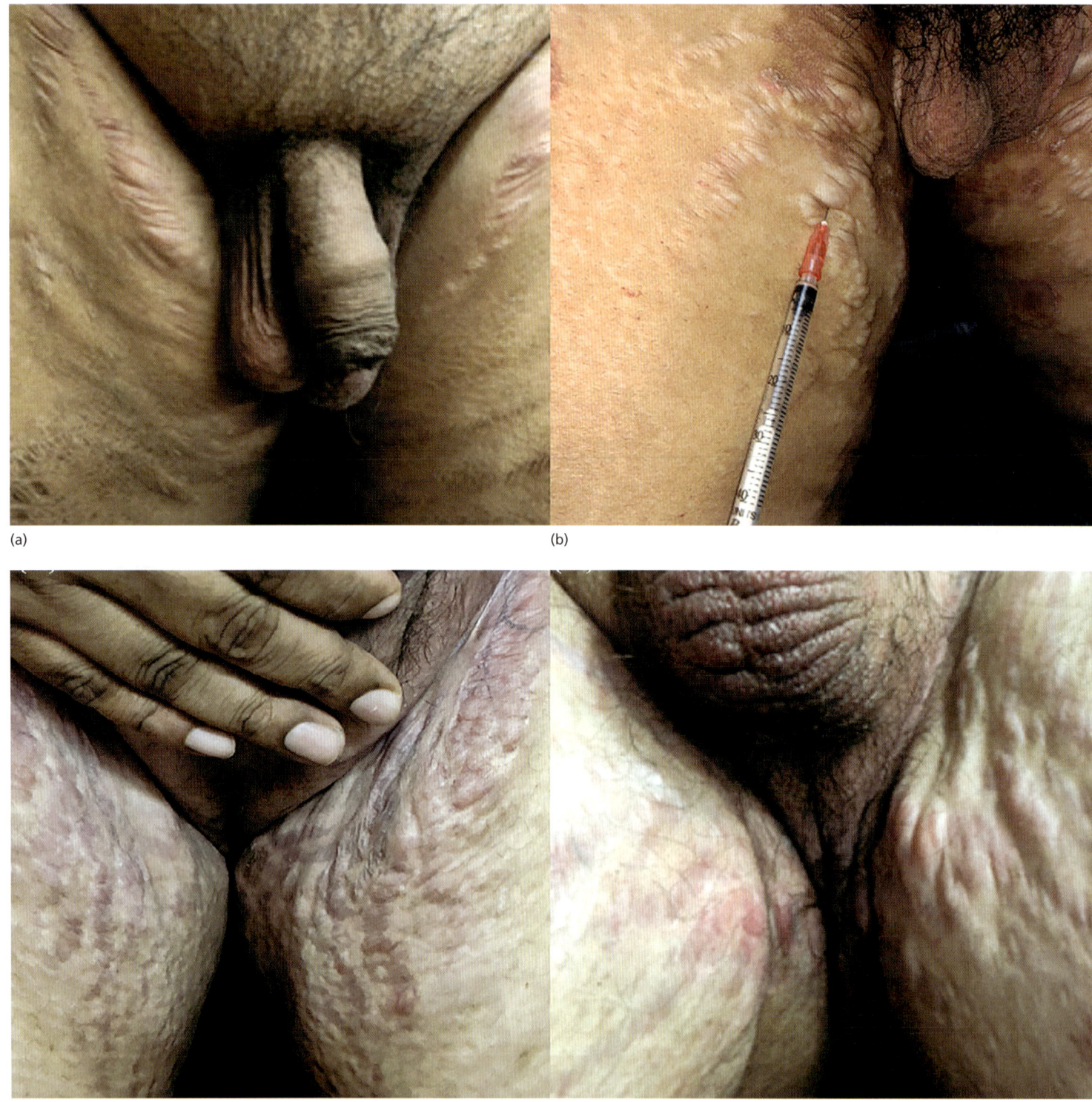

(a)

(b)

(c)

(d)

Figure 94.15 (a, c, d) Pseudoedematous-appearing striae with overlying skin atrophy. (b) Inability to draw fluid from the oedematous appearing striae. Reproduced from Verma *et al.* 2020 [27] with permission of John Wiley & Sons.

Some cases appear to respond to treatment with topical tretinoin cream (0.05% daily), which stimulates collagen synthesis, although weekly superficial dermabrasion is claimed to be better tolerated [21]. The vascular redness of 'younger' striae is claimed to respond to the 585 nm pulsed dye and Nd:YAG lasers, which may also stimulate collagen synthesis [22,23]. Fractional photothermolysis has been used in chronic striae [24]. The application of silicone gel may be beneficial [25]. Narrow-band UV light or 308 nm xenon chloride laser may enhance melanin production but these treatments have no effect on cutaneous atrophy [26].

There is no proven long-term benefit of treatments.

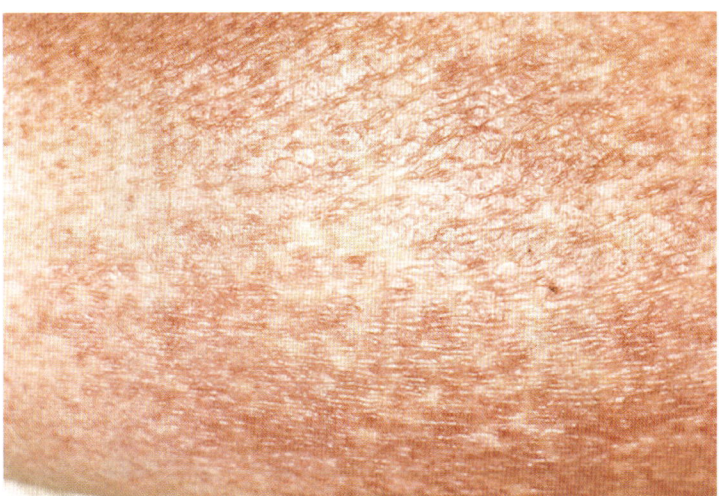

Figure 94.16 Poikilodermatous mycosis fungoides.

Acquired poikiloderma

Poikiloderma is a descriptive term, comprising atrophy, macular or reticulate pigmentation and telangiectasia. There may be associated areas of scaling, hypopigmentation and petechiae and signs of inflammation such as lichenoid papules. Congenital poikiloderma is a feature of several inherited disorders, including Kindler syndrome (Chapter 69), dyskeratosis congenita, Rothmund–Thomson syndrome and acrokeratotic poikiloderma of Weary (Chapter 75) and erythrokeratoderma variabilis (Chapter 63). More recently, a syndrome has been described comprising hereditary early-onset poikiloderma with scleroderma-like skin changes, tendon contractures and adult-onset pulmonary fibrosis [1].

Poikiloderma may occur as a pattern of cutaneous response to injury by cold, heat or ionising radiation [2]. So-called poikiloderma of Civatte (Chapter 86) is a similar reaction mediated by photosensitising chemicals in cosmetics. Some inflammatory dermatoses, such as lichen planus, may also give rise to poikilodermatous changes.

Poikiloderma is a feature of some systemic autoimmune diseases, and is a marker of disease severity in dermatomyositis [3]. It is also seen in lupus erythematosus and rarely in systemic sclerosis. Poikiloderma atrophicans vasculare is an early presenting feature of cutaneous T-cell lymphoma (mycosis fungoides), typically stage IA–IIA; it predominantly affects males. It usually responds well to phototherapy and has a good prognosis (Figure 94.16) [4].

Atrophic scars

Definition

These are scars resulting from the destruction of connective tissue by trauma or by inflammatory changes.

Introduction and general description

The distribution and character of the atrophic lesions may assist in determining diagnosis and further management, if necessary.

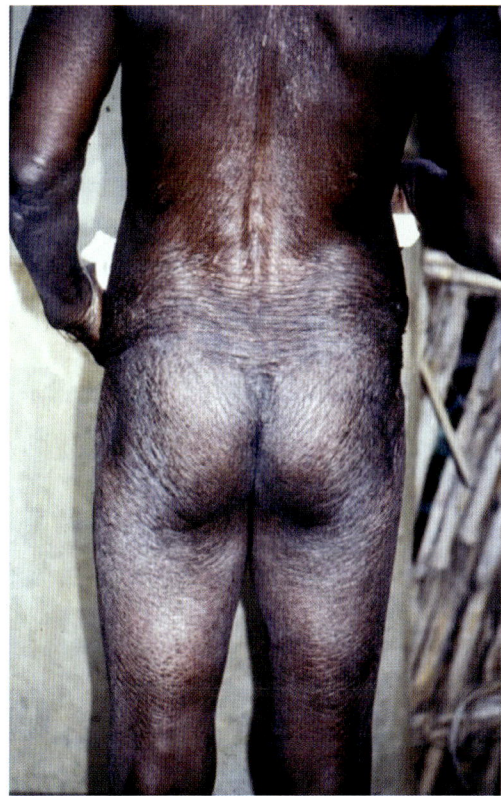

Figure 94.17 Atrophy due to onchocerciasis. Courtesy of Dr M. Murdoch.

Viral infections, such as varicella, can leave widespread small circular atrophic scars [1]. The scars left by tertiary syphilis, certain tuberculides and some deep mycoses, especially sporotrichosis, are usually completely atrophic. Onchocerciasis may result in extensive areas of dermal atrophy (Figure 94.17) [2]. Areas of cutaneous lupus erythematosus may also leave atrophy without clinical evidence of sclerosis. Lupus vulgaris, the chronic follicular pyodermas and some cases of lupus erythematosus leave a combination of atrophy and sclerosis, in which the latter predominates. Lesions that have been treated by intralesional steroid injections may also leave atrophic scars. Atrophic scarring may result from acne lesions (Chapter 88).

Exposure to ionising radiation gives rise to a very striking combination of atrophy, pigmentation and telangiectasia (poikiloderma).

The wide atrophic scars that follow injuries in Ehlers–Danlos syndrome (Chapter 70) emphasise the importance of constitutional factors in determining the pattern of dermal response to a known external injury.

Stellate pseudoscars are white, irregular or 'star-shaped' atrophic scars (Figure 94.18). They are common on light-exposed skin, particularly on the extensor aspects of the forearms, often in association with purpura. These are seen in 20% of patients aged 70–90 years, and a much less common presenile form occasionally occurs before the age of 50 years. These pseudoscars are secondary to mild trauma, and are usually preceded by haemorrhage into the dermis [3,4].

Stellate scars following trivial trauma can also occur in other conditions that cause fragile skin, for example porphyria cutanea tarda and prolonged use of potent topical steroids.

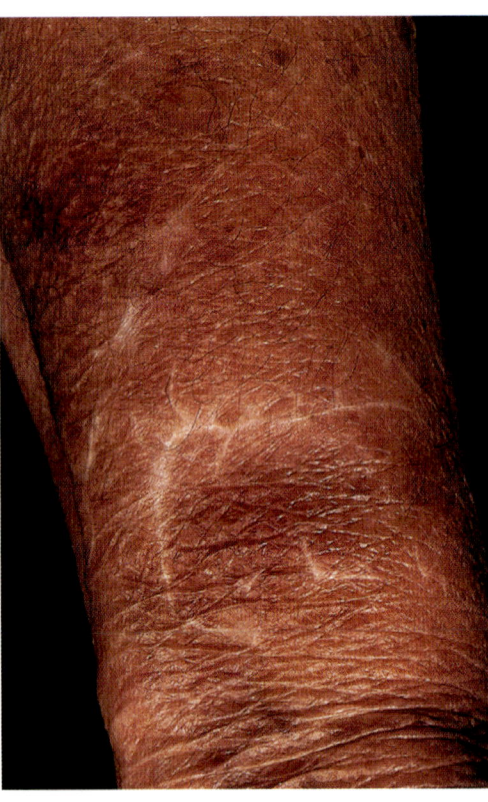

Figure 94.18 Stellate pseudoscars on the forearm of an elderly woman. There was no history of trauma.

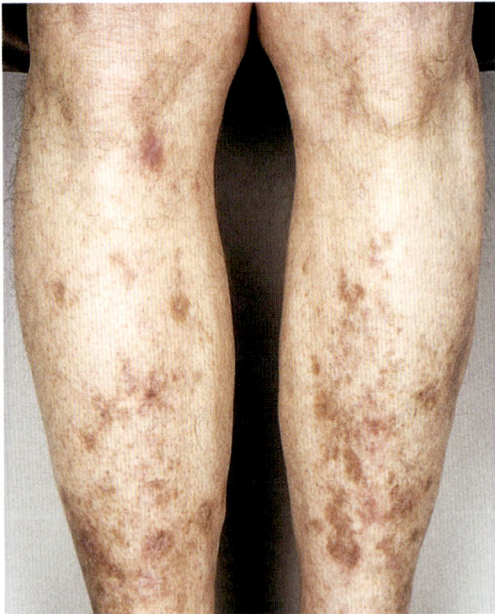

Figure 94.19 Brown pseudoscars of the legs due to diabetic dermopathy. There was no history of trauma.

Brown pseudoscars may also develop over the shins of diabetic patients, especially elderly men with no history of trauma (diabetic dermopathy) (Figure 94.19) (Chapter 62). Histology reveals that the pigmentation is due to dermal deposition of haemosiderin and melanin. Lesions may resolve spontaneously [5].

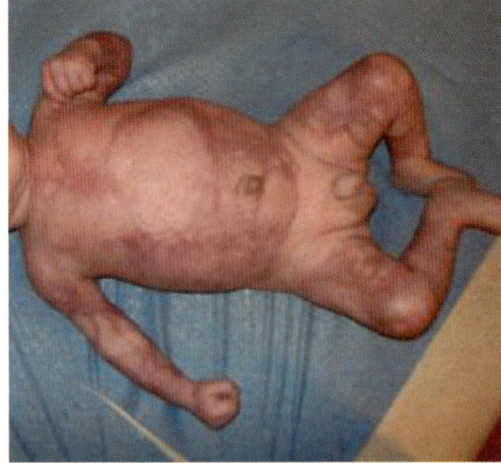

Figure 94.20 Congenital erosive and vesicular dermatosis with reticulate scarring. Reproduced from De Lange *et al.* 2009 [4] with permission of John Wiley & Sons.

Congenital erosive and vesicular dermatosis with reticulate scarring

This rare congenital condition, which was first described in 1985 [1], presents at birth with signs suggestive of congenital viral infection, including red skin, blistering, erosions and crusting often involving more than 75% of the skin surface. The skin heals over the course of a few months with soft reticulate scarring, which on the limbs tends to follow the long axis of the limbs (Figure 94.20). A review of 28 known cases [2] confirmed that it occurred predominantly in preterm infants (79%) and that there was often a history of maternal chorioamnionitis (43%). Neurodevelopmental problems were common. Histological examination in the early stages shows epidermal necrosis and subepidermal blistering but no evidence of viral infection or vasculitis. This is succeeded by scar formation with loss of appendageal structures, especially eccrine glands. The differential diagnosis includes Goltz syndrome, Rothmund–Thomson syndrome and aplasia cutis [2,3]. An infant was treated successfully using a silicone sheet dressing [4].

Spontaneous atrophic scarring of the cheeks

Synonyms and inclusions
- Varioliform atrophy
- Atrophia maculosa varioliformis cutis

This is a very rarely reported condition in which spontaneous scars develop on the cheeks (Figure 94.21) in young adults [1,2] or children [3]. It may, however, be much commoner than the lack of reports suggests. The shallow atrophic lesions have sharp margins and may be linear, curvilinear, rectangular or varioliform. They may be preceded by slight redness and scaling. Histology shows mild loss of collagen or elastic fibres; there may be thickening of the stratum corneum [4]. Most cases are sporadic, although familial cases are recorded [2,5]; inheritance is probably autosomal dominant [6]. The differential diagnosis includes atrophoderma

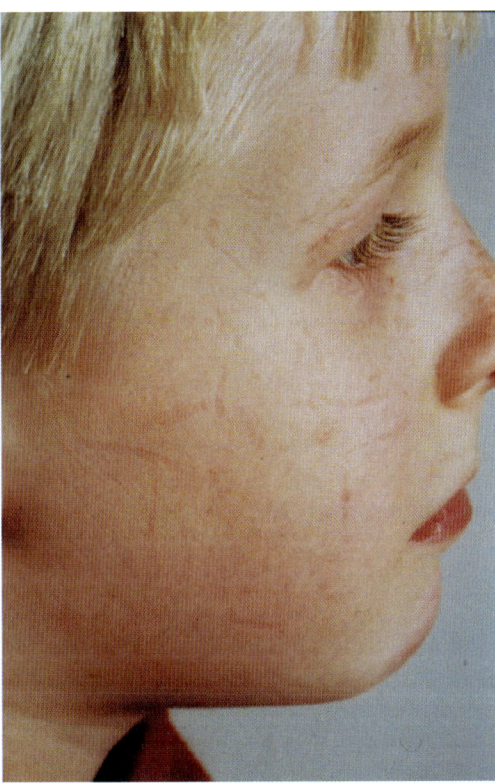

Figure 94.21 Spontaneous atrophic scarring of the cheeks (varioliform atrophy).

vermiculatum (Chapter 85), chickenpox scars and artefact. There is no evidence-based treatment, although topical retinoids have been used [7].

Acrodermatitis chronica atrophicans

Definition and nomenclature

This is a late skin manifestation of Lyme borreliosis (Chapter 26). It is characterised by the insidious onset of painless, dull-red nodules or plaques on the extremities, which slowly extend centrifugally for several months or years, leaving central areas of atrophy.

Synonyms and inclusions
- Chronic atrophic acrodermatitis
- Late-phase Lyme borreliosis

Introduction and general description

The condition is due to infection with a spirochaete, *Borrelia burgdorferi* (*sensu lato*), which is transmitted by ticks [1].

Epidemiology

Incidence and prevalence

This manifestation of borreliosis occurs mainly in northern or central Europe, Italy and the Iberian Peninsula. Occasional cases occur in other parts of Europe and Africa, but it is very rare in the UK,

America, Australia and Asia [2]. These geographical variations are related to different strains of the organism [3–5].

Age

It mostly occurs between the ages of 30 and 60 years, and is more common in female individuals.

Pathophysiology

Pathology [6]

During the early stages, there is non-specific dermal oedema with perivascular inflammatory infiltration. Subsequently, the epidermis becomes atrophic and the epidermal appendages are destroyed. Beneath a subepidermal zone of degenerate connective tissue lies a dense, band-like infiltrate, predominantly consisting of lymphocytes, histiocytes and plasma cells. Ultimately, the infiltrate is reduced to narrow bands between collagen fibres. In some patients, scleroderma-like changes may develop [7,8]. More typically, the dermis shows signs of atrophy; the swelling and homogenisation of collagen and elastic fibres is followed by their disappearance [9]. *Borrelia afzelii* has been cultured from the atrophic skin [7] but the culture is usually negative. *Borrelia afzelii* can be identified by polymerase chain reaction (PCR). The organism may be resistant to attack by the complement system and may lurk in immunologically protected areas such as fibroblasts and endothelial cells. Expression of pro-inflammatory cytokines, such as interferon γ (IFN-γ), is increased [10].

Causative organisms

Borrelia afzelii is the predominant species associated with acrodermatitis chronica atrophicans [11]. This species is transmitted by ticks in western Europe, but is rare in the USA, where *Borrelia burgdorferi* (*sensu stricto*) predominates [12].

Environmental factors

It is transmitted by bites from ticks, notably *Ixodes* spp., which favour bracken-covered hillsides and scrublands [12].

Clinical features

History

Most cases occur in country-dwellers. There is usually a history of a tick bite. The onset is usually insidious, and constitutional symptoms are exceptional [13].

Presentation

Dull-red or bluish-red oedematous nodules or plaques, more or less infiltrated, develop on the feet or legs, and less often on the forearms and hands. The lesions themselves are typically painless, but there may be associated acral pain or paraesthesiae. Erythema chronicum migrans (Chapter 26) may have been present at the same site some years earlier. Extension to the trunk and the greater part of the body, including the face, is sometimes seen. Single or multiple lesions may be present. They slowly extend centrifugally, the active inflammatory stage persisting for months, years or even decades. Marginal extension may continue once the central areas have already entered the atrophic phase, in which the skin is smooth, hairless and tissue-paper-like, dull red, pigmented or poikilodermatous (Figure 94.22).

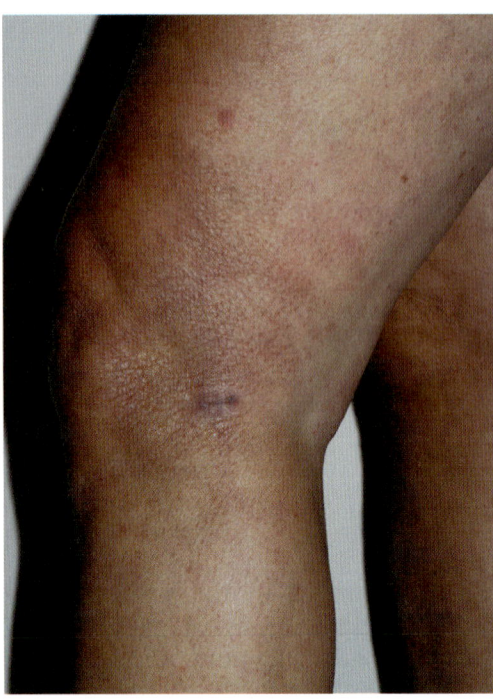

Figure 94.22 Acrodermatitis chronica atrophicans: image captured soon after the commencement of antibiotic therapy; note the atrophic wrinkled appearance of the skin at the side of the knee. Courtesy of Dr Ian Coulson.

Subcutaneous nodules may later develop around the knees or elbows, and fibrous bands along the ulnar margin of the forearms. Gaiter-like sclerosis of the lower third of the legs, often accompanied by ulceration, is a further complication. Morphoea of the trunk and lichen sclerosus (both genital and extragenital) have also been reported in association [2,14]. Conversely, *Borrelia* antibodies have been found in some patients with morphoea [14,15], although this does not appear to be a common finding [16]. Fifty per cent of patients develop peripheral neuropathy.

In some cases, involvement of the joint capsule or bone results in limitation of movement of the joints of the hands and feet, or of the shoulders.

Clinical variants
Occasional patients develop reddish plaques, clinically and histologically suggestive of mycosis fungoides [17].

Differential diagnosis
The early cutaneous phase of Lyme borreliosis, erythema chronicum migrans, may be confused with other annular erythemas, although a history of a recent tick bite at the site is often obtained. When it occurs on the lower legs, it may mimic venous insufficiency [18], with thick cyanotic itchy skin.

Complications and co-morbidities
Very rarely, squamous carcinoma has developed in the atrophic skin, and lymphoma has also been reported in non-affected skin, although it can be difficult to distinguish from the 'pseudolymphoma' lesions of borreliosis [16,19–21]. Other late manifestations of Lyme borreliosis (lymphocytoma, neurological, etc.) have been fully reviewed by Steere [1].

Disease course and prognosis
The bacteria can be eradicated with systemic antibiotics but some systemic features, such as neuroborreliosis, may persist.

Investigations
In the atrophic stage, diagnosis is usually readily made, and can be confirmed histologically. Immunoblotting using *Borrelia afzelii* flagellar antigen (41 kDa) is confirmatory [5]. Serology is used to confirm the diagnosis of Lyme disease, but false negative and false positive results are common. In chronic atrophic acrodermatitis, however, the antibody titre is very high. Serology may be positive on enzyme-linked immunosorbent assay (ELISA) but negative on immunoblotting, particularly in patients with neurological disease [22]. A high titre of antibodies may reflect occult central nervous system involvement, when the antibodies can also be demonstrated in colony-stimulating factor [23].

Management
Oral antibiotics should be given for 1 month, for example doxycycline or amoxicillin in standard doses [1]. Improvement occurs gradually and may not become apparent until several weeks after the course of treatment. There may be no improvement if treatment is delayed until atrophy has already developed. If the antibody titre is high or there are clinical features of systemic disease (e.g. neuroborreliosis), intravenous benzylpenicillin, ceftriaxone or cefotaxime should be given for 3 weeks [23,24]. There may be a case to be made for introducing public health measures such as prevention of enzoonotic transmission, chemoprophylaxis programmes or eventually a vaccine in endemic areas [25].

Elevated immunoglobulin G (IgG) and IgM antibodies may persist after treatment; this does not necessarily reflect treatment failure [26].

Treatment ladder for acrodermatitis chronica atrophicans

First line
- Oral antibiotics (e.g. doxycycline or amoxicillin)

Second line
- Intravenous antibiotics (e.g. benzylpenicillin if significant systemic manifestations)

Atrophodermas

Follicular atrophoderma

Definition
This distinctive abnormality manifests as dimple-like depressions at the follicular orifices and is usually associated with one of a small number of genetic syndromes but may be sporadic. It may be manifest at birth but may not become apparent until late in childhood.

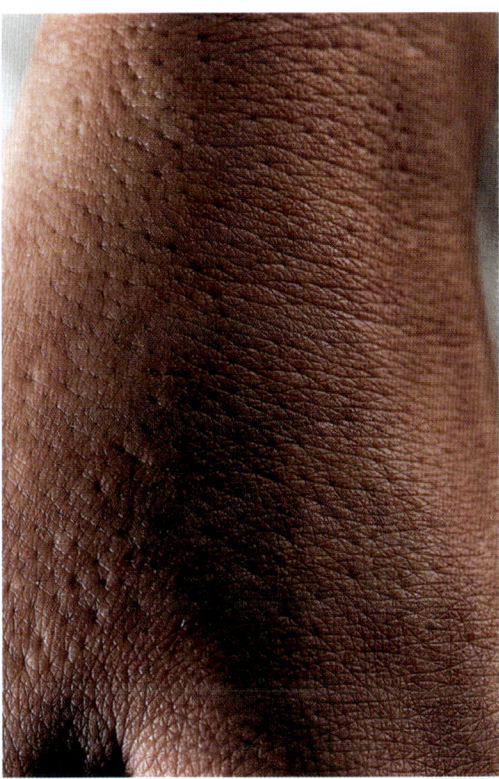

Figure 94.23 Follicular atrophoderma in Conradi syndrome.

It usually involves the backs of the hands (Figure 94.23) and the feet, and sometimes the elbow region. It may be associated with the following conditions [1]:
1 Conradi–Hünermann–Happle syndrome (calcifying chondrodysplasia) (Chapter 63) [2].
2 Bazex–Dupré–Christol syndrome (Chapter 66) [3].
3 Hyperkeratosis palmoplantaris, follicular keratosis or palmoplantar hyperhidrosis.
4 Ichthyosis and follicular atrophoderma with hypotrichosis and hypohidrosis [4].
It may also occur as an isolated defect of limited extent.

Pathophysiology
Pathology
Histology shows widened follicular ostia with thickening of the connective tissue sheath of the follicle.

Genetics
It appears to be associated with a variety of genetic defects. Variants of the ichthyosis-hypohidrosis syndrome are linked to mutations in the *ST14* gene, which encodes for matriptase [4].

Clinical features
Follicular atrophoderma present with follicular depressions on the backs of the hands (Figure 94.23), feet and occasionally elbows.

Management
There is no proven treatment.

Linear atrophoderma

Synonyms and inclusions
- Atrophoderma of Moulin

Introduction and general description
It is probable that this and atrophoderma of Pasini and Pierini are atrophic variants of morphoea [1].

Epidemiology
Incidence and prevalence
Cases are sporadic and worldwide.

Age
Most cases are described in childhood and adolescence.

Associated diseases
Leukonychia has been associated [2].

Pathophysiology
Pathology
Histologically, the epidermis is normal apart from hyperpigmentation in the basal layer. There is a perivascular lymphocytic infiltrate in the dermis [3]. The collagen bundles are normal or thickened and there is diminished periadnexal and subcutaneous fat [4].

Genetics
The condition may reflect mosaicism following a postzygotic mutational event [3,5].

Clinical features
History
Lesions are usually asymptomatic and insidious in onset.

Presentation
It presents with linear atrophic hyperpigmented plaques in the distribution of Blaschko lines, sometimes having a zosteriform appearance [4].

Differential diagnosis
Atrophic variants of morphoea strongly resemble this syndrome, and may be identical.

Investigations
Laboratory investigations are normal [4]. Skin biopsy is helpful if there is clinical doubt.

Management
One case of successful treatment with methotrexate is reported [6]. Unlike linear morphoea, linear atrophoderma is not associated with underlying joint contracture [5].

Atrophoderma of Pasini and Pierini

Definition
This condition is probably an atrophic variant of morphoea (Chapter 55) in which one or more patches of skin become bluish and sharply depressed, with no surrounding redness [1,2,**3**].

Epidemiology
Incidence and prevalence
Cases are mostly sporadic and rare.

Age
Most cases present in childhood or adolescence.

Associated diseases
There is a probable association with morphoea. Familial cases have been reported [4], together with an association with phenylketonuria [5].

Pathophysiology
Predisposing factors
The cause is unknown, although, as in morphoea, *Borrelia burgdorferi* has been implicated [6].

Pathology
The histological changes are often slight [**3**]. There may be increased pigmentation of the basal layer. During the earlier stages, the collagen in the lower dermis may be oedematous, and elastic tissue clumped and scanty. There may be a dermal perivascular infiltrate consisting of macrophages and T lymphocytes. Immunofluorescence studies may show IgM and C3 staining in the dermal blood vessels [7]. Later, the oedema subsides and there is some reduction in the total thickness of the dermis. Collagen bundles appear homogeneous and clumped in the reticular dermis. Eventually there may also be some epidermal atrophy.

Causative organisms
In common with morphoea, *Borrelia burgdorferi* has been implicated [6].

Genetics
No genetic factor has been reliably incriminated, although familial cases have been reported [4], and morphoea and atrophoderma of Pasini have occurred in siblings with phenylketonuria [5].

Clinical features
History
The lesions are generally asymptomatic.

Presentation [3,8,9]
The lesions, which may be single or multiple, range in size from 2 cm to many centimetres in diameter, and are round or oval in shape, but may become confluent to form irregular patches (Figure 94.24). They are smooth, slate-coloured or violet-brown, and are slightly depressed with a 'cliff drop' border [10] below the level of the entirely normal surrounding skin. The back is almost always involved, the chest and abdomen frequently, and the limbs occasionally.

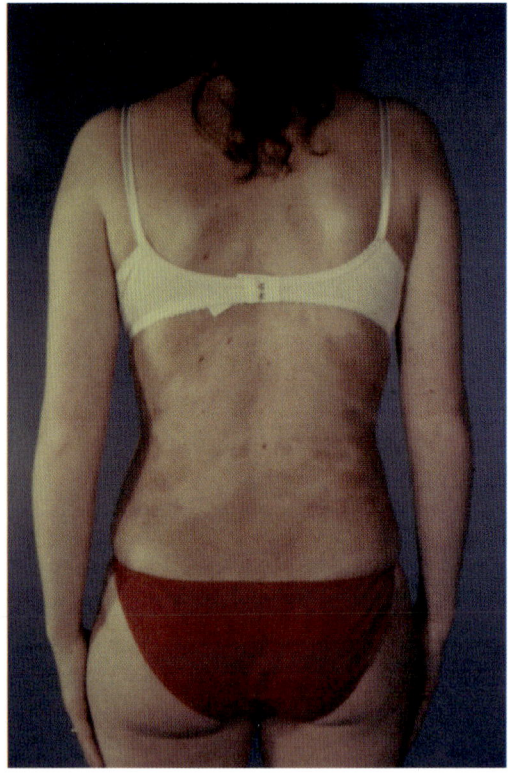

Figure 94.24 Atrophoderma of Pasini and Pierini.

Differential diagnosis
Atrophic morphoea and linear atrophoderma may represent the same condition. Clinical differentiation from morphoea, possibly an academic exercise, is based on the ivory-white indurated plaque with an oedematous lilac ring so characteristic of the latter. Histologically, sclerosis may be prominent in morphoea and is usually absent in atrophoderma. High-frequency ultrasound has been used as a non-invasive technique to aid diagnosis and to monitor disease progression [11].

Complications and co-morbidities
An overlap with juvenile idiopathic arthritis has been described [12].

Disease course and prognosis
The patches extend very slowly, increase in number for 10 years or more, and then usually persist unchanged. The eventual development of sclerodermatous changes within the patches has been observed, as has the presence in the same patient of lesions typical of atrophoderma and of morphoea.

Investigations
Serological tests for *Borrelia burgdorferi* are typically negative [**3**] although there are case reports of an association (for example, see [6]).

Management
No treatment is of proven efficacy, but psoralen and UVA (PUVA) has helped some patients. Topical calcineurin inhibitors are of limited value. Hydroxychloroquine has been used successfully [13].

Cases apparently associated with *Borrelia burgdorferi* have responded to penicillins and tetracyclines such as doxycycline [3,6].

Paroxysmal haematoma of the finger

Definition and nomenclature
This condition presents with the sudden spontaneous onset of one or more painful haematomas in the fingers (Figure 94.25).

Synonyms and inclusions
- Achenbach syndrome
- Acute idiopathic blue finger

Epidemiology
Age
It usually occurs in middle age.

Sex
There is a female predominance.

Associated diseases
There are no associated diseases.

Pathophysiology
Predisposing factors
The cause is unknown but has been hypothesised to be due to a localised acquired fragility of vascular connective tissue.

Pathology
There is no evidence of vasculitis or amyloid on skin biopsy.

Clinical features
History
There is a sudden onset of often painful haematoma.

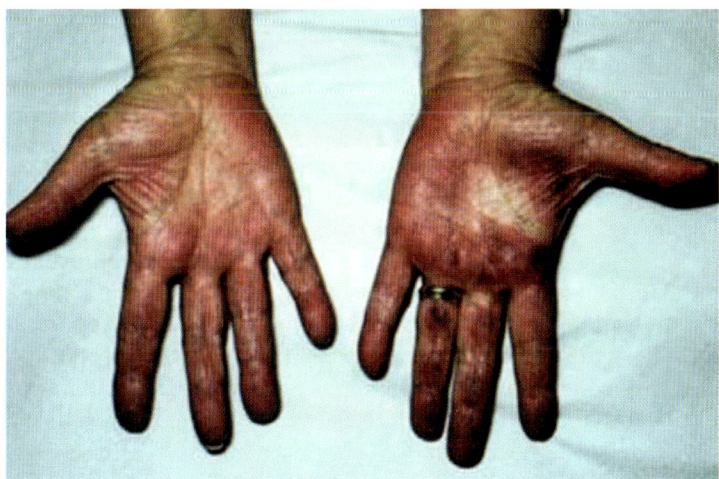

Figure 94.25 Paroxysmal haematoma of the finger. Courtesy of Dr J. Verbov.

Presentation
Sudden bruising of the volar aspect of a finger may occur spontaneously or after minor trauma; the bruising resolves within days and the patient is asymptomatic between flares [1–4]. The wrist may sometimes be involved [5]. There is no evidence of ischaemia [6].

Differential diagnosis
It may be mistaken for easy bruising due to steroid atrophy. The absence of ischaemic features and rapid improvement exclude occlusive vascular disease.

Complications and co-morbidities
There are no co-morbidities.

Disease course and prognosis
It may recur at intervals for several years [7]. Although troublesome, it is a benign condition.

Investigations
Although subtle angiographic abnormalities have been described [8], investigation of the patient for significant vascular disease is unnecessary [7,9,10].

Panatrophy

Definition
Local panatrophy is a rare disorder involving partial or total loss of subcutaneous fat and atrophy of the overlying skin, sometimes associated with atrophy or impaired growth of muscle or bone. A primary neurogenic disturbance has been postulated but not proved. The syndrome may represent the end result of more than one pathological process, but many cases may be due to a variant of morphoea. They are discussed further in Chapter 55.

The atrophic areas exhibit a reduced sympathetic response and aberrant production of non-esterified fatty acids after stimulation with norepinephrine (noradrenaline). It has been suggested that there may be a primary abnormality of the sympathetic nervous system [1].

Two groups of cases can be differentiated:
1 Panatrophy of Gower: in this rare condition no scleroderma or other sclerotic process accompanies or follows the loss of subcutaneous tissue. Most cases have occurred in women, usually in the second to fourth decades.
2 Sclerotic panatrophy: either typical morphoea or a similar sclerotic change in dermal collagen precedes the atrophy [2].

Clinical features
Clinical features of these two groups are as follows.

Panatrophy of Gower. Sharply defined areas of atrophy, irregular in size, shape and distribution, develop over a period of a few weeks, without preceding inflammatory stages [3,4]. In each affected area, the subcutaneous tissue disappears and the overlying skin appears atrophic and may be hypopigmented but is otherwise normal.

There may be a single area of atrophy or two or more. In size they range from 2 to 20 cm across, and in shape they are very variable but are sometimes triangular or quadrangular. Most lesions have occurred on the back, buttocks, thighs or upper arms, but some have involved the forearms or lower legs. The atrophy reaches its maximum extent within a few months and then remains unchanged indefinitely.

Sclerotic panatrophy. Atrophy of the subcutis, and sometimes of underlying muscle and bone, may follow clinically and histologically typical morphoea, especially when the process begins in childhood and involves a limb (Chapter 55). Sclerotic panatrophy may also occur in the absence of morphoea. The sclerosis involves subcutaneous tissue and muscle, and dense sclerotic, scar-like linear bands develop along a limb, or encircle the trunk in a metameric distribution, or encircle a limb. These lesions have also usually occurred in childhood. They cease to progress after a few months and, although new areas may be involved, most lesions have been solitary.

It is probable that Gower panatrophy and linear morphoea are at the ends of a continuous disease spectrum. The histology of linear morphoea reveals thickened bundles of collagen, which appear to be intact on B-scan ultrasound imaging [5].

In the differential diagnosis of panatrophy, the various forms of panniculitis must be excluded. The preceding inflammatory changes in the latter are the single most distinctive feature, but they are not always easy to distinguish. Some cases of panatrophy may have been misdiagnosed as steroid-induced atrophy [6].

Facial defects can be corrected by autologous fat grafting [7].

Facial hemiatrophy (Chapter 55)

Definition and nomenclature
Facial hemiatrophy is an atrophic dysplasia of the superficial facial tissues, but the underlying muscles, cartilage and bone may also be affected [1].

> **Synonyms and inclusions**
> • Parry–Romberg syndrome

Epidemiology
Age
This rare disease usually starts within the first two decades of life.

Sex
The sexes are equally affected.

Associated diseases
Some cases have been associated with syringomyelia, epilepsy or cerebrovascular disease, but in 90% of cases no such association is demonstrable.

Pathophysiology
Predisposing factors
The cause is unknown, but it may be a disorder of the sympathetic nervous system in some cases.

Genetics
There is no evidence that it is usually genetically determined, but it appears to be hereditary in a few pedigrees.

Clinical features
History
Occasionally, there may be premonitory muscle spasms or neuralgia [2] but often it is asymptomatic.

Presentation
The first manifestation is usually increased or decreased pigmentation in irregular patches on the cheeks, forehead or lower jaw. Progressive atrophy gradually develops in the affected sites, involving skin, subcutis, muscle and bone, and may extend in area – and sometimes in depth – for months or years with temporary remissions, eventually 'burning out'. Teeth on the affected side may be smaller, with short roots. The skin becomes dry, thin and atrophic, but may be scar-like and adherent in some areas. When the atrophy is fully developed, the contrast between the sunken, haggard, pigmented affected half of the face and the unaffected half is dramatic. The hair may be lost in the fronto-parietal region on the affected side but is often normal; occasionally, localised canities is an early change.

A variety of neurological signs have been reported, of which Horner syndrome is the most frequent. Heterochromia of the iris develops at the same time as the facial atrophy in about 5% of cases, and retinal changes may also be present [3], including central retinal artery occlusion [4]. There can be ipsilateral cerebral atrophy [5].

The degree of bone atrophy as established radiologically is usually much less than the clinical appearance suggests, and is severe only in some cases of early onset. In such cases, the cerebral cortex may also be affected, and contralateral epilepsy may result. Common findings on imaging include a variable degree of atrophy with obliteration of fat planes, ipsilateral deviation of the aero-digestive tract and enophthalmos due to loss of retrobulbar fat. Intracranial changes, where present, include discrete areas of subcortical calcification in the ipsilateral frontal lobe with areas of brain atrophy and abnormal white matter signalling [6].

Differential diagnosis
When the cutaneous involvement is early and conspicuous, the diagnosis presents few difficulties. Hypoplasia following radiotherapy given in infancy, perhaps in treatment of a naevus in the region of the temporo-mandibular joint, could cause confusion. If the skin changes are slight, or of later onset, physiological asymmetry, unilateral mandibular agenesis, hemihypertrophy and atrophy secondary to facial paralysis must be excluded. Hemihypertrophy is always congenital. When the limbs are involved, infantile hemiplegia and lipodystrophy (which is usually bilateral) must also be considered.

Lupus panniculitis results in subcutaneous atrophy which can be hemifacial. Atrophic morphoea of the 'coup de sabre' paramedian form may be associated with some degree of facial hemiatrophy, especially if it begins early in life. However, it is generally a more superficial process than progressive facial hemiatrophy. The skin in scleroderma is bound down and adherent, and loss of hair and pigmentary changes are conspicuous. In progressive facial hemiatrophy, the skin may remain mobile and grossly normal. The two processes have been confused frequently in the literature, and may coexist [7].

Complications and co-morbidities
There may be associated segmental vitiligo [8]. Spontaneous fracture of the jaw has also been reported [9]. Hemimasticatory spasm is a rare complication [10].

Disease course and prognosis
The atrophy may remain limited both in extent and depth. It may be confined to the distribution of one division of the trigeminal nerve or involve the whole of the side of the face, sharply demarcated at the midline. Rarely, it may be bilateral, and very rarely may involve half the body, usually on the same side as the face but exceptionally the opposite side in crossed hemiatrophy. The atrophy may, in such cases, begin on the trunk or a limb and only later involve the face.

Management
There are reports of clinical improvement following immunotherapy [6] although these may represent patients with linear morphoea. Plastic surgery offers cosmetic benefit once the disease appears to have stabilised. Serial autologous fat grafts can be beneficial for patients with mild to moderate disease [11,12]. Autologous lipoinjection may stimulate vascularity and tissue remodelling [13]. For patients with severe disease, free tissue transfer is the treatment of choice [12].

DISORDERS OF ELASTIC FIBRE DEGRADATION

Introduction and general description

The capacity of the skin to adapt to local or general changes in body size and contour, and to allow for movement of the head and limbs and a wide range of facial expression, depends upon its tension, elasticity and tensile strength. These properties may be congenitally defective or modified by ageing or disease [1–3]. Acquired disorders of elastic tissue have been reviewed in detail by Lewis et al. [4,5].

Elastic fibres are abundant in the skin, arteries, lungs and ligaments. They provide tissues with resilience and elasticity, enabling the skin to resume its original shape after deforming forces have ceased to act. Elastic fibres are comprised of an outer mantle of fibrillin-rich microfibrils surrounding a dense core of elastin. Elastin owes its remarkable elasticity to covalent crosslinks between tropoelastin monomers [6]. Although there is wide individual variation, elastic fibres tend to become less plentiful with age, when the skin becomes stiffer, with decreased viscoelastic recovery. Dermal fibroblasts become less responsive to mechanical stimuli with age; in contrast, the destruction of matrix proteins such as elastin by tissue metalloproteinases is increased [7]. Cutaneous elasticity is also reduced in a variety of skin disorders including cutis laxa. Additionally, elastic fibres provide adhesion for cells and play a role in regulating growth factors (e.g. transforming growth factor β (TGF-β)) [2].

Tensile strength
The tensile strength of the skin is the degree to which it can be elongated before it tears. It is greatest in infancy and decreases with age; it is also abnormally low in diseases associated with qualitatively or quantitatively abnormal collagen such as Ehlers–Danlos syndrome and Cushing syndrome [3].

Lax skin

Increased laxity of the skin due to ageing (accelerated by dermal photodegradation) is extremely common, but cutaneous laxity can occasionally result from marked weight loss (especially after gross obesity) or can follow recovery from severe oedema. Less commonly, the skin may become lax due to localised or generalised defects in elastic tissue resulting from other causes, and these may be grouped as follows:

1 Generalised elastolysis (cutis laxa):
 • Congenital (Chapter 70): this may be a component of inherited disorders including PXE, SCARF syndrome (skeletal abnormalities, cutis laxa, craniostenosis, ambiguous genitalia, retardation and facial abnormalities), de Barsy syndrome and geroderma osteodysplastica.
 • Acquired: there are numerous associated disorders, such as inflammatory skin disease, multiple myeloma, systemic lupus erythematosus, hypersensitivity reactions, complement deficiency and penicillamine therapy.
2 Localised elastolysis:
 • Anetoderma.
 • Blepharochalasis.
 • Chronic atrophic acrodermatitis (due to Borrelia; see earlier in this chapter).
 • Granulomatous slack skin (due to lymphoma).
 • Other localised lesions, including mid-dermal elastolysis, postinflammatory elastolysis and cutis laxa (PECL), elastic tissue naevi, etc.

It is probable that many of the above conditions are variations of the same disease, and there is considerable overlap. They share a similar pathological process, namely elastophagocytosis (the phagocytosis of elastic fibres by histiocytes and/or multinucleate giant cells) [1].

Acquired cutis laxa

Definition and nomenclature
Cutis laxa presents clinically as lax skin that hangs in folds, together with loss of dermal elastic tissue histologically. Congenital forms are discussed in Chapter 70.

Synonyms and inclusions
- Generalised elastolysis
- Generalised elastorrhexis
- Generalised dermatochalasia

Introduction and general description
Cutis laxa may be acquired following inflammatory skin disease [1] or following exposure *in utero* to drugs such as penicillamine [2]. An immunological pathogenesis has been suggested in many cases.

Epidemiology
Associated diseases
Acquired cutis laxa has been reported in association with urticaria and urticarial vasculitis [3,4], nephrotic syndrome [5], complement deficiency, sarcoidosis, syphilis, primary amyloidosis and multiple myeloma [6–8], drug hypersensitivity and the Klippel–Trenaunay syndrome [9]. Focal elastolysis can also occur in association with lupus erythematosus [10], severe rheumatoid arthritis [11] and coeliac disease [12]. D-penicillamine disrupts elastic fibre formation and may cause cutis laxa, elastosis perforans serpiginosa and pseudoxanthoma-like changes [13,14]. Congenital cutis laxa may also occur in offspring of mothers taking penicillamine [2].

Pathophysiology
Predisposing factors
These include immunological or chemical disruption of dermal elastic fibres.

Pathology
In acquired cutis laxa, dermal elastic tissue is markedly reduced, although collagen is normal. Fibroblasts express increased elastolytic activity (cathepsin G). Levels of serum α_1-antitrypsin and elastase inhibition are decreased [15].

Genetics
There may be an underlying genetic susceptibility, for example defects in the interaction of elastin and fibulin 5 results in elastic fibres that are more susceptible to degradation by matrix metalloproteinases [16].

Clinical features
History
Cutis laxa may rarely develop at any age following episodes of urticaria or angioedema, extensive inflammatory skin disease (such as systemic lupus erythematosus or erythema multiforme) or febrile illness (Figure 94.26). It may also follow hypersensitivity reactions such as penicillin allergy [17].

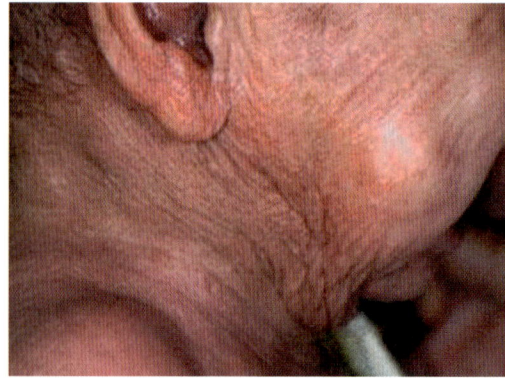

Figure 94.26 Acquired cutis laxa following a generalised inflammatory dermatitis in an 18-month-old child. Reproduced from Haider *et al.* [20] with permission of John Wiley & Sons.

Presentation
There may be widespread massive folds of lax skin, or the changes may be mild and confined to a limited area, in which case, it cannot be distinguished from anetoderma. Purpura may follow slight trauma and fibrotic nodules may form over bony prominences. Organs other than the skin may also be involved. Emphysema, gastric fibromas and tracheobronchomegaly have been reported [18].

Clinical variants
Postinflammatory elastolysis and cutis laxa (Marshall syndrome) (Figure 94.27) was originally described as a distinctive syndrome in African children but has subsequently been reported worldwide. Clinical features are intermediate between anetoderma and cutis laxa [19–21]. It is preceded by an inflammatory process, often with a neutrophilic component (e.g. Sweet syndrome [22,23]) or an insect bite. The preceding inflammatory lesions may be urticaria-like or multiple red papules, which slowly enlarge to form rings 2–10 cm in diameter [20]. PECL has been associated with α_1-antitrypsin deficiency, which may enable matrix metalloproteinases to destroy dermal elastin, and screening for this enzyme deficiency is recommended [23].

Differential diagnosis
The history should enable the condition to be distinguished from congenital cutis laxa. In Ehlers–Danlos syndrome, the skin is hyperextensible but not lax, and it recoils quickly. In PXE, the skin may be lax, but it is yellowish. The face is usually spared. It is distinguished histologically by the presence of calcification. There may be circumscribed folds of lax skin in neurofibromatosis, and loose folded skin may also occur in leprechaunism, Patterson syndrome and trisomy 18, but these conditions are distinguished by their associated features.

In severe actinic damage, there may be marked skin laxity due to damage to elastic fibres. There is doubtless considerable overlap with other elastolytic conditions described later.

Investigations
The diagnosis, which is suggested by finding loose skin that recoils only slowly after stretching, may be confirmed by histological confirmation of a reduction in elastic fibres. Investigations

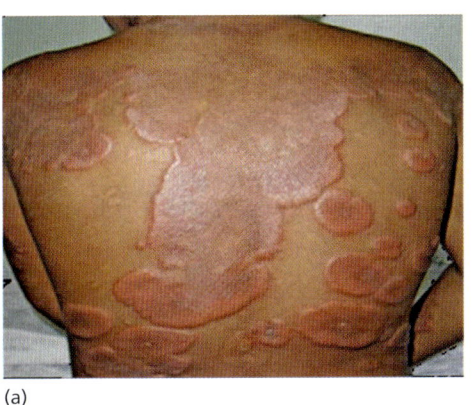 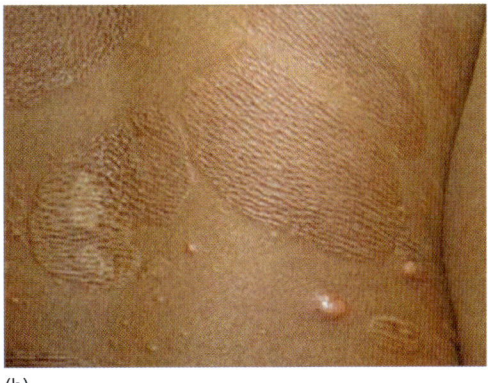 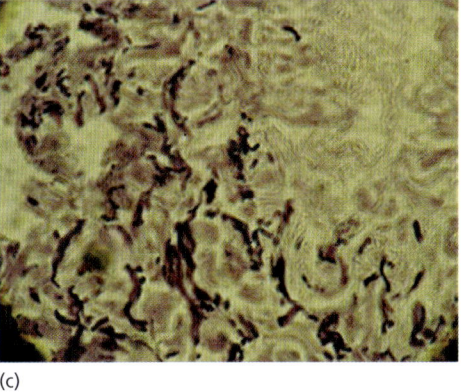

(a)   (b)   (c)

Figure 94.27 Postinflammatory elastolysis and cutis laxa (Marshall syndrome) in a 6-year-old boy showing (a) an acute inflammatory phase progressing to large plaques of lax wrinkled skin (b). (c) Histology shows shortened and fragmented elastic fibres in the reticular dermis. Reproduced from Fontenelle *et al.* 2013 [21] with permission of The Scientific Electronic Library Online (SciELO).

for emphysema may be indicated, with referral to a pulmonary physician if necessary. Underlying inflammatory disease may require investigation.

Management

Diphenyl sulfone appeared to prevent disease progression in a patient with cutis laxa associated with urticarial vasculitis [4]. Excision of redundant tissue ('face-lift') may substantially reduce the cosmetic disability [21,24].

Anetoderma

Definition and nomenclature

The term anetoderma (*anetos*: slack) refers to a circumscribed area of slack skin associated with a loss of dermal substance on palpation and a loss of elastic tissue on histological examination. 'Primary' anetoderma implies that there is no associated localised underlying cutaneous disease, whereas 'secondary' anetoderma can be attributed to some associated condition.

Synonyms and inclusions
• Macular atrophy

Introduction and general description

Previously, cases of 'primary' anetoderma were divided into the *Jadassohn–Pellizzari* type, in which the lesions are preceded by erythema or urticaria, and the *Schweninger–Buzzi* type, in which there are no preceding inflammatory lesions. This is now of historical interest only, because in the same patient some lesions may be preceded by inflammation and others may not, and the prognosis and histology are identical in the two types [1,2,3].

Epidemiology
Incidence and prevalence
Anetoderma is rare.

Age
It mainly occurs in patients aged 20–40 years, although is occasionally reported in infants and older patients.

Sex
It mainly occurs in women [2].

Associated diseases
Primary anetoderma is strongly associated with antiphospholipid syndrome [4–6] with or without features of systemic lupus. In older reports, this may have led to a misdiagnosis of syphilis in many cases, although there is a definite association with the disease and its treatment [7]. Secondary anetoderma has been reported in association with tuberculosis and leprosy [8,9], urticaria pigmentosa [10], pityriasis versicolor [11,12], granuloma annulare [13,14], Stevens–Johnson syndrome [15], B- and T-cell lymphoma [16–18] and other conditions. Some reported associations may be coincidental, but it is probable that many inflammatory diseases may occasionally be complicated by anetoderma.

Localised anetoderma may occur in premature infants, possibly due to the application of transcutaneous oxygen monitoring devices [19,20]. Localised anetoderma-like changes on histology have been reported in association with pilomatricoma [21], atrophic dermatofibroma and dermatofibrosarcoma protuberans [22,23], juvenile xanthogranuloma [24] and hamartomatous congenital naevi [25]. Lesions resembling anetoderma occur in PECL (Marshall syndrome) (Figure 94.27b). Penicillamine-induced anetoderma has also been reported [26].

Pathophysiology
Predisposing factors
Primary anetoderma. Recently, it has become apparent that 'primary' anetoderma is strongly associated with antiphospholipid antibodies, with or without a prothrombotic state (Figure 94.28) [4,5]. It is probable that these antibodies underlie the association historically noted with syphilis, and more recently with borreliosis [27] and systemic lupus.

In a few cases, there appears to be an underlying structural defect of connective tissue. Familial cases are reported [28–30] and there

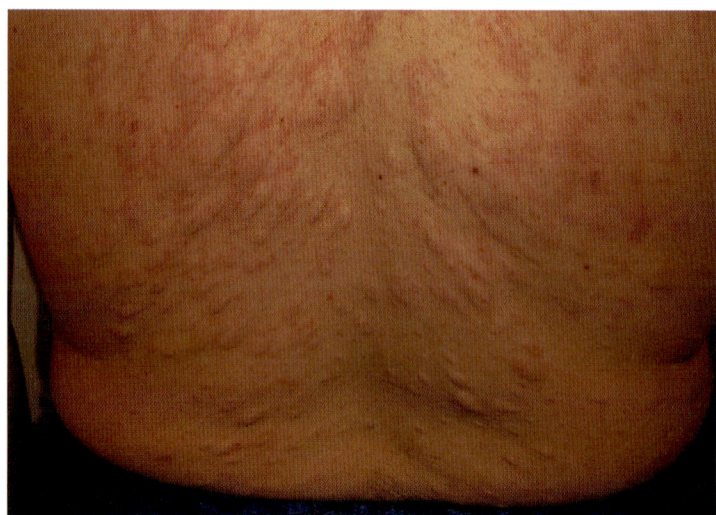

Figure 94.28 Primary anetoderma associated with antiphospholipid antibodies. Reproduced from Eungdamrong *et al.* 2012 [6] with permission of Regents of the University of California.

is an association with inherited bony or ocular abnormalities. The Blegvad–Haxthausen syndrome comprises anetoderma, blue sclerae and osteogenesis imperfecta.

The histology of anetoderma suggests that the basic abnormality is focal elastolysis [1,31,32]. This may be secondary to the release of elastase from inflammatory cells which are probably always present in the early stages. Metalloproteinases, notably MMP-2 and MMP-9, are increased in lesional skin [33,34].

Complement activation may be involved as C3 is deposited on the remaining elastic fibres [35]. It has been suggested that decay accelerating factor and vitronectin (an inhibitor of the membrane attack complex) may protect elastic fibres against this type of damage [36]. Abnormalities in the protective system could play a role in primary anetoderma.

Secondary anetoderma. This is seen in association with another identifiable disease, such as systemic [37] or chronic cutaneous lupus erythematosus [38], not always in relation to the lesions. Anetoderma is also associated with lupus profundus [39,40].

Some cases of primary anetoderma have direct immunofluorescence findings similar to those of either chronic cutaneous or systemic lupus erythematosus, even though there may be no other features of lupus erythematosus [41,42]. Biopsy shows a focal loss of elastic tissue, and a perivascular infiltrate with prominent plasma cells [1,2]. Generalised elastolysis (cutis laxa) has also occurred [43].

Antibodies have not been demonstrated against elastic fibres [42].

Pathology [2,27]

During the early stages, the dermis is oedematous, and a lymphocytic infiltrate (predominantly helper T cells) surrounds the blood vessels and appendages [1,32]. Plasma cells and histiocytes, with some granuloma formation, may also be seen. Later, the oedema and perivascular infiltrate subside and elastic fibres become scanty. The persistence of fine, irregular or twisted elastic fibres is common. The dermal collagen may also be diminished, but the fragmentation and disappearance of elastic tissue is the essential change,

beginning superficially in the subpapillary zone and extending downwards. Electron microscopy shows phagocytosis of elastic fibres by macrophages [44–46].

Causative organisms

Serological evidence of *Borrelia burgdorferi* infection has been observed in some cases [27].

Genetics

Familial cases are reported [28–30].

Environmental factors

It is perhaps more frequent in central Europe than elsewhere, which suggests a possible relationship to chronic atrophic acrodermatitis (due to *Borrelia* spp.) in some cases [27].

Clinical features

History

There may be a history of a previous inflammatory, perhaps urticated, lesion at the site. Often lesions are asymptomatic.

Presentation

In primary anetoderma crops of round or oval pink macules 0.5–1.0 cm in diameter develop on the trunk, thighs and upper arms, less commonly on the neck and face and rarely elsewhere. The scalp, palms and soles are usually spared. Each macule extends over a period of a week or two to reach a size of 2–3 cm. Sometimes, there are larger plaques of reddened skin, and nodules have also been reported as a primary lesion [47]. Slowly, each lesion fades and flattens from the centre outwards to leave a macule of wrinkled atrophic skin, which yields on pressure, admitting the finger through the surrounding ring of normal skin (Figure 94.29). The colour varies from skin colour to grey, white or blue. The number of lesions varies widely, from less than five to 100 or more. In a Korean series, indented lesions evolved into protuberant ones, reflecting more severe elastin loss [34].

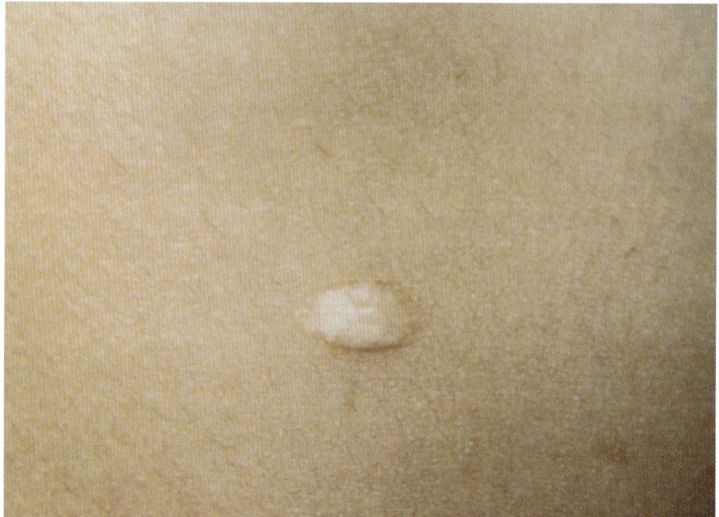

Figure 94.29 Secondary anetoderma in a chickenpox scar. Reproduced from Veraldi and Schianchi 2006 [51] with permission of John Wiley & Sons.

In some cases, the lesions are initially urticarial wheals, which, after a succession of exacerbations and remissions, perhaps continuing for many weeks, are succeeded by atrophy. They may become confluent, to cover large areas, especially at the roots of the limbs and on the neck.

The atrophic areas in secondary anetoderma do not always develop at the sites of the known inflammatory lesions. They are soft, round or oval areas, which occur mainly on the trunk.

Clinical variants

'Confetti-like macular atrophy' [48] may be a variant of anetoderma, although the lesions are not depressed or herniated. Hypopigmented, shiny, atrophic patches occur on the upper limbs and trunk. Histology shows an atrophic epidermis with disorganised, hyalinised coarse collagen bundles in mid-dermis, with elastic fibre loss and fragmentation in the upper dermis.

Differential diagnosis

Extragenital lichen sclerosus (Chapter 55) presenting as white spots around the base of the neck and shoulders should not be confused with anetoderma. Histological examination establishes the diagnosis if there is doubt. Focal dermal hypoplasia and atrophic scars must be also considered.

Aquired cutis laxa (see earlier) and anetoderma are closely related and may represent different forms of the same condition.

The diagnosis of 'primary' anetoderma can be established only by excluding the presence of any of the diseases known to be associated with 'secondary' atrophy such as perifollicular elastolysis (see later in this chapter).

Disease course and prognosis

The lesions remain unchanged throughout life and new lesions often continue to develop for many years. If the lesions coalesce they form large atrophic areas, which are indistinguishable from acquired cutis laxa [2].

Investigations

In patients with primary anetoderma it is important to test for antiphospholipid syndrome and treat appropriately, for example with aspirin or warfarin.

Management

No specific treatment exists. In the case of secondary anetoderma, treatment should be directed against underlying disease or infections.

Penicillin and the antifibrinolytic drug ε-aminocaproic acid have been advocated [49], but Venencie et al. [2] studied 16 patients and found no treatment was beneficial once the atrophy had developed. Colchicine may prevent some atrophic changes [50]. Ablative (e.g. carbon dioxide) lasers may reduce scarring [15].

Mid-dermal elastolysis

Definition and nomenclature

Idiopathic loss of the elastic fibres in the mid-dermis leads to widespread wrinkling of the crinkle type in otherwise healthy

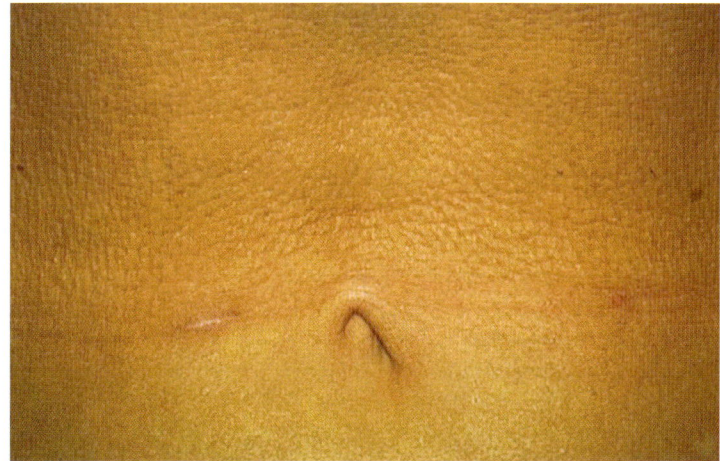

Figure 94.30 Idiopathic mid-dermal elastolysis. Courtesy of Dr L. Ostlere.

young or middle-aged women (Figure 94.30) [1,2]. The exact relationship between this condition and other elastolytic disorders such as acquired cutis laxa and anetoderma is uncertain. Localised areas may clinically resemble PXE, although they are histologically distinct [3–5].

Synonyms and inclusions
- Elastolysis mediodermalis
- Perifollicular elastolysis

Epidemiology
Incidence and prevalence
There are sporadic cases.

Age and sex
It mainly occurs in young to middle aged women.

Ethnicity
It occurs most commonly in fair-skinned people.

Associated diseases
Cases have been associated with a prothrombotic state [6], suggesting a similarity to anetoderma.

Pathophysiology
Predisposing factors
It has been reported to follow granuloma annulare [7] and other inflammatory conditions.

Pathology
Ultrastructural studies of mid-dermal elastolysis demonstrate elastic fibres engulfed by macrophages [8]. In the perifollicular variant, histology shows a non-inflammatory perifollicular loss of elastin fibres [9]. Immunological studies of affected skin show a non-specific profile of immune activation [10]. Cultured fibroblasts from lesional dermis exhibit increased elastolytic activity and reduced elastin mRNA compared with normal skin [11].

Maghraoui *et al.* [12] have distinguished postinflammatory elastolysis, with or without features of cutis laxa, from non-inflammatory elastolysis.

The histology of idiopathic mid-dermal elastolysis is similar to that of PECL (see earlier in this chapter). Those lesions are preceded by inflammatory lesions, but the lesions of idiopathic mid-dermal elastolysis may also occasionally be preceded by redness, urticaria or a burning sensation, and the two conditions are similar, if not identical.

Causative organisms

Elastase-producing strains *of Staphylococcus epidermidis* have been implicated in the perifollicular variant [13].

Environmental factors

Ultraviolet light may trigger elastophagocytosis [14]. The condition has also been reported in a patient receiving haemodialysis [15] and near the site of insertion of a pacemaker [16]. Inflammatory triggers may include UV radiation, insect bites, varicose veins, borreliosis and acute neutrophilic dermatosis [17,18].

Clinical features
History
The condition is typically asymptomatic.

Presentation
Presentation is with well-circumscribed or net-like areas of crinkly skin (cigarette paper-like fine wrinkling) that are up to 1 cm or more wide.

Clinical variants
Three variants have been described [19,20] as follows:
- Type 1: cigarette paper-like fine wrinkling (crinkle) affecting the trunk and upper arms.
- Type 2: perifollicular papules [9,13]. Lesions are small, grey-white, finely wrinkled, round or oval areas, each with a central hair follicle. Some exhibit a balloon-like bulge above the surface. They occur on the upper trunk, neck, earlobes and arms. Similar changes are more commonly seen in acne scars (Chapter 89).
- Type 3: reticular variant. Unlike other variants, this appears commoner in males [20]. Orange-red inflammatory papules precede net-like areas of atrophy, chiefly on the arms [5,16,19]. Localised areas may clinically resemble PXE, although they are histologically distinct [3,4]

In addition to these, a linear lumbar variant has also been described in a female [21].

Upper dermal elastolysis

Definition and nomenclature
Selective loss of elastic tissue in the papillary dermis was originally described in an otherwise healthy 86-year-old woman, who presented with numerous yellowish papules on the neck and upper trunk, and associated coarse wrinkles [1]. Since then, there have been several other reports, mostly in women aged 60–70 years [2,3,4]. This condition may be a unique variant or related to acquired PXE [4,5]. Although photodamage may be implicated, the condition has been described on the neck of a woman who wore a hijab [6].

Synonyms and inclusions
- Papillary dermal elastosis

Clinical features
Differential diagnosis
The histology of idiopathic mid-dermal elastolysis is similar to that of PECL, which occurs in young African girls (see earlier in this chapter). Those lesions are preceded by inflammatory lesions, but the lesions of idiopathic mid-dermal elastolysis may also occasionally be preceded by redness, urticaria or a burning sensation, and the two conditions are similar, if not identical.

Management
No definite treatment exists but topical retinoic acid (0.01% gel) has produced cosmetic improvement [7,8]. Reduction of degradation by metalloproteinases would be desirable, as in other elastophagocytic disorders [9].

Blepharochalasis

Definition and nomenclature
This is laxity of the eyelid skin due to a defect in the elastic tissue.

Synonyms and inclusions
- Ascher syndrome

Epidemiology
Incidence and prevalence
It is rare and mostly sporadic.

Age
It usually presents around the time of puberty.

Ethnicity
Most cases are reported in white people.

Associated diseases
Some cases may be a localised form of postinflammatory elastolysis or follow angioedema [1].

Pathophysiology
Predisposing factors
There is presumably an inflammatory stimulus to elastophagocytosis.

Pathology

In the early stages, there may be a mild dermal lymphocytic infiltrate, and in the later stages the elastic fibres in the lids fragment and decrease [2]. Normal elastin gene expression suggests other factors may be involved in elastic fibre loss [3]. IgA deposition may be detected on fibres, implying an immunopathogenic mechanism may be relevant [4]. Disintegration of collagen fibres has also been observed in one case [5].

Causative organisms

None is known.

Genetics

Some pedigrees show autosomal dominance, although most cases are sporadic.

Clinical features

History

There may be a history of previous transient episodes of painless eyelid swelling lasting for 2–3 days.

Presentation

Blepharochalasis is an uncommon condition that usually develops insidiously. Attacks of painless swelling of the eyelids are followed by laxity, atrophy, wrinkling and pigmentation, predominantly of the upper eyelids (Figure 94.31). There may be multiple telangiectases. These changes produce an appearance of tiredness, debauchery or premature ageing.

Reduplication of the mucous membrane of the upper eyelid is associated with blepharochalasis in about 10% of cases, and this may make the eyelids appear thick.

Clinical variants

Ascher syndrome is the association of blepharochalasis with progressive enlargement of the upper lip due to hypertrophy and inflammation of the labial mucosa [1–3,6–11,**12**,13,14]. The lip feels soft and lobulated and there may be excessive salivation. The lip abnormality is most noticeable when the patient speaks or smiles,

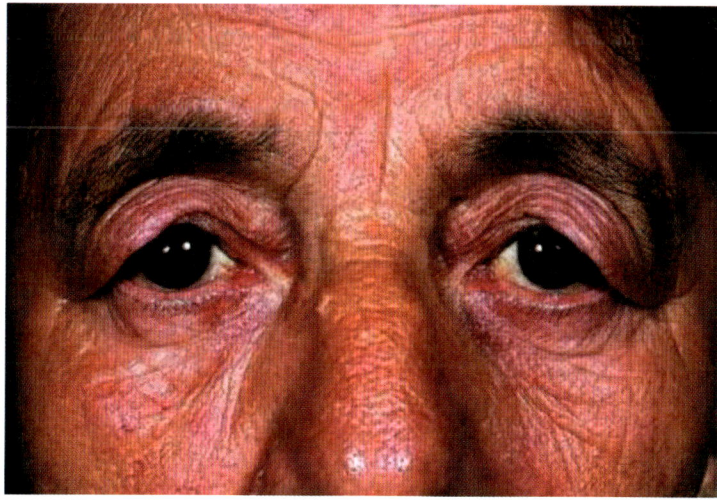

Figure 94.31 Blepharochalasis.

when the mucosal hyperplasia presents a 'cupid's bow' appearance. In some cases, the accessory lacrimal glands are also affected, with increased thickness of the eyelids. Goître (enlargement of the thyroid) [6] and autoimmune thyroiditis [15] have also been reported as part of the syndrome [6].

Differential diagnosis

The many other causes of eyelid swelling must be excluded (Chapter 107). Ptosis is easily distinguished because the skin appears normal. Blepharochalasis is occasionally a manifestation of generalised cutis laxa.

Laxity of the eyelid skin is most commonly an age-related phenomenon (dermatochalasis) due to degenerative changes in the connective tissue of the eyelid. Laxity also occurs in Ehlers–Danlos syndrome but other features of this syndrome will also be present. Occasionally laxity, particularly affecting the upper eyelid, occurs in otherwise healthy individuals [8].

Management

Various techniques of blepharoplasty can be performed, but the condition may recur [2,16]. Oral acetazolamide proved helpful in a patient with blepharochalasis and recurrent oedema [17].

Actinic granuloma and annular elastolytic giant cell granuloma

Definition and nomenclature

Actinic granuloma is an uncommon condition affecting actinically damaged skin that results from a low-grade reactive inflammatory process in which degenerate elastic fibres are phagocytosed by multinucleate giant cells and histiocytes. It is the commonest type of annular elastolytic giant cell granuloma (AEGCG), in which abnormal elastic fibres are progressively destroyed by an expanding ring of elastolysis and granulomatous inflammation.

Synonyms and inclusions
- Elastolytic actinic giant cell granuloma
- O'Brien granuloma
- Miescher granuloma of the face
- Atypical annular necrobiosis lipoidica of the face and scalp
- Granuloma multiforme

Introduction and general description

Annular elastolytic giant cell granuloma is an uncommon granulomatous cutaneous reaction pattern in which damaged dermal elastic fibres are slowly eliminated by a process of phagocytosis by multinucleate giant cells and histiocytes (Figure 94.32) [1]. The commonest form, actinic granuloma, occurs in sun-exposed skin and manifests as one or more slowly enlarging annular plaques with an elevated red margin, leaving behind a central area of atrophy devoid of elastic fibres (Figure 94.33) [2]. Actinic granuloma is associated with diabetes in up to 40% of cases: it has been postulated that hyperglycaemia may alter the immunogenicity of

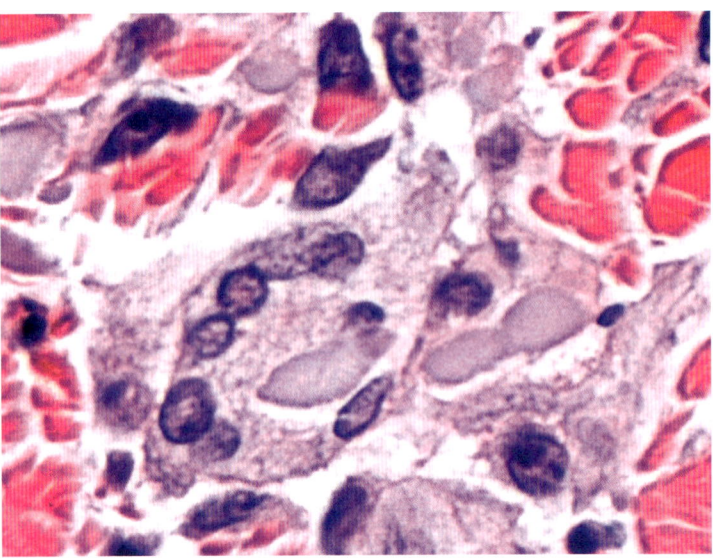

Figure 94.32 Annular elastolytic giant cell granuloma: high-power view showing fragments of degenerate elastic fibres engulfed by multinucleate giant cells. Courtesy of Professor Luis Requena.

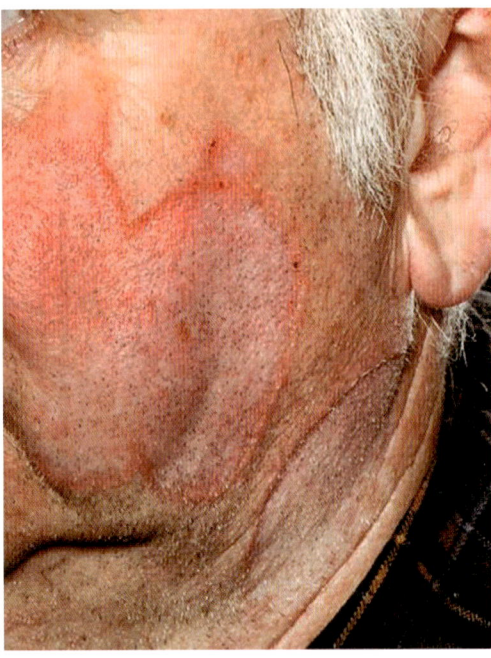

Figure 94.33 Typical actinic granulomas on the face and neck of an elderly man.

elastic fibres [1,3]. There are other less common variants of AEGCG including an annular form of sarcoidosis which typically presents around the temples and forehead and was originally described as atypical necrobiosis lipoidica [4,5]; AEGCG in sun-protected skin [6–8]; and AEGCG occurring in burn scars [9,10]. It has also been associated with prolonged doxycycline photosensitivity [11], prolonged sunbed exposure [12] and with the onset and recurrence of acute myeloid leukaemia [13]. In common with other granulomatous conditions, it has been associated with focal segmental glomerulosclerosis [14]. The common theme appears to be damage to elastic fibres provoking a granulomatous inflammatory response.

Epidemiology

Incidence and prevalence
The condition is more common in sunny countries.

Age
It usually occurs in people over the age of 30.

Ethnicity
People with Fitzpatrick skin type I are particularly susceptible.

Associated diseases
Diabetes is associated.

Pathophysiology

Pathology
The histological appearances are characteristic [1,2,15–19]. A biopsy taken radially across the thickened edge of the lesion and stained with elastic van Gieson stain shows three distinct zones in the dermis. In the external 'normal' skin, there is actinic elastosis. In the thickened annulus, there is a histiocytic and giant cell inflammatory reaction in relation to elastotic fibres (Figure 94.34), and in the centre, within the annulus, little or no elastic tissue remains. The cellular infiltrate slowly expands outwards, leaving behind a central area from which elastic fibres have been removed by 'elastoclasis'.

The epidermis may be normal, or it may show signs of actinic damage.

Environmental factors
Chronic photodamage may be involved.

Clinical features

History
Lesions are typically asymptomatic.

Presentation
Lesions may be single or multiple. They normally develop in sun-exposed skin such as the dorsa of the hands and forearms, the V of the neck or the bald scalp (Figure 94.35). Fair-skinned or freckled subjects are particularly susceptible. The lesions start insidiously as small pink papules, which slowly extend centrifugally to form a ring of firm, superficial dermal thickening which is smooth and slightly elevated (Figure 94.33). The ring initially measures a few millimetres across but gradually expands, often attaining a diameter of several centimetres. The centre may become slightly atrophic and variable depigmentation may occur. The lesions are usually asymptomatic, but a sunburn reaction may provoke severe redness and irritation. Hair growth is not affected (Figure 94.35).

Clinical variants
See the introduction; some cases of AEGCG may represent an annular form of cutaneous sarcoidosis [20]. Granuloma multiforme is a condition that many would regard as a variant of AEGCG (see next section).

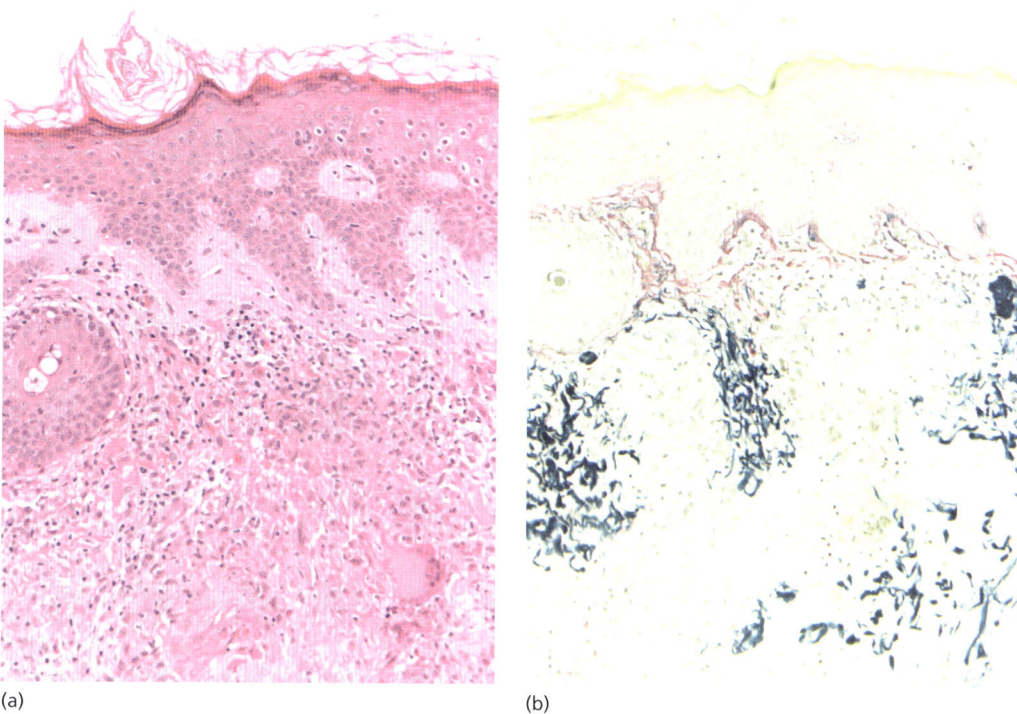

Figure 94.34 Annular elastolytic giant cell granuloma: (a) low-power view showing intense granulomatous inflammation and (b) elastorrhexis with a loss of elastic fibres. Courtesy of Dr Leigh Biddlestone.

(a)

(b)

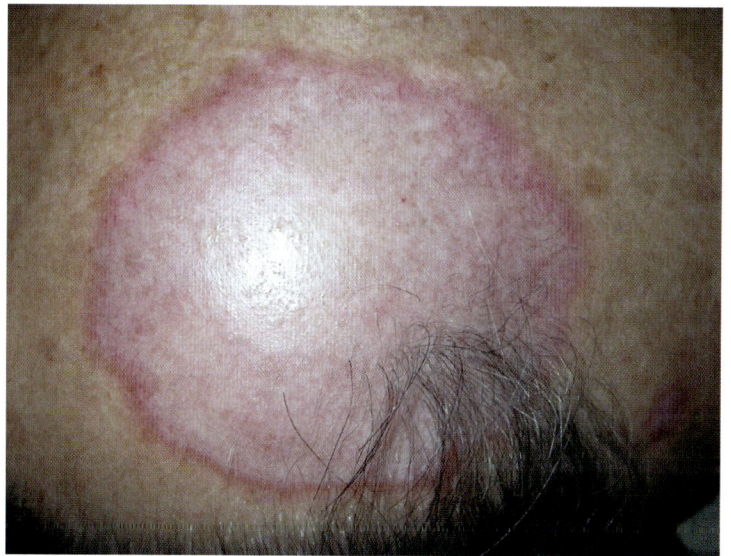

Figure 94.35 Actinic granuloma on a bald scalp. Courtesy of Professor Luis Requena.

Investigations
Skin biopsy should be performed.

Management
No treatment is of proven benefit. Topical steroids are generally unhelpful. In a series of 10 patients, hydroxychloroquine and photoprotection were beneficial [21].

Anecdotal reports of successful treatment include intralesional triamcinolone, isotretinoin (0.5 mg/kg/day) [22], doxycycline [23], acitretin 25 mg/day [24], oral prednisolone [25], dapsone, methotrexate and ciclosporin and topical tacrolimus [26]. A combination of pulsed dye laser and fractionated carbon dioxide laser has been used successfully [27], although AEGCG has been induced by pulsed dye laser therapy [28].

Differential diagnosis
- Granuloma annulare.
- Necrobiosis lipoidica.
- Elastosis perforans serpiginosa.
- Sarcoidosis.

Complications and co-morbidities
These may include diabetes.

Disease course and prognosis
The condition can improve with adequate sun protection.

Granuloma multiforme

Introduction and general description
Granuloma multiforme is a dermatosis reported in dark-skinned people mainly from Africa and India [1,2,3–8]. It shares many similarities with AEGCG in that it is characterised by annular plaques with giant cell granuloma formation at the periphery and loss of elastic tissue centrally [1]. As with AEGCG, it presents with papules that enlarge to form annular plaques with raised edges which may attain many centimetres in diameter. Histologically, the condition is difficult to distinguish from AEGCG except that focal necrobiosis and dermal mucin may be seen, which is not the case in AEGCG. Many authorities believe that granuloma multiforme should be regarded as a form of AEGCG [1].

PART 8: SPECIFIC CUTANEOUS STRUCTURES

Its importance lies in its superficial resemblance to tuberculoid leprosy, which is an important differential diagnosis. Leiker *et al.* [2,3,4] first described granuloma multiforme and distinguished it from tuberculoid leprosy. Leiker called it Mkar disease, after the town where it was first studied. The condition is endemic in certain villages in eastern Nigeria, where the local inhabitants refer to it in the Ibo tongue as 'Ununo Enyi' (elephant ringworm) [5,8]. The disease appears to occur predominantly in females over the age of 40 years [5,8,9]. Intense sun exposure over many years in people able to withstand acute photodamage appears to be a common feature. The difference in skin type and other unknown factors may explain the rather minor histopathological differences from AEGCG as seen in fair-skinned individuals.

Clinical features
Presentation
The upper, uncovered parts of the body are predominantly affected. The initial lesions are small flesh-coloured papules which become aggregated into plaques or form the elevated rims of annular lesions. In larger annular lesions, the central area is often hypopigmented. Pruritus may be prominent. The condition lasts for many months or years and may persist indefinitely.

Differential diagnosis
Leprosy is endemic in the same regions where granuloma multiforme is found and can look very similar. However, there is no loss of sensation or sweating, or other evidence of neural involvement in granuloma multiforme. Annular sarcoid, granuloma annulare and actinic granuloma can be distinguished histologically [10].

Management
No treatment is known to be effective, although a recent report describes a response to dapsone [11].

Other elastolytic conditions

Granulomatous slack skin is characterised by the slow development of pendulous folds of lax red skin, which on histological examination contain a dense granulomatous dermal infiltrate, with destruction of dermal elastic tissue. It is now considered to be a type of cutaneous T-cell lymphoma (mycosis fungoides) (Chapter 137) [1,2].

Acquired pseudoxanthoma elasticum-like syndromes

Perforating pseudoxanthoma elasticum

> **Synonyms and inclusions**
> - Perforating periumbilical calcific elastosis

Transepithelial elimination (TEE) of altered elastic fibres can occasionally occur in generalised hereditary forms of PXE (Chapter 70), but it can also occur as a localised acquired defect in patients who do not have the other features of PXE [1]. These localised lesions usually occur in the periumbilical area in obese, multiparous black or Asian women, and it is possible that this represents a response to repeated cutaneous stretching (e.g. ascites or previous abdominal surgery) [2–5]. Similar lesions on the breast have been reported in patients undergoing haemodialysis [2,6].

Clinically, asymptomatic yellow macules and papules coalesce into well-demarcated hyperpigmented plaques which slowly enlarge. The surface may be atrophic, grooved, fissured or verrucous, and compression of the edge of the lesion may produce a liquid discharge. Dermoscopic changes include yellowish brown structureless areas with curved or serpiginous lines, a few linear vessels and a keratotic plug with central crater [7].

It seems likely that most cases previously described as elastosis perforans serpiginosa in association with PXE were really examples of perforating PXE [8]. The histology of the two conditions is similar, but in perforating PXE there is transepidermal elimination of altered basophilic, calcified, elastic fibres [9], which are short, fragmented, curled and predominantly in the mid-dermis, whereas in elastosis perforans serpiginosa the fibres are abnormally large, non-calcified, eosinophilic and straight. The condition is similar or identical to upper dermal elastolysis (see earlier in this chapter) [10]. Spontaneous resolution has been reported [11].

Acquired pseudoxanthoma elasticum

> **Synonyms and inclusions**
> - Pseudo-pseudoxanthoma elasticum

Epidemiology
Iatrogenic causes
Skin changes that are virtually identical to those of PXE can rarely be produced by penicillamine (e.g. in the treatment of Wilson disease), although the systemic features do not occur [1,2]. The skin changes can be explained by the known effect of penicillamine in inhibiting collagen and elastin cross-linking, with the production of vastly increased amounts of abnormal elastin in the dermis [3]. Transepidermal extrusion of elastin has been reported in this condition [4].

Toxic causes
Lesions clinically resembling PXE are reported in the eosinophilia-myalgia syndrome; dermal calcification is absent on histology [5]. Eosinophilia-myalgia syndrome is defined by: (i) incapacitating myalgias; (ii) a blood eosinophil count greater than 1000 cells/µL; and (iii) no evidence of infection (e.g. trichinosis) or neoplastic conditions that could account for these findings. It is related to toxic oil syndrome, caused by the ingestion of contaminated L-tryptophan or other less well-characterised toxic substances (see Saltpetre disease).

Clinical features
Depositions

Yellowish papules and plaques resembling PXE are seen in some patients with amyloidosis; amyloid deposits are seen and, again, dermal calcification is absent [6,7].

Haematological disease

Pseudoxanthoma elasticum-like lesions are described in several haemoglobinopathies, including congenital anaemia, sickle cell disease and thalassaemia [8]. These patients may develop systemic manifestations such as peripheral vascular occlusive disease and retinal neovascularisation and haemorrhage [9].

Saltpetre disease

Saltpetre disease is a condition that resembles the skin changes of PXE clinically, histologically and ultrastructurally [1–3]. It has been described in a group of elderly farmers, who decades earlier had spread a fertiliser containing calcium-ammonium nitrate (Norwegian saltpetre). The patients developed cutaneous ulcers at sites of exposure (including antecubital fossae). These quickly healed to leave yellowish white papules and plaques. None of the patients had a positive family history or other signs of PXE.

Acrokeratoelastoidosis

Synonyms and inclusions
- Acrokeratoelastoidosis
- Focal acral hyperkeratosis
- Hereditary papulotranslucent acrokeratoderma
- Marginal papular acrokeratoderma

Acrokeratoelastoidosis is an uncommon asymptomatic disorder, which manifests as multiple, tiny, crateriform keratotic papules along the margins of the hands and feet, particularly in people of African descent (Figure 94.36). The name derives from the histological appearances which include not only epidermal acanthosis and hyperkeratosis but also fragmentation of the underlying dermal elastic fibres [1]. Fragmented elastic fibres resembling rooster crests are characteristic on scanning electron microscopy [2].

It is inherited in an autosomal dominant fashion but does not usually present until after puberty; sporadic cases also occur [3]. A potential linkage to chromosome 2 has been suggested [4]. As elastorrhexis cannot always be demonstrated, alternative names for clinically indistinguishable cases have been proposed: these include focal acral hyperkeratosis and marginal papular acrokeratoderma [5,6]. There is still controversy as to whether

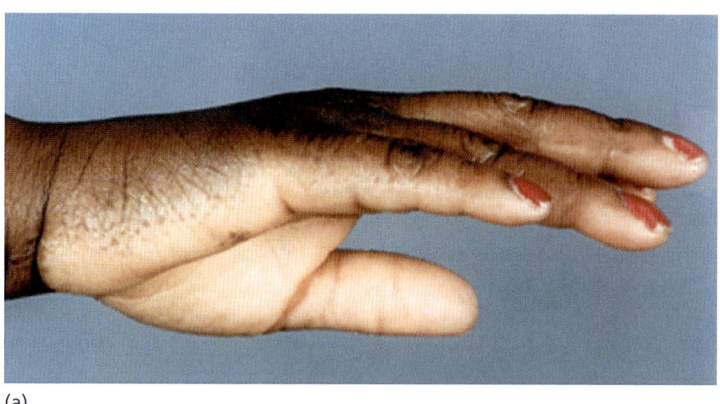

(a)

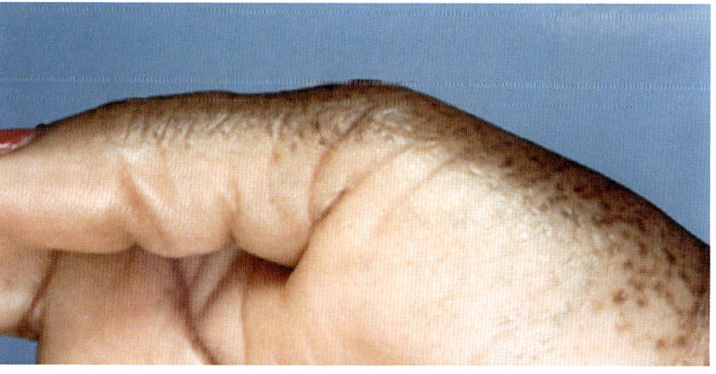

(b)

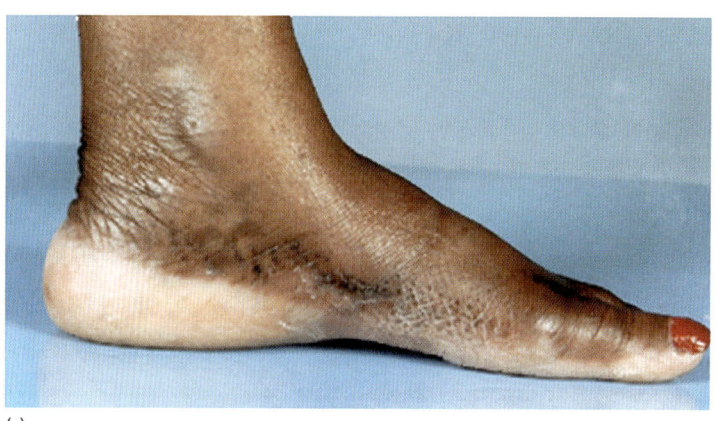

(c)

Figure 94.36 (a–c) Acrokeratoelastoidosis.

PART 8: SPECIFIC CUTANEOUS STRUCTURES

these should be regarded as separate entities [7,8]. In one patient, fragmented elastic fibres were demonstrated in clinically normal covered skin, suggesting a primary disorder of elastic fibres [9], although it is generally considered that this group of disorders represents variable expression of the same disease [5,8]. Systemic retinoids may be beneficial but this is offset by potential long-term toxicity and teratogenicity [8].

ACQUIRED DISORDERS OF ELASTIC TISSUE DEPOSITION

Linear focal elastosis

Definition and nomenclature

This condition is characterised by asymptomatic yellow linear bands arranged horizontally on the lower back [1,2–4]. It less commonly occurs on the legs and shoulders.

Synonyms and inclusions
• Elastotic striae

Introduction and general description

This condition may represent a keloidal reaction to striae distensae.

Epidemiology
Incidence and prevalence

Case reports are mostly sporadic. It may occur more frequently than reports suggest [5].

Age

It was initially reported in elderly males [1], although subsequently reported patients are chiefly adolescents [6–8].

Sex

It predominantly occurs in males.

Ethnicity

It is found in white, Asiatic and Afro-Caribbean people [6].

Pathophysiology
Predisposing factors

The lesions may be associated with a growth spurt, similar to adolescent growth striae [7]. Hereditary connective tissue disorders may have an aetiological factor in some cases [9].

Pathology

Ultrastructural studies reveal active elastogenesis. The middle and lower dermal collagen is separated by bluish grey fine fibrillar material, which is composed of thin wavy elastic fibres and fragmented elastic fibre bundles. Early lesions may, in contrast, show elastolysis, with decreased elastin and microfibrillar proteins [9]. The elastic fibres are near to or even in contact with fibroblasts [10].

Elastogenesis may occur in response to local trauma, UV light or perhaps following the development of striae distensae [11]. However, these mechanisms do not adequately explain the increasing number of cases reported, particularly in the young, and it may be that intrinsic defects of elastic fibre metabolism play a role [4].

Causative organisms
None is known.

Genetics

There may be an underlying defect of elastic tissue, as yet unidentified [4]. Familial cases are reported [6,12].

Clinical features
History

There is an insidious onset of asymptomatic lesions chiefly on the lower back.

Presentation

Superficially, the lesions resemble striae distensae, but they are palpable rather than depressed and yellow rather than purplish or white. Linear focal elastosis has been reported adjacent to striae distensae [11,13] and in one case following potent topical corticosteroids [14]. A recent case report presented focal linear elastosis in a patient with hypermobility syndrome [9]. Dermatoscopic features include linear and poorly defined yellow areas without a vascular component [15].

Differential diagnosis

This includes striae (which often coexist).

Classification of severity

This is of cosmetic importance only.

Complications and co-morbidities

Linear focal elastosis is associated with striae in many cases.

Disease course and prognosis

This is unknown. There is no effective treatment for linear focal elastosis. There was no clinical improvement seen in a retrospective case series of linear focal elastosis [5].

Investigations
None is needed.

Late-onset focal dermal elastosis

Yellowish papules with a peau d'orange appearance appear on the flexures. Clinically and histologically, the lesions resemble elastomas. This rare condition had only been reported in elderly Japanese men, however there are now case reports of female individuals presenting with multiple yellow papules on the dorsa of the hands [1,2–4]. Histopathology features include focal increases in thick, interlacing elastic fibres in the deep and mid-reticular dermis [4].

Elastofibroma dorsi

Elastofibroma occurs predominantly in elderly women. Most cases are reported from southern Japan [1]. There may be a history of prolonged manual labour. The painless or slightly tender swelling beneath the lower angle of the scapula, 2–10 cm in diameter, is often discovered fortuitously. It may enlarge slowly, displacing neighbouring structures, and it can be clinically confused with a sarcoma [2,3]. This is a benign lesion, however, despite the fact that it is poorly circumscribed. The growth is composed of mature fibrous tissue, containing fibres which stain as elastic fibres. The lesions may be solitary or multiple [4–9].

Histologically, the lesion contains abundant large elastic fibres, some broken into irregular masses, and large amounts of relatively acellular collagen. The elastic fibres are composed of true elastin surrounded by a large amount of hydrophilic material forming an orderly array of tubules [4]. It is generally regarded either as a type of reactive hyperplasia or as a hamartoma, arising either from dermis, subscapular connective tissue or periosteum [6]. Surgical excision is indicated if the patient develops symptoms from the lesion or if malignancy cannot be excluded [7,8]. There is a high complication rate after surgery; postoperative suction is recommended [9] and there is a risk of recurrence [9,**10**].

Elastoderma

Elastoderma is a very rare condition which is due to excessive elastogenesis, as distinct from acquired cutis laxa, where there is a loss of elastic tissue. A young woman developed a localised defect of the skin of one arm, which became pendulous and lax, but lost its elastic recoil. Histological and biochemical investigation showed this was due to accumulation of excessive elastin, with derangement of elastin fibrillogenesis [1].

In further cases, also affecting young women, clinically uninvolved skin showed thin elastic fibres on haematoxylin and eosin staining, without calcification [2]. Other areas of the skin reported to have been affected by elastoderma include the anterior neck in a teenage male patient [3]. Transmission electron microscopy showed irregular elastic tissue fibres with electron dense extensions; fibroblasts were abundant, possessing widened rough endoplasmic reticulum [4]. Despite the skin laxity, there is no joint hypermobility [4].

Papular elastorrhexis

This is a rare variant of connective tissue naevus. Adolescents or young adults present with multiple, non-follicular, oval, white or yellowish papules on the trunk or limbs; dermal elastic fibres are decreased and fragmented on histology. Most case reports are sporadic, with no family history and no extracutaneous manifestations [1–3]. A recent case report discussed the late-onset development of skin-coloured papules on the face of a female in her 60s. The histopathological findings were consistent with papular elastorrhexis [4].

The differential diagnosis includes acne scars, in which the papules are follicular, with decreased elastin but no elastorrhexis; familial cutaneous collagenoma is histologically similar, but cases of papular elastorrhexis are sporadic [5]. Similar lesions are seen in some patients with Buschke–Ollendorff syndrome (Chapter 73), in which osteopoikilosis is also a feature. To add to the confusion, abortive forms of Buschke–Ollendorff syndrome have been described, lacking osteopoikilosis [6]. A family has been described with this variant [7]. It is possible that papular elastorrhexis is not a separate entity [8]. Intralesional triamcinolone may be beneficial [9], if treatment is necessary [1–3].

FIBROMATOSES AND OTHER CAUSES OF DIFFUSE FIBROSIS

Introduction and general description

Fibrous overgrowth of dermal and subcutaneous connective tissue occurs most readily in certain sites and at certain ages, and some of the resulting syndromes are clinically and histologically distinctive and well defined. There are some cases, however, that defy precise classification, and others in which histological criteria may be a poor guide to prognosis. Invasiveness and a high local recurrence rate may or may not be associated with a tendency to metastasise. The borderline between simple overgrowth and a benign tumour may be equally difficult to define.

Abnormal fibrosis is a feature of many debilitating systemic disorders, such as cirrhosis and pulmonary fibrosis. A closer understanding of the myofibroblast and the regulatory pathways of cytokines and growth factors, such as TGF-β, should enable the development of effective and specific antifibrotic drugs [1].

Fibromatoses

Fibromatosis is a benign fibrous tissue proliferation, which is intermediate between benign fibroma and metastasising fibrosarcoma. The lesions of fibromatosis tend to infiltrate and recur when removed, but they do not metastasise. The term should not be applied to reactive fibrous proliferation, or to keloid, which is usually secondary to injury. The lesions in fibromatosis may be single or multiple, and the likelihood of recurrence after surgical removal varies with the location of the lesion and the age of the patient. The fibromatoses occur in two major groups:

1 Superficial fibromatoses (fascial fibromatoses):
   • Palmar (Dupuytren).
   • Plantar.
   • Penile (Peyronie).
   • Knuckle pads.
2 Deep fibromatoses (non-metastasizing fibrosarcoma). These are rapidly growing tumours that usually involve the musculature

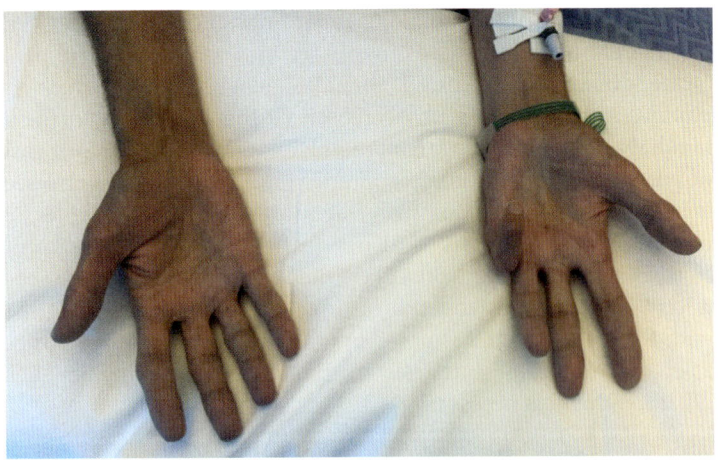

Figure 94.37 Palmar fascial fibromatosis: typical fixed contraction of the little finger of the left hand compared with the normal right hand, in a patient with palmar and plantar fascial fibromatosis. Reproduced from Newman and McQuaid 2019 [36] with permission of Irish Medical Organisation.

or aponeuroses. Their tendon-like consistency accounts for their alternative name of desmoid tumours. They are discussed in more detail in Chapter 136.

Palmar fascial fibromatosis

Definition and nomenclature

This is a fibromatous hyperplasia of the palmar aponeurosis, which is characterised by nodular thickening of the fascia with associated flexion contractures of one or more digits (Figure 94.37).

Synonyms and inclusions
• Dupuytren contracture

Introduction and general description

The condition seems to be due to a reactive proliferation of fibroblasts with no inflammatory component; the basic cause is obscure.

Epidemiology

Incidence and prevalence

The prevalence in the general adult population is around 2–6% [1], but it may approach 20% or more in elderly males [2,3,4], in diabetic patients and in patients with acquired immune deficiency syndrome (AIDS) [2].

Age

The age of onset is generally 30–60 years.

Sex

It is generally commoner in men. Some families are described in which there is a predominantly female expression [5].

Ethnicity

It is relatively uncommon in people of African or Asian descent.

Associated diseases

In about 5% of patients, the condition is associated with other fibromatoses such as knuckle pads or keloids. This has been termed the polyfibromatosis syndrome.

It occurs more commonly in patients with alcoholic cirrhosis, epilepsy [6] and diabetes [4,7], but the prevalence is decreased in rheumatoid arthritis [8]. Other conditions that have been less convincingly claimed to be associated include periarthritis of the shoulder, chronic lung disease, gout, trauma and ulnar nerve damage [9].

Phenytoin appears to stimulate fibrosis in the polyfibromatosis syndrome [10] and it may also cause gingival hypertrophy by stimulating fibroblasts and increasing collagen production [6,10,11]. There is one case report of a girl aged 14 years who developed Dupuytren contracture while receiving growth hormone therapy for hypopituitarism [12].

High alcohol consumption, smoking and trauma, notably the use of vibrating hand tools, have also been implicated [13].

Pathophysiology

Free radical production secondary to ischaemia may be involved: the concentration of hypoxanthine substrate capable of releasing free radicals is greatly increased in the affected tissue [14]. Localised ischaemia has been thought to play a part, and in animal studies allopurinol (a competitive inhibitor of xanthine oxidase) has been shown to limit the damage associated with acute ischaemia [15]. High concentrations of free radicals are toxic, but in low concentration they stimulate fibroblast proliferation [14]. The contractures, which are a late complication, appear to follow the conversion of the fibroblasts to contractile myofibroblasts [16].

The presence of CD3 lymphocytes and the expression of major histocompatibility complex (MHC) class II proteins in the affected tissue imply that palmar fascial fibromatosis is a T-cell mediated autoimmune disorder [17].

Pathology

Fibroblasts in affected fascia appear to be identical to those in normal palmar fascia but their density is increased and they tend to be clustered around narrowed small vessels [18,19]. In the early stages, there are nodules in the subcutaneous tissue or within the fascia: they are composed of proliferating fibroblasts (Figure 94.38) with irregular hyperchromatic nuclei but there is no excess of collagen. Later stages are characterised by the presence of myofibroblasts, which have a fibrillary cytoplasmic ultrastructure and seem to have some other properties of smooth muscle. The nuclei are deeply indented, possibly due to the contractile properties of the cell. The cells also have altered surface membrane properties which enable attachment to neighbouring cells and stroma. Cytokines including TGF-β, platelet-derived growth factor (PDGF) and interleukin 1 mediate changes involving α-actin when the fibroblasts are transformed to myofibroblasts [20]. Myofibroblasts have also been identified in the normal aorta and in granulation tissue, hypertrophic scars, keloids, liver fibrosis, dermatofibromas, etc. [16], in which their contractile properties may be important. The advanced stages of palmar fascial fibromatosis are characterised by dense fibrous connective tissue with a few elongated cells. An increased concentration of type III collagen is present in the nodules [21].

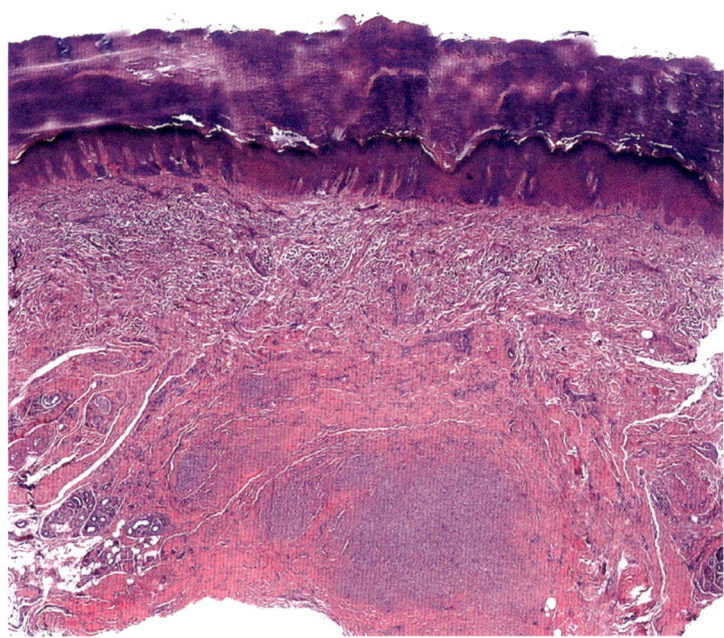

Figure 94.38 Low-power photomicrograph showing grossly thickened deep fascia with nodules of proliferating fibroblasts surrounded by dense collagen. Courtesy of Professor Luis Requena.

This may be due to decreased degradation resulting from increased levels of tissue metalloproteinase inhibitors in the lesions [22]. Structural abnormalities of glycosaminoglycans, notably dermatan sulphate, may predispose to abnormal fibrillogenesis [23].

Genetics

Palmar fascial fibromatosis is often familial and may be inherited as an autosomal dominant trait [24], in which case the onset tends to occur at an earlier age [25]. Genome-wide studies show increased expression levels of MMP-1, -3 and -16, fibroblast growth factor and several collagen genes [26]. Recent work has suggested that the *Wnt* pathway and transcription factor MafB may have key functions in the pathogenesis of palmar fascial fibromatosis [20].

Environmental factors

Occupational exposure to hand-transmitted vibration may be an exacerbating factor [13].

Clinical features

History

Nodules may be painful initially, although the condition typically develops insidiously over several months or years.

Presentation

The earliest sign is the development of a palmar nodule, usually in the ulnar half of the hand. There are usually no symptoms, but there may be a dull ache or tingling. Insidious progression of the fibrosis over several years causes flexion contractures of the affected fingers. There is often puckering of the overlying skin.

Clinical variants

Plantar and penile fibromatosis are closely related conditions.

Differential diagnosis

In most cases, the diagnosis is straightforward. There may be a histological resemblance to fibrosarcoma, but the latter is more pleomorphic, with larger nuclei and more mitoses. Juvenile aponeurotic fibroma may produce palmar or plantar nodules, but palmar fascial fibromatosis does not occur in young children.

Disease course and prognosis

The condition tends to progress more slowly in women [9]. Eventually, the function of the hand is impaired due to fixed flexion of one or more digits. If left untreated, there may be some improvement after many years.

Investigations

The possibility of one or more of the associated disorders, such as diabetes, should be considered and investigated if appropriate.

Management

The advice of an orthopaedic or hand surgeon should be sought. Traditionally, complete removal of the palmar aponeurosis has been recommended [27], although minimally invasive subtotal fasciectomy and direct closure is more generally favoured [28,29].

Initial encouraging placebo-contolled trials of collagenase injections [30] have been supported by subsequent experience, and the technique is now more widely practised [31].

Medical treatments are disappointing. Allopurinol may help by decreasing free radical production [14,32], and it has been suggested that vitamin C might prevent progression of the disease by acting as a free-radical scavenger [2].

Many other non-surgical approaches have been tried, including continuous slow skeletal traction, radiotherapy, dimethyl sulfoxide, vitamin E, steroid injections and interferon, although none has been proven to be clinically useful [33]. High-dose tamoxifen following minimally invasive surgery reduces the risk of recurrent fibrosis in the short term, but the effect is lost on discontinuing the drug [34]. Intriguing results have been reported from the use of relaxin gene therapy on Dupuytren myofibroblasts *in vitro*, with the potential for use *in vivo* [35].

Treatment ladder for palmar fascial fibromatosis

First line
- Minimally invasive partial fasciectomy

Second line
- Intralesional collagenase

Plantar fascial fibromatosis [1,2]

Definition and nomenclature

This is a rarer condition than palmar fascial fibromatosis, although they are often associated; a survey from Reykjavik found that 15% of men with the latter had plantar fibromatosis [3].

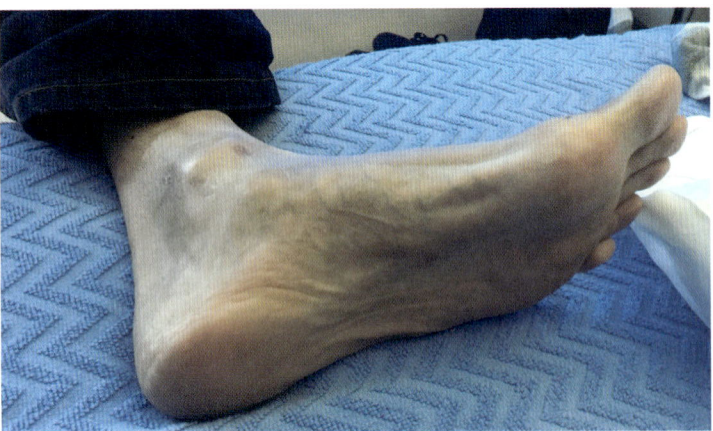

Figure 94.39 Plantar fascial fibromatosis in a patient with palmar and plantar fascial fibromatosis. Reproduced from Newman and McQuaid 2019 [4] with permission of Irish Medical Organisation.

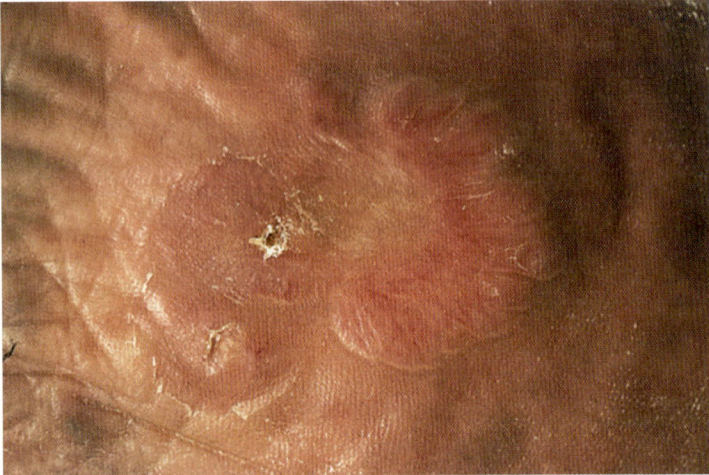

Figure 94.40 Plantar fibromatosis.

Synonyms and inclusions
- Ledderhose disease

Clinical features

It most commonly affects the medial half of the mid-foot (Figure 94.39), presenting as one or more nodules which may become painful and may ulcerate (Figure 94.40). In 25% of cases, it is bilateral. The fibromatosis rarely results in contractures but tends to be locally invasive and to recur. Up to 40% of cases seem to be associated with a background medical history of diabetes [4].

Differential diagnosis

The differential diagnosis includes keloid and fibrosarcoma. Magnetic resonance imaging may confusingly demonstrate the cerebriform pattern typically seen in fibromyxoid sarcoma [5].

In younger patients, aggressive infantile fibromatosis and aponeurotic fibroma must also be considered [6]. Complications are rare, although squamous carcinoma has been reported occurring within a lesion of plantar fibromatosis [7]. Similar nodules have been described symmetrically affecting the anteromedial aspects of the heel pad in children. They are asymptomatic and may resolve spontaneously [8,9]: surgery is contraindicated.

Management

Conservative management may be best in the early stages [4,9]. High-energy shockwave therapy reduces pain [10]. Radiotherapy may be considered in certain cases [4]. Total excision of the lesion and the entire plantar fascia seems to give the best results, with the lowest incidence of recurrence [4].

Penile fibromatosis

Definition and nomenclature

Penile fibromatosis is characterised by one or more irregular, dense fibrous plaques in the penile shaft. These commonly result in painful erections and curvature of the erect penis.

Synonyms and inclusions
- Peyronie disease
- Plastic induration of the penis
- Fibrous sclerosis of the penis

Epidemiology

Penile fibromatosis may occur as an isolated abnormality, or as one component of polyfibromatosis in association with palmoplantar fibromatosis, keloids and knuckle pads. The reported association with the use of α-adrenoreceptor-blocking drugs was probably attributable to concomitant atheroma [1,2]. The mode of inheritance is unclear. It is rare, with the highest incidence between 40 and 60 years.

Clinical features

Vasculitis in the areolar connective tissue beneath the tunica albuginea extends to adjacent structures. This is followed by fibroblastic proliferation, leading to a thickened plaque, which may calcify or ossify [3].

Presentation

The disease presents with painful erections and curvature of the erect penis due to a thickened subcutaneous plaque, usually on the dorsal aspect of the penis in its distal third (Figure 94.41), making penetration impossible. Fibrosis of the underlying cavernous erectile tissue may lead to a constriction or 'waisting' of the penile shaft, leading to flaccidity of the distal portion.

Disease course and prognosis

The course is unpredictable [4]. The pain generally subsides within a few months, but the fibrous plaque may resolve, remain unchanged or progress [5].

Management

Surgery is probably the treatment of choice, including penile straightening techniques [6].

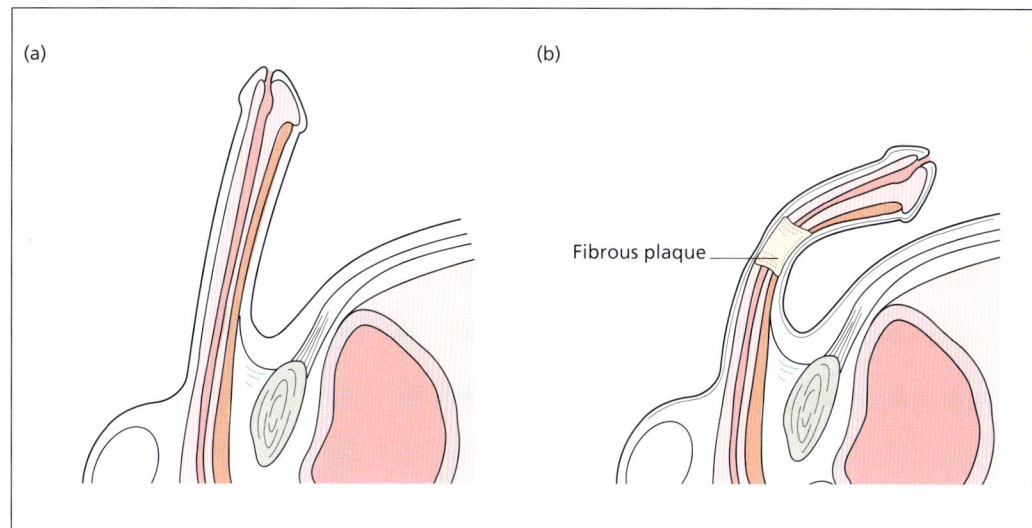

Figure 94.41 (a) Normal erect penis. (b) Erect penis with deformation from Peyronie disease showing a fibrous plaque causing 'waisting'.

Knuckle pads

Definition and nomenclature
Knuckle pads are circumscribed thickenings overlying the finger joints. The term is a misnomer as most lesions occur over the proximal interphalangeal rather than the metacarpophalangeal joints (knuckles).

Synonyms and inclusions
- Holoderma
- Pulvinus
- Subcutaneous fibroma

Introduction and general description
Knuckle pads were first described in the medical literature by Garrod [1] as an 'unusual form of nodule upon the joints of the fingers'. However, they are probably not so unusual, and they feature in several of Michelangelo's works, including the statues of *David* and the *Sleeping Slave* [1]. They should be distinguished from the 'pseudo-knuckle pads' associated with trauma.

Epidemiology
Incidence and prevalence
The condition is not rare but the true prevalence is uncertain, as most patients ignore the lesions. Mikkelsen reported a prevalence of 8.8% in the population of Haugesund, Norway, and of 44.3% in individuals with palmar fibromatosis [2].

Age
Onset is usually between 15 and 30 years of age; however, lesions typically develop slowly and asymmetrically and may not present significant cosmetic problems for several years.

Sex
Occurrence is probably equal between the sexes.

Ethnicity
It is mostly reported in white people.

Associated diseases
There is a strong association with other fibromatoses such as palmar fibromatosis [2,3,**4**]. An association between Dupuytren contracture and other fibromatous lesions has been recorded in some families. In one large family, knuckle pads were associated with sensorineural deafness and with leukonychia (Bart–Pumphrey syndrome) [5]. Knuckle pads have also been associated with epidermolytic palmoplantar keratoderma in a Chinese family due to keratin 9 mutations [6]. Another family has been described with knuckle pads in association with oesophageal cancer, hyperkeratosis and oral leukoplakia [7]. Knuckle pads have also been shown to be associated with an autosomal recessive condition called PLACK (peeling skin, leukonychia, acral punctate keratoses, cheiliti and knuckle pads) syndrome [8].

Pathophysiology
Predisposing factors
Although trauma has been implicated, this is more closely linked to 'pseudo-knuckle pads'. Familial cases are reported.

Pathology
The epidermis is grossly hyperkeratotic and acanthotic, with elongated rete ridges. The dermal connective tissue is hyperplastic; a proliferative phase is followed by a fibrotic phase. Individual collagen fibres may be obviously thickened and arranged in irregular bundles. Spindle-shaped myofibroblasts can be seen on electron microscopy [**4**,9,10]. Histologically, the changes resemble those of palmar fibromatosis.

Genetics
The condition is usually sporadic, but several pedigrees have shown an autosomal dominant inheritance, for example the Bart–Pumphrey syndrome [5]. The age of onset and the distribution of the lesions tend to be more or less constant in each family, but show interfamily variation. Similar single nucleotide

polymorphisms (SNPs) are found in familial Dupuytren contracture [11]. Knuckle pads are reported in families with palmoplantar keratodermas linked with keratin 9 mutations [6,12]. A family has been reported with familial knuckle pads but no associated conditions [4]. Patients with PLACK syndrome develop peeling skin, leukonychia, acral punctate keratosis, cheilitis and knuckle pads. There have been eight cases reported of this genetic condition [8]. Calpains are calcium-dependent cysteine proteases. In PLACK syndromes there are loss of function mutations in *CAST*, a gene that encodes calpastatin which inhibits calpains. *CAST* is found in stratified squamous epithelia including skin.

Environmental factors

Trauma is more probably relevant in 'pseudo knuckle pads'.

Clinical features

History

The history is usually asymptomatic, with insidious onset.

Presentation

Flat or convex, smooth, circumscribed nodules develop slowly and almost imperceptibly over the course of months or years, achieving 0.5–1.5 cm diameter. The lesions may be hypo- or hyperpigmented. In some patients, they become very much raised and obviously indurated, but in others the dermal component is not clinically apparent. They are most commonly seen over the dorsa of the proximal interphalangeal joints (Figure 94.42), but occasionally develop over the knuckles or the distal interphalangeal joints. Any single site or combination of sites may be involved [1,4,9].

Clinical variants

Sites other than the hands are not usually affected, but similar lesions on the knees were also present in one family [3].

Differential diagnosis

Knuckle pads should be distinguished from the 'pseudo knuckle pads' associated with occupational trauma, such as in carpet layers,

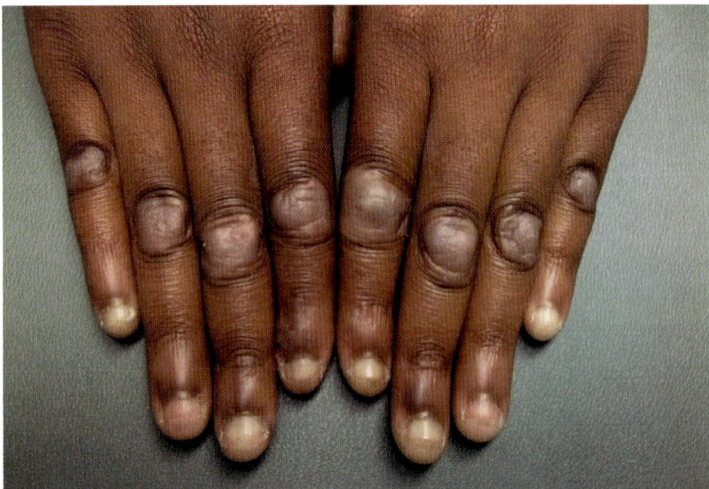

Figure 94.42 Knuckle pads. Reproduced from Hyman and Cohen 2013 [4] with permission of Regents of the University of California.

sheep shearers and tailors. Similar lesions are induced by children chewing or biting their fingers or 'knuckle cracking' [13] or playing video games [14]. Unlike true knuckle pads, these lesions tend to regress if the traumatic stimulus is removed, and may respond to topical keratolytics.

Heberden nodes of osteoarthritis, pachydermodactyly, granuloma annulare [15], erythema elevatum diutinum and rheumatoid nodules [16] should be excluded.

Classification of severity

These are of cosmetic significance.

Complications and co-morbidities

There is an association with other fibromatoses (as noted earlier).

Disease course and prognosis

Lesions gradually enlarge to a maximal size and tend to persist.

Investigations

None usually necessary, unless another inflammatory condition needs to be excluded by skin biopsy.

Management

If the lesions do not bother the patient, conservative management is appropriate. Recurrence and keloidal scarring are common following excision. Intralesional triamcinolone or cryotherapy are ineffective and often painful. Intralesional 5-fluorouracil inhibits fibroblast proliferation and shows promise clinically [17]. Topical cantharidin-podophyllotoxin-salicyclic acid has been used to successfully treat knuckle pads affecting an adolescent patient [18].

Treatment ladder for knuckle pads

First line
- Conservative management

Second line
- Consider intralesional 5-fluorouracil

Pachydermodactyly

Definition

This is a benign fibromatosis of the fingers.

Introduction and general description

This rare condition typically presents in adolescent males, who develop spade-like enlargement of the hands and occasionally the feet [1,2–9].

Epidemiology

Incidence and prevalence

Pachydermodactyly is rare and its incidence uncertain.

Age

It mainly occurs in young adults.

Sex

Males are mainly affected although it has been reported in women [4,5] and two young girls, one of whom had tuberous sclerosis and the other Ehlers–Danlos syndrome [6].

Associated diseases

It may be associated with bilateral carpal tunnel syndrome [2] and spontaneous atrophic scarring of the cheeks (see earlier in this chapter) [10].

Pathophysiology
Predisposing factors

It has been suggested that unconscious repeated rubbing and gripping of the fingers, repetitive movements or mechanical injury to the joints may contribute to the condition [3,6,11–13], but pachydermodactyly must be distinguished from occupational callosities and obsessive 'chewing pads'.

Pathology

Histology shows epidermal hyperplasia and marked dermal thickening, with extension of collagenous fibres into the subcutaneous tissue. Types III and V collagen are increased, and electron microscopy shows increased numbers of fine-diameter collagen fibres.

Genetics

Affected families have been reported [14].

Environmental factors

There is possible local repetitive trauma.

Clinical features
History

It is usually asymptomatic and insidious in onset. A few individuals describe pain of the long bones.

Presentation

It produces a symmetrical diffuse swelling of the skin around the dorsal and lateral aspects of the proximal interphalangeal joints of the index, ring and middle fingers (Figure 94.43). Pachydermodactyly seems to mimic inflammatory arthritis. Plain film radiography shows no abnormalities [13].

Clinical variants

A distal variant has been described in an elderly woman, who also presented with nodules over the extensor aspects of the elbows [15].

Differential diagnosis

Patients may be referred to the rheumatologist with a diagnosis of juvenile idiopathic arthritis [12,16]. It may be confused with knuckle pads [17,18], which may coexist [19].

Classification of severity

The condition is benign.

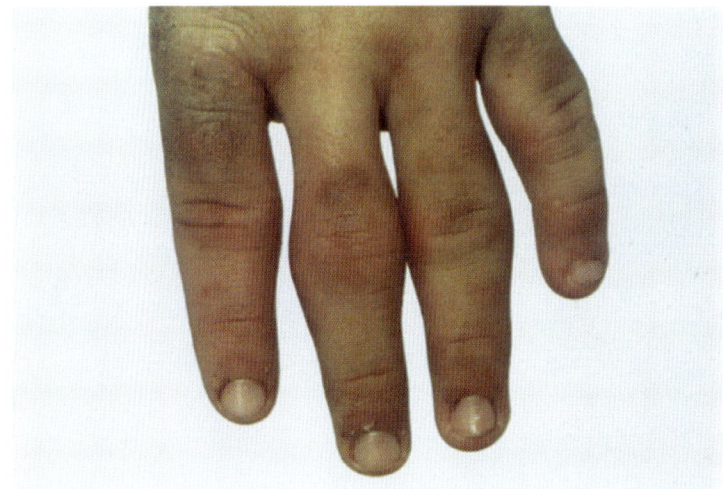

Figure 94.43 Pachydermodactyly. Courtesy of Dr A. Chamberlain.

Complications and co-morbidities

Knuckle pads and pachydermodactyly coexisted in one family [19].

Disease course and prognosis

The condition tends to persist.

Investigations

Patients with the condition can be spared the detailed investigations of a patient with suspected inflammatory arthritis [20].

Management

Most patients do not require treatment. Intralesional triamcinolone has been reported to be beneficial [21], although this is unlikely to be necessary.

White fibrous papulosis of the neck

Asymptomatic small white fibrous papules around the neck have been described in several Japanese [1,2], Iranian and European patients [3,4]. The number of papules ranges from 10 to 100; middle-aged to elderly men are predominantly affected, however the white fibrous papules have been reported to also develop in white women [5]. The papules are round to oval, clearly marginated and non-follicular (Figure 94.44). Histology is unremarkable, showing bundles of thickened collagen fibres in the mid-papillary dermis. Although lesions clinically resemble disorders of elastic tissue, such as anetoderma and Buschke–Ollendorff syndrome, elastic fibres are morphologically normal on histology. Acquired connective tissue naevi could exhibit similar features, although the late age of onset makes this diagnosis unlikely. The condition appears to have no prognostic significance and may be underreported. It may reflect intrinsic ageing or photoageing but aetiology is likely multifactorial [5,6].

It has been suggested that there may be a relationship between fibrous papulosis of the neck and acquired elastolysis of the papillary dermis [7,8]. Lesions of PXE-like upper dermal elastolysis coexisted in a patient with white fibrous papulosis, suggesting that they are part of the same disease spectrum [9]. These changes

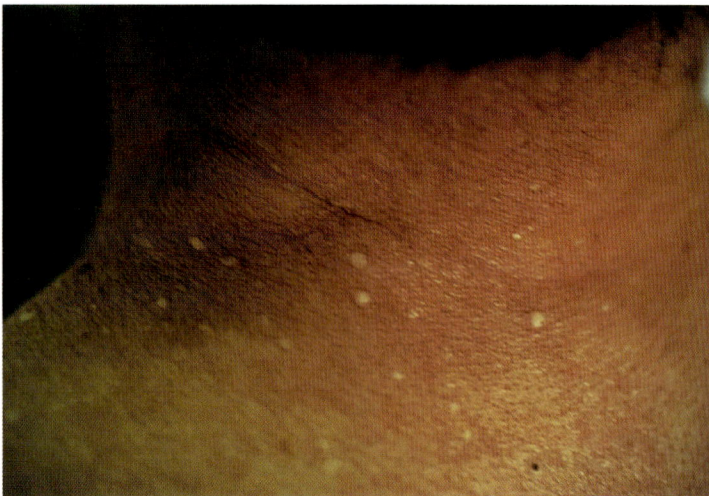

Figure 94.44 White fibrous papulosis of the neck. Courtesy of Professor H. Shimizu.

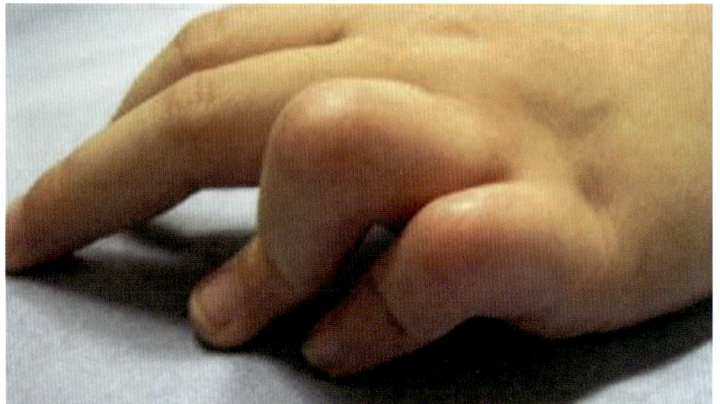

Figure 94.45 Camptodactyly in the ring and little fingers. Reproduced from Almeida *et al.* 2014 [17] with permission of The Scientific Electronic Library Online (SciELO).

are attributed to ageing or photoageing [6,10]. Treatment is not necessarily indicated. Topical treatment with topical retinoids has not demonstrated effectiveness [5]. Surgical excision and fractional non-ablative laser have been used successfully [5]. Currently, there is not sufficient evidence for specific treatments.

Camptodactyly

Definition

Camptodactyly is a non-traumatic flexion deformity affecting the proximal interphalangeal joint of one or more fingers (Figure 94.45) [1].

Introduction and general description

Camptodactyly should be distinguished from *clinodactyly*, which refers to bending or curvature of the finger in the plane of the hand. Camptodactyly is associated with numerous inherited disorders, the most important of which are described here. It is often depicted in Renaissance art [2].

Epidemiology

Incidence and prevalence

The prevalence of isolated camptodactyly is unclear. The commonest associated syndrome is microdeletion of *1p36*, which affects 1 : 5000 neonates [3,4].

Age

Most cases are congenital, although some familial cases present in adult life associated with an erosive arthritis [4].

Sex

There is probably equal sex incidence.

Ethnicity

All races may be affected.

Associated diseases

Camptodactyly may be a feature of a variety of syndromes of which several have had molecular defects identified. Dermatological associations are seen in Blau syndrome which encompasses familial camptodactyly, granulomatous arthritis, uveitis and a reddish skin eruption with phenotypic overlap with early-onset sarcoidosis [5]. In one family, taurinuria was associated [6]. Bilateral camptodactyly is also part of an autosomal recessive disorder (Crisponi syndrome) characterised by muscular contractions of the face, trismus, facial anomalies and death due to fevers. The syndrome is caused by *CRLF1* mutations and is allelic to cold-induced sweating syndrome type I [7].

Pathophysiology

Predisposing factors

There are several associated genetic disorders.

Pathology

The histology of the skin lesions may be unremarkable.

Genetics

Many cases are familial. Microdeletion of 1p36 is the most commonly associated abnormality. Mutations in *NOD2/CARD15* have been shown to confer susceptibility to several chronic inflammatory disorders, including Crohn disease, Blau syndrome and early-onset sarcoidosis [8]. CAP (or CACP (camptodactyly, arthropathy, coxa vara, pericarditis) syndrome is autosomal recessive, and related to the 1.9 cM interval in the human chromosome 1q25-31; this gene encodes for proteoglycan 4, a surface lubricant for tendons and joints [9]. CATSHL (camptodactyly, tall stature and hearing loss) syndrome is associated with mutation in *FGR3* [10], and Crisponi syndrome with a *CRLF1* mutation [7]. SLC29A3 disorder, involving a homozygous frameshift mutation in the *SLC29A3* gene, is associated with a spectrum of clinical features including H syndrome, pigmented hypertrichosis with insulin-dependent diabetes (PHID) and Faisalabad histiocytosis (FHC); these all involve camptodactyly [11].

Environmental factors

There are none apparent.

Clinical features

History

The deformity is asymptomatic.

Presentation

In most cases, the affected child will present with clinical features of a related syndrome.

Clinical variants

Streblodactyly [12,13] (*streblos* = crooked) is inherited as a sex-linked autosomal dominant character. The affected females show from birth a flexion deformity at the metacarpo-phalangeal joints of the thumbs and the proximal interphalangeal joints of the little fingers. Some fingers show swan-neck deformities and hyperextensible metacarpo-phalangeal joints. In one family, there was an abnormal amino aciduria.

Differential diagnosis

Dupuytren disease (palmar fibromatosis) is associated with fibrous scarring affecting the fascia. Juvenile chronic arthritis is typically erosive, whereas the arthritis in CACP syndrome and related disorders is non-erosive [14].

Classification of severity

Morbidity relates to the associated syndrome, if any.

Complications and co-morbidities

These relate to any associated syndrome.

Disease course and prognosis

Lesions are persistent.

Management

Treatment, if required, is surgical [1,15,16].

Juvenile fibromatoses

The term juvenile fibromatosis has been applied to a group of disorders occurring in infants and children, and is characterised by proliferative activity of the fibroblasts. There is a tendency to local recurrence but, unlike fibrosarcomas, they do not metastasise. The group includes a number of well-defined clinical entities that affect the skin as follows:
1 Infantile myofibromatosis.
2 Fibrous hamartoma of infancy.
3 Juvenile hyaline fibromatosis.
4 Infantile digital fibromatosis.
5 Calcifying aponeurotic fibroma.
6 Giant cell fibroblastoma.

Infantile myofibromatosis

Definition

Solitary or multiple fibrous nodules develop in infancy in the skin, striated muscle, bone and occasionally viscera [1,2].

Introduction and general description

Although rare, this is the commonest cause of fibrous nodules presenting in infancy. In around 50% of patients lesions are solitary, predominantly affecting the head and neck. Multiple lesions can occur, with or without visceral involvement.

Epidemiology

Incidence and prevalence

Infantile myofibromatosis is rare and its incidence unknown.

Age

Around 60% of lesions are present at birth, and around 80% by the age of 2 years.

Sex

There is a slight male predominance; around 60% of patients are boys [2].

Ethnicity

It may affect all races.

Pathophysiology

Predisposing factors

None is known.

Pathology

Histology of a lesion shows characteristic zoning, with peripheral spindle-shaped cells in bundles surrounding a central zone of less poorly differentiated round and polygonal cells. Staining is positive for vimentin and α-smooth muscle elastin, and negative for desmin and S-100 [1].

Genetics

Familial cases exhibit autosomal dominant inheritance. Mutations have been described in the *PDGFRB* [3–6] and *NOTCH3* [7] genes.

Environmental factors

None is known.

Clinical features

History

The lesions are typically asymptomatic.

Presentation

Solitary or multiple nodules occur mostly on the head and neck, more rarely on the arms, but can occur anywhere on the body. Multiple lesions may be associated with visceral involvement. Lesions may ulcerate. Cutaneous changes with hypopigmented macules have been described as the presenting feature in infantile myofibromatosis with visceral involvement [8].

Clinical variants

Solitary lesions on the upper eyelid may cause amblyopia [9].

Differential diagnosis

The solitary lesions of fibrous hamartoma of infancy usually affect the hand or foot, and histology is that of an organoid naevus containing mature adipose cells with a nodular aggregate of fibroblasts and interlacing collagen bands. Juvenile aponeurotic fibromatosis affects the fingers and palms of older children or adults; clinically, it may resemble Dupuytren disease (which is very rare in infants), but histology reveals large dark-staining nuclei in a background of bland fibrosis, with calcification. Bony lesions may be difficult to distinguish from fibrosarcoma.

Classification of severity

It has a benign process but the presence of systemic involvement considerably worsens the prognosis, with up to 30% mortality [2].

Complications and co-morbidities

These are dependent on systemic involvement.

Disease course and prognosis

Many solitary and even multiple cutaneous lesions involute sponta-neously [10,11]. Systemic involvement carries a worse prognosis.

Investigations

Histology is essential to differentiate this from other tumours and fibromatoses. Full clinical examination and chest and abdominal imaging are advisable in patients with multiple lesions.

Management
First line

Patients without systemic involvement can be managed conserva-tively. Debulking surgery, without attempting complete removal, may be necessary if there is a compromise of function by the tumour.

Second line

Systemic disease warrants chemotherapy, for instance with low-dose vinblastine and methotrexate [12].

Juvenile hyaline fibromatosis

Definition and nomenclature

This is an autosomal recessive disorder of glycosaminoglycan syn-thesis, which is characterised clinically by skin papules or tumours, gingival enlargement, osteolytic lesions and joint contractures, and histologically by deposition of amorphous hyaline material [1–3,4].

Synonyms and inclusions
- Molluscum fibrosum

Introduction and general description

This, together with systemic hyalinosis, is now regarded as part of the hyaline fibromatosis syndrome (Chapter 70).

Epidemiology
Incidence and prevalence

The disease is very rare and occurs sporadically, but it has occurred in siblings [5,6].

Age

Onset is in infancy.

Sex

There is a slight male predominance.

Ethnicity

Most case reports and series originate from the Indian subcontinent.

Pathophysiology
Predisposing factors

The cause is unknown, but increased chondroitin synthesis has been demonstrated in skin fibroblasts cultured from the tumour tissue [1].

Pathology [1–3,4,5,7]

The skin lesions contain 'chondroid' cells embedded in amorphous eosinophilic ground substance in the dermis. In the early lesions, this consists of glycosaminoglycans, but in the later lesions the matrix is mainly composed of chondroitin sulphate [8]. The dermal collagen is decreased and the collagen fibrils are fewer and thinner than in normal skin. The hyaline material may also be present in the muscles and bones. Absence of pro-α_2 chains and type III collagen has been demonstrated in affected skin [9].

Genetics

Inheritance is autosomal recessive. The gene has been mapped to 4q21; there are also mutations in the capillary morphogenesis factor 2 gene [10]. Infantile systemic hyalinosis has been associated with mutations of the *ANTXR2* gene [11,12].

Clinical features
History

The condition presents at birth or early infancy.

Presentation

There may be small pearly papules or nodules, particularly on the face or neck. Large subcutaneous tumours may also occur, particularly on the scalp. These may be hard or soft, fixed or mobile, and they may ulcerate. Gingival hypertrophy is commonly present, and flexion contractures of the fingers, elbows, hips and knees may develop. Osteolytic lesions can occur in the skull, long bones or phalanges. The musculature is poorly developed [1,9,13–17].

Clinical variants

Infantile systemic hyalinosis is probably an extreme variant, often leading to death in infancy.

Differential diagnosis

Other infiltrative disorders, such as lipoid proteinosis, may need to be excluded histologically.

Classification of severity

The condition is a severe disease, with considerable morbidity and reduced life expectancy.

Complications and co-morbidities

Joint contractures are disabling.

Disease course and prognosis

The condition persists into adult life. However, many patients die in infancy and rarely survive beyond the fourth decade [10].

Investigations

Histology is diagnostically helpful.

Management

No treatment is of proven benefit. Surgery may be the treatment of choice [7], although nodules may recur after excision [18]. The tumours do not respond to radiotherapy. Joint contractures may respond to intralesional steroid injections in the early stages and patients may benefit from systemic steroids and physiotherapy.

Other benign fibrous cutaneous nodules

Nodular fasciitis

In this condition, there is fibroblastic proliferation of one or more nodules, usually on the limbs or trunk. It is a benign self-limited condition which has pseudosarcomatous features [1]. If nodular fasciitis is rapidly increasing in size investigations including radiology may assist in making a clinical diagnosis. If such a lesion recurs after previous regression there may be an indication for surgical excision to exclude malignancy [2].

Collagenoma

Synonyms and inclusions
- Collagen naevi

Collagenoma (collagen naevus) is a form of connective tissue hamartoma (Chapter 70) which may manifest as a single or localised group of fibrous dermal papules or plaques: the shagreen patch of tuberous sclerosus is an example (Chapter 78). Multiple fibrous dermal nodules with coarse collagen fibres may develop as sporadic cases (eruptive collagenoma) or as a genetic disorder with a dominant inheritance (familial cutaneous collagenoma). Genetic disorders such as Birt–Hogg–Dubé syndrome and multiple endocrine neoplasia type 1 have cutaneous features including collagenomas [1,2] (Chapters 148 and 154).

Dominant dystrophic epidermolysis bullosa

Synonyms and inclusions
- Pasini syndrome

This rare form of epidermolysis bullosa [1,2] is characterised by the development of ivory-white papules (albopapuloid lesions). These occur chiefly on the trunk, in both clinical variants [1], in association with blistering, milia, nail dystrophy and atrophic, or more rarely, hypertrophic scarring (Chapter 69). Histologically changes of connective tissue hyperplasia are seen [3].

Buschke–Ollendorff syndrome

Extensive nodular fibrosis may occur in the Buschke–Ollendorff syndrome, in association with juvenile elastoma and osteopoikilosis.

Fibrous digital nodules

In addition to giant cell synovioma and infantile digital fibromatosis, fibrous nodules in the digits may be due to acquired digital fibrokeratoma, fibrous papule of the finger, dermatofibroma (Chapter 136) or the Koenen tumour (Chapter 93).

Nephrogenic systemic fibrosis

Definition and nomenclature

This is a rare fibrosing disorder that occurs in patients with renal impairment exposed to low-stability gadolinium-based contrast agents [1,2].

Synonyms and inclusions
- Nephrogenic fibrosing dermopathy
- Scleromyxoedema of renal disease

Introduction and general description

The condition was first described in 1997 as nephrogenic fibrosing dermopathy [1]. Initially thought to be restricted to the skin, there are several reports of involvement of internal organs including the lungs, myocardium and striated muscle, which contribute to a high mortality [3].

Epidemiology

Incidence and prevalence

It is rare. With the development of guidelines on the use of gadolinium-based contrast agents [4], it is hoped that the condition will become a matter of historical importance only. From 3% to 7% of patients with renal insufficiency can develop nephrogenic systemic fibrosis from use of gadodiamide [5].

Age

It occurs mostly in elderly adults but several cases have been reported in children [6].

Sex

There is equal sex incidence.

Ethnicity

All races may be affected.

Associated diseases

It is associated with renal impairment.

Pathophysiology
Predisposing factors
The condition is strongly associated with the prior administration of gadolinium-based magnetic resonance contrast agents, particularly in patients with severe renal disease, typically with a glomerular filtration rate below 30 mL/min/1.73 m^2 or on dialysis [7]. Gadolinium chelates stimulate an NLRP3 inflammasome-dependent inflammatory response, leading to fibroblast growth, synthesis and differentiation into myofibroblasts [8,9]. Non-ionic linear gadolinium-based contrast agents, particularly gadodiamide, are strongly implicated. Macrocyclic chelating agents, such as gadoterate, are more stable and considerably less likely to induce the syndrome [10]. While the development of nephrogenic systemic fibrosis after exposure to the newer gadolinium-based contrast agents is rare, the full risk of the more advanced contrasts is not yet clear [**11**].

Additional risk factors include an associated vascular repair (e.g. leaking aortic aneurysm), associated thrombosis or procoagulant state, and concurrent administration of intravenous iron [2]. High-dose erythropoietin is also implicated in some cases; it has a pro-inflammatory action, particularly in the presence of increased iron stores [12].

Pathology
Dermal mucin is detected with Alcian blue staining. Increased collagen and elastic fibres are laid down in haphazard bundles in the dermis and subcutis; there are increased numbers of CD68-positive fibroblasts in loose aggregates. Inflammatory changes may predominate, including a septal panniculitis [1,13].

Causative organisms
None is proven.

Genetics
There are no genetic associations.

Environmental factors
Gadolinium-based contrast agents are responsible.

Clinical features
History
A history should be obtained of exposure to gadolinium chelates, although the onset may be delayed by several years [8]. Patients may complain of myalgia.

Presentation
Irregular red or brownish indurated plaques, with amoeba-like projections and islands of sparing, occur chiefly on the lower trunk and legs (Figure 94.46). Typically, the face is spared. Sometimes the skin has a 'peau d'orange' texture, which can mimic carcinoma erysipeloides [14].

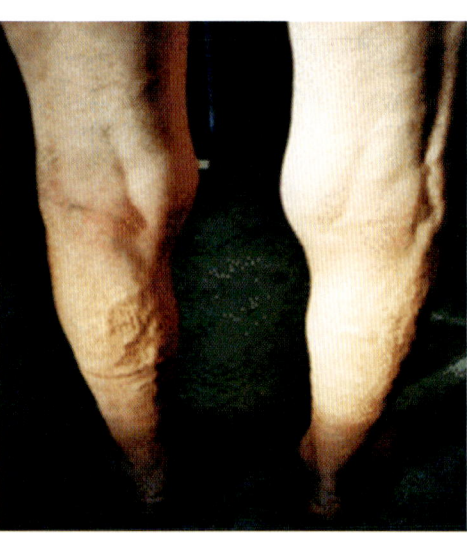

(a)

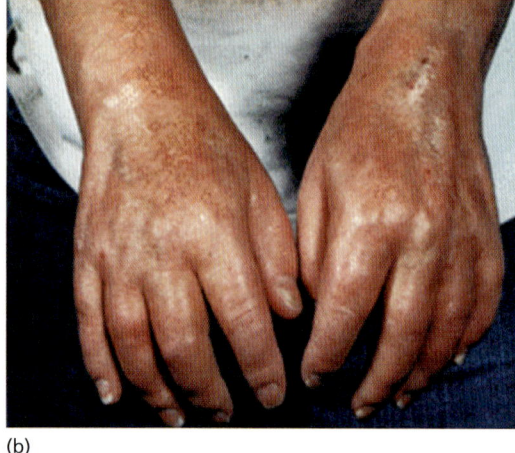

(b)

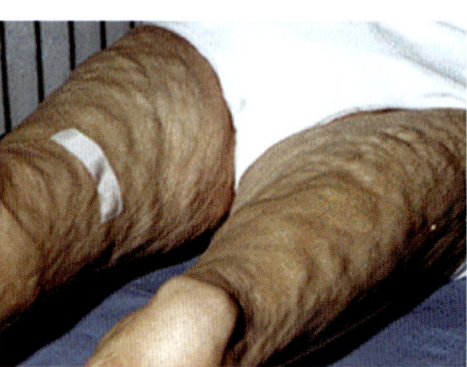

(c)

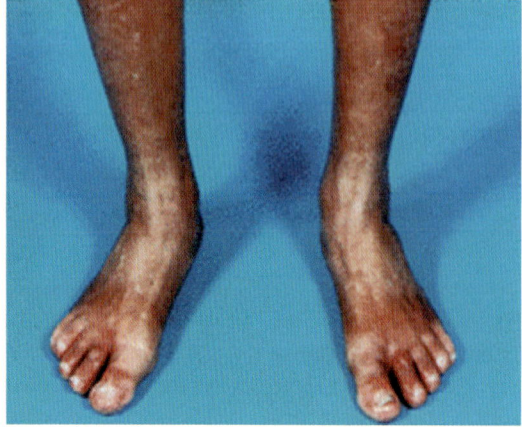

(d)

Figure 94.46 Nephrogenic systemic fibrosis. (a) Deep involvement where fibrosis pulls down a linear band of skin on the thighs. (b, d) Tightness and hardness of the hands (b) and feet (d) and joint contractures. (c) Firm nodules producing a cobblestone appearance. Reproduced from Elmholdt *et al.* 2011 [24] with permission of John Wiley & Sons.

Clinical variants

The extent of visceral involvement is variable; in some cases, the process may involve the testes, myocardium and dura.

Differential diagnosis

Although initially described as 'scleromyxoedema-like', the lesions have a different distribution and morphology, and there is no associated paraproteinaemia [3].

Classification of severity

The condition can be severe, occasionally fatal. In an effort to standardise the assessment and diagnosis of nephrogenic systemic fibrosis, a scoring system that incorporates clinical and histopathological findings was achieved by consensus with the Yale International Nephrogenic Systemic Fibrosis Registry [15].

Complications and co-morbidities

Fibrotic obstruction of structures, such as superior vena cava obstruction [16], may be a complicating factor. Associated metabolic abnormalities include hypophosphataemia [17]. It has been considered that co-morbidity with diabetes may be a protective factor against nephrogenic systemic fibrosis from exposure to gadolinium agents [18].

Disease course and prognosis

Usually, the condition is progressive, although it may remit spontaneously, particularly with the correction of renal abnormalities.

Investigations

A careful history, together with skin or muscle biopsy, can usually confirm the diagnosis. Investigations such as magnetic resonance imaging may be needed to determine the extent of macroscopic visceral involvement.

Management

The most important aspect of management is to maximise renal function. No other treatment is of proven benefit, but thalidomide [19], hydroxychloroquine [20], corticosteroids, immune modulators (e.g. etanercept and rituximab), PUVA, intravenous sodium thiosulphate and extracorporeal photopheresis [21] have been used empirically. Alefacept appears to improve the skin disease [22]. Therapeutic plasma exchange offers pain relief [23]. Renal transplantation is sometimes associated with remission [2].

Prevention should be achieved by adherence to guidelines for the use of gadolinium chelates in radiology [4].

Diabetic thick skin

Some patients with diabetes have thick, tight, waxy skin and limited joint mobility which is thought to be related to altered collagen. This topic is discussed in Chapter 62.

Environmental and drug-induced scleroderma

A variety of environmental triggers, including drugs and occupational toxins, may stimulate a localised or diffuse scleroderma-like reaction in a genetically susceptible host. Most of these damage the microvasculature in the skin by the release of free radicals [1]. Important causes are listed in Box 94.2. Scleroderma-like lesions are seen in a photosensitive distribution in porphyria cutanea tarda. Lesions resembling generalised morphoea are seen in chronic graft-versus-host disease and paraneoplastic scleroderma is associated with neoplasms such as carcinoid. In most cases, the fibrotic process continues after withdrawal of the external stimulus. Sometimes, the ensuing clinical pattern resembles idiopathic forms of morphoea or systemic sclerosis (Chapters 55 and 54, respectively).

Box 94.2 Scleroderma-like syndromes due to chemical exposure

- Vinyl chloride
- Silica dust
- Cocaine abuse

Organic solvents
- Aromatic hydrocarbons (e.g. toluene, benzene)
- Aliphatic hydrocarbons:
  - Chlorinated (e.g. trichlorethylene, perchlorethylene)
  - Non-chlorinated (e.g. naphtha-n-hexane)
- Acrylamide
- Epoxy resins
- Toxic oil syndrome
- Urea formaldehyde foam insulation
- Breast augmentation (paraffin, silicone) (unproven)

Drugs
- Reactions to local injection
- Phytomenadione, pentazocine, heparin
- Etanercept
- Reactions to systemic therapy
- Bleomycin
- L-tryptophan (eosinophilia–myalgia syndrome)
- Carbidopa and L-5-hydroxytryptophan
- Penicillamine
- Valproate sodium
- Cocaine
- Appetite suppressants (diethylpropion hydrochloride, amphetamine)
- Diltiazem
- Interferon α-2b

Several occupational disorders resembling systemic sclerosis have been reported. In a Belgian study, men in construction-related occupations (notably electricians) were 10 times more likely to have systemic sclerosis than the general population [2]. Exposure to *vinyl chloride monomer* occurs in workers involved in polyvinyl chloride (PVC) production. One-third of male operatives in a British factory developed a clinical syndrome that included Raynaud phenomenon, dyspnoea, cutaneous sclerosis, pulp atrophy and radiological evidence of acro-osteolysis (Figure 94.47) [3]. Genetic marker studies have demonstrated an increased incidence of human leukocyte antigen (HLA)-DR5 in affected individuals; severe disease is linked with -B8 and -DR3 [4]. A similar syndrome has been reported in gold miners exposed to silica dust [5], which is the commonest occupational association in the literature [6]. Organic

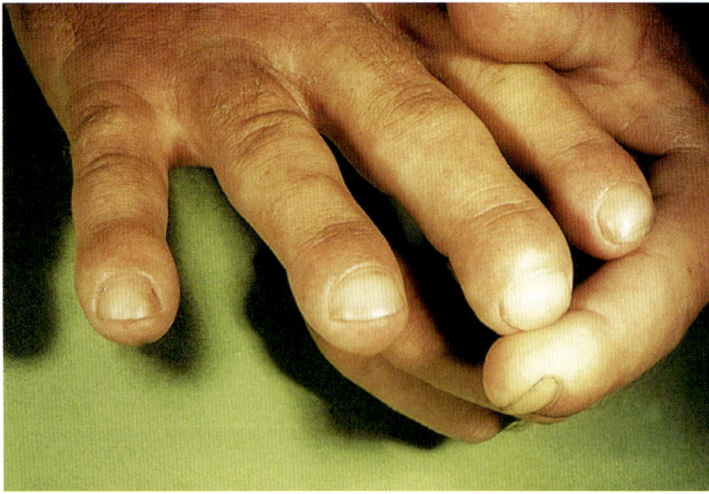

Figure 94.47 Vinyl chloride-induced osteolysis affecting the fingertips.

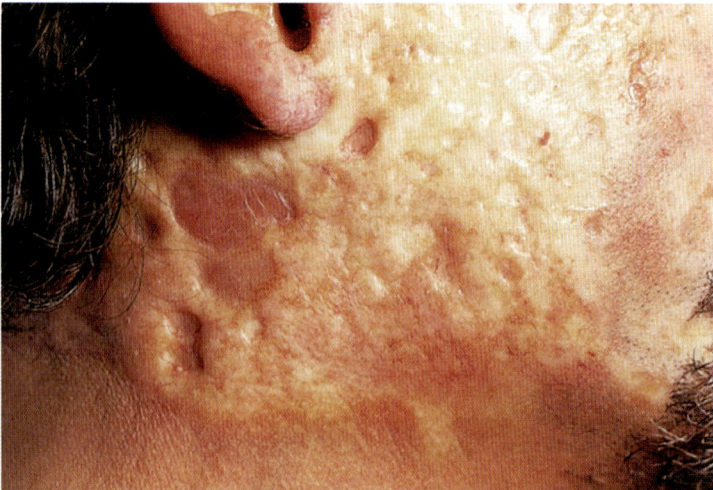

Figure 94.48 Scleroderma and scarring of the face due to porphyria cutanea tarda.

solvents, such as trichlorethylene [7] and perchlorethylene [8], which are structurally similar to vinyl chloride, have also been implicated. Exposure to epoxy resin results in an acute syndrome of cutaneous sclerosis, muscle weakness, arthralgia, impotence, lung and oesophageal involvement [9]. The causative agent appears to be a cyclohexylamine. Acrylamide has also been implicated [10].

Toxic oil syndrome is a multisystem illness, reported in Spain in 1981. Acute fever, severe but transient pulmonary oedema, myalgia and a pruritic exanthem and eosinophilia were followed after several months by widespread cutaneous sclerosis in 30% of cases [11,12]. The syndrome was probably due to ingestion of imported rapeseed oil mixed with an aniline denaturant, designed to make the oil unfit for human consumption. Toxic oil syndrome bears a striking resemblance to the *eosinophilia–myalgia syndrome* [13–15], linked with consumption of L-tryptophan; this was used as a 'food supplement' to treat insomnia and depression. The offending batches of L-tryptophan contained impurities similar to the contaminants in toxic oil [16,17].

In environmental fibrotic disorders, as in idiopathic scleroderma, subpopulations of fibroblasts appear to be activated to synthesise excess collagen; this property is perpetuated by fibroblasts *in vitro*, indicating that the elevated collagen gene expression is independent of extracellular stimuli [15]. Cytokines appear to stimulate the proliferation of these abnormal clones of fibroblasts; thus, TGF-β and PDGF are elevated in the eosinophilia–myalgia syndrome [18].

Numerous drugs have been reported to induce cutaneous sclerosis. Lesions resembling morphoea may follow injections of pentazocine [19], heparin [20] and vitamin K_1 (phytomenadione) [21–24]; in the case of vitamin K_1, the trigger may be a solvent rather than vitamin K_1 itself [25]. Morphoea-like plaques have also been reported in patients taking penicillamine [26], valproate [27] and etanercept, even in areas remote from the injection site [28]. The case is not proven that silicone breast implants are associated with scleroderma-like disease [29].

Diffuse scleroderma-like changes have been reported following bleomycin therapy [30,31]. A combination of L-5-hydroxytryptophan and carbidopa induced lesions resembling eosinophilia–myalgia syndrome [32]. Phenytoin and diltiazem both induce gingival hypertrophy [33,34]. A patient on phenytoin developed florid

hypertrophic retroauricular folds [35]. Thickened skin on the feet has been reported in a patient taking diltiazem [36]. Raynaud phenomenon, thickened facial and hand skin, sclerodactyly and telangiectasies with oesophageal involvement and positive antinuclear antibody developed in a patient who had a diagnosis of metastatic melanoma and received interferon α-2b following surgery [37].

Alcohol can provoke porphyria cutanea tarda, which can produce a sclerodermatous appearance in a photosensitive distribution (Figure 94.48).

Limited and diffuse scleroderma changes including skin ulceration, digital gangrene and scleroderma renal crisis were seen with patients who had inhaled cocaine for a number of years [38]. The use of other drugs including alcohol can confound the role of cocaine in drug-induced scleroderma.

Constricting bands of the extremities

Definition and nomenclature

Constricting bands occur around a digit or limb. The bands may be shallow, involving only the skin, or deeper, involving fascia or bone, and in some cases amputation may result. The term *ainhum* (an African word meaning 'to saw') [1] is applied to a specific type in which a painful constriction of the fifth toe occurs in adults, with eventual spontaneous amputation. *Pseudo-ainhum* is the term applied to other constricting bands which are congenital or secondary to another disease.

Synonyms and inclusions

- Ainhum (dactylolysis spontanea)
- Amniotic bands

Introduction and general description

Constricting bands characteristically present in infants. Patterson [2] has provided a classification of congenital constrictions. Type I

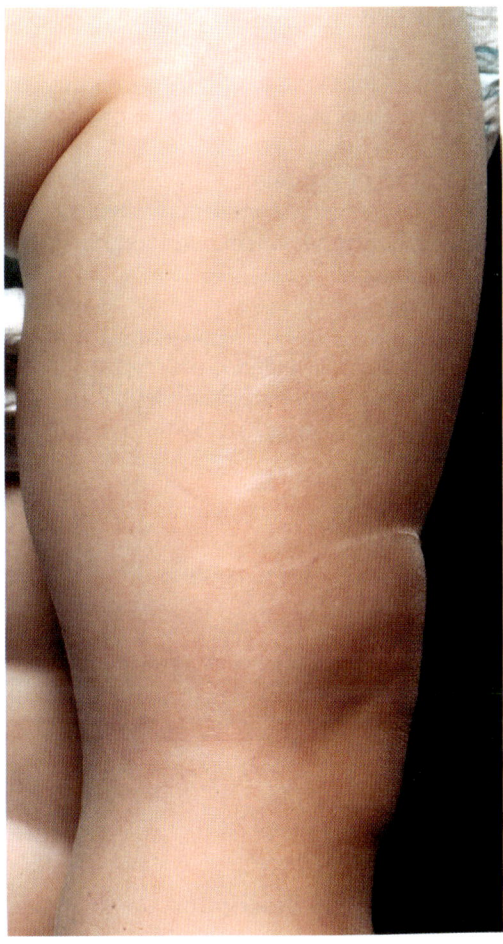

Figure 94.49 Type I constricting band across the thigh of a 6-month-old infant.

describes simple fibrotic rings; the limb distal to the ring is normal. In type II there is neurovascular or lymphatic disruption distal to the ring, causing atrophy, lymphoedema and maybe sensory deficit. Type III refers to acrosyndactyly (fenestrated syndactyly), where there is distal fusion of digits which are separated proximally, forming a 'window'. In type IV there is amputation of the digit or limb (ainhum).

Epidemioloqy
Incidence and prevalence
Sporadic cases of constricting bands occur rarely worldwide.

Age
Constricting bands typically present in infants and young children (Figure 94.49). Adults in resource-poor countries present with ainhum aged around 30–50 years, although the onset of the condition is probably in childhood [3–5].

Sex
Both sexes are affected.

Ethnicity
Ainhum has been reported chiefly in black Africans and African Americans.

Associated diseases
Constricting bands are often associated with other congenital abnormalities [6].

Pathophysiology
Extrinsic and intrinsic factors are probably equally important. Disruption of the development of the germinal disc in the embryo may predispose to fibrotic bands and associated congenital abnormalities. Rupture of the amnion may result in loss of amniotic fluid and extrusion of all or part of the fetus into the chorionic cavity, with resultant trapping of the limbs [6,7]. In adults with ainhum, vascular damage appears to be important, resulting in hypoxia. In some patients, arteriography has shown that the posterior tibial artery is attenuated at the ankle, and the plantar arch and its branches are absent [3].

Predisposing factors
Vascular damage secondary to smoking or diabetes may exacerbate ainhum in adults [3].

Pathology
Fibrosis may be associated with distal degenerative change and osteoporosis, particularly in ainhum.

Causative organisms
Tropical infections have been implicated in ainhum, but are probably coincidental [3,4].

Genetics
Most cases are sporadic, although familial cases of ainhum have been reported.

Environmental factors
Rupture of the amniotic membrane is likely to be an important factor in congenital constrictions. Mechanical factors, including trauma from walking barefoot, may precipitate the development of a groove in the ischaemic toe in ainhum.

Clinical features
Fibrous bands may be solitary or multiple, encasing the limb (usually the leg or foot).

Clinical variants
Ainhum represents the extreme form of the condition, resulting in spontaneous amputation of the digit.

Painful fissuring and hyperkeratosis on the medial aspect of the digit is followed by fibrosis, distal degeneration and osteoporosis. There may be secondary infection and osteomyelitis. The toe becomes dorsiflexed at the metatarso-phalangeal joint, and gradually becomes clawed. Rest pain, coolness and cyanosis of the digit distal to the groove suggest that ischaemia is present. Once the constricting band has encircled the toe, the condition tends to progress rapidly. The toe becomes globular, hangs by a thread of fibrous tissue and is eventually shed (Figure 94.50). Control of secondary infection and protection from trauma may prevent extension of the scarring process. If symptoms are severe, or the dangling digit is a disability, amputation is indicated.

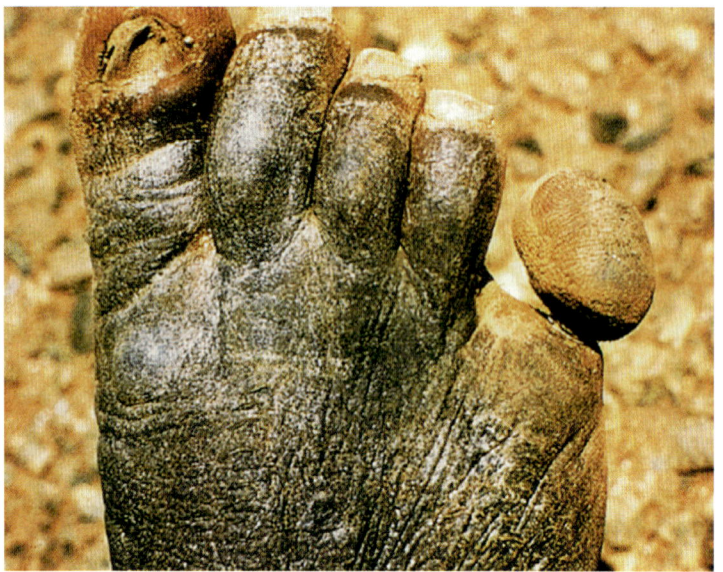

Figure 94.50 Ainhum, just before shedding of the fifth digit. Courtesy of Dr D. Burley.

Differential diagnosis

Congenital pseudo-ainhum. Congenital pseudo-ainhum may involve a digit, a limb or even the trunk, and it ranges in severity from a superficial groove to amputation *in utero* [6,8–10]. The cause is unknown, but familial cases have been reported. Some cases of pseudo-ainhum may be due to amniotic bands [11] or adhesions *in utero*, which may arise as a result of tearing of the amnion sometime after the 45th day of pregnancy [12]. Cases have occurred in Ehlers–Danlos syndrome and after amniocentesis [12,13]. Several cases are reported where raised limb bands develop in the postnatal period, not always associated with amniotic tears; other possible causes include an early teratogenic insult [1,14].

Histology of the affected digit or limb reveals broad, finger-like projections of collagen, and coarse elastic bundles that penetrate deep into the subcutaneous fat [10].

Congenital pseudo-ainhum must be distinguished from the following: *aplasia* of the limbs with rudimentary digits; *acromelia* (in which part of the limb does not develop); and *hypoplasia* (in which the parts, although formed, are poorly developed).

Acquired pseudo-ainhum. Pseudo-ainhum may be acquired as a result of infection (particularly leprosy), trauma, cold injury, neuropathy (especially congenital sensory neuropathy), systemic sclerosis [15] or chronic psoriasis [16], and it may occur in association with other hereditary diseases such as palmoplantar keratoderma, particularly Vohwinkel keratoderma (Figure 63.53b), pachyonychia congenita, erythropoietic protoporphyria [17,18] and Olmsted syndrome (Chapter 63). Factitial pseudo-ainhum has also been reported due to the self-application of a rubber tourniquet.

Multiple skin creases resembling constrictions may be seen in the Michelin tyre baby syndrome and in 'multiple benign annular creases of the extremity'.

Classification of severity

See the Patterson severity grading earlier in this section.

Complications and co-morbidities

Constricting bands may be associated with other congenital defects. In types II–IV, limb mutilation may be caused by fibrotic adhesions [6]. Ainhum results in spontaneous amputation of the digit.

Disease course and prognosis

Some children's constricting bands may involute spontaneously without functional deficit. Most will require surgery to prevent limb deformity or amputation.

Management

Surgical treatments include staged Z-plasty [19]. Good results have been obtained from two-stage sine plasty with removal of the fascial groove and fasciotomy, treating half the limb initially and the other half a week later [20].

ABNORMAL FIBROTIC RESPONSES TO SKIN INJURY

Keloids and hypertrophic scars

Synonyms and inclusions
- Cheloid

Introduction and general description

Keloids and hypertrophic scars represent an excessive connective tissue response to injury, which may be trivial. The term 'keloïde' was coined by Alibert in 1825, likening the lesion to a crab's claw. A keloid is a benign, well-demarcated overgrowth of fibrotic tissue which extends beyond the original boundaries of a defect (Figure 94.51a). A hypertrophic scar is similar, but remains confined to the original defect and tends to resolve after several months (Figure 94.51b). Both conditions may represent different stages of the same disorder [1].

Keloids and hypertrophic scars are nowadays cosmetically distressing but in some cultures they were deliberately induced as

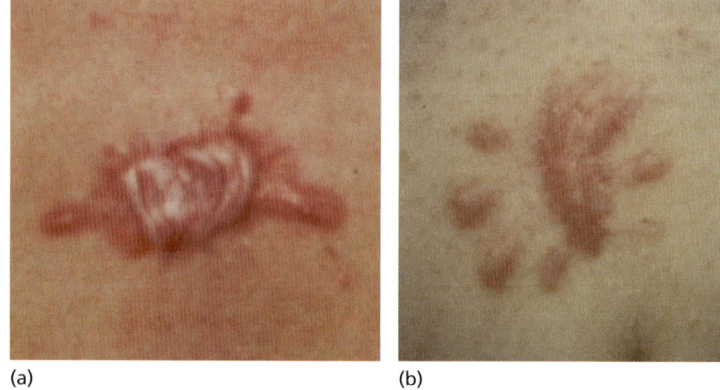

(a)   (b)

Figure 94.51 Contrast between two scars from the presternal area: (a) spontaneous keloid and (b) hypertrophic scar following excision of a benign mole; the former shows partial involution after the injection of triamcinolone.

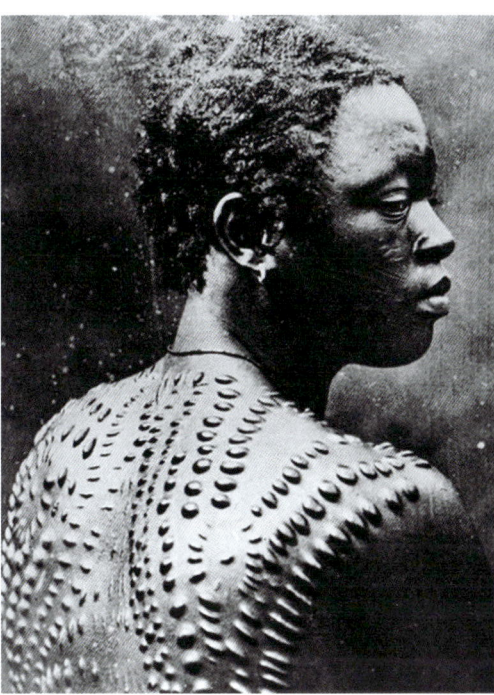

Figure 94.52 Deliberate keloid scarring as a scarification practice. Courtesy of Archives of the Missionaries of Africa.

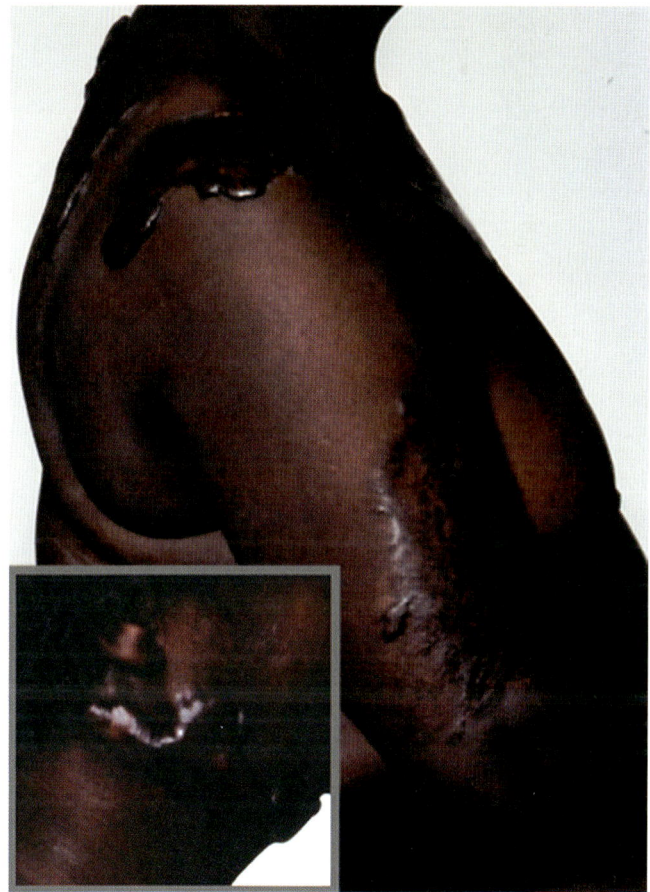

Figure 94.53 Extensive disfiguring keloids affecting an Afro-Caribbean woman.

ritual scarification (Figure 94.52) and regarded as a sign of beauty or strength, which may be why their incidence is higher in descendants from such populations (Figure 94.53). It was an evolutionary advantage for humans and warriors, in particular, to heal wounds rapidly in the setting of dirt and infections, over other species [2].

They may be painful or pruritic. They appear to be unique to humans, and the lack of an animal model has hampered studies into their pathogenesis. A scar at any site has the potential to become keloidal or hypertrophic, although the earlobes (especially after ear piercing) (Figure 94.54), and sites exposed to constant stretching, such as chin, neck, shoulders, upper trunk and lower legs, are especially vulnerable [3]. Burns, scars or tissue infection predispose to hypertrophic scarring. Lesions may follow trivial trauma or inflammatory conditions such as acne. Even chemical trauma, such as from irritant herbal remedies, can trigger keloid formation. Sometimes keloids appear to develop spontaneously, particularly on the upper chest.

The introduction of foreign material, either exogenous, such as suture material, or endogenous, such as embedded hairs, is another risk factor. Some African tribes introduce foreign bodies into tribal marks to induce scar hypertrophy. Scarring acne, particularly on the trunk, may become keloid-like (Figure 94.55).

Isotretinoin has been reported to delay wound healing and induce keloids in patients who received argon laser or dermabrasion for acne or rosacea, although there is debate as to whether the association is real [4].

Epidemiology
Incidence and prevalence
Keloids or hypertrophic scars occur in 4.5–16.0% of people of African or Hispanic descent. Racial factors appear to be more important than skin pigmentation; the incidence in individuals with albinism is similar to those with pigmented skin [5]. A survey of Taiwanese children reported a prevalence of keloids of 0.3–0.6% [6]. A positive family history is obtained in 5–10% of Europeans with keloids, particularly severe lesions. Family studies suggest an autosomal dominant inheritance with incomplete penetrance [7]. Keloids have been reported in identical twins [8].

Age
Keloids are rare in infancy and old age, occurring chiefly between puberty and age 30 years.

Sex
Women have a greater predisposition in some ethnic groups; keloids may appear or enlarge during pregnancy [9].

Ethnicity
Individuals of African, Hispanic or Asian descent are more prone to keloids (Figures 94.52 and 94.53) [5].

Associated diseases
Keloids are associated with other fibromatoses such as palmar fibromatosis (Dupuytren contracture) [10], together with genetic disorders such as Ehlers–Danlos syndrome, pachydermoperiostosis [11], Rubinstein–Taybi syndrome [12] and Dubowitz syndrome [13].

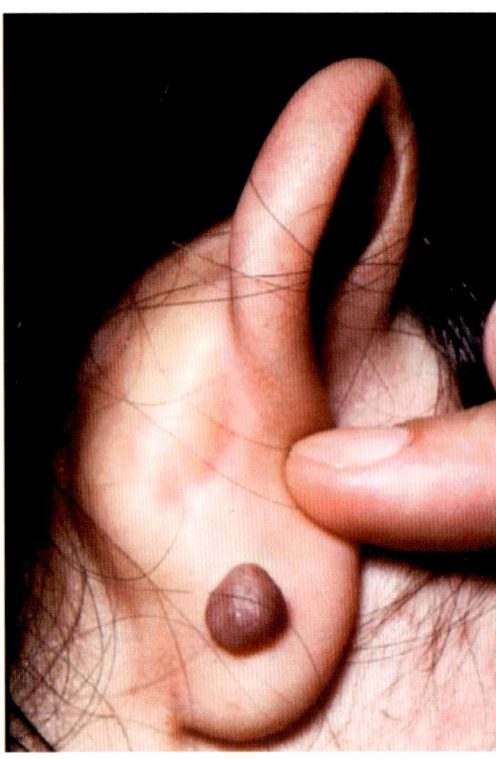 (a)

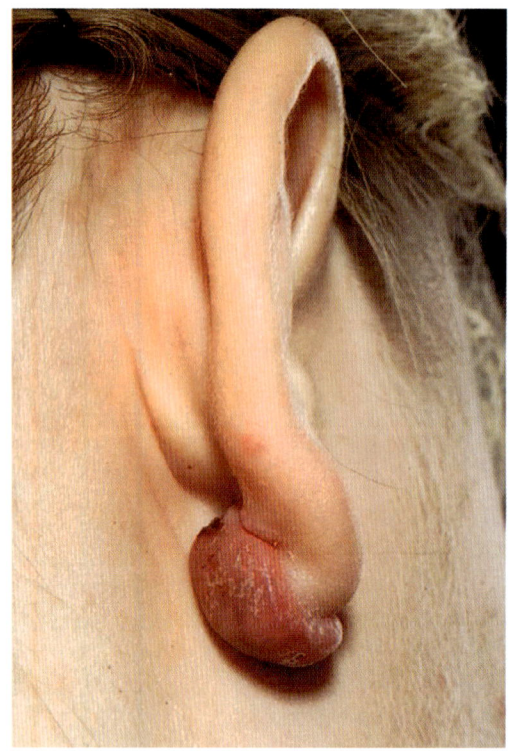 (b)

Figure 94.54 (a, b) Earlobe keloid.

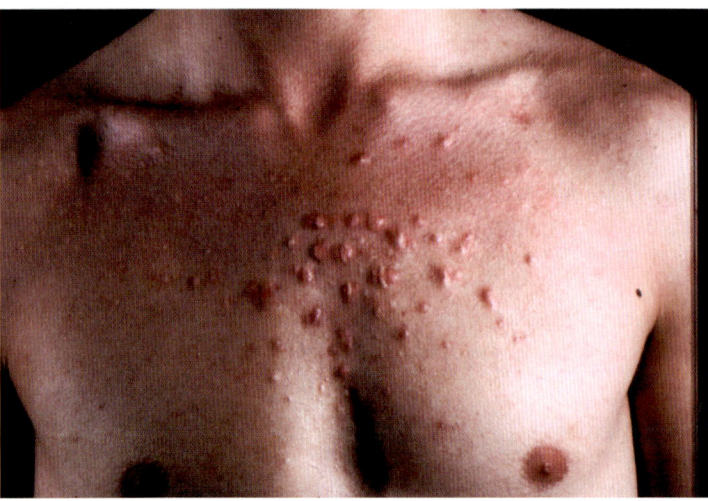

Figure 94.55 Keloid nodules secondary to acne.

Linear keloids occur in athletes abusing anabolic steroids [14]. They form readily in individuals with acromegaly and following thyroidectomy in young patients. It has been postulated that systemic hypertension may promote the development of keloids [15].

Pathophysiology

The locally invasive nature of keloids mimics a neoplastic process, although keloids do not metastasise. Suggested triggers include increased skin tension, local hypoxia (which favours the conversion of fibroblasts to myofibroblasts), a chronic inflammatory stimulus and vascular factors. Biochemical studies confirm that synthesis of type I and type III collagen is increased in both keloids and hypertrophic scars [16]. Keloids differ from healthy skin in that there is greatly increased dermal cellularity, the ratio of type I to type III collagen is increased and there is greater dermal expression of several extracellular matrix proteins including fibronectin, versican, elastin and tenascin; conversely, there is decreased expression of fibrillin 1 and decorin [17,18]. Hypertrophic scar collagen possesses the reducible keto cross-link, dehydrohydroxylysinonorleucine, normally associated with embryonic skin and granulation tissue [19].

Periostin may play an important role in pathogenesis: it is expressed by keloid fibroblasts in hypoxic conditions and, among other actions, stimulates collagen synthesis and angiogenesis [20]. Altered expression of proteoglycans may affect the three-dimensional organisation of collagen fibres [21]. Keloid fibroblasts, unlike those from hypertrophic scar tissue, are hyperresponsive to TGF-β, which is abundant in healing wounds [22], and to PDGF [23]. They also express increased levels of heat shock protein 47, another stimulus to collagen synthesis [24]. Neuropeptide-containing nerves are present [25] and the increased discomfort and itching which may be experienced in hypertrophic scars may be due to upregulation of opioid receptors [26].

Pathology

Histology may resemble normal wound healing in the early stages, with increased cellularity. In a keloid of recent onset, endothelial proliferation is surrounded by increased numbers of fibroblasts, which form large, irregular nodules or whorls of hyalinised collagen. Later, the lesion matures into an acellular core, made up of thick, poorly vascularised bands of immature collagen with loss of the boundary between the papillary and reticular dermis (Figure 94.56) [27]. There may be focal deposition of mucinous

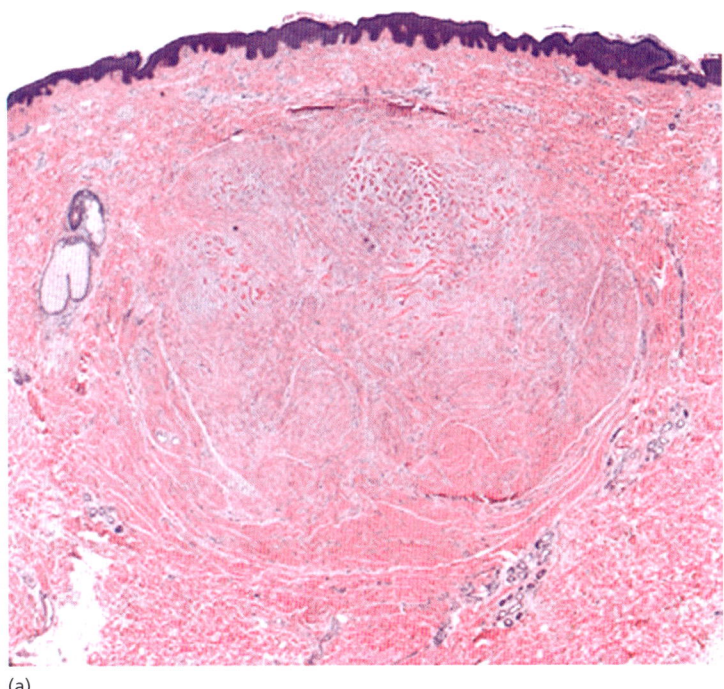

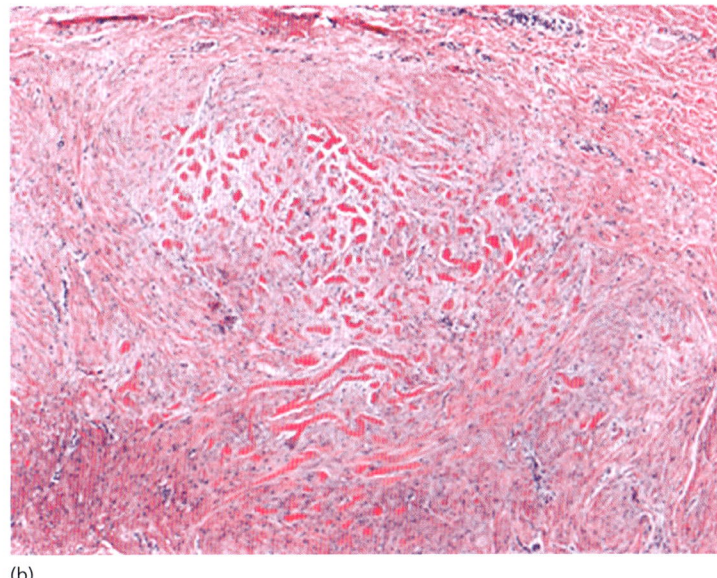

(a)   (b)

Figure 94.56 Keloid nodule: (a) a large, well-circumscribed dermal nodule sparing the papillary dermis; (b) a higher power view with haphazardly arranged thick sclerotic collagen surrounded by whorls of fibroblasts. Courtesy of Professor Luis Requena.

material in keloids, but not in hypertrophic scars. Mast cell numbers are increased in hypertrophic scars [28]. The epidermis is normal or thinned and flattened by the underlying lesion in keloids, but may be thickened in hypertrophic scars [29]. There is variable expression of α smooth muscle actin, a marker for myofibroblasts [17]. The fibroblasts have a stellate morphology on transmission electron microscopy [29,30]. Scanning electron microscopy reveals a more haphazard organisation of collagen bundles than in normal skin or mature scars, with collagen fibrils about half the diameter of those of normal skin.

Genetics
The genetic basis is unknown. Telomere shortening has been described in keloids, and attributed to oxidative stress [31].

Environmental factors
Local trauma, which may be trivial, can be a factor in keloid formation. Hypertrophic scars commonly follow deep burns. Tension on the scar and the presence of foreign material are aggravating factors in keloids.

Clinical features
History
Hypertrophic scars and keloids typically become raised and thickened within 3–4 weeks of the provocative stimulus, although keloids may develop up to a year later. Lesions are often pruritic and hypersensitive, and sometimes exquisitely tender. They may continue to grow for months or years.

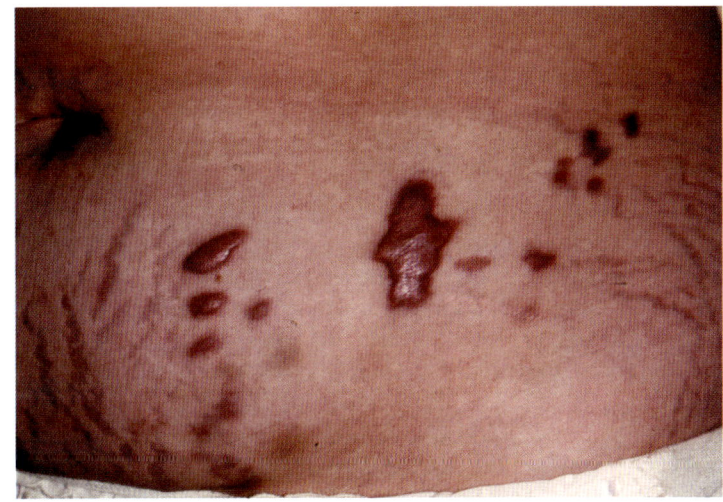

Figure 94.57 Fresh keloids arising in the striae gravidarum 3 years after pregnancy.

Presentation
Depending on skin colour, lesions may present as tender, firm, skin-coloured, pink or red plaques (Figure 94.57). Hypertrophic scars remain within the boundaries of the initial wound (Figure 94.51b), whereas keloids become smoother and rounder and extend outside the wound boundary (Figure 94.51a), often assuming a 'dumb-bell' configuration but sometimes becoming bizarre and irregular (Figure 94.53), particularly following an infected surgical wound [32]. The lesions may regress centrally, with loss of redness.

Clinical variants

Keloids on the beard area sometimes undergo central suppurative necrosis.

Differential diagnosis

The diagnosis is usually straightforward if there is a history of trauma or an inflammatory skin lesion. Keloid scarring may follow surgical treatment of BCC, and a sclerotic BCC can mimic a keloid. Other differential diagnoses include fibrosarcoma, dermatofibrosarcoma protuberans, keloidal atypical fibroxanthoma, a malignancy developing in a scar, keloidal morphoea or scar sarcoid. In endemic regions, blastomycosis and lobomycosis cause keloidal reactions.

Classification of severity

The Vancouver scar scale (VSS), recording pliability, height, vascularisation and pigmentation, is used to quantify disease severity and response to treatment [33].

Complications and co-morbidities

Malignant degeneration is reported [34], although a fibrosarcoma can mimic a keloid clinically.

Disease course and prognosis

Hypertrophic scars typically regress spontaneously, although it may take a few years. Regression of keloids is a much slower process, and keloids can expand gradually over years.

Investigations

A diagnostic skin biopsy is mandatory if the diagnosis is in doubt, particularly if malignancy is suspected.

Management

Non-essential surgery should be avoided in sites prone to keloids. Despite numerous small case series advocating a wide range of therapies, there is no level one evidence for any single treatment [35]. Enthusiastic reports should be assessed critically as there may be racial variation in response to treatment and some studies include both keloids and hypertrophic scars. The follow-up period may be brief, and keloids have a high recurrence rate. Some modalities of treatment may exacerbate the condition. The optimal approach may involve a combination of different modalities of treatment.

First line

Intralesional corticosteroids (most commonly triamcinolone acetonide) inhibit fibroblast proliferation and collagen synthesis. However, there is a risk of telangiectasia, atrophy and pigmentary change. Injections may need to be repeated monthly and recurrence rates can be up to 50% [36]. Corticosteroid impregnated tape may reduce recurrence after surgery for earlobe keloids.

Second line

Self-adherent silicone gel sheeting may be effective for keloids and hypertrophic scars [37]; they may maintain skin hydration by occlusion but a meta-analysis of 13 trials showed only a weak preventative effect [38]. A cream made of 20% silicone oil applied under occlusion may be beneficial where it is impracticable to use silicone sheeting [39].

Third line

Other treatments include the following:

- Mechanical pressure with custom-made devices or garments can be beneficial, particularly on the earlobe [40] and bras or body corsets for truncal lesions.
- Surgical excision runs the risk of recurrence of an even bigger keloid. Intralesional (core) excision is preferable; postsurgical intralesional steroids may prevent recurrence [41]. This topic is discussed in greater detail in Chapter 20.
- 5-fluorouracil (5-FU), a pyrimidine analogue, inhibits keloid growth *in vitro* and *in vivo*. Two double-blind studies have demonstrated that intralesional 5-FU (50 mg/mL) is more effective than silicone gel sheeting [42] and intralesional corticosteroids [43] in the treatment of keloids.
- A small case series has demonstrated benefit from bleomycin, using a multiple puncture injection method [44]. A Brazilian study reports favourable results from a combination of bleomycin (0.375 IU) and triamcinolone 4 mg injected 3-monthly [45]. Topical mitomycin C (0.4 mg/5 mL) applied before surgery may reduce the risk of recurrence after shave biopsy or excision [46]. Intralesional mitomycin may induce ulceration [47]. Similarly, topical imiquimod may reduce the risk of postsurgical recurrence [47].
- Photodynamic therapy has a cytotoxic effect on keloid fibroblasts. A small case series demonstrated reduced blood flow, increased pliability and decreased collagen levels with no recurrence after 9 months [48].
- In a recent randomised study, intralesional verapamil (2.5 mg/mL) gave comparable results to triamcinolone, and was well tolerated [49]. Verapamil inhibits collagen synthesis and may also have an anti-inflammatory mode of action; it can be used in combination with triamcinolone [47].
- Studies of *Botulinum* toxin have given conflicting results, although one randomised controlled trial showed it to be equally as effective, and well tolerated, as intralesional triamcinolone [47].
- Laser and light-based treatments give variable results [50]. Ablative (e.g. carbon dioxide) laser monotherapy carries a high recurrence rate. Pulsed dye and Nd:YAG lasers appear to be more effective, particularly in combination with intralesional corticosteroids or 5-FU. Lasers may be useful as tools for drug delivery [47]. Low-level red and infrared light-emitting diodes (LEDs) suppress fibroblast synthesis and achieve cosmetic improvement. Other physical therapies include degenerate wave electrical stimulation [51].
- Inhibitors of pro-inflammatory cytokines such as TGF-β analogues [52] and IFN-α [47,53] show promise, perhaps in conjunction with intralesional triamcinolone. Recent reviews suggest that a combination of surgery with adjuvant radiotherapy [54] or intralesional 5-FU or corticosteroids [55] is preferable to monotherapy.

- Activation of the renin–angiotensin system may induce fibrosis and there are encouraging reports of the use of angiotensin-converting enzyme (ACE) inhibitors (e.g. topical captopril or low-dose oral enalapril) in the treatment of keloids [56].

PERFORATING DERMATOSES

Definition

These are skin disorders in which material is eliminated from the dermis by extrusion through the epidermis to the skin surface by a process of transepidermal (transepithelial) elimination. The primary perforating disorders are particularly associated with diabetes and chronic renal failure in the case of acquired perforating dermatosis and heritable disorders of connective tissue or Down syndrome in the case of elastosis perforans serpiginosum.

Introduction and general description

There has been considerable confusion over the terminology used to describe the perforating disorders, with an array of different terms used to denote what is now thought to represent essentially the same underlying process: biopsies taken at different sites or times from the same patient may show a variety of different patterns depending on whether the lesion involves a follicle and whether it has been modified by excoriation. Perforation is a histopathological construct signifying that material, usually degenerate collagen or elastin, has breached or perforated an epithelium, usually the epidermis, in which case the process is usually referred to as transepidermal elimination (TEE).

The term perforating folliculitis continues to be used in the published literature as a disease entity, although several authorities have recommended that it should be abandoned [1,2]. The term acquired reactive perforating collagenosis fell out of favour some years ago, to be replaced by acquired perforating dermatosis when it was demonstrated that both collagen and elastin were commonly involved [2]. Similarly, the distinction between acquired perforating dermatosis and Kyrle disease is not clear-cut [3] and separation of the two is no longer felt to be valid.

Many dermatoses occasionally exhibit the phenomenon of TEE, in which material from the dermis is extruded through the epidermis to the exterior with little or no disruption of the surrounding structures [4]. The extruded material may include inflammatory cells, red cells, microorganisms and extracellular substances, such as mucin or degenerate collagen and elastin [4,5,6,7]. In most of these conditions, the TEE is secondary to some underlying disease, such as granuloma annulare or PXE. There is also a rare hereditary disorder, familial reactive perforating collagenosis, which is characterised by TEE of collagen from an early age (Chapter 70). The primary acquired perforating skin disorders which will be discussed here are therefore limited to acquired perforating dermatosis, which is strongly linked in the majority but not all cases to either diabetes, renal failure or both, and elastosis perforans serpiginosa, which is linked to heritable disorders of connective tissue and Down syndrome.

Acquired perforating dermatosis

Definition and nomenclature

This is an acquired disorder of TEE of degenerate collagen, elastin and other connective tissue components. It is strongly associated with diabetes and chronic kidney disease.

> **Synonyms and inclusions**
> - Acquired reactive perforating dermatosis
> - Acquired perforating collagenosis

Introduction and general description

Acquired perforating dermatosis is strongly linked with longstanding diabetes (Figure 94.58) and chronic kidney disease, often in association with haemodialysis [1,2–8]. It is characterised by TEE of both collagen and elastin and presents as a chronic pruritic dermatosis with multiple keratotic crusted papules and nodules.

Epidemiology
Incidence and prevalence
It is relatively frequent in the commonly affected populations with reported rates of 4–11% of patients on haemodialysis [7,8].

Age
It generally occurs in the fifth to sixth decades of life.

Sex
The female to male ratio is 3 : 1 [9,10].

Ethnicity
All races are affected.

Associated diseases
There is a strong association with chronic kidney disease and diabetes, and an association with chronic pruritus [11]. There are

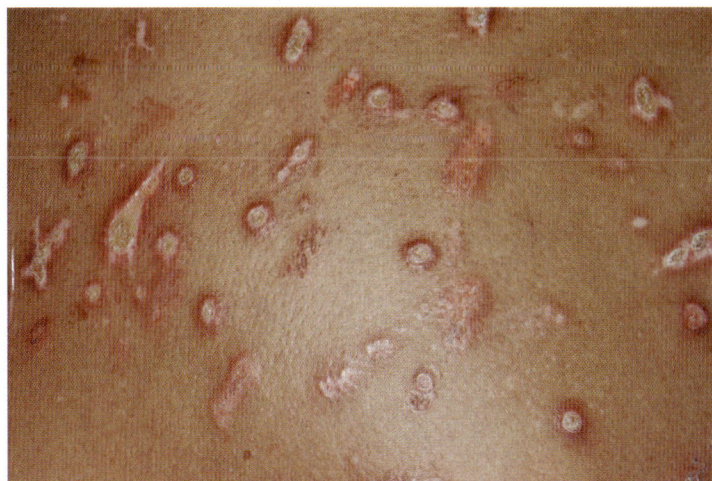

Figure 94.58 Acquired perforating dermatosis: close-up view of the back of a 65-year-old woman with longstanding diabetes.

PART 8: SPECIFIC CUTANEOUS STRUCTURES

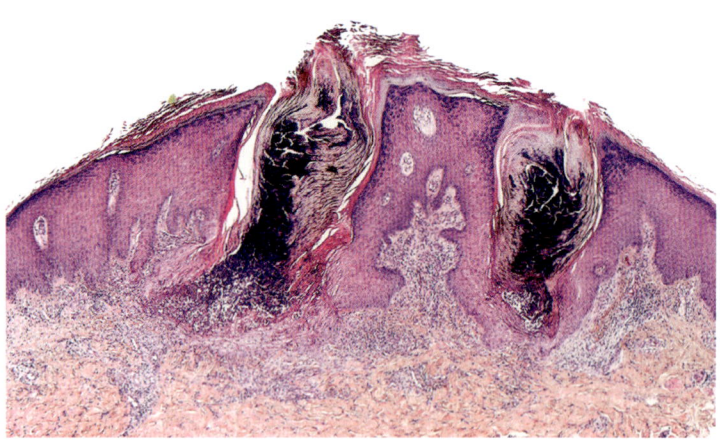

Figure 94.59 Acquired perforating dermatosis: invaginations of the epidermis enable columns of necrotic inflammatory debris to be extruded from the dermis. Courtesy of Professor Luis Requena.

case reports of an association with dermatomyositis [12] and drugs such as cetuximab, panitumumab and natalizumab [13–15].

Pathophysiology

The bulk of the coarse granular basophilic material which is extruded by TEE appears to derive from the nuclei of polymorphonuclear leukocytes [16]. It has been suggested that lysosomal enzymes derived from leukocytes might be responsible for the altered staining of collagen fibres, the degradation of elastic fibres and the impairment of keratinocyte adhesion, which allows TEE of dermal components [3].

Most patients have chronic renal disease and/or longstanding diabetes.

Pathology

Histology reveals cup-shaped invaginations of the epidermis, which is plugged with necrotic inflammatory debris. Collagen bundles are arranged vertically at the base of the lesion and there is TEE of collagen fibres (Figure 94.59) [17].

Causative organisms

Generally there are none, although there is one reported case associated with disseminated histoplasmosis [18].

Genetics

There are no known genetic factors.

Clinical features
History

Pruritus, which may be intractable, is a common symptom.

Presentation

Keratotic dome-shaped papules with central crusts develop anywhere on the body but primarily on the extensor aspects of the limbs and trunk (Figure 94.60). Dermoscopy with polarised light reveals bright white patches on a featureless grey background, surrounded by reticulate brown lines [**1**].

Clinical variants

Familial reactive perforating collagenosis. Familial reactive perforating collagenosis [2,9,16,19–21] is a rare inherited form of TEE in which collagen is extruded through the epidermis. It is usually precipitated by environmental cold or trauma. The basic defect seems to be a type of focal damage to collagen, which is then extruded as a result of necrolysis of the overlying epidermis [22].

The lesion originates in the papillary dermis where collagen is surrounded and engulfed by focal epidermal proliferation. The collagen appears normal on electron microscopy, but gives an abnormal staining pattern with trichrome and phosphotungstic acid haematoxylin. The central crater which develops contains inflammatory cells and keratinous debris. Elastic tissue is typically absent, and the abnormal collagen is eliminated by transepithelial migration [22–24].

It usually starts in early childhood as small papules on the extensor surface of the hands, elbows and knees following superficial trauma. Each skin-coloured papule increases to a size of about 6 mm over 3–5 weeks and then becomes umbilicated, with a ker-

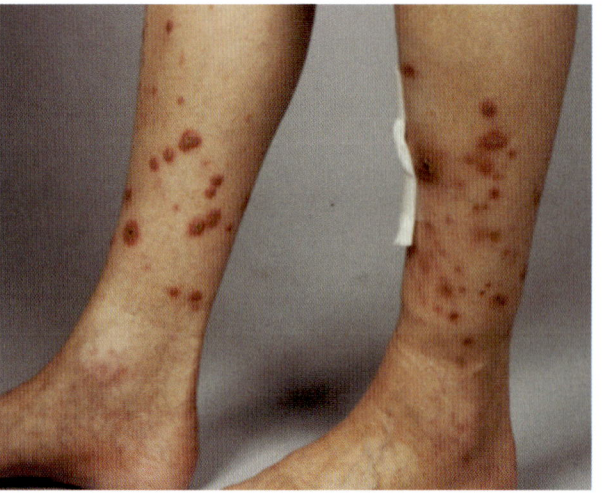

(a)

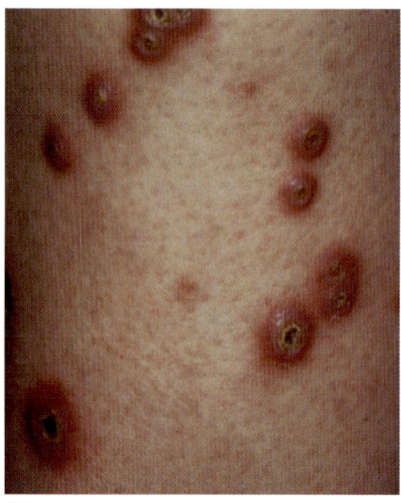

(b)

Figure 94.60 (a, b) Acquired perforating dermatosis: a 48-year-old woman with a 25-year history of type 1 diabetes with retinopathy and renal failure, and a 12-year history of skin ulceration with multiple, tender, crusted sores which were slow to heal.

atinous plug [22]. The lesions regress spontaneously in 6–8 weeks to leave a hypopigmented area or slight scar, but new lesions may appear. Lesions can be produced experimentally, and the Koebner phenomenon may result in linear lesions [25]. The papules can also be provoked by inflamed acne lesions, but deep incisions do not produce the lesions. The condition persists into adult life. In some cases, the disease is associated with intolerance to cold and improves in warm weather.

The nosological relationship between familial reactive perforating collagenosis and the acquired reactive perforating dermatosis of chronic kidney disease remains uncertain [26].

Verrucous perforating collagenoma. Verrucous perforating collagenoma [27–29] (synonym collagénome perforant verruciforme) is rarely reported and appears to be a reaction to the traumatic introduction of foreign materials including fibreglass, vegetable matter, calcium chloride and irritant drugs into the skin. Damaged collagen extruded to the surface by TEE is manifest as verrucous papules.

Perforating disease due to exogenous agents. Occasionally, a chemical that has been applied to the skin topically or by intradermal injection can be eliminated by the transepidermal route. Eight cases have been reported following occupational exposure to a caustic drilling fluid used in the petrochemical industry [30]. Each patient noted skin irritation following exposure to the fluid and 1 or 2 days later developed tender papules with central umbilication followed by ulceration and crusting. Histological examination demonstrated TEE of altered collagen and debris which stained for calcium.

It is possible that the lesions were due to follicular penetration by the calcium present in the drilling mud. The drilling fluids contain many additives, but calcium carbonate or calcium chloride are often present in high concentrations in the mud. Similar cases have been reported following the use of calcium-containing electroencephalography paste [31].

TEE of altered collagen has also been reported following the use of intradermal steroid injections [32,33].

Differential diagnosis

The condition may be mistaken clinically for molluscum contagiosum, papular urticaria or other perforating disorders, but the histology is characteristic [17,21].

Management

Some patients improve spontaneously, particularly if renal function can be improved [7,10]. No treatment is of proven benefit, although there are several reports of the use of allopurinol [34,35].

Topical retinoids may reduce the number of lesions. Other treatments which may help include oral isotretinoin, methotrexate, rifampicin, emollient creams, intralesional steroids and topical steroids under occlusion [5,9,26]. Narrow-band UVB [36], PUVA [37] and photodynamic therapy [38] have all been used. Associated uraemic pruritus may improve with amitriptyline [39]. Complete remission has been reported after the use of topical tacalcitol [40], however spontaneous resolution can occur.

Elastosis perforans serpiginosa

Definition and nomenclature

This is a perforating dermatosis in which the material extruded through the epidermis is derived from elastic fibres in the upper dermis [1]. It is closely associated with heritable disorders of connective tissue and Down syndrome.

Synonyms and inclusions
- Perforating elastoma
- Elastoma intrapapillare perforans

Epidemiology

Incidence and prevalence

It is rare.

Age

It usually presents between the ages of 5 and 20 years.

Sex

Males are predominantly affected.

Ethnicity

All races are affected.

Associated diseases

Some 40% of reported cases have been associated with heritable connective tissue disorders, such as PXE, Ehlers–Danlos syndrome, Marfan syndrome, osteogenesis imperfecta and acrogeria [2,**3**]. It has also been reported in otherwise healthy individuals and in association with Down syndrome [4–7]. Elastosis perforans serpiginosa has been reported as a paraneoplastic phenomenon [8].

It sometimes occurs in patients receiving penicillamine, which is known to cause the production of abnormal elastin [9–13], and there is an overlap with pseudo-PXE (see earlier in this chapter).

Pathophysiology

Predisposing factors

The altered elastin resembles that seen in experimental animals subjected to lathyrogens or copper deficiency. It is probable that the primary abnormality is in the dermal elastin, which provokes a cellular response that ultimately leads to extrusion of the abnormal elastic tissue. It may be significant that the lesions are commonly seen in areas subjected to wear and tear.

Pathology

The earliest detectable change is the focal development of elastotic-staining tissue and basophilic debris in the dermis. This is followed by a reaction of the overlying epidermis, which grows down to engulf the elastotic material. The epidermis surrounding the fully developed lesion is acanthotic and hyperkeratotic (Figure 94.61). The papule consists of a circumscribed area of epidermal hyperplasia traversed by a channel communicating directly with the dermis

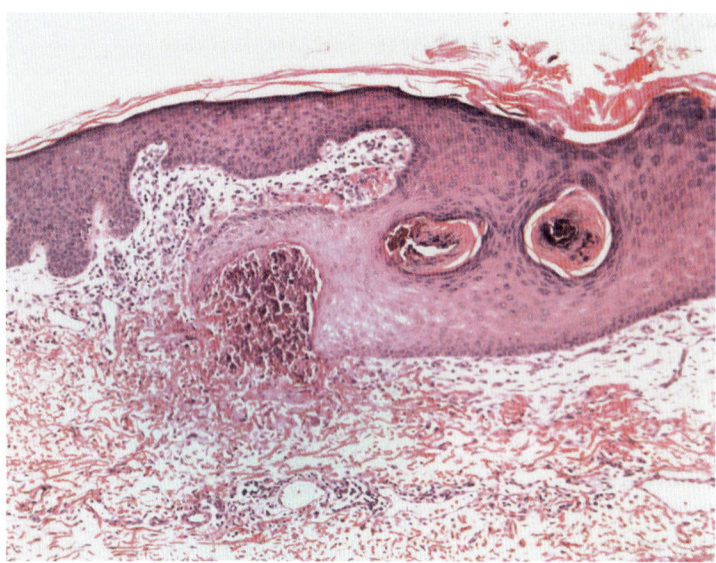

Figure 94.61 Elastosis perforans serpiginosa: note the acanthotic epidermis growing downward in order to surround and engulf a focus of basophilic elastotic debris. Courtesy of Dr Leigh Biddlestone.

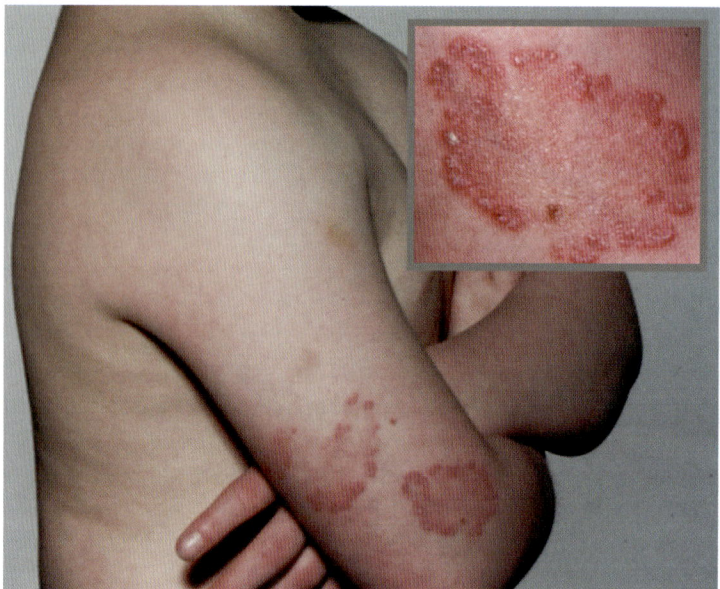

Figure 94.62 Elastosis perforans serpiginosa in a boy with Down syndrome.

PART 8: SPECIFIC CUTANEOUS STRUCTURES

and containing a mass of tissue, which projects above the surface. This plug consists of horny material in its upper third and of amorphous debris derived from elastin in its lower two-thirds [4,14–17]. In the dermis beneath and around the lesion, there is a foreign-body giant cell reaction. The elastotic material is finally extruded, to leave irregular scarring and warty thickening. Electron microscopy shows an increase in elastic fibres, with fine filaments on the surface similar to those seen in normal embryos. In penicillamine-induced cases the elastic fibres have a characteristic 'bramble bush' or 'lumpy-bumpy' morphology [11,18]. The hydroxylation of dermal collagen is similar to that of newborn skin [15].

Causative organisms
No specific organism has been identified.

Genetics
The cause is unknown, but a genetically determined defect of elastic tissue may be involved [1]. It is often associated with a known heritable disorder of connective tissue.

Environmental factors
The lesions may follow minor trauma such as an abrasion.

Clinical features
History
The lesions are generally asymptomatic.

Presentation
Small, horny or umbilicated papules are characteristically arranged in lines, circles or segments of circles in a serpiginous pattern (Figure 94.62). The individual papules may remain small or may enlarge slightly to assume a crateriform appearance with an elevated edge and a central plug, or enlarge further to leave an area of atrophic skin surrounded by smaller papules, each with a horny plug. The rings may reach a diameter of 15–20 cm but are usually

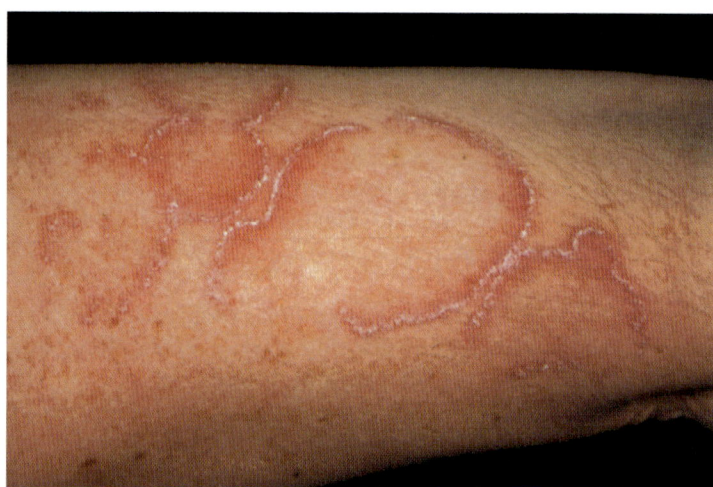

Figure 94.63 Elastosis perforans serpiginosa in a patient with vascular Ehlers–Danlos syndrome.

smaller (Figure 94.63). The back and sides of the neck are most commonly affected, but the lesions may also occur on the cheeks or on the arms or thighs, and are sometimes bilaterally symmetrical [1,17,19,20].

Differential diagnosis
The annular or linear arrangements of the papules and their distribution suggest the diagnosis, which is confirmed by the characteristic histology. Conditions that may cause confusion include porokeratosis of Mibelli, familial reactive perforating collagenosis and perforating granuloma annulare. A similar histological appearance can occur in acquired perforating dermatosis (see earlier in this chapter) [21].

Classification of severity
It is not of prognostic significance in its own right, but may reflect an underlying heritable disorder of connective tissue.

Complications and co-morbidities
There may be an associated connective tissue disease.

Disease course and prognosis
The lesions may persist for several years, but eventually involute spontaneously to leave reticulate atrophic scars.

Investigations
Skin biopsy is diagnostic, but biopsy scars readily become keloidal.

Management
The condition tends to be self-limiting, and no treatment is of proven benefit [19]. However, careful removal of the nodules with a curette under local anaesthesia may give a reasonable cosmetic result. Freezing has been recommended [19,22,23]. Excision should be avoided, and dermabrasion may make the condition worse [4]. In a child with Down syndrome and associated vitamin A deficiency, clinical improvement was observed with oral retinoid therapy, even though the treatment produced side effects [6]. Isotretinoin has been used successfully in a patient with penicillamine-induced disease [24]. It has been reported that acitretin has treated extensive elastosis perforans serpiginosa in a man with Down syndrome [25]. There are reports of improvement following Sellotape® stripping of the surface keratinous material [26], tazarotene [27], imiquimod [28] and calcipotriol [3]. Treatment with pulsed dye [29], ultrapulsed carbon dioxide [30,31] and Er:YAG [32] lasers have also been advocated [2].

Treatment ladder

First line
- Conservative management

Second line
- Trial of cryotherapy initially to test site

Third line
- Curettage

Key references

The full list of references can be found in the online version at https://www.wiley.com/rooksdermatology10e

Changes in dermal connective tissue due to ageing and photodamage
Introduction and general description
4 Battie C, Jitsukawa S, Bernerd F, Del Bino S, Marionnet C, Verschoore M. New insights in photoaging, UVA induced damage and skin types. *Exp Dermatol* 2014;23(Suppl. 1):7–12.

Wrinkles
4 Kligman AM, Zheng P, Lavker RM. The anatomy and pathogenesis of wrinkles. *Br J Dermatol* 1985;113:37–42.

Actinic elastosis
4 Sachs DL, Varani J, Chubb H *et al.* Atrophic and hypertrophic photoaging: clinical, histologic, and molecular features of 2 distinct phenotypes of photoaged skin. *J Am Acad Dermatol* 2019;81:480–8.

Collagenous and elastotic marginal plaques of the hands
5 Calderone DC, Fenske NA. The clinical spectrum of actinic elastosis. *J Am Acad Dermatol* 1995;32:1016–24.

Adult colloid milium and colloid degeneration of the skin
1 Mehregan D, Hooten J. Adult colloid milium: a case report and literature review. *Int J Dermatol* 2011;50:1531–4.

Other causes of cutaneous atrophy
Atrophy due to corticosteroids
1 Barnes L, Kaya G, Rollason V. Topical corticosteroid-induced skin atrophy: a comprehensive review. *Drug Saf* 2015;38:493–509.

Striae
20 Al-Himdani S, Ud-Din S, Gilmore S *et al.* Striae distensae: a comprehensive revision and evidence-based evaluation of prophylaxis and treatment. *Br J Dermatol* 2014;170:527–47.

Atrophic scars
3 Colomb D. Stellate spontaneous pseudoscars. Senile and presenile forms: especially those forms caused by prolonged corticoid therapy. *Arch Dermatol* 1972;105:551–4.

Spontaneous atrophic scarring of the cheeks
1 Marks VJ, Miller OF. Atrophia maculosa varioliformis cutis. *Br J Dermatol* 1986;115:105–9.

Acrodermatitis chronica atrophicans
25 Radolf JD, Strle K, Lemieux JE, Strle F. Lyme disease in humans. *Curr Issues Mol Biol* 2021;42:333–84.

Atrophodermas
Linear atrophoderma
1 De Golian E, Echols K, Pearl H *et al.* Linear atrophoderma of Moulin: a distinct entity? *Pediatr Dermatol* 2014;31:373–7.

Atrophoderma of Pasini and Pierini
3 Buechner SA, Rufli T. Atrophoderma of Pasini and Pierini. *J Am Acad Dermatol* 1994;30:441–6.

Disorders of elastic fibre degradation
4 Lewis KG, Bercovitch L, Dill SW *et al.* Acquired disorders of elastic tissue: Part 1. Increased elastic tissue and solar elastotic syndromes *J Am Acad Dermatol* 2004;51:1–21.
5 Lewis KG, Bercovitch L, Dill SW *et al.* Acquired disorders of elastic tissue: Part II. Decreased elastic tissue. *J Am Acad Dermatol* 2004;51:165–85.

Anetoderma
1 Venencie PY, Winkelmann RK. Histopathologic findings in anetoderma. *Arch Dermatol* 1984;120:1040–4.
2 Venencie PY, Winkelmann RK, Moore BA. Anetoderma: clinical findings, associations, and long term follow-up evaluations. *Arch Dermatol* 1984;120:1032–9.

Mid-dermal elastolysis
1 Brenner W, Gschnait FG, Konrad K *et al.* Non-inflammatory dermal elastolysis. *Br J Dermatol* 1978;99:335–8.

Upper dermal elastolysis
2 Newlove T, Tzu J, Meehan S. Papillary dermal elastosis. *Dermatol Online J* 2011;17:12.

PART 8: SPECIFIC CUTANEOUS STRUCTURES

Blepharochalasis

12 Ali K. Ascher syndrome: a case report and review of the literature. *Oral Surg Oral Med Oral Pathol Oral Radiol Endod* 2007;103:e26–8.

Actinic granuloma and annular elastolytic giant cell granuloma

1 Hanke CW, Bailin PL, Roenigk HH. Annular elastolytic giant cell granuloma: a clinicopathologic study of five cases and a review of similar entities. *J Am Acad Dermatol* 1979;1:413–21.

Granuloma multiforme

2 Leiker DL, Kok SH, Spaas JA. Granuloma multiforme: a new skin disease resembling leprosy. *Int J Lepr* 1964;32:368–76.

Acquired pseudoxanthoma elasticum-like syndromes
Perforating pseudoxanthoma elasticum

1 Premalatha S, Yesudian P, Thambiah AS. Periumbilical pseudoxanthoma elasticum with transepithelial elimination. *Int J Dermatol* 1982;10:604–5.

Acquired disorders of elastic tissue deposition
Linear focal elastosis

1 Burket JM, Zelickson AS, Padilla RS. Linear focal elastosis (elastotic striae). *J Am Acad Dermatol* 1989;20:633–6.

Late-onset focal dermal elastosis

1 Tajima S, Shimizu K, Izumi T, Kurihara S, Harada T. Late-onset focal dermal elastosis: clinical and histological features. *Br J Dermatol* 1995;133:303–5.

Elastofibroma dorsi

10 Karakurt O, Kaplan T, Gunal N *et al*. Elastofibroma dorsi management and outcomes: review of 16 cases. *Interact Cardiovasc Thorac Surg* 2014;18:197–201.

Elastoderma

3 Adil H, Walsh S. Elastoderma: case report and literature review. *Am J Dermatopathol* 2015;37:577–80.

Papular elastorrhexis

8 Ryder HF, Antaya RJ. Nevus anelasticus, papular elastorrhexis, and eruptive collagenoma: clinically similar entities with focal absence of elastic fibers in childhood. *Pediatr Dermatol* 2005;22:153–7.

Fibromatoses and other causes of diffuse fibrosis
Fibromatoses
Palmar fascial fibromatosis

3 Evans RA. The aetiology of Dupuytren's disease. *Br J Hosp Med* 1986;36:198–9.
20 Zhang AY, Kargel JS. The basic science of Dupuytren disease. *Hand Clin* 2018; 34:301–5.

Plantar fascial fibromatosis

3 Gudmundsson KG, Jónsson T, Arngrímsson R. Association of morbus ledderhose with Dupuytren's contracture. *Foot Ankle Int* 2013;34:841–5.

Penile fibromatosis

4 Gingell JC, Desai KM. Peyronie's disease. *BMJ* 1988;297:1489–90.

Knuckle pads

4 Hyman CH, Cohen PR. Report of a family with idiopathic knuckle pads and review of idiopathic and disease-associated knuckle pads. *Dermatol Online J* 2013; 19:18177.

Pachydermodactyly

1 Al Hammadi A, Hakim M. Pachydermodactyly: case report and review of the literature. *J Cutan Med Surg* 2007;11:185–7.

White fibrous papulosis of the neck

3 Cerio R, Gold S, Jones EW. White fibrous papulosis of the neck. *Clin Exp Dermatol* 1991;16:224–5.

Camptodactyly

1 Engber WD, Flatt AE. Camptodactyly: an analysis of sixty-six patients and twenty-four operations. *J Hand Surg Am* 1977;2(3):216–24.

Juvenile fibromatoses
Infantile myofibromatosis

2 Mashiah J, Hadj-Rabia S, Dompmartin A *et al*. Infantile myofibromatosis: a series of 28 cases. *J Am Acad Dermatol* 2014;71:264–70.

Juvenile hyaline fibromatosis

4 Finlay AY, Ferguson SD, Holt PJ. Juvenile hyaline fibromatosis. *Br J Dermatol* 1983;108:609–16.

Other benign fibrous cutaneous nodules
Nodular fasciitis

1 Luna A, Molinari L, Bollea Garlatti LA *et al*. Nodular fasciitis, a forgotten entity. *Int J Dermatol* 2019;58:190–3.

Nephrogenic systemic fibrosis

11 Lunyera J, Mohottige D, Alexopoulos AS *et al*. Risk for nephrogenic systemic fibrosis after exposure to newer gadolinium agents: a systematic review. *Ann Intern Med* 2020;173:110–19.

Environmental and drug-induced scleroderma

1 Murrell DF. A radical proposal for the pathogenesis of scleroderma. *J Am Acad Dermatol* 1993;28:78–85.

Constricting bands of the extremities

6 Cignini P, Giorlandino C, Padula F, Dugo N, Cafà EV, Spata A. Epidemiology and risk factors of amniotic band syndrome, or ADAM sequence. *J Prenat Med* 2012;6:59–63.

Abnormal fibrotic responses to skin injury
Keloids and hypertrophic scars

1 Köse O, Waseem A. Keloids and hypertrophic scars: are they two different sides of the same coin? *Dermatol Surg* 2008;34:336–46.
36 Gauglitz GG, Korting HC, Pavicic T *et al*. Hypertrophic scarring and keloids: pathomechanisms and current and emerging treatment strategies. *Mol Med* 2011; 17:113–25.

Perforating dermatoses

6 Akoglu G, Emre S, Sungu N, Kurtoglu G, Metin A. Clinicopathological features of 25 patients with acquired perforating dermatosis. *Eur J Dermatol* 2013;23:864–71.

Acquired perforating dermatosis

1 Ramirez-Fort MK, Khan F, Rosendahl CO, Mercer SE, Shim-Chang H, Levitt JO. Acquired perforating dermatosis: a clinical and dermatoscopic correlation. *Dermatol Online J* 2013;19:18958.

Elastosis perforans serpiginosa

3 Mehta RK, Burrows NP, Payne CM, Mendelsohn SS, Pope FM, Rytina E. Elastosis perforans serpiginosa and associated disorders. *Clin Exp Dermatol* 2001;26:521–4.

CHAPTER 95

Granulomatous Disorders of the Skin

John W. Frew[1] and Saleem M. Taibjee[2]

[1]Department of Dermatology, Liverpool Hospital, University of New South Wales, Sydney, Australia
[2]Departments of Dermatology and Pathology, Dorset County Hospital, Dorchester, Dorset, UK

Granuloma annulare

Definition

This is a disease of the skin and subcutaneous tissue characterised by granulomatous annular plaques, nodules or papules containing foci of altered collagen surrounded by histiocytes and lymphocytes.

Introduction and general description

Granuloma annulare (GA) is a distinctive condition presenting with annular indurated papules and/or plaques on the extremities [1,2]. These lesions may slowly enlarge before eventually flattening and fading over the course of months or years (Figure 95.1). GA may occur at any age and is more common in women. Several different clinical types are seen: localised, generalised, subcutaneous (deep) and perforating. The aetiology and pathophysiology are incompletely understood, although there are reports of associated infective and other triggers. The widely cited association with diabetes has not been fully substantiated; adequate controlled studies have not been performed to date. Treatment is often unnecessary given the self-limiting nature. In severe generalised disease many treatments have been reported to be effective although the evidence is largely anecdotal.

Epidemiology

Incidence and prevalence

The population prevalence is documented as 0.06% with an annualised incidence of 0.04% in North America [3]. GA has been estimated to account for approximately 0.1–0.4% of dermatology outpatient consultations in the UK [1,3].

Age

GA is most common in children and young adults but can occur at any age [1]. Generalised GA occurs more commonly in adults with a mean around 50 years of age in most series [4,5,6,7]. Subcutaneous (deep) GA is seen predominantly in children. Perforating GA has been reported in both adults and children.

Sex

GA is at least twice as common in women as in men [8].

Ethnicity

There does not appear to be any racial predilection for GA, except for perforating GA, which is more common among ethnic Hawaiians [9,10].

Associated diseases

GA is associated with an increased odds ratio of coexistent type 1 and type 2 diabetes mellitus [11,12], hyperlipidaemia and hypothyroidism. There have been suggestions that the rates of type 2 diabetes mellitus are probably *not* increased among patients with GA [13,14]. The majority of publications report retrospective surveys, in which some have suggested an association with type 1 diabetes [15–17]. One case–control study [14] showed a lack of association with type 2 diabetes, although it should be noted that psoriasis patients were used as controls. The recently recognised association between psoriasis and insulin resistance [18] casts doubt on the appropriateness of psoriasis as a control group in this study. The largest study to date involving 5137 individuals with GA [11] presented an adjusted odds ratio of 1.67; 95%CI 1.55–1.80.

Both localised and generalised GA have been reported in association with autoimmune thyroiditis and hypothyroidism in women [7,19–21], including in one case–control study [21]. Generalised GA has also been reported in a patient with a toxic adenoma of the thyroid (Plummer disease) [22]. Two papers suggest the possibility of an association between uveitis and GA [23,24].

The incidence of hyperlipidaemia has recently been reported to be four times higher among people with GA than in age-matched controls [25].

Although there are several reports of an association with malignancy, many of the cases were atypical (e.g. painful lesions of the palms and soles). Recent reviews of the literature have concluded that there is no convincing relationship, including with haematological malignancies [26,27], although older patients with atypical forms of GA may be exceptions.

Rook's Textbook of Dermatology, Tenth Edition. Edited by Christopher Griffiths, Jonathan Barker, Tanya Bleiker, Walayat Hussain and Rosalind Simpson.
© 2024 John Wiley & Sons Ltd. Published 2024 by John Wiley & Sons Ltd.

PART 8: SPECIFIC CUTANEOUS STRUCTURES

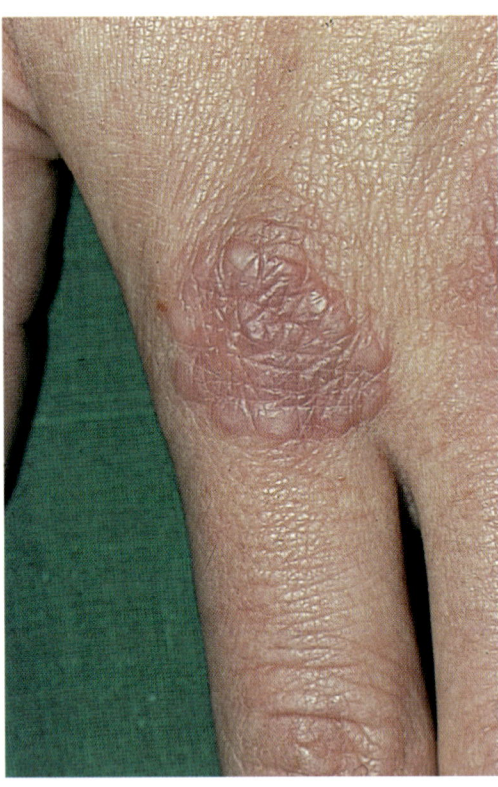

Figure 95.1 Granuloma annulare on the dorsum of the hand – a typical site.

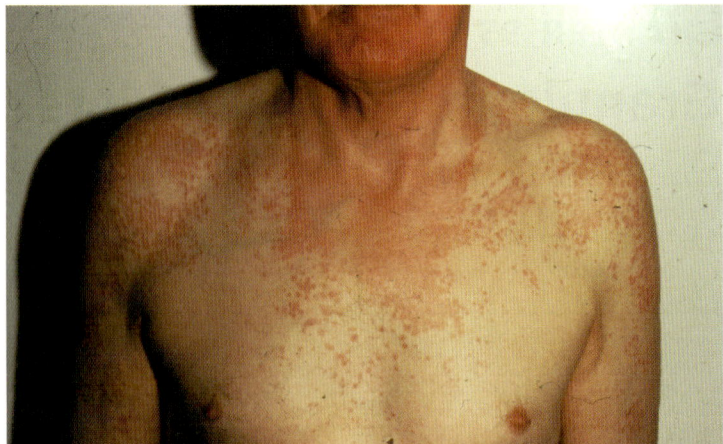

Figure 95.2 Generalised granuloma annulare showing a clear photo-distribution over the 'V' of the neck and shoulders.

There are isolated reports of the coincidence of temporal arteritis [28] and morphoea [29] in patients with GA. Coexistence with necrobiosis lipoidica [30–34] and sarcoidosis [35–38] has also been reported.

Pathophysiology

Immunological investigations have identified a mixed T-helper-1/T-helper-2/Janus kinase-driven immune response in lesional tissue of GA compared with healthy controls [39]. Cytokines including tumour necrosis factor α (TNF-α), interleukin 1B (IL-1B), Janus kinase 3, IL-4, IL-13, IL-31 and IL-12/23p40 are elevated in gene expression analysis [39]. This mixed inflammatory response likely represents a reaction pattern to a variety of triggering factors [8,40]. A miscellany of infections and infestations have been linked; these include scabies [41], hepatitis B [42], *Mycobacterium tuberculosis* [43,44], human papillomavirus [45], varicella/zoster [46–54], Epstein–Barr virus [55,56], parvovirus B19 [57], hepatitis C [58], HIV [59–70] and *Borrelia burgdorferi* [71–73]. The heterogeneity of associated organisms and lack of demonstration of persistent viral or bacterial DNA within lesions are likely to suggest a reactive inflammatory process rather than specific infection [51,59,73–76].

Traumatic triggers that have been linked to GA have included a variety of immunisations [77–81], tuberculin testing [82], animal and insect bites [83,84], waxing [85] and saphenectomy [86]. Perforating GA has also been reported in the red areas of tattoos [87,88].

Sunlight exposure has been implicated in seasonal GA [89,90] and, more obviously, in cases where there is a clear photo-distribution (Figure 95.2) [91–94]. Generalised GA following psoralen and UVA (PUVA) has also been reported [95]. Whether actinic granuloma is a distinct entity, or represents GA on sun-exposed skin, has been the subject of debate [96–104].

There are several reports of drug-induced GA, although some could alternatively represent examples of interstitial granulomatous drug reaction, the latter tending to show different clinical features and histology [105]. GA has been previously associated with immunosuppressant medications [106]. A recent publication from Greece reported that GA was found in almost 4% of rheumatology patients treated with TNF-α blockers [107]. There are also intriguing cases of association with immune checkpoint inhibitors for treatment of malignancy, in particular anti-PD1 blockade [108,109].

There is a report of disseminated GA occurring in the same sites as lesions of erythema multiforme [110].

It has been suggested that an immunoglobulin-mediated vasculitis is the cause of the necrobiotic granulomas in GA [111,**112**], but evidence from immunofluorescence studies is conflicting: some authors have demonstrated immunoreactants in vessel walls [111], whereas others have not [113,114]. An alternative view is that the pathogenetic mechanism is a delayed-type hypersensitivity response [**112**,114–118].

Gli-1, the glioma-associated oncogene homologue, is highly expressed in various granulomatous diseases including GA. The relevance to pathophysiology remains unclear, but this raises the possibility of inhibitors of gli-1 as a therapeutic target [119].

Pathology

The most characteristic histological feature in GA is the necrobiotic palisading granuloma, but there are three histological patterns that may occur: (i) necrobiotic palisading granulomas; (ii) an interstitial form; and (iii) granulomas of sarcoidal type [120]. There is some variation in the literature in relation to the prevalence of each of these types in the different clinical patterns of disease [6,121,122]. Observer variation and the existence of more than one pattern in the same section may have contributed to differences in the findings in these series.

Necrobiotic palisading granulomas (Figure 95.3) are typically situated in the superficial and mid-dermis, and separated by relatively normal tissue in GA, in contrast to necrobiosis lipoidica (see later).

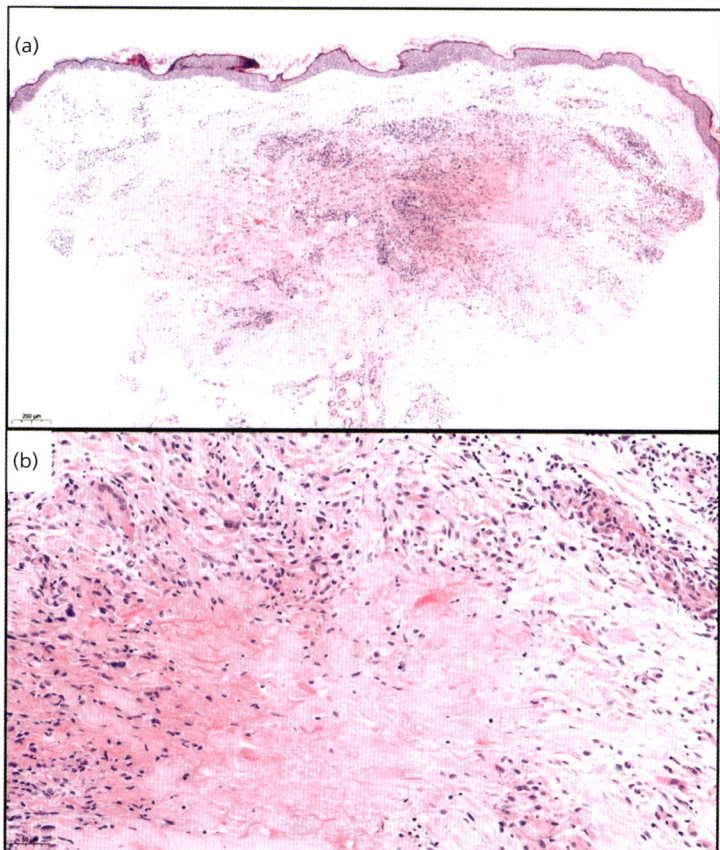

Figure 95.3 (a) Classical histology of GA; the dermis shows foci of necrobiotic palisading granulomas with perivascular lymphocytic inflammation. (b) Necrobiotic palisading granuloma characterised by degenerate collagen with increased mucin and surrounding radial arrangement of histiocytes and lymphocytes with occasional multinucleated giant cells.

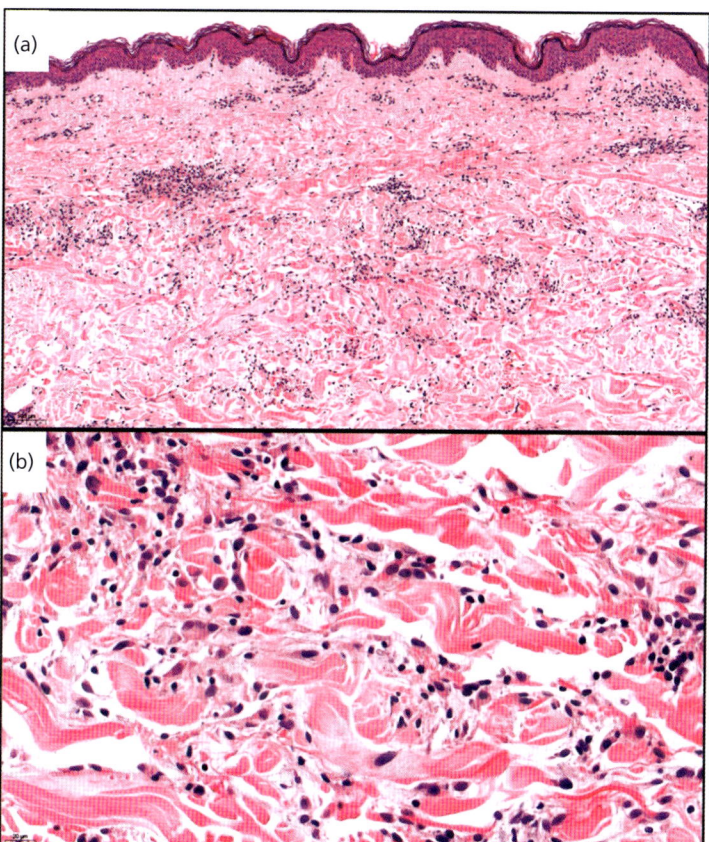

Figure 95.4 (a) Interstitial GA with impression of 'busy' dermis at low power. (b) Higher power shows swollen collagen bundles with interspersed histiocytes and lymphocytes and hint of increased mucin leading to separate of collagen bundles.

They are characterised by a central zone of degenerate (necrobiotic) collagen surrounded by histiocytes and lymphocytes, commonly in a radial or palisaded arrangement, with variable numbers of multinucleated giant cells. Histiocytes express the marker PG-M1 [123]. A useful clue to GA is often an additional perivascular lymphocytic component which comprises mainly T-helper phenotype (CD4+) [124–126], but in two cases associated with HIV infection a predominant CD8+ infiltrate was demonstrated [127,128]. A small number of skin-specific clones have been demonstrated together with many non-specific T cells [126], possibly attracted by a high local production of IL-2. In many instances the necrobiotic foci have a basophilic appearance due to the presence of mucin, also highlighted by Alcian blue or colloidal iron stains. Small deposits of lipid material may also be present. Collagen alteration, most commonly fragmentation of collagen bundles, was observed in 79% of cases of localised and 53% of cases of generalised GA [6]. There is also a marked reduction in or absence of elastic fibres [129,130]. Metalloproteinases are probably involved in the damage to collagen and elastic fibres [131,132].

The interstitial or diffuse pattern (Figure 95.4) is often the most challenging to diagnose histologically, in which well-formed areas of necrobiosis are lacking. There is a 'busy' dermis with histiocytes and lymphocytes around blood vessels and dispersed between swollen collagen bundles, and collagen fibres are separated by mucin. In some instances, additional levels may be required to reveal more typical features.

The sarcoidal pattern (Figure 95.5) is uncommon and may cause problems in differential diagnosis from true sarcoidosis which can also show overlapping clinical features. As the name implies, in this variant, histology shows well-formed epithelioid granulomas with inconspicuous necrobiosis. The presence of mucin and eosinophils can help to distinguish GA from sarcoidosis.

Subcutaneous (deep) GA is clinically and histologically similar to a rheumatoid nodule with large zones of necrobiosis. Alcian blue stained mucin is the most useful distinguishing feature, contrasting with a more eosinophilic degeneration of collagen with increased fibrin in a true rheumatoid nodule, although there are cases which are histologically indistinguishable [133].

In perforating GA (Figure 95.6), superficial zones of necrobiotic collagen are extruded through the epidermis or follicular infundibula, associated with varying degrees of reactive epidermal hyperplasia [120,134,135].

Vasculitic features have been described [136] but not found by others [137]. The different patterns of lipid deposition demonstrated by adipophilin staining have been reported to be helpful in distinguishing GA from necrobiosis lipoidica and sarcoidosis [138]. In GA there is both extracellular and intracellular adipophilin staining, whereas this is limited to extracellular areas in the zones

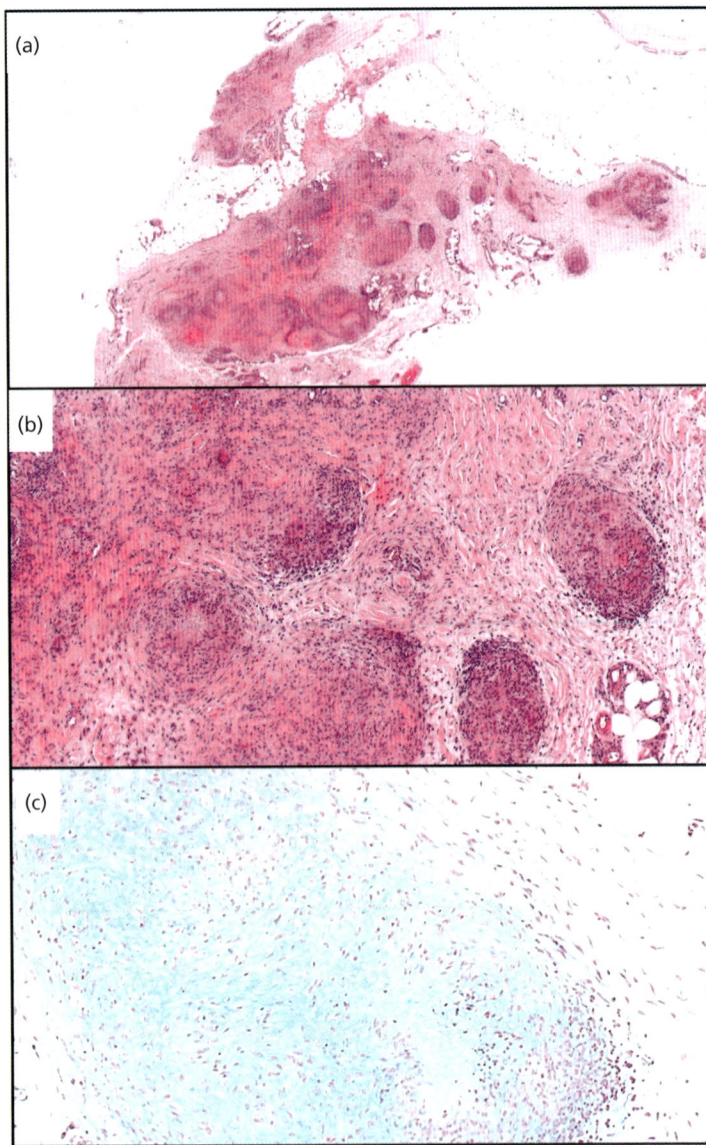

Figure 95.5 (a) An example of GA with sarcoidal pattern. This case shows overlap with subcutaneous (deep) GA. (b) Higher power shows well-formed epithelioid granulomas. There are subtle foci of central necrobiosis within some of the granulomas as a clue to distinguishing as GA rather than sarcoidosis. (c) Alcian blue demonstrates increased mucin within the subtle necrobiotic foci.

of damaged collagen in necrobiosis lipoidica and in sarcoidosis the staining tends to be intracellular. Epithelioid sarcoma, with its associated geographic necrosis, may show a passing resemblance to GA. However, it is usually distinguishable due to nuclear atypia and cellular pleomorphism, but it should be noted that the histiocytes in GA can sometimes show mitotic activity [123,139–141]. Other histological differential diagnoses include the interstitial variant of mycosis fungoides [142–145], interstitial granulomatous dermatitis (interstitial granulomatous dermatitis with arthritis; interstitial granulomatous dermatitis with plaques; palisaded neutrophilic granulomatous dermatitis) [146–152] and interstitial granulomatous drug reaction [153–156].

Causative organisms
There are no confirmed pathogenic organisms.

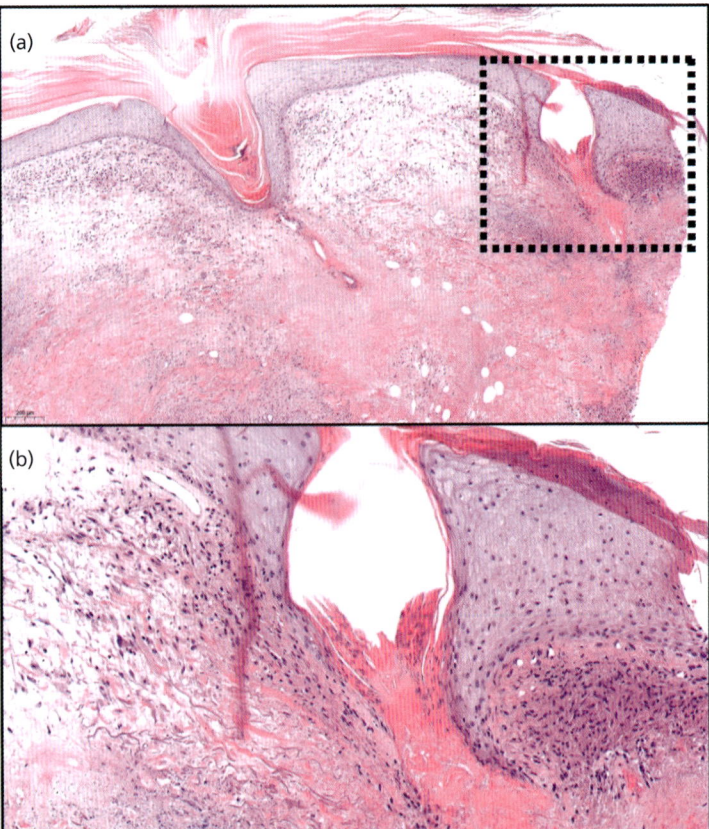

Figure 95.6 (a) Perforating GA; low power showing prominent dermal necrobiosis. (b) High power showing extrusion of necrobiotic collagen to the skin surface through a follicular infundibulum.

Genetics
There is an increased prevalence of HLA-Bw35 among individuals with generalised GA compared with controls or those with localised GA [157]. There are a few reports of familial cases [157–162].

Clinical features
History
Patients with subcutaneous GA may complain of tenderness and generalised GA may be itchy, but most patients are asymptomatic. Acute, painful, acral lesions have been described [163]. Commonly, the annular lesions will have been treated with antifungal agents before the correct diagnosis is reached.

Presentation and clinical variants
There are four commonly recognised clinical variants, which typically appear independently, although some patients may exhibit more than one variant [164,165].

Localised GA. This accounts for about three-quarters of cases and typically presents as a ring of small, smooth, flesh-coloured or reddish papules (Figure 95.7a). Stretching the skin enables the papules to be seen more readily (Figure 95.7b). The surface of the skin over the papules is intact and there is usually no scaling. Annular lesions tend to enlarge centrifugally before eventually clearing. They may be solitary or multiple, and may occur anywhere on the skin, although the dorsa of the hands (Figure 95.8a), knuckles

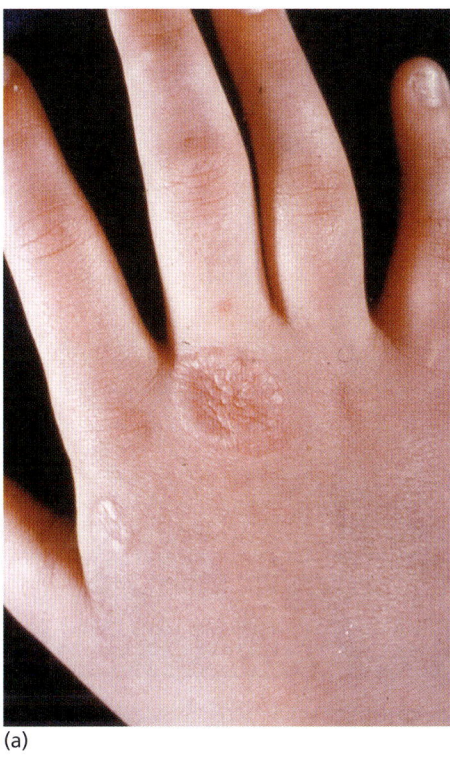

(a)

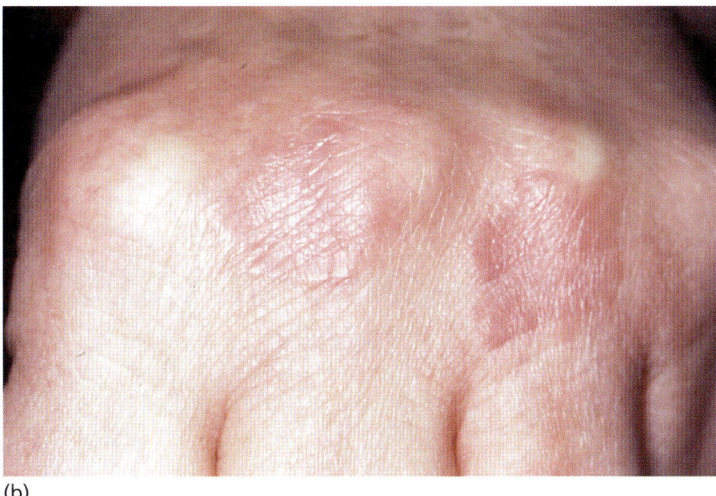

(b)

Figure 95.7 (a) Typical appearance of localised granuloma annulare over the knuckles. (b) Appearance of granuloma annulare over the knuckles on clenching the fist.

(Figures 95.1 and 95.7), fingers (Figure 95.8b) and feet (Figure 95.8c) are the commonest sites. Some, typically acral, lesions enlarge as nodules rather than as annular plaques.

Generalised or disseminated GA. Generalised or disseminated GA makes up 10–15% of cases [7,8], is seen predominantly in adults and is twice as common in females. Pruritus may be the presenting feature. Interestingly, it is the commonest form seen in HIV patients [166–168]. The lesions are often ill-defined with skin-coloured or reddish macules, papules and/or plaques in an annular pattern surrounding a faintly violaceous central area on the trunk and limbs (Figure 95.9) [7,168–171]. The sparing of vaccination sites in a case of generalised GA is an interesting phenomenon [172].

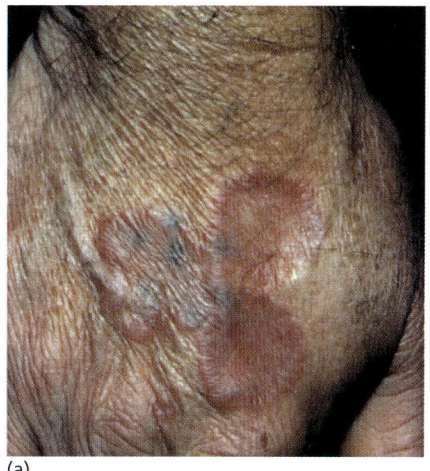

(a)

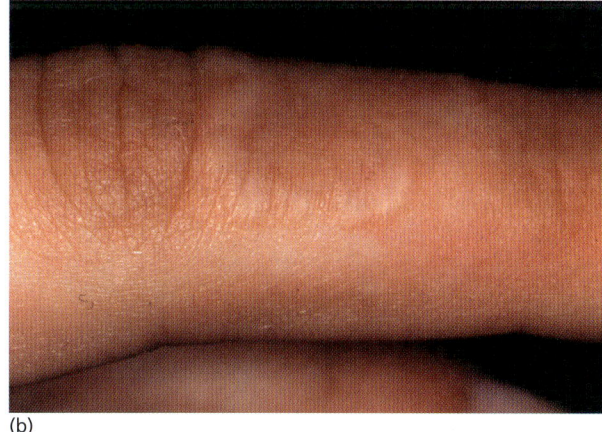

(b)

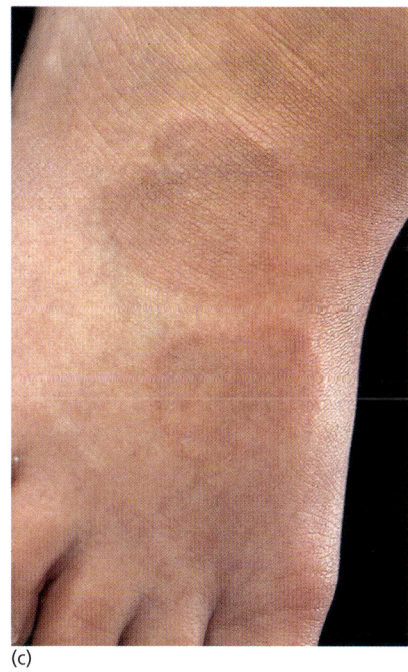

(c)

Figure 95.8 Common sites of localised granuloma annulare. (a) On the dorsum of the hand; note the atrophy in the centre of the lesions. (b) On the dorsum of a finger. (c) On the dorsum of a child's foot; this is often mistaken for tinea, but there is no scale and tinea in this site would be unlikely in a child.

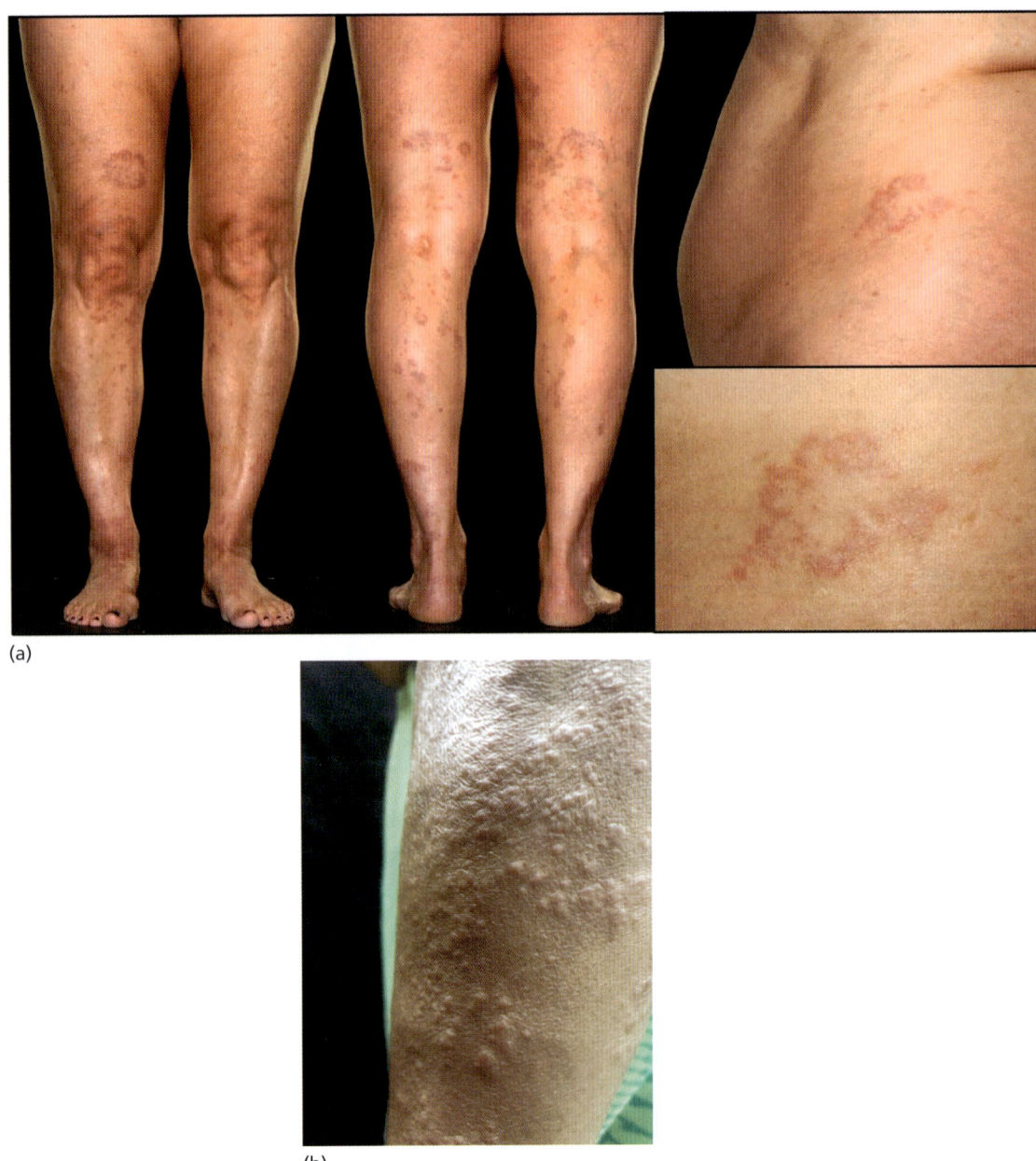

Figure 95.9 (a) Generalised granuloma annulare on the lower limbs and flank. (b) Generalised granuloma annulare on the arm and leg of a female patient with diabetes. Courtesy of Dr Shyam Verma.

Perforating GA. This is uncommon [173] but has been described in all ages including infancy [174] and in HIV [59]. Localised or generalised papules develop yellowish centres and discharge a little clear, viscous fluid that dries to form a crust, eventually separating to leave a hypo- or hyperpigmented scar (Figures 95.6 and 95.10) [135,175].

Subcutaneous GA. This is also uncommon. It occurs predominantly in children (Figure 95.11) and has been given a variety of names, including benign rheumatoid nodules [176], pseudorheumatoid nodules [177,178], deep GA [179,180], subcutaneous palisading granuloma [181], isolated subcutaneous granuloma and subcutaneous necrobiotic granuloma [182]. Lesions are nodular and occur predominantly on the scalp and legs, particularly in the pretibial region [159,183,184], but unusual locations include the periorbital area, palm [185,186] and penis [187]. Rarely, there may be subperiosteal lesions [188]. A congenital case has been recorded [189]. Magnetic resonance imaging features are diagnostically helpful [186–188].

Other reported variants of GA include a papular umbilicated form on the dorsa of the hands in children [190], a case of 'follicular pustulous' GA, in which palisading necrobiotic granulomas occurred in a perifollicular distribution [190], pustular generalised perforating GA, in which a dense infiltrate of neutrophils was present in areas of necrobiosis [191], linear GA [192,193], and 'patch' GA, in which erythematous patches occurred on the trunk and limbs [194]. Although some examples of linear GA may be truly Blaschkoid and underpinned by genetic mosaicism [195], other linear cases may overlap with interstitial granulomatous

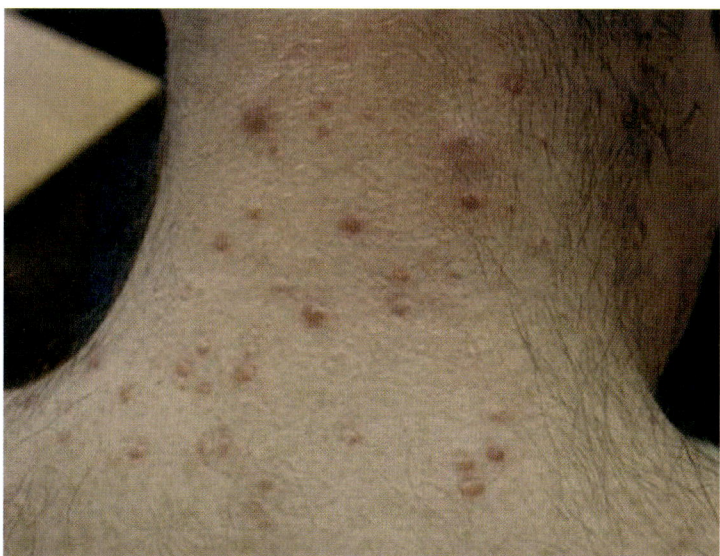

Figure 95.10 Perforating granuloma annulare on the neck.

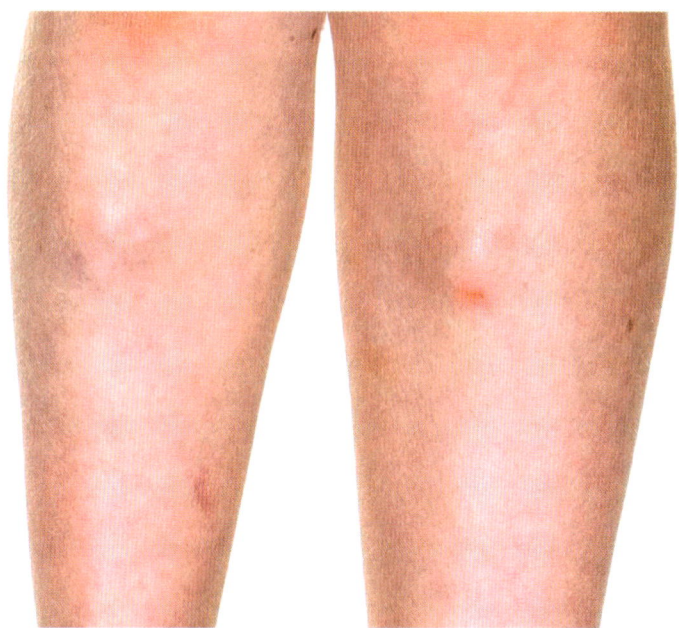

Figure 95.11 Subcutaneous granuloma annulare with palpable nodules in a classical location on this child's shins.

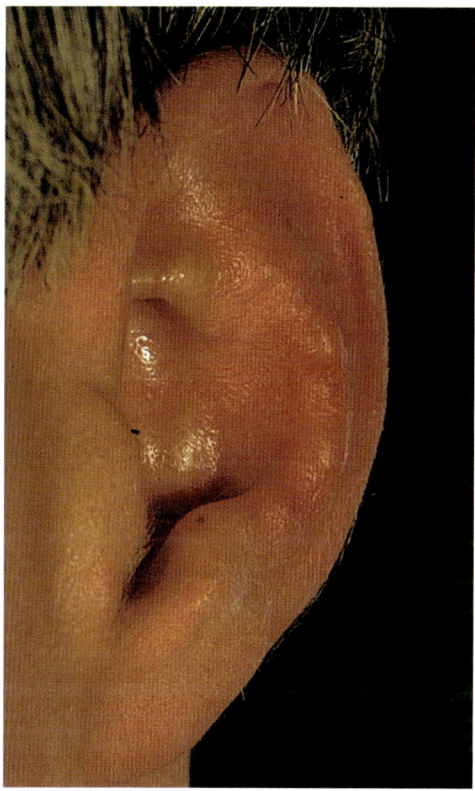

Figure 95.12 Granuloma annulare on the ear. Note the nodules overlying the auricular cartilage of the antihelix.

dermatitis, and those with 'patch' lesions may represent examples of interstitial granulomatous drug reaction [196].

Uncommon sites for lesions of GA are the ears (Figure 95.12), where the perforating variety may be encountered [197], penis [198–200], palms [201] and periocular regions [202–207]. Mucous membranes are generally spared, although there is a single report of involvement of the oral mucosa in a patient with HIV infection [67]. A destructive form has been described causing damage to soft tissues, tendons, bones and joints [208,209].

Differential diagnosis
Localised GA may be mistaken for tinea or erythema multiforme. Other annular lesions and granulomatous conditions may cause diagnostic confusion, including annular lichen planus, erythema annulare centrifugum, erythema migrans of Lyme disease, sarcoidosis, tuberculides [210] and tertiary syphilis [211]. The morphology and distribution of lesions may simulate mycosis fungoides [212].

The differential diagnosis of subcutaneous GA is extensive, including trauma, infection, tumours, sarcoidosis and rheumatoid nodules. A diagnostic biopsy will usually be necessary.

The differential diagnosis of perforating GA includes molluscum contagiosum [213], other perforating disorders (Chapter 94), sarcoidosis and papulonecrotic tuberculide [135,214]. Epithelioid sarcoma may also masquerade as perforating GA [123,139–141].

Mycobacterium marinum infection has histologically simulated interstitial GA [215]. Other histological differential diagnoses include granulomatous mycosis fungoides [216], interstitial granulomatous dermatitis and interstitial granulomatous drug reaction.

Complications and co-morbidities
There are reports of anetoderma secondary to generalised GA [217], and mid-dermal elastolysis occurring with GA [218,219] and subsequent to lesions resembling GA [220]. In another case, loss of elastic fibres was presumed to be responsible for the development of open comedones on the rim of GA lesions occurring on light-exposed areas [221].

Disease course and prognosis
A postal questionnaire survey carried out by Wells and Smith [1] revealed that in about 50% of patients the lesions resolved within 2 years. However, about 40% of those whose lesions cleared had a recurrence, in most cases at the same sites as the original lesions.

In this study, there did not appear to be any difference in prognosis between individuals with single lesions and those with multiple lesions, and although there is an impression that spontaneous resolution is less likely to occur with generalised GA there does not appear to be any documented confirmation of this.

Levin *et al.* [222] have discussed the resolution of lesions following biopsy and have noted the paucity of information relating to this phenomenon in the literature. There appears to be anecdotal evidence of its occurrence, but little documentation. However, it is of interest, in this context, that scarification is one form of physical treatment that has been advocated in the past [223–225].

Investigations

Biopsy may be necessary in nodular, subcutaneous, perforating, generalised and atypical forms. Investigation for diabetes, thyroid disease, malignancy and/or hyperlipidaemia is probably necessary if clinical history and examination are suggestive.

Management

In most cases, particularly in children, reassurance of eventual resolution is all that is needed. As with other conditions that spontaneously resolve, assessment of the efficacy of reported treatments is difficult. There is no high-quality evidence of the efficacy of any intervention for any form of GA and most recommendations rely on anecdotal case reports or small uncontrolled case series.

In persistent localised GA, a trial of topical steroid or tacrolimus/pimecrolimus is reasonable although often ineffective [226,227] even under occlusion. Cryotherapy and intralesional steroid injection [228] may be appropriate for symptomatic localised lesions although the risk of permanent scarring or atrophy is significant. Nitrous oxide has been reported in one study to give a better cosmetic result [229].

For generalised disease, PUVA appears to give the best results [230–238], with one retrospective study of 33 patients showing 50% clearance and a further 31% good to moderate improvement [239]. UVA1 has also been reported to be effective in two case series [240,241]. Of the systemic therapies, dapsone [242–244], retinoids [245–250], antimalarials [251–253], fumaric acid esters [254–256] and methotrexate [257,258] have been most extensively reported. None of these has been shown to be reliably beneficial. The potential toxicity of these agents [259] must be weighed against the benign nature of the disease.

Other agents that have been claimed to be effective in localised GA include imiquimod [260,261], isotretinoin [262], local injections of low-dose recombinant interferon-γ [263], photodynamic therapy [264], and pulsed dye [265], neodymium:yttrium-aluminium-garnet (Nd:YAG) [266], carbon dioxide [267] and excimer [268] lasers.

For generalised disease, potassium iodide has been shown to be ineffective [269]. There are anecdotal reports claiming efficacy for topical tacrolimus [270] and pimecrolimus [271], ciclosporin [272–275], low-dose chlorambucil [6,276–278], nicotinamide (niacinamide) [279], pentoxifylline [280], tranilast [281], clofazimine [282], topical vitamin E [283], a combination of vitamin E and a 5-lipoxygenase inhibitor [284], defibrotide [285] and oral calcitriol [286]. Infliximab [287,288], adalimumab [289–292], etanercept [293] and efalizumab [294] have also been reported to be effective; however, in a small series of patients reported by Kreuter *et al.* [295]

there was either no change or deterioration during therapy with etanercept. Treatment with secukinumab is associated with worsening of GA [296]. Janus kinase inhibitors including tofacitinib as well as IL-4/13 antagonism with dupilumab have been reported to be successful in GA [296,297]. However larger placebo-controlled trials are needed.

Most of the treatments mentioned here have been employed in patients with perforating lesions, with varying degrees of success [298,299]. Lesions of subcutaneous GA generally resolve spontaneously once the diagnosis has been confirmed [300].

Treatment ladder

First line
- No treatment/expectant
- Cryotherapy
- Intralesional corticosteroid
- Potent topical corticosteroid

Second line
- Topical tacrolimus
- Pimecrolimus
- Imiquimod
- Narrow-band UVB phototherapy
- PUVA[a]
- Dapsone
- Hydroxychloroquine/chloroquine
- Ciclosporin
- Fumaric acid esters
- Methotrexate

Third line
- Photodynamic therapy
- Pulsed dye laser
- 308 excimer laser

[a]Principally for generalised disease.

Resources

Patient resources

British Association of Dermatologists, patient information leaflet: https://www.bad.org.uk/shared/get-file.ashx?id=85&itemtype=document.

DermNet NZ, granuloma annulare: https://dermnetnz.org/topics/granuloma-annulare.

(Both last accessed November 2022.)

Necrobiosis lipoidica

Definition and nomenclature

Necrobiosis lipoidica is a distinctive skin disorder characterised clinically by well-demarcated waxy red-brown plaques with an atrophic centre, most commonly located on the shins, and histologically by full-thickness dermal lymphohistiocytic perivascular infiltration with extensive areas of necrobiosis.

Synonyms and inclusions
- Necrobiosis lipoidica diabeticorum

Introduction and general description

Necrobiosis lipoidica is a distinctive skin condition characterised by well-defined red-brown indurated plaques with an atrophic yellow centre [1] (Figure 95.13). It is most commonly seen on the legs and may ulcerate, causing considerable pain. Histologically, there is a full-thickness dermal lymphohistiocytic infiltrate with extensive necrobiosis of collagen. It is associated with diabetes (both type 1 and type 2) and glucose intolerance.

Epidemiology

Incidence and prevalence

Necrobiosis lipoidica is relatively uncommon. In patients with diabetes, reported prevalences range from 0.3% [2] to 1.2% [3]; it appears to be rare (0.06%) in childhood diabetes [4]. Its prevalence among non-diabetics is not well established.

Age

Necrobiosis lipoidica may occur at any age [1,3]. It is uncommon in childhood and is most commonly seen in young adults and in early middle age. When associated with type 1 diabetes, it is seen at a younger age (third decade) than in type 2 or those without diabetes (fourth decade).

Sex

The female to male ratio is 3 : 1 [1].

Associated diseases

There is no doubt that necrobiosis lipoidica is associated with diabetes, although only about 1% of diabetics develop it [1,2,3,4,5]. In a much-quoted study from a large, specialist, tertiary referral centre, two-thirds of 171 patients with necrobiosis lipoidica had known diabetes at presentation [1,2]. This is unlikely, however, to be a true reflection of the overall incidence of diabetes in patients with necrobiosis lipoidica. In another study, however, 55 of 65 patients with necrobiosis lipoidica (85%) had no evidence of diabetes or impaired glucose tolerance at presentation. Only 3 of 42 patients re-evaluated between 5 and 15 years after initial presentation were found to have abnormal glucose handling [6].

There is some evidence that diabetic patients who have necrobiosis lipoidica are at higher risk of retinopathy and nephropathy than diabetics who do not [7,8,9]. Necrobiosis lipoidica has also been described in association with a number of other conditions including ulcerative colitis [10], Crohn's disease [11] and after jejunal bypass surgery [12]. Reports of its occurrence with GA have been mentioned previously (see the section on Granuloma annulare). It has also been reported in association with sarcoidosis [13,14].

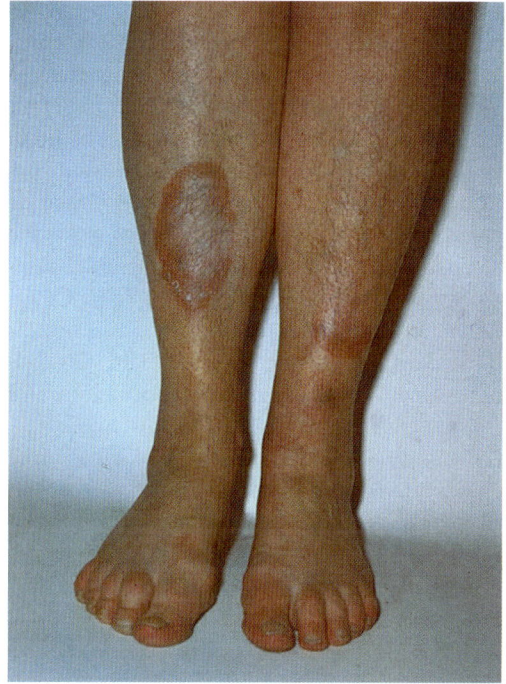

(a)

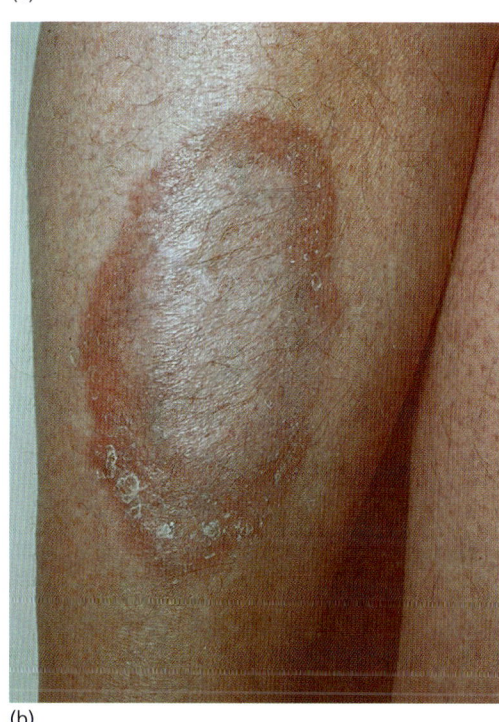

(b)

Figure 95.13 (a) Necrobiosis lipoidica of the shins in a 50-year-old woman. (b) Close-up view of the shin.

Pathophysiology

The precise pathogenesis of necrobiosis lipoidica remains unknown [15]. Some authors have considered microangiopathy to be important: this might explain the association with diabetes. An altered plasma protein profile [16], elevated factor VIII-related antigen [17] and fibronectin [18] have been proposed as contributory factors. However, in Muller and Winkelmann's histopathological study, vascular involvement was very mild in about a third of the cases [19]. Furthermore, studies investigating blood flow in plaques of necrobiosis have yielded conflicting results. Boateng *et al.* [20] reported reduced blood flow compared with healthy controls and Brungger [21] demonstrated reduced transcutaneous oxygen. However, Ngo *et al.* reported increased blood flow [22].

The possible role of an antibody-mediated vasculitis as an initiating event in necrobiosis lipoidica has also provoked debate as the results of immunofluorescence studies differ. Laukkanen *et al.* [23] did not demonstrate immunoreactants in lesional skin, but others have shown immunoreactants, principally IgM, C3 and fibrin, in vessel walls in the involved skin, and IgM, C3 and fibrinogen at the dermal–epidermal junction [24,25]. Dahl [26] has discussed immunofluorescence findings in necrobiosis lipoidica. Glut-1 is expressed by the fibroblasts in necrobiosis lipoidica, raising the possibility of abnormal glucose transport playing a role [27]. Gli-1, the glioma-associated oncogene homologue, is expressed in various granulomatous diseases including necrobiosis lipoidica. The precise role in aetiology remains unclear, but this raises the possibility of inhibitors of gli-1 as a therapeutic target (see the section on Granuloma annulare).

Predisposing factors
The link with diabetes is discussed in 'Associated diseases'.

Pathology [28–30]
The histological appearances are somewhat similar to those of GA, but with distinguishing features. Hyperkeratosis can be present. The epidermis may be otherwise normal or atrophic, or absent if there is ulceration. There are changes involving the full thickness of the dermis and these often extend into the subcutaneous fat, especially the septae (Figure 95.14). Early lesions show a perivascular and interstitial mixed inflammatory cell infiltrate. Areas

of necrobiosis are more common in necrobiosis lipoidica associated with diabetes and are usually more extensive and less well-defined than in GA [31]. There is degeneration of collagen and elastin within the lesions [32]. Histiocytes border the areas of necrobiosis. In the sarcoidal variant more commonly seen in non-diabetics, epithelioid granulomata predominate with conspicuous Langhans and foreign body-type giant cells. Necrobiosis is usually minimal in such cases and it may require multiple levels to identify. The perivascular inflammatory infiltrate often includes plasma cells, in contrast with GA. In one case report, the plasma cell infiltrate was monoclonal with an underlying monoclonal gammopathy identified [33]. Lymphoid nodules containing germinal centres may be present in the deep dermis or subcutaneous fat [34]. Rarely asteroid bodies may be seen. Lipid can be demonstrated in the necrobiotic areas with adipophilin immunohistochemistry, or oil red O or Sudan-IV on frozen section (see the section on Granuloma annulare for differences), and rarely cholesterol clefts may be present [35]. Mucin may be present in the dermis, but it is not as prominent as in GA.

Small superficial blood vessels are increased in number and are telangiectatic. Deeper dermal blood vessels often show intimal thickening (which can be highlighted by periodic acid–Schiff stain) and narrowing of the lumen (Figure 95.15). Comedo-like plugs and even perforating necrobiosis lipoidica may result from elimination of necrobiotic material through hair follicles [36,37]. Anaesthesia in the lesions appears to be related to destruction and reduced density of nerves highlighted by S100 [38]. In old atrophic lesions the dermis and subcutaneous fat may be replaced by extensive fibrosis. Lipomembranous fat necrosis may be evident.

Genetics
Familial cases are rare [39,40].

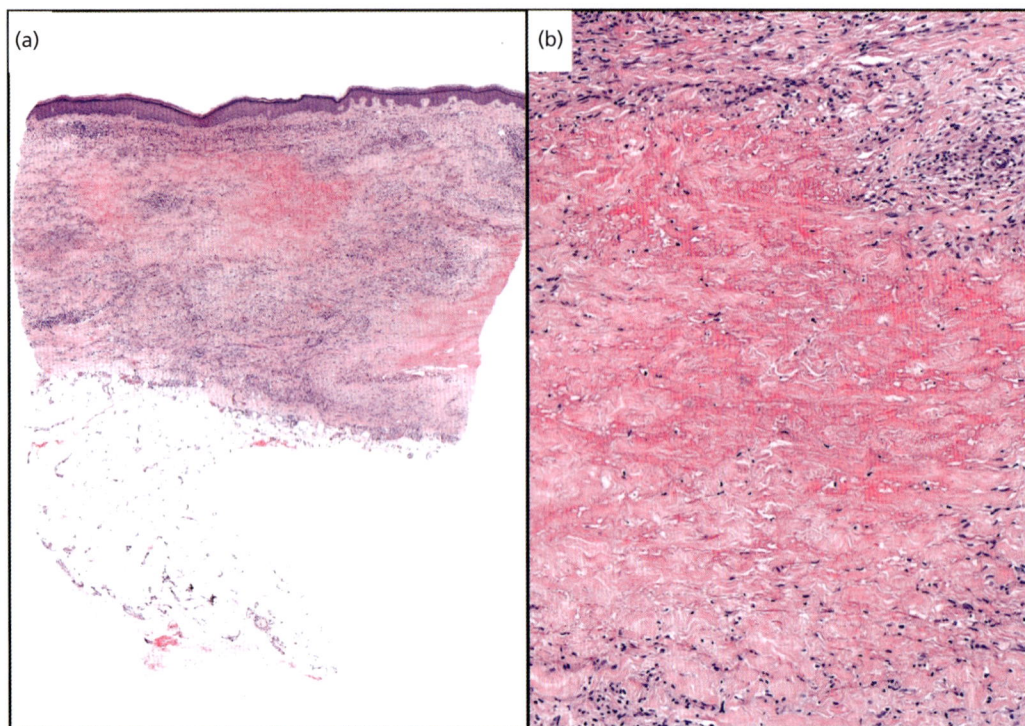

Figure 95.14 (a) Necrobiosis lipoidica showing extensive necrobiotic inflammation involving the full thickness of the dermis with focal extension into underlying subcutis. (b) Higher power showing a geographic zone of necrobiotic collagen with surrounding inflammatory cells.

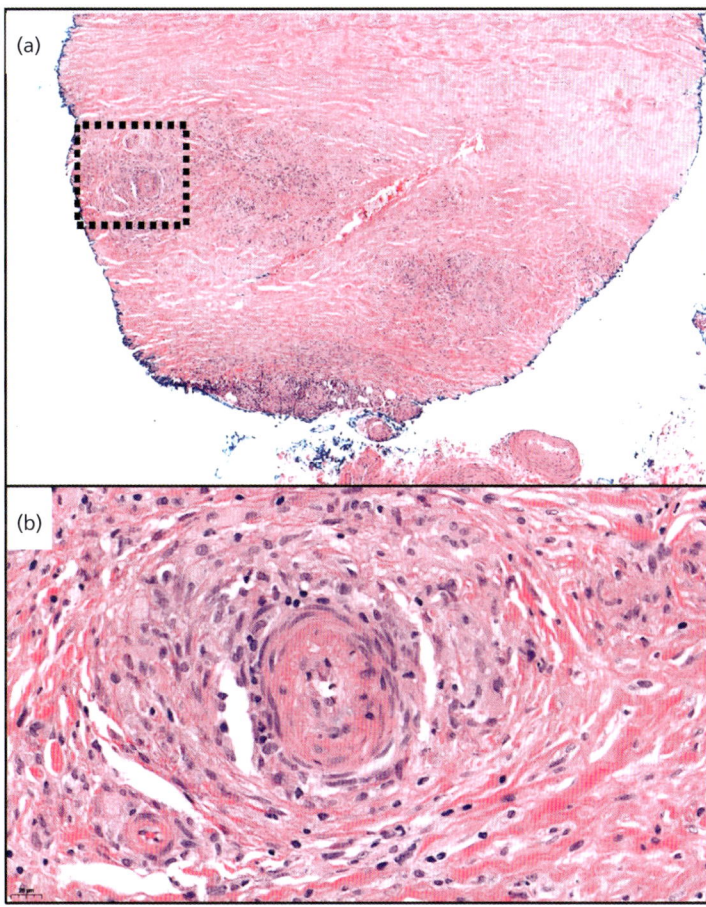

Figure 95.15 (a) Another case of necrobiosis lipoidica showing layers of fibrosis with intervening necrobiotic granulomatous inflammation. (b) Higher power shows a vessel with intimal thickening and narrowing of the lumen.

Clinical features
History
The lesions are normally asymptomatic unless ulcerated, which is generally a late feature of the condition.

Presentation [41–43]
Necrobiosis lipoidica may occur at any age, but usually develops in young adults and in early middle age. In insulin-dependent diabetics the age of onset is earlier than in non-insulin-dependent and non-diabetic individuals [44]. It is rare in childhood [45,46].

Typical lesions occur on the pretibial skin, and begin as a firm, dull red papule or plaque that enlarges radially to become a yellowish atrophic plaque with a red edge (Figures 95.13 and 95.16). The surface is often glazed in appearance and telangiectatic vessels may be prominent (Figure 95.17). Hypohidrosis and hypoaesthesia or anaesthesia may develop [42,47,48]. Comedo-like plugs may occur at the periphery of lesions [49]. In most cases lesions are bilateral, and they are similar in appearance whether occurring in diabetic or non-diabetic individuals [41]. They tend to be persistent and may ulcerate [50]: in one study [44], ulceration correlated with sensory impairment. Squamous cell carcinoma may develop in longstanding lesions [51–58].

Lesions can occur on other parts of the body, including the trunk [59] and penis [60,61], and rarely may be diffuse [62]. Koebnerisation

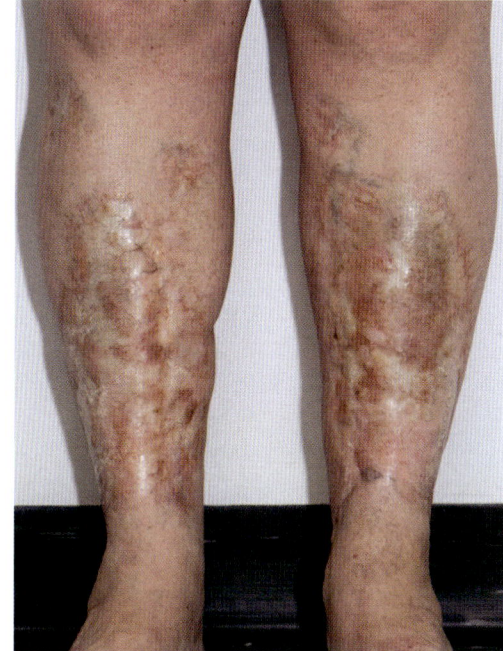

Figure 95.16 Chronic necrobiosis lipoidica (over a 20-year period) in a 41-year-old patient with insulin-dependent diabetes. Note the marked atrophy and telangiectasia.

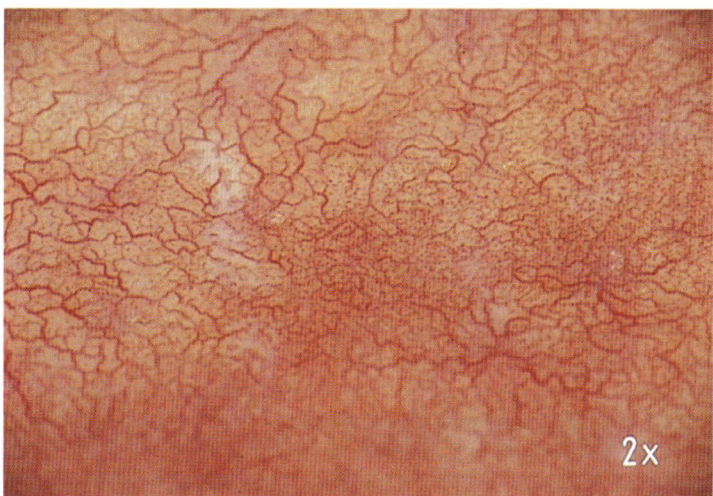

Figure 95.17 Prominent telangiectasia in an area of necrobiosis.

at sites of trauma may also occur (Figure 95.18) [63–66]. The number of lesions and their rate of progress are very variable.

Differential diagnosis
The histological differential diagnosis from GA is discussed earlier. However, there is a case report of necrobiotic reaction to a tattoo showing mixed features of GA and necrobiosis lipoidica [67]. A distinctive condition typically affecting the skin of the head and neck of middle-aged women previously described as 'atypical necrobiosis of the face and scalp margins' (Figure 95.19) [68] or Miescher granuloma [69] has now been accepted by most as being more closely related to O'Brien actinic granuloma [70]. In both conditions there is granulomatous inflammation affecting sun-exposed skin with prominent elastophagocytosis and complete loss of elastic

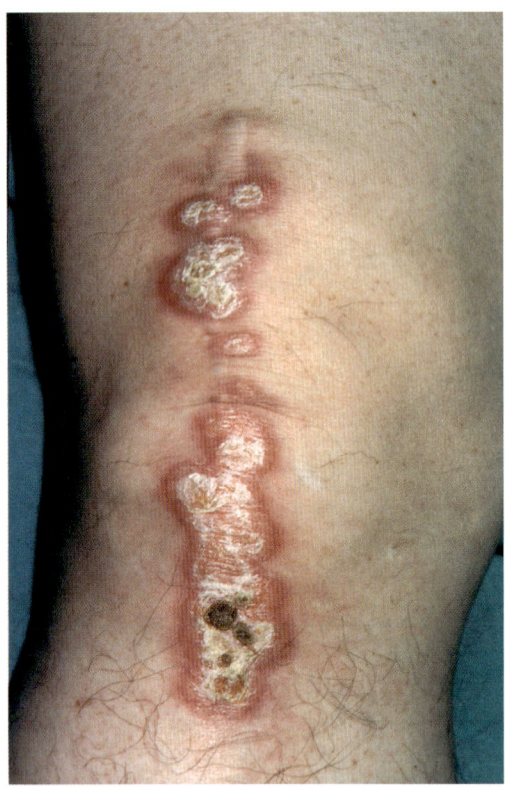

Figure 95.18 Necrobiosis lipoidica Koebnerising in a scar from previous knee surgery.

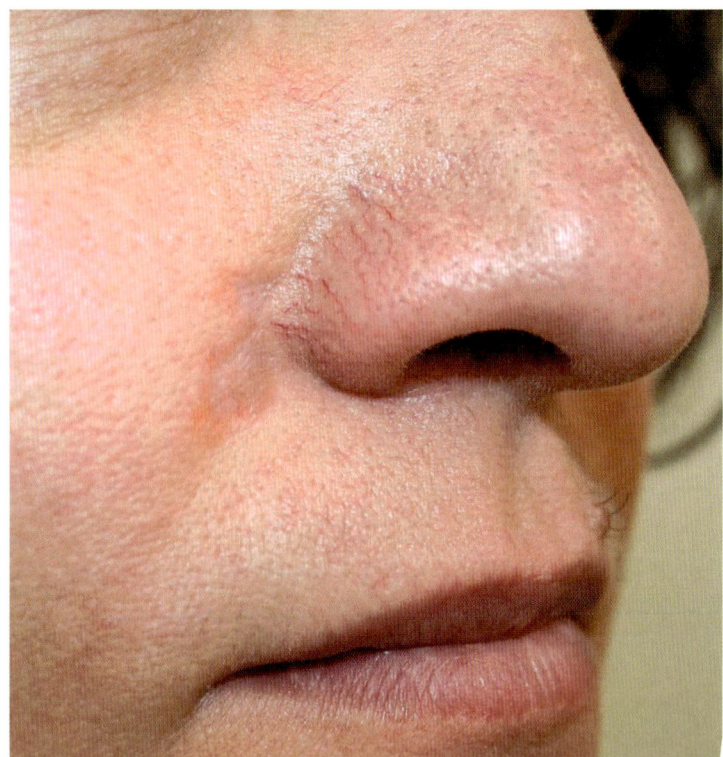

Figure 95.19 Atypical facial necrobiosis involving the nasolabial fold in a middle-aged female.

tissue. A unifying term of 'annular elastolytic giant cell granuloma' was proposed in 1979 by Hanke *et al.* [71] and has been widely adopted [72] (Chapter 94). There is also a case series in which patients presented with pretibial lesions suggestive of necrobiosis lipoidica, whereas histology showed features of venous insufficiency only. The name 'pretibial angioplasia' has been proposed for this entity [73].

Lesions with marked fatty infiltration, particularly when not on the legs, may be mistaken for xanthomas. Necrobiotic xanthogranuloma is a rare, destructive, non-Langerhans cell histiocytosis, in which red-orange or yellowish indurated plaques most frequently involve the periorbital regions and trunk [74,75]. It is associated with systemic lesions and a monoclonal gammopathy (Chapter 135). The presence of numerous cholesterol clefts, bizarre multinucleated giant cells and Touton-type giant cells are points of distinction histologically.

Complications and co-morbidities
Ulceration is the principal complication, affecting up to 35% of patients (Figure 95.20) [1]. Squamous cell carcinoma has also been reported but is rare [51–58].

Disease course and prognosis
Slow extension over many years is usual, but long periods of quiescence or resolution with variable atrophy and scarring may occur (Figure 95.21).

Investigations
Skin biopsy is not usually necessary except in atypical cases. Annual screening for diabetes is recommended.

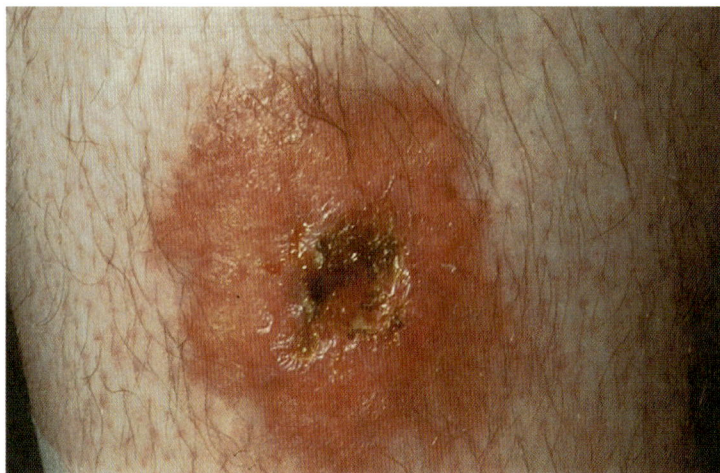

Figure 95.20 Ulcerated necrobiosis lipoidica in a 34-year-old woman with diabetes.

Management
The response of necrobiosis lipoidica to therapeutic intervention is generally disappointing. Many treatments have been reported to be effective but there are virtually no double-blind placebo-controlled clinical trials and no convincing evidence that any intervention significantly alters the course of the disease.

Potent topical corticosteroids, particularly if applied beneath an occlusive dressing and changed weekly, may help [76]. Locally injected triamcinolone delivered by needle or jet injector [77] can improve the appearance, but atrophy usually remains. As there is evidence of extension of the inflammatory infiltrate into apparently normal skin surrounding active lesions, the injection of steroids into

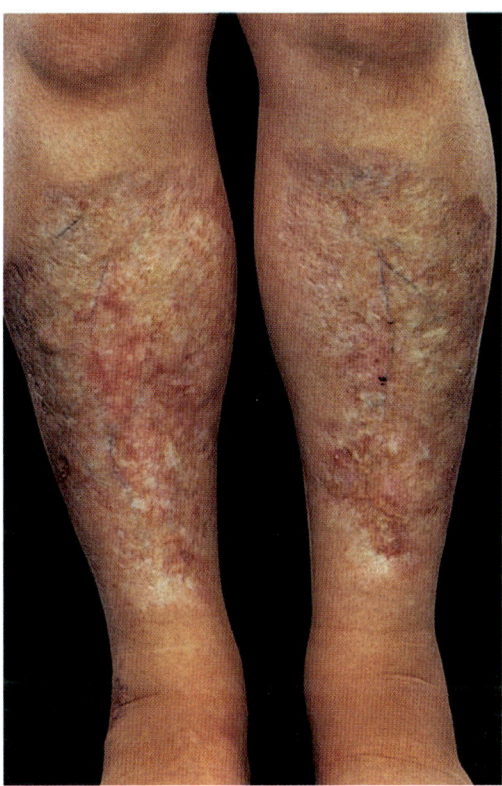

Figure 95.21 'Burnt out' necrobiosis lipoidica – marked atrophy is evident.

perilesional areas has been advocated to help limit progression [78]. The use of oral steroids may be of benefit [79,80]. Petzelbauer *et al.* [80] employed short-course steroid therapy that resulted in cessation of disease activity in all six patients treated and no recurrence in a mean follow-up period of 7 months.

There are reports of benefit from PUVA [81–87], topical tacrolimus [88], fumaric acid esters [89], thalidomide [90], chloroquine [91], photodynamic therapy [92], a combination of split-thickness autografting and immunomodulatory therapy [93]. The response to UVA1 phototherapy has been mixed [94].

Other treatments that have been advocated in the past include fibrinolytic agents [95], high-dose nicotinamide [96], clofazimine [97], pentoxifylline [98–101], tretinoin (0.05%) [102], prostaglandin E1 [103,104] and aspirin or an aspirin/dipyridamole combination [105–107]. Aspirin alone was subsequently shown to be ineffective [108,109] and, in a randomised double-blind comparison with placebo, patients treated with an aspirin/dipyridamole combination did not show any significant improvement [110].

Pulsed dye laser has been employed and may improve the telangiectatic and erythematous components [111] but skin breakdown can occur [112].

Ulcerated necrobiosis lipoidica has been treated by excision and grafting [113–115], although recurrence tends to occur unless the excision is deep [115]. Other treatments that have been advocated for this problem include oral steroids [116], ciclosporin [117–119], mycophenolate mofetil [120], topical granulocyte–macrophage colony-stimulating factor [121,122], etanercept [123], infliximab [124], intravenous immunoglobulin [125], hyperbaric oxygen [126,127], topically applied bovine collagen [128] and grafting with bioengineered dermal tissue [6,129,130]. Recent case reports of

ustekinumab [131] and Janus kinase inhibitors [132] have been described.

Treatment ladder

First line
- No treatment
- Topical steroids
- Intralesional steroids
- Topical tacrolimus

Second line
- PUVA
- UVA1

Third line
- Multiple therapies of uncertain value

Resources

Patient resources

British Association of Dermatologists, patient information leaflet: https://www.bad.org.uk/shared/get-file.ashx?id=109&itemtype=document.

Changing Faces: The Squire Centre, 33–37 University Street, London WC1E 6JN; www.changingfaces.org.uk.

DermNet NZ, necrobiosis lipoidica: https://dermnetnz.org/topics/necrobiosis-lipoidica.

(All last accessed November 2022.)

Cutaneous Crohn disease

Definition and nomenclature
This is a granulomatous inflammation of the skin in patients with underlying Crohn disease.

Synonyms and inclusions
- Granulomatous cheilitis
- Oro-facial granulomatosis
- Metastatic Crohn disease

Introduction and general description
Cutaneous disease is common in patients with Crohn disease but manifests most commonly as an associated reactive inflammatory disorder such as aphthous ulcers, erythema nodosum and pyoderma gangrenosum (Chapter 49) or from the effects on the skin of nutritional deficiency (Chapter 61).

Granulomatous involvement of the skin may occur by direct extension of Crohn disease particularly in the lips, perineum, umbilicus and at the sites of surgery or around a stoma. It is characterised by sinuses, abscesses, fissures, ulcers and indurated plaques

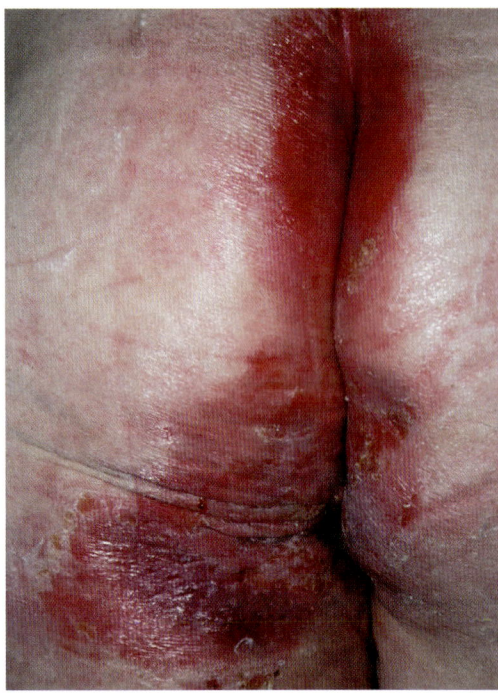

Figure 95.22 Severe perianal Crohn disease.

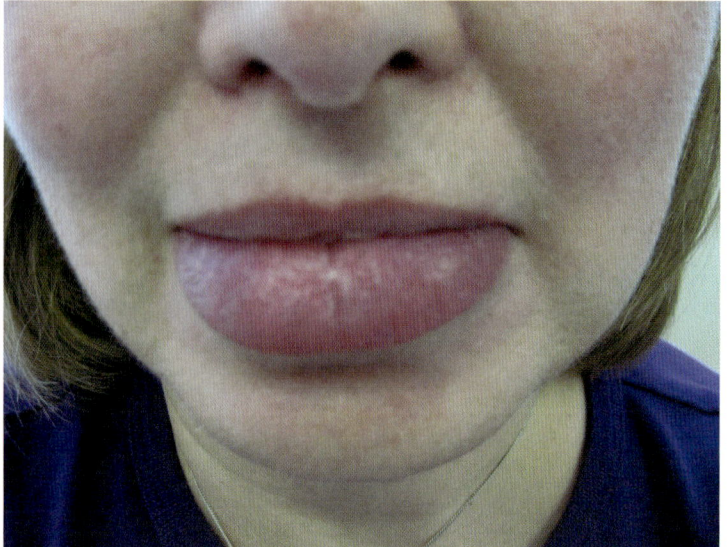

Figure 95.23 Lip swelling due to oro-facial granulomatosis developed in this patient some 5 years before she presented with severe intestinal Crohn disease. Courtesy of Dr E. P. Burova.

(Figure 95.22) (Chapter 153). It is usually seen in the presence of active underlying Crohn disease but may predate its diagnosis, particularly in children [1].

Oro-facial granulomatosis (Figure 95.23) may be associated with sarcoidosis or food allergy or be part of the Melkersson–Rosenthal syndrome (Chapter 108). When isolated, it is regarded by many as a localised form of Crohn disease. It may predate intestinal Crohn disease by many years.

Pathology [2–5]

Histologically, cutaneous Crohn disease typically shows ill-defined granulomatous inflammation in the superficial dermis (Figure 95.24), which may extend into deeper dermis or subcutis with additional perivascular mixed inflammation comprising lymphocytes and plasma cells, although eosinophils can sometimes be prominent [2,3]. It should be noted, however, that in a case series of vulval Crohn disease granulomas were present in only 5 of 13 (38%) patients, and the authors point out that granulomas should not be an absolute criterion for a diagnosis of metastatic Crohn disease [4].

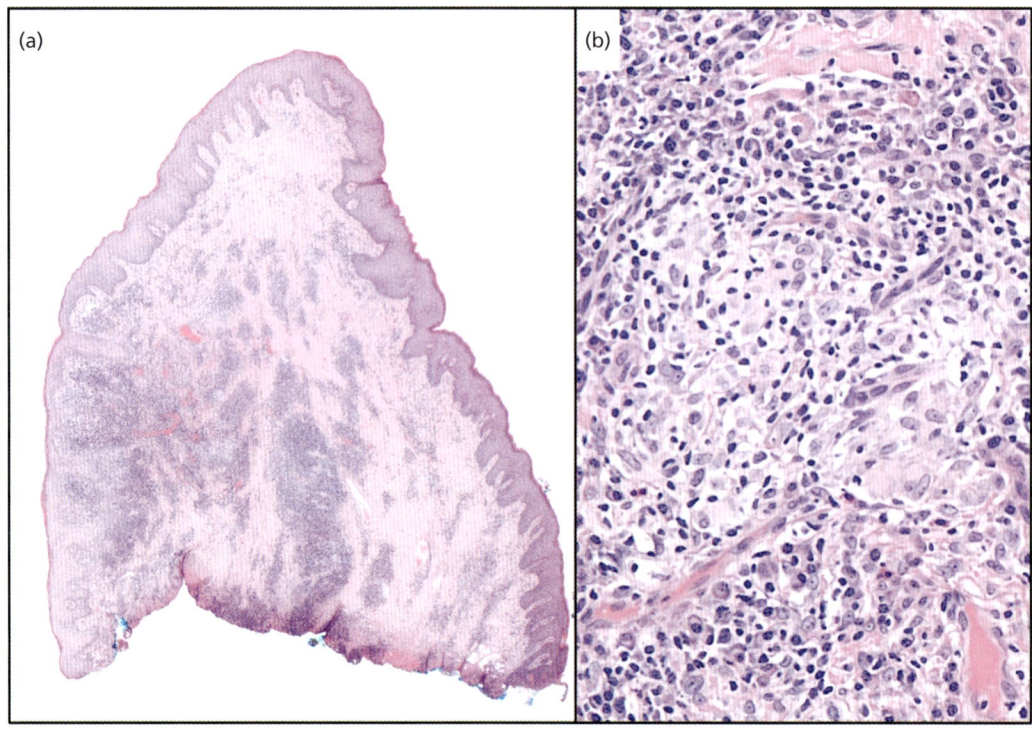

Figure 95.24 A patient with Crohn disease and perianal skin tags. (a) Low power shows a highly inflamed polypoid lesion. (b) Higher power demonstrates the granulomatous nature of the infiltrate.

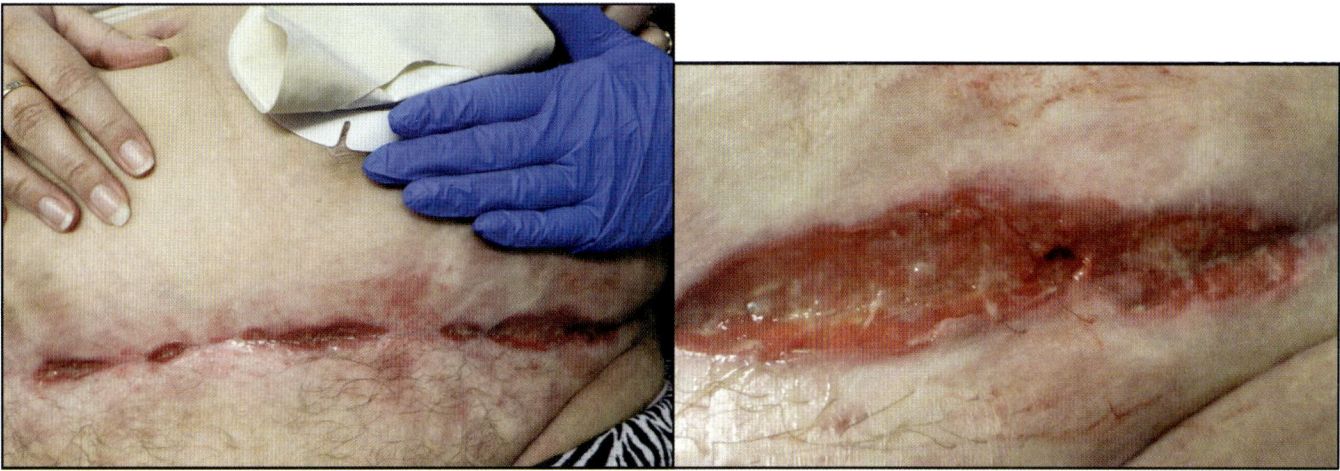

Figure 95.25 'Knife-cut' fissures seen in metastatic Crohn disease affecting the abdominal fold.

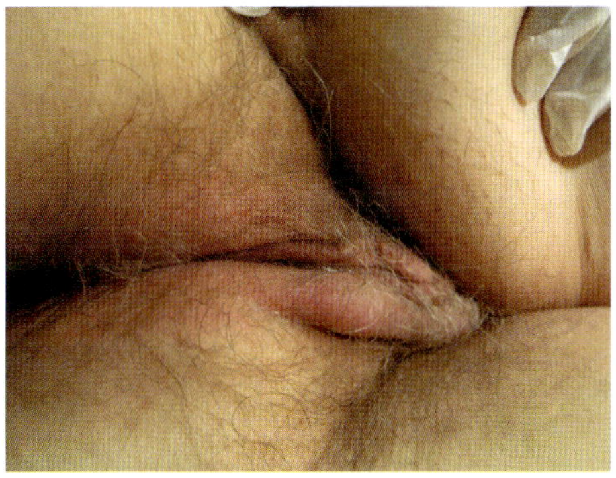

(a)

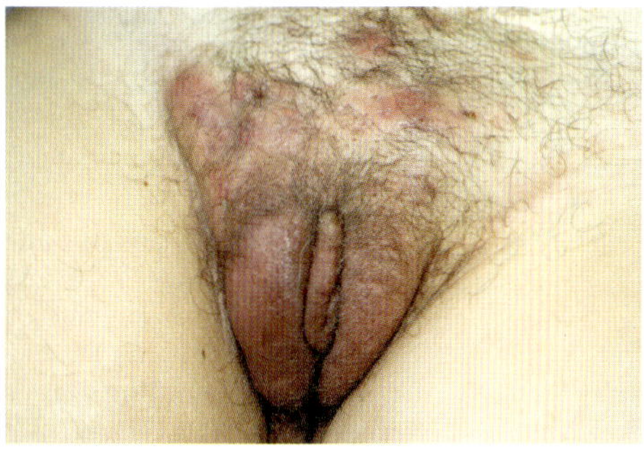

(b)

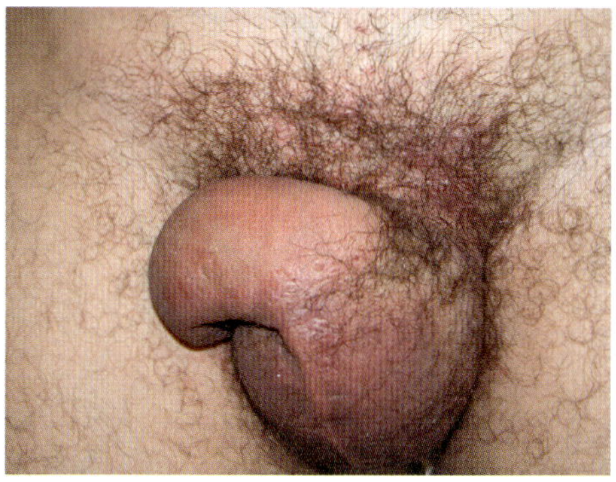

(c)

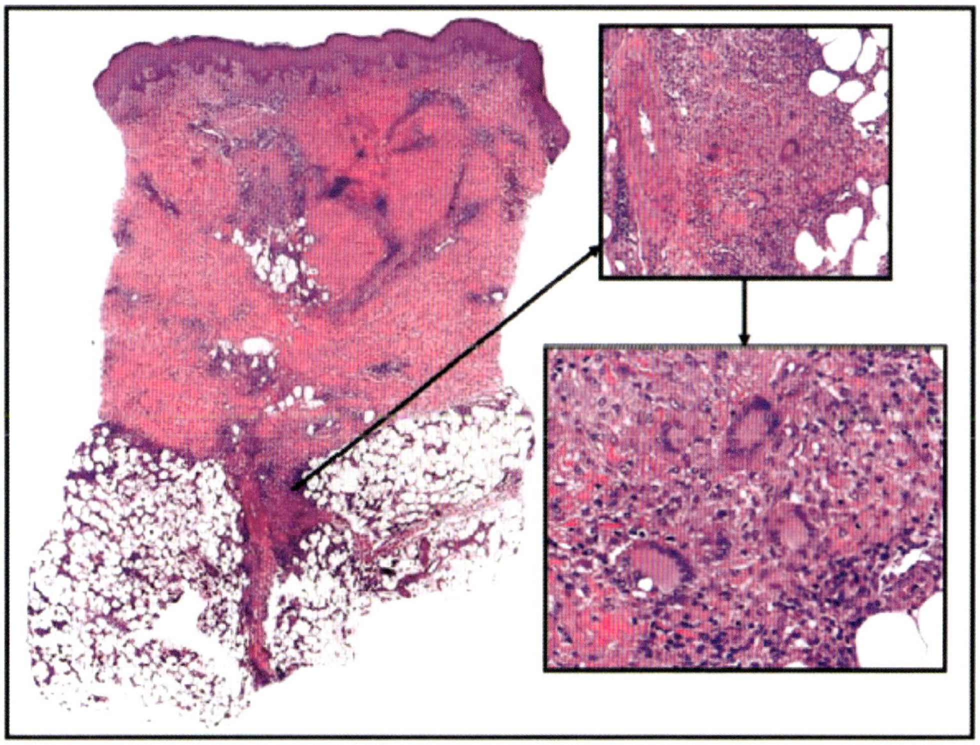

(d)

Figure 95.26 (a) Vulval swelling due to Crohn disease presented in the same patient as shown in Figure 95.23 about 1 year after she developed intestinal Crohn disease. (b) More advanced Crohn disease affecting the mons pubis and vulva; this developed 2 years after presentation with intestinal Crohn disease. (c) Peno-scrotal lymphoedema that presented together with perianal fistulae 5 years after the onset of intestinal Crohn disease. (d) Histology showing superficial and deep perivascular dermal infiltrates and a predominantly septal panniculitis. Higher power demonstrates the granulomatous nature of the infiltrate involving the subcutaneous septae. Granulomas are composed of epithelioid histiocytes and multinucleated giant cells arranged in a perivascular fashion. (a) Courtesy of Dr E. P. Burova. (c) and (d) Courtesy of Professor L. Requena.

In patients with orofacial granulomatosis and granulomatous cheilitis it has been noted that granulomas may bulge into and obstruct vessels [5] or even be truly intralymphatic [6]. Necrobiotic collagen has been described in a number of cases. Some cases may show leukocytoclasis with vasculitis falling within the spectrum of palisaded neutrophilic and granulomatous dermatitis [7].

Clinical features

The skin may also be involved at distant sites, sometimes referred to as metastatic Crohn disease. The presentation is variable, with ulcers, nodules, plaques, papules, pustules or abscesses. It has been reported at many body sites including the face, ears, nipples, palms, soles, lower limbs and abdomen [8]. Involvement of the perineum and genitalia without direct extension is sometimes considered in this category. 'Knife-cut fissures' are typical for metastatic Crohn disease (Figure 95.25). Such presentation can overlap with severe hidradenitis suppurativa. Metastatic Crohn disease may present with oedema and swelling of the perineum and/or genitalia (Figure 95.26). Several deep biopsies may be needed to confirm the diagnosis in such cases through the identification of granulomas, which may be only focally present (Figure 95.26d).

Management

Treatment of cutaneous Crohn disease is usually dictated by the severity of the intestinal involvement. For localised disease, topical tacrolimus has been reported to be of benefit [9] although systemic treatment along similar lines to that used in intestinal disease is likely to be necessary for satisfactory resolution. There is no consistent relationship between the appearance of skin lesions and the severity of the intestinal disease, and treatment of the intestinal disease does not necessarily affect the cutaneous features of Crohn disease [10,11] (Chapters 110 and 111).

Key references

The full list of references can be found in the online version at https://www.wiley.com/rooksdermatology10e

Granuloma annulare

1 Wells RS, Smith MA. The natural history of granuloma annulare. *Br J Dermatol* 1963;75:199–205.
2 Thornsberry LA, English JC, 3rd. Etiology, diagnosis, and therapeutic management of granuloma annulare: an update. *Am J Clin Dermatol* 2013;14:279–90.
6 Dabski K, Winkelmann RK. Generalized granuloma annulare: histopathology and immunopathology. Systematic review of 100 cases and comparison with localized granuloma annulare. *J Am Acad Dermatol* 1989;20:28–39.
7 Dabski K, Winkelmann RK. Generalized granuloma annulare: clinical and laboratory findings in 100 patients. *J Am Acad Dermatol* 1989;20:39–47.
8 Muhlbauer JE. Granuloma annulare. *J Am Acad Dermatol* 1980;3:217–30.
13 Cox NH. Diabetes and the skin: an update for dermatologists. *Expert Rev Dermatol* 2007;2:305–16.
27 Hawryluk EB, Izikson L, English JC, 3rd. Non-infectious granulomatous diseases of the skin and their associated systemic diseases: an evidence-based update to important clinical questions. *Am J Clin Dermatol* 2010;11:171–81.
112 Dahl MV. Speculations on the pathogenesis of granuloma annulare. *Australas J Dermatol* 1985;26:49–57.
239 Browne F, Turner D, Goulden V. Psoralen and ultraviolet A in the treatment of granuloma annulare. *Photodermatol Photoimmunol Photomed* 2011;27:81–4.

Necrobiosis lipoidica

2 Muller SA, Winkelmann RK. Necrobiosis lipoidica diabeticorum. A clinical and pathological investigation of 171 cases. *Arch Dermatol* 1966;93:272–81.
5 Reid SD, Ladzinski B, Lee K, Baibergenova A, Alavi A. Update on necrobiosis lipoidica: a review of etiology, diagnosis, and treatment options. *J Am Acad Dermatol* 2013;69:783–91.
6 O'Toole EA, Kennedy U, Nolan JJ et al. Necrobiosis lipoidica: only a minority of patients have diabetes mellitus. *Br J Dermatol* 1999;140:283–6.
7 Boulton AJM, Cutfield RG, Abouganem D et al. Necrobiosis lipoidica diabeticorum: a clinicopathologic study. *J Am Acad Dermatol* 1988;18:530–7.

Cutaneous Crohn disease

1 Keiler S, Tyson P, Tamburro J. Metastatic cutaneous Crohn's disease in children: case report and review of the literature. *Pediatr Dermatol* 2009;26:604–9.

CHAPTER 96

Sarcoidosis

Joaquim Marcoval[1] and Juan Mañá[2]

[1]Department of Dermatology, Bellvitge University Hospital and Barcelona University, Barcelona, Spain
[2]Department of Internal Medicine, Corachan and Sagrada Familia Clinics, Barcelona, Spain

Sarcoidosis

Definition, nomenclature and classification

Sarcoidosis is an antigen-mediated disease of unknown aetiology characterised by the presence of non-caseating epithelioid cell granulomas in multiple organs. It involves mainly the lungs, mediastinal and peripheral lymph nodes, eyes and skin. Less frequent but usually severe manifestations can occur in the liver, spleen, central nervous system, heart, upper respiratory tract and bones. Cutaneous lesions of sarcoidosis may be specific, showing histopathologically sarcoid granulomas, or non-specific, mainly erythema nodosum (EN). Cutaneous lesions are frequently the presentation of the disease and skin biopsy enables early diagnosis. Moreover, some types of lesions have prognostic significance and may help to predict the outcome of the systemic disease.

Classification links
- ICD-10: D86.3
- Snomed CT: 31541009
- Orphanet: ORPHA797
- Other: UMLS C0036202 MeSH D012507 MedDRA 10039486

Introduction and general description of sarcoidosis

Sarcoidosis is a multisystemic granulomatous disease of unknown ethiology that mainly involves the lungs, mediastinal and peripheral lymph nodes, eyes and skin. Specific cutaneous lesions are frequently the presentation of the disease. Skin biopsy is easy to perform, enabling early diagnosis with a minor invasive procedure. Some types of lesions have prognostic significance and may help to predict the outcome of the systemic disease. Although cutaneous lesions of sarcoidosis almost never cause significant morbidity or mortality, it may be grossly disfiguring and have a strong psychosocial impact.

Epidemiology

Incidence and prevalence

The incidence of sarcoidosis varies widely throughout the world [1,2]. Sarcoidosis seems to be most prevalent in developed countries, ranging from 10 to 40 per 100 000 in the USA and Europe [3,4]. The annual incidence is not known with certainty. Löfgren syndrome (the association of EN with bilateral hilar lymphadenopathy on chest radiograph) is more frequent in the northern European countries and Spain, and predominates during the spring months [2,5–7].

Age

Sarcoidosis occurs at all ages but it is more frequent in young and middle-aged adults with a peak age at diagnosis in men at 30–50 years and 50–60 years in women. It is less common in older people and is rare in children [8].

Sex

Sarcoidosis is slightly more common in women than in men [8]. In the subpopulation of Löfgren syndrome there is a clear predominance in white women [3,6,9].

Ethnicity

In the USA, a population-based study showed that the incidence of sarcoidosis was 3–17 times higher in African American people than in white people. Some studies have detected a high prevalence in Scandinavian people, in Puerto Rican people in New York and in Irish immigrants in England [1,3]. There is also a significant heterogeneity in disease presentation and course. In the USA, African American and Asian Indian people have more severe disease at diagnosis than their white counterparts [10,11], while asymptomatic cases and Löfgren syndrome are more common in white people [12].

Associated diseases

An increased risk of developing lymphoproliferative disease [13], mainly Hodgkin disease, has been reported in sarcoidosis [14].

The relationship between sarcoidosis and solid tumours is less clear-cut [15,16], although it has been suggested that immunological abnormalities mediated by sarcoidosis or the effects of treatment may increase the risk [17,18]. Several case reports have described the concomitant association of sarcoidosis with multiple immune-mediated diseases [19–28].

Pathophysiology
Pathology
The histopathological changes are similar in all organs affected by sarcoidosis [29]. The cardinal feature is the sarcoid granuloma, defined as aggregates of epithelioid cells with a sparse lymphocytic component [29,30], the so-called 'naked granuloma' (Figure 96.1a,b)

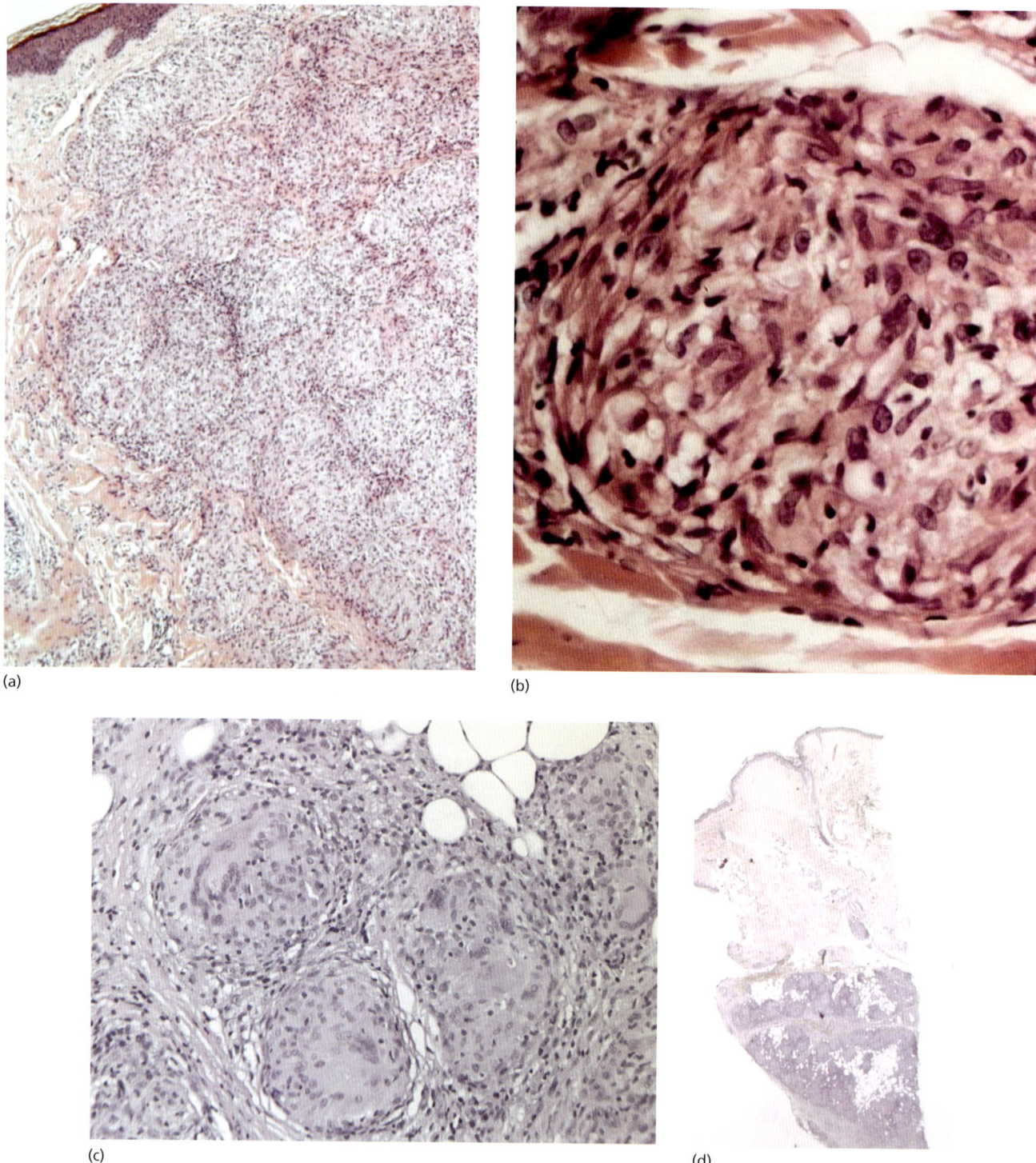

(a)

(b)

(c)

(d)

Figure 96.1 (a) Sarcoid granulomas in the dermis in a specific cutaneous lesion of sarcoidosis. (b) Sarcoid granulomas are mainly composed of epithelioid cells with sparse lymphocytic component, without necrosis. (c) Sarcoid granulomas with prominent giant cells. (d) Low-power view of subcutaneous sarcoidosis. The granulomatous infiltrate is limited to the subcutis and is mainly lobular with the appearance of a granulomatous lobular panniculitis.

[29,31,32]. In the skin, sarcoid granulomas are usually observed in the dermis but can also extend to subcutaneous tissue. There is no particular relation to skin appendages, although in some cases linear granulomas may follow dermal nerves [33]. Granulomas usually contain few or no giant cells, generally of Langhans type, that tend to be more abundant in old lesions (Figure 96.1c) [31]. In some cases, tuberculoid granulomas are also observed [33,34]. Although caseous necrosis is typically absent [29,35], discrete foci of fibrinoid or coagulation necrosis can be detected [33,36,37]. Palisading necrobiotic granulomas are rarely observed [33,38]. Although it is considered that the epidermis is usually normal, 49 of 62 cases in a series displayed epidermal abnormalities [39]. Lichenoid changes [33] and transepidermal elimination of granulomas have also been reported [33,38,40,41]. In subcutaneous sarcoidosis, the granulomatous infiltrate is limited to subcutaneous tissue, although minimal lower dermal involvement may be observed [42–44] (Figure 96.1d). It is predominantly lobular, appearing as a lobular panniculitis, but can also involve the septa [42,44]. Fibrosis is a frequent finding in subcutaneous sarcoidosis (75% of cases in a recent series), and although this may be intense, it is not associated with pulmonary fibrosis [42].

Giant cells can contain inclusion bodies. Schaumann bodies are basophilic, round or oval concentric, lamellar structures composed of lipomucoglycoproteins impregnated with calcium and iron [31,45]. Asteroid bodies are considered to be formed from trapped collagen bundles and have an eosinophilic central body surrounded by radiating spicules (Figure 96.2a) [46]. None of these bodies is specific to sarcoidosis; they have been observed in other granulomatous processes [29,30,47]. Polarisable foreign bodies (Figure 96.2) are observed in 22–58% of cutaneous sarcoidosis [33,37,48,49,50], suggesting that foreign bodies may be an inciting stimulus for granuloma formation in sarcoidosis [48,51,52].

CD4 helper/inducer T lymphocytes are present at the centre of the granuloma and a smaller population of CD8 suppressor/cytotoxic T lymphocytes at the periphery [53]. Immunofluorescence studies have shown, in some cases, immunoglobulin M (IgM) within blood vessel walls and at the dermal–epidermal junction, and IgG within and around the granuloma [54].

Histological differential diagnosis. Lupus vulgaris usually shows a marked lymphocytic infiltrate around granulomas and significant central necrosis [31]. Tuberculous leprosy granulomas follow nerves and therefore appear elongated and show small areas of central necrosis more often than sarcoidosis [31]. Although perineural granulomas are not uncommon in sarcoidosis [55–57], the nerves are intact and stains for acid-fast bacilli are negative [33]. Rosacea granulomas are usually perifollicular [31]. Lupoid leishmaniasis, Crohn disease and orofacial granulomatosis (Chapter 108) may also pose difficulties. Plasma cells and coagulative necrosis are features of syphilis [45]. Foreign-body granulomas can also resemble sarcoidosis. The presence of polarisable foreign bodies does not exclude sarcoidosis. Moreover, an exaggerated response to foreign bodies, coexistence with other types of skin lesions of sarcoidosis and the involvement of other organs favours sarcoidosis.

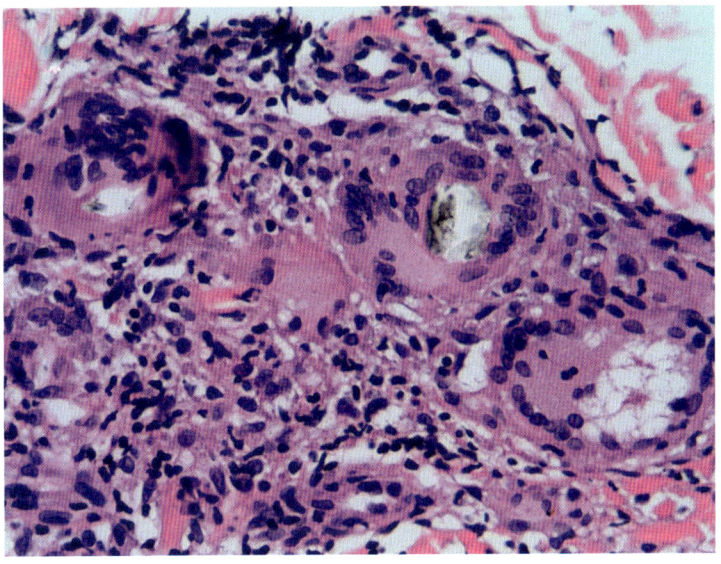

(a)

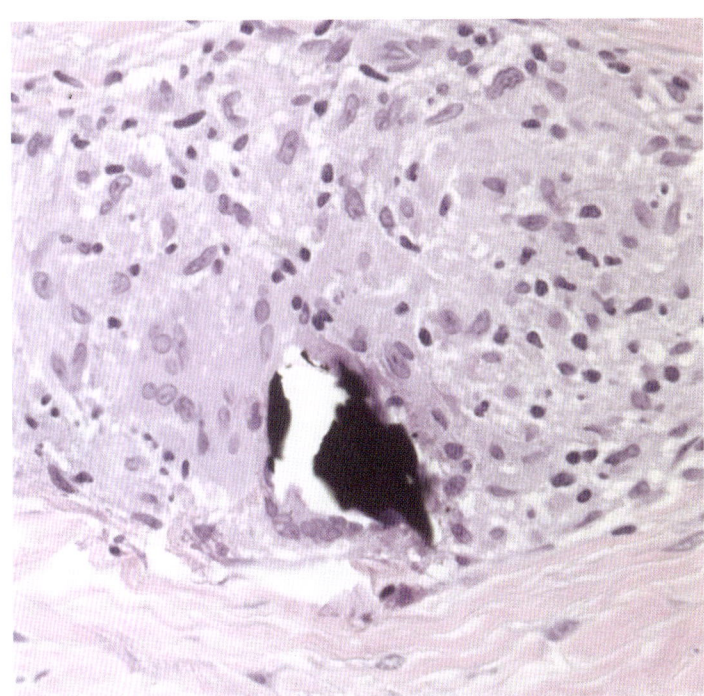

(b)

Figure 96.2 (a) An incipient asteroid body and two foreign bodies in a sarcoid granuloma. (b) A foreign body is observed in a sarcoid granuloma.

Immunopathogenesis

Most researchers agree that genetic factors, environmental antigens and a dysregulated immune system characterised by an exaggerated T helper 1 (TH1)] immune response are involved in causing sarcoidosis [2]. Multiple antigens, probably derived from infectious agents as well as organic and inorganic compounds that are not completely cleared by the immune system, may induce the antigen-presenting cells to produce high levels of tumour necrosis factor-alpha (TNF-α) and to present these antigens to CD4+ T-cells [58]. T helper cells differentiate into TH1 and TH17.1 effector cells that produce interferon-gamma (IFN-γ) and interleukin (IL)-17. Pro-inflammatory cytokines, such as TNF-α, IL-12, IL-18 and IL-6, and regulatory cytokines, such as transforming growth factor-beta (TGF-β) and IL-10, are also upregulated in affected tissues [2]. IFN-γ activates macrophages and induces transformation into giant cells while TNF-α induces its differentiation into epithelioid cells [59]. Macrophages also release IFN-γ, TNF-α and chemokines such as CXCL10, attracting additional T cells of CD4/TH1 phenotype [60,61]. It is postulated that IFN-γ inhibits apoptosis in macrophages through the expression of high levels of P21, which leads to granuloma perpetuation [62]. Incapacitation of Tregs is also a key feature of granuloma maintenance [58]. TNF-α is considered the main cytokine in the development and maintenance of the granuloma [63,64], and it is considered the cause of pulmonary fibrosis by stimulating fibroblast proliferation and collagen synthesis [65]. Anti-TNF-α agents are currently used in sarcoidosis as third line therapy, although cases of sarcoidosis paradoxically induced by TNF-α inhibitors are being reported [66].

It has been suggested that the accumulation of serum amyloid A in granulomas promotes amplification of TH1 immune responses [2]. Vimentin has been proposed as a potential autoantigen in sarcoidosis [2,58]. Recent studies have shown that the JAK–STAT pathway activation signatures are characteristic of the transcriptome of sarcoidosis and several cases of cutaneous sarcoidosis improving with JAK inhibitors have been reported [2,67].

Causative organisms

Histopathological similarities with tuberculosis led to extensive evaluation of *Mycobacterium tuberculosis* as a possible aetiological factor. Several studies have detected the presence of mycobacteria by different methods, while similar surveys have obtained negative results [68–75]. The presence of mycobacterial DNA/RNA has been reported in 0–80% of patients with sarcoidosis [76–98]. However, the absence of caseation necrosis, the negativity of the Mantoux test, and the lack of response to antituberculous treatment are arguments against mycobacterial involvement in sarcoidosis [95].

Propionibacterium acnes has been isolated from bronchial lavage in pulmonary sarcoidosis and DNA of propionibacteria has also been detected [89,93,99]. *Propionibacterium acnes* has been also observed by immunohistochemical methods in sarcoid granulomas [100,101]. However, it is known that *P. acnes* is a commensal in peripheral lung tissues and its presence does not appear to be specific for sarcoidosis [89,93,102]. Other infectious agents proposed by some studies but denied by others include *Rickettsia helvetica* [103,104], *Chlamydia pneumoniae* [105,106], *Borrelia burgdorferi* [107–110], leptospira species [58], mycoplasma species [58], *Pneumocystis jirovecii* [58], herpesvirus 8 [111–114] and Epstein–Barr virus [95]. Histoplasmosis and other fungi, which can produce sarcoid granulomas, have also been suspected as possible causes, but geographical limitations rule them out [45].

Genetics

A positive family history of sarcoidosis ranges from 2.7 to 17% [60] and having a first-degree relative with sarcoidosis increases 3.7–5- fold the risk [115,116]. The risk of developing sarcoidosis in the co-twin of an affected monozygotic brother was increased 80-fold while in dizygotic twins the risk was only sevenfold higher

[117]. However, sarcoidosis is not a disease of a single gene. The first reported association with specific gene products was the association between HLA-B8 antigens and acute sarcoidosis [118]. Later, HLA class II antigens were also related to sarcoidosis. The HLA-DR allele DRB1*1101 was significantly associated with sarcoidosis development in both African American and white people [119]. Other HLA genotypes predispose to the disease phenotype rather than to susceptibility. For example, HLA-DQB1*0201 and HLA-DRB1*0301 are strongly associated with acute disease and good prognosis [120–122]. HLA-DRB1*03 and C-C chemokine receptor 2 gene have been associated with Löfgren syndrome [123].

Genome-wide scanning for sarcoidosis susceptibility genes has identified several genes associated with increased susceptibility to the disease such as the butyrophilin-like 2 gene and annexin A11 [124–127]. In recent years, other genes have also been implicated [58,61].

Environmental factors

Several environmental agents (e.g. beryllium) may induce sarcoid granulomas [128]. For this reason and the tendency for sarcoidosis to involve organs exposed to the environment such as the lung, eyes and skin, an environmental cause for sarcoidosis has been suspected. Seasonal outbreaks of sarcoidosis also support this possibility [5,129–133]. Multiple environmental agents have been reported to confer increased risk of sarcoidosis, including exposure to tree pollen [134], inorganic particles [135], insecticides [136] and moulds [136,137]. Occupational studies have shown associations with US Navy personnel [138], metalworking [137], firefighters [139] and the handling of building supplies [140]. Also of interest is the fact that following the World Trade Center disaster, New York City firefighters developed 'sarcoid-like' granulomatous pulmonary disease at significantly higher than normal rates [141].

Sarcoidosis induced by drugs

Sarcoidosis has been reported in association with IFN-α for hepatitis C but also for melanoma [142–149]. It has been suggested that IFN-α increases IFN-γ and interleukin 2, promoting granuloma formation [144,146,150–152]. The development of cutaneous sarcoidosis as a paradoxical adverse effect of TNF-α and IL-17 blockers has also been reported [66,153–159].

More recently, multiple cases of sarcoidosis induced by inhibitors of CTLA-4, PD1-PDL-1 and BRAF/MEK, have been observed [160,161]. Downregulating peripheral tolerance using anti-CTLA-4 or anti-PD1-PDL-1 antibodies may propagate sarcoidosis inflammation [2]. The association with BRAF inhibitors could be explained by the increase of TNF-α and IFN-γ during BRAF inhibition treatment [160,161]. In a recent study, 22% of patients receiving nivolumab alone or in combination with ipilimimab developed a sarcoid-like reaction [162]. Although it is important to rule out the possibility of cancer metastasis [163,164], it is not mandatory to stop these drugs because sarcoidosis may remain stable even when therapy was maintained [160,162,164,165].

Sarcoidosis has been reported to be induced by dendritic cell vaccination immunotherapy in melanoma patients [166] and a sarcoid cutaneous reaction has been observed in patients treated with natalizumab [167] and with rituximab [168–170].

Clinical features

Systemic manifestations of sarcoidosis

Sarcoidosis is often discovered incidentally on a chest radiograph or thoracic computed tomography (CT) scan [171]. The clinical onset of sarcoidosis may be acute or insidious. Acute or subacute sarcoidosis develops over a period of weeks or a few months and it usually heralds a good prognosis [129,172]. One of the most typical forms of acute sarcoidosis is Löfgren syndrome [6,173]. An insidious onset for several months correlates with a chronic course and permanent organ damage [10,172,174–178].

Pulmonary sarcoidosis. Intrathoracic involvement occurs in 90% of cases [2,3]. Patients may be asymptomatic or present dry cough and dyspnea [171]. Associated bronchial hyperreactivity may be present. Hemoptysis is rare. Pulmonary sarcoidosis is classically divided into four stages on the basis of the chest radiograph (Table 96.1). Hilar bilateral and right paratracheal lymphadenopathy and bilateral reticulonodular infiltration with upper lung zones predominance is the most typical pattern [179]. Figure 96.3 shows a stage 2 chest radiograph. Atypical radiological findings include large nodules, alveolar infiltrates, hilar calcification, pleural effusion and pneumothorax [180–182]. Sarcoidosis-associated pulmonary hypertension is typically seen in advanced cases, with pulmonary fibrosis, destruction and obliteration of the pulmonary vasculature, and chronic hypoxemia [183–187].

Extrapulmonary sarcoidosis

Eye. Ocular involvement occurs in 15–20% of patients. Since it may be asymptomatic, slit-lamp and ophthalmoscopic examinations should be performed on every patient with sarcoidosis [188]. The most frequent findings are anterior or posterior uveitis, choroidoretinitis, periphlebitis, papilloedema and retinal hemorrhages. Conjunctival follicles, lacrimal gland involvement and keratoconjunctivitis sicca may be present as well [189–191]. Secondary glaucoma, cataract formation and blindness are late complications in untreated cases [192].

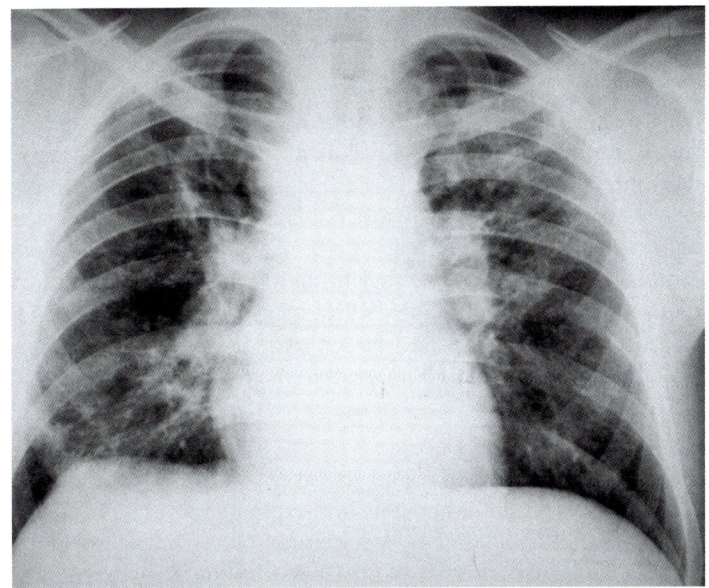

Figure 96.3 Chest radiograph showing stage II pulmonary sarcoidosis (bilateral hilar and right paratracheal lympadenopathy and pulmonary infiltrates with upper and middle lobe predominance).

Reticuloendothelial system. Peripheral lymphadenopathy involving the cervical, supraclavicular, epitrochlear, axillary and inguinal nodes may be present. In addition to intrathoracic, mesenteric chain and retroperitoneal lymph nodes may be present as well. Splenic involvement is frequent, although splenomegaly occurs only in 5–10% of cases and may result in hypersplenism and pancytopenia [193]. Bone marrow involvement is rare [1,3].

Liver. Mild hepatomegaly with slight cholestasis occurs in 20–30% of patients. Non-caseating granulomas are present in up to 75% of liver biopsies. Hepatic sarcoidosis affects the periportal areas. Severe chronic cholestasis syndrome, portal hypertension, and Budd–Chiari syndrome are rare. Multiple low-attenuation nodules in the liver on CT may be observed [194,195].

Neurosarcoidosis. Five to 10% of patients with sarcoidosis have clinically recognisable neurological involvement [1,3]. The disease has a predilection for the basal meninges, so cranial nerve involvement, particularly facial paralysis, are common. Other central nervous system manifestations include aseptic meningitis, seizures, pyramidal tract signs, optic nerve dysfunction, papilloedema, hypothalamic and pituitary lesions with diabetes insipidus or hypopituitarism, and cognitive impairment [196–199]. Spinal cord involvement is rare [200]. Gadolinium-enhanced magnetic resonance imaging (MRI) may reveal non-enhancing multifocal periventricular and subcortical white matter lesions mimicking those of multiple sclerosis, meningeal enhancement, space-occupying lesions and hydrocephalus [201]. Small fibre neuropathy was first reported in 2002. Fluctuating sensorineural hearing loss may also occur [202].

Musculoskeletal system. Transient or chronic polyarthralgias are common but frank arthritis is uncommon. Asymptomatic muscle involvement is also common but symptomatic diffuse or nodular

Table 96.1 Chest radiograph stages in pulmonary sarcoidosis.[a]

Chest radiograph stages	% at onset	% with resolution
Stage 0: normal chest radiograph	<10	
Stage I: bilateral hilar lymphadenopathy without pulmonary involvement	50	65; <10% progress to pulmonary involvement
Stage II: bilateral hilar lymphadenopathy with pulmonary involvement	30	20–50
Stage III[b]: Pulmonary involvement without bilateral hilar lymphadenopathy	10–15	<20

Adapted from Hunninghake et al. 1999 [3] © American Thoracic Society.

[a] Classification based on chest radiograph. Although high-resolution CT may suggest a different stage, it is not necessary to change the criteria since this test is indicated only in a limited number of patients.

[b] Stage III may be subclassified into stage IV, which includes cases with advanced pulmonary fibrosis (hilar retraction, coarse linear opacities, honeycombing, bullae, emphysematous changes, architectural distortion and pulmonary hypertension).

myopathy is rare. Bone lesions, usually osteolytic, are not frequent [1,3].

Heart. Clinical cardiac involvement occurs in 5% of patients. Supraventricular and ventricular arrhythmias, and aberrations of atrioventricular or intraventricular conduction, may result in complete heart block or sudden death; papillary muscle dysfunction and congestive heart failure may be present. Cor pulmonale is usually secondary to chronic pulmonary fibrosis. Cardiac MRI and cardiac positron emission tomography (PET) scans are the most useful tests for the diagnosis of cardiac sarcoidosis. Endomyocardial biopsy may reveal granulomas although the diagnostic yield may be low [203–207].

Other manifestations. Parotid involvement is frequent and may produce parotid enlargement and xerostomia. Hypercalcemia (5–10% of patients) and hypercalciuria (40%) are explained by increased production of 1.25-dihydroxyvitamin D by granulomas [208]. Interstitial granulomatous nephritis and renal failure have been reported [209,210]. Sarcoidosis may involve any structure of the upper respiratory tract, most frequently causing nasal stuffiness [211]. Gastrointestinal, genital, endocrine and mammary involvement are rare [1,3]. Fatigue, depression and cognitive impairment, sometimes associated with small fibre neuropathy, have been classified as 'parasarcoidosis' syndromes (non-granulomatous manifestations of sarcoidosis) [212–215]. Autoimmune thyroid disease may also be related [216].

Course and prognosis. In most patients, particularly those with an acute presentation, the disease resolves spontaneously without sequelae within 2–5 years. Löfgren syndrome has an excellent prognosis [6]. An insidious presentation usually correlates with a chronic course and permanent organ damage [10,172,174–178]. Ten to 30% of patients show active disease for more than 5 years and are classified as chronic sarcoidosis [7,217]. Some patients with chronic disease may show a mild degree of activity (smoldering sarcoidosis) [7]. Another subgroup of patients with chronic disease show a progressive course with moderate to severe organ damage, sometimes with irreversible fibrotic changes [3,129,176,177,184,187]. Occasionally, recurrence of sarcoidosis many years after spontaneous remission may occur, particularly in patients with Löfgren syndrome [218]. Pregnancy is not contraindicated except in severe chronic disease. Mortality is less than 5%.

Cutaneous manifestations of sarcoidosis

Cutaneous manifestations of sarcoidosis are extremely variable and sarcoidosis is considered one of the 'great imitators' in dermatology. Cutaneous lesions are the most frequent extrapulmonary manifestations of sarcoidosis [7]. They are classified as specific and non-specific [**219**]. Specific lesions are those that histopathologically display sarcoid granulomas [**219**,220]. The most frequent specific lesions are maculopapules, plaques, lupus pernio, scar-sarcoidosis and subcutaneous sarcoidosis [**219**,220–224]. The most important non-specific lesion is EN. Cutaneous lesions of sarcoidosis are more frequent in women than in men [2:1] and in African American people than in other ethnic groups [**219**].

Specific cutaneous lesions. Specific cutaneous lesions develop in 9–37% of patients with systemic sarcoidosis [10,220,222,225–231]. Although they can appear at any time, they are usually present at the onset of sarcoidosis [37,232,**233**,234,235]. In the initial evaluation of patients with suspected sarcoidosis the entire skin surface must be examined [220]. Because cutaneous biopsy is straightforward, it is a very useful diagnostic procedure that avoids aggressive diagnostic techniques [220] and shortens the diagnosis time of sarcoidosis [236].

The presence or absence of specific cutaneous lesions as a whole lacks prognostic significance in the progression of sarcoidosis [220,232,237,**238**]. However, some types of cutaneous lesions are associated with acute forms of sarcoidosis and others with chronic forms with a less favourable prognosis.

The clinical appearance is due to the presence of epithelioid cell granulomas in the dermis [45]. Specific lesions are red-brown or red-violaceous in colour. In patients with skin of colour the lesions tend to be more violaceous and can develop a hypopigmented surface. Specific lesions are generally multiple and they do not cause symptoms. Diascopy reveals the subtle brown-yellow or 'apple jelly' colour characteristic of granulomatous diseases (Figure 96.4),

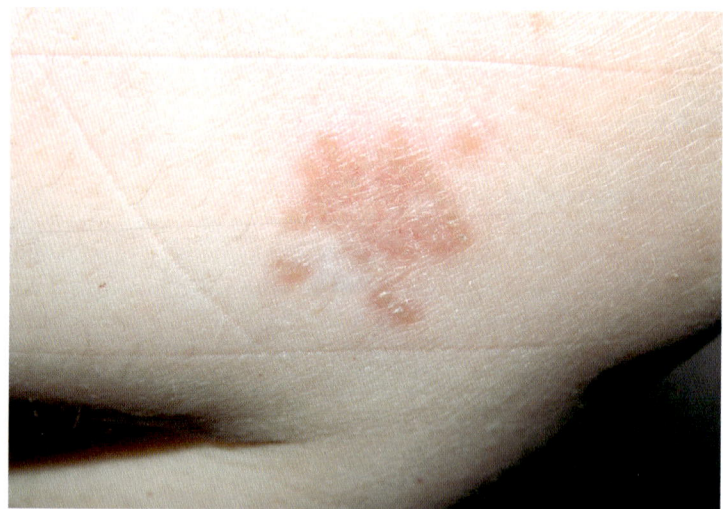

(a)

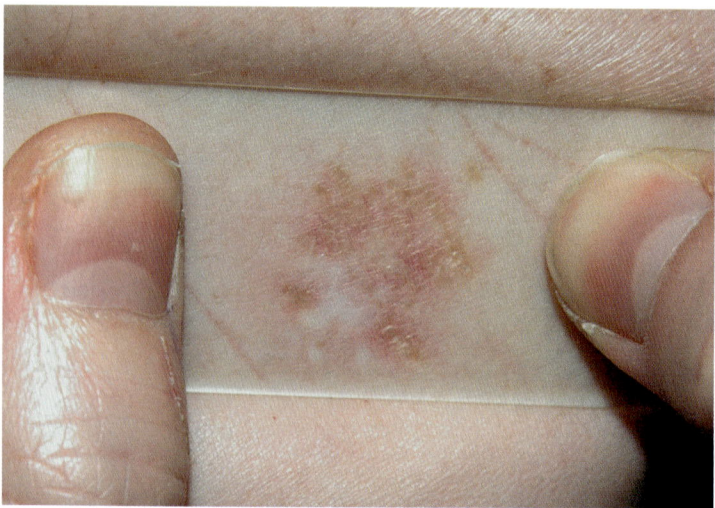

(b)

Figure 96.4 Sarcoid granulomas (a) revealed under diascopy as 'apple-jelly nodules' (b).

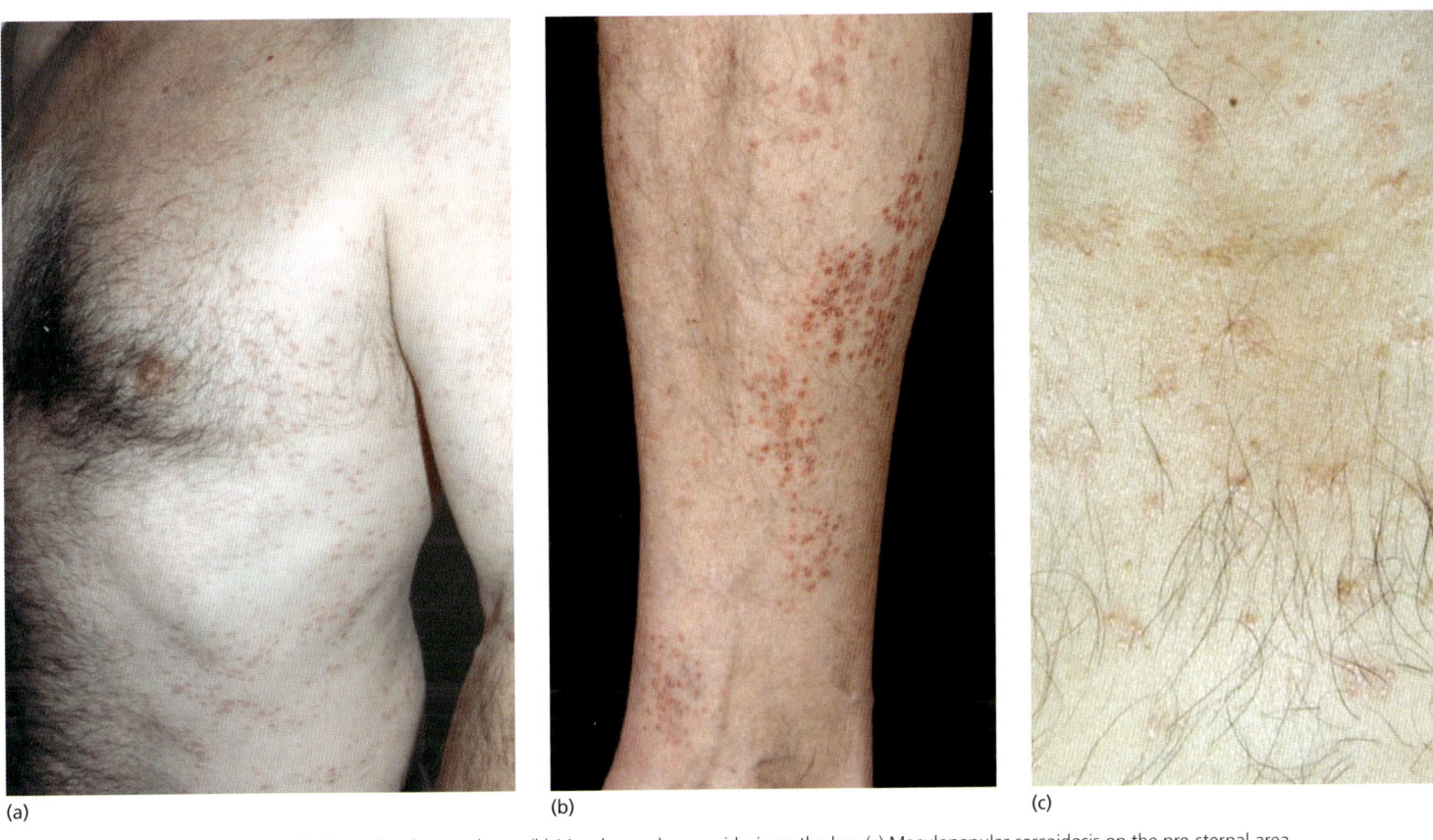

(a)   (b)   (c)

Figure 96.5 (a) Maculopapular sarcoidosis on the chest and arm. (b) Maculopapular sarcoidosis on the leg. (c) Maculopapular sarcoidosis on the pre-sternal area.

usually more opaque than in lupus vulgaris [219]. However, differential diagnosis may be difficult [239]. Diverse types of lesion may coexist in the same patient.

At dermoscopy the typical findings consist of translucent, yellowish or yellowish-orange areas. Vascular structures are another relevant dermatoscopic feature that includes linear vessels, branching vessels or arborising vessels [240,241].

Maculopapular sarcoidosis. Macules and papules are the most common specific lesion in some studies [**219**,220,223,242]. This form includes patients with slightly infiltrated patches as well as patients with multiple infiltrated lesions <10 mm (Figure 96.5). They are usually located on the face, mainly around the eyes and in the nasolabial folds, although the occipital area of the neck, trunk, extremities and even mucous membranes may be involved [**219**,221,222]. They may simulate xanthelasma, rosacea, secondary syphilis, lupus erythematosus, trichoepitheliomas, sebaceous adenoma, granuloma annulare, lichen nitidus, and syringomata [243–245]. They are usually transient and appear to herald the onset of the disease [221]. In some cases, papules can enlarge or coalesce to form plaques [**219**,246]. Maculopapular lesions often resolve either spontaneously or with treatment in less than 2 years without significant scarring. They are commonly associated with acute forms of systemic sarcoidosis [222,238,247] and connote a more favourable prognosis than other forms of specific cutaneous lesions [220,**233**].

A particular type of papular lesion involving the extensor surface of the knees has been reported. The papules are grouped over the

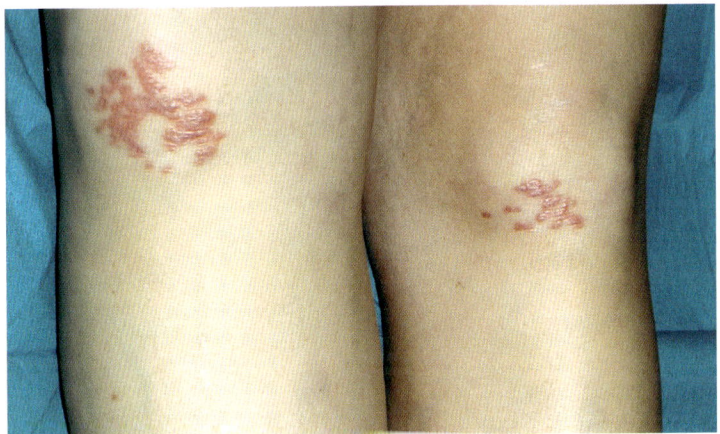

Figure 96.6 Papular sarcoidosis of the knees.

knees frequently with a linear arrangement that confers a lichenoid appearance (Figure 96.6) [50,248]. Polarisable foreign bodies are present in a high proportion of biopsies (up to 58%) [50]. These lesions are usually transient and may easily be overlooked. For this reason, the knees should always be examined when sarcoidosis is suspected [50,248].

Nodular and plaque sarcoidosis. This form is almost as common as maculopapular sarcoidosis in some studies and more frequent in others [220,234,249]. It usually presents as multiple, round or oval infiltrated lesions with red-brown colouration (Figure 96.7) [**219**,220]. They are larger than 10 mm in diameter and tend to be

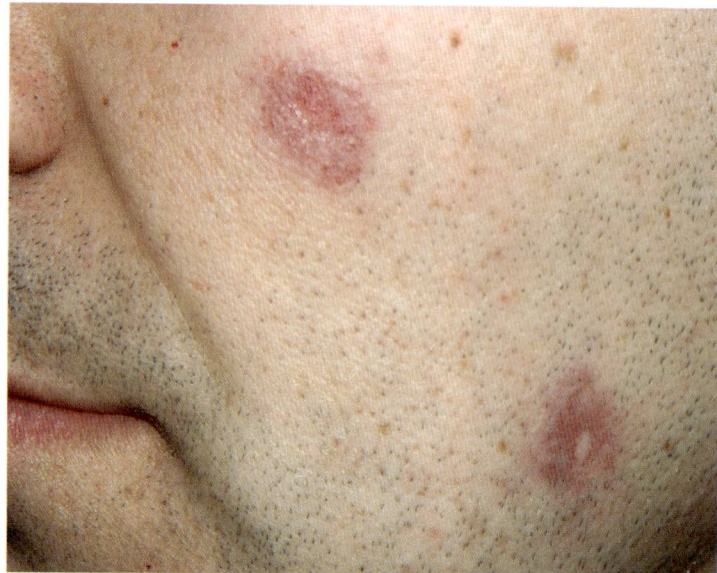

Figure 96.7 Sarcoid plaques on the cheek.

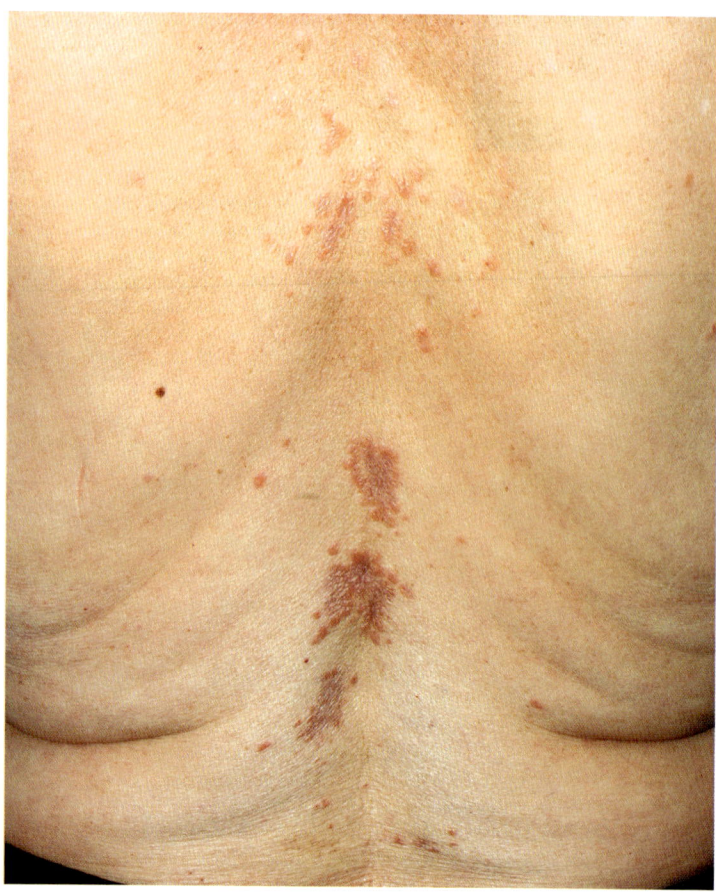

Figure 96.8 Plaque sarcoidosis on the back.

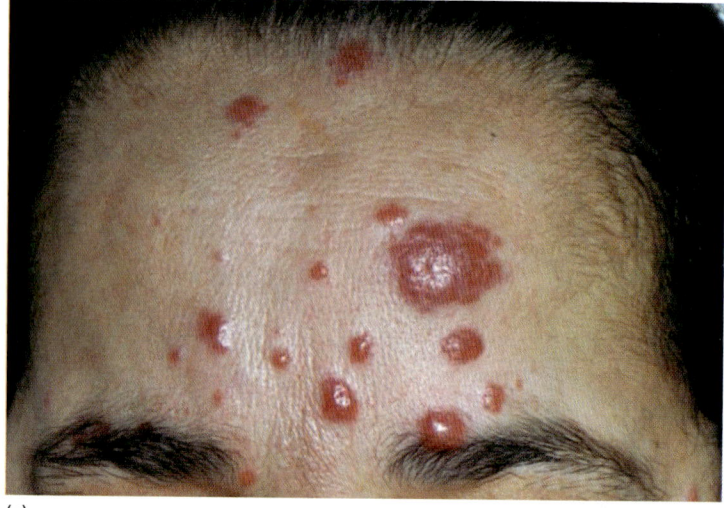

(a)

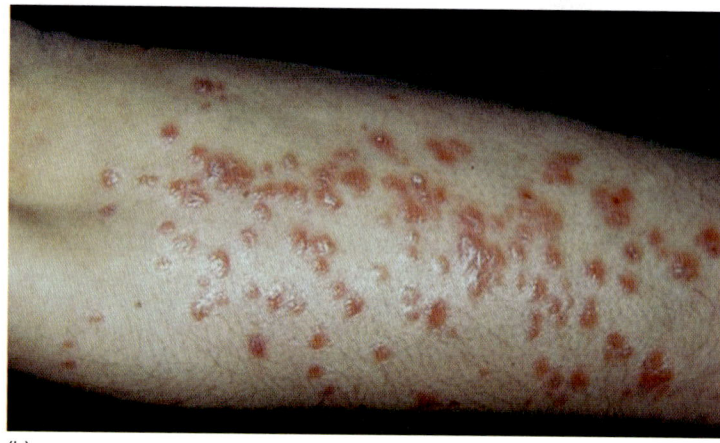

(b)

Figure 96.9 Dermal plaque and nodules on the forehead (a) and nodules on the forearm (b).

neck (Figure 96.11) [222,**238**]. Plaques can simulate lupus vulgaris, necrobiosis lipoidica, morphoea, leprosy, leishmaniasis, discoid lupus erythematosus and granuloma annulare [243,250]. After treatment plaques tend to recur; when they do resolve they can leave permanent scarring [**219**,221,222,237,251]. They are associated with chronic forms of sarcoidosis such as pulmonary fibrosis, peripheral lymphadenopathy, splenomegaly and chronic uveitis [220,237,**238**,242,247,252]. In patients with plaque-type lesions the activity of the systemic disease usually persists for more than 2 years [220,**233**,**238**]. However, unlike lupus pernio, plaques are not associated with bony cysts nor sarcoidosis of the upper respiratory tract [221].

Lupus pernio. Lupus pernio is the most characteristic cutaneous lesion of sarcoidosis [220]. In reported case series of lupus pernio it tends to appear in older people more than other forms of cutaneous sarcoidosis and is especially frequent in women of African American background [3,223,253]. Also, according to the case series reported, the incidence in white people varies widely according to the country of origin of the study [**233**,**238**,254]. Infiltrated erythematoviolaceous plaques involve the nose, cheeks, ears, lips, forehead and fingers [45,**219**] (Figure 96.12). On the cheeks, a prominent

thicker and more indurated and persistent than papules and are sometimes mammillated (Figure 96.8). Plaques can be associated with nodular dermal lesions (Figure 96.9). They can be located on the face, scalp, back, buttocks, and extremities (Figure 96.10) [220]. Plaques can adopt an annular appearance by means of peripheral extension and central cleaning, mainly in the forehead and

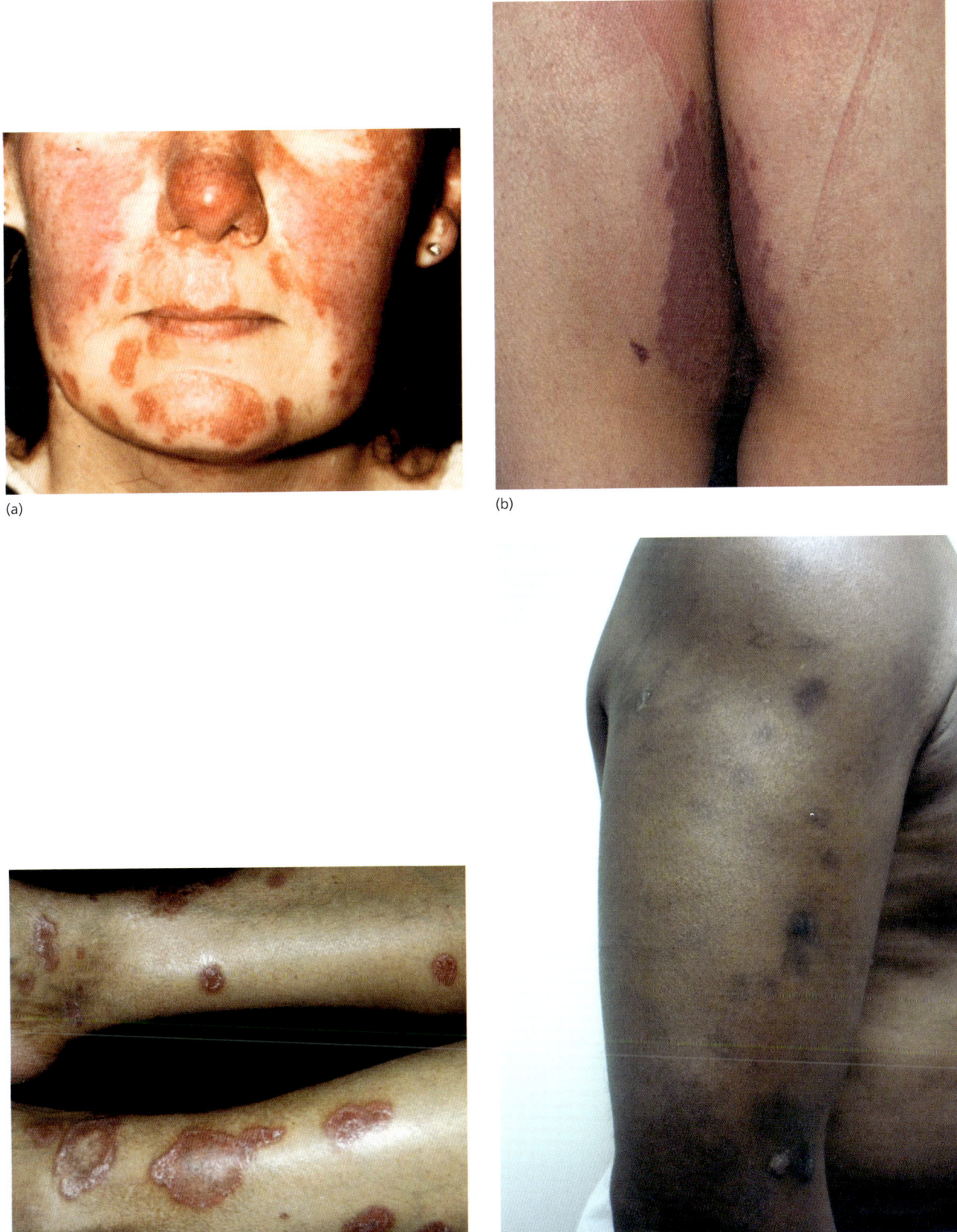

(a)

(b)

(c)

(d)

Figure 96.10 (a) Extensive coalescing plaques of sarcoidosis on the face. (b) Plaque sarcoidosis extending from perianal skin to the buttocks. (c) Plaque sarcoidosis of the lower extremities resembling necrobiosis lipoidica. Courtesy of the copyright holder Dr J. E. Bothwell, Barnsley District General Hospital, Barnsley, UK) (d) Plaque sarcoidosis on arm in patient with skin of colour. Courtesy of Professor Dedee Murrell.

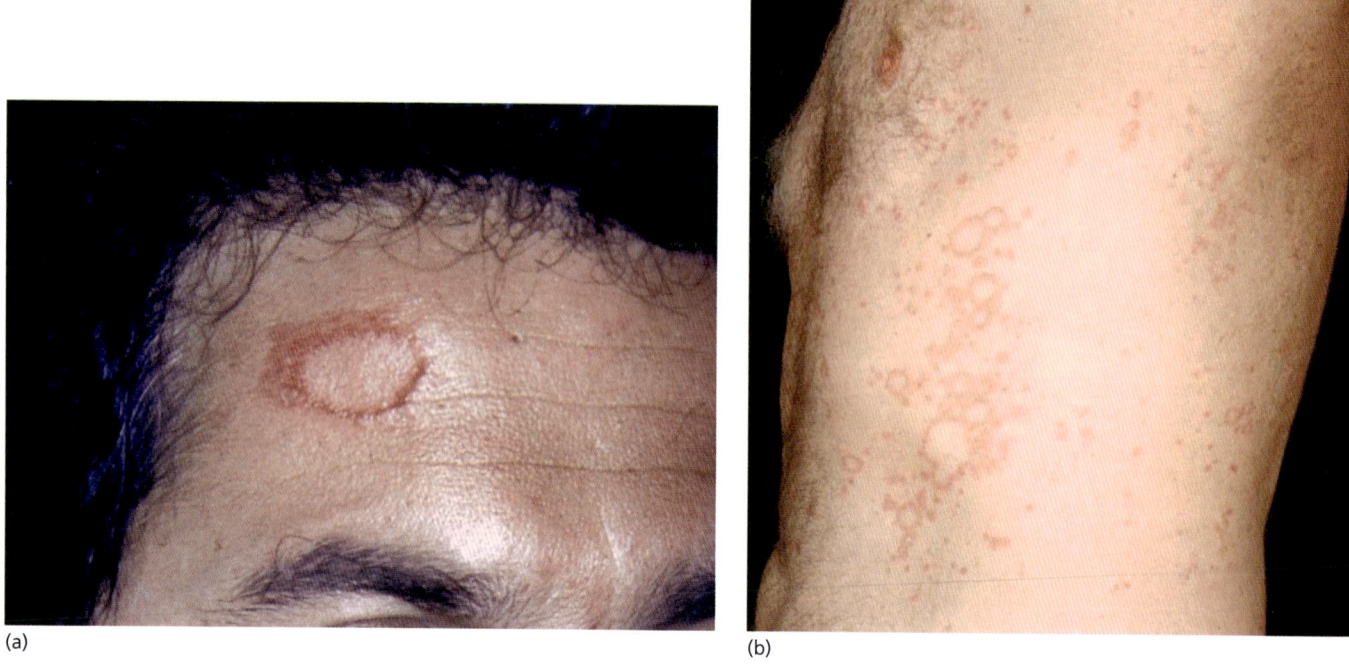

(a)

(b)

Figure 96.11 (a) Annular sarcoidosis on the forehead. (b) Extensive truncal annular sarcoidosis.

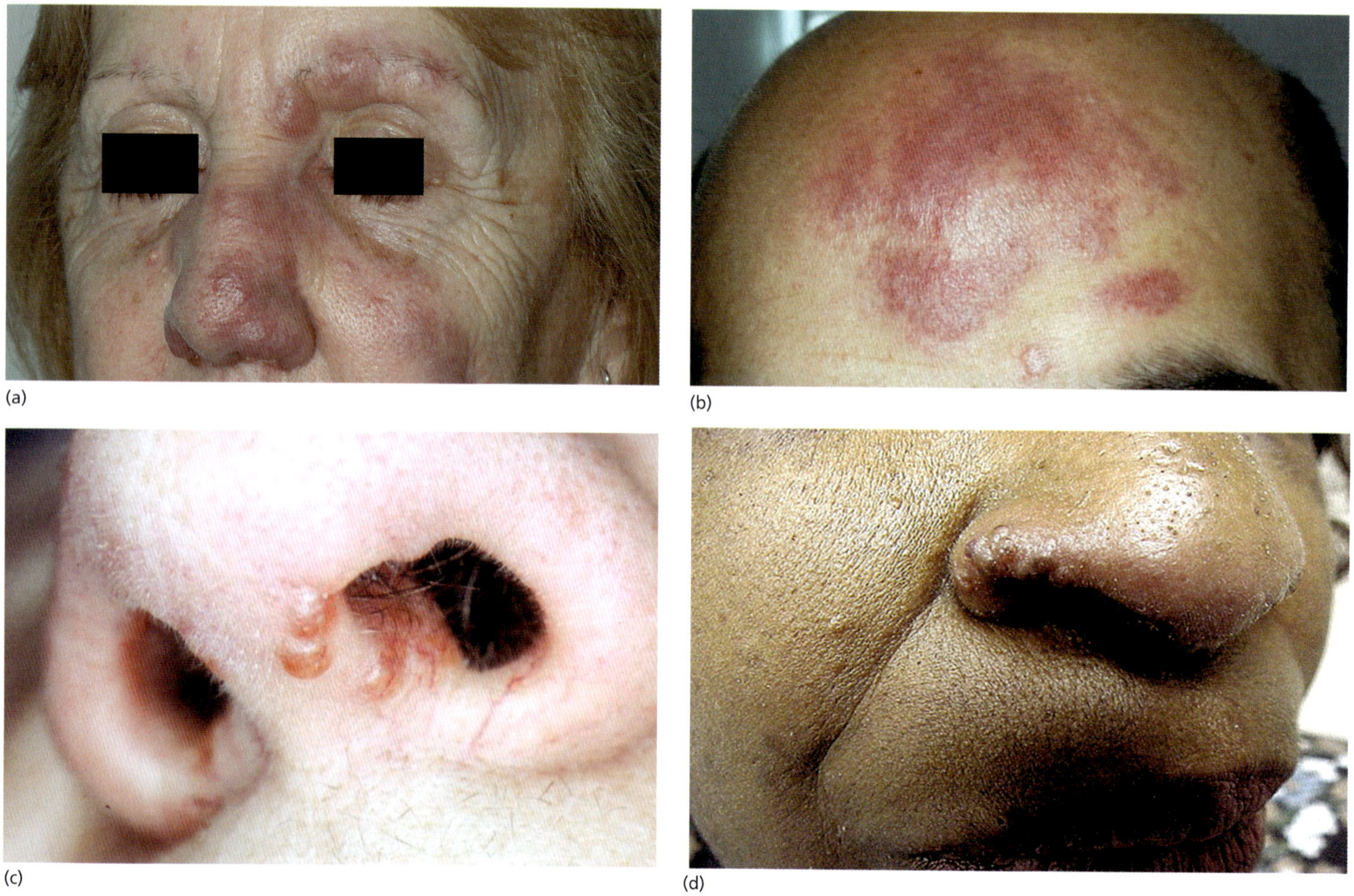

(a)

(b)

(c)

(d)

Figure 96.12 (a) Lupus pernio involving the nose, cheek, and eyebrow. (b) Lupus pernio involving forehead. (c) Sarcoid nodules on columella. (d) Nodules on the nose of female patient with skin of colour. Courtesy of Professor Dedee Murrell.

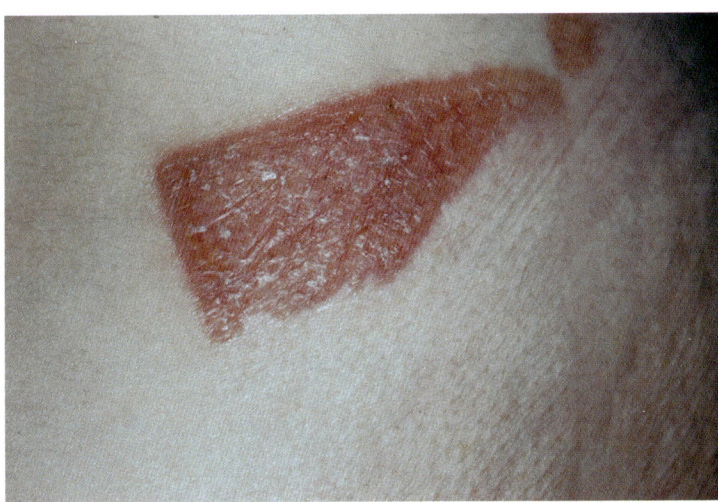

Figure 96.13 Scar sarcoidosis in a burn on the buttock.

telangiectatic component is characteristic. Lupus pernio is usually painless and does not tend to ulcerate [3], and it is not as mutilating as lupus vulgaris [45]. However, unlike other forms of sarcoidosis, lupus pernio can be disfiguring [255,256]. It may simulate rosacea, lupus vulgaris and discoid lupus erythematosus [250].

In more than half of cases, lupus pernio is associated with sarcoidosis of the upper respiratory tract [238,253,257,258], especially in patients with involvement of the nasal rims [259]. It is typically associated with pulmonary fibrosis, chronic uveitis and bony cysts [221,253]. The fingers affected by lupus pernio usually present bony cysts [**219**] and when the terminal phalange is involved the nails are usually dystrophic [260]. Lupus pernio usually follows an extremely chronic course (from 2 to 25 years) [221,247] and is associated with chronic systemic disease [217,**238**,261,262].

Scar-sarcoidosis. Scar-sarcoidosis can involve scars resulting from surgery, trauma, acne, venipuncture, vaccinations, herpes zoster or the Mantoux test [45,263–267]. In scar-sarcoidosis the old scars become infiltrated and red, showing sarcoid granulomas histopathologically (Figure 96.13). Scar-sarcoidosis has been observed in 9% of cutaneous sarcoidosis patients [249] and is frequently located in the knees [45]. The scar infiltration tends to persist according to the activity of the disease [**219**,222,237,247]. Scar-sarcoidosis can appear at the beginning of the disease and must be looked for whenever a diagnosis of sarcoidosis is considered [45]. However, with greater frequency it is associated with long-lasting pulmonary and mediastinal involvement, uveitis, peripheral lymphadenopathy, bony cysts and parotid infiltration [221,222,249].

Tattoo sarcoidosis may be considered a variant of scar-sarcoidosis that may occur decades after tattoo placement [222,268–274]. Sarcoidosis should be excluded in cases of granulomatous tattoo reaction even if the reaction is restricted to one colour [274].

It has been suggested that foreign material frequently present in the scars can act as an antigenic stimulus for the induction of granuloma in the scar [**48**,49,263,275]. Even the smallest amount of oil used as lubricant in blood sampling needles can induce granulomas in sarcoidosis patients [266].

Subcutaneous sarcoidosis. Subcutaneous sarcoidosis must be differentiated from nodular dermal lesions with extension into subcutaneous fat [43,276]. It has been observed in 1.4–6% of patients with systemic sarcoidosis [44,227,277] and represents 12–38% of specific cutaneous lesions [44,278]. Most cases occur in white women, mainly in the fifth and sixth decades of life [279]. The lesions are painless, indurated, and covered by normal-appearing skin [**219**,220,280]. In most patients the lesions involve the forearms,

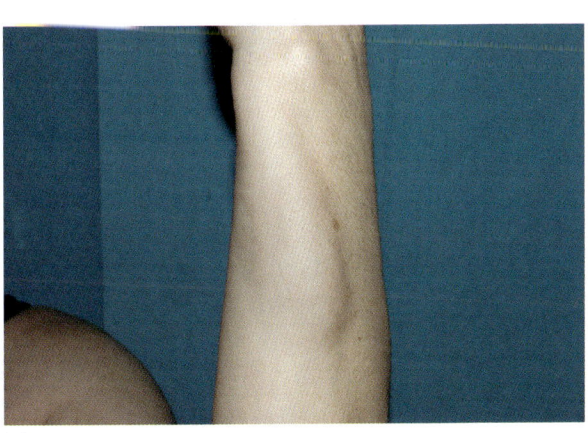
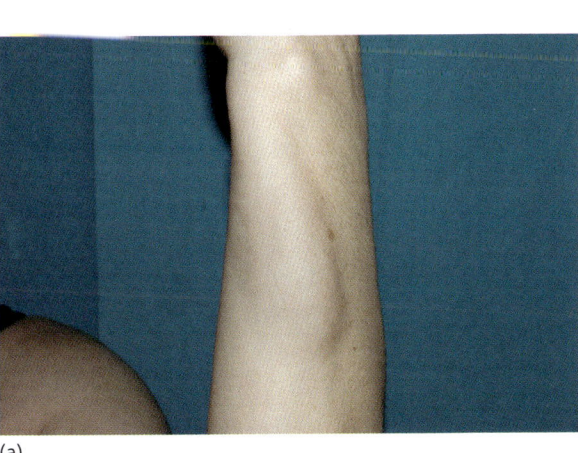
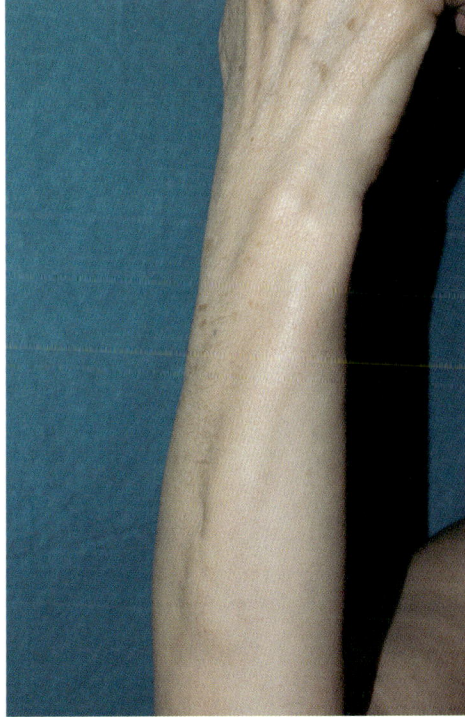

Figure 96.14 (a,b) Subcutaneous sarcoidosis in the arm with indurated linear bands from the elbow to the hand.

(a)   (b)

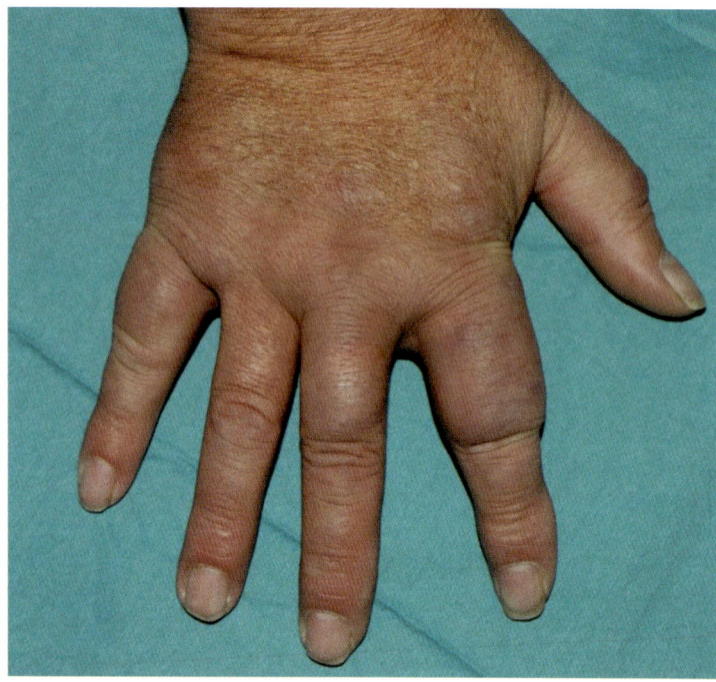

(a)

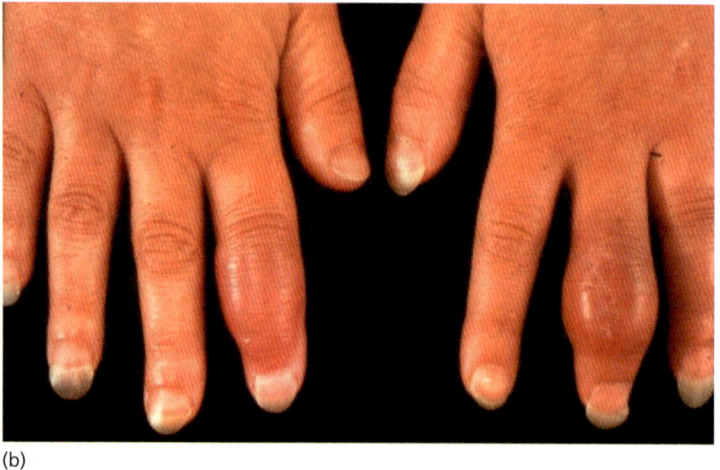

(b)

Figure 96.15 (a,b) Sarcoid dactylitis.

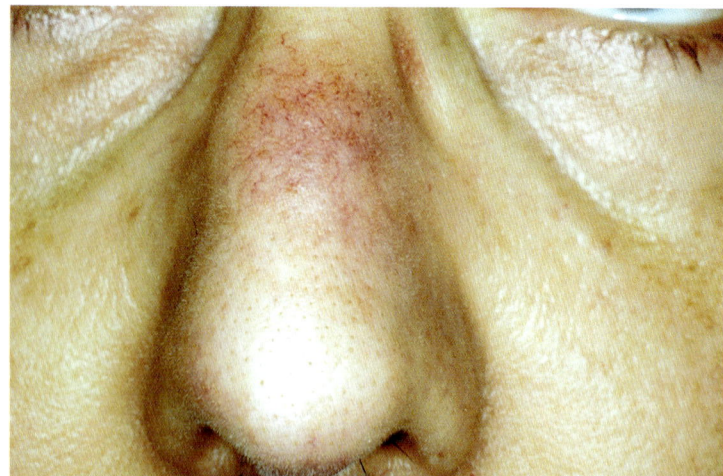

Figure 96.16 Angiolupoid sarcoidosis in the bridge of the nose.

diagnosis [44]. It is associated with stage I on chest radiograph and with less than 2 years' activity of systemic sarcoidosis [**233**].

Less frequent specific cutaneous lesions.

Angiolupoid sarcoidosis. It typically presents in women as a single raised plaque on the bridge of the nose (Figure 96.16), central face, ears or scalp [250,289]. It has been observed in 8% of patients with cutaneous sarcoidosis in an Indian series [290], and while rare in Europe and America, is the most frequent form in Taiwan, where it is often associated with eye involvement [291].

Hypopigmented sarcoidosis. Hypopigmented, well-demarcated, round-to-oval patches are mainly observed on the limbs [219,292]. In a series of 145 patients with sarcoidosis, the hypopigmented variant was observed in only eight individuals, most of whom were of Afro-Caribbean ethnicity (Figure 96.17) [227]. It must be differentiated from leprosy, postinflammatory hypopigmentation, idiopathic hypomelanosis guttate and pityriasis lichenoides chronica [45]. The presence of an interphase dermatitis associated with granulomas may explain the hypomelanosis [293].

tend to be spindle-shaped, and may form indurated lineal bands from the elbow to the hand (Figure 96.14) [44,281–284]. In some cases the dorsa of the hands are infiltrated and the fingers develop asymptomatic, firm, fusiform swelling (sarcoid dactylitis) (Figure 96.15) [44,285,286]. In Japanese patients the lower extremities are the most common location [278,287]. Differential diagnosis includes epidermal cysts, lipomata, calcinosis, rheumatoid nodules, morphoea, cutaneous metastasis, tuberculosis and deep mycoses [280,286]. Cases of subcutaneous sarcoidosis simulating breast carcinoma have also been reported [288]. It is not unusual for subcutaneous sarcoidosis to coexist with or appear shortly after EN [44]. However, subcutaneous sarcoidosis lesions are non-tender, flesh coloured and more persistent [277,284].

Subcutaneous sarcoidosis usually appears at the onset of sarcoidosis [44,276,278–280] and is frequently the main complaint at

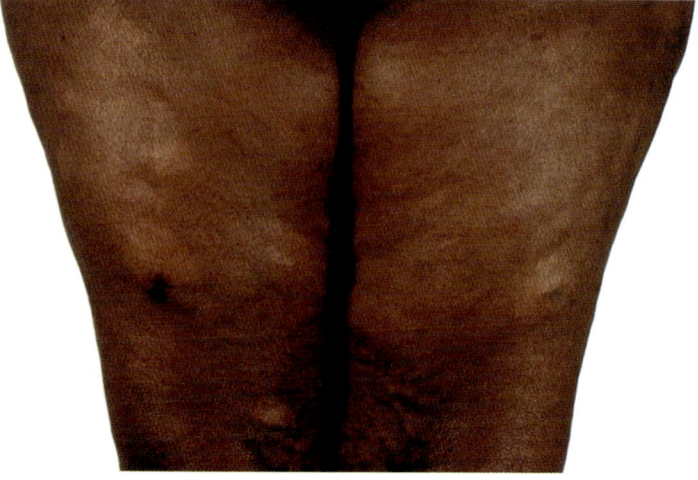

Figure 96.17 Hypopigmented sarcoidosis. Courtesy of the copyright holder Dr S. Walsh, King's College Hospital, London, UK.

Lichenoid sarcoidosis. This is more frequent in children [294–300] and is estimated to account for 1–2% of cases of cutaneous sarcoidosis [301]. Multiple 1–3 mm, flat-topped or dome-shaped red or skin-coloured papules may involve extensive areas of the trunk, limbs and face [298,299]. The differential diagnosis includes lichen planus, lichen nitidus, lichenoid drug eruptions, lupus erythematosus and papular mucinosis (lichen myxoedematosus) [298]. Wickham striae are absent [299].

Ulcerative sarcoidosis. This usually develops in papulonodular or atrophic lesions on the lower legs and heals with scarring [302–304]. It has been reported in 1.1–4.8% of skin sarcoidosis [**238**,303] and is more frequent in black and Japanese people [302,304,305]. Subjacent granulomatous vasculitis has been reported in some cases [305–307]

Psoriasiform sarcoidosis. Well-demarcated, red, scaly plaques that may be clinically indistinguishable from psoriasis [250,308,309] are found in 0.9% of patients with cutaneous sarcoidosis [249]. However, psoriasis lesions have a redder colour and larger scales, and heal without scarring [251]. Most cases have been reported in dark-skinned patients [310].

Verrucous sarcoidosis. This presents as well-demarcated, hyperkeratotic, papillomatous lesions usually located on the lower extremities [311–313]. Most reported cases have been male patients of African descent with long-standing systemic disease [314,315]. It may resemble warts, nodular prurigo, hypertrophic lichen planus, keratoacanthoma, squamous cell carcinoma or deep fungal infections [312,315,316], and may appear at the site of cosmetic tattoos [317].

Necrobiosis-lipoidica-like lesions. Pink to violaceous plaques of sarcoidosis with depressed centres located on the shins may resemble necrobiosis lipoidica [250,318–322]. Sarcoidosis must be considered in the differential diagnosis of necrobiosis lipoidica in non-diabetic patients [323]. The granulomatous nature of both diseases may explain this resemblance. On the other hand, sarcoidosis and necrobiosis lipoidica have been reported to coexist in some patients [321,322].

Ichthyosiform sarcoidosis. This is characterised by adherent, polygonal, grey or brown 0.1–1 cm scales most commonly located on the lower extremities of patients of African descent [324–327]. Biopsy reveals both sarcoid granulomas and compact orthokeratosis with a diminished granular layer, mimicking ichthyosis vulgaris [325,327,328]. Ichthyosiform sarcoidosis may be misdiagnosed as xerotic skin and may be more prevalent than previously estimated [329].

Erythrodermic sarcoidosis. Slightly infiltrated, red plaques coalesce over large areas. In contrast to classic erythroderma, some areas of skin are spared [250,330]. Some patients with prominent scaling have been reported as acquired ichthyosiform erythroderma. Histopathological evaluation may be necessary to exclude more common causes of erythroderma [157,331,332].

Morphoeaform sarcoidosis. Indurated and atrophic plaques, usually located on the thighs, have also been described in sarcoidosis [333,334]. Some cases show a linear distribution resembling linear morphea [334,335]. In addition to epithelioid granulomas, dermal sclerosis is observed histopathologically [333,335,336].

Livedo. Sarcoidosis may rarely present with livedo. Most reported cases are Japanese women [337,338]. Biopsy specimens usually reveal epithelioid cell granulomas around blood vessels conditioning luminal narrowing [337,339,340]. Sarcoidosis with livedo is characterised by a high frequency of ophthalmologic and central nervous system involvement [337,338].

Other. Less common specific lesions which have been described in cutaneous sarcoidosis may resemble discoid lupus erythematosus [341–343], lichen sclerosus [344], lipodermatosclerosis [345], cellulitis [346] or breast carcinoma en cuirasse [347,348]. Other reported variants include pseudotumoral sarcoidosis [349,350], follicular sarcoidosis [351], photo-induced sarcoidosis [352–354] and variants presenting as palmar erythema [355] or as lower limb oedema, which is generally unilateral [356,357].

Special locations of specific cutaneous lesions

Alopecia. Scarring alopecia is more common, although non-scarring alopecia has also been reported [358]. In reported case series of scarring alopecia secondary to sarcoidosis, most cases were women of African American background [341,358–365]. Scale is usually absent, although follicular plugging may be present [341]. Differential diagnoses include lichen planopilaris, discoid lupus erythematosus, folliculitis decalvans and central centrifugal cicatrizal alopecia [358,364]. Advanced lesions may be indistinguishable from pseudopelada of Brocq [250]. However, other cutaneous signs of sarcoidosis are often present [360]. Response to therapy is usually poor [358].

Nails. Splinter haemorrhages, thinning, pitting, thickening, transverse layering, longitudinal ridging, onycholysis, subungual hyperkeratosis, paronychia, pterigium, trachyonychia, longitudinal erythronychia and red or brown discoloration of the nail bed have all been reported in sarcoidosis [366–371]. In advanced cases, granulomatous infiltration of the nail matrix can result in total loss of the nail [369]. Nail sarcoidosis is associated in most reported cases with bony cysts in the underlying terminal phalanx [369,372] and a chronic disease course [45,369].

Oral. Oral mucosa lesions are infrequent in sarcoidosis [373,374]. They often appear at the beginning of the disease and may be similar in morphology, shape and size to their cutaneous counterparts [375]. They usually present as a diffuse submucous enlargement or a firm nodular solitary lesion more frequently located in the tongue, followed by the lips, oral mucosa, palate and gingiva (Figure 96.18) [373,374,376–378]. Papules, superficial ulcerations [373,379] and strawberry gums [380] have also been reported. Differential diagnosis includes oro-facial granulomatosis and Crohn disease [381].

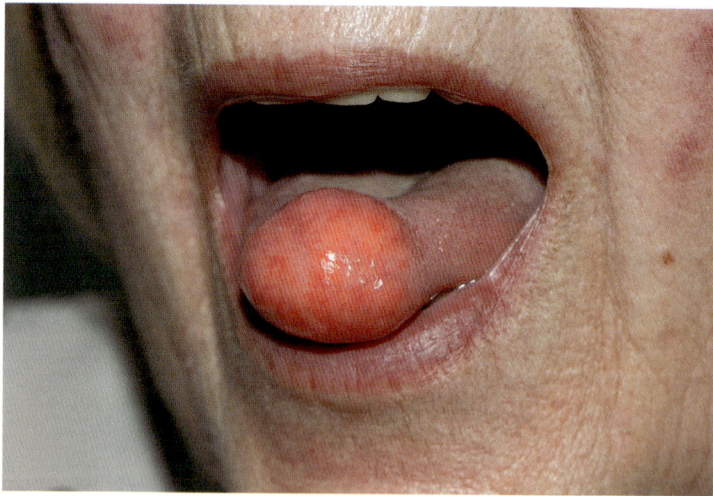

Figure 96.18 Sarcoidosis involving the tongue.

Genital. In the male genitalia sarcoidosis usually presents with testicular or epididymal masses without cutaneous lesions [382,383]. However, several patients with indurated papules, painful nodules or swelling involving the scrotum or penis have been reported [382,384–387]. Vulval sarcoidosis is rare [388,389]. It may present with semi-translucent reddish brown papules and nodules, pruritic infiltrated plaques or ulcerated vulval lesions that must be distinguished from tuberculosis, Crohn disease, syphilis, foreign body reactions and lymphogranuloma venereum [389–392].

Non-specific lesions. EN is the most common non-specific lesion of sarcoidosis and is frequently the initial manifestation of the disease (Figure 96.19). It is the marker of acute and benign sarcoidosis and tends to affect younger people than infiltrative cutaneous lesions [238]. The prevalence of EN in sarcoidosis is between 20% and 40% [7,229,249].

The association of EN with bilateral hilar and right paratracheal adenopathies, with or without pulmonary infiltrates, is known as Löfgren syndrome [393–396]. It is more frequent in young women from northern Europe [228,395,397–399] and is one of the most frequent forms of sarcoidosis in Spain [6,231,400]. The prognosis is very good and it usually resolves spontaneously in 1 year [6,396,398,401–403].

When sarcoidosis is associated with EN it usually evolves as a benign and self-limited disease [399,402,404–406]. In multivariate analysis, the presence of EN proved to be the strongest predictive factor for a favourable prognosis [404]. However, the good prognosis of sarcoidosis presenting with EN seems to be limited to white patients [407].

On the other hand, sarcoidosis is one of the most frequent causes of EN since 10–22% of EN cases were considered to be caused by sarcoidosis [408].

Less frequent non-specific lesions are erythema multiforme [219,409], prurigo [410–413], cutaneous calcinosis [414–418] and digital clubbing, which is considered a poor prognostic sign [419–426]. Pseudo-clubbing originated by granulomatous phalangeal involvement has been reported and must be

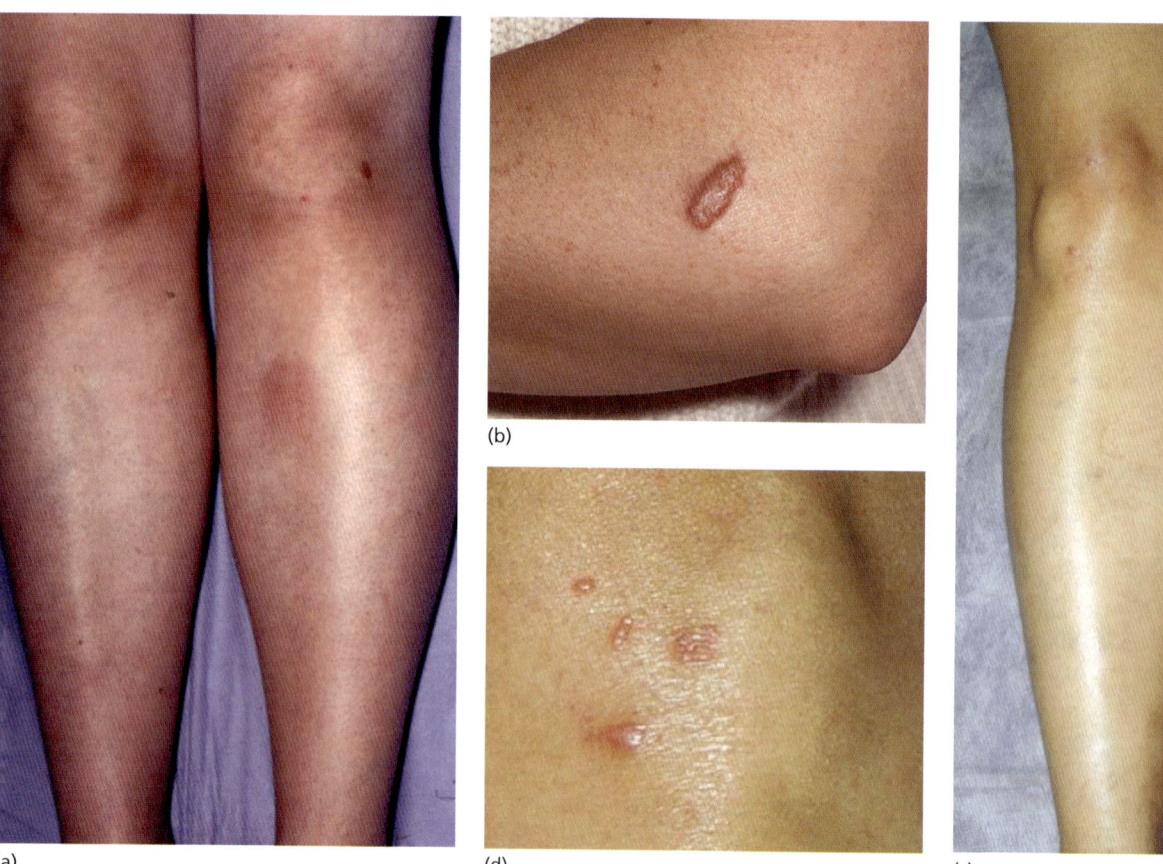

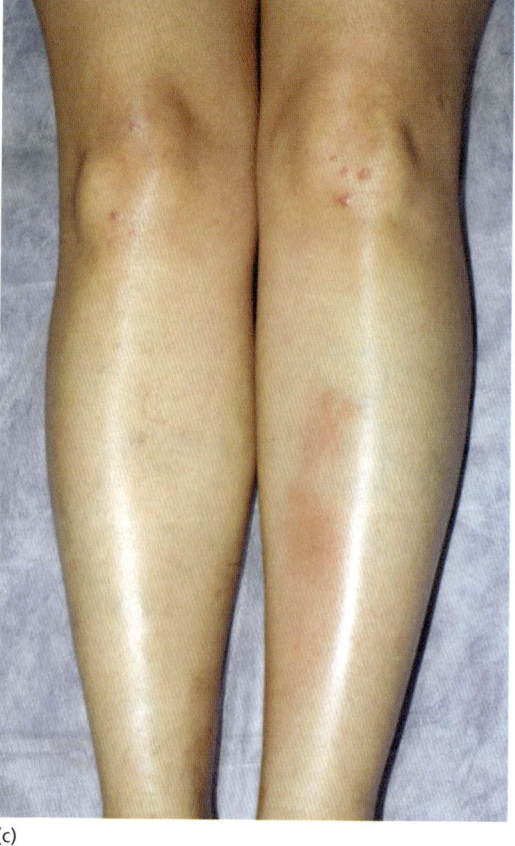

Figure 96.19 (a,c) Erythema nodosum in two patients with Löfgren syndrome with associated specific lesions of sarcoidosis in a scar on the elbow (b) and papular sarcoidosis of the knees (c,d).

differentiated from true digital clubbing [427,428]. The association of Sweet syndrome with sarcoidosis has been reported in several patients [429–439]. Sweet syndrome is mostly associated with acute sarcoidosis [438] and usually appears at the beginning of the disease [437]. Pyoderma gangrenosum has been exceptionally associated with sarcoidosis [440–444] and, although this association may be fortuitous, one case showed a clear-cut relation between biopsy of EN and the development of pyoderma gangrenosum [444].

Investigations

A workup for systemic sarcoidosis should be undertaken in all patients with cutaneous sarcoid granulomas [445–448]. Box 96.1 lists recommended essential investigations to be carried out.

Box 96.1 Recommended basic assessment of patients with sarcoidosis at presentation

- History: family sarcoidosis, occupational and environmental exposures (beryllium and others)
- Respiratory and extrarespiratory symptoms
- Physical examination
- Ophthalmological examination (slit lamp and ophthalmoscopic examination)
- Chest radiograph (thoracic CT if atypical chest radiograph)
- Standard haematological and biochemistry profiles (including urine and serum calcium level, hepatic enzymes and renal function tests), and serum angiotensin converting enzyme level
- ECG
- Pulmonary function tests (including spirometry and DL_{co})
- Mantoux test or interferon-gamma release assay for tuberculosis (QuantiFERON-TB Gold In-Tube assay)
- Biopsies (including culture for mycobacteria and fungus)

At diagnosis, at least 60% of patients have increased serum angiotensin converting enzyme level, although it is not specific. Pulmonary function tests may reveal decreased forced vital capacity and diffusing capacity for carbon monoxide. Thoracic high resolution CT is useful in patients with atypical radiological findings on chest radiograph [179,182]. The demonstration on bronchoalveolar lavage of a lymphocytic alveolitis with a proportion of CD4/CD8 >3.5 has a sensitivity of 53% and a specificity of 94%. Mantoux test is negative in more than 80% of patients [129]. Apart from the assessment of cardiac sarcoidosis, PET with ^{18}F-fluorodeoxyglucose (^{18}F-FDG PET) is useful for assessing disease activity and extension of sarcoidosis (Figure 96.20). ^{18}F-FDG PET/CT is particularly helpful in the detection of occult granuloma sites for biopsy and in evaluating treatment efficacy [449]. However, a positive ^{18}F-FDG PET/CT finding, by itself, is not an indication for treatment [450]. Other exams and appropriate biopsies should be performed according to the suspected organ involvement [451].

Diagnostic criteria

The diagnosis of sarcoidosis is based on a compatible clinical and radiological picture, demonstration of non-caseating granulomas with negative cultures for mycobacteria and fungus and exclusion of other granulomatous diseases [3,452]. When the clinical and radiological findings are not typical, particularly with a stage 0 chest radiograph, it is recommended that at least two positive biopsies are obtained. On the other hand, some clinical and radiological pictures, such as in Löfgren syndrome, are so typical of sarcoidosis that histological confirmation is not considered necessary [2,4,6].

Management

Oral corticosteroids are the treatment of choice for systemic sarcoidosis [3]. The recommended dose in pulmonary sarcoidosis is prednisolone 30–40 mg per day, with gradual reduction to 5–10 mg per day or 10–20 mg every other day for at least 1 year [3,220]. In patients with severe uveitis, neurosarcoidosis or symptomatic cardiac involvement, a dose of 1 mg/kg/day or intravenous high dose metilprednisolone pulse therapy may be required [3]. When corticosteroids cannot be withdrawn, other drugs such as chloroquine or cytotoxic drugs can be considered [3].

Cutaneous lesions usually respond to the treatment administered for the systemic disease but frequently recur when tapering corticosteroids [243,453]. When there is not significant visceral involvement to justify oral corticosteroid treatment, the options for cutaneous lesion treatment are not completely effective and therapeutic recommendations are usually supported by isolated case reports or short series [243,454,455]. For patients with cosmetically insignificant and asymptomatic cutaneous lesions, treatment may be unnecessary.

Patients with sarcoidosis should avoid tattoos, fillers and probably also platelet-rich plasma dermal infiltrations [52,456]. Treatments with drugs that may induce or worsen sarcoidosis should be used with caution in these patients.

Two instruments for measuring the severity of cutaneous sarcoidosis have been validated to assess the response to therapy [457–459].

First line

Mild to moderate disease. Cutaneous lesions may respond to potent topical corticosteroids with few adverse effects [460,461]. Intralesional injections of triamcinolone acetonide at concentrations of 5–20 mg/mL repeated every 3–4 weeks may be more effective [462–465].

Severe disfigurement or lupus pernio. Prednisolone 20–60 mg/day is administered until there is a clinical response (usually 1–3 months) and then tapered by 5–10 mg/week to the lowest dose that prevents relapse [453,463,465]: corticosteroid-sparing agents are indicated when a dose of at least 10 mg of prednisolone daily is required for this [466]. The mechanism of osteoporosis is multifactorial in sarcoidosis and all patients on chronic corticosteroids should have a baseline bone density study. For patients without hypercalcaemia or nephrolithiasis, oral calcium supplements may be used. The addition of vitamin D is less clear-cut. Calcium levels should be checked in the summer months to detect hypercalcaemia. Bisphosphonates have been shown to be useful in treating corticosteroid-induced osteoporosis [467].

Second line

Antimalarials, methotrexate or tetracycline can be used as second line therapy for mild to moderate disease and as corticosteroid-sparing agents in patients with severe disfigurement or lupus

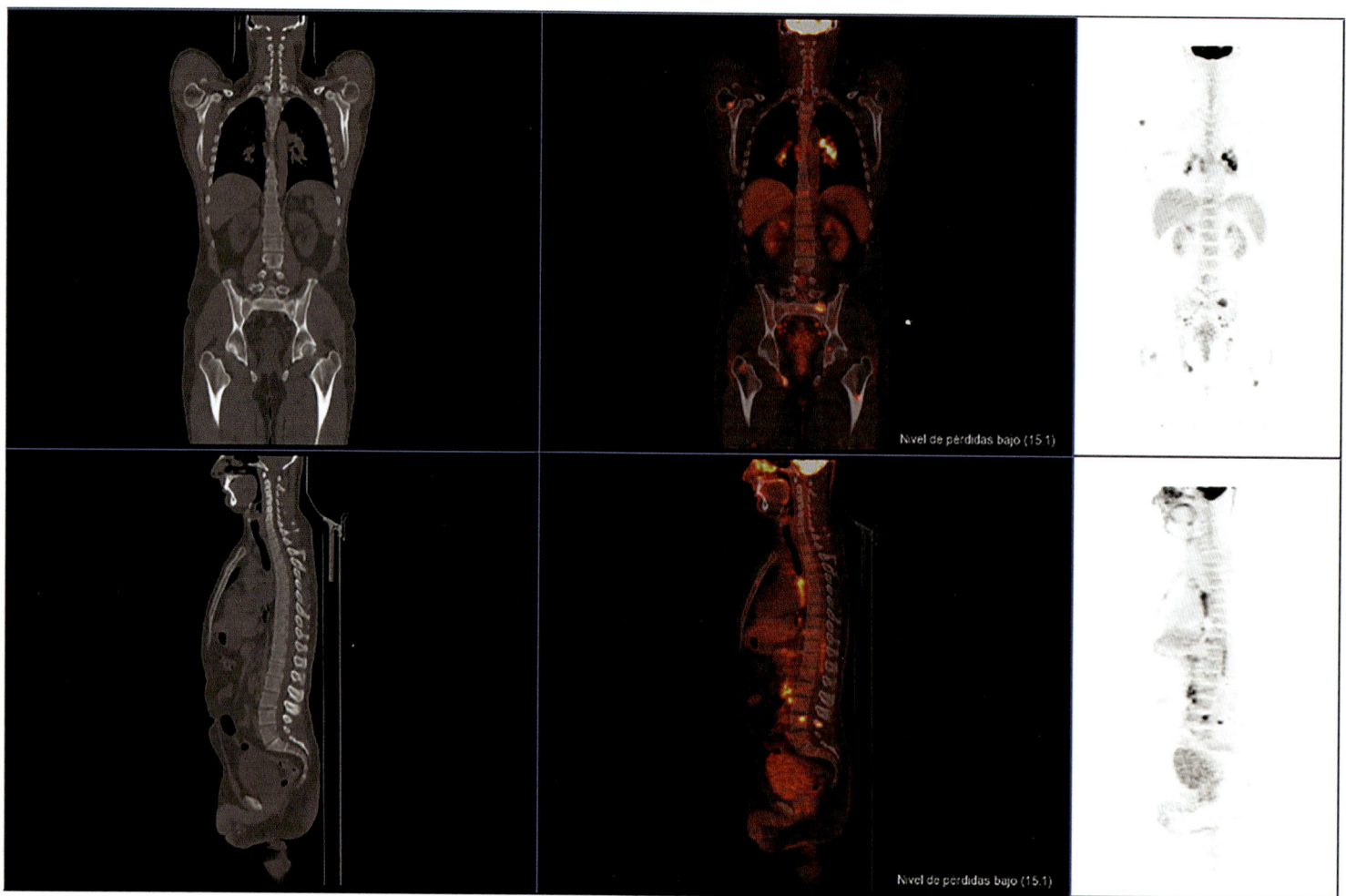

Figure 96.20 Whole body PET/CT with ^{18}F-fluorodeoxyglucose (^{18}F-FDG). High metabolic activity in the nasal mucosa, at thoracic and extrathoracic lymph nodes, in both lungs, spinal cord, and in several bones of the axial skeleton, with a predominance of lumbosacral and pelvic involvement.

pernio. They may be the first option when systemic corticosteroids are contraindicated [455].

Antimalarials. Hydroxychloroquine (200–400 mg daily) and chloroquine (250– 500 mg daily) are among the most commonly prescribed drugs [468–470]. They are particularly useful in chronic cutaneous lesions and can be used as corticosteroid-sparing agents in severe cases (Figure 96.21) [220]. In a review, 57 of 78 reported patients improved with hydroxychloroquine or chloroquine alone [471]. Hydroxychloroquine has a lower risk of retinopathy but chloroquine seems to be more effective [467,470,472]. Baseline ocular fundus examination, a dose of hydroxychloroquine ≤5 mg/kg and annual ophthalmologic evaluation after 5 years of therapy is recommended [473].

Methotrexate. Methotrexate has been the most widely studied non-steroidal therapy for systemic sarcoidosis [467]. The overall response rate appears to be greater than 80% for skin lesions [467,474,475]. It is used either for recalcitrant skin disease or as a corticosteroid-sparing agent [476] that can be effective for both pulmonary and cutaneous disease [453,475,477,478]. Patients need to be monitored for neutropenia, renal function, and liver and pulmonary

toxicity. Nausea can be reduced with folic acid supplementation [467,479] (Chapter 19). The response to methotrexate may take at least 6 months to achieve [476]. In a recent prospective study, patients receiving methotrexate have more improvement in cutaneous sarcoidosis activity and morphology instrument compared with the hydroxychloroquine and tetracycline groups [480].

Tetracycline. Several non-randomised studies suggest the utility of tetracyclines in cutaneous sarcoidosis [465,481–483]. Minocycline 100 mg twice daily achieved complete resolution of chronic cutaneous lesions in eight of 12 patients and partial response in two [481]. A recent study suggests that the response to minocycline is associated with the detection of *Propionibacterium acnes* in sarcoid cutaneous granulomas by immunochemistry [484]. However, poor response to tetracycline has been reported in lupus pernio [**485**]. Although the mechanism of action is unclear, an anti-inflammatory action of minocycline has been suggested [467]. Because of the relatively benign safety profile of tetracycline, proposed therapeutic strategies include initiating treatment with minocycline for 3 months; if the response is unsatisfactory, hydroxychloroquine can be added, and if the desired improvement is not achieved, methotrexate may then be added to the regimen [455].

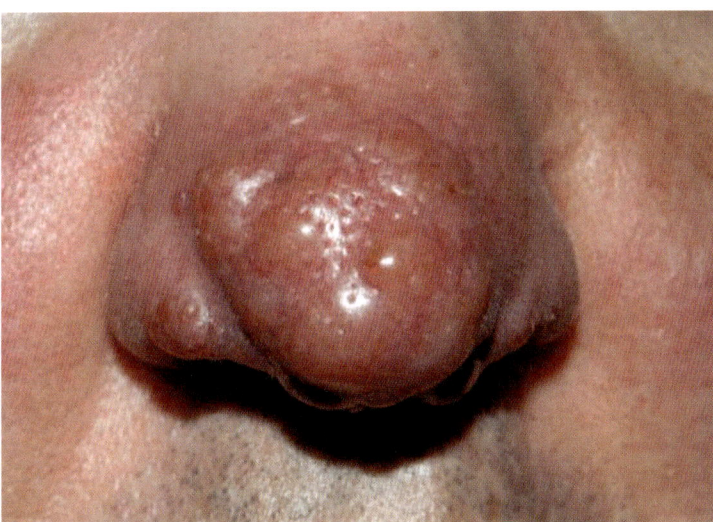

(a)

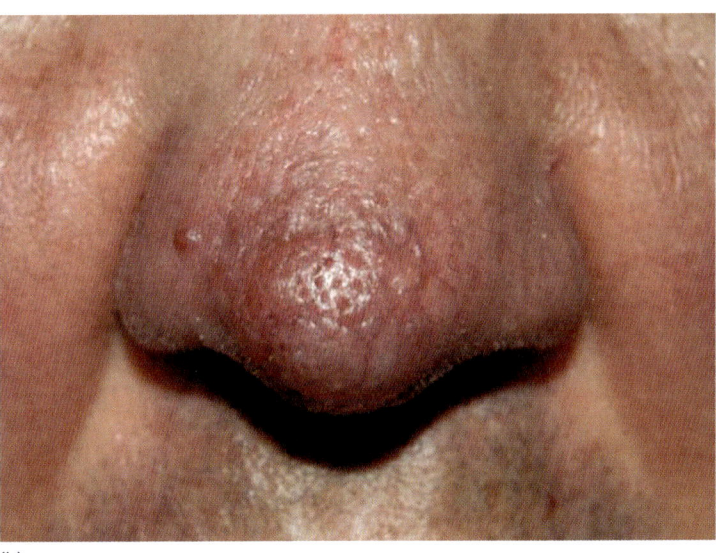

(b)

Figure 96.21 (a,b) Lupus pernio before and after treatment with hydroxychloroquine.

Third line

TNF-α antagonists. Although multiple cases of sarcoidosis induced by anti-TNF therapy have been reported [66,154,486–495], several studies support the use of infliximab as third line treatment for resistant cutaneous specific lesions of sarcoidosis [185,496–506], including a recent randomised clinical trial [507]. Screening for tuberculosis is mandatory before initiating TNF-α inhibitors and latent tuberculosis has to be treated. Not all TNF-α antagonist are effective in sarcoidosis. Several studies have also reported successful use of adalimumab [495,501,506,508–512]. Etanercept is generally not recommended [511,513–515].

Other reported treatments

Non-systemic. Non-systemic treatments claimed to be useful in isolated cases include topical tacrolimus [516–519], topical pimecrolimus [520,521], topical psoralen gel and ultraviolet A [522], surgical treatment [255,523–527] and topical photodynamic therapy [528–531]. Pulsed dye laser is the most used laser in cutaneous sarcoidosis [532–537]. Radiotherapy has rarely been used [538].

Systemic treatments. Isotretinoin [539–541], mycophenolate [542], allopurinol [543–547], pentoxiphylline [548], tacrolimus [549], fumaric acid esters [550,551], psoralens and ultraviolet A (PUVA) [453,552,553], tranilast [554,555], apremilast [556], chlorambucil [465,557], leflunomide [465,557,558] and melatonin [559,560] have occasionally been used with apparent benefit. The use of ciclosporin is controversial [465,557]. Thalidomide has been reported to be effective in patients unresponsive to other treatments [561–566]. However, its use is limited because of its teratogenicity and high risk of neuropathy [566,567], and a recent randomised trial does not encourage its use [568]. Antimycobacterial therapy reduced the diameter of lesions and disease severity of chronic cutaneous sarcoidosis in a recent survey [569]; however, the same treatment did not result in significant improvement in pulmonary sarcoidosis [570].

Several cases of cutaneous sarcoidosis responding to rituximab, JAK inhibitors (tofacinib and ruxolitinib) and tocilizumab have been recently reported [307,571–576].

Treatment ladder for cutaneous sarcoidosis

First line
- Mild to moderate disease
  - Potent topical corticosteroids
  - Intralesional triamcinolone acetonide 5–20 mg/mL every 3–4 weeks
- Severe disfigurement or lupus pernio
  - Prednisolone 20–60 mg/day until clinical response (usually 1–3 months), then tapered by 5–10 mg/week
  - Consider corticosteroid sparing agents when prednisolone cannot be lowered below 10 mg/day

Second line
- Minocycline 100 mg twice daily
- Hydroxychloroquine 200–400 mg/day
- Methotrexate 15 mg/week
  (All the above can be combined)

Third line
- TNF-α antagonists (for example, infliximab 5 mg/kg per week for 2 weeks, then once a month)

Cutaneous sarcoid reaction

The histopathological differential diagnosis between cutaneous lesions of systemic sarcoidosis and cutaneous sarcoid granulomas of other aetiology may be very difficult. For this reason, the detection of non-caseating granulomas in the skin is not sufficient to confirm the diagnosis of sarcoidosis in the absence of other organ involvement [3]. Those cases with cutaneous sarcoid granulomas of unknown aetiology are better considered as idiopathic sarcoid reactions. These patients should be followed up because some of them will develop involvement of other organs and thus fulfil the diagnostic criteria for sarcoidosis. Covid-induced sarcoid-like reaction has been recently reported [577].

Key references

The full list of references can be found in the online version at https://www.wiley.com/rooksdermatology10e

2 Grunewald J, Grutters JC, Arkema EV *et al*. Sarcoidosis. *Nat Rev Dis Primers* 2019;5–45.

3 Hunninghake GW, Costabel U, Ando M *et al*. ATS/ERS/WASOG Statement on sarcoidosis. *Sarcoidosis Vasc Diffuse Lung Dis* 1999;16:149–73 / *Am J Respir Crit Care Med* 1999;160:736–55.

4 Valeyre D, Prasse A, Nunes H *et al*. Sarcoidosis. *Lancet* 2014;383:1155–67.

48 Marcoval J, Mañá J, Moreno A *et al*. Foreign bodies in granulomatous cutaneous lesions of patients with systemic sarcoidosis. *Arch Dermatol* 2001;137:427–30.

219 Elgart ML. Cutaneous sarcoidosis: definitions and types of lesions. *Clin Dermatol* 1986;4:35–45.

233 Marcoval J, Mañá J, Rubio M. Specific cutaneous lesions in patients with systemic sarcoidosis: relationship to severity and chronicity of disease. *Clin Exp Dermatol* 2011;36:739–44.

238 Veien NK, Stahl D, Brodthagen H. Cutaneous sarcoidosis in caucasians. *J Am Acad Dermatol* 1987;16:534–40.

452 Crouser ED, Maier LA, Wilson KC *et al*. Diagnosis and detection of sarcoidosis. An official American Thoracic Society clinical practice guideline. *Am J Respir Crit Care Med* 2020;201:e26–e51.

485 Stagaki E, Mountford WK, Lackland DT, Judson MA. The treatment of lupus pernio: results of 116 treatment courses in 54 patients. *Chest* 2009;135:468–76.

507 Baughman RP, Judson MA, Lower EE *et al*. Infliximab for chronic cutaneous sarcoidosis: a subset analysis from a double-blind randomized clinical trial. *Sarcoidosis Vasc Diffuse Lung Dis* 2016;32:289–95.

CHAPTER 97

Panniculitis

Luis Requena[1] *and Lorenzo Cerroni*[2]

[1]Department of Dermatology, Fundación Jiménez Díaz, Universidad Autónoma, Madrid, Spain
[2]Department of Dermatology, Medical University of Graz, Graz, Austria

Anatomy and physiology of subcutaneous fat

Introduction

In order to appreciate how subcutaneous fat responds to inflammation, it is important to understand its structure and function. Subcutaneous tissue (subcutis) is composed predominantly of fat cells embedded in a connective tissue framework (Figure 97.1). Subcutaneous fat is present almost universally over the body surface between the skin and the deep fascia and, in the normal state, constitutes about 10% of body weight (Figure 97.2). It forms a specialised, closely regulated metabolic reserve capable of storing or rapidly releasing energy, typically providing sufficient for about 40 days' requirements [1]. Subcutaneous fat acts as an insulating layer against heat loss and a protective cushion against external injury. It also provides structural support to the overlying skin and has a cosmetic function, for example in the contours of the face.

Subcutaneous fat is absent from the eyelids and the male genitalia. There are obvious sexual differences in the distribution of fat around the body surface, with an increase in thickness resulting in the rounded contours of the female trunk, breasts, hips, pubis and thighs. Subcutaneous fat also varies in thickness with the race, age and endocrine and nutritional status of the individual.

Brown fat in particular has a very important thermoregulatory role and acts by increasing the basal metabolic rate [2]. This is particularly important in infancy, and heat production in response to cold exposure is maximal in neonates, who have large quantities of brown fat.

Cellular composition of subcutaneous tissue [3,4]

The first fat-containing cell, the pre-adipocyte, appears in the mesenchyme around the 14th week of fetal life. The primitive mesenchymal cell that forms the determined pre-adipocyte is also capable of maturing to form a fibrocyte, myocyte, chondrocyte or osteoblast. Pre-adipocytes can terminally differentiate into either brown adipocytes or white adipocytes.

Brown fat is a special type of granular fat that differs from white fat in its distribution, histology and function. It is multilocular and is metabolically very active with many mitochondria, so that it is capable of transferring energy from food to produce heat. As it has

Rook's Textbook of Dermatology, Tenth Edition. Edited by Christopher Griffiths, Jonathan Barker, Tanya Bleiker, Walayat Hussain and Rosalind Simpson.
© 2024 John Wiley & Sons Ltd. Published 2024 by John Wiley & Sons Ltd.

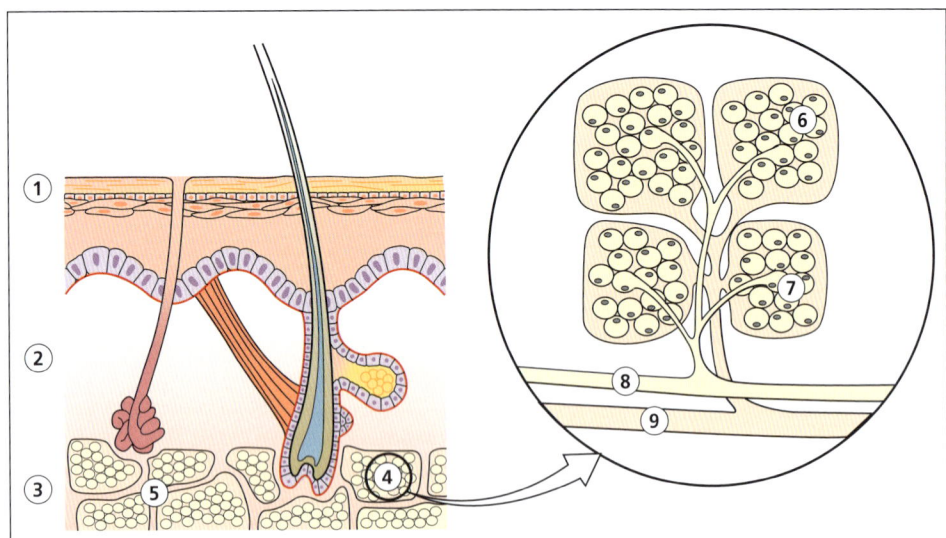

Figure 97.1 Schematic representation of the anatomy of subcutaneous fat with detailed view showing the vascular supply to the fat lobule and its constituent microlobules. 1, epidermis; 2, dermis; 3, subcutis; 4, fat lobule; 5, connective tissue septum; 6, adipocyte; 7, arteriole; 8, artery; 9, vein.

a much greater capillary network surrounding it compared with white fat (which is partly responsible for the brown colour), heat can be rapidly transferred into the circulation. It is most prominent in the neck and upper thorax of the fetus, and it may be homologous to the hibernating gland fat found in some animals [5]. Brown fat is now known to persist into adult life [6], and it may have a role in preventing obesity [6]. Warm patches develop in the skin 1 h after taking ephedrine orally, and these warm patches may indicate the site of thermogenic brown fat. Brown and white fat may be distinguished using ^{18}F fluorodeoxyglucose positron emission tomography (FDG-PET) [7].

Brown fat adipocyte mitochondria uniquely express uncoupling protein 1 (UCP-1), allowing confirmation that brown fat is present in adult white fat depots in variable amounts, and that transdifferentiation from white to brown adipocytes can occur. Development of brown fat begins at the 20th week of gestation, reaches its maximum at birth and then diminishes so that there are no large collections of brown fat in the adult, though FDG-PET suggests that some adults have supraclavicular areas of brown fat [8]. Evidence for cold induction by brown fat as an adaptive response in humans is at present equivocal [8].

White fat adipocytes are the largest connective tissue cells in the body, with a diameter of up to 100 µm. Much of their differentiation occurs soon after birth. The mature adipocyte has a characteristic signet-ring appearance, because the flat, oval nucleus is displaced to the side by a single, large, intracellular, fat-containing vacuole, which is surrounded by perilipin. Originally thought of as an inert store for emergency supplies of energy when necessary, it is now realised that the white adipocyte has a huge array of functions, secreting factors (adipokines) that affect lipid and glucose metabolism, endocrine functions, blood pressure control, coagulation, fibrinolysis, angiogenesis and inflammation. For a full review the reader is referred to Frühbeck [4].

Anatomy of subcutaneous tissue

Subcutaneous tissue is widely distributed throughout the body, forming a true organ as regards both structure and function [1]. Groups of adipocytes are arranged in lobules, each measuring approximately 1 cm in diameter; they are separated from each other by interlobular septa composed of collagen and reticulin fibres. Each lobule may be subdivided into 1 mm diameter microlobules, which represent the functional unit of the subcutaneous fat. Each microlobule is composed of a group of adipocytes arrayed around a central arteriole and surrounded by capillaries and postcapillary venules. Arteries and veins of the subcutis run along the septa (Figure 97.1). Each individual fat lobule is supplied by a small muscular artery (250–500 µm diameter) branching from the septa to form arterioles (up to 100 µm diameter) that supply every individual microlobule. Each arteriole branches to form a network of capillaries that surrounds each individual adipocyte. In addition to an abundant blood supply, subcutaneous fat also contains a rich lymphatic plexus, which receives vessels from the dermis. These lymph vessels traverse the subcutaneous layer parallel to the skin surface for some distance, before eventually penetrating the deep fascia and draining into the regional lymph nodes. The nature of the adipocyte and its relationship to blood vessels and lymphatics has been reviewed in detail by Ryan and Curri [9]. Both white fat and brown fat are innervated by noradrenergic fibres of the sympathetic nervous system and parasympathetic fibres.

The adipocytes may comprise only 25% of the total cell population of a lobule; the remainder, the stroma–vascular fraction, are macrophages, fibroblasts, mast cells, pericytes, endothelial cells and pre-adipocytes, enabling considerable cross-talk between cells by means of locally secreted cytokines including leptin and adiponectin (see later in this chapter).

All fat tissue is composed of lobules of fat cells with their supporting connective and stroma–vascular tissue. In addition to the subcutaneous fat, approximately 20% of fat tissue occurs internally, in the mediastinal and retroperitoneal tissues, the mesentery and the bone marrow and in and around individual organs, including blood vessels. This tissue, although it is widely scattered throughout the body, forms a true organ as regards both structure and function [1] but in which depot-specific differences occur [10]. For example, increases in subcutaneous upper body and visceral fat are associated with an increased cardiovascular and metabolic

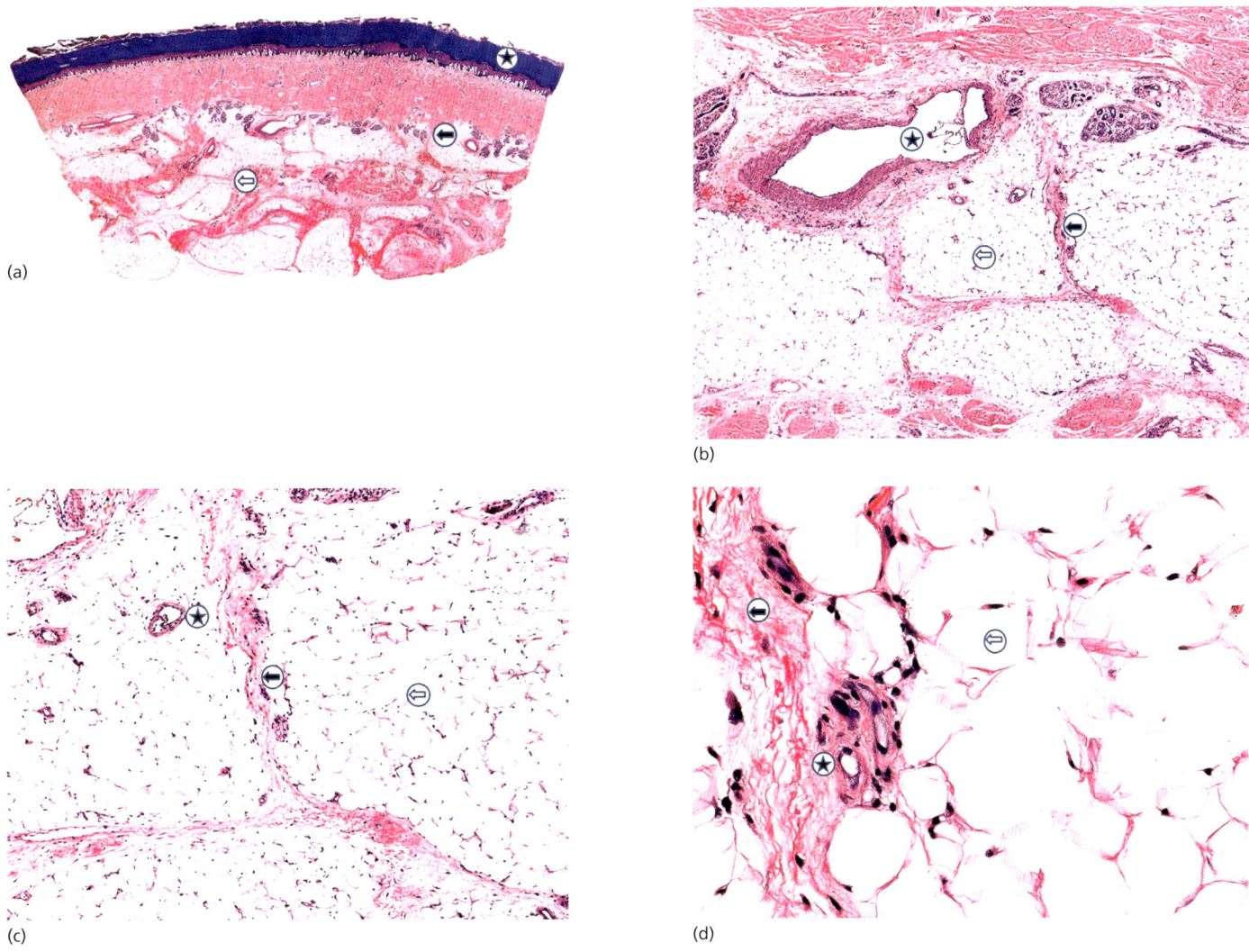

Figure 97.2 (a) Scanning power view of the normal skin of the sole. The epidermis is covered by a thick, compact, orthokeratotic horny layer (star). Numerous eccrine units are seen along the interface between the deep reticular dermis and subcutis (black arrow). The subcutis is organised into lobules of adipocytes and connective tissue septa (white arrow) surrounding and demarcating each fat lobule, and associated vessels and nerves. (b) At higher magnification, a large vein (star) may be identified in the deeper dermis because of the presence of valves within its lumen. The subcutis is composed of thin connective tissue septa (black arrow), which delimit lobules of adipocytes (white arrow). (c) At even higher magnification, a small venule is seen within the fat lobule (star), as well as the thin septa of connective septa (black arrow) and mature adipocytes of the fat lobule (white arrow). (d) Still higher magnification shows that the connective tissue septa are mostly composed of thin collagen bundles (black arrow). A capillary is seen at the periphery of the fat lobule (star). With H&E stain, adipocytes appear as empty cells with signet-ring morphology. This is due to the fact that the lipid content dissolves in routinely processed specimens and the flat spindle nucleus is displaced to the periphery of the cell by a single, large, intracytoplasmic vacuole, which contains fat (white arrow).

risk but increases in gluteo-femoral subcutaneous fat are not [11]. In addition, perivascular adipose tissue shows increased angiogenesis compared with subcutaneous fat [12]. The fact that some genetic lipodystrophy patients lose peripheral fat but fat padding for absorption of mechanical pressure is maintained, is further evidence for depot-specific differences.

The combination of the obesity epidemic and the advent of liposuction has rekindled interest in the structure of subcutaneous fat with magnetic resonance imaging (MRI) scanning [13] and ultrasound [14] as investigative tools. Subcutaneous fat is divided by the superficial fascia into two compartments: superficial and deep. The fat mass in the superficial (areolar) layer is compartmentalised into lobules by vertical and oblique fibrous septal planes and bands, while that of the deeper (lamellar) layer has its septae more horizontally positioned. The superficial layer is fairly constant, but the

deeper is more variable, with an increase in fat mass accumulating between the split horizontal septae. In females, subcutaneous fat is most abundant in the gluteo-femoral region and breasts, resulting in the so-called gynaecoid distribution, whereas in males the android distribution of shoulders and upper arms, neck and lumbo-sacral area predominates.

Physiology of adipose tissue

Traditionally, adipose tissue was regarded as an inert energy store with insulating and padding properties. While storage is still a major function, there is now an appreciation that adipocytes and their stroma–vascular tissue have many other highly complex and dynamic actions, including energy homeostasis, adipogenesis, insulin sensitivity and influences on immune and inflammatory responses [3,4,15–18] (Chapter 150).

Energy homeostasis

A major function of white adipose tissue is to store energy at times of calorie excess and release it when needed, such as during exercise or starvation. The synthesis (anabolism) and catabolism of fat in the subcutaneous depot depends on many factors, including nourishment and endocrine and neural activity. The role of the autonomic nervous system in regulating fat metabolism is now well established [19], being particularly important for rapid energy need compared with the slower control exerted by neuroendocrine factors [20]. A decrease in parasympathetic activity results in increased lipolysis, as does an increase in sympathetic activity, with the opposites stimulating lipogenesis [21]. Hormones that may affect the energy metabolism of fat cells include insulin, cortisol, norepinephrine (noradrenaline) and several pituitary hormones, including somatotrophin, adrenocorticotrophic hormone (ACTH), thyrotrophin, lipotrophin and natriurietic peptide [22].

The fats contained within adipocytes are predominantly triglycerides (triacylglycerols), especially those of palmitic and stearic acids and the unsaturated oleic acid. All the fatty acids have an even number of carbon atoms, predominantly C16 and C18, with a few C14 and C12. Adipose tissue contains 10–30% of water with a small proportion of lipochromes, and less than 2% cholesterol. Fat-soluble substances are also present in varying amounts. These include fat-soluble vitamins and traces of chlorinated hydrocarbons (e.g. aldrin, dieldrin) ingested with the diet, as well as drugs such as acitretin. Adipose tissue *in vitro* has a metabolic rate similar to that of kidney tissue, and approximately half that of liver. Approximately half the triglyceride in the adipose tissue of rats and mice is catabolised and reconstituted in the course of a week or so.

The fat for storage enters the adipocyte as fatty acids, having been converted from lipoproteins by the extracellular enzyme lipoprotein lipase (Figure 97.3). The fatty acids combine with coenzyme A, using the energy of adenosine triphosphate (ATP), to form the corresponding acetyl coenzyme A compounds. Some of these are then oxidised to provide energy for the regeneration of ATP, but most are converted to triglyceride by combination with glycerol-3-phosphate derived from glucose.

The adipocyte is one of the few cells to express the insulin-dependent glucose transporter receptor 4 (GLUT-4), which mediates the passage of glucose into the cell and thus facilitates triglyceride formation within the adipocyte via *de novo* lipogenesis, the latter providing only a small contribution to the pool. At the same time, insulin inhibits hydrolysis and breakdown of triglyceride, conserving the energy store.

When the body requires energy, lipolysis occurs. Triglyceride is hydrolysed in the adipocyte, converted to non-esterified fatty acids (NEFAs) and glycerol, the rate-limiting enzyme being hormone-sensitive lipase (HSL). The NEFAs are conveyed in the blood to tissues such as the liver and muscle, in which fatty acid oxidation readily takes place. In both tissues, the essential part of the process consists of the oxidation in the mitochondria of the long-chain fatty acids. The glycerol of the triglyceride molecule reacts with ATP to form glycerol phosphate, which is oxidised to glyceraldehyde-3-phosphate. This in turn may either be converted to glycogen by reversal of glycolysis, or it may be converted to pyruvate. Skeletal muscle readily oxidises fatty acids but glucose, if available, is preferentially used. In cardiac muscle, fatty acids are a major source of energy. Lipolysis is regulated predominantly through insulin and catecholamines. The latter, elevated during a sudden energy demand, bind to β-adrenergic receptors on the adipocyte and activate HSL through the classic adenosine monophosphate–protein kinase A (AMP- PKA) pathway.

Role of leptin

Leptin is an adipokine involved in energy homeostasis that may have evolved to help adaptation from the starved to the adequately nourished state rather than to prevent obesity [23]. Leptin, a product of the *ob* gene, is a 16 kDa polypeptide comprising 167 amino

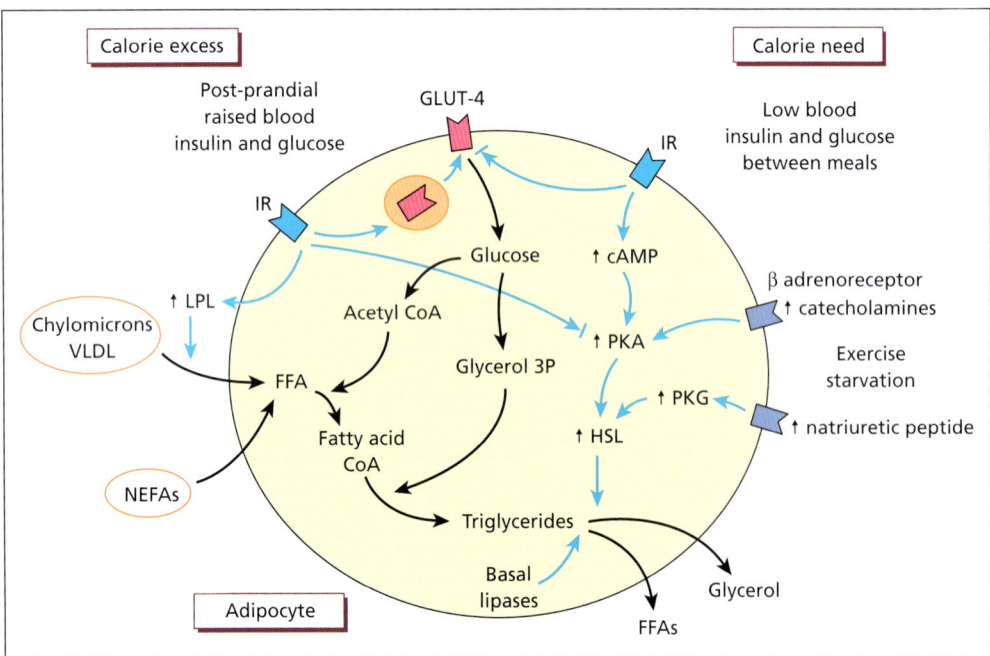

Figure 97.3 Simplified outline of lipogenesis in an adipocyte during energy excess and lipolysis during calorie need. The effects of hormones and enzymes are in blue. cAMP, cyclic adenosine monophosphate; CoA, coenzyme A; FFA, free fatty acid; GLUT-4, glucose transporter receptor 4; HSL, hormone-sensitive lipase; IR, insulin resistance; LPL, lipoprotein lipase; NEFAs, non-esterified fatty acids; 3P, 3-phosphate; PKA, protein kinase A; PKG, protein kinase G; VLDL, very low-density lipoprotein.

acids with a structural homology similar to other cytokine proteins such as tumour necrosis factor α (TNF-α) and interleukin 6 (IL-6). It is secreted by adipocytes predominantly, but also by the stomach, aiding immediate appetite control. Leptin receptors are present in the hypothalamus, on adipocytes, skeletal muscle, liver, pancreatic β cells, ovary and endometrium. The main effect of leptin is via the satiety centres in the hypothalamus. If excess energy is being stored, rising leptin levels stimulate the satiety centres to reduce appetite. Conversely, during starvation low leptin levels stimulate appetite. Circulating levels of leptin correlate with increasing body mass index (BMI), but have little effect on the satiety centres, indicating an apparent leptin resistance. Leptin also influences several other functions, including neuroendocrine and reproductive functions, insulin secretion and blood pressure. Patients with congenital leptin deficiency (Chapter 72) have gross obesity, hyperphagia, delayed pubertal development, abnormal T-cell number and function, and altered thyroid and growth hormone function [24]. In addition, leptin has a role in immune function and inflammation [25]. There is increased expression in chondrocytes and leptin may have a part to play in articular degenerative disease.

Adipogenesis

Adipogenesis refers to the recruitment from multipotent stem cells in the mesenchyme and stroma–vascular tissue, and proliferation of pre-adipocytes followed by their differentiation into mature fat cells. Culture of cell lines has led to the elucidation of many of the transcriptional factors involved in adipogenesis, the major ones being peroxisome proliferator-activated receptor γ (PPAR-γ) and the CCAAT enhancer binding proteins (C/EBPs). The precise contribution of adipogenesis towards enlargement of the fat organ at different stages of human development and life changes is uncertain, but it seems maximal before and around birth before diminishing, then possibly continuing at a low rate throughout adult life. Glucocorticoids, growth hormone and insulin stimulate cells to terminal differentiation, but when mature fat cells reach a certain size, recruitment occurs so that the fat organ enlarges through hyperplasia (increased numbers of cells) rather than hypertrophy (increase in size of cells). Control of this hyperplastic response may come from local adipocytes through paracrine effects involving local growth factors. During adipogenesis the local extracellular matrix also changes, the effects of which might play their own role in differentiation. This is supported by the fact that fat tissue repair is improved if elements of this matrix are included with the donor adipocytes.

Insulin sensitivity

Insulin secretion, stimulated by raised blood glucose levels after meals to reverse hyperglycaemia, has two major effects. It facilitates glucose uptake into most of the body's cells (liver, skeletal muscle and adipocytes) and it suppresses glucose output by the liver. Insulin resistance occurs when a target organ fails to respond normally to insulin, resulting in hyperinsulinaemia. The effect may be incomplete suppression of hepatic glucose output in the liver and/or impaired insulin-mediated glucose uptake in peripheral tissues, including adipocytes. If increased insulin secretion cannot prevent hyperglycaemia, type 2 diabetes results. Adipocytes secrete

many factors, some of which have direct and indirect effects on insulin sensitivity.

Adiponectin

Adiponectin is a 30 kDa protein composed of 244 amino acids with some structural similarity to both collagen and complement C1q and is currently thought to be secreted exclusively by adipocytes [26–28]. It has autocrine/paracrine effects locally within adipose tissue as well as endocrine effects distantly. Locally, it can promote pre-adipocytes to become mature fat cells, which with increasing cell size downregulate their adiponectin secretion to exert some feedback control. Adiponectin receptors are present in many tissues as well as adipocytes. It is likely that adiponectin receptor-activated AMPK (AMP-activated protein kinase) leads to enhanced insulin signalling and therefore insulin sensitivity. If BMI is elevated, the expression of adiponectin is reduced in visceral adipose tissue (VAT) adipocytes in comparison with that in subcutaneous adipose tissue (SAT). Serum adiponectin levels fall with weight gain and rise with weight loss.

Additionally, adiponectin exerts protective anti-inflammatory effects both locally and distantly. Local effects are mediated by inhibiting secretion of IL-6, IL-8, macrophage inflammatory protein 1 and monocyte chemotactic protein 1. It also has distant effects by its direct action on a range of cells including monocytes/ macrophages, endothelial cells, hepatocytes and muscle cells, and indirectly by inhibition of TNF-α production.

There is an as yet unexplained paradox concerning adiponectin and its anti-inflammatory effects. Obesity is associated with macrophages in VAT that generate factors, particularly TNF-α, that suppress adiponectin secretion. However, low levels of adiponectin promote inflammation, generating a self-sustaining loop: thus, in obesity, adiponectin levels are inversely correlated with levels of inflammatory markers. In autoimmune states such as rheumatoid arthritis and systemic lupus erythematosus, adiponectin levels are raised, the level positively correlating with inflammatory markers. To explain this, it has been suggested that the adiponectin system has evolved as a mechanism for adaptation to starvation, a catabolic state [29]. It is therefore raised in other catabolic states such as autoimmune disease and inflammatory bowel disease, and did not evolve as a protective device against insulin resistance.

Other adipokines

Many other adipokines have been described [4,18] and most are still being evaluated for their relevance to human biology. The stroma–vascular tissue itself is also responsible for a variety of cytokines. Macrophages secrete TNF-α, IL-1, IL-6, IL-8, IL-10, monocyte chemoattractant protein 1 (MCP-1), macrophage migration inhibitory factor (MIF), angiotensinogen and endothelial and vascular growth factors. Therefore, as well as affecting energy homeostasis, insulin sensitivity and adipocyte differentiation, the fat organ has influences on inflammation, immune function, vascular inflammation and neoangiogenesis. All of this lends credence to the concept of the fat organ being an endocrine organ in its own right. While these discoveries are of the utmost importance for worldwide obesity-associated morbidity and mortality, their relevance in disorders of subcutaneous fat other than lipodystrophies is unclear.

PANNICULITIS

Introduction and general description

Inflammatory diseases involving the subcutaneous fat comprise a heterogeneous group of disorders named generically panniculitis. These diseases have been classically considered diagnostically challenging both for clinicians and dermatopathologists; the reasons for this difficulty are varied. Firstly, dermatologists usually evaluate different morphological aspects of the skin anomalies to reach a specific diagnosis, but subcutaneous tissue is too deep to be visible to the examining eye. Moreover, cutaneous lesions of panniculitis usually show a disappointing monotony with completely different diseases involving the subcutaneous tissue showing the same clinical morphology, namely reddish nodules located preferentially on the lower extremities. Secondly, because the lesions are situated deep in subcutaneous tissue, large incisional biopsies are necessary for diagnosis, which is usually based on the correct evaluation of the pattern of the inflammatory infiltrate and the involvement of blood vessels. This requires at the very least that the biopsy specimen should include a fat lobule and its surrounding connective tissue septa, but many dermatologists perform superficial or small biopsies which are not diagnostic. Thirdly, many panniculitides are also histopathologically unsatisfactory, because subcutaneous fat has a limited range of responses and a variety of insults and panniculitic processes of entirely different aetiologies may produce very similar histopathological changes. Moreover, before an accurate histopathological diagnosis may be established, it must be remembered that panniculitides, like other inflammatory cutaneous disorders, are dynamic processes in which both the distribution and composition of the inflammatory cells of the infiltrate may change rapidly over the course of a few days: when biopsies are taken from late or resolving lesions, especially in predominantly lobular panniculitis, they may show completely non-specific findings. For the aforementioned reasons, some authorities have considered that 'the histological septal–lobular dichotomy is sometimes diagnostically useful, but more often there is a mixed picture that adds to interpretative difficulties' [1].

Despite these potential pitfalls, serial sections of an adequate biopsy enable the dermatopathologist in most cases to classify the panniculitic process as either a predominantly septal or a predominantly lobular panniculitis. This first classification step into one of the two general categories of panniculitis is very helpful for diagnostic purposes. However, classification of a panniculitis into a predominantly septal or predominantly lobular panniculitis is no more than an initial descriptive working classification and it should be followed by a search for additional histopathological clues to help reach a more specific, clinically relevant, final diagnosis. Thus, the next diagnostic step requires assessment of whether vasculitis is or is not present and, when it is present, of the size and nature of the involved blood vessels. The final diagnostic step requires the microscopic identification of the composition of the inflammatory

infiltrate involving the septa and/or the fat lobule, the type of adipocyte necrosis and a search for additional histopathological features to enable a specific diagnosis to be reached. Table 97.1 provides a working classification of the panniculitides using this approach for diagnosis [2,3].

There is probably no individual cell of the human body with a better vascular supply than the adipocyte. Postcapillary venules drain into veins which also run along the septa. In each microlobule, the arteriole occupies a central position, whereas the venule runs along the periphery [4]. As a consequence, interference with the arterial supply results in dramatic necrotic changes within the fat lobule (predominantly lobular panniculitis), while venous disorders manifest by alterations in the septal and paraseptal areas (predominantly septal panniculitis) [5]. This peculiar distribution of the vascularisation in subcutaneous tissue explains why large-vessel vasculitis involving the septal vessels is usually accompanied by little inflammation of the fat lobules, whereas vasculitis involving small blood vessels of the lobule usually causes extensive necrosis of the centrilobular adipocytes and a dense inflammatory response. In contrast with the dermal vascular network, the blood supply of each subcutaneous microlobule is terminal, implying there are no vascular connections between adjacent microlobules or between the dermis and subcutaneous fat. The septa of the subcutaneous fat also contain a prominent lymphatic plexus, which comes from the dermis and traverses the subcutis, first, parallel to the surface of the skin, and then vertically penetrating the underlying fascia and draining into regional lymph nodes. The connective tissue septa, which are contiguous with the overlying reticular traverses and with the underlying fascia, provide stability to the subcutaneous tissue by compartmentalising it. The normal septa are thin, from 200 to 300 μm, and are composed mostly of collagen bundles and thin elastic and reticulin fibres.

Mature, normal individual adipocytes are relatively large cells with a diameter up to 100 mm and, in formalin-fixed and haematoxylin and eosin (H&E) stained sections, appear as empty cells with signet-ring morphology. This is due to the fact that the lipid and triglyceride content dissolves in routinely processed specimens and the single, large intracytoplasmic vacuole displaces the flat spindle nucleus without discernible nuclear features to the periphery of the cell. Frozen sections and special stains such as oil red O or Sudan B are required to demonstrate the lipid contents within the cytoplasm of mature adipocytes, but are not necessary for diagnostic purposes.

Perivascular adipocytes have been also demonstrated to be powerful endocrine cells capable of responding to metabolic changes and transducing signals to adjacent blood vessels. Cross-talk between perivascular adipose tissue and blood vessels is now being intensely investigated. There is evidence suggesting that perivascular adipose tissue regulates vascular function through a variety of mechanisms and plays an important role in inflammation and vasoreactivity in subcutaneous tissue [6]. Adipocytes also interact with the immune system. Normal subcutaneous fat contains T lymphocytes located between adipocytes of the fat lobule. They differ from those of other tissues and vary between different regions of the body [7]. It has recently been demonstrated that cytotoxic T lymphocytes precede the accumulation of macrophages during the process of inflammation of the fat lobule. *In vitro* co-cultures have shown a vicious cycle of interaction between cytotoxic T lymphocytes, macrophages and

Table 97.1 Classification of the panniculitides.

Diagnostic feature	Disorder
Predominantly septal panniculitides	
With vasculitis	
Veins	Superficial migratory thrombophlebitis
Arteries	Cutaneous polyarteritis nodosa (cutaneous arteritis)
No vasculitis	
Lymphocytes and plasma cells predominantly:	
With granulomatous infiltrate in septa	Necrobiosis lipoidica
No granulomatous infiltrate in septa	Deep morphoea
Histiocytes predominantly (granulomatous):	
With mucin in centre of palisaded granulomas	Subcutaneous granuloma annulare
With fibrin in centre of palisaded granulomas	Rheumatoid nodule
With large areas of degenerate collagen, foamy histiocytes and cholesterol clefts	Necrobiotic xanthogranuloma
Without mucin, fibrin or degeneration of collagen, but with radial granulomas in septa	Erythema nodosum
Predominantly lobular panniculitides	
With vasculitis	
Small vessels: venules	Erythema nodosum leprosum
	Erythema induratum of Bazin
Large vessels: arteries	Erythema induratum of Bazin
No vasculitis	
Few or no inflammatory cells:	
Necrosis at the centre of the lobule	Sclerosing panniculitis (lipodermatosclerosis)
With vascular calcification	Calcific uraemic arteriolopathy (calciphylaxis)
Lymphocytes predominant:	
With superficial and deep perivascular dermal infiltrate	Cold panniculitis
With lymphoid follicles, plasma cells, clusters of plasmacytoid dendritic cells and nuclear dust of lymphocytes	Lupus panniculitis Panniculitis associated with dermatomyositis
Neutrophils predominant:	
Extensive fat necrosis with saponification of adipocytes	Pancreatic panniculitis
With neutrophils between collagen bundles of deep reticular dermis	α_1-antitrypsin deficiency panniculitis
With bacteria, fungi or protozoa	Infective panniculitis
With foreign bodies	Factitious panniculitis
Neutrophilic lobular panniculitis	Subcutaneous Sweet syndrome
	Drug-induced (checkpoint inhibitor drugs) panniculitis
Histiocytes predominant (granulomatous):	
No crystals in adipocytes	Subcutaneous sarcoidosis
	Traumatic panniculitis
With crystals in histiocytes or adipocytes	Subcutaneous fat necrosis of the newborn
	Poststeroid panniculitis
	Sclerema neonatorum
	Gouty panniculitis
	Fungal panniculitis due to zygomycosis, mucormycosis and aspergillosis
With cytophagic histiocytes	Cytophagic histiocytic panniculitis, subcutaneous gamma/delta T-cell lymphoma and some cases of subcutaneous panniculitis-like T-cell lymphoma[a]
With sclerosis of the septa	Sclerosing postirradiation panniculitis

[a] Although these disorders are characterised by a neoplastic proliferation of cytotoxic or gamma/delta T lymphocytes rather than an authentic panniculitic process, they are included in the classification of the panniculitides because they may mimic panniculitis both clinically and histopathologically.

adipocytes, suggesting that adipocytes activate cytotoxic T lymphocytes with subsequent recruitment and activation of macrophages [8]. That there is an interaction between adipocytes and lymphocytes is also supported by the demonstration on human adipocytes of the inflammatory receptor CD40, which contributes to intercellular cross-talk between adipocytes and lymphocytes [9]. Co-cultures of adipocytes and lymphocytes have also shown upregulation of pro-inflammatory cytokines, including IL-6, MCP-1 and plasminogen activator inhibitor 1 (PAI-1), but downregulation of leptin and adiponectin [9].

Immunohistochemically, adipocytes express S-100 protein, with staining around the periphery of the cell, and vimentin [10]. In contrast with the multivacuolated cytoplasm of sebocytes and foamy histiocytes, which express adipophilin, the single large cytoplasmic vacuole of the adipocyte is adipophilin negative [11,12].

Pattern-based histopathological classification of panniculitis with large-vessel vasculitis also requires ascertainment of whether the involved vessel is an artery or a vein. A peculiarity of the veins in the subcutaneous fat of the lower limbs is that they have a thick muscular layer, conferring upon them an 'arterial' appearance [13]. However, it is usually possible to establish this distinction with confidence from H&E preparations, because the middle layer of subcutaneous veins is composed of several muscular fascicles separated by tiny unstained elastic fibres, whereas arteries show a more compact muscular layer. Nevertheless, many authors continue to promote the misleading notion that arteries of the subcutaneous fat of the lower legs have a thicker muscular layer than veins, when in fact veins often have a thicker muscular layer than arteries [13]. In difficult cases, elastic tissue staining allows definite discrimination between artery and vein, because arteries have a well-demarcated, thick and sharp internal elastic membrane, whereas veins have an ill-defined, thin and multilayered internal elastic lamina and tiny elastic fibres interspersed between muscular fascicles of the middle layer of the vessel wall. Some authors, however, believe that when inflammation is present within and around the wall of the vessel, all of the studied histological features become less reliable, and that the interobserver reliability of distinguishing arteritis from thrombophlebitis is low [14].

Types of necrosis of the adipocytes

The appearance of necrotic adipocytes is polymorphous and different from other necrotic cells [15–17]. In classic histopathology, nuclear abnormalities such as pyknosis, karyorrhesis and karyolysis are signs of cellular necrosis. In contrast, necrotic adipocytes, regardless of the aetiology of the cell death, show great variability and may appear as either anucleate cells or with complete disintegration of the cellular structure. Unfortunately, these distinctive forms of adipocyte necrosis have little value for diagnostic specificity.

Often, the only sign of necrosis of the adipocytes is the lack of nuclei in the involved cells, and dead fat cells appear as round empty bags with no inflammatory infiltrate among them. The most frequent type of adipocyte necrosis is *lipophagic necrosis*, which consists of the replacement of necrotic adipocytes by foamy macrophages formed by the engulfing of lipid products released from dead adipocytes by macrophages. These lipophages appear quite different from normal adipocytes, with large, pale, microvacuolated or granular-like cytoplasm and round, central, vesicular nuclei.

Lipophagic granulomatous inflammation, however, is entirely non-specific and many lobular panniculitides show this pattern of fat necrosis at their late or resolving stages. It is usually seen in lipodermatosclerosis and traumatic panniculitis, but may also be present in erythema nodosum and erythema induratum of Bazin.

In contrast, *liquefactive fat necrosis* is a more specific pattern of adipocyte necrosis and it is more often seen in α_1-antitrypsin deficiency panniculitis and in pancreatic panniculitis. Necrotic adipocytes injured by this mechanism appear as granular wisps of amphophilic detritus and their cellular structures are no longer evident. Enzymatic fat necrosis is a specific type of liquefactive fat necrosis characteristically observed in pancreatic panniculitis. It is due to saponification of the adipocyte lipid contents by pancreatic lipase, with secondary deposition of calcium salts, resulting in so-called ghost adipocytes that consist of adipocytes with no nuclei and granular basophilic cytoplasm.

Hyalinising fat necrosis is characteristically observed in lupus panniculitis and panniculitis associated with dermatomyositis. In this pattern, necrotic adipocytes appear as mummified anucleated cells, which are surrounded by glassy homogeneous proteinaceous material, effacing the architecture of the fat lobule.

Membranous fat necrosis is also a late-stage and non-specific type of necrosis of adipocytes, in which a leathery eosinophilic or amphophilic rim of collapsed cellular organelles with a crenulated or arabesque appearance is seen: periodic acid–Schiff (PAS) and Sudan III staining is positive. When membranous fat necrosis is extensive, formation of cystic structures devoid of cellular components and lined by hyaline-crenulated membrane can be observed. Membranous and membrano-cystic fat necrosis are almost always seen in lipodermatosclerosis, but like other types of fat necrosis, they may also be seen in late-stage lesions of several types of panniculitis.

Ischaemic fat necrosis is more frequently seen at the centre of fat lobules and is characterised by pallor of adipocytes, which are smaller than normal due to severe impairment of blood supply. Later stages of ischaemic necrosis also show lipophagic granulomas. Ischaemic fat necrosis is frequently seen in erythema induratum of Bazin, but may also be observed in other panniculitides, including calcific uraemic arteriolopathy (calciphylaxis), infectious panniculitis and cutaneous polyarteritis nodosa.

Finally, *basophilic fat necrosis* results from the necrosis of adipocytes intermingled with nuclear dust of neutrophils and granular basophilic material, which represent aggregations of bacteria, and is characteristically seen in cases of infectious panniculitis.

There are some disorders that should no longer be considered as specific variants of panniculitis. *Weber–Christian disease* is the term that has been classically used to refer to cases of predominantly lobular panniculitis without vasculitis in association with systemic manifestations including fever and involvement of visceral fat tissue. Additional terms such as idiopathic nodular panniculitis, nodular panniculitis and relapsing febrile non-suppurative nodular panniculitis have been used as synonyms for Weber–Christian disease. However, many cases originally considered as examples of Weber–Christian disease were later reclassified when other variants of lobular panniculitis, including erythema induratum of Bazin (nodular vasculitis), pancreatic panniculitis and α_1-antitrypsin deficiency panniculitis, were separated as specific diseases. White and Winkelmann [18] reviewed the clinical and histopathological features of 30 cases of panniculitis previously diagnosed as Weber–Christian disease at the Mayo Clinic and most of the cases could be reclassified: 12 cases as erythema nodosum, six cases as superficial thrombophlebitis (STP), five cases as factitious panniculitis, three cases as traumatic panniculitis and individual cases as cytophagic histiocytic panniculitis, subcutaneous 'panniculitic' lymphoma and subcutaneous involvement by leukaemia. The authors concluded that the term Weber–Christian disease should be abandoned as a diagnosis for cases of lobular panniculitis because now a more specific diagnosis may be reached in the majority of cases. The same is true for *Rothmann–Makai disease*, a term that was used previously to describe cases of relapsing nodular panniculitis similar to that of Weber–Christian disease but with no fever or other systemic manifestations. These are now considered obsolete terms that should be no longer used.

Superficial migratory thrombophlebitis

Introduction and general description
Superficial thrombophlebitis is an inflammation and thrombosis of the superficial veins that presents as painful induration with red areas of skin, often in a linear or branching configuration forming cords (Figure 97.4) [1,2]. The clinical features are fully described in Chapter 101.

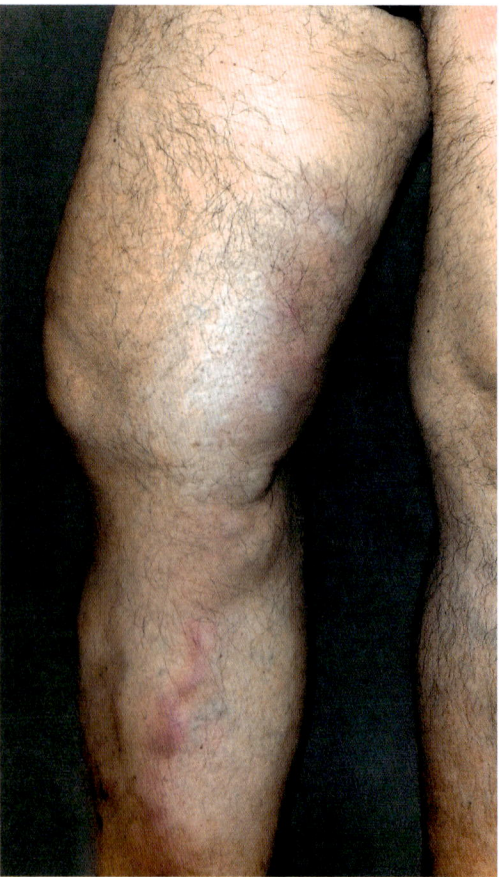

Figure 97.4 Superficial thrombophlebitis. Varicosities and red nodules with linear arrangement involving the right lower extremity.

Pathophysiology
Predisposing factors
Superficial thrombophlebitis results from a hypercoagulable state, either primary [3] or secondary [4] (Box 97.1). The causes of secondary hypercoagulable states are varied, but in the majority of cases venous insufficiency of the lower extremities is the only precipitating factor.

Box 97.1 Primary and secondary hypercoagulable states that cause superficial thrombophlebitis

Primary hypercoagulable states
- Antiphospholipid syndrome
- Deficiencies of:
  - Protein C
  - Protein S
  - Heparin cofactor II
  - Antithrombin III
  - Factor XII
  - Tissue plasminogen activator
  - Factor V Leiden [3]

Secondary hypercoagulable states
- Paraneoplastic superficial migratory thrombophlebitis (Trousseau syndrome) [1,5]
- Behçet syndrome [6]
- Buerger disease [7]
- Pregnancy [8]
- HIV-associated immune reconstitution syndrome (IRIS) [9]
- Secondary syphilis [10,11]
- Infectious suppurative thrombophlebitis in children due to *Staphylococcus aureus, Escherichia coli, Pseudomonas aeruginosa* or fungi [12–14]
- Oral contraceptive pills
- Sepsis, intravenous injections or catheterisations
- Complications of venous sclerotherapy [4]

Histopathology
Histopathologically, cutaneous lesions of STP involve large veins of the septa in the upper subcutaneous tissue. The affected vein exhibits luminal thrombosis and an inflammatory infiltrate within its wall (Figure 97.5). In early lesions, the inflammatory cell infiltrate is composed mostly of neutrophils, whereas in later stages there are lymphocytes, histiocytes and occasional multinucleated giant cells. Granulomatous infiltration participates in the recanalisation of the thrombus. A striking feature is that, in spite of the intense damage of the involved vein with dense inflammatory infiltrate in its wall and with marked septal thickening, there is little or no involvement of the adjacent fat lobule, and the process is more vasculitic than panniculitic. Intramural microabscesses in the wall of the involved vein have been described as characteristic of STP associated with Buerger disease [15].

Clinical features
Patients with STP should be appropriately investigated to rule out hypercoagulable states, paraneoplastic processes (Trousseau sign)

and Behçet disease, although by far the most common cause of STP is chronic venous insufficiency of the lower limbs.

Differential diagnosis
The main histopathological differential diagnosis for STP is cutaneous polyarteritis nodosa. In contrast to STP, cutaneous polyarteritis nodosa is characterised by involvement of the small arteries and arterioles of the subcutaneous septa. The process is more inflammatory than thrombotic, with prominent fibrinoid necrosis of the tunica intima, resulting in the so-called target-like arteritis, in which an eosinophilic ring of fibrinoid necrosis replaces the intima of the affected arteriole. In doubtful cases, elastic tissue stain usually resolves any uncertainty, because in cutaneous polyarteritis nodosa the involved artery shows sharp and prominent internal elastic lamina, whereas in STP the damaged vessel is a vein with little or no discernible internal elastic membrane [16,17]. Some authors, however, believe that when inflammation is present within and around the wall of the vessel, the identification of the internal elastic lamina of the involved vessel is less reliable even with elastic tissue stains, and the smooth muscle pattern has the highest sensitivity and specificity for distinguishing arteries from veins [18]. The recently described type of tuberculid, nodular granulomatous phlebitis, may clinically resemble STP, but this tuberculid is histopathologically characterised by tuberculoid granulomas and multinucleate giant cells involving the walls of the veins of subcutaneous tissue [19,20].

Management
Treatment of STP is conservative with the application of a support stocking on the involved limb. In chronic and recurrent cases, especially those associated with malignancy, heparin and fibrinolytic drugs may be used. Patients with a high risk of pulmonary embolism should receive fondaparinux 2.5 mg/day subcutaneously for 45 days. Phlebectomy may be necessary in recurrent cases due to large varicosities.

Cutaneous polyarteritis nodosa (cutaneous arteritis)

Introduction and general description
This is a cutaneous vasculitis of poorly understood aetiology affecting the subcutaneous arteries and arterioles (Figure 97.6). In contrast to systemic polyarteritis nodosa, there is little or no evidence of systemic disease [1,2]. So-called macular lymphocytic arteritis [3] is now considered by most authors as a mild variant of cutaneous polyarteritis nodosa characterised by macular rather than nodular lesions [4]. Cutaneous polyarteritis nodosa is fully described in Chapter 100.

Pathophysiology
The serum of patients with cutaneous polyarteritis nodosa is usually negative for both myeloperoxidase (MPO) antineutrophil cytoplasmic antibodies (ANCA) (p-ANCA) and proteinase 3 (PR3) ANCA (c-ANCA) by direct enzyme-linked immunoabsorbent assay (ELISA) and capture ELISA but 84% of the patients reveal p-ANCA positivity by indirect immunofluorescence. Serum

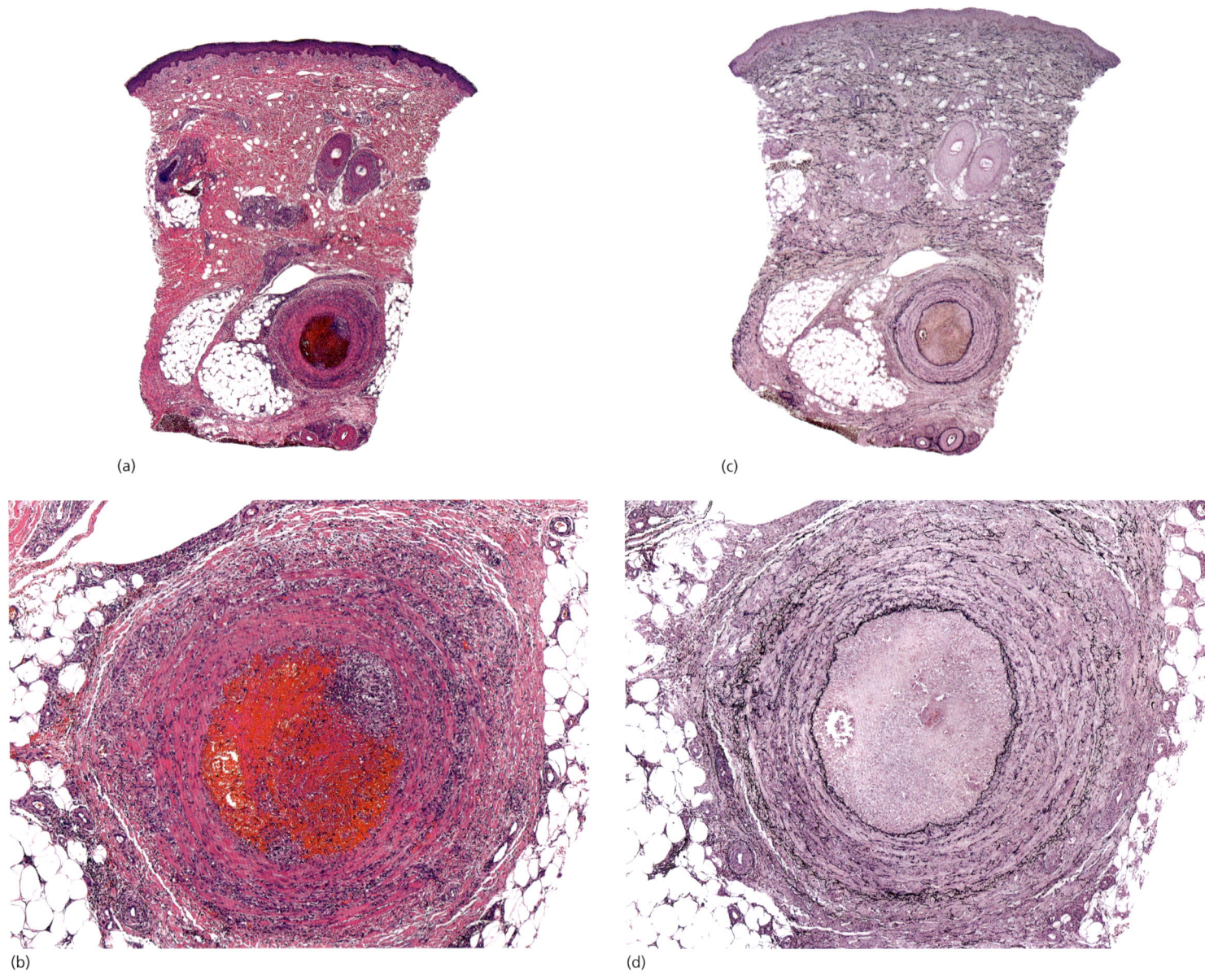

(a)

(c)

(b)

(d)

Figure 97.5 Histopathological features of superficial thrombophlebitis. (a) Scanning view showing involvement of a large vein in the septa of subcutaneous tissue. (b) The involved vein shows thrombosis of its lumen. (c) The same specimen stained for elastic tissue. (d) Several layers of internal elastic lamina are seen around the luminal thrombus.

antilysosomal-associated membrane protein 2 (anti-LAMP-2) antibody levels in cutaneous polyarteritis nodosa patients with p-ANCA are significantly elevated compared with those with negative p-ANCA, which suggests that anti-LAMP-2 antibodies might play an important role in the pathogenesis of the condition [5]. Immunoglobulin G (IgG) antiphosphatidylserine–prothrombin complex (anti-PS/PT) antibodies and/or IgG anticardiolipin antibodies have also been detected in the serum of some patients with cutaneous polyarteritis nodosa [6].

A recently identified, genetically determined form of polyarteritis nodosa has a broad spectrum of disease. Loss-of-function mutation in the adenosine deaminase type 2 gene (known as ADA2 deficiency) is linked to autosomal recessive, childhood-onset disease with features similar to those of classic polyarteritis nodosa. It shows considerable variability in severity and ranges from cutaneous to systemic vasculopathy [7,8].

Histopathology

Cutaneous lesions exhibit vasculitis involving medium-sized arteries and arterioles at the septa of the upper subcutis (Figure 97.7). Direct immunofluorescence studies of lesions of cutaneous polyarteritis nodosa have demonstrated IgM and complement deposition in the involved vessel walls and consistent absence of IgG [9]. The involved vessel appears with a thickened wall, within which an inflammatory infiltrate is seen. Its composition varies with the stage of evolution of the process. In early lesions, a neutrophilic infiltrate and leukocytoclasis are often seen, in some cases eosinophils may be prominent [10]. Characteristically, the intima of the involved artery exhibits an eosinophilic ring of fibrinoid necrosis, giving a target-like appearance to the damaged vessel. In older lesions, lymphocytes are predominant, and in a still later stage there is fibrosis of the entire thickness of the vessel wall, leading to the obliteration of its lumen. A rare complication

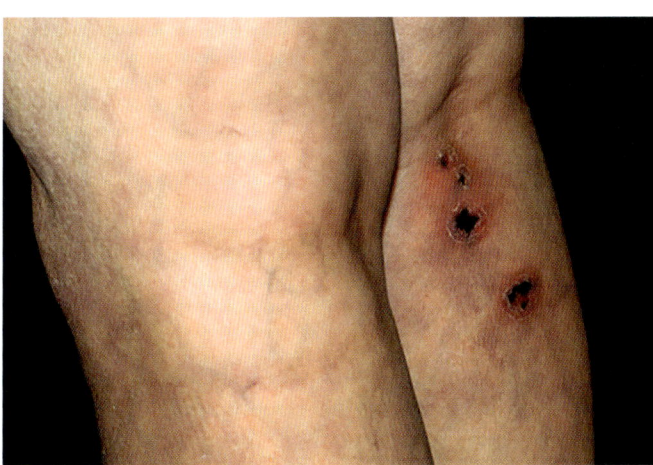

Figure 97.6 Clinical appearance of cutaneous polyarteritis nodosa showing livedo reticularis of the lower extremities with ulcerated nodules on the right calf of a middle-aged woman.

is the formation of periosteal new bone beneath the cutaneous lesions [10]. Although luminal thrombi may be present, they are less frequent than in lesions of superficial thrombophlebitis. Often, arterial involvement is segmental and serial sections throughout the entire specimen are required to demonstrate the pathology. As is the case in superficial thrombophlebitis, lesions of cutaneous polyarteritis nodosa show little or no involvement of the adjacent fat lobule, and the process is exclusively a septal arteritis.

Management
Usually, cutaneous polyarteritis nodosa follows a benign clinical course. Topical or intralesional corticosteroids may be helpful in localised involved areas. Extensive disease may warrant systemic corticosteroids. Symptomatic relief may also be achieved with non-steroidal anti-inflammatory drugs (NSAIDs).

Necrobiosis lipoidica

Introduction and general description
Necrobiosis lipoidica is an uncommon skin condition in which degenerated dermal collagen is surrounded by a granulomatous inflammatory response to produce shiny, red-brown or yellowish plaques in the skin, particularly on the shins (Figure 97.8). In severe cases, the affected skin may ulcerate. It is associated in the majority of but not all cases with underlying diabetes, the onset of which it may precede. It is fully described in Chapter 95. It may involve the subcutis but does not cause a true panniculitis because the palisading granulomatous process involving the subcutis is always a deep extension of the dermal process and, to our knowledge, there are no descriptions of necrobiosis lipoidica involving only subcutaneous fat.

Pathophysiology
Histopathology
Histopathologically, lesions of necrobiosis lipoidica involve the full thickness of the dermis, and often extend to the superficial

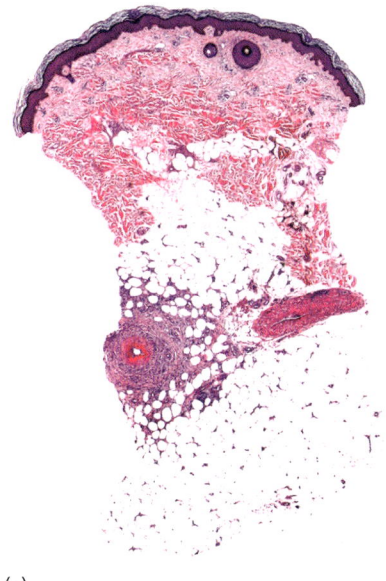

(a)

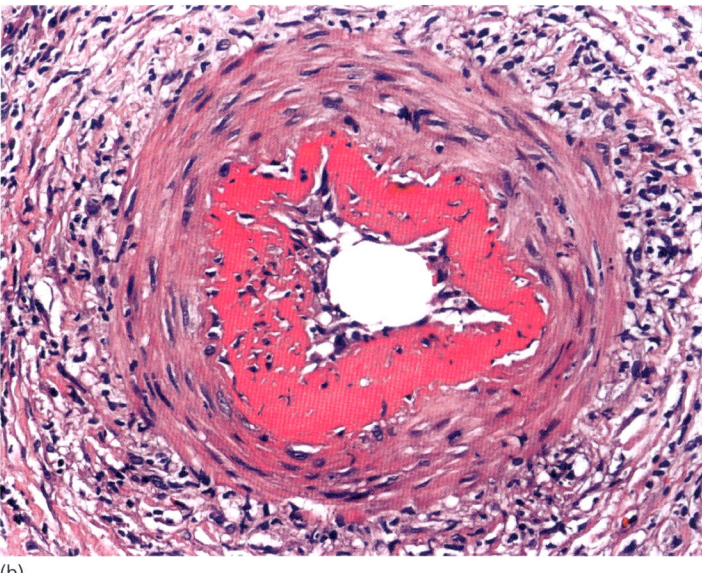

(b)

Figure 97.7 Histopathological features of cutaneous polyarteritis nodosa. (a) Scanning view of a punch biopsy showing involvement of a vessel of the septa of subcutaneous fat. (b) Higher magnification showing fibrinoid necrosis of the intima, giving a target-like appearance to the involved arteriole.

subcutaneous tissue causing septal panniculitis (Figure 97.9) [1]. There are palisading granulomas with histiocytes surrounding areas of degenerate collagen within widened septa. The most characteristic feature supporting a diagnosis of necrobiosis lipoidica as the cause of an inflammatory process involving the subcutis is the coexistence of similar lesions in the dermis, with alternating horizontal bands of inflammatory cells and fibrosis involving the entire dermis [2].

Early lesions show an inflammatory infiltrate composed predominantly of neutrophils scattered within the septa, whereas in later lesions, histiocytes, lymphocytes and plasma cells, sometimes with lymphoid follicle formation [3], are predominant. Multinucleated giant cells involving the septa are sometimes prominent and in these cases histopathological findings resemble erythema nodosum.

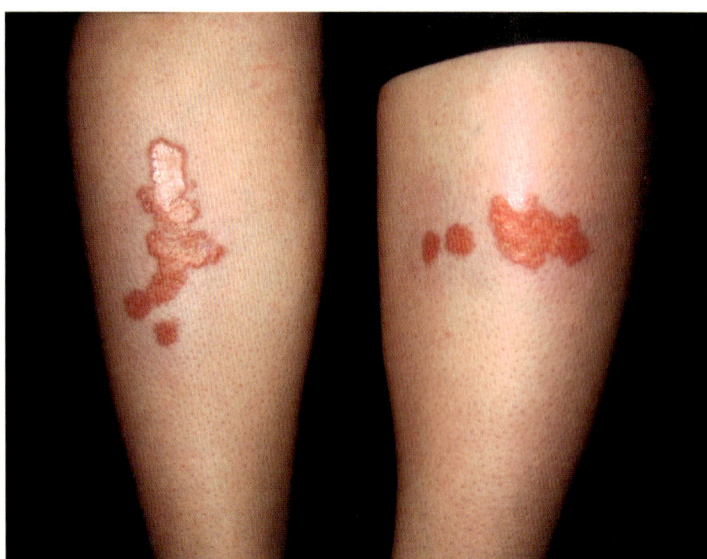

Figure 97.8 Necrobiosis lipoidica showing yellowish indurated plaques on the anterior aspect of the legs in a diabetic woman.

Differential diagnosis is, however, straightforward because in the latter condition there are no significant dermal changes other than a perivascular lymphocytic infiltrate.

In chronic longstanding lesions, the dermis and the superficial subcutaneous tissue are replaced by horizontal fibrosis with sclerotic collagen bundles arranged parallel to the epidermis and scattered with plasma cells, closely resembling the findings seen in morphoea. In these late-stage lesions, features of necrobiosis are no longer evident and elastic tissue stains demonstrate a dramatic loss of elastic fibres. Some authors have postulated that the finding of vasculitis and leukocytoclasis in lesions of necrobiosis lipoidica is indicative of an underlying systemic disease [4]. Membranous fat necrosis has also been described in late-stage lesions of necrobiosis lipoidica extending to the subcutaneous tissue [5].

Direct immunofluorescence studies have demonstrated IgM and complement in the blood vessels of some lesions of necrobiosis lipoidica, suggesting that this process is an immune complex vasculitis [6], but extensive histopathological studies identified vascular involvement in only 30% of the cases [7]. The finding of GLUT-1 immunohistochemical expression in areas of sclerotic collagen of necrobiosis lipoidica raises the possibility that a disturbance in glucose transport by fibroblasts may contribute to the histogenesis of necrobiosis lipoidica [8].

Management

There is no effective treatment for necrobiosis lipoidica. Spontaneous remission after several years occurs rarely. Potent topical corticosteroids (including under occlusion) and intralesional corticosteroids for early lesions are the most commonly used therapies. In some cases, topical tacrolimus 0.1% ointment has led to improvement. Pentoxifylline, stanozolol, nicofuranose and ticlopidine hydrochloride have been tried with variable results. Additional anti-inflammatory drugs, including antimalarials, niacinamide, mycophenolate mofetil, doxycycline, colchicine, methotrexate, thalidomide, TNF-α inhibitors and ciclosporin have been described as beneficial in anecdotal cases. Improvement has been also achieved in some patients with topical ultraviolet A1 (UVA1) and psoralen and UVA (PUVA) phototherapy.

Deep morphoea

Introduction and general description

This is a group of related diseases of poorly understood aetiology affecting principally the skin and subcutaneous tissue and characterised by variable fibrosis, sclerosis and cutaneous atrophy (Figure 97.10). Within the deep morphoea group, three closely related processes are included, namely morphoea profunda,

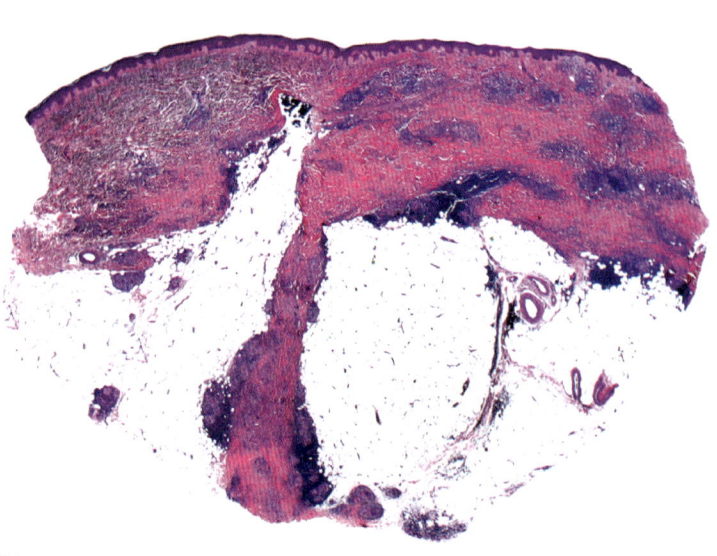
(a)

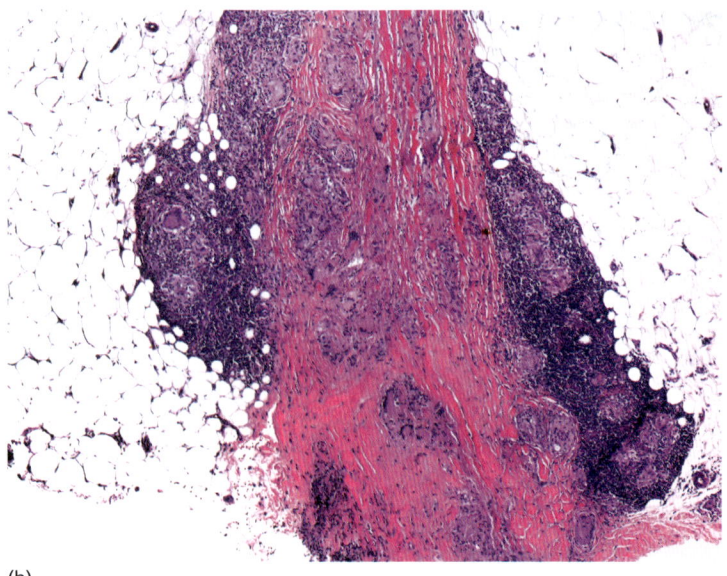
(b)

Figure 97.9 Histopathological features of necrobiosis lipoidica extending to subcutaneous tissue. (a) Scanning power showing involvement of the full thickness of the dermis and extension to the subcutaneous tissue throughout the septa. (b) Granulomas involving the thickened fibrous septa of the subcutaneous tissue.

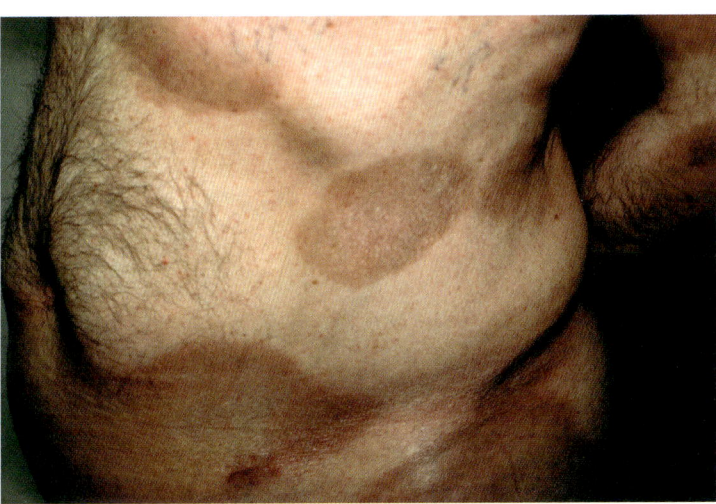

Figure 97.10 Morphoea profunda. The lesions consisted of indurated, hyperpigmented and slightly depressed plaques.

eosinophilic fasciitis and disabling pansclerotic morphoea of children [1]. Although classic morphoea often extends from the deep dermis to the subcutaneous tissue, morphoea is sometimes an entirely panniculitic process with no involvement of the epidermis, cutaneous adnexa or dermis. The process is known variously as morphoea profunda, nodular scleroderma or keloidal scleroderma. These conditions are fully described in Chapter 55.

Pathophysiology
Histopathology
Histopathologically, the lesions show a marked fibrous thickening of the septa of subcutaneous fat (Figure 97.11). As a consequence of thickening, collagen also replaces the fat normally present around and below the eccrine coils, giving the misleading impression that the sweat glands have ascended into the dermis. When the sclerotic process involves both the dermis and subcutis, the full thickness of the specimen appears homogeneously eosinophilic. Inflammatory infiltrate is present only in active lesions, consisting of aggregates of lymphocytes surrounded by plasma cells at the interface between the thickened septa and the fat lobules. Plasma cells may be also present arranged interstitially between the sclerotic collagen bundles [2–4]. Active lesions of deep morphoea usually show denser infiltrate than dermal morphoea [4–6].

Eosinophilic fasciitis (Shulman syndrome) is regarded as a variant of deep morphoea in which the thick and sclerotic septa and the fascia show inflammatory infiltrate of lymphocytes, histiocytes, plasma cells and abundant numbers of eosinophils [7–14]. Histopathological study of the early stages of eosinophilic fasciitis shows oedema and infiltration by eosinophils, lymphocytes and plasma cells between the collagen bundles of the connective tissue septa of the subcutis and subcutaneous fascia. Lymphoid aggregates may be also present. In the later stages, there is fibrosis and hyalinisation of the involved tissues [11]. The presence of eosinophils in the blood and fascia and a focal loss of CD34 staining are more suggestive of eosinophilic fasciitis than deep morphoea [15].

Disabling pansclerotic morphoea in children is an aggressive clinical variant of morphoea which appears before 14 years of age [16], although adult onset has been also described [17]. The process

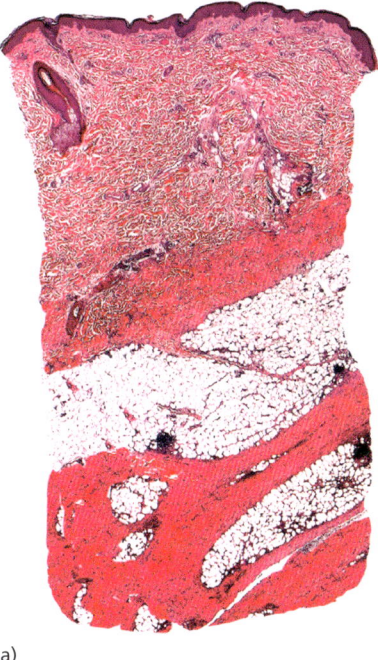
(a)

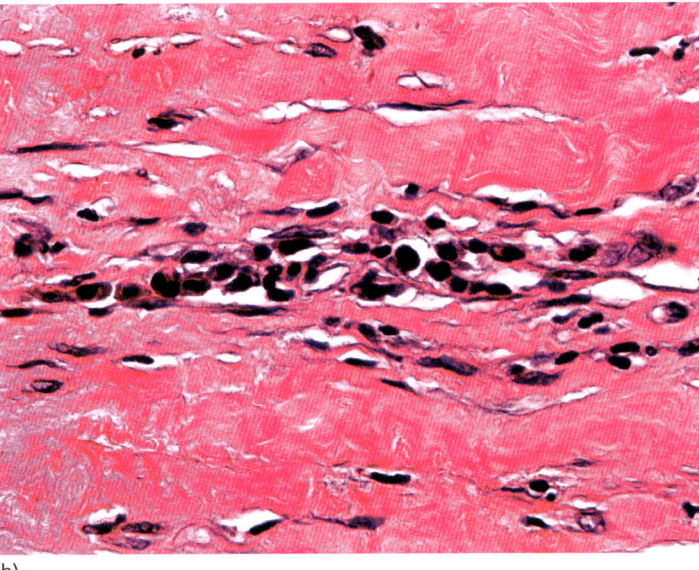
(b)

Figure 97.11 Histopathology of deep morphoea. (a) Scanning power showing sclerosis of the deeper reticular dermis and the septa of subcutaneous tissue. Note that the superficial and mid-dermis were spared. (b) Thickened sclerotic collagen bundles with interstitial lymphocytes and plasma cells.

involves not only the full thickness of the skin, but also the subcutaneous tissues, muscle and bone. Histopathological findings in cutaneous lesions of disabling pansclerotic morphoea show sclerotic replacement of the full thickness of the dermis and subcutaneous fat and the process extending to the underlying fascia. In active lesions, a variable infiltrate of lymphocytes and plasma cells is seen between the sclerotic collagen bundles [16].

Management
In patients with progressive disease and disseminated forms of disease, systemic therapy is indicated. The most commonly used

therapies include combinations of pulsed intravenous and/or oral steroids with methotrexate as the first line treatment.

Subcutaneous granuloma annulare

Introduction and general description

Subcutaneous granuloma annulare is a rare clinicopathological variant of granuloma annulare, characterised by subcutaneous nodules that may appear alone or in association with the classic dermal papular lesions (Figure 97.12) [1,2]. It typically presents in children or young adults [3,4] and is fully described in Chapter 95.

Pathophysiology

An immunoglobulin-mediated vasculitis has been proposed as the underlying mechanism for necrobiotic areas in granuloma annulare [5], although direct immunofluorescence studies failed to demonstrate immune deposits within the vessels walls [6]. Additional postulated pathogenic mechanisms include a cell-mediated immune response with increased helper/inducer T cells and CD1a-positive Langerhans cells [7], a Th1 inflammatory reaction with interferon γ (IFN-γ) producing lymphocytes eliciting matrix degradation [8], increased collagen synthesis [9] and elastic tissue degeneration [10]. The inflammatory cells release cytokines, including macrophage inhibitor factor, which cause histiocytes to accumulate in the necrobiotic areas and release lysosomal enzymes resulting in degenerate connective tissue [11]. Usually, subcutaneous granuloma annulare is a true panniculitic process with no dermal involvement, although in 25% of patients subcutaneous nodular lesions coexist with the classic presentation of superficial papules [12,13]. In rare instances, subcutaneous granuloma annulare may extend to involve deeper soft tissues and producing a destructive arthritis and limb deformity [14].

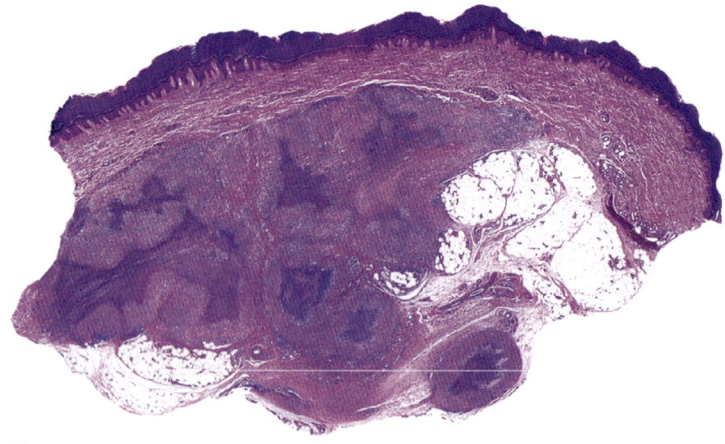

(a)

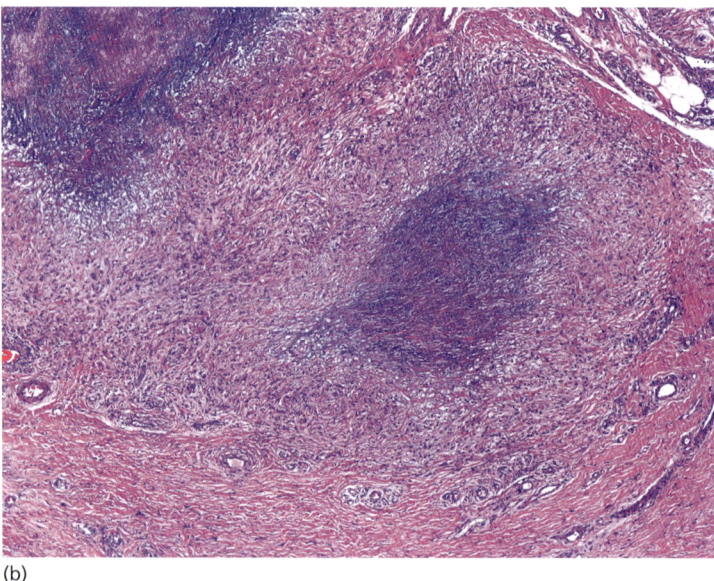

(b)

Figure 97.13 Histopathological findings in subcutaneous granuloma annulare. (a) Scanning power showing the involvement of deeper dermis and subcutaneous tissue. (b) There are several areas of basophilic degeneration of collagen bundles surrounded by a palisade of histiocytes.

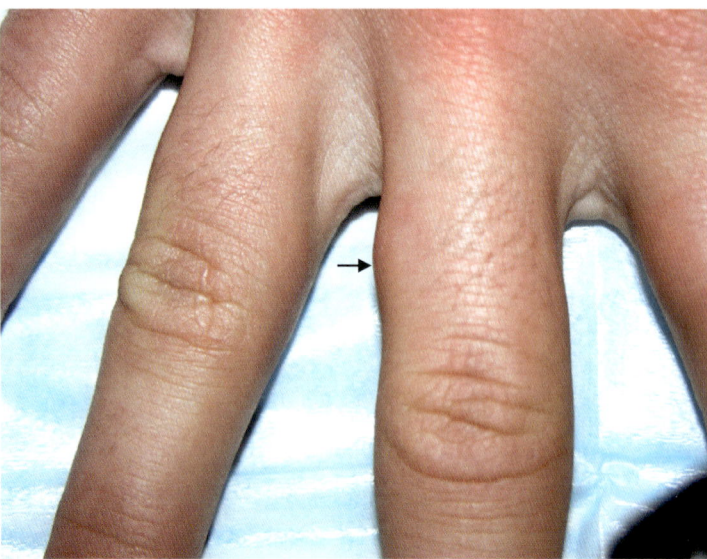

Figure 97.12 Subcutaneous granuloma annulare involving the lateral aspect (arrow) of the first phalanx of the third right finger in a 14-year-old boy.

Histopathology

The histopathological changes seen in subcutaneous granuloma annulare consist of areas of basophilic degeneration of collagen bundles with peripheral palisading granulomas involving the connective tissue septa of the subcutis (Figure 97.13). Usually, the areas of collagen degeneration are larger than in the dermal counterpart of the process. The central necrobiotic areas contain increased amounts of connective tissue mucin and nuclear dust from neutrophils between the degenerated collagen bundles. Elastic tissue is usually absent within the foci of degenerate collagen. The peripheral ring is composed of epithelioid histiocytes arranged in a palisade fashion and multinucleated giant cells may also be seen [15,16]. Eosinophils are more common in subcutaneous granuloma annulare than in the dermal superficial lesions [16]. The interstitial histopathological variant of granuloma annulare is characterised by histiocytes interstitially arranged between collagen bundles, with mucin deposition but no areas of degenerate collagen. This histopathological pattern, more frequent than the necrobiotic one in dermal lesions, has yet to be described in subcutaneous granuloma annulare and all reported patients with deep forms of the process showed the classic palisading necrobiotic pattern [17]. Immunohistochemical studies showed intense expression of CD68/PGM1 in the histiocytic population and a variable one of lysozyme. T-cell markers (CD3, CD4 and CD8) have been detected mainly in the perivascular lymphocytic infiltrate, with CD4+ T lymphocytes predominating over CD8+ [18].

Clinical features
Differential diagnosis
Histopathological differential diagnosis of subcutaneous granuloma annulare includes rheumatoid nodule, necrobiosis lipoidica and epithelioid sarcoma.

In contrast to subcutaneous granuloma annulare, which usually exhibits a pale and mucinous centre with a tendency to be basophilic, the central necrobiotic areas of rheumatoid nodules appear homogeneous and eosinophilic with abundant fibrin deposits. Sometimes, however, the differential diagnosis between subcutaneous granuloma annulare and rheumatoid nodule may be impossible on histopathological grounds alone. Old rheumatoid nodules may show extensive fibrosis in which necrobiotic areas persist.

Lesions of necrobiosis lipoidica involve the full thickness of the dermis and the subcutaneous involvement is just a deep extension from the dermis into the connective tissue septa of the subcutis. Plasma cells, aggregations of histiocytes and multinucleated giant cells are more common in necrobiosis lipoidica than in subcutaneous granuloma annulare. In the late stages of necrobiosis lipoidica, there is extensive fibrosis and degenerate collagen is no longer seen.

Epithelioid sarcoma (Chapter 136) is a neoplastic process in which central areas of degenerate collagen are surrounded by epithelioid cells with hyperchromatic and pleomorphic nuclei, some of them showing atypical mitotic figures. Immunohistochemical studies demonstrate that, in contrast to the inflammatory cells in subcutaneous granuloma annulare, the neoplastic cells in the palisades of epithelioid sarcoma express immunoreactivity for low- and high-molecular-weight cytokeratins, epithelial membrane antigen and CD34; furthermore, their nuclei show no expression of integrase interactor 1 [19–21].

Management
Because the lesions may regress spontaneously, assessment of the efficacy of reported treatments is difficult. Intralesional corticosteroids are the first choice treatment for solitary symptomatic lesions.

Rheumatoid nodule

Introduction and general description
Rheumatoid nodules are one of the extra-articular manifestations of rheumatoid arthritis. They are usually found in proximity to joints or extensor surfaces (Figure 97.14) and other areas subjected

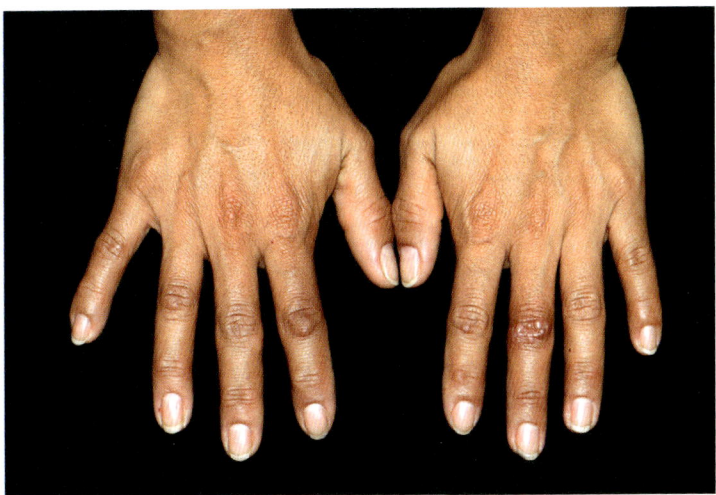

Figure 97.14 Rheumatoid nodules involving the dorsum of the fingers in an adult woman with seropositive rheumatoid arthritis.

to mechanical pressure. They can also develop elsewhere, including in the pleura and meninges. Nodules vary in size and consistency and are rarely symptomatic. They are described more fully in Chapter 155.

Pathophysiology
The pathogenesis of rheumatoid nodules remains unknown. Because the lesions develop at sites of trauma and pressure, mechanical factors have been postulated as pathogenic factors. Some genetic factor may also be involved, because patients with human leukocyte antigen (HLA) DRB1 present with severe rheumatoid arthritis and frequent rheumatoid nodules, whereas those with HLA-DRw2 have a mild articular disease and infrequent rheumatoid nodules [1–4]. Recently, microchimerism has been demonstrated in almost 50% of the cases of rheumatoid nodules of patients with rheumatoid arthritis. Since microchimerism is genetically disparate, it is possible that microchimerism in rheumatoid nodules serves as an allogeneic stimulus or allogeneic target [5]. Pro-inflammatory cytokines and cell adhesion molecules are very similar in rheumatoid nodules and the synovial lining in rheumatoid joints. The cytokine profile identified within the rheumatoid nodule showed the presence of IFN-γ, but not IL-2, and prominent expression of IL-1β and TNF-α together with IL-12, IL-18, IL-15 and IL-10. These findings support the hypothesis that the formation of rheumatoid nodules is driven by Th1 lymphocytes [6]. An immune complex-mediated mechanism has also been postulated: IgG and IgM have been detected by direct immunofluorescence in the vessel walls of rheumatoid nodules, suggesting that a vasculitic process may be involved [7,8]. The mechanism for the central degeneration of the collagen bundles is also unknown. Although apoptosis has been demonstrated throughout the entire nodule [9], it seems that the proteases, collagenases and other chemotactic factors (e.g. granulocyte–macrophage colony-stimulating factor and fibronectin) secreted by lesional monocytes and macrophages are the main factors inducing the degeneration of collagen, mucin deposition and palisading granuloma formation [7,10].

PART 8: SPECIFIC CUTANEOUS STRUCTURES

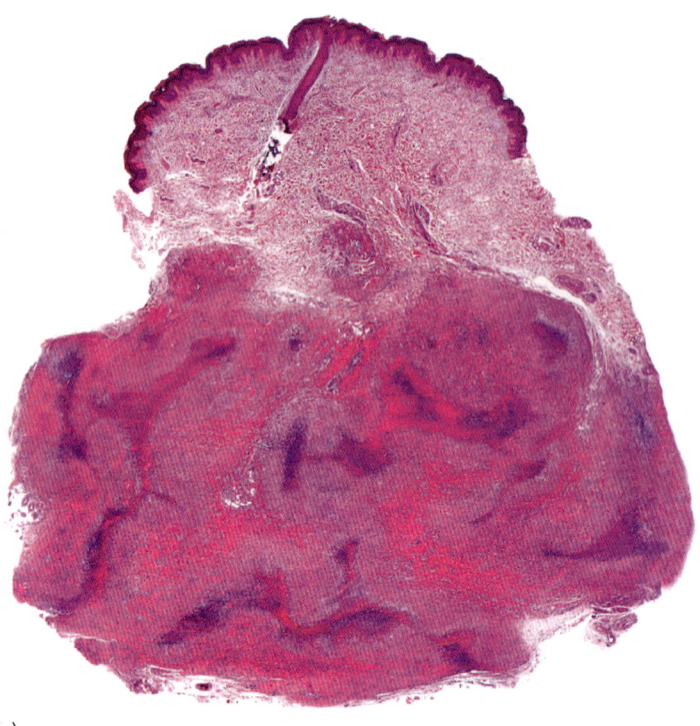

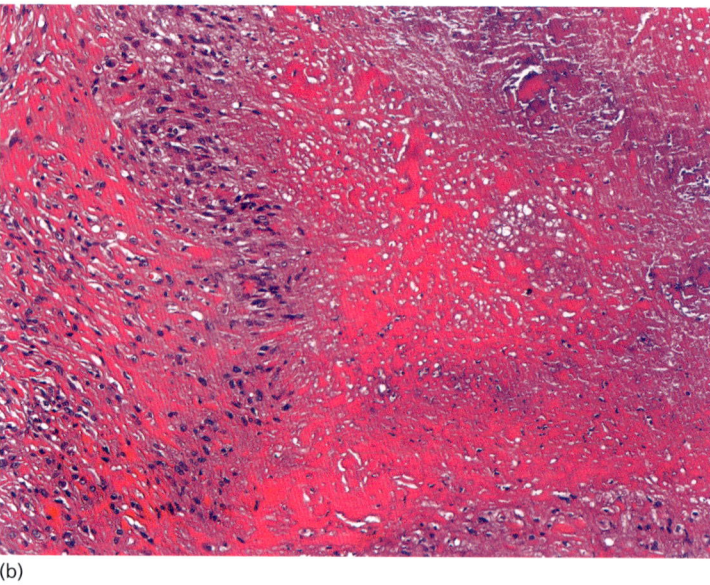

(a)   (b)

Figure 97.15 Histopathological features of rheumatoid nodule. (a) Scanning power showing a diffuse replacement of subcutaneous tissue by a fibrotic process with scattered areas of degenerate collagen. (b) The eosinophilic fibrinoid areas are surrounded by a palisade of histiocytes.

Histopathology

Histopathological findings in rheumatoid nodules vary according to the age of the lesion. Early lesions show microscopic features of granulation tissue surrounded by mononuclear cells and fibroblasts [11]. In later stages, the lesions show a central area of degenerate collagen admixed with fibrinoid material and surrounded by a palisade of elongated mononuclear histiocytes (Figure 97.15). The inner central degenerated zone appears as intensely eosinophilic amorphous, granular or fibrillary material containing collagen fibrils, fibrin and cellular debris. Multinucleated giant cells, T lymphocytes, plasma cells, mast cells and eosinophils may also be seen at the periphery. Uncommonly, features of acute vasculitis have been described in the surrounding vessels and sometimes a necrotic blood vessel associated with nuclear debris and sparse neutrophils may be seen at the centre of necrobiotic areas, although these findings probably represent secondary vasculitis. In rare instances, superficial nodules may perforate the epidermis [12]. Longstanding rheumatoid nodules exhibit extensive fibrosis in which clefts and cystic degeneration appear due to liquefactive degeneration of the contents of the nodules [13].

Clinical features
Clinical variants

Accelerated rheumatoid nodulosis (ARN) is the term used to describe the development of new painful rheumatoid nodules in patients with chronic rheumatoid arthritis under treatment with methotrexate. These new nodules develop preferentially on the hands, feet and ears [14–18]. It seems that there is an individual susceptibility

to ARN, because it develops more frequently in patients with HLA-DRB1 and seropositive rheumatoid arthritis [1,18]. Genetically predisposed patients appear to be protected against the development of methotrexate-induced ARN by the concomitant administration of hydroxychloroquine [19], D-penicillamine [20], colchicine [21] or sulfasalazine [22]. The pathogenesis of ARN is unknown, although an adenosine A1 receptor promotion of multinucleated giant cell formation by human monocytes has been postulated [23]. ARN is not exclusively related to methotrexate therapy and identical lesions have also been reported in patients with rheumatoid arthritis receiving treatment with azathioprine [24], etanercept [25,26], infliximab [27], leflunomide [23,28] and tocilizumab [29]. Neither is ARN found exclusively in rheumatoid arthritis: similar lesions have been described in patients with psoriatic arthritis [30] and systemic lupus erythematosus [31–34]. ARN has also been described in seropositive, polyarthritic-onset juvenile rheumatoid arthritis after methotrexate treatment [35,36]. In all these patients, the condition causes minimal symptoms and regresses after methotrexate is withdrawn; it does, however, recur when methotrexate is reintroduced.

Differential diagnosis

Histopathological differential diagnosis of rheumatoid nodules includes other palisading granulomas, mainly necrobiosis lipoidica and subcutaneous granuloma annulare. Table 97.2 summarises the main differential diagnostic features among these three necrobiotic disorders. Palisading necrobiotic granulomas have been classified into 'blue' and 'red' granulomas according to the colour of the

Table 97.2 Histopathological differential diagnosis of rheumatoid nodules, subcutaneous granuloma annulare and necrobiosis lipoidica.

	Rheumatoid nodule	**Subcutaneous granuloma annulare**	**Necrobiosis lipoidica**
Location	Subcutaneous septa	Subcutaneous septa, often upper and mid reticular dermis involvement	Full thickness of the dermis with extension into subcutaneous septa
Pattern	Massive areas of degenerate collagen with fibrin deposition (eosinophilic necrobiotic granuloma)	Discrete foci of degenerate collagen with mucin deposition (basophilic necrobiotic granuloma)	Fibrosis and ill-defined areas of collagen degeneration (eosinophilic necrobiotic granuloma)
Collagen degeneration	Complete	Complete	Indistinct, elongated areas of degenerate collagen
Fibrosis	Common	Uncommon	Common
Histiocytes	Well-defined palisades of histiocytes	Well-defined palisades of histiocytes	Interstitial histiocytes, no palisading
Inflammatory components	Tuberculoid and sarcoid reaction common	Tuberculoid and sarcoid reaction uncommon	Tuberculoid and sarcoid reaction common
Vascular anomalies	Capillary hyperplasia at the periphery	Perivascular lymphocytes	Capillary wall thickening
Mucin	Variable	Common	Variable
Fibrin	Common	No	Variable

Adapted from Hewitt and Cole 2005 [39].

central area of degenerate collagen stained with H&E [37,38]. Blue granulomas, which show a basophilic centre due to mucin deposition and the presence of neutrophils and nuclear dust, are usually seen in subcutaneous granuloma annulare. Red granulomas exhibit an eosinophilic necrobiotic central area due to fibrin deposition and are seen predominantly in rheumatoid nodules (Figure 97.15). Necrobiosis lipoidica usually shows a more fibrotic pattern and the process always involves the dermis.

Management
Often, cutaneous nodules wax and wane with treatment of the associated rheumatoid arthritis. Rituximab has proved to be a beneficial treatment. Intralesional corticosteroids may be indicated in solitary symptomatic lesions. It must be remembered that some drugs, including methotrexate and anti-TNF agents, may exacerbate the lesions (accelerated rheumatoid nodulosis).

Necrobiotic xanthogranuloma

Introduction and general description
Necrobiotic xanthogranuloma is a rare histiocytic disorder that causes progressive destruction of the involved cutaneous and extracutaneous tissues. It most commonly presents as multiple, indurated, yellow-red (Figure 97.16) or violaceous plaques or nodules, preferentially involving periorbital skin. Paraproteinaemia is detected in 82.1% of the patients, most often IgG-κ, and a malignant condition in 25.1% of the patients, most often multiple myeloma [1]. It is described in detail in Chapter 135.

Pathophysiology
The pathogenesis of necrobiotic xanthogranuloma is poorly understood. One proposed mechanism is that the monoclonal paraprotein behaves as a lipoprotein, binding to monocyte lipoprotein receptors to form xanthomas [2]. Intracellular accumulation of lipoprotein-derived lipids in skin macrophages may result from activation of monocytes [3], with both the paraprotein and

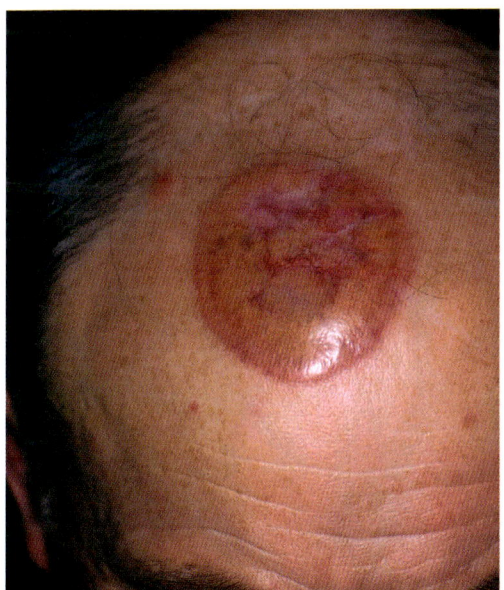

Figure 97.16 Necrobiotic xanthogranuloma. A plaque with yellowish hue involving the scalp.

immune complexes inducing granuloma formation [4]. It has been suggested that the central areas of necrobiosis in lesions of necrobiotic xanthogranuloma may be the consequence of ischaemia [5]. Another proposed pathogenetic mechanism is that an increase in circulating macrophage colony-stimulating factor (M-CSF) levels activates monocytes and favours the accumulation of large amounts of lipid and xanthoma formation [6–8]. The finding of *Borrelia* organisms in six of seven cases of necrobiotic xanthogranuloma using focus-floating microscopy has led some authors to propose an infectious aetiology for this process [9].

Histopathology
From the histopathological point of view, necrobiotic xanthogranuloma is not a true panniculitis but a deeper extension of a predominantly dermal process (Figure 97.17). The most characteristic findings consist of a diffuse involvement of the dermis by

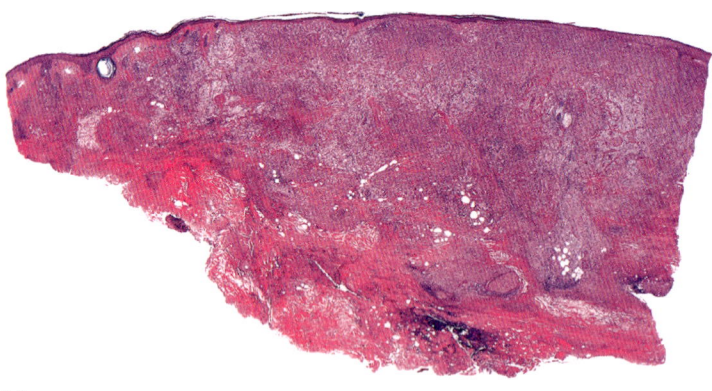

(a)

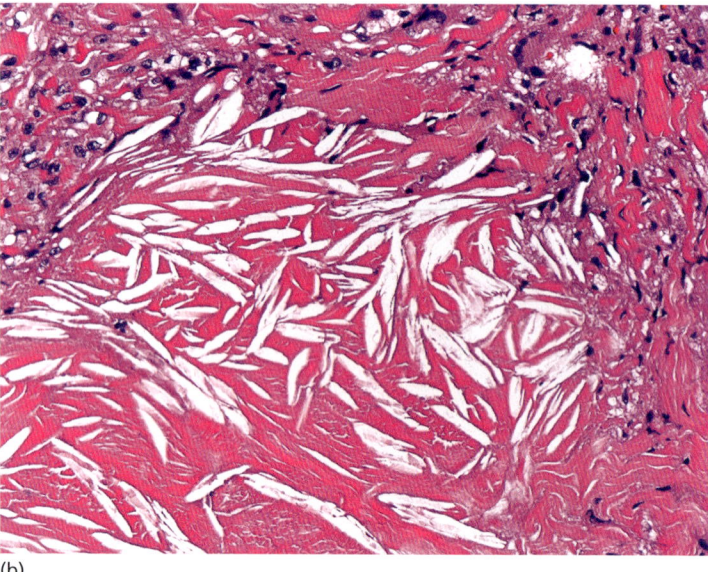

(b)

Figure 97.17 Histopathological features of necrobiotic xanthogranuloma. (a) Scanning power showing diffuse involvement of the entire thickness of the dermis and extension to subcutaneous tissue. (b) Areas of degenerate collagen with abundant cholesterol clefts.

foamy histiocytes and some Touton-like multinucleated giant cells. From the dermis, the infiltrate extends through the connective tissue septa of the subcutis and underlying soft tissues. Areas of degenerate collagen bundles and cholesterol clefts are often seen within the diffuse infiltrate [10,11]. A palisading granuloma of epithelioid histiocytes is present, at least focally, around the areas of degenerate collagen [12]. Lymphoid aggregates, sometimes with germinal centre formation, and numerous plasma cells at the periphery are often seen around the deeper areas of collagen degeneration [13]. Although there is a diffuse infiltration of the dermis and subcutaneous tissue, some cases exhibit a multinodular pattern [14]. From the immunohistochemical point of view, histiocytes and foamy macrophages express immunoreactivity for lysozyme, CD68, CD163 and CD11b [15]. In one case, intense histiocytic expression of CD10 was also observed [16].

Immunohistochemistry has demonstrated that, although necrobiotic xanthogranuloma is frequently associated with paraproteinaemia, the skin lesions represent reactive inflammation because the plasma cells present in the cutaneous lesions are polyclonal [17]. Vasculitis is not usually seen, although some lesions may show leukocytoclasis and thrombosis [14,18]. Transepidermal and transfollicular elimination of degenerate collagen and cholesterol clefts have also been reported [19]. Reports of granuloma annulare with subsequent evolution into necrobiosis lipoidica or necrobiotic xanthogranuloma raise the possibility of a general granulomatous process accompanying paraproteinaemia [20,21]. The coexistence of normolipaemic plane xanthoma and necrobiotic xanthogranuloma in the same patient also suggests that these two processes represent part of a spectrum of xanthomatous dermal reactions associated with paraproteinaemia and that they may be more closely related than previously recognised [22].

Clinical features
Differential diagnosis
The histopathological differential diagnosis of necrobiotic xanthogranuloma includes necrobiosis lipoidica, subcutaneous granuloma annulare, juvenile xanthogranuloma and deep xanthomas [6,12]. Subcutaneous granuloma annulare occurs mainly in children and does not tend to ulcerate. Usually, mucin deposits are evident at the centre of degenerate collagen; lymphoid follicles and cholesterol clefts are absent. Necrobiosis lipoidica may extend to subcutaneous tissue and then the differential diagnosis may be challenging. However, xanthomatisation, lymphoid follicles and cholesterol clefts are less frequently seen than in necrobiotic xanthogranuloma. Juvenile xanthogranuloma and deep xanthomas do not show large areas of degenerate collagen as seen in necrobiotic xanthogranuloma.

Management
Due to the rarity of the condition, there is no consensus regarding the optimal treatment. Therapies directed to the associated paraproteinaemia have shown variable response of the cutaneous lesions. Melphalan, with or without prednisolone, achieved temporary improvement of cutaneous lesions, Intralesional corticosteroids, chlorambucil, IFN-α, cyclophosphamide, methotrexate, hydroxychloroquine, azathioprine, intravenous immunoglobulin and thalidomide have been used in isolated cases with variable results. More agressive therapies, including radiotherapy and carbon dioxide laser, should be considered in individual cases.

Erythema nodosum

Introduction and general description
Erythema nodosum is the most common panniculitis. The process usually shows an acute onset and self-limited course. It is clinically characterised by the sudden eruption of several red, tender, non-ulcerating nodules and plaques, typically located on the shins. The condition normally resolves spontaneously without ulceration, scarring or atrophy, but recurrent episodes are common. Erythema nodosum is a cutaneous reactive process that may be triggered by a wide variety of infectious and inflammatory disorders and, less commonly, by malignant neoplasms and medications (Table 97.3) [1–9,**10**,11–78,**79**,80–150]. The most common triggers are bacterial infections, sarcoidosis and inflammatory bowel disease.

Table 97.3 Aetiological factors in erythema nodosum [1–9,**10**,11–78,**79**,80–150].

Infections

Bacterial infections

Atypical mycobacterial infections [1]
Bartonella henselae [2]
Borrelia burgdorferi infections [3]
Boutonneuse fever [4]
Brucellosis [5]
Campylobacter infections [6]
Cat-scratch disease [7]
Chancroid [1]
***Chlamydia psittaci* infections** [8]
Chlamydophila pneumoniae [9]
Corynebacterium diphtheriae infections [1]
Escherichia coli infections [**10**]
Gonorrhoea [11]
Klebsiella pneumoniae infections [12]
Leprosy [13]
Leptospirosis [14]
Lymphogranuloma venereum [15]
Melioidosis [16]
Meningococcemia [17]
Moraxella catarrhalis infections [18]
***Mycoplasma pneumoniae* infections** [19]
Pasteurella pseudotuberculosis infections [20]
Propionibacterium acnés [21]
Pseudomona aeruginosa infections [22]
Q fever [23]
Rickettsiae [24]
***Salmonella* infections** [25]
***Shigella* infections** [26]
Staphylococcus xylosus [27]
Streptococcal infections [28]
Syphilis [29]
Tuberculosis [30]
Tularaemia [31]
***Yersinia* infections** [32]

Viral infections

Covid-19 infection [33]
Cytomegalovirus [34]
Epstein–Barr virus infection after living-donor liver transplantation [35]
Hepatitis B [36]
Hepatitis C [37]
Herpes simplex [1]
HIV infection [38]
Infectious mononucleosis [39]
Measles [40]
Orf [41]
Parvovirus B19 [42]
Varicella [43]

Fungal infections

Aspergillosis [44]
Blastomycosis [45]
Coccidioidomycosis [46]
Dermatophytes [47]
Histoplasmosis [48]
Sporotrichosis [49]

Protozoal infections

Amoebiasis [50]
Ascariasis [51]
Giardiasis [52]
Hookworm infestation [1]
Hydatidosis [53]
Sparganum larva [54]

Protozoal infections *(cont.)*

Toxoplasmosis [55]
Trichomoniasis [56]
Visceral larva migrans [57]

Drugs

Acetaminophen [58]
Actinomycin-D [58]
All-*trans* retinoic acid [59]
Aminopyrine [1]
Amiodarone [58]
Amoxicillin [**10**]
Ampicillin [**10**]
Antimony [1]
Arsphenamine [11]
Azathioprine [58]
BRAF inhibitors [60]
Bromides [61]
Busulfan [58]
Cabergoline [62]
Capecitabine [63]
Carbamazepine [58]
Carbenicillin [58]
Carbimazole [64]
Cefdinir [58]
Certolizumab [65]
Chlordiazepoxide [58]
Chlorotrianisene [58]
Chlorpropamide [58]
Ciprofloxacin [58]
Clomiphene [58]
Codeine [58]
Cotrimoxazole [58]
D-penicillamine [66]
Dabrafenib and trametinib [67]
Dapsone [58]
Diclofenac [58]
Dicloxacillin [58]
Diethylstilbestrol [58]
Disopyramide [58]
Echinacea herbal therapy [68]
Enoxacin [58]
Erythromycin [**10**]
Etanercept [69]
Everolimus [70]
Fluoxetine [58]
Furosemide [58]
Glatiramer acetate [71]
Glucagon [58]
Gold salts [72]
Granulocyte colony-stimulating factor [73]
Hepatitis B vaccine [74]
HPV vaccine [75]
Hydralazine [58]
Ibuprofen [58]
Imatinib mesylate [76]
Indomethacin [58]
Infliximab [77]
Interleukin-2 [78]
Iodides [58]
Ipilimumab [**79**]
Isotretinoin [80]
Leukotriene modifying agents (zileuton and rafirlukast) [81]

(continued)

Table 97.3 (*continued*)

Drugs (cont.)	**Levofloxacin** [58]
	Lidocaine [82]
	Meclofenamate [58]
	Medroxyprogesterone [58]
	Meprobamate [58]
	Mesalamine [58]
	Methicillin [58]
	Methimazole [58]
	Methyldopa [58]
	Mezlozillin [58]
	Minocycline [83]
	Naproxen [58]
	Nifedipine [58]
	Nitrofurantoin [1]
	Nivolumab [84]
	Norethindrone acetate, ethinyl estradiol and ferrous
	    fumarato combination therapy [85]
	Oestrogens [58]
	Ofloxacin [58]
	Olaparib [86]
	Omeprazole [87]
	Oral contraceptives [88]
	Oxacillin [58]
	Paroxetine [58]
	Penicillin [58]
	Phenylbutazone [58]
	Phenytoin [58]
	Piperacillin [58]
	Progestins [58]
	Propylthiouracil [89]
	Pyritinol [11]
	Rabies vaccine [90]
	Serotonin reuptake inhibitors [91]
	Sparfloxacin [58]
	Streptomycin [58]
	Sulfamethoxazole [58]
	Sulfasalazine [58]
	Sulfisoxazole [58]
	Sulfonamides [92]
	Thalidomide [93]
	Ticarcillin [58]
	Trimethoprim [94]
	Typhoid vaccination [95]
	Valproate [96]
	Vedolizumab [97]
	Verapamil [58]
		Malignant diseases (cont.)
		
		Miscellaneous diseases
			Lung cancer [104]
			Myelodysplastic syndrome [105]
			Non-Hodgkin lymphoma [106]
			Pancreatic carcinoma [107]
			Parathyroid carcinoma [108]
			Post-radiotherapy for pelvic carcinoma [109]
			Renal carcinoma [78]
			Sarcoma [11]
			Stomach cancer [**10**]
			
			Acne fulminans [110]
			Acupuncture therapy and flu-like infection [111]
			Adult-onset Still disease [112]
			Ankylosing spondylitis [113]
			Antiphospholipid antibody syndrome [114]
			Autoimmune atrophic gastritis [115]
			Behçet disease [116]
			Breast abscesses [117]
			Chronic active hepatitis [118]
			Coeliac disease [119]
			Colon diverticulosis [120]
			Crohn disease [121]
			Cryopyrin-associated periodic syndrome [122]
			Diverticulitis [120]
			Eosinophilic oesophagitis [123]
			Exercise [124]
			GATA-2 deficiency [125]
			Granulomatosis with polyangiitis [150]
			Granulomatous mastitis [126]
			IgA nephropathy [127,128]
			Immune-mediated necrotising myopathy [129]
			Intestinal bypass syndrome [130]
			Jellyfish sting [131]
			Kawasaki disease [132]
			Large-vessel giant cell arteritis [133]
			Lupus erythematosus [134]
			Polyarteritis nodosa [135]
			Pregnancy [136]
			Primary biliary cirrhosis [137]
			Radiotherapy [138]
			Reactive arthritis [140]
			Relapsing polychondritis [139]
			Rheumatoid arthritis [141]
			Sarcoidosis [142]
			Sjögren syndrome [143]
			Smoke inhalation in a house fire [144]
			Sweet syndrome [145]
			Systemic lupus erythematosus-like syndrome due
			    to C4 deficiency [146]
			Takayasu arteritis [147]
			Ulcerative colitis [148]
			Vogt–Koyanagi disease [143]
			Whipple disease [149]

Malignant diseases	Adenocarcinoma of the colon [98] Carcinoid tumour [99] Carcinoma of the uterine cervix [100] Hepatocellular carcinoma [101] Hodgkin disease [102] Leukaemia [103]		

The most well-documented associations are shown in bold.

HIV, human immunodeficiency virus; HPV, human papillomavirus; IgA, immunoglobulin A.

Epidemiology

Incidence and prevalence

The population prevalence of erythema nodosum in a semirural area of England over a 2-year period was 2.4 cases per 1000 population per year [151]. Erythema nodosum accounted for about 0.5% of new cases seen in departments of dermatology in England [109] and about 0.38% of all patients seen in a department of internal medicine in Spain [152]. The average annual incidence of biopsy-proven erythema nodosum in persons aged 14 years or more at a hospital in northwestern Spain was 52 cases per million population served [10], although this almost certainly underestimated the real incidence of the disease, because only biopsy-confirmed cases were included. Most cases of erythema nodosum occur within the first half of the year [10], probably due to the increased frequency of streptococcal infections in this period; there is no difference in incidence between urban and rural areas [153]. Familial cases are usually attributable to infection; simultaneous occurrence in monozygotic twin sisters has been reported [154].

Age

Erythema nodosum may occur at any age, but most cases appear between the second and fourth decades of life, with the peak between 20 and 30 years of age, probably due to the high incidence of sarcoidosis at this age [155]. Racial and geographical variations in incidence may be explained by differences in the prevalence of aetiological factors.

Sex

Several studies have demonstrated that erythema nodosum occurs three to six times more frequently in women than in men [156], although the incidence before puberty is approximately equal in both genders [157].

Associated diseases

Concomitant presentation of Sweet syndrome and erythema nodosum has been repeatedly reported in the literature [12,158–169]. The simultaneous occurrence of these two reactive processes has been associated with sarcoidosis [159], throat infection [159,160], acute myelogenous leukaemia [161,162] and Crohn disease [162]. The association has been described in up to 15–30% of the patients in some series of biopsy-proven erythema nodosum [163–166], which suggests a common underlying pathogenetic mechanism for both processes [163,169].

Pathophysiology

There are numerous recognised triggers of erythema nodosum (Table 97.3). Aetiological factors show considerable geographical variation related to specific endemic infections. In Europe, streptococcal infections, sarcoidosis and inflammatory bowel disease are important causes. In a significant percentage of cases (ranging between 37% and 60% in reported series), the aetiology of erythema nodosum cannot be determined despite extensive clinical and laboratory investigation [10,43,157,170–173].

A previous episode of upper respiratory infection by group A β-haemolytic *Streptococcus* is a frequent cause for erythema nodosum in children and young adults. Erythematous subcutaneous nodules usually develop 2–3 weeks after the throat infection and are accompanied by an elevation of the antistreptolysin O (ASO) titre; by the time cutaneous lesions appear, the cultures from throat swabs usually fail to detect microorganisms [10,28]. Tuberculosis is a common cause of erythema nodosum in areas of high endemicity. This used to apply to many parts of Europe but no longer does so [10,170,174]. Erythema nodosum, when triggered by tuberculosis, presents mainly in children at the time of primary pulmonary infection and concomitant with the conversion of the tuberculin test [28].

Many medications have been implicated as the cause of erythema nodosum, although their real pathogenetic role is difficult to establish with confidence. Historically, sulfonamides, bromides and oral contraceptive pills have been the most commonly associated medications but a large number of drugs have been reported as triggers (Table 97.3). Oral contraceptive pills have become a rare cause since their oestrogen content was greatly reduced. Where erythema nodosum has arisen in patients receiving antibiotics for infections it is difficult to discern whether the cutaneous reaction is due to the antibiotic or the infectious process.

Sarcoidosis is one of the commonest disorders associated with erythema nodosum in adults [170]. Hilar adenopathy, arthritis around the ankles and erythema nodosum is characteristic of Löfgren syndrome [175]. However, erythema nodosum and bilateral hilar adenopathy do not occur exclusively in sarcoidosis but may also be seen in lymphomas, tuberculosis, streptococcal infections, coccidioidomycosis, histoplasmosis and acute infections by *Chlamydophila pneumoniae* [176,177].

In adults, erythema nodosum is often associated with a flare of inflammatory bowel disease, although the cutaneous eruption may sometimes precede the bowel disease. Crohn disease [121] is more frequently associated than ulcerative colitis [148].

The large list of very disparate processes that may be associated with erythema nodosum indicates that this disorder is a cutaneous reactive process and that the skin has a limited response capacity to very different triggers. Most probably, erythema nodosum results from immune complex deposition in and around veins of the connective tissue septa of the subcutis. In support of this hypothesis is the demonstration of circulating immune complexes [178], complement activation [179,180] and deposits of immunoglobulins in the blood vessels walls of the septa of subcutaneous fat in patients with erythema nodosum [181,182]. Some investigators have, however, failed to demonstrate circulating immune complexes in erythema nodosum patients and a type IV delayed hypersensitivity reaction has been proposed as a possible pathogenetic mechanism [183].

Early lesions of erythema nodosum show a predominantly neutrophilic infiltrate. Recent investigations have demonstrated that patients with erythema nodosum have a fourfold higher percentage of reactive oxygen intermediates (ROIs) produced by activated neutrophils in their peripheral blood compared with healthy volunteers. The percentage of ROI-producing cells correlates with the clinical severity of erythema nodosum and ROIs may play their pathogenic role by oxidative tissue damage and by promoting tissue inflammation [184].

Patients with sarcoidosis-associated erythema nodosum secrete an uncommon TNF-α II due to a nucleotide exchange (G-A) at position -308 in the human TNF-α gene promoter, whereas patients with erythema nodosum without underlying sarcoidosis do not have this genomic anomaly [185]. Conversely, polymorphism of the macrophage *MIF* gene at position -173 has been associated with a significantly increased risk of developing sarcoidosis in patients with erythema nodosum [186]. These investigations support the hypothesis that sarcoidosis-associated erythema nodosum might be pathogenically linked to altered TNF-α or MIF production due to a genetic promoter polymorphism.

Other investigators have found that the pro-inflammatory cytokine pattern, both in infectious and non-infectious disease related erythema nodosum, is characterised by raised IL-6 serum concentrations [146]. High expression of Th1 cytokines (IL-2 and IFN-γ) has also been demonstrated in most skin lesions and in the peripheral blood of patients with erythema nodosum, whereas this cytokine gene expression pattern was absent or only minimally present in the skin and peripheral blood of control subjects. These results directly demonstrate that a polarised Th1 immune response occurs in the skin lesions of erythema nodosum patients regardless of the wide variety of provoking agents [187].

Recently, it has been demonstrated that adipocytes play an important role in activating inflammatory systems and adaptive immune systems, destroying pathogens throughout the secretion of multiple adipokines and adipocytokines [188]. This immunological role may explain why both coccidioidomycosis [189] and sarcoidosis appear to be less severe and of shorter duration in those patients who develop erythema nodosum, especially if they are carriers of the HLA-DRB1*03-positive leukocyte antigen [190].

Histopathology

Histopathologically, erythema nodosum is the prototype of a predominantly septal panniculitis without vasculitis. The connective tissue septa of the subcutis appear thickened and oedematous and are infiltrated by inflammatory cells that involve mainly the interface between the septa and the fat lobule. Usually, a mild, superficial and deep perivascular inflammatory infiltrate composed predominantly of lymphocytes is also present in the overlying dermis.

As with other panniculitides, erythema nodosum is a dynamic process and the composition of the inflammatory cells involving the septa varies with the stage of the condition. Early lesions of less than 48 h duration show oedema and haemorrhage at the septa and numerous neutrophils arranged interstitially between collagen bundles (Figure 97.18) [172]. In some early lesions most cells are represented by 'histiocytoid' cells, which in fact are immature neutrophils similar to those observed in histiocytoid Sweet syndrome. Sometimes, if these early lesions show extension of the infiltrate to the periphery of the fat lobule surrounding individual adipocytes in a lace-like fashion, the process may be misinterpreted as a predominantly lobular panniculitis. However, in contrast with a true lobular panniculitis, necrosis of the adipocytes at the centre of the fat lobule is never seen in erythema nodosum. In rare instances, eosinophils may be numerous in early lesions: this finding does not, however, correlate with any specific aetiological factor [191].

A histopathological hallmark of erythema nodosum is the presence of so-called Miescher radial granulomas [192,193,**194**], that consist of small, well-defined nodular aggregates of small histiocytoid cells around a central stellate or banana-shaped cleft (Figure 97.19). The nature of the central cleft is unknown and,

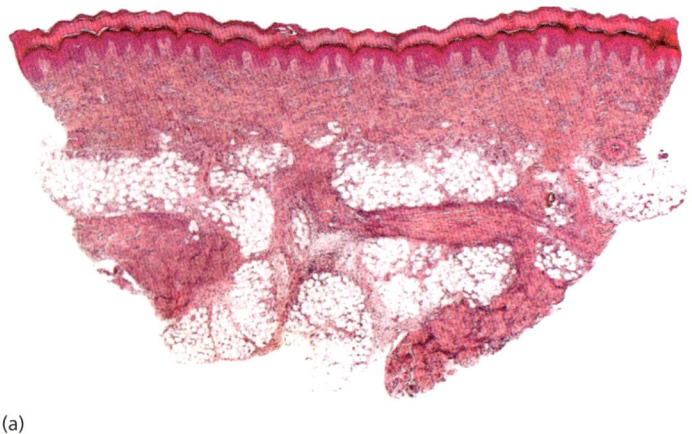

(a)

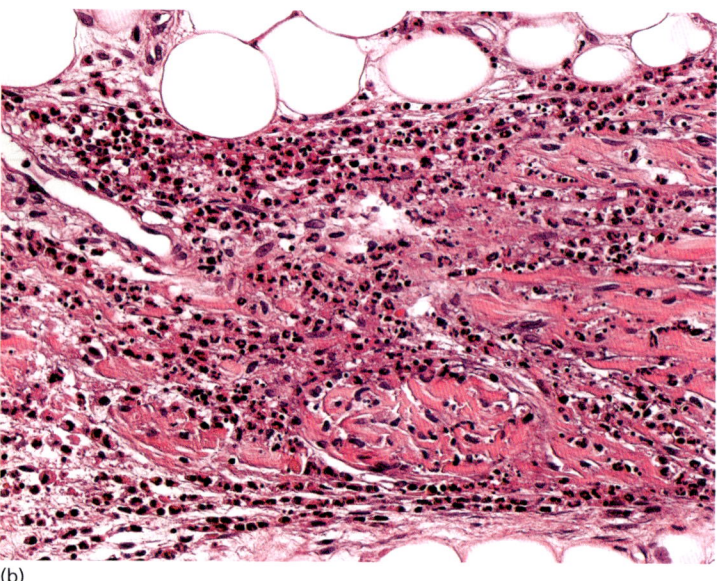

(b)

Figure 97.18 Histopathological features of an early lesion of erythema nodosum. (a) Scanning power showing a mostly septal panniculitis with thickened connective tissue septa of the subcutis. (b) The infiltrate at the septa is mostly composed of neutrophils interstitially arranged between collagen bundles.

although some authors have considered them to be lymphatic spaces, immunohistochemical and ultrastructural studies have failed to demonstrate any endothelial cell lining. In early lesions, these granulomas are scattered in the septa and are surrounded by neutrophils. In older nodules, histiocytic cells group to form multinucleated giant cells, many of which still retain in their cytoplasm the stellate central cleft as found in Miescher radial granulomas.

Sometimes Miescher radial granulomas are conspicuous in the septa. Occasionally, however, serial sections are required to identify them: if carefully sought, they can be found in almost all stages of erythema nodosum lesions and such a search should always be undertaken to establish a specific diagnosis [**194**]. However, some authors consider that similar granulomas may be found in subcutaneous Sweet syndrome, erythema induratum of Bazin, Behçet disease and necrobiosis lipoidica [200]. Recent immunohistochemical studies have demonstrated that the cells around the central clefts of Miescher radial granulomas express MPO [195] in a similar way to those of the small, elongated, twisted-appearing

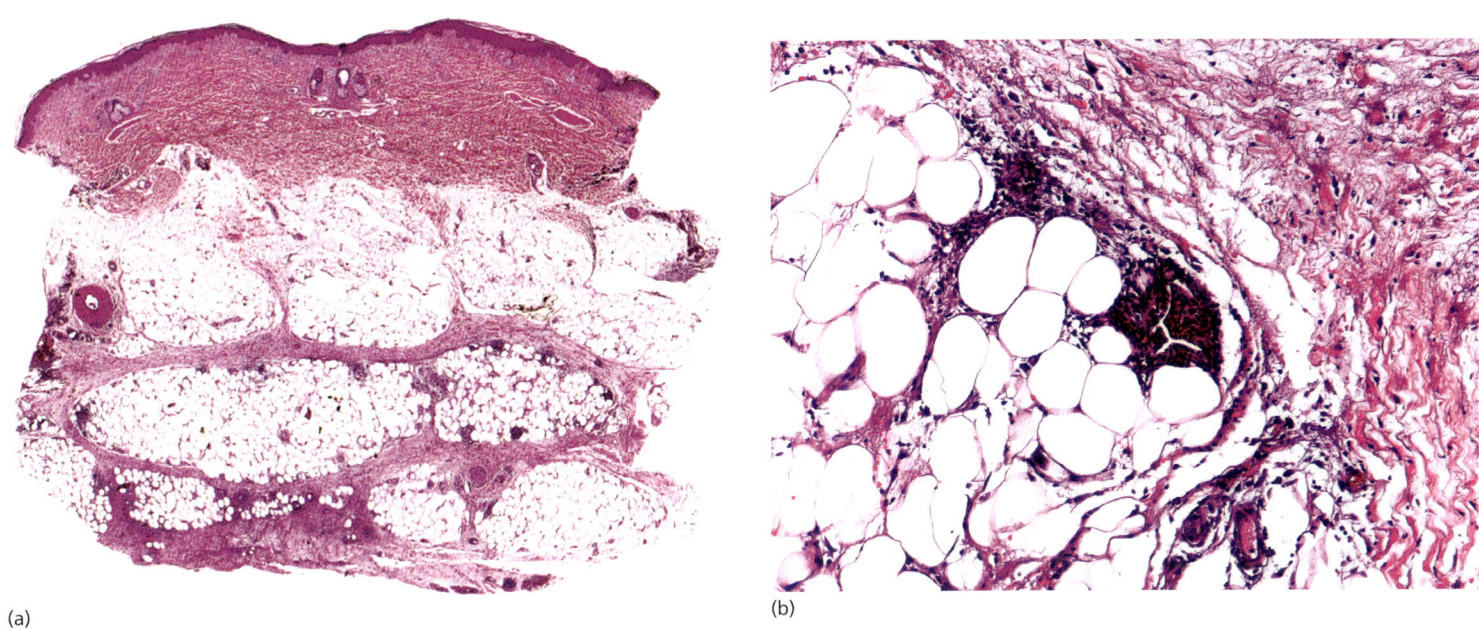

(a)

(b)

Figure 97.19 Histopathological features of a fully developed lesion of erythema nodosum. (a) Scanning power showing thickened septa of the subcutaneous tissue. (b) Higher magnification shows the characteristic features of Miescher radial granuloma: aggregations of small histiocytes around a central cleft.

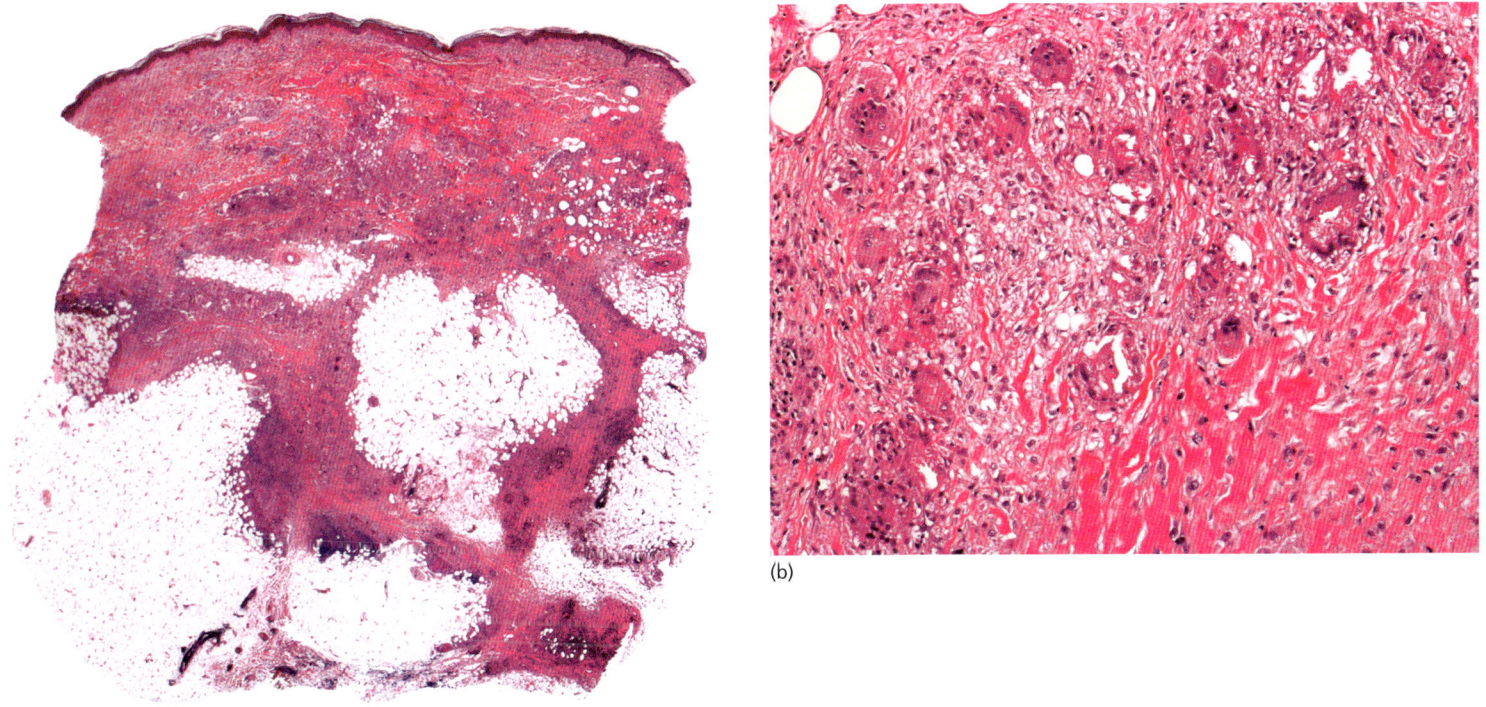

(b)

(a)

Figure 97.20 Histopathological features of a late-stage lesion of erythema nodosum. (a) Scanning power showing a mostly septal panniculitis. (b) Numerous multinucleated giant cells are present in the infiltrate at the septa.

mononuclear cells of the infiltrate in so-called histiocytoid Sweet syndrome [196,197]. These findings demonstrate that the mononuclear cells that make up Miescher radial granuloma, and those seen in the so-called histiocytoid Sweet syndrome, are actually immature myeloid cells, providing a link between erythema nodosum and Sweet syndrome, two conditions in which neutrophils participate.

Late-stage lesions of erythema nodosum show septal fibrosis and periseptal granulation tissue, partially replacing the fat lobules, with an infiltrate composed of lymphocytes, histiocytes and multinucleated giant cells (Figures 97.20 and 97.21). Despite this fibrotic process involving the septa, it is striking that erythema nodosum resolves completely after some weeks or months.

PART 8: SPECIFIC CUTANEOUS STRUCTURES

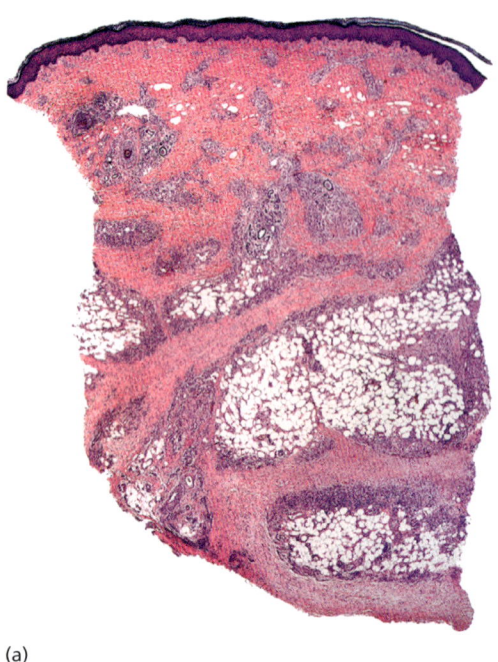

(a)

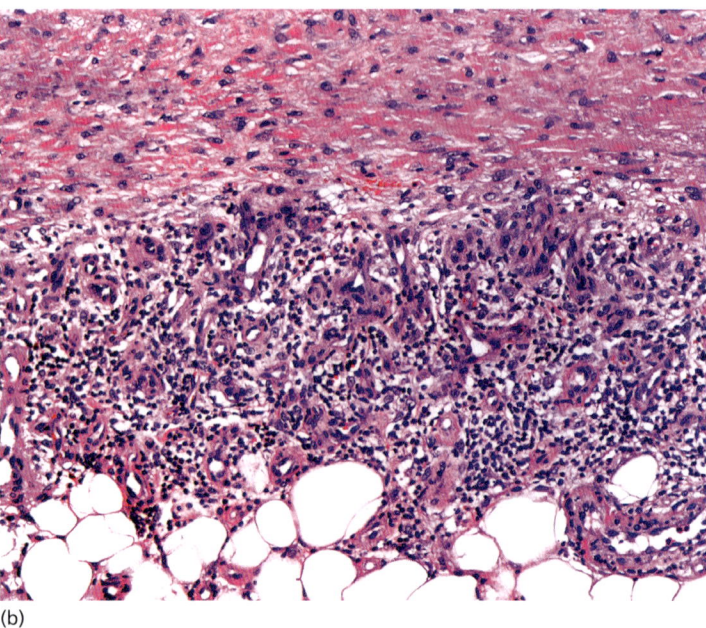

(b)

Figure 97.21 Histopathological findings of a very late-stage lesion of erythema nodosum. (a) Scanning power showing very thick connective tissue septa at the subcutis. (b) The infiltrate at the interface shows features of granulation tissue.

Vasculitis is not normally seen at any stage in the course of ery-thema nodosum, although in rare cases a necrotising small-vessel vasculitis with fibrinoid necrosis of the small vessels in the septa has been described [198]. In a detailed histopathological study of a series of 79 cases of erythema nodosum, true leukocytoclastic vasculitis was not found [194]. The cases described as erythema nodosum with lobular neutrophilic panniculitis and vasculitis involving medium-size arteries are better interpreted as examples of STP because the involved vessels were medium-size veins rather than arteries [199]. Ultrastructural studies have also failed to demonstrate true vasculitis in lesions of erythema nodosum

[200,201]. Lipomembranous or membranocystic panniculitis [202] and encapsulated fat necrosis ('mobile encapsulated lipoma') [203] may be seen in late-stage lesions of erythema nodosum.

Clinical features
Presentation
Clinically, the eruption is quite characteristic and consists of a sudden onset of symmetrical, bilateral, tender, red, warm nodules and raised plaques usually involving the shins (Figure 97.22), ankles and knees. The nodules range from 1 to 5 cm or more in diameter and may become confluent resulting in red plaques. Occa-sionally, lesions of erythema nodosum may appear in other areas, including the thighs, extensor aspects of the arms, neck and even the face. Early lesions show a bright red colour and are raised slightly above the skin. After a few days, they become flat, with a livid red or purplish colour. Finally, they show a yellow or greenish appearance, often taking on the look of a deep bruise, and for that reason the process was classically named 'erythema contusiformis'. Nodules of erythema nodosum never ulcerate and the lesions regress with-out atrophy or scarring. Often, acute bouts of erythema nodosum are associated with a fever of 38–39°C, fatigue, malaise, arthralgia, headache, abdominal pain, vomiting, cough or diarrhoea. Episcleral lesions and phlyctenular conjunctivitis may also accompany the cutaneous lesions. Rare clinical manifestations associated with erythema nodosum include lymphadenopathy, hepatomegaly, splenomegaly and pleuritis [171]. The eruption persists for 3–6 weeks and regresses leaving no residual marks. Recurrences are

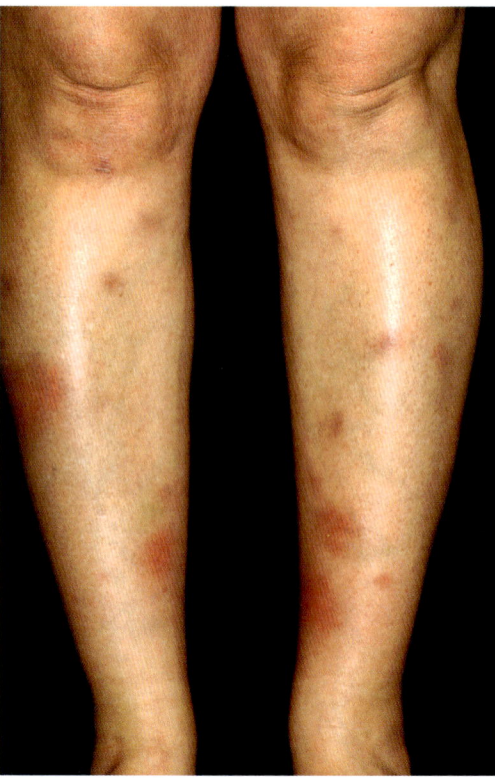

Figure 97.22 Characteristic eruption of erythema nodosum with lesions in different stages of evolution involving the anterior aspect of the legs of an adult woman. Some early lesions consist of bilateral red nodules and plaques, whereas later stage lesions show a bruise-like appearance.

common. Duration of erythema nodosum in children is shorter than in adults and arthralgias and fever are less frequent in paediatric cases [204–206].

Clinical variants

The processes described under the names of erythema nodosum migrans [207–210], subacute nodular migratory panniculitis of Vilanova and Piñol [211,212] and chronic erythema nodosum [174] are now all thought to be expressions of different stages of the evolution of erythema nodosum rather than separate entities [213]. In children, there is a rare variant of erythema nodosum characterised by unilateral red nodules involving the palms or soles that appear after physical activity [214–217]. Histopathological study of these palmoplantar lesions shows features of classic erythema nodosum.

Differential diagnosis

Besides authentic erythema nodosum, patients with Behçet disease may present with eruptions that clinically resemble erythema nodosum [116]. However, histopathological study demonstrates that these are not erythema nodosum but show a predominantly lobular panniculitis with leukocytoclastic or lymphocytic vasculitis [218,219]. Furthermore, the frequency of thrombophlebitis is higher in the erythema nodosum-like lesions of patients with Behçet disease compared with individuals with idiopathic erythema nodosum.

Investigations

To identify the responsible aetiological factor in a patient with erythema nodosum, a rational, cost-effective diagnostic approach should be initiated. A complete clinical history should include enquiry about previous diseases, medications, foreign travels, pets and hobbies, and possible familial cases. Initial laboratory investigations should include complete blood count, erythrocyte sedimentation rate, ASO titre, urinalysis, throat culture, intradermal tuberculin test and/or chest X-ray. When the aetiology is unclear, serological tests for those bacterial, viral, fungal or protozoal infections most prevalent in the area should be undertaken. The results of the tuberculin test should be evaluated in the context of the local prevalence of tuberculosis: where tuberculosis is endemic, a significant percentage of healthy adults show positive results for the tuberculin test. A stronger relationship with tuberculosis may be established using an IFN-γ release assay.

When the clinical and laboratory findings are characteristic, a tentative diagnosis of erythema nodosum may be established, but diagnostic confirmation requires biopsy.

Management

Most cases of erythema nodosum regress spontaneously in 3–4 weeks, but relapses are common. Recurrent episodes of erythema nodosum are more frequent in patients with idiopathic erythema nodosum and erythema nodosum associated with streptococcal upper respiratory tract infections. Complications are uncommon, although cases of retrobulbar optic nerve neuritis during the acute episode of erythema nodosum [220] and erythema nodosum coexisting with erythema multiforme, lichen planus and concomitant reactivation of hepatitis C viral replication [221] have each been described.

Treatment primarily includes identification and management of the underlying cause, especially if infectious. Usually, nodules of erythema nodosum regress spontaneously within a few weeks: limiting physical exercise and bed rest should be recommended. Aspirin, as well as several other NSAIDs, such as indometacin 100–150 mg daily [222] or naproxen 500 mg daily [223], are helpful for pain and for hastening resolution. NSAIDs are contraindicated in patients with inflammatory bowel disease.

In more persistent cases, potassium iodide 400–900 mg daily or a saturated solution of potassium iodide, 2–10 drops in water or orange juice three times per day, may be administered [224–226]. The mechanism of action of potassium iodide in erythema nodosum is unknown, but it probably induces mast cells to release heparin, which suppresses delayed hypersensitivity reactions. The reported response in some patients with erythema nodosum to heparinoid ointment under occlusion also supports this mechanism of action [227]. In addition, potassium iodide inhibits neutrophil chemotaxis [228]. It should be remembered that potassium iodide is contraindicated during pregnancy because it may induce goitre in the fetus. Severe hypothyroidism secondary to exogenous intake of iodide has also been described in patients with erythema nodosum treated with potassium iodide [229].

Systemic corticosteroids are not usually indicated in erythema nodosum and they should not be commenced unless an infectious aetiology has been excluded. When administered, prednisolone in a dosage of 40 mg/day is followed by resolution of the nodules in a few days. Intralesional injection of triamcinolone acetonide at a concentration of 10 mg/mL into the centre of the nodules may also be helpful in solitary persistent lesions.

Some patients have responded to a course of colchicine, 0.6–1.2 mg twice a day [230,231], and to hydroxychloroquine in a dosage of 200 mg twice a day [232].

Recently, cases of erythema nodosum have responded to treatment with anti-TNF biological agents including etanercept [233], adalimumab [234] and infliximab in patients treated with these drugs for inflammatory bowel disease [235]. Paradoxically, however, etanercept [69] and infliximab [77] have been reported to produce erythema nodosum as a cutaneous side effect.

Erythema nodosum leprosum

Definition

Erythema nodosum leprosum is a type II leprosy reaction that is characterised by a necrotising vasculitis involving small- to medium-size vessels of the deep dermis and subcutis. It is provoked by an immune complex-mediated response to the release of mycobacterial antigens from effete bacilli in patients with multibacillary leprosy (lepromatous and borderline lepromatous), usually after initiation of treatment (Figure 97.23). Leprosy reactions are described in detail in Chapter 28.

Introduction and general description

Type II reactions are due to the formation and deposit of immune complexes in association with excessive humoral reaction: the tissue expression of cytokines is mostly of IL-4 and IL-10. Erythema

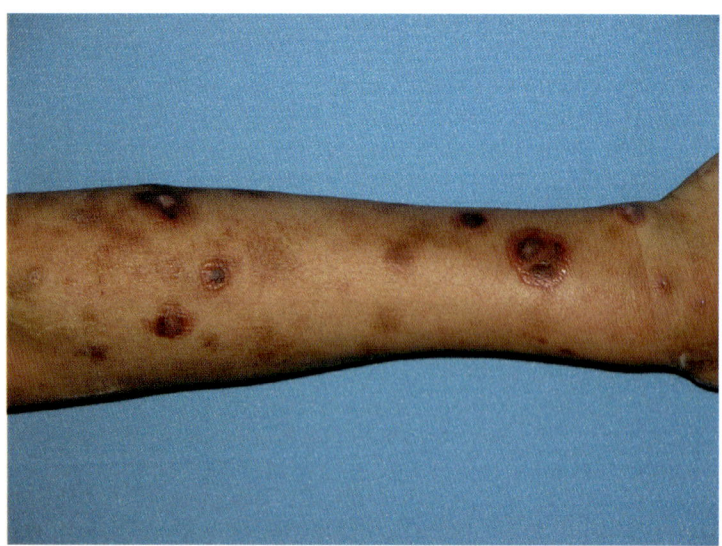

Figure 97.23 Clinical features of erythema nodosum leprosum. Acute onset of erythematous nodules involving the left upper extremity in a patient with lepromatous leprosy.

nodosum leprosum occurs only in patients with lepromatous or borderline lepromatous leprosy and usually occurs during treatment. It represents an immune complex-mediated vasculitis secondary to the deposition of large amounts of mycobacterial antigen, immunoglobulins and complement in the vessel walls [1]. During this type of reaction, patients show an increased CD4/CD8 ratio due to an increase in T-helper and a decrease in T-suppressor lymphocytes, accompanied by a specific increase in Th2 lymphocytes, which induce plasma cell proliferation and release of immunoglobulins [2,3]. In addition, these patients show a temporary recovery of Langerhans cell antigen-presenting function [4], which is directly proportional to the severity of the leprosy reaction [5,6].

The term 'erythema nodosum leprosum' is inadequate because it may easily be confused with true erythema nodosum, the prototype of septal panniculitis without vasculitis. Erythema nodosum leprosum is a predominantly lobular panniculitis with vasculitis involving the large vessels of the subcutis [7,8].

Pathophysiology
Histopathology
Histopathological findings in erythema nodosum leprosum vary according to the age of the lesions. Early nodules show oedema of the papillary dermis and a neutrophilic infiltrate with necrotising vasculitis. Although the process is mostly centred in the dermis, it may occasionally extend to subcutaneous tissue, appearing as a predominantly lobular panniculitis with vasculitis involving vessels of the subcutis (Figure 97.24). Later stage lesions exhibit a lymphohistiocytic infiltrate in which foamy macrophages with numerous mycobacteria are seen within the fat lobule [7–9].

Lucio phenomenon is an uncommon variant of type II leprosy reaction with a unique clinical morphology [8,10–12]. It occurs almost exclusively in Mexican and Central American patients with untreated, diffusely infiltrated, non-nodular lepromatous leprosy and is characterised by multiple haemorrhagic necrotic skin infarcts. It does not result in panniculitis and subcutaneous tissue is

not usually involved. Histologically, there is a necrotising vasculitis involving the superficial and mid dermis [8,12].

Management
Erythema nodosum leprosum is difficult to treat. It often requires systemic therapy with high-dose corticosteroids (80 mg/day, (tapered down rapidly) or thalidomide (400 mg/day). Improvement has been also described in some patients with clofazimine (300 mg/day).

Erythema induratum of Bazin

Synonyms and inclusions
- Nodular vasculitis
- Bazin disease
- Erythema induratum of Whitfield

Introduction and general description
Erythema induratum is a chronic, recurrent, reactive disorder characterised by subcutaneous nodules located preferentially on the posterior aspects of the lower legs of adult women. The nodules commonly develop after exposure to cold and may break down to form irregular ulcers (Figure 97.25). Its clinical features are discussed in greater detail in Chapter 27.

Erythema induratum has historically been regarded as a tuberculid linked to the presence of a distant focus of tuberculosis and, when this is the case, the condition has been referred to as erythema induratum of Bazin. *Mycobacterium tuberculosis* is not implicated in all cases, however, and the terms erythema induratum of Whitfield and nodular vasculitis have both been used to differentiate such cases from those linked to tuberculosis [1–9]. Whether it makes sense to maintain different terms for what is essentially an identical reactive process is open to question. Although there are still authors who regard erythema induratum of Bazin and nodular vasculitis as separate entities [10,11], no significant clinicopathological differences have been consistently demonstrated between cases related to tuberculosis and those which are not. In recent years, most authors thus consider erythema induratum of Bazin and nodular vasculitis to be a single reactive process that may be provoked by a number of different mechanisms, one of which is active tuberculosis [12]. Box 97.2 shows other suspected aetiological associations that have been reported [13–24,**25**,26–29].

Pathophysiology
Histopathology
As in other panniculitides, the histopathological findings in the lesional skin of erythema induratum vary with the age of the lesions. It is the prototype of a predominantly lobular panniculitis with vasculitis, but the histopathological picture and the composition of the infiltrate in the fat lobule greatly depend on the stage at which the biopsy was taken [10,30–32]. In early stages, the fat lobules are punctuated throughout by discrete collections of inflammatory cells, mostly neutrophils. There may be extensive necrosis

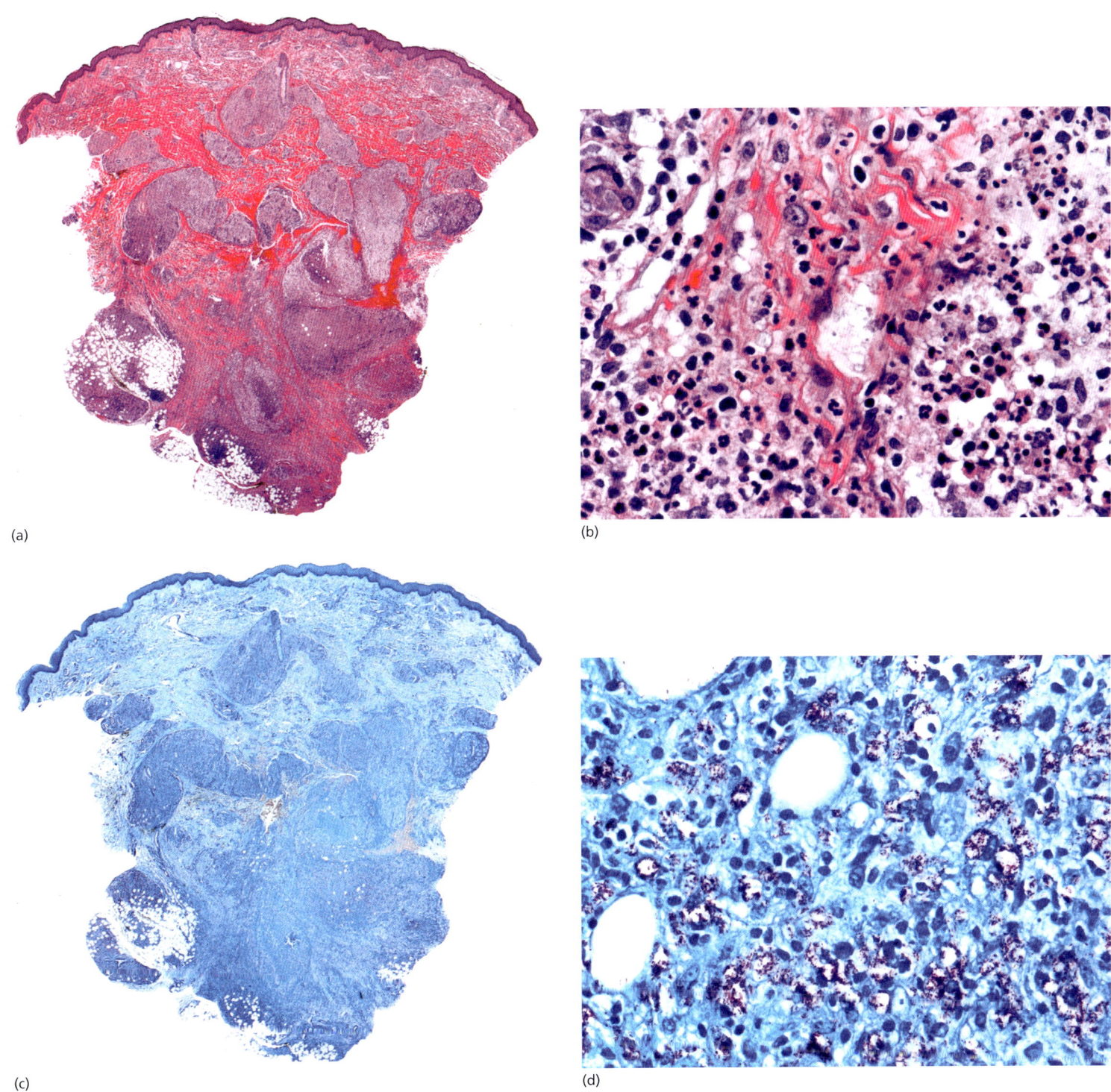

(a)

(b)

(c)

(d)

Figure 97.24 Histopathological features of erythema nodosum leprosum. (a) Scanning power showing dense nodular infiltrates in the dermis and a mostly lobular panniculitis. (b) Some of the small capillaries of the fat lobule show fibrin deposits and neutrophils involving their vessel walls. (c) A section of the same case stained with Ziehl–Neelsen stain. (d) Higher magnification of numerous microorganisms of *Mycobacterium leprae* within the cytoplasmic vacuoles of the histiocytes.

of the adipocytes of the fat lobule (Figure 97.26). These necrotic adipocytes elicit a response from histiocytes, which phagocytose lipid and become lipophages. In fully developed lesions, epithelioid and foamy histiocytes, Langhans type or foreign-body multinucleated giant cells and lymphocytes contribute to the granulomatous appearance of the inflammatory infiltrate (Figure 97.27). When intense vascular damage occurs, large areas of caseous necrosis

appear and the lesions show all the histopathological attributes of a tuberculoid granuloma. However, stains for acid-fast bacilli, such as Ziehl–Neelsen or Fite, and immunohistochemical stains for mycobacteria are negative. Caseous necrosis may extend to the overlying dermis and secondarily involve the epidermis with ulceration and discharge of liquefied necrotic fat. Previously, the presence of tuberculoid granulomas around the eccrine coils was

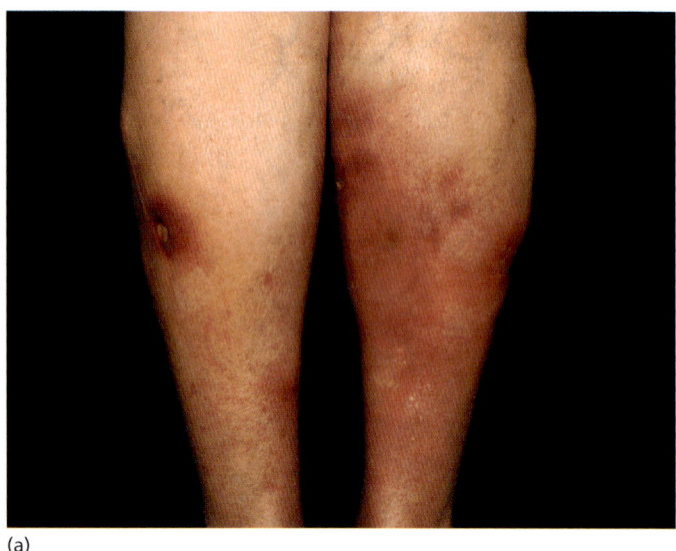

(a)

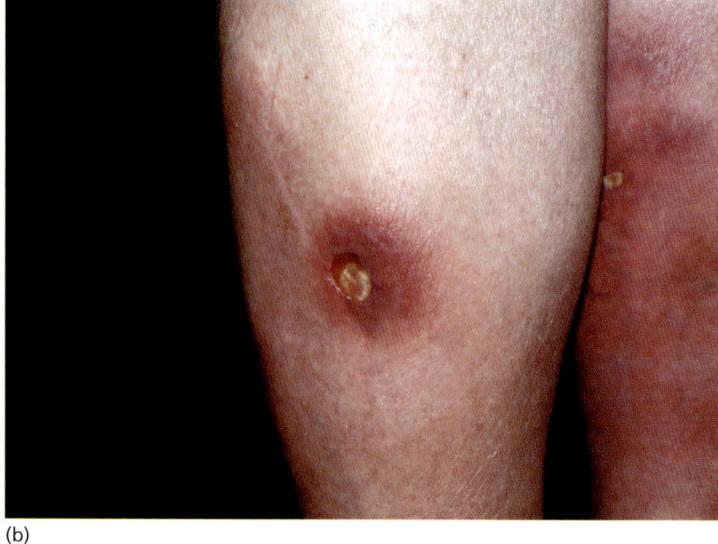

(b)

Figure 97.25 Clinical features of erythema induratum. (a) Erythematous nodules and plaques on the posterior aspect of the legs of an adult woman. (b) Some of the lesions are ulcerated.

Box 97.2 Aetiological associations of erythema induratum other than tuberculosis

- Chronic hepatitis C [13–15]
- Ulcerative colitis [16]
- Brucellosis [17]
- Paraneoplastic process [18]
- *Nocardia* infections [19]
- Propylthiouracil [20]
- Systemic lupus erythematosus [21]
- Pneumonia due to *Chlamydophila pneumoniae* [22]
- Bacille Calmette–Guérin (BCG) vaccination [23]
- Aortic valve stenosis [24]
- Hepatitis B [25]
- Crohn disease [25]
- Leukaemia [25]
- Rheumatoid arthritis [25]
- Hypothyroidism [25]
- Cold weather [25]
- Chronic venous insufficiency [25]
- Tumor necrosis factor antagonist therapy [26]
- Takayasu arteritis [27]
- Lung adenocarcinoma [28]
- Cobimetinib and vemurafenib therapy [29]

---

regarded as suggestive of a tuberculous aetiology [33], but these findings may also be seen in non-tuberculous cases.

In the literature, considerable controversy persists about whether or not vasculitis is a required histopathological criterion for establishing a diagnosis of erythema induratum. Furthermore, there is no agreement about the nature of the vessels involved in the vasculitis, because some authors have failed to report their nature or size [34], and even when the nature of the involved vessel was specifically stated there has been disagreement as to whether it is arteries [35,36], veins [37,38] or both [39–43] that are affected. In a recent large study of 101 skin biopsies from 86 patients with a clinicopathological

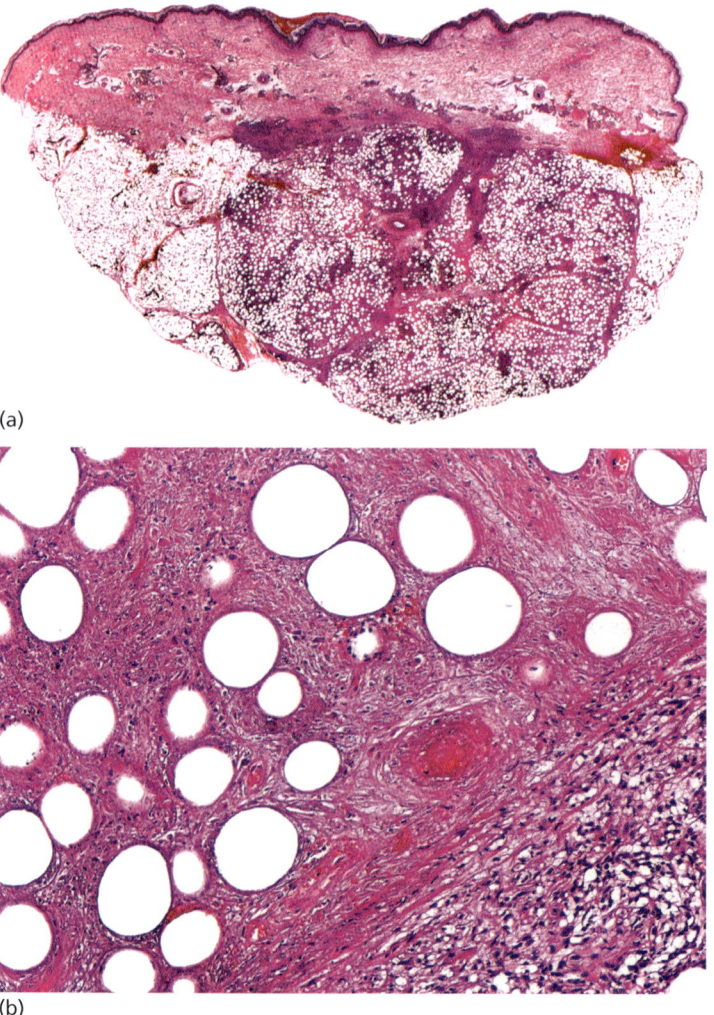

(a)

(b)

Figure 97.26 Histopathological features of an early lesion of erythema induratum. (a) Scanning power showing a mostly lobular panniculitis. (b) Higher magnification showing necrotic adipocytes without nuclei and luminal thrombosis of a small blood vessel.

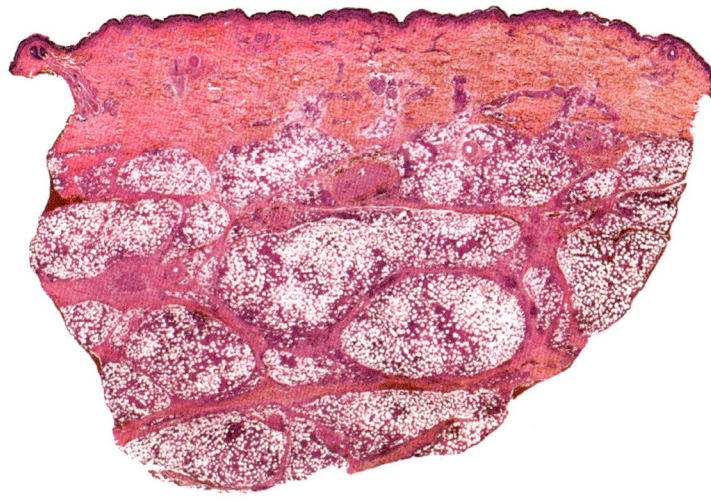

(a)

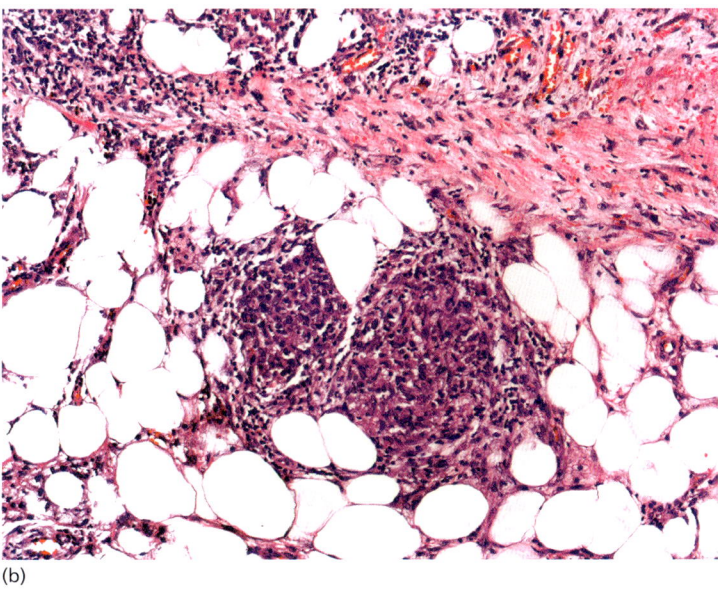

(b)

Figure 97.27 Histopathological features of a fully developed lesion of erythema induratum. (a) Scanning power showing a mostly lobular panniculitis. (b) Small granulomas involving the fat lobule.

diagnosis of erythema induratum, vasculitis was, however, present in 90% of cases (Box 97.3) [25].

Box 97.3 Vascular involvement in erythema induratum

- Small venules of the fat lobule (46.5% of cases)
- Both large veins of the connective tissue septa and small venules of the fat lobule (12.8% of cases)
- Only large veins of the connective tissue septa (11.8% of cases)
- Large veins and arteries of the connective tissue septa and small venules of the fat lobule (9.9% of cases)
- Large veins and arteries of the connective tissue septa (8.9% of cases)
- No evidence of vasculitis (9.9% of cases)

Adapted from Segura et al. 2008 [25].

Although vasculitis can be demonstrated in the majority of cases, there are some cases with all the other clinicopathological attributes of erythema induratum where vasculitis cannot be demonstrated despite a careful search. Therefore its presence should not be considered as an essential criterion for its histopathological diagnosis [25].

Clinical features
Presentation

From soon after its original description, the relationship between erythema induratum and *M. tuberculosis* has been a controversial issue, because mycobacteria cannot be cultured from the cutaneous lesions. Thus, evidence for the aetiological role of *M. tuberculosis* in erythema induratum has had to be established indirectly from a range of clinical and epidemiological data, including the strong hypersensitivity reaction to tuberculin [25], the presence of concomitant active distant (usually pulmonary) tuberculous infection [30,44], the occasional coexistence in the same patient of erythema induratum and another tuberculid [45,46], the frequent personal or family history of tuberculosis [47,48] and the favourable response to antituberculous chemotherapy [49]. It has been suggested that adipose tissue might constitute a reservoir where the *M. tuberculosis* bacillus could persist for long periods of time and avoid both killing by antimicrobials and recognition by the host immune system [50]. It has, however, never been possible to isolate *M. tuberculosis* from lesions of erythema induratum [51].

Several recent polymerase chain reaction (PCR) studies have demonstrated the presence of *M. tuberculosis* DNA in cutaneous lesions of erythema induratum, with frequencies ranging from 25% to 77% of cases, supporting the pathogenic role of *M. tuberculosis* [52–56]. However, in a Spanish study of patients from a region with a high prevalence of tuberculosis, *M. tuberculosis* DNA was detected by PCR in only 14% of cases of erythema induratum [57]. Other investigators have failed to demonstrate the presence of DNA from *M. tuberculosis* or from any other *Mycobacterium* in lesions of erythema induratum [58], supporting the contention that there are likely to be other triggers than tuberculosis.

It has been suggested that erythema induratum results from an immune complex-mediated vasculitis [10], but most authors believe that the disorder results from a type IV cell-mediated response to an antigenic stimulus [59]. Supporting a delayed hypersensitivity reaction is the presence of an abundant number of S-100-positive dendritic cells within the granulomatous infiltrate, which are probably presenting antigens to T cells [60,61]. The presence in the lesional skin of *M. tuberculosis* DNA but not viable tuberculous bacilli suggests that erythema induratum is a hypersensitivity reaction to fragments of tuberculous bacilli.

Management

In those cases in which positive QuantiFERON-TB Gold in Tube® (QFT-GIT) or PCR studies have demonstrated the presence of *M. tuberculosis* DNA in cutaneous lesions of erythema induratum, full specific antituberculous therapy should be given according to current recommended guidelines for systemic tuberculosis. No monotherapy should be administered as has been recommended in the past because drug resistance is likely to develop. In patients with negative results for QFT-GIT or PCR for *M. tuberculosis* DNA, simple measures such as resting, NSAIDs and compression bandaging may be helpful. As in erythema nodosum, potassium iodide 400–900 mg/daily or a saturated solution of potassium iodide, 2–10 drops in water or orange juice, three times per day, may be administered in more persistent cases.

Sclerosing panniculitis

Definition and nomenclature

Sclerosing panniculitis is a relatively common form of long-term chronic panniculitis associated with chronic venous insufficiency and typically affecting the lower extremities of middle-aged or elderly women. This is manifested as a diffuse sclerosis and pigmentation of the skin and subcutaneous tissue (lipodermatosclerosis) (Figure 97.28). It is discussed in more detail in Chapter 101.

> **Synonyms and inclusions**
> - Lipodermatosclerosis

Pathophysiology
Histopathology

Often, clinicians are reluctant to biopsy lesions of sclerosing panniculitis because it is not unusual to induce a chronic ulcer with poor healing at the site of the biopsy [1,2]; most biopsies are thus obtained in the later stages of the disease. However, when a biopsy is performed at the early stages of the process, microscopic study demonstrates a sparse inflammatory infiltrate of lymphocytes in the septa and areas of ischaemic necrosis at the centre of the fat lobules. Necrosis of fat in these early stages is characterised by small, pale, anucleate adipocytes. The small blood vessels of the fat lobule appear congested, with extravasated erythrocytes, haemosiderin deposits

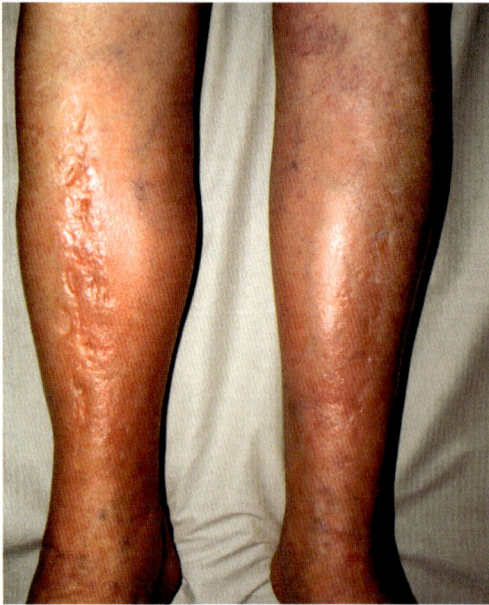

Figure 97.28 Late-stage sclerosing panniculitis showing depressed hard areas with woody induration involving the lower legs.

and necrosis of endothelial cells [3]. In fully developed lesions, the septa show marked thickening and fibrosis, whereas lobules appear atrophic, often with lipophagic granulomas at their periphery. In this stage, the inflammatory infiltrate is composed of lymphocytes, histiocytes and foamy macrophages. Blood vessels appear prominent in the septa at all stages.

In late-stage lesions, the inflammatory infiltrate is sparse or absent, septal sclerosis is prominent and fat lobules appear atrophic, with microcysts and focal lipomembranous (membranocystic) changes (Figure 97.29). The latter consist of cystic structures lined by a lipomembrane, which appears as feathery amorphous eosinophilic material, sometimes with a crenellated or arabesque pattern. The thickened undulating membrane is PAS positive, stains for Sudan black and Luxol fast blue, and expresses immunoreactivity for CD68 and lysozyme [4–6], suggesting the contribution of these macrophage-derived enzymes in its histogenesis. Histopathological findings of pseudomembranous or membranocystic changes involving the dermis have been described as a clue for early lesions of lipodermatosclerosis [7]. These changes are not, however, specific for sclerosing panniculitis because they may be seen in longstanding lesions of various forms of septal and lobular panniculitis. Box 97.4 summarises the conditions in which lipomembranous fat necrosis has been described in the literature [4–6,8–42]. Calcification and elastic tissue degeneration, sometimes with fragmented and calcified elastic fibres resembling those of pseudoxanthoma elasticum (PXE), may be seen in longstanding lesions [43]. These PXE-like fibres are positive for both von Kossa and Verhoeff–van Gieson stains and may develop metaplastic ossification [44]. Elastic fibres with PXE-like changes are not specific for sclerosing panniculitis because they have also been described in uraemic and non-uraemic calcific arteriolopathy (calciphylaxis) [45,46], erythema nodosum, granuloma annulare, morphoea profunda [13,42] and nephrogenic systemic fibrosis [47].

The overlying superficial dermis shows venous stasis changes, with lobules of capillaries and venules of slightly thick-walled vessels in concert with extravasated erythrocytes and haemosiderin deposition. Increased melanin pigment along the basal layer of the epidermis as well as within melanophages in the superficial dermis also contribute to the characteristic hyperpigmentation [48].

Histopathological differential diagnosis of sclerosing panniculitis includes panniculitis of scleroderma and deep morphoea, but these conditions show predominantly septal panniculitis and, although lipodystrophy and lipophagic changes adjacent to the septa may be seen, they are not prominent. Panniculitis of scleroderma and deep morphoea do no show stasis changes in the superficial dermis.

Clinical features
Presentation

The aetiological role of venous hypertension in the pathogenesis of sclerosing panniculitis is undisputed. Venous hypertension increases capillary permeability, which results in leakage of fibrinogen and its polymerisation to form fibrin rings around vessels, with impedance of oxygen exchange and tissue anoxia [49]. Other factors such as trauma and recurrent episodes of cellulitis may also play a role [1,50]. In a study of 128 patients with systemic sclerosis, patients with sclerosing panniculitis had pulmonary hypertension at a significantly higher incidence than

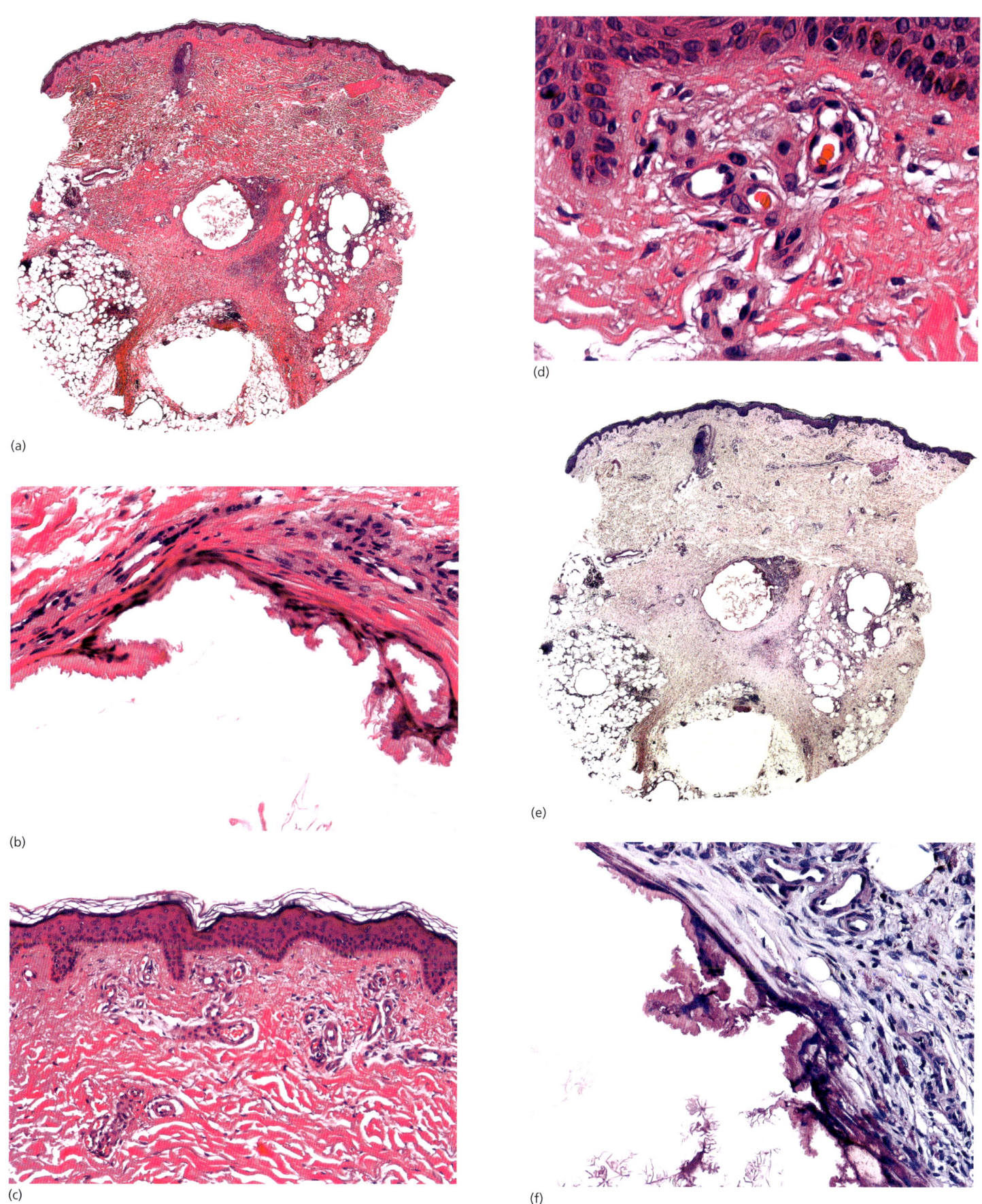

Figure 97.29 Histopathological findings in sclerosing panniculitis. (a) Scanning power showing thickened septa and cystic spaces replacing the fat lobules. (b) A cystic structure lined by a lipomembrane with a crenellated border. (c) Superficial dermis shows stasis changes. (d) Proliferation of thick-walled capillaries and venules in the superficial dermis. (e) A section of the same case stained with periodic acid–Schiff (PAS). (f) PAS positivity of the pseudopapillae with feathery projections into the cystic cavity.

Box 97.4 Panniculitides and other disorders with lipomembranous fat necrosis reported in the literature

Vascular disorders
- Venous insufficiency (lipodermatosclerosis) [3,4,9,14,25]
- Arteriosclerosis [11,12]
- Thromboangiitis obliterans [11]
- Thrombophlebitis [9,13]
- Diabetes [9,13–15]

Connective tissue disease/autoimmune disease
- Lupus panniculitis/discoid lupus erythematosus [4,8,9,14,16,17,27,30]
- Morphoea/scleroderma [8,13,18,31,32]
- CREST syndrome [8]
- Dermatomyositis-associated panniculitis [19,25]
- Vasculitis [9,14,21]
- Behçet disease [17,22]

Inflammatory panniculitis
- Erythema nodosum [4,13,14]
- Erythema induratum [4]
- Traumatic panniculitis [4,23]
- Necrobiosis lipoidica [4,14]
- Pancreatic panniculitis [4]
- Factitial panniculitis [16]
- Nodular fat necrosis [33]

Infections
- Atypical mycobacteria [23]
- Erysipelas [4,14]

Neoplastic panniculitis
- Subcutaneous panniculitic-like T-cell lymphoma [24,34]

Miscellaneous conditions
- Splinter granuloma [35]
- Chemotherapy for leukaemia [36]
- Chemotherapy for breast cancer [37]
- Testicular torsion [38]
- Subcutaneous elemental mercury injections [39]
- Mature cystic teratomas of the ovary [40]
- Myospherulosis [41]
- Breast after radiotherapy [42]

Adapted from Segura and Pujol 2008 [10].
CREST, calcinosis, Raynaud phenomenon, oesophageal dysfunction, sclerodactyly and telangiectasia.

those without. The authors suggested that thrombosis caused by venous hypertension of the leg may be the main cause of pulmonary hypertension in patients with systemic sclerosis and sclerosing panniculitis [51].

Reported findings that may be of pathogenetic relevance in sclerosing panniculitis include increased plasminogen activation in the affected tissue [52–54], increased expression of vascular endothelial growth factor receptor 1 (VEGFR-1) and angiopoietin 2 (Ang-2) [55], deficiencies of protein C and S [56] and local increased synthesis of collagen [57,58].

Differential diagnosis

Because initial stages of the disease involve only one leg, it may be confused clinically with bacterial cellulitis or erysipelas, although in the latter situation there is accompanying heat on palpation, fever or other systemic symptoms [59]. Early lesions may also mimic erythema nodosum [60]. In longstanding lesions, the differential diagnosis is with other sclerodermiform processes, but the absence of histopathological findings of dermal sclerosis, the peculiar distribution affecting only the distal part of one or both legs and the presence of features of chronic venous stasis exclude morphoea, scleroderma and acrodermatitis chronica atrophicans. A rare case of sarcoidosis clinically mimicked sclerosing panniculitis [61].

Management

There is no effective treatment for sclerosing panniculitis. Compression bandaging may achieve transitory results in early cases. In more chronic cases, multilayer lymphoedema compression bandaging is a better therapy. Improvement has been reported with the anabolic steroid stanozolol, mostly in the earlier stages of the disorder, but this medication is no longer commercially available. Danazol has been successfully administered as a substitute. However, this drug may cause severe side effects, including sodium retention, lipid profile abnormalities, hepatotoxicity and virilisation in women. Oxandrolone is an anabolic steroid with less androgenic effects and hepatotoxicity and may be another therapeutic option. Other described therapies that have been reported with variable results include ultrasound, pentoxifylline, fasciotomy and phlebectomy.

Calcific uraemic arteriolopathy

Synonyms and inclusions
- Calciphylaxis

Introduction and general description

Calcific arteriolopathy (calciphylaxis) is strongly associated with end-stage chronic kidney disease and renal transplantation, particularly in diabetics, although a small proportion of cases arise in the absence of renal disease. It typically presents as irregular, exquisitely tender patches of mottled, dusky, livedoid red skin with pale greyish areas of devitalisation before progressing to full-thickness infarction of the skin with consequent necrotic ulceration. These changes commonly extend deeply into subcutaneous fat. Although the most common areas of involvement are the lower extremities and abdomen, the process may also involve other areas (Figure 97.30) including the genitalia. The condition is discussed fully in Chapter 59.

Pathophysiology

Three-dimensional studies in calcific arteriolopathy have shown vascular mural calcification as an early feature, which probably precedes endovascular fibrosis [1]. Recent studies have revealed the presence of the matrix Gla protein, osteopontin and bone

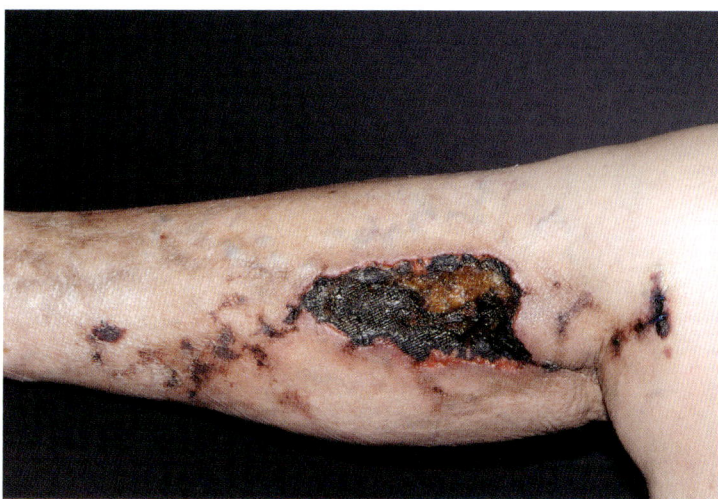

Figure 97.30 Calciphylaxis involving the inner arm in a patient with end-stage renal disease.

morphogenic protein 2 (BMP-2) in pathologically calcified arteries [2,3]. In involved skin, a significant upregulation of BMP-2, its target gene *Runx2* and its indirect antagonist sclerostin, as well as increased expression of inactive uncarboxylated matrix Gla protein (Glu-MGP), have been detected. The upregulation of osteogenesis-associated markers is accompanied by an increased expression of osteopontin, fibronectin, laminin and collagen I indicating an extensive remodelling of the subcutaneous extracellular matrix. Electron dispersive X-ray analysis has revealed calcium/phosphate accumulations in the subcutis of patients with calcific arteriolopathy. Widespread medial calcification in cutaneous arterioles is associated with destruction of the endothelial layer and partial exfoliation of the endothelial cells. CD31 immunostaining has revealed aggregates of endothelial cells contributing to intraluminal obstruction and the consequent malperfusion which results in the clinical picture of ulcerative necrosis. These data indicate that vascular calcification in calciphylaxis is an active osteogenic process involving upregulation of BMP-2 signalling, hydroxyapatite deposition and extensive matrix remodelling of the subcutis [4]. Matrix Gla protein is vitamin K dependent and inhibits vascular calcification. Therefore, oral anticoagulant therapy with warfarin, a vitamin K antagonist, favours vascular calcification in these patients [5]. Other triggering factors that have been recognised as inducers of vascular calcification in calcific arteriolopathy include low levels of albumin, arterial hypertension, obesity, administration of systemic corticosteroids, vitamin D supplementation, blood transfusions, oral phosphate binders, metallic salts, calcitriol, local trauma, UV light treatment, malnutrition with weight loss and insulin injections [6–12].

Histopathology

The most characteristic histopathological finding in calcific arteriolopathy consists in small and medium-sized vessel calcification (Figure 97.31). Small arteries, arterioles and venules may be involved. Vascular calcification is usually extensive within the vessel walls and often exhibits a concentric, circumferential, ring-like pattern. Detailed histopathological studies, however, have demonstrated that the earliest sites of calcification are the media and/or

intima of cutaneous arterioles [13]. Vascular calcification in the arterioles of the deeper reticular dermis or subcutaneous tissue is usually evident with H&E staining but von Kossa stain may help to highlight these deposits. Sometimes the involved vessels also show luminal thrombosis. The affected vessels develop intimal hyperplasia with endovascular endothelial proliferation and intimal fibrosis, resulting in ischaemia of the areas they supply [13,14]. Secondary ischaemic changes include epidermal ulceration and degeneration of dermal collagen. Focal lobular panniculitis is frequently seen [14], although some biopsies show few or no inflammatory infiltrate in the fat lobule adjacent to the calcified vessel. Some authors, however, have described a predominantly septal panniculitis in calcific arteriolopathy [13]. Since vascular calcification may be seen in cutaneous biopsies from other disorders (Box 97.5), additional features may be needed to support a histological diagnosis of calcific arteriolopathy: these include interstitial deposition of calcium in the dermis, fine calcium deposits in and around the adipocytes [15], epidermal and hair follicle calcification [16], perineural calcium deposits [17], calcified elastic fibres with a PXE-like appearance [18,19] and association with diffuse dermal angiomatosis [20]. Perieccrine calcium deposition has been reported as a highly specific histopathological finding in calcific arteriolopathy [21].

Box 97.5 Disorders associated with cutaneous vascular calcification

Renal failure and hyperparathyroidism
- Atherosclerosis [23]
- Liver disease (alcoholic cirrhosis) [24–26]
- Crohn disease [27]
- Malignancies: metastatic breast carcinoma [28], cholangiocarcinoma [29], malignant melanoma [30], osteosclerotic myeloma [31], chronic myelomonocytic leukaemia [32]
- Rheumatoid arthritis on long-term steroid and methotrexate treatment [33,34]
- Protein S deficiency [25,33]
- AIDS [35]
- Antiphospholipid antibody syndrome [36]
- POEMS syndrome [37]

Cutaneous vascular calcification as an incidental histopathological finding
- Calcinosis cutis secondary to injections
- Sclerosing panniculitis (lipodermatosclerosis)
- Erythema induratum
- Leukocytoclastic vasculitis
- Traumatic ulcer
- Basal cell and squamous cell cutaneous carcinomas
- Scars

Adapted from Dauden *et al*. 2002 [15] and Dauden and Oñate 2008 [38]. AIDS, acquired immune deficiency syndrome; POEMS, polyneuropathy, organomegaly, endocrinopathy, monoclonal protein and skin changes.

Calcific arteriolopathy should be distinguished from metastatic cutaneous calcification, which is a rare phenomenon involving the

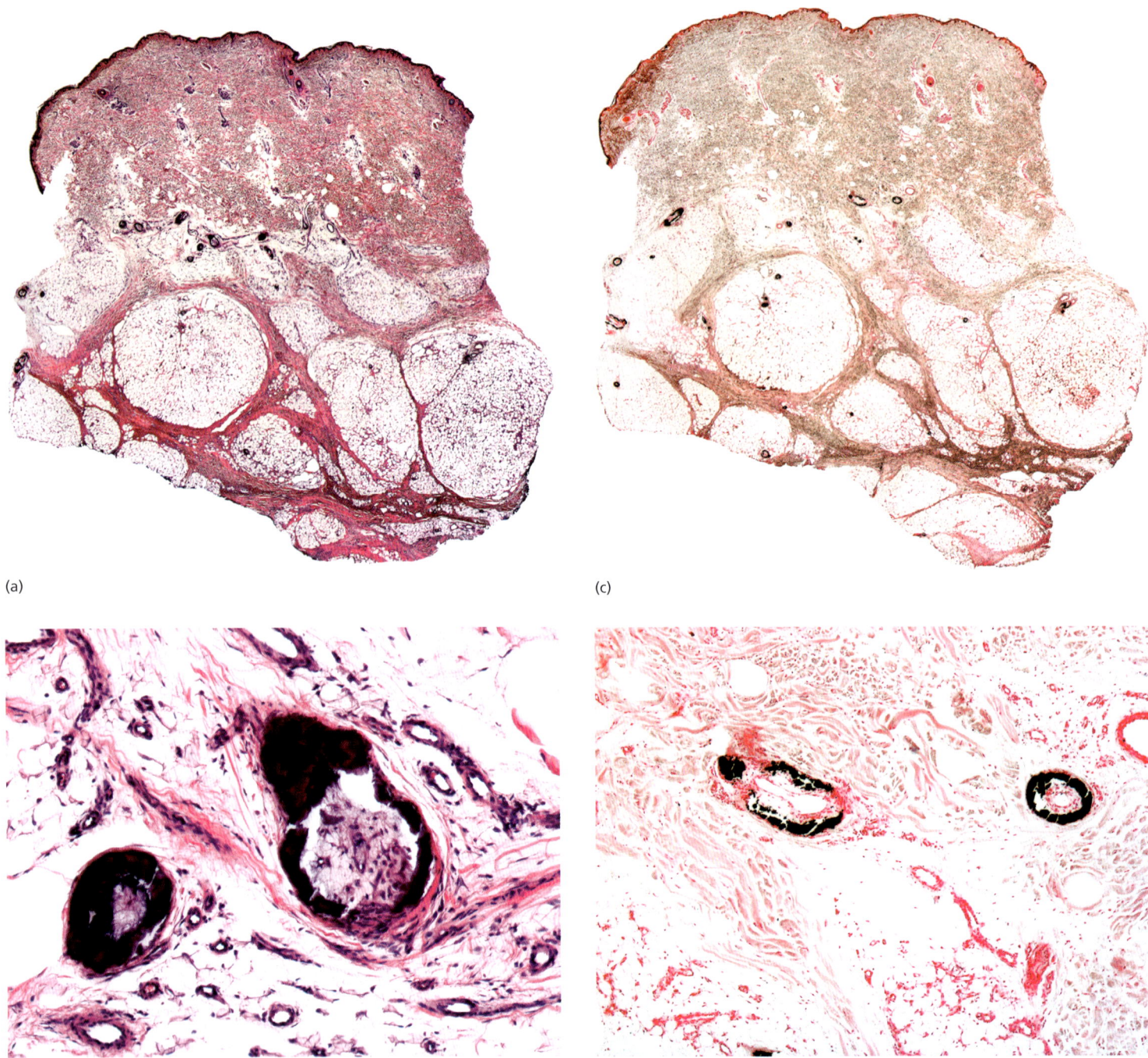

Figure 97.31 Histopathological features of calcific arteriolopathy. (a) Scanning power view showing involvement of the vessels of deeper reticular dermis. (b) Calcification of the vessel walls and occlusion of the vascular lumina. (c) A section of the same case stained with von Kossa stain. (d) Calcification of the vessel walls is positive with von Kossa stain.

dermis and subcutis and affecting predominantly uraemic patients with combined hyperphosphataemia and hypercalcaemia, often in the context of hyperparathyroidism (Chapter 59). It typically presents as firm papules, nodules or plaques in the dermis or subcutis, particularly around large joints or flexural sites. Unlike calciphylaxis, metastatic cutaneous calcification does not lead to tissue necrosis; histopathologically, deposits of calcium, appearing blue with H&E and black with von Kossa stains, are seen in the dermis and subcutis with variable surrounding inflammatory infiltrate, but the vessel walls are spared [22].

Management

Precipitating factors such as calcium supplementation and vitamin D intake should be identified and addressed. In patients with end-stage renal insufficiency, the frequency and duration of dialysis should be increased, in addition to a low phosphate diet and phosphate binders. Cinacalcet or etelcalcetide may be administered in patients with hyperparathyroidism, whereas parathyroidectomy should be reserved for those who fail to respond. There are multiple reported cases of the successful use of sodium thiosulfate; for patients in haemodialysis, the proposed intravenous dose is 25 g thrice weekly (during the last hour of haemodialysis). Although very painful, intralesional sodium thiosulfate is a beneficial treatment that should be kept until the resolution of erythema and purpura. In patients with extensive ulcerations, intensive wound care is required. Surgical debridement is usually followed by improvement and significantly better long-term survival, although there are also reports of the onset of new lesions and worsening of the disease after surgical debridement. Isolated cases have improved under treatment with hyperbaric oxygen therapy.

Cold panniculitis

Introduction and general description
Cold panniculitis is a form of injury to subcutaneous fat induced by exposure to cold, either environmental [1] or as cold objects applied to the skin (e.g. ice packs) [2–3]. Infants are particularly susceptible. It is not uncommon in children in regions subject to low temperatures [4].

Pathophysiology
Predisposing factors
Cold panniculitis was originally described by Hochsinger in 1902 as submental nodules and plaques in children after cold exposure [5]. Lemez, in 1928, demonstrated infants to be more susceptible to fat necrosis by exposure to cold than adults [6]. Haxthausen, in 1941, described similar cases on the cheeks of infants after cold temperatures and named the condition 'adiponecrosis e frigore' [7]. Adams et al. in 1954 clarified the pathogenesis of cold panniculitis demonstrating that pigs fed with a diet rich in saturated fatty acids showed higher cold susceptibility due to the higher ratio of saturated to unsaturated fatty acids, resulting in an elevated freezing point of fat [8]. In 1965 Hirsch confirmed than saturated fats solidified at a higher temperature than unsaturated fats [9]. Solomon and Beerman, in 1963, reported the occurrence of panniculitis in a 28-year-old Jamaican woman within hours of cold exposure with lesions which were readily inducible with local applications of ice [10]. Rotman reported similar cases involving the cheeks in two infants of 5 and 8 months of age [11]. A similar process was described under the name 'popsicle panniculitis' on the cheeks of children a few hours after eating ice lollies [1,2,12]. The most extensive histopathological study of cold panniculitis was performed by Duncan et al. in 1966, who studied serial skin biopsies after exposing the skin of the child to ice for 2–4 min and performing sequential punch biopsies. Increased duration of ice exposure was required to produce cold panniculitis as the child aged and the reaction no longer occurred at the age of 22 months [3].

Histopathology
Histopathologically, cold panniculitis consists of a predominantly lobular panniculitis [13], although a variable septal component is usually present [14]. Inflammation is denser in the lower reticular dermis and dermal–hypodermal interface (Figure 97.32) and the process is more a dermatitis than a panniculitis. The infiltrate is composed mostly of lymphocytes and some histiocytes involving the fat lobules. The overlying dermis shows a superficial and

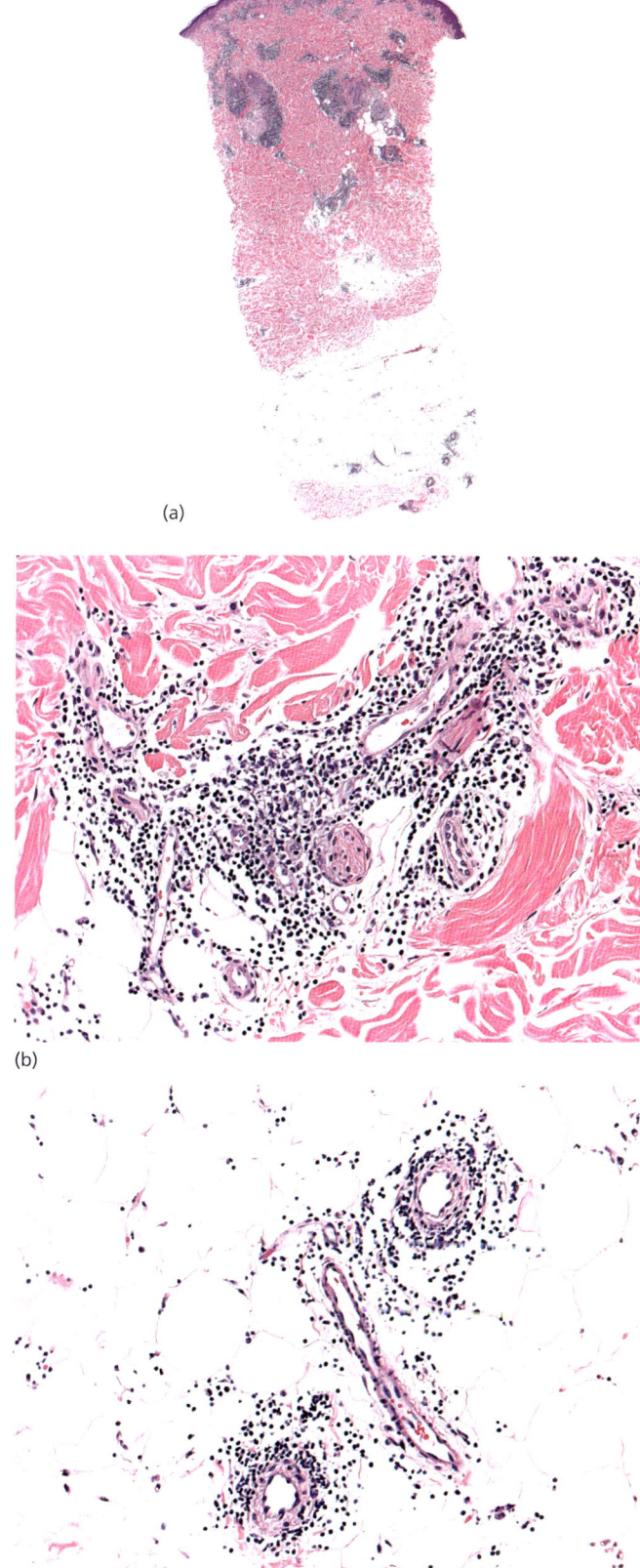

(a)

(b)

(c)

Figure 97.32 Histopathology of equestrian chilblain. (a) Scanning power showing dense nodular infiltrates in reticular dermis. (b) Dense deep dermal perivascular lymphocytic infiltrate. (c) Sparse perivascular lymphocytic infiltrate in the fat lobule.

deep perivascular lymphocytic infiltrate with no vasculitis [13]. Blood vessels of both septa and fat lobules may exhibit endothelial swelling and intramural oedema, but there are no fibrin deposits or nuclear dust as would be seen in a true vasculitis. Interstitial mucin deposition may also be seen with a histopathological picture closely resembling lupus panniculitis [15].

Duncan *et al.* described the 'lives of lesions' of cold panniculitis in a 6-month-old black male infant by applying an ice cube to his buttocks and taking serial punch biopsies at 30 min, 6 h, 24 h, 48 h, 72 h, 6 days and 2 weeks [3]. The earliest changes were seen in the 24 h specimen, which showed a mild perivascular lymphohistio-cytic infiltrate mostly located at the dermal–hypodermal interface, without associated fat necrosis. The changes were more intense in the specimens taken at 48 and 72 h, which showed a denser mixed infiltrate, composed of lymphocytes, scattered neutrophils, histio-cytes and foamy macrophages mostly involving the fat lobule. At this time, features of adipocytic necrosis were evident in the form of lipophagic granulomas surrounding small cystic spaces. The inflammatory reaction progressively increased in biopsies taken in the next 2–3 days and then slowly decreased to regress com-pletely by 2 weeks. The subcutaneous nodules regressed leaving no residual lesion.

In adults, histopathological findings of the so-called cold panni-culitis are similar to those of perniosis, with variable oedema of the superficial dermis and superficial and deep dermal perivascular lymphocytic infiltrate that may extend to underlying fat lobules, but usually involvement of the subcutis is no prominent.

Clinical features
Presentation
Neonatal and infantile cold panniculitis. Neonates are particu-larly susceptible to cold panniculitis. This is thought to be because subcutaneous fat in newborns is rich in saturated fatty acids, particularly palmitic and stearic acids, which have a higher freezing point than unsaturated fatty acids [9,16] so that a small decrease in an infant's temperature may result in crystallisation of subcu-taneous fat [1]. The risk in neonates may be increased by cooling for management of birth asphyxia or for infants undergoing car-diac surgery [1,17,18]. Cold panniculitis has also been reported in neonates who are administered ice packs to control neonatal supraventricular tachycardia [19,20]. Over the first 2 years of life the subcutaneous fat of children rapidly becomes less saturated, with an increase in the oleic acid content and a consequent lowering of the freezing point and lessening of the risk of cold injury.

In young children, the most commonly involved areas are the cheeks and chin, because they are rich in subcutaneous fat and are normally more exposed to the cold than other body areas. The lesions consist of indolent red or violaceous indurated plaques or nodules with no systemic manifestations. The child is otherwise healthy and the lesions regress without treatment within weeks.

Cold panniculitis in adults (equestrain chilblain). Adult patients with cold panniculitis are typically obese and predominantly female. The most commonly affected areas are the lateral upper thighs and gluteal region (Figure 97.33). The distribution of the lesions in adults has been postulated to be attributable to the effects of tight-fitting clothing compromising the blood flow in the upper

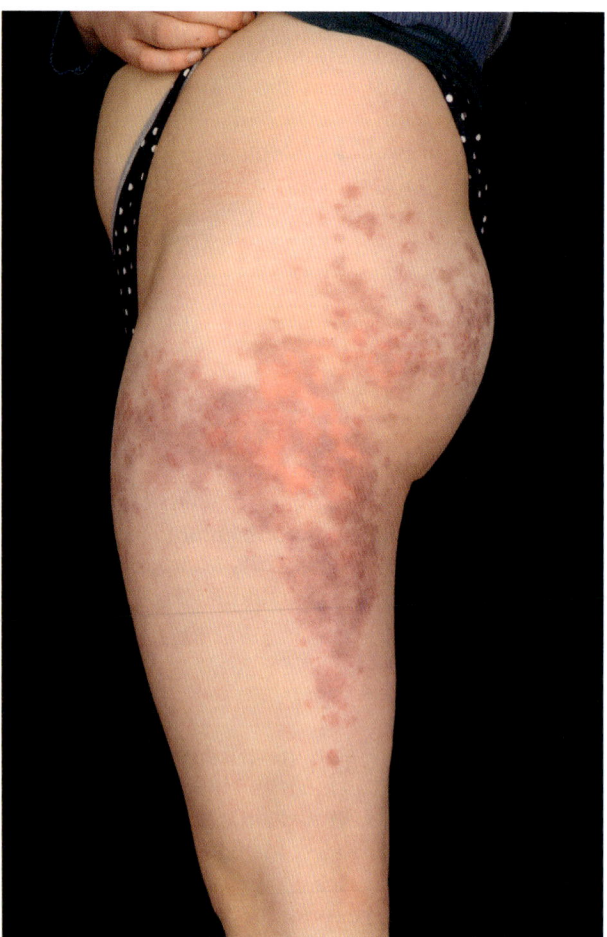

Figure 97.33 Red nodules on the gluteal region and outer side of the thigh of a woman with equestrian chilblain.

lateral thighs, rendering the ischaemic fat more susceptible to cold injury [21]. These patients often have very cold skin in the affected areas even when they are seen in clinic and perhaps a more plau-sible explanation is that the skin and immediately subjacent fat is insulated from core body temperature by a thick layer of interven-ing fat. The tight-fitting clothing offers little protection from low external environmental temperature and the lesions are usually accompanied by some degree of vasodilatation as one would expect with perniosis. It has also been suggested that a diet rich in satu-rated fatty acids would result in a subcutaneous fat similar to that of a newborn [22]. Some such patients have been found to have cryofibrinogenaemia, which probably predisposed them to cold panniculitis [23].

Cold panniculitis has also been described in healthy adult women with lesions involving the lateral upper thighs after prolonged horse-riding in cold weather. This variant may be regarded as a form of perniosis and has been named 'equestrian chilblain' or horse rider's pernio [21]. Symptoms have been reported to be more pro-nounced in older women and appear to be aggravated by heavy smoking, by wearing tight riding clothes and by longer riding times [24]. Similar cases have been described in obese women engaged in sporting activities such as cycling and motorcycling in conditions of humidity and wind [25], or riding on open, slow-moving vehicles in similar weather conditions [26].

Prolonged application of ice directly to the skin can produce local injury in a manner similar to popsicle panniculitis: 'ice pack dermatosis' has been described on the lower back of adults using ice packs for the alleviation of chronic low back pain [27].

Differential diagnosis

The clinicopathological differential diagnosis of cold panniculitis in children includes subcutaneous fat necrosis of the newborn, sclerema neonatorum, lupus panniculitis and poststeroid panniculitis, whereas in adults lupus erythematosus tumidus, perniosis and frostbite are the main differential diagnoses.

Subcutaneous fat necrosis of the newborn usually appears in the first days of life and has a predilection for the thighs, buttocks, cheeks, back and arms. It may occasionally be associated with symptomatic hypercalcaemia. This panniculitis may be associated with hypothermia, obstetric trauma, maternal diabetes and maternal pre-eclampsia. Histopathology shows a lobular panniculitis with a mostly histiocytic infiltrate including multinucleate giant cells, and adipocytes and histiocytes contain needle-shaped clefts that result from lipid crystallisation [17,18,28,29].

Sclerema neonatorum is an extremely rare disorder which was described in premature or debilitated children who developed a diffuse board-like stiffness due to generalised fat necrosis. The condition appeared in the first days after birth and was usually fatal. Histologically, the adipocytes contain needle-shaped clefts in radial arrays with no inflammatory response [13,30]. There have been no recent reports of sclerema neonatorum and it is likely that the problem has disappeared in places with proper facilities for neonatal care of premature and debilitated newborns.

Lupus panniculitis is rare in children and the few described paediatric cases [31–35] do not differ significantly from lupus panniculitis in adults. Histopathology shows a mostly lobular panniculitis, with an infiltrate composed predominantly of lymphocytes and plasma cells, lymphoid aggregates with germinal centre formation and sclerotic collagen bundles at connective tissue septa. The process is chronic and longstanding lesions show hyaline necrosis of the fat lobule, which is not seen in the more acute and self-resolving process of cold panniculitis.

Poststeroid panniculitis occurs in children receiving high doses of systemic corticosteroids when the dose is rapidly decreased or suddenly withdrawn. The lesions appear as small painful nodules on the cheeks and posterior neck, the areas in which corticosteroid therapy has induced fat deposition. The histopathological picture is identical to that of subcutaneous fat necrosis of the newborn [14,29].

Chilblains appear following cold exposure as bluish macules, papules and plaques involving mostly the acral areas of the skin, but they can also be found on the thighs and buttocks. Histopathologically, the picture may be very similar to cold panniculitis; in adults although chilblains usually show oedema of the papillary dermis, the lymphocytic infiltrate is mostly arranged around eccrine coils and some cases show features of lymphocytic vasculitis in dermal blood vessels. Extension to subcutaneous fat is uncommon in chilblains [35,36], except in lesions involving the thighs and buttocks.

Lupus erythematosus tumidus may be also very similar to cold panniculitis, although usually there is no oedema in the superficial dermis and interstitial mucin deposits are often prominent.

In early frostbite, there are reddish and oedematous plaques that may be painful or anaesthetic. In fully developed severe frostbite there is blistering and necrosis. Histopathology shows subepidermal oedema with blister formation, necrosis of epidermal keratinocytes and a superficial and deep perivascular lymphocytic infiltrate involving the full thickness of the dermis [35].

Management

Treatment of cold panniculitis is not usually required because the condition resolves spontaneously. Prevention of infantile cold panniculitis in children is achieved by avoiding cold exposure and direct contact with ice products [10,18]. For equestrian cold panniculitis in adult women, the use of loose, warm clothing should be recommended when riding, with avoidance of tight-fitting clothes and, where possible, cold exposure [21,37]. Nifedipine has been shown to be ineffective [37]. In one case, a dramatic response to tetracycline was observed, which was also effective prophylactically [38].

Lupus panniculitis

Definition and nomenclature

Lupus panniculitis is characterised by a destructive inflammation of subcutaneous fat.

Synonyms and inclusions
- Lupus erythematosus profundus
- Subcutaneous lupus erythematosus

Pathophysiology

Histopathology

Histopathologically, lupus panniculitis is a predominantly lobular panniculitis in which the infiltrate in active lesions involves mainly the fat lobule [1]. Some authors find difficulty in classifying lupus panniculitis as predominantly lobular panniculitis because of the prominent septal component [2–4]. The septal component, however, consists of thickening and sclerosis of the collagen bundles in the septa, whereas most of the infiltrate is found in the fat lobule. Active lesions exhibit a picture of a predominantly lymphocytic panniculitis with numerous plasma cells. Longstanding lesions show hyaline necrosis of the fat lobule with little or no infiltrate and replacement by diffuse eosinophilic glassy remnants of adipocytes [5,6–8]. Lymphoid aggregates, sometimes with germinal centre formation, are also frequently seen in the septa or at the periphery of the fat lobules (Figure 97.34). These lymphoid follicles, although characteristic, are not pathognomonic of lupus panniculitis because they may also be seen in deep morphoea, erythema nodosum, erythema induratum, necrobiosis lipoidica, panniculitis associated with dermatomyositis and necrobiotic xanthogranuloma [9].

Additional histopathological findings consist in calcification, interstitial mucin deposition and features of discoid lupus erythematosus in the overlying epidermis. An uncommon but, when seen, distinctive feature is the presence of nuclear dust within the infiltrate [4,10,11]. Eosinophils are not usually prominent in lesions

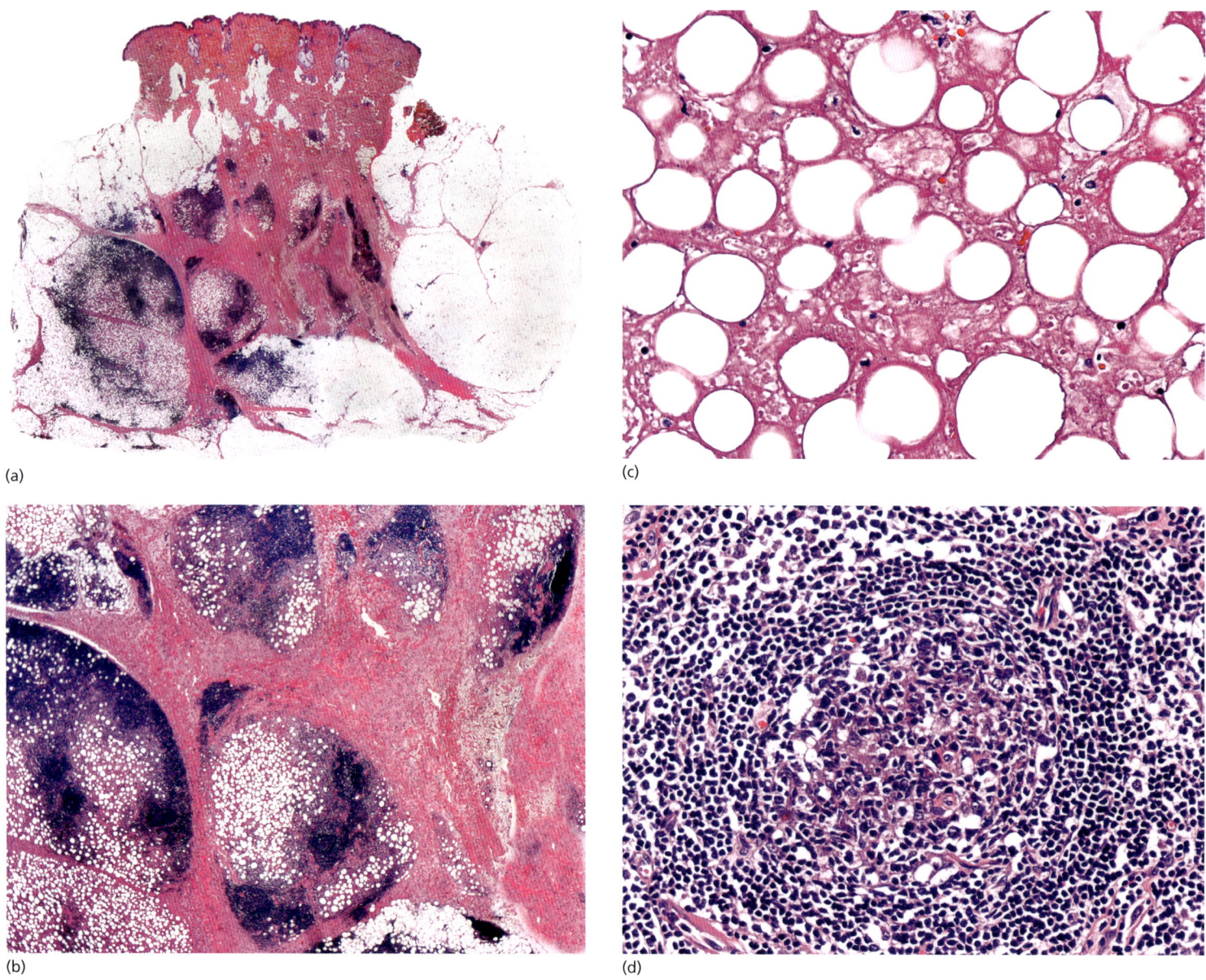

Figure 97.34 Histopathological features of lupus panniculitis. (a) Scanning magnification showing a predominantly lobular panniculitis. (b) Dense lymphoid aggregations at the interphase between the fat lobule and the thickened septa. (c) Hyaline necrosis involving the fat lobule. (d) Reactive germinal centre formation within the lymphoid aggregates.

of lupus panniculitis [5,7] but, in contrast with other forms of cutaneous lupus erythematosus in which eosinophils are characteristically absent, the infiltrate of lupus panniculitis may contain some eosinophils [12].

As with other lobular panniculitides, longstanding and residual lesions of lupus panniculitis may show lipomembranous changes [13]. Lymphocytic vasculitis has been described in lupus panniculitis with variable frequency [14–16]. This vasculitis consists of the presence of lymphocytes in and around the vessel walls, mural fibrin deposition, luminal thrombosis and nuclear dust. Some authors consider that hyaline necrosis of the fat lobule results from the ischaemic process secondary to this lymphocytic vasculitis [17].

Histopathological features of discoid lupus erythematosus at the dermal–epidermal junction in lesions of lupus panniculitis have been described in varying proportions, ranging from 20% to 75% of cases [1,5,6,8,18,19]. These changes include epidermal

atrophy with hyperkeratosis, follicular plugging, vacuolar alteration of the basal layer of the epidermis and basement membrane thickening. Additional features of discoid lupus erythematosus are interstitial mucin deposition, telangiectasia and superficial and deep perivascular dermal lymphocytic infiltrate. Calcification is also a frequent finding in chronic lesions of lupus panniculitis and consists of individual calcification of elastic fibres or large masses of calcium within the lobules and septa [8,20].

Only a few direct immunofluorescence studies have been performed in lesions of lupus panniculitis. The lupus band test at the dermal–epidermal junction is often positive [21]. Additional findings consist of IgG deposition at the periphery of adipocytes and around the vessels [19,22].

Immunohistochemical studies have demonstrated that the infiltrate in lupus panniculitis is composed mostly of T lymphocytes, with a slight preponderance of CD4 over CD8 lymphocytes. All of

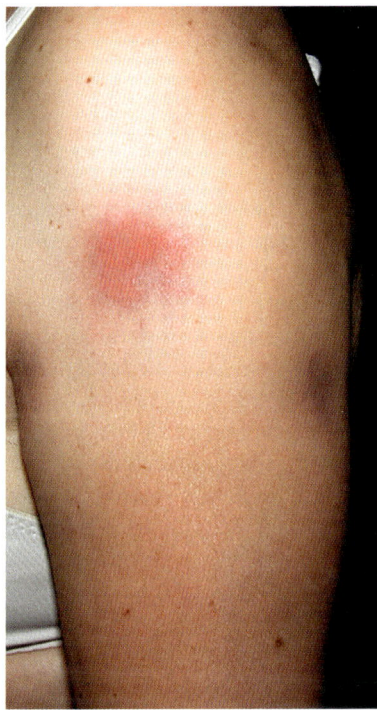

Figure 97.35 Clinical features of lupus panniculitis showing an active red subcutaneous nodule and areas of hyperpigmented lipoatrophy secondary to regressed lesions.

them show α/β immunophenotype. Small aggregates of B lymphocytes are also present at the periphery of the lymphoid aggregates. PCR analyses for *TCRγ* gene rearrangement in the infiltrate has demonstrated its polyclonal nature in most cases [4,22–25]. Because of the presence of cytotoxic CXCR3+ lymphocytes in the fat lobules, it has been suggested that lupus panniculitis may be due to a type I interferon Th1-driven immune response [26].

Clinical features
Presentation
Clinically, lesions consist of indurated plaques that resolve with localised lipoatrophy. Depending on the intensity of inflammation a patient may first present with lipoatrophy rather than induration. The overlying skin may show changes of chronic cutaneous lupus erythematosus. The face, upper arms (Figure 97.35), upper trunk, breasts, buttocks and thighs are most commonly affected. The clinical features are described in detail in Chapter 51.

Differential diagnosis
Panniculitis associated with dermatomyositis shares identical histopathological findings with lupus panniculitis [27–39]. Histopathological differential diagnosis of lupus panniculitis also includes cold panniculitis, deep morphoea, persistent nodules after injection of vaccines containing aluminium, panniculitis at the injection sites of glatiramer acetate and subcutaneous panniculitis-like T-cell lymphoma (SPTCL). Differential diagnosis with cold panniculitis is discussed earlier in this chapter.

Deep morphoea may also display lymphoid nodules at the connective tissue septa of the subcutis, but in contrast with lupus panniculitis the process involves exclusively the septa and the fat lobule is spared.

Persistent nodules at injection sites of a vaccine containing aluminium show similar features to lupus panniculitis, including hyaline necrosis of the fat lobules and lymphoid aggregates, but the correct diagnosis may be suspected by the presence of histiocytes containing fine basophilic granules of aluminium and abundant number of eosinophils [40]. In addition, unlike lupus panniculitis, the infiltrate in vaccine-associated panniculitis is centred around an area of degenerated collagen representing the site of injection.

Several patients receiving daily glatiramer acetate injections for the treatment of multiple sclerosis developed localised panniculitis at the injection sites. The lesions consisted of a mostly lobular panniculitis, with lipophagic granulomas, namely histiocytes engulfing the lipids from necrotic adipocytes. In many areas, scattered neutrophils and eosinophils were seen both in the septa and in the fat lobules. Connective tissue septa showed widening and fibrosis in conjunction with many lymphoid follicles, presenting with germinal centre formation. Immunohistochemically, the inflammatory infiltrate of the fat lobule consisted of CD68-positive histiocytes and suppressor/cytotoxic T lymphocytes. In contrast, the lymphoid follicles in the septa and at the interface between the septum and fat lobule were mainly composed of B lymphocytes. The clinical history with lesions localised only at the injection sites rules out lupus panniculitis [41,42].

The most difficult histopathological differential diagnosis of lupus panniculitis is SPTCL and overlapping cases of lupus profundus and SPTCL have been described. SPTCL is a peculiar α/β T-cell lymphoma, usually CD8+, which involves subcutaneous fat without epidermal and/or dermal involvement, and mimics a panniculitic process (Chapter 139). Magro *et al.* [23] reviewed 32 cases of lymphocytic lobular panniculitis and classified them into three groups: lupus panniculitis, SPTCL and a third group with intermediate features that they named 'indeterminate lymphocytic lobular panniculitis'. Lesions of this third group showed the involvement of subcutaneous fat by atypical lymphocytes with pleomorphic and hyperchromatic nuclei. The same group has recently proposed the term 'atypical lymphocytic lobular panniculitis' for these intermediate cases [43]. The infiltrate showed deletion of one or more pan-T-cell markers (CD3, CD5 and/or CD7) and monoclonal *TCRγ* gene rearrangement by PCR. The authors introduced the concept of subcutaneous lymphoid dyscrasia to encompass cases with overlapping findings of lupus panniculitis and SPTCL. More recently, Pincus *et al.* [44] reported on five patients and Bosisio *et al.* [45] described 11 patients with SPTCL who were unusual in that they also exhibited features of lupus erythematosus. In all cases, attributes indicating SPTCL included an infiltrate of lymphocytes with pleomorphic nuclei involving subcutaneous lobules exhibiting a cytotoxic T-cell (CD3/CD8/βF1) immunophenotype. Additionally, a high proliferation rate and a monoclonal *TCRγ* gene rearrangement were observed in most cases. The manifestations of lupus erythematosus in these patients included a spectrum of clinical and histopathological abnormalities. The clinical manifestations consisted of subcutaneous nodules that healed with lipoatrophy on the face and serological and/or extracutaneous end-organ abnormalities as seen in patients with systemic lupus erythematosus. Histopathological evidences of lupus erythematosus included vacuolar change at the dermal–epidermal interface, interstitial deposition of mucin in the reticular dermis, clusters of

CD20+ B cells partially arranged within germinal centres, a few small clusters of CD123+ plasmacytoid dendritic cells within the adipose tissue and a positive direct immunofluorescence test on clinically uninvolved and lesional skin. The authors concluded that some patients show overlap between SPTCL and lupus panniculitis and that patients with lupus panniculitis should be monitored for possible evolution into SPTCL. This recommendation is also supported by other reports of T-cell lymphomas with subcutaneous tissue involvement, probably cutaneous γ/δ T-cell lymphomas, with histopathological features similar to those of lupus panniculitis, including vacuolar interface dermatitis and dermal mucinosis [46–48]. In fact, one of these cases was erroneously diagnosed as lupus panniculitis [23]. Recently, it has been proposed that these 'overlapping' cases represent examples of lupus panniculitis with focal atypical lymphoid infiltrates rather than true subcutaneous panniculitis T-cell lymphomas [49].

The most useful criteria now for distinguishing lupus panniculitis from SPTCL are the presence in lupus panniculitis of epidermal involvement, superficial and deep perivascular lymphocytic infiltrate in the dermis, lymphoid follicles with reactive germinal centres, a mixed infiltrate with numerous plasma cells, clusters of B lymphocytes, clusters of CD123+ plasmacytoid dendritic cells [2,50], low proliferative index in lymphocytes [51], few or no lymphocytes with immunohistochemical positivity for c-Myc [52] and polyclonal *TCRγ* rearrangement [5].

Management

Oral antimalarials drugs usually improve cutaneous lesions of lupus panniculitis. Isolated lesions may be handled with intralesional corticosteroids. Systemic corticosteroids are more effective in early phases of the disease. Other systemic therapies reported with variable results include dapsone, mycophenolate mofetil, cyclophosphamide, thalidomide and intravenous immunoglobulins. In facial residual lesions of lipoatrophy cosmetic improvement may be achieved with intralesional fillers, although these injections may be followed by reactivation of apparently non-active lesions.

Dermatomyositis-associated panniculitis

Clinical features

Presentation

Panniculitis is less frequent in dermatomyositis than in lupus erythematosus and systemic sclerosis [1–15]. In a series of 55 adult patients with dermatomyositis and cutaneous lesions studied histopathologically, panniculitis was only found in five cases [1]. Panniculitis has also been described in juvenile dermatomyositis [8,11]. When the inflammation settles it leaves areas of lipoatrophy [4].

In some patients, panniculitis is associated with other characteristic cutaneous lesions of dermatomyositis [8,16], whereas in others panniculitis is the only cutaneous manifestation of the disease [3,9]. Conversely, there is a report of a patient presenting with panniculitis and vesiculo-bullous skin lesions but no evidence of muscle involvement [15]. The clinical features of dermatomyositis are discussed in detail in Chapter 52.

Pathophysiology

Histopathology

The histopathological features of dermatomyositis-associated panniculitis are similar to those of lupus panniculitis and consist of a predominantly lobular panniculitis with lymphocytes and plasma cells among the adipocytes. The septal collagen bundles show hyaline sclerosis, and there is progressive replacement of fat with fibrous tissue [2]. Additional histopathological findings include thickening of the blood vessels of the fat lobule, neutrophilic vasculitis with fibrinoid necrosis or lymphocytic vasculitis involving the arterioles of the septa, and calcification [16]. Lymphoid follicles, with or without reactive germinal centre formation, have also been described [5], although this finding is less frequent than in lupus panniculitis or deep morphoea. As in lupus panniculitis, there may be vacuolar change at the dermal–epidermal junction and, in the late stages of the process, membranocystic changes [9,12].

Direct immunofluorescence studies have been reported in only three cases: the results were negative in one case [5]; the second case had deposits of IgM, C3 and fibrinogen in the blood vessels walls of the dermis, but not at the dermal–epidermal junction [9]; and the third case showed deposits of C3 at the basement membrane zone of the dermal–epidermal junction and around the dermal blood vessels, but in the subcutaneous fat only deposits of fibrinogen were detected [5]. As with lupus panniculitis, patients with dermatomyositis-associated panniculitis seem to be a subgroup with a generally good prognosis and no obvious increase in the incidence of malignancy [10,16]. In fact, malignancy has been reported in only one patient with dermatomyositis-associated panniculitis [3].

More common than pure dermatomyositis-associated panniculitis is panniculitis occurring in association with calcification of the muscle and deep tissue. In these cases, the fat lobule shows lipophagic granulomas, calcification and various degrees of acute and chronic inflammation [2].

Management

There is a clear discordance between response of the muscle disease to therapy and response of the skin disease. Cutaneous lesions of dermatomyositis-associated panniculitis respond better to immunosuppressive therapy than other cutaneous lesions of dermatomyositis. If muscle disease is confirmed, then systemic corticosteroid therapy should be initiated in doses aimed at the control of the myositis. In amyopathic dermatomyositis, systemic corticosteroids are not traditionally utilised. Oral antimalarial drugs are less effective in dermatomyositis-associated panniculitis than in lupus panniculitis. Other treatments that have been administered in patients with dermatomyositis-associated panniculitis include low-dose weekly methotrexate, mycophenolate mofetil, intravenous immunoglobulins, dapsone, tofacitinib and thalidomide. In contrast with lupus panniculitis, the face is usually spared in dermatomyositis-associated panniculitis and no cosmetic fillers are usually necessary for the treatment of lipoatrophic residual lesions.

Pancreatic panniculitis

Synonyms and inclusions
- Enzymatic fat necrosis

Introduction and general description

Pancreatic panniculitis was originally described by Chiari in 1883 [1], but it was not until 1961 that Szymanski and Bluefarb reported the first case in the English literature [2]. There are only a few published series of patients with pancreatic panniculitis [3,4–7], and most reports include descriptions of no more than one or two cases.

Epidemiology
Incidence and prevalence

Pancreatic panniculitis is uncommon and appears in only about 2–3% of all patients with pancreatic disease [8], although its incidence is higher among males with alcoholism [9,10].

Pathophysiology

The pathogenesis of pancreatic panniculitis remains unclear, but the release of pancreatic enzymes, such as lipase, trypsin and amylase, seems to be the most important aetiological factor. It is not completely clear how pancreatic proenzymes become activated in the tissues to produce fat necrosis [11], but trypsin may increase the permeability of the microcirculation within the lymphatic vessels [6], allowing lipase and amylase to enter the peripheral circulation. Within the fat lobules these enzymes hydrolyse neutral fat to form glycerol and free fatty acids, which results in adipocyte necrosis and an inflammatory response [12,13]. This theory is supported by the finding of elevated enzyme levels in the blood, urine and skin lesions, even in the absence of detectable pancreatic disease [12], and by the positive intracellular immunostaining of adipocytes with a monoclonal antibody to pancreatic lipase in lesions of pancreatic fat necrosis [14]. However, other factors apart from pancreatic enzymes must also play some pathogenetic role because there is clear discrepancy between the small number of cases of pancreatic panniculitis compared with the great number of patients with pancreatitis and pancreatic carcinoma who have increased serum levels of pancreatic enzymes but no panniculitis [13,15]. Conversely, some patients with pancreatic panniculitis have had normal serum levels of all pancreatic enzymes [5]. Furthermore, *in vitro* investigations have failed to reproduce pancreatic panniculitis when normal human fat has been incubated with the serum of patients with high levels of pancreatic lipase, trypsin and amylase [5]. Other proposed mechanisms implicate vascular damage [12,16], immune complexes [17], and adipocyte-generated cytokines and adipokines released in response to high levels of free fatty acids. Resistin and leptin have been shown to be potential markers of extrapancreatic fat necrosis [18].

Histopathology

Histopathology of pancreatic panniculitis is almost pathognomonic, consisting of a predominantly lobular panniculitis without vasculitis [6,17]. However, some authors have proposed that the earliest feature in pancreatic panniculitis is a predominantly septal panniculitis resulting from enzymatic damage to endothelial cells lining septal blood vessels. These damaged endothelial cells allow pancreatic enzymes to cross from the blood to fat lobules, resulting in necrosis of adipocytes [3,6]. Regardless of this, early states of pancreatic panniculitis show a predominantly neutrophilic infiltrate, with occasional eosinophils and, as the most characteristic finding, ghost adipocytes resulting from coagulative adipocyte necrosis. These ghost adipocytes lose their nuclei and show a finely granular and basophilic material within their cytoplasm because of calcification. Often, ghost adipocytes group in small clusters at the centre of the fat lobule, whereas the neutrophilic infiltrate is present at the periphery (Figure 97.36) [19]. Dystrophic calcification in ghost adipocytes results from the hydrolytic action of pancreatic enzymes on fat cells with subsequent calcium deposition, a process known as saponification [5,6]. Often, adjacent lobules show a different stage in the histopathological evolution of the process. In late stages, fat necrosis and ghost adipocytes are less evident and the inflammatory infiltrate is more granulomatous, containing foamy histiocytes, multinucleate giant cells and haemosiderin deposits [11]. Residual lesions show fibrosis and lipoatrophy. Although ghost adipocytes are very characteristic of pancreatic panniculitis, they are not pathognomonic and similar findings may be seen in mucocutaneous mucormycosis [20] and cutaneous aspergillosis [21]. It has been shown that fungi of the family Mucoraceae produce remarkable amounts of extracellular lipases [22,23] and thus it is likely that the ghost adipocytes result from the local effect of these lipases.

Most patients, although not all, show elevated serum levels of amylase, lipase or trypsin though often one enzyme is within normal levels while the others are elevated [10]. There is no correlation between the serum levels of pancreatic enzymes and the severity of the cutaneous lesions [24]. In rare instances, patients with pancreatic panniculitis may show high serum levels of pancreatic lipase with no evidence of underlying pancreatic disease [25,26]. A leukaemoid reaction and eosinophilia in the peripheral blood are also common haematological abnormalities, particularly in patients with pancreatic carcinoma [26,27]. Other tumour markers such as carcinoembryonic antigen or Ca 19.9 are often elevated in these patients.

Clinical features
Presentation

Clinically, cutaneous lesions of pancreatic panniculitis consist of tender, red or red-brown nodules that may spontaneously ulcerate, draining an oily brown, sterile and viscous material that results from liquefactive necrosis of adipocytes (Figure 97.37). These lesions show a predilection for the distal parts of the lower extremities, mostly around the ankles. Venous stasis may promote this process, although lesions in other areas including the knees, thighs, buttocks, arms, abdomen, chest and scalp may also be seen [28]. Ulceration and fistulisation of necrotic fat to the skin surface are frequent clinical features in pancreatic panniculitis, but they may also occur in other panniculitides. Although there are no specific clinical findings, it seems that the panniculitis associated with pancreatic carcinoma tends to be more persistent, with more frequent recurrences and a greater tendency to ulceration, fistulisation

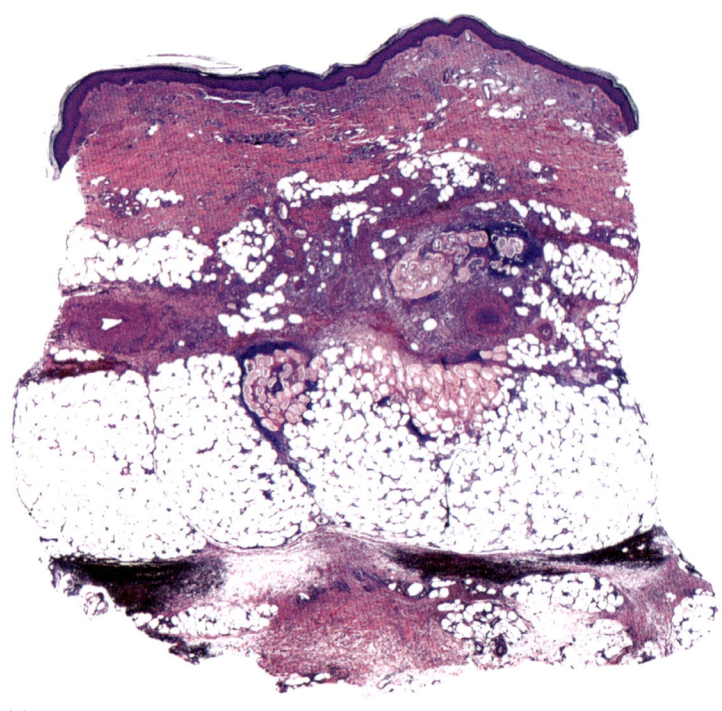

(a)

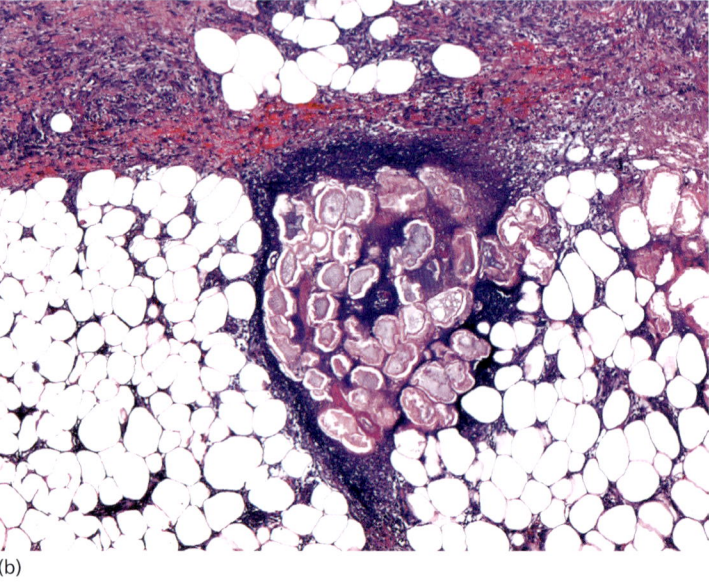

(b)

Figure 97.36 Histopathological features of pancreatic panniculitis. (a) Scanning power showing a mostly lobular panniculitis. (b) A group of ghost adipocytes surrounded by neutrophils is seen at the periphery of the fat lobule.

and involvement of cutaneous areas beyond the lower extremities than that related to inflammatory pancreatic disease [10]. Cases of pancreatic panniculitis with a single cutaneous nodule have, however, also been reported [29]. The association of panniculitis with fever, polyarthritis and abdominal pain should raise suspicion of pancreatic disease.

Enzymatic fat necrosis induced by pancreatic enzymes is not confined to the subcutaneous fat and often patients have other foci of fat necrosis. When this involves periarticular fat it may cause a mono- or oligoarticular arthritis [10,25], which may be symmetrical

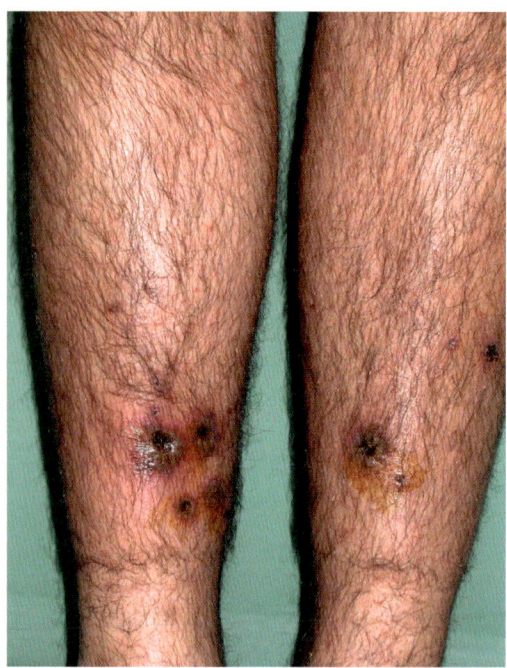

Figure 97.37 Pancreatic panniculitis in an alcoholic male showing nodular lesions, many of them ulcerated around the ankles.

and can be intermittent, migratory or persistent [16], causing the so-called pancreatitis, panniculitis and polyarthritis syndrome (PPP syndrome) [30]. This enzymatic arthritis usually involves the small joints of the hands, wrists and feet, but also may affect larger joints such as the elbows, knees and ankles. Aspiration of the involved joint yields a creamy, purulent, sterile fluid with a few white cells [31]. Joint fluid may also contain lipid crystals with increased levels of amylase, lipase, free fatty acids, triglycerides and cholesterol [31]. In rare instances, this may progress to chondronecrosis and osteonecrosis of the involved joints [32]. Other less common extra-pancreatic sites involved by enzymatic fat necrosis rarely cause symptomatology, but autopsies of patients with pancreatic carcinoma and panniculitis have demonstrated fat necrosis in abdominal fat [33] and bone marrow [34]. Radiological images are characteristic, showing osteolytic lesions, moth-eaten bone destruction and periostitis of the involved bone of the extremities due to extensive areas of bone marrow fat necrosis and trabecular bone destruction [35]. The association of panniculitis, polyarthritis and eosinophilia in a patient with pancreatic cancer is known as the Schmid triad and usually carries a poor prognosis [16].

Skin lesions may be the first sign of pancreatic disease and therefore represent an important clue for the diagnosis [1,16,36]. In the literature, there are several reports in which cutaneous nodules of pancreatic panniculitis preceded the detection of pancreatic carcinoma by several months, and the development of panniculitis may also predict progressive or metastatic malignant disease [37]. However, the most frequent underlying associated pancreatic disease is not pancreatic carcinoma, but acute [6] or chronic [38,39] pancreatitis caused by alcohol abuse [6], trauma [40,41] or cholelithiasis [42]. After acute and chronic pancreatitis, pancreatic carcinoma is the next most common cause of pancreatic panniculitis. Rarer disorders that may also cause this type of panniculitis are listed in Box 97.6 [**3**,6,13,16,17,25,37,40–78].

Box 97.6 Disorders associated with pancreatic panniculitis

Acute or chronic pancreatitis
- Pancreatitis secondary to alcohol abuse [6]
- Pancreatitis secondary to trauma [40,41]
- Pancreatitis secondary to cholelithiasis [42]
- Pancreatic pseudocyst [43,44]
- Acute fatty liver of pregnancy and pancreatitis [45]

Malignancy
- Acinar cell pancreatic carcinoma [3,13,37,46–51]
- Islet cell pancreatic carcinoma [17,37,52–57]
- Acinar cell pancreatic cystadenocarcinoma [16]
- Liver carcinoma [25]
- Adenocarcinoma of unknown origin [58]
- Cancer-associated fasciitis–panniculitis syndrome [59]
- Pancreatic adenosquamous carcinoma [60]
- Pancreatic neuroendocrine carcinoma [61]

Postprocedural
- Following renal or simultaneous pancreas and kidney transplantation [62–65]
- After endoscopic retrograde cholangiopancreatography [66]

Pancreatic anomalies
- Vascular pancreatic fistulae [67]
- Pancreas divisum [68–71]

Miscellaneous
- Systemic lupus erythematosus [72,73]
- Association with HIV infection and haemophagocytic syndrome [74]
- Hypertriglyceridaemia and nephrotic syndrome [75]
- Sulindac therapy [76]
- Following L-asparginase treatment for acute lymphoblastic leukaemia [77,78]

Differential diagnosis

Clinically, the main differential diagnoses are erythema induratum, α_1-antitrypsin deficiency panniculitis and infectious panniculitis [3,12,17]. Histopathology usually resolves any doubt by finding ghost adipocytes in the saponified fat lobule [12]. Lobular panniculitis at the site of subcutaneous IFN-β injections for the treatment of multiple sclerosis may histologically mimic pancreatic panniculitis [79].

Management

Treatment of pancreatic panniculitis should be directed to the underlying pancreatic disease and usually the cutaneous lesions heal once the acute inflammatory pancreatic process has resolved or the pancreatic anomaly has been surgically corrected [3,13,64,80]. Administration of the somatostatin analogue octreotide, a synthetic polypeptide that inhibits pancreatic enzyme production, has been reported to result in a significant improvement in pancreatic panniculitis in some [13,47,81] but not all [17,39,46,57] patients with pancreatic carcinoma. Corticosteroids, NSAIDs and immunosuppressive drugs are usually not effective treatments for pancreatic panniculitis [35].

Alpha-1 antitrypsin deficiency panniculitis

Introduction and general description

Alpha-1 antitrypsin deficiency is a genetic disorder that manifests as pulmonary emphysema, liver cirrhosis and, rarely, as cutaneous panniculitis. It is characterised by low serum levels of α_1-antitrypsin, the main protease inhibitor in human serum.

Warter *et al.*, in 1972, were the first authors to describe panniculitis in association with α_1-antitrypsin deficiency, although these authors considered the process to be a manifestation of familial Weber–Christian disease [1]. Rubinstein *et al.*, in 1977, described the first two cases of α_1-antitrypsin deficiency-related panniculitis as a specific manifestation of this autosomal recessive inborn error of metabolism [2].

Epidemiology

Panniculitis associated with α_1-antitrypsin deficiency is rare, with a female preponderance of 71% among the reported cases [3] and the age of presentation ranging from 7 to 73 years, with a mean age of 39.7 years [4], although children may also be affected [5].

Pathophysiology
Genetics

Alpha-1 antitrypsin is the most important serine protease inhibitor produced in the liver. Its principal function is to inhibit trypsin activity, but it also acts as a potent inhibitor of chymotrypsin, plasmin, thrombin, neutrophilic elastase, pancreatic elastase, serine proteases, collagenase, factor VIII, kallikrein, urokinase and cathepsin G. It may also inhibit complement activation, both through a direct effect on complement-related proteases and by inhibiting the neutrophil proteases that activate enzymes of the complement system. Additionally, it is thought to help regulate protease-stimulated activation of lymphocytes and phagocytosis by macrophages and neutrophils. It is an acute phase reactant which is released in stress situations.

Alpha-1 antitrypsin consists of 394 amino acids organised into three β sheets and nine α helices. The active site of the protein is a reactive central loop composed of 20 amino acids, which, when in contact with a serine protease, induces conformational changes resulting in inactivation of both α_1-antitrypsin and protease [6]. The gene that encodes this protein, *SERPINA 1* (formerly known as *PI*), is located at 14q32.1. More than 120 allelic variants have been described to date [6]. The most frequent allele, PiM, defined by its protein isoelectrophoretic mobility (M = medium mobility), is associated with a homozygous PiMM phenotype and normal serum levels of α_1-antitrypsin (120–200 mg/dL) [7]. Two alleles, PiS (S = slow mobility) and PiZ (Z = very slow mobility), each caused by a single nucleic acid substitution, are considered to be involved in pathological manifestations. In the Z variant, glutamic acid replaces lysine at position 342 [8]. Homozygosity for the Z allele (PiZZ) is associated with very low serum levels of α_1-antitrypsin (20–45 mg/dL), whereas the heterozygous phenotypes PiMZ or PiMS result in a moderate reduction of α_1-antitrypsin serum levels. A null allele variant, without any apparent gene alteration, but with no detectable mRNA produced, has also been described.

In individuals who are homozygous for Pi null/null mutations, serum α_1-antitrypsin is not detectable at all [9]. Heterozygosity for pathogenic α_1-antitrypsin mutations (PiMS, MZ, SZ) is estimated to occur in about 10% of the general population [10], with 2% heterozygous for the Z allele [11]. The prevalence of the homozygous PiZZ phenotype is only about 1 in 3500 in northern Europe populations [8]. In heterozygous carriers of the S or Z allele, α_1-antitrypsin production and function are apparently normal but only a small amount of α_1-antitrypsin enters the circulation from its production site in the liver. Both mutations result in a high tendency for the protein to polymerise, especially in the Z variant. In both homozygous and heterozygous phenotypes, polymerised α_1-antitrypsin cannot as a result be released from the liver. Z-type α_1-antitrypsin polymers have been detected in lesional skin, which supports the inflammatory pathogenesis of panniculitis and the potential pro-inflammatory role of polymers [12].

In situations causing tissue injury, such as smoking for emphysema, trauma for panniculitis or hepatotoxins for cirrhosis, the absence or deficiency of α_1-antitrypsin results in uncontrolled activation of lymphocytes and macrophages, a lack of inhibition of the complement cascade including C3a–C5a neutrophilic chemotactic factors, and the accumulation of neutrophils with a release of proteolytic enzymes and secondary tissue damage [13]. The special susceptibility of subcutaneous fat to proteolytic degradation when not protected by α_1-antitrypsin is due to its high fatty acid content. Fatty acids modify elastin conformation and render fat more susceptible to proteolytic degradation [14].

Severe α_1-antitrypsin deficiency is associated with a variety of clinical manifestations including disorders of blood coagulation and fibrinolysis, anomalies in the phagocytic mechanism of the immune response and anomalies in the activation of zymogens and the release of hormonal peptides in addition to its effect on the lung, liver and subcutaneous fat.

Alpha-1 antitrypsin deficiency panniculitis is most severe in homozygous PiZZ individuals. It can, however, also develop in heterozygotes with PiMS [6,14], PiMZ [15] and PiSZ [16] genotypes and in homozygotes with PiSS [17] and PiM_1M_1 [18] genotypes. This suggests that factors other than α_1-antitrypsin deficiency may be involved in the pathogenesis. Furthermore, some authors believe that there are patients with the phenotypic features of α_1-antitrypsin deficiency but normal serum levels of α_1-antitrypsin who develop panniculitis because of mutations that do not induce polymerisation but that affect the reactive centre loop, resulting in the production of non-functional protein [6,16].

Histopathology

Histopathological study of α_1-antitrypsin deficiency panniculitis shows a predominantly lobular panniculitis with no vasculitis. In the early stages, the presence of neutrophils extending into the lower reticular dermis in an interstitial pattern between collagen bundles ('splaying of neutrophils') has been proposed by some authors as a specific clue for the diagnosis [19]. This is, however, a non-specific finding that may be found in any neutrophilic lobular panniculitis. A more specific finding consists in the focal nature of the damage with large clusters of normal adipocytes adjacent to areas of necrosis and dense neutrophilic and histiocytic infiltrates (Figure 97.38) [20,21]. Occasionally, the

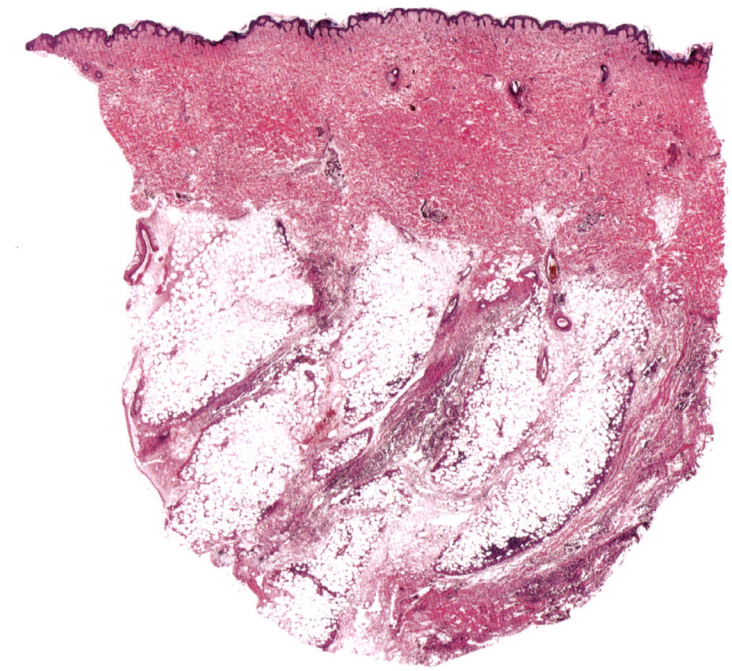

(a)

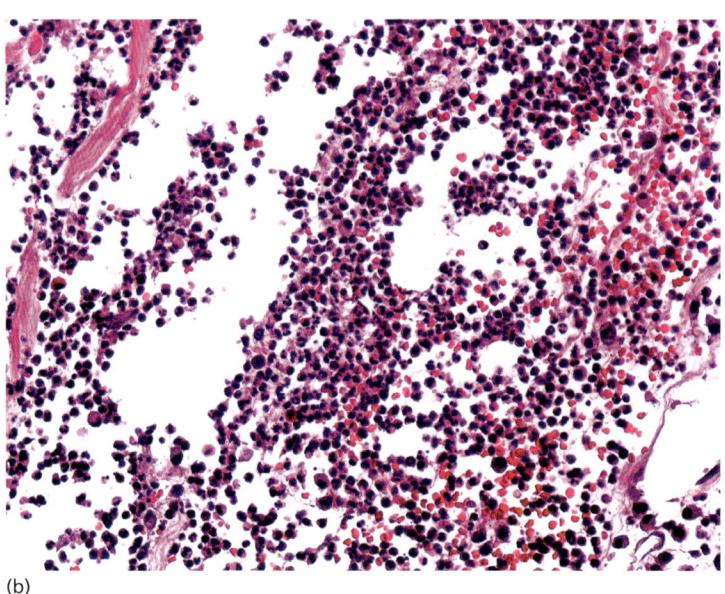

(b)

Figure 97.38 Histopathological features of α_1-antitrypsin deficiency panniculitis. (a) Scanning power showing involvement at the septa and the periphery of the fat lobules. (b) Neutrophilic infiltrate and nuclear dust but no evidence of vasculitis.

intense neutrophilic infiltrate may cause collagenolysis and elastic tissue destruction at the connective tissue septa and then necrotic fat lobules appear to be 'floating' and surrounded by neutrophils [22]. Transepidermal elimination of liquefied dermis may occur as a secondary phenomenon [23]. In late-stage lesions, neutrophils and necrotic adipocytes are less evident and the histopathological picture is dominated by non-specific lipophagic granulomas replacing fat lobules. Some macrophages may engulf nuclear dust of neutrophils and dystrophic calcification may develop [15]. Direct immunofluorescence studies have revealed deposits of complement

C3 and IgM around the dermal blood vessels: these are of uncertain significance [14,20].

Laboratory anomalies include absence or significantly reduced levels of α_1-globulin on plasma protein electrophoresis and abnormally reduced levels of α_1-antitrypsin. Sometimes an isoelectrophoretic mobility study for α_1-antitrypsin may demonstrate an abnormal phenotype with normal serum levels. Therefore, α_1-antitrypsin levels measured outside of the acute phase (α_1-antitrypsin is an acute-phase reactive protein that may be elevated in the setting of inflammation) as well as α_1-antitrypsin phenotyping and genotyping should be requested in suspicious cases. In chronic cases, normocytic normochromic anaemia and hypoalbuminaemia are frequently found [24].

Clinical features

Presentation

Dermatologically, panniculitis is the most important clinical manifestation of α_1-antitrypsin deficiency. Inflammation of subcutaneous fat may be the first sign of the disease, although subcutaneous nodules usually appear when other manifestations of the disorder have already developed. The panniculitis presents as red nodules and plaques mainly located on the trunk and around the shoulders and hips [14]. The head and extremities may sometimes also be involved [20]. The earliest lesions resemble cellulitis [11] and show a tendency to ulcerate and exude oily material derived from necrotic adipocytes (Figure 97.39) [20]. Healing of lesions leaves atrophic scars. A chronic relapsing course is characteristic. Antecedent trauma at the site of the lesion [14], surgical debridement [20], cryosurgery [25] or injections [24] can precipitate new lesions. Postpartum flares of the process have been attributed to an oestrogen-stimulated increase in proteinase inhibitor levels during

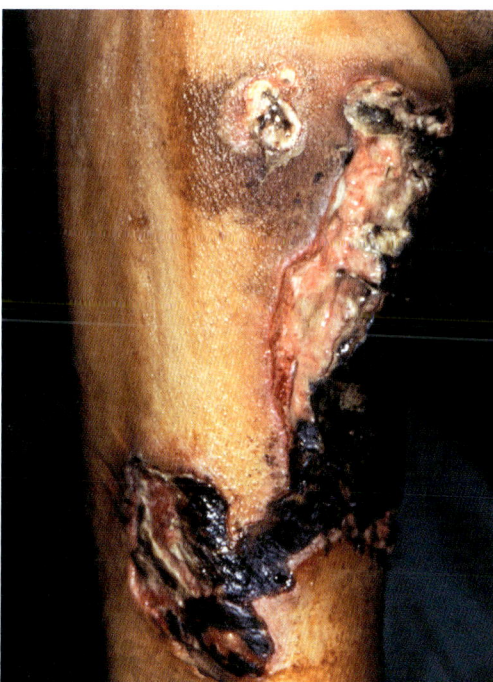

Figure 97.39 Panniculitis associated with α_1-antitrypsin deficiency. Necrotic ulcers exudate oily material that result from necrotic adipocytes.

pregnancy, followed by a precipitous decline to subnormal levels postpartum [26]. Uncommon cutaneous manifestations associated with α_1-antitrypsin deficiency include vasculitis and acquired angioedema [7,27,28]. Visceral extension is uncommon, but the involvement of perinephric fat as well as hepatic and splenic sterile abscesses have been reported [17].

Differential diagnosis

Differential diagnosis of α_1-antitrypsin deficiency panniculitis includes other neutrophilic panniculitides with a tendency to ulceration and fistula formation such as the early stages of erythema induratum, pancreatic panniculitis, factitial panniculitis and infective panniculitis. Most of these panniculitides show specific histopathological findings. When neutrophilic lobular panniculitis is found without indications of other specific diagnoses, measurement of serum levels of α_1-antitrypsin and electrophoretic mobility studies should be undertaken.

Complications and co-morbidities

Systemic manifestations of α_1-antitrypsin deficiency include panacinar emphysema, neonatal hepatitis, cirrhosis and liver disease resulting from retention of the abnormal polymerised protein within the liver, pancreatitis, membranoproliferative glomerulonephritis, c-ANCA-positive vasculitis and angioedema due to deficiency of a protease inhibitor [14,24]. Approximately 50% of ZZ patients will die from emphysema-related complications and 10% will develop liver disease; the MZ phenotype is associated with a slightly higher risk of both lung and liver disease; and no increased likelihood of either lung or liver disease is seen in MS patients [6]. The null/null phenotype is usually accompanied by emphysema but no liver disease because there is no α_1-antitrypsin synthesis and accumulation in the liver cannot therefore occur [9].

Management

Trauma and surgical debridement should be avoided, as should smoking or exposure to hepatotoxins. Reduction of alcohol intake should be recommended. Several treatments including corticosteroids [14], immunosuppressive drugs, colchicine [25], danazol and antimalarials have shown poor or no response. The first line of treatment is based on doxycycline or minocycline in a dose of 200 mg daily for at least 3 months, which may be effective in mild cases as tetracyclines have anticollagenase activity which may partly re-establish protease–antiprotease homeostasis [10]. Dapsone has also shown to be effective because it inhibits the migration of neutrophils [14,17]. For severe cases with liver and lung involvement, the best option is replacement of α_1-antitrypsin using human pooled plasma from normal donors (Prolastin®). Intravenous infusions in a dosage of 60–100 mg/kg per week, depending on the severity of the deficiency, over a period of 3–7 weeks is recommended [3,8,23,29–35]. Recurrence after discontinuation of therapy is common, but there is a good response to reinfusion [31]. Other interventions that have been used include plasma exchange [36] and liver transplantation [37]. In one patient α_1-antitrypsin deficiency panniculitis appeared after liver transplant and was successfully treated with retransplant [38]. The role of genetic engineering in producing α_1-antitrypsin is being investigated [39–41].

Infective panniculitis

Pathophysiology

Histopathology

The histopathological features of infective panniculitis consist of a predominantly lobular neutrophilic panniculitis without vasculitis [1–3], although in some cases small-vessel vasculitis has been described [1]. Apart from the neutrophilic infiltrate in the fat lobule, additional features suggestive of an infective aetiology of a lobular panniculitis are haemorrhage, proliferation of vessels, foci of basophilic necrosis and necrosis of sweat glands [1]. Special stains, including Gram, PAS, Ziehl–Neelsen and methenamine-silver, as well as tissue cultures should be performed.

Rarely, infective panniculitis may resemble SPTCL, as was reported in a case due to *Borrelia burgdorferi* where the lobular infiltrate was composed of atypical lymphocytes with cytotoxic immunophenotye. *B. burgdorferi* aetiology was, however, proven by positive PCR findings, serology and a favourable response to antibiotics [4].

The histopathological findings in panniculitis caused by mycobacterial infections vary according to the organism involved and the immune state of the host. In most cases, the histopathological picture, as in other bacterial panniculitides, is a neutrophilic lobular panniculitis, but mycobacterial panniculitides often contain suppurative granulomas (Figure 97.40) [5–8] or frank tuberculoid granulomas [5,9,10]. Caseous necrosis is suggestive of tuberculous panniculitis [9].

In Q fever due to *Coxiella burnetii*, a 'doughnut-like' lobular granulomatous panniculitis, similar to the changes found in the liver and bone marrow, has been described [11].

Ghost adipocytes reminiscent of pancreatic panniculitis have been documented in cases of mucormycosis [12] and aspergillosis [13] involving subcutaneous fat.

Different histopathological patterns have been described according to the inoculation route of the microorganisms into the skin. Primary cutaneous infections arise either from direct physical inoculation or at the site of an occlusive dressing over an indwelling catheter, whereas secondary cutaneous infections develop either from direct extension to the chest wall in pulmonary infections or from haematogenous dissemination. In primary cutaneous infections, the epicentre of the inflammation is the superficial dermis, and thrombosed vessels do not contain intravascular organisms. In contrast, in secondary cutaneous infections, the epicentre of the inflammation is more deeply seated and involves only the deep reticular dermis and subcutaneous fat. The blood vessels are thrombosed and dilated with masses of organisms expanding their lumina [14]. In immunosuppressed patients, microorganisms are numerous and they may be easily identified in tissue sections with routine H&E staining or with special stains. However, in immunocompetent patients, microorganisms are sparse and may be difficult to detect. In these latter cases, the diagnosis may be established only from culture [1,15]. In cases with few microorganisms, immunohistochemical staining with anti-bacille Calmette–Guérin (anti-BCG) antibody was proposed as a helpful tool for screening because this commercially available polyclonal antibody showed

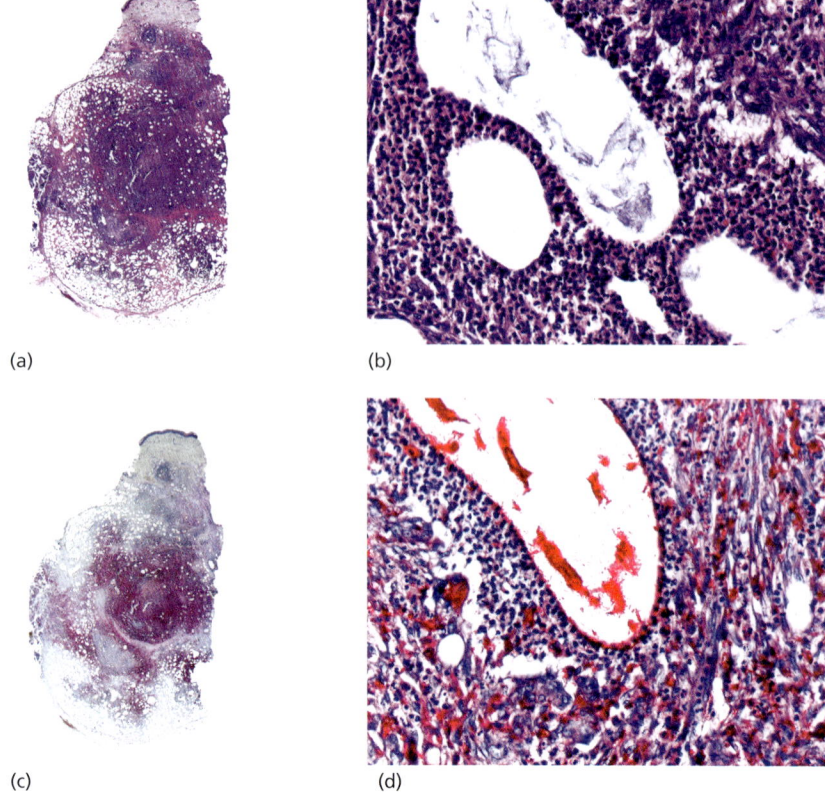

(a)

(b)

(c)

(d)

Figure 97.40 Histopathological features in a cutaneous infection by *Mycobacterium chelonae*. (a) Scanning power showing involvement of the reticular dermis and subcutaneous fat. (b) Suppurative granuloma involving the fat lobule, with granular basophilic material that corresponds to mycobacteria. (c) A section of the same case immunostained with the anti-BCG antibody. (d) Clusters of anti-BCG-positive mycobacteria are seen within the holes of the abscess.

cross-reactivity with many bacteria, mycobacteria and fungi, and produced minimal background staining; it might therefore identify microorganisms that could not be seen using conventional stains [16]. However, due to overpurification by the manufacturer in recent years, anti-BCG antibody no longer has the original wide sensitivity for bacteria and fungi and currently it should be restricted to the search for mycobacteria in formalin-fixed and paraffin-embedded samples. PCR-based methods are also available to test formalin-fixed tissue for specific agents.

Causative organisms

Several bacterial and fungal infections may cause panniculitis as their main clinical manifestation.

Bacteria implicated in subcutaneous panniculitis include *Streptococcus pyogenes* [1], *Staphylococcus aureus* [1], *Pseudomonas* spp. [1,17,18], *Klebsiella* [1], *Nocardia* spp. [1,19], *Brucella* [2] and *Borrelia burgdorferi* [4,20]. Cutaneous lesions in patients with sepsis due to *Stenotrophomonas maltophilia* may also show a lobular panniculitis with macrophages engulfed by microorganisms [21]. Most cases of mycobacterial panniculitis reported in the literature have been caused by non-tuberculous mycobacteria [6,7,9,22–29], especially rapidly growing mycobacteria such as *Mycobacterium chelonae* [5,6,27,28] and *M. fortuitum* [7,29], and less frequently by slow-growing mycobacteria such as *M. avium intracellulare complex* [23–25] and *M. marinum* [9,22–25]. There are exceptional cases due to *M. tuberculosis* [6,7,9,26–30] and panniculitis caused by *M. leprae* is extremely rare [31]. *M. ulcerans* causes a well-defined clinicopathological entity known as Buruli ulcer, which involves predominantly subcutaneous fat [32–37]. Specific cutaneous involvement in Whipple disease (disorder of the small intestine due to infection with *Tropheryma whippelii*) is extremely rare. The few described cases presented subcutaneous nodules on their legs which histopathologically consisted of a mostly septal panniculitis with infiltration of the septa by foamy macrophages containing PAS-positive intracellular granules [38–41]. In some patients, erythema nodosum-like lesions appeared in treated Whipple disease as a sign of immune reconstitution inflammatory syndrome [42–44].

Fungal infections of the subcutaneous fat may be classified into two main categories: (i) panniculitis in the setting of a disseminated fungal infection; and (ii) classic subcutaneous mycosis. These two groups differ in their causative microorganisms, their pathogenesis, the setting in which they appear, their prognosis and their treatment. The most common disseminated fungal infections causing panniculitis are *Candida* spp. [1,45,46], *Aspergillus* spp. [18], *Fusarium* spp. [1] and *Histoplasma capsulatum* [47,48]. The most common classic subcutaneous mycoses are sporotrichosis due to *Sporothrix schenckii*, eumycetoma caused by *Madurella mycetomatis* [20,49] and chromoblastomycosis caused by pigmented fungi, the most common being *Phialophora verrucosa*, *Fonsecaea pedrosoi*, *F. compacta* and *Cladophialophora carrionii* [50,51]. Uncommon subcutaneous fungal infections include phaeohyphomycosis, lobomycosis, rhinosporidiosis and subcutaneous zygomycosis. A case of septal panniculitis caused by cytomegalovirus infection with many cytomegalovirus inclusions in endothelial cells has been described in an immunosuppressed patient [52] and another case of neutrophilic lobular panniculitis due to acanthamoebiasis has been reported in a patient with acquired immune deficiency syndrome (AIDS) [53].

Clinical features
Presentation

With the exception of the classic subcutaneous mycoses, most of these infective panniculitides occur in immunosuppressed patients and are uncommon in immunocompetent hosts. The immunosuppressed population, which has been increasing in recent decades due to human immunodeficiency virus (HIV) infection, organ transplantation and the widespread use of immunosuppressive drugs, is at risk not only of common cutaneous infections but also of opportunistic infections with atypical clinical presentations [54,55].

Bacterial panniculitis may appear in the setting of septicaemia, as the consequence of direct inoculation or by direct spread from an underlying infection. In patients with sepsis, solitary or multiple nodules and abscesses appear as a consequence of the haematogenous dissemination of bacteria. Constitutional symptoms are often absent, but the general condition of the patient is impaired by the underlying disease.

The clinical features of subcutaneous mycobacterial infections vary according to the immune state of the patient. In immunocompromised patients, lesions tend to be widespread due to haematogenous dissemination. Sporotrichoid spread is not uncommon in these patients (Figure 97.41) [3,15,56] and spread to internal organs may occur [23,56]. In immunocompetent patients, the infection is usually localised and related to trauma, such as penetrating injury, surgical procedures, acupuncture, injections or postepilation folliculitis [6,24,25].

Panniculitis in immunosuppressed patients with disseminated fungal infection presents as multiple, reddish, subcutaneous nodules, pustules or fluctuant abscesses [14,45,47]. In subcutaneous mycoses, the fungus enters the skin from the soil, plants or wood via a penetrating injury and the lesions are localised mostly to

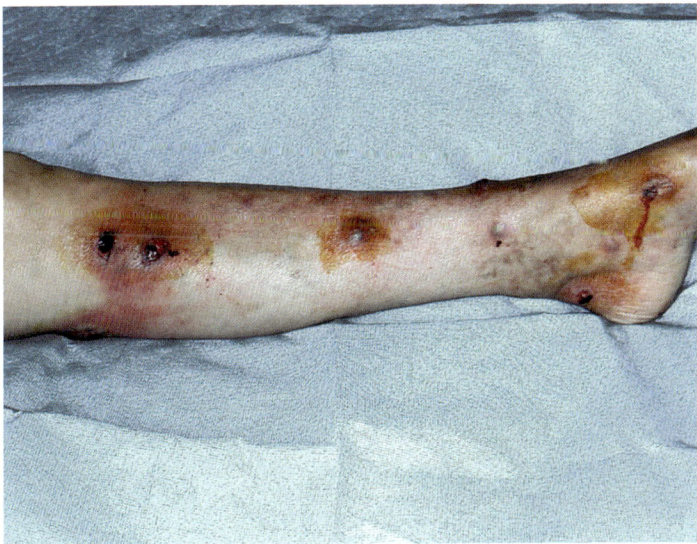

Figure 97.41 Sporotrichoid arrangement of subcutaneous nodules, several of them ulcerated and draining serous or oily discharge in an immunocompromised patient. Cultures isolated *Mycobacterium chelonae*.

exposed areas of the skin, such as the face, hands, arms or feet [49]. These lesions consist of a solitary painless nodule that spreads slowly; with time, secondary nodules and papules may develop in adjacent skin and may be accompanied by sinuses exuding a serous or oily discharge.

Management

Treatment of infective panniculitis consists of appropriate antimicrobial therapy. Surgical excision may be necessary for isolated lesions due to grain-forming fungi or bacteria, such as mycetoma or botryomycosis.

Factitious panniculitis

Introduction and general description

Factitious or artefactual panniculitides result from external injury to subcutaneous fat. Aetiological factors may be mechanical trauma, chemical substances and thermal injury; the reasons for the injury may be accidental, intentional or iatrogenic. Traumatic and cold panniculitis are covered in other sections of this chapter. Often factitious panniculitis is a manifestation of underlying psychiatric disorders [1]. In other instances, the process results from iatrogenic injections of drugs or immunisation agents.

Pathophysiology
Histopathology

The histopathological findings in factitious panniculitis vary depending on the causal agent. In most cases, early lesions show features of a predominantly neutrophilic lobular panniculitis, with severe fat necrosis and an intense inflammatory infiltrate. In some instances, eosinophils may be abundant [2], especially in panniculitis arising at the site of cancer vaccines [3], and in sclerosing lipogranulomas of the genitalia [4]. Superimposed infection often complicates self-induced panniculitis. Fully developed lesions show granulomatous infiltrates involving the fat lobule, whereas longstanding lesions are characterised by lipophagic granulomas and surrounding fibrosis. In some cases, polarised light will reveal the birefringent foreign bodies responsible for the panniculitis. In panniculitis due to injected substances, the dermis is also involved by the inflammatory process, which may be a clue to the correct diagnosis.

Sometimes, specific histopathological findings may be helpful in identifying the nature of the foreign material. *Paraffinoma* is characterised by a predominantly lobular panniculitis in which the subcutaneous fat exhibits a 'Swiss-cheese' appearance, with cystic spaces of variable size and shape, surrounded by foamy histiocytes and multinucleated giant cells; intense fibrosis with sclerotic collagen bundles is seen surrounding the cystic spaces [5]. Similar findings have been described in the penis following a grease gun injury [6]. Exogenous oils may be highlighted by special stains such as oil red O and osmium tetroxide [7].

Histopathological findings in local reactions to implants of *silicone* are variable depending mainly on the form of the injected silicone.

Solid elastomer silicone induces an exuberant foreign-body granulomatous reaction, whereas silicone oil and gel induce a sparser inflammatory response. Silicone particles appear as groups of round, empty vacuoles of different sizes between collagen bundles or within macrophages. Silicone particles are not birefringent under polarised light, but sometimes translucent angulated foreign bodies that represent impurities in the silicone are also found [8]. Granulomas from polymethylsiloxane fillers consist of irregularly shaped cystic spaces containing translucent, jagged 'popcorn', non-birefringent particles of varying size dispersed in a sclerotic stroma, surrounded by abundant multinucleated foreign-body giant cells [9].

Granulomas from collagen-based cosmetic fillers containing *polymethylmethacrylate* microspheres show a nodular or diffuse granulomatous infiltrate surrounding rounded vacuoles of similar shape and size, which mimic normal adipocytes and correspond to the implanted microspheres [10].

Injections of lipomas with *phosphatidylcholine*-containing substances induce an early reaction characterised by neutrophilic infiltration with partially destroyed fat cells. Late lesions show infiltration of T lymphocytes and macrophages with foamy histiocytes, accompanied by thickened septa and pseudocapsule formation surrounding the inflamed area [11].

Persistent reactions to aluminium at the site of injection of hyposensitisation vaccines show abundant lymphoid follicles in the subcutaneous tissue with germinal centre formation. They may mimic lupus profundus, pseudolymphoma or deep morphoea, but the abundant eosinophils and the identification of characteristic histiocytes with basophilic granular cytoplasm are the key distinctive features allowing the correct diagnosis [12]. These macrophages contain lysosomes filled with aluminium salts that can be demonstrated with X-ray dispersion microanalysis.

Pentazozine panniculitis is manifested as sclerodermoid plaques that result from the thrombosis of small vessels, endarteritis, granulomatous inflammation, lipophagic granulomas and pronounced fibrosis of the dermis and subcutaneous fat [13,14].

Panniculitis secondary to *vitamin K* injections is also characterised by prominent sclerosis of the collagen bundles of the connective tissue septa of the subcutis and an inflammatory infiltrate of lymphocytes, mast cells and plasma cells, which raises the histopathological differential diagnosis with morphoea [15,16]. In contrast with deep morphoea, vitamin K_1 panniculitis usually also involves the fat lobule with lipophagic granulomas.

Povidone panniculitis shows granulomatous infiltration of the fat lobule with focal haemorrhage and necrosis. Many macrophages contain grey-blue foamy material in their cytoplasm, which is positive for Congo red and chlorazol-fast pink [17].

Extravasation of *cytotoxic drugs* shows lobular panniculitis, abundant adipocyte necrosis with little inflammatory infiltrate together with epidermal lesions attributable to direct cytotoxicity. More chronic cases show marked fibrosis and lipomembranous changes [18,19].

Panniculitis secondary to *subcutaneous glatiramer acetate* injections for the treatment of multiple sclerosis (Figure 97.42) consists of a predominantly lobular panniculitis, with lipophagic granulomas

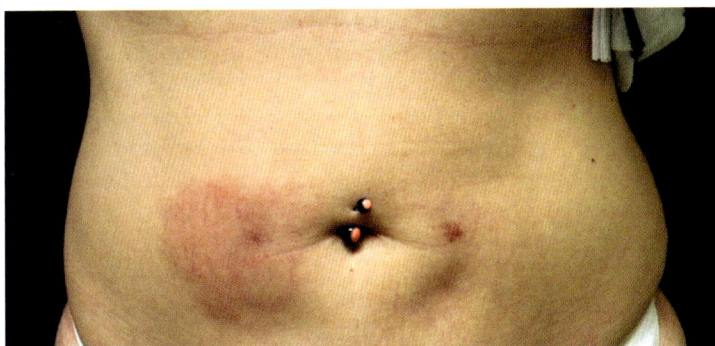

Figure 97.42 Panniculitis on the anterior abdominal wall secondary to subcutaneous glatiramer acetate injections for the treatment of multiple sclerosis.

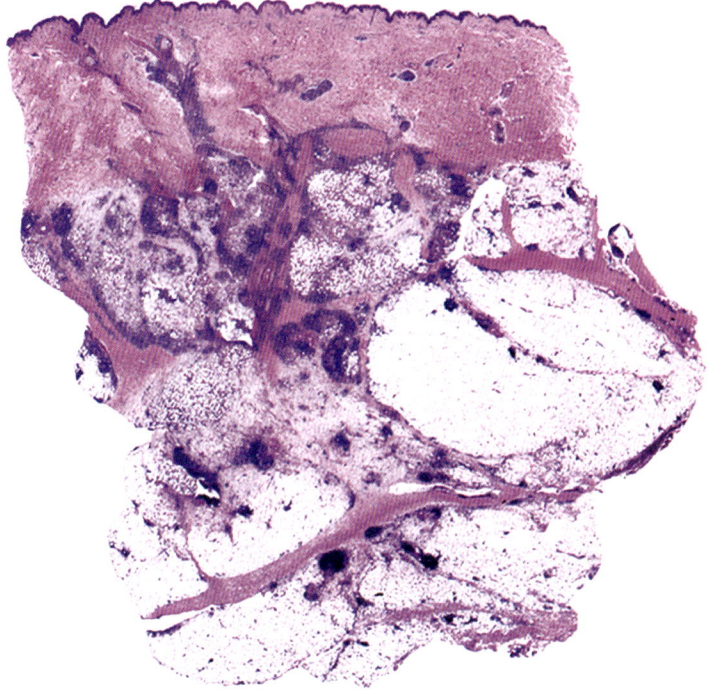

(a)

and scattered neutrophils and eosinophils both in the septa and in the fat lobules. The connective tissue septa show widening and fibrosis in conjunction with many lymphoid follicles, some with reactive germinal centres (Figure 97.43). Immunohistochemistry demonstrates that the inflammatory infiltrate of the fat lobule consists of CD68-positive histiocytes and suppressor/cytotoxic T lymphocytes. In contrast, the lymphoid follicles in the septa and at the interface between the septum and fat lobule are mainly composed of B lymphocytes [20].

Factitious panniculitis due to repeated *trauma* shows organising haematomas, focal granulomas and haemosiderin deposition [21].

Causative organisms

Recently, the use of injectable filler agents has become widespread in aesthetic dermatology and plastic surgery for the treatment of wrinkles and soft-tissue augmentation. Biodegradable or resorbable agents may induce severe complications but these will usually disappear spontaneously in a few months. Slowly biodegradable or non-resorbable fillers may give rise to severe reactions that show little or no tendency to spontaneous improvement. They may appear several years after the injection, when the patient does not remember which product was injected. Previously, factitious panniculitis frequently resulted from subcutaneous injection of oily materials including mineral oil (paraffin) or vegetable oils (cottonseed and sesame oils) [7]. These products were used over many years to augment the size of breasts or genitalia but often induced subcutaneous foreign-body reactions known as paraffinoma or sclerosing lipogranuloma. Fortunately, most such fillers have now been abandoned by medical professionals, although complications may appear a long time after the injections, even 30 years later, and it still is possible to see cases of paraffinoma or sclerosing granuloma [8]. Although cosmetic fillers currently used for tissue augmentation, such as bovine collagen, silicone, polymethylmethacrylate microspheres (Artecoll®), polymethyl-siloxane (Bioplastique®) and hydroxyethylmethacrylate particles in hyaluronic acid (Dermalive®), are better tolerated, they may also sometimes induce factitious panniculitis [10,22–25]. In recent years, injections with Lipostabil®, a phosphatidylcholine-containing substance, have become a popular therapeutic technique for the

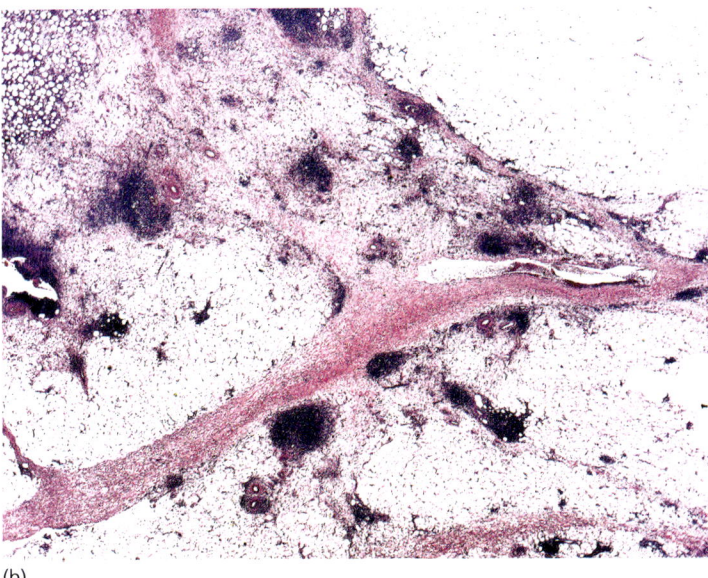

(b)

Figure 97.43 Histopathological features of panniculitis secondary to subcutaneous glatiramer acetate injections for the treatment of multiple sclerosis (a) Scanning power showing a mostly lobular panniculitis. (b) Numerous lymphoid aggregates are seen at the periphery of the fat lobules.

treatment of localised fat accumulation and lipomas, causing factitious panniculitis of the injected fat tissue [11]. Mesotherapy injections in an attempt to produce reduction of the thickness of hypertrophic subcutaneous fat produce a granulomatous panniculitis with some cystic fat necrosis [26]. Panniculitis has also been reported at the sites of injection of several therapeutic drugs (Box 97.7) [3,12,13,15,20,27–34].

Box 97.7 Medications causing panniculitis at the sites of injection

- Pethidine [13]
- Pentazocine [27]
- Methadone [28]
- Povidone [29]
- Gold salts (aurothioglucose) [30]
- Phytomenadione (vitamin K₁) [15]
- Glatiramer acetate for the treatment of multiple sclerosis (Figure 97.42) [20]
- Tetanus antitoxoid vaccination and antihepatitis vaccines [31]
- Hyposensitisation vaccination with vaccines containing aluminium [12]
- Anticancer vaccines such as gangliosides for melanoma and carcinoembryonic antigen and mucin-1 (MUC1) for pancreatic cancer [3]
- Interferon β [32]
- Granulocyte colony-stimulating factor [33]
- Interleukin 2 [34]

The extravasation of cytostatic agents during antineoplastic chemotherapy also presents as a severe panniculitis [18,35]. Cupping and acupuncture techniques for the relief of pain may induce factitious panniculitis on the limbs [36,37]. Finally, patients with psychiatric disorders may present with self-inflicted panniculitis due to subcutaneous injections of a wide range of substances including acids, alkalis, farming products, mustard, milk, microbiologically contaminated material, urine and faeces [1,2].

The exact mechanisms involved in factitious panniculitis are uncertain, but vasoconstriction with tissue ischaemia at injection sites, a local inflammatory response elicited by direct contact with drugs or noxious injected substances, immune mechanisms and trauma due to repeated injections may be implicated.

Clinical features
Presentation
The clinical features of factitious panniculitis are variable, depending upon the causative agent. Self-induced factitious panniculitis usually occurs in young adults or middle-aged women with a history of drug addiction or psychiatric disorders (Chapter 84). Lesions tend to be localised to areas easily accessible to the hands, such as the buttocks and thighs, and they are usually solitary or few; when multiple they tend to be grouped. The clinical appearance is bizarre and suspicions should be raised when they do not fit with any well-defined dermatosis. Lesions due to blunt trauma often appear bruised and frequently involve the arm or hand [21]. A particular presentation of self-induced traumatic panniculitis is the so-called Secretan syndrome (l'oedème bleu) [38,39], which consists of a factitious oedema of the hand caused by the frequent application of a tourniquet or repeated trauma. The course is chronic and recurrent, leading to progressive fibrosis of the dorsum of the hand [40].

Self-inflicted injections with contaminated material produce an acute suppurative panniculitis, often with systemic symptoms [41]. Early lesions manifest as inflammatory nodules and plaques secondary to fat necrosis and suppuration. Some cases may show abscess formation and lymphangitic spread. A case of factitious panniculitis masquerading as florid pyoderma gangrenosum was reported in a depressed woman [42]. There is a risk of progression to granulomatous inflammation and fibrosis in longstanding lesions. Sclerosing lipogranuloma is the term used for factitious lesions of the male genitalia secondary to injections of liquid paraffin intended to augment the size of the penis [43]. Often, these patients deny previous injections, making diagnosis difficult. Lesions similar to sclerosing granuloma may appear in other locations such as the eyelids, lips or gluteal region after the injection of liquid silicone [44].

Diagnosis of panniculitis secondary to the injection of drugs is usually easy and the location of the lesions provides a clue to their cause. Pentazocine abuse has been described in patients with chronic pain or addiction: repeated injections may induce panniculitis and myositis. Pentazocine panniculitis presents as multiple nodulo-ulcerative lesions of long duration located bilaterally on the buttocks and shoulders [27]. These nodules slowly progress to fibrosis resulting in sclerodermoid plaques that extend to the underlying fascia and muscle [45]. Texier disease is another iatrogenic panniculitis due to vitamin K₁ injections [15]: early lesions have an eczematous appearance, but longstanding reactions mimic morphoea [16]. Procaine povidone was used to treat chronic pain with local infiltrations. Povidone is a synthetic product now widely used in skin care products such as hair sprays and as a dispersing or suspending agent in drugs such as procaine and hormones. Povidone polymers cannot be excreted by the kidney and they are phagocytised and stored permanently in macrophages, resulting in the so-called 'povidone storage disease' [17]. In addition to panniculitis at the sites of injection, povidone may cause pulmonary lesions, lymphadenopathy and visceromegaly [29].

Subcutaneous extravasation of cytotoxic agents causes severe, painful, necrotic reactions of the subcutis and underlying muscles, which may disable a patient for months. Clinical lesions show red-brown painful oedema that may evolve into necrotic plaques that heal with sclerotic, indurated scars which may become bound to underlying muscle and bone [35].

Management
Early lesions of factitious panniculitis should be treated with systemic antibiotics to cover a wide spectrum of microorganisms. If artefact is suspected, the affected area may be occluded for a week with a bandage: improvement would support a suspicion of self-induced factitious panniculitis, for which appropriate social and psychiatric care should be offered. Regrettably, these offers are usually rejected by patients.

Panniculitis secondary to cosmetic fillers usually requires intralesional steroids and, if possible, removal of the implanted material. Panniculitis secondary to injection of drugs usually requires only supportive care and withdrawal of the responsible drug.

Neutrophilic lobular panniculitis

Neutrophilic lobular panniculitis incorporates a range of different panniculitides in which the fat lobule infiltrate is mostly composed of neutrophils (Box 97.8). According to Cohen, 'neutrophilic lobular panniculitis is not a distinct entity but has a concise pathologic description of specific changes in the subcutaneous fat that have been observed in association with several conditions' [1]. Some of these entities have been covered in other sections of this chapter. Included here is a small group of rare disorders characterised by neutrophilic lobular panniculitis [2]. It must be underlined that an infectious aetiology must always be ruled out before making the histopathological diagnosis of a neutrophilic lobular panniculitis.

Box 97.8 Types of neutrophilic lobular panniculitis

- Alpha-1 antitrypsin deficiency panniculitis
- Pancreatic panniculitis
- Infective panniculitis
- Factitious panniculitis
- Neutrophilic lobular panniculitis/subcutaneous Sweet syndrome
- Neutrophilic/pustular panniculitis of rheumatoid arthritis
- Erythema nodosum-like lesions of Behçet disease
- Bowel bypass dermatosis
- Iatrogenic neutrophilic panniculitis
- Drug-induced neutrophilic panniculitis
- Neutrophil-rich lupus panniculitis [79]
- Neutrophilic variant of subcutaneous fat necrosis of the newborn [80]

Adapted from Guhl and García-Díez 2008 [22].

Subcutaneous Sweet syndrome (Chapter 49)

Introduction and general description

Acute febrile neutrophilic dermatosis or Sweet syndrome is a neutrophilic dermatosis characterised by an acute onset of oedematous, red papules and plaques, often accompanied by fever and malaise, which was first described by Sweet in 1964 [3]. Histopathologically, cutaneous lesions show oedema of the papillary dermis and a dense band-like infiltrate of neutrophils involving mostly the superficial dermis, with no vasculitis [4]. Usually, Sweet syndrome is mainly a dermal process, but even in the original series Sweet reported that the neutrophilic infiltrate may extend into the underlying subcutaneous tissue with an associated neutrophilic panniculitis [3]. Subcutaneous involvement in classic Sweet syndrome is not rare and it has been described in some series with frequencies ranging from 25% to 50% of cases [5–9]. A diagnosis of subcutaneous Sweet syndrome should be made, however, only in those cases in which the neutrophilic infiltrate involves exclusively the subcutaneous tissue with few or no neutrophils in the dermis.

Only a few patients have been described with this peculiar variant of Sweet syndrome with exclusively subcutaneous involvement. Cullity *et al.* [10] were the first authors to use the term 'Sweet's panniculitis' or 'acute febrile neutrophilic panniculitis' to describe this entity, although similar cases had been previously reported [5,11]. Most of the cases show a neutrophilic lobular panniculitis, although in rare instances a septal component may be predominant [12]. To date, only 27 well-documented cases of subcutaneous Sweet syndrome have been reported [10–32]. Several features support the relationship of neutrophilic lobular panniculitis to Sweet syndrome. In some cases, subcutaneous Sweet syndrome

was followed by classic dermal Sweet syndrome [5], whereas another patient presented simultaneously with classic Sweet syndrome and Sweet panniculitis [18]. As in classic Sweet syndrome, many patients with subcutaneous Sweet syndrome had associated myelodysplastic syndromes and haematological neoplasms [10,13–15,19,20,24,25,27–34], and their cutaneous lesions showed an excellent response to systemic corticosteroids.

Pathophysiology
Histopathology

Histopathological study of the lesions demonstrates a dense infiltrate of mature neutrophils involving subcutaneous tissue. The neutrophilic infiltrate may involve the septa, lobules or both [1], but in most cases the lobular component predominates (Figure 97.44) [10,12,13,15–18]. Vasculitis is usually absent in all cases, but in two patients leukocytoclasia was noted [10,13]. The dermis is, by definition, spared in all patients. Occasionally, some mononuclear cells may be found in the subcutaneous tissue [10,14]. Rarely, infiltration of myeloperoxidase-positive immature granulocytes has been described [21], representing the subcutaneous counterpart of the so-called histiocytoid Sweet syndrome [35].

In summary, Sweet syndrome may involve subcutaneous tissue with two different patterns: (i) with a mostly septal panniculitis and occasionally granulomatous infiltrate, as in classic erythema nodosum associated with Sweet syndrome [36]; and (ii) with a neutrophilic infiltrate mostly involving the fat lobules, as is the case in subcutaneous Sweet syndrome.

Clinical features
Presentation

Subcutaneous Sweet syndrome, like classic Sweet syndrome, has a median age of onset during the sixth decade of life but appears not to show the female preponderance of the latter [4,9]. Clinically, the lesions consist of red nodules [11–15,17,18] or plaques [10,12] (Figure 97.45). Often the nodules are tender or painful [15]. Frequently, the onset of subcutaneous nodules is preceded or accompanied by systemic symptoms such as fever and malaise [5,10,12,14,16,17]; leukocytosis was found in several patients [12–14,16,17]. The most frequent locations are the lower extremities [11–15,17,18], followed by the upper extremities [12,13,15], trunk [10,12,13,15] and head [10]. In one patient, the lesions were associated with all-*trans*-retinoic acid chemotherapy for promyelocytic leukaemia [19]; another patient presented associated dacryoadenitis [20]; and another developed the condition when administered pegylated granulocyte colony-stimulating factor (GCSF) [26].

Management

Most patients with subcutaneous Sweet syndrome show dramatic response to systemic corticosteroids, such as prednisolone [10,11,14–16]. Dapsone has also been administered successfully in one patient [17].

Behçet disease (Chapter 48)

In the differential diagnosis of subcutaneous Sweet syndrome are the 'erythema nodosum-like' lesions which occur in approximately 30% of patients with Behçet disease [37,38]. They consist of nod-

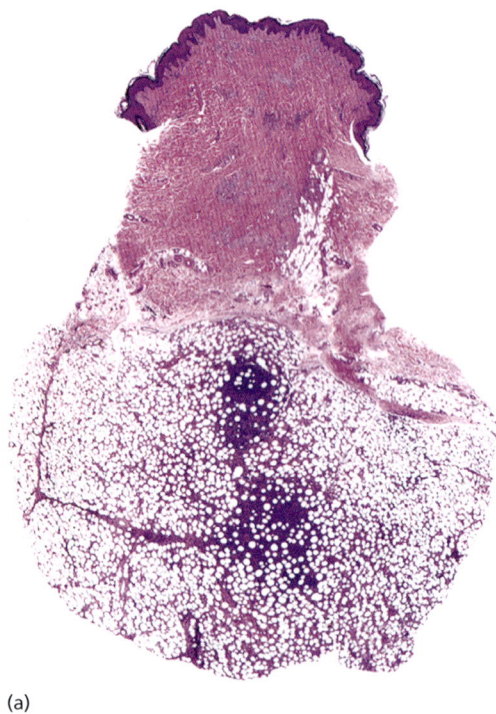

(a)

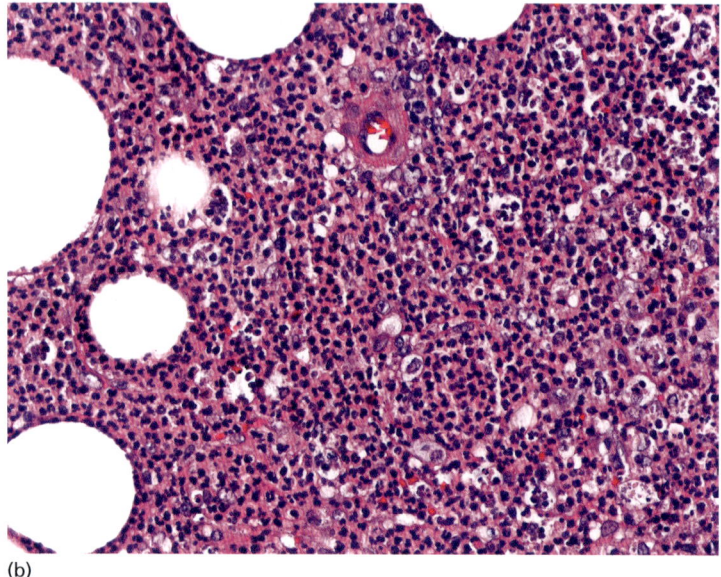

(b)

Figure 97.44 Histopathological features of neutrophilic lobular panniculitis. (a) Scanning power showing a predominantly lobular panniculitis. (b) The lobular infiltrate is composed mainly of neutrophils.

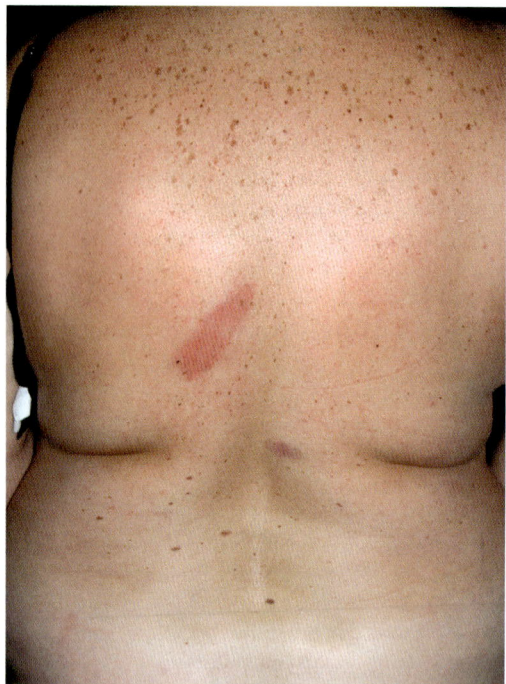

Figure 97.45 Neutrophilic lobular panniculitis showing red plaques and nodules on the back of an adult woman.

Rheumatoid arthritis (Chapter 155)

Several cases of neutrophilic (pustular) panniculitis have been described in patients with rheumatoid arthritis [43–54]. In these patients, subcutaneous nodules are mostly located on the lower extremities and they show a tendency to form draining fistulae with a yellowish discharge [46–50]. Histopathologically, these lesions are characterised by a lobular infiltrate of neutrophils accompanied by lymphocytes, macrophages and multinucleate giant cells [45,47,48]. Fat necrosis has been found in nearly all cases [42,43,47,48] and leukocytoclastic vasculitis was described in some [43,48].

Bowel-associated dermatosis–arthritis syndrome (Chapter 153)

The bowel-associated dermatosis–arthritis syndrome is characterised by recurrent fever, arthralgia and skin lesions after intestinal bypass or bariatric surgery [55,56]. The most frequent skin lesions consist of red papules or vesiculopustules. Lobular neutrophilic panniculitis with tender subcutaneous nodules on the lower extremities has, however, rarely been described in these patients [55,56].

Drug-induced neutrophilic panniculitis

In addition to drug-induced erythema nodosum and panniculitis induced by drugs at the sites of injection (see earlier), some recently introduced drugs may induce neutrophilic septal or lobular panniculitis beyond the sites of injection [57–78], with red subcutaneous nodules mostly involving the upper and lower limbs (Table 97.4; Figures 97.46 and 97.47). These drug-induced panniculitides usually appear after an average of 30 days from the onset of treatment. They are often associated with systemic symptoms, such as fever or arthralgia. Lesions are usually mild and do not require withdrawal of the responsible drug.

ules on the lower extremities [38–42], and sometimes also on the arms [38,39], identical to those of classic erythema nodosum [37]. However, histopathological study demonstrates involvement of both the septa and fat lobules [38,39], with necrotising leukocytoclastic vasculitis involving the arterioles and venules [37–40]. In some cases, neutrophilic abscesses are found within the fat lobules [37]. A variable degree of fat necrosis is nearly always present [37]. Therefore, the histopathological findings rule out a diagnosis of erythema nodosum and the vasculitis component allows subcutaneous Sweet syndrome to be ruled out [38].

Table 97.4 Drug-induced panniculitis.

Drug	Histopathological patterns reported
Immune checkpoint inhibitors (e.g. ipilimumab, erythema nivolumab, pembrolizumab)	Granulomatous/sarcoid-like, nodosum-like
BRAF inhibitors (e.g. vemurafenib, dabrafenib)	Erythema nodosum-like, neutrophilic lobular
Tyrosine kinase inhibitors (e.g. imatinib, dasatinib)	Neutrophilic lobular
Bruton tyrosine kinase (BTK) inhibitors (e.g. ibrutinib, acalabrutinib, zanubrutinib)	Neutrophilic lobular
TNF inhibitors (e.g. etanercept, infliximab, adalimumab)	Erythema nodosum-like, lupus profundus-like
Hypomethylating agents (e.g. azacitidine, decitabine, guadecitabine)	Neutrophilic lobular

TNF, tumour necrosis factor.

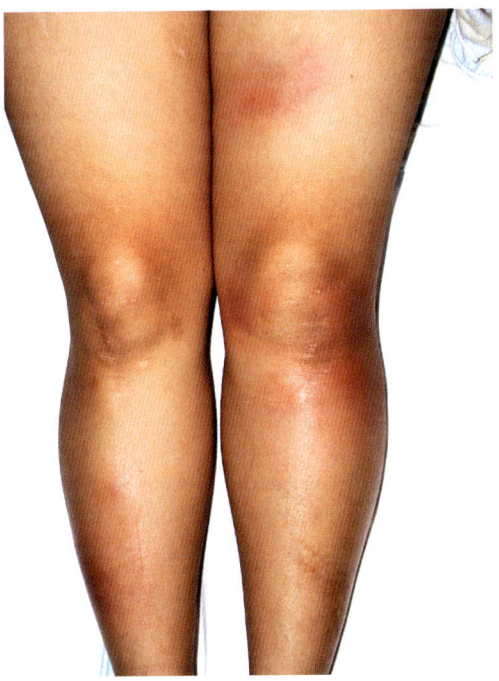

Figure 97.46 Panniculitis on the anterior aspect of the lower extremities in a woman with metastatic melanoma receiving treatment with nivolumab.

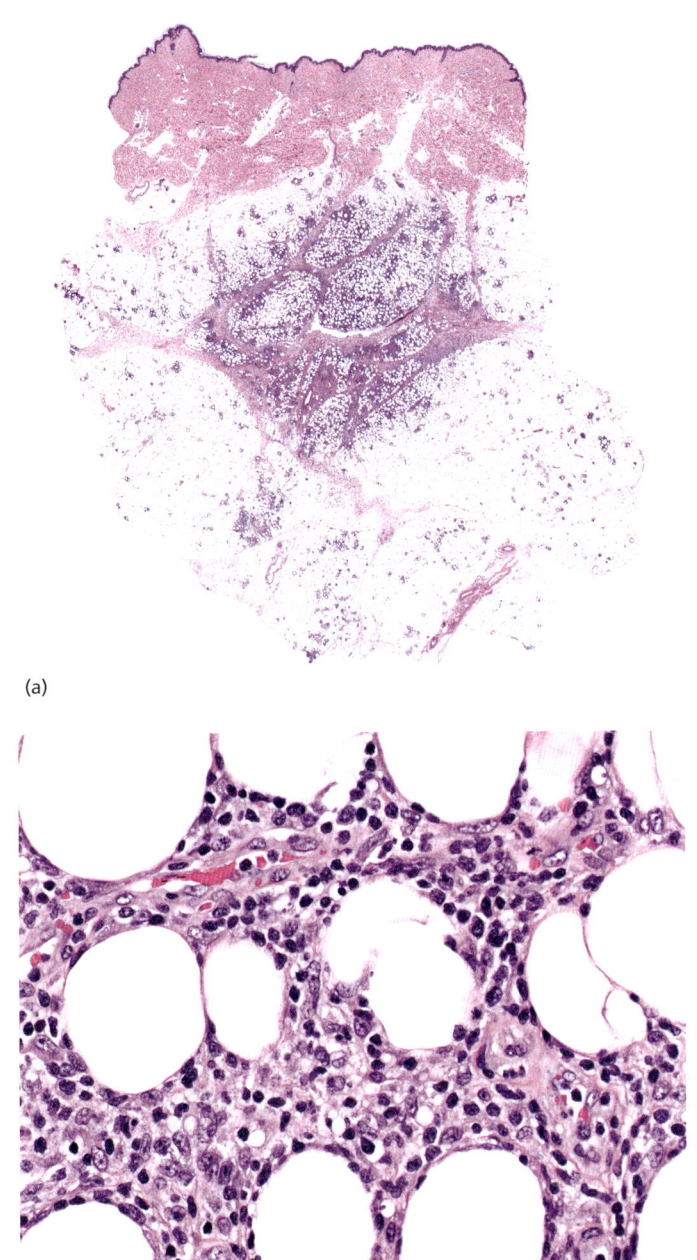

(a)

(b)

Figure 97.47 Histopathological features of panniculitis induced by nivolumab. (a) Scanning power showing a predominantly lobular panniculitis. (b) The lobular infiltrate is composed mainly of histiocytes and lymphocytes.

Subcutaneous sarcoidosis

Synonyms and inclusions
- Darier–Roussy sarcoid

Introduction and general description
Minimal dermal involvement is acceptable for a histopathological diagnosis of subcutaneous sarcoidosis [1], but subcutaneous sarcoidosis is considered a specific clinicopathological variant of sarcoidosis involving exclusively the subcutaneous fat. It should be differentiated from nodular dermal lesions of sarcoidosis with deep extension into the subcutaneous tissue [2]. Mostly, subcutaneous sarcoidosis is associated with systemic sarcoidosis, although with an indolent and non-aggressive form of the disease [3].

The most frequent subcutaneous disorder associated with sarcoidosis is not subcutaneous sarcoidosis, but classic erythema nodosum [3]. However, patients with systemic sarcoidosis may also develop sarcoidal granulomas involving the subcutaneous tissue as a specific cutaneous lesion (Figure 97.48); this is referred to as subcutaneous sarcoidosis. Subcutaneous sarcoidosis is a rare form of cutaneous sarcoidosis [3–6] (Chapter 96).

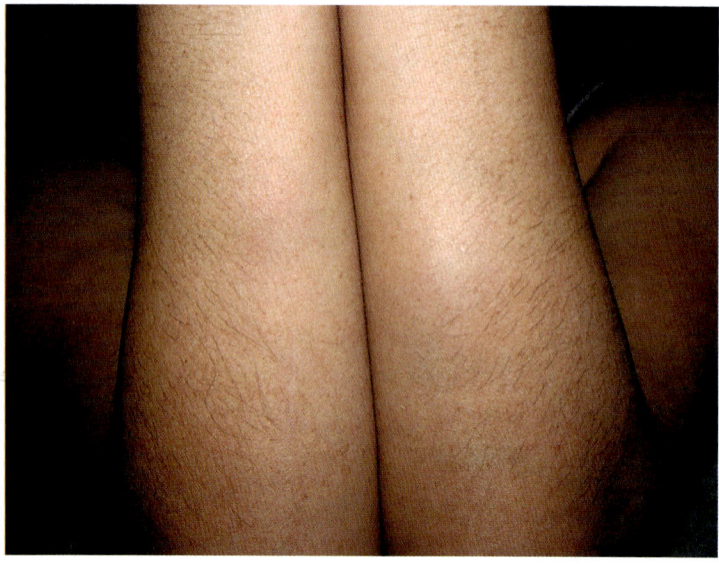

Figure 97.48 Subcutaneous sarcoidosis. Subcutaneous firm nodules on the forearms covered by normal-appearing skin.

Epidemiology
Incidence and prevalence
Subcutaneous sarcoidosis is the least common specific cutaneous manifestation of sarcoidosis. Its frequency varies, ranging in different series between 1.4% and 6% of patients with systemic sarcoidosis [7] and represents 11.76% of specific cutaneous lesions [8]. Its clinical features are described in detail in Chapter 96.

Pathophysiology
Histopathology
Histopathologically, subcutaneous sarcoidosis is characterised by non-caseating granulomas involving fat lobules (Figure 97.49) [3,8]. At low-power magnification, the process appears as a predominantly lobular panniculitis, with minimal or no septal involvement. Sarcoidal granulomas in subcutaneous tissue are usually small, uniform in size and mainly composed of epithelioid histiocytes, with limited numbers of multinucleate giant cells and a sparse lymphocytic component. Fibrosis is a frequent finding in subcutaneous sarcoidosis, and although it may be intense, it is not associated with pulmonary fibrosis or with long-term persistence of systemic sarcoidosis activity [9]. Occasionally, small foci of eosinophilic necrosis may appear in the centre of regressing sarcoid granulomas [10], raising the differential diagnosis of tuberculosis [11]. In rare instances, caseating necrosis may be extensive [11]. The development of calcification in these sarcoidal granulomas has also been reported [12]. Foreign refractile particles under polarised light have been detected in some cases of subcutaneous sarcoidosis and this finding should not exclude the diagnosis [13–15].

Management
Corticosteroids, in either topical, intralesional or systemic form, are the mainstay of therapy for subcutaneous sarcoidosis. For extensive lesions, the usual dose is 0.5–1 mg/kg/day for 4–6 weeks, followed by a slow taper. For solitary cutaneous lesions, topical or intralesional corticosteroids may suffice. Alternative non-steroidal systemic medications include hydroxychloroquine (200–400 mg/day), chloroquine (250–500 mg/day), minocycline (200 mg/day), methotrexate (10–25 mg weekly) and thalidomide (50–300 mg/day). Improvement of both systemic and cutaneous sarcoidosis has been observed with TNF-α inhibitors, including infliximab and adalimumab.

Traumatic panniculitis

Introduction and general description
Traumatic panniculitis refers to the damage of subcutaneous tissue induced by physical and chemical agents. The physical injuries may

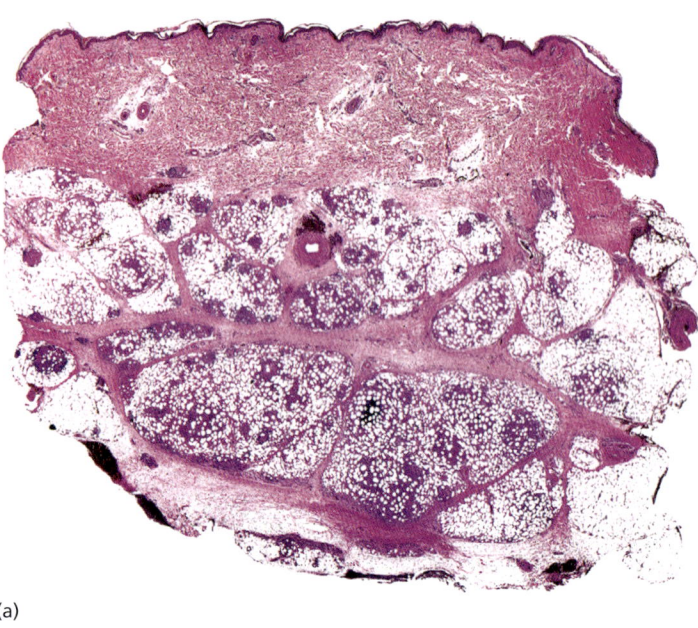

(a)

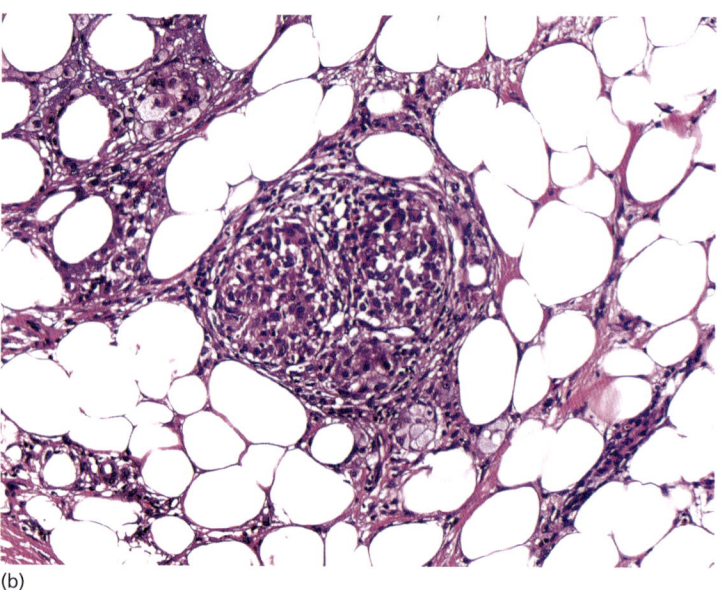

(b)

Figure 97.49 Histopathological features of subcutaneous sarcoidosis. (a) Scanning power showing a predominantly lobular panniculitis. (b) Small non-caseating granulomas involving the fat lobule.

PART 8: SPECIFIC CUTANEOUS STRUCTURES

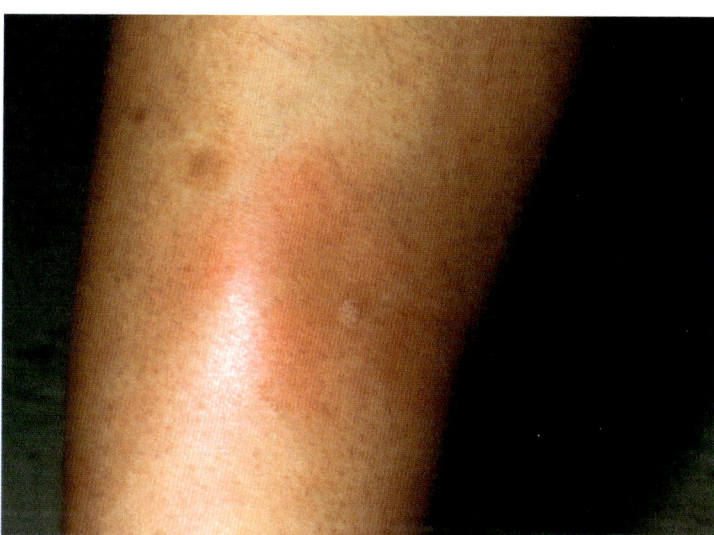

Figure 97.50 Traumatic panniculitis involving the shin.

be from trauma, cold, electricity or chemicals. Cold panniculitis and chemical factitious panniculitis have been covered in other sections of this chapter. In general, there is no direct relationship between the severity of the injury and the severity of the resultant panniculitis: even minor trauma often causes nodules of panniculitis on the shins (Figure 97.50).

Pathophysiology
Histopathology
The histopathological findings in traumatic panniculitis are not specific. Early lesions show intense haemorrhage and an inflammatory infiltrate, mostly composed of lymphocytes and macrophages arranged around septal vessels. Fully developed lesions are associated with cystic areas of fat necrosis surrounded by histiocytes, lipophagic granulomas scattered with haemosiderophages, and

some neutrophils and eosinophils. Late lesions show fibrotic replacement of the fat lobule with residual cystic fat necrosis surrounded by macrophages and foreign-body multinucleate giant cells. Lipomembranous changes are also common in late-stage lesions of traumatic panniculitis [1]. Dystrophic calcification may appear in longstanding nodules.

Biopsy from semicircular atrophy shows inflammatory perivascular changes in early lesions. Nodular–cystic fat necrosis shows extensive necrosis of the fat lobules, with cystic fat necrosis and lipomembranous changes, and as the most characteristic finding a thick, eosinophilic, peripheral, fibrotic pseudocapsule with hyaline appearance encircling the nodule and separating it from the surrounding tissues (Figure 97.51) [2].

Clinical features
Presentation
A specific form of traumatic panniculitis is common in women with large pendulous breasts. Large breast masses can form and may be misinterpreted as breast cancer [3].

Another peculiar variant of traumatic panniculitis is the so-called semicircular lipoatrophy that is probably induced by repeated microtrauma [4–9] (Chapter 98). These patients, generally adult women, develop horizontal band-like or circular depressions around the anterolateral aspects of the thighs. Lipoatrophy in these areas develops over several weeks without symptoms. Trauma is the most probable cause because the affected areas of the thighs are vulnerable to repetitive trauma from sitting at desks and tables.

Post-traumatic panniculitis may present as a solitary nodule or as multiple subcutaneous nodules caused by traumatic separation and consequent devascularisation of pieces of subcutaneous fat from its blood supply. The resultant walling off of the necrotic fat by fibrous tissue results in so-called encapsulated fat necrosis, otherwise termed nodular cystic fat necrosis or mobile encapsulated lipoma [10–19].

PART 8: SPECIFIC CUTANEOUS STRUCTURES

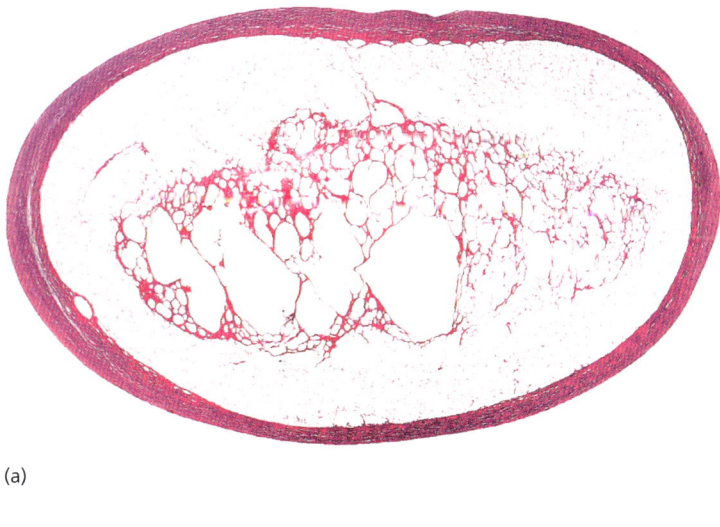

(a)

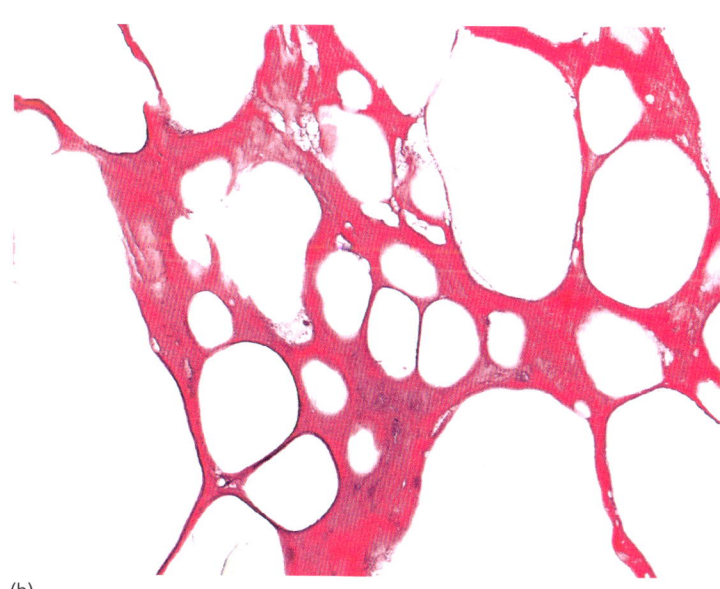

(b)

Figure 97.51 Histopathological features of encapsulated fat necrosis. (a) Scanning power showing an enucleated and very well-circumscribed lesion. (b) Necrotic adipocytes surrounded by hyaline material.

Electrical injuries appear at the point of contact of different electrodes causing skin burns with superficial subcutaneous involvement.

Management

Traumatic panniculitis is usually a self-limiting disorder and considerable improvement occurs with time.

Lipoatrophic panniculitis of the ankles in childhood

Introduction and general description

Lipoatrophic panniculitis characteristically involving the ankles was initially reported by Shelley and Izumi in 1970 and they coined the expression 'annular atrophy of the ankles' to name this process [1]. Since then, only a handful of cases have been reported [2–19], some of them under the heading of connective tissue panniculitis [3]. A recently published small series proposed the term 'recurrent lipoatrophic panniculitis in children' as the best name for this paediatric form of panniculitis [20].

Pathophysiology

Histopathology

In all except one case in which histopathology has been reported, a mainly lobular inflammation of the subcutaneous tissue has been described, with predominance of histiocytes, lipophagic granulomas and a smaller number of lymphocytes, neutrophils, plasma cells and eosinophils (Figure 97.52) [1–4,9–18]. Neutrophils and myeloid cells are more prominent in early lesions, whereas macrophages predominate in late stages, leading to lipophagia and lipoatrophy [20]. Immunohistochemistry shows positive staining for myeloperoxidase around the necrotic adipocytes in the early stages and CD68/PGM1 macrophages in the late stages. Intense STAT1 staining has been observed in the inflammatory infiltrate [20].

One reported case was remarkable for the relative abundance of lymphocytes, some of them mildly atypical [19]. Immunohistochemistry in this case demonstrated that most lymphocytes were positive for CD3 and CD7, with only occasional CD20+ B lymphocytes, and approximately equal numbers of CD4 and CD8 cells. A PCR study for B- and T-cell clonality yielded polyclonal results [19]. The authors concluded that their findings of a mostly lymphocytic panniculitis in that case were due to a biopsy performed in an earlier stage of evolution of the lesions of the panniculitic process, compared with previously reported cases [19]. The partial 'rimming' of necrotic adipocytes by lymphocytes, as well as the relatively high proliferative activity disclosed by MIB-1, raised the differential diagnosis of SPTCL, but the other immunohistochemical results and PCR studies ruled out that diagnosis.

Clinical features

Presentation

Many of the reported patients with lipoatrophic panniculitis of the ankles are children with antinuclear antibodies, autoimmune

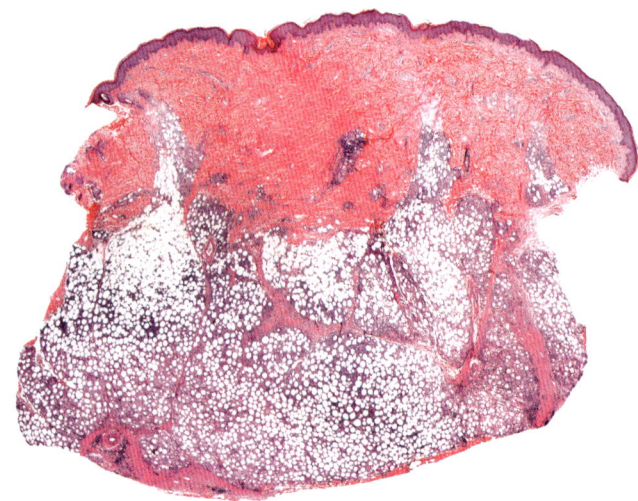

(a)

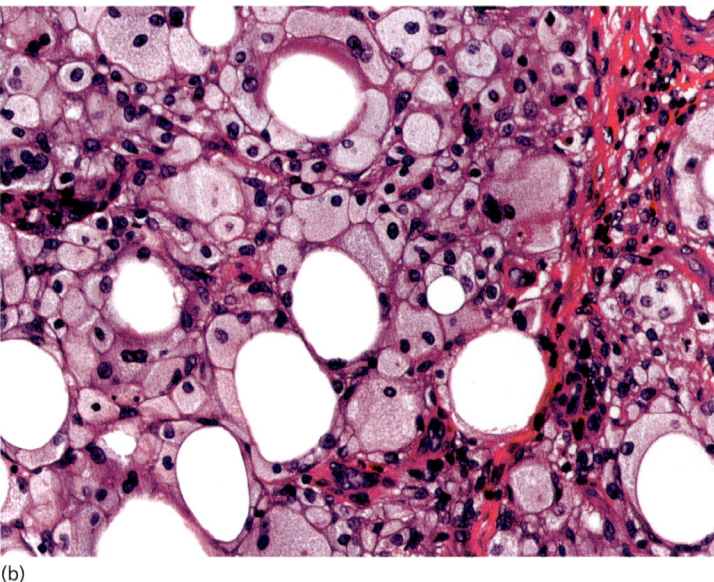

(b)

Figure 97.52 Histopathological findings in lipoatrophic panniculitis of the ankles in children. (a) Scanning power showing a mostly lobular panniculitis. (b) The fat lobule is replaced by a diffuse histiocytic infiltrate. Many histiocytes show a foamy cytoplasm as a consequence of phagocytosis of lipids, resulting in a lipophagic granuloma.

conditions or both, so that this disorder has been included under connective tissue panniculitis, together with morphoea, lupus panniculitis and dermatomyositis [4,10].

Clinically, the characteristic annular or semicircular involvement of the ankles makes this a distinctive condition with few if any differential diagnoses. The lesions are tender and the onset of subcutaneous nodules is accompanied by fever, malaise and arthralgia of the ankles. Red nodules and plaques resolve with annular scaling leaving lipoatrophy around the ankles (Figure 97.53). In some cases, the lesions may extend to other areas of the lower and upper limbs and even the face may be involved. Lipoatrophy is the characteristic residual lesion of the affected areas [20].

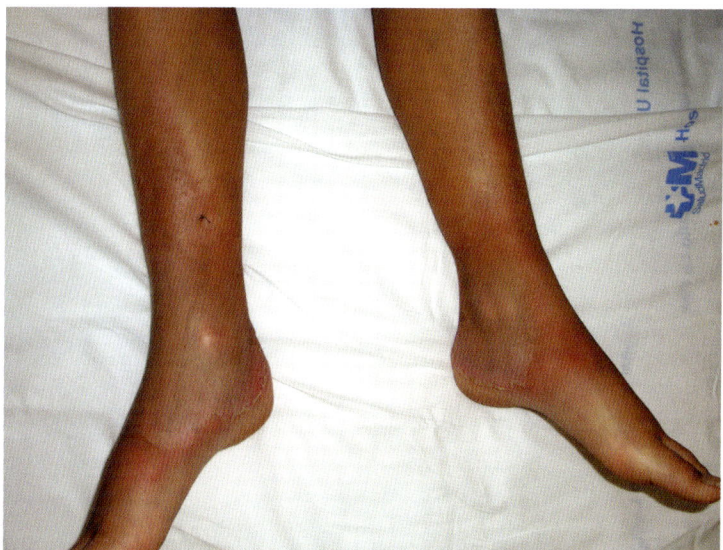

Figure 97.53 Lipoatrophic panniculitis of the ankles in a 12-year-old boy.

Laboratory abnormalities include increased acute phase reactants, leukocytosis with mild neutrophilia, microcytic anaemia and elevated liver enzymes [20]. The clinicopathological presentation of this variant of panniculitis shares features with other autoinflammatory disorders [20].

Management
Symptomatic treatment with NSAIDs provides analgesia and helps resolution. Oral prednisolone usually leads to marked improvement, but some cases have recurred on tapering, and then other drugs such as hydroxychloroquine, methotrexate and azathioprine have been administered with good effect. Residual lipoatrophy of the ankles tends to improve slowly with time. In a recent small series of five cases, all patients improved with a combined therapy of methotrexate and corticosteroids [20].

Subcutaneous fat necrosis of the newborn

Pathophysiology
Predisposing factors
The pathogenesis of this disorder is unknown. In many cases, perinatal complications are recorded, such as Rh factor incompatibility, meconium aspiration, umbilical cord prolapse, placenta praevia, birth asphyxia, seizures, congenital heart disease, intestinal perforation, hypothermia, sepsis, anaemia, obstetric trauma, gestational diabetes, pre-eclampsia or maternal abuse of drugs [1–12], but in many instances there is no history or any other associated anomaly. It has been suggested that localised and transient hypoxia may be an aetiological factor [13]. Cold may also play a role, because there are several reports of subcutaneous fat necrosis of the newborn in children who have had cardiac surgery and the lesions appeared after cutaneous applications of ice to induce hypothermia [10,14–17]. Cases of subcutaneous fat necrosis

of the newborn have been described after whole body cooling in an infant with polycythaemia and hypocalcaemia [18] and in other newborns after hypothermia treatment of hypoxic ischaemic encephalopathy [19].

Another important predisposing factor may be the particular subcutaneous fat composition in neonates, with a relatively high concentration of saturated fatty acids compared with unsaturated fatty acids, which results in a higher melting point for neonatal fat that confers on it a greater propensity to undergo crystallisation under cold temperatures, resulting in adipocyte necrosis [20]. It has also been suggested that newborns with subcutaneous fat necrosis might have a transitory protease inhibitor deficiency due to liver immaturity, similar to α_1-antitrypsin deficiency [21]. The histopathological findings of subcutaneous fat necrosis of the newborn are, however, entirely different from those of α_1-antitrypsin deficiency-associated panniculitis, which militates against this theory. Other authors have proposed that subcutaneous fat necrosis of the newborn is a disorder of brown fat, which is present in the most frequently involved areas [12].

Subcutaneous fat necrosis of the newborn has also been described after the administration of prostaglandin E_1 for the treatment of congenital heart disease, which supports some pathogenic role of prostaglandin E_1 [22].

Approximately 25% of infants with subcutaneous fat necrosis of the newborn present with hypercalcaemia for unknown reasons: this anomaly is more frequent in infants with extensive lesions and when the trunk is involved [23]. The origin of this hypercalcaemia is not known, but increased calcium absorption due to extrarenal hyperproduction of 1,25-dihydroxyvitamin D_3 (calcitriol) has been detected in several granulomatous processes, including sarcoidosis and subcutaneous fat necrosis of the newborn [23–27]. Elevated parathormone levels have been detected in some cases [28], but autopsy studies failed to reveal any parathyroid hyperplasia. Elevated urinary excretion of prostaglandin E_1 suggests an increased calcium resorption from bone as the explanation for the hypercalcaemia [29,30].

Histopathology
Histopathologically, subcutaneous fat necrosis of the newborn shows a predominantly lobular panniculitis, with a dense inflammatory infiltrate composed of lymphocytes, histiocytes, lipophages, multinucleate giant cells and sometimes eosinophils interspersed among the adipocytes of the fat lobule. A neutrophilic variant mimicking infective panniculitis has been described, which probably corresponds to early stages of this disorder [31]. Many adipocytes are replaced by cells with finely eosinophilic granular cytoplasm that contain doubly refractile, narrow, needle-shaped clefts radially arranged, which represent triglyceride crystallisation within adipocytes and stain with oil red O (Figure 97.54) [32]. Some of these refractile clefts may also be found within the cytoplasm of multinucleate giant cells. The latter may also contain eosinophilic granules in their cytoplasm [33–35] and their origin from degranulating eosinophils has been postulated [33]. Fibrotic obliteration of small arterioles and calcium deposits in necrotic fat have also been described [36–39]. In late-stage lesions, there is septal fibrosis and areas of calcification and lipoatrophy may appear within the fat lobule [11]. Adipocytes containing needle-shaped clefts

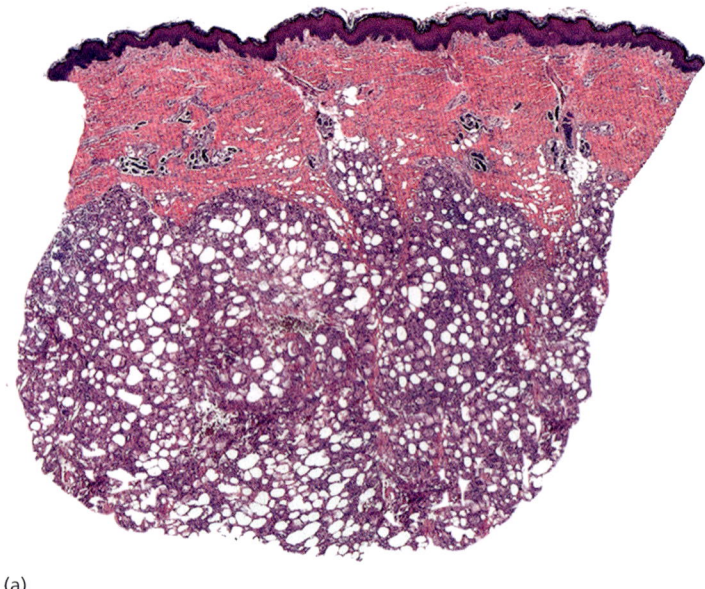

(a)

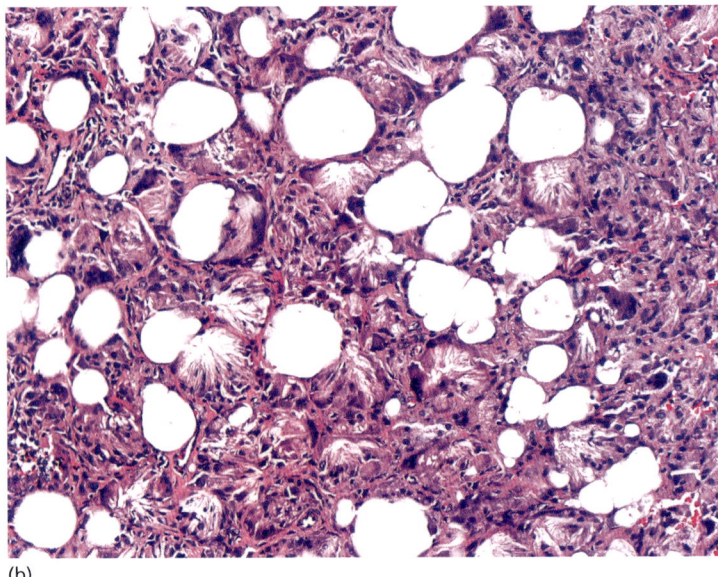

(b)

Figure 97.54 Histopathological features of subcutaneous fat necrosis of the newborn. (a) Scanning power showing a lobular panniculitis. (b) The fat lobule is replaced by a histiocytic infiltrate with some multinucleated giant cells. Many necrotic adipocytes and multinucleated giant cells contain needle-shaped clefts radially arranged.

radially arranged have been also found during autopsy studies in ventilator-associated tracheobronchitis [4,8]. In some cases, the diagnosis was established using touch preparation, which was prepared by pressing a fresh sample biopsy against a glass slide, and fine-needle aspiration techniques [40,41].

Clinical features
Presentation
Clinically, the lesions consist of multiple, symmetrically distributed, indurated, smooth, non-pitting, mobile, subcutaneous red or violaceous nodules or plaques that appear in the first few weeks of life. The most common locations are the shoulders and buttocks, but lesions on the face, thighs, back and distal areas of the extremities have been also described [42,43]. These lesions tend to spare the anterior trunk. In rare instances, the nodules may ulcerate, discharge their oily contents and heal leaving atrophic scars. Confluence of the nodules results in extensive red indurated plaques.

Complications and co-morbidities
Most children remain otherwise healthy as the subcutaneous nodules develop, but approximately 25% develop complicating hypercalcaemia [23–30,44–46]. The hypercalcaemia may persist for several weeks after the subcutaneous lesions have regressed, which requires calcium levels to be monitored and associated endocrinological disorders to be ruled out. Other reported laboratory anomalies include transient thrombocytopenia, probably due to platelet sequestration [5,12,13,47], hypoglycaemia due to maternal diabetes and hypertriglyceridaemia [48]. In rare instances, the condition may be fatal, particularly when visceral fat is involved [4]. Nephrocalcinosis persisting several years after resolution of the skin nodules has been reported as a rare complication [49].

Management
In most children with subcutaneous fat necrosis of the newborn, treatment is not required because the problem tends to resolve

spontaneously. The main goals are the detection and treatment of hypercalcaemia [23–30,44,45] with avoidance of calcium and vitamin D_3. Etidronate, a bisphosphonate that decreases bone resorption of calcium, has been helpful in the management of the associated hypercalcaemia [27,28,42–44]. It should be used as a second line drug because its effects on bone production, growth plates and mineralisation in infants are as yet unknown. Pamidronate is also helpful for the treatment for hypercalcaemia and may reduce the risk of nephrocalcinosis [50,51]. Calcitonin and citrate may be used as second line therapy for resistant cases.

Poststeroid panniculitis

Introduction and general description
In 1956, Smith and Good [1] reported 11 children with acute rheumatic fever receiving high doses of corticosteroids with rapid taper, of whom five developed red subcutaneous nodules.

Poststeroid panniculitis is a rare panniculitis of children and infants on prolonged systemic corticosteroid treatment and is related to a rapid decrease or a sudden withdrawal of steroid therapy. Only about 20 cases have been described in the literature [2–15]. It develops in an older age group than sclerema neonatorum and subcutaneous fat necrosis of the newborn, with reported ages ranging from 20 months to 14 years [3]. Although the process is mostly seen in children, there are also a few reported cases in adults [12,13,15]. In one adult patient, the lesions involved the arms and legs and were painless [15].

Pathophysiology
Histopathology
Histopathological findings in poststeroid panniculitis lesions are identical to those of subcutaneous fat necrosis of the newborn.

They consist of a mostly lobular panniculitis with an inflammatory infiltrate of foamy histiocytes and lymphocytes involving the fat lobules [6]. Often, doubly refractile narrow needle-shaped clefts radially arranged are found within the cytoplasm of some histiocytes and necrotic adipocytes, although usually they are not as numerous as in subcutaneous fat necrosis of the newborn.

Clinical features

The lesions vary in size from 0.5 to 4 cm and consist of asymptomatic firm subcutaneous nodules, often with overlying redness, and tend to be localised in those areas where there is the greatest accumulation of fat from steroid therapy, such as the face, arms and posterior neck [5]. They usually appear 1–10 days after the cessation of high doses of systemic corticosteroids.

The disorders for which treatment with high doses of corticosteroids have been administered are varied, including rheumatic fever, leukaemia, nephrotic syndrome, acute exacerbation of chronic obstructive pulmonary disease, erythema nodosum leprosum, autoimmune enteropathy, Sjögren syndrome and brain tumours. Conversely, different oral or intravenous corticosteroid drugs, including prednisolone and dexamethasone, have been associated with this panniculitis. Usually, reinstitution of corticosteroid administration induces improvement of panniculitis, although some authors believe that this is not necessary for its resolution [3].

Management

Lesions of poststeroid panniculitis usually disappear gradually without residual scarring over the course of weeks or months, even without resuming steroid therapy and therefore no treatment is usually necessary. However, readministration of high doses of systemic corticosteroid and a slower and more gradual decrease of the dose is followed by a faster improvement and resolution of the lesions.

Sclerema neonatorum

Introduction and general description

Sclerema neonatorum is an uncommon condition that typically affects gravely ill, preterm neonates in the first week of life. It manifests as a diffuse hardening of skin and subcutaneous tissue such that the skin cannot be pitted or picked up and pinched into a fold. Histologically, there is minimal inflammation with extensive fat necrosis. It is associated with a high mortality (Chapter 114).

Pathophysiology
Histopathology

Histopathologically, there is a striking contrast at low-power magnification between the severe damage in the subcutaneous fat and the sparse inflammatory response (Figure 97.55) [1–3]. Most fat lobules appear to be replaced by amphophilic granular detritus and the cellular structures of the adipocytes are no longer evident. Surprisingly, there is sparse or no inflammatory infiltrate in spite of the intense fat necrosis. The most characteristic histopathological feature consists of the presence of radially arranged needle-shaped refractile clefts in adipocytes and, occasionally, in the few multinucleate giant cells, which result from crystallisation of the lipid contents of the adipocytes. X-ray diffraction studies have demonstrated that the clefts in the fat cells are due to crystallisation of triglycerides [4]. In late-stage lesions, thickened connective tissue septa may be the only anomaly [3].

Clinical features
Presentation

Sclerema neonatorum is an extremely uncommon process and almost always appears during the first week of life, although there are also reports of infants born preterm with low birth weight who developed this condition later. In most cases, sclerema neonatorum

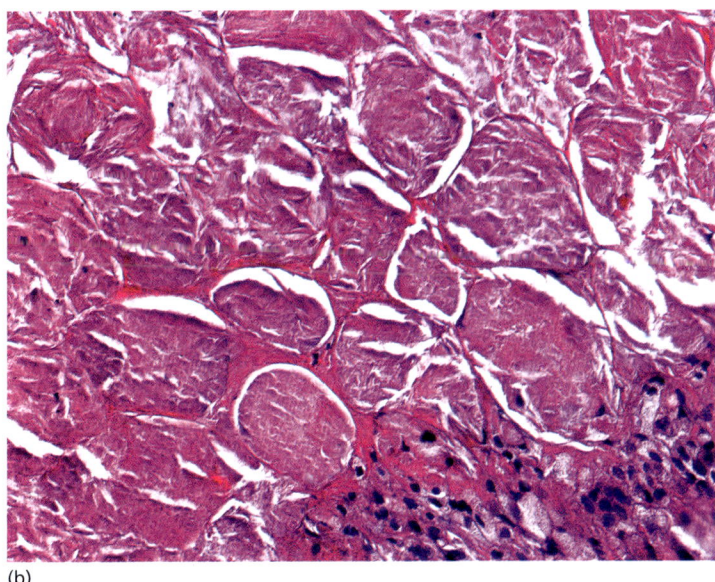

(a)   (b)

Figure 97.55 Histopathological features of sclerema neonatorum. (a) Scanning power showing necrosis of the entire fat lobules and thickened connective tissue septa. (b) An entire fat lobule is replaced by granular detritus and the cellular structures of the adipocytes are no longer evident. Many necrotic adipocytes contain needle-shaped clefts.

PART 8: SPECIFIC CUTANEOUS STRUCTURES

is a grave illness and it has been associated with a mortality of up to 75% [5–7]. However, most case series date from 40 or more years ago, and now the process is very uncommon, probably due to better neonatal care. Prematurity and placental insufficiency have been proposed as pathogenetic factors for its development [7,8]. Affected infants are almost always severely ill from conditions such as septicaemia or other disseminated infections, congenital heart disease, pneumonia, diarrhoea, dehydration, intestinal obstruction or other congenital developmental defects [7]. In a multivariate analysis of risk factors for sclerema neonatorum in preterm neonates in Bangladesh, lower maternal education, signs of jaundice and poor feeding on admission were the main risk factors, although the diagnosis in that study was not histopathologically confirmed [9]. Cold injury has also been proposed as an aetiological factor [10], but it does not appear to be important in most cases.

Lipolytic immaturity in infants born preterm [11] and the different composition of subcutaneous fat in newborns, with a higher proportion of saturated (palmitic and stearic) to unsaturated (oleic) fatty acids, may also be predisposing factors [1,12] because they favour solidification of subcutaneous fat if there is a fall in the temperature of subcutaneous tissue as a result of peripheral circulatory collapse [2]. Sclerema neonatorum is characterised by increased blood lipid peroxidation and diminished superoxide dismutase activity, which raises the possibility that free radicals may also play some role in the pathogenesis of the process [13].

Clinically, infants with sclerema neonatorum typically appear severely ill from birth and during the first days of life they develop generalised woody induration of the skin [2,14]. Usually, the process begins on the buttocks and thighs but rapidly extends to involve almost the entire skin surface with the exception of the palms, soles and genitalia. The involved skin has a hard consistency, is non-pitting and is cold to the touch; it is yellowish white in colour, often with purplish mottling. There is immobility of the extremities and the face shows a mask-like expression. The prognosis is poor and most affected infants die within a few days. However, if the infant survives, the skin recovers its normal appearance and there are no long-term complications such as calcification.

Differential diagnosis

The main differential diagnosis of sclerema neonatorum is subcutaneous fat necrosis of the newborn. This is important because they represent two distinctive clinicopathological processes with very different prognoses [14]. There is a single reported case of coexistence of both disorders in the same infant, but that is a doubtful case because histopathological study was lacking [15]. Usually this differential is straightforward, because subcutaneous fat necrosis of the newborn, which is a localised and self-healing process, does not develop in the first days of life and has characteristic histopathology consisting of a dense histiocytic infiltrate in the fat lobules with radially arranged needle-shaped refractile clefts within adipocytes and histiocytes.

Histopathological changes similar to those of sclerema neonatorum have been described in a patient with gemcitabine-associated livedoid thrombotic microangiopathy. The cutaneous biopsy showed small-vessel occlusion by intravascular fibrin and leukocytes, vessel wall thickening and endothelial cell swelling and some structures arranged radially with needle-shaped clefts resembling those of sclerema neonatorum [16].

Sclerema neonatorum should be not confused with scleroedema neonatorum, an entirely different process seen in premature infants with congenital heart disease, which is characterised by distended skin with wax-like appearance that results from dermal oedema with increased amounts of mucin [14].

Management

Treatment of sclerema neonatorum is mainly directed to the underlying disease. Systemic corticosteroids have been demonstrated not to be effective [6]. Repeated exchange transfusions may substantially reduce mortality [17,18], but the diagnosis in those cases was not histopathologically confirmed. Intravenous immunoglobulins were used in a newborn with sclerema neonatorum and sepsis, with transitory improvement of the skin induration, but the patient died of respiratory failure [19].

Gouty panniculitis

Definition

Panniculitis is a very uncommon complication of tophaceous gout (Chapter 155).

Pathophysiology

Histopathology

Histopathology shows a lobular, sometimes neutrophilic, panniculitis with deposition of needle-shaped refractile crystals within adipocytes (Figure 97.56) [1]. Frequently, histiocytes and multinucleate giant cells form a palisade around the urate crystals. Ultrasound scans may be helpful for diagnosis and monitoring of the disorder [2].

Clinical features

Presentation

The usual clinical presentation consists of painful ulcerating nodules on the lower legs (Figure 97.57) [1,3–10]. In most reported cases, patients had already sustained severe joint damage by the time panniculitis manifested as subcutaneous nodules, but in some cases panniculitis may be the first manifestation of hyperuricaemia [1]. One of the patients reported also had involvement of bone marrow fat [10].

Management

In gouthy tophi, the usually administered systemic drugs including colchicine, allopurinol and febuxostat block uric acid production, but they have little or no effect in cutaneous and subcutaneous tophi. Symptomatic lesions may improve with NSAIDs.

Fungal panniculitis due to zygomycosis, mucormycosis and aspergillosis

A predominantly lobular panniculitis with fine needle-shaped refractile crystals within adipocytes has been described in subcutaneous fungal infections including zygomycosis [1], mucormycosis [2]

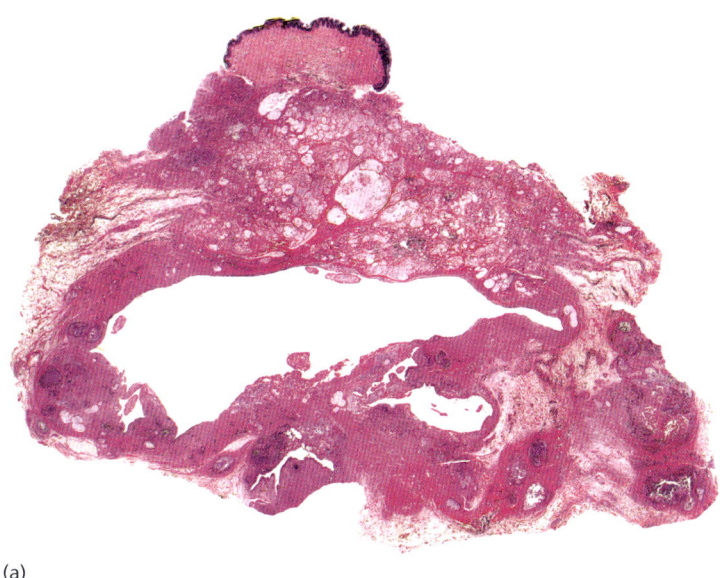

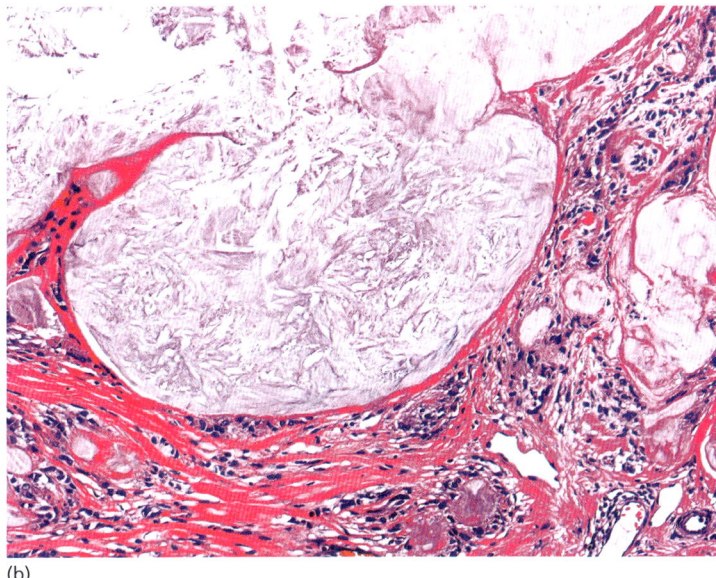

(a)

(b)

Figure 97.56 Histopathology of gouty panniculitis. (a) Scanning power showing involvement of the subcutaneous tissue, whereas the dermis is spared. (b) Basophilic amorphous deposits, which are fine needle-like shaped urate crystals, appear surrounded by histiocytes.

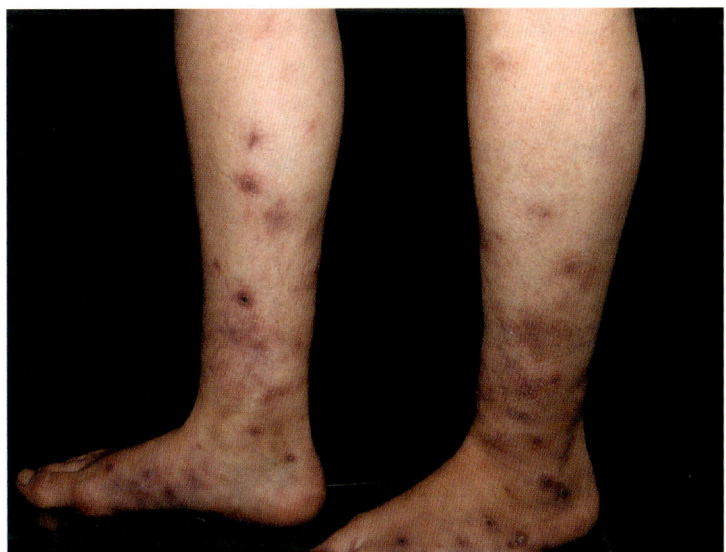

Figure 97.57 Gouty panniculitis. Ulcerated nodules on the lower legs of a patient with hyperuricaemia.

and aspergillosis [3] (Chapter 32). The presumed urate crystals are similar to those found in gouty panniculitis but the mechanism by which they are formed is unknown.

Cytophagic histiocytic panniculitis, subcutaneous γ/δ T-cell lymphoma and subcutaneous panniculitis-like T-cell lymphoma

Introduction and general description

The term cytophagic histiocytic panniculitis was introduced to describe a rare entity characterised by the development of subcutaneous nodules containing lobular infiltrates of macrophages which had phagocytosed lymphocytes, erythrocytes and nuclear debris [1]. With the benefit of modern immunohistochemistry and genetic techniques, it has become evident that most patients who are found to have cytophagic histiocytic panniculitis have one of two types of primary lymphoma affecting the subcutaneous tissue [2]: SPTCL or primary cutaneous γ/δ T-cell lymphoma. The former is a homogeneous entity with an α/β+ T-cell phenotype, indolent biological behaviour and good prognosis, whereas patients with the latter and a γ/δ+ T-cell phenotype are more heterogeneous and show a very aggressive clinical course with poor prognosis [3–7]. Both entities are discussed in detail in Chapter 139. This section focuses on SPTCL.

Although most cases of cytophagic histiocytic panniculitis represent examples of one of the subcutaneous lymphomas, it seems that there is still a group of patients in whom a definitive diagnosis of lymphoma cannot be made and in whom molecular studies fail to demonstrate monoclonal rearrangements of infiltrating lymphocytes. Nevertheless, the prognosis within this group is often poor, with pancytopenia and fatal outcome from haemophagocytic syndrome involving liver, spleen and bone marrow [8].

Pathophysiology
Histopathology
Histopathologically, SPTCL and cytophagic histiocytic panniculitis may be indistinguishable, and only after immunohistochemical and molecular studies can they be differentiated. At low power both disorders mimic a predominantly lobular panniculitis. The fat lobule is involved by small and medium-sized atypical lymphocytes with hyperchromatic nuclei. Numerous macrophages are also intermingled with the atypical lymphocytes. A characteristic finding in favour of the diagnosis of SPTCL consists in the sparing of the epidermis and dermis (Figure 97.58). In some areas, atypical lymphocytes are arranged in a circle around necrotic adipocytes, although this rimming is not entirely specific for SPTCL and it may

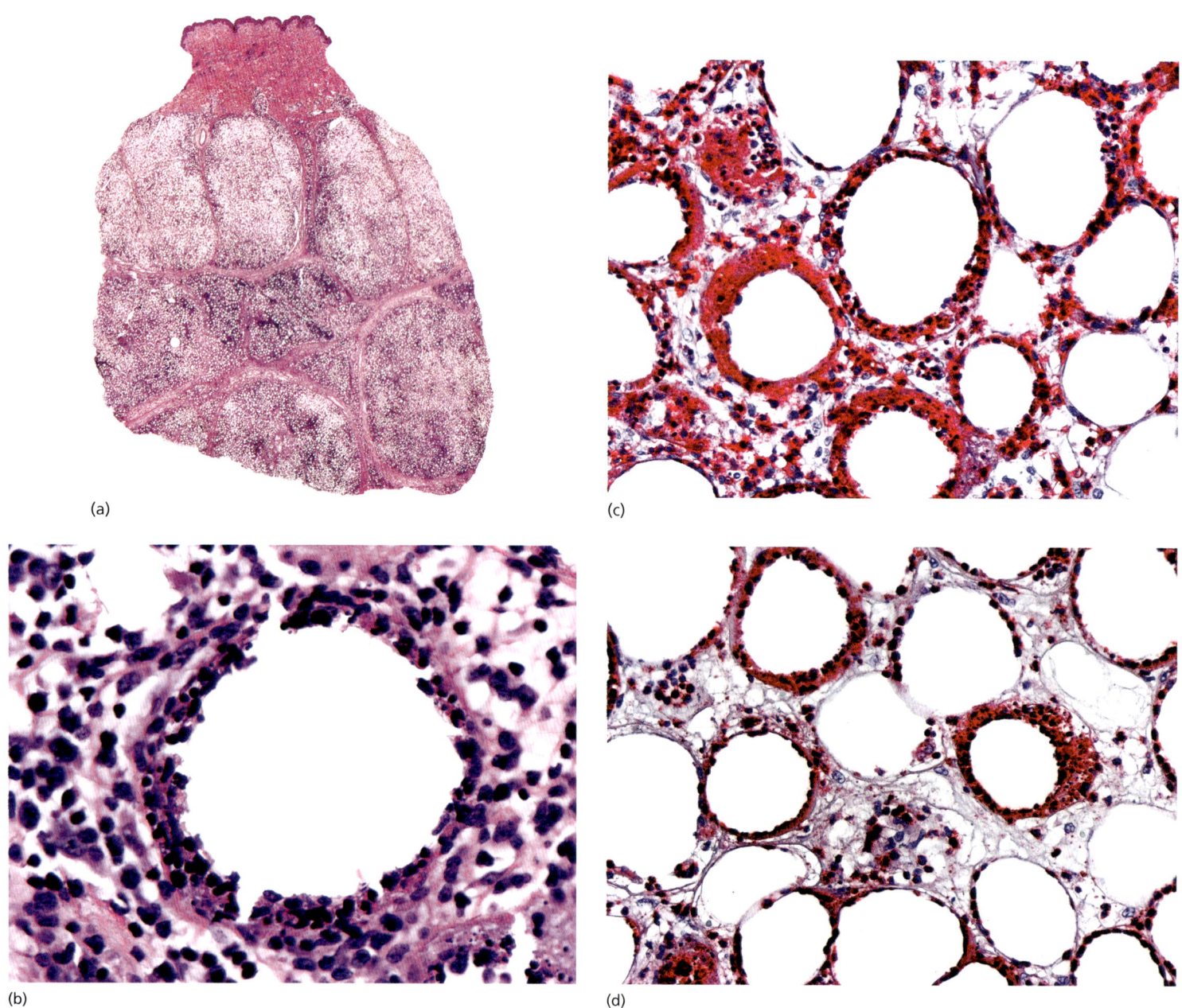

Figure 97.58 Histopathological features of subcutaneous panniculitis-like T-cell lymphoma. (a) Scanning power showing features simulating a lobular panniculitis. (b) Atypical lymphocytes arranged in a circle around necrotic adipocytes. (c) Neoplastic lymphocytes show CD8 immunopositivity. (d) Neoplastic lymphocytes express also positivity for TIA-1.

also be seen in other lymphoid processes involving subcutaneous fat [9]. The presence of macrophages with cytophagic activity containing lymphocytes, neutrophils and nuclear debris within their cytoplasm is also a frequent finding in both processes, the so-called 'bean bag' cells. Foamy histiocytes are also frequently found in areas of fat necrosis.

A diagnosis of SPTCL can usually be established with confidence using immunohistochemistry and molecular techniques. Immunohistochemical studies have demonstrated that lymphocytes involving the fat lobules in SPTCL have a TCR-α/β+, CD3+, CD4–, CD8+, T-cell intracellular antigen 1+ (TIA-1+), perforin+, granzyme B+, CD30– T-cell immunophenotype. There is no evidence of Epstein–Barr virus (EBV) infection, either using PCR amplification to detect EBV-encoded RNA and EBV DNA or by

immunohistochemical staining for latent membrane protein 1. As a consequence of its α/β+ T-cell phenotype, SPTCL expresses βF1 but is negative for TCRγ and TCRδ, in contrast with primary cutaneous γ/δ+ T-cell lymphoma and other lymphoproliferative processes involving subcutaneous fat. Monoclonal rearrangement of γ or β genes can usually be detected in lesions of SPTCL using molecular analyses, whereas these rearrangements are not found in patients with cytophagic histiocytic panniculitis.

Clinical features
Presentation
Subcutaneous panniculitis-like T-cell lymphoma is rare, accounting for less than 1% of all primary cutaneous T-cell lymphomas, with equal incidence in both genders and preferentially involving

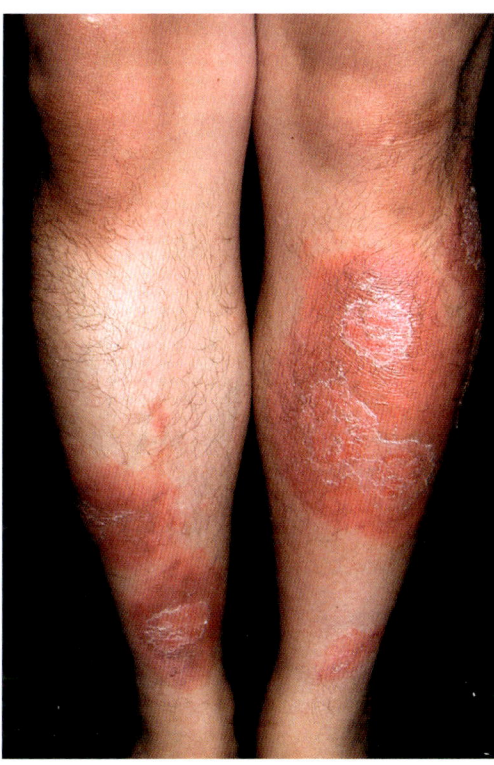

Figure 97.59 Subcutaneous pannicultis-like T-cell lymphoma. Red plaques involving the anterior aspects of the lower extremities.

adult patients, although there are also cases described in children. Clinically, patients present with red subcutaneous nodules that may group into large plaques typically involving the lower extremities (Figure 97.59). A common feature consists of areas of lipoatrophy when the lesions resolve. Less commonly, SPTCL may involve the trunk, head or upper extremities. Approximately, 50% of patients have B symptoms, including fever, fatigue and weight loss; cytopenia and elevation of liver enzymes are frequently found, but a frank haemophagocytic syndrome is rare [10].

Management
Conservative immunosuppressive regimens based on systemic corticosteroids and ciclosporin may be effective in patients with subcutaneous panniculitic T-cell lymphopma without an associated hemophagocytic syndrome. In patients presenting with solitary lesions, local radiotherapy may suffice.

Sclerosing postirradiation panniculitis

Synonyms and inclusions
• Postradiotherapy panniculitis

Introduction and general description
Sclerosing postirradiation panniculitis is a rare clinicopathological variant of panniculitis that appears months or years after radiotherapy in the irradiated skin. Clinically, lesions consist of subcutaneous indurated nodules.

In 1993, Winkelmann *et al.* [1] described the first four cases of pseudosclerodermatous panniculitis after irradiation and, since then, only 10 additional cases have been published [2–9]. This process represents an unusual variant of panniculitis which may rarely occur as a cutaneous complication of radiotherapy.

Pathophysiology
Histopathology
The histopathological findings in sclerosing postirradiation panniculitis include a predominantly lobular panniculitis with necrosis of the adipocytes at the centre of the fat lobule and dense inflammatory infiltrates composed mainly of foamy histiocytes. Lipophagic granulomas involving the periphery of the fat lobules and thickening and sclerosis of the connective tissue septa are the most characteristic features in the subcutaneous tissue (Figure 97.60).

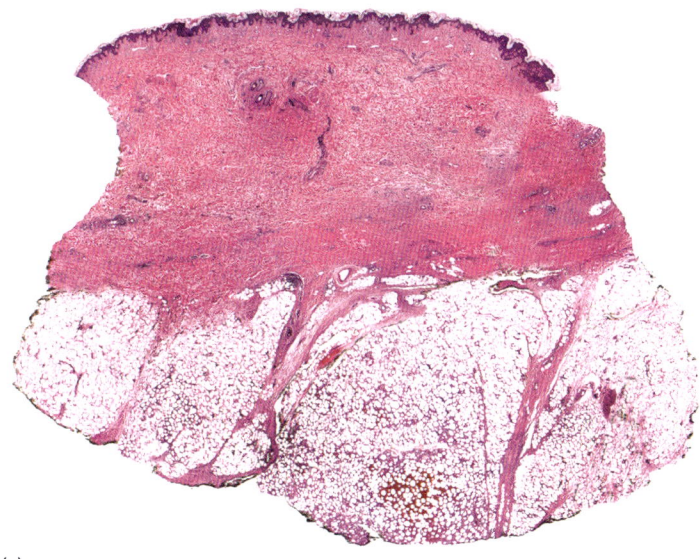

(a)

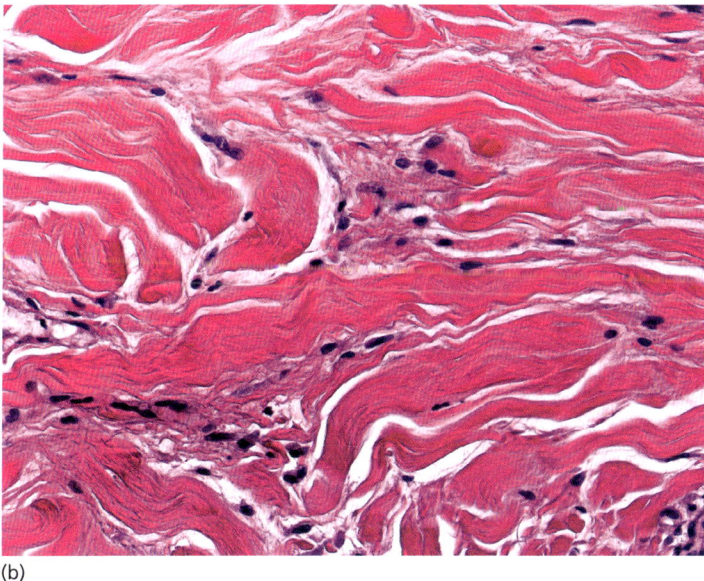

(b)

Figure 97.60 Histopathological features of sclerosing postirradiation panniculitis. (a) Scanning power showing a mostly lobular panniculitis. (b) Sclerotic collagen bundles at the septa of connective tissue of the subcutis.

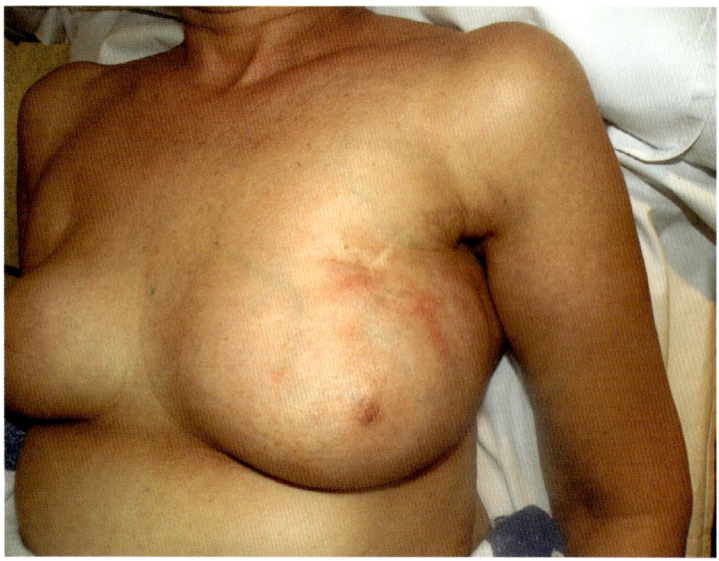

Figure 97.61 Sclerosing postirradiation panniculitis showing a depressed and indurated nodule on the previously irradiated area of the skin.

These histopathological findings may or may not be accompanied by dermal changes secondary to radiotherapy [10–12], namely sclerosis of the papillary dermis, atypical star-shaped fibroblasts scattered among dermal collagen bundles and dilated thrombosed blood vessels with endothelial cell swelling and hyaline sclerosis of their walls.

Clinical features
Presentation
Clinically, sclerosing postirradiation panniculitis presents as an indurated, asymptomatic, subcutaneous nodule or plaque with little or no change in the epidermis and dermis at the site of previous radiotherapy (Figure 97.61). The most common location is the anterior chest wall following treatment for breast cancer. However, it may appear in any previously irradiated area of the skin [2,6,7]. The interval between the radiotherapy and the presentation of the condition varies from months to several years [1–5].

Differential diagnosis
The histopathological differential diagnosis includes other diseases showing a septal or lobular panniculitis with sclerosis of the connective tissue septa of the subcutis, such as deep morphoea [13–15] and lupus panniculitis [16]. Deep morphoea consists histopathologically of a septal panniculitis without significant lobular involvement in which there are sclerotic collagen bundles and aggregates of lymphocytes and especially plasma cells at the interface between the connective tissue septa and the fat lobules. In contrast with sclerosing postirradiation panniculitis, deep morphoea does not show lobular involvement and the inflammatory cells within the thickened septa are mainly plasma cells. Lupus panniculitis is a mostly lobular panniculitis with sclerotic septa,

but, in contrast with sclerosing postirradiation panniculitis, the inflammatory infiltrate involving the lobules is mostly composed of lymphocytes and plasma cells.

Management
Treatment of sclerosing postirradiation panniculitis is not required and biopsy and subsequent histopathological study are only performed when the possibility of a subcutaneous metastasis from the previously excised and/or irradiated breast cancer is raised.

Key references

The full list of references can be found in the online version at https://www.wiley.com/rooksdermatology10e

Panniculitis
Introduction and general description
2 Requena L, Sánchez Yus E. Panniculitis. Part I. Mostly septal panniculitis. *J Am Acad Dermatol* 2001;45:163–83.
3 Requena L, Sánchez Yus E. Panniculitis. Part II. Mostly lobular panniculitis. *J Am Acad Dermatol* 2001;45:325–61.

Cutaneous polyarteritis nodosa (cutaneous arteritis)
1 Jennette JC, Falk RJ, Bacon PA *et al.* 2012 revised international Chapel Hill consensus conference nomenclature of vasculitides. *Arthritis Rheum* 2013;65:1–11.
2 Sunderkötter CH, Zelger B, Chen KR *et al.* Nomenclature of cutaneous vasculitis: dermatologic addendum to the 2012 revised international Chapel Hill consensus conference nomenclature of vasculitides. *Arthritis Rheumatol* 2018;70:171–84.

Deep morphoea
15 Onajin O, Wieland CN, Peters MS, Lohse CM, Lehman JS. Clinicopathologic and immunophenotypic features of eosinophilic fasciitis and morphea profunda: a comparative study of 27 cases. *J Am Acad Dermatol* 2018;78:121–8.

Erythema nodosum
10 García-Porrúa C, González-Gay MA, Vázquez-Caruncho M *et al.* Erythema nodosum. Etiologic and predictive factors in defined population. *Arthritis Rheum* 2000;43:584–92.
79 Tetzlaff MT, Jazaeri AA, Torres-Cabala CA *et al.* Erythema nodosum-like panniculitis mimicking disease recurrence: a novel toxicity from immune checkpoint blockade therapy – report of 2 patients. *J Cutan Pathol* 2017;44:1080–6.
194 Sanchez Yus E, Sanz Vico MD, de Diego V. Miescher's radial granuloma. A characteristic marker of erythema nodosum. *Am J Dermatopathol* 1989;11:434–42.

Erythema induratum of Bazin
25 Segura S, Pujol RM, Trindade F, Requena L. Vasculitis in erythema induratum of Bazin: a histopathologic study of 101 biopsy specimens from 86 patients. *J Am Acad Dermatol* 2008;59:839–51.

Lupus panniculitis
5 Massone C, Kodama K, Salmhofer W *et al.* Lupus erythematosus panniculitis (lupus profundus): clinical, histopathological, and molecular analysis of nine cases. *J Cutan Pathol* 2005;32:396–404.

Pancreatic panniculitis
3 Dahl PR, Su WP, Cullimore KC, Dicken CH. Pancreatic panniculitis. *J Am Acad Dermatol* 1995;33:413–17.

CHAPTER 98

Non-inflammatory Disorders of Subcutaneous Fat

Grace L. Lee[1], Amit Garg[2] and Amy Y.-Y. Chen[3]

[1]Department of Dermatology, Baylor College of Medicine, Houston, TX, USA
[2]Department of Dermatology, Donald and Barbara Zucker School of Medicine at Hofstra Northwell, Hempstead, NY, USA
[3]Central Connecticut Dermatology, Cromwell, CT, USA

Introduction

This chapter addresses principally non-inflammatory acquired disorders of subcutaneous fat with an emphasis on acquired lipodystrophy, fat hypertrophy, subcutaneous lipomatosis and lipoedema. While some of the entities discussed are very common, such as cellulite and obesity, most are much rarer. Panniculitis and genetic disorders of subcutaneous fat are addressed in Chapters 72 and 97, respectively.

ACQUIRED LIPODYSTROPHY

Acquired lipodystrophy refers to a heterogeneous group of disorders in which there is localised, partial or generalised loss of subcutaneous fat (lipoatrophy), in certain cases accompanied by fat accumulation in other body sites.

Acquired generalised lipodystrophy

Definition and nomenclature
Acquired generalised lipodystrophy (AGL) is a rare disease characterised by a selective loss of adipose tissue from large regions of the body, occurring after birth [1].

Synonyms and inclusions
- Lawrence syndrome
- Lawrence–Seip syndrome

Introduction and general description
After its initial report by Ziegler in 1928 [2], AGL was described in more detail through autopsy findings by Lawrence in 1946 [3]. Although loss of adipose tissue in AGL most often occurs during childhood and adolescence, a few cases report AGL in individuals over the age of 65 years [4,5]. The pattern and extent of fat loss in AGL are variable. Most patients have generalised loss of fat, though fat may be spared in some areas, such as retro-orbital fat. In addition to the loss of adipose tissue, patients often develop severe hepatic steatosis and fibrosis, severe insulin resistance and hyperinsulinaemia, hypertriglyceridaemia and low serum high-density lipoprotein (HDL) levels [6–9].

Epidemiology
Incidence and prevalence
AGL is a rare disease and thus its incidence and prevalence are difficult to estimate. Fewer than 100 cases were identified in a literature review published in 2003 [10]. In 2012, it was estimated that AGL affects approximately 1 in 100 000 people in the European Union.

PART 8: SPECIFIC CUTANEOUS STRUCTURES

Age
Most patients with AGL present during childhood or adolescence.

Sex
Women are affected three times more often than men [10].

Ethnicity
In a case series, the majority of patients reported have been white although AGL has also been reported in Hispanic and East Asian patients [10,11].

Associated diseases
Most AGL patients have some degree of metabolic derangement, including fasting and/or postprandial hyperinsulinaemia, hypertriglyceridaemia, low serum levels of HDL, and low leptin and adiponectin [6–9,10]. Diabetes most often occurs subsequent to the onset of AGL, although in some it may present before or at the time of onset [10]. AGL patients usually do not develop diabetic ketoacidosis [12]. Patients may also have increased basal metabolic rate and complain of fatigue and voracious appetite [10].

Hepatomegaly occurs in 70–100% of AGL patients. Hepatic steatosis or non-alcoholic steatohepatitis results in mild to moderate elevation of serum transaminases. Splenomegaly may result from portal hypertension and cirrhosis [10].

Cardiomyopathy may be associated with AGL. In a 2011 study of left ventricular mass in 13 patients with AGL, three had mild and three had moderate ventricular hypertrophy. Abnormalities were seen in 5 of 11 AGL patients whose electrocardiogram was available for analysis [13].

Muscle and neurological involvement have rarely been reported [5,11].

Reproductive capacity is normal in male patients with AGL. Female AGL patients may have normal reproduction although irregular menses are common [10]. Primary or secondary amenorrhoea rarely occurs [10,14,15]. Single [16] or multiple [17,18] bone lucencies and cysts have been reported in AGL patients, although the clinical significance of these lesions is not clear [18]. Lymphadenopathy has also been reported in some [7,18–20]. Recently, there have been five cases of patients with AGL who developed lymphoma, particularly peripheral T-cell lymphoma with possible association to metreleptin therapy [21].

Pathophysiology
The mechanism of fat loss in AGL is unknown. Despite reports of a variety of preceding infections, it is not clear that these infections directly cause AGL [22,23]. The classic complement pathway is postulated to be involved in the pathogenesis among AGL patients with autoimmune hepatitis and low serum complement [24,25]. Antibody-mediated destruction or cell-mediated lysis of adipocytes has also been considered [26]. Specifically, anti-adipocyte antibodies against perilipin 1 (PLIN1) were found to be present in the serum of five patients with AGL [27].

The consequences are that there is an insufficient mass of adipose tissue to store excess energy, which is stored instead as triglyceride in the liver and skeletal muscle, and that there is a perpetual elevation of plasma free fatty acid (FFA), resulting in an impaired β-cell response to glucose and insulin resistance [28–31]. Low serum leptin and adiponectin levels, reflecting the low amount of body fat in these patients, may further contribute to severe insulin resistance and the metabolic complications observed in AGL [32–35].

Pathology
AGL is a clinical diagnosis, although histopathology may help confirm the diagnosis. Tissue examination demonstrates a complete or near-complete absence of subcutaneous fat, with the dermis and fascia in direct apposition. If adipocytes are present, they are markedly reduced in number and size and they are arranged in small groups surrounded by abundant connective tissue [36].

Genetics
No known genetic mutation or familial cluster has been identified.

Clinical features
Presentation
In contrast to congenital lipodystrophy, patients with AGL have normal fat density and distribution at birth. The onset of fat loss is typically insidious over months to years (Figure 98.1), although rapid progression over weeks has been observed [10]. Rarely, the process of fat destruction may occur rapidly in one area and stay quiescent over months to years, only to become active again later and result in generalised fat loss [2,10]. The extent and degree of fat loss are variable. Usual sites of involvement include the face (Figure 98.1a), trunk, abdomen and extremities. Underlying veins and musculature become prominent with severe fat loss (Figure 98.1b). In some, loss of fat may also involve the palms, soles and abdominal cavity. Generally, marrow and retro-orbital fat are preserved. Clinically, AGL and HIV-associated lipodystrophy can present similarly (see later).

Acanthosis nigricans of the axillae, groin, neck, umbilicus and nipples is noted in 45–64% of AGL patients [10]. Other less common dermatological findings include localised [37,38] or generalised hyperpigmentation [39,40], telangiectasia [19] and hyperkeratosis of the palms and soles [16]. Women with AGL may have mild hirsutism [10,39,41,42]. Rarely, virilisation with temporal recession of hair and acne has been reported [14,43]. Alopecia [6] and curly hair [17,10,16,22,39,42,44] have also been observed. Acromegaloid facial features with large hands and feet may rarely be seen [9,10].

In 2003, Misra and Garg proposed new diagnostic criteria applicable to the broad spectrum of AGL patients. Essential criteria include selective loss of body fat affecting large regions of the body, beginning after birth but usually before adolescence. Supportive clinical criteria include loss of subcutaneous fat from the palms and soles, a preceding history of tender subcutaneous nodular swellings, histological confirmation from involved tissue, acanthosis nigricans, hepatosplenomegaly and the presence of other autoimmune diseases.

Supportive laboratory criteria include impaired glucose tolerance, severe fasting and/or postprandial hyperinsulinaemia, hypertriglyceridaemia, low serum HDL, low serum leptin and/or adiponectin, and evidence by magnetic resonance imaging (MRI) of fat loss from large regions of the body with preserved bone marrow fat [10]. The number of these secondary clinical or laboratory

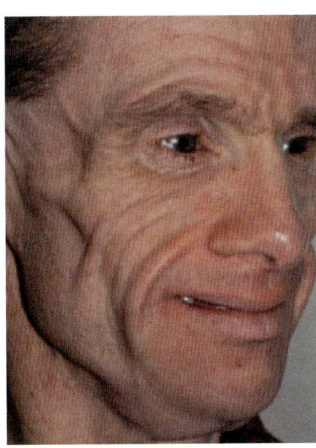 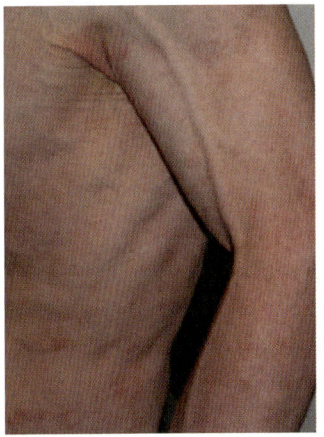 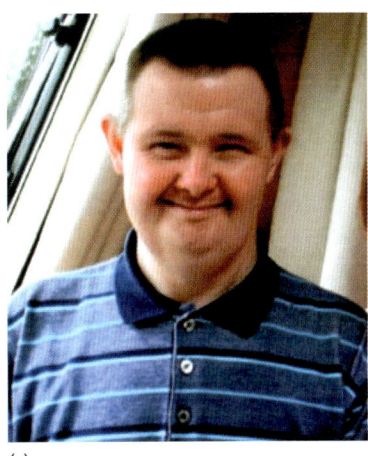

Figure 98.1 Physical examination revealed (a) lipoatrophy of the face and (b) generalised lipoatrophy of the torso with visible subcutaneous veins. (c) A photograph of the patient taken 5 years earlier, in 2008, is shown for comparison. Reproduced from Aslam *et al*. [56] with permission of John Wiley & Sons.

(a)　　　　　　　　　(b)　　　　　　　　(c)

criteria needed to support a diagnosis of AGL has not been formally established.

Clinical variants

AGL is subdivided into three types:

i. *Type I AGL*, in which initially localised panniculitis precedes generalised fat loss, accounts for approximately 25% of cases [1].

ii. *Type II AGL*, which accounts for another 25% of cases, is associated with autoimmune diseases including haemolytic anaemia, chronic autoimmune hepatitis, Hashimoto thyroiditis, juvenile rheumatoid arthritis, juvenile dermatomyositis and vitiligo [6,24,37,38,45–47]. Juvenile dermatomyositis may have the strongest association with AGL [10].

iii. *Type III (idiopathic) AGL*, the most common subtype, in which no triggers or associated diseases are identified.

More recently, anti-PD-1 immune checkpoint inhibitor (nivolumab or pembrolizumab) associated AGL has been reported [48–50].

Differential diagnosis

Some AGL patients may initially present with localised or partial lipodystrophy and hence may be misclassified as having acquired partial lipodystrophy or localised lipodystrophy.

AGL patients are differentiated from *congenital generalised lipodystrophy* (CGL) patients who have near-complete generalised fat loss at birth (Chapter 72). Furthermore, CGL patients have advanced bone age and intellectual disability. As with AGL, CGL patients may have acromegaloid features, lytic bone lesions and cardiomyopathy [10]. Lytic bone lesions are, however, more common and the cardiomyopathy more severe in CGL [10,13]. MRI studies of CGL patients show an absence of 'metabolically active' fat in intra-abdominal and intrathoracic regions, and in bone marrow, while marrow fat is preserved in AGL patients [10,51]. Genetic analysis for known mutations may aid in the confirmation of CGL.

While patients with *mandibuloacral dysplasia* may have generalised fat loss, these patients also have skeletal anomalies (Chapter 72). The identification of associated genetic mutations can help to confirm this diagnosis.

Family histories as well as genotyping will also help differentiate AGL from *autosomal dominant familial partial lipodystrophy* (Chapter 74) [1].

Complications and co-morbidities

Patients with AGL may suffer complications from metabolic disturbances and other associated co-morbid conditions in association with type II AGL. Retinopathy, nephropathy and neuropathy are common complications because of the patients' longstanding diabetes. Hypertriglyceridaemia may lead to eruptive xanthomas, lipaemia retinalis and acute pancreatitis [10]. These metabolic abnormalities also predispose AGL patients to premature atherosclerosis and coronary heart disease [6,10].

Disease course and prognosis

The loss of subcutaneous fat tissue in AGL patients is permanent. The prognosis of AGL patients largely depends on the course and management of co-morbidities.

Investigations

Laboratory and ancillary testing are pursued to establish the presence and monitor the course of co-morbid diseases. While serum leptin is not useful for establishing the diagnosis, it may predict response to replacement therapy with the synthetic recombinant analogue of human leptin, metreleptin [1].

Management

There is no established management algorithm for AGL. Subcutaneous fat loss is irreversible. To the extent feasible, cosmetic procedures such as filler injections, autologous adipose tissue transfer and muscle tissue transfers may help correct volume losses [1,52,53]. Optimal management of co-morbid conditions requires collaboration between primary care physicians and several specialists.

In one trial, which included three AGL patients amongst others with various lipodystrophies, 4 months of twice-daily subcutaneous metreleptin injections were shown to be safe and effective. There was a significant decrease in fasting blood glucose level and glycosylated haemoglobin in two patients. In three patients with hypertriglyceridaemia, fasting levels of plasma triglycerides decreased by 83%. In these patients, fasting plasma triglycerides increased soon after discontinuation of the injections and were corrected once again after reinitiation of the therapy [54]. Furthermore, liver volume and serum transaminases decreased significantly during metreleptin therapy, suggesting that it reduced hepatic steatosis [55]. Metreleptin is approved in both the European Union and USA for the treatment of complications of leptin deficiency in patients with CGL or AGL.

Acquired partial lipodystrophy

Definition and nomenclature

Acquired partial lipodystrophy (APL) is a rare disease characterised by symmetrical fat loss, usually occurring before the age of 15 years [1,2].

Synonyms and inclusions
- Barraquer–Simons syndrome
- Progressive cephalothoracic lipodystrophy

Introduction and general description

APL was first reported by Mitchell [3] and later by Barraquer [4] and by Simons [5]. Although rare, APL is the most common of the non-localised lipodystrophies, other than HIV-associated lipodystrophy. It is characterised by symmetrical and insidious although progressive fat loss starting from the face and scalp and gradually progressing downwards, to involve the neck, shoulders, upper extremities, thoracic region and upper abdomen. Involvement of the lower extremities is uncommon [1,2].

Epidemiology
Incidence and prevalence

Because it is rare, the incidence and prevalence of APL is difficult to estimate. By 2000, there were approximately 250 cases reported in the English literature [1].

Age

Onset is typically before the age of 15 years, with a median of 8 years [1,2].

Sex

Women are affected approximately three times more commonly than men [1].

Ethnicity

In a case series, most reported patients have been white [1].

Associated diseases

Approximately one-third of patients develop mesangiocapillary glomerulonephritis (MCGN), usually more than 10 years after the onset of lipodystrophy [1]. Systemic lupus erythematosus has been associated with APL and has occurred 2–28 years after the onset of lipodystrophy [6–9]. Other autoimmune diseases, such as dermatomyositis [10], leukocytoclastic vasculitis [11], dermatitis herpetiformis and coeliac diseases [12], hypothyroidism, pernicious anaemia [13], rheumatoid arthritis [8] and temporal arteritis, have also been reported. More recently, APL has been reported in the setting of chronic sclerodermatous graft-versus-host disease,

POEMS (Polyneuropathy, Organomegaly, Endocrinopathy, Monoclonal gammopathy and Skin changes) syndrome and extrinsic allergic alveolitis, as well as central nervous system (CNS) disorders including epilepsy, sensorineural deafness and intellectual disability (Chapter 149) [14,15–17].

Pathophysiology

There is evidence to support an autoimmune-mediated destruction of adipocytes in APL. Approximately 80–90% of APL patients have a serum immunoglobulin G named C3 nephritic factor [18,19]. This blocks the degradation of the enzyme C3 convertase, which leads to excessive consumption of C3. As a result, serum C3 levels are low in more than 80% of APL patients [20]. Levels of C1q, C4, C5 and C6 and factors B and P are usually normal, suggesting selective activation of the alternative complement pathway [21,22]. Lysis of adipocytes may be related to the expression of several complement proteins such as factors D (adipsin), B, H and P [23,24,25]. For example, *in vitro* studies suggest that the C3 nephritic factor causes lysis in adipocytes expressing factor D [23]. Heterogeneity of factor D expression in adipose tissue in different anatomical locations has been postulated to explain the selective loss of upper body fat in APL [24].

In those APL patients without C3 nephritic factor, other immune abnormalities are postulated to be relevant pathogenetic factors. In a paediatric APL patient without C3 nephritic factor, serum tumour necrosis factor α (TNF-α) and interleukin 6 (IL-6) were noted to be elevated [26]. TNF-α has been shown to cause apoptosis in adipocyte cultures, and IL-6 stimulates lipolysis in human adipocytes [27,28]. TNF-α also influences the complement pathway by controlling factor D production in adipocytes [26].

Pathology

APL is a clinical diagnosis based on the presentation and progression of disease. Histopathology, in common with AGL, shows complete or near-complete absence of subcutaneous fat, with the dermis and fascia in direct apposition. If adipocytes are present, they are markedly reduced in number and size, and they are arranged in small groups surrounded by abundant connective tissues [29].

Causative organisms

Although fat loss has been preceded by infection in some reported cases of APL, the relationship between APL and infection is unclear [24].

Genetics

LMNB2 mutations have been reported in five patients with APL, although some of these had atypical presentations [30].

Clinical features
Presentation

Fat loss in APL occurs symmetrically, starting on the face and scalp, then gradually spreading to involve the neck, shoulders, upper extremities, thoracic region and upper abdomen (Figure 98.2). Involvement of the inguinal region or thighs is uncommon. Fat in the hips and lower extremities is unaffected. In fact, affected women frequently accumulate excess fat in these regions after puberty. Fat loss typically progresses over a period of about 18 months,

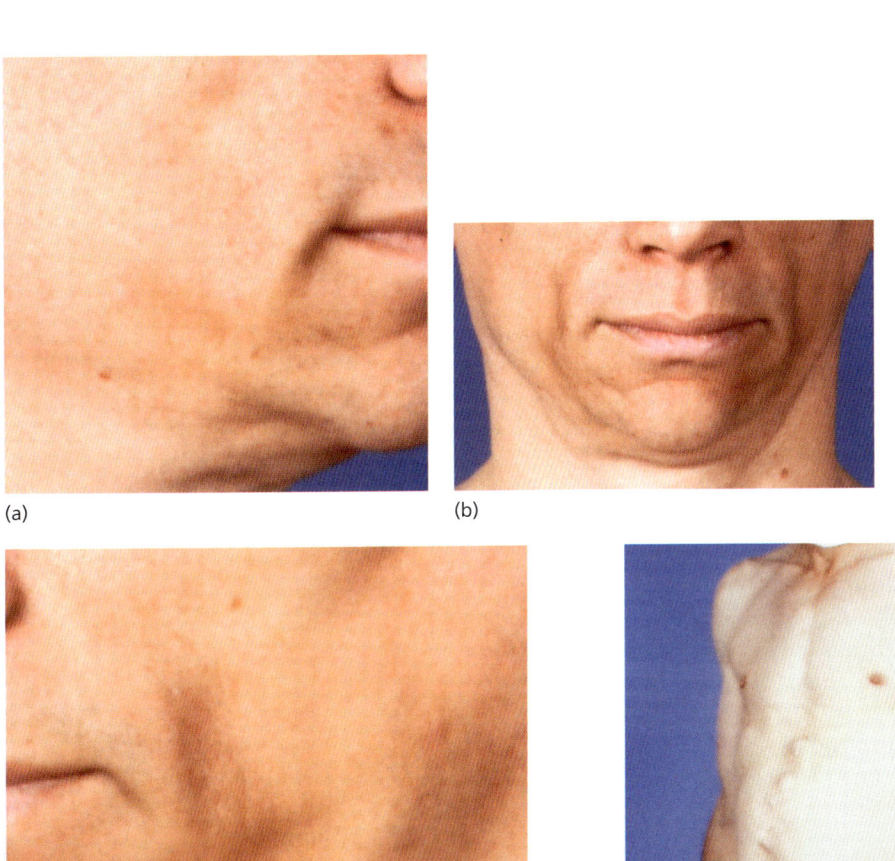

(a)

(b)

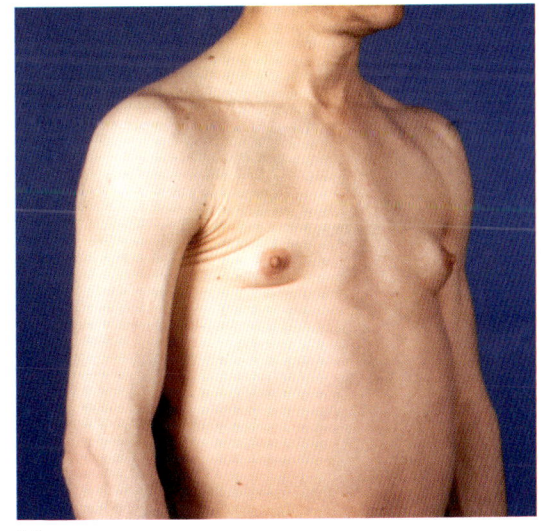

(c)

(d)

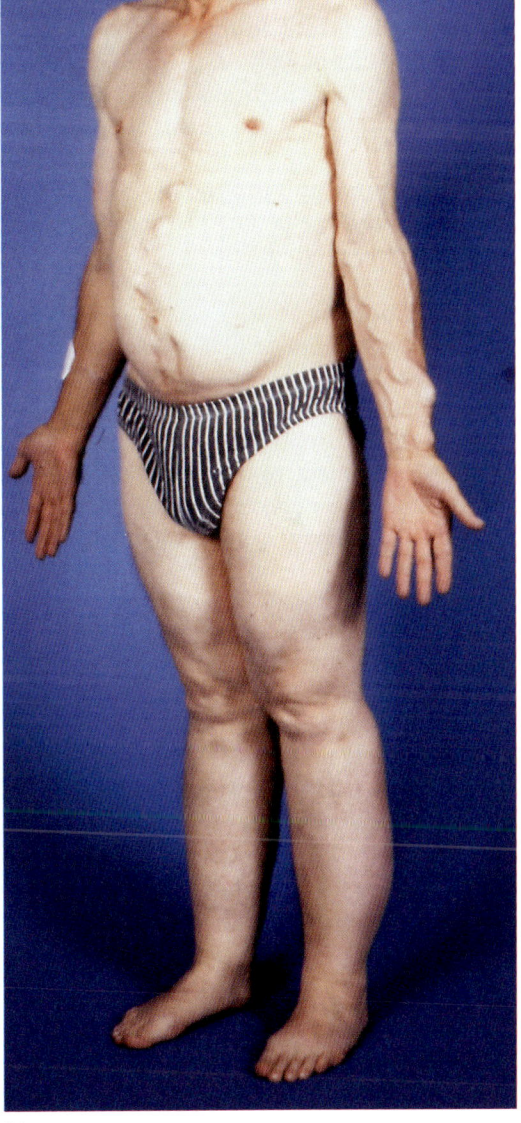

(e)

Figure 98.2 Acquired partial lipodystrophy (APL); (a–c) marked loss of facial fat resulting in a prematurely aged appearance and (d) prominence of arm veins, sternomastoid muscles and breast tissue resulting from subcutaneous fat loss in a 31-year-old man with APL and renal failure; (e) note preservation of subcutaneous fat in the lower half of the body contrasting with dramatic loss of subcutaneous fat in the upper half of the body in a 50-year-old man whose longstanding APL was not recognised until he presented with accelerated hypertension secondary to APL-related glomerulonephritis.

PART 8: SPECIFIC CUTANEOUS STRUCTURES

although it may continue for several years. Orbital, mediastinal, gluteal, intramuscular, intraperitoneal, perirenal and bone marrow fat is usually unaffected [1,2].

Clinical variants
Three phenotypic subtypes have been recognised: (i) upper body fat loss; (ii) upper body fat loss with hypertrophy of adipose tissue in the lower half of the body; and (iii) hemilipodystrophy in which only one side of the face or body is affected.

Differential diagnosis
APL is differentiated from familial partial lipodystrophy in which there is a family history of similar lipodystrophy, variations in clinical presentation of fat loss and identified genetic mutations. A history of trauma and medication history can help differentiate other forms of acquired lipodystrophy from APL. APL is differentiated from AGL based on the extent of involvement as well as sparing of the intra-abdominal fat.

Complications and co-morbidities
Unlike in patients with AGL, insulin resistance, diabetes, dyslipidaemia, acanthosis nigricans, hirsutism or menstrual abnormalities are less common in APL patients [1].

Disease course and prognosis
Fat loss is irreversible in APL. Overall prognosis is driven by the presence of co-morbidities.

Investigations
The initial evaluation of APL patients should include serum C3 level and C3 nephritic factor, as well as baseline screening for metabolic derangements with a comprehensive metabolic panel, fasting glucose, lipid panels and insulin level. Evaluation should also include assessment of associated co-morbid conditions. Periodic and continued monitoring for renal disease and autoimmunity is warranted. MRI may demonstrate the extent of fat loss if needed.

Management
There is no established management algorithm for APL. Subcutaneous fat loss is irreversible. To the extent feasible, cosmetic procedures such as filler injections, autologous adipose tissue transfer and muscle tissue transfers may help correct volume losses. However, the durable efficacy and safety of these approaches have not been extensively investigated. The identification of neutralising antibodies against C3 nephritic factors in intravenous immunoglobulin (IVIg) has led to treatment of patients who have C3 nephritic factors and type II MCGN with IVIg with encouraging results [31,32]. Optimal management of co-morbid conditions requires collaboration between primary care physicians and several specialists.

HIV-associated lipodystrophy

Definition and nomenclature
Lipodystrophy in patients affected with human immunodeficiency virus (HIV) is associated with highly active antiretroviral therapy

(HAART) regimens containing protease inhibitor (PI) or nucleoside reverse transcriptase inhibitor (NRTI). It is now the most prevalent type of lipodystrophy, in which both lipoatrophy and lipohypertrophy may be observed (Chapter 31).

> **Synonyms and inclusions**
> - Pseudo-Cushing syndrome
> - Fat redistribution syndrome
> - Maldistribution syndrome
> - Protease inhibitor-associated lipodystrophy syndrome

Introduction and general description
The first report of fat redistribution in an HIV-infected individual undergoing antiretroviral therapy including a PI was in 1997 [1]. Lipodystrophy in HIV-infected patients usually appears after patients have been receiving PI- or NRTI-containing HAART regimens for at least 2 years [2]. Currently, there is no consensus on the definition or diagnostic criteria for lipodystrophy in the HIV-infected patient [3]. In 2003, Carr *et al.* established a diagnostic model that included the variables of age, sex, known duration of HIV infection, HIV disease stage, waist to hip ratio, anion gap, serum HDL cholesterol level and trunk to peripheral fat ratio [4]. Although follow-up prospective studies confirmed its high diagnostic sensitivity, the complexity of the model is thought to impede its use in daily clinical practice [5].

Epidemiology
Incidence and prevalence
Lipodystrophy in HIV-infected patients is the most prevalent among lipodystrophies. Due to limitations in the definition, selection of study population and duration of follow-up, there are considerable differences in its reported incidence and prevalence. Prevalence ranges from 8% to 84% with an average of 42% [6]. Average incidence ranges from 7.3 to 11.7 per 100 patient-years [7,8]. Generally, higher prevalence is reported among patients receiving long-term therapy. In pooled analyses, the prevalence is 17% among adults treated with PI-containing therapy for less than 1 year and 43% in those treated for more than 1 year [6]. Each additional 6 months of treatment with HAART is associated with a 1.57 times increased risk of lipodystrophy [7]. It is expected that the prevalence will increase in the future with longer follow-up and continued use of HAART [6].

Age
The risk of developing HIV-associated lipodystrophy increases with age [6,9]. Children receiving PI-containing HAART therapy exhibit a similar redistribution of body fat and metabolic derangements, although children may have a relatively smaller increase in visceral fat in the trunk [10–13].

Sex
Female sex is associated with an increased risk in some studies [3].

Ethnicity
White and East Asian races have been linked to having an increased risk of HIV-associated lipodystrophy in a Canadian cohort

study [14]. It was also found that white males have more peripheral lipoatrophy whereas white females have more central lipohypertrophy. According to the same study, women of African descent are most vulnerable to developing lipodystrophy [14].

Associated diseases
Patients with HIV-related lipodystrophy may develop hypertriglyceridaemia, although diabetes is less common [2]. There may also be a predisposition to coronary artery disease [15].

Pathophysiology
While the exact cause of HIV-associated lipodystrophy is unknown, both PIs and NRTIs are implicated in the pathogenesis. Because these drug classes are often given together as part of HAART, the individual effects of these drugs on the specific lipodystrophy phenotype remains unclear. It is speculated that while PIs induce peripheral lipodystrophy and metabolic abnormalities, NRTIs may be responsible for the fat accumulation in certain regions such as the buffalo hump [2].

First and second generation PIs have been shown to inhibit adipocyte differentiation and lipogenesis *in vitro* [16]. PIs may also induce insulin resistance by inhibiting glucose transporter-4 expressions [17]. NRTIs, especially zidovudine and stavudine, have been proposed to induce fat loss by inhibiting mitochondrial polymerase γ and causing mitochondrial toxicity [18,19]. This results in production of reactive oxygen species (ROS), which have been linked to lipoatrophy [20]. Excess adipocyte apoptosis was also observed in *ex vivo* fat samples from lipoatrophic areas [21].

The mechanism for the increased amounts of visceral adipose tissue (VAT) observed in HIV-associated lipodystrophy is also unclear. VAT and subcutaneous adipose tissue (SAT) differ in their metabolism, gene expression and inflammatory status [22]. As a result, adipocytes or other cells in VAT and SAT may respond to stimuli (e.g. PIs) in different ways, resulting in hypertrophy in one area and atrophy in another [3].

Predisposing factors
Several factors have been postulated to influence the risk of developing HIV-associated lipodystrophy, including age, gender, ethnicity, duration and status of HIV infection, as well as exposure to both PI- and non-PI-containing HAART [3,6]. Both high and low CD4 counts have been reported in affected patients [23,24,25].

There is some evidence that first generation unboosted PIs, such as indinavir, are associated with a higher risk of lipodystrophy than are booster PIs [3]. In one study, the incidence of lipoatrophy was lower in patients treated with ritonavir-boosted atazanavir than in those who received unboosted atazanavir [14]. In another study, patients treated with ritonavir-boosted lopinavir developed lipodystrophy by 96 weeks of treatment less frequently than those who received efavirenz, regardless of the type of NRTI used [26].

Genetics
Polymorphisms in genes involved in adipocyte apoptosis and metabolism have also been implicated [3], including ones involved in the pyrimidine pathway or encoding potentially relevant enzymes, cytokines or peptides such as polymerase γ, matrix met-alloproteinase 1, TNF-α, IL-1β, IL-6, resistin and mitochondrial haplogroups.

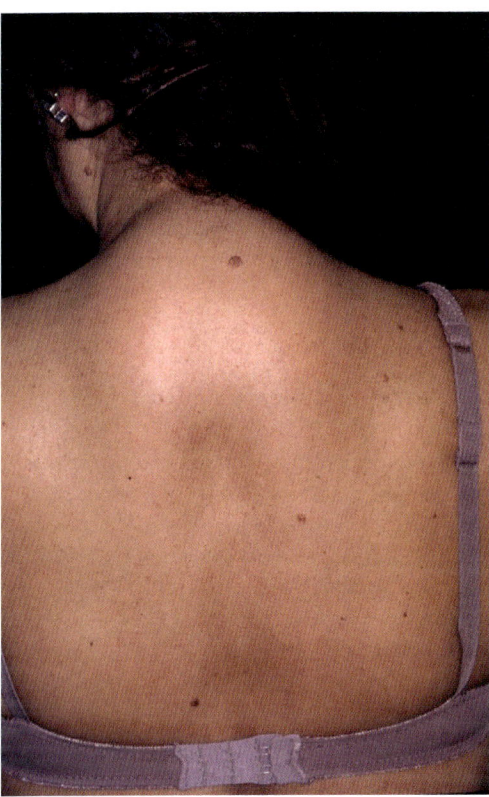

Figure 98.3 Buffalo hump appearance in an HIV patient with lipodystrophy. Courtesy of Professor L. Requena, Universidad Autónoma de Madrid, Spain.

Clinical features
Presentation
Most patients present with a gradual loss of subcutaneous fat from the face, arms and legs. Facial involvement is present in 38–52% of HIV patients with lipodystrophy [3]. Fat loss from the suprazygomatic and temporal regions of the face can be severe enough to impart a stigmatising emaciated appearance. Patients may also accumulate excess fat over the chin, breasts and waist, as well as over the upper back, producing a so-called buffalo hump (Figure 98.3) [6].

Differential diagnosis
Generalised loss of body fat is commonly seen in HIV-infected patients with AIDS wasting syndrome. Patients with AIDS wasting syndrome have decreased body weight and lean body mass, without accumulation of excess fat over the chin, upper back, breasts or waist. Those with AIDS wasting syndrome also do not develop glucose intolerance or hyperinsulinaemia, although they may have hypertriglyceridaemia [6]. Other differential diagnoses to consider include Cushing syndrome and iatrogenic lipodystrophy related to testosterone therapy.

Classification of severity
Scoring systems have been developed to quantify facial lipoatrophy. In one, the score ranges from 0 (absent) to 4 (severe), depending on the degree of malar depression, presence or absence of buccal extension and defined melolabial ridge [27]. Other scoring methods involve the use of various imaging modalities which may not be practical in the clinical setting [3].

Complications and co-morbidities

Complications are related to co-morbidities, including dyslipidaemia, impaired glucose intolerance, insulin resistance and coronary artery disease.

Disease course and prognosis

Lipodystrophy is progressive with ongoing HAART therapy [2]. While the possibility of subcutaneous fat recovery exists, it is typically slow and incomplete [3].

Management

There is no established algorithm for the management of HIV-associated lipodystrophy. Management is challenging and requires multidisciplinary input from infectious disease specialists, endocrinologists, nutritionists and primary care physicians. The stigma associated with facial lipodystrophy particularly may have a profound psychosocial impact and psychological support may be required.

Modification of previously successful antiretroviral therapy may increase the risk of treatment failure and must be done in consultation with an infectious disease specialist. Modest improvement in lipoatrophy has been reported with the removal of NRTIs [28]. While metabolic derangements such as dyslipidaemia and insulin resistance seem to be partly reversible if PI therapy is discontinued, lipodystrophy is usually unchanged [3].

Low-calorie or low-fat, high-fibre diets combined with aerobic exercise may improve central fat accumulation [29], although there is little evidence that diet or exercise significantly improves lipoatrophy [29–31]. Thiazolidinediones, which have been shown to induce adipocyte differentiation and increase subcutaneous fat mass, have been tried as pharmacological agents to treat lipoatrophy in HIV-infected patients with inconsistent results [32]. Uridine and pravastatin have been reported to improve lipoatrophy in small, randomised trials, but these results need further confirmation [33,34]. Facial fillers such as injectable poly-L-lactic acid as well as autologous fat transfers have both been used to correct severe facial lipoatrophy [35,36].

Switching or discontinuing antiretroviral therapy has not been shown to reduce VAT [37,38]. Since growth hormone deficiency has been associated with visceral adiposity in the general population as well as in HIV patients with lipodystrophy, growth hormone supplementation with doses ranging from 0.33 to 6 mg daily has been tried [39,40]: patients with abdominal lipohypertrophy achieved a 10–20% reduction in VAT and 6–7% reduction in SAT in two studies involving the administration of growth hormone [41,42]. The improvement was lost once therapy was discontinued. Treatment with tesamorelin, a growth hormone-releasing hormone analogue that closely mimics the physiological dose and function of its physiological counterpart, showed a 15.2% reduction in VAT, compared with a 5% increase in VAT in the placebo group ($P < 0.001$), at 6 months in a large, randomised, double-blind, placebo-controlled study [43].

Surgical interventions such as liposuction have been used to remove excess fat from the anterior neck, breasts and abdominal compartment [44–46]. However, liposuction cannot remove intra-abdominal visceral fat. Furthermore, approximately 25% of patients will experience recurrence of lipohypertrophy after liposuction.

Lipodystrophy associated with total body irradiation and haematopoietic stem cell transplant

Definition and nomenclature

Development of partial lipodystrophy following total body irradiation (TBI) and haematopoietic stem cell transplant (HSCT) is now a recognised entity in the literature. Patients who have undergone TBI as part of the conditioning regimen prior to HSCT are predisposed to endocrinapthies [1].

Introduction and general description

Endocrine disorders, including growth hormone deficiency, hypothyroidism and metabolic syndromes, can develop as long-term sequelae from TBI and HSCT [2]. Lipodystrophy associated with TBI and HSCT was first described by Adachi in 2013 [3]. Both lipoatrophy and lipohypertrophy are observed in these patients [3].

Epidemiology

Incidence and prevalence

Partial lipodystrophy associated with TBI and HSCT is rare. A total of 11 cases was identified in the literature published in 2020, but the prevalence is likely higher [2]. A cross-sectional survey conducted at a children's hospital in Japan showed a prevalence of 9.2% among those who underwent TBI and HSCT [1].

Age

Most patients with lipodystrophy associated with TBI and HSCT were adolescents [2].

Sex

Men and women are equally affected [2].

Ethnicity

White and Asian patients have been reported [2].

Associated diseases

Patients with lipodystrophy associated with TBI and HSCT frequently have concomitant insulin resistance, diabetes, hypertriglyceridaemia and fatty liver disease [1].

Pathophysiology

The exact pathophysiology is unknown. Patients with lipodystrophy associated with TBI and HSCT have decreased adiponectin levels. It is postulated that inflammatory cytokines may be involved, although the level of TNF-α following HSCT is not different from those without HSCT. TBI and intensive chemotherapy may also cause damage to the subcutaneous adipose tissue expandability, which in turn forces lipids to accumulate in ectopic locations [3,4].

Genetics

No known genetic mutation has been identified.

Clinical features
Presentation
Lipodystrophy typically develops 10 years after HSCT in those who received HSCT during infancy with a rigorous chemotherapy regimen [3]. Proposed diagnostic criteria include presence of abnormal fat distribution favouring lipohypertrophy in the cheek and/or neck and lipoatrophy in the buttocks, along with presence of fatty liver disease and/or diabetes. Unlike patients with obesity, body mass index (BMI) is normal or low [3].

Differential diagnosis
Dunnigan-type familial partial lipodystrophy (FPLD2) should be considered.

Complications and co-morbidities
Patients with lipodystrophy associated with TBI and HSCT may have complications similar to those of patients with FPLD2, including premature atherosclerosis, associated hypertriglyceridemia and insulin-resistant diabetes [1,4]. Patients are also at a higher risk for developing hypertension, elevated LDL-c, insulin resistance and fatty liver disease [3]. Cancer recurrence and multiple HSCTs are more common in those with lipodystrophy than those without [1].

Disease course and prognosis
Due to underlying malignancy, lipodystrophy associated with TBI and HSCT runs a complicated course because patients may develop graft-versus-host disease [2]. The changes in subcutaneous adipose tissue are likely permanent.

Investigations
Patients should be evaluated for metabolic derangements and fatty liver with a comprehensive metabolic panel, fasting glucose, lipid panels and insulin levels. Regular blood pressure monitoring is recommended [3].

Management
There is no established algorithm for the management of lipodystrophy associated with TBI and HSCT. Metreleptin may improve the hyperinsulinaemia and underlying metabolic derangement [4].

Localised lipoatrophy and/or lipodystrophy

Localised lipoatrophy and/or lipodystrophy is a heterogeneous group of disorders presenting as one or multiple depressions of various sizes, ranging from a few centimetres to greater than 20 cm in diameter.

Semicircular lipoatrophy

Definition and nomenclature
Semicircular lipoatrophy (SL) is characterised by localised, often bilateral, symmetrical, transverse, semicircular depressions across the anterolateral aspects of the thighs due to atrophy of the underlying subcutaneous fat.

Introduction and general description
First described in the German literature in 1974 [1], SL is characterised by localised, symmetrical and often bilateral, transverse, semicircular depressions over the anterolateral thighs [1,2,3].

Epidemiology
Incidence and prevalence
SL is probably commoner than the small number of reported cases (about 100) would suggest [2,4,5].

Age
Most SL cases present in the third or fourth decades of life [6], although it has also been reported among children and the elderly [4].

Sex
The majority of cases occur in women [3].

Pathophysiology
The aetiology of SL is unclear. An older theory related the presence of SL to impaired circulation in the upper leg as a consequence of a congenital abnormality in the lateral femoral circumflex artery [7]. However, patients with arteritis or those whose quadriceps artery has been ligated do not develop SL [8]. An anomaly of fat metabolism in these patients has also been proposed [8,9].

A current and more plausible explanation associates SL with repeated mechanical pressure as a form of microtrauma to the thighs [10,11]. Suggested mechanisms include repeatedly standing or sitting in an unvarying position in which the affected area is constantly compressed by or knocked against various objects [1,12]. Wearing constricting jeans or use of an elastic girdle has also been implicated [3,13,14,15].

In cases where clusters of co-workers are affected in the same company, repetitive pressure against desk furniture has been identified. In those cases, the height of the depression on the leg measured from the floor plus the height of the shoe heel were constant and the same as the height of the desk [12,16]. In a recent company-wide case–control study, the only statistically significant variables for SL development are female sex and leaning of thighs against the edge of the table [6].

Pathology
The histopathology findings in SL are non-specific. There is partial or complete loss of fat in the affected area with replacement by newly formed collagen [5,17].

Clinical features
Presentation
SL is characterised by localised, transverse, semicircular depressions, 2–4 cm in width, that are often symmetrical and bilateral. These depressions may also appear band-like, and when more than one is present, they may appear in a parallel arrangement [2,3].

There is no preceding inflammation and the overlying skin is normal. The anterolateral thighs are commonly affected bilaterally. Unilateral cases have been described as well [2,10,11,18]. Multilocular and progressive lesions affecting the trunk and limbs were seen in one patient [19]. Although SL is usually asymptomatic, some patients complained of heavy legs, a burning sensation, cramps or pain after exercising [2,10,18,20].

Differential diagnosis

The differential diagnosis of SL includes other forms of localised lipoatrophy or lipodystrophy as described elsewhere in this chapter.

Disease course and prognosis

SL has an excellent prognosis as most cases resolve gradually upon withdrawal of repetitive trauma.

Investigations

SL is a clinical diagnosis and further investigation is rarely required [3,6].

Management

There are no established management guidelines for SL. However, lesions usually regress spontaneously after the removal of microtrauma over months to as long as 8 years [12]. Recurrences are possible, however [7,9].

Localised lipoatrophy due to injected drugs

Localised loss of subcutaneous fat can occur after intradermal, subcutaneous or intramuscular injection of certain drugs. The two most commonly implicated agents are insulin and corticosteroids and these are discussed in detail. Other injected medications or substances that have been implicated as causes of localised lipoatrophy include benzathine penicillin, vasopressin, human growth hormone, methotrexate, iron dextran and diphtheria–pertussis–tetanus (DPT) vaccine [1–4].

Insulin-induced localised lipoatrophy

Definition

Insulin-induced localised lipoatrophy is the loss of subcutaneous fat at the site of insulin injection [1].

Introduction and general description

Insulin-induced localised lipoatrophy was a common complication of insulin therapy prior to the development of purified insulin in the 1970s [2,3]. With the advent of human insulin, the incidence of lipoatrophy has decreased dramatically [4].

Epidemiology
Incidence and prevalence

Prior to the introduction of purified human insulin, lipoatrophy occurred in 25–55% of patients using insulin. Since the introduction of highly purified insulin, it is estimated that fewer than 10% of patients are affected [5,6], although lipoatrophy is still reported with the use of recombinant human insulin, rapid-acting insulin analogues and continuous subcutaneous insulin infusion [4,7–9,10,11,12].

Age

Insulin-induced lipoatrophy occurs predominantly in children and young adults [13–15].

Sex

The risk is greater in females than males [16,17].

Pathophysiology

The pathogenesis of insulin-induced lipoatrophy is not completely understood. Lipolytic components or impurities in certain insulin preparations may have resulted in local allergic or immunological reactions. For example, a local immune reaction to insulin crystals with resultant dedifferentiation of adipocytes has been suggested [14,18]. An immune-mediated inflammatory process with release of lysosomal enzymes promoting lipoatrophy has also been proposed [19]. It has also been suggested that mast cells may play a pathogenetic role [12]: in one case series involving five patients with human insulin analogue-induced lipoatrophy, an elevated number of tryptase-positive, chymase-positive degranulated mast cells were seen in the subcutaneous tissue.

Predisposing factors

This form of lipoatrophy is more common among those with prior dermal reactions to insulin [1]. The use of older, less purified forms of insulin such as bovine or porcine insulin conveys a higher risk of lipoatrophy [20]. Repeated use of the same injection site also increases the risk.

Pathology

Histopathology shows lobules of small adipocytes and lipomembranous changes [21]. A discrete lymphoid infiltration abutting the blood vessels in the hypodermis may also be observed [22].

Clinical features
Presentation

Insulin-induced lipoatrophy presents as a depressed plaque due to loss of subcutaneous fat at the site of insulin injection (Figure 98.4). The overlying and surrounding skin appears normal. Lipoatrophy normally presents after 6–24 months of insulin treatment [1]. Interestingly, there is concomitant lipohypertrophy in approximately 25% of patients [23].

Differential diagnosis

Other forms of localised lipoatrophy should be considered.

Complications and co-morbidities

Because insulin absorption from the lipoatrophic area is erratic, continued injection of insulin into affected areas may result in poor glycaemic control [22].

Management

The risk of lipoatrophy may be reduced by regular rotation of insulin injection sites. The importance of this should be explained to all patients who require insulin. Once lipoatrophy develops, continued injection into the lipoatrophic site should be avoided due to erratic absorption of insulin. Spontaneous resolution of established insulin-induced localised lipoatrophy is rare.

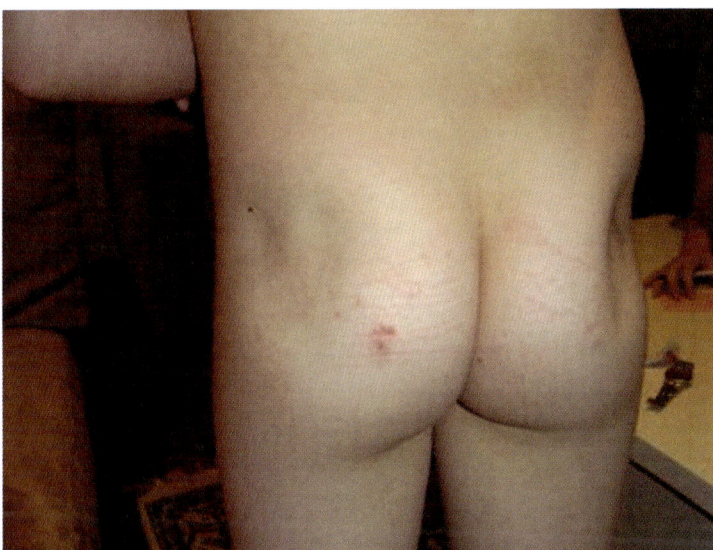

Figure 98.4 Depressed plaques over bilateral hips due to subcutaneous fat atrophy at the site of insulin injections. Courtesy of Denise Metry, MD, Texas Children's Hospital, USA.

There is no generally agreed management algorithm but, if feasible, a change to purified human insulin is recommended. Several authors describe success in restoring fat by co-administration of a corticosteroid such as dexamethasone with the insulin [4,18,24–27]. Other strategies have included using an insulin jet-injection device [28] or a continuous insulin infusion pump [29], although lipoatrophy with the latter has also been reported [7,8]. Twice-daily application of 4% sodium cromoglycate prepared in petrolatum has been claimed to reverse early lipoatrophy and prevent new lesions in one small case series [12].

Localised lipoatrophy due to injected corticosteroid

Definition
Localised lipoatrophy due to injected corticosteroid is the localised loss of subcutaneous fat that occurs after intramuscular or intralesional injection of corticosteroids [1].

Introduction and general description
Injected depot preparations of corticosteroids have been widely used for their sustained systemic antiallergic and anti-inflammatory action for more than half a century. It was recognised at an early stage that corticosteroids were capable of producing profound lipoatrophy if they were injected into subcutaneous fat.

Epidemiology
Incidence and prevalence
An overall incidence of local reactions following intralesional corticosteroid injection is reported to be 0.5%. These reactions include pain, panniculitis, haemorrhage, secondary infection, pigment alteration, hypersensitivity and atrophy [2]. Of all the persistent local reactions due to corticosteroids, atrophy is the most common [3].

Sex
Women appear to be at significantly greater risk than men [1,4]. In one early study, it was observed that lipoatrophy occurred in 6 of 14 women but in none of 13 men who received repeated intramuscular or deep subcutaneous injections of triamcinolone diacetate [4].

Pathophysiology
The exact pathogenesis is not clear but several factors are thought to be involved. It is believed that intramuscular injection of triamcinolone has a direct traumatic and a hormonally mediated destructive effect on fat cells [5]. In addition, decreased type I collagen and glycosaminoglycan synthesis has been noted following the injection of corticosteroid [6]. One common finding from histological analyses is the identification of a granular basophilic material in the dermis, thought to represent altered ground substance associated with deposits of corticosteroid crystals [5,7,8]. Cutaneous atrophy has been noted to resolve in parallel with the gradual disappearance of corticosteroid crystals from the tissue [7].

Predisposing factors
Compounds with low solubility, such as triamcinolone acetonide, injected at higher concentrations appear to be associated with greater risks of atrophy. One group of investigators noted that intralesional injections of triamcinolone acetonide at concentrations above $5\,mg/cm^3$ were associated with increased risks of cutaneous atrophy [9]. However, no lipoatrophy was observed at 6 and 12 weeks after injection in a series of 14 patients with dermatological conditions who had received one or two 30 mg or 60 mg doses of intramuscular triamcinolone acetonide [10].

Pathology
In addition to the presence of granular basophilic material associated with the deposition of corticosteroid, other histological findings include epidermal atrophy, homogenisation of collagen, degeneration of sebaceous glands, decreased elastin and involution of subcutaneous fat lobules with small lipocytes separated by hyaline material [1,5,7,8]. Inflammatory cells are not usually prominent although a sparse mononuclear cell infiltrate can be observed. There is no vascular inflammation [1].

Clinical features
Presentation
Patients present with an oval or circular depressed plaque at the site of prior injection (Figures 98.5 and 98.6). The overlying epidermis is usually normal, although telangiectasia, hypopigmentation or alopecia may occur [3]. There is no associated redness or tenderness. Atrophy generally begins within weeks to 3 months after injection. The time course and extent of the atrophy depend on several factors, including the solubility and concentration of the corticosteroid used and the depth and anatomical location of the injection [5].

Differential diagnosis
Other forms of localised lipoatrophy should be considered.

Disease course and prognosis
The lipoatrophy may resolve spontaneously over the course of 1–2 years [11–14], although it may persist for longer in some cases [15].

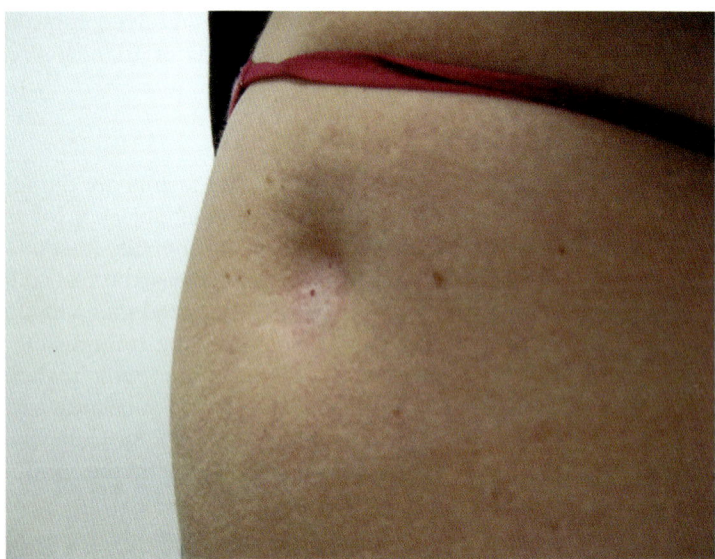

Figure 98.5 Delling of the skin over the right hip due to subcutaneous fat atrophy at the site of depot corticosteroid injection.

Management

There is no established management guideline. In one small case series, four patients were treated by infiltration of the affected area with normal saline. All four patients demonstrated complete resolution of lipoatrophy and restoration of surface contour after 4–8 weekly injections. The injected volume ranged from 5 to 20 cm^3 per treatment session, depending on the size to be treated. The authors speculated that the efficacy of the treatment may be due to resuspension and redistribution of the poorly soluble corticosteroid crystals by saline solution [3].

Localised lipodystrophy secondary to panniculitis

Localised lipodystrophy may be secondary to inflammation of the subcutaneous fat, of which there are several aetiologies (Chapter 97).

Centrifugal lipodystrophy

Definition and nomenclature

Centrifugal lipodystrophy (CLD) is a form of localised lipodystrophy in which atrophic plaques extend centrifugally.

Synonyms and inclusions
- Lipodystrophia centrifugalis abdominalis infantilis

Introduction and general description

CLD is characterised by localised lipoatrophy that expands centrifugally. Most cases of CLD have been reported from a single region of Japan. The condition predominantly affects children who are otherwise well. Because there have been a few cases of adult onset as well as of involvement of areas other than the abdomen, the term CLD may be more appropriate than lipodystrophia centrifugalis abdominalis infantilis.

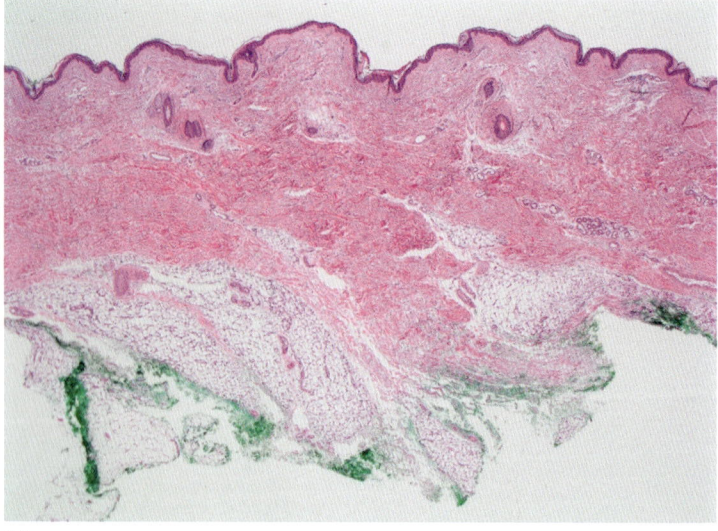

(a)

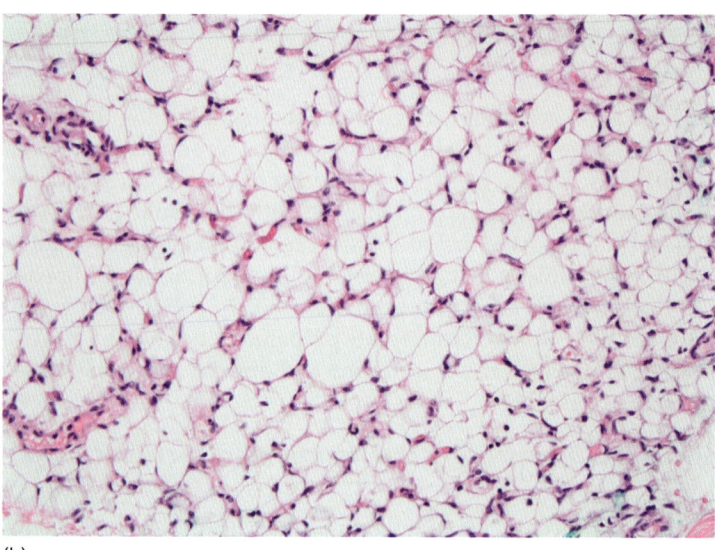

(b)

Figure 98.6 Histopathology of localised lipoatrophy secondary to corticosteroid injection. The sections show variably sized diminution of adipocytes without inflammation. (a) 20× (b) 200×. Courtesy of Catherine Chung, MD, The Ohio State University, USA.

Epidemiology
Incidence and prevalence
CLD is rare: approximately 170 cases have been described [1] since its initial report in 1971 by Imamura *et al*. [2].

Age
The majority (90%) of CLD patients develop the condition in the first 4 years of life with a mean of 2.4 years and a median of 2 years [1]. Very few patients have developed their initial lesions as an adult [1,3].

Sex
Girls outnumber boys by approximately 2 : 1 [1].

Ethnicity

CLD is reported almost exclusively among children of Asian descent, especially of Japanese origin [1,4–6]. There have been a few white patients reported from the USA [7], the UK [8,9], France [10], Italy [11], Germany [12] and Spain [13].

Associated diseases

Most CLD patients exhibit no other signs or symptoms of systemic illness. However, immunological abnormalities that have been reported include positive antinuclear antibodies [1], rheumatoid factor [10], antigliadin antibodies [12] and partial IgA deficiency [10,12].

Pathophysiology

The cause of CLD is unknown. It has been suggested that apoptosis may play a part in the fatty tissue degeneration of CLD, but it is unclear whether this is a primary event [14]. Fibrous long-spacing collagen has been observed on ultrastructural studies of lesional skin, although the relation of their presence to disease pathogenesis remains to be elucidated [15]. So far, no abnormalities of serum leptin levels have been reported [1].

Pathology

The epidermis and dermis in CLD are unaffected but there is markedly reduced or absent subcutaneous tissue in the affected areas. In the inflamed periphery of the plaque, the loss of subcutaneous fat is accompanied by a moderate mononuclear cell infiltrate. Rarely, multinucleated giant cells, foam cells, swelling of blood vessels, vasculitis and thrombosis have been observed [1].

Genetics

CLD has occurred in one pair of dizygotic twins and in one pair of affected siblings, which has raised the possibility of a genetic component of the disease [1].

Environmental factors

Although various external factors such as hernia, congenital dislocation of the hip, external pressure, injection or previous skin infection at the sites were reported in about 10% of the cases, no clear relationship has been established between CLD and environmental insults [1].

Clinical features

Presentation

Most cases of CLD begin with a single depressed plaque involving the groin (80%), axillae (20%) or neighbouring regions. Interestingly, in all reported non-Japanese cases, the initial plaque developed exclusively in or near the groin [1]. Less common areas of involvement include the neck, lower chin, retroauricular area or scalp [16–18]. The periphery of the atrophic plaque is typically red while the centre is of normal colour or may have a violaceous or bluish hue. Ulceration of the plaques has been reported to occur rarely [1,19]. Plaques beginning in the groin area may expand to involve the genital region, abdominal wall or even the chest wall. Plaques developing in the axillary region may also extend to the chest wall and abdominal wall. During the initial enlargement period, the atrophy may be multifocal. Although most lesions are asymptomatic, some patients report mild discomfort or tenderness [1]. Regional lymph nodes are enlarged in 65% of cases. When the lesion stops expanding, the red rim and lymphadenopathy tend to resolve.

Differential diagnosis

Differential diagnosis of CLD includes other localised lipodystrophies.

Complications and co-morbidities

Patients with CLD usually do not suffer from any complications and co-morbidities, except for rare instances of ulceration involving plaques [1,19]. A case of angioblastoma developing in a non-regressing CLD lesion lasting into adulthood has been reported. The angioblastoma responded to resection followed by radiation therapy [20].

Disease course and prognosis

The atrophic area slowly enlarges centrifugally for 3–8 years, often stopping with the onset of puberty. By 13 years, 82% of cases show no residual inflammation at the periphery and 65% no longer have regional lymphadenopathy.

The atrophic portion may subsequently improve but may remain depressed [1]. Hair regrowth has been observed in cases of scalp involvement [16–18].

Investigations

Results of routine laboratory tests are unremarkable.

Management

There is no established guideline for the management of CLD. Many topical therapies have been tried including topical steroids, pimecrolimus, vitamin A cream and dimethyl sulfoxide. Various systemic therapies have been attempted including corticosteroids, chloroquine, penicillin, vitamin E and ibuprofen. None of these has been effective in preventing enlargement, although topical and systemic steroids occasionally reduced the inflammation at the periphery of the plaque [1]. Psoralen with UVA was reported to be effective in softening the skin and preventing further enlargement in one case [4].

FAT HYPERTROPHY

Fat hypertrophy is a circumscribed expansion of subcutaneous fat and is particularly associated with insulin injection sites. Less commonly, growth hormone and pegvisomant (growth hormone receptor antagonist) injections can also cause fat lipohypertrophy [1,2]. Injection site rotation or discontinuation of the injections should be instituted. Fat hypertrophy is distinguished from lipomatosis in that the latter involves the formation of multiple foci of proliferating adipocytes.

Insulin-induced localised fat hypertrophy

Definition and nomenclature

Insulin-induced fat hypertrophy is a circumscribed increase in subcutaneous fat at the site or sites of repeated insulin injection by insulin-dependent diabetics.

Synonyms and inclusions
- Insulin-induced lipohypertrophy

Introduction and general description

Insulin-induced fat hypertrophy was, and still is, the most common cutaneous complication of insulin therapy [3]. It is thought to be due to the direct local anabolic and lipogenic effects of insulin on adipocytes.

Epidemiology

Incidence and prevalence

With highly purified human insulin, the prevalence of fat hypertrophy is approximately 30% in patients with type 1 diabetes and less than 5% in patients with type 2 diabetes [4].

Age

No specific age of onset has been identified, although the condition is generally believed to be associated with a young age [4].

Pathophysiology

The fat hypertrophy is thought to be secondary to the anabolic and lipogenic effect of insulin [3,4]. Although insulin antibodies are associated with fat hypertrophy in children and adolescents with type 1 diabetes, it is not known whether they play a role in its pathogenesis [5,6].

Predisposing factors

Several factors have been associated with the development of fat hypertrophy. These include recent insulin initiation, low BMI, use of the abdomen as the injection site and infrequent rotation of the injection site [4].

Pathology

Histological examination shows lobules of large mature adipocytes. Electron microscopy has revealed discrete populations of small adipocytes, suggesting differentiation or proliferation [7].

Clinical features

Presentation

The disorder presents as soft subcutaneous swellings at the sites of insulin injection (Figure 98.7). The overlying epidermis is normal. Because the involved skin tends to be hypoaesthetic relative to uninvolved skin, patients often continue to inject insulin preferentially into affected sites [3].

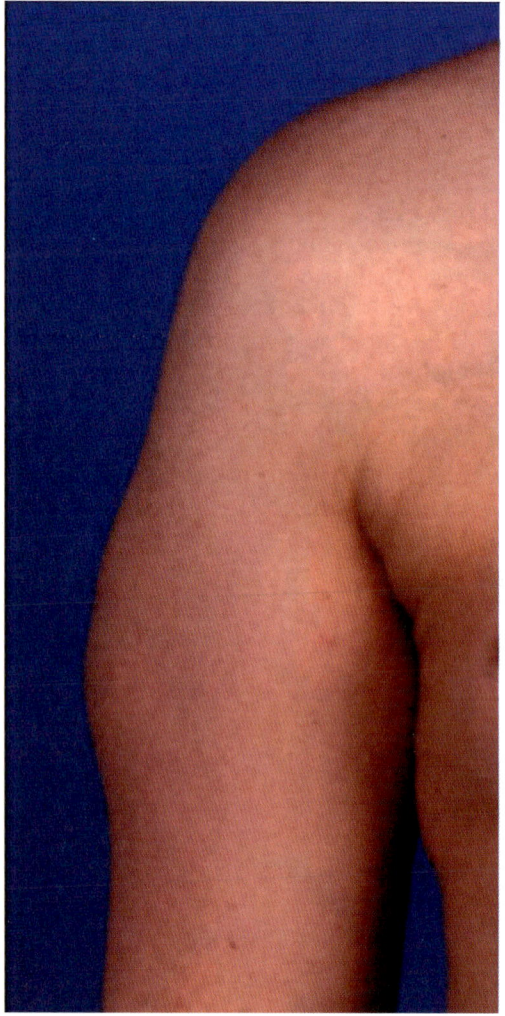

Figure 98.7 Insulin-induced fat hypertrophy of the lateral aspect of the upper arm.

Differential diagnosis

Localised cutaneous amyloidosis has been associated with insulin injection sites and may be mistaken for insulin-induced fat hypertrophy [8]. Furthermore, insulin *per se* has been identified as one of the proteins that can form amyloid fibrils [9]. Affected skin feels firmer on palpation than that overlying insulin-induced fat hypertrophy and is unlikely to improve after changing the insulin injection site [3].

Complications and co-morbidities

Because the lipohypertrophic nodules have decreased vascularity, impaired insulin absorption at these sites may result in poor glycaemic control [3,10–12].

Disease course and prognosis

Regression of insulin-induced lipohypertrophy is possible once management is instituted.

Management

To prevent the development of fat hypertrophy, patients requiring insulin injections should be advised of the importance of changing injection sites regularly [4]. No universal treatment guideline has been established in the management of this condition. Rotation of injection sites is recommended with the anticipation that existing nodules will regress [3]. Most patients requiring insulin will nowadays be prescribed biosynthetic human insulin analogues, which carry a lower risk of inducing fat hypertrophy. If they are not, changing to human insulin, particularly the short-acting, rapidly absorbed preparations, may help to reverse the condition [13]. Changing the insulin delivery method from injection to continuous subcutaneous infusion using a pump has also been advocated. This method of administration reduces overall insulin requirements and is therefore thought to lessen the overall stimulus to lipogenesis [3]. If the above strategies fail, some patients will demand removal of the excess fat. Liposuction has achieved good cosmetic results [14,15].

SUBCUTANEOUS LIPOMATOSIS

Benign symmetrical lipomatosis

Definition and nomenclature

Benign symmetrical lipomatosis (BSL) is an uncommon condition characterised by multiple, symmetrical, unencapsulated fatty tissue deposits throughout the body.

Synonyms and inclusions
- Madelung disease
- Multiple symmetrical lipomatosis
- Launois–Bensaude adenolipomatosis

Introduction and general description

What subsequently came to be known as Madelung disease was first mentioned by Brodie in 1846 [1]. Madelung described a series of patients with the lipomatosis in 1888 [2] and Launois and Bensaude reported it again 10 years later [3]. More recently, the term benign symmetrical lipomatosis has been preferred for this uncommon condition. It is characterised by multiple, symmetrical, unencapsulated fatty tissue deposits involving multiple areas of the body, particularly the neck, shoulder girdle and the proximal upper and lower extremities.

Epidemiology
Incidence and prevalence

The exact incidence and prevalence of BSL are not known. The incidence in Italy has been estimated to be 1 : 25 000 [4]. There are, however, fewer than 300 cases reported in the literature since its initial description [5].

Age

The age of onset ranges from 30 to 60 years [6]. However, a few paediatric cases have been reported [7,8].

Sex

Benign symmetrical lipomatosis is a disorder that predominantly affects males, with a reported male : female ratio as high as 31 : 1 [1,6,9–11].

Ethnicity

Historically, BSL has been linked to people of Mediterranean descent [1]. However, cases from non-Mediterranean ethnicities have been described [5,12,13].

Associated diseases

Many conditions are associated with BSL. These include alcohol abuse, chronic hepatic disorders possibly related to the underlying alcohol abuse, lipid abnormalities, arterial hypertension, chronic obstructive pulmonary disease (COPD), gynaecomastia, hypothyroidism, peripheral neuropathy, diabetes, hyperuricaemia and myoclonic epilepsy and ragged red fibres (MERRF) syndrome [1,7,8,10,14–16]. In one study of 22 patients from Spain, 95.5% of the patients had high alcohol intake and 59.1% had some form of hepatic disease. Furthermore, 77% of these patients were reported to be regular smokers. Statistics of reported associations include 41% with dyslipidaemia, 27% with gynaecomastia, 23% with arterial hypertension, 23% with COPD, 14% with hyperuricaemia, 9% with hypothyroidism and 4.5% with type 2 diabetes [1].

Peripheral neuropathy, polyneuropathy and autonomic dysfunction are also common findings among BSL patients [11,17–19,20] and it may be the presenting symptom in some [21]. However, there is controversy as to whether these neurological manifestations are directly related to BSL or are the result of alcoholism.

Compression symptoms affecting the respiratory and digestive tracts are thought to be directly due to fatty masses in the anterior neck and, in one case series, were the symptoms that in all cases occasioned their patients' initial consultation [1].

Pathophysiology

While many theories on the pathogenesis of BSL exist, a role for brown fat in BSL has garnered attention. Although, grossly and histologically, the accumulated adipose tissue in BSL is indistinguishable from mature fat [1], ultrastructural analysis of adipose tissue deposits in BSL suggests that it resembles brown fat [22]. Further support for the role of brown fat in BSL came from another study that demonstrated mRNA expression of brown adipose tissue-specific uncoupling protein-1 (UCP-1) in a lipoma of a patient with BSL, but not in the normal subcutaneous fat from the same patient [23]. Brown fat hypertrophy has been proposed to result from functional sympathetic denervation [22], or from alterations in the synthesis of intracellular cyclic adenosine monophosphate (cAMP) under noradrenergic stimulation [24,25].

Pathology

Lipomatous tissue in BSL consists of small adipocytes with no atypical features and a slight increase in vascular and fibrous elements. The lipomas are typically not encapsulated and may infiltrate across fasciomuscular and neurovascular planes [26].

Genetics

Genetic alternations in mitochondrial DNA have been demonstrated in BSL patients [18,27]. Most reported BSL cases have been

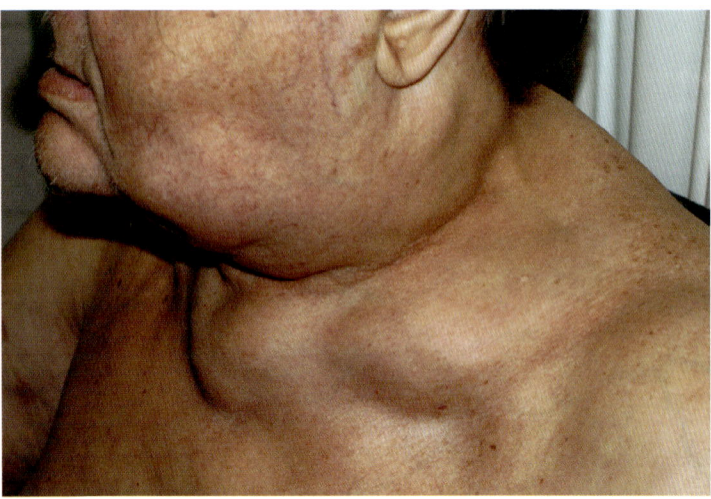

Figure 98.8 Non-tender fatty deposits around the neck in a patient with benign symmetrical lipomatosis. Courtesy of Professor L. Requena, Universidad Autónoma de Madrid, Spain.

sporadic, although a very small number of familial cases exist for which autosomal recessive inheritance has been proposed [28].

Clinical features

Presentation

Fatty masses develop most commonly on the neck (Figure 98.8), shoulder girdle and proximal upper and lower extremities. Other less common locations include the retroauricular and submandibular areas [29], tongue [21], mammary region [22], abdomen [7] and perineum or scrotum [30]. Although rare, laryngeal involvement resulting in a compromised airway has been described [12,31–34]. The fatty deposits are slow growing and progressive over many years. In contrast to Dercum disease, the fatty growths in BSL are not tender or painful.

Clinical variants

Enzi's classification of BSL is the most widely accepted [6]. In type I BSL, fatty deposits are mainly distributed around the neck, shoulders, supraclavicular fossa and proximal regions of the upper extremities. In type II BSL, more caudal regions of the body are involved, while the neck is unaffected. As a consequence, type II BSL patients may appear similar to obese patients.

Differential diagnosis

Differential diagnosis of BSL includes obesity, Dercum disease, familial multiple lipomatosis and less likely angiolipoma and liposarcoma. Genetic syndromes presenting with multiple lipomas such as Cowden syndrome, Bannayan–Riley–Ruvalcaba syndrome, multiple endocrine neoplasia type 1 (MEN1) and Gardner syndrome can be differentiated from BSL by the presence of other disease-specific clinical features.

Complications and co-morbidities

Respiratory or digestive symptoms may develop if the lipomatosis from the anterior neck is significant enough to compress vital structures. There have been a few cases of head and neck cancer, especially squamous cell carcinoma, reported in patients with BSL [9,35]. However, it is possible that this simply reflects the increased alcohol and tobacco consumption observed among BSL patients. Malignant transformation of lipoma into liposarcomas in BSL has been reported only twice [36,37].

Disease course and prognosis

The lipomatous masses are slow growing and progressive. There are few long-term follow-up data on BSL patients. In one study, however, in which 31 BSL patients were observed for up to 26 years, three of the eight deaths observed were sudden and occurred in patients with autonomic neuropathy in the absence of coronary artery disease or history of cardiac disease [20].

Investigations

The diagnosis of BSL is based on clinical presentation and disease history. Chest radiographs may show abnormal symmetrical mass lesions due to accumulations of adipose tissue. MRI is the best diagnostic tool in evaluation of the spread of adipose tissue, presence of tracheal compression, vascular topography within the fat mass and exclusion of synchronous malignant disease [37,38].

Management

There is no established guideline for the management of BSL. A thorough clinical review, especially for respiratory symptoms, should be carried out at each visit to check for signs of compression or for the rare occurrence of malignant transformation.

Medical treatments have been tried with generally poor results. Oral salbutamol, which induces lipolysis by adrenergic stimulation, has been tested on BSL patients but the results have been disappointing [24]. Fibrate has been claimed to stop the growth or even reduce the volume of fatty masses in BSL patients [39]. Among BSL patients who reported alcohol abuse, abstinence from alcohol has had mixed results in preventing the progression or recurrence of the lesions after surgical treatment [1,40]. General weight loss does not seem to be effective in reducing fatty masses [1].

Open surgery, lipectomy and liposuction, with or without ultrasound assistance, have been tried with varying success rates. Liposuction is less traumatic, has a lower complication rate and produces less scarring than open surgery [41–45,46]. However, because the fatty deposits are unencapsulated and diffusely infiltrate muscles and vessels without a clear plane for dissection, open surgery with direct observation of important structures is a safer approach in certain anatomical regions where liposuction may be too dangerous [1,46]. Some authors advocate ultrasound-assisted liposuction which can treat multiple areas in a single session and produces limited scarring.

Regardless of the mode of surgical intervention, multiple procedures are often required, especially given the high rates of recurrence [1,47,48]. In one study, BSL patients underwent an average of 3.3 open surgical procedures with a 51% recurrence rate. Isolated lipoaspiration had a 95% recurrence rate in the same study. Recurrence rates vary by anatomical site and are highest following procedures on the arms and pectoral region. The average time taken for fat to reaccumulate after a surgical intervention is approximately 21 months [1].

Emergency intervention is needed when compression symptoms develop. In rare cases where the fatty tissue deposits extend to the mediastinum and compress the trachea, a tracheostomy may be required [20].

Dercum disease

Definition and nomenclature
Dercum disease is a rare disease characterised by generalised over-weight status or obesity and pronounced pain in the adipose tissue with or without the presence of lipomas.

Synonyms and inclusions
- Adiposis dolorosa
- Morbus Dercum
- Adiposalgia
- Lipomatosis dolorosa
- Adipose tissue rheumatism
- Neurolipomatosis

Introduction and general description
Dercum disease was first described in 1888 [1]. The disease is characterised by diffuse or localised pain involving adipose tissue, usually affecting those who are overweight or obese. Patients experience a number of other somatoform symptoms, and management of the condition is a challenge.

Epidemiology
Incidence and prevalence
The exact incidence and prevalence of Dercum disease are not known.

Age
Dercum disease most commonly presents between the ages of 35 and 50 years [2,3]. While it was initially proposed that Dercum disease affects postmenopausal women, a recent survey revealed that 86% of patients developed their symptoms prior to the menopause [3].

Sex
Dercum disease is 5–30 times more common in women than in men [3,4].

Ethnicity
No known ethnic predilection has been identified.

Associated diseases
Although various symptoms or diseases have been observed in these patients, none is consistently associated. These include easy bruising, sleep disturbances, impaired memory, depression, difficulty concentrating, anxiety, rapid heart rate, shortness of breath, diabetes, bloating, constipation, fatigue, weakness and joint and muscle aches [3,5].

Pathophysiology
While the exact aetiology of Dercum disease is not known, many theories have been proposed. A local defect in lipid metabolism has been considered. One study showed a difference in the formation of long-chain monounsaturated fatty acids between the painful adipose tissue and the unaffected adipose tissue in the same patient [6]. Another study showed that the proportion of monosaturated fatty acids was significantly higher in Dercum disease patients than in healthy controls [7].

Recently, a study identified seven patients with Dercum disease with preceding infections which include histoplasmosis, coccidiomycosis or Lyme disease. It is postulated that these infections may lead to altered lymphatics and subsequently development of Dercum disease [8].

Painful adipose tissue from a Dercum disease subject was found to have a significantly lower conversion rate of glucose to neutral glycerides than non-painful adipose tissue from the same subject [9]. *In vitro* analysis demonstrated that painful adipose tissue had reduced responsiveness to norepinephrine and lack of response to the antilipolytic effect of insulin compared with non-painful adipose tissue [10].

Roles of various inflammatory factors have also been investigated. Higher levels of IL-13 and significantly lower macrophage inflammatory protein 1β and fractalkine expression were seen in Dercum disease patients. Fractalkine is a unique chemokine that is constitutively expressed by neurons. When fractalkine receptors are occupied, pain and resistance to opioid analgesia are promoted, which is in concordance with symptoms in Dercum disease [11].

Other theories for pain in Dercum disease have included endocrine dysfunction [10,12–17] as well as autonomic nervous system dysfunction [18] and stretching of and pressure on nerves by the growing fatty masses [19,20].

The significance of these observations is, however, unclear and their contribution to disease pathogenesis remains to be elucidated.

Pathology
When lipomas are present, they show the typical histological features of lipomas without inflammation or vascular abnormalities [21].

Genetics
The majority of cases occur sporadically [5]. An autosomal dominant inheritance with variable expression has also been reported [2,22,23,24,25,26]. HLA typing has not been revealing [10]. A to G mutation at position A8344 of mitochondrial DNA, which is sometimes associated with familial multiple lipomas, is not detected [25,27].

Clinical features
Presentation
The main symptom in Dercum disease is the either abrupt or indolent onset of pain in adipose tissue [1]. Lipomas may or may not be present in these patients, who are typically obese. Patients have most commonly described the pain as burning or aching of the subcutaneous tissue. Some experience spontaneous paroxysmal

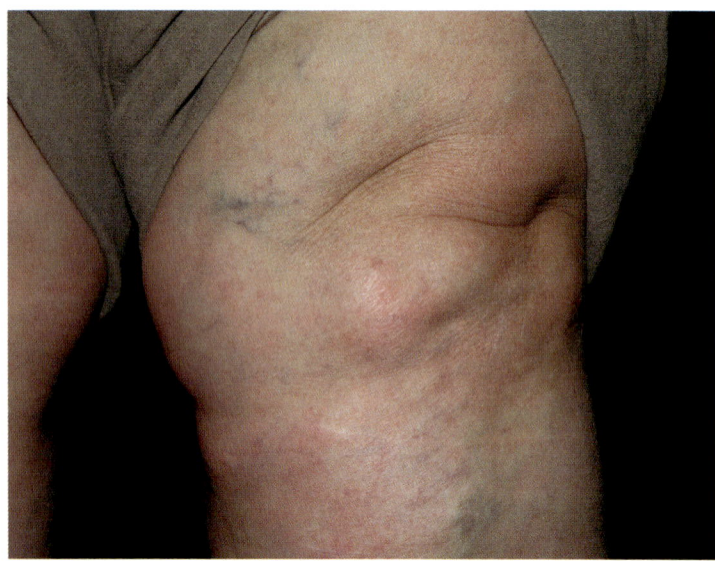

Figure 98.9 Painful lipomas on the lower extremity of a patient with Dercum disease. Courtesy of Professor L. Requena, Universidad Autónoma de Madrid, Spain.

attacks of pain [5,28]. The most common locations of painful fat and lipomas are the extremities (Figure 98.9), trunk, pelvic area and buttocks [3]. The head and neck are spared [28]. Interestingly, patients experience more pain in the medial aspects of the involved extremities [5]. Lipomas, when present, vary in size and firmness [3].

While fatigue and psychiatric manifestations were initially included as cardinal symptoms of Dercum disease [29], subsequent literature has not supported this claim. Certainly, not all patients with Dercum disease exhibit psychiatric symptoms [30,31]. More recently, an association between BMI and anxiety and personality disorders has been noted [32]. It has also been proposed that pain and obesity in Dercum disease may contribute to the psychiatric manifestations seen in some patients [5].

Clinical variants
Various classifications have been proposed over the years [5,17,28,29]. In 2012, Hansson and colleagues proposed the following classification [5]:
  I. Generalised diffuse form: widespread painful adipose tissue without clear lipomas.
  II. Generalised nodular form: general pain in adipose tissue and intense pain in and around multiple lipomas.
  III. Localised nodular form: pain in and around multiple lipomas.
  IV. Juxta-articular form: pain in solitary deposits of excess fat, for example at the medial aspect of the knee.

Differential diagnosis
Many diseases have similar symptoms to those of Dercum disease. For the generalised diffuse form, fibromyalgia, lipoedema, panniculitis and primary psychiatric disorders may be considered in the differential.

Other types of Dercum disease must be differentiated from conditions that may include solitary or multiple lipomas, as they may also sometimes be painful. These include multiple symmetrical lipomatosis, familial multiple lipomatosis, adipocytic

tumours, neurofibromatosis type 1, MEN1 and MERRF syndrome. MERRF syndrome is a disease of mitochondria which is sometimes accompanied by non-painful lipomas.

Complications and co-morbidities
The lipomas in Dercum disease may in rare instances become necrotic [33] or may compress visceral organs [34,35]. Other co-morbidities are mostly related to the associated obesity or the psychiatric morbidity.

Disease course and prognosis
Very little is known about the natural progression of Dercum disease. Several case reports suggest that the pain gets worse over time [26]. However, in one long-term study of patients with the condition, pain seemed to be relatively constant over the 5-year study period [36].

Investigations
Diagnosis is based on clinical criteria after a thorough physical examination and exclusion of the differential diagnoses discussed earlier [5]. There are no laboratory markers for the condition and laboratory tests for inflammatory and autoimmune disease are typically negative [3,37–39].

Management
Overall, there is little evidence on which to base treatment of Dercum disease. Management may be best achieved through a multidisciplinary approach involving multiple specialists including dermatologists, surgeons, pain specialists, psychiatrists and psychologists.

Pain in this setting has been observed to be refractory to traditional analgesics and non-steroidal anti-inflammatory drugs (NSAIDs) [8,21,24,40–47]. However, this experience has been challenged recently after a study found that pain diminished in 89% of patients when treated with NSAIDs and in 97% when treated with narcotics [3].

Topical lidocaine with or without prilocaine [39,48,49], intralesional lidocaine [50] and intravenous lidocaine [8,37,41,43,51–53] have also been tried with varying degrees of success. Pain relief from intravenous lidocaine infusion lasted from 10 h [51] to 12 months [41]. A recent case report of deoxycholic acid injection to the lipomas provided subjective reduction in pain in a patient with Dercum disease at his 3-month follow-up [54].

Systemic corticosteroids have been reported to improve pain in some [16,24,55], while worsening it in other patients [56]. Two patients with juxta-articular Dercum disease treated with intralesional corticosteroids experienced dramatic improvement of pain [57]. Methotrexate alone [26] and in combination with infliximab [58], pregabalin or oxacarbazepine [17,38,59,60], has also been used. Two patients with concurrent Dercum disease and hepatitis C were successfully treated with interferon-α-2b [61].

A small pilot study involving 10 patients showed that rapid cycling hypobaric pressure may decrease pain [62].

Procedure-based approaches with suction-assisted liposuction [36] and lipectomy [4,19–21,63,64,65] have also been tried. However, pain often recurs after these procedures.

Infiltrating lipomatosis of the face

Definition and nomenclature
Infiltrating lipomatosis of the face is a congenital disorder where the unilateral overgrowth of unencapsulated benign and mature but invasive adipocytes involves the lower two-thirds of the face.

Synonyms and inclusions
• Congenital infiltrating lipomatosis of the face (CIL-F)

Introduction and general description
Infiltrating lipomatosis of the face (IL-F) is a disorder characterised by unilateral overgrowth of unencapsulated benign and mature but invasive adipocytes involving the lower two-thirds of the face. Although it usually presents at birth (congenital infiltrating lipomatosis of the face) it may present in adolescence or early adulthood. Somatic mutation in the *PIK3CA* gene have been identified in patients with IL-F [1]. It is associated with soft tissue and bony hypertrophy [2,3]. IL-F patients have normal psychomotor development [4].

Epidemiology
Incidence and prevalence
Infiltrating lipomatosis of the face is a rare disorder with approximately 65 cases reported in the world literature [2–4,5,6–13,14, 15–19,20,21,22,23–25,26,27,28].

Age
Although most cases present at birth, adolescent and early adulthood presentations have also been reported. All reported cases presented during the first three decades of life [24].

Sex
There is no gender predilection [4].

Ethnicity
There is no racial predilection.

Pathophysiology
IL-F is caused by somatic mutation in the *PIK3CA* gene and it is now considered one of the conditions in the *PIK3CA*-related overgrowth spectrum (PROS) along with Congenital Lipomatous Overgrowth, Vascular malformation, Epidermal nevi, Scoliosis/skeletal (CLOVES) and Klippel–Trenaunay syndrome [1]. *PIK3CA* regulates cellular growth, survival and proliferation in the *PIK3CA*/AKT/mTOR pathway. Dysregulation in this pathway leads to overgrowth of tissues that are the hallmark of conditions in this group of disorders [29].

Pathology
In the initial case description, Slavin *et al.* described the histopathological features of IL-F, which include infiltration of mature benign adipocytes into adjacent soft tissue with hypertrophy of the underlying skeleton. They also emphasised the absence of malignant characteristics and lipoblasts, but found an increase in fibrous elements with focal fibrosis affecting nerve bundles and vessels with unifocally thickened muscular walls [3].

Causative organisms
Two patients with IL-F have been found to have cytomegalovirus inclusions within the secretory cells of the parotid gland. However, the relationship between cytomegalovirus and IL-F remains unclear [7,9].

Genetics
Non-inheritable somatic mutation in the *PIK3CA* gene.

Clinical features
Presentation
Patients with IL-F present with unilateral facial swelling that is typically present at birth or in early childhood although it may be delayed until early adult life [24]. The facial swelling is due to the proliferation of unencapsulated benign and mature adipocytes as well as associated soft tissue and bony hypertrophy. There is a wide range of clinical presentations depending on the extent of involvement of the underlying tissue. The lower two-thirds of the face is most commonly involved [2].

Macroglossia and mucosal neuromas on the tongue and buccal mucosa have also been reported [14,20,22], as have dental abnormalities such as abnormal tooth formation [8], root hypoplasia [24] and early eruption of deciduous and permanent teeth on the affected side [14,21,22,24]. A cutaneous capillary blush, usually occurring after resection, has also been reported [14].

Differential diagnosis
Differential diagnosis of IL-F includes other hamartomatous or overgrowth syndromes such as Proteus syndrome, vascular or lymphatic malformations and trauma, as well as benign and malignant neoplasms of the bone and/or soft tissue. MEN2b, Bannayan–Riley–Ruvalcaba syndrome and Cowden syndrome should be considered since they are also associated with mucosal neuromas [14,22]. Congenital hemifacial hyperplasia shares some features with IL-F but this condition does not involve lipocytic infiltration [14,22]. Conditions causing contralateral hypoplasia, such as hemifacial microsomia and progressive hemifacial atrophy (Romberg syndrome), should be excluded [21]. Other disorders of fat tissue infiltration such as liposarcoma or lipoblastomatosis may be ruled out based on histological findings [16,17].

Complications and co-morbidities
Complications and co-morbidities arising from IL-F depend on the extent of involvement of the underlying soft tissue and bone. The lipomatosis itself is benign, although cosmesis may be significantly altered. Resection of IL-F risks injury to vital structures such as the facial nerve.

Investigations
Imaging with MRI provides the best delineation [14].

Management
Management of IL-F involves resection of the tumour followed by reconstruction. The resection is almost always subtotal due to the

infiltrative nature of the tumour into vital structures and carries a risk of injury to the facial nerve. On average, IL-F patients undergo at least three surgical procedures [10] with a recurrence rate that is as high as 62.5% with surgical resection alone [15].

The timing of surgery remains controversial. While earlier reports advocated early and wide local excision to prevent extensive lipomatous infiltration [3,10], more recent literature favours delayed resection with temporising measures such as liposuction, excision of mucosal neuromas and surgery to the upper lip to restore facial symmetry [14]. By delaying the resection until early adulthood it is believed that the chances of facial nerve damage and the total number of debulking procedures required are diminished [6]. It has also been conjectured that growth hormone may play a role in recurrences, implying that mass reduction attempts prior to the end of adolescence may be more likely to fail [14]. Recently, a case of IL-F demonstrating C-KIT and platelet-derived growth factor receptor oncogene expression was treated with imatinib after subtotal surgical resection. At 18 months follow-up, the patient showed no disease progression [2]. *PIK3CA*-inhibitors may offer a new treatment paradigm for PROS which includes IL-F.

Encephalocraniocutaneous lipomatosis

Definition and nomenclature
Encephalocraniocutaneous lipomatosis (ECCL) is a rare, neurocutaneous syndrome characterised by profound intellectual disability, early onset of seizures, unilateral temporofrontal lipomatosis, ipsilateral cerebral and leptomeningeal lipomatosis, cerebral malformation and calcification, and lipomas of the skull, eye and heart.

> **Synonyms and inclusions**
> - Haberland syndrome
> - Fishman syndrome

Introduction and general description
ECCL is a rare, sporadic, neurocutaneous syndrome involving tissues of ectodermal and mesodermal origin. It is associated with profound intellectual disability, early onset of seizures, unilateral temporofrontal lipomatosis, ipsilateral cerebral and leptomeningeal lipomatosis, cerebral malformation and calcification, and lipomas of the skull, eye and heart [1,2]. The hallmark skin finding is naevus psiloliparus, which is a fatty hamartomatous malformation of the scalp [3]. The condition is typically present at birth or shortly after birth.

Epidemiology
Incidence and prevalence
ECCL is a rare disorder with about 60 cases reported in the English literature.

Age
Cutaneous and eye findings are usually present at or shortly after birth. Neurological manifestations may present at a later time.

Sex
There is no gender predilection.

Ethnicity
There is no racial or ethnic predilection.

Pathophysiology
ECCL is caused by activating mutations in the *FGFR1* gene which is involved in production of the fibroblast growth factor receptor. This receptor is involved in the signalling pathway for normal development of multiple organs including the brain, eyes and skin [4].

Pathology
The histopathology of naevus psiloliparus shows focal dermal fibrosis with subcutaneous fat in the reticular dermis.

Clinical features
Presentation
Patients with ECCL present with a wide spectrum of clinical manifestations. Naevus psiloliparus of the scalp is the most common skin finding and was present in 44 of 54 patients studied [5]. Unilateral or bilateral subcutaneous fatty masses are often seen in the frontotemporal or zygomatic region and they are rarely seen outside the craniofacial region (Figure 98.10). Patchy or linear alopecia which is typically non-scarring is commonly observed: it may follow the lines of Blaschko or occasionally be scarring. Fibromas, lipomas and fibrolipomas present typically as ipsilateral skin tag-like cutaneous polyps on the eyelid or following a line from the outer canthus to the tragus. Less common cutaneous manifestations include irregular or disrupted eyebrows and café-au-lait macules [5].

Choristomas, with or without other eye anomalies, were observed in 43 of 54 patients [5] but other ocular abnormalities may also be seen.

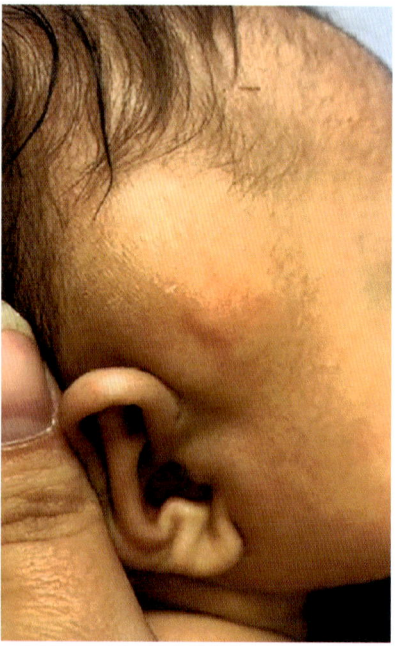

Figure 98.10 Unilateral subcutaneous fatty mass over right temple in a neonate with encephalocraniocutaneous lipomatosis. Courtesy of Megan Craddock, MD, Texas Children's Hospital, USA.

Brain anomalies primarily involve the tissue surrounding the brain including blood vessels [6]. Intracranial lipomas are the most prominent feature; other features include meningeal and meningovascular anomalies and spinal cord lipomas, which may be extensive. CNS findings are frequently confined to the same body side as the cutaneous lesions. The spectrum of neurological manifestations of ECCL patients is broad, ranging from normal development to intellectual impairment of various degrees to intractable seizures. Less commonly, skeletal system involvement with jaw tumours or lytic bone lesions may be present; these may be progressive [7–11].

Congenital heart malformation, particularly aortic coarctation, is seen in about 10% of ECCL patients [5].

Differential diagnosis

This includes the Proteus syndrome, oculoectodermal syndrome, oculocerebrocutaneous syndrome and epidermal naevus syndrome [12–16].

Complications and co-morbidities

Complications and co-morbidities depend on the extent of organ system involvement.

Investigations

Investigations for suspected ECCL include a biopsy of suspected naevus psiloliparus lesions or 'skin tags' around the eye. Ophthalmological examination is required to detect associated ocular anomalies. Neuroimaging studies may characterise and assess the extent of CNS involvement [5]. Since fatty masses can involve the spinal cord, it is recommended that MRI of the spine be performed [5]. An electrocardiogram and an echocardiogram may help screen for cardiac problems.

Management

Treatment is symptomatic and requires multidisciplinary care.

LIPOEDEMA

Lipoedema is the term used to describe swelling of tissues due to abnormal accumulation of subcutaneous fat rather than fluid as seen in lymphoedema, with which it may be confused or coexist (lipo-lymphoedema). In the majority of cases, lipoedema affects the lower extremities but it may also affect the upper extremities and the scalp. Hereafter the term lipoedema, if unqualified, will be used to denote lipoedema of the lower limbs.

Lipoedema of the lower limbs

Definition

Lipoedema is characterised by progressive, symmetrical and bilateral enlargement of involved areas due to subcutaneous deposition of fat.

Introduction and general description

Lipoedema, first described in 1940 [1], is characterised by progressive, symmetrical and bilateral enlargement due to subcutaneous deposition of fat occurring anywhere from the buttocks to the ankles, with sparing of the feet [1,2]. Lipoedema occurs independently of lymphatic stasis or venous insufficiency. Imaging studies verify that oedema is minimal and the swelling is in fact due to homogenous enlargement of the subcutaneous compartment [3–6,7,8]. Its principal clinical features are summarised in Box 98.1 [2].

Epidemiology

Incidence and prevalence

The exact incidence and prevalence of lipoedema are unknown. It is probably underreported and often misdiagnosed due to unfamiliarity with this disorder [9–12]. In lymphoedema clinics, up to 15% of referred patients were diagnosed with lipoedema [13,14].

Box 98.1 Clinical characteristics of lipoedema

- Occurrence is almost exclusively in women
- Bilateral and symmetrical nature with minimal involvement of the feet
- Minimal pitting oedema
- Pain, tenderness and easy bruising
- Persistent enlargement despite elevation of the affected extremities or weight loss

---

Age

Onset occurs during or soon after puberty [15].

Sex

Lipoedema occurs almost exclusively in women [1,2,9,16]. The condition has been reported only rarely in men [9,17].

Ethnicity

There is no racial or ethnic predilection.

Associated diseases

Most lipoedema patients do not have elevated lipids or other abnormal laboratory values [9,18]. One group of investigators found elevated plasma lipids as well as an abnormal fatty acid composition of tissue triglycerides in lipoedema patients relative to controls. However, the clinical significance of this finding is unclear [19].

Pathophysiology

The aetiology of lipoedema is unknown. Hormones appear to play a role in the development of lipoedema, given that it occurs almost exclusively in women with a typical onset near puberty or during periods of significant hormonal changes [1,2,9,16]. Moreover, male lipoedema cases occurred in those receiving hormonal therapy for prostate carcinoma or with hepatic cirrhosis [12,20].

The anatomy of the lymphatic vessel system in lipoedema patients has been found to be normal or sufficient, as far as the large lymph vessels are concerned [15]. The degree of insufficiency in lipoedema

Table 98.1 Differential diagnosis of lipoedema.

	Lipoedema	Lymphoedema	Obesity	Chronic venous insufficiency
Sex	Female	Both	Both	Both
Family history	Frequent	Rare (except for Milroy disease)	Frequent	In some cases
Effect of leg elevation	Little to none	Initially with moderate improvement[a]	No effect	Marked improvement[b]
History of cellulitis	None	Frequent in secondary lymphoedema	None	Frequent
History of ulcers	None	None	None	Very frequent
Symmetry	Present	Absent	Present	Present or absent
Involvement of feet	No	Yes	Yes	Yes
Tenderness to palpation	Yes	No	No	Yes
Pitting oedema	None or minimal initially[c]	Present with varying severity	Absent	Marked[b]
Tissue consistency	May be soft, fat or firm	Doughy, similar to gelatine	Soft, like fat	Soft, pitting

[a] Longstanding lymphoedema may not show improvement with leg elevation.
[b] Longstanding venous insufficiency may be complicated by lymphoedema, in which case this may not apply.
[c] Longstanding lipoedema may have pitting oedema.

patients, if present, never however reached the level of true chronic venous insufficiency or lymphoedema [10,11,21,22]. The lymphatic transport in lipoedema decreases as the body ages and the fibrosis increases [15]. As a result, in longstanding cases, lipoedema and lymphoedema often coexist [12].

Predisposing factors
Although obese patients may be overrepresented, individuals with normal weight are also affected [1,2,9,**16**].

Pathology
No histological abnormalities have been identified by haematoxylin and eosin (H&E) stains, fat stains or electron microscopy [9,10,13,14,**16**,17–19].

Genetics
A significant portion (16–64%) of affected women have a self-reported positive family history of lipoedema [1,11,14]. *Pit-1* mutation was identified in female members of one family with multiple anterior pituitary hormone deficiency and lipoedema [23]. However, no other genetic mutations have been identified.

Clinical features
Presentation
The onset of symmetrical and bilateral gradual fat deposition starts around puberty in most cases. However, it may also develop during other periods of hormonal changes such as pregnancy or menopause [24].

Enlargement of the lower extremities is disproportionate in relation to the trunk, upper extremities, face and neck [15], even among obese patients [2,13]. Feet are generally spared. Fat deposition of lipoedema begins abruptly above the malleoli, causing a sharp demarcation between the normal and abnormal tissue at the ankles, which is known as the 'cuff sign'. The only sign during early stages of disease may be the disappearance of the retromalleolar sulcus. As the disease progress, this characteristic physical sign becomes more prominent. If the upper extremities are affected, a similar cuff sign that ends sharply above the wrists is seen with sparing of the hands [15]. Although the non to minimal pitting oedema component is mild initially, prominent oedema may eventually develop [15].

Patients often complain of heaviness and discomfort of the involved areas with sensitivity to pressure. The swelling and aching are aggravated by exercise and warm weather [15].

Clinical variants
A classification based on the location of involved areas has been proposed [25]:
  I. Mostly buttocks.
  II. Buttocks to knees.
 III. Buttocks to malleoli.
  IV. Mainly arms.
  V. Mainly lower legs.

Differential diagnosis
Differential diagnosis of lipoedema includes lymphoedema, obesity, chronic venous insufficiency and lipohypertrophy (Table 98.1) [12,15,26]. In contrast to lipoedema, patients with lymphoedema have a positive Stemmer sign where there is an inability to pinch a fold of skin at the base of the second toe due to thickening and fibrosis of the subcutaneous tissue. In obesity, the increase in subcutaneous fat is generalised and pain is not usually a feature; furthermore, the typical sparing of the feet is not seen in obese patients. Chronic venous insufficiency is associated with hyperpigmentation and, initially, pitting oedema that can be relieved by leg elevation; with time, however, lymphoedema may supervene. The main difference between lipohypertrophy and lipoedema is the absence of oedema and pain in lipohypertrophy [15]. Other differential diagnoses include Dercum disease and benign symmetrical lipomatosis.

Complications and co-morbidities
Mobility can be significantly impaired.

Disease course and prognosis
Lipoedema is a progressive lifelong disorder.

Investigations
Lipoedema remains a clinical diagnosis. MRI may be used to verify that the swelling is due to homogenous enlargement of the

subcutaneous compartment [3–6,7,8]. Dynamic lymphoscintigraphy can rule out true lymphoedema. Since venous disease can present concomitantly, duplex ultrasound is advocated by some if patients' complaints cannot be fully explained by lipoedema [15]. No specific abnormalities have been found in phlebograms or arteriograms from lipoedema patients [16,18,19].

Management

Management includes strategies to address the physical as well as psychological impact of the disease and, as such, a multidisciplinary approach is necessary [15].

Management of diet is important because additional fat laid down in lipoedematous limbs may be abnormally resistant to control by dieting and exercise and will also compound the difficulties of taking adequate exercise, causing further frustration and low self-esteem [15,20,27]. Because BMI and total body weight may not accurately reflect obesity status in lipoedema patients, some authors advocate the use of waist circumference as an indicator for 'healthy weight' [15,28].

Diuretics and leg elevation do not help patients with lipoedema [11,13], although they may benefit patients with concomitant lymphoedema.

Complex physical decongestion therapy, which combines manual lymphatic drainage and compression therapy, is widely accepted as a conservative therapeutic approach [13,20,29,30]. While manual lymphatic drainage reduces the actual volume, compression by stocking or bandage is used to minimise recurrence. Compression therapy may improve, in part, the symptoms of lipoedema and also mitigate the progression of the lymphatic component. Certainly, patients with concomitant chronic venous insufficiency and/or lymphoedema will benefit from compression therapy [15]. In lipoedema patients, however, despite lifelong decongestion therapy, the amount of subcutaneous tissue increases and the disease overall progresses over time.

Tumescent liposuction has become an integral part in the management of lipoedema. Ideally, it should be performed early, and multiple sessions are often required [15]. Patients experience significant improvement in swelling, pain, mobility, appearance and quality of life [24,25,31–33]. Decongestion therapy should remain an integral part of post-liposuction management [24].

Lipo-lymphoedema

Definition

Lipo-lymphoedema is the coexistence of lipoedema and secondary lymphoedema.

Introduction and general description

Secondary lymphoedema may coexist in patients with longstanding lipoedema and the distinction between the two entities can be a challenge. The increased pressure from expansion of fat tissues in lipoedema contributes to the development of lipo-lymphoedema by causing mechanical obstruction of small lymphatic vessels.

Pathophysiology

The lymphatic system in lipoedema is thought to be normal or sufficient, at least as far as the large lymph vessels are concerned. However, the increased pressure from the expansion of fat tissues may cause mechanical obstruction of the small lymphatic vessels in the septa, resulting in mild lymphostasis and oedema of the subcutaneous tissue. Furthermore, lymphatic transport in lipoedema also decreases as fibrosis increases with age, and this can exacerbate the secondary lymphoedema [1].

Pathology

No distinct histological abnormalities have been identified in lipo-lymphoedema by H&E, fat stains or electron microscopy [2–4].

Clinical features

Presentation

In addition to the physical examination findings in lipoedema, patients with lipo-lymphoedema may have a positive Stemmer sign – the inability to pinch a skin fold at the base of the second toe due to oedema or fibrosis of the skin. Stemmer sign is often present in lymphoedema patients but is usually absent in lipoedema patients [5].

Disease course and prognosis

Lipo-lymphoedema has a chronic and progressive course.

Investigations

Lipo-lymphoedema is a clinical diagnosis. Table 98.2 describes imaging modalities that may assist in identifying lipo-lymphoedema [5].

Management

The lymphatic oedema component of lipo-lymphoedema may improve initially with leg elevation and compression. See also the management section for lipoedema of the lower limbs.

Table 98.2 Imaging characteristics of lipoedema and lymphoedema.

Imaging modality	Lipoedema	Lymphoedema
Lymphangiogram	Normal	Abnormal
Lymphoscintigram	Normal, with mild lymphatic delay in some	Abnormal with delayed lymphatic flow, subdermal collateralisation and dermal backflow
Computed tomography	Diffuse and homogenous lipomatous hypertrophy of subcutaneous tissue	Thickening of the calf subcutaneous tissues and perimuscular aponeurosis Increased fat density Honeycomb appearance due to fibrous and oedematous stranding of fat
Magnetic resonance imaging	Normal skin thickness, increased fatty tissue	Thickening of the skin and subcutaneous tissue Honeycomb appearance

PART 8: SPECIFIC CUTANEOUS STRUCTURES

Lipoedema of the scalp and lipoedematous alopecia

Definition and nomenclature

Lipoedema of the scalp and lipoedematous alopecia are characterised by the presence of a thick, boggy scalp due to a prominent increase in subcutaneous adipose tissue, which may be associated with varying degrees of hair loss.

Synonyms and inclusions
- Lipoedematous scalp
- Lipoedematous alopecia

Introduction and general description

Lipoedema of the scalp is a rare condition of unknown aetiology where a thick, boggy scalp develops due to a prominent increase in subcutaneous adipose tissue. It can be associated with scarring or non-scarring hair loss, when it is known as lipoedematous alopecia [1]. Lipoedema of the scalp was first described by Cornbleet in 1935 [2] and lipoedematous alopecia was first described by Coskey *et al.* in 1961 [3]. There is some debate as to whether lipoedema of the scalp and lipoedematous alopecia represent clinical variants of the same entity or two different disorders [1]. Since they are both very rare, they will be grouped together for the purposes of this discussion.

Epidemiology
Incidence and prevalence

These are rare conditions with only approximately 45 cases of lipoedema of the scalp and 30 cases of lipoedematous alopecia reported in the literature [1,**4**].

Age

Lipoedema of the scalp and lipoedematous alopecia are reported most commonly in adults [2,3,5–11,**12**,13,**14**,15,**16**,17,**18**,19–24,**25–28**,29–31].

Sex

Among reported cases, there is an approximate female to male ratio of 5:1 [2,3,**4**,5–11,**12**,13,**14**,15,**16**,17,**18**,19–24,**25–28**,29].

Ethnicity

Both lipoedema of the scalp and lipoedematous alopecia have been described in all ethnicities [2,3,**4**,5–11,**12**,13,**14**,15,**16**,17,**18**,19–24,**25–28**,29].

Associated diseases

Several conditions have been reported in association with lipoedema of the scalp or lipoedematous alopecia but there is no consistent link with any of them [3,5,8,**12**,13,15,**16**,17,**18**,19,21,23].

Pathophysiology

The exact aetiology is unknown. A failure to maintain the integrity of the dermal–subcutaneous interface with an expansion and invasion of subcutaneous fat into the dermis is likely to be of relevance [27]. Some have speculated that female sex hormones may play a role, since these conditions have a predilection for women [29].

Hair cycle disturbance could occur as a result of lymphangiectasia [1,**16**,21,24] or oedema [1,9], both of which have been observed histologically in lipoedema of the scalp and lipoedematous alopecia. Alternatively, the fat itself might invade and destroy the hair follicle [**27**].

Pathology

The main pathological feature in both lipoedema of the scalp and lipoedematous alopecia is an approximate doubling in scalp thickness resulting from expansion of the subcutaneous fat layer [1]. Dilated lymphatic vessels have been observed in both conditions [1,**16**,21,24]. In lipoedematous alopecia there is also a loss of hair follicles without any inflammation. Perifollicular fat cells in direct continuity with underlying subcutaneous fat lobules are noted in the dermis, together with fibrous tracks [**27**] and fragmentation of dermal elastic fibres [1,11].

Genetics

No genetic mutation has been identified in patients with lipoedema of the scalp and lipoedematous alopecia. However, a lipoedema of the scalp mother–lipoedematous alopecia daughter pair has been reported [23].

Environmental factors

One group of Egyptian investigators observed that all of their patients wore a special tight head scarf called a mandil [19]. The associations between lipoedema of the scalp, lipoedematous alopecia and other headwear have not been reported by others.

Clinical features
Presentation

Although lipoedema of the scalp and lipoedematous alopecia are usually asymptomatic, some patients may experience pain, pruritus, paraesthesiae or headache [**27**]. While lipoedematous alopecia patients may present earlier due to alopecia, most patients with lipoedema of the scalp were not aware of their condition and presented for other reasons [1].

Patients with lipoedema of the scalp and lipoedematous alopecia present with boggy thickening of the scalp, predominantly over the vertex, parietal and occipital scalp (Figure 98.11) [**12**]. The bogginess may gradually extend to the entire scalp. The condition is more easily palpable than visible [1]. The consistency of the scalp has been likened to cotton wadding as used in quilting and upholstering [**27**]. The involved scalp is easily pressed down to the underlying bone but returns to its original form immediately after pressure is removed [19].

Hair loss in lipoedematous alopecia is variable and both scarring and non-scarring alopecia have been reported. Hairs do not exceed 2 cm in length and tend to break off easily [3]. Sometimes the hair in the affected area can have a lighter colour than hair from the surrounding unaffected scalp [**4**].

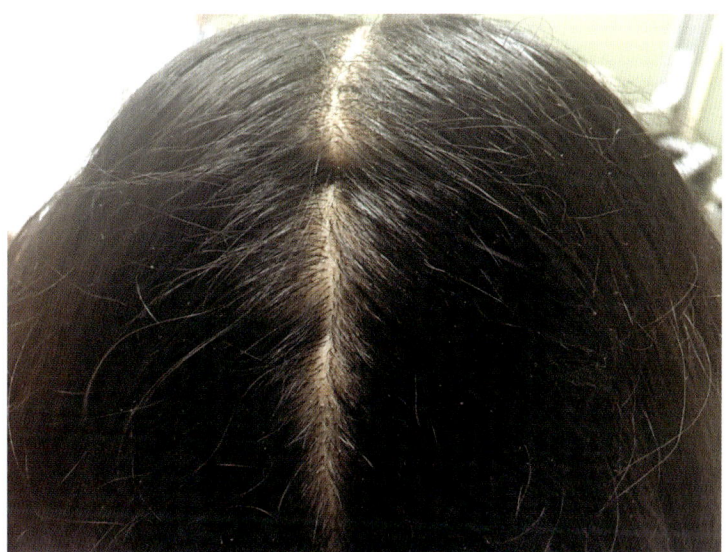

Figure 98.11 Boggy thickening of the scalp over scalp vertex seen in lipoedema of the scalp. Courtesy of Soo Jung Kim, MD, Baylor College of Medicine, USA.

Of note is the fact that none of the lipoedema of the scalp and lipoedematous alopecia patients reported to date has had concurrent lipoedema of the legs.

Differential diagnosis

Differential diagnosis of lipoedema of the scalp and lipoedematous alopecia includes naevus lipomatosus superficialis of the scalp, cutis verticis gyrata and encephalocraniocutaneous lipomatosis. Naevus lipomatosus superficialis is usually present at birth and may have solitary or multiple lesions [20]. The scalp in cutis verticis gyrata is furrowed and on biopsy demonstrates closely packed hair follicles and considerable thickening of the collagen bundles of the dermis and subcutaneous tissue [25]. Encephalocraniocutaneous lipomatosis is associated with ophthalmological and neurological abnormalities.

Disease course and prognosis

Both lipoedema of the scalp and lipoedematous alopecia are chronic and persistent conditions.

Investigations

Ultrasound or MRI of the involved scalp area can confirm subcutaneous tissue thickening [27]. The average scalp thickness in healthy individuals was 5.8 ± 0.12 mm [31]. In contrast, the scalp thickness in lipoedema of the scalp and lipoedematous alopecia patients ranged from 8.5 to 16 mm with an average of 11.4 mm [25]. Biopsy of the affected area may also support the diagnosis.

Management

There is no specific and effective management guideline for lipoedema of the scalp and lipoedematous alopecia. Pain, pruritus and paraesthesia are managed symptomatically. Surgical excision of lipoedema of the scalp has been reported in one patient. At 12-month follow-up, there was no recurrence although residual alopecia remained [27]. Topical minoxidil solutions have not been helpful in regrowing hair [27].

MISCELLANEOUS DISORDERS OF SUBCUTANEOUS FAT

Cellulite

Definition and nomenclature

Cellulite is an architectural disorder of human adipose tissue. It is characterised by the dimpled and nodular appearance of the skin in cellulite-prone areas in postpubertal females [1].

Synonyms and inclusions
- Adiposis oedematosa
- Status protusus cutis
- Dermopanniculosis deformans
- Nodular liposclerosis
- Gynoid lipodystrophy
- Oedematofibrosclerotic panniculopathy

Introduction and general description

The term cellulite was first introduced in the French literature 150 years ago [2]. Cellulite is nowadays among the more common concerns of patients presenting to dermatologists. It is a localised metabolic disorder of subcutaneous tissue that results in a readily visible alteration in the appearance of the female body. Cellulite presents as a change of skin topography evident by skin with dimpling and nodularity that principally involves the pelvic region, lower limbs and abdomen of women. The topographical alteration is caused by herniations of subcutaneous fat through its fibrous connective tissue support matrix.

Epidemiology
Incidence and prevalence

It is estimated that between 85% and 98% of postpubertal females display some degree of cellulite [1].

Age

It first appears after puberty.

Sex

It is almost exclusive to women [1].

Ethnicity

White women are affected more frequently than women of other races [3].

Pathophysiology

The exact pathophysiology of cellulite is not fully understood; many theories seek to explain the structural, architectural, metabolic and biochemical differences between cellulite and non-cellulite fat. In a study performed by Rosenbaum *et al.* [4], biopsies from women with and without cellulite showed an irregular and discontinuous dermal–subcutaneous interface that was characterised by fat protrusion into the dermis. In contrast, the dermal–subcutaneous and connective tissue interface was smooth and continuous in male subjects. These findings suggest that there is a sexual dimorphism in the structural characteristics of subdermal connective tissue that predisposes women to the development of cellulite. Women with cellulite have a higher percentage of thinner, perpendicularly orientated, dermal septa: this appears to facilitate herniation of adipose tissue into the reticular dermis [5,6]. Furthermore, a recent anatomical study from cadavers comparing gender differences in gluteal subcutaneous architecture and biomechanics found that the force required to break the septae is significantly greater in the male cadavers than in female cadavers ($P = 0.021$) [7].

There are also regional differences in both the hormonal responsiveness and metabolic activity of human adipose tissue. For example, adipocytes in the gluteal–femoral region are larger and are influenced by female sex hormones. The gluteal–femoral adipocytes are also metabolically more stable and resistant to lipolysis [1]. Although it has been conjectured that deterioration of the dermal vasculature with oedema and deposition of glycosoaminoglycans in the dermal capillary walls could result in cellulite [3], this observation has not been supported by others [5,6,8]. Similarly, the role of inflammation in the pathogenesis of cellulite remains controversial [2,5,9,10–12].

Predisposing factors
Excessively high carbohydrate diets provoke hyperinsulinaemia and lipogenesis, leading to an increase in total body fat content, and thereby predispose to cellulite [1,12]. Prolonged periods of sitting or standing may impede normal blood flow and lead to stasis, which alters microcirculation and may increase the risk of cellulite. Finally, fluid retention and the hormonal environment in pregnancy may also be contributory [1].

Pathology
Cellulite is a clinical diagnosis. Tissue sampling is not required for the diagnosis. Histopathological specimens demonstrate indentations of subcutaneous fat into the dermis [5].

Genetics
There seems to be a genetic predisposition to the development of cellulite as most women with cellulite report its occurrence in other family members [13]. However, no specific genetic mutation has been identified.

Clinical features
Presentation
Cellulite presents almost exclusively in postpubertal females and involves the skin of the pelvic region, lower limbs and abdomen. The skin appears dimpled, like the surface of a mattress or of orange peel [1,5]. This surface irregularity is especially apparent when the skin is pinched. Cellulite can affect individuals with both high and low BMI [1].

Differential diagnosis
Obesity is differentiated from cellulite in that obesity is characterised by hypertrophy and hyperplasia of adipose tissue that is not necessarily limited to the pelvis, thighs and abdomen [1]. The skin is not dimpled in obesity.

Classification of severity
Cellulite has been divided into three grades of severity [1]:

Grade I	Skin dimpling is apparent on pinching but not otherwise.
Grade II	Skin dimpling is apparent on standing but not on lying down.
Grade III	Skin dimpling is apparent both on standing and on lying down.

Complications and co-morbidities
There is no associated morbidity or mortality [1].

Disease course and prognosis
Cellulite can be progressive.

Management
Although cellulite is a very common complaint, treatments proposed for it have lacked substantial proof of efficacy. There is no single treatment or treatment combination that has been shown to be reliably effective. The best currently available treatments have resulted in mild to moderate improvement at best. Most of any improvement obtained is not sustained over time and maintenance treatment is often needed.

Weight gain may accentuate the visibility of cellulite. Weight reduction may reduce but, ironically, may also sometimes increase its prominence. One group of investigators has shown, however, that, on average, cellulite severity decreases following weight loss. This is especially true for those with higher BMI and greater cellulite severity grading [14].

Various over-the-counter and prescription topical therapies have been advocated for cellulite. Topical application of 0.3% retinol for 6 months or more has been claimed to improve cellulite [15]. So-called mesotherapy, whereby a variety of substances including phosphatidylcholine, caffeine, theophylline and herbal extracts are injected into subcutaneous tissue in an attempt to dissolve fat, has been widely promoted but, not surprisingly, has not been shown to have any useful place in managing cellulite [15–17]. A 2019 phase IIa, randomised, double-blind placebo-controlled study ($n = 375$) of women with cellulite treated with collagenase *Clostridium histolyticum* 0.84 mg showed improvement in the Clinician Reported Photonumeric Cellulite Severity Scale and Patient Reported Photonumeric Cellulite Severity Scale scores from placebo [18].

Many non-invasive devices have been promoted for the treatment of cellulite. These include a skin-kneading device, unipolar and bipolar radiofrequency devices, ultrasound devices and selective cryolysis [15].

More invasive procedures such as subcision and liposuction have also been attempted. While subcision may temporarily improve cellulite appearance, long-term efficacy remains to be demonstrated. Liposuction for the treatment of cellulite carries risk. While liposuction reduces fat deposits deeper in the subcutaneous fat, cellulite adipose tissue is deposited more superficially. When liposuction is performed at more superficial levels, there is an increased risk of necrosis and poor cosmetic outcome. Laser-assisted liposuction and/or laser-assisted lipoplasty, which are less invasive than traditional liposuction and offer simultaneous skin tightening, may be the preferred treatment [1].

In the search for a novel approach to managing cellulite, various investigators have looked at peroxisome proliferator-activated receptors (PPARs), which are found on adipocytes and are thought to have an effect on the extracellular matrix, as possible targets for the treatment of cellulite, but there is no evidence to date that they are likely to be effective [15,19–23].

The ideal management for this condition, which so many women find distressing and for the treatment of which considerable sums have been expended, has yet to be found.

Obesity and the skin

Rates of people being overweight and obese (BMI $>25 \, \text{kg/m}^2$) have been rising at an alarming rate in many countries of the world in recent years: in England, for instance, 62% of adults are currently overweight or obese [1]. The prevalence of obesity (BMI $>30 \, \text{kg/m}^2$) in adult men and women rose over the 20 years from 1993 to 2013 from 13.2% and 16.4% to 26.0% and 23.8%, respectively [1]. Nearly 10% of all children entering English schools (at age 4–5 years) were classified as obese (weight $\geq$95th centile for age) [1].

Obesity not only exposes people to well-known metabolic and cardiovascular consequences including type 2 diabetes, but also has significant effects on other body systems including the skin [2].

Physiological consequences of obesity on the skin. Subcutaneous fat insulates the body core from the external environment. Whilst this may be of benefit in protecting the body from the effects of exposure to cold, it also means that it is harder for the obese to dissipate heat from the core out to the skin surface. This increases the reliance on sweating for thermoregulation in obese people, who tend to sweat more profusely than those who are not overweight [3]. Paradoxically, however, transepidermal water loss is increased in obese people, who are prone to xerosis [4].

Mechanical problems contributing to skin disease in the obese. Friction, sweating and maceration within body folds frequently lead to a painful erosive intertriginous dermatitis with secondary candidiosis. Obese women with restricted mobility are more likely to have problems with urinary incontinence, which can contribute further to inflammation, with an irritant contact dermatitis affecting the genito-crural folds [5]. Stretch marks (striae distensae) are common, particularly if weight gain has been rapid [2,5,6]. They tend to be located in the axillary folds, upper thighs, buttocks and abdomen.

The mechanical effects of obesity may impede lymphatic drainage not only in the lower extremities but also elsewhere, for example in abdominal apron folds, resulting in lymphoedema [3]. The chronic high pressure exerted on the skin of the soles of the feet may result in plantar hyperkeratosis and postmenopausal plantar keratoderma (keratoderma climactericum) [2,6].

Peripheral vascular and lymphovascular disorders in the obese. Obesity puts strain on the vascular system. Lower limb venous hypertension from whatever cause may be exacerbated in the obese by high intra-abdominal pressures and by immobility. The risks

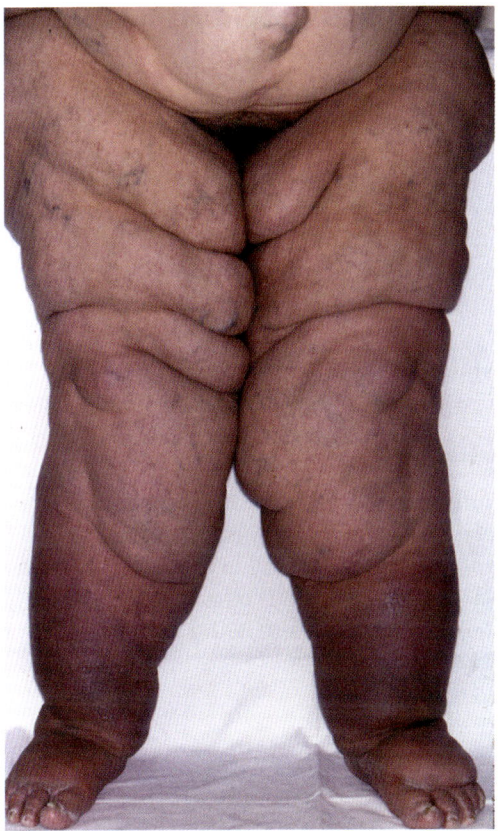

Figure 98.12 Gross obesity with bilateral lymphoedema of lower legs.

of venous eczema and venous ulceration are increased and they may be more difficult to manage. Chronic lymphoedema frequently supervenes (Figure 98.12) [2].

Cutaneous infections and obesity. The prevalence of superficial skin infections such as candidosis, dermatophytosis and erythrasma is raised in the obese [2]. Pyogenic infections such as folliculitis and furunculosis are also more frequently seen and may be recurrent. In a large study of patients requiring operative treatment of skin and soft tissue infections by community-acquired methicillin-resistant *Staphylococcus aureus* (MRSA), obese patients were more than three times likely to need further surgical intervention within a year than non-obese patients [7]. Lymphoedema in the obese is commonly complicated by streptococcal cellulitis. Obesity also increases the risk of surgical wound infection and of necrotising fasciitis [8].

Cutaneous consequences of immunological and endocrine dysregulation in the obese. It is increasingly recognised that adipose tissue has multiple, complex regulatory and hormonal functions in addition to its role as an energy store (see Chapter 97 for anatomy and physiology of subcutaneous fat); these functions may be disturbed in the obese. Altered adipocytokine secretion may have an effect on inflammation in the obese [9,10]: for instance, delayed-type hypersensitivity responses are increased in obesity and decline with weight reduction [11]. Adipocytokines may also play a role in the well-recognised link between severe psoriasis and obesity, with evidence that weight reduction, including that achieved by bariatric surgery, can produce significant improvement in psoriasis [2,12,13]. There is also some evidence of a link between obesity and atopy including atopic eczema [2,14].

The hyperinsulinaemia associated with obesity increases androgen production from adipose tissue and reduces the production of sex-hormone-binding globulin, thus increasing circulating free androgen levels. This manifests as increased risks of acne, hirsutism, androgenetic alopecia and polycystic ovary syndrome in the obese [2,15]. Type 2 diabetes is a common complication of obesity and is associated with a variety of specific skin disorders (Chapter 62).

Genetic disorders associated with obesity. Obesity is a component of a number of genetic disorders of which Prader–Willi syndrome is one of the best known. These are discussed in Chapter 72.

Other skin disorders in the obese. Dercum disease (see earlier in this chapter) is strongly associated with obesity. The presence of obesity may aggravate a variety of other skin disorders including hidradenitis suppurativa and pilonidal sinus. Surgical wound healing is impaired in the obese with an increased risk of incisional hernia [16].

Key references

The full list of references can be found in the online version at https://www.wiley.com/rooksdermatology10e

Acquired lipodystrophy
Acquired generalised lipodystrophy

1 Garg A. Clinical review: lipodystrophies: genetic and acquired body fat disorders. *J Clin Endocrinol Metab* 2011;96:3313–25.
10 Misra A, Garg A. Clinical features and metabolic derangements in acquired generalized lipodystrophy: case reports and review of the literature. *Medicine (Baltimore)* 2003;82:129–46.
13 Lupsa BC, Sachdev V, Lungu AO, Rosing DR, Gorden P. Cardiomyopathy in congenital and acquired generalized lipodystrophy: a clinical assessment. *Medicine (Baltimore)* 2010;89:245–50.
21 Brown RJ, Chan JL, Jaffe ES *et al*. Lymphoma in acquired generalized lipodystrophy. *Leuk Lymphoma* 2016;57:45–50.
23 Garg A. Lipodystrophies. *Am J Med* 2000;108:143–52.
27 Corvillo F, Aparicio V, Lopez-Lera A *et al*. Autoantibodies against perilipin1 as a cause of acquired generalized lipodystrophy. *Front Immunol* 2018;9:2142.
48 Haddad N, Vidal-Trecan T, Baroudjian B *et al*. Acquired generalized lipodystrophy under immune checkpoint inhibition. *Br J Dermatol* 2019;182:477–80.
49 Falcao C, Cabral M, Mota J *et al*. Acquired lipodystrophy associated with nivolumab in a patient with advanced renal cell carcinoma. *J Clin Endocrinol Metab* 2019;104:3245–8.
50 Bedrose S, Turin CG, Lavis VR *et al*. A case of acquired generalized lipodystrophy associated with pembrolizumab in a patient with metastatic malignant melanoma. *AACE Clin Case Rep* 2020;6:e40–e45.
54 Oral EA, Simha V, Ruiz E *et al*. Leptin-replacement therapy for lipodystrophy. *N Engl J Med* 2002;346:570–8.

Acquired partial lipodystrophy

1 Garg A. Lipodystrophies. *Am J Med* 2000;108:143–52.
2 Garg A. Clinical review: lipodystrophies: genetic and acquired body fat disorders. *J Clin Endocrinol Metab* 2011;96:3313–25.
14 Spranger S, Spranger M, Tasman AJ, Reith W, Voigtlander T, Voigtlander V. Barraquer-Simons syndrome (with sensorineural deafness): a contribution to the differential diagnosis of lipodystrophy syndromes. *Am J Med Genet* 1997;71:397–400.

20 Misra A, Peethambaram A, Garg A. Clinical features and metabolic and autoimmune derangements in acquired partial lipodystrophy: report of 35 cases and review of the literature. *Medicine (Baltimore)* 2004;83:18–34.
21 Sissons JG, West RJ, Fallows J *et al*. The complement abnormalities of lipodystrophy. *N Engl J Med* 1976;294:461–5.
22 Corvillo F, Nozal P, Lopez-Lera A *et al*. Evidence of ongoing complement activation on adipose tissue from an 11-year-old girl with Barraquer-Simons syndrome. *J Dermatol* 2020;47:1439–44.
24 Mathieson PW, Peters DK. Lipodystrophy in MCGN type II: the clue to links between the adipocyte and the complement system. *Nephrol Dial Transplant* 1997;12:1804–6.
26 Oswiecimska J, Ziora K, Geisler G, Dyduch A. Acquired partial lipodystrophy in an 11-year-old girl. *Pediatr Int* 2008;50:714–16.
31 Baccjo VF, Maillet F, Berian L *et al*. Neutralising antibodies against C3NeF in intravenous immunoglobulin. *Lancet* 1992;340:63–4.
32 Levy Y, George J, Yona E *et al*. Partial lipodystrophy, mesangiocapillary glomerulonephritis, and complement dysregulation. An autoimmune phenomenon. *Immunol Res* 1998;18:55–60.

HIV-associated lipodystrophy

2 Garg A. Clinical review: lipodystrophies: genetic and acquired body fat disorders. *J Clin Endocrinol Metab* 2011;96:3313–25.
3 Domingo P, Estrada V, Lopez-Aldeguer J, Villaroya F, Martinez E. Fat redistribution syndromes associated with HIV-1 infection and combination antiretroviral therapy. *AIDS Rev* 2012;14:112–23.
6 Chen D, Misra A, Garg A. Clinical review 153: lipodystrophy in human immunodeficiency virus-infected patients. *J Clin Endocrinol Metab* 2002;87:4845–56.
14 Andany N, Raboud J, Walmsley S *et al*. Ethnicity and gender differences in lipodystrophy of HIV-positive individuals taking antiretroviral therapy in Ontario, Canada. *HIV Clin Trials* 2011;12:89–103.
25 Podzamczer D, Ferrer E, Sanchez P *et al*. Less lipoatrophy and better lipid profile with abacavir as compared to stavudine: 96-week results of a randomized study. *J Acquir Immune Defic Syndr* 2007;44:139–47.
28 Hansen BR, Haugaard SB, Iversen J, Nielsen JO, Andersen O. Impact of switching antiretroviral therapy on lipodystrophy and other metabolic complications: a review. *Scand J Infect Dis* 2004;36:244–53.
36 Guaraldi G, Fontdevila J, Christensen LH *et al*. Surgical correction of HIV-associated facial lipoatrophy. *AIDS* 2011;25:1–12.
38 Moyle G, Moutschen M, Martinez E *et al*. Epidemiology, assessment, and management of excess abdominal fat in persons with HIV infection. *AIDS Rev* 2010;12:3–14.
46 Nelson L, Stewart KJ. Plastic surgical options for HIV-associated lipodystrophy. *J Plast Reconstr Aesthet Surg* 2008;61:359–65.

Lipodystrophy associated with total body irradiation and hematopoietic stem cell transplant

1 Adachi M, Oto Y, Muroya K *et al*. Partial lipodystrophy in patients who have undergone hematopoietic stem cell transplantation during childhood: an institutional cross-sectional survey. *Clin Pediatr Endocrinol* 2017;26:99–108.
2 Lorenc A, Hailton-Shield J, Perry R, Stevens M. Body composition after allogeneic haematopoietic cell transplantation/total body irradiation in children and young people: a restricted systematic review. *J Cancer Surviv* 2020;14:624–42.
3 Adachi M, Asakura Y, Muroya K *et al*. Abnormal adipose tissue distribution with unfavorable metabolic profile in five children following hematopoietic stem cell transplantation: a new etiology for acquired partial lipodystrophy. *Clin Pediatr Endocrinol* 2013;22:53–64.
4 Adachi M, Muroya K, Hanakawa J, Asakura Y. Metreleptin worked in diabetic woman with a history of hematopoietic stem cell transplantation (HSCT) during infancy: further support for the concept of 'HSCT-associated lipodystrophy'. *Endocr J* 2021;68(4):399–407.

Localised lipoatrophy and/or lipodystrophy

Semicircular lipoatrophy

1 Gschwandtner WR, Munzberger H. [Lipoatrophia semicircularis. Linear and circular atrophy of the subcutaneous fat in the extremities.] *Hautarzt* 1974;25:222–7.
2 De Groot AC. Is lipoatrophia semicircularis induced by pressure? *Br J Dermatol* 1994;131:887–90.

4 Gomez-Espejo C, Perez-Bernal A, Camacho-Martinez F. A new case of semicircular lipoatrophy associated with repeated external microtraumas and review of the literature. *J Eur Acad Dermatol Venereol* 2005;19:459–61.

5 Nagore E, Sanchez-Motilla JM, Rodriguez-Serna M, Vilata JJ, Aliaga A. Lipoatrophia semicircularis – a traumatic panniculitis: report of seven cases and review of the literature. *J Am Acad Dermatol* 1998;39:879–81.

6 Reinoso-Barbero L, Gonzalez-Gomez MF, Belanger-Quintana D *et al*. Case-control study of semicircular lipoatrophy, a new occupational disease in office workers. *J Occup Health* 2013;55:149–57.

10 Mallett R, Champion R. Lipoatrophia semicircularis. *Br J Dermatol* 1989;121:94–5.

12 Senecal S, Victor V, Choudat D, Hornez-Davin S, Conso F. Semicircular lipoatrophy: 18 cases in the same company. *Contact Dermatitis* 2000;42:101–2.

15 Ogino J, Saga K, Tamagawa M, Akutsu Y. Magnetic resonance imaging of semicircular lipoatrophy. *Dermatology* 2004;209:340–1.

16 Gruber PC, Fuller LC. Lipoatrophy semicircularis induced by trauma. *Clin Exp Dermatol* 2001;26:269–71.

17 Rongioletti F, Rebora A. Annular and semicircular lipoatrophies. Report of three cases and review of the literature. *J Am Acad Dermatol* 1989;20:433–6.

Localised lipoatrophy due to injected drugs

1 Underwood LE, Voina SJ, Van Wyk JJ. Restoration of growth by human growth hormone (Roos) in hypopituitary dwarfs immunized by other human growth hormone preparations: clinical and immunological studies. *J Clin Endocrinol Metab* 1974;38:288–97.

2 Dahl PR, Zalla MJ, Winkelmann RK. Localized involutional lipoatrophy: a clinicopathologic study of 16 patients. *J Am Acad Dermatol* 1996;35:523–8.

3 Kayikcioglu A, Akyurek M, Erk Y. Semicircular lipoatrophy after intragluteal injection of benzathine penicillin. *J Pediatr* 1996;129:166–7.

4 Bauerschmitz J, Bork K. Multifocal disseminated lipoatrophy secondary to intravenous corticosteroid administration in a patient with adrenal insufficiency. *J Am Acad Dermatol* 2002;46(Suppl. 5):S130–2.

Insulin-induced localised lipoatrophy

7 Griffin ME, Feder A, Tamborlane WV. Lipoatrophy associated with lispro insulin in insulin pump therapy: an old complication, a new cause? *Diabetes Care* 2001;24:174.

8 Ampudia-Blasco FJ, Hasbum B, Carmena R. A new case of lipoatrophy with lispro insulin in insulin pump therapy: is there any insulin preparation free of complications? *Diabetes Care* 2003;26:953–4.

9 Felner EI. Human insulin-induced lipoatrophy. *J Pediatr* 2003;142:448.

12 Lopez X, Castells M, Ricker A, Velazquez EF, Mun E, Goldfine AB. Human insulin analog-induced lipoatrophy. *Diabetes Care* 2008;31:442–4.

Subcutaneous lipomatosis
Benign symmetrical lipomatosis

1 Brea-Garcia B, Cameselle-Teijeiro J, Couto-Gonzalez I, Taboada-Suarez A, Gonzalez-Alvarez E. Madelung's disease: comorbidities, fatty mass distribution, and response to treatment of 22 patients. *Aesthetic Plast Surg* 2013;37:409–16.

20 Enzi G, Busetto L, Ceschin E, Coin A, Digito M, Pigozzo S. Multiple symmetric lipomatosis: clinical aspects and outcome in a long-term longitudinal study. *Int J Obes Relat Metab Disord* 2002;26:253–61.

46 Martinez-Escribano JA, Gonzalez R, Quecedo E, Febrer I. Efficacy of lipectomy and liposuction in the treatment of multiple symmetric lipomatosis. *Int J Dermatol* 1999;38:551–4.

Dercum disease

3 Herbst KL, Asare-Bediako S. Adiposis dolorosa is more than painful fat. *Endocrinologist* 2007;17:326–34.

8 Beltran K, Wadeea R, Herbst K. Infections preceding the development of Dercum disease. *IDCases* 2020;19:e00682.

24 Brodovsky S, Westreich M, Leibowitz A, Schwartz Y. Adiposis dolorosa (Dercum's disease): 10-year follow-up. *Ann Plast Surg* 1994;33:664–8.

64 Held JL, Andrew JA, Kohn SR. Surgical amelioration of Dercum's disease: a report and review. *J Dermatol Surg Oncol* 1989;15:1294–6.

65 Devillers AC, Oranje AP. Treatment of pain in adiposis dolorosa (Dercum's disease) with intravenous lidocaine: a case report with a 10-year follow-up. *Clin Exp Dermatol* 1999;24:240–1.

Infiltrating lipomatosis of the face

2 Tracy JC, Klement GL, Scott AR. Interdisciplinary management of congenital infiltrating lipomatosis. *Int J Pediatr Otorhinolaryngol* 2013;77:2071–4.

3 Slavin SA, Baker DC, McCarthy JG, Mufarrij A. Congenital infiltrating lipomatosis of the face: clinicopathologic evaluation and treatment. *Plast Reconstr Surg* 1983;72:158–64.

4 Urs AB, Augustine J, Kumar P, Arora S, Aggarwal N, Sultana N. Infiltrating lipomatosis of the face: a case series. *J Nat Sci Biol Med* 2013;4:252–7.

14 Padwa BL, Mulliken JB. Facial infiltrating lipomatosis. *Plast Reconstr Surg* 2001;108:1544–54.

20 Pires Fraga MF, Mello D, Jorge D, Perin LF, Helene A. Congenital infiltrating lipomatosis. *J Plast Reconstr Aesthet Surg* 2009;62:e561–4.

22 Kim JE, Gottschall JA, Bachman RP, Nemzer L, Puligandla B, Schauer G. Facial infiltrating lipomatosis: physical, radiological, and histopathological findings. *Arch Otolaryngol Head Neck Surg* 2010;136:301–3.

26 Keramidas T, Lagogiannis G, Vlachou V, Katsikeris N. Congenital infiltrating lipomatosis of the face with associated involvement of the TMJ structures. Case report and review of the literature. *J Craniomaxillofac Surg* 2012;40:750–6.

28 Serpa MS, Sully C, Molina VA *et al*. Infiltrating lipomatosis of the face: case series and literature review. *Oral Maxillofacial Path* 2017;123:e99–e105.

Encephalocraniocutaneous lipomatosis

7 Moog U, Roelens F, Mortier GR *et al*. Encephalocraniocutaneous lipomatosis accompanied by the formation of bone cysts: harboring clues to pathogenesis? *Am J Med Genet A* 2007;143A:2973–80.

8 Savage MG, Heldt L, Dann JJ, Bump RL. Encephalocraniocutaneous lipomatosis and mixed odontogenic tumors. *J Oral Maxillofac Surg* 1985;43:617–20.

9 Hauber K, Warmuth-Metz M, Rose C, Brocker EB, Hamm H. Encephalocraniocutaneous lipomatosis: a case with unilateral odontomas and review of the literature. *Eur J Pediatr* 2003;162:589–93.

10 Andreadis DA, Rizos CB, Belazi M, Peneva M, Antoniades DZ. Encephalocraniocutaneous lipomatosis accompanied by maxillary compound odontoma and juvenile angiofibroma: report of a case. *Birth Defects Res A Clin Mol Teratol* 2004; 70:889–91.

11 Zielinska-Kazmierska B, Grodecka J, Jablonska-Polakowska L, Arkuszewski P. Mandibular osteoma in the encephalocraniocutaneous lipomatosis. *J Craniomaxillofac Surg* 2005;33:286–9.

Lipoedema
Lipoedema of the lower limbs

7 Dimakakos PB, Stefanopoulos T, Antoniades P, Antoniou A, Gouliamos A, Rizos D. MRI and ultrasonographic findings in the investigation of lymphedema and lipedema. *Int Surg* 1997;82:411–16.

16 Rudkin GH, Miller TA. Lipedema: a clinical entity distinct from lymphedema. *Plast Reconstr Surg* 1994;94:841–7; discussion 8–9.

Lipo-lymphoedema

2 Stallworth JM, Hennigar GR, Jonsson HT, Jr, Rodriguez O. The chronically swollen painful extremity. A detailed study for possible etiological factors. *JAMA* 1974;228:1656–9.

3 Dennison J, Edolglass JW. Lipedema – the non-lymphatic masquerader. *Angiology* 1984;35:506–10.

4 Rudkin GH, Miller TA. Lipedema: a clinical entity distinct from lymphedema. *Plast Reconstr Surg* 1994;94:841–7; discussion 8–9.

Lipoedema of the scalp and lipoedematous alopecia

4 Zeng YP, Ma DL, Wang BX. Lipedematous scalp with heterochromia of scalp hair in a boy. *Eur J Dermatol* 2011;21:144–5.

12 Scheufler O, Kania NM, Heinrichs CM, Exner K. Hyperplasia of the subcutaneous adipose tissue is the primary histopathologic abnormality in lipedematous scalp. *Am J Dermatopathol* 2003;25:248–52.

14 Mohsin RM. Lipedematous scalp, a rare form of diffuse hair loss. *J Am Acad Dermatol* 2004;50:P90.

16 Martin JM, Monteagudo C, Montesinos E, Guijarro J, Llombart B, Jorda E. Lipedematous scalp and lipedematous alopecia: a clinical and histologic analysis of 3 cases. *J Am Acad Dermatol* 2005;52:152–6.

PART 8: SPECIFIC CUTANEOUS STRUCTURES

18 Rowan DM, Simpson A, Wong KP. Lipedematous scalp in a child. *Pediatr Dermatol* 2006;23:276–8.

25 Gonzalez-Guerra E, Haro R, Angulo J, Del Carmen Farina M, Martin L, Requena L. Lipedematous alopecia: an uncommon clinicopathologic variant of nonscarring but permanent alopecia. *Int J Dermatol* 2008;47:605–9.

26 Kavak A, Yuceer D, Yildirim U, Baykal C, Sarisoy HT. Lipedematous scalp: a rare entity. *J Dermatol* 2008;35:102–5.

27 Yip L, Mason G, Pohl M, Sinclair R. Successful surgical management of lipoedematous alopecia. *Australas J Dermatol* 2008;49:52–4.

28 Martinez-Moran C, Sanz-Munoz C, Miranda-Sivelo A, Torne I, Miranda-Romero A. [Lipedematous scalp.] *Actas Dermosifiliogr* 2009;100:69–72.

Miscellaneous disorders of subcutaneous fat
Cellulite

5 Nurnberger F, Muller G. So-called cellulite: an invented disease. *J Dermatol Surg Oncol* 1978;4:221–9.

9 Draelos ZD, Marenus KD. Cellulite. *Etiology and purported treatment. Dermatol Surg* 1997;23:1177–81.

CHAPTER 99

Purpura

Nick J. Levell

Norwich Medical School, Norfolk and Norwich University Hospital, Norwich, UK

Introduction

Purpura and bruising, terms to describe bleeding into the skin, may be due to fragility or occlusion of blood vessels or haematological disturbance. It may be localised to one area or more generalised if part of a systemic disorder. Purpura is seen by haematologists when due to platelet and coagulation disorders and as part of cutaneous vasculitis which may be limited to the skin or part of a systemic vasculitis. Vasculitis also causes other cutaneous lesions with a purpuric component, including urticarial lesions, nodules, ulcers, livedo and skin necrosis. These lesions also occur in disorders in which vessels are occluded. Morphology and biopsy of a lesion less than 48 hours old can aid diagnosis [1].

Management of purpura involves a multidisciplinary approach including haematology, general medicine, nephrology, rheumatology and dermatology.

Classification of purpura is challenging, as similar clinical patterns may arise from different causes, including vasculitic and non-vasculitic. Aetiology of purpura or vasculitis may be impossible to determine. Classifications based on morphology or aetiology have limitations. Capillaritis may be idiopathic, drug-induced or a manifestation of cutaneous T-cell lymphoma. Purpura due to idiopathic thrombocytopenic purpura may have more than one mechanism [2]. Although microvascular occlusion may initially be less inflamed than vasculitis, secondary inflammation may lead to palpable lesions with a similar appearance and histology to vasculitis.

Haematological causes (thrombocytopenia and clotting factor abnormalities) can often be rapidly evaluated by full blood count and laboratory measures of clotting times. More complex haematological disorders (e.g. thrombophilias or abnormal platelet function) [3], vessel wall defects (both structural and others) [4], infections, immunological disorders and thrombotic microvascular occlusion disorders should be considered.

The differential diagnosis of purpura is based on history and morphology [1]. It is important to differentiate whether early lesions are inflammatory or non-inflammatory [5] as inflammation can point towards a diagnosis of vasculitis.

Purpura is discoloration of the skin or mucous membranes due to extravasation of red blood cells. Petechiae are small, 1–2 mm, purpuric lesions. Ecchymoses (bruises) are larger extravasations of blood. The causes of petechiae and ecchymoses overlap. Thrombocytopenia usually causes petechiae but very low platelet counts can cause more extensive bleeding. Coagulation disorders cause ecchymoses rather than petechiae [6,7]. Haemophilias may present as bleeding from the umbilical cord or gingivae, or as haematomas or haemarthroses, although haemorrhagic subcutaneous nodules may be the first sign of an inherited haemophilia [8]. Gingival bleeding, epistaxis or internal bleeding may occur with platelet or coagulation disorders.

Rook's Textbook of Dermatology, Tenth Edition. Edited by Christopher Griffiths, Jonathan Barker, Tanya Bleiker, Walayat Hussain and Rosalind Simpson.
© 2024 John Wiley & Sons Ltd. Published 2024 by John Wiley & Sons Ltd.

PART 9: VASCULAR DISORDERS

Extravasated blood is broken down to pigments derived from haem in 2–3 weeks. Colour changes include red, blue and purple in the first 5 days, green after 5–7 days and yellow after 7–14 days [9]. Darker pigmented skin may show brown or black discoloration. Individual factors and the injury determine the time scale: age, sex, skin colour, body site, amount of blood extravasated, depth of bruising and medications that alter bruise dispersion. Superficial, purpuric lesions may be orange or brown in colour due to residual haemosiderin.

Box 99.1 Causes of purpura and ecchymosis

Platelet disorders
- Thrombocytopenia
- Abnormal platelet function
- Thrombocytosis

Coagulation disorders
- Inherited, e.g. haemophilia or acquired factor deficiency or dysfunction (e.g. antibody inhibitor)
- Drugs, e.g. anticoagulants
- Localised, e.g. heparin injection sites, some insect bites
- Metabolic, e.g. vitamin K deficiency, hepatic failure (decreased synthesis of clotting factors)
- Thrombophilias, e.g. protein C deficiency, protein S deficiency
- Disseminated intravascular coagulopathy and purpura fulminans
- Secondary to systemic disease (often multifactorial, e.g. macrophage activation syndrome)

Other intravascular causes of purpura/microvascular occlusion
- Dysproteinaemias, e.g. hypergammaglobulinaemic purpura (Waldenström), Sjögren syndrome
- Cryoproteinaemias
- Emboli: crystal, fat, myxoma, infective

Mechanical vascular causes of purpura
- Raised intravascular pressure:
  - Coughing, vomiting, Valsalva manoeuvre, tourniquets, non-accidental injury
- Decreased support for blood vessels:
  - Actinic ('senile') purpura
  - Corticosteroid purpura
  - Scurvy
  - Amyloidosis
- Inherited disorders of connective tissue (pseudoxanthoma elasticum, Ehlers–Danlos syndrome)
- Abnormal vasculature
- Purpura around vascular lesions, e.g. targetoid haemosiderotic haemangioma, tufted angioma, aneurysmal fibrous histiocytoma

Purpura with inflammation
- Vasculitis
- Non-thrombocytopenic toxin- and drug-induced purpura
- Contact purpura
- Purpura associated with infections
- Capillaritis (pigmented purpuric dermatoses):
  - Idiopathic
  - Drug-induced
  - Pre-mycotic
- Associated with other inflammatory dermatoses that are not usually purpuric

- Solar purpura

External and other causes of purpura or ecchymosis
- Physical and artefactual causes
- Easy bruising syndrome and purpura simplex
- Paroxysmal finger haematoma (Achenbach syndrome)
- Painful bruising (autoerythrocyte sensitisation, Gardner–Diamond syndrome)
- Stigmata

The assessment of traumatic ecchymoses may be important in suspected non-accidental injury of children or adults.

Unlike purpura, increased intravascular blood in the skin can be blanched by pressure, typically using diascopy. Not all telangiectatic lesions can be emptied in this way. Small angiomas (e.g. in angioma serpiginosum or multiple minute Campbell de Morgan spots) and angiokeratomas may cause confusion [10]. Observation over several days may be necessary. Capillary microscopy or dermoscopy may help determine whether blood is intravascular or extravascular.

Classification of purpura

An aetiological classification of purpura is provided in Box 99.1.

A simple pathogenetic classification of purpura can divide mechanisms of extravascular bleeding into three groups:
1 Simple haemorrhage.
2 Inflammatory haemorrhage.
3 Occlusion/ischaemia.

Simple haemorrhage presents as non-inflammatory purpuric macules (Box 99.2), or as subcutaneous haemorrhage palpable as a haematoma. Inflammatory causes of haemorrhagic lesions usually evolve with increasing erythema in the first 24–36 h, along with increasing purpura. Palpable purpura syndromes may uncommonly produce lesions with retiform or stellate patterning, with accompanying early erythema. By 48 h, erythema and palpability begin to fade in both types of lesions, although the purpura may persist for several days. By contrast, occlusion/ischaemia usually begins with minimal or no erythema and is not usually palpable unless eschar forms. Erythema may develop if necrosis induces a wound healing response. Occlusive syndromes tend to manifest retiform or branching patterns of purpura (non-inflammatory retiform purpura), sometimes with accompanying localised livedo reticularis, or as necrotic plaques with minimal erythema.

PURPURA DUE TO THROMBOCYTOPENIA OR PLATELET DEFECTS

Thrombocytopenia

Platelets are an essential component of the haemostatic process. Thrombocytopenia or abnormal platelet function from any cause may therefore produce purpura or a bleeding tendency [**1**,2,3,**4**,5–8,**9**].

Box 99.2 Diagnosis of macular non-retiform haemorrhage/petechiae/ecchymosis by size

Lesions <4 mm
- Thrombocytopenia:
  - Immune thrombocytopenic purpura
  - Thrombotic thrombocytopenic purpura
  - Disseminated intravascular coagulation (DIC)
  - Other causes (see Box 99.3)
- Abnormal platelet function:
  - Congenital/hereditary
  - Acquired: drug, systemic disease
  - In myeloproliferative disease
  - Other causes (see Box 99.3)
- With normal platelets:
  - Raised intravascular pressure
  - Trauma
  - Scurvy (perifollicular pattern)
  - Hypergammaglobulinaemic purpura (Waldenström)

Intermediate-sized lesions
- Hypergammaglobulinaemic purpura (Waldenström)
- Infection in patients with thrombocytopenia or immune compromise
- Early lesions of vasculitis (sometimes)

Lesions >1 cm (all involve a degree of minor trauma)
- Procoagulant defect:
  - Anticoagulation
  - Liver failure
  - Vitamin K deficiency
  - Disseminated intravascular coagulation (DIC) (some)
- Poor dermal support:
  - Actinic and corticosteroid purpura
  - Scurvy
  - Hereditary (Ehlers–Danlos syndrome)
  - Amyloidosis
- Platelet deficiency or functional defect
- Other causes:
  - Hypergammaglobulinaemic purpura (Waldenström)
  - Capillaritis
  - Easy bruising syndrome, purpura simplex
  - Physical and artefactual causes
  - Gardner–Diamond syndrome
  - Stigmata

Platelets exposed to damaged endothelium adhere to one another, collagen and other subendothelial components. Complex interactions occur, involving von Willebrand factor and its glycoprotein receptor, various integrin adhesion molecules, thrombospondin, fibronectin, laminin, phospholipases and adenosine diphosphate released from damaged cells, as well as collagen and platelets. Platelet activation causes the release of serotonin and thromboxane A_2, which cause vasoconstriction, and increases platelet adhesiveness and aggregation leading to platelet plug formation. This process is aided by the presence of plasma fibrinogen and thrombin. The production of prostacyclin, a powerful vasodilator and inhibitor of platelet aggregation, is decreased because of endothelial damage. Developing platelet plugs are reinforced by fibrin strands formed due to activation of the plasma clotting system by platelet factor 3, exposed by alterations in the surface characteristics of aggregated platelets.

Purpura due to platelet defects can be divided into three groups, the second and third of which are discussed in this chapter:
1. Thrombocytopenia, i.e. decreased platelet numbers.
2. Abnormalities of platelet function.
3. Thrombocytosis, i.e. increased platelet numbers.

Abnormalities of platelet function

There are several haemorrhagic syndromes with abnormal platelet function, although the total count may be normal [1,2–4,5,6]. These may be inherited, idiopathic or secondary to drugs or other illnesses, including thrombopathia, thrombasthenia, von Willebrand disease, severe anaemia, chronic renal failure and fibrinogen defects. Hermansky–Pudlak syndrome consists of a bleeding diathesis due to storage pool disorder, with oculocutaneous albinism and pigment-containing cells in the bone marrow [6].

Drugs that may cause abnormal platelet function with clinical bleeding include those listed in Box 99.3 [3,4,5].

Thrombocytosis

Abnormally high platelet counts may be due to essential thrombocythaemia or other myeloproliferative disorders, or secondary to a variety of other disease processes (Box 99.3). This may lead to platelet plugging and thrombosis or, paradoxically, to a bleeding tendency (particularly when the platelet count exceeds $1000 \times 10^9/L$ with a clonal platelet defect such as in storage pool disease). Many cases of thrombocytosis do not have this high platelet count and are unlikely to cause purpura, unless there are additional reasons related to the causative disorder (such as lymphoma or other malignant disease).

Box 99.3 Platelet disorders causing purpura

Thrombocytopenia
- Defective platelet production:
  - Bone marrow abnormality:
    - Aplasia: toxic, immunological, idiopathic
    - Neoplasia: leukaemia, myeloma, carcinomatosis
    - Replacement: myelofibrosis, radiation damage, sarcoidosis
  - Other impaired production: Wiskott–Aldrich syndrome, vitamin B_{12} or folate deficiency
  - Metabolic: uraemia, alcohol, drugs
  - Infections
- Diminished platelet survival:
  - Platelet alloantibodies:
    - Neonatal
    - Post-transfusion
    - Antilymphocyte globulin
  - Platelet autoantibodies:

- Idiopathic (immune) thrombocytopenic purpura
- Marrow transplant
- Antiphospholipid antibodies
- Systemic lupus erythematosus
- Mechanical: prosthetic heart valves
- Drugs and vaccines
- Infections, sepsis syndrome
- Excessive platelet consumption:
  - Disseminated intravascular coagulation
  - Haemangioma (Kasabach–Merritt)
  - Hereditary haemorrhagic telangiectasia ('mini-Kasabach–Merritt')
  - Thrombotic microangiopathies:
    - Haemolytic–uraemic syndrome
    - Thrombotic thrombocytopenic purpura
- Sequestration:
  - Splenomegaly
  - Hypothermia

Abnormal platelet function
- Inherited and congenital:
  - Von Willebrand disease and defects of the platelet von Willebrand factor receptor
  - Hereditary haemorrhagic telangiectasia (often with platelet dysfunction too)
  - Bernard–Soulier disease (GpIb/IX/V receptor defect with low platelet count)
  - GpIa deficiency
  - Glanzmann thrombasthenia (GpIIb/IIIa deficiency)
  - MYH9-related disorders (e.g. May–Hegglin abnormality)
  - α-granule disorders
  - Dense granule (δ-granule) disorders (Hermansky–Pudlak syndrome, Chediak–Higashi syndrome, storage pool disease)
  - Abnormalities of signal transduction pathways
  - Membrane phospholipids abnormalities (e.g. Scott syndrome)
  - Wiskott–Aldrich syndrome (δ-granule abnormality) and X-linked thrombocytopenia (WASP gene mutations)
- Drug-induced (almost any drug may occasionally cause purpura but some more common causes listed):
  - Aspirin
  - P2Y12 platelet receptor antagonists (clopidogrel, cangrelor, ticagrelor, prasugrel)
  - Selective prostacyclin (IP) receptor antagonists (selexipag)
  - Phosphodiesterase 3 inhibitors (cilostazol, dipyridamole, milrinone, amrinone)
  - Glycoprotein IIb/IIIa antagonists (abciximab, eptifibatide, tirofiban)
  - Protease-activated receptor antagonist (vorapaxar)
  - Non-steroidal anti-inflammatory drugs (NSAIDs)
  - Some penicillin and β-lactam antibiotics (especially high-dose penicillin)
  - Some cardiovascular drugs (nitrates, calcium channel blockers, quinidine)
  - Tricyclic antidepressants and phenothiazines
  - Some chemotherapeutic agents (mitomycin and daunorubicin)
  - Volume expanders (dextran or hydroxyethyl starch)
  - Radiocontrast media
  - Fibrinolytic agents (e.g. streptokinase, alteplase)
  - Agents that increase platelet cAMP levels (iloprost or prostacyclin)
  - Natural and herbal remedy agents including fish oil, garlic, cumin, turmeric, Gingko biloba and black tree fungus
- Uraemia

- Cardiac bypass
- Platelet antibodies:
  - Idiopathic (immune) thrombocytopenic purpura
  - Systemic lupus erythematosus/antiphospholipid syndrome
- Myeloproliferative disorders
- Dysproteinaemias (especially IgA myeloma and macroglobulinaemia)
- Cold-stored (blood bank) platelets

Thrombocytosis
- Essential thrombocythaemia
- Other myeloproliferative syndromes
- Medical diseases and other causes:
  - Blood loss, trauma, burns
  - Post-splenectomy
  - Malignant disease
  - Tuberculosis
  - Sarcoidosis

Dermatological manifestations and associations of thrombocythaemia include purpura with or without necrosis, livedo reticularis, acrocyanosis, purple (blue) toe syndrome, Raynaud phenomenon, erythromelalgia, other vascular symptoms including gangrene, and associated disorders such as pyoderma gangrenosum [1,2–6,7]. Many of these presentations are also seen in other hyperviscosity and dysproteinaemic conditions.

Platelet hyperreactivity is not usually a dermatological consideration, but it is a factor in peripheral arterial disease and thrombotic emboli [8]. It may be more common in females, who have higher mean platelet levels [9].

NON-THROMBOCYTOPENIC VASCULAR CAUSES OF PURPURA AND SYNDROMES OF PRIMARY ECCHYMOTIC HAEMORRHAGE

RAISED INTRAVASCULAR PRESSURE

Gravitational purpura. Gravity and venous stasis commonly cause purpura due to raised intravascular pressure. Many dermatoses on the lower leg, especially in the elderly, can become purpuric due to a combination of gravitational changes with vascular damage. Rapid development of lower leg oedema may cause eczema with purpura [1].

Acroangiodermatitis. Acroangiodermatitis (of Mali, or pseudo-Kaposi sarcoma) may mimic a pigmented purpuric dermatosis, but the purpura is due to abnormal vasculature and not capillaritis. Occuring more often in men than in women, it is associated with venous insufficiency or with vascular anomalies such as Klippel-Trenaunay syndrome. It may occur as a stump dermatosis in amputees [2], and it has been linked with a thrombophilic prothrombin mutation [3].

Acroangiodermatitis lesions occur mainly on the lower legs but may extend onto the dorsa of the feet and toes, and over dilated varicosities on the thighs. Individual minute purpuric macules may coalesce to form irregular plaques, which may be several centimetres in diameter. Follicular lesions may occur. The colour is not usually the purple of fresh purpura but varying shades of yellow (ochre) and brown from haemosiderin and other breakdown products. The epidermis may be normal or show mild eczematous changes. Oedema, sclerosis, ulceration and other signs of venous insufficiency may be associated but may be entirely absent even in cases of long duration.

Differential diagnosis includes gravitational eczema, Schamberg disease and Kaposi sarcoma. CD34 antigen stains perivascular spindle cells in Kaposi sarcoma but only the endothelial cells in acroangiodermatitis [4].

Treatment for acroangiodermatitis is unsatisfactory but support hosiery seems logical.

Exercise-induced purpura. Exercise-induced purpura is common. Histologically, it is a form of leukocytoclastic vasculitis [5]. There may be coexisting venous disease. The typical presentation of exercise-induced pin point purpura, which may resemble capillaritis or be urticarial, is on the lower legs after prolonged standing or exercise (many descriptions are in golfers, clubbers or festival goers after dancing, marathon runners or long-distance walkers), often worse in hot weather. It may occur in all ages and has been described in a child with recurrent purpura on the trunk after vigorous exercise [6]. Compression stockings may help exercise-induced purpura.

ABNORMAL OR DECREASED SUPPORT OF BLOOD VESSELS

Several disorders are associated with abnormal collagen, elastic or other structural proteins, leading to abnormal vessels and/or poor dermal support (Table 99.1). Examples are Ehlers–Danlos syndrome (collagen), pseudoxanthoma elasticum (elastic) and amyloidosis (abnormal protein).

Actinic purpura. Actinic purpura (also known as Bateman purpura or senile purpura) is the most common purpura due to lack of support in blood vessels [1,2]. It occurs in skin altered by both age and solar radiation and may occur in premature ageing syndromes. Damage to the connective tissue of the dermis by sun exposure results in decreased support for blood vessels. Minor, often unnoticed, trauma leads to purpuric macules, commonly on the forearms, hands, face and neck. These resolve after 1–3 weeks sometimes with residual hyperpigmentation. Further damage is reduced by clothing or sunscreen with UVA and UVB protection [3]. Topical retinoids may help.

Corticosteroid purpura. Corticosteroid purpura due to topical, oral, endogenous (Cushing syndrome) or inhaled corticosteroids [4] is common and may coexist with actinic purpura, with a similar presentation. Macular purpura occurs after minor trauma in atrophic skin, often on the hands, forearms or legs. Usually asymptomatic,

Table 99.1 Some dermatologically relevant non-thrombocytopenic causes of purpura, easy bruising or cutaneous bleeding.

Type of disorder	Examples
Inherited defects affecting structural components of the dermis and/or vascular wall	Ehlers–Danlos syndrome[a]
	Marfan syndrome[a]
	Osteogenesis imperfecta
	Pseudoxanthoma elasticum
Acquired defects affecting structural components of the dermis and/or vascular wall	Deposition disorders, e.g. amyloidosis[b]
	Solar damage (solar/actinic purpura)
	Scurvy
Haemangiomatous disorders	Cavernous haemangioma[b]
	Hereditary haemorrhagic telangiectasia[a,b]
Clotting factor and related inherited or acquired deficiencies	Haemophilias
	Von Willebrand disease
	Vitamin K deficiency
	Other nutritional deficiencies (often mixed)
Non-thrombocytopenic platelet abnormalities	See Box 99.3
Biochemical (congenital or acquired)	Homocystinuria
	Hyperhomocystinaemia[a,b]
	Diabetes
	Cushing syndrome
Connective tissue disorders	Systemic sclerosis
	Dermatomyositis
Paraproteinaemias and hyperviscosity	Waldenström macroglobulinaemia[a]
	Other paraproteinaemias[a]
Intra- or perivascular inflammation	Capillaropathies
	Vasculitides
	Behçet disease
	Many inflammatory dermatoses
Microvascular occlusion	See section 'Disorders of cutaneous microvascular occlusion' later
Infection	Septicaemia, measles, meningococcal infections
Increased pressure within vessels	Valsalva manoeuvre
	Cough purpura
	Distal to a sphygmomanometer cuff
	Non-accidental injury (self-induced or external)
Physical	Simple trauma
	Venous rupture (Achenbach syndrome)
	Artefactual
	Chemical and mechanical contact irritants
Drugs	Drugs altering vascular permeability or causing direct endothelial damage
	Antiangiogenic drugs
Others	Malignant hypertension
	Autoerythrocyte sensitisation

[a] May also have platelet dysfunction.
[b] May also have clotting factor abnormalities.

lesions vary in size from a few millimetres to several centimetres; they may be linear or have a geometric shape. There is no inflammation, the lesions are usually dark purple, persist for several weeks and may leave residual hyperpigmentation.

Paroxysmal finger haematoma. Also known as Achenbach syndrome, paroxysmal finger haematoma is more common than the number of reported cases suggests [5]. It may be confused with Raynaud phenomenon or acute connective tissue diseases and investigated unnecessarily [6]. In paroxysmal finger haematoma

PART 9: VASCULAR DISORDERS

there are recurrent episodes of painful bruising on the palms and palmar aspects of the fingers. The syndrome probably represents venous rupture, due to frictional trauma.

Scurvy. In scurvy, altered collagen for the blood vessels causes either petechiae, especially on the legs, or small or large bruises on the limbs following mild trauma [7]. Large, deep bruises may lead to woody induration, usually of the legs. Perifollicular purpura is typical but is not diagnostic and frequently absent. Diagnosis is established by the associated symptoms and signs (twisted 'corkscrew' hairs, gingival bleeding), dietary history, laboratory tests and therapeutic response.

Physical and artefactual bleeding

Definition and nomenclature
This is bruising due to trauma.

> **Synonyms and inclusions**
> - Black heel and palm
> - Talon noir
> - Calcaneal petechiae

Introduction and general description
Bruising due to trauma may be revealed by taking a good history, except when it occurs as an artefact or in elder or child abuse. Bizarre patterns of purpura may be caused by suction, for example vacuum extractors in the neonate, electrocardiogram leads or around the mouth after sucking out the air from a glass [1]. Cultural remedies such as cupping, coin rubbing (Cao Gio) and spooning (Quat sha) produce unusual patterns of purpura [2]. Black heel (talon noir) is a form of purpura due to frictional shearing of vessels. It is pigmentation of the heel (or palm) secondary to extravasation of red blood cells [3].

Epidemiology
Incidence and prevalence
Black heel and palm is common and can occur in athletic people of any age or sex. Football, basketball, tennis and squash players are often affected. The condition can occur on the hands of weightlifters.

Pathophysiology
Pathology
In black heel, extravasated erythrocytes may be found in the dermal papillae [1]. In older lesions, the histological changes are limited to the stratum corneum, where amorphous yellow-brown material may be found in rounded collections having undergone transepidermal elimination. This material is often negative with Perls' (haemosiderin) stain but gives a positive benzidine reaction, showing that it is from haemoglobin [4].

Clinical features
History
Black heel or palm results from shear–stress rupture of papillary capillaries, for example during athletic sport where repeated jumping and sudden stopping or twisting occur. In abuse, an empathetic approach and evidence gathering from other sources may help to explain recurrent unexplained traumatic lesions.

Presentation
In black heel or palm, loosely aggregated groups of bluish black specks occur suddenly at the back or side of the heel just above the hyperkeratotic edge of the foot or palm. The metatarsal area is rarely involved. The lesion may resemble a tattoo or a melanoma [5]. Abuse should be considered when atypical purpuric lesions possibly due to gripping, trauma or shaking are seen.

Differential diagnosis
When there is sudden appearance of the pigmented lesions at a typical site after activity, diagnosis of black heel and palm is rarely in doubt. Viral warts can produce a similar appearance due to red cell extravasation, but skin surface is abnormal. Melanoma or atypical melanocytic hyperplasia [6] may sometimes need to be excluded.

Investigations
With black heel, the patient and physician can usually be reassured by carefully paring the affected stratum corneum, removing the abnormality. There are specific features on dermoscopy and epiluminescence microscopy [7].

Management
The condition is usually asymptomatic, and its importance lies in its resemblance to melanoma. When in doubt, carefully paring may remove the pigment.

Dysproteinaemic and Waldenström hypergammaglobulinaemic purpura

Definition and nomenclature
A syndrome with essential features of purpura with polyclonal hypergammaglobulinaemia. Descriptions in the literature appear to represent a collection of different diseases producing these end features. In time the term may be dropped or refined as it is probably not a specific entity.

> **Synonyms and inclusions**
> - Benign hypergammaglobulinaemic purpura

Introduction and general description
Waldenström hypergammaglobulinaemic purpura was first described in 1943, in three women with chronic relapsing purpura, hypergammaglobulinaemia, an elevated erythrocyte sedimentation rate (ESR) and mild anaemia [1]. Purpura may be the presenting and only symptom. It has been described at exposed skin sites in cryoproteinaemia and may occur due to monoclonal hypergammaglobulinaemia in myeloma. In such instances there may be platelet dysfunction, but clinical bleeding is usually related to the hyperviscosity syndrome rather than to the altered platelet function.

Epidemiology

Age

In younger patients, Waldenström hypergammaglobulinaemic purpura may be thought to be primary. Over time many patients manifest an underlying disease.

Pathophysiology

Predisposing factors

Waldenström hypergammaglobulinaemic purpura was originally thought to imply an idiopathic phenomenon but in fact two of Waldenström's three cases had sicca symptoms, one with sarcoidosis [1]. Waldenström is linked with sarcoidosis, lupus erythematosus, Sjögren syndrome and other autoimmune conditions [2,3,4]. Some patients have positive antinuclear antibody and anti-SSA (Ro) or anti-SSB (La) antibodies [5]. It has been associated with severe infective lung disease with a poor prognosis. Other associations include arthropathy, renal tubular acidosis, lymphopenia and immune hypersensitivity pneumonitis.

Pathology

Hypergammaglobulinaemic purpura is usually polyclonal with a high presence of specific circulating immune complexes containing IgG or IgA rheumatoid factor. Histologically, lesions may be characterised by simple haemorrhage, or by mild perivascular lymphocytic infiltrate or leukocytoclastic vasculitis [6,7].

Causative organisms

A high antigenic load due to chronic lung infection may be a cause of hypergammaglobulinaemic purpura.

Clinical features

Presentation

Hypergammaglobulinaemic purpura is characterised by recurring crops of petechiae and larger purpuric macules, which commonly burn or sting. It may appear suddenly, mainly affects the lower legs, and is exacerbated by prolonged standing or by tight garments or footwear. Other cutaneous features of paraproteinaemia include various patterns of vasculitis, neutrophilic dermatosis, cryoglobulinaemia, urticaria and systemic capillary leak syndrome, abnormalities of lipid metabolism (such as diffuse plane xanthomatosis), subcorneal pustular dermatosis, scleromyxoedema, amyloidosis, and features due to hyperviscosity (purpura, mucous membrane bleeding, retinopathy and neurological disturbance) [8,9].

Differential diagnosis

The condition may be due to many underlying disorders which should be considered. In palpable purpura one should consider cutaneous small-vessel vasculitis (Chapter 100).

Complications and co-morbidities

The complications and co-morbidities of all possible underlying conditions (as described earlier) should be considered.

Disease course and prognosis

This depends on any underlying disease. In some, hypergammaglobulinaemic purpura can be primary, where lesions usually resolve in about a week, or may become confluent and permanent. The disease may be secondary to many underlying conditions with consequent variable prognosis.

Investigations

Laboratory evaluation typically reveals polyclonal hypergammaglobulinaemia and an elevated ESR. Specific tests for IgG and IgA rheumatoid factor may be performed. Where anti-Ro (SS-A) and anti-La (SS-B) antibodies are present, this may indicate a higher likelihood of developing an associated autoimmune connective tissue disease [5]. Other tests for associated conditions should be guided by clinical findings.

Management

In the benign form, treatment may not be required for Waldenström hypergammaglobulinaemic purpura. However, if underlying disease is present this will require specific treatment. There have been descriptions of the use of prednisolone, NSAIDs, hydroxychloroquine and etamsylate (ethamsylate). Support stockings may help or exacerbate symptoms, depending on the underlying cause. Avoidance of prolonged standing may help. Where the disease is secondary, treatment should be targeted at the underlying disease.

PIGMENTED PURPURIC DERMATOSES

Five main morphological variants of idiopathic pigmented purpuric dermatosis exist [1,2,3,4,5,6–9]:

1 Schamberg disease (about 50% of cases).
2 Itching purpura (eczematid-like purpura of Doucas and Kapetanakis) (about 10%).
3 Pigmented purpuric lichenoid dermatosis of Gougerot and Blum (about 5%).
4 Lichen aureus (about 10%).
5 Purpura annularis telangiectodes (Majocchi disease) (about 5%).

Variations of these may contain granulomatous histology or be segmental. Favre–Chaix purpura is associated with pigmentation, oedema, cyanosis and sclerosis of the lower limb and is a manifestation of venous disease. About 20% of cases are unclassifiable [2] and many drugs, systemic diseases or local skin inflammation in the setting of venous hypertension may lead to localised, mild purpura with haemosiderin deposition and secondary melanin pigmentation [6].

Pigmented purpuric dermatosis

Synonyms and inclusions
- Capillaritis
- Purpura progressiva pigmentosa

PART 9: VASCULAR DISORDERS

Introduction and general description

The pigmented purpuric dermatoses are a set of diseases, characterised by capillaritis [7]. They are usually benign and of unknown aetiology, but have rarely been described secondary to underlying disorders. Distinctive pupuric lesions occur with petechial haemorrhage (or extravasation or erythrocytes in the skin with marked haemosiderin deposition). The term 'purpura simplex' is best avoided because it has been applied to this group of disorders but also to other mild, unexplained and morphologically different patterns of purpura such as easy bruising.

Epidemiology

Incidence and prevalence

Schamberg disease is the most common form, occurring in around 50% of cases. Other conditions are rare, while granulomatous pigmented purpura is extremely rare.

Age

Adults are mainly affected. Schamberg disease is seen rarely in children, while linear pigmented purpura can occur in children and adolescents, and purpura annularis telangiectodes occurs in adolescents and young adults, especially women [1,8].

Sex

Schamberg disease is most often seen in middle-aged to older men, as are itching purpura and pigmented purpuric lichenoid dermatitis of Gougerot and Blum.

Pathophysiology

Predisposing factors

The identification of pigmented purpuric dermatoses secondary to a systemic cause is discussed later. Gravity and increased venous pressure are important localising factors. Exercise may be a provoking factor.

Pathology

There is inflammation and haemorrhage of capillaries and other superficial papillary dermal vessels. There is no association with coagulation abnormality.

These disorders are characterised by narrowing of the lumen and endothelial swelling of superficial small vessels, accompanied by perivascular T-lymphocytic infiltration, extravasation of erythrocytes and haemosiderin deposits in macrophages. An appearance termed 'ectasising endocapillaritis' has been reported in a study which divided 22 cases into those that were papular (with an upper dermal bandlike infiltrate), macular (with a perivascular infiltrate) or eczematous (with exocytosis and spongiosis) [6], but this has not improved understanding. The cellular infiltrate contains CD4+ T cells in close contact with CD1a+ Langerhans cells [7], suggesting cell-mediated immune mechanisms. Strong expression of the endothelial cell adhesion molecules ICAM-1 (intercellular adhesion molecule 1) and ELAM-1 (endothelial cell leukocyte adhesion molecule 1) may determine the pattern of the infiltrate [7]. Immune complex deposition has been reported but

direct immunofluorescence is usually negative. An IgA-associated lymphocytic vasculopathy was described in six cases with clinical and histological features of a pigmented purpuric dermatosis [7] who had a preceding or associated condition: viral infection, Henoch–Schönlein purpura, undifferentiated connective tissue disease, lupus erythematosus profundus, Degos disease and Buerger disease, suggesting a non-specific reaction pattern to a variety of triggers.

Clinical features

Presentation

The key characteristics of pigmented purpuric dermatoses are clusters of petechial haemorrhages. The background is often yellow-brown from haemosiderin deposition; brown or black in darker skin. Each subtype has a particular morphology and location (Table 99.2).

Differential diagnosis

Differential diagnoses include stasis dermatitis, fixed drug eruption, contact dermatitis and purpura secondary to haematological disorders. The petechial haemorrhage of lesions may lead to misdiagnosis of thrombocytopenia or vasculitis.

Complications and co-morbidities

These dermatoses are typically asymptomatic with no systemic findings. Pruritus is prominent in itching purpura.

Disease course and prognosis

Most are chronic, but two-thirds may improve or clear eventually [5].

Investigations

Histology can be helpful but may not be necessary in uncomplicated asymptomatic cases. Usually, no further investigations are necessary.

Management

Consider medication causes and try discontinuing for several months. Some try avoiding food preservatives and artificial colouring agents for several months.

Lesions may clear spontaneously, but they may persist for many years and are resistant to therapy. Explanation without active intervention, or support hosiery, is often the best approach. Topical corticosteroids may be of some help for itch, but prolonged use is best avoided. Emollients can help itching. A rapid response of lichen aureus to topical pimecrolimus has been reported [1]. Psoralen and UVA (PUVA) has proven effective in treating capillaritis of Schamberg, Gougerot–Blum and lichen aureus patterns [10]. Narrow-band UVB (TL01) has been reported to help Schamberg disease [5] and Gougerot–Blum pigmented purpuric lichenoid dermatitis [1]. Ciclosporin has been effective in individual reports [8].

Table 99.2 Presentation of different pigmented purpuric dermatoses.

Syndrome	Clinical features	Location
Schamberg disease	Orange-red flat patches with 'cayenne pepper' spots on the borders	Usually lower legs; also involves trunk, arms, thighs and buttocks
	Old lesions become yellow-brown patches	
	Oval or irregular outline pinpoint petechiae inside patches	Irregularly distributed on both sides with few or many patches
	Successive crops	
Itching purpura	Pruritic, scaly petechial or purpuric macules, papules and patches	Usually lower extremities
	Appears similar to Schamberg disease	
Pigmented purpuric lichenoid dermatosis of Gougerot and Blum	Combination of Schamberg-like and purpuric red-brown lichenoid thickened papules	Usually lower extremities
	Chronic, can be pruritic	
Lichen aureus	Isolated, persistent patch	Usually lower extremities
	Varying colour, purple-brown to golden or rust	Commonly overlies a varicose vein
Purpura annularis telangiectodes (Majocchi disease)	Annular brown plaques, 1–3 cm in size	Trunk, lower extremities (proximal)
	Plaques gradually spread outwards	
	Punctuate telangiectases and petechiae inside border	
Contact allergy	Scaling, erythema, vesicles	Only affects skin in contact with material responsible (e.g. clothing dye, rubber)
Exercise-induced	Crops of small red spots following prolonged or vigorous exercise	Commonly on ankles
	Fade to brown and disappear within days	
	Possible burning sensation accompanies new lesions	

DISORDERS OF CUTANEOUS MICROVASCULAR OCCLUSION

Platelet plugging: heparin necrosis

Definition and nomenclature

There are two types of heparin-induced thrombocytopenia (HIT). Type I is a benign condition, not due to immune factors, with a mild, transient reduction in platelets. HIT type II is an autoimmune condition leading to low platelet counts and blood clotting. This occurs in 1–5% of patients, usually 5–10 days after starting heparin. HIT usually refers to type II heparin-induced necrosis. Ulceration related to heparin may be due to other mechanisms causing heparin-induced necrosis [1]. A similar process to HIT has been postulated as a cause of sometimes life-threatening thrombosis after Covid-19 vaccinations.

Synonyms and inclusions

- Heparin-induced thrombocytopenia syndrome with heparin-reactive antibodies
- Heparin-induced thrombocytopenia associated thrombosis
- Heparin-associated thrombocytopenia with thrombosis (HATT) syndrome

---

Introduction and general description

Heparin necrosis may occur after subcutaneous or intravenous heparin administration. It is a rare but important iatrogenic syndrome first described in the 1970s. HIT is characterised by platelet factor 4 (PF4)/heparin-reactive antibodies (HIT antibodies). In 90% of patients with HIT there is an absolute or relative thrombocytopenia and evidence of venous or arterial thrombosis with heparin necrosis in the skin [2].

Incidence and prevalence

Heparin-induced thrombocytopenia is an uncommon response to heparin and occurs in 1–5% of adults exposed to heparin, with up to 30% of these developing subsequent thrombosis [3]. In children on intensive care units the incidence of thrombosis was 2.3%.

Sex

F > M [4].

Pathophysiology
Predisposing factors

Unfractionated heparin is three times more likely to trigger HIT than low-molecular heparin and is more common with bovine-derived unfractionated heparin than the porcine variety [2]. It is caused by an antibody, which binds to PF4 tetramers, platelet surface proteins.

HIT is more common in postsurgical patients requiring heparin than in medical and obstetric settings [2].

Pathology

Heparin necrosis is usually mediated by IgG [5], although IgA and IgM antibodies may play a role. These antibodies can be directed at heparin and other polyanions when bound to tetrameric PF4, exposing new epitopes. This may trigger further antibody production. Antiheparin/PF4 antibodies bind with heparin/PF4 complexes on the surface of platelets resulting in platelet activation and aggregation. Other antibodies associated with HIT bind to chemokines or cytokines, including neutrophil-activating peptide-2 (NAP-2) and interleukin 8, leading to platelet activation [2,5,6].

Clinical features
History

People with HIT often develop an absolute or relative thrombocytopenia (90%) with venous or arterial thromboses or heparin necrosis in the skin [2]. A better indicator of early heparin-induced platelet aggregation is a proportional drop of over 50% in platelet number from the pre-treatment count rather than an absolute thrombocytopenia of $100–150 \times 10^9/L$ [2]. If heparin has been received within the past 10 days, this may occur immediately on administration. However, two-thirds of patients have a fall in platelet count 5–10 days after heparin administration, with significant thrombocytopenia taking up to 7–14 days to develop. Occasionally, HIT may develop several days after stopping heparin therapy (delayed-onset HIT). A history of HIT does not necessarily predict a second episode if there has been over 100 days between treatments.

Presentation

Cutaneous findings include haemorrhage with echymoses and occasionally urticaria or infiltrated plaques [7]. Rarely there is cutaneous microvasular occlusion. Some cases present with sharply demarcated, purpuric, tender plaques, with marginal retiform extensions, accompanied by erythema. These lesions are most common at subcutaneous injection sites (Figure 99.1), although they can occur elsewhere, and often develop between day 5 and day 10 of heparin therapy [8]. Patients already sensitised to heparin may develop heparin necrosis much earlier. There is a subset of delayed-onset heparin necrosis, which may take up to 3 weeks.

Differential diagnosis

People on heparin may develop thrombocytopenia for other reasons, while patients without thrombocytopenia may develop arterial or venous thromboses [2]. A history as to whether heparin has been given is therefore very important in patients who develop retiform purpura or bland necrosis, with or without thrombocytopenia.

Management

Stopping heparin is important. Substituting heparin with warfarin can lead to venous limb gangrene. Low-molecular-weight heparin is much less likely to cause HIT but may be contraindicated in patients with HIT due to other types of heparin.

If patients with a previous history of HIT have not received heparin within 100 days, their antibodies may disappear, allowing them to be retreated with heparin. The anticoagulants used to treat HIT are typically a direct thrombin inhibitor such as argatroban or bivalirudin in people undergoing percutaneous coronary intervention [9].

Platelet plugging: thrombocytosis

Introduction and general description

Thrombocytosis can be due to essential thrombocythaemia (ET) linked to a myeloproliferative disorder or polycythaemia vera (PV) [1]. However, transient thrombocytosis is a common finding with a wide range of primary and secondary causes such as infection.

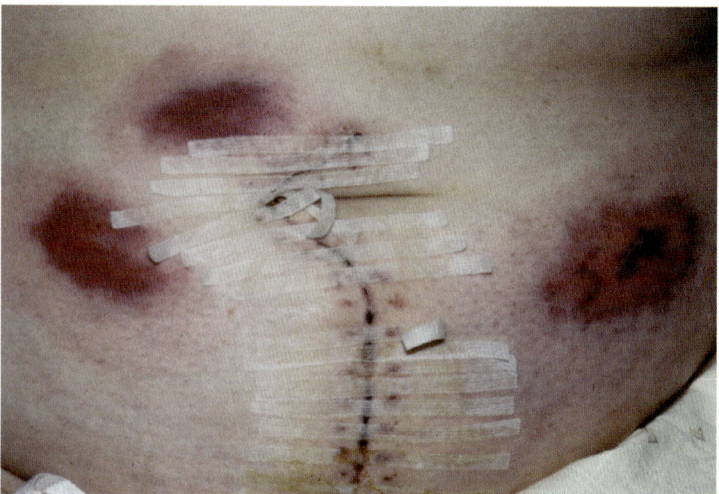

(a)

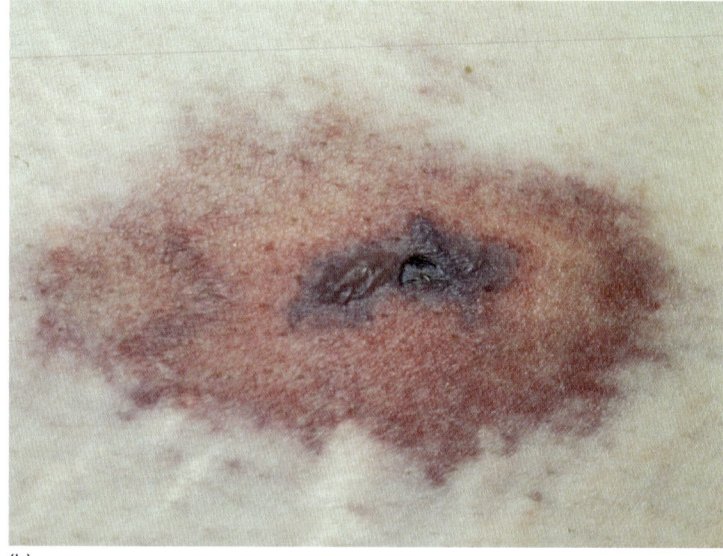

(b)

Figure 99.1 (a) Heparin necrosis at sites of subcutaneous heparin injection. (b) Close-up of a 15 cm lesion on the left abdomen. The lesion is a non-palpable haemorrhage with retiform margins, minimal erythema and central retiform-intense haemorrhage, early necrosis and bullae formation. From Robson and Piette 1999 [**11**]. Reproduced with permission of Elsevier.

Epidemiology

Incidence and prevalence

ET and PV are rare but are the first and second most common causes of persistent elevated platelet counts, with an increased frequency of thrombotic events and of erythromelalgia [2]. ET has a 14% risk of thrombosis over 10 years [3].

Pathophysiology

Reactive or post-splenectomy thrombocytosis at any level is not associated with blood vessel occlusion, suggesting that thrombosis in the setting of myeloproliferative disease is not a function of thrombocytosis alone. JAK2, CALR or myeloproliferative leukaemia mutations are found in 90% of patients with ET and JAK2 mutations in all with PV [4].

Predisposing factors

Acquired von Willebrand factors in myeloproliferative disease have been associated with both bleeding and thrombotic complications. Anticardiolipin antibodies, factor V Leiden mutations, abnormal endothelial cell function, and decreased levels of protein C and protein S may be synergistic for thrombosis in chronic myeloproliferative diseases [5,6]. In addition to high platelet counts, abnormal platelet function occurs in myeloproliferative or myelodysplastic disease, although whether this can lead to vascular occlusion at platelet counts of fewer than 1000×10^9/L is controversial. Thrombotic events have been reported at platelet counts of below 600×10^9/L in patients with essential thrombocytosis, including some events in those with normal platelet counts [7].

Pathology

PV causes elevation of haemoglobin, haematocrit and red cell mass. All syndromes may show elevations in white cell count, but this is characteristic of chronic granulocytic leukaemia, especially in association with elevated eosinophil and basophil counts. Biopsy findings are variable, but livedo reticularis and acral infarcts may be associated with microvascular occlusion.

Clinical features
Presentation

Cutaneous lesions are common in ET and other myeloproliferative disorders. Paradoxically, patients with myeloproliferative thrombocytosis may both bleed and clot abnormally. Skin lesions in 22% of 268 people with ET [8] included urticaria, livedo reticularis, petechiae, ecchymoses, haematomas, erythromelalgia, Raynaud phenomenon, recurrent superficial thrombophlebitis, necrotising vasculitis, leg ulceration and gangrene. Tender erythematous facial plaques and palmar violet macules and papules were reported as manifestations of platelet plugging in atypical chronic myeloproliferative disease with a history of Budd–Chiari syndrome, another known thrombotic complication of myeloproliferative disease [9]. Ruddy cyanosis is characteristic of PV.

Erythromelalgia can occur as a primary or secondary syndrome. This intensely uncomfortable burning associated with paroxysmal erythema of the distal extremities can be triggered by skin contact with a warm surface. The association of purpuric or necrotic areas on the hands and feet with dysaesthetic erythema is seen with myeloproliferative or myelodysplastic thrombocytosis [10].

Complications and co-morbidities

People with ET and PV have a higher risk of thrombotic complications [1]. Anaemia and altered red cell morphology can occur over time, and these diseases may progress to dyspoiesis, severe anaemia, leukaemia or myelofibrosis. Splenomegaly may be seen in all forms of myeloproliferative syndromes.

Disease course and prognosis

Median survival is 14 years for PV and 20 years for ET. In PV, there are two risk categories for thrombosis: high (age over 60 or history of thrombosis) and low (absence of both risk factors). In ET, thrombosis risk increases with age over 60, JAK2 mutation and history of thrombosis. Leukaemic transformation rates at 10 years are estimated to be less than 1% for ET and 3% for PV [4].

Investigations

The diagnosis of ET requires a sustained thrombocytosis with platelet counts of greater than 400×10^9/L, with the exclusion of reactive causes. The blood film will show thrombocytosis with platelet anisocytosis. There may be an elevated white blood cell count. Bone marrow examination remains the basis of diagnosis for PV and ET supported by genetic testing.

Management

Therapy in both PV and ET aims to prevent thrombotic and haemorrhagic complications. People with PV receive phlebotomy to keep the haematocrit below 45% and aspirin. Low-risk ET is given aspirin. Cytoreductive therapy is recommended for high-risk ET and PV using hydroxyurea first line with second line interferon α or busulfan. Ruxolutinib, a selective JAK1 and JAK2 inhibitor, can help PV with severe and protracted pruritus or marked splenomegaly [4].

Because of the platelet origin of occlusion and vascular symptoms in thrombocythaemic erythromelalgia, aspirin administration may be effective in clearing lesions and alleviating burning pain, whereas it is much less effective in primary and other secondary forms of erythromelalgia.

Cryogelling/cryoagglutination disorders

Introduction and general description

Disorders of cryogelling or cryoagulation, due to type 1 cryoglobulins, cyrofibrinogen or cold agglutinins (uncommon), are occlusive syndromes in the skin triggered by cold exposure.

Cryoglobulins are immunoglobulins that reversibly precipitate or gel in the cold. They were first reported in 1933 and named cryoglobulins in 1947 [1,2,3,4]. In 1974, Brouet et al. [1] proposed the classification of cryoglobulins into types I, II and III. Type I (single molecule) cryoglobulins are single monoclonal immunoglobulins. Types II and III, termed mixed cryoglobulins, are multiple molecule proteins, typically immune complexes, that gel under laboratory conditions (2–4°C). Cryofibrinogen deposits consist of a complex of fibrinogen, fibrin and fibronectin that forms on cold exposure [5].

Cold agglutinins are immunoglobulins that can agglutinate red blood cells below normal body temperatures.

Although the precipitation of cryoglobulins is primarily related to reversible cold-induced denaturation of protein, other factors such as cryoglobulin concentration in the microvascular environment, pH and non-covalent binding factors also influence the likelihood and intensity of precipitation.

Epidemiology
Incidence and prevalence

Type I account for 10–15% of cryoglobulins. Cryofibrinogens and cold agglutinins are rarely the cause of occlusive syndromes triggered by cold exposure, despite being often detected in patients with various illnesses [6].

Age

The median age at diagnosis of cryoglobulinaemia is the early to middle sixth decade.

PART 9: VASCULAR DISORDERS

Sex
Female : male 2 : 1 [2].

Associated diseases
Type I cryoglobulins are often associated with an underlying lymphoproliferative disorder, especially multiple myeloma or Waldenström macroglobulinaemia [5]. Unless they gel at temperatures close to body temperature, type I and II cryoglobulins are much more likely to cause disease as immune complexes than as cryoproteins, but they can cause disease through either or both mechanisms in any given patient. Rheumatoid factor activity (defined by anti-Fc binding) is detectable in the sera of 87–100% of patients with mixed cryoglobulinaemia [3].

Antibodies to hepatitis C virus (HCV) have been found in more than 50% (42–98%) of patients with type II and III cryoglobulins [2,3,4]. Conversely, 13–54% of people with HCV have mixed cryoglobulins detected in the laboratory, and the majority of these are type III cryoglobulins (67–91%). Of HCV-infected individuals with cryoglobulins, only 27% had clinical signs consistent with the syndrome of cryoglobulinaemia [2]. The reasons why only a fraction of HCV-infected and cryoglobulin-positive people develop symptomatic cryoglobulinaemia are unknown.

Although type I cryoglobulinaemia is usually associated with lymphoproliferative disease, it is a much less common type than II and III. The latter two types account for the majority of cryoglobulinaemia-associated lymphoproliferative disease in regions with a high endemic rate of HCV and mixed cryoglobulinaemia [2].

Other syndromes are also associated with cryoglobulins detectable in serum. Patients with connective tissue disease have higher rates of cryoglobulinaemia, including patients with systemic lupus erythematosus (SLE), systemic sclerosis, active rheumatoid arthritis and Sjögren syndrome [2]. In addition to HCV, other chronic infections such as Lyme disease, subacute bacterial endocarditis, Q fever, hepatitis A and B, hantavirus, cytomegalovirus, human T-cell leukaemia virus I and HIV have been reported [2,7]. Chronic inflammatory disease, such as liver cirrhosis from any cause, is also associated with a higher-than-expected rate of detectable cryoglobulins.

Cryofibrinogenaemia may be idiopathic or can be associated with malignant disorders (especially haematological), thromboembolic disease, IgA nephropathy or various inflammatory, connective tissue or infectious syndromes including Covid-19 [8–10].

Monoclonal cold agglutinins are idiopathic or secondary to malignant lymphoproliferative diseases. Polyclonal cold agglutinins are usually associated with infection, especially due to *Mycoplasma pneumoniae*, and less often with HCV, parvovirus B19 or leptospiral infections.

Pathophysiology
Predisposing factors
The presence of cryoglobulins in serum does not invariably predict disease. In fact, despite detectable serum cryoglobulins in the patient groups mentioned, most will not develop symptomatic cryoglobulinaemia [2].

Pathology
Type I cryoglobulins are single monoclonal immunoglobulins, usually IgG or IgM, less commonly IgA, and rarely Bence–Jones protein.

Type II cryoglobulins are composed of monoclonal proteins of IgM, IgG or occasionally IgA class that bind to an antigen present in the blood, most commonly the Fc portion of polyclonal IgG molecules. Those that bind immunoglobulin (usually IgG) by anti-Fc affinity are also, by definition, rheumatoid factors, although only the IgM/anti-IgG rheumatoid factors are recognised by standard rheumatoid factor testing. In up to 95% of type II cryoglobulins with IgM as the antirheumatoid factor immunoglobulin, the IgM contains a κ light chain [3]. Type III mixed cryoglobulins are also most commonly rheumatoid factors, but the IgM, IgG or IgA anti-Fc antibodies in this group are polyclonal rather than monoclonal. In people with mixed type II and III cryoglobulins, complement levels are usually reduced, especially C4 component.

Acquired dysfibrinogenaemia may rarely mimic a cryofibrinogen syndrome by acral occlusion, including gangrene. This subset of dysfibrinogenaemia appears to act by greatly increasing red cell aggregation, mimicking occlusion-inducing cold agglutinins. Blood smear preparations show marked rouleaux formation.

In cases of cold agglutinin-related cutaneous occlusion, the agglutination of red blood cells depends on binding of antibody to more than one cell at a time. Pentavalent IgM is almost exclusively responsible for this phenomenon. As with cryoglobulins, there are both monoclonal and polyclonal cold agglutinins, usually directed at the I, i or Pr antigens of erythrocytes [11].

Clinical features
History
The patient will have undergone exposure to cold temperatures.

Presentation
Occlusion syndromes triggered by cold exposure are suggested by an acral distribution of lesions of necrosis or purpura, often with retiform features, and sometimes associated with acral livedo reticularis. An acral distribution must be distinguished from a dependent distribution of lesions. Both patterns may involve hands and feet, but with a dependent pattern there are typically many more lesions on the feet and legs than on the hands.

Recurrent showers of dependent palpable purpura, sometimes with burning or itching, frequently associated with arthritis or arthralgia, is the classic presentation of mixed (type II and III) cryoglobulinaemia (the combination of purpura, asthenia and arthralgia is termed Meltzer's triad). Patients with symptomatic cryoglobulinaemia of any type most often present with cutaneous lesions, usually purpura (in 55–100%, especially if HCV associated) [3,12]. Ulceration, haemorrhagic crusts or cutaneous infarction are seen in 10–25%, most often with type I cryoglobulins. Cold-induced acrocyanosis of acral areas and non-inflammatory retiform purpura are also more typical of type I cryoglobulinaemia. Other reported cutaneous findings include acral cyanosis, Raynaud phenomenon, urticarial lesions, ulceration and livedo reticularis [4,13].

Non-cutaneous clinical findings include involvement of the joints, peripheral nerves, kidneys and liver [2,3,4].

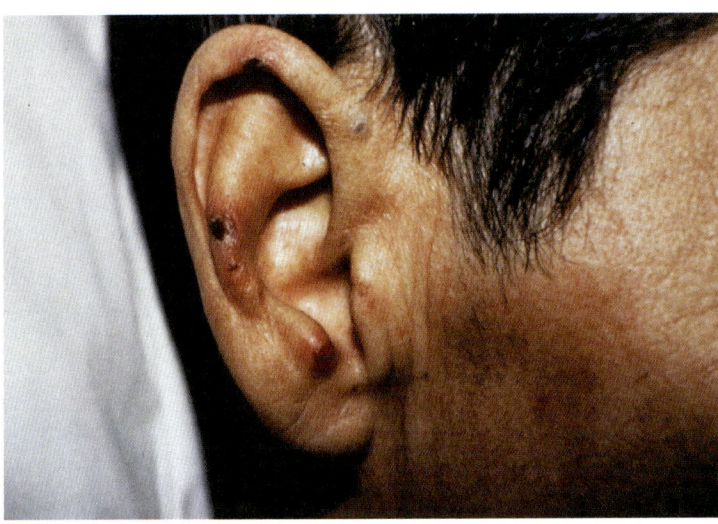

(a)

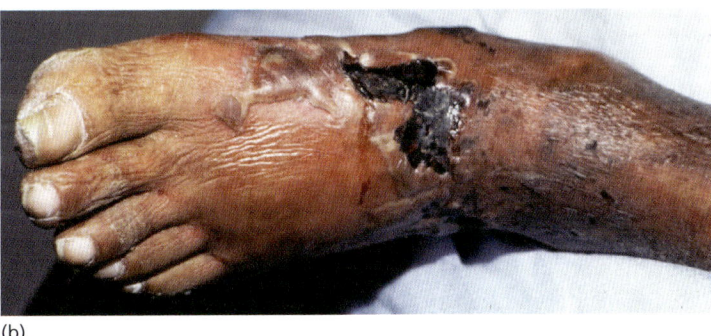

(b)

Figure 99.2 Cold-induced lesions due to cryofibrinogenaemia, (a) on the ear and (b) on the foot. An acral location is typical for cryogelling. The foot lesion shows minimal erythema, retiform bullae and haemorrhage with necrosis.

The most common cutaneous findings in cryofibrinogenaemia are cold intolerance, purpura, necrosis, livedo reticularis, gangrene and ulceration (Figure 99.2) [9,14]. The purpura, or necrosis, typically has a non-inflammatory retiform morphology. In 67% of Covid-19-related acral chilblain-like presentations, cryofibrinogens were detected [10].

Clinical variants
The acral distribution of cryo-occlusion syndromes often includes the ears and nose.

Differential diagnosis
A dependent distribution of lesions suggests immune complex-mediated disease that usually presents as palpable purpura or occasionally as inflammatory retiform purpura, not as non-inflammatory purpura or necrosis. Although an acral distribution is also characteristic of erythema multiforme, this presents with target lesions, atypical target lesions or classic palpable purpura, rather than livedo reticularis, non-inflammatory retiform purpura or necrosis. Chilbains usually develop slowly and rarely have acute purpura or necrosis [6].

Although ill, supine patients with immune complex vasculitis may develop dependent lesions on the posterior portions of the ears; their other lesions are typically in dependent areas as well, and cold exposure does not usually precipitate lesions.

Distal occlusion syndromes (cholesterol emboli, acral antiphospholipid antibody syndrome) may have a similar presentation but lack a history of cold exposure and lesions on the nose and ears.

Complications and co-morbidities
There are two ways in which cryoglobulins can result in disease. The first is by precipitation within the vascular lumen, typically cold induced, with hyaline plug formation and minor early phase inflammation. Typical clinical lesions are characterised by minimally inflammatory cutaneous infarction, with or without associated livedo reticularis, or non-inflammatory retiform purpura. Since there is little evidence that cryogelling of monoclonal antibody induces complement activation, cryogelling is the mechanism for vascular lesions for type I cryoglobulins [15]. The second mechanism is that of immune complex vasculitis. Nearly all type II and III cryoglobulins are immune complexes. Some may induce an immune complex vasculitis, although many do not. Those that cryoprecipitate near body temperature may cause vascular injury by simple occlusion, although most gel at temperatures well below 37°C. Cryofibrinogenaemia is common as a laboratory abnormality but rarely causes symptomatic clinical disease [16].

As with many cryoglobulins and most cryofibrinogens, cold agglutinins are most likely to be asymptomatic. When responsible for disease, reversible acrocyanosis secondary to cold-induced acral agglutination is most common. Livedo reticularis, Raynaud phenomenon, cold urticaria and rarely cutaneous necrosis may occur. In addition to acral lesions on environmental cold exposure, cold intravenous infusions can also trigger localised cutaneous necrosis [17]. Cold agglutinins can induce complement activation after cold-induced binding to red blood cells, followed by lysis and haemolytic anaemia, independent of occlusive syndromes from agglutination.

Investigations
A biopsy of early lesions less than 48 hours old, before necrosis has had time to trigger a secondary vasculitic histology, should show non-inflammatory occlusion of dermal vessels with cryoprotein or agglutinated red cells. Early lesions may show a mixture of erythema and purpura, partially blanching on pressure.

Careful handling of serum and plasma allows identification of cryogelling proteins because those most likely to cause disease gel at temperatures close to normal body temperature. The identification of cryoproteins or cryoagglutinins does not prove a cryo-occlusion syndrome, because these may either gel at temperatures that are not relevant to typical cold exposure or may simply represent incidental findings. The latter is especially true of cryofibrinogens and cold agglutinins [2,3].

Despite the presence of monoclonal protein, polyclonal gammopathy is the most frequent finding on serum protein electrophoresis of serum samples (not cryoprecipitate specimens) in patients with type II cryoglobulinaemia [2]. A more sensitive technique, such as immunofixation, is needed to identify the presence of a clonal protein.

Histological demonstration of non-inflammatory hyaline thrombosis is more common in patients with type I cryoglobulinaemia, but some patients have been reported to have cutaneous vasculitis, possibly due to biopsy of later lesions with secondary changes [12].

Since cryofibrinogens can be cleaved to form fibrin, plasma rather than serum must be tested to detect these cryogelling proteins. Cryoglobulins should be present in both plasma and sera [5,14]. Biopsy specimens from skin lesions typically show thrombi in small vessels with dermal necrosis [8]. Leukocytoclastic vasculitis has been reported, but is probably due to secondary ischaemic necrosis [9]. Fibronectin may be a major component of vascular plugs in patients with cryofibrinogenaemia alone, whereas vascular occlusion in patients with both cryofibrinogens and cryoglobulins shows a predominance of cryoglobulin deposition [9].

Management

Treatment of cryoglobulinaemia is often challenging. Prospective, controlled trials are rare [3,4]. If symptoms are mild, no treatment may be needed. If symptoms of acral lesions are precipitated by cold, then the protection of affected areas may be sufficient. Measures to reduce the concentration of a type I cryoglobulin, such as plasmapheresis, plasma exchange or cytotoxic therapy, are occasionally effective, but usually only in the short term. For immune complex-related disease, corticosteroids, cytotoxic agents or plasmapheresis may be effective, but relapse is typical once therapy is stopped. Interferon α has been used to treat HCV-associated cryoglobulinaemia, with or without ribavarin [3,4]. Treatment with these agents has resulted in partial or complete remissions of vasculitis, but relapse often follows cessation of therapy. The therapy itself may trigger vasculitis. In mixed cryoglobulinaemia with recurrent cutaneous vasculitic lesions, colchicine or dapsone may reduce frequency and severity of episodes.

Treatment of cryofibrinogenaemia should be aimed at the underlying disease, where possible, and at protection from cold exposure [18]. Stanozolol, an androgenic steroid with fibrinolysis-enhancing effects, has been used for treatment of cryofibrinogenaemia, as have other fibrinolytic androgenic steroids [19]. Those with cold-induced agglutination syndromes must avoid cold exposure. Therapies such as corticosteroids, cytotoxic agents, danazol, rituxan or interferon α have been occasionally beneficial [18].

ORGANISMS IN VESSELS

Cutaneous infections can produce purpuric lesions such as:
- Ecthyma gangrenosum, caused by *Pseudomonas aeruginosa* (Chapter 32).
- *Aspergillus* and *Mucor* fungal infections (Chapter 26).
- Disseminated strongyloides infection (Chapter 33).
- Lucio phenomenon (erythema necroticans) (Chapter 28).

EMBOLI

Cholesterol embolus

Definition and nomenclature

Cholesterol emboli resulting from the ulceration of arteriosclerotic plaques and the subsequent release of cholesterol crystals can cause disease of the skin, particularly in the lower extremities.

Synonyms and inclusions
- Blue toe syndrome

Introduction and general description

The most diagnosed cutaneous embolic syndrome is cholesterol embolus, which occurs secondary to fragmentation of ulcerated arteriosclerotic plaques, with distal cutaneous and visceral vessel obstruction.

Epidemiology

Incidence and prevalence

The incidence of cholesterol embolisation syndrome (CES) following vascular procedures has ranged from 0.15% to 30%, with large retrospective studies reporting figures of 0.6–0.9% [1,2]. Autopsy studies have shown cholesterol emboli in 77% of patients who underwent aortic aneurysm resection [2]. A prospective study of 1786 consecutive people aged over 40 years who underwent left heart catheterisation found an incidence of cholesterol embolus of 1.4% [1]. Patients with cutaneous findings (livedo reticularis, blue toe syndrome or digital gangrene) were considered to have definite CES. In-hospital mortality was 16% of those with CES and was associated with progressive renal dysfunction.

Age and sex

Cholesterol embolus is a syndrome reported primarily in men aged 50 years or older.

Associated diseases

Cholesterol embolus is associated with peripheral vascular disease and the known risk factors for atherosclerosis such as diabetes, hypertension and smoking [3]. Blue toe syndrome associated with warfarin use is a syndrome of cholesterol embolus and not of warfarin-induced skin necrosis.

Pathophysiology

Predisposing factors

Although cholesterol embolus may be spontaneous, known triggers include angiography, angioplasty, vascular surgery, intra-aortic pump placement, cardiopulmonary resuscitation (all inducing traumatic rupture of plaques, usually within hours or days), thrombolytic therapy (acute clot lysis in plaque with release of friable plaque within hours or days) and anticoagulation (slow reduction of clot with release of plaque fragments, usually after at least 2 months of therapy) [3,4].

Pathology

Histology shows the skin arterioles, usually at the dermal–subcutaneous junction, with elongated clefts and thrombi within small-vessel lumina [5]. The clefts result from fixation-related dissolving of cholesterol crystals. In experimentally produced cholesterol embolus, a mixed inflammatory infiltrate in the arterial walls occurs within 24–48 h, followed by multinucleated histiocytes within 3–6 days, and subsequent occasional intimal fibrosis.

Clinical features

Presentation

There are two 'classic' clinical triads of cholesterol embolus. The first comprises leg or foot pain, livedo reticularis and preservation of good peripheral pulses [4]. The second comprises livedo reticularis, renal insufficiency and eosinophilia [6]. Cutaneous findings in cholesterol embolus include livedo reticularis, gangrene, cyanosis, ulceration, nodules and purpura. Systemic findings include fever, myalgia, altered mental status, sudden-onset arterial hypertension, gastrointestinal ulceration and renal insufficiency that may progress to renal failure [4,6].

Investigations

Eosinophilia occurs in up to 80% of those with CES, possibly due to C5 complement [1,7]. Pre-procedure elevation in serum C-reactive protein has been associated with an increased risk of post-procedure CES [1]. There may be leukocytosis, thrombocytopenia, pyuria, eosinophiluria, blood-positive urine or stool, elevated values of ESR, creatinine, urea and amylase, and decreased serum levels of complement [3,7].

Management

The risk of further embolisation should be minimised (removal of remaining plaque or stenting of an atheromatous segment of a major vessel) to reduce end-organ damage. Aim to slow progression of atheromatous disease. Statins, iloprost (prostacyclin analogue), pentoxifylline (oxpentifylline) and steroids have limited success in minimising organ damage [2,8]. Limit anticoagulant use in known CES to reduce precipitation of further cholesterol emboli [2,9]. Some types of cardiac surgery that may precipitate CES also require postoperative anticoagulation [4,9].

Oxalate embolus, cardiac embolus and other emboli

Introduction and general description

Oxalate crystals are a rare cause of emboli but can mimic the cutaneous findings of cholesterol embolism. Primary (type I) hyperoxaluria is rare but the most common cause of oxalate crystal embolus. Atrial myxomas, marantic endocarditis and septic endocarditis are associated with cutaneous emboli. Fat emboli can produce petechiae, which may be few or very numerous [1].

Clinical features

Presentation

Primary hyperoxaluria oxalate crystal embolisation causes livedo reticularis, acrocyanosis, peripheral gangrene, purpura or ulcers [2]. Secondary hyperoxaluria, especially when due to long-term dialysis, causes extravascular cutaneous deposits of oxalate, producing calcified cutaneous nodules, or firm miliary papules often on the palmar aspect of the fingers [3].

Constitutional symptoms of atrial myxomas may mimic those of infectious endocarditis, connective tissue disease, vasculitis or rheumatic fever, with fever, malaise, arthralgia or weight loss.

Obstruction of intracardiac blood flow may mimic valvular disease and emboli may occur.

Lentigines may be a cutaneous finding in the hereditary NAME (naevi (meaning birthmarks or moles), atrial myxoma, myxoid neurofibromas and ephelides (freckles)) or LAMB (lentigines, atrial and mucocutaneous myxomas and multiple blue naevi) syndromes, which are associated with cardiac myxomas.

Cutaneous findings of myxomatous emboli include livedo reticularis, splinter haemorrhages, Raynaud phenomenon, an acral papular eruption with claudication, serpiginous or annular purpuric lesions of the fingertips, red-violet malar flush, petechiae of hands and feet, or toe necrosis [4].

Marantic endocarditis results in the attachment of fibrin vegetations to heart valve leaflets, like those seen in acute rheumatic endocarditis and Libman–Sacks (antiphospholipid syndrome) valve disease, and these vegetations can embolise [5]. Infective endocarditis can also produce emboli from vegetations, but these are usually associated with acute bacterial endocarditis. Cutaneous lesions in subacute bacterial endocarditis may be from either emboli or immune complex-related vasculitis. Idiopathic hypereosinophilic syndrome is associated with intracardiac mural thrombi, which can produce emboli [6] causing splinter haemorrhages, non-blanching livedoid discoloration, necrotic, blistering or purpuric lesions [7].

Crystal globulin vasculopathy is rare and usually associated with IgG or light-chain paraproteins, which can produce intravascular occlusion by spontaneous crystallisation [8]. This results in rapidly progressive renal failure, polyarthropathy, peripheral neuropathy and skin lesions. Cutaneous lesions include ulcers, petechiae, ecchymoses, with intravascular thrombus and crystalline deposits [9].

Investigations

Histology can confirm myxomatous emboli but finding the emboli may require serial sectioning and multiple biopsies [4,5]. An echocardiogram is useful.

Systemic coagulopathies: protein C/ protein S-related disease including warfarin necrosis and purpura fulminans

Synonyms and inclusions

- Warfarin-induced skin necrosis: severe acquired protein C deficiency which may exacerbate inherited protein C or rarely protein S deficiency
- Neonatal purpura fulminans: homozygous protein C or protein S deficiency
- Sepsis-related purpura fulminans with disseminated intravascular coagulation: acquired severe protein C deficiency and acquired severe protein S dysfunction
- Idiopathic or postinfectious purpura fulminans: protein S deficiency

Introduction and general description

Several systemic coagulopathies have a predilection for the cutaneous microvasculature. Cutaneous lesions may be a minor feature of a multiorgan syndrome, a prominent finding of multiorgan involvement or the sole target of occlusion. Recognising these syndromes is critical to begin early, and sometimes syndrome-specific, therapy.

The term 'purpura fulminans' has been used by physicians for three different situations. It was originally coined in 1887 to describe a syndrome occurring days to a few weeks after some preceding infection, especially varicella-zoster or streptococcal infections (now termed idiopathic 'postinfectious purpura fulminans') [1]. The term purpura fulminans has subsequently been used for widespread cutaneous haemorrhage in patients with sepsis triggered disseminated intravascular coagulation (DIC), including infection with *Neisseria meningitidis*, *Staphylococcus aureus*, groups A and B β-haemolytic streptococci, *Streptococcus pneumoniae*, *Haemophilus influenzae* and *H. aegyptius* [2]. The term neonatal purpura fulminans describes a disease seen in neonates due to homozygous or complicated heterozygous protein C or protein S deficiency.

Epidemiology
Incidence and prevalence
The frequency of homozygous protein C deficiency causing neonatal purpura fulminans is estimated at 1 in 250 000–500 000 births [3]. Sepsis-induced purpura fulminans is the most common type seen in around 10–20% of people with meningococcal septicaemia. Idiopathic, postinfectious purpura fulminans is very rare.

Age
The peak incidence of warfarin-induced skin necrosis is between the sixth and seventh decades. Neonatal purpura fulminans occurs in the first 5 days of life. Sepsis or idiopathic purpura fulminans can occur at any age [2,4].

Sex
Female : male 4 : 1.

Homozygous deficiency of either protein C or protein S is associated with cerebral and ophthalmic vessel thrombosis.

The most common associated infections in cases of postinfectious purpura fulminans are varicella-zoster and *Streptococcus*. This syndrome has been associated with lupus anticoagulant activity and with autoantibodies to protein S [2,4].

Pathophysiology
Predisposing factors
Two natural anticoagulant pathways exist in humans. The antithrombin III–heparin/heparan pathway is important for primarily venous large-vessel thrombosis. The only cutaneous lesions related to antithrombin III disorders are stasis ulcers secondary to recurrent venous thrombosis with venous insufficiency. By contrast, disorders of the thrombomodulin–protein C/S anticoagulant pathway are important causes of severe cutaneous occlusion syndromes.

The end point of the coagulation cascade is the conversion of prothrombin to thrombin, which catalyses the conversion of fibrinogen to fibrin and clot formation. When thrombin fails to bind to procoagulant sites on membranes and binds instead to the membrane protein receptor thrombomodulin, this powerful prothrombotic molecule undergoes a transformation. Bound to thrombomodulin, thrombin becomes ineffective at binding and

activating clotting factors, and instead rapidly converts protein C in the plasma to activated protein C. Activated protein C, stabilised by certain phospholipids and by protein S, downregulates clotting by cleaving circulating activated clotting factors, including factor VIIIa and factor Va, thus it exerts an anticoagulant effect. Therefore, deficiency of protein C, or of its co-factor protein S, creates a procoagulant tendency.

Protein C and S deficiencies can be inherited autosomally with variable penetrance. Homozygous deficiency leads to neonatal purpura fulminans. People who are heterozygous for the deficiency may develop repeated venous thrombosis or pulmonary embolism early in adult life or may be asymptomatic [1]. One variable affecting thrombosis risk in protein C and S deficiencies is co-inheritance of homozygous or heterozygous factor V Leiden mutations [5,6].

The factor V Leiden mutation is present in 5% of UK and North American populations. This reduces cleavage of the factor V Leiden molecule by activated protein C (APC resistance). Activated factor V Leiden remains longer in the plasma enhancing coagulation. In some groups of protein C-deficient families, the additional presence of the factor V Leiden mutation predicts those who develop large-vessel thrombosis in individuals with similar levels of protein C deficiency.

The risk of warfarin necrosis is increased if loading doses (10 mg or more) of warfarin are used and if a second form of anticoagulation such as heparin therapy is not used to cover the initial phase of anticoagulant therapy [7].

The therapeutic effect of warfarin is due to inhibition of γ-carboxylation of the vitamin K-dependent coagulant factors II, VII, IX and X. Although these factors are still in plasma, without γ-carboxylation they are dysfunctional. Protein C and protein S are also vitamin K-dependent plasma factors affected by warfarin, and their inhibition can lead to a prothrombotic state. Protein C and factor VII, with half-lives of roughly 5 h, are particularly vulnerable to early inhibition, whereas protein S and the remaining procoagulant factors with much longer half-lives remain active for a considerably longer period [7]. There is thus a period after administration of warfarin when the anticoagulant effect of protein C has been inhibited and there is an excess of uninhibited procoagulant clotting factors. Although up to one-third of patients with warfarin-induced skin necrosis may have partial protein C deficiency, most cases appear unrelated to inherited deficiencies of protein C [8].

Clinical features
Presentation
Retiform (stellate) purpura and necrosis result from thrombosis within the cutaneous microvasculature. In neonatal pulmina fulminans, skin lesions typically begin within a few hours to 5 days after birth, and on the extremities, abdomen, buttocks and scalp; they may localise to sites of pressure or previous trauma [3,9].

Warfarin necrosis usually presents as the sudden onset of cutaneous pain 3–5 days after beginning warfarin therapy, followed by well-demarcated erythema progressing to haemorrhage, necrosis and often haemorrhagic bullae or eschar [10]. Warfarin necrosis may rarely involve acral areas, but acral cutaneous purpura in patients on warfarin is more likely to be due to cholesterol embolus (see earlier) – so-called purple (blue) toe syndrome. Warfarin necrosis is commoner in areas with more fat, such as the breast, hip, buttocks and thigh [8,10].

Cutaneous microvascular occlusion in sepsis with DIC presents clinically as non-inflammatory (bland) haemorrhage, usually with a retiform, stellate or branching configuration, with rapid transition to necrosis and eschar [11,12].

Differential diagnosis
Haemorrhage in patients with DIC may be due to septic vasculitis, simple bleeding or microvascular thrombosis. The patterns of cutaneous haemorrhage for each of these different mechanisms are distinctive and can be a guide to pathophysiology and therapy [13].

Disease course and prognosis
In the absence of appropriate therapy, warfarin necrosis and skin lesions in purpura fulminans can progress to full-thickness cutaneous necrosis.

Investigations
Laboratory findings in sepsis purpura fulminans are consistent with DIC, with evidence of the consumption of clotting factors (prolonged partial thromboplastin time, PTT), clot lysis (elevated fibrin split products) and often thrombocytopenia.

Early biopsy of retiform purpuric lesions showed microvascular occlusion with fibrin, and perivascular haemorrhage with minimal to no inflammation; these findings correlated with severe protein C deficiency [12]. This was not true of other forms of purpura in sepsis with DIC.

Management
Warfarin skin necrosis is managed by stopping warfarin. Heparin can be used for anticoagulation in the short term if this is essential. If there is severe or life-threatening coagulation, then protein C concentrates can be helpful. The areas of skin necrosis may require skin grafting.

All forms of purpura fulminans require adequate hydration and supportive care to reduce end organ damage. Treatment of neonatal purpura fulminans is with fresh frozen plasma to replace deficient protein C or S, or protein C concentrates. Management of idiopathic or postinfectious purpura fulminans is similar.

In adult sepsis-related purpura fulminans, early antibiotic treatment of the infective agent is essential. IVIg and activated protein C may be given. Anticoagulation is dependent on the presence of DIC [14–18].

Systemic coagulopathies: antiphospholipid antibody/lupus anticoagulant syndrome

Introduction and general description
Another major cluster of systemic coagulopathies with cutaneous microvascular occlusion are those related to lupus anticoagulant activity and antiphospholipid syndrome (APLS) (Chapter 51). APLS (Hughes syndrome), continues to be redefined [1], most recently by the addition of anti β_2-glycoprotein I (β_2-GPI) antibodies to the laboratory criteria for diagnosis (Box 99.4) [2].

Box 99.4 Criteria for antiphospholipid antibody syndrome (definitive diagnosis requires at least one clinical and one laboratory criterion) [2]

Clinical criteria
- Vascular thrombosis: one or more clinical episodes of arterial, venous or small-vessel thrombosis
- Complications of pregnancy:
  - One or more unexplained deaths of morphologically normal fetuses at or after 10 weeks of pregnancy *or*
  - One or more premature births of morphologically normal neonates at or before 34 weeks of gestation *or*
  - Three or more unexplained consecutive spontaneous pregnancy losses before 10 weeks of gestation

Laboratory criteria
- Anticardiolipin antibodies, IgG or IgM, present at moderate or high levels on two or more occasions at least 12 weeks apart
- Lupus anticoagulant antibodies on two or more occasions at least 12 weeks apart
- Anti β_2-glycoprotein I (>99th centile) antibodies on two or more occasions at least 12 weeks apart

---

Antiphospholid antibodies (aPL) bind to $\beta2$GPI on cell surfaces. The binding activates endothelial cells, monocytes and platelets, and leads to proinflammatory, prothrombotic changes and complement activation [2]. This leads to thrombosis. There is neutrophil involvement with tissue factor (TF) expression and neutrophil extracellular traps. Rapamycin target (mTOR) upregulation on endothelial cells may contribute to the aPL-related vasculopathy. Prothrombotic effects include acquired protein C resistance, TF pathway inhibitor inhibition and inhibition of tissue plasminogen inhibitor [3].

Epidemiology
Incidence and prevalence
APLS may occur as a primary or secondary disorder. In one study, primary APLS comprised 53% of cases, lupus-associated APLS 36%, lupus-like APLS 5% and other disease associations with APLS 6%, with catastrophic APLS occurring in 0.8% of cases [4].

Age
In a large study the mean age was 42 ± 14 years at study entry, and the onset of symptoms was most often in young to middle-aged patients (2.8% before age 15 years, 12.7% after age 50) [4].

Sex
Female : male 4 : 1 [4].

Associated diseases
Compared with primary syndrome patients, those with lupus APLS are more likely to have arthritis, livedo reticularis, thrombocytopenia or leukopenia [4].

Pathophysiology

Predisposing factors

Precipitating factors include infections, surgical procedures, drugs and the discontinuation of anticoagulation.

Pathology

β_2-GPI (apolipoprotein H) has five domains and binds anionic phospholipids as part of the physiological disposal of apoptotic cells [5]. Infections (such as leprosy, leishmaniasis, leptospirosis) may trigger anti β_2-GPI antibodies, as may childhood atopic eczema. These antibodies may differ from those that trigger thrombosis by binding to domain V of the β_2-GPI molecule, rather than to the domain I region of the thrombogenic subset [6]. Infection-related antibodies, especially in leprosy, are more often IgM than IgG type. IgM and IgA anti β_2-GPI and anticardiolipin antibodies are seldom implicated in thrombotic events, except in cerebral stroke. IgG antibodies to β_2-GPI are the most likely to be thrombogenic [7].

Clinical features

Presentation

APLS can present with a variety of cutaneous findings (Box 99.5) [8]. Livedo is common but is not specific since this and retiform purpura or necrosis occur in other microvascular occlusion disorders [10]. In one study, the frequency of these findings was livedo reticularis 24%, leg ulcers 5.5%, pseudovasculitis 3.9%, digital gangrene 3.3%, cutaneous necrosis 2.1% and splinter haemorrhages 0.7% [4]. Thrombosis may lead to swollen red ears [9] (Figure 99.3).

Box 99.5 Cutaneous findings in the antiphospholipid antibody syndrome

- Livedo reticularis, with or without retiform purpura or retiform necrosis
- Sneddon syndrome (this may be a subgroup of antiphospholipid syndrome)
- Livedoid vasculopathy/atrophie blanche
- Raynaud phenomenon
- Anetoderma-like lesions with thrombosis
- Behçet-like lesions
- Nailfold ulcers
- Widespread cutaneous necrosis (catastrophic antiphospholipid antibody syndrome)
- Leg ulcers, secondary to recurrent thrombosis with stasis, or from conditions in this list
- Cholesterol embolus-like proximal livedo reticularis, with or without distal retiform purpura
- Acral livedo
- Degos (malignant atrophic papulosis)–like lesions
- Pseudo-Kaposi sarcoma
- Vasculitis-like lesions
- Pyoderma gangrenosum-like ulcers
- Splinter haemorrhages
- Superficial thrombophlebitis migrans

Clinical variants

Catastrophic APLS is an uncommon variant with widespread cutaneous necrosis and multiorgan failure, especially renal and pulmonary.

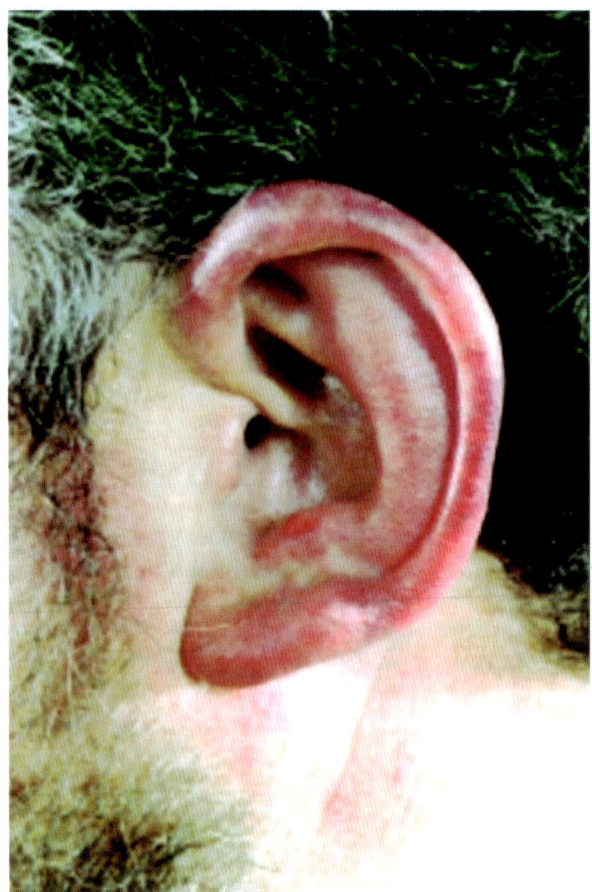

Figure 99.3 Thrombosis producing bilateral swollen red ears in antiphospholipid syndrome. Reproduced from O'Gradaigh et al. [9] with permission from BMJ Publishing Group Ltd.

Common extracutaneous manifestations of APLS include deep-vein thrombosis, pulmonary embolus, central nervous system abnormalities and pregnancy loss.

Investigations

Serological markers are usually detected as antibodies against phospholipids (especially cardiolipin) in combination with antigens from a co-factor molecule (e.g. β_2-GPI, prothrombin, annexin V, plasmin, tissue plasminogen activator, thrombin), or as an inhibitor of an *in vitro* coagulation test. The detection of antiphospholipid antibodies is roughly five times more common than the detection of lupus anticoagulant [10].

Mechanisms of coagulation in APLS are most often detected as anti β_2-GPI antibodies, lupus anticoagulant or antiphospholipid antibodies. The lupus anticoagulant activity is detected, often incidentally, by prolongation of the activated partial thromboplastin time (aPTT), the dilute Russell viper venom time (dRVVT) or the kaolin clotting time [7]. Activation of the intrinsic pathway can be tested by either aPTT or kaolin clotting time and direct activation of factor X (dRVVT).

Antiphospholipid antibody activity is detected by one of several antibody assays, the most common being enzyme-linked immunosorbent assay screens for IgG or IgM antibody affinity for cardiolipin, a negatively charged phospholipid molecule found in mitochondrial membranes.

Management

Thrombotic and pregnancy complication risk is assessed using antibody characteristics and other clinical factors. Definitions of 'high risk' vary, but generally include lupus anticoagulant with or without high-titre anticardiolipin or anti β_2-GPI autoantibodies. IgG autoantibodies are more thrombogenic than IgM or IgA. EULAR management recommendations [11] for APLS define high risk by the presence of multiple antibodies with high titres. Pregnancy morbidity risk assessments consider autoantibodies and history of thrombosis, diagnosis of SLE, elevated homocysteine, lower age, low complement and abnormal uterine artery Doppler velocimetry [2].

Asymptomatic APLS without underlying lupus may be left untreated. Low-dose aspirin therapy is of uncertain benefit but may be given to those with a high-risk profile. Most people after APLS-provoked venous or arterial thrombosis receive acute and often long-term anticoagulation. This is with either standard or low-molecular-weight heparin initially followed by warfarin [5]. Studies of DOACS (direct oral anticoagulants) to date have not showed benefits. Antimalarial therapy may help atrophie blanche-like or Degos-like syndromes in lupus patients; evidence suggests a protective effect in lupus patients against arterial or venous thromboses [1]. There is evidence that hydroxychloroquine may interfere with the binding of IgG–β_2-GPI complexes on phospholipid bilayers or to a line of cultured human monocytic leukaemia cells, which may provide some rationale for possible prophylactic benefit in APLS for high-risk patients [12]. Inconclusive data suggest a possible role for statins in high-risk patients [2].

VASCULAR COAGULOPATHIES

Sneddon syndrome

Introduction and general description

This syndrome comprises livedo racemosa with cerebrovascular lesions that cause focal neurological symptoms or signs [1,2,3,4,5]. Livedo racemosa is usually the first manifestation, initially affecting the lower trunk and proximal part of the legs but becoming more generalised. Livedo racemose (or broken livedo) has a network pattern with breaks producing incomplete circles in places (Figure 99.4). Associated Raynaud phenomenon or acrocyanosis may occur, and may be the presenting feature [1,2]. Various conditions, including APLS, may produce this presentation and have been reported as Sneddon syndrome, but Sneddon syndrome is thought to be a specific genetic disorder or group of disorders. In an affected family with three siblings with Sneddon syndrome a compound heterozygous mutation in the CECR1 gene segregated those with the condition [6].

Epidemiology
Incidence and prevalence

This may be confused by overlap with other conditions such as APLS or SLE but has been estimated at four cases per million people per year [3], and it is usually sporadic, although familial Sneddon syndrome has been reported.

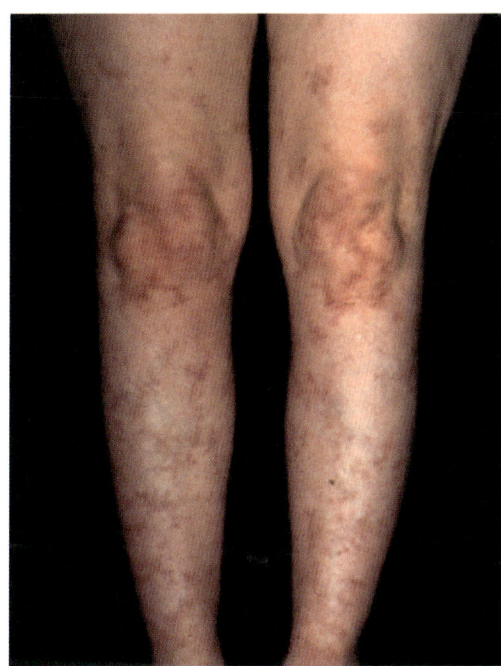

Figure 99.4 Sneddon syndrome showing a typical, broad, racemose livedo patterning.

Age

Sneddon syndrome typically presents in the fourth or fifth decade of life.

Sex

Female : male 2 : 1.

Pathophysiology

The CECR1 gene produces adenosine deaminase 2, which when blocked produces changes in endothelial cells triggering coagulation. The presence of antinuclear antibodies or of antiphospholipid antibodies/lupus anticoagulant has been reported [4], but probably represents APLS with a higher risk of seizures, mitral regurgitation and thrombocytopenia [5]. Reported cases reflect a spectrum of disease from APLS to SLE. Antiprothrombin antibodies were demonstrated in 57% of 46 patients in one series [7], and there are reports of platelet activation in a patient with persistently elevated levels of circulating PF4 [8] and increased levels of antithrombin III [9], factor V Leiden mutation [10] and activated protein C resistance [11]. In the future, genetic testing should clarify this condition.

Pathology

As a range of conditions have been reported as Sneddon syndrome, not surprisingly the reported histology is variable. Biopsies may show an endarteritis of dermal arterioles. The most informative biopsies are from the clinically normal centre of any network area rather than from the peripheral 'watershed' area of livedo, and taking multiple biopsies increases the sensitivity [12]. Initial changes are endothelial swelling with a mixed inflammatory infiltrate, progressing to vascular plugging, subendothelial proliferation and eventual vascular occlusion, fibrosis and disappearance of the inflammatory component [13].

Clinical features

Presentation

In addition to the cutaneous livedo, there may be non-specific neurological prodromal symptoms such as headache, migraine, dizziness or vertigo. Transient ischaemic attacks are reported more often than completed stroke [14].

Clinical variants

This represents various diseases reported as Sneddon syndrome. Peripheral nerves may be affected and hypertension present, sometimes aggravated by pregnancy or the use of oral contraceptives. There may be renal or cardiac involvement, including valve defects such as mitral regurgitation, although internal organ involvement other than neurological is often asymptomatic [3]. Other features such as shortened digits have been reported.

Differential diagnosis

The differential diagnosis is wide, including other causes of livedo and microvascular occlusion syndromes as well as vasculitis (e.g. polyarteritis nodosa). Other patterns of livedo with anticardiolipin antibodies are associated with cerebral microthrombosis such as livedo with summer ulceration or livedo with pyoderma gangrenosum [15].

Disease course and prognosis

Later neurological features include focal paresis or hemiparesis, focal sensory or hemisensory symptoms, fits and visual defects, and later cognitive changes. Hypertension confers a worse prognosis if untreated.

Investigations

Genetic testing should take place. Magnetic resonance imaging (MRI), electroencephalography and arteriography may help to confirm the neurological component; skin biopsy (as earlier) and exclusion of other causes of livedo are necessary. Cases with positive antiphospholipid antibodies more commonly have infarcts in the distribution of the main cerebral arteries on MRI, whereas those with negative antibodies have small lacunar infarcts [16] and progressive leukoencephalopathy [14].

Management

There is no very effective treatment, reflecting the non-inflammatory nature of the disease. There is no good evidence for corticosteroids or other immunosuppressives to which response may be difficult to assess, due to the intermittent nature of the neurological disease. The avoidance of smoking and oral contraceptives, and treatment of hypertension, hyperlipidaemia and diabetes, are important. Thrombolytic agents and vasodilators have been used in acute situations, and antiplatelet agents may be effective in some cases [5].

Livedoid vasculopathy/atrophie blanche

Synonyms and inclusions

- Livedo reticularis with summer ulceration
- Segmental hyalinising 'vasculitis'

Introduction and general description

This syndrome can be either an idiopathic or secondary syndrome [1]. It is the association of persistent painful ulceration of the lower limbs with atrophie blanche and livedo racemosa (broken livedo). Any vasculitis changes are secondary to blood vessel occlusion. Cases described are probably due to a range of underlying disorders including APLS leading to vessel occlusion in the setting of venous hypertension. Cutaneous vasculitis can cause similar clinical appearances [2].

Epidemiology

Differential diagnosis

The porcelain white skin changes of atrophie blanche associated with chronic venous hypertension and varicosities of any cause are a common finding, but are not preceded by small painful ulcerations, nor with surrounding livedo reticularis. Common venous stasis-related atrophie blanche is distinct from other forms of the syndrome.

Pathophysiology

The pathogenesis of livedoid vasculopathy is thought to be various causes of blood vessel occlusion in the setting often of venous hypertension. APLS can produce this syndrome [3]. Abnormalities implicated include platelet activation, factor V Leiden, altered fibrinolysis, antiphospholipid antibodies and hyperhomocystinaemia [1,3,4,5]. In one series of 32 patients, heterozygous factor V Leiden mutation was found in 2 of 9 patients tested (22%), decreased protein C or protein S activity in 2 of 15 (13%), prothrombin G20210A mutation in 1 of 12 (8%), lupus anticoagulant in 5 of 28 (18%), anticardiolipin antibodies in 8 of 29 (29%) and elevated homocysteine levels in 3 of 21 (14%) [6], suggesting a clinical syndrome with many possible causes.

Pathology

The most characteristic histological findings are thickening or hyaline changes in the walls of superficial dermal vessels, and luminal fibrin deposition [1,7]. Red cell extravasation and perivascular lymphocytic infiltrates are expected findings. In a series of 45 skin biopsies from 32 patients, all but one showed intraluminal thrombus and direct immunofluorescence was positive in 86% [6].

Clinical features

Presentation

Persistent, very painful and often punched-out ulcerations of the legs, especially around the malleoli, in women are typical of atrophie blanche [7] (Figure 99.5). The disease is bilateral in most cases. When accompanied by surrounding livedo reticularis, the term 'livedoid vasculitis' has been incorrectly applied. Retiform or stellate purpura or ulcer extension can occur. Healing results in a porcelain-white scar, frequently surrounded by telangiectasia – the characteristic appearance of atrophie blanche. Besides venous hypertension and antiphospholipid antibody-related syndromes, sickle cell ulcers can show the same porcelain-white scar of atrophie blanche.

Investigations

A skin biopsy may be helpful.

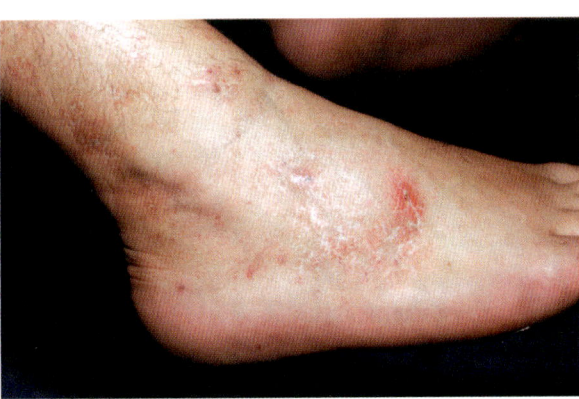

Figure 99.5 Atrophie blanche. Reproduced from Bilgic *et al.* 2021 [2] with permission from Elsevier.

Management

Treatment depends on the underlying cause. In idiopathic disease, antiplatelet, anticoagulant and fibrinolytic therapies have been used, as well as danazol and stanozolol [3]. PUVA therapy has been reported as effective [8]. In lupus with atrophie blanche, antimalarial therapy may help. Intravenous immunoglobulins may rapidly relieve pain [9], perhaps due to improved perfusion. Good response to lipoprostaglandin E_1 with essential cryoglobulinaemia [10] has been reported. There are reports of response to tetracyclines [11] and dapsone in those with underlying myeloproliferative syndromes.

Malignant atrophic papulosis

Definition and nomenclature

Malignant atrophic papulosis is a progressive vasculopathy causing occlusion of small and medium-sized arteries [1].

Synonyms and inclusions

- Degos disease
- Kohlmeier–Degos disease
- Lethal cutaneous and gastrointestinal arteriolar thrombosis

Introduction and general description

Malignant atrophic papulosis is characterised by skin and gastrointestinal lesions, but neurological features are also frequent and postmortem studies show widespread organ involvement. Skin lesions are usually the first feature and may be the only manifestation over many years. Whether this represents a truly 'benign' variant is uncertain. However, it is suggested that the disease should be classified into a malignant systemic form and a benign, cutaneous one [2].

Epidemiology
Incidence and prevalence

It is rare; a review in 1995 suggested that about 120 cases had been reported [3].

Age

It is mainly a disease of young adults, although it can affect any age group [4].

Sex

M > F.

Ethnicity

It is mainly reported in white people.

Associated diseases

Cases have been reported with HIV infection, but a causal association is unproven.

Pathophysiology

The pathogenesis probably involves abnormal coagulation, although the precise mechanism is uncertain. Platelet and fibrin thrombi are present in dermal, mesenteric and nervous system blood vessels, with abnormal platelet aggregation and inhibition of fibrinolysis [4–6]. However, most have no evidence of systemic coagulopathy, suggesting that the thrombotic tendency is at the microvascular level. Antiphospholipid antibodies have been documented in a small number of patients, usually in the context of SLE, although also in so far benign cutaneous cases [7].

Lesions resembling malignant atrophic papulosis occur in some patients with SLE, rheumatoid arthritis, scleroderma or dermatomyositis [8–11]. Antiendothelial antibodies may be found but are probably not pathogenic [4]. Circulating immune complexes, or deposition of immune complexes or complement, are not usually demonstrated [2,12]. Although there can be a prominent lymphocytic infiltrate in later lesions, especially around venules, true arteritis and leukocytoclasis are not found [4,13].

Abnormal mucin deposits, which may be thrombogenic, are commoner in later lesions [4,13] possibly induced by activated T cells. A viral aetiology was proposed as electron microscopic structures resembling viral inclusions were seen in endothelial cells, but these are seen in other disorders, including SLE, and can be induced by interferon [4].

Pathology

The histological picture in Degos disease depends upon lesion duration. Early lesions show a superficial and deep perivascular, perineural and periappendageal chronic inflammatory cell infiltrate [13]. Deep dermal vessels show endovascular inflammation, proliferation and thickening with thrombosis [14]. Mucin deposition is seen at all stages [2,3,13] and fibrin deposition may be demonstrated; fibrinoid necrosis of vessel walls may occur [14]. Immunofluorescence is occasionally positive for IgG or C3. Lymphocytes in damaged vessel walls have led to some classifying Degos disease as a lymphocytic vasculitis [15], although this is probably not the primary abnormality and is secondary to vessel occlusion. Later lesions show a 'wedge-shaped' sclerotic change in the dermis, which is only sparsely cellular. Between these stages there is a phase with neutrophilic and eosinophilic infiltrate around adnexae and a dense perivascular lymphocytic infiltrate [13]. The epidermis, initially showing a mild vacuolar reaction, becomes atrophic with slight scaling, resembling lichen sclerosus and corresponding with the porcelain-white colour seen clinically. There may be associated pigmentary incontinence.

Panniculitis resembling that in lupus profundus has been reported [16]. Similar changes occur in the intestinal wall, particularly the submucosa. The muscularis mucosae is intact. Blood vessels are thickened and disorganised, with fibrinoid degeneration; platelet–fibrin thrombi are more prominent than in skin biopsy material. Microaneurysms of the bulbar conjunctival vessels have been described. Renal changes include thickening of the afferent glomerular arterioles and of the capillary basement membrane.

Genetics
Familial cases have been reported [17].

Clinical features
Presentation
Crops of cutaneous lesions usually precede systemic manifestations by months to years. These are usually asymptomatic, although they may be preceded by slight burning. Skin lesions typically affect the trunk and proximal limbs with sparing of the face, palms and soles. Although they may evolve gradually, and the number of lesions may vary considerably, about 30–40 active lesions are usually present [5]. Oral mucosal lesions are rare but penile lesions may occur [18]; the bulbar conjunctiva is often affected by lesions, which appear as sharply demarcated avascular areas [3]. Peristomal lesions have been reported.

Early skin lesions are pink or red, dome-shaped papules, usually 2–5 mm in size, but sometimes up to about 15 mm. Papules soon become necrotic and umbilicated with a central porcelain-white pallor and scaling, and the pink oedematous border becomes telangiectatic. Most heal slowly to leave a small white scar, often surrounded by telangiectases, as in atrophie blanche. Urticaria-like, ulceropustular and gumma-like nodules have been reported. New crops of lesions may continue for several years. Similar lesions occur in many organs. Gastrointestinal lesions are the most important as perforation of the gut is a cause of death [19]. Neurological symptoms are also relatively common.

For features in different systems see Box 99.6.

Differential diagnosis
There can be a resemblance to atrophie blanche or to guttate lichen sclerosus, although the evolution of lesions is different. Identical lesions have been described in various connective tissue diseases [8–11] and in Crohn disease [20]. The characteristic features are usually hard to confuse with those of other syndromes once the diagnosis is considered. Another disorder termed 'cutaneous–intestinal syndrome with oropharyngeal ulceration' [21] included a combination of macular, blistering and crusting lesions of the skin, with oro-pharyngeal ulceration and death from perforation of one of many intestinal ulcers. This differed clinically and histologically from Degos disease. Patients in whom systemic disease precedes skin lesions may cause diagnostic problems.

Disease course and prognosis
Although probably overestimated by reporting bias and acknowledging that there does appear to be a benign cutaneous ('skin-limited') variant, a mortality of 50% within 2–3 years is reported, and prognosis in males appears to be worse than in females. Systemic manifestations can develop years after the appearance of the skin lesions, including bowel perforation and peritonitis, thrombosis of the cerebral arteries, meningitis, encephalitis and myelitis [22].

Management
There is no consistently effective treatment [2,3]. Systemic corticosteroids do not help, although some benefit in neurological symptoms has been suggested. Aspirin, antiplatelet agents, fibrinolytic agents and pentoxifylline, alone or in combination, may lead to remission in the cutaneous disease [2,3,4,7,23]. Heparin may produce short-term benefits. There is one report of a good response to transdermal nicotine patches [24]. Warfarin, dextrans, chloroquine, immunosuppressive agents and plasma exchange have all been tried. Surgery to treat intestinal perforation may resolve acute situations but as there are usually multiple lesions, there may be little long-term benefit.

Box 99.6 Features of Degos disease in different systems [3]

Gastrointestinal
- Dyspepsia
- Abdominal pain or distension
- Bleeding
- Perforation
- Peritonitis
- Fistulae (enteroenteral or enterocutaneous)
- Obstruction
- Pancreatitis

Neurological
- Cerebral infarction (causing headache, aphasia, dementia, focal epilepsy, hemiparesis, pseudobulbar palsy)
- Cord infarction (paraplegia/quadriplegia, transverse myelopathy)
- Peripheral nerve (cauda equina syndrome, mononeuritis multiplex)
- Various sites (sensory disturbance)

Ocular
- Ptosis
- Diplopia
- Nystagmus
- Ophthalmoplegia
- Optic neuritis
- Papilloedema
- Visual field loss
- Pupillary reaction defects
- Conjunctival avascular lesions
- Posterior subcapsular cataract

Cardiovascular
- Renal artery occlusion
- Pericardial effusion
- Constrictive pericarditis
- Ventricular wall defects

Pulmonary
- Pleuritis

Calcific uraemic arteriolopathy

Synonyms and inclusions
- Calciphylaxis

Introduction and general description

Calcific uraemic arteriolopathy or calciphylaxis is usually seen in end-stage renal disease on dialysis. It is also seen at earlier stages of renal disease with normal kidney function when it is termed non-uraemic calciphylaxis [1]. It has a 1-year mortality rate of 45–80% and is characterised by painful skin ulceration [2,3,4].

Epidemiology

Incidence and prevalence
It is rare but appears to be increasing in prevalence, possibly due to better awareness [5].

Age
The disease is most common in the fifth decade but can be seen in children and the elderly [1].

Sex
Female : male 2 : 1.

Associated diseases
Diabetes and obesity are commonly reported co-morbidities. It very rarely occurs in autoimmune diseases such as SLE. Hypercoagulable problems such as protein C and S deficiencies may be associated. Liver disease may lead to protein C or S deficiency [1,2].

Pathophysiology

The pathogenesis remains obscure. Earlier animal models involving parathyroid hormone and vitamin D are considered unhelpful. Risk factors of obesity, diabetes, hypercalcaemia, hyperphosphataemia and hyperparathyroidism are common in renal disease but calciphylaxis is rare. It appears to be the common end point of a heterogeneous group of stimuli. Theories include uraemic-induced defects in the nuclear factor-kB (RANK), RANK ligand and osteoprotegerin; chronic inflammation-induced reduction of fetuin-A, a liver-produced inhibitor of calcification; and upregulation of BMP-2 triggering osteogenesis.

Predisposing factors

One large institutional study showed that, compared with other patients on dialysis, risk factors included obesity, liver disease, corticosteroid use, elevated calcium–phosphate product and elevated aluminium levels [2]. Hypoalbuminuria (or albumin infusions), recent rapid weight loss, protein C or protein S deficiency, warfarin treatment and hypotension may be risk factors.

Pathology

There is calcification in the medial layer of the wall of small subcutaneous vessels, with necrosis of overlying tissue [2,3,4]. Calcification may occur in dermal vessels, subcutaneous fat septae and adipocytes. Thrombosed vessels are presumably secondary to the calcification of small-vessel walls, which extends more widely than the thrombotic change or the extravascular calcification [4]. Dermal inflammation may be present without ulceration and bullae sometimes occur.

Clinical features

Presentation

Early lesions tend to present as painful purpuric plaques, often with a retiform or stellate pattern, and may show blistering or central necrosis. Some may become semiconfluent as a 'broken' livedo. Ninety per cent of lesions are on the lower extremities. The abdomen, thigh and hips are typical sites, but the breasts may be involved. In some patients the disease is mainly distal below the knee. Uncommon sites include the penis and tongue [6] as well as the muscles and internal organs [3]. Woody induration with extending ulcer and eschar formation develops. Peripheral pulse detection may distinguish calciphylaxis from atherosclerotic peripheral vascular disease.

Disease course and prognosis

The prognosis is generally poor, with a 1-year mortality of 45–80%, although there are occasional reports of a more benign course [2]. Cutaneous lesions may develop into skin necrosis with sepsis. Internal involvement may lead to organ failure, infarction and gastrointestinal haemorrhage.

Investigations

A deep skin biopsy for histopathology is usually undertaken to confirm the diagnosis. Plain radiographs show vascular calcification in a net-like pattern. Investigations include full coagulation assessment, amylase, parathyroid hormone, cryoglobulins and cryofibrinogens, and investigations for vasculitis including ANCA, ANA and hepatitis C.

Management

Give good wound care, pain management and treat infection. Consider removal of possible trigger factors such as parenteral iron, calcium, vitamin D and warfarin. Reduce elevated calcium–phosphorus product with low-calcium dialysate fluids and non-calcium oral phosphate binders. Sodium thiosulphate infusions [7] increase the solubility of calcium deposits and have an antioxidant function, but may produce an anion gap metabolic acidosis requiring adjustment of dialysate bicarbonate. Correct hypercoagulability disorders. In hyperparathyroidism, cinacalcet [8] and parathyroid surgery may be useful. Hyperbaric oxygen, skin grafting and iloprost infusions can be useful adjuncts [9].

Solar purpura

The term 'solar purpura' describes rapid development of purpuric lesions after exposure to sunlight. This condition is distinct from

PART 9: VASCULAR DISORDERS

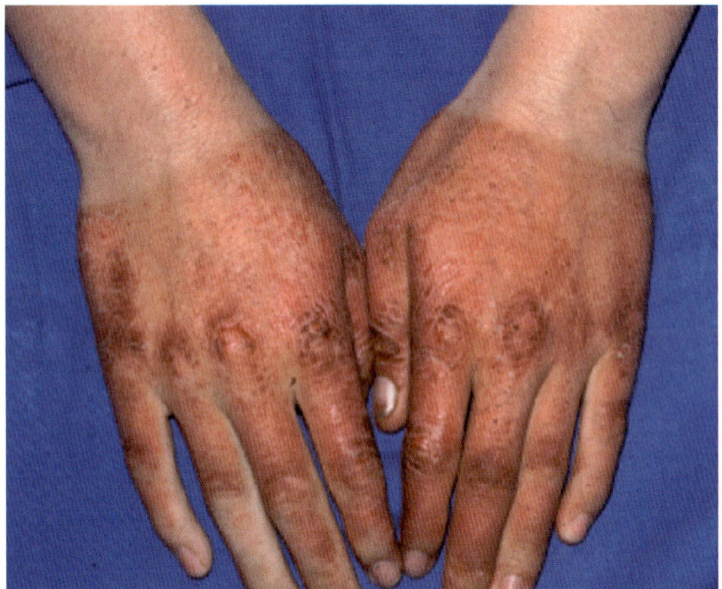

Figure 99.6 Erythropoietic protoporphyria showing marked purpura with sharp cut-off after sunlight exposure.

actinic purpura, due to cumulative sunlight-induced ageing of the skin. The nature of solar purpura is uncertain. It may be a variant of polymorphic light eruption or arising from solar capillaritis [1,2]. It is distinct from erythropoietic protoporphyria, which can cause purpura (Figure 99.6). Some cases may be due to profound inflammation, which has allowed purpura to develop in dermatoses which are not usually purpuric.

Key references

The full list of references can be found in the online version at https://www.wiley.com/rooksdermatology10e

Introduction

1 Piette WW. The differential diagnosis of purpura from a morphologic perspective. *Adv Dermatol* 1994;9:3–23.
4 Thornsberry LA, LoSicco KI, English JC, 3rd. The skin and hypercoagulable states. *J Am Acad Dermatol* 2013;69:450–62.
9 Maguire S, Mann M. Systematic reviews of bruising in relation to child abuse – what have we learnt: an overview of review updates. *Evid Based Child Health* 2013;8:255–63.

Purpura due to thrombocytopenia or platelet defects
Thrombocytopenia

1 Shenkman B, Einav Y. Thrombotic thrombocytopenic purpura and other thrombotic microangiopathic hemolytic anemias: diagnosis and classification. *Autoimmun Rev* 2014;13:584–6.
4 Handin RI. Inherited platelet disorders. *Hematology (Am Soc Hematol Educ Program)* 2005;2005:396–402.
9 Hassan AA, Kroll MH. Acquired disorders of platelet function. *Hematology (Am Soc Hematol Educ Program)* 2005;2005:403–8.

Abnormalities of platelet function

1 Handin RI. Inherited platelet disorders. *Hematology (Am Soc Hematol Educ Program)* 2005;2005:396–402.
5 Shen Y-MP, Frenkel EP. Acquired platelet dysfunction. *Hematol Oncol Clin North Am* 2007;21:647–61.

6 Diz-Küçükkaya R. Inherited platelet disorders including Glanzmann thrombasthenia and Bernard-Soulier syndrome. *Hematology (Am Soc Hematol Educ Program)* 2013;2013:268–75.

Thrombocytosis

1 Champion RH, Rook A. Idiopathic thrombocythemia: cutaneous manifestations. *Arch Dermatol* 1963;87:302–5.
7 Kaszewski S, Czajkowski R, Protas-Drozd *et al*. Sweet's syndrome with idiopathic thrombocythemia. *Postepy Dermatol Alergol* 2014;31:47–52.
8 Bray PF. Platelet hyperreactivity: predictive and intrinsic properties. *Hematol Oncol Clin North Am* 2007;21:633–45.

Non-thrombocytopenic vascular causes of purpura and syndromes of primary ecchymotic haemorrhage
Raised intravascular pressure

2 Trindade F, Requena L. Pseudo-Kaposi's sarcoma because of suction-socket lower limb prosthesis. *J Cutan Pathol* 2009;36:482–5.
5 Ramelet AA. Exercise-induced purpura. *Dermatology (Basel)* 2004;208:293–6.

Abnormal or decreased support of blood vessels

1 Bick R. Vascular thrombohemorrhagic disorders: hereditary and acquired. *Clin Appl Thrombosis Hemostasis* 2001;7:178–94.
3 Kaya G, Saurat JH. Dermatoporosis: a chronic cutaneous insufficiency/fragility syndrome. Clinicopathological features, mechanisms, prevention and potential treatments. *Dermatology* 2007;215:284–94.
6 Thies K, Beschorner U, Noory E *et al*. Achenbach's syndrome revisited. *Vasa* 2012;41:366–70.

Physical and artefactual bleeding

1 Metzker A, Merlob P. Suction purpura. *Arch Dermatol* 1992;128:822–4.
3 Lao M, Weisshar A, Siegfried E. Talon noir. *J Pediatr* 2013;163:919.
7 Saida T, Oguchi S, Ishihara Y. In vivo observations of magnified features of pigmented lesions on volar skin using video microscope. *Arch Dermatol* 1995;131:248–304.

Dysproteinaemic and Waldenström hypergammaglobulinaemic purpura

1 Waldenström J. Three new cases of purpura hyperglobulinaemica. A study of a long-standing benign increase in serum globulin. *Acta Med Scand* 1952;266(Suppl.):931–46.
2 Miyagawa S, Fukumoto T, Kanauchi M *et al*. Hypergammaglobulinaemic purpura of Waldenström and Ro/SSA autoantibodies. *Br J Dermatol* 1996;134:919–23.
7 Lewin JM, Hunt R, Fischer M *et al*. Hypergammaglobulinemic purpura of Waldenstrom. *Dermatol Online J* 2012;18:2.

Pigmented purpuric dermatoses

1 Tristani-Firouzi P, Meadows KP, Vanderhooft S. Pigmented purpuric eruptions of childhood: a series of cases and review of literature. *Pediatr Dermatol* 2001;18:299–304.
3 Jensen AL, Vanderhooft SL. Pigmented purpuras. In: Harper J, Oranje AP, Prose N, eds. *Textbook of Pediatric Dermatology*, 3rd edn. Oxford: Blackwell Science, 2011:165.1–6.
5 Sardana K, Sarkar R, Seghal VN. Pigmented purpuric dermatoses: an overview. *Int J Dermatol* 2004;43:482–8.

Disorders of cutaneous microvascular occlusion
Platelet plugging: heparin necrosis

9 Cuker A, Arcpally GM, Chong BH *et al*. American Society of Hematology 2018 guidelines for management of venous thromboembolism: heparin-induced thrombocytopenia. *Blood Adv* 2018;2:3360–92.

Platelet plugging: thrombocytosis

1 Harrison CN, Bareford D, Butt N *et al*. Guideline for investigation and management of adults and children presenting with a thrombocytosis. *Br J Haematol* 2010;149:352–75.

4 Tefferi A, Barbui T. Polycythemia vera and essential thrombocythemia: 2019 update on diagnosis, risk-stratification and management. *Am J Hematol* 2019;94:133–43.

Cryogelling/cryagglutination

2 Ramos-Casals M, Stone JH, Cid MC *et al*. The cryoglobulinaemias. *Lancet* 2012;379(9813):348–60.

11 Lauchli S, Widmer L, Lautenschlager S. Cold agglutinin disease: the importance of cutaneous signs. *Dermatology* 2001;202:356–8.

16 Michaud M, Pourrat J. Cryofibrinogenemia. *J Clin Rheumatol* 2013;19:142–8.

Emboli

Cholesterol embolus

2 Bashore T, Gehrig T. Cholesterol emboli after invasive cardiac procedures. *J Am Coll Cardiol* 2003;42:217–18.

4 Pennington M, Yeager J, Skelton H, Smith K. Cholesterol embolization syndrome: cutaneous histopathological features and the variable onset of symptoms in patients with different risk factors. *Br J Dermatol* 2002;146:511–17.

6 Saric M, Kronzon I. Cholesterol embolization syndrome. *Curr Opin Cardiol* 2011;26:472–9.

Oxalate embolus, cardiac embolus and other emboli

1 Akhtar S. Fat embolism. *Anesthesiol Clin* 2009;27:533–50.

2 Blackmon JA, Jeffy BG, Malone JC *et al*. Oxalosis involving the skin: case report and literature review. *Arch Dermatol* 2011;147:1302–5.

4 Greeson D, Wright J, Zanolli M. Cutaneous findings associated with cardiac myxomas. *Cutis* 1998;62:275–80.

Systemic coagulopathies: protein C/protein S-related disease

3 Marlar RA, Montgomery RR, Broekmans AW. Diagnosis and treatment of homozygous protein C deficiency. Report of the Working Party on Homozygous Protein C Deficiency of the Subcommittee on Protein C and Protein S, International Committee on Thrombosis and Haemostasis. *J Pediatr* 1989;114:528–34.

7 Kakagia DD, Papanas N, Karadimas E *et al*. Warfarin-induced skin necrosis. *Ann Dermatol* 2014;26:96–8.

11 Robson K, Piette W. The presentation and differential diagnosis of cutaneous vascular occlusion syndromes. *Adv Dermatol* 1999;15:153–82.

Systemic coagulopathies: antiphospholipid antibody/lupus anticoagulant syndrome

1 Lim W. Antiphospholipid syndrome. *Hematology (Am Soc Hematol Educ Program)* 2013;2013:675–80.

5 Chaturvedi S, McCrae KR. Recent advances in the antiphospholipid antibody syndrome. *Curr Opin Hematol* 2014;21:371–9.

6 Giannakopolulos B, Krills SA. The pathogenesis of the antiphospholipid syndrome. *N Engl J Med* 2013;368:1033–44.

Vascular coagulopathies

1 Sneddon IB. Cerebro-vascular lesions and livedo reticularis. *Br J Dermatol* 1965;77:180–5.

3 Aladdin Y, Hamadeh M, Butcher K. The Sneddon syndrome. *Arch Neurol* 2008;65:834–5.

5 Caldas CA, de Carvalho JF. Primary antiphospholipid syndrome with and without Sneddon's syndrome. *Rheumatol Int* 2011;31:197–200.

Livedoid vasculopathy/atrophie blanche

1 Chang D, Patel RM. Livedoid vasculopathy. *Cutis* 2012;90:179.

3 Acland K, Darvay A, Wakelin S, Russell-Jones R. Livedoid vasculitis: a manifestation of the antiphospholipid syndrome? *Br J Dermatol* 1999;140:131–5.

6 Kerk N, Goerge T. Livedoid vasculopathy – current aspects of diagnosis and treatment of cutaneous infarction. *J Dtsch Dermatol Ges* 2013;11:407–10.

Malignant atrophic papulosis

1 Degos R. Malignant atrophic papulosis. *Br J Dermatol* 1979;100:21–36.

2 Theodoridis A, Konstantinidou A, Makrantonaki E *et al*. Malignant and benign forms of atrophic papulosis (Kohlmeier-Degos disease): systemic involvement determines the prognosis. *Br J Dermatol* 2014;170:110–15.

22 Theodoridis A, Makrantonaki E, Zouboulis CC. Malignant atrophic papulosis (Kohlmeier-Degos disease) – a review. *Orphanet J Rare Dis* 2013;8:10.

Calcific uraemic arteriolopathy

1 Nigwekar SU, Kroshinsky D, Nazarian RM *et al*. Calciphylaxis: risk factors, diagnosis, and treatment. *Am J Kidney Dis* 2015;66:133–46.

2 Weenig RH, Sewell LD, Davis MPD *et al*. Calciphylaxis: natural history, risk factor analysis, and outcome. *J Am Acad Dermatol* 2007;56:569–79.

3 Hayashi M. Calciphylaxis: diagnosis and clinical features. *Clin Exp Nephrol* 2013;17:498–503.

9 Ong S, Coulson IH. Diagnosis and treatment of calciphylaxis. *Skinmed* 2012;10:166–70.

Solar purpura

2 Waters AJ, Sandhu C, Green CM *et al*. Solar capillaritis as a cause of solar purpura. *Clin Exp Dermatol* 2009;34:e821–4.

PART 9: VASCULAR DISORDERS

CHAPTER 100

Cutaneous Vasculitis

Nick J. Levell and Chetan Mukhtyar

Norwich Medical School, Norfolk and Norwich University Hospital, Norwich, UK

Introduction

Definition

Cutaneous vasculitis is inflammation of dermal blood vessel walls, resulting in purpura, which may be painful and palpable. Tissue loss can cause infarction and rarely ulceration. Nomenclature of the vasculitides is based upon the size of blood vessel affected (Box 100.1) [1].

Introduction and general description

Vasculitis is usually a multisystem disorder that presents in a myriad of ways. Diagnosis is based on a detailed history and careful examination. Patients may present to different specialties and their care should be led by a multidisciplinary team involving physicians with a specialist interest in vasculitis.

Vasculitis can be classified by aetiology or by calibre of the vessel involved. The accepted nomenclature was defined at an international consensus meeting held in 2012 in Chapel Hill, USA [1]. The meeting did not involve dermatologists, and all cutaneous vasculitides were considered under the umbrella of 'single-organ vasculitis'. In 2018 a European skin vasculitis task force published a cutaneous vasculitis nomenclature [2]. It should be recognised that names and classifications will change in the future with greater understanding of the underlying disease mechanisms.

The treatment of primary vasculitis involves immunosuppression. The balance between disease severity and adverse effects of therapy requires expertise and experience in the management of these rare conditions. Secondary vasculitis can be due to infection, drugs, malignancy or inflammatory disease; treatment of the underlying condition may resolve the vasculitis.

Epidemiology

See the specific diseases.

Pathophysiology

The pathophysiology and histopathology vary according to the specific disease.

Clinical features

History

The management of patients presenting with cutaneous vasculitis should begin with a full history. Questions about systemic disease include (i) complications of vasculitis; (ii) potential malignant and infectious triggers; and (iii) systemic features of systemic vasculitides (Box 100.2). The history should consider diseases that may present with secondary vasculitis including rheumatological diseases (such as systemic lupus erythematosus), thrombo-occlusive disorders and other inflammatory dermatoses.

Rook's Textbook of Dermatology, Tenth Edition. Edited by Christopher Griffiths, Jonathan Barker, Tanya Bleiker, Walayat Hussain and Rosalind Simpson.

PART 9: VASCULAR DISORDERS

Box 100.1 Classification of cutaneous vasculitis adapted from the 2012 Chapel Hill Consensus nomenclature [1]

Single-organ (skin) small-vessel vasculitis
- Cutaneous small-vessel vasculitis (see Figure 100.1)
- Urticarial vasculitis (excluding immune complex disease)
- Erythema elevatum diutinum (see Figure 100.8)
- Acute haemorrhagic oedema of infancy
- Recurrent cutaneous necrotising eosinophilic vasculitis (controversial entity)
- Granuloma faciale (see Figure 100.10)

Cutaneous vasculitis associated with systemic disease or variable vessel size
- Behçet syndrome
- Lupus vasculitis
- Sarcoid vasculitis
- Rheumatoid vasculitis

Small-vessel immune complex-associated vasculitis
- IgA vasculitis (Henoch–Schönlein purpura) (see Figure 100.12)
- Cryoglobulinaemic vasculitis (see Figure 100.13)
- Hypocomplementaemic urticarial vasculitis (HUV)
- Antiglomerular basement membrane vasculitis (anti-GBM/Goodpasture syndrome)

Small-vessel ANCA-associated vasculitis
- Microscopic polyangiitis (MPA)
- Granulomatosis with polyangiitis (GPA) (see Figure 100.18a)
- Eosinophilic granulomatosis with polyangiitis (EGPA/Churg–Strauss syndrome)

Medium-vessel vasculitis
- Polyarteritis nodosa (PAN) (including cutaneous PAN – now referred to as cutaneous arteritis[a]) (see Figure 100.3 and Figure 100.22)
- Kawasaki disease

Large-vessel vasculitis
- Giant cell arteritis (GCA)
- Takayasu arteritis

[a] In the classification [1] cutaneous PAN is recognised as cutaneous arteritis (single-organ vasculitis), whereas in this chapter it is considered with PAN.
ANCA, antineutrophil cytoplasmic antibody; IgA, immunoglobulin A.

Box 100.2 Areas in the history of a patient with cutaneous vasculitis that may give clues indicating systemic disease

- Weight loss, fatigue, fever
- Arthralgia, myalgia, arthritis
- Dry eyes, dry mouth
- Red eye, eye pain, vision loss
- Nasal or sinus congestion
- Ear pain
- Oral/nasal ulcers
- Chest pain/dyspnoea
- Abdominal pain, blood in faeces
- Blackouts, weakness, fits

A full drug history, taken from the patient, the case notes and other relevant clinicians, should focus on medication changes in the days, weeks and months prior to the onset of vasculitis. Occasionally, drugs taken for many years may precipitate reactions. Drugs purchased from pharmacies or borrowed from relatives, herbal treatments, tonics and vitamins should also be considered. Patients may be unwilling to reveal recreational drugs, drugs causing addiction or drugs taken for bodybuilding or sexual purposes. The reason for any drug change should be established.

Vasculitis may be secondary to infection. A history should be taken of infections, both acute and chronic, and their treatments.

Presentation

On general examination, establish if the patient is acutely unwell; patients with systemic vasculitis may have life-threatening internal organ involvement requiring prompt management. All the skin and the mouth should be examined. Cutaneous vasculitis often results in painful, palpable purpura (Figure 100.1). Leakage of blood from the vasculature into the interstitium causes purpura, which is identified by a failure to blanch on diascopy (pressure with a glass slide). Increased pressure in the venous circulation increases blood vessel leakage and may worsen damage to the vessel walls. Purpura is therefore most apparent on the lower limbs. Prolonged standing

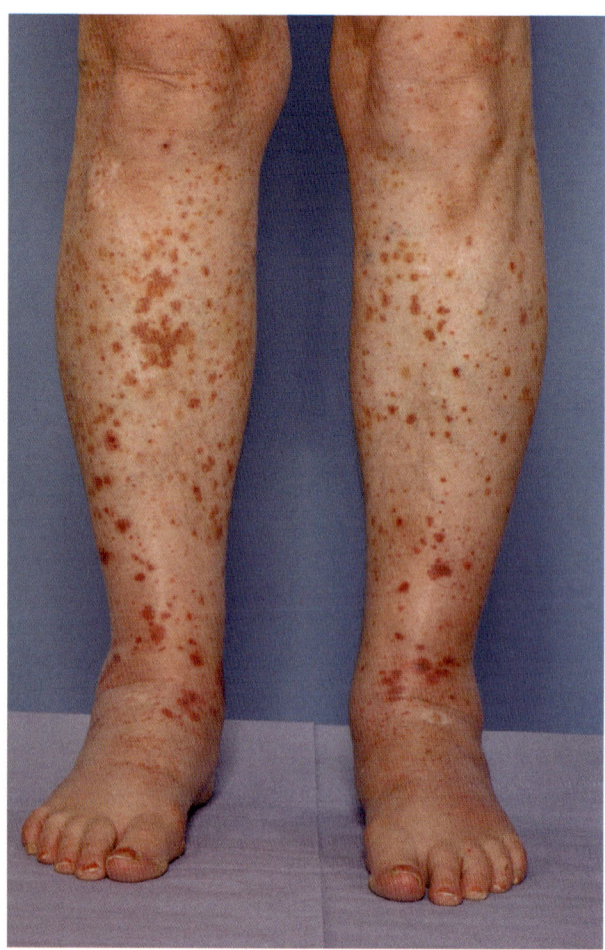

Figure 100.1 Cutaneous small-vessel vasculitis producing palpable purpura. Courtesy of Andrew Carmichael.

exaggerates venous hypertension and thus increases blood leakage and purpura.

The physical signs are determined to some extent by the size of vessel involved (Table 100.1). Severe cutaneous vasculitis will result in painful ischaemia of the skin. Lesional skin will become haemorrhagic (Figure 100.2) and then necrotic and will eventually detach, leaving erosions or ulcers (Figure 100.3), most commonly on the lower limbs. These ulcers may then become secondarily infected. The ulcers may be slow to heal, even after resolution of the vasculitis, due to venous stasis, malnutrition, anaemia, lymphoedema, prolonged infection or old age.

In people with more pigmented skin, vasculitis lesions may appear dark brown to black in colour.

Table 100.1 Physical signs may give clues as to the predominant vessel size involved in the vasculitis.

Blood vessel size	Physical signs
Small blood vessels	Purpuric macules and papules, haemorrhagic vesicles, urticarial plaques Necrosis not usually a major feature
Medium-sized blood vessels	Broken livedo (net/reticulate) pattern, infarction, ulceration, deep nodules

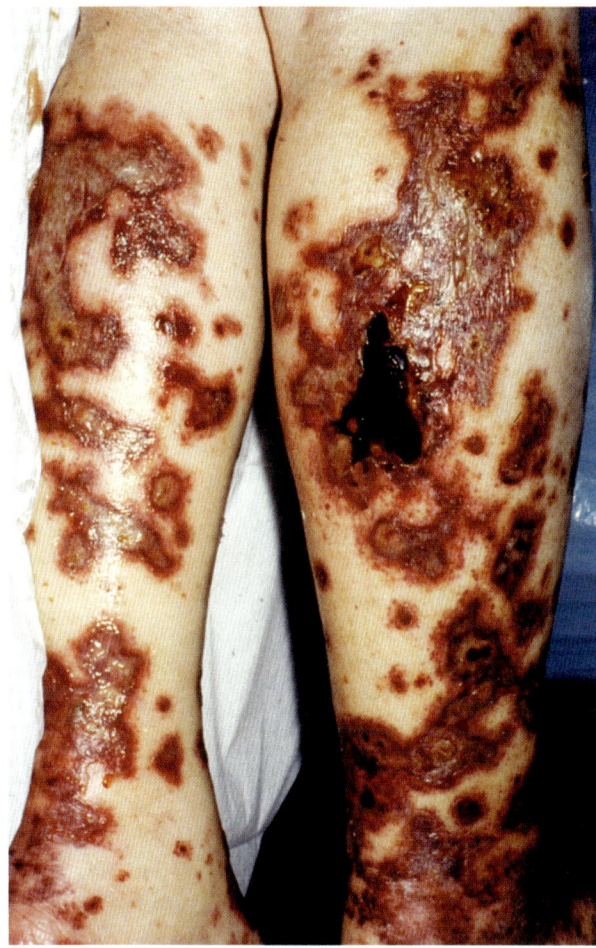

Figure 100.3 Ulcerated necrotic lesions in a livedo distribution suggestive of medium-vessel disease. Courtesy of Andrew Carmichael.

The extent of systemic examination will depend on the history and on the overall assessment of the patient. Systemic examination may reveal an underlying infection or malignancy acting as a trigger for the vasculitis. Signs of a systemic primary vasculitis may be found (Box 100.3). Other underlying diseases that may cause secondary vasculitis such as rheumatoid arthritis or systemic lupus erythematosus may be apparent.

> ### Box 100.3 Examination and bedside investigation for systemic vasculitis
>
> - Haematuria, proteinuria (urinalysis), oedema, hypertension
> - Congestive cardiac failure, pericardial rub, oedema
> - Cough, haemoptysis (examine sputum), wheeze, crepitations
> - Abdominal tenderness, melaena, nausea, vomiting, hepatosplenomegaly
> - Paraesthesiae, numbness, weakness, abnormal reflexes, psychiatric signs

Clinical variants

The size of purpuric lesions varies according to the disease. Areas of purpura that are flat and less than 5 mm in diameter are called petechiae, those larger than 1 cm are ecchymoses; non-palpable

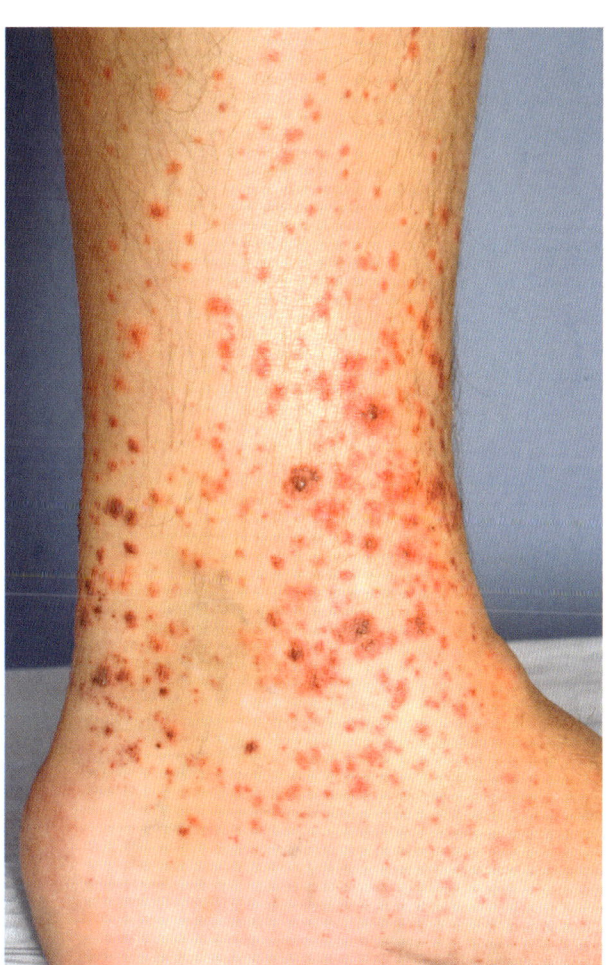

Figure 100.2 Cutaneous small-vessel vasculitis demonstrating a haemorrhagic vesicle. Courtesy of Andrew Carmichael.

Table 100.2 The purpura pattern may give clues as to the disease.

Pattern of purpura	Diseases to consider
Pinpoint, cayenne pepper macular purpura, typically <5 mm	Capillaritis, exercise-induced purpura ('runners' legs'), coughing, ligatures
	Purpura in contact dermatitis (e.g. rubber), venous hypertension, suction induced, fixed drug eruptions, cutaneous T-cell lymphoma
Macular purpura of any size	Purpura due to infections, platelet disorders and thrombocytopenia, other clotting disorders, mild small-vessel vasculitis
	Trauma/artefact
Large macular purpura, typically over 2 cm	Purpura of old age, topical, inhaled or systemic corticosteroid-induced purpura, scurvy
Painful palpable purpura of any size	Cutaneous vasculitis of all types, pityriasis lichenoides, thrombo-occlusive disorders of all types, secondary purpura in tuberculosis or leprosy reactions, neutrophilic disorders, atypical benign or malignant cutaneous growths (e.g. haemangiosarcoma, Kaposi sarcoma, amelanotic melanoma with haemorrhage)
Livedo pattern purpura	Antiphospholipid syndromes, vasculitis in medium-sized blood vessels (e.g. polyarteritis, ANCA vasculitides), thrombo-occlusive disorders of all types including cryoglobulins, chilblains

ANCA, antineutrophil cytoplasmic antibody.

purpura are somewhere between the two. Raised, non-blanching lesions are palpable purpura. A reticulate (like a net) livedo pattern is seen in some vasculitides and thrombo-occlusive disorders (Table 100.2). A broken livedo (incomplete net) (Figure 100.3) is said to be a feature of vasculitis disorders but may also be seen in thrombo-occlusive disease.

Differential diagnosis

Thrombo-occlusive disorders, trauma, inflammatory dermatoses with disordered clotting, purpura due to prolonged running, neutrophilic disorders, erythema ab igne, cellulitis (particularly in the elderly with oedematous legs), platelet disorders, insect and snake bites are often confused with vasculitis.

Disease course and prognosis

See specific diseases.

Investigations

The investigation of vasculitis is dependent on the history and examination findings. A thorough assessment may clarify the likely cause and limit the need for extensive investigations. However, investigations are necessary for two main purposes. First, it is important to establish if the vasculitis is primary or secondary. Investigations should be directed to identify underlying rheumatological disease, malignancy, infection or a primary vasculitis. Second, investigations should be performed to demonstrate the presence of vasculitis involving internal organs. Urinalysis to exclude renal disease is useful in most patients.

Skin biopsy in vasculitis, if needed, should be taken from a fresh lesion less than 48 h old. Patients may find it difficult to remember the age of lesions, particularly if there is widespread disease, so a useful clinical guide is to seek out lesions with a mixture of purpura and inflammation, which partially lose their

Table 100.3 Vasculitis investigations. The 'vasculitis screen' is dependent on the history and examination findings. In acute vasculitis with an obvious infection or drug trigger, investigations may be minimal. The purposes of investigation are threefold: to look for (i) complications of vasculitis; (ii) causes of vasculitis; and (iii) differential diagnoses of vasculitis, such as thrombo-occlusive disorders.

Investigation	Notes
Blood and urine tests	
Urinalysis	Haematuria and proteinuria in renal involvement
Urea and electrolytes	Raised creatinine and urea in renal involvement
Full blood count	Raised white cells in infection/cryoglobulinaemia Thrombocytopenia may cause purpura
Liver function	Low albumin in renal disease
Erythrocyte sedimentation rate	May be raised in systemic vasculitis, infection and malignancy
C-reactive protein	May be raised in infections
Antineutrophil cytoplasmic antibody (ANCA)	May be present in systemic vasculitides – see text
Antinuclear antibodies	May be present in autoimmune connective tissue disease
Specialist haematological tests for thromboembolic disease such as lupus anticoagulant and anticardiolipin antibodies	If thrombo-occlusive disease is possible from the history, examination or histology
Cryoglobulins	If there is skin, kidney and joint vasculitis. Not necessarily triggered by cold
Tissue tests	
Skin biopsy from early lesion (less than 48 h old) for histopathology	Indicate if vasculitis or thromboembolic disorder Indicate size of blood vessel involvement and predominant cell type Indicate presence of granulomas Indicate certain infections, e.g. mycobacteria
Skin biopsy from early lesion for direct immunofluorescence	Indicate if IgA vasculitis
Skin biopsy for culture	May be useful for chronic infections, e.g. TB
Infection	
Infection screen: cultures, serology and radiology	Depends on age, history of travel and country of residence, history and examination. Screen for acute and/or chronic infections
Malignancy	
Malignancy screen: blood tests and radiology for malignancy	Relevant tests depend on the age of patient, history and examination
Inflammatory disease	
Investigations for other systemic inflammatory disease	If diseases (e.g. inflammatory bowel disease, rheumatoid arthritis) are suspected from history and examination

red colour with pressure (the 'partial blancher'). Older vasculitic lesions may develop secondary thrombosis making it difficult to differentiate from a thrombo-occlusive disorder. Older lesions of thrombo-occlusive disorders may develop secondary vasculitis.

A skin biopsy for direct immunofluoresence should be taken if immunoglobulin A (IgA) vasculitis is suspected. A 'lupus band' of IgG and complement at the dermal–epidermal junction is of little value as a diagnostic test and is no longer recommended. A vasculitis screen may be used by inexperienced clinicians as a substitute for taking a history and examination and then applying logic. A list of tests is given in Table 100.3, but these should be used in support of clinical findings and careful reflection, and not as a substitute.

Management

The management of vasculitis is dependent on the diagnosis and the severity and presence of systemic vasculitis. Triggering drugs should be stopped, underlying infections treated and malignancy or associated rheumatological diseases managed. If systemic vasculitis or vasculitic disease is identified, then the treatment is described under the specific diseases in this book. The correction of venous stasis by elevation of the legs, treatment of secondary infection, appropriate dressings in ulcerated areas and pain relief are required.

In systemic vasculitis a multidisciplinary team approach is appropriate. Specialists may be required to deal with disease in almost any organ. In the UK, rheumatologists with an interest in vasculitis often lead or coordinate teams of other specialists to manage complex patients. Early referral is desirable to avoid potentially treatable disease in other organs causing irreversible damage.

SINGLE-ORGAN SMALL-VESSEL VASCULITIS

Cutaneous small-vessel vasculitis

Definition and nomenclature

Cutaneous small-vessel vasculitis (CSVV) is a single-organ vasculitis producing leukocytoclastic angiitis of cutaneous vasculature [1,2].

Synonyms and inclusions

- Allergic cutaneous vasculitis
- Allergic cutaneous angiitis
- Hypersensitivity angiitis
- Hypersensitivity vasculitis
- Cutaneous leukocytoclastic angiitis
- Cutaneous leukocytoclastic vasculitis
- Cutaneous allergic vasculitis

Introduction and general description

The American College of Rheumatology (ACR) has produced classification criteria for CSVV. The presence of three of the following five criteria has 84% specificity for CSVV: (i) age greater than 16 years at disease onset; (ii) history of taking a medication at the onset that may have been a precipitating factor; (iii) the presence of palpable purpura; (iv) the presence of a maculopapular rash; and (v) a biopsy demonstrating granulocytes around an arteriole or venule [3].

CSVV is a single-organ vasculitis and therefore by definition does not have systemic manifestations. However, the diagnosis should prompt ongoing surveillance because it may be a first manifestation of a more generalised vasculitis indicating another disease. CSVV is a clinical syndrome that encompasses vasculitis due to a variety of causes.

Epidemiology

Incidence and prevalence

The annual global incidence of CSVV is reported to be between 15 and 30 per million [4,5].

Age

The mean age at onset is between 36 and 56 years [4,6,7]. However, the age range is wide and extends from the second to the eighth decade of life.

Sex

In a Spanish cohort, men were more commonly affected with a ratio of 1.6 : 1 [4], but in a Singapore cohort there was a female dominance of 2.1 : 1 [6].

Associated diseases

By definition the condition is localised to the skin, but it may be a precursor for other systemic vasculitides.

Pathophysiology

Predisposing factors

There are many causes of cutaneous vasculitis, but most CSVV is idiopathic [6]. This is a consequence of vasculitis classification systems. For example, if patients with CSVV are found to have viral hepatitis and cryoglobulinaemia, they are no longer classifiable as CSVV. There are factors that are thought to contribute to a pure CSVV, which are listed in Box 100.4 [8–31].

Box 100.4 Aetiological triggers for cutaneous small-vessel vasculitis (with relevant references)

- Acenocoumarol [8]
- Staphylococcal protein A column immunoadsorption therapy [9–11]
- Anisoylated plasminogen activator complex [12]
- Food allergies [13]
- Propylthiouracil [14]
- Interferon 1B [15]
- Ibuprofen [16]
- Methotrexate [17]
- Warfarin [18]
- Granulocyte colony-stimulating factor [19]
- Ant bite [20]
- Procainamide [21]
- Infliximab [22]
- Maprotiline [23]
- Omeprazole [24]
- Exercise [25]
- Insulin [26]
- Imipenem-cilastatin [27]
- Gabapentin [28]
- Lamotrigine [28]
- Coumarin [29]
- Atenolol [30]
- Solid-organ malignancies [31]

Pathology

Leukocytoclastic vasculitis with segmental inflammation in an angiocentric pattern, swelling of the endothelium, fibrinoid necrosis

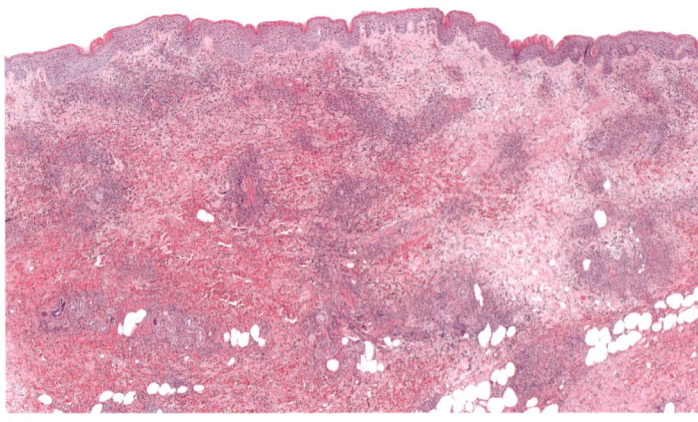

(a)

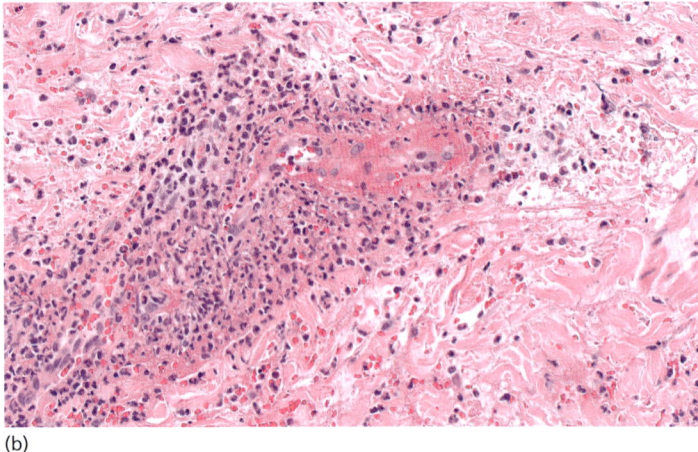

(b)

Figure 100.4 Leukocytoclastic vasculitis. (a) Low-magnification photomicrograph showing perivascular infiltrates and fibrinoid deposits within the vessels of the upper dermis. (b) Higher magnification demonstrating nuclear dust, fibrinoid deposits, vascular alteration and collagen degeneration. Courtesy of Dr Eduardo Calonje.

of vessel walls, extravasation of erythrocytes and an infiltrate of neutrophils with karyorrhexis of the nuclei (i.e. leukocytoclasia) are major features of CSVV (Figure 100.4). In superficial dermal papillary vessels, perivascular deposits of IgM or complement C3 are demonstrated in up to 80% of fresh lesions [32]. Some studies state lower proportions, but this may depend on the timing of the biopsy and because IgM is relatively poor at fixing complement. IgG is found less often.

Causative organisms
In most patients, CSVV is idiopathic, but a small number of cases (4/138) [33] may be related to a bacterial infection. There have been case reports of CSVV following Covid-19 vaccination [34].

Genetics
The genetics are not known.

Clinical features
History
The skin lesions of CSVV typically arise as a simultaneous 'crop', resulting from exposure to an inciting stimulus. The formation of new lesions can continue for several weeks although they usually resolve within several weeks or a few months; approximately 10% of patients will have recurrent disease. There are no known risk factors to predict relapses.

Presentation
Lesions typically occur in areas prone to stasis, commonly including the ankles and lower legs (Figures 100.1 and 100.5a), and typically sparing intertriginous regions. CSVV is often asymptomatic although pruritus, pain or burning may be experienced, as well as systemic symptoms including fever, arthralgia, myalgia and anorexia. The major cutaneous manifestation of CSVV is palpable purpura, ranging in size from 1 mm to several centimetres (Figure 100.5b, c). Sometimes macular in the early stages, such purpura may progress to a wide array of lesions including papules, nodules, vesicles, plaques, bullae or pustules, with secondary findings of ulceration, necrosis and postinflammatory hyperpigmentation (Figure 100.6).

Clinical variants
Other cutaneous findings include oedema, livedo reticularis and urticaria. The presence of the latter two should prompt consideration of cutaneous polyarteritis nodosa and urticarial vasculitis, respectively.

Differential diagnosis
The differential diagnosis of CSVV includes many more specifically defined disorders, which are discussed in this chapter and in other publications [2,3,8,9,33,35,36]. CSVV is a diagnosis of exclusion. Cutaneous vasculitis should prompt a search for a wide array of differential diagnoses, including systemic vasculitides, cancer, infections, allergies, chemical exposures, etc.

Classification of severity
There is no validated biomarker for quantifying disease severity in patients with CSVV. Histopathology is not a good surrogate for severity of disease [35]. The Birmingham Vasculitis Activity Score (BVAS) v3 has been validated to quantify the activity of systemic vasculitis [36]. The validation cohort of BVAS v3 included patients with cutaneous vasculitis and it can be used to create a tangible activity score.

Complications and co-morbidities
Hyperpigmentation and haemosiderosis can take months to resolve. Ulcerated lesions may become infected, adding to the morbidity.

Investigations
Investigation of CSVV is guided by the history and examination findings; the range of tests chosen will range from nothing to extensive blood testing, scanning and organ biopsies. The purpose of investigation is twofold: firstly, to look for evidence of vasculitis in other organ systems, and secondly, to look for evidence of a disease that is predisposing towards CSVV, such as infection or malignancy.

Management
Treatment of CSVV is often unnecessary as the disease may be self-limiting. The evidence for efficacy of therapy is derived from

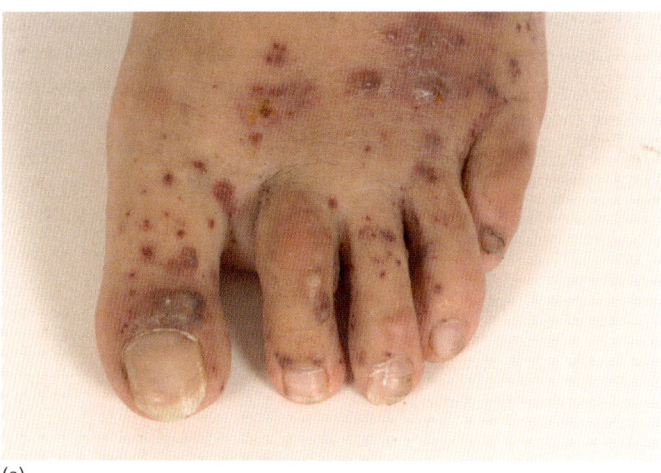

(a)

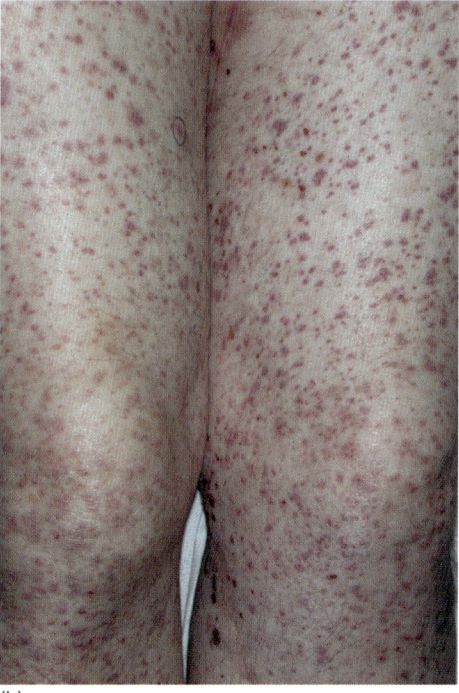

(b)

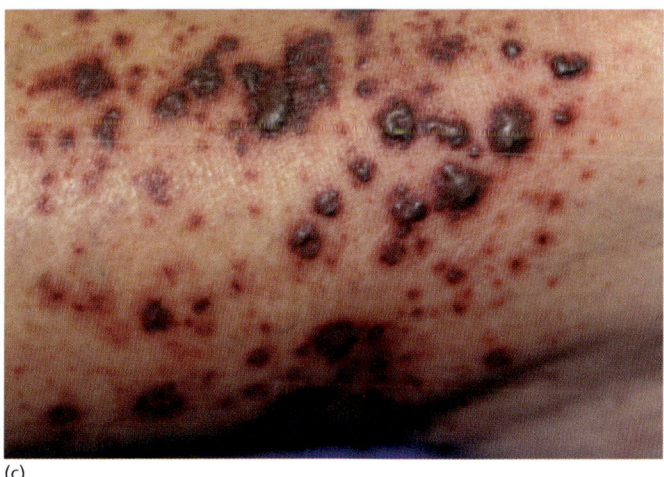

(c)

Figure 100.5 Cutaneous small-vessel vasculitis (CSVV). (a) Vesicles in a dependent area on the foot. (b) Purpura on the thighs; there was similar involvement on the lower legs. (c) CSVV progressing to blistering.

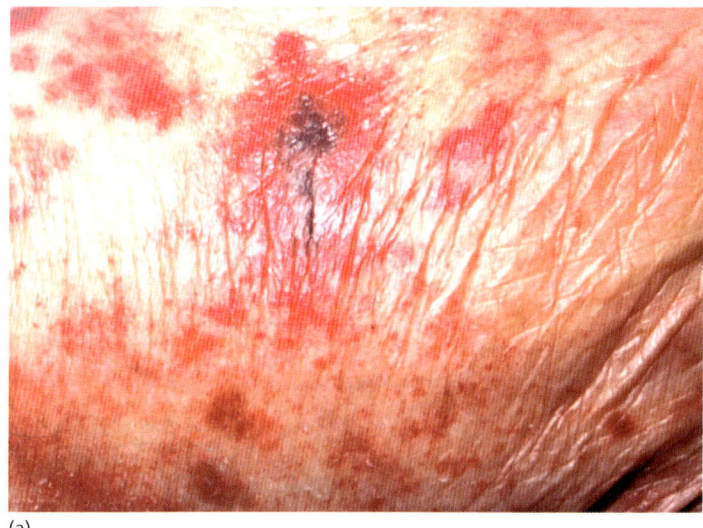

(a)

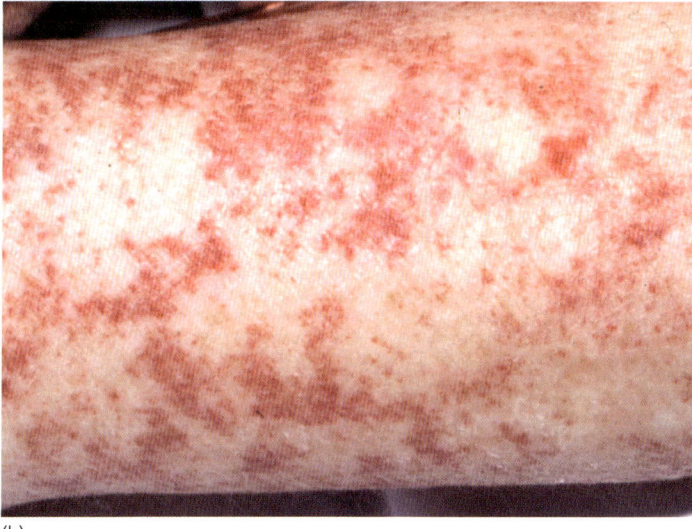

(b)

Figure 100.6 Vasculitis due to sepsis, in a patient with impaired level of consciousness. The necrotic lesion in (a) and the reticulate pattern on the leg in (b) are clues to the involvement of deeper vessels. Histologically, vasculitis due to infection may involve vessels at all levels of the dermis.

clinical experience rather than controlled trials. If a triggering agent is identified, such as a drug or infection, it should be removed or treated. Efforts to minimise stasis, such as use of compression hosiery and the elevation of dependent areas, as well as the use of non-steroidal anti-inflammatory drugs (NSAIDs) and antihistamines, may reduce symptoms [35] although they do not alter the course of the disease.

First line
Oral prednisolone 30–80 mg once daily, tapered over 2–3 weeks, often gives symptom control, although no controlled trials have been carried out to evaluate the treatment of CSVV with oral corticosteroids. Corticosteroid use may be of particular benefit in cases with painful progressive cutaneous lesions. No data support the use of topical corticosteroids or antibiotics in CSVV although such therapies are commonly used.

PART 9: VASCULAR DISORDERS

Second line
Colchicine 0.6 mg twice daily has been shown to be of benefit by anecdotal evidence and open-label studies [11–13]. Dapsone 50–150 mg daily may be advantageous in the treatment of CSVV [14–17].

Third line
In patients with disease refractory to the above therapies, cytotoxic agents may be considered. Such agents include azathioprine (1–2 mg/kg/day) and methotrexate (15–25 mg/week). The use of ciclosporin (2.5–4 mg/kg/day) and cyclophosphamide is almost never indicated for purely cutaneous disease.

Erythema elevatum diutinum

Definition and nomenclature
Erythema elevatum diutinum (EED) is a rare, chronic, cutaneous eruption. The first descriptions were by Hutchinson and Bury in the 1880s, and the condition was later named in 1894 by Radcliffe-Crocker and Williams. It is characterised by fibrosing plaques with histological evidence of leukocytoclastic vasculitis. The condition in younger women has been called Bury disease after the early report. Hutchinson's original cases were described in older men. Some early reports make this distinction although the conditions are considered synonymous.

Epidemiology
Incidence and prevalence
Erythema elevatum diutinum is very rare with only a few hundred cases described. There are small case series published but most reports are of single cases only. Few dermatologists have looked after more than a handful of cases.

Age
Erythema elevatum diutinum is most commonly seen in adults in the fourth to seventh decades although occasional childhood cases are reported [1].

Sex
It occurs equally in males and females.

Ethnicity
There has been no description of predilection in any ethnic groups.

Associated diseases
Erythema elevatum diutinum has been associated with autoimmune diseases such as rheumatoid arthritis, coeliac disease, inflammatory bowel disease and type 1 diabetes. Associations with infections, including *Streptococcus*, hepatitis and syphilis, have also been suggested [2–5,**6**,**7**,**8**,**9**,**10**,11]. Lesions characteristic of EED have been induced by injection of streptococcal antigen into the dermis [12–15], and have occurred at sites of mosquito bites [**10**]. EED has been associated with human immunodeficiency virus (HIV) infection. As lesions of EED have responded to antiretroviral

and dapsone treatment in HIV-positive patients, it is now recognised as one of the defined reactive dermatoses associated with HIV [16]. EED has been associated with hypergammaglobulinaemia and IgA monoclonal gammopathies, as well as with myelodysplasia, pyoderma gangrenosum and relapsing polychondritis. The association with haematological abnormalities, such as multiple myeloma, is strong; however, EED may precede the haematological disease by several years [**17**].

Pathophysiology
Although the exact aetiology is unknown, EED is thought to be related to an Arthus-type reaction with immune complex deposition and subsequent inflammation.

Predisposing factors
See the associated diseases.

Pathology
Acute lesions of EED are characterised by leukocytoclastic vasculitis, with little fibrin deposition (Figure 100.7). Eosinophils may also be present in the upper and mid dermis. Depending on the degree of oedema and infiltration into the dermis, unaffected collagen may

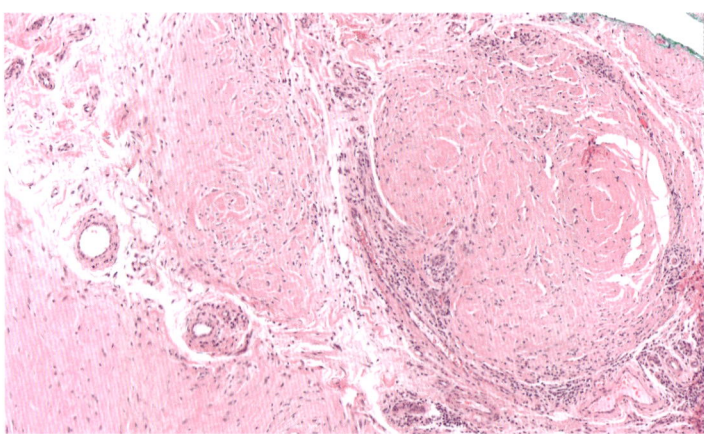

(a)

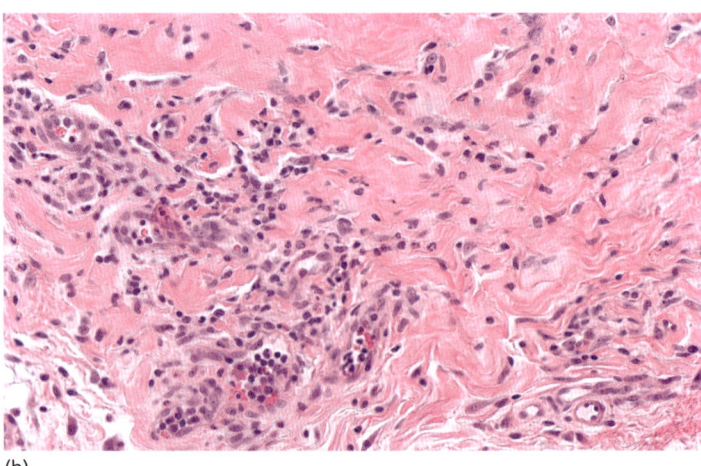

(b)

Figure 100.7 Erythema elevatum diutinum. (a) Prominent, often concentric, fibrosis is seen in the background. (b) Higher magnification showing a perivascular inflammatory cell infiltrate with neutrophils and nuclear dust. Fibrin is often missing or minimal. Courtesy of Dr Eduardo Calonje.

be present just under the epidermis. Chronic lesions demonstrate angiocentric eosinophilic fibrosis, capillary proliferation and infiltration of macrophages, plasma cells and lymphocytes. Cholesterol deposits in histiocytes and in the extracellular tissue (the latter in a pattern that has been termed 'extracellular cholesterolosis') may be present in older lesions [18]. Dermal nodules of EED contain spindle cells and fibrosis [19].

Clinical features

History
Although they are generally asymptomatic, the lesions of EED may be painful.

Presentation
Lesions of EED most commonly appear chronically in a symmetrical fashion over the dorsa of the hands, knees, buttocks and Achilles tendons (Figure 100.8). They are red-violaceous, red-brown or yellowish papules, plaques or nodules. Occasionally, the face and ears are also affected by EED. Initially the lesions are soft, but eventually they fibrose and later leave atrophic scars.

Differential diagnosis
Erythema elevatum diutinum may be difficult to distinguish from CSVV on histology but the clinical presentation enables accurate diagnosis. EED and Sweet syndrome are both described as neutrophilic dermatoses. However, EED differs from Sweet syndrome by the character of the lesions and their distribution, as well as by histopathological features. The classic assumption that lesions from patients with Sweet syndrome lack histopathological fibrinoid necrosis of the vessel walls has been challenged. In one series, 29% of patients had biopsy specimens showing leukocytoclastic vasculitis [20], although this may have been secondary changes in older lesions. Clinically, the lesions in Sweet syndrome are acute, more often asymmetrical and located on the arms, face and neck [21]. By contrast, EED lesions are chronic, symmetrical and classically located over the dorsum of the hands and knees, buttocks and Achilles tendons. Although leukocytoclastic vasculitis has now been reported as a possible feature of Sweet lesions [2], it is not always present and the fibrosis seen in lesions of EED correlates with the clinical chronicity. Granuloma faciale has been considered in the same group of disorders as EED, but may have features of the IgG4-related sclerosing diseases, such as storiform fibrosis, which is histologically absent in EED [22].

Complications and co-morbidities
Although the lesions can be painful and heal with scarring, complications are rare.

Disease course and prognosis
Erythema elevatum diutinum may last from 5 to 35 years, with crops of new lesions developing every few weeks to months.

Investigations
The demonstration of IgA antineutrophil cytoplasmic antibodies (ANCA) (with various specificities) in 6 of 10 cases of EED has been suggested to be of some diagnostic value [23]; in this series, 7 of the 10 patients had raised IgA levels (monoclonal in three).

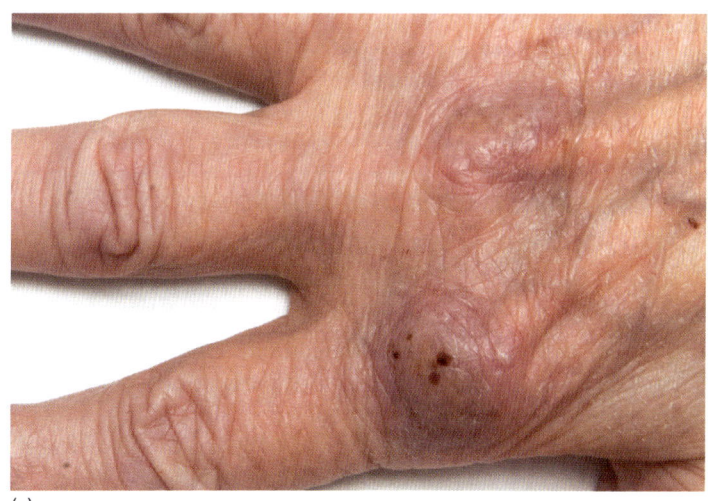
(a)

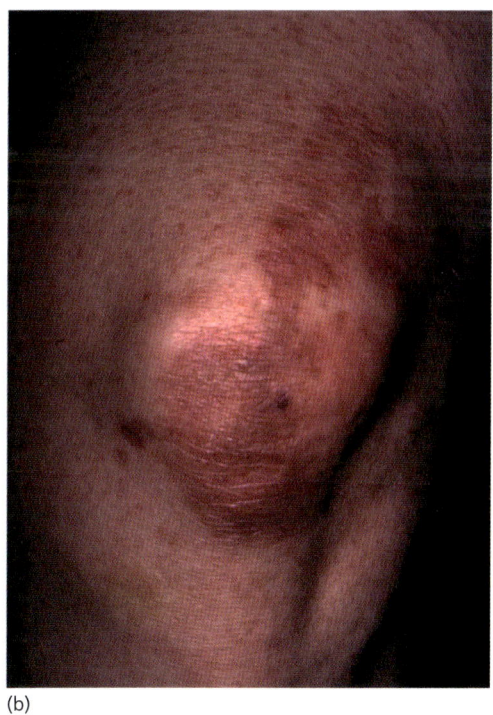
(b)

Figure 100.8 Erythema elevatum diutinum (EED). (a) On the hands. (b) Early non-fibrotic lesions at a typical site on the knee. This patient also had EED on the hands, and pyoderma gangrenosum.

Management
Treatment of an associated disorder such as HIV infection or paraproteinaemia may be effective [24].

First line
Dapsone is usually effective in EED [15], although relapse on stopping may occur.

Second line
Niacinamide has also been used with good effect [25]. High-potency topical, or intralesional, corticosteroids may minimise the size of lesions in patients with limited disease; 5% topical dapsone gel has been described as effective [26].

PART 9: VASCULAR DISORDERS

Third line
Other therapies used for CSVV may also be effective in treating patients with EED.

Recurrent cutaneous necrotising eosinophilic vasculitis

Definition and nomenclature
This is a relatively recently described and rare vasculitis consisting of a predominantly centripetal purpuric papular rash, angioedema, peripheral blood eosinophilia and an eosinophilic necrotising vasculitis of small vessels [1,2]. It can be argued that this is a pathological subdivision of CSVV rather than a distinct entity.

Synonyms and inclusions
- Recurrent cutaneous eosinophilic necrotising vasculitis

Epidemiology
Incidence and prevalence
This is a very rarely described disease with only a few cases in the literature.

Age
The condition has been described in adults aged 17–81 years.

Sex
Either sex may be affected.

Ethnicity
There is no known association.

Associated diseases
Association with connective tissue diseases and with rheumatoid arthritis has been reported [3,4].

Pathophysiology
The cause is unknown. As in other strongly eosinophilic disorders, eosinophil cytokines such as interleukin 5 (IL-5) and toxic eosinophil granule proteins such as the major basic protein have been demonstrated in serum and tissues, respectively, and presumably play a part in the tissue damage. Neutrophil elastase is prominent around vessels, and mast cell degranulation occurs. Eosinophilic vasculitis has also been reported in a patient with the hypereosinophilic syndrome; in this patient, CD40 (a glycoprotein of the tumour necrosis factor (TNF) receptor family) was considered to be important in pathogenesis [5].

Predisposing factors
There are no known predisposing factors.

Pathology
Histopathology shows fibrinoid deposition and necrosis of small dermal vessels with an infiltrate of eosinophils and absent or minimal leukocytoclasis. Small epidermal vesicles containing eosinophils may be present. Immunoglobulin deposition is not a feature. This eosinophilic small-vessel vasculitis may be distinct from other vasculitides such as eosinophilic granulomatosis with polyangiitis (previously known as Churg–Strauss syndrome), in which predominantly medium vessels are affected; and from most drug-induced vasculitis in which eosinophils are generally less prominent.

Causative organisms
There is no known association with causative organisms.

Genetics
The genetics of the condition are unknown.

Environmental factors
There are no reported environmental triggers.

Clinical features
History
Patients may initially present with pruritic papules over the lower limbs. The course is long and recurrent, but fever, arthralgia and visceral involvement are absent.

Presentation
Recurrent pruritic papules and urticarial lesions occur at any site, especially the lower limbs, head and neck, with angioedema of the face and extremities. Digital occlusions manifesting as Raynaud phenomenon or digital gangrene have been reported in patients with cutaneous eosinophilic vasculitis associated with the hypereosinophilic syndrome [5,6], but they can also occur in the hypereosinophilic syndrome in the absence of cutaneous eosinophilic vasculitis [7,8].

Clinical variants
An eosinophilic vasculitis, typically with hypocomplementaemia, also occurs in connective tissue diseases [9].

Differential diagnosis
This condition was recently distinguished from other eosinophilic vasculitides that affect medium-sized vessels (eosinophilic granulomatosis with polyangiitis; see separate section this chapter) and from eosinophilic disorders in which pruritic papules and/or angioedema may occur such as hypereosinophilic syndrome, episodic angioedema with eosinophilia, dermatitis herpetiformis, Wells syndrome, polymorphic eruption of pregnancy or drug eruptions.

Complications and co-morbidities
Ulceration and secondary infection of necrotic lesions may occur. By contrast with eosinophilic granulomatosis with polyangiitis, systemic features are not reported.

Disease course and prognosis
A good response to corticosteroids is reported.

Investigations
Investigations are guided by history and clinical examination and will be needed to exclude the differential diagnoses.

Management
First line
The few cases described have been treated with oral corticosteroids with good effect, intermittently or as prolonged maintenance therapy depending on response [10].

Second line
Secondary infection of ulcerated lesions may require topical or systemic antibiotics according to sensitivities.

Granuloma faciale

Definition and nomenclature
Granuloma faciale is an uncommon condition typified by asymptomatic cutaneous nodules occurring primarily on the face, with occasional extrafacial involvement. Granuloma faciale is limited to the skin, without any systemic manifestations.

Synonyms and inclusions
- Eosinophilic granuloma (not to be confused with Langerhans cell histiocytosis)

Introduction and general description
Granuloma faciale is an uncommon condition of unknown aetiology that is characterised by the presence of benign, purely CSVV. In 1945, Wigley described a 46-year-old woman with recurrent, multiple, raised, discrete, smooth, greyish brown facial lesions. The histology demonstrated pleomorphic infiltrate with predominant eosinophils, but also polymorphs and plasma cells. In the absence of any bony involvement, this was diagnosed as an eosinophilic granuloma [1]. The term 'granuloma faciale' and 'facial granuloma with eosinophilia' was first used by Boersma in 1951 [2].

Epidemiology
Incidence and prevalence
Granuloma faciale is a rare condition.

Age
It is seen most commonly in 40–60-year-olds [3,4].

Sex
It is commoner in males [3].

Ethnicity
Granuloma faciale has been reported from various parts of the world and does not seem to have any ethnic predilection.

Associated diseases
As noted by Wigley [1], the dermal infiltrate consists of eosinophils and plasma cells. Cesinaro *et al.* reported a storiform fibrotic pattern and the presence of large amounts of IgG4-staining deposits [5]. This raises the possibility that some patients with granuloma faciale may have IgG4-related disease.

Pathophysiology
Although the aetiology is unclear, this disease is considered to be a histological variant of leukocytoclastic vasculitis with a prominent eosinophilic infiltrate and confined to the skin [4]. The presence of plasma cells and IgG deposition in and around the dermal vasculature has been demonstrated, indicating that granuloma faciale may be immune complex mediated [5]. The reporting of T cells in the tissue is variable. Smoller and Bortz reported large numbers of CD4+ cells that stain strongly for IL-2R antibodies [6], and Cesinaro *et al.* found T-cell subsets to be variable but with a predominance of GATA-3 lymphocytes [5].

Pathology
Granuloma faciale is a misnomer. The one pathological finding that is almost always absent is a granuloma [7]. It is characterised by a mixed inflammatory infiltrate with a predominance of eosinophils and plasma cells as part of a pleomorphic infiltrate, mainly in the upper half of the dermis but with occasional spread into the lower dermis and subcutaneous tissue (Figure 100.9). A band of normal collagen referred to as a Grenz zone typically separates the inflammatory infiltrate from the epidermis and pilosebaceous appendages. Nuclear dust (fragmented neutrophil nuclei) may be observed near capillaries. The vascular changes may be mild (perivascular distribution of inflammatory cells) to florid (leukocytoclastic vasculitis with fibrinoid necrosis). Perivascular storiform fibrosis and obliterative venulitis have been observed.

Clinical features
History
Lesions of granuloma faciale commonly occur on the face (Figure 100.10); multiple lesions are present in about a third of cases but extrafacial involvement is uncommon, occurring in 5 of 66 patients in one study [4]. They are almost always asymptomatic, although some patients may describe itching, burning or pain associated with the lesions.

Presentation
The nodules or plaques are soft and red-brown. They are smooth, with prominent follicular orifices and telangiectatic surface changes or scaling. The lesions never ulcerate. Dermoscopy shows parallel, arborising blood vessels, brown dots and globules and dilated follicular openings [8].

Clinical variants
Extrafacial granuloma faciale is rare, but it has been reported on the scalp, back, shoulders, arms, breast and trunk [9–12]. In a study of 66 patients, only five patients had extrafacial lesions [4]; all these lesions coexisted with facial lesions. Intranasal lesions have been reported.

Eosinophilic angiocentric fibrosis is thought to be a mucosal variant of granuloma faciale that may occur in the nasal passages or upper airways in conjunction with skin lesions of granuloma faciale [13,14]. Eosinophilic angiocentric fibrosis may cause fibrotic stenosis of the affected site with localised extension and damage [15].

PART 9: VASCULAR DISORDERS

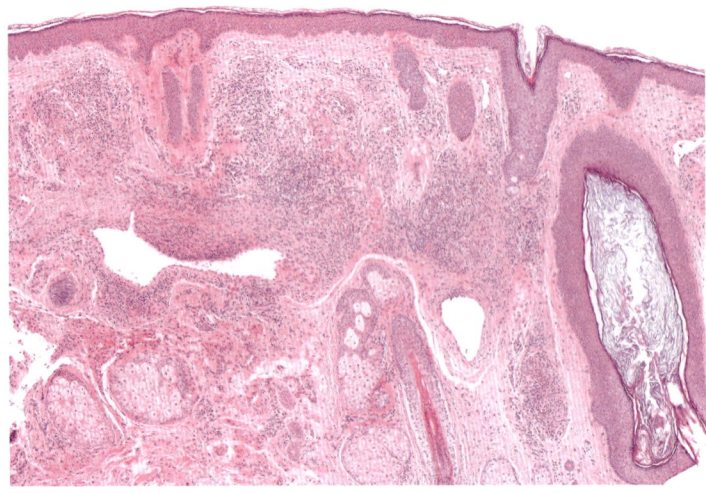

(a)

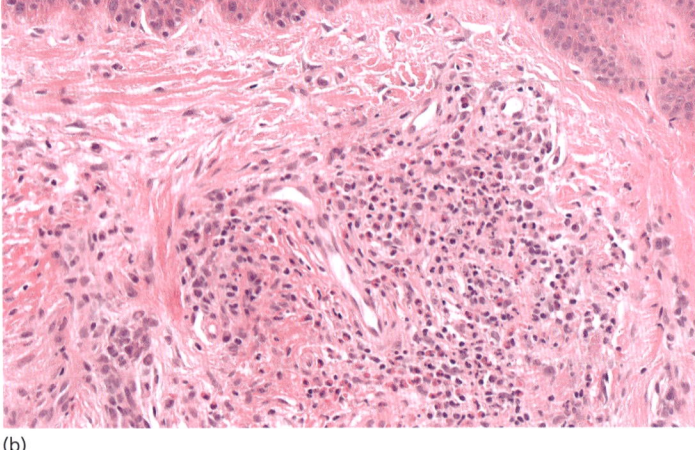

(b)

Figure 100.9 Granuloma faciale. (a) Low-power magnification showing a prominent perivascular inflammatory cell infiltrate. (b) Higher magnification where eosinophils, neutrophils with nuclear dust and plasma cells are noted. Courtesy of Dr Eduardo Calonje.

For example, epiphora and proptosis have been reported in patients with obstructive sino-nasal eosinophilic angiocentric fibrosis [16].

Differential diagnosis
Granulomatous rosacea does not have vasculitis on histology. Sarcoid, tuberculosis, cutaneous lupus erythematosus and rarely EED may present with solitary cutaneous lesions.

Disease course and prognosis
Granuloma faciale is a chronic disease with intermittent acute flares that is notoriously resistant to treatment.

Investigations
A definitive diagnosis of granuloma faciale requires clinically consistent lesions and a confirmatory biopsy. Although most laboratory studies are normal, mild peripheral blood eosinophilia may be present [10].

Management
Management of granuloma faciale may be challenging and difficult to treat.

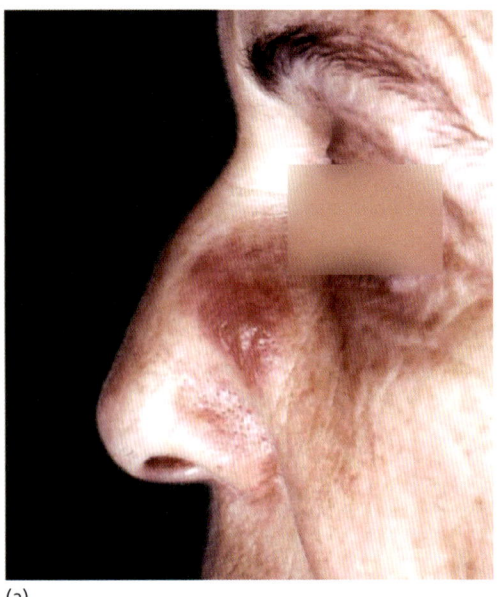

(a)

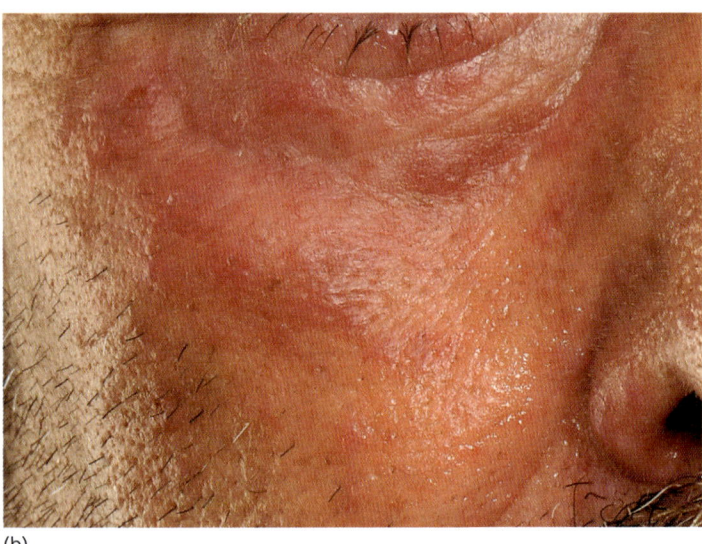

(b)

Figure 100.10 Granuloma faciale. (a) Reddish brown plaque on the nose. (b) Close up of a facial plaque. (a) Courtesy of Dr G. Dawn, Monklands Hospital, UK.

Treatment ladder

First line
- Topical tacrolimus 0.03% or 0.1%

Second line
- Topical or intralesional corticosteroids

Third line
- Dermabrasion [17], laser treatments of various types [17–19], electrosurgery [17], cryosurgery [20], psoralen with ultraviolet A (PUVA) and other systemic treatments including dapsone [21] and tacrolimus [22]
- Some cases have been treated with surgical excision [12]

SMALL-VESSEL IMMUNE COMPLEX-ASSOCIATED VASCULITIS

IgA vasculitis

Definition and nomenclature

IgA vasculitis is an immune complex vasculitis characterised by IgA1-dominant immune deposits affecting small vessels (predominantly capillaries, venules or arterioles). It often involves the skin and gastrointestinal tract, and frequently causes arthritis. Glomerulonephritis indistinguishable from IgA nephropathy may occur [1].

Synonyms and inclusions
- Henoch–Schönlein purpura (HSP)
- Anaphylactoid purpura
- Rheumatoid purpura
- Allergic purpura
- Haemorrhagic vasculitis
- Purpura haemorrhagica
- Non-thrombocytopenic purpura

Introduction and general description

William Heberden, in the 1780s, described two children with petechiae, purpura and ecchymosis in conjunction with arthritis. One of the two boys also had abdominal pain, melaena and haematuria [2]. In the 19th century, Johann Schönlein and Eduard Henoch independently characterised the condition, which bore their name until the renaming of eponymous vasculitides in 2012 [1].

For the purposes of homogeneity and classification, there are two sets of classification criteria in use. The ACR proposed classification criteria in 1990: if any two of the following four criteria were satisfied, the case could be classified as IgA vasculitis: (i) palpable purpura; (ii) bowel angina; (iii) age <20 years at onset; and (iv) the presence of granulocytes in the vessel wall on biopsy [3]. These criteria were modified in a combined effort by the European League Against Rheumatism and the Paediatric Rheumatology Society for classifying childhood-onset vasculitis. The presence of any one of the following four features in the presence of palpable purpura satisfies a classification of IgA vasculitis: (i) diffuse abdominal pain; (ii) any biopsy demonstrating predominant IgA deposition; (iii) any acute arthritis or arthralgia; and (iv) renal involvement in the form of haematuria or proteinuria [4].

Epidemiology

Incidence and prevalence

The annual incidence of IgA vasculitis is 10–20/100 000 in children [5–7,8], and about 1–1.5/100 000 in adults [9,10]. The incidence of nephritis in conjunction with IgA vasculitis is lower in children, at about 3.5/100 000 [11]. A peak incidence of 70.3/100 000 children between 4 and 6 years of age has been observed [8].

Age

The peak incidence is between the ages of 4 and 6 years [8]. Children developing nephritis are typically slightly older. In one study,

children >8 years of age had an odds ratio of 2.7 for developing nephritis [12]. Adult-onset IgA vasculitis can occur at any age.

Sex

There may be a mild male preponderance with reported ratios of 1.8 : 1 [13].

Ethnicity

There is a higher incidence of IgA vasculitis reported from Scotland (20.3–26.7/100 000) [5] than in Taiwan (12.9/100 000) [6] or the Czech Republic (10.2/100 000) [7]. IgA-related nephritis has been more commonly reported in American Indians as compared with Hispanics [14].

Associated diseases

Pathologically, IgA vasculitis in the kidney is indistinguishable from IgA nephropathy. Patients with IgA vasculitis are typically younger and have more extrarenal manifestations [15].

There may be an association of IgA vasculitis with familial Mediterranean fever (FMF). *MEFV* (familial Mediterranean fever) gene mutations have been observed in IgA vasculitis more commonly than the general population [16,17]. The clinical syndrome of IgA vasculitis has been observed more commonly in patients with FMF than in the general population, and some consider it to be a feature of FMF [17–19].

Pathophysiology

Predisposing factors

IgA vasculitis appears to be commoner in the spring, autumn and winter as compared with the summer months [6,20–22]. Respiratory infections may be a precursor in a small number of cases and may be the second hit in patients with a genetic predisposition [21,23]. Streptococcal infections are the most commonly observed predisposing infections [24,25]. It has been reported with Covid-19 infection [26].

Pathology

IgA is thought to be key in the pathogenesis. Increased levels of IgA in the serum (in 50% with active disease), circulating immune complexes containing IgA, and the deposition of IgA in blood vessel walls and in the renal mesangium are associated with IgA vasculitis (Figure 100.11). In IgA vasculitis, IgA1 rather than IgA2 is the main IgA subclass deposited in skin lesions [27,28]. Diminished glycosylation of the proline-rich hinge region of the IgA1 heavy chain is thought to be an important factor in allowing the IgA to be deposited in the mesangium and in activating the alternative pathway of complement in IgA, as it makes such IgA1 molecules more prone to forming macromolecular complexes [29]. Other IgA antibodies that occur in IgA vasculitis include IgA ANCA, although this finding is very variable between studies. IgA rheumatoid factor and IgA anticardiolipin antibodies are also sometimes present, as are IgA antiendothelial cell antibodies.

The activation of several cytokines is documented although these are unlikely to be a primary cause. Levels of TNF-α in the peripheral blood are increased, and it can be detected in skin lesions. IL-6, IL-8, transforming growth factor β (TGF-β) and vascular endothelial growth factor (VEGF) levels are all increased in active IgA

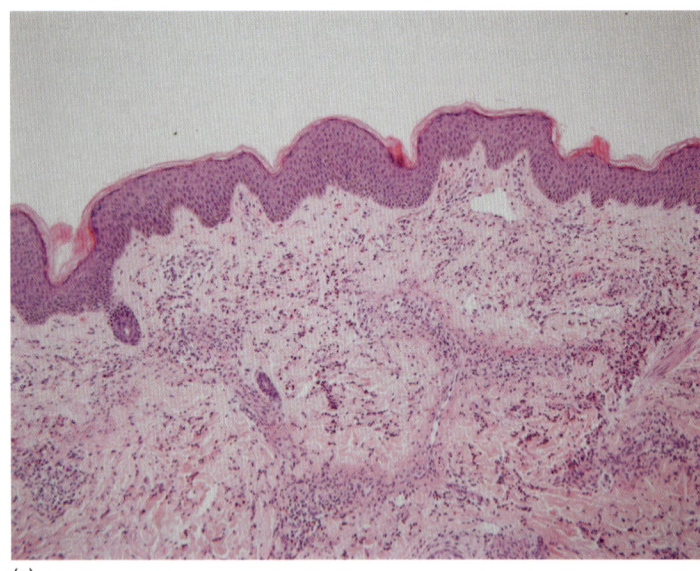

(a)

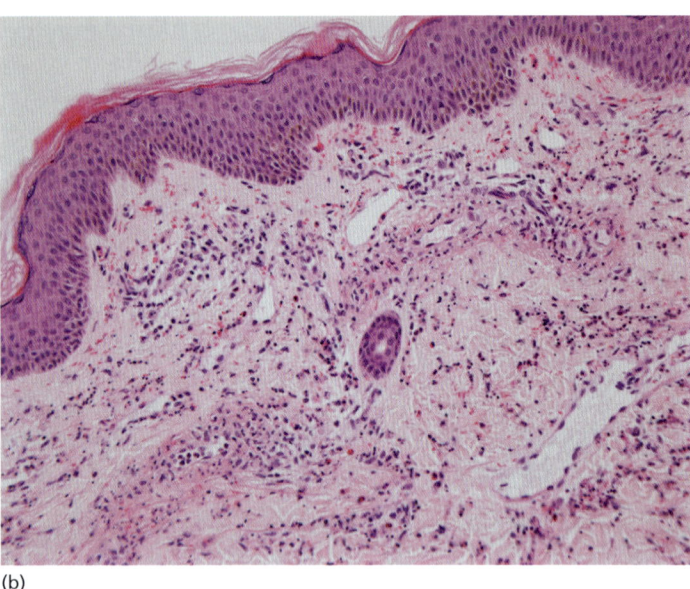

(b)

Figure 100.11 IgA vasculitis at (a) lower and (b) higher magnifications. There is perivascular leukocytoclasis and fibrin deposition, and eosinophils are present. Courtesy of Dr Laszlo Igali, Norfolk and Norwich University Hospital, Norwich, UK.

vasculitis. TGF-β is of particular interest as blood levels of T cells that produce this cytokine are increased, and it is known to enhance IgA1 responses. Neutrophil activation, elevated nitric oxide levels, reactive oxygen species and increased urinary leukotriene are all documented.

Causative organisms

There are no definitive causative organisms for IgA vasculitis. Streptococcal infections predispose to IgA vasculitis, and antistreptolysin O titre positivity confers a 10-fold risk of IgA vasculitis [25] but the exact role of the bacteria is unknown. It is likely to be a complex interplay between genetic predisposition, bacterial infection and perhaps other environmental factors. *Bartonella* and *Haemophilus* have been implicated [30,31]; *Helicobacter* antibodies have been reported in adults with IgA vasculitis [32].

Genetics

There is no definite association of any genes with IgA vasculitis. Human leukocyte antigen (HLA) class I genes may be of relevance [33]. *MEFV* gene mutations have been observed to be commoner in patients with IgA vasculitis than in the general population [16,17].

Clinical features

History

Most commonly, IgA vasculitis manifests at the outset with the classic findings of purpura, arthralgia and abdominal pain. Individual lesions usually fade within 5–7 days but crops of lesions can recur for a few weeks to several months.

Presentation

The cutaneous findings are typically red urticarial papules, which may evolve within 24 h into palpable purpura with haemorrhage. Urticaria, vesicles, bullae (Figure 100.12a) and necrotic ulcers (Figure 100.12b) may develop. A retiform pattern within lesions is characteristic, but not always present. The presentation may be identical to CSVV (see Figure 100.1). Although it typically involves the extensor aspects of the limbs (especially the elbows and knees) and buttocks in a symmetrical fashion, IgA vasculitis may also affect the trunk and face. Renal involvement with IgA vasculitis is common, occurring in approximately 40–50% of patients; 25% have gross haematuria and the remainder microscopic haematuria. Proteinuria occurs in 60% of these but is uncommon in the absence of haematuria. Gastrointestinal involvement is common (65%), with frank gastrointestinal bleeding in 30% of patients with IgA vasculitis. Painful arthritis is seen in about 75% of patients, most frequently affecting the knees and ankles. Less common manifestations of IgA vasculitis include orchitis (in 10–20% of boys), intussusception, pancreatitis, neurological abnormalities, uveitis, carditis and pulmonary haemorrhage.

Clinical variants

Rarely, gastrointestinal involvement and arthritis can occur in the absence of skin disease.

Differential diagnosis

This includes IgA nephropathy, idiopathic thrombocytopenic purpura, septic shock, acute abdomen and systemic lupus erythematosus (SLE).

Classification of severity

The BVAS v3 system has been validated to assess the severity of IgA vasculitis alongside several other forms of systemic vasculitides. The tool can describe the nature of the clinical involvement, with higher scores suggestive of more severe disease, and is responsive to changes in clinical activity [34].

Complications and co-morbidities

End-stage renal disease is uncommon but, if it occurs, may need renal transplantation. Renal transplant survival is over 80% at 5 years. Uncommonly, IgA vasculitis may recur in the graft and cause graft rejection [35].

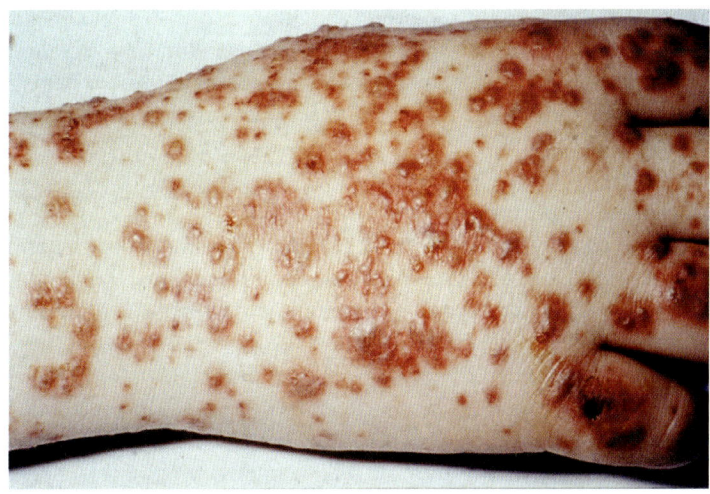

(a)

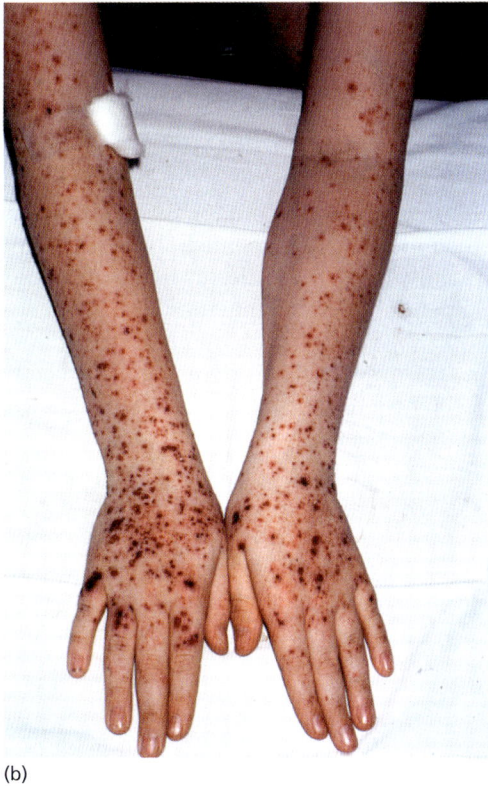

(b)

Figure 100.12 IgA vasculitis. (a) Haemorrhagic vesicles present on the hand. (b) Vasculitis extending onto the arms. (a) Courtesy of Andrew Carmichael, South Tees Hospitals NHS Trust, UK.

Disease course and prognosis

About 25% of patients will relapse, and typically the relapse is mild and easily treated [36]. IgA vasculitis can become chronic in 5–10% of patients, the cutaneous involvement usually lasting between 6 and 16 weeks. Only 1–3% of these patients progress to end-stage renal disease, although one-third to one-half of patients have renal abnormalities on long-term follow-up [13,37]. The presence of nephrotic or nephritic-nephrotic phenotype and the presence of crescents carry an adverse prognosis [38]. IgA vasculitis is not a benign disease in those above the age of 50 years. The 5-year survival for those under the age of 21, aged 21–50 and those over 50 is 100%, 94% and 40%, respectively [39].

Investigations

IgA vasculitis is a clinical diagnosis, with confirmation by direct immunofluorescence and routine histology. Perivascular IgA deposits are characteristic of IgA vasculitis and can help to distinguish it from other vasculitides including CSVV, granulomatosis with polyangiitis, eosinophilic granulomatosis with polyangiitis and microscopic polyangiitis. In one study, all individuals with IgA vasculitis had deposits of galactose-deficient IgA1 [40]. IgA immune complexes are not specific to IgA vasculitis, but can be seen in a variety of patients including those with SLE, endocarditis, dermatitis herpetiformis, alcoholism, IgA nephropathy, inflammatory bowel disease, ankylosing spondylitis, Sjögren syndrome, rheumatoid arthritis, some cancers and in some drug hypersensitivity reactions. No laboratory tests are specific for IgA vasculitis, but the serum levels of galactose-deficient IgA1 may be higher in all individuals with IgA vasculitis, especially those with nephritis [41].

Management

In children, the treatment of IgA vasculitis is supportive because the condition may be self-limiting. There are no controlled studies of any drugs used in IgA vasculitis. Glucocorticoid agents may be of value in children with renal involvement and in most adults. Pulsed intravenous methylprednisolone, ciclosporin A, cyclophosphamide, azathioprine and mycophenolate mofetil have all been tried in open-label fashion. There are no convincing data for any of them [42]. The recognition of poor prognosis in adults, especially those with renal involvement, does suggest the need for greater immunosuppression with first line glucocorticoids and cyclophosphamide. The use of rituximab for refractory cases appears to be safe and effective but has not been subject to randomised controlled trials [43].

Cryoglobulinaemic vasculitis

Definition and nomenclature

Cryoglobulins are abnormal immunoglobulins that precipitate spontaneously when serum is cooled to a temperature below 37°C. Cryoglobulinaemia is the condition characterised by the presence of circulating cryoglobulins; the accompanying vasculitis that affects the small vessels is due to cryoglobulins deposited as immune complexes. It is mainly the skin glomeruli and peripheral nerves that are affected. Not all cryoglobulinaemia is associated with symptoms. This chapter only deals with the vasculitis manifestations; details of the history, aetiology and pathogenesis of cryoglobulinaemia are provided in Chapter 124.

Synonyms and inclusions

- Type II and type III cryoglobulinaemia
- Mixed essential cryoglobulinaemia
- Cryoglobulinaemia

Introduction and general description

Cryoglobulinaemic vasculitis is a small-vessel vasculitis affecting the skin, joints, peripheral nerves and kidneys. About 80% of cases are secondary to hepatitis C infection [1]. Other causes include B-cell lymphoproliferative disorders, autoimmune diseases like Sjögren syndrome, other viral disorders (e.g. hepatitis B, HIV) and essential mixed cryoglobulinaemia.

Cryoglobulins may be divided into three main subtypes:

1 Monoclonal immunoglobulin, usually IgG or IgM, accounts for about 10–25% of cases and is usually associated with lymphoproliferative disease, especially multiple myeloma or Waldenström macroglobulinaemia.

2 Mixed polyclonal (usually IgG) immunoglobulin and monoclonal (usually IgM-κ) immunoglobulin, the latter having rheumatoid factor activity, account for about 25% of cases.

3 Polyclonal IgM with rheumatoid factor activity and polyclonal IgG with antigenic activity account for about 50–65% of cases.

Epidemiology

Incidence and prevalence

Cryoglobulinaemic vasculitis is a rare disease, and its incidence and prevalence are not known.

Age

The condition is seen usually in adults and is very rare in children.

Associated diseases

Hepatitis C is responsible for about 80% of cryoglobulinaemic vasculitis. The other common associations are Sjögren syndrome and B-cell lymphoproliferative disorders.

Pathophysiology

The mechanism to produce cryoglobulins by a clonally expanded B-cell population is ill understood. Since most patients with hepatitis C do not develop vasculitis, but have circulating cryoglobulins, there may be a failure of a separate mechanism responsible for the disease manifestations. There are significantly lower circulating T-regulatory cells in patients who develop vasculitis as compared with those with just cryoglobulinaemia [2].

Typically, a polyvalent IgM rheumatoid factor binds to antigen (although other monovalent immunoglobulins can also be responsible) to produce immune complexes that activate complement resulting in endothelial activation and tissue damage.

Predisposing factors

Cold and immobility may precipitate acute episodes.

Pathology

Cryoglobulinaemic vasculitis affects capillaries, arterioles and venules. In the skin, it produces a pan-dermal leukocytoclastic vasculitis that may extend into the subcutis. Eosinophilic periodic acid–Schiff (PAS) positive globular immune complex deposits and PAS-negative intraluminal fibrin deposits can be visualised. More chronic lesions develop a mononuclear-predominant infiltrate and may become granulomatous. Changes in other organs include membranoproliferative glomerulonephritis, immune complex deposition in the lungs causing bronchiolitis obliterans organising pneumonia, and vasa nervosa vasculitis causing a peripheral neuropathy.

Causative organisms

The main aetiological factor in mixed cryoglobulinaemia is hepatitis C virus (HCV) infection, which accounts for about 80% of cases. However, although cryoglobulinaemia can be detected in about 50% of subjects with HCV, immune complex vasculitis occurs in less than 5% [3].

Environmental factors

Exposure to cold and immobility can trigger gelling in cryoglobulinaemia, resulting in cutaneous necrosis.

Clinical features

History and presentation

The classic 'Meltzer triad' of arthralgia, purpura and weakness was described in 1966, but is seen in less than a third of patients [4]. Myalgia, headache, fever and weight loss are common. Palpable purpura, the commonest presenting feature, is nearly universal (Figure 100.13). Sensorimotor neuropathy and mononeuritis multiplex are both commonly documented. Pulmonary involvement is rare. Renal involvement is usually in the form of membranoproliferative glomerulonephritis, and presents with nephrotic range proteinuria [5]. A smaller proportion of patients may present with proliferative mesangial lesions or thrombotic lesions [5]. The Raynaud phenomenon may be seen in patients with associated connective tissue disease.

Differential diagnosis

Cryoglobulinaemic vasculitis should be distinguished from other causes of CSVV because corticosteroid therapy, although sometimes necessary in the short term, may in the longer term worsen the underlying infection that is present in the majority of

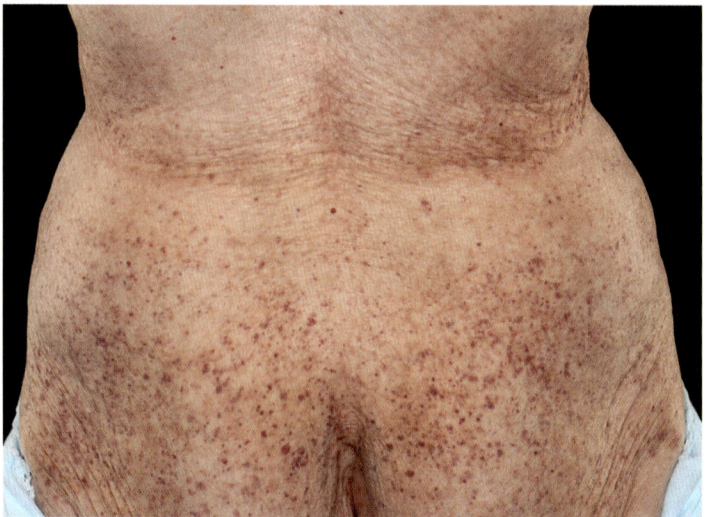

Figure 100.13 Cryoglobulinaemic vasculitis.

cases. Most other causes of leukocytoclastic vasculitis appear as a more superficial vasculitis in biopsy specimens, and if cryoglobulin deposits are seen histologically then the diagnosis is usually suspected (although this is much commoner in type I cryoglobulinaemia). Clinically, head and neck involvement, significant livedo, acrocyanosis, Raynaud phenomenon or larger-vessel occlusion are all more suggestive of type I cryoglobulinaemia.

Complications and co-morbidities

In patients with HCV-induced disease, the complications are those of liver involvement. Associated glomerulonephritis is common and important and may be more frequent in those with hepatitis C [6]. There is an increased risk of myeloproliferative disorders, particularly a B-cell non-Hodgkin lymphoma [7]. This appears to be fourfold greater in patients without hepatitis C [8]. Sjögren syndrome has been reported in up to 20% of patients [4].

Disease course and prognosis

Cryoglobulinaemic vasculitis *per se* does not confer a significant mortality risk. In patients with HCV-induced disease, the viral disease will determine the prognosis. In patients without hepatitis C, renal involvement is associated with greater morbidity. There are no large cohort studies to predict outcomes.

Investigations

A pivotal consideration when testing for cryoglobulinaemic vasculitis is transport of the specimen. The greatest care should be taken to ensure that the blood is transported to the laboratory at 37°C to ensure that the tests are not falsely negative. The demonstration of cryocrit in patients with clinical evidence of small-vessel vasculitis is probably the gold standard for the diagnosis (Figure 100.14). A low complement C4 level with a near normal C3 is nearly universal. Rheumatoid factor is positive in high titres. Evidence of viral hepatitis should be looked for. Inflammatory markers will be elevated.

Urine analysis can range from normal to nephrotic range proteinuria. A renal biopsy will often be positive in the presence of significant renal disease, although occasionally the lesions may be due to minimal change disease [5]. A cutaneous biopsy will demonstrate leukocytoclastic vasculitis.

Management

Treatment will depend on the underlying cause. In patients with hepatitis C infection, the treatment should be coordinated with a hepatologist and will need a combination of glucocorticoids, antiviral therapy and immunomodulatory agents [9]. The HCV genotype will dictate the exact choice and duration of the antiviral agent. Interferon α in combination with ribavirin is beneficial, but relapses are common, necessitating long-term treatment [9]. Rituximab may be of benefit in this group of patients [10].

There is little evidence for the management of non-hepatitis C cryoglobulinaemic vasculitis. Consensus from the European League Against Rheumatism recommends a combination of immunomodulatory agents and glucocorticoid treatment based on the model of treating the other small-vessel vasculitides, such as the ANCA-associated vasculitides [9].

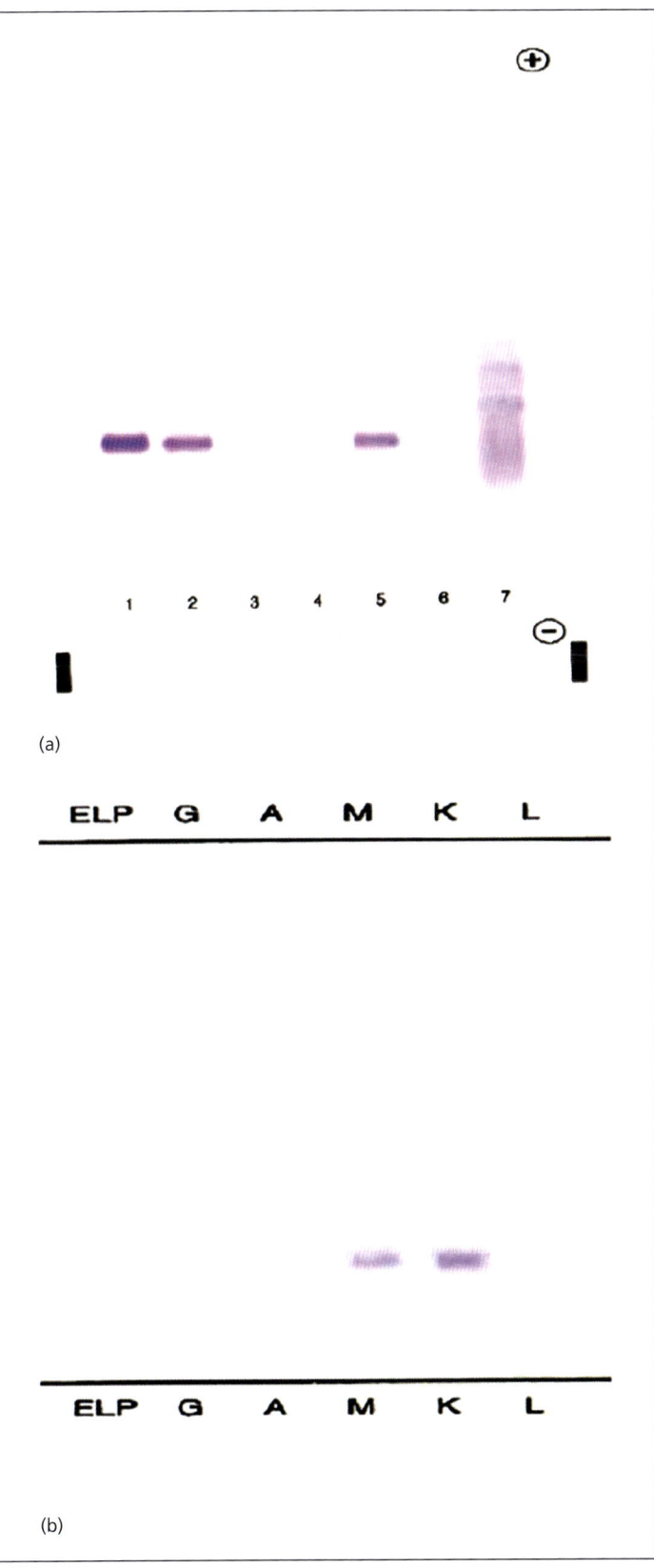

(a)

(b)

Figure 100.14 Serum protein electrophoresis. (a) Demonstrating a clear band in lanes 1, 2 and 5. Lanes 3 and 4 are negative controls and lane 5 is a urine control from a nephrotic specimen. The sample was run on an enhanced urine programme and gel for greater demonstration of the migration of low protein concentrations. (b) Demonstrating the same sample as an IgM-κ band. Courtesy of Ian Thirkettle and Karen Ashurst.

Hypocomplementaemic urticarial vasculitis

Definition and nomenclature

This section deals with hypocomplementaemic urticarial vasculitis (HUV); other forms of urticarial vasculitis are discussed in Chapter 44. HUV is defined as vasculitis affecting small vessels (i.e. capillaries, venules or arterioles), accompanied by urticaria and hypocomplementaemia and associated with anti-C1q antibodies. Glomerulonephritis, arthritis, obstructive pulmonary disease and ocular inflammation are common [1].

> **Synonyms and inclusions**
> - Anti-C1q vasculitis
> - MacDuffie hypocomplementaemic urticarial vasculitis
> - MacDuffie syndrome

Introduction and general description

The condition is very rare and is characterised by persistent urticarial lesions lasting for longer than 24 h with circulating anti-C1q autoantibodies. Arthritis, glomerulonephritis, pulmonary and ocular disease, leukocytoclastic vasculitis, ocular inflammation and abdominal pain are associated.

Epidemiology

Incidence and prevalence

Hypocomplementaemic urticarial vasculitis is very rare with only a few hundred cases described. The annual incidence in Sweden is 0.7/million [2].

Age

The most common presentation is when a person is in their thirties, but childhood cases have been described.

Sex

It is commoner in females [3,4].

Ethnicity

There are no associations.

Associated diseases

It may be associated with SLE [4] and may be linked with increased susceptibility to pyogenic infections.

Pathophysiology

The sera of patients with HUV contains polyclonal IgG with C1q precipitin activity contained within the Fab fragments [5]. These IgG antibodies are directed against the collagen-like region of C1q, resulting in a reduction of C1q in the serum with subsequent activation of the complement pathway [6].

Predisposing factors

These are unknown.

Pathology

Lesions of urticarial vasculitis are typically viewed as showing a leukocytoclastic vasculitis. HUV shows many interstitial neutrophils rather than the pleomorphic infiltrate of normocomplementaemic vasculitis [7]. The deposition of immune complexes is present in normal and lesional skin in HUV, as opposed to only lesional skin in normocomplementaemic vasculitis [4,7].

Clinical features

History

Hypocomplementaemic urticarial vasculitis is characterised by weals, which are characteristically painful but can be itchy, and persist for more than 24 h. In HUV, weals resolve with areas of discoloration. Angioedema is common and may be a presenting feature.

Presentation

Cutaneous lesions of both the hypocomplementaemic and normocomplementaemic forms of UV are red indurated weals that may contain purpuric foci (Figure 100.15). Angioedema and macular erythema may also occur. Livedo reticularis, nodules and bullae may be evident, and may also contain purpuric foci. Patients with the hypocomplementaemic form may have constitutional symptoms.

Differential diagnosis

Hypocomplementaemic urticarial vasculitis has features similar to SLE and may overlap. Signs such as ocular inflammation, angioedema and chronic obstructive pulmonary disease may help distinguish the two processes. Pre-bullous pemphigoid, erythema multiforme, Sweet syndrome, other causes of vasculitis and urticaria coexisting with various forms of eczema should be considered, as should mixed cryoglobulinaemia, Muckle–Wells syndrome, Cogan syndrome and Schnitzler syndrome.

Classification of severity

There is no classification.

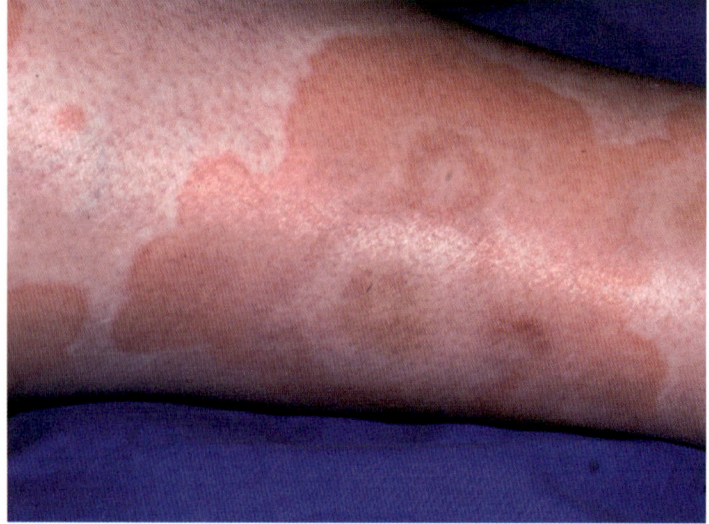

Figure 100.15 Urticarial vasculitis.

Complications and co-morbidities

Cough or dyspnoea may indicate pleural and pericardial effusions, emphysema or chronic obstructive pulmonary disease (seen in 20–50%). Proteinuria or haematuria may indicate glomerulonephritis, which may progress to end-stage renal failure, particularly in those with childhood onset. Gastrointestinal symptoms (abdominal discomfort, nausea, vomiting and diarrhoea), arthritis, episcleritis, uveitis, conjunctivitis, aseptic meningitis, nerve palsies and transverse myelitis may occur.

Investigations

If urticarial lesions last for longer than 24 h (which can be determined by drawing around their margin), then they are not ordinary urticaria (except delayed pressure urticaria) and a skin biopsy should be considered. Pain rather than itch, or the presence of purpura, also suggests urticarial vasculitis. History, physical examination and laboratory studies, including C3, C4 and antinuclear antibody, should help to establish the extent of disease and to exclude underlying disease (e.g. hepatitis C) and to evaluate for SLE. Some patients may demonstrate an elevated erythrocyte sedimentation rate (ESR), hypocomplementaemia, a low-titre positive antinuclear antibody and haematuria. A biopsy may help to confirm the diagnosis and to exclude other disorders.

Management

The evidence for the treatment of HUV is anecdotal. Systemic corticosteroids are effective. Steroid-sparing agents should be considered, but the evidence for their use is restricted to case reports for cyclophosphamide [8], methotrexate [9], dapsone [10], colchicine [11] and hydroxychloroquine [12]. Some patients require oral antihistamines for the control of angioedema and urticaria-like lesions in addition to therapies directed at the vasculitis.

First line

Although no single treatment is effective for all cases of urticarial vasculitis, most patients respond to systemic corticosteroids.

Second line

Drugs that have been shown to be effective for the treatment of urticarial vasculitis include dapsone (100–200 mg once daily), colchicine (0.6 mg twice to three times daily) and hydroxychloroquine (200 mg once to twice daily).

Third line

For patients with refractory disease, there is limited evidence for the use of cyclophosphamide or mycophenolate mofetil [8,13].

Antiglomerular basement membrane vasculitis

Definition and nomenclature

Antiglomerular basement membrane (anti-GBM) vasculitis affects glomerular capillaries or pulmonary capillaries, or both, with GBM deposition of anti-GBM autoantibodies. Lung involvement causes pulmonary haemorrhage, and renal involvement causes glomerulonephritis with necrosis and crescents [1].

> **Synonyms and inclusions**
> - Anti-GBM syndrome
> - Goodpasture syndrome
> - Lung purpura with nephritis

Introduction and general description

In 1919, Ernest Goodpasture described two men who he thought had a viral influenza. One of them had the classic changes that came to bear the eponymous diagnosis of Goodpasture syndrome – alveolar haemorrhage and glomerulonephritis with arteriolar vasculitis [2]. The name was formally changed by international consensus to anti-GBM disease in 2012 [1]. The consensus name is flawed because the antibodies bind to pulmonary alveolar capillary basement membranes as well. Cutaneous involvement is not common, although there are anecdotal reports of non-vasculitic skin changes with immune deposition [3]. Patients may present to dermatologists with pallor.

Epidemiology
Incidence and prevalence

There are about 0.5 cases/million population per year [4]. The prevalence is unknown.

Age

The disease is known to occur in children [5]; but the peaks seem to occur in the third and seventh decades [6].

Sex

In children the male to female ratio is 1 : 2 [7], whereas this is reversed in those older than 65 years with a ratio of 1.9 : 1 [8].

Ethnicity

The relative ethnic differences are unknown.

Pathophysiology

The condition is due to immune complexes composed of autoantibodies directed against the NC1 domain of the α3 chain of type IV collagen [9]. The distribution of this molecule restricts the condition to the lung and kidney.

Pathology

Perivasculitis and anti-IgM and C3 antibodies at the basement membrane zone in cutaneous lesions have been described in one case [3].

Genetics

Familial instances of the disease have been described including in a pair of identical twins with exposure to hydrocarbon fumes [10].

Environmental factors

It is most common in late spring and early summer.

PART 9: VASCULAR DISORDERS

Clinical features
History and presentation
Haemoptysis, fatigue, dyspnoea and cough may be presenting features. Pallor, oedema, chest signs, heart murmurs and hepatomegaly may be present. Discrete, red, macular lesions on the instep of the foot have been described [3].

Clinical variants
Respiratory features predate renal disease by up to a year in two-thirds of cases, and there may be a gap of up to 12 years.

Differential diagnosis
Granulomatosis with polyangiitis, eosinophilic granulomatosis with polyangiitis, IgA vasculitis and microscopic polyangiitis may all present with renal failure and pulmonary haemorrhage. Identification of anti-GBM antibodies helps diagnosis.

Disease course and prognosis
Untreated outcome is very poor, with near 100% mortality. With treatment, 1-year survival depends on early renal function: there is 100% survival if the serum creatinine is <500 μmol/L, but 65% survival in dialysis-dependent cases [11]. In a French cohort of 119 individuals treated with a combination of renal replacement therapy, plasmapheresis and immunosuppression, the 5-year survival was 92% [12]. Poor prognostic markers include oliguria or anuria, hypertension, dyslipidaemia or need for mechanical ventilation on presentation; glomerulosclerosis, tubular atrophy or interstitial fibrosis on biopsy; and advancing age [12,13].

Investigations
Investigations should exclude other systemic vasculitides. ANCA may be positive but antinuclear antibody is usually negative. Specific testing should be done for anti-GBM antibodies.

Management
First line
Treatment is with corticosteroids, cyclophosphamide and plasma exchange.

Second line
Patients may require renal dialysis if in renal failure or respiratory support if there is severe pulmonary haemorrhage. Rituximab has been used safely in small series [14].

SMALL-VESSEL ANCA-ASSOCIATED VASCULITIS

Microscopic polyangiitis

Definition and nomenclature
Microscopic polyangiitis (MPA) is a necrotising vasculitis, with few or no immune deposits, predominantly affecting small vessels (i.e. capillaries, venules or arterioles). Necrotising arteritis involving small and medium arteries may be present. Necrotising glomerulonephritis is very common and pulmonary capillaritis often occurs. Granulomatous inflammation is absent [1]. Historically, MPA was grouped with polyarteritis nodosa and the two terms were often used interchangeably. It was defined and classified as a separate condition in 1994 at the first Chapel Hill Consensus Conference [2].

Synonyms and inclusions
- Microscopic polyangiitides

Introduction and general description
Friedrich Wohlwill described two cases with glomerulonephritis and non-granulomatous inflammation of small vessels in 1923 [3]. However, it was not until 1994 that MPA was formally defined by an international consensus [2]. MPA is part of a group of conditions termed ANCA-associated vasculitis (AAV). The other two conditions in this group are granulomatosis with polyangiitis (GPA) and eosinophilic granulomatosis with polyangiitis (EGPA). They are united by their association with antibodies directed against proteinase 3 (PR3) and myeloperoxidase (MPO). PR3 and MPO are proteins that serve as antigens inside the azurophilic granules in the cytoplasm of a neutrophil. Phenotypically, MPA and GPA are very similar in presentation, with the prime difference being the absence of granulomatous inflammation in MPA.

Epidemiology
Incidence and prevalence
The annual incidence of MPA is 2.5–10/million [4,5]. However, this rises to 45/million per year in the population over the age of 65 years [6]. The point prevalence figures vary from 25 to 100/million population [7–9].

Age
The peak incidence is in populations aged over 65 years [6].

Sex
No predilection is known.

Ethnicity
White people are more commonly affected [10]. In Japan, the overall incidence of AAV is similar to that in the western European population, but the AAV is exclusively MPA, with almost no GPA [6].

Associated diseases
No associations are known.

Pathophysiology
The exact mechanism of the production of vascular inflammation is not known, but ANCA has a prime role in the pathogenesis. Murine models have demonstrated the pathogenicity of MPO ANCA in producing glomerulonephritis and pulmonary haemorrhage [11,12]. ANCA can induce degranulation of neutrophils primed by TNF-α [13]. Primed neutrophils exhibit MPO on their surface. The MPO ANCA can induce a respiratory burst leading to degranulation and the release of toxic oxygen radicals and intracytoplasmic enzymes, which may lead to vascular inflammation [13,14].

Predisposing factors

Farming may predispose to pANCA positivity and MPA [15].

Pathology

Histological specimens from MPA lesions demonstrate segmental vascular necrosis. Neutrophils and monocytes permeate vessel walls, causing leukocytoclasis, the accumulation of fibrin and haemorrhage. Biopsy specimens from lesions of palpable purpura demonstrate leukocytoclastic vasculitis. Focal segmental glomerulonephritis with extracapillary crescents is a characteristic finding in renal biopsies. The presence of glomerulosclerosis is suggestive of the duration of disease and dictates the renal impairment.

Genetics

No culprit genes have been identified but the geographical distribution of the disease is suggestive of a genetic influence.

Environmental factors

Exposure to farming may be associated with MPA [15].

Clinical features

History

Many patients with MPA initially experience constitutional symptoms, including fever, weight loss, myalgia and arthralgia. These may be present for several weeks before the onset of the pulmonary and renal disease that often occurs in patients with MPA.

Presentation

About 40% of patients have palpable purpura on dependent skin sites upon presentation [16]. Mouth ulcers, necrotic lesions on the fingers or toes, splinter haemorrhages and livedo reticularis can all be present. The presence of nodules and livedo reticularis is commoner in polyarteritis nodosa; 80% of patients will have renal involvement. The presentation may be explosive with rapidly progressive glomerulonephritis or pulmonary haemorrhage (Figure 100.16). Peripheral neuropathy is common and is usually sensorimotor. Mononeuritis multiplex and even cranial nerve involvement are not unusual.

Differential diagnosis

Microscopic polyangiitis should be distinguished from other ANCA-associated vasculitides and polyarteritis nodosa. The diagnosis of MPA can be made only in the absence of cardinal features of EGPA and GPA. Significant peripheral eosinophilia, extravascular eosinophils, nasal or paranasal sinus involvement, endobronchial involvement, granulomas on a biopsy, fixed pulmonary infiltrates, cavitating nodules on a chest X-ray, asthma and mastoidal or retro-orbital disease all lead away from a diagnosis of MPA.

Similarly, the absence of blood, protein or red cell casts in the urine leads away from the diagnosis of MPA.

Alternate conditions that can produce a pulmonary renal syndrome include thrombotic thrombocytopenic purpura and anti-GBM disease. Anti-GBM disease does not cause skin involvement. The absence of ANCA and a haemolytic anaemia would suggest thrombotic thrombocytopenic purpura.

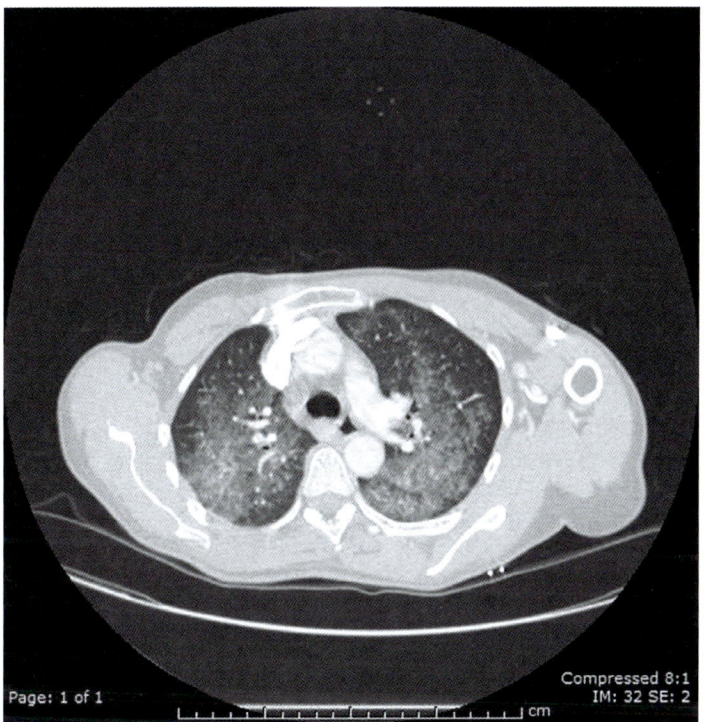

Figure 100.16 Computed tomography of the thorax demonstrating pulmonary haemorrhage affecting both lung fields in microscopic polyangiitis.

Classification of severity

The diagnosis of MPA is associated with significant morbidity and mortality. Previous classifications of severity were based around need for cyclophosphamide. But now all individuals with MPA should be treated as having an organ or life-threatening disease.

Complications and co-morbidities

Microscopic polyangiitis can be associated with renal failure or life-threatening pulmonary haemorrhage. Pulmonary haemorrhage occurs in about 10% of patients and carries a high risk of death [17,18]. In the long term, there is a raised risk of coronary artery disease and hypertension. At 5 years, there is a 16% incidence of cardiovascular events (myocardial infarctions, cerebrovascular accidents or coronary revascularisation procedures) [19]. MPO ANCA positivity confers a higher risk of cardiovascular events compared with PR3 ANCA positivity.

Disease course and prognosis

Relapse is common and increases with time. In separate studies it has been documented to be 8% at 18 months [20] and 34% at 70 months [16]. Survival at 12 months is 82–92%, falling to 45–76% at 5 years.

Investigations

Anaemia of chronic disease and laboratory markers of an acute phase response predominate. Urine analysis provides big clues. Most patients will have a blood and protein leak to varying extents. ANCA directed against PR3 or MPO are present in nearly all patients. Imaging helps to establish the extent and severity of disease in patients with lung involvement. Chest X-ray followed by computed tomography (CT) scanning identifies alveolar haemorrhage or pulmonary fibrosis. Histopathology is the gold standard for diagnosis and, when possible, the kidneys should be biopsied on suspicion of MPA. Other tissues that may provide an answer are the sural nerve, muscle and skin.

Management [21]

Recommendations for the management of MPA have been proposed by the European League Against Rheumatism [22] and the British Society for Rheumatology [23]. Immunosuppressive therapies, including oral or intravenous glucocorticoids, are the mainstay of treatment.

Remission induction

Pulsed intravenous cyclophosphamide (15 mg/kg every 2–3 weeks) or daily oral cyclophosphamide (2 mg/kg/day) forms the mainstay of treatment for most patients with MPA. Intravenous cyclophosphamide has the advantage of lower cumulative dose and lower risk of adverse events, but carries a greater risk of relapse [24,25]. Pulsed intravenous rituximab (1 g twice, 2 weeks apart) can also be used for remission induction. The authors prefer cyclophosphamide over rituximab as a first line agent unless there is a contraindication to the use of cyclophosphamide. Rituximab changes the B-cell repertoire irreversibly and can affect the production of antibodies long term. In the context of vaccine responses, this is an extremely important consideration since the beginning of the SARS-CoV-2 pandemic. Oral prednisolone usually 40 mg daily is commonly used as an adjunct to cyclophosphamide, with the aim of reducing the dose to 10–15 mg/day at 3 months [22]. At the physician's discretion, intravenous methylprednisolone can be added to speed up the induction of remission at the commencement of cyclophosphamide. Standard practice would be to add 1 g intravenously per day for up to 3 days in those needing mechanical ventilation or renal replacement therapy. Avacopan is a complement C5a inhibitor and in one clinical trial a dose of 30 mg BD appeared to be as effective when used instead of prednisolone 60 mg [26]. Further evaluation will be necessary before its exact role in managing ANCA-associated vasculitis is understood.

Relapsing and refractory disease

For relapsing disease, pulsed intravenous rituximab is superior to pulsed intravenous cyclophosphamide [27,28]. Refractoriness to cyclophosphamide or rituximab is rare and should prompt re-evaluation of diagnosis and disease activity. But in the rare event of true refractoriness to cyclophosphamide (progressive disease after three pulses), a switch should be made to rituximab. Conversely, true refractoriness to rituximab can be treated with a switch to cyclophosphamide [21]. Methotrexate (20–25 mg/week subcutaneously), mycophenolate mofetil (2–3 g daily in divided doses) and leflunomide (20–30 mg daily) can be used when it is not safe or possible to use cyclophosphamide or rituximab.

Remission maintenance

Post-cyclophosphamide. Due to the cumulative toxicity of cyclophosphamide, azathioprine (2 mg/kg/day) is preferred to maintain remission [20]. The switchover can happen either at the end of six pulses of intravenous cyclophosphamide or after 3–6 months of oral cyclophosphamide. Methotrexate 20–25 mg/week subcutaneously can be used in the case of intolerance to azathioprine if the renal function will allow.

Post-rituximab. In patients where rituximab is used to induce remission it can be continued in a dose of 500–1000 mg every 6 months for 2 years [21,29,30]. Hypogammaglobulinaemia following the use of long-term rituximab can lead to serious, persistent, unexpected and resistant infections (SPUR infections). Consensus recommendations have been published that advocate monitoring of immunoglobulin levels and the judicious use of antibiotics and intravenous immunoglobulin (IVIg) [31].

Granulomatosis with polyangiitis

Definition and nomenclature

Granulomatosis with polyangiitis is a necrotising granulomatous inflammation usually involving the upper and lower respiratory tract, and necrotising vasculitis affecting predominantly small to medium vessels (e.g. capillaries, venules, arterioles, arteries and veins). Necrotising glomerulonephritis is common [1].

> **Synonyms and inclusions**
> * Wegener granulomatosis

Introduction and general description

Friedrich Wegener published three cases in 1937 of patients in their thirties who had a 4–7-month history of spiking temperatures with negative septic screens, raised ESR, predominant upper respiratory tract inflammation with nasal septal involvement and active urinary sediment, resulting in death [2]. Sven Johnsson first used the term Wegener granulomatosis as a distinct diagnosis [3]. The name was changed to granulomatosis with polyangiitis by international consensus in 2013 [1].

The ANCA-associated vasculitides are a group of conditions characterised by their association with the presence of antibodies directed against PR3 and MPO. PR3 and MPO are intracytoplasmic enzymes of neutrophils. GPA is the archetypal ANCA-associated vasculitis, incorporating most of the clinical features of the other two AAVs – MPA and EGPA.

Epidemiology
Incidence and prevalence

The incidence of GPA is 3–10/million per year [4–6,7]. There may be a distinct latitudinal divide, with GPA being commoner in the northern latitudes than in the southern latitudes [6]. The point prevalence of GPA is 24–112/million [8–10].

Age

In children, the median age of onset is 14 years [11,12]. In adulthood, the median age of onset is 50–59 years [10,13,14].

Sex

The condition affects males and females equally.

Ethnicity
It is reported all over the world. GPA is rare in Japan [15], and may be rare in Inuits [16].

Pathophysiology
The exact mechanism of the production of vascular inflammation and granulomas is not known, but ANCA has a prime role in the pathogenesis. Murine models have demonstrated the pathogenicity of MPO ANCA in producing glomerulonephritis and pulmonary haemorrhage [17,18]. There is some evidence of *in vitro* pathogenicity of PR3 ANCA [19]. ANCA can induce the degranulation of neutrophils primed by TNF-α [20]. Primed neutrophils exhibit PR3 on their surface. The PR3 ANCA can induce a respiratory burst leading to degranulation and release of toxic oxygen radicals and intracytoplasmic enzymes, which may lead to vascular inflammation [20,21].

There may be a role for a bacterial infection (e.g. *Staphylococcus aureus*), which stimulates autoreactive PR3-producing B cells within granulomas [22,23]. In the autoinflammatory process, granuloma formation occurs prior to vasculitis. The granulomas in GPA have a high proportion of granulocytes, which serve as a source of PR3 [24], which in turn help to continue driving a Th1 cytokine response to further the inflammatory process.

Predisposing factors
Farming and occupational solvent exposure may predispose to GPA [25].

Pathology
Skin histology in GPA may show perivascular lymphocytic infiltrates; however, such non-specific infiltrates may not be related to disease pathogenesis. More specific findings such as leukocytoclastic vasculitis and/or granulomatous inflammation may be present in up to 50% of skin biopsy specimens (Figure 100.17). Granulomatous inflammation around vessels and palisading necrotising granulomas are uncommonly demonstrated in skin lesions.

Causative organisms
Clinical observation points to *Staphylococcus aureus* as a potential trigger in some patients. The incidence of chronic nasal carriage of *S. aureus* is significantly higher in patients with GPA compared with healthy individuals and constitutes a risk factor for disease relapse [26,27].

Genetics
There is evidence that GPA has an association with HLA-DP, although this may be an association with PR3 ANCA rather than the syndrome of GPA [28,**29**].

Clinical features
History
Features of the classic triad of GPA, including the skin, respiratory tract and kidneys, are not always present early in the course of the disease, sometimes making the diagnosis difficult. In up to 80% of patients, symptoms involving the upper or lower respiratory tract are present, and at presentation approximately 73% of patients will have nasal, sinus, tracheal or ear involvement.

Less than half present with pulmonary infiltrates or nodules. Overt renal disease is initially present in only 18%, although approximately 77% will eventually develop glomerulonephritis. Although 40% will eventually manifest skin findings, cutaneous manifestations and oral ulcers are only found in 13% and 6% of patients at initial presentation, respectively.

Presentation
The most common cutaneous manifestation of GPA is palpable purpura on dependent skin sites (Figure 100.18a); digital infarcts (Figure 100.18b), tender subcutaneous nodules, papules, vesicles and petechiae, as well as non-specific ulcers or pyoderma gangrenosum-like lesions may occur. Cases previously diagnosed as having malignant pyoderma may have had lesions secondary to GPA. Nodular or papulonecrotic lesions occur on the extremities and sometimes on the face and scalp. These may be differentiated from rheumatoid nodules in that they ulcerate, whereas rheumatoid nodules do not.

Oral ulcers are the second most common mucocutaneous sign of GPA. The upper respiratory tract is commonly affected, with otitis, epistaxis, rhinorrhoea and sinusitis as frequent presenting features. A saddle nose deformity may result from necrotising granulomas of the nasal mucosa. Lower respiratory signs and symptoms include cough, dyspnoea, chest pain and haemoptysis. Nodules, which may be cavitating, may be visible on imaging (Figure 100.19). Ulcerative lesions in GPA are shown in Figure 100.20.

Differential diagnosis
Granulomatosis with polyangiitis must be differentiated from the other types of AAV. Destructive upper respiratory involvement and severe glomerulonephritis are unusual in EGPA, which typically has asthma and eosinophilia, along with paranasal polypoidal involvement. MPA has predominant renal involvement and is more likely to be associated with MPO ANCA. Granulomatous disease involving midline structures can be seen in sarcoidosis and lymphomas.

Classification of severity
Granulomatosis with polyangiitis was historically classified as being classic or localised. Clinical trials used this classification to restrict exposure to cyclophosphamide. However, this classification was not based on good evidence [30]. All patients with newly diagnosed GPA should be treated in the same way as those suffering with organ or life-threatening disease.

Complications and co-morbidities
Granulomatosis with polyangiitis or its treatment (especially cyclophosphamide) has a twofold increase in the risk of cancer including acute myeloid leukaemia, bladder cancer and non-melanoma skin cancers [**31**,32]. The risk of bladder cancer has been mitigated by the use of concurrent mercaptoethane sulfonate sodium (MESNA). GPA also predisposes to increased cardiovascular morbidity [33].

Disease course and prognosis
Remission can be achieved in up to 90% of patients [**34**]. At 2 years, the relapse rate is between 18% and 40% [**34**]. Untreated GPA has a

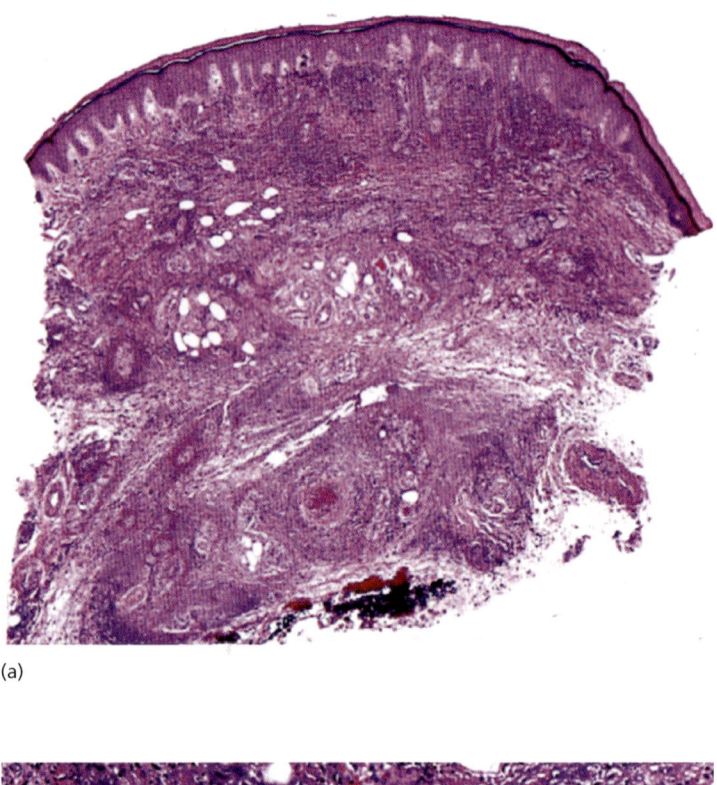

(a)

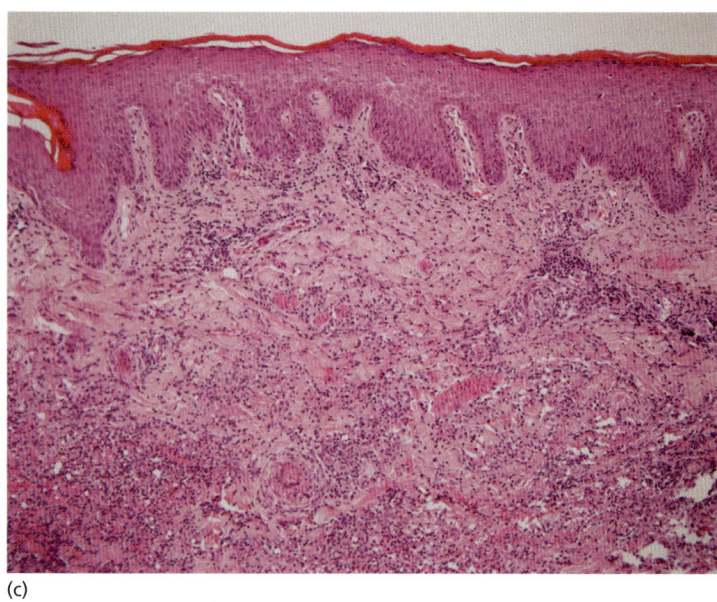

(c)

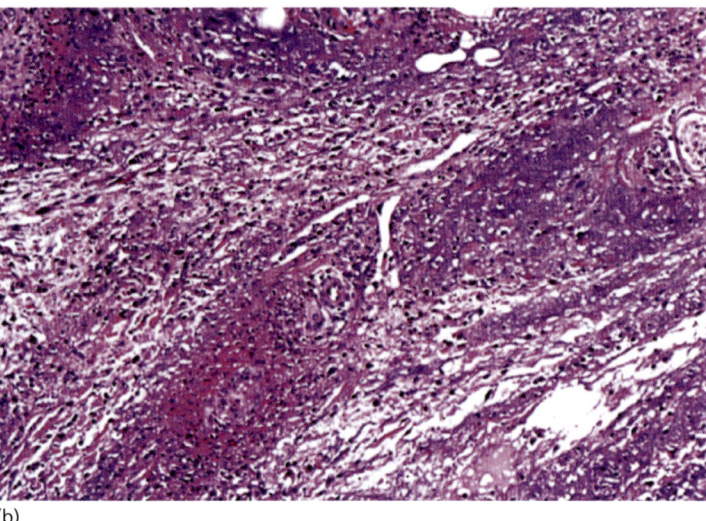

(b)

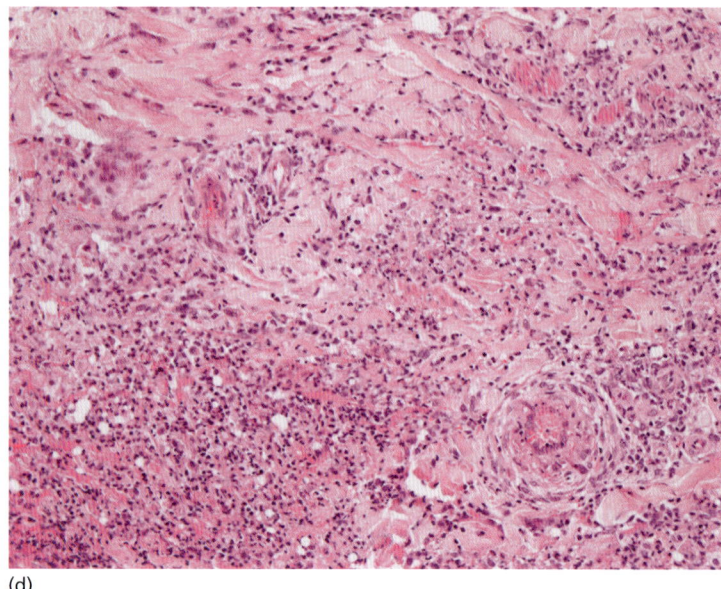

(d)

Figure 100.17 Granulomatosis with polyangiitis. (a) There is extensive leukocytoclastic vasculitis involving the entire dermis. (b) Note the extensive area of collagen degeneration, destruction of vessels and mixed inflammatory infiltrate. (c, d) There is a necrotising vasculitis with fibrin deposition, red blood cell extravasation and a granulomatous reaction, at lower (c) and higher (d) magnifications. (a, b) courtesy of Dr Omar Sangueza, Wake Forest University School of Medicine, Winston-Salem, NC, USA. (c, d) Courtesy of Dr Laszlo Igali, Norfolk and Norwich University Hospital, Norwich, UK.

1-year mortality of 83%; the survival of treated disease at 1 year is >80% [35]. End-stage renal disease occurs in 7% at 12 months, rising to 14% at 5 years and 23% at 10 years [36]. Cancer risk is as discussed earlier.

Investigations
Investigations are as in MPA.

Management [37]
Recommendations for the management of GPA have been proposed by the European League Against Rheumatism [30] and the British Society for Rheumatology [38]. Immunosuppressive therapy including oral or intravenous glucocorticoid is the mainstay of treatment.

First line
This is as for MPA.

Second line
This is as for MPA.

Third line
15-Deoxyspergualin and IVIg have a role in refractory and persistent disease [39,40].

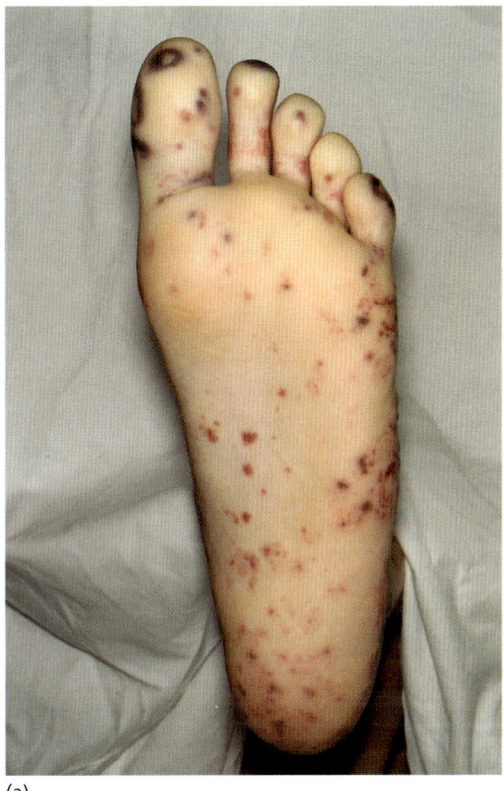
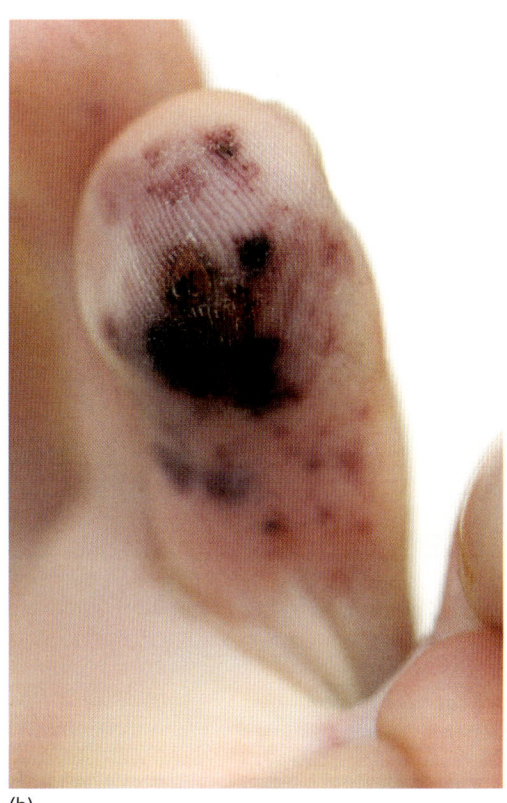

Figure 100.18 Granulomatosis with polyangiitis. (a) Cutaneous infarction. (b) Digital infarction. (a)   (b)

Remission maintenance
This is as for MPA.

Eosinophilic granulomatosis with polyangiitis

Definition and nomenclature
Eosinophilic granulomatosis with polyangiitis is a very rare systemic disorder characterised by an eosinophil-rich and necrotising granulomatous inflammation, often involving the respiratory tract, and necrotising vasculitis predominantly affecting small to medium vessels. There is an association with asthma and eosinophilia. ANCA is more frequent when glomerulonephritis is present [1].

Synonyms and inclusions
- Churg–Strauss syndrome
- Allergic granulomatous angiitis
- Churg–Strauss vasculitis
- Allergic angiitis and granulomatosis
- Allergic granulomatosis
- Allergic granulomatosis and angiitis
- Eosinophilic granulomatous vasculitis
- Allergic angiitis
- Granulomatous allergic angiitis

Introduction and general description
This is a rare systemic vasculitis characterised by asthma, peripheral blood and tissue eosinophilia (especially in the respiratory tract) and necrotising vasculitis with extravascular granulomas. The majority of patients have cutaneous findings in the active phase of the disease. It was originally described by Rackemann and Greene in 1939 as an allergic disease and was not classified as periarteritis nodosa; Churg and Strauss later described the syndrome and its histopathological characteristics in 1951 [2]. The condition was renamed EGPA in 2012 by the Chapel Hill Consensus Conference on the Nomenclature of Vasculitides [1]. EGPA is associated with antibodies directed against MPO and PR3, and, along with GPA and MPA, forms the group of conditions termed ANCA-associated vasculitis.

Epidemiology
Incidence and prevalence
The incidence is 1–2.5 per million [3,4,5] with a prevalence of 10–15 per million [6,7]. The incidence of EGPA in known asthma sufferers may be up to 67/million per year [8].

Age
It is most common in those aged 15–70 years with a peak incidence around the age of 50. It is very rare in children.

Sex
There may be a slight male predilection.

Ethnicity
No connection is recognised.

Associated diseases
It is associated with atopy, particularly asthma and allergic rhinitis.

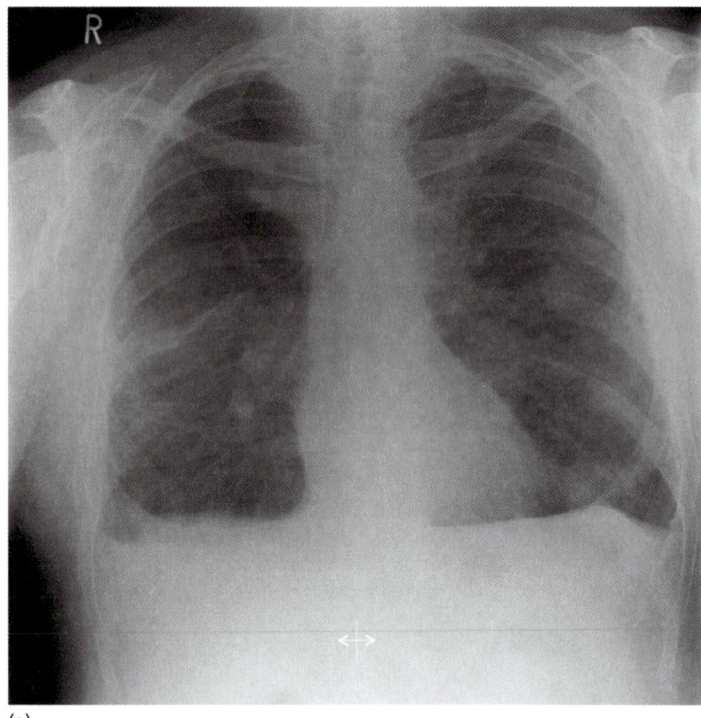

(a)

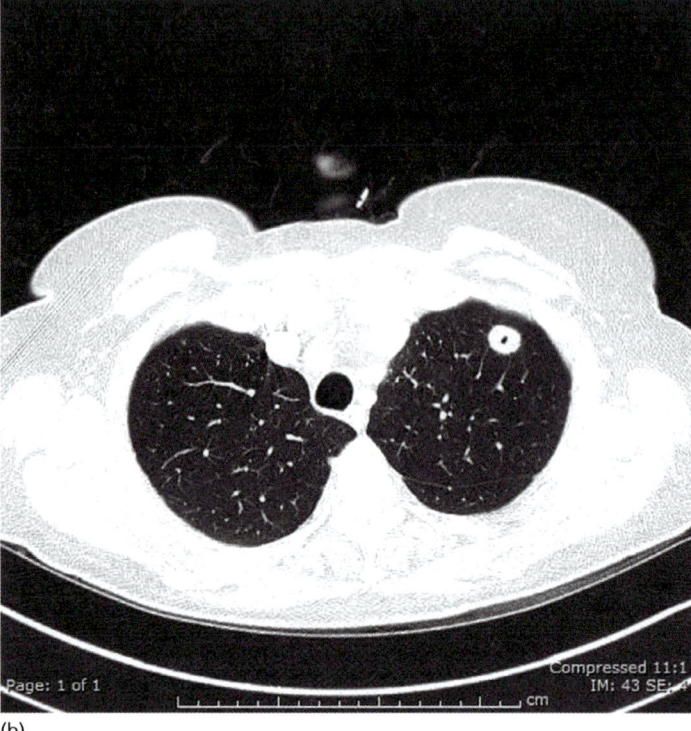

(b)

Figure 100.19 Granulomatosis with polyangiitis. (a) X-ray showing bilateral nodules. (b) Computed tomography of the thorax demonstrating a thick-walled cavity in the right lung field.

Pathophysiology

The pathogenesis of EGPA is not precisely known. Allergy probably plays a central role, but the disease is almost certainly multifactorial. As the allergy association might suggest, the inflammatory response is primarily Th2 in nature, although Th1 and Th17 responses are

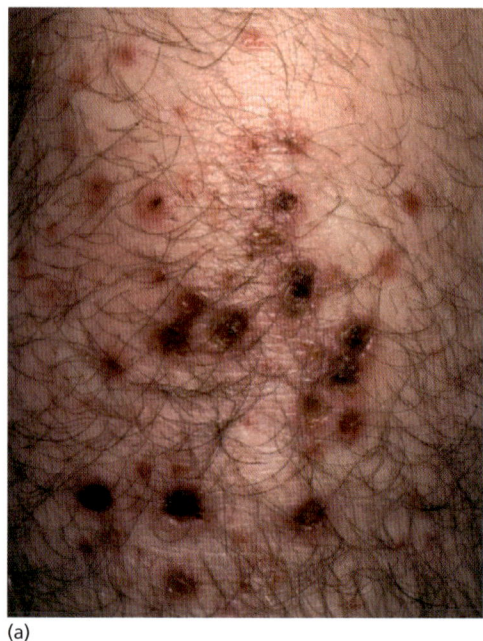

(a)

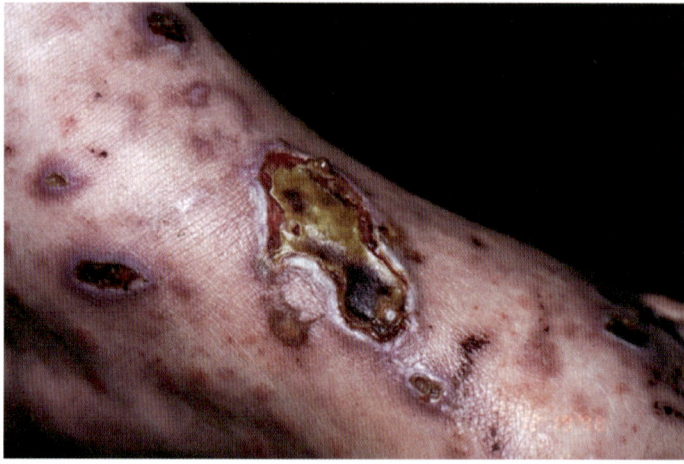

(b)

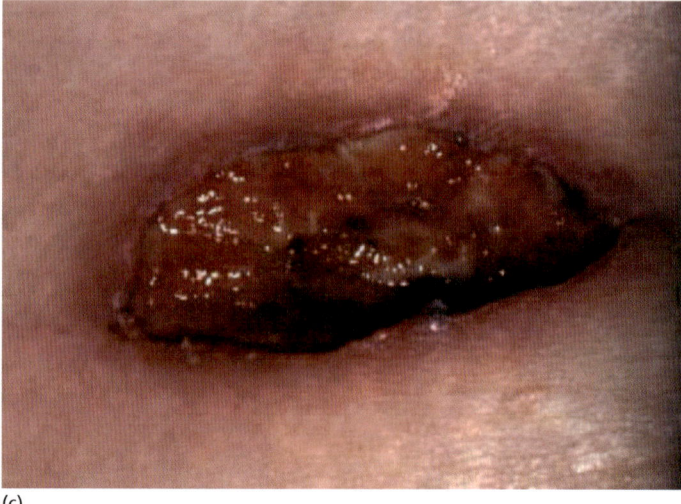

(c)

Figure 100.20 Granulomatosis with polyangiitis. (a) Ulcerated lesions of cutaneous small-vessel vasculitis. (b) Larger ulcerated lesions with background vasculitis. (c) Deep skin ulcer in a person with nasal symptoms.

seen [**9**,10,**11**]. The Th2 response has been thought to be responsible for eosinophilic activation and prolonged eosinophil survival. The products of eosinophilic and neutrophilic degradation have been observed in inflamed tissues and are probably responsible for tissue injury [12,13]. The association with ANCA probably suggests a B-cell involvement as well. The role of ANCA in producing vasculitis has been discussed in the GPA and EGPA sections.

Predisposing factors
None is known.

Pathology
Eosinophilic granulomatosis with polyangiitis has three key histopathological features: eosinophilic infiltration of tissue, formation of extravascular granulomas in visceral and cutaneous tissues, and vasculitis involving both arteries and veins. The histology of a cutaneous lesion in EGPA may demonstrate any one, if not all, of these features [**14**]. The granulomas contain necrotic polymorphonuclear leukocytes, eosinophils, severe fibrinoid and fibrillar collagen degeneration and a proliferation of granulomatous tissue.

Causative organisms
None is known.

Genetics
The genetics of EGPA may be stratified by the ANCA status. Those individuals who are ANCA positive appear to have an association in the HLA-DQ region. Those who are ANCA negative appear to have HLA and non-HLA associations [15]. This probably suggests that EGPA may have syndromic variants within the spectrum of hypereosinophilic syndromes.

Environmental factors
Environmental allergens are associated with more severe asthma.

Clinical features
History
Three phases of EGPA are recognised:
1 The first phase, which may continue for years, consists of asthma with allergic rhinitis and nasal polyps. The asthma typically begins in adulthood in contrast to allergic asthma.
2 The second phase is that of rising peripheral and tissue eosinophilia.
3 The third phase is the predominantly vasculitic phase of EGPA, which may affect almost all organ systems including the cutaneous, cardiac, pulmonary, nervous, gastrointestinal, renal, genito-urinary and musculoskeletal systems. Cardiac involvement is the primary cause of death in patients who do not respond to conventional corticosteroid therapy.

Presentation
In all phases of the disease there may be cutaneous manifestations, with approximately 5% demonstrating cutaneous vasculitis [**14**]. Palpable purpura and infiltrated nodules (typically located on the scalp or limbs) are the most common skin manifestations, but livedo reticularis, necrotising livedo (i.e. retiform purpura), migratory

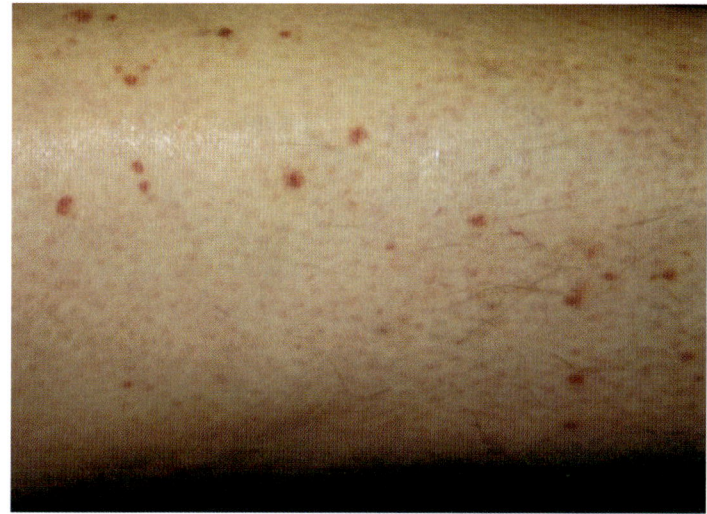

Figure 100.21 Relatively subtle vasculitis on the legs in eosinophilic granulomatosis with polyangiitis. The patient also had eosinophilia and rapidly developed a mononeuritis multiplex.

redness of the skin, new-onset Raynaud phenomenon, aseptic pustules or vesicles, or infiltrated papules may also be present.

In the vasculitis phase of EGPA, 50–70% of patients have vasculitic skin lesions, most commonly on the lower limbs (Figure 100.21).

Differential diagnosis
Nasal polyp disease is common in patients with allergic rhinitis. The demonstration of vasculitis and systemic involvement is essential for a diagnosis of EGPA. Hypereosinophilic syndrome, Samter triad and allergic rhinitis should all be considered. None of them is known to cause skin involvement.

Disease course and prognosis
Remission is common in EGPA and is achieved in >90% of patients [16]. Relapse rates rise from 10% at 12 months to 20% at 4 years [16]. Survival is better than in the other AAVs. In a pooled analysis, survival at 1 and 5 years was 94% and 60–97%, respectively [17].

Investigations
Peripheral blood eosinophilia is a requisite for the diagnosis of EGPA. Inflammatory markers will be raised and IgE is often elevated. ANCA directed against MPO or PR3 is positive in 30% of patients [18,19]. A urine microscopy demonstrates active urinary sediment in patients with glomerulonephritis. Renal involvement is more likely in ANCA-positive patients [18]. Chest radiographs demonstrate infiltrates. CT scans of the paranasal sinuses are often abnormal and demonstrate mucosal thickening, but rarely bone involvement; the latter is more a feature of GPA. The gold standard remains a biopsy of the affected organ.

Management
There are no randomised controlled trials of any treatment for EGPA. Knowledge of its treatment comes from open-labelled trials and from international consensus-based recommendations [**20**,21]. General management principles are as for MPA and GPA.

PART 9: VASCULAR DISORDERS

Remission induction
This is as for MPA and GPA.

Remission maintenance
This is as for MPA and GPA.

Relapsing and refractory disease
Mepolizumab is a humanised monoclonal antibody that targets IL-5. There is one clinical trial that has demonstrated that in combination with glucocorticoid therapy it is more effective than placebo in inducing and maintaining remission [22]. Its exact place in the management of EGPA is as yet undefined.

MEDIUM-VESSEL VASCULITIS

Polyarteritis nodosa and cutaneous arteritis (cutaneous polyarteritis nodosa)

Definition and nomenclature
Polyarteritis nodosa (PAN) is a rare necrotising arteritis of medium or small arteries without glomerulonephritis and without vasculitis in the arterioles, capillaries or venules. It is not associated with ANCA [1]. Cutaneous PAN is a single-organ vasculitis affecting the skin. It is better termed cutaneous arteritis. It can be considered a limited expression of PAN and does not exhibit systemic involvement [1,2].

> **Synonyms and inclusions**
> - Benign cutaneous periarteritis nodosa
> - Periarteritis nodosa
> - Kussmaul–Maier disease
> - Necrotising arteritis
> - Essential polyarteritis

Introduction and general description
A condition described as periarteritis nodosa was described by Adolf Kussmaul and Rudolf Maier in 1866. The first use of the phrase 'polyarteritis nodosa' denoting the pathological extent of the disease involving the arterial wall may have been in 1945 [3]. PAN was used as a term to cover a large variety of vasculitides. In 1994, the label was uniquely applied to a condition that spared small-calibre vessels [4].

This chapter considers cutaneous arteritis as a variant of PAN that is limited to the skin [5]. It may progress to become classic PAN [1], but conversion is exceedingly rare [2]. Although a distinct entity as described by Lindberg in 1931, the diagnosis of cutaneous arteritis should not be made until systemic disease is excluded.

Epidemiology
Incidence and prevalence
The annual incidence of classic PAN is 1–2.5/million [6,7]. The point prevalence has been reported to be 30 per million [8,9]. Cutaneous arteritis is much rarer and there are no formal reports on the incidence and prevalence of this variant.

Age
The peak age is between 40 and 60 years. However, it can be observed in all ages, including in children.

Sex
There is no specific predilection.

Ethnicity
No racial predilection has been described.

Associated diseases
Hepatitis B was described as an association in 1970 [10]. PAN can be the first manifestation of hepatitis B and occurs in most cases within 6 months of infection. Successful treatment of hepatitis B results in the cure of PAN with disappearance of any aneurysms [11].

Pathophysiology
Predisposing factors
Viral infections have been implicated in provoking classic PAN. Besides hepatitis B virus, Epstein–Barr virus [12], HIV [13], erythrovirus (parvovirus B19) [14] and cytomegalovirus [15] have been reported in new cases of PAN. Other microbial associations reported have been streptococcal infections [16] and coxsackie B4 [17].

Streptococcal infections [18], erythrovirus (parvovirus B19) [19] and *Mycobacterium fortuitum* [20] have been reported in association with cutaneous arteritis. Minocycline has been reported to induce classic PAN-like vasculitis [21] as well as cutaneous arteritis [22].

Pathology
Early in the disease course there is a predominantly neutrophilic inflammatory infiltrate in the walls of medium-sized arteries and arterioles of septae in the upper portions of the subcutaneous fat. The involved vessels classically demonstrate a target-like appearance resulting from an eosinophilic ring of fibrinoid necrosis. Later in the disease process the infiltrate becomes less neutrophilic, consisting predominantly of lymphocytes and histiocytes. Complement and IgM deposits in vessel walls of lesions of cutaneous arteritis from some patients may be demonstrated by direct immunofluorescence. Unlike those of systemic PAN, lesions of cutaneous arteritis do not typically involve arterial bifurcations.

Genetics
Recessively inherited missense mutations in *CECR1* (cat eye syndrome chromosome region, candidate 1), encoding adenosine deaminase 2 (ADA2), have been observed in nine unrelated cases from eight families [23]. Similar mutations were found in a separate study of 19 patients of Georgian Jewish descent [24].

Clinical features
History
Although some patients with cutaneous arteritis may report constitutional symptoms, along with mild involvement of the muscles and nerves, cutaneous manifestations are the most striking feature of the disease.

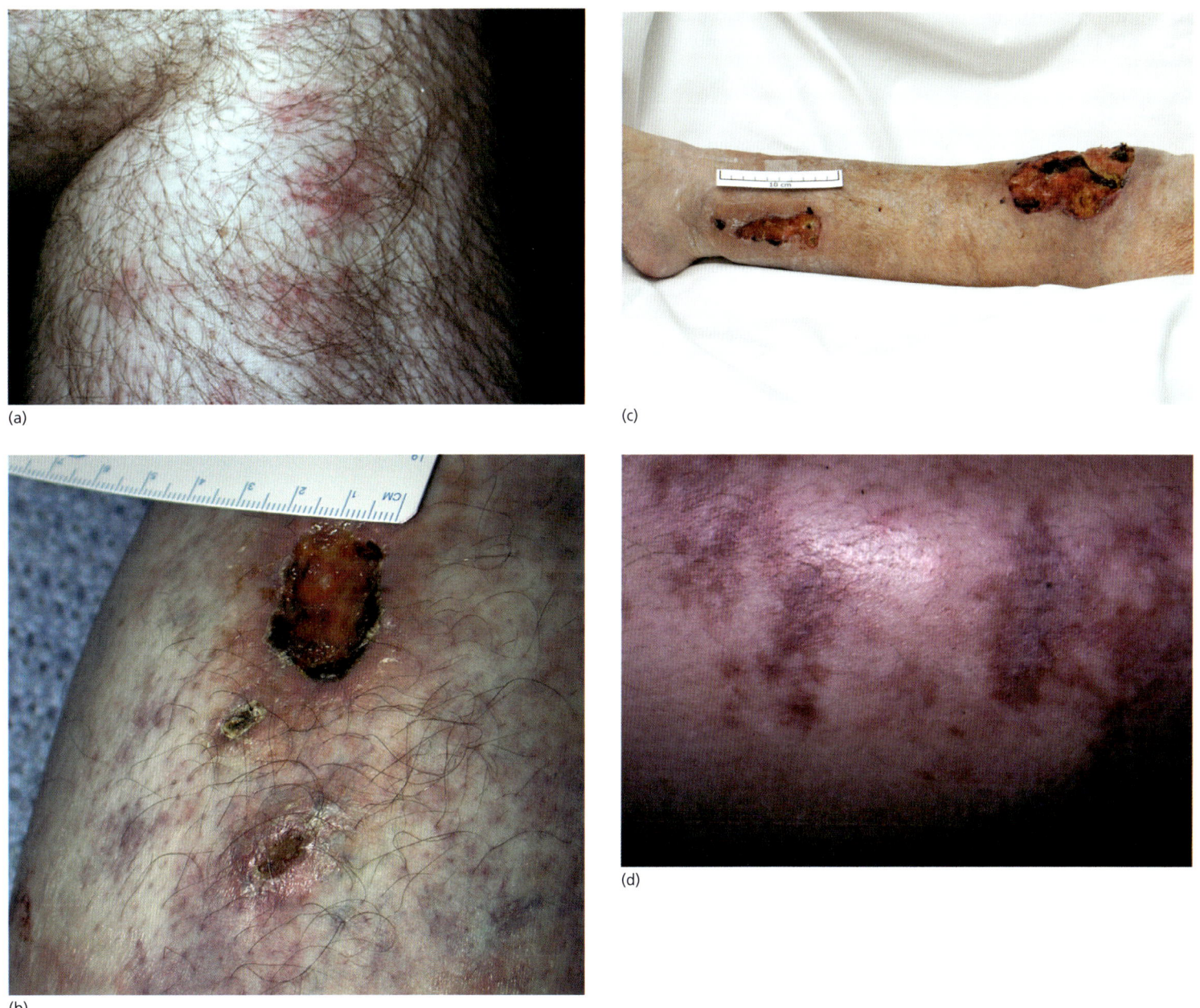

Figure 100.22 Cutaneous polyarteritis nodosa. (a) Red lesions on the leg. (b) Nodules and ulceration on the leg. (c) Ulcerating lesions on the leg. (d) Livedo of the leg.

Presentation

Dermal or subcutaneous nodules are mostly located on the distal lower extremities near the malleoli (Figure 100.22a) and may extend proximally to the thighs, buttock, arms or hands. Patients may report tenderness associated with the nodules, which may ulcerate (Figure 100.22b, c) or more commonly demonstrate necrotising livedo reticularis, also referred to as retiform purpura (see Figure 100.3). Gangrene of the digits can ultimately occur, most commonly in children with cutaneous arteritis, but this finding should trigger an aggressive search to exclude systemic features of PAN.

Differential diagnosis

Recurrent spiking fevers, polyarthralgia and a macular upper extremity eruption are symptoms shared by both PAN and adult-onset Still disease (AOSD) and can sometimes create a diagnostic challenge. The presence of livedo reticularis (Figure 100.22d) and the finding of a characteristic skin biopsy appearance with PAN help to differentiate it from AOSD.

Those with necrotising lesions of livedo reticularis must be evaluated for vasculitis or vasculopathy (e.g. antiphospholipid antibody syndrome, cholesterol emboli or other factors that can produce non-vasculitic vessel occlusion; see Chapter 99).

ANCA-associated vasculitis should also be considered as a differential diagnosis [25].

If nodules are present, they should be biopsied by incisional biopsy methods to assess for a pan-arteritis of muscular arteries which would confirm a diagnosis of PAN.

Cutaneous arteritis is best considered a variant of PAN, so evaluation by history, physical examination, screening laboratory tests and ongoing follow-up for systemic features are required.

A multidisciplinary team approach helps accurate diagnosis and limits the chances of missing or undertreating potentially life-threatening systemic features of PAN.

Classification of severity

Cutaneous arteritis is considered to have a more benign prognosis than PAN with systemic features.

Disease course and prognosis

Gastrointestinal tract, renal, heart and central nervous system involvement are associated with higher mortality [26].

Investigations

Laboratory investigations are usually non-specific, revealing an acute phase response. Screening for potential infective triggers should be undertaken. Diagnosis of PAN requires histological evidence of medium-sized artery vasculitis if possible. Biopsies should be from symptomatic organs. Skin, muscle and nerve histology offer higher diagnostic yield and may be safer. If biopsies are unsupportive, visceral angiography may identify multiple micro-aneurysms suggesting PAN.

Management

There should be screening for infection (see the section on predisposing factors) and consideration should be given to a trial of discontinuing medication that predates disease. If associated with hepatitis B infection, antiviral therapies form the focus of treatment in combination with immunosuppressive treatment.

First line

Non-steroidal anti-inflammatory drugs and salicylates can be an effective treatment for symptoms of cutaneous arteritis. High-dose corticosteroids followed by tapering of the dosage over 3–6 months may occasionally be necessary for some patients. Also, without evidence from controlled trials, but based on a strong association with streptococcal infection, penicillin is often used for treatment and prophylaxis in children with cutaneous arteritis. Screening for recent streptococcal infection with anti-DNAse B or other tests may guide this decision.

Other treatments documented in anecdotal reports include the use of dipyridamole, sulfapyridine, pentoxifylline and dapsone. Low-dose weekly methotrexate (7.5–20 mg/week) has been successful in some patients with skin lesions unresponsive to corticosteroids given topically, intralesionally and orally [27]. Chronic leg ulcers resistant to treatment with high-dose corticosteroids have been successfully treated with granulocyte–macrophage colony-stimulating factor (GM-CSF) [28].

Second line

There is international consensus that PAN requires treatment with a combination of cyclophosphamide and corticosteroids which achieves sustained remission but probably does not alter survival [29]. For patients with hepatitis B-associated PAN, the recommendation is to start with high-dose corticosteroids for 2 weeks followed by antiviral treatment and plasma exchange [29]. This treatment should be supervised at a specialist centre in conjunction with a hepatologist.

Third line

There are case reports for the use of rituximab in refractory disease [30,31].

Kawasaki disease

Definition and nomenclature

The 2012 Chapel Hill Consensus defined Kawasaki disease as an arteritis associated with the mucocutaneous lymph node syndrome and predominantly affecting medium and small arteries. Coronary arteries are often involved; the aorta and large arteries may be involved. It usually occurs in infants and young children [1].

Synonyms and inclusions
- Mucocutaneous lymph node syndrome arteritis
- Mucocutaneous lymph node syndrome
- Kawasaki syndrome
- Infantile polyarteritis

Introduction and general description

Kawasaki disease occurs typically in infants and children less than 5 years of age. It was first recognised in 1967 and thought to be a benign, febrile illness associated with mucocutaneous inflammation and lymphadenopathy, until the demonstration of associated coronary arteritis in 1975 [2]. It is thought to be the commonest cause of acquired heart disease in children. Prompt diagnosis with treatment with aspirin and IVIg reduces heart complications [3,4].

Epidemiology
Incidence and prevalence

The annual incidence per 100 000 children aged under 5 years was 8.4 in England in the period 1998–2003 [5]. In a series of epidemiological surveys, Nakamura *et al.* have established that the incidence was rising in Japan every year and had peaked at 240/100 000 in 2010 [6].

Age

The disease almost always occurs in children.

Sex

There is a mild male predilection.

Ethnicity

The disease is much more common in Asia, particularly in Japan.

Associated diseases

Associated diseases include coronary vessel aneurysms and myocardial infarction.

Pathophysiology

Kawasaki disease is thought to be due to an intense inflammatory response to an unidentified infectious agent in genetically susceptible hosts.

Pathology

The angiitis of Kawasaki disease affects nearly all organs, with a very high frequency of cardiac involvement. It is predominantly a vasculitis of medium-sized arteries but can involve any smaller and larger calibre blood vessels. Initially, there is medial oedema associated with neutrophilic infiltration. The inflammatory processes lead to the breakdown of internal and external elastic laminae, resulting in aneurysms and thrombosis. The inflammatory processes heal with scarring and resultant stenosis of the affected blood vessel.

Causative organisms

The disease is thought to be triggered by as yet unidentified infectious agents.

Genetics

A functional polymorphism of the *ITPKC* (inositol-1,4,5-trisphosphate 3-kinase C) gene on chromosome 19q13.2 is significantly associated with a susceptibility to Kawasaki disease and coronary artery aneurysms [7]. Single nucleotide polymorphisms of interest have been found on the *CD40LG* gene [8] and *CASP3* gene [9]. Genome-wide association studies have identified further loci of interest around the FAM167A-BLK region at 8p22-23, the HLA region at 6p21.3 and the CD40 region at 20q13 and the IgG receptor gene *FCGR2A* [10,11].

Clinical features
History

Patients present with at least 5 days of fever, irritability, vomiting, anorexia, cough, diarrhoea, runny nose, weakness and abdominal and joint pain.

The disease typically has an initial acute, febrile stage lasting up to 2 weeks, a second phase lasting 4–6 weeks when the risk of death from coronary aneurysms is greatest, followed by a convalescent phase lasting up to 3 months and characterised by a reduction in the ESR and C-reactive protein (CRP) levels to normal. Larger aneurysms may expand leading to myocardial infarction in the convalescent phase. Those with established heart disease may enter a chronic phase with a risk of late aneurysm rupture even in adult life.

Presentation

The fever is typically spiking and unresponsive to paracetamol. There is acral and perianal redness and acral oedema, bilateral conjunctivitis with anterior uveitis, fissured lips and a strawberry tongue, and cervical lymphadenopathy, typically a single large cervical node.

Clinical variants

Incomplete Kawasaki disease should be considered in children who do not have all the features of the full disease. Typical echocardiographic features should lead to consideration of treatment as Kawasaki disease in the absence of external clinical features [12].

Differential diagnosis

Scarlet fever, systemic-onset juvenile idiopathic arthritis and erythema multiforme can mimic Kawasaki disease, as can other localised and systemic infections. The diagnosis should be suspected in a child with prolonged fever.

Classification of severity

The Harada score has been used in some countries as an indication for IVIg therapy [13]. Four of the following seven criteria are needed: (i) white blood count >12 000/mm^3; (ii) platelet count <35 × 10^4/mm^3; (iii) CRP >3; (iv) haematocrit <35%; (v) albumin <3.5 g/dL; (vi) age <12 months; and (vii) male sex.

Complications and co-morbidities

There may be hepatic, renal and gastrointestinal dysfunction, myocarditis and pericarditis.

Disease course and prognosis

Deaths may occur due to myocarditis, dysrhythmias, pericarditis, rupture of aneurysms and occlusion of coronary arteries; there is also an increased risk of atherosclerosis due to endothelial cell dysfunction. Coronary aneurysms are demonstrated in around 20% of patients (and in 90% of those who die); some will regress (potentially with stenosis) but giant aneurysms (>80 mm) may require bypass surgery. Clinical factors that predict a higher risk of coronary artery arteritic lesions or aneurysms, or that predict a poor response to treatment, include age below 1 year, low serum albumin, low haemoglobin, high CRP, abnormal liver function and, especially, duration of fever before treatment. Peripheral blood eosinophilia (>4%) after treatment is also associated with treatment resistance. Early IVIg reduces the coronary aneurysm risk from around 25% to less than 5%. Delaying IVIg beyond day 10 of fever increases the risk of death, particularly in boys under 1 year old.

Investigations

There are no diagnostic tests and Kawasaki disease remains a clinical diagnosis.

Management

Patients should be treated in a specialist paediatric unit. Aspirin and IVIg are the mainstay of treatment.

First line

Intravenous immunoglobulin and aspirin should be given early. Aspirin 100 mg/kg/day is given initially until the fever has settled and is then reduced to 3–5 mg/kg/day for 6–8 weeks in those with no cardiac abnormality, but longer in those with coronary aneurysms. All children should receive IVIg, usually given as a single dose of 2 g/kg over 12 h [4].

Second line

For children who remain febrile 36 h after the first dose of IVIg, a further dose of 2 g/kg can be given. Patients who are unresponsive to IVIg [14] can be treated with high-dose prednisolone

PART 9: VASCULAR DISORDERS

2 mg/kg/day, which should be tapered after normalisation of the CRP [15].

LARGE-VESSEL VASCULITIS

Giant cell arteritis

Definition and nomenclature

Giant cell arteritis (GCA) is an arteritis, often granulomatous, usually affecting the aorta and/or its major branches, with a predilection for the branches of the external carotid and subclavian arteries. The onset is usually in patients older than 50 years.

Synonyms and inclusions
- Horton disease
- Temporal arteritis
- Cranial arteritis
- Giant cell aortitis

Introduction and general description

This is a disease of the elderly, often associated with shoulder girdle stiffness, which presents with headaches and tender palpable arteries, including the temporal and facial arteries. It can rarely cause cutaneous infarction, so presenting to dermatologists [1].

Epidemiology
Incidence and prevalence

The highest mean annual incidence of GCA in people over the age of 50 years was recorded at 32.8/100 000 in southern Norway [2]. The age-adjusted (>50 years) annual incidence per 100 000 population was 18.8 in Olmsted county, Minnesota, USA [3] and 22.0 in the UK [4].

Age

This affects people over the age of 50 years. The age-specific incidence per 100 000 population rises from 2.2 in the sixth decade to 51.9 in the ninth decade [3].

Sex

The disease is 2–3 times more common in women than men [3].

Ethnicity

Giant cell arteritis is considered a disease that particularly targets people who have northern European ancestry.

Associated diseases

Symptoms of polymyalgia rheumatica are commonly seen in GCA and it is hypothesised that the two conditions may have a similar aetiology or lie on a disease spectrum. It is equally possible that the shoulder girdle involvement because of the subclavian artery and its branches may be mistaken for polymyalgia rheumatica.

Pathophysiology

The disease is thought to represent an inflammatory response in predisposed individuals towards an environmental factor. Local dendritic cells recruit and activate CD4 cells in the adventitia. Cytokine cascades involving Th1 and Th17 pathways dominate in the early phase, followed by a chronic smouldering arteritis led by chronic Th1 activation. The result is a stenosing arteritis.

Predisposing factors

These are unknown. But there is a possibility that individuals with diabetes may be protected against GCA [5,6].

Pathology

Lesions can be found in all layers of the affected branches of the aorta, particularly the carotid branches. These show segmental and focal pan-arteritis with polymorphic cell infiltrates along with T cells, macrophages and multinucleated giant cells, as well as intimal hyperplasia with a fragmented internal elastic lamina (Figure 100.23).

Causative organisms

None is known.

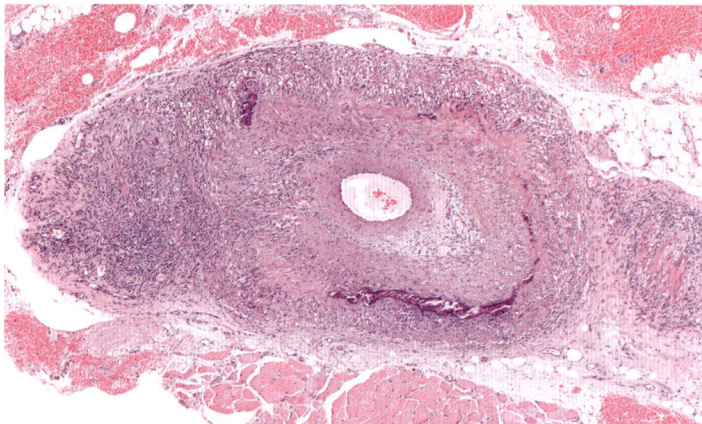

(a)

(b)

Figure 100.23 Giant cell arteritis at (a) lower and (b) higher magnification showing involvement of the vessel wall by a granulomatous reaction. Dystyrophic calcification is also seen. Courtesy of Dr Eduardo Calonje.

Genetics

There is no known genetic association.

Clinical features

History

Fever and weight loss may occur, and GCA is associated with shoulder girdle stiffness in about 50% of patients. Headache may be localised to the area of the affected artery that is temporal with temporal arteritis and occipital with occipital arteritis. The headache may start abruptly. Facial pain may occur on chewing due to claudication of the jaw muscles because of maxillary arteritis. Sudden, permanent visual loss is related to involvement of the branches of the ophthalmic artery causing either anterior ischaemic optic neuropathy or central retinal artery occlusion. Transient monocular loss of vision (amaurosis fugax) may precede permanent loss. Vertebrobasilar artery involvement may cause posterior cerebral circulation or a cerebellar stroke.

Presentation

Patients may present with a new headache on the background of feeling generally unwell or with painless loss of vision. Very rarely, GCA may present with skin infarction. The temporal arteries may be tender, thickened and pulseless. A bruit may be heard over affected arteries (e.g. the axillary artery).

Clinical variants

Isolated involvement of the extracranial arteries is well recognised with a phenotype that is not unlike Takayasu arteritis.

Differential diagnosis

The temporal artery can be involved in other vasculitides, such as ANCA-associated vasculitides [7,8]. Cancer should always be looked for when the diagnosis of GCA cannot be established beyond doubt [9].

Complications and co-morbidities

Permanent visual loss can be a presenting feature. There is a risk of aortic aneurysms developing as a late complication [10].

Disease course and prognosis

Following a diagnosis of GCA there is a slight excess mortality over 2 years (standard mortality rate 1.52; 95% confidence interval 1.20–1.85), but not with longer follow-up [11]. The excess mortality was greater in women and in those aged ≤70 years.

Investigations

International recommendations advocate an imaging modality like ultrasonography as the first line of investigation. In those where this is negative, but there is a high suspicion, a temporal artery biopsy may be offered. The ESR or CRP is almost always elevated. A normochromic, normocytic anaemia, thrombocytosis and raised alkaline phosphatase may all be present. Colour Doppler ultrasound of the temporal and axillary arteries (Video 100.1) in steroid-naïve patients commonly reveals intramural inflammatory change – the halo sign (Figure 100.24) [12]. Positron emission tomography with 18-fluorodeoxyglucose is of value in demonstrating aortitis [13].

Management

Treatment should be started as soon as the diagnosis is suspected in order to avoid complications; if the diagnosis turns out to be incorrect, the corticosteroids can be withdrawn [14]. Intravenous methylprednisolone 500–1000 mg daily for 3 days, followed by oral prednisolone, could be considered in individuals with threatened visual loss in the absence of any contraindications.

First line

Corticosteroids, for example prednisolone 40–60 mg daily, are used for GCA [15]. The dose can usually be reduced slowly in small steps every month, providing that the CRP and ESR levels remain controlled. Treatment is usually for about 2 years [16].

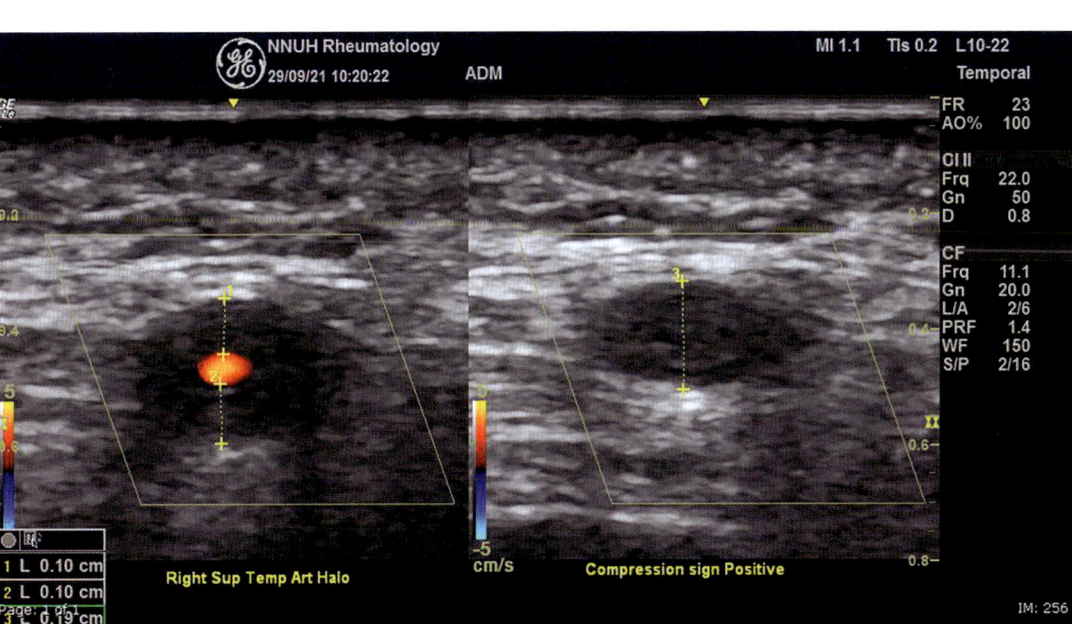

Figure 100.24 Ultrasonographic image of the superficial temporal artery demonstrating (on the left) concentric hypoechoic thickening of the intima–media complex and (on the right) the compression sign, where it is possible to eradicate the lumen on pressure, but not the hypoechoic thickening. The image was taken with a GE Logiq™ e ultrasound machine with a 10–22 MHz linear probe. Courtesy of Georgina Ducker.

PART 9: VASCULAR DISORDERS

Second line

Methotrexate 20 mg/week subcutaneously can be used in addition to prednisolone for individuals with relapsing disease [17]. Toclizumab 162 mg/week subcutaneously has been shown to be highly effective in reducing the need for prednisolone in individuals with GCA. The authors usually reserve this as a third line treatment or as second line in those where methotrexate is contraindicated or not tolerated [18].

Takayasu arteritis

Definition and nomenclature

Takayasu arteritis is often granulomatous and predominantly affects the aorta and/or its major branches. The onset is usually in those younger than 50 years [1].

Synonyms and inclusions
- Takayasu disease
- Takayasu syndrome
- Pulseless disease
- Aortic arch syndrome
- Aortitis syndrome
- Occlusive thromboarteriopathy

Introduction and general description

Mikito Takayasu, a Japanese ophthalmologist, is credited with the eponym, but the earliest convincing clinical and pathological description in literature of this disease was provided by William Savory's account of a 22-year-old woman's 13-month hospital stay and postmortem examination that demonstrated widespread large arterial inflammation [2].

Epidemiology
Incidence and prevalence

The annual incidence of Takayasu arteritis in Europe and the USA is 0.5–2.5/million [3,4,**5**]. The incidence in Japan is believed to be much higher [6].

Age

The disease is seen in younger people, typically below the age of 50 years, and is found also in children.

Sex

The disease is commoner in females than males.

Ethnicity

It is found in all populations but is commoner in Asians.

Pathophysiology
Pathology

The aorta and its branches are targeted and skip lesions can occur. During the acute phase, a pan-arteritis is present. The inflammatory infiltrate may be predominantly around the vasa vasorum, and fibrosis gradually replaces the inflammatory infiltrates. The vessel lumen may be narrowed secondary to the fibrosing stenotic lesions and/or by intraluminal thrombosis. In older patients there may be superimposed atherosclerosis, and calcification in the wall may occur as a late feature.

Genetics

IL-12B on chromosome 5, MLX on chromosome 17, FCGR2A/FCGR3A on chromosome 1 and HLA-B*52:01 are known associations [7,8]. Two independent susceptibility loci have been identified in the HLA region (HLA-DQB1/HLA-DRB1 and HLA-B/MICA) [8].

Clinical features
History

Headache, malaise and fever are common presenting symptoms in children. Cutaneous lesions are present in around one-third of patients.

Presentation

Hypertension, pyrexia and pulseless disease are common findings in children. Skin lesions have been reported in up to a third of cases and may comprise erythema nodosum, erythema induratum and pyoderma gangrenosum, as well as ulcerated subacute nodular lesions, papulonecrotic eruptions, red papular lesions of the hands and fingers, facial lupus-like rashes and panniculitis [**9**]. Cutaneous necrotising vasculitis has been described resembling nodular vasculitis/erythema induratum. The skin lesions do not appear to relate to the distribution of vascular involvement in any way.

Complications and co-morbidities

Renal artery stenosis, increased arterial stiffness and increased sensitivity of the carotid sinus reflex all contribute to the hypertension. Involvement of the renal arteries can also cause renal dysfunction, and abdominal pain, bleeding or perforation may result from ischaemia or infarction of a viscus. Involvement of the aortic arch and its branches can lead to the 'aortic arch syndrome' with arm claudication, absent radial or brachial pulses (hence 'pulseless disease') or subclavian artery bruits. Aortic regurgitation, coronary artery ischaemia with angina or myocardial infarction, pulmonary hypertension, stroke, syncope and visual disturbances can occur.

Disease course and prognosis

Most patients with Takayasu arteritis will need vascular surgery [10], although restenosis is common [**11**]. The disease and its treatment both lead to an impairment in quality of life even for patients believed to be in remission [10].

Investigations

Positron emission tomography using 18-fluorodeoxyglucose has replaced conventional angiography as the gold standard for the diagnosis of Takayasu arteritis. However, due to the high radiation dose, magnetic resonance angiography could be used for follow-up monitoring. The ESR and CRP are usually elevated but this may be modest.

Management

There are no proven treatments in Takayasu arteritis.

First line

Prednisolone 1 mg/kg/day is the usual favoured first line treatment [12].

Second line

Tocilizumab 162 mg/week subcutaneously is added to the prednisolone in individuals with relapsing or refractory disease [13].

Video legend

Video for this chapter is available on the companion website (https://www.wiley.com/rooksdermatology10e).

Video 100.1 Colour Doppler ultrasound of the temporal and axillary arteries in steroid-naïve patients with giant cell arteritis commonly reveals an intramural inflammatory change – the halo sign.

Key references

The full list of references can be found in the online version at https://www.wiley.com/rooksdermatology10e

Single-organ small-vessel vasculitis
Cutaneous small-vessel vasculitis
2 Jennette JC, Falk RJ, Bacon PA *et al.* 2012 revised International Chapel Hill Consensus Conference Nomenclature of Vasculitides. *Arthritis Rheum* 2013;65:1–11.
3 Calabrese LH, Michel BA, Bloch DA *et al.* The American College of Rheumatology 1990 criteria for the classification of hypersensitivity vasculitis. *Arthritis Rheum* 1990;33:1108–13.
4 Garcia-Porrua C, Gonzalez-Gay MA. Comparative clinical and epidemiological study of hypersensitivity vasculitis versus Henoch-Schonlein purpura in adults. *Semin Arthritis Rheum* 1999;28:404–12.
5 Watts RA, Jolliffe VA, Grattan CE, Elliott J, Lockwood M, Scott DG. Cutaneous vasculitis in a defined population – clinical and epidemiological associations. *J Rheumatol* 1998;25:920–4.
7 Martinez-Taboada VM, Blanco R, Garcia-Fuentes M, Rodriguez-Valverde V. Clinical features and outcome of 95 patients with hypersensitivity vasculitis. *Am J Med* 1997;102:186–91.
32 Boom BW, Mommaas AM, Vermeer BJ. Presence and interpretation of vascular immune deposits in human skin: the value of direct immunofluorescence. *J Dermatol Sci* 1992;3:26–34.
33 Garcia-Porrua C, Gonzalez-Gay MA. Bacterial infection presenting as cutaneous vasculitis in adults. *Clin Exp Rheumatol* 1999;17:471–3.
34 Kharkar V, Vishwanath T, Mahajan S, Joshi R, Gole P. Asymmetrical cutaneous vasculitis following COVID-19 vaccination with unusual eosinophil preponderance. *Clin Exp Dermatol* 2021;46:1596–7.
35 Cribier B, Couilliet D, Meyer P, Grosshans E. The severity of histopathological changes of leukocytoclastic vasculitis is not predictive of extracutaneous involvement. *Am J Dermatopathol* 1999;21:532–6.
36 Mukhtyar C, Lee R, Brown D *et al.* Modification and validation of the Birmingham Vasculitis Activity Score (version 3). *Ann Rheum Dis* 2009;68:1827–32.

Erythema elevatum diutinum
6 Planagumá M, Puig L, Alomar A *et al.* Pyoderma gangrenosum in association with erythema elevatum diutinum: report of two cases. *Cutis* 1992;49:201–6.
8 Creus L, Salleras M, Sola MA *et al.* Erythema elevatum diutinum associated with pulmonary infiltrate. *Br J Dermatol* 1997;137:652–3.
10 Sangüeza OP, Pilcher B, Sangüeza JM. Erythema elevatum diutinum: a clinicopathological study of eight cases. *Am J Dermatopathol* 1997;19:214–22.
17 Yiannias JA, el-Azhary RA, Gibson LE. Erythema elevatum diutinum: a clinical and histopathologic study of 13 patients. *J Am Acad Dermatol* 1992;26:38–44.
18 LeBoit PE, Yen TS, Wintroub B. The evolution of lesions in erythema elevatum diutinum. *Am J Dermatopathol* 1986;8:392–402.
22 Cesinaro AM, Lonardi S, Faccheti F. Granuloma faciale: a cutaneous lesion sharing features with IgG4-associated sclerosing diseases. *Am J Surg Pathol* 2013;27:66–73.

23 Ayoub N, Charuel J-L, Diemerte M-C *et al.* Antineutrophil cytoplasmic antibodies of IgA class in neutrophilic dermatoses with emphasis on erythema elevatum diutinum. *Arch Dermatol* 2004;140:931–6.
24 Chow RKP, Benny WB, Coupe RL *et al.* Erythema elevatum diutinum associated with IgA paraproteinaemia successfully controlled with intermittent plasma exchange. *Arch Dermatol* 1996;132:1360–4.
25 Kohler IK, Lorincz AL. Erythema elevatum diutinum treated with niacinamide and tetracycline. *Arch Dermatol* 1980;116:693–5.
26 Frieling GW, Williams NL, Sim SJ. Novel use of topical 5% dapsone gel in erythema elevatum diutinum: safer and effective. *J Drugs Dermatol* 2013;12:381–4.

Recurrent cutaneous necrotising eosinophilic vasculitis
2 Chen KR, Pittelkow MR, Su D *et al.* Recurrent cutaneous eosinophilic necrotizing vasculitis: a novel eosinophil-mediated syndrome. *Arch Dermatol* 1994;130:1159–66.
5 Jang KA, Lim YS, Choi JH *et al.* Hypereosinophilic syndrome presenting as cutaneous necrotizing eosinophilic vasculitis and Raynaud's phenomenon complicated by digital gangrene. *Br J Dermatol* 2000;143:641–4.
10 Li W, Cao W, Song H *et al.* Recurrent cutaneous necrotizing eosinophilic vasculitis: a case report and review of the literature. *Diagn Pathol* 2013;8:135.

Granuloma faciale
1 Wigley JE. Eosinophilic granuloma. Sarcoid of Boeck. *Proc R Soc Med* 1945;38:125–6.
3 Marcoval J, Moreno A, Peyr J. Granuloma faciale: a clinicopathological study of 11 cases. *J Am Acad Dermatol* 2004;51:269–73.
5 Cesinaro AM, Lonardi S, Facchetti F. Granuloma faciale: a cutaneous lesion sharing features with IgG4-associated sclerosing diseases. *Am J Surg Pathol* 2013;37:66–73.
8 Lallas A, Sidiropoulos T, Lefaki I, Tzellos T, Sotiriou E, Apalla Z. Photoletter to the editor: Dermoscopy of granuloma faciale. *J Dermatol Case Rep* 2012;6:59–60.
17 Dinehart SM, Gross DJ, Davis CM, Herzberg AJ. Granuloma faciale. Comparison of different treatment modalities. *Arch Otolaryngol Head Neck Surg* 1990;116:849–51.
18 Apfelberg DB, Maser MR, Lash H, Flores J. Expanded role of the argon laser in plastic surgery. *J Dermatol Surg Oncol* 1983;9:145–51.
19 Ludwig E, Allam JP, Bieber T, Novak N. New treatment modalities for granuloma faciale. *Br J Dermatol* 2003;149:634–7.
20 Zacarian SA. Cryosurgery effective for granuloma faciale. *J Dermatol Surg Oncol* 1985;11:11–13.
21 Van de Kerkhof PC. On the efficacy of dapsone in granuloma faciale. *Acta Derm Venereol* 1994;74:61–2.
22 Caldarola G, Zalaudek I, Argenziano G, Bisceglia M, Pellicano R. Granuloma faciale: a case report on long-term treatment with topical tacrolimus and dermoscopic aspects. *Dermatol Ther* 2011;24:508–11.

Small-vessel immune complex-associated vasculitis
IgA vasculitis
1 Jennette JC, Falk RJ, Bacon PA *et al.* 2012 revised International Chapel Hill Consensus Conference Nomenclature of Vasculitides. *Arthritis Rheum* 2013;65:1–11.
3 Millo JA, Michel BA, Bloch DA *et al.* The American College of Rheumatology 1990 criteria for the classification of Henoch-Schonlein purpura. *Arthritis Rheum* 1990;33:1114–21.
8 Gardner-Medwin JM, Dolezalova P, Cummins C, Southwood TR. Incidence of Henoch-Schonlein purpura, Kawasaki disease, and rare vasculitides in children of different ethnic origins. *Lancet* 2002;360:1197–202.
12 Jauhola O, Ronkainen J, Koskimies O *et al.* Renal manifestations of Henoch-Schonlein purpura in a 6-month prospective study of 223 children. *Arch Dis Child* 2010;95:877–82.
13 Trapani S, Micheli A, Grisolia F *et al.* Henoch Schonlein purpura in childhood: epidemiological and clinical analysis of 150 cases over a 5-year period and review of literature. *Semin Arthritis Rheum* 2005;35:143–53.
27 Yang YH, Chuang YH, Wang LC, Huang HY, Gershwin ME, Chiang BL. The immunobiology of Henoch-Schonlein purpura. *Autoimmun Rev* 2008;7:179–84.
33 Peru H, Soylemezoglu O, Gonen S *et al.* HLA class 1 associations in Henoch Schonlein purpura: increased and decreased frequencies. *Clin Rheumatol* 2008;27:5–10.
36 Deng F, Lu L, Zhang Q, Hu B, Wang SJ, Huang N. Henoch-Schonlein purpura in childhood: treatment and prognosis. Analysis of 425 cases over a 5-year period. *Clin Rheumatol* 2010;29:369–74.

PART 9: VASCULAR DISORDERS

42 Zaffanello M, Brugnara M, Franchini M. Therapy for children with Henoch-Schonlein purpura nephritis: a systematic review. *Sci World J* 2007;7:20–30.

Cryoglobulinaemic vasculitis

1 Terrier B, Cacoub P. Cryoglobulinemia vasculitis: an update. *Curr Opin Rheumatol* 2013;25:10–18.

9 Mukhtyar C, Guillevin L, Cid MC *et al*. EULAR recommendations for the management of primary small and medium vessel vasculitis. *Ann Rheum Dis* 2009;68:310–17.

10 De Vita S, Quartuccio L, Isola M *et al*. A randomized controlled trial of rituximab for the treatment of severe cryoglobulinemic vasculitis. *Arthritis Rheum* 2012;64:843–53.

Hypocomplementaemic urticarial vasculitis

3 Dincy CV, George R, Jacob M, Mathai E, Pulimood S, Eapen EP. Clinicopathologic profile of normocomplementemic and hypocomplementemic urticarial vasculitis: a study from South India. *J Eur Acad Dermatol Venereol* 2008;22:789–94.

11 Ashida A, Murata H, Ohashi A, Ogawa E, Uhara H, Okuyama R. A case of hypocomplementaemic urticarial vasculitis with a high serum level of rheumatoid factor. *Australas J Dermatol* 2013;54:e62–3.

13 Enriquez R, Sirvent AE, Amoros F, Perez M, Matarredona J, Reyes A. Crescentic membranoproliferative glomerulonephritis and hypocomplementemic urticarial vasculitis. *J Nephrol* 2005;18:318–22.

Antiglomerular basement membrane vasculitis disease

2 Goodpasture EW. Landmark publication from the American Journal of the Medical Sciences: the significance of certain pulmonary lesions in relation to the etiology of influenza. *Am J Med Sci* 2009;338:148–51.

7 Bayat A, Kamperis K, Herlin T. Characteristics and outcome of Goodpasture's disease in children. *Clin Rheumatol* 2012;31:1745–51.

8 Cui Z, Zhao J, Jia XY, Zhu SN, Zhao MH. Clinical features and outcomes of anti-glomerular basement membrane disease in older patients. *Am J Kidney Dis* 2011;57:575–82.

Small-vessel ANCA-associated vasculitis
Microscopic polyangiitis

1 Jennette JC, Falk RJ, Bacon PA *et al*. 2012 revised International Chapel Hill Consensus Conference Nomenclature of Vasculitides. *Arthritis Rheum* 2013;65:1–11.

5 Mohammad AJ, Jacobsson LT, Westman KW, Sturfelt G, Segelmark M. Incidence and survival rates in Wegener's granulomatosis, microscopic polyangiitis, Churg-Strauss syndrome and polyarteritis nodosa. *Rheumatology (Oxford)* 2009;48:1560–5.

10 Lane SE, Watts R, Scott DG. Epidemiology of systemic vasculitis. *Curr Rheumatol Rep* 2005;7:270–5.

20 Jayne D, Rasmussen N, Andrassy K *et al*. A randomized trial of maintenance therapy for vasculitis associated with antineutrophil cytoplasmic autoantibodies. *N Engl J Med* 2003;349:36–44.

22 Mukhtyar C, Guillevin L, Cid MC *et al*. EULAR recommendations for the management of primary small and medium vessel vasculitis. *Ann Rheum Dis* 2009;68:310–17.

23 Ntatsaki E, Carruthers D, Chakravarty K *et al*. BSR and BHPR guideline for the management of adults with ANCA-associated vasculitis. *Rheumatology (Oxford)* 2014;53:2306–9.

27 Stone JH, Merkel PA, Spiera R *et al*. Rituximab versus cyclophosphamide for ANCA-associated vasculitis. *N Engl J Med* 2010;363:221–32.

28 Jones RB, Tervaert JW, Hauser T *et al*. Rituximab versus cyclophosphamide in ANCA-associated renal vasculitis. *N Engl J Med* 2010;363:211–20.

Granulomatosis with polyangiitis

1 Jennette JC, Falk RJ, Bacon PA *et al*. 2012 revised International Chapel Hill Consensus Conference Nomenclature of Vasculitides. *Arthritis Rheum* 2013;65:1–11.

7 Watts RA, Mooney J, Skinner J, Scott DG, Macgregor AJ. The contrasting epidemiology of granulomatosis with polyangiitis (Wegener's) and microscopic polyangiitis. *Rheumatology (Oxford)* 2012;51:926–31.

29 Lyons PA, Rayner TF, Trivedi S *et al*. Genetically distinct subsets within ANCA-associated vasculitis. *N Engl J Med* 2012;367:214–23.

30 Mukhtyar C, Mills J, Scott DGI. The nose is an organ too. *Rheumatology (Oxford)* 2020;59:1196–7.

31 Faurschou M, Sorensen IJ, Mellemkjaer L *et al*. Malignancies in Wegener's granulomatosis: incidence and relation to cyclophosphamide therapy in a cohort of 293 patients. *J Rheumatol* 2008;35:100–5.

34 Mukhtyar C, Flossmann O, Hellmich B *et al*. Outcomes from studies of antineutrophil cytoplasm antibody associated vasculitis: a systematic review by the European League Against Rheumatism systemic vasculitis task force. *Ann Rheum Dis* 2008;67:1004–10.

35 Mukhtyar C, Hellmich B, Jayne D, Flossmann O, Luqmani R. Remission in antineutrophil cytoplasmic antibody-associated systemic vasculitis. *Clin Exp Rheumatol* 2006;24(Suppl. 43):S93–8.

37 Yates M, Watts RA, Bajema IM *et al*. EULAR/ERA-EDTA recommendations for the management of ANCA-associated vasculitis. *Ann Rheum Dis* 2016;75:1583–94.

Eosinophilic granulomatosis with polyangiitis

1 Jennette JC, Falk RJ, Bacon PA *et al*. 2012 revised International Chapel Hill Consensus Conference Nomenclature of Vasculitides. *Arthritis Rheum* 2013;65:1–11.

2 Churg J, Strauss L. Allergic granulomatosis, allergic angiitis, and periarteritis nodosa. *Am J Pathol* 1951;27:277–301.

3 Lane SE, Scott DG, Heaton A, Watts RA. Primary renal vasculitis in Norfolk – increasing incidence or increasing recognition? *Nephrol Dial Transplant* 2000;15:23–7.

9 Vaglio A, Buzio C, Zwerina J. Eosinophilic granulomatosis with polyangiitis (Churg-Strauss): state of the art. *Allergy* 2013;68:261–73.

11 Jakiela B, Sanak M, Szczeklik W *et al*. Both Th2 and Th17 responses are involved in the pathogenesis of Churg-Strauss syndrome. *Clin Exp Rheumatol* 2011;29(Suppl. 64):S23–34.

14 Davis MD, Daoud MS, McEvoy MT, Su WP. Cutaneous manifestations of Churg-Strauss syndrome: a clinicopathologic correlation. *J Am Acad Dermatol* 1997;37:199–203.

20 Mukhtyar C, Guillevin L, Cid MC *et al*. EULAR recommendations for the management of primary small and medium vessel vasculitis. *Ann Rheum Dis* 2009;68:310–17.

Medium-vessel vasculitis
Polyarteritis nodosa and cutaneous polyarteritis nodosa

1 Jennette JC, Falk RJ, Bacon PA *et al*. 2012 revised International Chapel Hill Consensus Conference Nomenclature of Vasculitides. *Arthritis Rheum* 2013;65:1–11.

2 Daoud MS, Hutton KP, Gibson LE. Cutaneous periarteritis nodosa: a clinicopathological study of 79 cases. *Br J Dermatol* 1997;136:706–13.

5 Ishiguro N, Kawashima M. Cutaneous polyarteritis nodosa: a report of 16 cases with clinical and histopathological analysis and a review of the published work. *J Dermatol* 2010;37:85–93.

6 Mohammad AJ, Jacobsson LT, Westman KW, Sturfelt G, Segelmark M. Incidence and survival rates in Wegener's granulomatosis, microscopic polyangiitis, Churg-Strauss syndrome and polyarteritis nodosa. *Rheumatology (Oxford)* 2009;48:1560–5.

11 Darras-Joly C, Lortholary O, Cohen P, Brauner M, Guillevin L. Regressing microaneurysms in 5 cases of hepatitis B virus related polyarteritis nodosa. *J Rheumatol* 1995;22:876–80.

12 Caldeira T, Meireles C, Cunha F, Valbuena C, Aparicio J, Ribeiro A. Systemic polyarteritis nodosa associated with acute Epstein-Barr virus infection. *Clin Rheumatol* 2007;26:1733–5.

24 Navon Elkan P, Pierce SB, Segel R *et al*. Mutant adenosine deaminase 2 in a polyarteritis nodosa vasculopathy. *N Engl J Med* 2014;370:921–31.

26 Guillevin L, Lhote F, Gayraud M *et al*. Prognostic factors in polyarteritis nodosa and Churg-Strauss syndrome. A prospective study in 342 patients. *Medicine (Baltimore)* 1996;75:17–28.

29 Mukhtyar C, Guillevin L, Cid MC *et al*. EULAR recommendations for the management of primary small and medium vessel vasculitis. *Ann Rheum Dis* 2009;68:310–17.

30 Krishnan S, Bhakuni DS, Kartik S. Rituximab in refractory cutaneous polyarteritis. *Int J Rheum Dis* 2012;15:e127.

Kawasaki disease

3 Baumer JH, Love SJ, Gupta A, Haines LC, Maconochie I, Dua JS. Salicylate for the treatment of Kawasaki disease in children. *Cochrane Database Syst Rev* 2006;Issue 4:CD004175.

4 Newburger JW, Takahashi M, Gerber MA *et al*. Diagnosis, treatment, and long-term management of Kawasaki disease: a statement for health professionals from the Committee on Rheumatic Fever, Endocarditis, and Kawasaki Disease, Council on Cardiovascular Disease in the Young, American Heart Association. *Pediatrics* 2004;114:1708–33.

14 Kobayashi T, Inoue Y, Takeuchi K *et al*. Prediction of intravenous immunoglobulin unresponsiveness in patients with Kawasaki disease. *Circulation* 2006;113:2606–12.

15 Kobayashi T, Saji T, Otani T *et al*. Efficacy of immunoglobulin plus prednisolone for prevention of coronary artery abnormalities in severe Kawasaki disease (RAISE study): a randomised, open-label, blinded-endpoints trial. *Lancet* 2012;379:1613–20.

Large-vessel vasculitis
Giant cell arteritis

1 Baum EW, Sams WM, Jr, Payne RR. Giant cell arteritis: a systemic disease with rare cutaneous manifestations. *J Am Acad Dermatol* 1982;6:1081–8.

2 Haugeberg G, Paulsen PQ, Bie RB. Temporal arteritis in Vest Agder County in southern Norway: incidence and clinical findings. *J Rheumatol* 2000;27:2624–7.

4 Smeeth L, Cook C, Hall AJ. Incidence of diagnosed polymyalgia rheumatica and temporal arteritis in the United Kingdom, 1990–2001. *Ann Rheum Dis* 2006;65:1093–8.

15 Mukhtyar C, Guillevin L, Cid MC *et al*. EULAR recommendations for the management of large vessel vasculitis. *Ann Rheum Dis* 2009;68:318–23.

Takayasu arteritis

5 Watts R, Al-Taiar A, Mooney J, Scott D, Macgregor A. The epidemiology of Takayasu arteritis in the UK. *Rheumatology (Oxford)* 2009;48:1008–11.

9 Frances C, Boisnic S, Bletry O *et al*. Cutaneous manifestations of Takayasu arteritis. A retrospective study of 80 cases. *Dermatologica* 1990;181:266–72.

11 Maksimowicz-McKinnon K, Clark TM, Hoffman GS. Limitations of therapy and a guarded prognosis in an American cohort of Takayasu arteritis patients. *Arthritis Rheum* 2007;56:1000–9.

CHAPTER 101

Dermatoses Resulting from Disorders of the Veins and Arteries

Portia C. Goldsmith[1] and Christina George[2]

[1] Barts Health and Homerton University Hospital, London, UK
[2] Imperial College Healthcare NHS Trust, London, UK

ARTERIAL AND ARTERIOLAR DISORDERS

Vasculogenesis, angiogenesis and arteriogenesis

Vasculogenesis is the first step in the development of blood vessels and is the process by which endothelial cells differentiate from their mesodermal precursors. Vasculogenesis leads to the formation of a primary capillary plexus and occurs mainly in embryonal development [1]. Angiogenesis is the process by which new capillaries are formed from existing vessels by sprouting, expanding and remodelling [2]. It is a normal process essential to growth and development. It is pivotal in wound healing, but it is also a key element in the pathogenesis of disease [3]. The establishment and remodelling of blood vessels require a complex orchestration of molecular regulators. In order for angiogenesis to occur, there exists an imbalance in angiogenic growth factors compared with angiogenesis inhibitors. Initially, there is an upregulation of angiogenic growth factors which are released to nearby tissues. The growth factors bind to specific receptors on adjacent vascular endothelial cells leading to cellular activation. The endothelial cells proliferate and secrete matrix metalloproteinases (MMPs) which degrade the extracellular matrix. This permits migration of budding endothelial cells under the influence of angiogenic stimuli, particularly the family of vascular endothelial growth factors (VEGF) A, B, C, D and E, plus placental growth factor and their tyrosine kinase receptors, VEGFR-1, VEGFR-2 and VEGFR-3. Stabilisation and maintenance of newly formed vessels occur mainly as a consequence of the angiopoietins [4], Ang1 (expressed by pericytes, smooth muscle cells and fibroblasts) and Ang2 (from endothelial cells) through their Tie receptors. There are many other angiogenic growth factors which are variously important in health and disease such as basic fibroblast growth factor, interleukin-8, platelet-derived growth factor, transforming growth factor β and tumour necrosis factor α [3].

Differentiation into arteries, veins and capillaries is the responsibility of angiogenesis. Neoangiogenesis is an important cause of recurrent varicose veins after stripping [5]. Arteriogenesis produces rapid circumferential growth in the pre-existing collateral vessels, which are less perfused under normal flow conditions. While local tissue ischaemia or hypoxia stimulates angiogenesis, arteriogenesis is mainly induced by inflammation and sheer stress [6].

Rook's Textbook of Dermatology, Tenth Edition. Edited by Christopher Griffiths, Jonathan Barker, Tanya Bleiker, Walayat Hussain and Rosalind Simpson.
© 2024 John Wiley & Sons Ltd. Published 2024 by John Wiley & Sons Ltd.

PART 9: VASCULAR DISORDERS

Arterial disease and peripheral ischaemic disorders

Definition and nomenclature

Disorders where the arterial blood supply to the limb (usually the leg) is damaged by any disorder which restricts flow to the lower limb – typically atherosclerosis, a chronic disorder that can result in intravascular thrombosis that leads to damage and death of the tissues, but may include arterial embolisation of thrombi, cholesterol emboli and other causes.

Synonyms and inclusions
- Atherosclerosis
- Peripheral ischaemia
- Peripheral vascular disease

Introduction and general description to atherosclerotic peripheral vascular disease

Atherosclerosis of the lower limb is a condition most frequently managed by vascular surgeons, but patients may present to dermatologists when peripheral ischaemia leads to infarction and ulceration of the skin.

Epidemiology

Atherosclerosis is responsible for more than 90% of all arterial disease in the Western world. Approximately 202 million people worldwide are living with arterial disease of the lower extremity, and the numbers continue to rise with a 23% increase in incidence in the past 10 years. It commonly develops after the age of 50, with the rate increasing exponentially after the age of 65, going on to affect approximately 20% of those aged 80 and above [1]. Smoking is an important modifiable risk factor, with the association of lower extremity arterial disease reducing considerably after 10 years of cessation, although it continues to persist [2]. Other important risk factors include hypertension, dyslipidaemia, diabetes and family history of arterial disease.

Pathophysiology

This is a multifactorial disorder, but it is thought that the underlying mechanism is immunological [3]. Evidence suggests that cardio-vascular risk factors induce endothelial injury and endothelial dysfunction. Monocytes recruited to the inflamed endothelium of blood vessels differentiate into phagocytic macrophages which scavenge modified lipids to produce foam cells. This is the basis for the development of the lipid-rich atheroma core. In time, there is further influx and inflammation leading to unstable atherosclerotic plaques which can eventually ulcerate through the endothelial lining, exposing a highly thrombogenic surface. Platelets adhere to the ulcerated plaque and platelet aggregates (platelet thrombi) may embolise distally or may initiate local thrombosis. Inadequate collaterals, or occlusion by thrombosis or embolism, will lead to tissue infarction (e.g. peripheral gangrene).

Clinical features

The clinical features of peripheral vascular disease are described in Table 101.1

Investigations

The most important investigations are summarised in Tables 101.2 and 101.3. Radiological investigations aim to provide a detailed assessment of the anatomy of the arterial tree. Choosing the appropriate tests should be made with the guidance of vascular surgeons and interventional radiologists [5].

Management

Once the diagnosis of peripheral vascular disease is made, the patient is best managed by a vascular surgeon who can address the underlying cause. Table 101.4 outlines the basic management

Table 101.1 Clinical features of peripheral vascular disease.

History	Claudication: cramping pain on walking, usually in the posterior calf, relieved with rest
	Rest pain at night usually in the foot: indication of critical ischaemia
	Skin ulceration
	Poor healing of wounds on the extremities
Presentation	Erythematous or dusky mottled hue to legs; elevation of the leg leads to a white foot (Figure 101.1)
	Trophic changes (including dry skin, cracks, loss of hair, thickened nails) (Figure 101.2)
	Platelet emboli can lodge in the vasculature causing areas of discoloration in the toes and sole of the foot and can appear 'vasculitic-like' (Figure 101.3)
	Ulceration of skin at pressure points and the dorsum of the foot (Figure 101.4)
Clinical variants	N/A
Differential diagnosis	Buerger disease
	Embolism leading to acute ischaemia
	External arterial compression (popliteal entrapment or cervical rib)
	Dissecting aneurysms
	Ergot alkaloid poisoning
	Coagulation disorders (polycythaemia, thrombocytosis)
	Vasculitis
	Calciphyllaxis
	Fabry disease
Classification of severity	Mild, moderate and severe peripheral vascular disease (see the ankle–brachial Doppler pressure index in Table 101.2)
Risk factors	Tobacco smoking (present or past), hypertension, dyslipidaemia, diabetes, history of peripheral vascular disease, chronic kidney disease, sedentary lifestyle, poor diet, family history of cardiovascular or peripheral vascular disease, autoimmune conditions (such as systemic lupus erythematosus, rheumatoid arthritis)
	Examination of skin (colour, temperature, trophic changes, vasculitic-like appearance)
Physical examination	Palpation of peripheral pulses
	Cardiovascular: atrial fibrillation and other dysrhythmias, murmurs, heart failure, aortic aneurysm and bruits over stenosed vessels
	Fundi (may show hypertensive changes or cholesterol emboli)
	Peripheral neuropathy
Disease course and prognosis	90% have coronary artery disease and the extent of this determines the overall survival of the patient rather than the peripheral vascular disease [4]

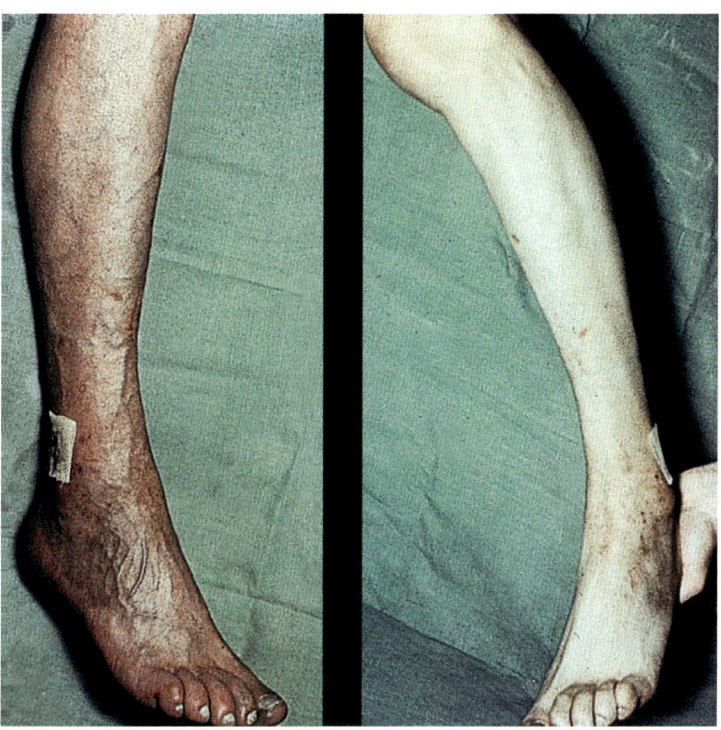

Figure 101.1 Buerger test showing postural colour change in an ischaemic foot – white when the foot is elevated (right) and red when lowered (left).

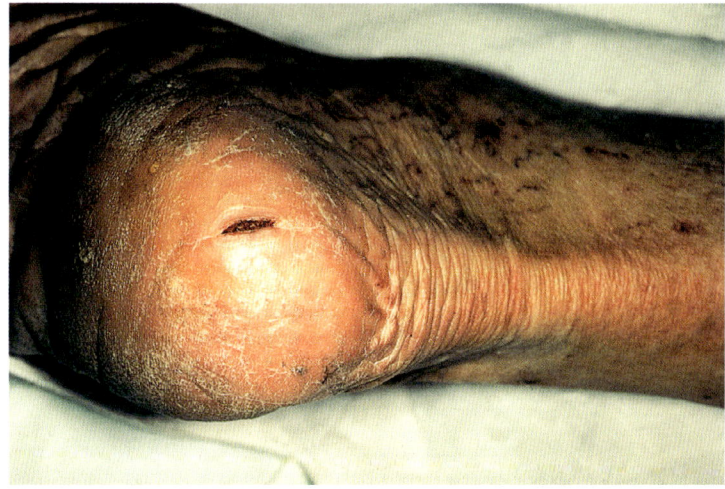

Figure 101.2 Trophic changes including dry skin, cracks, loss of hair and thickened nails (the latter two not shown in figure).

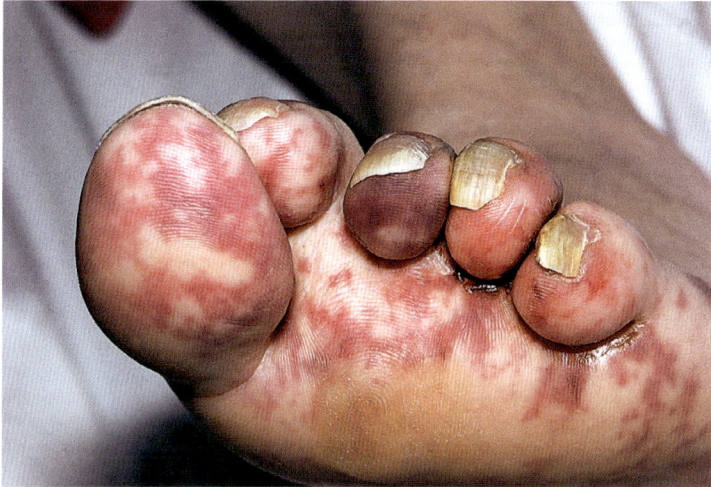

Figure 101.3 Platelet emboli can lodge in the vasculature causing areas of discoloration in the toes and sole of the foot, and can appear 'vasculitic-like'.

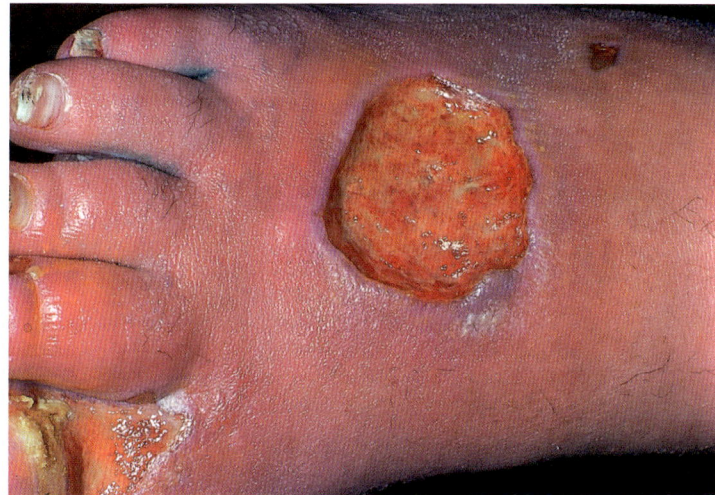

Figure 101.4 Ulceration of the skin at pressure points.

2017 ESC Guidelines on the Diagnosis and Treatment of Peripheral Arterial Diseases, in collaboration with the European Society for Vascular Surgery (ESVS); endorsed by the European Stroke Organisation (ESO)

Patient resources
https://patient.info/heart-health/peripheral-arterial-disease-leaflet
(All last accessed March 2022)

strategies. Treatment options differ for patients presenting with claudication, rest pain or gangrene and acute limb ischaemia.

Resources

Further information
Lower limb peripheral arterial disease; diagnosis and management, NICE guideline February 2018, http://guidance.nice.org.uk/CG147
Percutaneous laser atherectomy as an adjunct to balloon angioplasty (with or without stenting) for peripheral arterial disease, NICE guideline November 2012, http://guidance.nice.org.uk/IPG433

Thromboangiitis obliterans

Definition and nomenclature
This is a non-atherosclerotic segmental inflammatory disease of the small- and medium-sized arteries of the distal extremities of predominantly young male smokers [1]. These patients are normally seen by vascular surgeons but may present to dermatologists with redness and/or ulceration of the skin of the fingers and toes.

Synonyms and inclusions
• Buerger disease

PART 9: VASCULAR DISORDERS

Table 101.2 Investigations for patients with suspected peripheral vascular disease.

Doppler ultrasound to measure the ankle–brachial Doppler pressure index	After the Doppler ultrasound probe has been used to locate the dorsalis pedis or posterior tibial vessel, a sphygmomanometer cuff is placed around the limb above the ankle and inflated (Figure 101.5). The red cells flowing past the tip of the ultrasound probe deflect the beam, creating an audible noise. As the cuff is inflated above systolic pressure, flow in the artery ceases and the noise disappears. This ankle–brachial systolic gradient is normally 1.0. A fall in ankle pressure results in a reduction of the pressure index. Falsely high indices may be obtained in some limbs if the vessels are very calcified and fail to compress at systolic pressure. This is especially true for diabetic limbs. In such circumstances a more accurate means of assessment is to measure the Doppler pressures at the toe Ratio >1.4 = calcification may be present Normal result = 1.0–1.4 Ratio 0.8–1.0 = no significant/mild peripheral vascular disease Ratio 0.5–0.8 = moderate peripheral vascular disease Ratio <0.5 = severe peripheral vascular disease Ratio <0.3 = usually associated with critical ischaemia and gangrene
Toe systolic BP, toe–brachial index (TBI) and transcutaneous oxygen pressure (TCPO$_2$)	Useful in cases of lower extremity arterial disease with calcinosis and incompressible arteries; TBI considered abnormal if <0.70. TCPO$_2$ determinant of healing capacity after amputation (<10 mmHg = wound healing unlikely)
Blood tests	Full blood count (to exclude anaemia and polycythaemia), urea and electrolytes (to monitor renal function), haemoglobinA1C/fasting glucose, fasting lipid profile, C-reactive protein (as a marker of inflammation), homocysteine; enzyme/genetic tests if Fabry disease suspected (Chapters 79 and 154)
Cardiovascular and respiratory investigations	Electrocardiogram (to investigate for ischaemic heart disease and cardiac dysrhythmias), chest radiograph (for heart failure, cardiomegaly)
Treadmill test	Useful for unmasking intermitted claudication of the lower limbs

Table 101.3 Radiological investigations for patients with suspected peripheral vascular disease.

Duplex ultrasound	Duplex ultrasound is often the initial investigation and is used as a screening test to confirm the major sites of stenosis or occlusion in the vascular tree [6,7]. A duplex ultrasound scan provides both a B-mode image of the artery and a measurement of blood velocity; these can be combined to provide a map of stenoses and occlusions within the arterial tree from the aorta to the crural (calf) vessels. The greater the velocity, the tighter the stenosis
Digital subtraction angiography	Often used to aid interventional procedures; however, it is invasive and comes with risk of complication. It is useful in cases of discrepancy with non-invasive imaging techniques
Computed tomography angiography (CTA)	Non-invasive and widely available, providing essential imaging for planning interventional procedures. Disadvantages include radiation of exposure and risk of nephrotoxicity from iodinated contrast
Magnetic resonance angiography	Useful alternative for cases unsuitable for CTA imaging, for example those with kidney disease. However, there is a greater risk of motion artefact and may be contraindicated in those with pacemakers and implantable cardioverter defibrillators

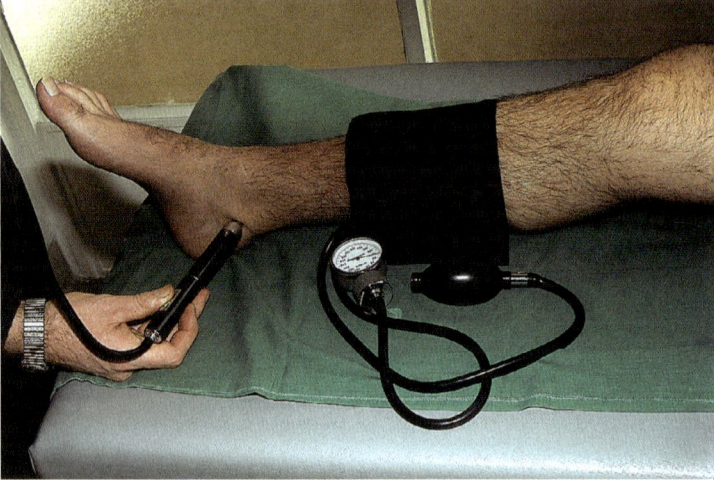

Figure 101.5 Doppler ultrasound to measure the ankle–brachial Doppler pressure index.

Introduction and general description

Thromboangiitis obliterans (Buerger disease) appears to be a distinct condition separate from other forms of vascular occlusion [2,3], with differences in the pathological appearance of the vessel wall, and in the population affected, compared with other arterial diseases [2]. It was first described by Felix von Winiwarter in 1879. In 1908, Buerger published a pathological description of 11 amputated limbs in young male smokers [4].

Epidemiology

Incidence, prevalence and ethnicity

The prevalence is higher in the Mediterranean, the Middle East, India and the Far East and less common in Western Europe and North America.

In Western Europe the prevalence varies, affecting between 0.5% and 5.6% of the population. By contrast, in Korea and Japan it affects 15–66%, and 45–63% in India [5]. These differences are thought to reflect smoking habits and in particular the use of homemade cigarettes.

The prevalence is falling in the USA, from 104/100 000 in 1947 to 13/100 000 in 1986 [6], and in Thailand, the prevalence in one clinic has halved from 1988 to 1995, while the prevalence of peripheral vascular disease doubled in the same time period [7]. This is thought to be due to a decline in the numbers of cigarette smokers.

Age

Most are under the age of 45.

Sex

The condition is much more common in males, with 70–91% of those diagnosed being male [8]. The number of women with the condition

Table 101.4 Treatment options for patients with peripheral ischaemia.

Claudication: aim of treatment is to relieve symptoms	**First line (conservative)** as only 5% of patients go on to develop rest pain or gangrene *Modify risk factors* Smoking, hypertension, dyslipidaemia, diabetes *Supervised exercise programme* To encourage the development of collateral blood vessels. This is effective and improves symptoms and quality of life *Pharmacotherapy* Antihypertensive agents reduce the risk of cardiovascular events and are preferred as they cause peripheral arterial dilatation. Verapamil in particular is preferred as it has been shown to increase walking distance in those with peripheral arterial disease [8] Statins are indicated in all patients with peripheral vascular disease. Lipid-lowering agents reduce major adverse cardiovascular events by 17% and significantly reduce risk of stroke [9] Single antiplatelet therapy is indicated if patients are symptomatic or have undergone revascularisation; clopidogrel is the preferred treatment of choice [10] Drugs such as naftidrofuryl oxalate, cilostazol, pentoxifylline, buflomedil and carnitine may be trialled; however, the benefit is variable and limited. Patients taking naftidrofuryl oxalate should be assessed for improvement after 3–6 months **Second line** *Revascularisation* Endovascular therapy and open surgery can be beneficial for symptomatic relief; hybrid procedures with endarterectomy/bypass and endovascular therapy may indicated in cases of ilio-femoral lesions Importantly, endovascular therapy is associated with significant mortality, morbidity and has limited durability. Potential complications of endovascular therapy include arterial rupture, aneurysm formation, thrombosis and dissection. Therefore, these procedures should be limited to those who do not respond to conservative measures Open surgery is associated with greater durability but higher complication rates
Rest pain and gangrene: aim of treatment is to prevent amputation, relieve pain and preserve life	**First line** Manage complicating conditions such as diabetes, dehydration, infection, polycythaemia and anaemia Effective wound care with analgesia and treatment of secondary infections *Revascularisation* Endovascular therapy is preferable in short, stenotic occlusions, or long occlusions where there is a risk of open surgery In long occlusions where patients are fit for surgery, bypass is considered first line **Second line** If these interventions fail, amputation is considered
Acute limb ischaemia: aim of treatment is to prevent amputation, relieve pain and preserve life	**First line** Treatment with unfractionated heparin [11] Ensure adequate analgesia Urgent angiography to confirm the diagnosis (consider embolism if patient is in atrial fibrillation, has had recent myocardial infarction or if the vascular flow in the other limbs is normal. The cardiac dysrhythmia should be managed) *Revascularisation* If any evidence of neurovascular compromise, urgent revascularisation is essential and should not be delayed by imaging [12] If embolic: balloon angioplasty with or without stenting and sometimes with percutaneous laser atherectomy as an adjunct Peripheral arterial disease: balloon catheter embolectomy with or without stenting and sometimes with percutaneous laser atherectomy and thrombolysis and anticoagulation If stenotic: thrombolysis often via an intra-arterial catheter, followed by anticoagulation. Angioplasty, stenting or surgery may be necessary Platelet emboli should be managed by antiplatelet medication **Second line** Amputation

PART 9: VASCULAR DISORDERS

is rising but is about 11% in the USA [6], and fewer than 3% reported in Thailand [7].

Pathophysiology
Predisposing factors
The aetiology of this condition is unknown although tobacco addiction is invariably a major contributing factor [8], and a failure to overcome this addiction is associated with progressive occlusion of the vessels.

Pathology
Circulating autoantibodies have been identified, in particular antiendothelial cell antibodies are present in high titre in active disease [9]. Antibodies have a pathogenic role and can be used to monitor disease activity [2]. The full thickness of the vessel wall is invaded by lymphocytes, eosinophils, plasma cells and monocytes which disrupt the internal elastic lamina. There is luminal occlusion from thrombosis which is highly cellular. Accompanying nerves and veins may become involved in the inflammatory process.

All changes are segmental or focal. At a later stage in the disease, fibrosis occurs, which spreads to involve surrounding structures [2]. Prothrombotic factors may also be contributory, with anticardiolipin antibodies implicated in more severe disease [10].

Although smoking is known to contribute to the development and progression of the condition, its precise role in the pathophysiology of the condition is unknown. It is postulated that it causes a delayed hypersensitivity reaction or toxic angiitis, triggering the release of cytokines which contributes to the inflammatory process [11].

Causative organisms

Rickettsial infections have been postulated to play a role but evidence is lacking [12]. Chronic anaerobic periodontal infection has also been postulated to play a role, with approximately two-thirds of patients with thrombophlebitis obliterans having severe infection [13]. However, this may be confounded by the fact that many chronic heavy smokers also have this condition concurrently.

Genetics

No confirmed genetic basis has been found though studies have been looking at the role of polymorphisms in the T allele of endothelial nitric oxide synthase [14,15].

Environmental factors

Ambient temperature may be relevant; two studies have reported that thromboangiitis obliterans is worse in the winter and better in warmer weather [16,17].

Clinical features

The clinical features are summarised in Table 101.5.

Investigations

There are no diagnostic tests. Often the diagnosis can be made on clinical grounds with other causes excluded. The erythrocyte sedimentation rate (ESR) may be elevated and blood tests should be undertaken to exclude collagen vascular disorders and coagulation abnormalities. Angiography may be used to identify and establish the extent of the disease, showing arterial occlusion and the development of corkscrew collaterals (Figure 101.7).

Management

These patients are best managed by vascular surgeons. Treatment is difficult and many different modalities have been tried (Table 101.6) but evidence for their success is limited.

NEUROVASCULAR DISORDERS

Erythromelalgia

Definition and nomenclature

This is a rare neurovascular disorder in which the extremities are episodically painful and red (Chapter 82). A sensation of burning is associated with vasodilatation of the small blood vessels in the affected area.

Table 101.5 Clinical features of thromboangiitis obliterans.

History	Pain in the upper and lower limbs with cold extremities
	• Intermittent claudication (classically in the arch of the foot)
	• Rest pain
	• Neuropathic pain and increased sensitivity to cold
	• Athralgia/arthritis – may be the first indication of disease
Presentation	Ulcers: at the sites of trauma and often the sides of the nails or the tips of the digits
	Gangrene (occurs early) (Figure 101.6)
	Trophic changes
	Red or cyanotic peripheries
	Oedema
	Venous thrombosis and thrombophlebitis migrans
	Proximal pulses are present, but dorsalis pedis, posterior tibial and brachial pulses are lost early
	Other organ ischaemia
Diagnostic criteria	Age less than 45
	History of smoking
	Distal extremity ischaemia
	Findings supported by arteriography
	Other conditions such as autoimmune, thrombophilia, diabetes, embolic sources excluded
Differential diagnosis	Early onset atherosclerosis
	Multiple emboli
	Trauma or local lesions (such as entrapment)
	Collagen vascular disease
	Diabetic vasculopathy
	Hypercoagulable states
	Ergotism, cocaine/amphetamine abuse
Classification of severity	N/A
Complications and co-morbidities	Ulcers and gangrene can lead to sepsis and digital/limb loss
Disease course and prognosis	If patients continue to smoke, the prognosis is poor as most will require multiple amputations

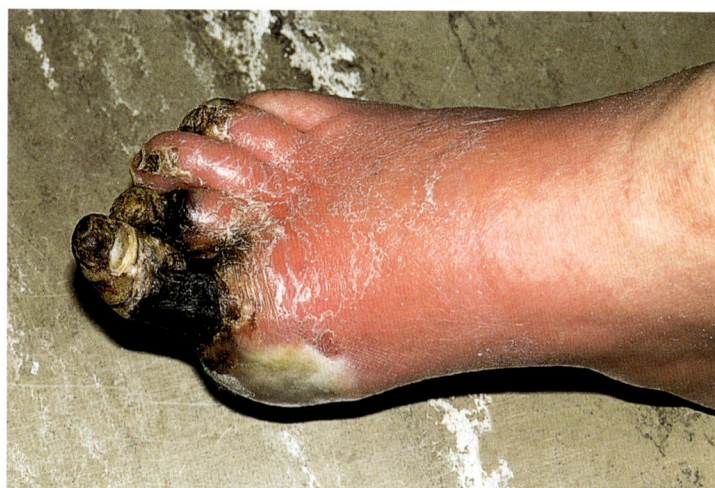

Figure 101.6 Ischaemic toes in thromboangiitis obliterans.

Synonyms and inclusions
- Mitchell disease (after Silas Weir Mitchell)
- Acromelalgia
- Red neuralgia
- Erythermalgia

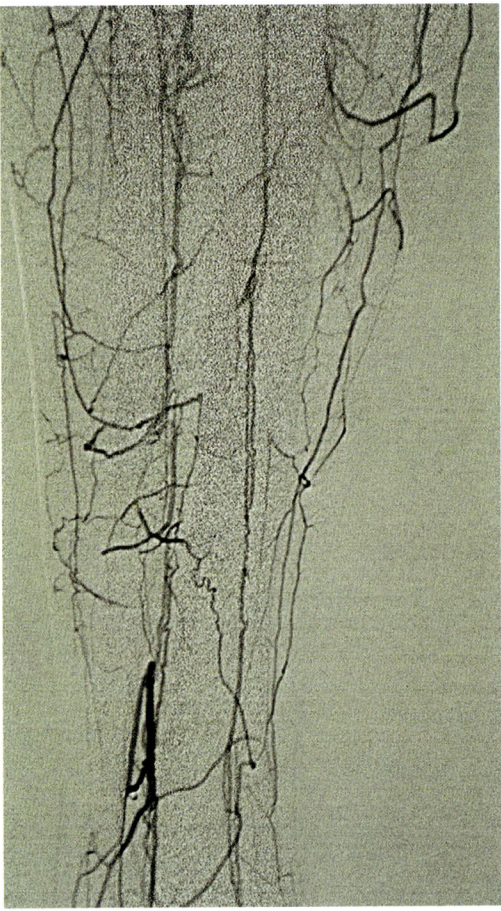

Figure 101.7 Angiography in thromboangiitis obliterans showing vascular occlusion and corkscrew collaterals.

Table 101.6 Management of thromboangiitis obliterans.

First line	Cessation of smoking. This is the only intervention of proven value and is most beneficial if undertaken before the onset of gangrene or tissue loss [1]
Second line	Surgical: • revascularisation if possible (most occlusions are not amenable because they are too distal or diffuse and segmental) • amputation for gangrene Medical: prostacyclin analogue infusions, phosphodiesterase inhibitors, calcium channel blockers, thrombolytics, anticoagulants Sympathectomy: spinal cord stimulators Stimulating angiogenesis through autologous bone marrow cells rich in endothelial progenitor cells

Introduction and general description

Erythromelalgia is derived from the Greek *erythros* = red, *melos* = limb and *algos* = pain. The painful burning attacks typically affect the hands or feet but can involve the face and ears. It is a disabling disorder which may be primary idiopathic, primary hereditary (15% of patients have been shown to have a mutation in the *SCNA9A* gene) or secondary to a number of underlying conditions. It is poorly understood although advances are being made, but unfortunately treatment is often unsuccessful. There are primary and secondary forms of this condition, and the aetiology and management of these conditions differ.

Epidemiology
Incidence and prevalence

There is not much data on the incidence of this rare condition. One study from the USA suggested a rate of 1.3/100 000 of the general population having both primary and secondary erythromelalgia, with 5% of those having the primary inherited form [1]; other studies from Norway [2] and Sweden [3] have found the incidence to be even lower. A study from the Mayo Clinic recorded the incidence as 1 case per 40 000 patients attending the hospital [4]. As there have been more recent discoveries of genetic causes of primary erythromelalgia resulting in a change in classification for some patients, the previous reports may not represent the true incidence of this condition. Dermatologists see this condition rarely even in specialist centres, although the incidence may be higher in reality as this condition is often underrecognised.

Age

Age of onset is variable. The primary form is generally thought to have a younger age of onset; however, although earlier reports from the Mayo Clinic suggested a median onset age in the primary form of 10 years, later studies have shown a wide range of onset: 5–91 years, with a median age of 60 overall [1]. In Norway, the range of onset is from 7 to 76 years in the primary group and 18 to 81 years in the secondary group [2]. In a paediatric case series of 32 patients at the Mayo clinic, the mean age was 14 years, with an age range of 5–18 years [5].

Sex

There is a small female predominance [1,2].

Ethnicity

There is no current evidence that this is relevant.

Associated diseases in secondary erythromelalgia

This diagnosis was initially associated with myeloproliferative disorders, with figures reporting between 20% and 25% [6]. However, a case series of 168 patients with erythromelalgia has found this association in fewer than 10% of cases at presentation, with only 1.3% going on to develop a myeloproliferative disorder subsequently.

Erythromelalgia is now recognised to be associated with a number of other conditions including connective tissue diseases, malignancies, metabolic conditions (such as diabetes and hypercholesterolaemia), infection, musculoskeletal conditions, neuropathies, and drug reactions [7]. It is associated with a significant decrease in mortality and morbidity in the US general population compared with age and sex-matched non-affected equivalents [8].

Pathophysiology
Primary erythromelalgia

Erythromelalgia is the first condition in which an ion channel mutation has been associated with chronic pain [9]. In 15% of cases genetic mutations have been identified. Other cases are thought to have a non-genetic cause or may be mediated by mutations in one or more as yet unidentified genes. Since 2004, at least 20 mutations in the *SCN9A* gene have been identified in erythromelalgia [**10**,11–20].

The *SCN9A* gene codes for the α-subunit of a sodium channel called NaV1.7. Sodium channels transport positively charged sodium ions into cells. They act as threshold sensors and initiate action potentials. The mutations alter the activation profile to produce channels that are open for a longer period of time, leading to more prolonged changes in the membrane potential. NaV1.7 sodium channels are found in nociceptors in the dorsal root ganglion and sympathetic ganglion neurons. The hyperexcitability of the C-fibres in the dorsal root ganglion leads to the burning pain that characterises erythromelalgia. In the sympathetic system, there is hyporeactivity [14] resulting in altered vascular responses to stimuli such as heat and exercise, which causes persistent vasodilatation of the affected skin. It has been shown that the shift in a patient's mutation hyperpolarisation activation was less great in milder late-onset primary type erythromelalgia than in a patient with severe early-onset primary erythromelalgia [21].

It is unknown why the pain episodes associated with erythromelalgia occur mainly in the hands and feet.

Secondary erythromelalgia

In cases associated with thrombocythaemia, biopsies have revealed arteriolar fibrosis and vascular occlusion due to platelet thrombi [22]. It is thought the abnormally functioning platelets in thrombocythaemia clump in vessels and induce neurovascular damage by triggering inflammation. The pathophysiology of cases associated with other underlying conditions remain unknown.

Pathology

There are no diagnostic histopathological findings.

Causative organisms

There have been epidemic outbreaks of erythromelalgia reported in students in rural China. The cause is unknown but poxviruses were isolated from throat swabs of several patients in different areas and at different times of the year [23–25].

Genetics

The primary idiopathic form may occur sporadically but when familial it is inherited in an autosomal dominant manner.

Environmental factors

Eating certain fungi, such as *Clitocybe acromelalgia* (Japan) and *Clitocybe amoenolens* (France), has led to reports of mushroom-induced erythromelalgia which has persisted for up to 5 months following ingestion [26]. In medication-induced erythromelalgia, calcium-channel blockers and bromocriptine can trigger the condition.

Clinical features

Patients may present to general physicians, paediatricians, rheumatologists, vascular surgeons and dermatologists. There may be no abnormal signs at the consultation since the condition is episodic. Consequently, it often takes some time before a diagnosis is made.

The Thompson criteria can be helpful in making the diagnosis. This includes burning pain of the extremities, symptoms exacerbated by warmth and relieved by cooling, redness and warmth of the affected area [27].

The clinical features erythromelalgia are shown in Table 101.7.

Table 101.7 Clinical features of erythromelalgia.

History	Intense burning associated with erythema and increased warmth of the extremities (hands, feet, arms, legs, face and/or ears)
	Triggers of attacks may include heat (often wake the patient at night), movement, exercise and emotional distress
	Attacks last from a few minutes to several hours
	During attacks, patients are desperate to cool the affected area
Examination	During attacks, the affected part is very red
	Initially, between attacks, the affected area appears normal. Over time dusky discoloration and acrocyanosis persist and the skin become shiny (Figure 101.8)
Differential diagnosis	Complex regional pain syndrome (reflex sympathetic dystrophy) following trauma
	Thromboangiitis obliterans
	Vasculitis
	Gout
	Lipodermatosclerosis
	Acrocyanosis
Classification of severity	N/A
Complications	Skin changes such as irritant dermatitis (Figure 101.9a) and fissuring (Figure 101.9b) secondary to chronic immersion in cold water to relieve symptoms
	Vascular occlusion in erythromelalgia secondary to thrombocythaemia can lead to ulceration, necrosis and gangrene
	Tendency to avoid using the affected limbs leading to oedema and atrophy
	Psychological issues due to chronic pain
Disease course and prognosis	Secondary erythromelalgia due to myeloproliferative disease will respond if the underlying condition is treated successfully
	Primary erythromelalgia is a chronic disorder which is generally unremitting

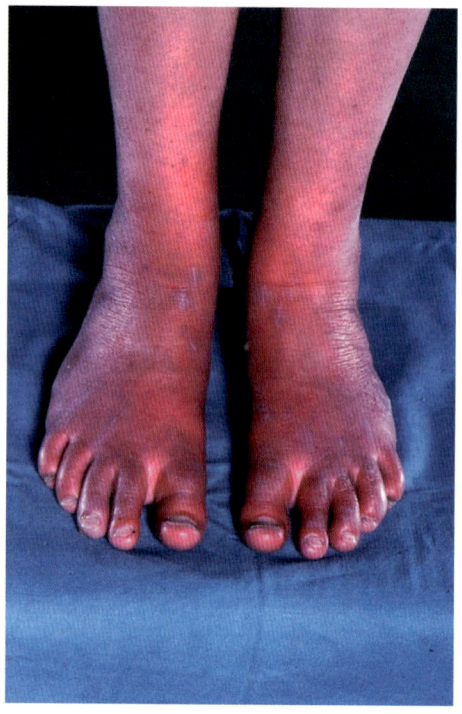

Figure 101.8 Patient during an attack of erythromelalgia.

Table 101.8 Investigations for a patient with suspected erythromelalgia.

Blood tests	To exclude underlying conditions including myeloproliferative disorders, collagen vascular disorder, gout, diabetes; if no haematological abnormalities are identified, serial blood tests following the diagnosis should be considered
Nerve conduction studies	If a peripheral neuropathy is suspected
Genetic testing - if primary erythromelalgia suspected	For *SCNA9A* gene mutation

Table 101.9 Management of erythromelalgia.

Conservative measures	Advice on avoiding exacerbating factors
	Advise patient against cold water immersion to relieve symptoms
General treatment	Psychological support
	Selective serotonin reuptake inhibitors such as venlafaxine, antiepileptic agents, calcium channel blockers, tricyclic antidepressants such as amitriptyline, neuropathic agents such as gabapentin and pregabalin [33]
	Lidocaine patch [34]
	Capsaicin cream (can cause exacerbations)
	Referral to pain specialist clinic
Primary erythromelalgia specific treatment	Mexiletine can be effective
	Ranolazine (one case report)
Secondary erythromelalgia specific treatment	Treat underlying condition
	If due to myeloproliferative disorder, refer to haematologist
	Aspirin for thrombocythaemia [35]

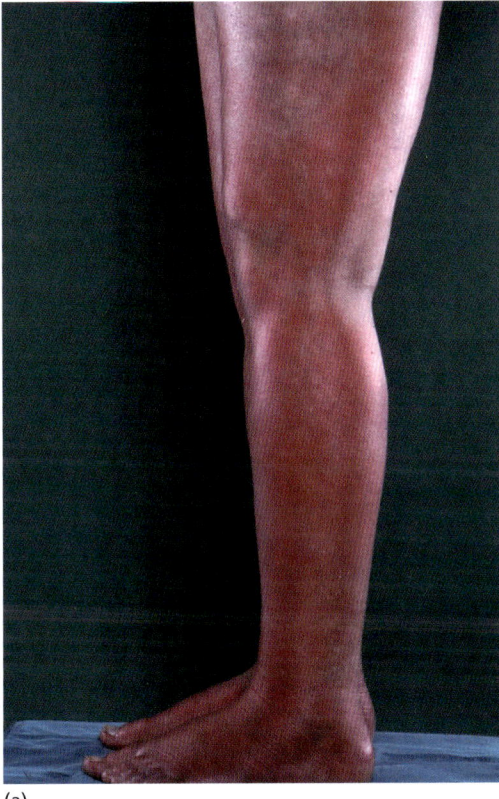

(a)

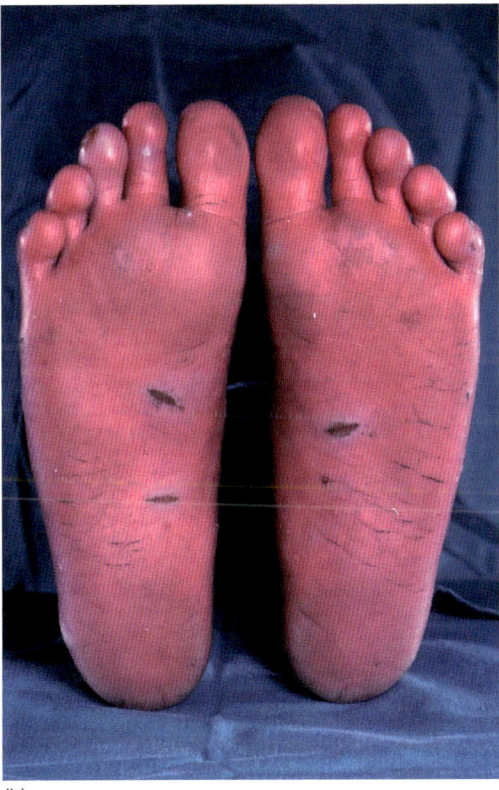

(b)

Figure 101.9 Secondary changes in erythromelalgia due to immersion in water to relieve symptoms (a) irritant contact dermatitis, and (b) fissuring. Courtesy of Professor Pauline Dowd, University College London Hospital, London, UK.

Investigations

The diagnosis of erythromelalgia remains a clinical one, and investigations should be undertaken to exclude secondary causes and for other conditions which can give painful red extremities (Table 101.8). Provocation by immersing affected areas in hot water can be helpful on occasion. Skin biopsies are not diagnostic, and may show non-specific changes, such as increased or decreased nerve density in primary erythromelalgia [28], and thrombi in the secondary form associated with haematological abnormalities.

Once the diagnosis has been made, it should be classified into primary or secondary. Firstly, causes of secondary erythromelalgia should be excluded. Importantly, myeloproliferative disorders can follow by a median of 2.5 years, and therefore serial blood tests should be considered [29]. If primary erythromelalgia is suspected, genetic testing can be undertaken to look for mutation of the *SCNA9A* gene. This can be requested directly by dermatologists for NHS patients meeting the eligibility criteria [30].

Management

Treatment is largely symptomatic. There are no large trials comparing supportive measures. Treatment of the underlying condition in secondary erythromelalgia yields variable results. Response to supportive treatment is also highly variable. In primary erythromelalgia, mexiletine has been shown to normalise the biophysical properties of the mutated NaV1.7 sodium channels and is very effective in some cases [31]. In one case report, ranolazine has also shown efficacy by a similar mechanism [32].

The management of erythromelalgia is outlined in Table 101.9.

PART 9: VASCULAR DISORDERS

TELANGIECTASES

Definition and nomenclature

Telangiectases (Latin: *tel* = end + Greek: *angos* = vessel + ectasis from Greek: *ektasis* = expansion) are chronically dilated capillaries or venules.

Synonyms and inclusions
• Telangectasia

Introduction and general description

Telangiectases appear on the skin and mucous membranes as small, dull red, linear, stellate or punctate macules or papules which blanche on palpation. They represent dilatations (expansion, stretching) of pre-existing vessels without any apparently new vessel growth (angiogenesis) occurring. As such, telangiectases can be bracketed with spider angioma (spider naevi) and capillary aneurysm–venous lakes, whereas vascular malformations represent anomalies of embryological development (disturbances in vasculogenesis or angiogenesis). Hamartomas include proliferation of other tissue elements, for example melanocytic or eccrine cells, and are not solely vascular [1].

Pathophysiology

The telangiectases are a heterogeneous group of disorders. They can be broadly divided into primary and secondary according to their aetiology, although one of the commonest naevi (spider naevi) can be both (Table 101.10). They have varying clinical appearances and are different structurally (Table 101.11).

Table 101.10 Causes of telangiectases.

Primary telangiectases	Secondary telangiectases
Generalised essential telangiectasia	Prolonged vasodilatation (rosacea, venous disease, calcium-channel blocking drugs, smoking)
Hereditary benign telangiectasia	
Hereditary haemorrhagic telangiectasia	
Unilateral naevoid telangiectasia	Chronic UV exposure (ageing skin) and post-irradiation
Ataxia–telangiectasia	
Bloom syndrome	Post-traumatic
Vascular naevi (naevus flammeus)	Atrophy (poikiloderma and steroid-induced)
Angiomas and angiokeratomas	Collagen vascular disease
Angioma serpiginosum	Raynaud phenomenon, CREST syndrome, scleroderma, morphoea lupus erythematosus
Mycosis fungoides and angiotrophic lymphoma	
Spider naevi	Dermatomyositis
Naevus anaemicus with telangiectatic vessels	Mastocytosis: telangiectasia macularis eruptiva perstans
Cutis marmorata telangiectatica	HIV infection
Solitary plaque-like telangiectatic glomangioma	Miscellaneous genodermatoses
	Spider naevi

CREST: calcinosis, Raynaud phenomenon, oesophageal dysmotility, sclerodactyly and telangiectasia.

Table 101.11 Telangiectases with their underlying histology.

Naevus flammeus (Figure 101.10)	Ultrastructure of the collecting venules shows ectopic development of small valve-containing collecting veins
Cherry angiomas (Figure 101.12)	Interconnecting dilated capillaries in the superficial dermis
Angiokeratomas of Fabry and Fordyce (Figure 101.13)	Microvascular arteriovenous anastomoses
Generalised essential telangiectasia (Figure 101.17)	Dilatation of the postcapillary venules of the upper horizontal (subpapillary) plexus
Hereditary haemorrhagic telangiectasia (Figure 101.19)	Spherical and tubular dilatations of capillary loops in the dermal papillae with tortuous cross-connections between individual loops
Telangiectasia macularis eruptiva perstans	Subtle increase in mast cell numbers; mast cells loosely arranged around the dilated vessels of the superficial plexus

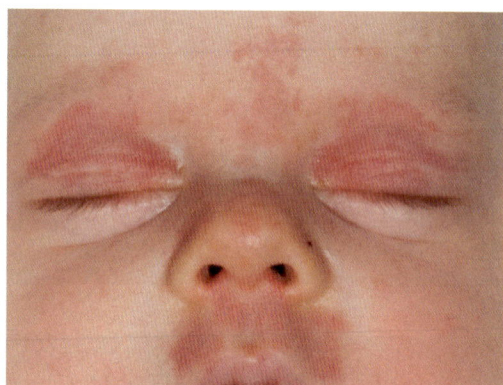

Figure 101.10 Naevus flammeus.

Spider telangiectases

Definition and nomenclature

These are common small vascular lesions found on the skin of the upper body which are benign. They have a characteristic appearance which can resemble a spider.

Synonyms and inclusions
• Arterial spider
• Spider naevus
• Naevus araneus
• Spider angioma

Introduction and general description

Spider telangiectases may be solitary or multiple. Their characteristic appearance is due to a central red arteriole (which resembles the body of the spider) surrounded by a circular pattern of thin-walled capillaries (which look like the multiple legs of a spider).

Epidemiology

Incidence and prevalence

Spider telangiectases occur in up to 15% of healthy people [1].

Age

They are a frequent finding in healthy children [6].

Sex

Commoner in women (especially when pregnant or on the oral contraceptive pill).

Ethnicity

No difference in racial groups has been reported but the lesions are much more visible in patients with less pigmented skins.

Associated diseases

Spider naevi are associated with states of excessive oestrogen and may occur in large numbers during pregnancy – one or more spider naevi are found in two-thirds of all pregnant women with white skin and 11% of those with skin of colour [7]. They may appear in the first few months but tend to increase in number until term; they usually disappear within 6 weeks of delivery but may persist or recur in the same sites in subsequent pregnancies. They are also characteristically found in patients with liver disease, when they can be a presenting sign [8] and again this is thought to be due to a state of oestradiol excess relative to free testosterone [9]. They are more common in alcohol-induced disease than that due to viral hepatitis and the number correlates with disease severity [10]. They are also found in association with use of the oral contraceptive pill, and in states of thyrotoxicosis.

Pathophysiology
Pathology

The main vessel of the spider telangiectasis is an arteriole. The blood flows from this to the periphery, and then passes into a capillary network [11]. The pressure in spider telangiectases rises to 40 mmHg. The lesions consist of a central, ascending, spiral, thick-walled arteriole which ends in a thin-walled ampulla just beneath the epidermis. From the ampulla, thin-walled branching channels

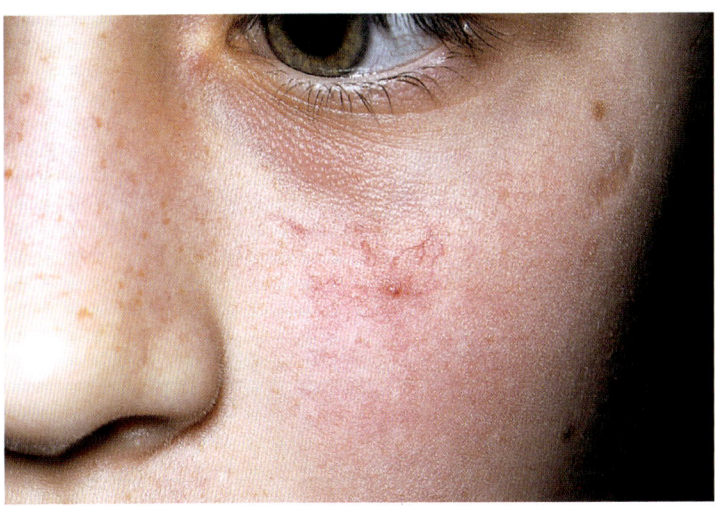

Figure 101.11 Spider telangiectases. Classically, when the central arteriole is compressed, the skin blanches and the lesion temporarily vanishes but rapidly returns when the pressure is released.

radiate peripherally in the papillary dermis. Glomus cells have been described in the wall of the central arteriole [12]. Therefore, these lesions actually resemble microarteriovenous malformations. The high oestrogen states that predispose to the lesions (pregnancy and liver disease) are thought to induce vasodilatation of the central arteriole [13]. Other substances implicated in the pathogenesis of spider naevi include vascular endothelial growth factor (VEGF), basic fibroblastic growth factor (bFGF) [14] and substance P [15].

Clinical features

The clinical features of spider telangiectases are described in Table 101.12.

Investigations

An approach to investigating patients with spider telangiectases is outlined in Table 101.13.

Table 101.12 Clinical features of spider telangiectases.

History	Lesions appear suddenly. They are asymptomatic but can be a cosmetic issue
Presentation	Single or multiple
	1–1.5 mm in diameter
	The central body may be raised, and is usually pulsatile on diascopy
	Found on upper body: neck, face, arms and chest, etc. (in the territory of the superior vena cava)
	Often on the hands and fingers in children
	Sometimes at sites of trauma
	May be unilateral [2]
	Classically, when the central arteriole is compressed, the skin blanches and the lesion temporarily vanishes but rapidly returns when the pressure is released (Figure 101.11)
Clinical variants	Can rarely occur on the mucous membranes of the lips and nose
Differential diagnosis	The typical morphology, with a central pulsating vessel, does not occur in other conditions
	In hereditary haemorrhagic telangiectasia, the lesions are macular, punctate or linear; when they are stellate they do not pulsate
Complications and co-morbidities	Trauma may cause bleeding, but this stops with simple pressure
	Liver disease
	Number of telangiectases (>20), size (>15 mm) and atypical distribution of lesions (lower body) can predict severity of liver disease and risk of complications such as bleeding varices [3–5]
Disease course and prognosis	Lesions can spontaneously resolve in healthy adults and children
	Lesions may disappear at the end of the pregnancy or with resolution of the liver disorder

Table 101.13 Investigation of patients with spider telangiectases.

Phenotype	Investigations
Healthy children and adults with single lesions or only a few typical lesions	No investigations needed
Multiple lesions: examine for clinical signs of pregnancy, liver disease, thyrotoxicosis, or use of oral contraceptive pill or topical oestrogen use	When concerned about underlying disease: • Blood tests: full blood count, urea and electrolytes, liver function tests, autoantibody screen, hepatitis viral serology, thyroid function tests, α-fetoprotein • Liver: ultrasound if clinical examination and/or blood tests suggests liver disease

Table 101.14 Management of spider telangiectases.

First line	Conservative approach (especially in children and pregnant patients) Many lesions resolve spontaneously Identify and treat underlying disease Cosmetic camouflage
Second line	Electrodesiccation (small risk of a depressed scar if overtreated and may recur if undertreated) Laser: 585 nm pulsed dye laser produces a high rate of initial clearance [16] but may recur and require a second treatment. Laser is non-scarring but produces purpura KTP 532 nm laser is also highly effective with no post-treatment purpura [17,18] Multi-wavelength laser treatment has recently shown efficacy [18]

Management

Spider telangiectases are asymptomatic and may resolve spontaneously. They may also resolve through treating the underlying condition. When on the face, they can be a cosmetic issue. Management is outlined in Table 101.14.

Cherry angiomas

Definition and nomenclature

These are very common, cherry red papules seen in the skin due to abnormal vascular proliferations.

Synonyms and inclusions
• Cherry haemangioma
• Campbell de Morgan spots
• Senile angiomas

Introduction and general description

Cherry angiomas are the commonest angiomas seen in the skin. They are entirely benign and increase in numbers with age.

Epidemiology
Incidence and prevalence

The actual incidence of cherry angiomas is not known. They are very common. One study reported that cherry angiomas were observed in 5% of adolescents and 75% of adults over 75 years of age [1].

Age

They normally spontaneously appear in middle age and increase in number with age, although they can first appear in the second decade of life.

Sex

There is no difference between the sexes in the prevalence of cherry angiomas.

Ethnicity

They occur in all ethnic groups, although are more obvious in patients with less pigmented skins.

Associated diseases

There are no significant disease associations, although they have been reported to appear in pregnancy [2].

Pathophysiology
Pathology

Cherry angiomas are true capillary haemangiomas, formed by numerous, newly formed capillaries with narrow lumens and prominent endothelial cells arranged in a lobular pattern in the papillary dermis. The pathogenesis of these lesions remains poorly understood. One study has suggested a possible molecular basis for their pathogenesis. The level of MicroRNA424 is reduced in cherry angiomas when compared with normal skin. This is thought to lead to increased expression of MEK1 and Cyclin E1 which *in vitro* causes endothelial cells to proliferate and could possibly result in the vascular proliferations which make up cherry angiomas [3]. In a case series of 10 cherry angioma samples, 50% displayed oncogenic mutations in GNAQ and GNA11 (also found in other vascular conditions such as congenital haemangiomas and port-wine stains), although the relevance of these findings remains unclear [4].

Environmental factors

Exposure to chemicals such as bromides, solvents and mustard gas has been associated with the development of cherry angiomas [5–7].

Clinical features
History

They appear as small asymptomatic red dots on the skin usually in the third and fourth decade of life. They often start as pin prick sized lesions which gradually grow. They increase in number with increasing age.

Presentation

They may be single or multiple lesions predominantly on the upper trunk and arms [2]. However, they can arise anywhere on the skin, although rarely on the hands and feet, and not on the mucous membranes. Typically, they appear as round to oval, bright red, dome-shaped papules and pinpoint macules varying from less than 1 mm in diameter and up to several millimetres in diameter (Figure 101.12). The larger lesions may be purple in colour.

Differential diagnosis

This includes angiokeratomas, infantile haemangiomas, bacillary angiomatosis, blue rubber bleb naevus syndrome and amelanotic melanoma.

PART 9: VASCULAR DISORDERS

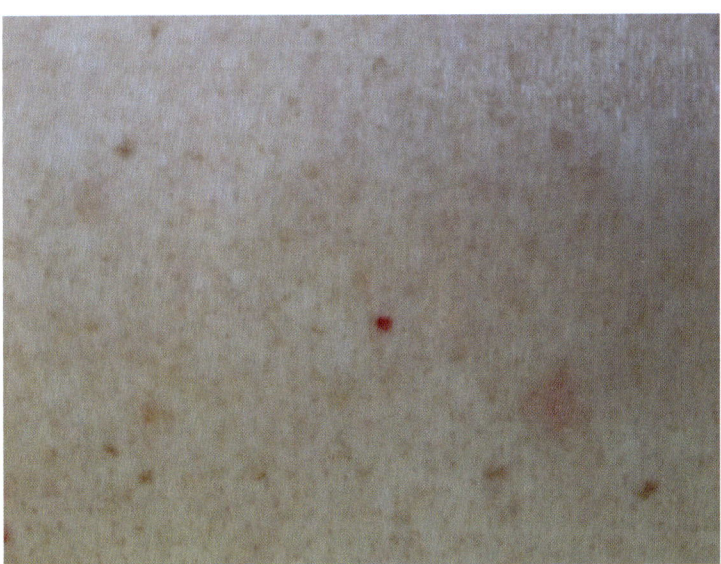

Figure 101.12 Cherry angioma.

Complications and co-morbidities
If traumatised, cherry angiomas may bleed. They are not associated with underlying disease.

Disease course and prognosis
These lesions are benign and increase in number with age.

Investigations
The diagnosis is usually made clinically, but a biopsy can be confirmatory in doubtful cases.

Management
No treatment is needed in most cases as cherry angiomas are benign and asymptomatic. For lesions that are bleeding, or cosmetically troubling, treatment options include shave excision, hyfrecation, cryotherapy and pulsed dye laser and intense pulsed light [9].

Resources

Further information
http://www.pcds.org.uk/clinical-guidance/cherry-angioma-syn.-campbell-de-morgan-spot

Patient resources
https://patient.info/doctor/campbell-de-morgan-spot
(All last accessed March 2022.)

Angiokeratomas

Definition
These are small benign cutaneous vascular lesions which present as red/blue or purple papules.

Introduction and general description
Angiokeratomas are not true angiomas but occur in existing vessels and are characterised by superficial vascular ectasia and overlying acanthosis or hyperkeratosis. They may be solitary or diffuse. There are many different clinical types with similar histology. The main ones are as follows:

- Angiokeratoma of Mibelli – acral skin.
- Angiokeratoma of Fordyce – scrotal or vulval skin (Chapter 109).
- Angiokeratoma corporis diffusum – seen in Fabry disease (Chapters 79 and 154).
- Angiokeratoma circumscriptum – usually congenital, associated with naevus flammeus and cavernous haemangioma.
- Solitary or multiple angiokeratomas.

Angiokeratoma circumscriptum

These are usually solitary and asymptomatic benign lesions.

Epidemiology
Incidence and prevalence
This is not known, although they are much rarer than other telangiectases such cherry angiomas and spider naevi.

Age
The lesions may be congenital or acquired and therefore can be present at birth. They are more frequently seen in childhood and early adulthood. Angiokeratomas of the vulva usually develop between the age of 20 and 40 years [1], and in general, the Fordyce subtype is most prevalent in those over 40.

Sex
They are commoner in females than males (3 : 1 ratio).

Ethnicity
There is no known ethnic variation in this condition.

Associated diseases
Angiokeratoma circumscriptum may coexist with other types of angiokeratomas and with Klippel–Trenaunay syndrome (KTS), naevus flammeus, cavernous haemangiomas and traumatic arteriovenous fistulae.

Pathophysiology
Pathology
There is a thin layer of hyperkeratosis with papillomatosis and slight acanthosis of the overlying epidermis. There are dilated thin-walled vascular spaces encircled by elongated rete ridges filled with red blood cells. There may be associated telangiectasia in the subcutis.

Genetics
These are *not* thought to be genetically determined, unlike the lesions characteristic of Fabry disease (angiokeratoma corporis diffusum)

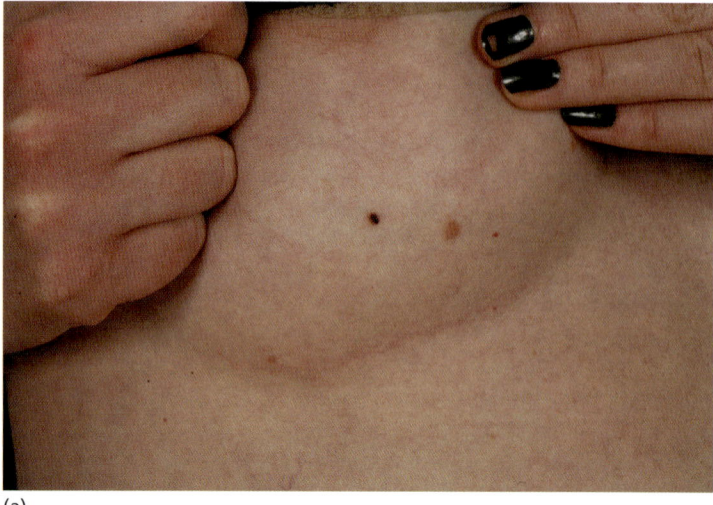

(a)

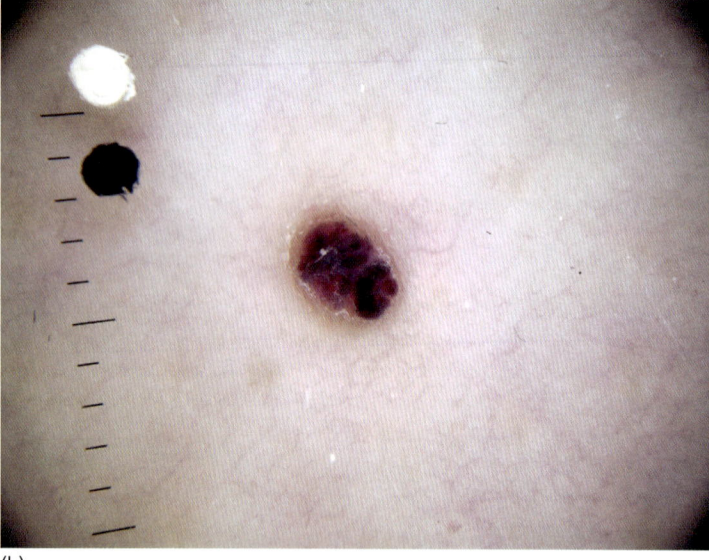

(b)

Figure 101.13 (a) Angiokeratoma; (b) dermoscopic view of angiokeratoma.

Clinical features

History
Generally, these lesions are solitary (although multiple lesions may occur in adulthood) and usually occur on the lower extremities. However, they can occur anywhere on the skin including the tongue and may be multiple and even distributed in band-like formation. They are largely asymptomatic but patients usually present because the lesion has turned very dark or black in colour and there is a concern about it being a malignant melanoma.

Presentation
Angiokeratomas are usually red/blue or purple in colour, sometimes with a slightly rough surface (Figure 101.13). They may appear black if they have thrombosed or if they have been traumatised and bled. Lesions vary from small papules to larger plaques. Dermoscopy can be helpful in revealing blood-filled vascular spaces, known as lacunae (Figure 101.13b). A number of subtypes of angiokeratoma exist (Table 101.15).

Differential diagnosis
This includes other angiokeratomas, malignant melanoma and cherry angiomas.

Complications and co-morbidities
Trauma may lead to bleeding and/or thrombosis.

Disease course and prognosis
The lesions are benign and generally resolve spontaneously.

Investigations
No investigations are needed for isolated lesions. If there are multiple lesions, Fabry disease should be considered and genetic testing undertaken.

Management
None is needed if the lesions are asymptomatic. In cases of diagnostic uncertainty, they can be surgically excised. Other treatment modalities that can be adopted are hyfrecation for superficial and small lesions, curettage and cautery and cryotherapy. Different lasers have been used (argon, carbon dioxide, erbium) but the KTP laser or 800 nm diode laser appears to be both effective and the least scarring thus giving the best cosmetic result [2].

Resources

Further information
https://www.pcds.org.uk/clinical-guidance/angiokeratoma

Patient resources
http://dermnetnz.org/vascular/angiokeratoma.html
(All last accessed March 2022.)

Venous lakes

Definition and nomenclature
Venous lakes are composed of dilated venules. They are dark purple/blue papules that appear on the face, lips and ears of elderly patients.

Synonyms and inclusions
• Phlebectases

Introduction and general description
Though venous lakes are entirely benign they can clinically mimic melanoma.

Epidemiology
Incidence and prevalence
The incidence of venous lakes is unknown. A study from a dermatology clinic in Italy identified the prevalence of venous lakes of the lips as 3.7% over a 10-month period [1].

Table 101.15 Subtypes of angiokeratoma.

Subtype	Age (years)	Sex	Association	Presentation
Angiokeratoma of Mibelli	Childhood/adolescence	F>M	Association with chilblains Familial variant described	Often acral skin, often over bony prominences; can be warty [3] Multiple May bleed with trauma
Angiokeratoma of Fordyce	Over 40	M>F	None known	Most commonly scrotal skin; also penis, vulva and groin Single or multiple Asymptomatic, but may bleed with trauma
Angiokeratoma corporis diffusum [4]	Often prior to puberty	M>F	Fabry disease and a variety of other lysosomal enzyme deficiencies Also reported in healthy individuals [5]	Multiple Mainly lower trunk/groin 'bathing suit area'
Angiokeratoma circumscriptum	Usually at birth, can occur later in life	F>M 3 : 1	Numerous including naevus flammeus, cavernous haemangioma, Klippel–Trenaunay syndrome, traumatic arteriovenous fistulae, Cobb syndrome	Solitary, asymptomatic Often unilateral Initially red and macular; become darker red/blue and raised/warty/hyperkeratotic with time
Sporadic angiokeratomas	Over 40	M>F	None known	Often solitary Any body area can be affected, often lower limbs

Age

Venous lakes occur mainly in the elderly. The mean age has been reported to be variously 65 [2] and 76.7 years [1].

Sex

They are commoner in men; early studies suggested 95% occurred in men [2] though a more recent report found the male to female ratio to be 1.5 : 1 [1]. Women may present for treatment more readily than men.

Ethnicity

There is no known racial predilection for this condition.

Associated diseases

Menni *et al.* [1] showed a significant increase in solar keratoses in patients with venous lakes.

Pathophysiology
Pathology

Venous lakes are dilated venules. The lesions consist of a single layer of flattened endothelial cells and a thick wall of fibrous tissue. There is often elastosis in the surrounding tissue.

Environmental factors

Sunshine and ageing have been thought to be triggers, and possibly smoking [1,2].

Clinical features
History

The patient usually presents with a painless dark purple/blue papule often on the lip (Figures 101.14 and 101.15) which bleeds if traumatised.

Presentation

The papule is soft and compressible. They are usually single but multiple lesions can occur. The commonest sites are the ears, face and lips [2]. When they occur on the lips, the lower lip is the commonest site [1].

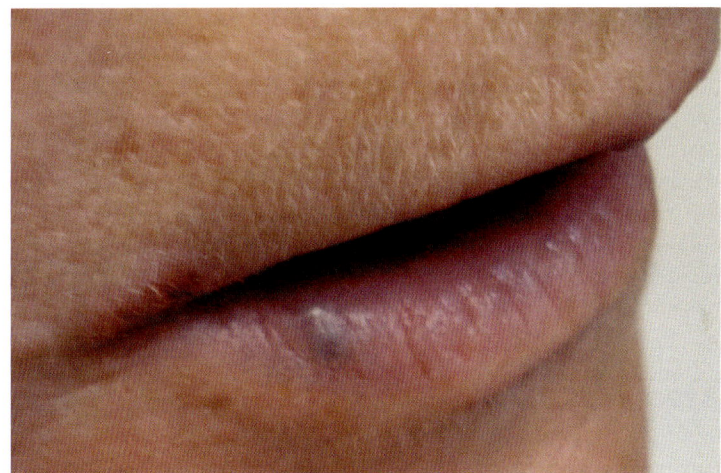

Figure 101.14 Small venous lake.

Differential diagnosis

The fact that they can be emptied by compression usually excludes malignant melanoma on clinical grounds. Blue naevi may appear similar, but again cannot be emptied by compression, and rarely occur on the face. Cherry angiomas and angiokeratomas can be similar clinically.

Complications and co-morbidities

Venous lakes are benign and usually asymptomatic but occasionally when traumatised they will bleed. Cosmetically they can be an issue for patients.

Disease course and prognosis

Untreated venous lakes persist.

Investigations

None are necessary but biopsy can be confirmatory if the diagnosis is in doubt.

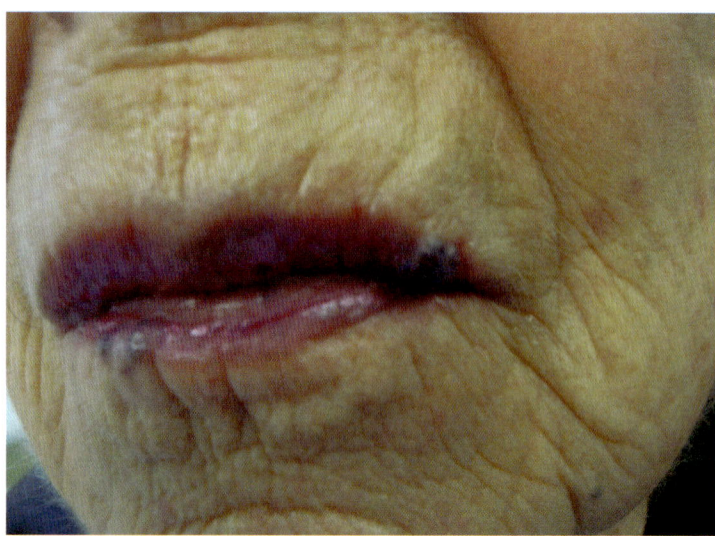

Figure 101.15 Larger venous lakes on upper and lower lips.

Management

Treatment is only needed if the patient is having problems with bleeding or finds the lesions cosmetically troubling. The lesions can be excised, or treated with cryotherapy or laser [3–5]. Many different lasers have been used (such as argon, carbon dioxide, pulsed dye and potassium titanyl phosphate lasers). The more destructive the laser treatment, the more likely it is to be effective; however, the risks of scarring are increased. Intralesional radiofrequency ablation has also shown good results with minimal scarring and recurrence [6]. Sclerotherapy is another therapeutic option which has shown efficacy [7].

Resources

Further information

http://www.pcds.org.uk/clinical-guidance/venous-lake (last accessed March 2022).

Primary telangiectasia

A summary of primary telangiectasias described can be found in Table 101.16.

Angioma serpiginosum

Definition

Angioma serpiginosum is a rare naevoid disorder affecting the small vessels of the upper dermis. It has been proposed that this condition be classified as a capillary naevus, although there is ongoing debate surrounding its classification [1].

Introduction and general description

This is a benign, asymptomatic vascular condition characterised by small red puncta that cluster together in linear, serpiginous or gyrate patterns, chiefly on the lower limbs in females. It can also occur on acral sites [2] and disseminated forms have also been reported, although this is very rare [3].

Epidemiology

Incidence and prevalence

This is not known.

Age

The condition may be present at birth and often starts in childhood. Eighty per cent of cases occur before the age of 20 years. A late onset case at 35 years of age has been described [4].

Sex

Ninety per cent of cases occur in females.

Ethnicity

There is no racial predilection for this condition.

Associated diseases

There is one report of a family whose members had oesophageal papillomatosis associated with angioma serpiginosum, inherited in an X-linked dominant fashion with the genetic defect linking to Xp11.3-Xq12 [5].

Pathophysiology

Pathology

Generally, it is thought that the condition results from a vascular malformation or neoplasm and is not just a simple telangiectasia. A recent case report describes histology with positive immunohistochemistry for Wilms Tumour-1 [6]. This is an endothelial marker of angiogenesis found in vascular tumours, suggesting that this condition is a vascular proliferation in origin [7]. The classical puncta of angioma serpiginosum are caused by either congenital hyperplasia or ectasia of pre-existing superficial dermal capillaries. Histology shows that the affected papillae are distended by a large single ectatic capillary, lined by flattened endothelial cells of normal appearance. Inflammatory changes are not present. Sometimes the vascular spaces disappear due to thrombosis.

Genetics

Most cases are sporadic. However, both autosomal dominant and X-linked dominant inheritance has been recorded and *PORCN* gene mutations or deletions have been reported [8,9].

Clinical features

These are described in Table 101.17.

Investigations

If the diagnosis is in doubt, skin biopsy and imaging can be performed.

Management

Angioma serpiginosum is benign and asymptomatic. It tends to persist, and treatment is only indicated for cosmetic reasons. Cosmetic camouflage can be helpful and treatment with pulsed dye laser can be effective [13].

Table 101.16 Summary of primary telangiectases described.

Skin condition	History	Examination	Clinical variants	Investigations	Co-morbidities	Disease course	Treatment
Spider telangiectasia	Age of onset: any age Sex: commoner in females Asymptomatic	Small spider-like appearance Solitary or multiple Site: mainly upper body	N/A	Solitary: none required Multiple: Blood tests Liver ultrasound if appropriate Pregnancy test	Liver disease, pregnancy, thyrotoxicosis, use of oral contraceptive pill	May resolve spontaneously	Treat underlying disease For cosmesis: cosmetic camouflage
Cherry angioma	Age of onset: at any age, common in middle-age, increase in number with age Sex: equal in males/females Asymptomatic	Single or multiple Oval, bright red papules/pinpoint macules Site: predominantly upper trunk/limbs	N/A	None	None	Benign, increase with age May bleed if traumatised	If symptomatic: shave excision, hyfrecation, cryotherapy, laser
Angiokeratoma	Age of onset: varies according to subtype History varies according to subtype Asymptomatic	Red/blue or purple papules Varies according to subtype	Solitary/ multiple angiokeratomas Angiokeratoma of Mebilli Angiokeratoma of Fordyce Angiokeratoma coroporis diffusum Angiokeratoma circumscriptum	Solitary do not require investigations	According to subtype (see Table 101.15)	Lesions often persist	If symptomatic: hyfrecation, curettage and cautery, cryotherapy, lasers
Venous lake	Age of onset: elderly Sex: commoner in males Asymptomatic	Painless dark purple/blue compressible papule Site: often on the lip Empties on compression	N/A	None	None	Lesion persists May bleed if traumatised	If symptomatic: excision, cryotherapy, laser
Angioma serpiginosum	Age of onset: at birth or in childhood Sex: commoner in females Asymptomatic	Pinpoint violaceous/ red macules Grouped in areas May be annular/ serpiginous /linear Site: mainly lower legs Diascopy: does not blanch	N/A	None	None	Lesions persists	For cosmesis: camouflage, pulsed dye laser
Generalised essential telangiectasia	Age of onset: late childhood/ adolescence Sex: commoner in females Asymptomatic	Red confluent sheets comprising of blanching telangiectasias Site: predilection for lower body	N/A	None	None	Lesions persist	For cosmesis: camouflage, lasers
Hereditary benign telangiectasia	Age of onset: childhood Asymptomatic	Extensive telangiectases resembling generalised essertial telangiectasia Site: sun exposed sites more common	N/A	None	Arteriovenous anastomoses	Lesions persist	For cosmesis: camouflage; lasers; intense pulsed light

Table 101.17 Clinical features of angioma serpiginosum.

History	Onset usually in early childhood
	Asymptomatic
	One or more small lesions that grow over a period of months or years
	Growth is irregular with little dots that form satellites that later coalesce
	Predominantly found on the lower limbs and extremities, but can be extensive [10]
	Not reported on the hands or mucosae
Examination	Pinpoint violaceous or red macules (may be non-blanching)
	Grouped in areas a few centimetres across, or sometimes form large sheets
	May be annular, serpiginous or linear (Figure 101.16)
	No bleeding, inflammation or pigmentation
	Dermoscopy: well-demarcated red oval or round lagoons can be seen [11]
Clinical variants	Rarely natural resolution leads to atrophic areas [12]
Differential diagnosis	Capillary haemangioma
	Angiokeratomas
Complications and co-morbidities	None
Disease course and prognosis	Lesions often stop growing at puberty and remain unchanged
	Occasionally, they may partially resolve spontaneously

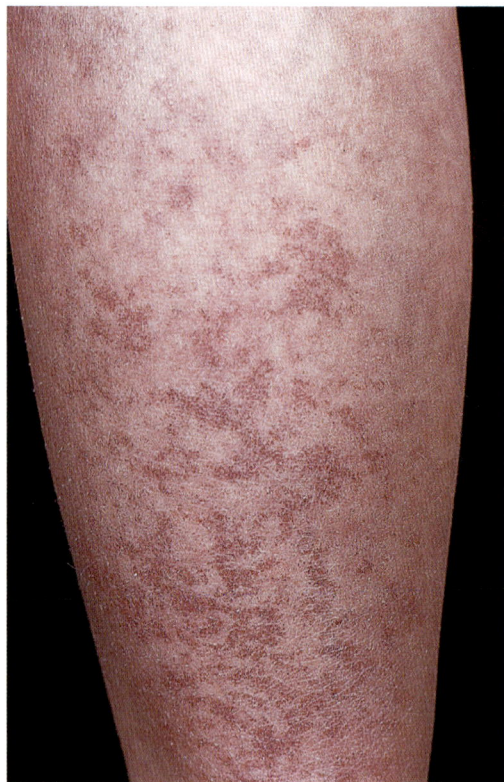

(a)

Resources

Patient resources

https://dermnetnz.org/topics/angioma-serpiginosum/ (last accessed March 2022).

Generalised essential telangiectasia

Definition
This is a syndrome of primary acquired telangiectases with a widespread cutaneous distribution of lesions.

Introduction and general description
This is a benign, non-inherited condition chiefly distinguished from hereditary haemorrhagic telangiectasia by the distribution of the lesions, their arrangement into sheets and the usual lack of bleeding from the lesions.

Epidemiology
Incidence and prevalence
This not known. It is not commonly reported in the literature.

Age
It commonly starts in late childhood or early adult life, although one report of 13 patients found the mean age of onset to be 38 years [1].

Sex
It is much commoner in women (in one study, 10 out of 13 were females [1]).

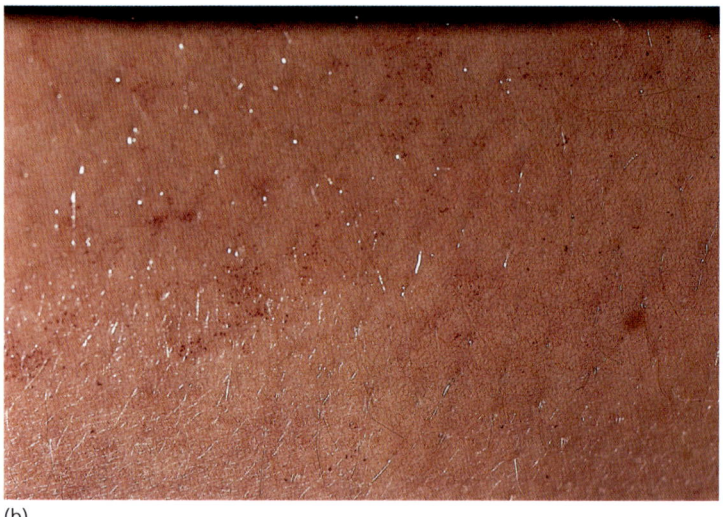

(b)

Figure 101.16 Angioma serpiginosum: (a) grouped lesions, and (b) close up appearance.

Ethnicity
There is no known racial predilection for this condition. Reported cases have largely been in patients with less pigmented skin which may just reflect the fact that the telangiectasia are less noticeable in darkly pigmented skins.

Associated diseases
No known disease associations occur with this condition.

Pathophysiology

The aetiology and pathogenesis of this condition is unknown.

Pathology

There is chiefly dilatation of the capillaries with some dilated post-capillary venules of the upper horizontal (subpapillary) plexus. There are no associated epidermal or dermal changes.

Genetics

There is no known genetic basis for this condition.

Environmental factors

The role of environmental factors in unknown but female hormones, trauma and UVB have been postulated to be of importance [2,3].

Clinical features

History

The eruption frequently starts on the lower limbs as individual lesions, and then spreads to form red confluent sheets comprised of blanching telangiectasia. It is usually asymptomatic but tingling and numbness have occasionally been reported.

Presentation

The eruption is usually symmetrical. Early lesions are small, red, or pink linear telangiectases with occasional larger macules arranged in groups. The lesions spread over the skin to become large erythematous sheets and individual telangiectasia can be difficult to distinguish (Figure 101.17). There is a predilection for the lower body, but they can occur anywhere; occasionally mucosal and conjunctival lesions have been reported [4]. The sheeted telangiectases are usually fixed but will blanch on pressure.

Differential diagnosis

This includes hereditary haemorrhagic telangiectasia, hereditary benign telangiectasia, telangiectasia triggered by calcium channel blockers and cutaneous collagenous vasculopathy.

Disease course and prognosis

This benign condition is progressive and the lesions become fixed with time.

Investigations

None are needed.

Management

Treatment is largely for cosmetic issues. Skin camouflage creams can be helpful, but laser (pulsed dye and ND-Yag) treatment is often attempted. However, the lesions are often so widespread that multiple treatments are needed and those on the lower leg are often very resistant to treatment [5]. Sclerotherapy is not feasible due to the size and number of lesions. Single cases have reported positive responses to treatment with a tetracycline [6], oral acyclovir [7], ketoconazole [8] and 6-mercaptopurine [9].

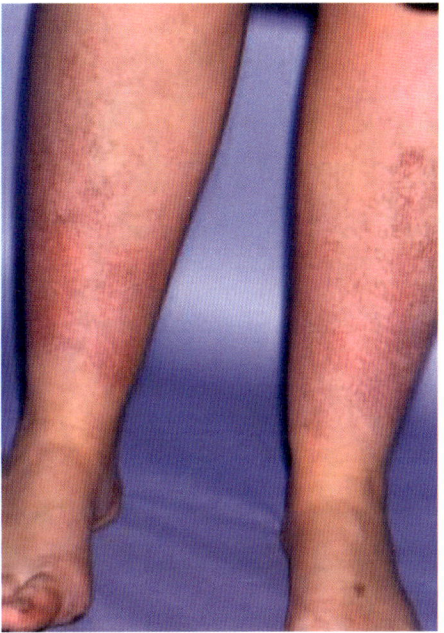

(a)

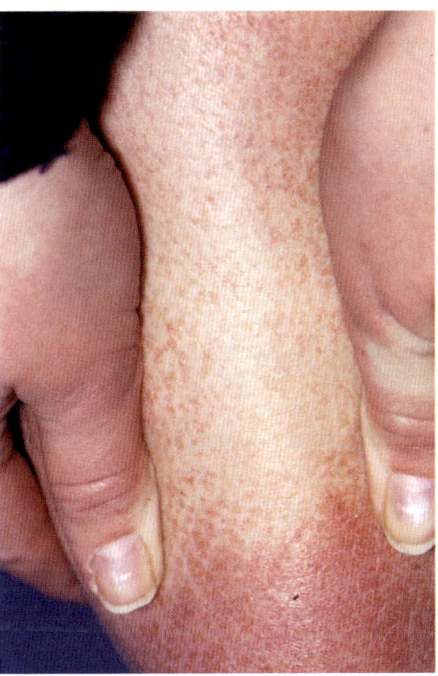

(b)

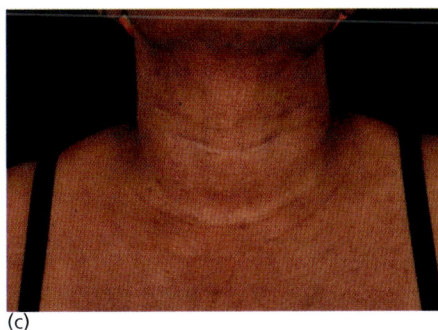

(c)

Figure 101.17 (a) Generalised essential telangiectasia; (b) generalised essential telangiectasia showing blanching with pressure; (c) generalised essential telangiectasia in pigmented skin.

PART 9: VASCULAR DISORDERS

Hereditary benign telangiectasia (formerly Osler–Weber–Rendu disease)

This disorder has autosomal dominant inheritance [1] However, it has also been described in cases without positive family history [2–4]. It is characterised by the presence of extensive telangiectases, resembling generalised essential telangiectasia, which start in childhood and occur without systemic lesions (Figure 101.18) [5,6]. Less commonly, the telangiectases may be present at birth [7]. They tend to occur more in light-exposed skin including the lips. Histology and electron microscopy have been used to distinguish this condition from hereditary haemorrhagic telangiectasia [8], which is the most important differential diagnosis (Figure 101.19). The distinction is dependent on the lack of bleeding and systemic involvement, although lesions do appear related to arteriovenous anastomoses as in hereditary haemorrhagic telangiectasia [9].

Unilateral naevoid telangiectasia syndrome

Definition and nomenclature

A condition of telangiectases occurring in a Blaschkoid distribution on the skin.

Synonyms and inclusions
- Unilateral dermatomal superficial telangiectasia
- Unilateral spider naevus
- Linear telangiectasia

Introduction and general description

This condition was first described by Blaschko in 1899. It may be congenital or acquired and runs a benign course.

Epidemiology
Incidence and prevalence

This is not known. There have been around 100 reported cases to date [1]. However, it is not thought to be that uncommon, and is likely to be under-reported due to its benign course [2].

Age

The congenital form appears during or shortly after the neonatal period. The acquired form often starts at puberty or during pregnancy but can occur at any time. Of the reported cases, the age of onset ranges from birth to 69 years [3].

Sex

The congenital form is commoner in males, but the acquired form is much commoner in females.

Ethnicity

There is no racial predilection reported.

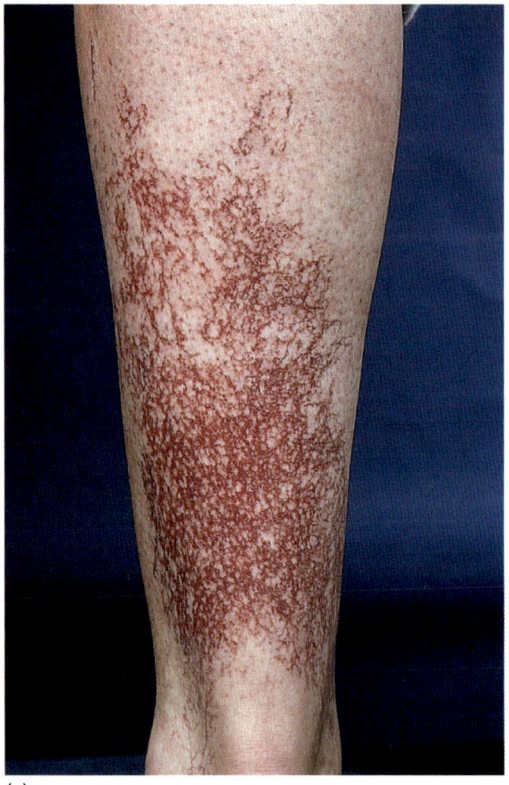

(a)

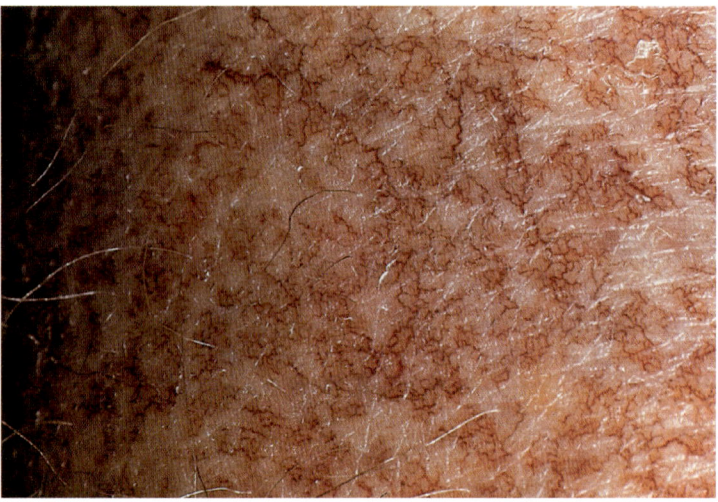

(b)

Figure 101.18 Benign essential telangiectasia: (a) arborising pattern, and (b) close up appearance.

Environmental factors

The occurrence of the acquired form of this condition has been reported to be associated with states of oestrogen excess. Increased oestrogen and progesterone receptors in the affected skin have been found by one research group [4]. This finding has not been repeated.

Associated diseases

Often there are no associated diseases, but in the acquired form it has been seen in patients with liver disease, hyperthyroidism and during pregnancy. This is hypothesised to be due to the

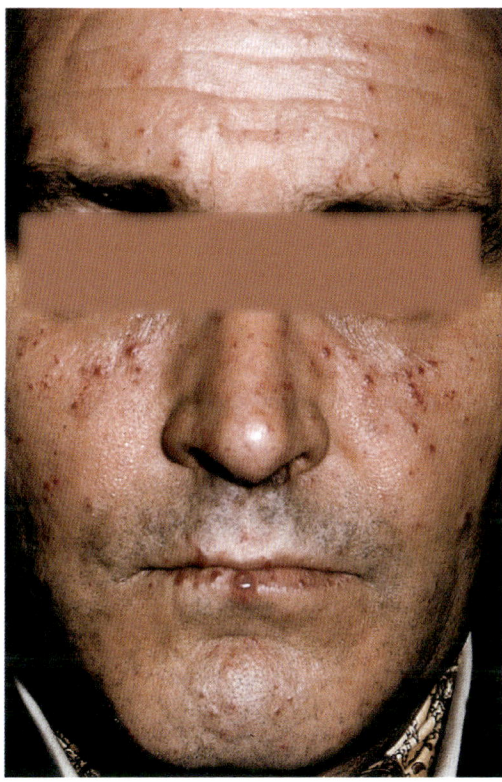

Figure 101.19 Hereditary haemorrhagic telangiectasia.

hyper-oestrogenic state, with a similar pathogenesis to spider naevi, although this remains a subject of debate.

Pathophysiology

The pathogenesis is not understood. The Blaschkoid distribution of the lesions suggests that there is genetic mosaicism that leads to the development of the telangiectasia.

Pathology

Biopsy of lesions shows multiple, dilated, thin-walled vessels lined by pump endothelial cells in the papillary and upper reticular dermis.

Genetics

The congenital form has been reported to be inherited in an autosomal dominant fashion.

Clinical features

These are summarised in Table 101.18.

History

Patients develop asymptomatic unilateral telangiectases.

Presentation

The telangiectases are often distributed in the third and fourth cervical dermatomes in a Blaschkoid distribution (Figure 101.20). The lesions are most commonly seen on the upper body especially on the face, neck, shoulder and arm. Sometimes there is a pale ring ('anaemic halo') in the skin surrounding the telangiectases. The lesions blanch on pressure.

Table 101.18 Summary of clinical features of unilateral naevoid telangiectasia syndrome.

History	Onset of congenital form: neonatal period
	Onset of acquired form: most commonly puberty/pregnancy
	Can occur at any time
	Asymptomatic
Examination	C3/C4 dermatome in Blaschkoid distribution
	Mainly upper body
	Sometimes pale ring is visible around the lesions
	Dermoscopy: tortuous capillaries in reticulated pattern
	Diascopy: does not blanch
Clinical variants	Congenital or acquired
Differential diagnosis	Angioma serpiginosum
Investigations	None required
	Liver function tests and pregnancy test if appropriate
Complications and co-morbidities	None
Disease course and prognosis	Lesions remain fixed
Treatment	None required
	Pulsed dye laser
	Cosmetic camouflage

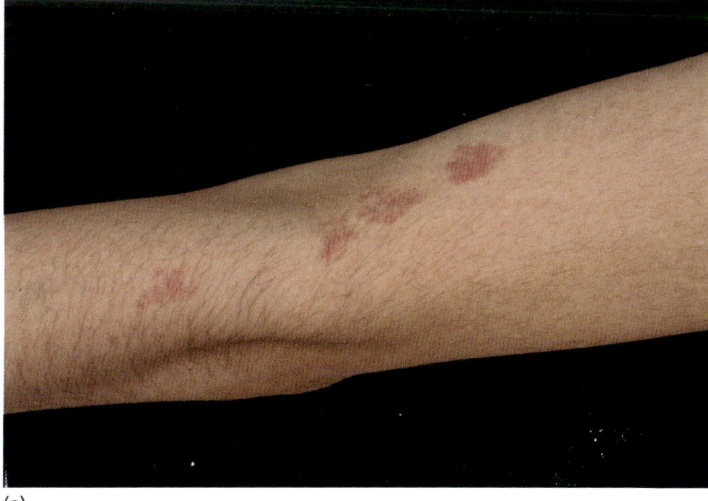

(a)

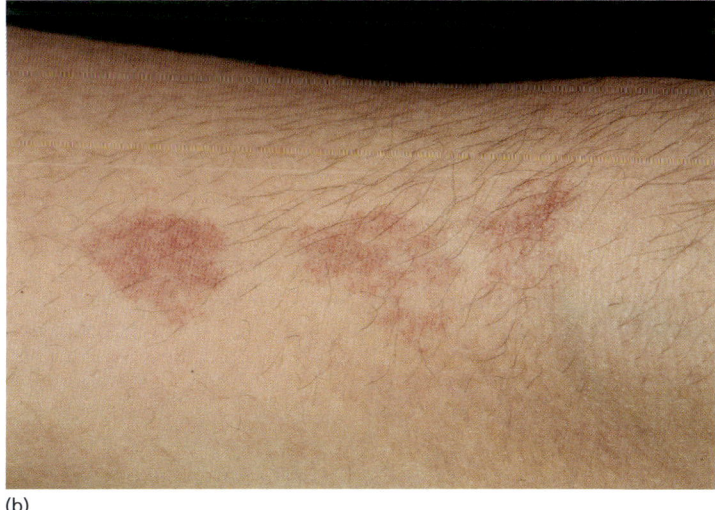

(b)

Figure 101.20 (a) Unilateral naevoid telangiectasia, and (b) showing grouped lesions in close up.

PART 9: VASCULAR DISORDERS

Differential diagnosis

Benign essential telangiectasia, angioma serpiginosum.

Complications and co-morbidities

Unilateral naevoid telangiectasia is asymptomatic and benign. There are no complications but it can be associated with high oestrogen states, such as liver disease.

Disease course and prognosis

In most cases of the acquired and congenital form, the lesions are fixed and persist. However, occasionally if the condition is associated with pregnancy or the oral contraceptive pill, the lesions resolve or improve once the patient's oestrogen levels have fallen.

Investigations

None are necessary but liver function tests and a pregnancy test may be helpful if there are clinical indications of those underlying conditions. Dermoscopy characteristically shows red, tortuous, reticulated capillaries. The lesion blanches with diascopy, differentiating it from angioma serpiginosum [5]. A skin biopsy may help if there are diagnostic difficulties.

Management

No treatment is necessary for this benign condition unless the patient finds it cosmetically disabling. Cosmetic camouflage can be helpful. If the patient is pregnant or on the contraceptive pill then waiting to see what happens when the oestrogen levels normalise is advised. Pulsed dye laser can be effective but some authors have reported recurrence [6,7].

MALFORMATIONS

Arteriovenous malformations

Definition and nomenclature

Arteriovenous malformations are fast-flow vascular lesions composed of malformed arterial and venous vessels connected directly to one another without an intervening capillary bed [1,2].

Synonyms and inclusions
- AV malformations
- AVMs
- Arteriovenous anomalies

Introduction and general description

Arteriovenous malformations can occur throughout the body in many different organs and can be fatal in certain instances. For instance, brain arteriovenous malformations account for 1–2% of all strokes. Dermatologists are more likely to encounter arteriovenous malformations when the vasculature affected involves the skin or mucosal surfaces, or as an association of hereditary haemorrhagic telangiectasia (Table 101.19).

Epidemiology

Incidence and prevalence

This is not known for arteriovenous malformations involving the skin but the incidence of brain arteriovenous malformations is ~1/100 000 per year in unselected populations, and the point prevalence in adults is ~18/100 000 [1].

Age

Approximately half are visible in the neonatal period and others become apparent during childhood and adolescence [2]. They often worsen with puberty and pregnancy.

Sex

There is equal incidence in females and males [2].

Ethnicity

There is no known racial variance in this condition.

Associated diseases

See Table 101.19.

Table 101.19 Conditions associated with arteriovenous malformations.

Condition	Clinical features	Sites of arteriovenous malformations
Familial cases of capillary malformations associated with arteriovenous malformations Autosomal dominant inheritance (inactivating mutation in *RASA1*)	Multiple cutaneous capillary malformations	Subcutaneous, intramuscular, intraosseous and/or cerebral
Parkes Weber syndrome	Soft-tissue and bony hypertrophy associated with the overlying arteriovenous malformation	On an extremity (usually limbs)
Hereditary haemorrhagic telangiectasia (autosomal dominance inheritance)	Epistaxis – spontaneous, recurrent nose bleeds Telangiectases – multiple, at characteristic sites (lips, oral cavity, fingers, nose) Visceral lesions such as gastrointestinal telangiectasia	Lungs, liver, gastrointestinal tract and central nervous system (these may result in massive visceral haemorrhage and death)
Cobb syndrome (cutaneomeningospinal angiomatosis)	Capillary malformation on the skin along the midline of the back	Intraspinal corresponding to the dermatomal distribution of the overlying capillary malformation which may lead to spinal cord damage
PTEN mutation syndromes: Bannayan–Riley–Ruvalcaba syndrome, Cowden syndrome, *PTEN* hamartoma tumour syndrome	Dependent on syndrome: ectopic fat overgrowth, hamartomas, intracranial developmental issues, macrocephaly	Intramuscular AVMs

Pathophysiology
Pathology

Arteriovenous malformations consist of arteries connecting directly to veins without the intervening capillary bed. Where they connect is called the nidus. The feeding arteries have a deficient muscularis layer and the draining veins dilate due to the high-velocity blood flow they receive. It is not known how these abnormal connections arise. It is postulated that during early fetal development there is a failure of regression of arteriovenous channels in the primitive plexus that allows these lesions to form, which may be due to an aberration in the transforming growth factor β signalling pathway [3]. Elevated levels of vascular endothelial growth factor (VEGF) have also been found in the plasma, and the nidus and adjacent cells of cerebral arteriovenous malformations suggesting this may also play a role in the pathogenesis [4].

Genetics

Although most cases of arteriovenous malformations are sporadic, there are a few inherited syndromes whose molecular genetics have been elucidated. Approximately 5% cases are autosomal dominant, most commonly in association with conditions such as hereditary haemorrhagic telangiectasia, and the capillary malformation-AVM syndrome [5]. A mutation in the gene *RASA1* has been identified on chromosome 5q in families with capillary malformations associated with arteriovenous malformations [6].

Environmental factors

None are known but existing lesions may progress during puberty and pregnancy.

Clinical features

See Table 101.20.

Investigations

1 To confirm the diagnosis and monitor the response to treatment: ultrasound with colour Doppler examination shows low resistance high-velocity arterial flow, with high diastolic flux, and pulsatile venous flow below the baseline. Arteriovenous shunting is seen within tortuous vessels.

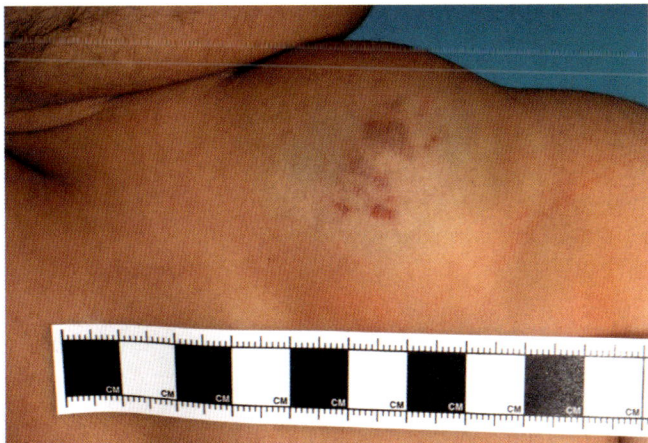

Figure 101.21 Infant with an arteriovenous malformation.

Table 101.20 Clinical features of arteriovenous malformations.

History	40–60% are visible at birth
	30% become apparent during childhood
	More common in the head and neck area
	Excessive warmth in the area
	Unusual pain
	Bleeding episodes
Examination	Overlying skin feels warm
	Prominent vessels (Figure 101.21)
	Possible palpable thrill
	Auscultation of the lesion should detect a machinery murmur
Clinical variants	Parkes Weber and Cobb syndromes
Differential diagnosis	Other vascular birthmarks and vascular malformations such as capillary malformations (increased warmth and prominent blood vessels should help make the diagnosis)
	Vascular tumours
	Kaposi sarcoma
Classification of severity (Schobinger staging system)	*Stage I* (quiescent phase)
	Asymptomatic
	May be clinically not apparent, or
	May resemble a port-wine stain or involuting haemangioma
	Stage II (progressive stage)
	Vascular lesions enlarge and darken
	Lesions deform the integument
	Overlying skin becomes warm
	A pulse or thrill can be palpated
	Audible bruit may be present
	Stage III (same as stage II plus the following):
	Deep destruction of tissues occurs with spontaneous necrosis
	Chronic ulceration, pain and haemorrhage
	Stage IV (same as stage III plus the following):
	Cardiac decompensation due to high-output cardiac failure
	Patients usually start in stage I in childhood and may remain that way throughout life. Triggers for progression are puberty, pregnancy and trauma. Approximately 84% may progress to stage II [5]
Complications	Haemorrhage
	Ischaemia
	Chronic venous insufficiency
	Pain
	Cosmetic deformity
	Limb growth asymmetry
	High output cardiac failure
	Problems related to site of lesion such as impaired vision, difficulty eating or breathing, limb fracture
Disease course and prognosis	Arteriovenous malformations grow with the child
	They do not regress
	It is not known how to predict which patients will go on to stage III and IV
	Morbidity and mortality depend on location, size of lesion (both determine its treatability), presence of severe complications such as heart failure

2 To evaluate the extent of the arteriovenous malformation: magnetic resonance imaging (MRI) and magnetic resonance angiography (MRA) demonstrate a collection of vascular flow voids which are the fast-flow vessels that do not enhance with contrast (no tumour aspect); the arteriovenous malformations and its network can be delineated.

3 Catheter-based angiography is useful for planning and implementing endovascular procedures.

4 If the patient is bleeding, full blood count and clotting studies should be undertaken

Management

A multidisciplinary approach is essential with specialist vascular surgeons, interventional radiologists and paediatricians where appropriate [7]. Management is challenging. Treatment may be curative but is frequently palliative. Sclerotherapy, embolisation and surgery are all options.

Arteriovenous malformations often recur following embolisation and surgical resection, because incomplete destruction of the lesion leads to rapid recruitment of new vessels from adjacent arteries to supply the nidus, with resultant growth and recurrence of the lesion.

Surgery

The aim of surgery is curative and may be possible for small and accessible lesions. Sometimes embolisation is performed beforehand to reduce intraoperative bleeding.

Embolisation

The aim is to temporarily occlude the nidus with either ethanol, glue, ethylene vinyl alcohol copolymer or coils [8]. This is usually palliative for bleeding, pain or the control of heart failure or prior to surgery.

Sclerotherapy

Alcohol is injected into the nidus. Sclerotherapy tends to be palliative and is generally reserved for low flow lesions [9]. It can be used as an adjunct to embolisation or surgical resection [10].

When to treat

For stage I and II arteriovenous malformations in infancy and early childhood, there is no treatment; just monitoring is recommended (see later for staging system). When the child is older, some clinicians offer surgical resection if the cosmetic result is predicted to be acceptable and the lesion amenable. Follow-up is essential as there is a high rate of recurrence.

For stage II later in childhood, and stage III and IV, surgical treatment (excision and reconstruction) where possible should be considered. However, often the lesions are too deep or extensive for cure, and management is only palliative using embolisation and partial resection.

Venous malformations

Solitary venous malformations

Definition and nomenclature

Venous malformations are slow-flow, non-proliferating vascular birthmarks. They are composed of anomalous ectatic venous channels.

Synonyms and inclusions
- Venous angioma
- Cavernous angioma
- Phlebangioma

Introduction and general description

These are the commonest of all vascular anomalies. They are classified as 'slow-flow' lesions. They vary enormously clinically, ranging from single small superficial lesions to deep extensive lesions. They may be single or multiple and can arise in the skin and mucosae and can involve the limbs, the gastrointestinal tract and cranio-facial area. They may be asymptomatic or a major problem for patients with pain, bleeding and disfigurement being the commonest complications.

Epidemiology

Incidence and prevalence

Venous malformations are relatively common and the incidence has been reported to be 1 in 2000–5000 births [1].

Age

The lesions are always present at birth but may not become clinically noticeable until later in childhood as they grow with the child.

Sex

There is no sex difference in venous malformations.

Ethnicity

There is no known racial difference.

Clinical features

Cutaneous venous malformations can be classified into a number of subtypes: common/sporadic, familial cutaneo-mucosal, glomuvenous and blue rubber bleb naevus syndrome [1].

The clinical features of venous malformations are outlined in Table 101.21.

Associated diseases

In blue rubber bleb naevus syndrome (Bean syndrome), there are cutaneous and gastrointestinal venous malformations which typically become apparent with age. There may be a risk of severe gastrointestinal haemorrhage. Maffucci syndrome is a rare condition characterised by venous malformations usually on the extremities and dyschondroplasia resulting in enchondromas. Patients with Turner syndrome may have venous malformations of the intestine and feet.

Pathophysiology

The pathogenesis of venous malformations remains poorly understood. It is thought that the slow flow of blood through the malformed vessels results in coagulation [2] which can lead to acute pain and localised intravascular coagulopathy [3].

Pathology

The vascular channels of venous malformations are irregular, have narrow lumens lined with flattened endothelial cells and lack smooth muscle cells. The basement membranes are thin and there is no expression of vascular endothelial growth factor or basic fibroblast growth factor.

Table 101.21 Clinical features of venous malformations.

History	Usually visible at birth sometimes as a blue/purple mark
	May appear more obvious at a later age
	They grow with the child
Presentation	Typically soft blue compressible masses
	More prominent with exercise or when the affected area is held in a dependent position
	No palpable thrill
Clinical variants	*Common/sporadic:*
	Typical presentation as above
	Not genetically inherited
	Cutaneo-mucosal:
	Multiple small lesions affecting skin and oral mucosa
	Autosomal dominant
	Glomuvenous malformations (glomangioma):
	Small firmer blue papules or larger pebbly plaques
	Tender to touch
	Pathology: anomalous venous channels lined by cuboidal glomus cells
	Often familial (autosomal dominant) with variable clinical appearance
	Associated syndromes:
	Blue rubber bleb naevus syndrome:
	Multiple cutaneous and gastrointestinal venous malformations
	Gastrointestinal venous malformations may bleed and cause anaemia
	Small dark raised lesions on palms and soles
	Maffucci syndrome:
	Rare sporadic condition
	Venous malformations usually on the extremities
	Dyschondroplasia resulting in enchondromas
	Increased risk of malignancy
Differential diagnosis	Haemangiomas (venous malformations do *not* spontaneously regress or go through rapid proliferation phases)
Classification of severity	N/A
Complications and co-morbidities	Pain
	Thrombosis (phleboliths may form even under the age of 2 years)
	Bleeding
	Localised intravascular coagulopathy
	Cervico-facial lesions can cause airway obstruction, speech and dental abnormalities and sinus pericranii
	Limb lesions can be deep and involve muscle, bones and joints with functional difficulty, deformity and pain
Disease course and prognosis	Never regress spontaneously
	Prognosis depends on the lesions' depth and extent, and involvement of other organs

Table 101.22 Investigations for venous malformations.

Blood tests:	Full blood count
should be undertaken in extensive lesions and if there is bleeding	Coagulation screen including D-dimers – if raised then suggestive of localised intravascular coagulopathy
Plain X-ray	For phleboliths
Direct intralesional injection of contrast	Can outline the vascular anomaly with faint opacification of the draining veins and filling defects at the site of phleboliths
MRI	Most helpful for diagnosis and showing extent of lesion
	Characteristically lobulated margins and round signal voids (due to phleboliths). Contrast enhances lesional tissue and allows differentiation from unenhancing lymphatic malformations
CT scan	Phleboliths seen
	CT with contrast also demonstrates lesion enhancement
Doppler ultrasound	Confirms lesion is 'slow flow'
	Assess patency of deep venous system

Genetics

Most cases of venous malformations are sporadic. There have been familial cases of patients with multiple mucosal and cutaneous venous malformations. Genetic analysis has found a mutation in the gene that encodes for the tyrosine kinase domain of the endothelial cell receptor *TIE2* which has an important role in vascular proliferation and maturation [4].

Somatic mutations on the angiopoietin receptor gene *TEK* (which encodes *TIE2*) have been identified in the different subtypes of venous malformation including sporadic (mutation in 50% cases [5], cutaneomucosal venous malformations and blue rubber bleb naevus syndrome [6,7]. Glomulovenous malformations have been found to be related to mutations in the glomulin gene, which is important for vascular smooth muscle cell differentiation [8].

Environmental factors

Venous malformations do not regress but may expand with trauma, pregnancy and puberty.

Investigations

These are outlined in Table 101.22.

Management

The management of venous malformations depends on the size, depth and complications arising from the lesions. In many cases, the treatment is not curative but supportive. Patients with complex lesions are best managed by multidisciplinary teams in specialist centres. Small localised lesions can be managed with supportive care. Compression garments can prevent malformations on the limbs from growing and may reduce pain. Trunk and limb venous malformations are often difficult to manage.

Treatment modalities for venous malformations are outlined in Table 101.23. Often treatment modalities may be combined. For instance, for extensive cervico-facial lesions, the lesions may be treated with sclerotherapy, surgical excision and laser. The mammalian target of rapamycin (mTor) inhibitors are emerging as a possible therapeutic option. Sirolimus has shown some efficacy in a small group of patients who were refractory to other treatments, with improvement in pain, function and quality of life [9].

Resources

Patient resources

https://www.gosh.nhs.uk/conditions-and-treatments/conditions-we-treat/venous-malformations (last accessed March 2022).

Table 101.23 Treatment options for venous malformations.

Compression garments (supportive care)	In limb lesions these can do the following: • Reduce pain • Protect the overlying skin • Limit swelling • Decrease localised intravascular coagulation
Sclerotherapy (supportive care)	Usually under general anaesthetic by an interventional radiologist Multiple sessions are often needed Larger lesions usually injected with 95% ethanol Smaller lesions injected with 1% sodium tetradecyl sulphate
Laser Nd:YAG or endovenous laser	This is often used for mucosal lesions
Surgery	Clotting studies and D-dimers should be measured before surgery due to risk of disseminated intravascular coagulopathy during surgery; treat with low molecular weight heparin prior to surgery [10] Surgery may be curative in small lesions Or to debulk larger lesions
Analgesia	Lose dose aspirin Anti-inflammatory medications Low-molecular weight heparin if evidence of localised intravascular coagulopathy

Verrucous haemangioma

Synonyms and inclusions
• Verrucous venous malformation

Definition
This is a congenital vascular anomaly made up of a dermal and sub-cutaneous capillary vascular component with an overlying warty surface. There has been some debate as to whether it should be classified as a vascular neoplasm, though evidence supports the original view that it should be regarded as a vascular malformation [1].

Introduction
Verrucous haemangioma was first described in 1967 by Imperial and Hedwig [2], who reported 21 cases and distinguished it from other variants of angiokeratoma and considered it to be a vascular malformation.

Epidemiology [3–5]
Incidence and prevalence
This is a rare condition but the prevalence is unknown.

Age
It is usually noted at birth but can appear during the first 2 years.

Sex
The condition is equal in males and females.

Ethnicity
There is no known racial predilection.

Pathophysiology
The pathogenesis is not understood. The lesions show overlying epidermal hyperkeratosis, papillomatosis and irregular acanthosis with underlying dilated capillary vascular channels in the dermis and also often in the subcutis (Figure 101.22b, c). The vessels are organised in a diffuse or lobular pattern. Most studies show positive staining for GLUT-1 and WT-1, suggesting it is a type of vascular tumour [2]. However, a large study of 74 patients found most were negative for WT-1 staining, supporting the clinical view that these lesions behave like vascular malformations [5]. Recently, a somatic mutation in the *MAP3K3* gene has been associated with this condition. This gene is important for vascular development, again supporting the notion that these are vascular malformations [6].

Clinical features
History
Over 70% occur on the lower limb but lesions can involve the upper limb and more rarely the trunk; most are solitary.

Presentation
The lesions initially are non-keratotic, soft and bluish-red in colour. They are well-circumscribed linear vascular plaques and vary from a few centimetres to 25 cm in diameter. Over time the surface becomes hyperkeratotic and verrucous (Figure 101.22a). Over 50% are asymptomatic. However, the lesions may be painful and itchy.

Differential diagnosis
Angiokeratomas, circumscribed lymphangioma.

Complications and co-morbidities
They may ulcerate and become infected.

Disease course and prognosis
Unlike infantile haemangiomas they do not undergo spontaneous regression and grow in proportion to the child's growth.

Investigations
Skin biopsy and magnetic resonance imaging should be undertaken to confirm the diagnosis and to evaluate the extent of the lesion.

Management
Surgery is the treatment of choice. Most can be excised in a single procedure or in stages. However, if lesions are deep and excision is incomplete, recurrence may be a problem. Where excision is not possible, Nd:YAG laser for plaques and pulsed dye laser for patches can help improve the appearance and relieve symptoms. Recently, sirolimus has emerged as a potentially effective treatment option [7]. Intralesional bleomycin has also been reported as a potential successful treatment modality for localised lesions, although the duration of efficacy remains unknown [8].

Disorders associated with cutaneous vascular malformations

A number of disorders exist which are associated with cutaneous vascular malformations (Chapter 71). These were outlined in the

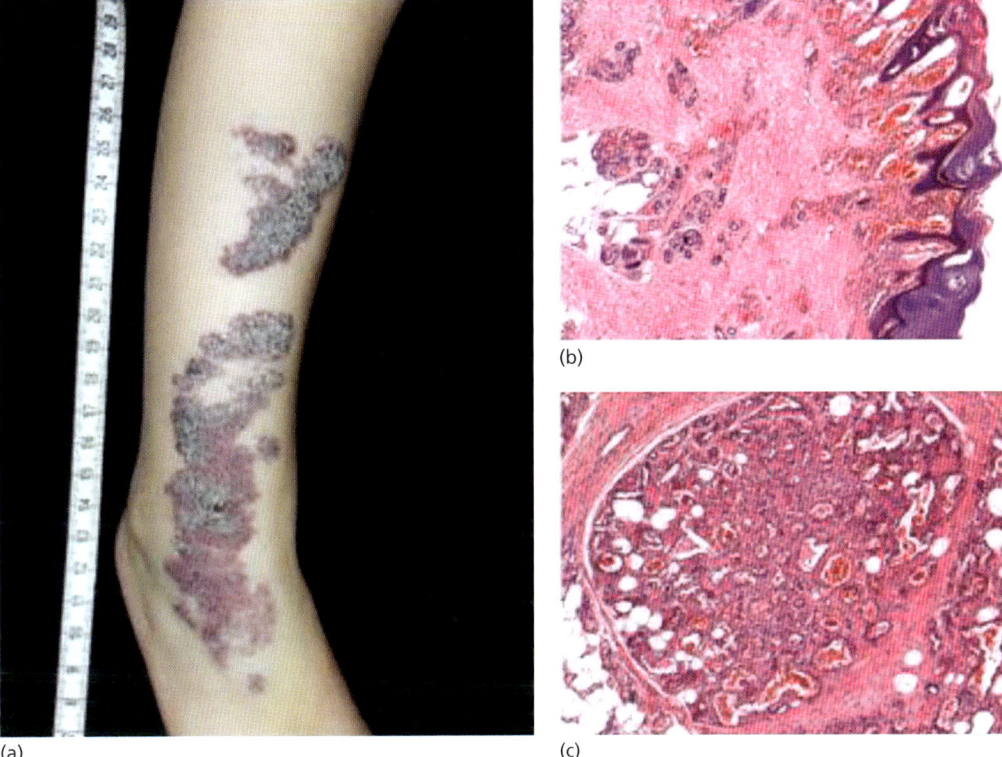

Figure 101.22 Verrucous haemangioma. (a) A linear congenital hyperkeratotic plaque on the lower leg and ankle of a child. (b) Dilated vessels in the superficial dermis and verrucous epidermal hyperplasia. (c) Lobules of capillaries in the subcutaneous tissue. Reproduced from Hoeger and Colmenero 2014 [1]. Reproduced with permission from John Wiley & Sons.

(a)

(b)

(c)

2018 classification of the International Society for the Study of Vascular Anomalies [1] (Table 101.24).

Klippel–Trenaunay syndrome

Definition
KTS is characterised by three features: (i) a capillary malformation (port-wine stain) of the skin associated with (ii) a soft tissue and bone overgrowth and hypertrophy in combination with (iii) varicose veins, with or without deep venous and lymphatic abnormalities. It can be diagnosed if only two of the three features are present.

Introduction and general description
KTS was first described in 1900, when Maurice Klippel and Paul Trenaunay reported two patients with a capillary malformation, varicosities and hypertrophy of soft tissue and bone in their lower limb [1]. In 1907, Frederick Parkes Weber independently reported several cases similar to those described by Klippel and Trenaunay, although his cases were caused by multiple congenital arteriovenous malformations [2]. KTS most commonly involves the lower limbs, followed by the arms, the trunk and rarely the head and neck. KTS is a congenital condition of unknown aetiology, the management of which is largely supportive [2].

Epidemiology
Incidence and prevalence
It is rare with an incidence <1 : 10 000.

Age
It is a congenital anomaly present at birth but clinically may present later in childhood.

Sex
There is no sex difference in the incidence of KTS.

Ethnicity
There is no known racial predilection.

Pathophysiology
The pathogenesis of KTS is not elucidated. Increased angiogenesis appears to be pivotal.

Pathology
The capillary malformations consist of ectatic capillaries with superficial dilated dermal venules corresponding to nodular lesions within the port-wine stains. When there are lymphatic malformations they appear to be due to lymphatic hypoplasia resulting in lymphatic macrocysts on the pelvis or trunk, and microcysts on the abdominal wall, gluteal region and/or limbs. The atypical varicose veins are persistent embryonic veins of the superficial venous system which lack valves and are long and tortuous. The deep venous system is abnormal in 25% of patients with KTS. Abnormalities include aneurysmal dilatations, duplications, hypoplasia, aplasia and external compression from anomalous vessels or fibrotic bands. Some patients get perianal and perirectal varicose veins, and suprapubic varicose veins can be a sign of atresia of the iliac vein.

Genetics
Most cases of KTS are sporadic. Many cases have shown postzygotic gain-of-function somatic mutations in the *PIK3CA* gene [3–5], which results in increased cell proliferation and angiogenesis. This has been similarly identified in syndromes such as MCAP

PART 9: VASCULAR DISORDERS

Table 101.24 Disorders associated with cutaneous vascular malformations.

Syndrome	Associated abnormalities
Klippel–Trenaunay syndrome	Capillary malformations, venous malformations, limb overgrowth, lymphatic malformations
Parkes Weber syndrome	Capillary malformations, arteriovenous fistulae, limb overgrowth
Servelle–Martorelle syndrome	Venous malformations of the limb, bone overgrowth
Sturge–Weber syndrome	Facial/leptomeningeal capillary malformations, eye anomalies, bone/soft tissue overgrowth
Limb capillary malformation and congenital non-progressive limb overgrowth	As described
Macro/microcephaly-capillary malformation syndrome	Macrocephaly/microcephaly, capillary malformation, asymmetry/overgrowth, developmental delay, syndactyly/polydactyly
Mafucci syndrome	Venous malformations, spindle cell haemangioma, echondroma
CLOVES syndrome	Lymphatic malformation, venous malformation, capillary malformation, arteriovenous fistulae, lipomatous overgrowth
Proteus syndrome	Capillary malformation, venous malformation, lymphatic malformation, asymmetrical somatic overgrowth
Bannayan–Riley –Ruvalcaba syndrome	Arteriovenous malformation, venous malformation, macrocephaly, lipomatous overgrowth
CLAPO syndrome	Lower lip capillary malformation, face/neck lymphatic malformation, asymmetry, partial/generalised overgrowth

CLAPO, Capillary vascular malformation of the lower lip, Lymphatic malformations of the head and neck, Asymmetry and Partial or generalized Overgrowth; CLOVES, Congenital Lipomatous asymmetric Overgrowth, Vascular malformations, Epidermal naevi and Skeletal and spinal abnormalities.

(megalencephaly capillary malformation syndrome) and CLOVES (congenital lipomatous asymmetric overgrowth, vascular malformations, epidermal naevi and skeletal and spinal abnormalities), suggesting that these are all in a group of *PIK3A*-related overgrowth spectrum disorders.

There have also been reports of a defect in the angiogenic factor VG5Q [6], *RASA1* mutations [7] and a *de novo* supernumerary ring chromosome 18 in KTS patients [8]. A case report of KTS in a monozygotic twin with an unaffected twin suggests the possibility of paradominant inheritance, although this remains rare [9].

Clinical features (Figure 101.23)
The clinical features are described in Table 101.25.

Differential diagnosis
- Diffuse capillary malformation with overgrowth (DCMO) – these cases do not have lymphatic involvement and overgrowth tends to be proportionate rather than progressive [10].
- Other PIK3A-related overgrowth spectrum disorders.
- Parkes Weber syndrome.

Investigations
KTS is often diagnosed based on the history and examination alone. Physical examination should include auscultation and palpation of the involved area to assess for the presence of an arteriovenous

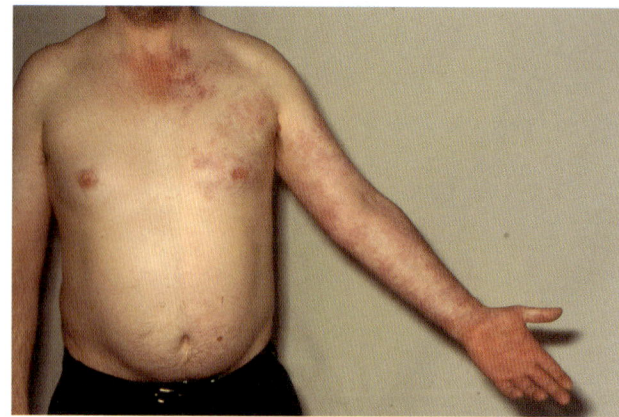

(a)

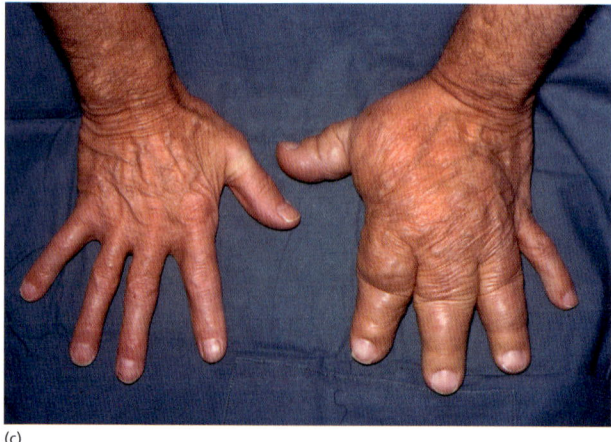

(b)

(c)

Figure 101.23 Klippel–Trenaunay syndrome: (a) with capillary/venular malformation; (b,c) abnormal veins and soft-tissue overgrowth.

Table 101.25 Clinical features of Klippel–Trenaunay syndrome (KTS).

History	Capillary/venular malformation (port-wine stain) in 98% of cases; usually present at birth; when deep can cause visceral haemorrhage
	Abnormal veins in 72% cases; often not visible until the child is walking; can cause pain, ulceration, thrombosis
	Hypertrophy in 67% cases; usually present at birth, 63% have all three features, and 37% have two out of the three features
Presentation	Capillary/venular malformation (port-wine stain) • Pink or reddish stain with linear borders, may darken with age to purple • 10% are nodular • Does not cross the midline • May be deep and involve underlying organs Venous abnormalities • Dilated tortuous veins • Can lead to skin ulcers and scarring if deep venous system involved Hypertrophy • Increase in limb girth and/or length • Bony and soft-tissue enlargement • May have hand and feet abnormalities (macrodactyly, syndactyly, ectodactyly, clinodactyly and camptodactyly) Lymphoedema
Clinical variants [2]	Simple KTS • Blotchy or segmental port-wine stain • Venous malformations and hypertrophy Complex KTS • Geographic port-wine stain • Venous malformations and hypertrophy • Higher risk of lymphatic involvement • Increased risk of complications
Differential diagnosis	Proteus syndrome Bannayan–Riley–Ruvalcaba syndrome Maffucci syndrome Parkes Weber syndrome Diffuse capillary malformation with overgrowth (DCMO) Other *PIK3A*-related overgrowth spectrum disorders
Complications and co-morbidities	Skin • Stasis dermatitis • Ulcers • Secondary infection Veins • Thrombosis • Thrombophlebitis • Haemorrhage • Pulmonary emboli Hypertrophy of a limb • May lead to subsequent vertebral scoliosis • Gait problems • Impaired function • Premature onset of degenerative joint disease Lymphoedema Pain – multifactorial aetiology • Rarer complications depend on the site and depth of the lesions • Genitourinary haemorrhage • Gastrointestinal haemorrhage • Haemothorax • Pulmonary emboli secondary to venous thrombosis • Heart failure • Central nervous system involvement with haemorrhage, infection, hemimegalencephaly, hydrocephalus, atrophy, epilepsy
Disease course and prognosis	Risks of thrombosis and venous complications tend to increase with age

malformation to rule out Parkes Weber syndrome. Duplex ultrasound scanning is the study of choice to evaluate for superficial and deep venous anomalies and can also be used in differentiating vascular tumours from vascular malformations and arteriovenous fistulae. MRI scans are effective for visualising the extent of tissue overgrowth of lesions and infiltration of deeper tissues. X-rays may show increased thickness or abnormal density of the affected soft tissue as well as phleboliths. Venograms may be required to delineate the venous abnormality and to exclude deep-vein agenesis. Blood tests, including full blood count, D-dimer and coagulation screen, should be performed as a baseline, prior to surgery and during pregnancy, due to the higher risk of thromboembolism [11]. Genomic testing on skin biopsy is not done routinely but can be helpful if there is diagnostic uncertainty [12].

Management

The treatment of KTS is conservative and aimed at relieving the symptoms and preventing the complications of the condition. Patients are often managed best by a multidisciplinary team consisting of the following specialists: paediatricians, dermatologists, vascular surgeons, orthopaedic surgeons, interventional radiologists and pain specialists. The treatment modalities for KTS are outlined in Table 101.26.

Table 101.26 Management of Klippel–Trenaunay syndrome (KTS).

Compression garments (not helpful in patients with a hypoplastic deep venous system)	To prevent/treat: • Chronic venous insufficiency • Lymphoedema • Recurrent cellulitis/bleeding
Orthotics	To manage asymmetry in the limbs
Orthopaedics	• For small difference in limb length heel inserts can be used • Larger differences may need osteotomy, epiphysiodesis, epiphyseal stapling
Avoidance of the oral contraceptive pill	Females with KTS should not use the oral contraceptive pill
Anticoagulation	Consider anticoagulation prophylaxis for patients prior to surgical procedures/long haul flights, etc.
Pain management	Pain can be a difficult symptom to relieve and referral to a pain clinic should be considered
Sirolimus	Recently shown to have modest benefit in reducing overgrowth, however associated with significant side effect profile [13]
Laser	• To treat the capillary malformation (port-wine stain) use pulsed dye laser for cosmesis • For treating ulceration • To treat the greater saphenous vein to manage varicosities, an endovenous laser can be used
Surgery	Treatment of venous malformations and varicosities by venous stripping, ligation, excision and sclerotherapy. This therapy is controversial because there is a high risk of complications and 90% chance of recurrence: • It should only be undertaken if the deep system is normal or shows mild to moderate reflux • It may help heaviness and recurrent bleeding Amputation is a last resort for intractable bleeding, pain or ulceration

PART 9: VASCULAR DISORDERS

Resources

Patient resources

https://www.gosh.nhs.uk/conditions-and-treatments/conditions-we-treat/
    klippel-trenaunay-syndrome
Patient support group: https://k-t.org
(All last accessed March 2022.)

Parkes Weber syndrome

Definition
This syndrome was first described by Sir Frederick Parkes Weber in 1907. It is a combined vascular malformation, similar to KTS, characterised by an arteriovenous fistula with varicosities and hypertrophy of the affected extremity. It differs from KTS because of the presence of the arteriovenous fistula and the absence of the following associations: an overlying vascular naevus, a marginal vein malformation and lymphatic malformations. The musculoskeletal involvement is often less prominent than in KTS [1].

Epidemiology
Incidence and prevalence
This is a rare condition but the prevalence is unknown.

Age
It is present from birth.

Sex
The condition is equal in males and females.

Ethnicity
There is no known racial predilection.

Pathophysiology
The pathogenesis is not fully understood. The pathology of the arteriovenous malformation is described under arteriovenous malformations above.

Genetics
Most cases are sporadic. A mutation in the gene *RASA1* has been identified on chromosome 5q in families with capillary malformations associated with arteriovenous malformations [2].

Clinical features
These are described in Table 101.27

History
Over 70% occur on the lower limb, but Parkes Weber syndrome can involve the upper limb and the head and neck. The tissue overgrowth leads to limb enlargement that continues past puberty and gets progressively worse. There is frequently bone involvement rather than just soft tissue overgrowth. The arteriovenous malformation may not appear until puberty or after trauma.

Presentation
An obvious pulsatile swelling may be visible with discoloration of the overlying skin and large veins radiating from it. The overlying skin feels warm; there are prominent vessels with a possible

Table 101.27 Clinical features of Parkes Weber syndrome.

Clinical features	Large capillary malformation on extremity
	Arteriovenous fistula with varicosities
	Hypertrophy of bone and soft tissue of the affected extremity
History	Present from birth
	Over 70% occur on lower limb, but can involve upper limb/head/neck
	Limb enlargement continues beyond puberty and gets progressively worse
	Frequent bone involvement
	Arteriovenous malformation may not appear until puberty or after trauma
Presentation	Pulsatile swelling may be visible with discoloration of overlying skin and large radiating veins
	Overlying skin feels warm
	Prominent vessels with possible palpable thrill
	Machinery murmur on auscultation
	Hypertrophy and asymmetry of affected extremity
	Musculoskeletal involvement often less prominent than in Klippel–Trenaunay syndrome
Clinical variants	Capillary malformation – arteriovenous malformation
	CLOVES syndrome
Differential diagnosis	Klippel–Trenaunay syndrome
	Proteus syndrome
Complications and co-morbidities	Main complications due to arteriovenous fistula: • Tissue ischaemia • Ulceration • Cellulitis • Blood loss and anaemia due to bleeding • High output cardiac failure
Disease course and prognosis	Depends on type, location and severity of the arteriovenous malformation

CLOVES, Congenital Lipomatous asymmetric Overgrowth, Vascular malformations, Epidermal naevi and Skeletal and spinal abnormalities.

palpable thrill. Auscultation of the lesion should detect a machinery murmur. There may be obvious asymmetry of the affected limbs.

Clinical variants

- Capillary malformation – arteriovenous malformation, a new clinical and genetic disorder caused by *RASA1* mutations [2].
- CLOVES syndrome (congenital lipomatous overgrowth, vascular malformations, epidermal naevi and scoliosis, seizures and spinal and skeletal abnormalities) [3].

Differential diagnosis

- Klippel–Trenaunay syndrome.
- Proteus syndrome.

Classification of severity
The classification of the severity of arteriovenous malformations is described in Table 101.16.

Complications and co-morbidities
The main risks are complications of the arteriovenous fistula such as tissue ischaemia and high output cardiac failure.

Disease course and prognosis

This is dependent on type, location and severity of the arteriovenous malformation.

Investigations

The capillary malformation in Parkes Weber syndrome cannot be distinguished clinically from that in KTS. Imaging with ultrasound, MRI and MRA are helpful in distinguishing the two conditions.

To confirm the diagnosis and monitor the response to treatment. Ultrasound with colour Doppler examination which shows low-resistance, high-velocity arterial flow, with high diastolic flux, and pulsatile venous flow below the baseline and arteriovenous shunting within tortuous vessels.

To evaluate the extent of the arteriovenous malformation. MRI and MRA demonstrate a collection of vascular flow voids which are the fast-flow vessels that do not enhance with contrast (no tumour aspect). The arteriovenous malformation and its network can be delineated.

Management

A multidisciplinary approach is essential with specialist vascular surgeons, invasive radiologists and paediatricians where appropriate. Management is challenging, and treatment is frequently palliative. Sclerotherapy, embolisation and surgery are all options. Orthotics and compression garments may help with limb involvement.

VENOUS DISORDERS

Anatomy [1–7]

Most veins contain semi-lunar valves; these are usually in pairs, but some veins only contain one valve leaflet and sometimes three (tricuspid) valve leaflets are present. These valves are lined by endothelium and are found especially in the smaller veins and at the junction of these veins with larger branches. They prevent the reflux of blood and are particularly important in the leg, where their integrity, and that of the calf muscle pump (the venous heart), counters the gravitational hydrostatic pressure.

There are three venous systems: the deep veins, the superficial veins and the perforating veins (or perforators). The perforating veins are numerous and inconstant, and connect the other two systems. During muscular activity, blood is directed from the superficial to the deep system, up from the foot to the thigh and thence to the abdomen, before venous blood returns towards the heart. Bicuspid valves are found in all three systems. The smallest veins contain valves which lie at the dermal subcutaneous junctions [4] and the valves are extremely variable. Valves may become damaged, thickened or degenerate with age [5]. Thrombosis also causes valvular destruction; the re-canalised post-thrombotic vein is valveless, anatomically distorted and functionally inefficient [5]. The most important perforating veins are considered to be on the medial side of the calf. Incompetence of the valves in these veins has been thought to be important in the causation of venous ulceration [5].

The superficial venous system of the leg begins from the veins on the dorsum of the foot, which join the greater saphenous vein (GSV) (originally called the long saphenous vein) and the short saphenous vein (SSV). They form a dorsal arch, which connects the territory of the SSV with that of the GSV. On the plantar side of the foot, the same venous network joins to a plantar venous arch that also joins both saphenous veins [6,7].

Physiology: the venous macrocirculation [1,2]

Veins act as the capacitance vessels of the circulation. The 'venous return' is the blood returning to the heart via the great veins. Venous return from the lower limbs is achieved by the pumping action of the foot and calf muscles, associated with competent valves that prevent backflow [1].

The venous system of the legs contains a volume of 300–350 mL in a healthy standing subject. The venous wall contracts in response to filling, and its function is called 'venous tone'. This acts as counter-pressure and automatically changes to attempt to maintain venous pressure at a constant level. The superficial veins drain through the communicating (perforating) veins into the deep system, and only 10% of the venous blood flow from the lower limb passes through the saphenofemoral junction (SFJ).

The deep veins are compressed by each muscle contraction, shifting the blood column towards the heart against the pressure of gravity. The venous valves prevent backflow during muscle relaxation. This mechanism is the 'calf muscle pump'. Other muscle groups such as those of the foot also compress veins and aid venous return, but the calf muscle pump is the most important muscle pump of the leg.

Venous thrombosis

Deep-vein thrombosis

Definition

A deep-vein thrombosis (DVT) is a blood clot that forms within the deep veins usually of the leg, but can occur in the veins of the arms [1] and in the mesenteric and cerebral veins.

Introduction and general description

Deep-vein thrombosis is a common and important disease. It is part of the venous thromboembolism disorders which represent the third most common cause of death from cardiovascular disease after heart attacks and stroke [2]. Even in patients who do not get pulmonary emboli, recurrent thrombosis and 'post-thrombotic syndrome' are a major cause of morbidity.

Epidemiology

Incidence and prevalence

Deep-vein thrombosis and pulmonary emboli are common and often 'silent' and thus go undiagnosed or are only picked up at post-mortem. Therefore, their incidence and prevalence is often underestimated. It is thought that there are approximately 900 000 cases of DVT in the USA each year, although the precise numbers remain unknown. Between 60 000 and 100 000 Americans die of venous thromboembolism each year. In the UK, 1–2 per 1000 people have venous thrombosis each year. A third of those with DVT have ongoing complications as a result [3].

Age

Deep-vein thrombosis is rare in children and the risk increases with age, most occurring in the over 40s.

Sex

There is no consensus about whether there is a sex bias in the incidence of DVT, although some reports suggest that the incidence is higher in men [4].

Ethnicity

There is evidence from the USA that there is an increased incidence of DVT and an increased risk of complications in African American and white people when compared with Hispanic and Asian people [5,6].

Associated diseases

The risk factors for DVT are listed in Table 101.28. In hospital the most commonly associated conditions are malignancy, congestive heart failure, obstructive airways disease and patients undergoing surgery.

Pathophysiology

Pathology

In 1856, Virchow postulated that the main causes of thrombus formation were damage to the vessel wall, alterations in blood flow and hypercoagulability. This is called 'Virchow's triad' and is still valid today.

Maintenance of the fluidity and circulation of the blood and its ability to thrombose are essential for the maintenance of life and are governed by extremely complex homeostatic mechanisms. Thrombosis is a protective mechanism which prevents loss of blood and seals off damaged blood vessels. Fibrinolysis counteracts or stabilises the thrombosis. The triggers of venous thrombosis are frequently multifactorial, with the different parts of the Virchow triad contributing in varying degrees in each patient, but all resulting in early thrombus interaction with the endothelium. This then stimulates local cytokine production and causes leukocyte adhesion to the endothelium, both of which promote venous thrombosis. Depending on the relative balance between the coagulation and thrombolytic pathways, thrombus propagation occurs.

DVT is commonest in the lower limb below the knee and starts at low-flow sites, such as the soleal sinuses, behind venous valve pockets.

Table 101.28 Risk factors for deep-vein thrombosis (DVT).

Reduced blood flow	Immobility (bed rest, general anaesthesia, operations, stroke, long haul flights)
Increased venous pressure	Mechanical compression or functional impairment leading to reduced flow in the veins (neoplasm, pregnancy, stenosis, or congenital anomaly which increases outflow resistance)
Mechanical injury to the vein	Trauma, surgery, peripherally inserted venous catheters
	Previous DVT
	Intravenous drug abuse
Increased blood viscosity	Polycythaemia
	Thrombocytosis
	Dehydration

Increased risk of coagulation

Genetic	Deficiencies in protein C, S or antithrombin III, factor V Leiden
Acquired	Cancer
	Sepsis
	Myocardial infarction
	Heart failure
	Vasculitis, systemic lupus erythematosus and lupus anticoagulant
	Inflammatory bowel disease
	Nephrotic syndrome
	Burns
	Oral oestrogens
	Smoking
	Hypertension
	Diabetes
Constitutional factors	Obesity
	Pregnancy
	Increasing age

Causes

The risk factors for DVT are shown in Table 101.28. The most important ones are previous DVT (up to 25% of patients give a previous history of a DVT), active cancer, being postoperative and immobilisation. There is now an increasing understanding that the risk factors for DVT often overlap with those of atherothrombosis and that there is a common pathophysiology that includes inflammation, hypercoagulability and endothelial injury [2].

Clinical features

These are outlined in Table 101.29. Deep-vein thrombosis may be 'silent' in 5% of cases, at times making the diagnosis challenging as many patients do not have the classical signs or symptoms; and some of those with 'classical' features do not have DVT when investigated.

Investigations

These are outlined clearly in the National Institute for Health and Care Excellence (NICE) guidelines with a helpful algorithm [7]. Investigations that are performed are D-dimers (very sensitive but not very specific) and proximal leg vein ultrasound which when positive indicates that the patient should be treated as having a DVT (Table 101.30).

Deciding how to investigate is determined by the risk of DVT. The first step is to assess the clinical probability of a DVT using the Wells scoring system (Table 101.31). For patients with a score of 0–1 the

Table 101.29 Clinical features of deep-vein thrombosis (DVT).

History	Pain (50% of patients)
	Redness
	Swelling (70% of patients)
	Usually of the lower limb but can occur in the arms
Examination	Limb oedema may be unilateral or bilateral if the thrombus is extending to pelvic veins
	Red and hot skin, with dilated veins
	Tenderness
	Pain on dorsiflexion of the foot (the Homans sign)
Clinical variants	In upper limb DVTs
	• 80% have swelling
	• 30% have pain
	• Only 15% have redness
Differential diagnosis	Cellulitis
	Post-thrombotic syndrome (especially venous eczema and lipodermatosclerosis)
	Ruptured Baker cyst
	Trauma
	Superficial thrombophlebitis
	Peripheral oedema, heart failure, cirrhosis, nephrotic syndrome
	Venous or lymphatic obstruction
	Arteriovenous fistula and congenital vascular abnormalities
	Vasculitis
Classification	*Provoked*
	Due to acquired states (surgery, oral contraceptives, trauma, immobility, obesity, cancer)
	Unprovoked
	Due to idiopathic or endogenous reasons
	More likely to suffer recurrence if anticoagulation is discontinued
	Proximal (above the knee: affecting the femoral or iliofemoral veins)
	Much more likely to lead to complications such as pulmonary emboli
	Distal (below the knee)
Complications and co-morbidities	Pulmonary emboli (paradoxical emboli if an atrioseptal defect is present)
	Post-thrombotic syndrome
Disease course and prognosis	Many DVTs will resolve with no complications
	Post-thrombotic syndrome [6] occurs in 43% cases 2 years post-DVT (30% mild, 10% moderate, 3% severe)
	Risk of recurrence of DVT is high (up to 25%)
	Death occurs in approximately 6% of DVT cases and 12% of pulmonary embolism cases within 1 month of diagnosis
	Early mortality after venous thromboembolism is strongly associated with presentation as pulmonary embolism, advanced age, cancer and underlying cardiovascular disease [6]

Table 101.30 Investigations for deep-vein thrombosis (DVT).

D-dimers	These are specific cross-linked products of fibrin degradation and are raised in patients with venous thromboembolism
	Sensitivity is high but specificity poor
Compression duplex ultrasound	Sensitivity 97% for proximal and 73% for distal vein thrombosis compared with phlebography
	Non-invasive, simple, easy to repeat, relatively inexpensive and free of complications
	Two main disadvantages:
	• Calf vein thrombosis can be missed, especially when the examination is limited to the popliteal and femoral veins
	• Small isolated thrombi in the iliac and superficial femoral veins or within the adductor canal can be difficult to detect and are therefore easily overlooked [8]
Radiology	Magnetic resonance venography and CT venography may be useful adjuncts but are expensive and not always available
General investigations	Chest X-ray, routine blood tests (full blood count, liver function tests, urea and electrolytes), urinalysis
If DVT is 'unprovoked' in patients over the age of 40	Mammogram and abdominal pelvic CT scan to look for malignancy
	Antiphospholipid antibodies in patients who have had unprovoked DVT if stopping anticoagulation treatment is planned
	Test for hereditary thrombophilia in patients who have had unprovoked DVT and who have a first-degree relative who has had DVT, if stopping anticoagulation treatment is planned

Table 101.31 Two-level deep-vein thrombosis (DVT) Wells score. DVT is likely with a score of 2 or more.

Clinical feature	Points
Active cancer (treatment ongoing, within 6 months, or palliative)	1
Paralysis, paresis or recent plaster immobilisation of the lower extremities	1
Recently bedridden for 3 days or more or major surgery within 12 weeks requiring general or regional anaesthesia	1
Localised tenderness along the distribution of the deep venous system	1
Entire leg swollen	1
Calf swelling at least 3 cm larger than asymptomatic side	1
Pitting oedema confined to the symptomatic leg	1
Collateral superficial veins (non-varicose)	1
Previously documented DVT	1
An alternative diagnosis is at least as likely as DVT	−2

clinical probability is low, but for those with 2 or above the clinical probability is high.

If a patient *scores 2 or above,* a proximal leg vein ultrasound scan should be carried out within 4 hours of being requested and, if the result is negative, a D-dimer test should be undertaken. If imaging is not possible within 4 hours, a D-dimer test should be undertaken and an interim 24-hour dose of anticoagulation should be given. Then a proximal leg vein ultrasound scan should be carried out within 24 hours of being requested.

In the case of a positive D-dimer test and a negative proximal leg vein ultrasound scan, anticoagulation should be stopped, and the proximal leg vein ultrasound scan should be repeated 6–8 days later for all patients. If the patient *does not score 2* on the DVT Wells score but the D-dimer test is positive, the patient should have a proximal leg vein ultrasound scan carried out within 4 hours of being requested. Again, if this is not possible, the patient should receive an interim 24-hour dose of anticoagulation and a proximal leg vein ultrasound scan should then be carried out within 24 hours of being requested.

In all patients diagnosed with DVT, treat as if there is a positive proximal leg vein ultrasound scan.

Management

The aims of treatment of DVT are to prevent pulmonary embolism, reduce morbidity and prevent or minimise the risk of developing

PART 9: VASCULAR DISORDERS

Table 101.32 Treatment of proximal deep-vein thrombosis (DVT).

Anticoagulation	Anticoagulation for at least 3 months, taking into account co-morbidities/contraindications/patient preference
	Apixaban or rivaroxaban first line
	If neither apixaban or rivaroxaban suitable, consider LMWH for at least 5 days prior to dabigatran/edoxaban. Alternative is LMHW with vitamin K antagonist for at least 5 days, until INR >2 for 24 h (unfractionated heparin for patients with renal failure and increased risk of bleeding)
	In patients with cancer consider anticoagulation for 3–6 months
	In patients with unprovoked DVT consider anticoagulation beyond 3 months [12]
Thrombolysis	If there is:
	• Symptomatic iliofemoral DVT
	• Symptoms of <14 days duration
	• Good functional status
	• Life expectancy of 1 year or more
	• Low risk of bleeding
Inferior vena cava filters	If anticoagulation is contraindicated
	If emboli are occurring despite adequate anticoagulation

INR, international normalised ratio; LMWH, low molecular weight heparin.

the post-thrombotic syndrome. The cornerstone of treatment is anticoagulation. NICE guidelines only recommend treating proximal DVT (*not* distal) and those with pulmonary emboli. In each patient, the risks of anticoagulation need to be weighed against the benefits. The current guidelines recommend treatment for 3 months following diagnosis of DVT. The direct oral anticoagulants rivaroxaban and apixaban are now first line. However, low molecular weight heparin (LMWH) and unfractionated heparin are still used based on the patient's comorbidities (Table 101.32).

The greatest area of improved clinical care has been in identifying those at increased risk of thromboembolism in hospital and providing thromboembolism prophylaxis. This includes preventing dehydration, improving mobilisation, prescribing anti-embolic stockings, using intermittent pneumatic compression in stroke patients. and pharmacological prophylaxis with either LMWH or fondaparinux sodium unfractionated heparin [9]. In the case of elective hip or knee surgery, NICE guidelines recommend either venous thromboembolism prophylaxis with LMWH followed by aspirin, LMWH with anti-embolic stockings, or a direct oral anticoagulant such as rivaroxaban, apixaban or dabigatran [10]. Treatment of proximal DVT is outlined in Table 101.32.

Resources

Further information

https://www.nice.org.uk/guidance/ng158https://www.nice.org.uk/guidance/ng89 (last accessed March 2022).

Superficial venous thrombosis

Definition and nomenclature

This is common condition where there is the formation of a thrombus in the veins near the surface of the skin and is usually associated with inflammation of the walls of the vein.

Introduction and general description
Superficial venous thrombosis is an uncomfortable but self-limiting condition. It is often seen on the lower leg associated with varicose veins and in hospitals at the sites of intravenous cannulae. However, it can be associated with deep thrombosis and the serious consequences of venous thromboembolism.

Epidemiology
Incidence and prevalence
Superficial venous thrombosis is a common condition. The actual prevalence and incidence is unknown. However, it is reported to be more common than deep-vein thrombosis [1]. Up to 25–35% of all hospitalised patients are thought to experience superficial phlebitis at the site of venous cannulae [2].

Age
The mean age of onset is 60 [3].

Sex
It is commoner in females (55–70% occurring in women).

Ethnicity
There is no known racial predilection.

Associated diseases
Migratory thrombophlebitis may be associated with an underlying carcinoma (such as pancreatic cancer), states of hypercoagulability [4], thromboangiitis obliterans, and Behçet disease. Concurrent DVT is reported to be present in up to 53% of cases and the incidence of concurrent PE is reported to range between 1% and 33% [5].

Pathophysiology
Pathology
The pathogenesis of superficial venous thrombosis is similar to that of DVT, although trauma to the vein is thought to be the predominant trigger in the Virchow triad (stasis, increased coagulability and vessel wall injury). Several studies have described an association between superficial venous thrombosis and venous thromboembolism. Superficial venous thrombosis located in the main trunk of the saphenous vein has the strongest association with venous thromboembolism [3,6]. Superficial venous thrombosis usually develops in the lower limbs. In 60–80% of cases, the great saphenous vein system is involved, and in 10–20% the small saphenous vein system [7]. The main cause of superficial venous thrombosis of the lower limbs is varicose veins, which are present in 70% of cases [8]. The main cause of superficial venous thrombosis in the upper limb is iatrogenic, for example intravenous catheters or infusion of drugs such as chemotherapy or heroin. Mondor disease may also be a form of superficial venous thrombosis.

Table 101.33 Clinical features of superficial venous thrombosis (Figure 101.24).

History	Gradual onset of localised tenderness
	Redness along the path of a superficial vein
	May have had intravenous catheter at the site
	May have varicose veins
Examination	Overlying skin may be red and hot
	Oedema may be present
	A tender firm cord extending along the vein on palpation
	If it occurs within varicose veins there may be bleeding
	Low grade fever sometimes present
Clinical variants	Migratory thrombophlebitis
	Thrombophlebitis of the superficial veins of the breast and anterior chest wall (Mondor disease)
Differential diagnosis	Cellulitis
	Panniculitis
	Insect bites
	DVT
	Lymphangitis
	Neuritis
	Chronic venous insufficiency
	Baker's cyst
	Haematoma
Complications and co-morbidities	Extension into the deep venous system (DVT and pulmonary embolism)
	If thrombosed veins do not re-canalise, patient can develop post-thrombotic syndrome
	Post-inflammatory hyperpigmentation over the affected vein
	Persistent firm subcutaneous nodule at the site
	Secondary infection possibly leading to septic emboli, abscesses and septicaemia
Disease course and prognosis	Prognosis is usually good in uncomplicated disease and symptoms usually resolve within 3–4 weeks
	Recurrence is a risk with superficial venous thrombosis in association with varicose veins

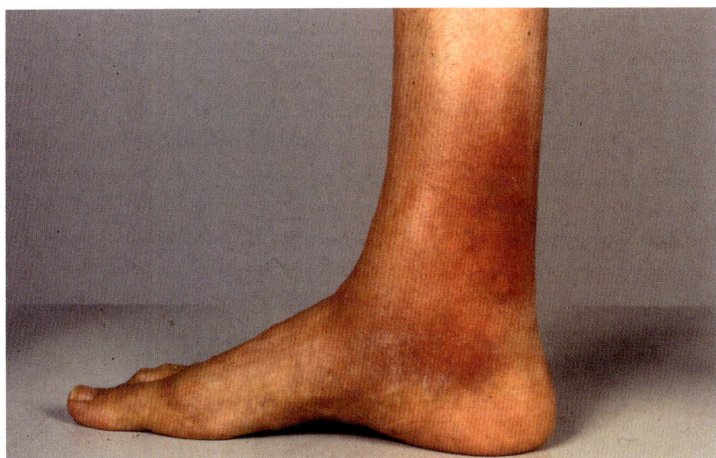

Figure 101.24 Superficial venous thrombosis.

Table 101.34 Investigations for superficial venous thrombosis.

Imaging To detect the location and extent of the superficial venous thrombosis and to exclude deep-vein thrombosis (DVT)	Duplex and compression ultrasonography (up to 53% may have proximal DVTs, although the superficial venous thrombosis will be contiguous with the proximal DVT in less than 50% of cases) [9]
Consider tests for underlying malignancy If there is migratory thrombophlebitis	Blood tumour markers, chest X-ray and CT abdomen/pelvis, mammogram in females
Consider tests for underlying coagulopathy If there is no obvious trigger	Factor V Leiden, protein C and S deficiency, antithrombin III deficiency, antiphospholipid antibodies

Predisposing factors

The risk factors are similar to those for DVT [6] (see Table 101.28). Venous stasis, which can be caused by DVT, as well as due to varicose veins and venous excision/ablation amongst others, also predisposes to the condition.

Clinical features

The clinical features of superficial venous thrombosis are outlined in Table 101.33.

Investigations

The aims of the investigations are to establish the extent of the thrombosis and to exclude involvement of the deep venous system. In patients without obvious risk factors for superficial venous thrombosis, studies to exclude hypercoagulability should be considered. In migratory thrombophlebitis, investigations to exclude an underlying internal malignancy should be considered. These are outlined in Table 101.34.

Management

The treatment of superficial venous thrombosis is outlined in Table 101.35. Initial treatment is supportive and aims to reduce the change of propagation of thrombus. The limb should be elevated, non-steroidal anti-inflammatory drugs (NSAIDS) given, compression therapy considered, and the patient encouraged to remain ambulatory.

Resources

Patient resources

https://patient.info/heart-health/varicose-veins-leaflet/superficial-thrombophlebitis (last accessed March 2022).

Thrombophlebitis migrans [1–4]

Synonyms and inclusions
- Migratory superficial thrombophlebitis
- Trousseau syndrome

Definition

This is a form of superficial venous thrombosis which is recurrent and diffuse affecting the large and small veins throughout the body.

Introduction and general description

This is a rare disorder which is important because it is often associated with underlying disease such as internal malignancy (Trousseau syndrome), Behçet disease and Buerger disease.

Epidemiology
Incidence and prevalence

This is not known but it is rare. In one study of 1500 cases of thrombophlebitis, 31 of 77 occurring in association with malignancy were

Table 101.35 Treatment of superficial venous thrombosis of the lower limb.

Medication	**Anticoagulation**
	Should be considered if there is increased risk of venous thromboembolism; prophylactic or treatment dosing dependent on location, extent of thrombosis and individual patient risk
	Non-steroidal anti-inflammatory drugs
	Similar in efficacy to low molecular weight heparin but easier to administer [3]; effective in reducing pain associated with inflammation
	Antibiotics: only of help in suppurative thrombophlebitis
Surgery	**Excision and ligation**
	When a thrombus is found in or near the saphenofemoral junction or saphenopopliteal junction (especially if it extends as free-floating thrombus extending into the common femoral vein or popliteal veins) it should be treated by surgical removal, combined with ligation and stripping and patient started on anticoagulation
	Sclerotherapy and stripping of any varicose veins should only be performed some months after the acute superficial venous thrombosis has settled
	Puncture and evacuation
	The thrombus can be squeezed out of the vein through a needle puncture
Compression hosiery or bandages	Used as an adjunct to medical and surgical treatments

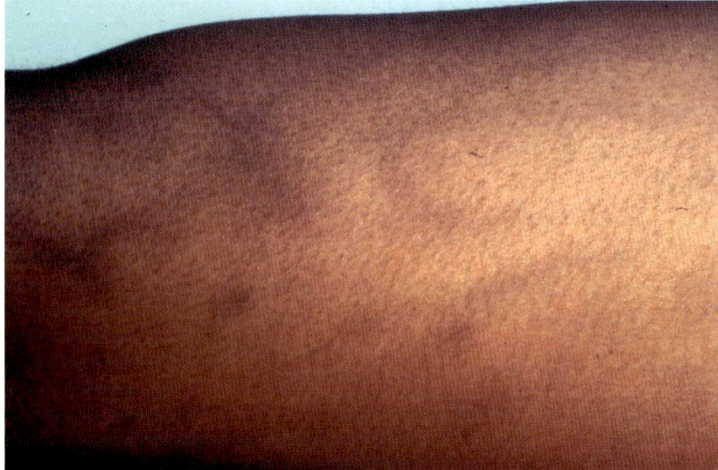

Figure 101.25 Thrombophlebitis migrans.

of a migratory type [1]. In this study, carcinomas of the lung and pancreas were the most common sites for the primary tumours, although carcinomas of the breast, colon and stomach were also reported [1]. Other associated diseases are Behçet (between 2% and 20% of all cases; Chapter 48) and Buerger disease (one study found thrombophlebitis migrans in up to 65.4% of 86 patients [2]). There is no known gender or racial predilection.

Pathophysiology
This is not fully understood. As with superficial venous thrombosis, the mechanism is thought to be within the Virchow triad (stasis, increased coagulability and vessel wall injury). In the thrombophlebitis migrans associated with malignancy, some have suggested that there is a state of chronic disseminated intravascular coagulation [3,4].

Clinical features
History
Patients develop crops of painful red lumps and streaks in the skin. These may resolve and then new ones develop. The lesions appear on the legs, arms, abdominal wall and flanks.

Presentation (Figure 101.25)
The lesions are hot and tender and can be linear or oval subcutaneous lumps or streaks. The overlying skin usually remains intact.

Differential diagnosis
This is wide as there are no pathognomonic features and includes cellulitis, panniculitis, DVT and states with increased coagulability.

Investigations
Ultrasound to confirm the diagnosis, clotting studies and tests to look for an underlying malignancy are all advised. CT scanning, ultrasound, MRI and positron emission tomographic (PET) scans of the abdomen may be necessary to pick up a pancreatic carcinoma.

Management
Treatment is generally conservative, and patients should be treated with adequate anticoagulation. Lowering triglycerides may be advisable and exercise is good for prophylaxis. Medical elastic compression stockings or bandages may alleviate symptoms. In Behçet disease, immunosuppressive medication is given (Chapter 48)

Mondor disease

Definition
This is a form of superficial venous thrombosis in the chest wall and affects veins that include the lateral thoracic vein, the superior epigastric vein and the thoracoepigastric vein [1,2]. Similar cases have been reported in the antecubital fossa, inguinal area, axilla, penis [3], abdomen and lower limbs.

Introduction and general description
This is a rare, self-limiting and benign condition that was first described in 1939 [1].

Epidemiology
Incidence and prevalence
The incidence and prevalence of this rare condition are unknown. Less than 500 cases have been published in the literature [2]. Penile Mondor disease is rarer still and accounts for fewer than 10% of cases. The incidence after breast surgery is estimated to be 1% [3].

Age
Typically the patients are between 30 and 60 years old.

Sex
The sex ratio is 3:1 female:male.

Ethnicity
There is no known racial bias.

Pathophysiology
The pathogenesis of Mondor disease is not understood. As with superficial venous thrombosis the mechanism is thought to be within the Virchow triad (stasis, increased coagulability and vessel wall injury).

In the *chest wall type*, a study of pooled cases of the disease found one-third of cases were idiopathic; most of the rest were related to trauma (injury, muscular strain, poorly fitting bras, surgery, breast prosthesis, etc.). Rare causes were underlying breast cancer, hypercoagulable states and connective tissue disorders [2].

In the *penile type*, surgical trauma, excessive sexual activity, sexual vacuum practices, use of constrictive elements during sexual activity, intravenous drug abuse, prolonged sexual abstinence, local or distant infection, venous obstruction due to bladder distension and pelvic tumours have all been reported [2].

Pathology [4]
It is a two- stage process: initially there is a dense inflammatory cell infiltrate and usually a thrombus occluding the lumen of the affected veins. Thereafter, connective tissue proliferation occurs in the vessel leading to a hard cord which resolves when the vessel canalises.

Clinical features (Figure 101.26)
The features are described according to the latest clinical classification of the disease, outlined in Table 101.36 [2].

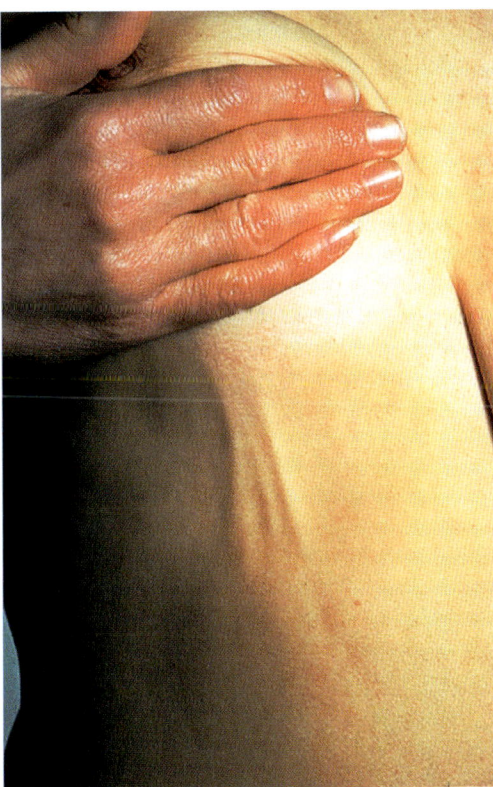

Figure 101.26 Mondor disease.

Mondor disease of the chest wall. The lesions appear and may be painful or asymptomatic. On examination, the lesions may involve any subcutaneous vein on the upper anterolateral chest wall and produce a fibrous painful cord with skin retraction. However, unlike classical superficial venous thrombosis there is *no* overlying cutaneous inflammation.

Mondor disease involving other venous territories. The most usual site of involvement is the penis. A fibrous painful cord with local preputial inflammation but without skin retraction is seen. Other possible sites include the brachial, femoral and calf veins but, unlike chest wall Mondor disease, local inflammation is present.

Mondor disease after breast surgery. This is a subtype described in association with axillary lymph node dissection in breast cancer, and is characterised by retractile scarring of the fascia. Some authors call it axillary web syndrome. It manifests with palpable cords with 'bowstringing' across the axilla, creating a web of skin. The cords are painful and restrict shoulder movement. They can extend into the ipsilateral arm, and even the forearm, creating linear grooves. There is usually no concomitant superficial venous thrombosis.

Differential diagnosis
The differential diagnosis is wide and includes cellulitis, erythema nodosum, skin metastatic carcinoma, lymphangiectasia and lymphangioma.

Disease course and prognosis
This depends on the site and type of disease.

In *Mondor disease on the chest wall*, this is generally benign and self-limiting with spontaneous resolution usually with 2–8 weeks [2] and only 13% recurrence is reported in one series [5] and none in another [6].

In *Mondor disease involving other venous territories*, the natural history is less well known and, as with other conditions with superficial venous thrombosis, can be associated with deeper thrombosis.

In *Mondor disease after breast surgery*, this usually spontaneously resolves.

Investigations
Diagnosis is largely clinical. Ultrasound examination can diagnose superficial thrombus and exclude a deep thrombus. Mammography can be helpful if there is suspicion of an underlying carcinoma.

Management
This depends on the type of Mondor disease.

In *Mondor disease on the chest wall*, as this is generally benign and self-limiting, no anticoagulation is needed and simple analgesia can be given if the patient is in pain.

In *Mondor disease involving other venous territories*, anticoagulation is recommended and sometimes in penile disease the superficial dorsal vein of the penis is treated with thrombectomy or excision.

In *Mondor disease after breast surgery*, no anticoagulation is needed. If the fascial fibrous bands persist, they can be manually ruptured with immediate return of function and reduction in pain [7].

PART 9: VASCULAR DISORDERS

Table 101.36 Subtypes of Mondor disease.

Subtype	Mondor disease of the chest wall	Mondor disease involving other venous territories	Mondor disease after breast surgery
Clinical features	Lesions may be painful or asymptomatic May involve any subcutaneous vein on the upper anterolateral chest wall Present as a fibrous painful cord with skin retraction No overlying cutaneous inflammation	Penis is most usual site of involvement A fibrous painful cord with local preputial inflammation but without skin retraction is seen Other possible sites include the brachial, femoral and calf veins Local inflammation is present	Associated with axillary lymph node dissection in breast cancer Retractile scarring of the fascia Palpable cords which 'bowstringing' across the axilla, creating a web of skin. Cords are painful and restrict shoulder movement Usually no concomitant superficial venous thrombosis
Disease course	Benign and self-limiting Spontaneous resolution within 2–8 weeks in most cases	Disease course less known Can be associated with other thromboses	Usually spontaneously resolves
Management	Simple analgesia if needed	Anticoagulation is recommended Penile disease may be treated with thrombectomy or excision	Fascial fibrous bands can be manually ruptured if persistent

Varicose veins

Definition and nomenclature
These are visible, dilated and tortuous elongations of the larger superficial venous trunks and their tributaries.

Synonyms and inclusions
- Venous varicosity

Introduction and general description
Varicose veins are very common and their characteristics and management were described by Hippocrates and Galen [1]. Over the millennia, they have been the subject of controversy and remain so today with much research still being needed to identify their pathogenesis and optimum treatment [2].

Epidemiology
Incidence and prevalence
Varicose veins are common. The incidence of varicose veins is unknown but several studies have reported the prevalence to be high (varying from 10% to 50% of the adult population). Each year, around 7% of those with varicose veins develop secondary skin-related changes. Of those with skin changes secondary to varicose veins, 1–2% go on to develop ulceration of the lower limbs [3]. The condition affects a third of those aged between 18 and 64 years old [4]. The prevalence in pregnant women is as high as 72%, and occurs due to compression on the pelvic veins and hormonal-related dilatation of veins [5]. Most cases resolve after pregnancy; however, a significant proportion go on to develop varicose veins later in life.

Age and sex
The prevalence increases with age and the condition is commoner in females. By 20 years of age, the prevalence of varicose veins is 10%; by the age of 40 years, it is 40% in women and 25% in men. Varicose veins are present in about 70% of 80-year-old women and 60% of 80-year-old men.

Ethnicity
There is no known ethnic variation in varicose veins, although there is some evidence that there is an increased prevalence in white people [6].

Risk factors
Older age, female sex, pregnancy, obesity, poor mobility, white race

Associated diseases
Klippel–Trenaunay syndrome, where there is a congenital malformation leading to varicose veins.

Pathophysiology [7]
In the healthy venous system, there is venous blood flow through the superficial system into the deep system and back to the heart. One-way valves exist in both systems, and in the perforating veins, which connect the two. Incompetence in any of the valves can disrupt the normal flow of the blood and cause venous hypertension. The pathogenesis of varicose veins is not fully understood. Valvular incompetence and venous hypertension are thought to be important and interdependent, but how they occur remains to be fully elucidated.

Varicose veins can be divided into primary and secondary. The mechanical issues of valve incompetence and raised pressure can occur in both and lead to complex molecular and histopathological alterations in the vessel wall and the extracellular matrix (Table 101.37).

Pathology
The chief findings in varicose veins are intimal hypertrophy, subendothelial fibrosis, luminal dilatation and wall thickening.

Genetics
A genetic basis has been thought to be possibly relevant in the pathogenesis of varicose veins, since familial clustering of cases occurs. Genetic studies in twins suggests that *FOXC2* plays a critical role in valve development and function, and that mutations in *FOXC2* may promote varicose veins. Other studies have suggested a link

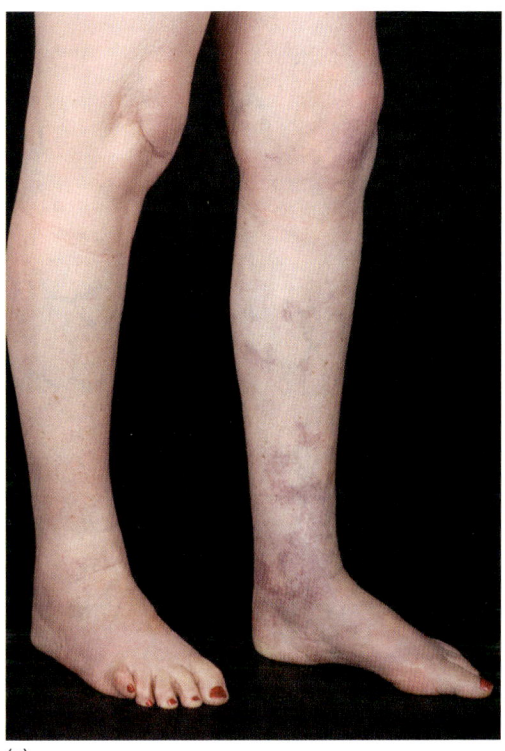
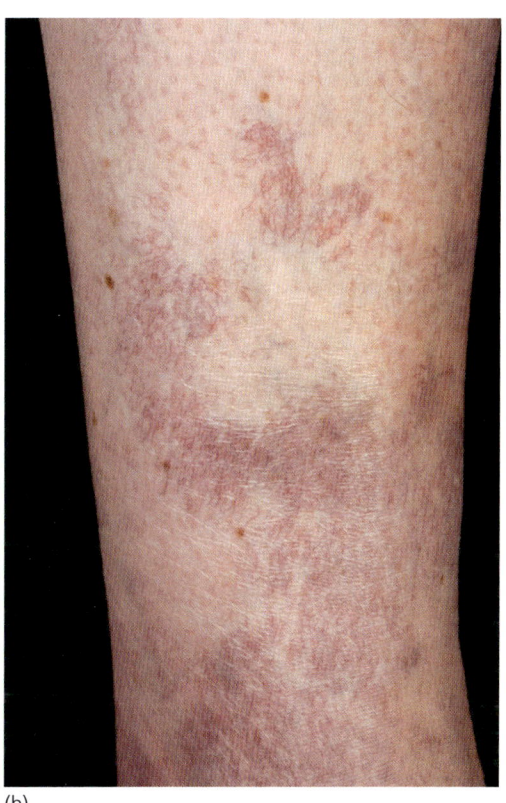

Figure 101.27 (a) Varicose veins in the left leg, and (b) with superficial telangiectasia.

(a)   (b)

Table 101.37 Pathogenesis of varicose veins.

	Pathogenetic features
Primary varicose veins	
No known underlying cause	No uniform valvular abnormality found
Associated with valvular incompetence	Intrinsic and structural abnormalities of vein walls are seen
Secondary varicose veins	
Raised endoluminal venous pressure (venous hypertension) due to thrombosis, pregnancy, trauma	Raised venous pressure is thought to cause: • Stretching of the endothelium • Expression of cytokines and adhesion molecules • Activation of extracellular signal-related kinases • Free radical production • Dysregulation of transforming growth factor β • Altered fibroblast activity

with varicose veins and mutations in the *NOTCH3* gene (thrombomodulin promoter), mutations in the *NDP* gene (which cause Norrie disease) and in the transforming growth factor β receptor 2 gene. More recently, over 30 genetic loci have been identified, and a strong genetic correlation between varicose veins and DVT has been discovered [8].

Environmental factors
A population-based cross-sectional survey in Germany of 3072 participants found that the prevalence of varicose veins was twice as high in an urban population as in a rural population [9].

Clinical features (Figure 101.27)
The severity of symptoms does not necessarily correlate with the size or extent of the visible varices and that in turn does not always correlate with the degree of reflux or severity of venous hypertension. The clinical features of varicose veins are described in Table 101.38.

Investigations
Colour duplex Doppler ultrasound scanning is used to investigate patients with varicose veins as it provides an anatomical picture of the venous system. It is the investigation of choice for detecting deep vein reflux. Duplex scanning is also essential to investigate patients with skin changes attributed to venous hypertension. There is some evidence that the incidence of recurrent varicose veins is lower after duplex assessment has been used to plan surgery.

Management
Patients with varicose veins are largely managed by vascular surgeons. The management of varicose veins is outlined in Table 101.39 and is based on the latest NICE guidelines [2,10].

Resources

Further information
NICE guidelines: http://guidance.nice.org.uk/CG168

Patient resources
https://patient.info/heart-health/varicose-veins-leaflet
(All last accessed March 2022.)

Table 101.38 Clinical features of varicose veins.

History	Often asymptomatic but unsightly
	Sometimes there is aching, which is worse on standing
	Ankle swelling
	Symptoms of chronic venous insufficiency: skin discoloration in a gaiter pattern, itching, chronic swelling, pain due to ulceration
Presentation	Visible palpable dilated and tortuous veins in the subcutis
	Reticular veins
	Telangiectases (spider veins)
	Signs of chronic venous insufficiency may accompany varicose veins: pigmentation, eczema, lipodermatosclerosis, ulceration
Differential diagnosis	Thrombophlebitis
	DVT
Classification of severity	CEAP classification [11,12]
	Clinical: C_0–C_6 (from no signs to active venous ulcer); S = symptomatic, A = asymptomatic
	Etiological: Ec, congenital; Ep, primary; Es, secondary; En, no venous cause found
	Anatomical: As, superficial veins; Ap, perforator veins; Ad, deep veins; An, no venous location identified
	Pathophysiological: Pr, reflux; Po, obstruction; Pr,o, obstruction; Pn, no venous pathophysiology identifiable
Complications and co-morbidities	Thrombophlebitis
	Bleeding
	DVT and chronic venous insufficiency
Disease course and prognosis	Approximately 4% of patients with varicose veins progress to more severe clinical stages per annum [13]
	3–6% of patients with varicose veins will develop venous leg ulcers in their lifetime [2]
	There is a suggestion that obesity, increasing age and genetic factors may be relevant. NICE has recommended that large observational prospective cohort studies are needed to identify the factors that influence progression [2]

NICE, National Institute for Health and Care Excellence.

Table 101.39 Management of varicose veins. Based on [2].

Patient advice and information	Discuss the cause and natural history of varicose veins
	Give advice about weight control
	Advise light to moderate physical activity
	Advise leg elevation where possible
Referral to a vascular unit	Refer if any of the following:
	Bleeding varicose veins
	Primary or symptomatic recurrent varicose veins
	Lower limb skin changes, such as pigmentation or eczema, thought to be caused by chronic venous insufficiency
	Superficial vein thrombosis (characterised by the appearance of hard painful veins) and suspected venous incompetence
	An active or healed venous leg ulcer
Assessment in a vascular unit	Use duplex ultrasound:
	To confirm the diagnosis of varicose veins
	To identify the extent of truncal reflux
	To plan treatment for people with suspected primary or recurrent varicose veins
Interventional treatment: for people with confirmed varicose veins and truncal reflux	Offer endothermal ablation and endovenous laser treatment of the long saphenous vein
	If endothermal ablation is unsuitable, offer ultrasound-guided foam sclerotherapy
	If ultrasound-guided foam sclerotherapy is unsuitable, offer surgery. If incompetent varicose tributaries are to be treated, consider treating them at the same time
	If offering compression bandaging or hosiery for use after interventional treatment, do not use for more than 7 days
Non-interventional treatment	Do not routinely offer compression hosiery to treat varicose veins unless interventional treatment is unsuitable
Management during pregnancy	Explain that pregnancy exacerbates varicose veins and that following pregnancy they may improve
	Do not carry out interventional treatment for varicose veins during pregnancy other than in exceptional circumstances
	Consider compression hosiery for symptom relief of leg swelling associated with varicose veins during pregnancy

Chronic venous insufficiency

Venous insufficiency

Definition and nomenclature

This is a state which occurs when the blood no longer flows in the correct path from the superficial system into the deep venous system and then back to the heart. This results in venous congestion and impairment of the venous system. Chronic venous insufficiency may be classified anatomically into three categories:

1 *Superficial vein insufficiency*: this is indicated by the presence of visible, tortuous, truncal varicose veins. It arises from primary valve failure or when the superficial veins become distended, causing the valves to become secondarily incompetent.

2 *Perforating vein insufficiency*: this is a rare condition in isolation, when it is caused by primary valve insufficiency. Secondary perforating vein insufficiency often occurs in combination with deep-vein insufficiency (post-thrombotic limb).

3 *Deep-vein insufficiency*: reflux is the most common type of abnormality. However, in approximately 10% of cases a functional obstruction from thrombosis (non-recanalised thrombosis) will be present, in which case it is likely to be associated with the post-thrombotic syndrome. Avalvulosis is rare unless associated with a mutation of the *FOXC2* gene [1].

If untreated, venous insufficiency in either the deep or superficial system causes the progressive syndrome of chronic venous insufficiency.

Synonyms and inclusions
- Post-thrombotic syndrome
- Postphlebetic syndrome

Introduction and general description

Chronic venous insufficiency is common and can be disabling. It is a major aetiological factor globally in the development of leg ulcers.

Epidemiology

Those with superficial venous insufficiency usually present with varicose veins initially. Chronic deep venous insufficiency is most frequently post-thrombosis, and occurs in fewer than half of patients after DVT [2].

Incidence and prevalence

Varicose veins and chronic venous insufficiency are common. One large study in 30 000 subjects found a prevalence of 7% for varicose veins and 0.86% for 'symptomatic' chronic venous insufficiency [3]. Another screened 1566 subjects and found chronic venous insufficiency in 9.4% of men, and 6.6% of women. Prevalence rose significantly with age: 21.2% in men >50 years and 12.0% in women >50 years [4].

Serious chronic venous insufficiency leading to venous ulcers has an estimated prevalence of approximately 0.3%, although active or healed ulcers are seen in up to 1% of the adult population [5]. In the USA, it is thought that approximately 2.5 million people have chronic venous insufficiency and about 20% of those develop venous ulcers [6]. The risk factors are summarised in Table 101.40.

Age

Chronic venous insufficiency prevalence increases with age.

Sex

Varicose veins are more common in females, but studies differ on the sex difference in the prevalence of severe chronic venous deficiency.

Ethnicity

There is not thought to be any racial difference in the prevalence of chronic venous insufficiency. However, it occurs more commonly in Western society and this probably reflects lifestyle differences such as sedentary or standing occupations, higher rates of obesity and generally reduced levels of physical activity.

Environmental factors

A sedentary lifestyle reduces the efficiency of the muscle pump and thus leads to reduced venous return; occupations with prolonged standing act to increase the risk of higher venous pressures in the legs.

Pathophysiology

Changes occurring in the macrocirculation lead to microvascular abnormalities and chronic inflammation which are thought to lead to the physical manifestations of chronic venous insufficiency.

Pathophysiology of venous reflux and chronic venous insufficiency

It is thought that there are two elements to the pathophysiology; the first is abnormal venous blood flow with reflux, and the second occurs at the microvascular level and is a chronic inflammatory process which leads to the skin changes seen in chronic venous insufficiency. Venous reflux is regarded as the major cause of venous disorders. Reflux is the presence of retrograde flow in a vein in response to a stimulus such as a calf squeeze. It occurs during standing when the valves are incompetent. It can occur in the superficial, deep and perforating veins of the lower extremity. An elevated and sustained ambulatory venous pressure (venous hypertension) is indicative of chronic venous insufficiency. This may be caused by valvular incompetence, venous outflow obstruction or poor muscle pump function (Table 101.41). Venous outflow obstruction occurs in some patients after a DVT; it is more serious than reflux and more difficult to treat. In this situation, when the leg muscles contract, the venous pressure increases, rather than the usual lowering of venous pressure that occurs during ambulation when the vein is not obstructed. Such heightened pressure is transmitted distally as far as the capillary system of the skin,

Table 101.40 Risk factors for chronic venous insufficiency.

Older age
Family history of venous disease
Female sex
Pregnancy
Smoking
Higher body mass index
Prolonged standing
Prior venous thrombosis
Prior trauma to the lower extremities
Hereditary conditions such as Klippel–Trenaunay syndrome

Table 101.41 Causes of chronic venous insufficiency.

Venous disease	Superficial venous incompetence (varicose veins)
	Deep venous incompetence
	Primary deep venous obstruction (rare)
	Previous deep-vein thrombosis
	External compression
Impaired calf muscle pump function	Immobility
	Joint disease
	Paralysis
	Obesity (immobility, femoral vein compression, high abdominal pressures)
Congestive cardiac failure	Multiple causes

PART 9: VASCULAR DISORDERS

Table 101.42 Pathogenesis of chronic venous disease.

Leukocytes accumulate in leg when there is chronic high venous pressure	Leukocytes are activated by plasminogen activator
	Activated leukocytes shed L-selectin into the plasma and express members of the integrin family (CD11b, which binds to intercellular adhesion molecule 1)
	Integrin binding promotes firm adhesion of leukocytes
	Leukocytes start their migration out of the vasculature and undergo degranulation
	Increased levels of activated leukocytes occur both locally and systemically in patients with chronic venous disease
Degradation of extracellular matrix proteins leads to breakdown of extracellular matrix causing reduced healing and promotes ulceration	Vascular cells and inflammatory cells (e.g. macrophages) produce proteolytic enzymes
	Proteolytic enzymes, including matrix metalloproteinases and serine proteinases, are released as inactive proenzymes and activated by other proteinases, including those produced by mast cells
Capillary proliferation and increased permeability; skin capillaries are elongated and there is tortuous proliferation of the capillary endothelium	Vascular endothelial growth factor, which is likely to be involved in these changes, has been shown to increase microvascular permeability
Dermal tissue fibrosis: feature of lipodermatosclerosis and ulceration	It is postulated that activated leukocytes migrate out of the vasculature and release transforming growth factor. Transforming growth factor is a fibrogenic cytokine, stimulating collagen production by dermal fibroblasts resulting in dermal fibrosis
Increased capillary permeability and extravasation of red blood cells leads to skin pigmentation, which induces the development of a microenvironment that exacerbates tissue damage and delays healing	This leads to elevated levels of ferritin and ferric iron in affected skin
	There is oxidative stress and matrix metalloproteinase activation

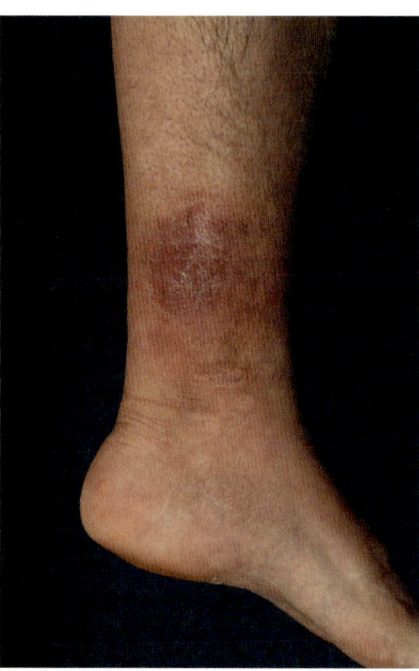

Figure 101.28 Venous eczema.

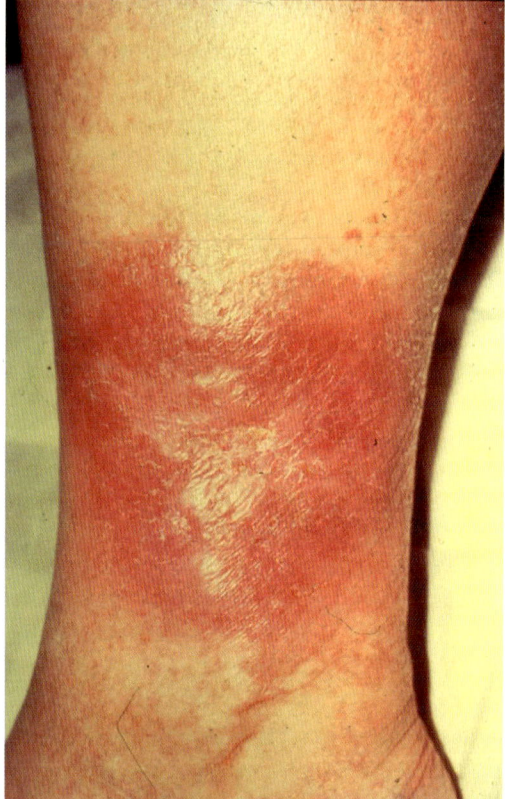

Figure 101.29 Lipodermatosclerosis.

causing capillary hypertension, and eventually leading to destruction of the nutritive capillaries [7]. The current theories on the mechanisms for the pathogenesis of the chronic inflammation in venous disease are outlined by Bergan *et al*. [8] and summarised in Table 101.42.

Genetics

A genetic basis has been thought to be relevant in the pathogenesis of varicose veins, since familial clustering of cases does occur. Genetic studies in twins suggests that *FOXC2* plays a critical role in valve development and function, and that mutations in *FOXC2* may promote varicose veins. Chronic venous insufficiency may also be a feature of Klippel–Trenaunay syndrome.

Clinical features
History

The clinical features of chronic venous insufficiency vary from mild oedema to severe incapacitating leg ulceration (outlined in Table 101.43). Patients with superficial venous insufficiency may complain of burning, swelling, throbbing, aching, cramping and heaviness in the legs. Those with deep venous insufficiency almost always have pain. The symptoms are often improved by elevation and rest of the legs.

Table 101.43 Clinical features of chronic venous insufficiency.

Feature	Description	Pathology
Swelling (oedema)	Pitting oedema (especially around the ankle) Worst at the end of the day Usually disappears at night May complain of a tight feeling Night cramps	The capillary filtration rate increases as a consequence of the increased ambulatory venous (and consequently capillary) pressure and overwhelms lymph drainage. This oedema always has a low protein content
Corona phlebectatica paraplantaris (ankle flare) (see Figure 101.31)	Presence of abnormally visible cutaneous blood vessels at the ankle with several components: 'venous cups', blue and red telangiectases and capillary 'stasis spots'	A direct consequence of increased capillary pressure, which causes these vessels to expand
Hyperpigmentation (see Figure 101.32)	Pigmentation in the 'gaiter skin' Pinpoint or patchy pigmentation may be minimal but may also extend over large indurated skin areas	Haemosiderin accumulates after extravasation of erythrocytes (red cells) Melanin can also be deposited as part of post-inflammatory hyperpigmentation following venous eczema and ulceration
Pressure erythema	Grouped, confluent, very small telangiectasiae develop Often found near incompetent perforating veins. Pressure erythema is often one of the first signs of evolving venous insufficiency	Direct result of increased venous pressure causing vascular dilatation
Venous eczema (see Figure 101.28) Synonyms: stasis dermatitis, hypostatic eczema, dermatitis veineuse	Starts around varicosities at the medial ankle Relatively sharply demarcated Papules and vesicles, which may also extend beyond the main area of eczematous skin Scaling and itching develop Chronic lichenified eczema may develop with time May lead to secondary spread onto adjacent and distant non-contact sites. Itching may develop at any site including the palms and soles Can be complicated by secondary infection Other types of eczema may also occur: • *Irritant and allergic contact dermatitis* due to locally applied treatments • *Asteatotic dermatitis* (synonym: eczema craquelé). Frequent washing may cause extreme dehydration of the skin. Morphologically similar to eczema with a 'crazy paving' pattern appears	Histopathological features of eczema Aetiology is not completely clear. Homing of activated T lymphocytes appears to be the most reasonable explanation
Lipodermatosclerosis (see Figure 101.29) Pathognomonic of venous and lymphatic hypertension Known to be associated with an increased risk of leg ulcer development	Often found just above the medial malleolus, at the level of the Cockett perforating veins, which are usually incompetent, as is the great saphenous vein When the small saphenous vein is incompetent, the lipodermatosclerosis often affects the lateral side of the calf Early stage lipodermatosclerosis may feel a little indurated and often has an inflamed erythematosus appearance It is also quite often tender and painful (can be confused with erysipelas, superficial venous thrombosis or even deep-vein thrombosis) In longstanding disease, there is a 'woody' hardness to the skin and subcutaneous tissues with pigmentation	Increased matrix turnover is caused by a chronic inflammatory reaction The most characteristic histological findings are dermal and subcutaneous fibrosis, with fat degeneration
Atrophie blanche	Atrophic ivory-white depressed skin lesion often located on the lower legs Usually multiple lesions (diameter 0.5–15 cm) Contains many centrally enlarged capillaries that are visible as red dots Often asymptomatic; however, associated ulceration can be very painful (see Figure 101.30) Not unique to venous insufficiency May also be seen in association with other disorders including lupus erythematosus, scleroderma, vasculitides, cryoglobulinaemia, polycythaemia and leukaemia	The result of decreased capillary density caused by microthrombi and matrix degradation causing hypoxia There is an atrophic epidermis and a thickened, scleroderma-like dermis with proliferative dilated capillaries One or more capillaries are often occluded with fibrinoid material
Varicosities (see section on Varicose veins)	Dilated and tortuous veins May be primary varicosities May be secondary, following deep-vein thrombosis	See section on Varicose veins
Secondary (high output) Lymphoedema	May develop in patients with longstanding chronic venous insufficiency Develops when the previously healthy local lymphatic system fails in the face of an overwhelming filtration load, with eventual structural obliteration of lymphatic routes	
Ulceration (end stage of chronic venous insufficiency)	See Chapter 102	See Chapter 102

PART 9: VASCULAR DISORDERS

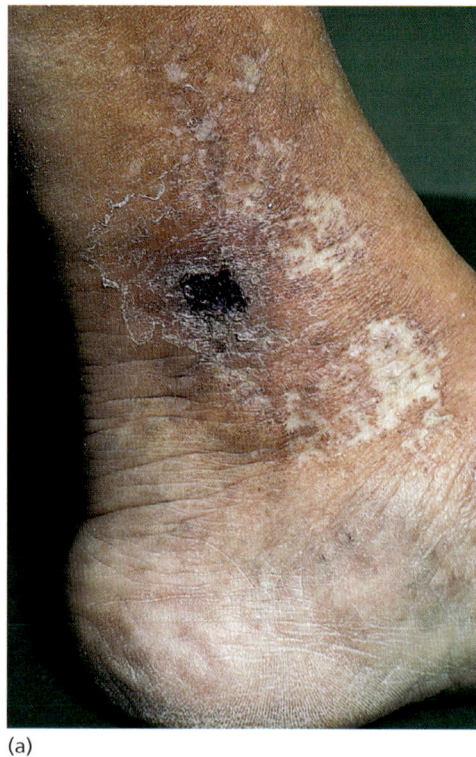

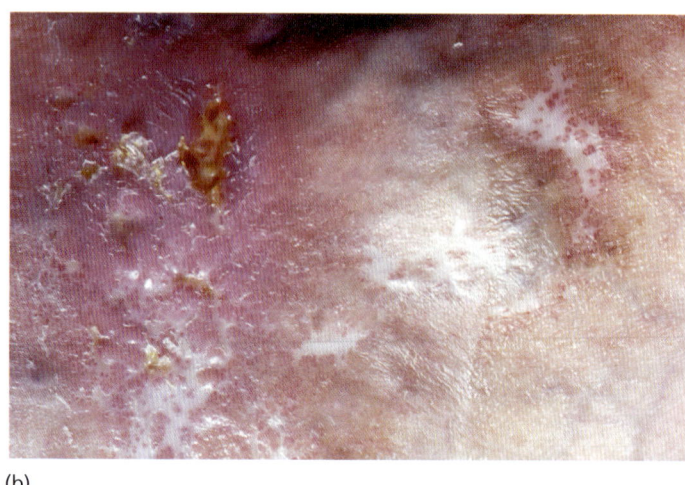

(a)   (b)

Figure 101.30 (a) Atrophie blanche: white scars with a central ischaemic ulcer and telangiectasia at the edge of the white areas. (b) Venous ulceration with atrophie blanche.

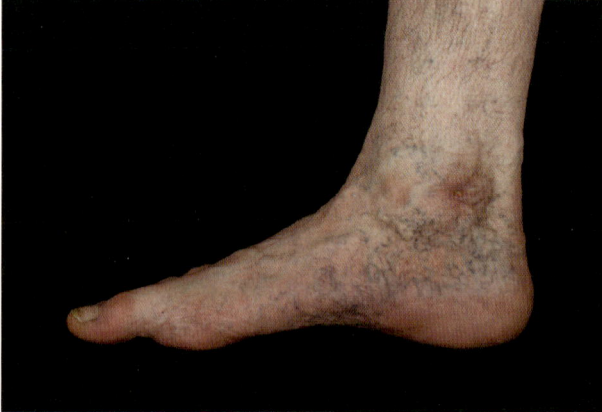

Figure 101.31 Corona phlebectatica paraplantaris.

Classification of severity

The CEAP classification is the most widely used classification for severity of chronic venous insufficiency, as it is for varicose veins (see Table 101.31 for explanation).

Complications and co-morbidities

These include thromboembolic disease, venous ulceration and secondary lymphoedema.

Disease course and prognosis

It is not known overall how many patients with chronic venous insufficiency progress to end-stage venous ulceration. Progression and disease severity appear to correlate with the severity of venous valve incompetence [9]. Approximately 4% of patients

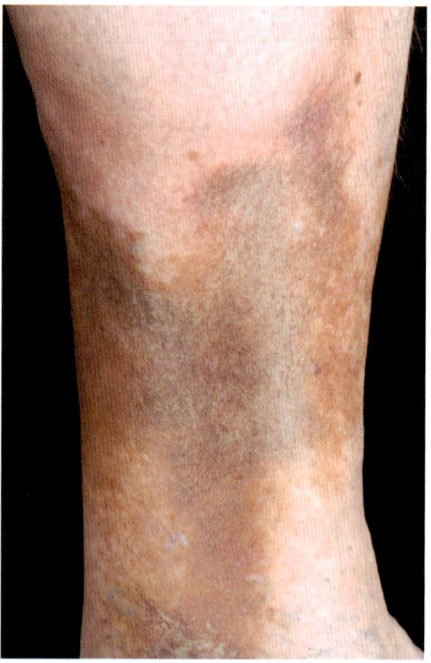

Figure 101.32 Hyperpigmentation secondary to venous insufficiency.

with varicose veins progress to more severe clinical stages per annum. Of patients with varicose veins, 3–6% will develop venous leg ulcers in their lifetime [10]. Patients with lipodermatosclerosis have an increased risk of venous ulceration. Approximately 3% of patients with DVT will go on to develop severe chronic venous insufficiency.

Table 101.44 Investigations for chronic venous insufficiency.

Duplex ultrasonography	The investigation of choice
Colour flow duplex imaging uses doppler information to colour code the two-dimensional sonogram	Duplex gives excellent information on venous anatomy and reflux
Accurate but very 'operator dependent'	Allows the communications between deep and superficial veins to be directly assessed
	Indications include: recurrent varicose veins, signs of deep-vein pathology, analysis of the popliteal fossa veins/perforating veins, preoperative marking of varicose veins, assessment of venous malformations, surveillance after treatment, duplex-guided sclerotherapy, evaluation before endovenous interventions, diagnosis of deep-vein thrombosis and follow-up after treatment
MRI venography (non-invasive venographic technique)	Most sensitive and specific test for the assessment of deep and superficial venous disease in the lower legs and pelvis
	Also helpful at excluding unsuspected non-vascular causes of leg pain
Phlebography (venography)	Invasive
Contrast is injected into a foot vein, and is driven into the deep veins by an ankle tourniquet	Largely replaced by MRI venography
Venous pressure measurement	Provides a direct measurement of the severity of chronic venous insufficiency, since it actually measures pressure
A vein in the foot is cannulated	
The patient stands up and down on tiptoes 10 times. The venous pressure drops and the pressure drop is measured. This is defined as the *ambulatory venous pressure* (should be below 40 mmHg or at least 50% of standing venous pressure)	
The patient stands still until the pressure returns; the time taken for the pressure to return is defined as the *venous refill time* (normally >25 s)	
Air plethysmography	Provides overall assessment of venous competence
Measures volume changes in the limb as a result of changes in posture and activity; measured by pressure changes in a cuff wrapped around the calf	Cannot localise sites of reflux
	Most often used to assess results of venous interventions and as a research tool
Photoplethysmography	Bays *et al.* found in chronic venous insufficiency a positive predictive value of venous refill time examined with venous plethysmography of 77% and a negative predictive value of 100% [12]
Photoelectric plethysmographic method of measuring the skin circulation	
The intensity of light reflected from the skin red cells correlates with the blood volume in the skin	
Venous refill time after a standardised exercise is measured	

Table 101.45 Treatment for chronic venous insufficiency.

General advice	Leg elevation
	Exercise
	Optimise analgesia
Graduated compression	Options include elastic stockings, bandages, intermittent pneumatic compression
	Improves venous dynamics during the day. They can be removed or a lower class of compression worn at night
	In varicose veins and lipodermatosclerosis, compression helps to relieve symptoms
	Compliance may be an issue due to difficulty getting the stockings on
	Consider 4-layer bandaging when legs are ulcerated and/or very swollen; patients with severe arterial disease can often not tolerate compression
Interventional treatments [17]	Aim to correct the venous insufficiency by removing the major reflux pathways
	Offer endothermal ablation and endovenous laser treatment of the long saphenous vein
	If endothermal ablation is unsuitable, offer ultrasound-guided foam sclerotherapy
	If ultrasound-guided foam sclerotherapy is unsuitable, offer surgery
	If incompetent varicose tributaries are to be treated, consider treating them at the same time as surgery

Investigations

The diagnosis of chronic venous insufficiency is made on clinical and symptomatic grounds. The purpose of investigation is to detect venous occlusion, acute or chronic thrombosis, post-thrombotic changes, and patterns of obstructive flow and reflux. The most useful and universal investigation is duplex ultrasonography [11]. The chief tools of investigation of chronic venous insufficiency are outlined in Table 101.44.

Management

The aims of treatment are to relieve the symptoms of chronic venous insufficiency and if possible to correct the underlying cause. These are outlined in Table 101.45. Patients should be referred to a vascular unit for assessment. Compression therapy remains the cornerstone of management, as this compresses varicose veins, reduces reflux and improves calf muscle function. This can take the form of elastic stockings (class 2, 30–40 mmHg; or class 3, >40 mmHg), non-elastic and elastic bandages (short- and long-stretch), and intermittent pneumatic compression. A Cochrane meta-analysis of 22 trials [13] showed that compression stockings were more effective than no compression in healing venous ulcers and higher compression pressures were more effective than lower ones; multilayer compression bandaging was superior to single-layer bandaging. Progressive graduated compression stockings (higher pressure at the calf than ankle) have been reported as having greater efficacy in symptoms and they are easier to apply. Intermittent pneumatic compression has been suggested for use in patients with refractory oedema and significant/persistent ulceration when other conservative measures have failed [14].

Interventional treatments are usually undertaken by vascular surgeons or interventional radiologists. These include endovenous techniques such as endovenous thermal ablation, non-thermal ablation and foam sclerotherapy. These are less invasive and as effective as open surgery [15]. A landmark study in 2018 has shown that in the presence of venous ulcers, early endovenous ablation of superficial venous reflux resulted in faster healing of ulcers and greater time free of further ulceration [16]. This should encourage clinicians to refer vascular surgeons early for timely treatment.

Key references

The full list of references can be found in the online version at https://www.wiley.com/rooksdermatology10e

Arterial and arteriolar disorders
Arterial disease and peripheral ischaemic disorders
5 Aboyans V, Ricco JB, Bartelink MEL *et al*. 2017 ESC Guidelines on the Diagnosis and Treatment of Peripheral Arterial Diseases, in collaboration with the European Society for Vascular Surgery (ESVS) *Eur Heart J* 2018;39:763–816.

Neurovascular disorders
Erythromelalgia
10 Yang Y, Wang Y, Li S *et al*. Mutations in SCN9A, encoding a sodium channel alpha subunit, in patients with primary erythromelalgia. *J Med Genet* 2004;41:171–4.
27 Thompson GH, Hahn G, Rang M. Erythromelalgia. *Clin Orthop Relat Res* 1979;144:249–54.

Telangiectases
Primary telangiectasia
Angioma serpiginosum
1 Happle R. Capillary malformations: a classification using specific names for specific skin disorders. *J Eur Acad Dermatol Venereol* 2015;29:2295–305.

Generalised essential telangiectasia
1 McGrae JD, Winkelmann RK. Generalised essential telangiectasia. *JAMA* 1963;185:909–13.

Malformations
Arteriovenous malformations
3 Vikkula M, Boon LM, Mulliken JB, Olsen BR. Molecular basis of vascular anomalies. *Trends Cardiovasc Med* 1998;8:281–92.

Venous malformations
1 Wassef M, Blei F, Adams D *et al*. Vascular anomalies classification: recommendations from the International Society for the Study of Vascular Anomalies. *Pediatrics* 2015;136:e203–14.

Venous disorders
Venous thrombosis
Deep-vein thrombosis
7 NICE (National Institute for Health and Care Excellence). *Venous Thromboembolic Diseases: Diagnosis, Management and Thrombophilia Testing*. NICE Clinical Guideline (March 2020). https://www.nice.org.uk/guidance/ng158 (last accessed March 2022).

Varicose veins
8 Fukaya E, Flores AM, Lindholm D *et al*. Clinical and genetic determinants of varicose veins: prospective, community-based study of ≈500 000 individuals. *Circulation* 2018;138:2869–80.

Chronic venous insufficiency
8 Bergan JJ, Schmid-Schönbein GW *et al*. Chronic venous disease. *N Engl J Med* 2006;355:488.

CHAPTER 102

Ulceration Resulting from Disorders of the Veins and Arteries

Jürg Hafner[1] and Eberhard Rabe[2]

[1]Department of Dermatology, University Hospital of Zurich, Zurich, Switzerland
[2]Department of Dermatology, University Hospital of Bonn, Bonn, Germany

Introduction

Leg and foot ulcers represent a serious burden of disease. Their impact – both physically and psychologically – is underestimated, on both the sufferer and their families and friends. Chronic wounds cause considerable economic burden and are estimated to be around 1% of total health care expenses in western countries, and even more (2–3%) when indirect costs are included. Pain is very common, to the detriment of sleep and quality of life [1–6].

Nevertheless, surprisingly, many patients suffering from leg and foot ulcers never receive an adequate clinical, vascular and laboratory examination and a rational treatment plan based on a valid diagnostic assessment. The majority of patients with chronic ulcers can be treated effectively and healed, and those with refractory lesions can be helped with palliative measures. This, however, requires standardised work-up and treatment planning [7,8,9–13,14,15].

There are four major categories of leg ulcers: venous leg ulcers (VLUs); mixed venous and arterial leg ulcers (MLUs); arterial leg ulcers (ALUs); and hypertensive ischaemic leg ulcers (HYTILUs) (Figure 102.1). These groups cover 80% of the underlying causes of leg and foot ulcers [16,17]; other aetiologies are shown in Box 102.1.

Peripheral arterial disease is categorised as asymptomatic, claudication or chronic critical limb ischaemia [18–20]. The majority of leg ulcer patients with concomitant peripheral arterial disease are above the threshold for chronic critical limb ischaemia [21].

Chronic venous disease is categorised with the CEAP classification which covers clinical stage, aetiology, anatomy and pathophysiology [22]. Atypical (i.e. non-venous and non-arterial leg ulcers) can often only be correctly diagnosed through histology, microbiology and laboratory work [17,23].

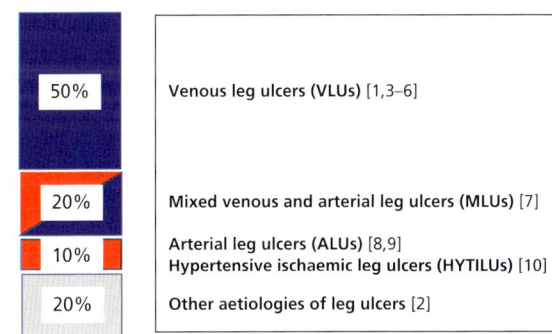

Figure 102.1 Aetiologies of leg ulcers.

50% — Venous leg ulcers (VLUs) [1,3–6]

20% — Mixed venous and arterial leg ulcers (MLUs) [7]

10% — Arterial leg ulcers (ALUs) [8,9]
Hypertensive ischaemic leg ulcers (HYTILUs) [10]

20% — Other aetiologies of leg ulcers [2]

Venous leg ulcer

Definition and nomenclature

Venous leg ulcers are chronic skin ulcers of the gaiter area that result from chronic peripheral venous hypertension [22,24–27]. They represent the most advanced grade of chronic venous disease (CVD) [24,28].

Synonyms and inclusions

- Stasis ulceration
- Venous ulcer
- Gaiter ulcer

Introduction and general description

Venous leg ulcers are the most extreme manifestation of CVD, which results from chronic peripheral venous hypertension caused

PART 9: VASCULAR DISORDERS

Box 102.1 Other aetiologies of leg ulcers [2]

- Vasculitis[a]
- Pyoderma gangrenosum[a]
- Ecthyma[a] and necrotising bacterial infections
- Klinefelter syndrome[b]
- Livedoid vasculopathy[b]
- Leg ulcers in patients with collagen vascular diseases
- Embolia cutis (cholesterol emboli, embolia cutis medicamentosa, septic embolism)
- Lacerations (skin tears) and deep dissecting hematoma in skin atrophy
- Physical traumas (radionecrosis, cryonecrosis, stings)
- Hydroxyurea associated
- Ulcerated skin cancers

[a] Risk of confounding with hypertensive ischaemic leg ulcer.
[b] Risk of confounding with venous leg ulcer.

---

by venous reflux and/or obstruction [29,30], or by neuromusculoskeletal dysfunction of the leg [31–34]. Venous pathologies involve the deep vein system and/or the superficial vein system and perforator veins [9–12,35–40]. The 'C' grading of the CEAP classification system of venous disease describes the insidious development of chronic venous insufficiency resulting from ankle oedema (C3) and reversible morphological skin changes, such as stasis eczema (C4a), through partly reversible morphological changes, such as lipodermatosclerosis (C4b) and atrophie blanche (C4b), to active (C6) or healed (C5) VLUs [22].

Epidemiology

Incidence and prevalence

The lifetime incidence of leg ulcers is around 1%, with a point prevalence of 0.1% [41–49]. Approximately half of all leg ulcers are VLUs, thus their lifetime incidence can be calculated at 0.5%, and point prevalence at 0.05%. The incidence of leg ulcers rises to 4% in the population aged over 80 years of age [45].

Age

Venous leg ulcers primarily affect individuals aged over 65 years although they can occur in younger adults. The incidence increases with every decade [45,48].

Sex

The advanced stages (C4–C6 including VLUs) occur equally in women and men. Pregnancy and a family history of varicosities create a predisposition for varicose veins (C1–C3), but not for advanced chronic venous disease and VLU (C4–C6) [41,43,45,46].

Ethnicity

While occurring in all countries and populations, the incidence and prevalence have been investigated mostly in western nations. Since VLUs occur more often in the obese and in people with standing occupations, western lifestyles create a predisposition. A body mass index (BMI) >30 increases the risk of chronic venous disease (OR 6.5 for women and 3.1 for men) [49], and a BMI >40 can cause advanced stages (C4–C6) of chronic venous disease even in the absence of

anatomical changes in the venous system [50]. Increased abdominal pressure hampers venous outflow which results in peripheral venous hypertension [51].

Associated diseases

Box 102.2 lists a number of the associated diseases.

Box 102.2 Disorders associated with venous leg ulcers

- Venous thromboembolism
- Superficial venous thrombosis
- Varicose veins
- Chronic venous disease
- Stasis dermatitis
- Lipodermatosclerosis
- Acroangiodermatitis
- Obesity
- Ankle joint ankylosis
- Rheumatoid arthritis
- Neuromuscular diseases with impact on venous calf pump ejection

---

Pathophysiology

Chronic venous disease and VLUs result from peripheral venous hypertension or chronic ambulatory venous hypertension [24–27,52]. They exclusively occur in humans. Gravitation, upright locomotion and dysfunctional venous ejection during leg motion or dysfunctional venous drainage due to obstruction (e.g. chronic occlusion, obesity, pregnancy) are prerequisites for the development of CVD and VLUs. Venous reflux can occur at the deep venous system – primarily or secondarily after deep venous thrombosis [29,30,53] – or at the superficial venous system (long and/or short saphenous vein) [9–12,29,35–40,54,55]. Perforator vein insufficiency rarely occurs in an isolated fashion and contributes less to chronic venous insufficiency and VLUs than previously suspected [56–58]. Congenital valvular aplasia is a rare condition leading to severe chronic venous insufficiency and VLU early in life [59,60]. All forms of neuromuscular diseases and/or ankle and knee joint dysfunction can induce CVD and VLUs [31–34]. Obesity raises the intra-abdominal pressure, which impedes venous drainage [49–51]. The May–Thurner syndrome describes an endovenous septum at the site where the right common iliac artery crosses the left common iliac vein. It predisposes to CVD and VLU of the left leg, with or without accompanying iliac vein thrombosis [61–70].

Venous hypertension induces changes that remain reversible in the early stages of CVD, such as stasis dermatitis and early lipodermatosclerosis (grade C4a in the CEAP classification). In later stages there are irreversible changes, such as severe forms of lipodermatosclerosis (with a leg shape of an inverted champagne bottle) and atrophie blanche (grade C4b). Chronic and recurrent protein-rich oedema and aseptic inflammation induce fibrosis and tissue hypoxia. Dermal and epidermal hypoxia causes skin breakdown and VLU (grade C6) [52,71,72]. Healed VLUs are classified as C5 [22].

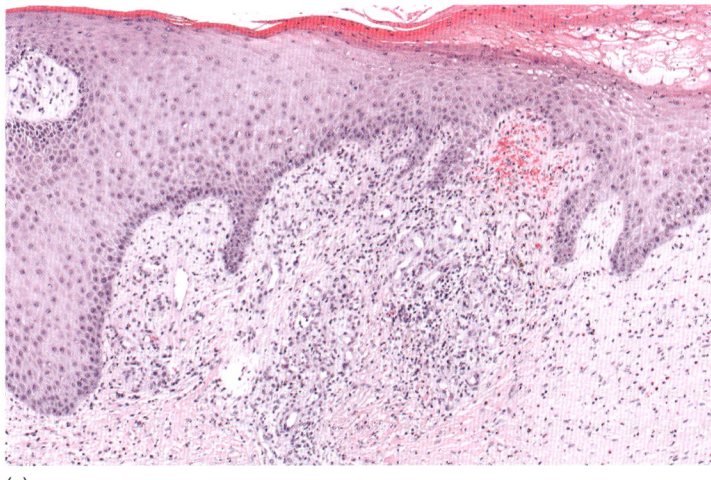

(a)

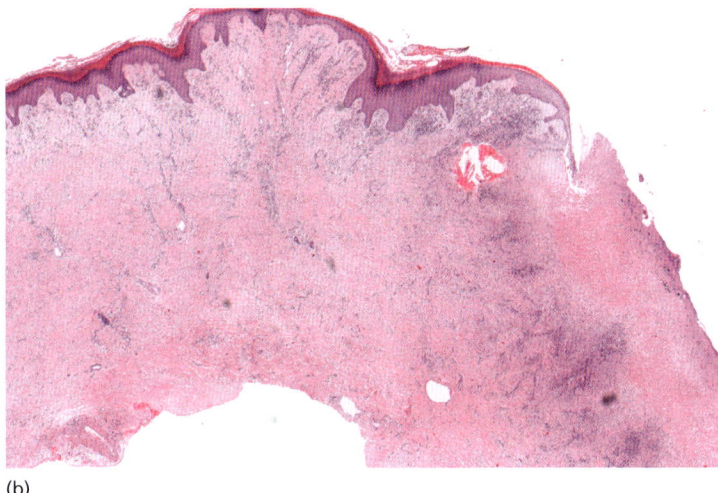

(b)

Figure 102.2 Histology of a venous leg ulcer. (a) Fibrotic dermis and subcutis with an apparent increase of vessels (venules) at the level of the subpapillary plexus. The apparent increase in vessels is caused by multiple cross-sections through tortuous subpapillary venules. The vessels have thick walls, changes caused by chronic venous hypertension. (b) Extensive fibrosis extends into the subcutis.

Predisposing factors

Predisposing factors include family history [45], obesity [49–51], standing occupation [73], venous thromboembolism [29,30,53], varicose veins [9–12,35–40], ankle joint ankyloses and neuro-muscular diseases with an impact on venous calf pump ejection [31–34].

Pathology

There is sclerosing panniculitis [74,75] with non-specific skin ulceration. The epidermis is acanthotic, while the dermis is thickened and fibrotic. The subpapillary veins are elongated with thickened walls (pseudo-increased due to more cross-sections of tortuous vessels) (Figure 102.2) and haemosiderin deposits. The chronically inflamed and fibrotic dermis expands, to the cost of the subcutis [75]. The fascia is thickened and fibrotic; the leg muscles may show fatty degeneration [76–78]. The ulceration itself is non-specific, exposing fibrin and/or biofilm layers, granulation tissue and a mixed inflammatory infiltrate.

Clinical features
History
There is frequently a family history of CVD and VLU [45] and a personal history of venous thromboembolism [29,30,53] and/or varicose veins [9–12,35–40].

Presentation
Chronic skin ulcers are common in the medial gaiter area, embedded in trophic skin changes attributed to CVD (stasis dermatitis, lipodermatosclerosis, pigmentation, induration, leg shape of an inverted champagne bottle) [7,8,10,15,16]. VLUs are less commonly located in the lateral retromalleolar area (related to deep and short saphenous vein reflux) [16,60].

Clinical variants
These ulcers may be semicircumferential or circumferential in extensive cases [76,79,80]. Patients with an insufficient deep venous system and an insufficient short saphenous vein may develop CVD at the lateral dorsum of the foot and the dorsum of the toes [16,60].

Differential diagnosis
This includes MLU, ALU, HYTILU and vasculitic leg ulcer [81–84], particularly in patients with chronic hepatitis C with cryoglobulinaemia [85–87] and males with Klinefelter syndrome [88,89].

Classification of severity
The CEAP system classifies active VLU as C6 and healed VLU as C5 [22]. The venous clinical severity score (VCSS) [90] and other score systems are also used [1–4,91].

Complications and co-morbidities
These include chronic pain and impairment of quality of life [1–6], local wound infection, systemic infection and sepsis [92], infestation with maggots (fly larvae) [93], secondary squamous cell carcinoma [94–97] and secondary lymphoedema (peri-ulcer lymphoedema and/or foot and toe lymphoedema) [98,99].

Disease course and prognosis
Venous leg ulcers are chronic and recurrent unless patients receive an accurate diagnostic assessment on which to base treatment and secondary prevention [29,100].

Investigations
Recommended investigations are summarised here.

Vascular investigations. These include assessment of peripheral arterial diseas and venous pathologies:
- Assessment of peripheral arterial disease: assessment of *systolic ankle blood pressure* and calculation of the *ankle brachial index* (ABI) [7,8,9,10,15,16,20].
- Assessment of venous pathologies: the *superficial venous reflux* can be detected with simple continuous wave Doppler ultrasound (if the operator is sufficiently experienced). *Deep venous reflux/obstruction and/or post-thrombotic findings* can only be examined with duplex ultrasound [7,8,9–13,**14**,15,35–40]. Magnetic resonance venography gives good morphological information, particularly on the iliac veins and inferior vena cava [62–70].

Wound documentation. The wound size and its morphological qualities should be documented at every visit. Electronic photographic documentation systems along with their software allow for photometric wound surface area measurement to objectify the healing process [101].

Microbiology. In the presence of clinical signs of critical colonisation and/or bacterial cellulitis and/or sepsis, wound microbiology must be analysed. A swab from the wound base (after the removal of fibrin layers and biofilms) or a small tissue biopsy from the wound base – if feasible – yields more representative microbiology results than superficial swabs from necrotic material [102,103].

Wound histology. If there is a suspicion of ulcerating malignant skin tumour, vasculitis, pyoderma gangrenosum or hypertensive ischaemic leg ulcer, or with any refractory chronic leg ulcer showing no improvement after 3 months of optimised standard treatment, a biopsy should be performed [15,94–97]. A punch biopsy from the wound border is sufficient to rule out malignancy [15], but the optimal way to perform a wound biopsy is a matter of debate. The French literature, for example, recommends diagnosing a hypertensive ischaemic leg ulcer exclusively on clinical grounds [104–106]. Our policy is to perform 4 mm wide, 3 cm long, cutaneous–subcutaneous biopsies from the surrounding skin into the wound [107]. Tumescent local anaesthesia guarantees analgesia. The 3 cm long, but narrow, biopsy wound can be easily closed with absorbable braided sutures. The risk of iatrogenic damage is small and justifiable. The body of the biopsy sent for histology should be left intact and sectioned lengthwise in order to obtain a histological profile from vital skin to the ulceration, extending from the epidermis to the deep subcutis. Punch biopsies are not suitable for diagnosing panarteritis nodosa cutanea or hypertensive ischaemic leg ulcer. Sampling error can lead to erroneous overdiagnosis of pyoderma gangrenosum or leukocytoclastic vasculitis [107,108].

Assessment of malnutrition. Total protein, albumin and lymphocyte count are sufficient to indicate malnutrition in the vast majority of cases [109,110]. More costly vitamin and/or zinc measurements should be restricted to specific situations [111,112].

Pain assessment. Pain should be assessed at regular (e.g. 4-week) intervals, with reproducible methods such as the visual analogue scale (VAS) [113,114].

Assessment of quality of life. The use of a standardised quality of life questionnaire (e.g. the more general SF36, or the more specific EQ-5D-3L or CIVIQ-20) is recommended [1–6].

Management

Compression therapy, either using bandages [115,116] or stockings [115,117], is the mainstay in the treatment of VLUs (Figure 102.3). Manual or mechanical lymph drainage (intermittent pneumatic compression) can be used as an adjunct [98,99,118,119]. Wound bed preparation considers *tissue* quality (T), *infection/*inflammation (I), *moisture* balance (M) and *edge* advancement (E), according to the TIME concept [120]. There is a large array of synthetic dressings and none is noticeably superior [121]. Dressings have to be selected according to the stage of wound healing and the TIME policy [120]. Initially, it is important to remove necrotic tissue and biofilm [93,122]. Most superinfected or critically colonised wounds benefit from local antiseptics. Povidone iodine [123,124] and sodium hypochlorite solution [124,125] are among the best investigated products. The use of local antibiotics can cause bacterial resistance and lead to allergies [126,127]. Systemic antibiotics are rarely involved in the treatment of chronic leg ulcers. Clinical signs of invasive infection, a swollen and red wound border and/or purulent discharge, with or without bacteraemia, are indications for bed rest and systemic administration of systemic antibiotics [126,127]. Negative pressure wound treatment (NPWT) is particularly effective in improving heavily infected wounds which have been debrided [128,129]. For optimal healing conditions, chronic wounds should be slightly moist. Therefore, heavily exuding wounds need highly absorbable synthetic dressings and frequent dressing changes, whereas dry wounds need hydrogels and semi-occlusive dressings to maintain an optimal moisture balance [120]. Ultimately, edge advancement is the result of optimal wound care. A variety of physical wound treatments with low-frequency pulsed current [130,131–133], low-dose high-frequency ultrasound [134], cold atmospheric argon plasma [135] or fluorescence biomodulation [136] have shown moderate, although statistically significant, enhancement of wound healing. Some chronic wounds fail to heal despite optimal management. A series of acellular and cellular matrices, or living skin equivalents, summarised as advanced therapies [137] in wound management, can be used to accelerate healing of refractory leg ulcers. Autologous skin grafts, such as punch grafts [138–143] or split-skin grafts [79,80,144,145], are a more invasive, but simple and proven alternative to treat hard-to-heal chronic wounds.

Approximately half of patients with VLU suffer from superficial venous reflux which can be abolished by a variety of methods (flush ligation and stripping, endovenous thermoablation, foam sclerotherapy) [29,35–40,54,55], whereas patients with predominantly deep venous reflux have less or no benefit from superficial vein surgery [29,54]. Longstanding VLUs that are located in areas of extensive dermatoliposclerosis benefit from tangential fibrosectomy followed by larger surface split-skin grafts (shave operation of VLU [77,79,80,145]; Figure 102.4). Recurrence of a healed VLU is common (30% in 12 months) if no preventative measures are taken. Consistent compression therapy [100] and the elimination of superficial venous reflux [29,54] are key to prevention.

An algorithm of management is summarised in Figure 102.5.

Mixed leg ulcer

Definition and nomenclature

Mixed leg ulcers are VLUs in a leg with concomitant peripheral arterial disease (PAD) [7,8,9,16,17,146–150]. They are harder to heal than VLUs and are indistinguishable on clinical appearance alone [16]. Diagnosis can only be made after vascular assessment. Bimalleolar (both medial and lateral) ulcer location is more common in MLUs than in VLUs [21]. Clinical grading of chronic venous

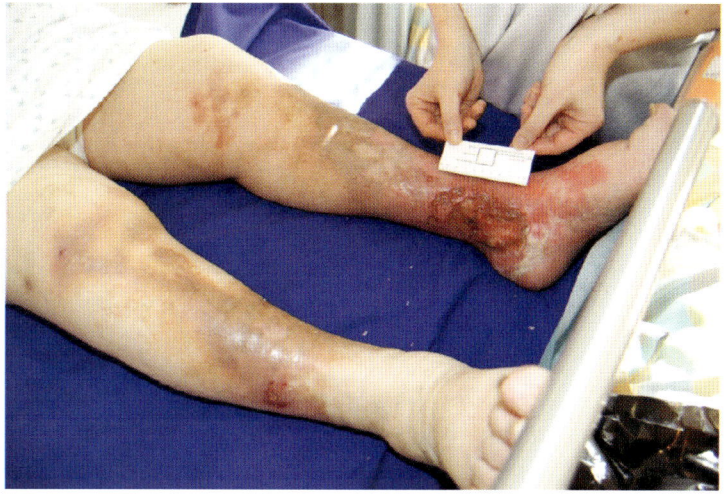

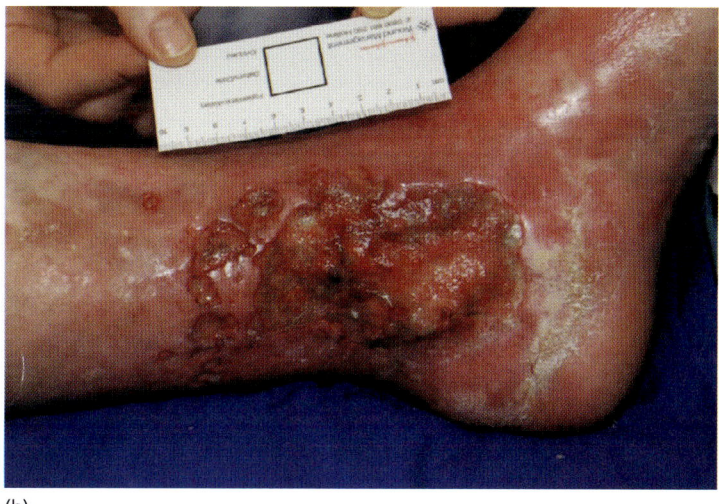

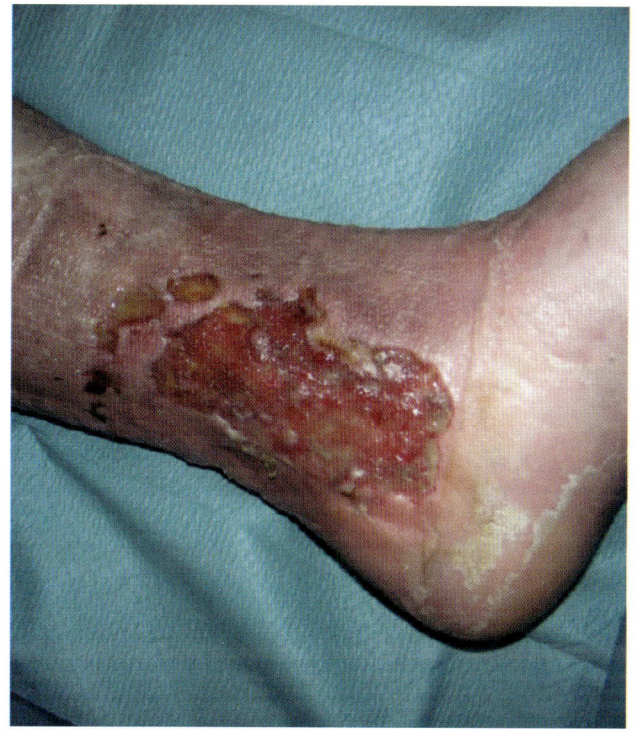

Figure 102.3 Venous leg ulcer. (a) A 77-year-old patient with chronic venous disease following recurrent venous thromboembolism. There was uncontrolled oedema and non-infectious redness of the skin; vascular assessment showed deep reflux of the superficial femoral and popliteal veins and segmental reflux of the long saphenous vein and side branches. There was no peripheral arterial disease. (b) Close-up view of the ulcer. (c) The same patient after 7 days of compression therapy with multilayer bandaging. The oedema and redness are under control, and there is early re-epithelialisation. This demonstrates the effectiveness of compression therapy.

insufficiency follows the CEAP classification [22], and PAD is graded after the Fontaine classification and the concept of chronic critical limb ischaemia (CLI) [18–20]. Most patients with MLU have Fontaine grade 2 PAD and do not meet the criteria of CLI [146–150].

Synonyms and inclusions
- Mixed venous and arterial leg ulcer

Introduction and general description

Approximately 20% of all leg ulcers are MLUs [16,17]. Since MLU patients with more advanced PAD do not tolerate compression therapy well, management primarily focuses on improving arterial inflow, mostly by the use of balloon catheter angioplasty (percutaneous transluminal angioplasty (PTA)), thereby transforming the MLU into a VLU [16,146–150]. As soon as the arterial

inflow is restored, management follows the algorithm for VLU (Figure 102.5).

Epidemiology
Incidence and prevalence
The lifetime incidence of leg ulcers is around 1% [41–49], with a point prevalence of 0.1%. Approximately 20% of all leg ulcers are MLUs, thus their lifetime incidence can be calculated as 0.2%, and point prevalence as 0.02%. The incidence of leg ulcers rises to 4% in the population aged over 80 years [45].

Age
Mixed leg ulcers at a young age are rare since PAD mainly affects people aged 50 years and older, thus MLUs primarily occur in this older age group [146–150].

Sex
Mixed leg ulcers occur equally in women and men [41,43,45,46, 146–150].

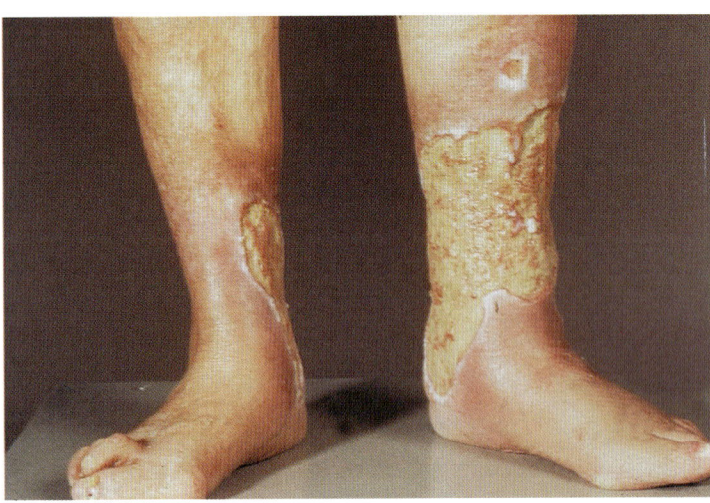

(a)

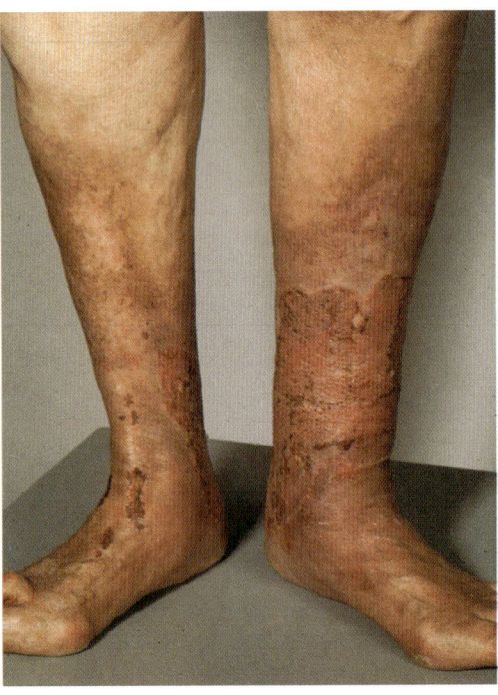

(b)

Figure 102.4 Post-thrombotic syndrome. (a) An 80-year-old patient with recurrent venous thromboembolism where the right leg shows a large chronic venous leg ulcer (VLU) at the medial ankle, the typical location. The left leg has a longstanding (approximately 30 years) circumferential VLU. (b) The same patient after a 'shave' operation with split-skin grafting in one procedure.

Ethnicity

Mixed leg ulcers occur in any country and population. The incidence and prevalence, however, have exclusively been investigated in western nations. Western lifestyle increases the risk for both CVD and PAD.

Associated diseases

Box 102.3 lists a number of the associated diseases.

Pathophysiology

Pathophysiology combines the pathophysiology of VLU [8–13] and PAD [18–20].

Venous leg ulcer (VLU)

↓

Vascular assessment:

Arterial examination and **venous** examination (see text)

↓

Exudate management according to the **TIME** concept

Management of **critical colonisation** or overt **infection**

Compression therapy (bandages or hosiery as practicable)

↓

Refluxive truncal veins: endovenous thermoablation or surgery

Feeder veins (side branches): US-guided foam sclerotherapy

Iliac vein stenosis-obstruction: recanalisation and stent

↓

No trend to healing (after 12 weeks):

A Wound biopsy (long, narrow, spindle-shaped biopsy): change management accordingly if alternative diagnosis occurs

B Punch grafts or **skin equivalents** (cellular/acellular)

or **shave therapy** and **split-skin graft** *or*

ulcer excision, negative pressure wound treatment and **graft**

↓

Prevention of recurrence:

Continue compression hosiery as long as underlying factors prevail

Figure 102.5 Algorithm of the management of venous leg ulcers. US, ultrasound.

Box 102.3 Disorders associated with mixed leg ulcers

- Venous thromboembolism
- Superficial venous thrombosis
- Varicose veins
- Chronic venous disease
- Stasis dermatitis
- Lipodermatosclerosis
- Acroangiodermatitis
- Obesity
- Smoking
- Diabetes
- Hyperlipidaemia
- Hypertension
- Coronary heart disease
- Stroke

Predisposing factors

Predisposing factors include family history [45], obesity [49,50], a standing occupation [73], venous thromboembolism [9,29,53,80], varicose veins [40,80], smoking [18–20], diabetes [18–20], hyperlipidaemia [18–20], hypertension [18–20], coronary heart disease [151,152], stroke [151,152], neuromuscular disease and joint disease [33,34].

Pathology
This is identical to VLU [72,74–78].

Clinical features
History
There is frequently a family history of CVD and VLU [45] and a personal history of venous thromboembolism [53,62,66,70] and/or varicose veins [9–12,36–40]. There are also cardiovascular risk factors: coronary heart disease, stroke and PAD [18–20,151,152].

Presentation
Mixed leg ulcers are clinically indistinguishable from VLUs [16,17,146] although a bimalleolar location (both medial and lateral skin ulcers on the same leg) occurs more frequently in MLUs (Figure 102.6) [16].

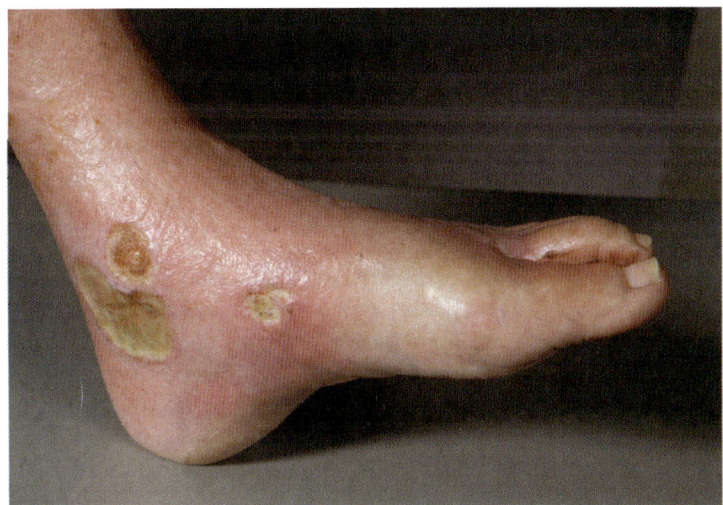

(a)

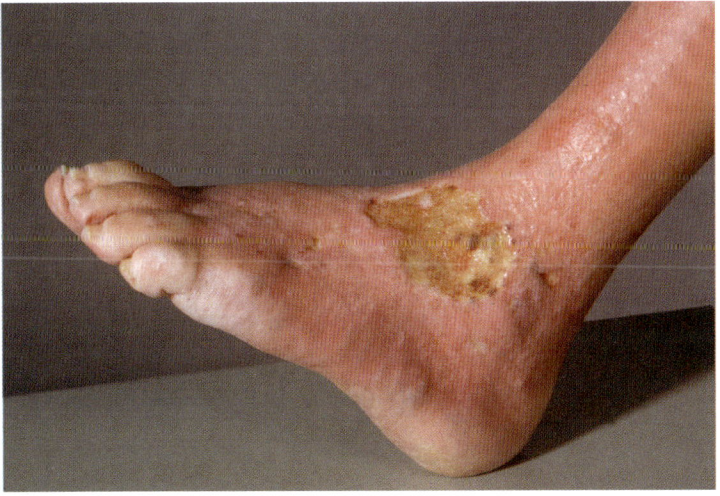

(b)

Figure 102.6 Mixed leg ulcer. (a) An 80-year-old patient with chronic venous disease with lipodermatosclerosis and chronic leg ulceration at the medial ankle region. Vascular assessment demonstrated insufficiency of the superficial femoral, popliteal and posterior tibial veins, as well as peripheral arterial disease (ankle pressure 104 mmHg, ankle brachial index 0.7). (b) The same patient with a chronic leg ulcer at the lateral ankle region (i.e. bimalleolar leg ulcers).

Clinical variants
These ulcers may be semicircumferential or circumferential in extensive cases [76,79,80], with CVD at the dorsum of the foot in such cases [16,17,146–153].

Differential diagnosis
This includes VLU, ALU, HYTILU and vasculitic leg ulcer [81–84] (particularly in patients with chronic hepatitis C with cryoglobulinaemia [85–87]) and males with Klinefelter syndrome [88,89].

Classification of severity
The CEAP system classifies active VLU as C6 and healed VLU as C5 [22]. The Fontaine classification of PAD and the concept of chronic CLI are also used [18–20] (see the section on arterial leg ulcers later in this chapter).

Complications and co-morbidities
These include chronic pain and impairment of quality of life [1–6], local wound infection, systemic infection and sepsis [92], infestation with maggots (fly larvae) [93], secondary squamous cell carcinoma [94–97], secondary lymphoedema (peri-ulcer lymphoedema and/or foot and toe lymphoedema) [98,99] and extensive tissue necrosis requiring major surgery or amputation [16,146–153,**154**].

Disease course and prognosis
There is a high risk of recurrence (50% in 12 months) [16,17,146–150]. Consistent compression therapy and angiological follow-up to quickly detect and re-treat PAD are key to reducing the frequency of recurrence [9,16,146–153,**154**]. Intermittent pneumatic compression (IPC) effectively treats both CVD and PAD. Therefore, IPC can be particularly beneficial to patients with MLU [119].

Investigations
Recommended investigations correspond to those for VLUs (see earlier section in this chapter) and work-up for detection and evaluation of PAD [7–20,146–153,**154**].

Management
An algorithm of management is summarised in Figure 102.7.

Arterial leg ulcer

Definition and nomenclature
Arterial leg ulcers are chronic skin ulcers primarily caused by skin ischaemia due to advanced PAD [16,**21**].

Synonyms and inclusions
- Ischaemic leg ulcer
- Leg ulcer in peripheral arterial disease

Introduction and general description
Arterial leg ulcers originate from local skin ischaemia in advanced PAD. They may occur spontaneously or after minor trauma to an

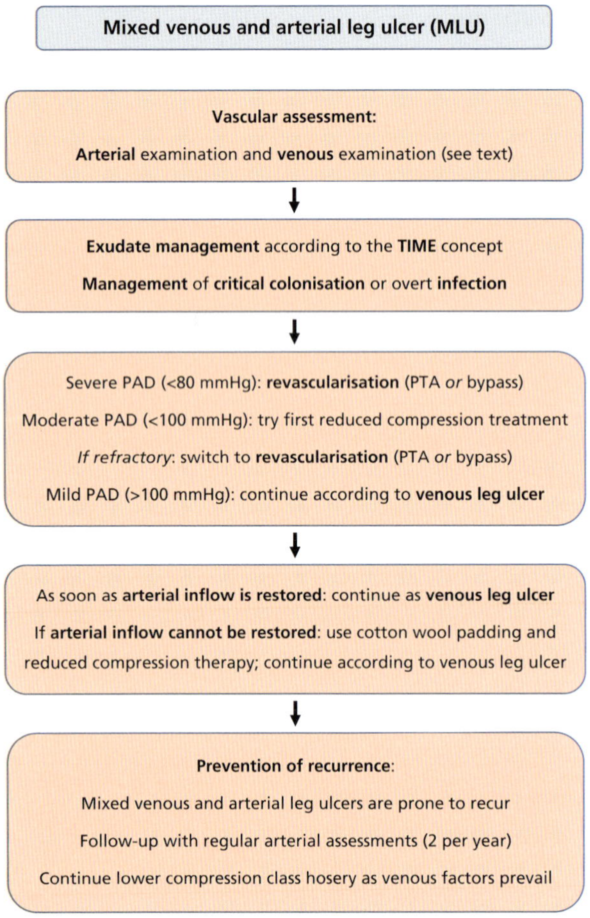

Figure 102.7 Algorithm of the management of mixed leg ulcers. PAD, peripheral arterial disease; PTA, percutaneous transluminal angioplasty.

area of ischaemic skin that is at risk of ulceration. Initially, they present as a black eschar or poorly granulating skin ulceration with a necrotic, black wound border. Delineation is sharp, and the wound border is generally steep. The surrounding skin does not exhibit signs of CVD, but looks unchanged and normal [16,17,21]. Distinction between ALU and HYTILU (see later in this chapter) can be challenging. Histology from debridement material or wound biopsy from ALU is non-specific and lacks subcutaneous arteriolosclerosis with medial calcification. Otherwise, by definition, HYTILU would be found in a leg with PAD [107,143,155].

The measurement of systolic ankle pressure (AP) and the calculation of the ankle brachial index (ABI) typically exhibit values of 70–100 mmHg AP, which corresponds to an ABI of 0.4–0.7, depending on the systolic blood pressure at the arm [21]. The criteria for CLI are rarely met: systolic AP <50 mmHg (or <70 mmHg in the presence of trophic skin lesions), systolic toe pressure <30 mmHg (or <50 mmHg in the presence of trophic skin lesions) and transcutaneous oxygen pressure ($tcPO_2$) <30 mmHg [18–20].

Epidemiology
Incidence and prevalence
The lifetime incidence of leg ulcers is around 1%, with a point prevalence of 0.1% [41–49]. Since ALUs and HYTILUs together account for approximately 10% of all leg ulcers, the lifetime incidence

of HYTILUs and ALUs can be calculated as 0.1%, and the point prevalence as 0.01%.

Age
Arterial leg ulcers generally affect people aged 50 years and above [21]. Since PAD mainly occurs in individuals older than 50 years, ALU is very rare in young adulthood.

Sex
Arterial leg ulcers occur equally in women and men [21].

Ethnicity
These ulcers occur in any country and population. The incidence and prevalence, however, have exclusively been investigated in western nations [7,8,17,21]. Western lifestyle increases the risk for ALUs.

Associated diseases
These include obesity, smoking, diabetes, hyperlipidaemia, hypertension, coronary heart disease and stroke [151,152].

Pathophysiology
Peripheral arterial disease leads to tissue ischaemia. The angiosome concept describes how each of the three calf arteries supplies arterial blood to well-delineated segments of the leg [156]. Occlusion of one or several branches of an atherosclerotic calf artery may directly and irreversibly shut down the skin circulation of a well-circumscribed area. The affected skin becomes cyanotic and then necrotic, a process accompanied by severe ischaemic pain. It remains to be shown if the lateral and pretibial skin circulation is less abundant and collateralised than at the medial and dorsal aspect of the leg, which would explain the proneness of these locations to be affected by ALUs.

Predisposing factors
Predisposing factors include smoking, diabetes, hyperlipidaemia, hypertension, coronary heart disease and stroke [151,152].

Pathology
The histology of ALU is non-specific. It shows tissue necrosis and – in the case of critical colonisation – dense inflammatory infiltrates with polymorphonuclear leukocytes.

Clinical features
History
There is a history of cardiovascular risk factors and often symptoms of atherosclerosis of other vascular territories (coronary heart disease, stroke, renal artery stenosis) [151,152].

Presentation
Arterial leg ulcers arise spontaneously as areas of painful skin necrosis (eschar), generally at the lateral or pretibial aspect of the leg (Figure 102.8). Typically, an ALU develops within normal-looking skin. Wound pain is intense or excruciating. The ulcer surface area tends to grow progressively. Clinically, there is a well-delineated zone of skin necrosis covered with eschar or remnants of necrotic

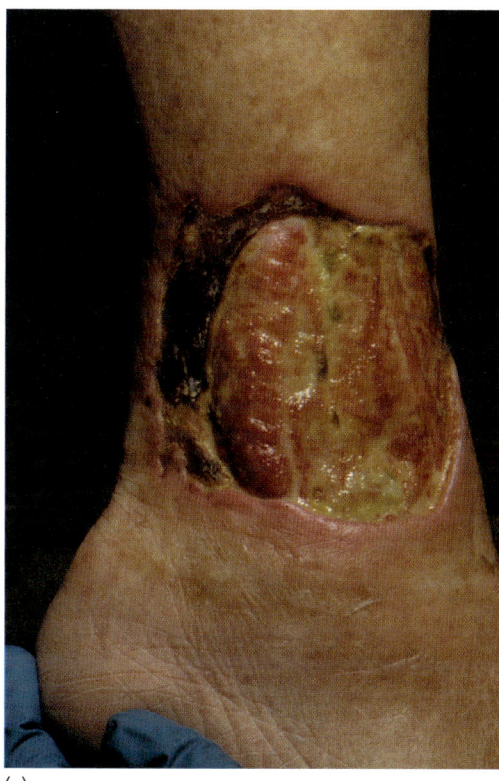

(a)

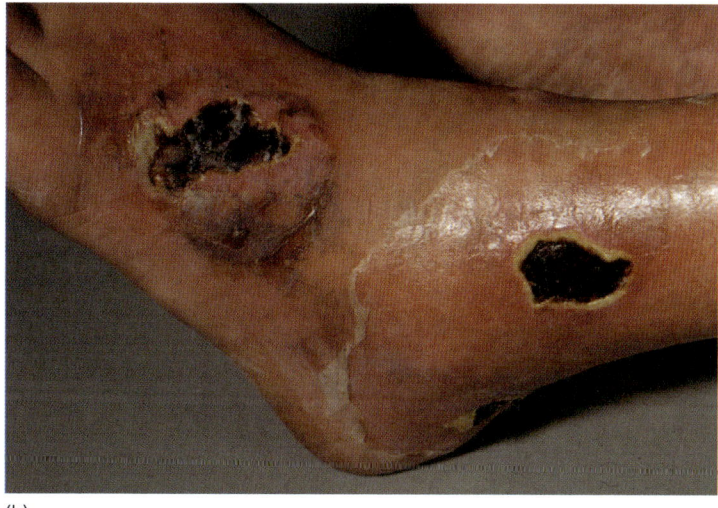

(b)

Figure 102.8 Arterial leg ulcer. (a) An 80-year-old patient with spontaneous and rapidly progressive, painful skin ulceration at the right lateral ankle region. Vascular assessment showed advanced peripheral arterial disease (ankle pressure 72 mmHg, ankle brachial index (ABI) 0.5). (b) A 51-year-old diabetic patient with skin necrosis with an eschar at the left lateral ankle and dorsum of the foot. Vascular assessment showed critical leg ischaemia (ankle pressure 54 mmHg, ABI 0.4, tcPO_2 21 mmHg).

wound border. Steep ulcer margins are usual, with a white or black wound base, with virtually no granulation tissue [21]. Smaller ALUs are round in shape and have a 'punched-out' appearance. Larger ALUs are polycyclic and figurated.

Clinical variants
Arterial ulcers at the dorsum of the foot usually occur in very advanced PAD, in a leg that typically meets the criteria of CLI [18–20]. ALUs can occur at a medial or dorsal location, however, this is unusual.

Differential diagnosis
This includes HYTILU [107,143,**157**] (in some situations discriminating between ALU and HYTILU is difficult), necrotising vasculitis [81–84], necrotising cutaneous embolism [158,159], pyoderma gangrenosum [160–162], necrotising cutaneous infections [163] and deep dissecting haematoma [164].

Classification of severity
Peripheral arterial disease can cause intermittent claudication (Fontaine grade 2), rest pain (Fontaine grade 3) and toe and/or forefoot necrosis (gangrene; Fontaine grade 4). The higher grades 3 and 4 of PAD commonly fulfil the criteria of chronic CLI, which are defined by systolic ankle pressure (<50 mmHg) and toe pressure (<30 mmHg) and tcPO_2 (<30 mmHg) [18–20]. ALUs do not fit well into the Fontaine classification, but approximately 90% correspond to Fontaine grade 2, even if they do not exhibit intermittent claudication, due to impaired mobility [21].

Complications and co-morbidities
These include chronic pain and impairment of quality of life [1–6], local wound infection, systemic infection and sepsis [102,103,163], infestation with maggots (fly larvae) [93] and extensive tissue necrosis requiring major surgery or amputation [18–20].

Disease course and prognosis
If PAD is amenable to PTA (balloon catheter angioplasty) or bypass surgery, prognosis is favourable [16,18–20,**21**]. Restored arterial inflow alleviates pain almost immediately [**21**]. Not all ALUs, however, heal spontaneously after revascularisation. The majority benefit from an early skin graft to speed up wound healing and to terminate wound pain [**21**]. The recurrence of ALUs is exceptional (unlike VLUs and MLUs) [**21**]. In patients who are not amenable to revascularisation, iloprost perfusions can add some benefit [18–20], and IPC helps improve microcirculation in PAD [119]. Wounds should be kept debrided, and occlusive wound dressings are contraindicated. Courses of antibiotic treatment may be required to treat critical colonisation, to reduce periwound oedema and to improve the chances of healing. Split-skin grafts should be tried even under suboptimal local conditions (e.g. little granulation tissue) [**21**].

Investigations
Work-up is required for the detection and evaluation of PAD [7–20].

Management
Percutaneous transluminal angioplasty (balloon angioplasty) or bypass surgery restores sufficient arterial inflow in the majority of cases [16,18–20,**21**]. As a result, wound pain improves dramatically, although the wounds do not necessarily start to heal [**21**]. Most patients still require a skin graft to speed up wound healing [**21**]. Recurrences of ALUs are exceptional [**21**].

An algorithm of management is summarised in Figure 102.9.

PART 9: VASCULAR DISORDERS

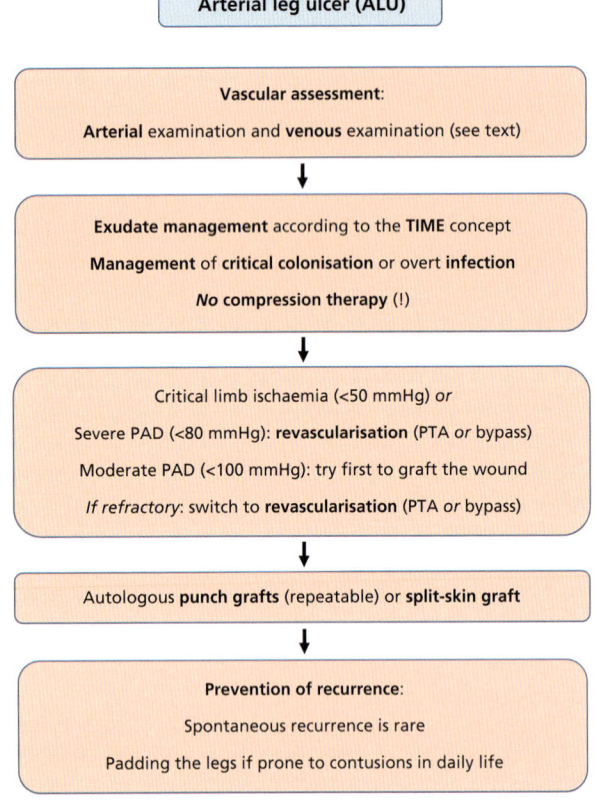

Figure 102.9 Algorithm of the management of arterial leg ulcers (ALUs). PAD, peripheral arterial disease; PTA, percutaneous transluminal angioplasty.

Hypertensive ischaemic leg ulcer

Definition and nomenclature

Hypertensive ischaemic leg ulcers represent a skin infarction due to ischaemic, subcutaneous arteriolosclerosis occurring in a patient with hypertension. Fifty-sixty per cent of patients have concomitant diabetes type 2 [107,165,166].

Synonyms and inclusions

- Martorell hypertensive ischaemic leg ulcer
- Ulcus hypertonicum Martorell
- Angiodermite nécrotique
- Martorell hypertensive ischaemic leg ulcer

Introduction and general description

First defined by Martorell in 1945 [167], and by Farber and Hines in 1946–47 [168], HYTILUs represent a form of skin infarction due to occlusive subcutaneous arteriolosclerosis [107,157,166–169]. Wound location is highly characteristic. In 80–90% of patients the eschar or wound is located at the laterodorsal aspect of the leg and/or over the Achilles tendon [107,143,155,170,171]. All patients have hypertension, and 60% have type 2 diabetes [107,165,166]. Clinically, HYTILU can be confused with pyoderma gangrenosum, vasculitic skin necrosis or ecthyma [107,108].

Epidemiology

Incidence and prevalence

The lifetime incidence of leg ulcers is around 1%, with a point prevalence of 0.1% [41–49]. Since ALUs and HYTILUs together account for approximately 10% of all leg ulcers [16,17], the lifetime incidence of HYTILUs and ALUs can be calculated as 0.1%, and the point prevalence as 0.01%.

Age

It is exceptional to see HIYTILUs at a young age, since longstanding hypertension and diabetes mainly affect individuals aged 50 years and older. Therefore, HYTLU typically occurs in patients aged over 50 years [107,143,157,165].

Sex

These ulcers occur equally in women and men [107,143,157,165].

Ethnicity

These ulcers occur in any country and population. The incidence and prevalence, however, have exclusively been investigated in western nations [107,143,157,165]. Western lifestyle increases the risk for HIYTILUs.

Associated diseases

Associated diseases include obesity, smoking, diabetes, hyperlipidaemia, hypertension, coronary heart disease and stroke [21,151,152,165].

Pathophysiology

An HYTILU is an ischaemic skin infarction caused by subcutaneous arteriolosclerosis (Figure 102.10) [107,157,166–169]. The arterioles regulate blood pressure, and hypertensive arteriolosclerosis is an expression of longstanding hypertension [107,165,167,168]. Most patients with HYTILUs have been treated for hypertension for many years and have controlled hypertension with normal blood pressure values. Antihypertensive treatment prevents large numbers of strokes and myocardial infarctions, leaving an increasingly large elderly population without any macrovascular complications of longstanding hypertension. This increases the likelihood that some well-treated hypertensive persons will develop HYTILUs as late complication of hypertension [107,172].

Hypertension and diabetes type 2 are the two undisputed risk factors of HYTILU. Oral anticoagulation with vitamin K antagonists may represent a further driver of disease. Calciphylaxis and HYTILU share striking morphological similarities, which suggests a common pathophysiology [173]. It has been shown that dysfunction of fetuin A and α_2-HS (Heremans–Schmid) glycoprotein A (matrix GLA) – two vitamin K-dependent proteins that protect tissues from calcification – can cause vascular calcification [165,174–178]. For the pathophysiology of calciphylaxis, medial calcification (and subintimal hyalinosis) is no longer believed to happen passively as a result of an elevated Ca × PO$_4$ product [172,173]. Recent research suggests that active biochemical cascades orchestrate simultaneous osseous break down and extraosseous calcification, summarised as chronic kidney disease–mineral bone

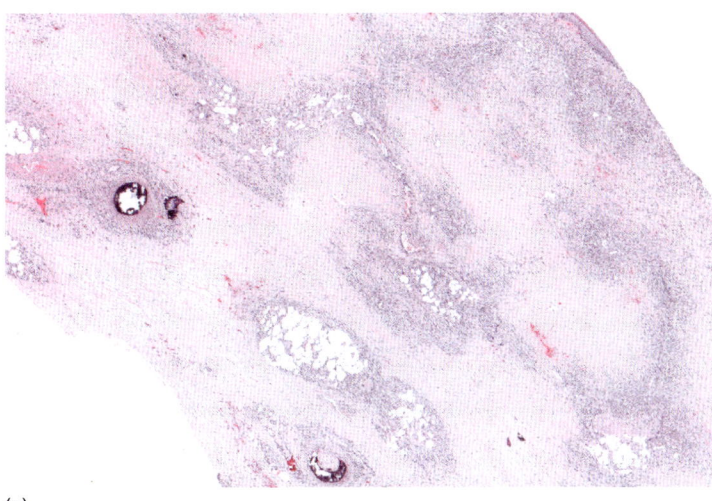

(a)

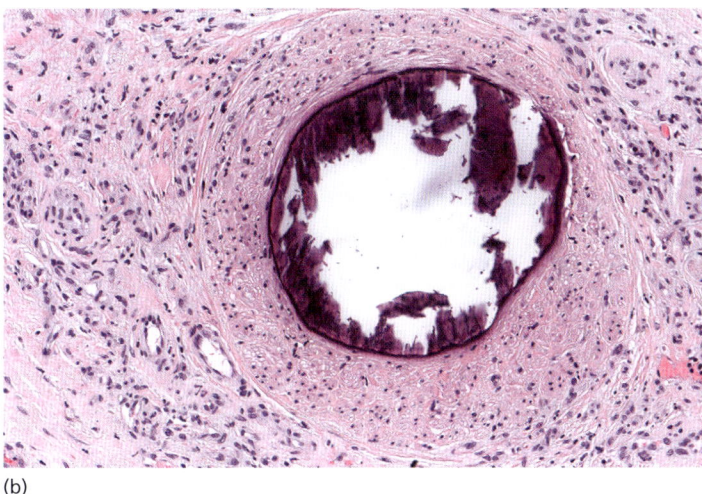

(b)

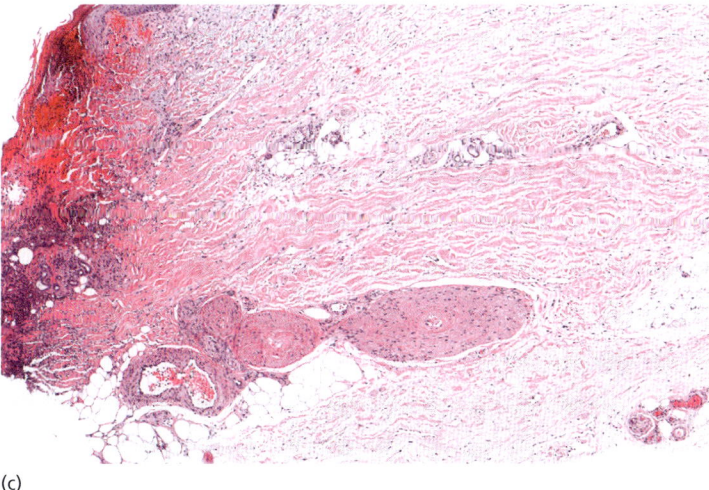

(c)

Figure 102.10 Subcutaneous arteriolosclerosis. (a, b) Skin biopsy showing subcutaneous arteriolosclerosis with medial calcification. (c) Skin biopsy showing stenotic subcutaneous arteriolosclerosis without medial calcification.

disorder (CKD-MBD) [179–182]. The better understanding of the pathophysiology of calciphylaxis can probably not be directly transferred to HYTILU, since HYTILU excludes by definition patients with advanced kidney disease (specifically KDIGO 4–5). Otherwise they would suffer calciphylaxis [172].

Predisposing factors
Predisposing factors include hypertension, diabetes type 2 [**107**, 165,166] and probably oral anticoagulation with vitamin K antagonists [165,172].

Pathology
The histology of HYTILUs is highly characteristic. The muscularis of the subcutaneous arterioles is greatly thickened at the expense of a narrow lumen [**107,157**,166–169]. Recently, however, the specificity of an increased wall-to-lumen ratio has been challenged. The wall-to-lumen ratio of subcutaneous arterioles does not significantly differ between various types of chronic leg ulcers, including VLU [166]. It can also be found coincidentally in any kind of skin biopsy from the leg, at a prevalence rising with patient age [106]. Arteriolar subendothelial hyalinosis (93%), medial calcinosis (76%) and decreased cellularity (Figure 102.10a, b) are the highly specific histological hallmarks of HYTILU [**107**,166]. Ring-shaped calcifications can be found in 35% of arterioles, horse-shaped in 26%, spotted in 9%, and 30% are completely calcified. Up to now extravascular calcification was considered specific to calciphylaxis. Recent work, however, has detected extravascular calcification in 85% of HYTILU sections as well. Alizarin Red S stain yields higher detection rates than haematoxylin and eosin (H&E) or von Kossa stains [169].

Clinical features
History
A history of longstanding and well-controlled hypertension, diabetes type 2 and atherosclerosis of other vascular territories (coronary heart disease, stroke, renal artery stenosis) is common [**21**,151,152].

Presentation
This ulcer usually starts as violaceous spot that rapidly turns black. Small lesions tend to remain more superficial, involving the epidermis and dermis, and can heal spontaneously. Larger lesions show a black eschar at the centre and a rapidly progressive violaceous undermined border. This circumscribed form of skin infarction commonly causes excrutiating pain. The classic location is at the laterodorsal aspect of the leg and/or over the Achilles tendon (Figure 102.11) [**107,157**,170–172]. In larger lesions, the necrosis comprises all skin levels and extends down to the fascia.

Clinical variants
There is overlap in localisation patterns, although the classic laterodorsal ulcer presentation prevails (80–90%). Mediodorsal (10–20%) and ventral (pretibial) (10%) location can occur simultaneously or as the sole manifestation [171]. HYTILUs are typically located at the mid-leg (more distant from the sole) compared with, for example, VLUs, MLUs or ALUs, which are typically located around the ankles [171]. A few patients (10%) exhibit isolated

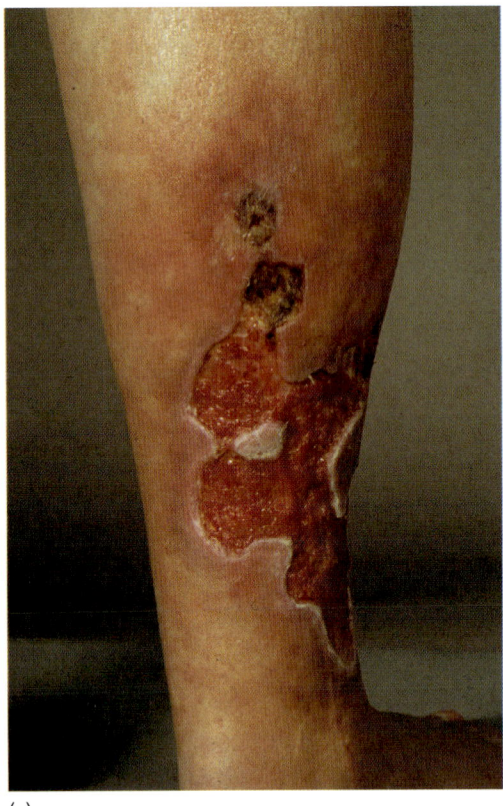

(a)

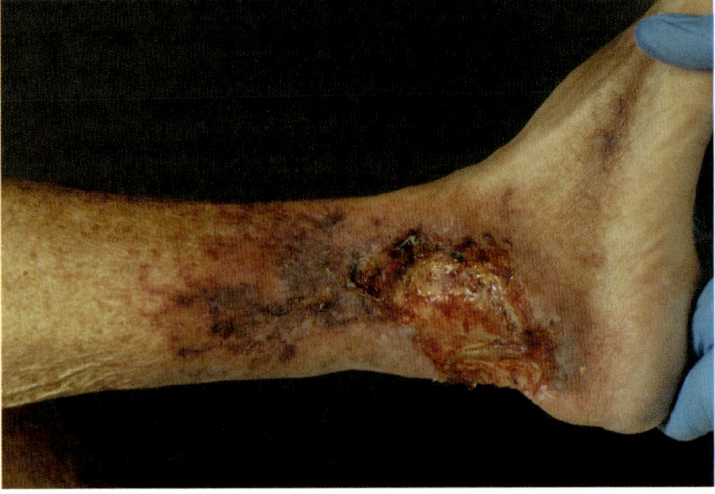

(b)

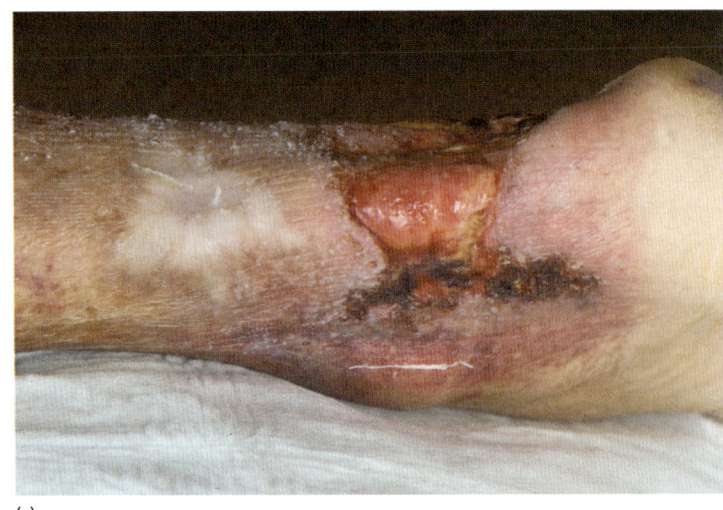

(c)

Figure 102.11 (a) A 65-year-old patient with hypertension (well controlled), diabetes (well controlled) and a polycyclic, figurated, painful ulcer at the laterodorsal aspect of the right leg. Vascular assessment showed no peripheral arterial disease (ankle pressure 132 mmHg, ankle brachial index (ABI) 1.0). (b) A 73-year-old patient with hypertension, no diabetes and skin necrosis at the right lateral ankle region, extending to the Achilles tendon. Vascular assessment showed no peripheral arterial disease (ankle pressure 146 mmHg, ABI 0.9). (c) The same patient as Figure 102.3 showing skin ulceration at the left Achilles tendon.

skin necrosis over the Achilles tendon as the sole manifestation [107,170–172].

Differential diagnosis

This includes pyoderma gangrenosum [160–163], vasculitic leg ulcer [81–84] and ecthyma [102,103].

Classification of severity

Different grades of severity exist, but up to now they have not been standardised.

Complications and co-morbidities

These include chronic pain and impairment of quality of life, local wound infection, systemic infection and sepsis, and exceptionally death [107,157,165]. Extensive tissue necrosis may require major surgery or, exceptionally, amputation.

Disease course and prognosis

Prognosis is good even though HYTILU represents a severe disease in older people. Half of patients require not only one, but several, skin grafts to completely heal all their wounds. Even if skin grafts do not 'take', pain often gets immediately alleviated and controlled [107,143,155].

Investigations

Recommended investigations correspond to those in ALUs (see earlier section in this chapter). The need to perform a wound and edge biopsy is a matter of debate [105–106,107]. As a rule these authors perform spindle biopsies of 3 × 0.4 cm for larger HYTILUs that require wound surgery at some point of treatment or in cases of diagnostic uncertainty. Laboratory work should rule out end-stage kidney disease (KDIGO 4–5). Patients with progressive skin necrosis and/or acral gangrene who have end-stage kidney disease (KDIGO 4–5) probably suffer from calciphylaxis. They urgently

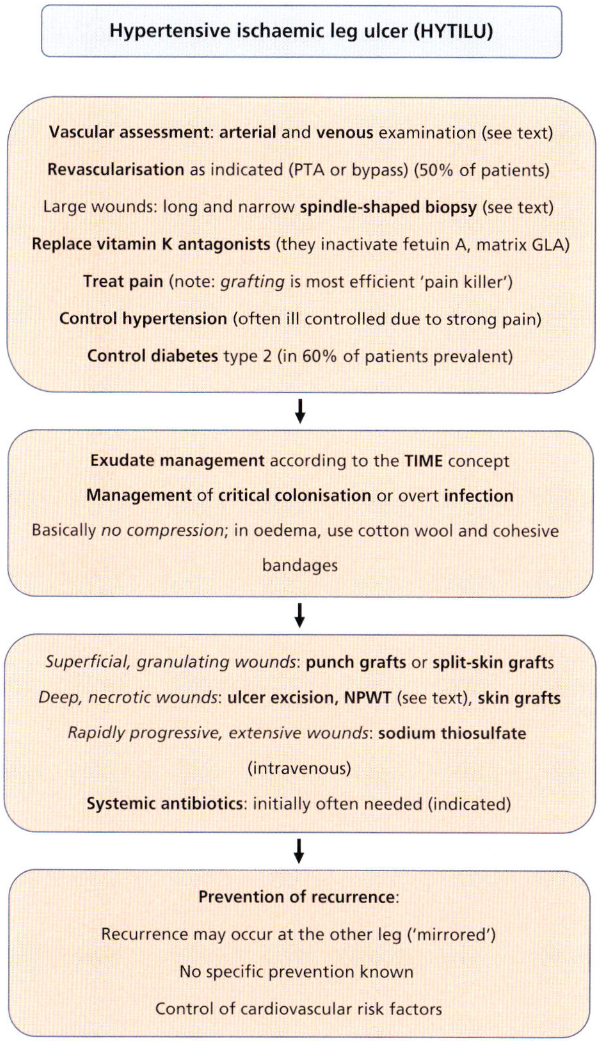

Figure 102.12 Algorithm of management of hypertensive ischaemic leg ulcers. GLA, glycoprotein A; NPWT, negative pressure wound treatment; PTA, percutaneous transluminal angioplasty.

need nephrology assessment. Relevant local or systemic infection requires microbiology, including tissue cultures.

Management

Pain control is the first thing to achieve. Skin grafts offer the most effective form of pain control [107,143,155], however their successful use requires some preparatory steps. Oral anticoagulation with vitamin K antagonists should be stopped [165,173] and replaced with other forms of anticoagulation, depending on indication, co-morbidities and co-medication. PAD (arterial macroangiopathy of the leg) should be searched for and, if necessary, treated [107]. Small HYTILUs do not require wound biopsy since this carries a risk of iatrogenic damage. Cautious superficial debridement combined with punch grafts may accelerate healing. Larger, progressive HYTILUs require an active surgical approach. Most patients benefit from systemic antibiotic treatment, early debridement, NPWT and early skin grafting [107,155]. Often, skin grafts take in the centre of the wound, whereas the wound borders continue to become necrotic and to expand. In such cases, serial debridements and skin grafts usually are the most effective way to end the ongoing process of skin infarction. Most extensive cases of HYTILU benefit from intravenous sodium thiosulfate [172,183], although this remains to be better studied in clinical trials [183–185].

An algorithm of management is summarised in Figure 102.12.

Key references

The full list of references can be found in the online version at https://www.wiley.com/rooksdermatology10e

8 Singer AJ, Tassiopoulos A, Kirsner RS. Evaluation and management of lower-extremity ulcers. *N Engl J Med* 2017;377:1559–67.

14 Wittens C, Davies AH, Baekgaard N *et al*. Editor's choice – Management of chronic venous disease: clinical practice guidelines of the European Society for Vascular Surgery (ESVS). *Eur J Vasc Endovasc Surg* 2015;49:678–737.

21 Hafner J, Schaad I, Schneider E *et al*. Leg ulcers in peripheral arterial disease (arterial leg ulcers): impaired wound healing above the threshold of chronic critical limb ischemia. *J Am Acad Dermatol* 2000;43:1001–8.

23 Isoherranen K, O'Brien JJ, Barker J *et al*. Atypical wounds. Best clinical practice and challenges. *J Wound Care* 2019;28(Suppl. 6):S1–92.

55 Gohel MS, Heatley F, Liu X *et al*. A randomized trial of early endovenous ablation in venous ulceration. *N Engl J Med* 2018;378:2105–14.

107 Hafner J, Nobbe S, Partsch H *et al*. Martorell hypertensive ischemic leg ulcer: a model of ischemic subcutaneous arteriolosclerosis. *Arch Dermatol* 2010; 146:961–8.

120 Schultz GS, Barillo DJ, Mozingo DW *et al*. Wound bed preparation and a brief history of TIME. *Int Wound J* 2004;1:19–32.

130 Piaggesi A, Lauchli S, Bassetto F *et al*. Advanced therapies in wound management: cell and tissue based therapies, physical and bio-physical therapies, smart and IT based technologies. *J Wound Care* 2018;27(Suppl. 6a):S1–137.

154 Obermayer A, Gostl K, Walli G *et al*. Chronic venous leg ulcers benefit from surgery: long-term results from 173 legs. *J Vasc Surg* 2006;44:572–9.

157 Vuerstaek JD, Reeder SW, Henquet CJ *et al*. Arteriolosclerotic ulcer of Martorell. *J Eur Acad Dermatol Venereol* 2010;24:867–74.

PART 9: VASCULAR DISORDERS

CHAPTER 103

Disorders of the Lymphatic System

Peter S. Mortimer and Kristiana Gordon

St George's Hospital, London, UK

PART 9: VASCULAR DISORDERS

Introduction

Basic principles

The lymphatic system is the body's cleansing and drainage system as well as being a transport route for immune cells and fat [1]. It is often described as the body's second circulation after the blood circulation. It consists of lymphatic vessels operating as a one-way drainage system (containing lymph) and the lymphoid organs (the role of which is mainly in host defence). It behaves like a one-way drainage system such as a river. Tissue fluid is absorbed by blind-ending lymphatic capillaries otherwise known as initial *lymphatic vessels* (like the tentacles on sea anemones) to become lymph. Lymph flows through increasingly bigger lymphatic vessels towards lymph nodes. After absorption by initial lymphatics, lymph enters the larger *collecting lymphatics* which are invested by smooth muscle to enable pumping. Collecting lymphatics contain valves that enable unidirectional flow. The lymphatic vessels are lined by endothelial cells. Lymph flows through a series of lymphoid organs such as lymph nodes before finally discharging back into the blood circulation via the thoracic duct. Lymph is interstitial (tissue)

Rook's Textbook of Dermatology, Tenth Edition. Edited by Christopher Griffiths, Jonathan Barker, Tanya Bleiker, Walayat Hussain and Rosalind Simpson.
© 2024 John Wiley & Sons Ltd. Published 2024 by John Wiley & Sons Ltd.

fluid, originally formed from a plasma ultrafiltrate, containing salts, proteins, fat and immune cells particularly lymphocytes and dendritic cells.

Lymphoid organs/tissues are organised structures within the lymphatic system that support immune responses through the receipt of antigen-presenting cells (APCs) and lymphocyte activation. Lymph nodes are secondary lymphoid organs (bone marrow and thymus are primary lymphoid organs and the sites of lymphocyte production). Lymph node-like structures such as mucosa-associated lymphoid tissue are also secondary lymphoid organs. The main cell of any lymphoid organ is the lymphocyte but also present are macrophages, vascular endothelium in the form of high endothelial venules and lymphoid stromal cells which include the specialised reticular and dendritic cells. These cells express cytokines and adhesion molecules, as well as other factors required for the migration, homeostasis and survival of immune cells. Adaptive immunity occurs within the secondary lymphoid organs.

Lymphatic dysfunction interferes with tissue immunity as well as fluid and fat homeostasis, resulting in a predilection to infection, oedema and disturbances in fat absorption and peripheral fat deposition.

Immunity and the lymphatic system

Many figures in publications on immune cell trafficking do not feature the lymphatics yet it is the lymphatic endothelial cells that provide the traffic light signals to direct immune cells towards, and into, the lymphatic vessels for transport to the lymph nodes, and other secondary lymphoid organs, which are the engine room for adaptive immunity. Trafficking of lymphocytes and dendritic cells via lymphatic vessels, with processing in lymph nodes, provides an important immunosurveillance function. Cells of the innate immune system, including dendritic cells, neutrophils and monocytes, as well as the adaptive immune system, including activated lymphocytes such as T and B cells, use lymphatic vessels to migrate from tissues into lymph nodes [2,3]. Lymphatic vessels are the primary route of communication from the skin to the immune system [4]. Dendritic cells such as Langerhans cells acting as APCs play an essential sentinel function by taking up antigen and transporting it via the lymphatics to the lymph nodes for T-cell recognition and the priming of immune responses (Figure 103.1) [5,6].

The inflammasome is a multiprotein intracellular complex that detects pathogenic microorganisms and sterile stressors, and activates the highly pro-inflammatory cytokines interleukin-1b (IL-1b) and IL-18. It is involved in the recycling of immune cells in lymph nodes. Dysregulation of inflammasomes is associated with a number of autoinflammatory syndromes and autoimmune diseases [7,8].

Fluid homeostasis, oedema and the lymphatic system

Fluid released from blood vessels into tissues is then drained away in the lymph and not, as was previously thought, removed by venous reabsorption [9]. It is therefore lymph drainage that mainly controls tissue fluid volume. This has implications for tissue fluid and plasma volume homeostasis.

All chronic peripheral oedema (i.e. subcutaneous oedema persisting for at least 3 months) is caused by either an absolute reduction in lymph transport, as in lymphoedema, or by lymph drainage being

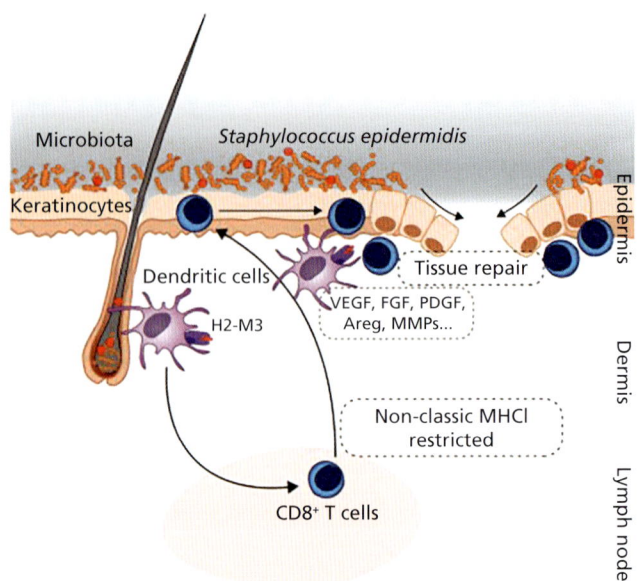

Figure 103.1 Microbiota induce a form of adaptive immunity that couples antimicrobial function with tissue repair. Areg, amphiregulin; FGF, fibroblast growth factor; MHCl, major histocompatibility complex (MHC) class I; MMPs, metalloproteinases; PDGF, platelet-derived growth factor; VEGF, vascular endothelial growth factor. Adapted from Lineham *et al*. 2018 [6].

overwhelmed by a fluid (lymph) load, such as occurs with higher venous pressures from heart failure or venous disease. Therefore, chronic oedema always represents lymph drainage failure and as it is easy to identify and has the same physiological effects, it can be considered a surrogate for lymphoedema.

Any chronic oedema represents lymphatic failure. If impaired lymph drainage is predominantly responsible, then lymphoedema results. This produces characteristic skin changes known as elephantiasis as well as fibrosis and increased fat deposition. Impaired immune cell trafficking results in an increased risk of infection, particularly cellulitis (erysipelas), which often becomes recurrent. This chapter describes the clinical consequences of lymphatic dysfunction and in particular the impact on the skin and subcutaneous tissues. The sections are divided according to common clinical presentations.

Fat homeostasis, nutrition and peripheral fat

Intestinal lymphatics (lacteals) are responsible for most fat absorption and consequently absorption of fat-soluble vitamins including vitamin D. Peripheral lymphatics are important for the return of extravascular lipoproteins to the blood. Reverse cholesterol transport is a multistep process resulting in the net movement of cholesterol from peripheral tissues back to the liver by first entering the lymphatic system. If lymph drainage is impaired, fat, as much as fluid, builds up in peripheral tissues [10]. This can influence subcutaneous fat accumulation and therefore obesity.

Lymphatic involvement in skin disease

The role of the lymphatic system in skin disease has not been specifically studied but much can be deduced from our knowledge of lymphatic function in general. *Inflammatory skin disease* inevitably will have increased blood flow and increased vascular permeability. The result will be increased microvascular filtration of fluid which then percolates through tissue and drains as lymph. Therefore, inflammation increases lymph load. This will apply to *eczematous dermatitis* where inflammatory fluid collects as spongiosis in the epidermis, in *urticaria* where fluid collects to form wheals before draining away in the lymph, and in *psoriasis* where lymphatic vessels as well as blood vessels are altered. The thickened plaque is as much to do with the upper dermal oedema as the keratinocyte hyperplasia [1]. Biological therapies aimed at blocking certain cytokines (e.g. IL-17 in psoriasis) may also exert parts of their anti-inflammatory effects by modulating the lymphatic vasculature [2]. In the dermis of psoriasis plaques, some elements of lymph node structure are contained in dermal aggregates, otherwise known as a tertiary lymphoid tissue or structure which may perpetuate the disease [3]. Tertiary lymphoid structures in cutaneous melanoma are postulated to serve as dynamic centres for the initiation of robust antitumour responses within affected regions of active disease [4].

The skin is a complex and dynamic ecosystem containing microbes – the microbiota. These microbes not only contribute to the development and function of the immune system but are also continuously sensed by the immune system via the lymphatic system. The constant feed of information by skin-resident APCs to lymphocytes within the lymph nodes results in a population of highly diverse T cells within the skin. The result of this dialogue is the induction of cognate, non-inflammatory B- and T-cell responses that control various aspects of skin function. One function of this homeostatic immunity between the skin and lymphoid organs is to identify and react to pathogens, but another role is to identify and tolerate non-pathogenic commensal microbes. Certain strains of *Staphylococcus aureus* are not only associated with more severe atopic dermatitis but are also sufficient to induce skin inflammation independent of host genetic predisposition [5]. In addition to their well-recognised importance in adaptive immunity, lymph nodes are reported to efficiently filter microbes and orchestrate innate immune responses that contain and kill pathogens [6].

B cells are sensitised in the lymph node to respond to antigens carried from the skin via the lymphatics. Without initial sensitisation via the lymphatics, immunoglobulin E (IgE)-mediated allergy would not occur. The lymphatic system appears to be important for self-tolerance in that it polices for self-antigens involving regulatory T cells.

The growth of new lymphatic vessels (lymphangiogenesis) accelerates *wound healing* and is required for local fluid homeostasis, granulation tissue formation, leukocyte trafficking and matrix remodelling. Poor lymph drainage results in oedema, fibrosis and lipid deposition, all of which have the potential to impair wound healing. Defective healing of chronic wounds in diabetic patients can be attributed, in part, to a deficiency in lymphatic regenerative potential.

Diagnosis of lymphoedema

A failure of lymph drainage results in a build-up of lymph within the body's tissues. If this affects peripheral tissues, it is called lymphoedema. Lymph is interstitial fluid formed from a blood capillary filtrate that would normally drain via the lymphatic system.

Chronic oedema

Definition and nomenclature

Oedema simply means swelling (Greek *oídēma*, a swelling) but implies a build-up of fluid within tissues. Interstitial fluid is reabsorbed almost entirely by the lymphatic vessels. Contrary to popular belief, venous reabsorption of interstitial fluid cannot be maintained for any length of time in peripheral tissues [1]. Therefore, all peripheral oedema represents lymphatic failure. Most chronic oedemas arise from increased microvascular filtration overwhelming the lymph drainage. Chronic peripheral oedema means excess fluid within skin and subcutaneous tissues that is of more than 3 months' duration.

Synonyms and inclusions
- Oedema
- Lymphoedema (primary and secondary)
- Venous oedema
- Phlebolymphoedema
- Elephantiasis
- Dependency oedema

Difference between chronic oedema and lymphoedema

There is little difference in composition between tissue fluid and lymph. Tissue fluid becomes lymph once it has entered the lymphatic system. All chronic oedema is a dynamic state balancing the inflow of fluid from blood vessels (lymph production or lymph load) with the outflow from lymph drainage. Chronic oedema is a clinical sign but lymphoedema is a diagnosis. In physiological terms chronic oedema always represents lymph drainage failure, and as it is easy to identify and has the same physiological effects, it can be considered a surrogate for lymphoedema. Both are due to lymph drainage failure, have the same pathophysiology and can be treated in the same way.

Epidemiology

Using chronic oedema as a surrogate for lymphoedema, the crude community prevalence was found to be as high as 3.93 per 1000 in an East Midlands population of the UK [2]. The prevalence increased with age and was twice as common in women as in men. The prevalence among hospital in-patients was 28.5%. Only 3% of patients in the community population had oedema related to cancer or cancer treatment but 40% had a concurrent leg ulcer.

A previous study using the same methodology in southwest London had determined a prevalence of 1.33/1000 population with a prevalence of 5.4/1000 in subjects aged over 65 years (i.e 1 in 200). In only a quarter did the oedema arise from cancer treatment [3].

Pathophysiology

Oedema develops when the microvascular (capillary and venular) filtration rate exceeds lymph drainage for a period of time. For

Table 103.1 Causes of chronic oedema.

Increased capillary filtration			Reduced lymph drainage	
↑ **Capillary pressure**	↓ **Plasma proteins**	↑ **Capillary permeability**	**Primary lymphatic insufficiency**	**Secondary lymphatic insufficiency**

↑ Venous pressure:
Right heart failure
DVT
Venous obstruction
Calcium channel antagonists
Dependency
Overtransfusion:
Salt and water overload
Advanced renal failure
↑ Blood flow:
Inflammation
Arteriovenous fistula
	↑ Loss:
	Nephrotic syndrome
	Protein-losing enteropathy
	↓ Synthesis:
	Cirrhosis
	Advanced cancer
	Malabsorption
	Malnutrition
		Inflammation:
		Varicose eczema
		Psoriasis
		Chronic infection
		Urticaria and angio-oedema
		Drugs
			Germline mutation:
			Genes known (Milroy disease,
			  lymphoedema, distichiasis)
			Genes unknown (Meige
			  disease)
			Mosaic mutation:
			Lymphatic malformation
			Overgrowth spectrum
				Iatrogenic:
				Surgery
				Radiotherapy
				Cancer
				Infection:
				Filanasis
				Cellulitis
				Accidental trauma
				Obesity
				Immobility
				Sustained lymph load:
				Venous disease
				Heart failure
				Venous obstruction
				DVT

DVT, deep-vein thrombosis.

oedema to develop either the microvascular filtration rate (lymph production) is high, the lymph flow is low, or there is a combination of the two.

The filtration rate is governed by the Starling principle of fluid exchange. Microvascular filtration of fluid from the capillary into the interstitium is driven by the hydraulic (water) pressure gradient across the blood vessel wall $(P_c - P_i)$ in which P_c indicates capillary pressure and P_i indicates interstitial pressure, and is opposed by the osmotic pressure gradient $(\pi_p - \pi_i)$ in which π_p indicates plasma osmotic pressure and π_i indicates interstitial osmotic pressure from tissue proteins. This is the suction force retaining fluid within the vessel. The colloid osmotic pressures influencing filtration across both fenestrated and continuous capillaries are exerted across the endothelial glycocalyx; the osmotic pressure of the interstitial fluid does not directly determine transendothelial fluid exchange. There is substantial evidence that with important exceptions such as the renal cortex and medulla, downstream microvessels are not in a state of sustained fluid absorption as traditionally depicted. Although doggedly persistent in textbooks and teaching, the traditional view of a filtration–reabsorption balance has little justification in the microcirculation of most tissues. Tissue fluid balance thus depends critically on lymphatic function in most tissues. Unlike the circulation where the heart pumps the blood around, lymph flow depends entirely on changes in local tissue pressures to drive fluid into and then along the initial lymphatics (lymph capillaries).

Most forms of chronic oedema derive from increased lymph production overwhelming the capacity of lymph drainage. Higher venous pressures in venous disease and heart failure change the Starling pressures and force more fluid from the blood vessels into the tissues, overwhelming the capacity of the lymph drainage to respond. In protein-losing states such as nephrotic syndrome and protein-losing enteropathy, the lower plasma osmotic pressure also encourages the escape of fluid from the blood vessels to increase lymph load. Dependency oedema is when gravitational forces increase venous pressures during standing and sitting to increase lymph load but limited movement results in no compensatory increase in lymph drainage (Table 103.1). Inflammatory oedema occurs from increased blood flow and increased vascular permeability raising lymph production. This can be seen with profound dermatitis.

In cases of sustained blood capillary filtration and thus high lymph load, the lymphatic vessels can eventually fail so that even if the increased lymph load is corrected the lymph drainage is permanently damaged and chronic oedema/lymphoedema remains. A good example is chronic venous disease which progresses to phlebolymphoedema.

Clinical features

Interstitial fluid volume must increase by over 100% before oedema is clinically detectable through pitting or indentation of the skin from pressure. Dermal oedema manifests as 'peau d'orange' due to expansion of the interfollicular dermis by fluid, whereas subcutaneous oedema gives rise to pitting. Pitting is a sign where pressure on the skin pushes fluid away to leave an indentation or pit when the pressure is removed.

Chronic oedema of the lower limbs due to high venous pressures will improve considerably overnight in bed if leg elevation allows venous pressures to drop and thereby reduce lymph production. However, lymphoedema does not reduce much overnight owing to the fact that elevation does not improve lymph drainage. Diuretics do not have much impact on chronic oedema where the dominant cause is impaired lymph drainage because they do not improve lymph flow. Diuretics work by reducing lymph production in circumstances of increased microvascular filtration secondary to salt and water overload (e.g. heart failure).

Investigations

Any chronic oedema should be assessed through a full history and examination followed by investigation. Causes of increased lymph production such as heart failure, venous disease and inflammation can be judged clinically.

The following blood tests should be considered:

- B-type natriuretic peptide (BNP) estimation is a useful screen for cardiac failure. The main clinical utility of either BNP or N-terminal pro-BNP (NT-proBNP) is that a normal level rules out cardiac failure.
- Plasma albumin should be measured and if low a search for loss (e.g. nephrotic syndrome or protein-losing enteropathy) or failure of synthesis (e.g. liver disease or malnutrition) should be considered.
- Local inflammation (e.g. infection, dermatitis or underlying arthritis) can be suspected if there are elevated levels of white blood cell count, erythrocyte sedimentation rate (ESR), C-reactive protein (CRP) and complement.

Venous or lymphatic obstruction may require ultrasound, computed tomography (CT) or magnetic resonance imaging (MRI). The gold standard investigation for chronic venous disease is colour Doppler duplex ultrasound and for lymph drainage abnormalities it is lymphoscintigraphy.

Management

If swelling is due to fluid, it is best not to approach a lower limb chronic oedema clinically by trying to pigeonhole the diagnosis into 'cardiac failure', 'venous oedema', 'lymphoedema', etc. A far better approach is to consider if the oedema represents pure lymphatic drainage failure, or, as is most common, increased lymph production overwhelming the lymph drainage capacity.

Most cases of chronic oedema have more than one factor contributing to the impaired lymph drainage and increased capillary filtration. Consequently, treatment of chronic oedema should aim to enhance lymph drainage and address any factors causing increased lymph production.

If lower limb oedema is unilateral or asymmetrical then local factors should be considered such as pelvic lymph or venous obstruction, post-thrombotic syndrome or inflammation from dermatitis or infection. Bilateral lower limb oedema suggests systemic factors such as hypoproteinaemia or high central venous pressure (e.g. heart failure). In an obese person, several factors contribute: increased intrabdominal pressure obstructs flow, and the weight of a huge abdominal apron when sitting causes obstruction of lymph and venous drainage in the thigh or groin; therefore weight loss is always helpful [4].

Poor mobility results in no enhancement of lymph drainage. Sitting with legs dependent causes periods of high venous pressure and consequently high microvascular fluid filtration (falling asleep in a chair without leg elevation is particularly bad). Sleep apnoea syndrome leads to periods of arterial and pulmonary hypertension and fluid retention [5].

Treatment of increased lymph production will depend on the cause. There is no drug or universally approved surgery for improving lymph drainage. Standard care is physically based therapy to stimulate lymph flow through a combination of movement combined with compression, with prudent use of massage techniques.

Lymphoedema

Definition
Lymphoedema occurs when lymph collects in tissues to cause swelling.

Introduction and general description
Strictly, lymphoedema is caused solely by impaired lymph drainage, but in practice lymphoedema can have multiple causes with an ever-changing balance between lymph production and lymph drainage. Lymphoedema is a common clinical condition encountered in all ages but is not often diagnosed except in well-recognised circumstances such as following cancer surgery.

Epidemiology
Reliable incidence and prevalence data for lymphoedema have been elusive or non-existent. Published prevalence estimates for the population generally derive from extrapolations related to the soft data surrounding the relevant cancers and infections that predispose to acquired lymphoedema.

Lymphoedema is not often diagnosed unless presenting in well-recognised circumstances such as after breast cancer treatment, where one in five women treated develops arm swelling [6], or presenting as elephantiasis in an area endemic for filariasis. Consequently, primary lymphoedema is often missed and so perceived as uncommon. However, of 120 million people infected, 40 million are considered disfigured and incapacitated by lymphatic disorders [7]. Chronic oedema is clinically recognisable and, being physiologically no different, has been used as a surrogate for lymphoedema in epidemiological studies. Using these criteria, lymphoedema encompassing all causes is common ranging from 1.33 to 3.93 per 1000 population in the UK [2].

Pathophysiology
There are many different causes of impaired lymph drainage. Primary lymphoedema is when there is an inborn or constitutional deficiency in the structure or function of the lymph draining routes. Genetic forms of lymphoedema fall into this category (Table 103.1). Secondary lymphoedema refers to those forms where there has been an identifiable injury to lymph draining routes such as occurs following cancer surgery where lymph glands are removed.

Impaired lymph drainage leads to fibrosis, fat deposition and cellular infiltrate. Long-term lymph accumulation can induce chronic tissue inflammation, progressive fibrosis, impaired homeostasis, altered remodelling of adipose tissue, impaired regenerative capacity and immunological dysfunction [8].

The underlying pathogenesis of lymphoedema involves a dysfunction in lymphatic transport, but there is evidence of lymphocyte involvement. Lymphoedema results in a mixed T-helper cell and T-regulatory cell (Treg) inflammatory response. Prolonged T-helper cell biased immune responses in lymphoedema regulate the pathology of this disease by promoting tissue fibrosis, inhibiting the formation of collateral lymphatics, decreasing lymphatic vessel pumping capacity and increasing lymphatic leakiness. These

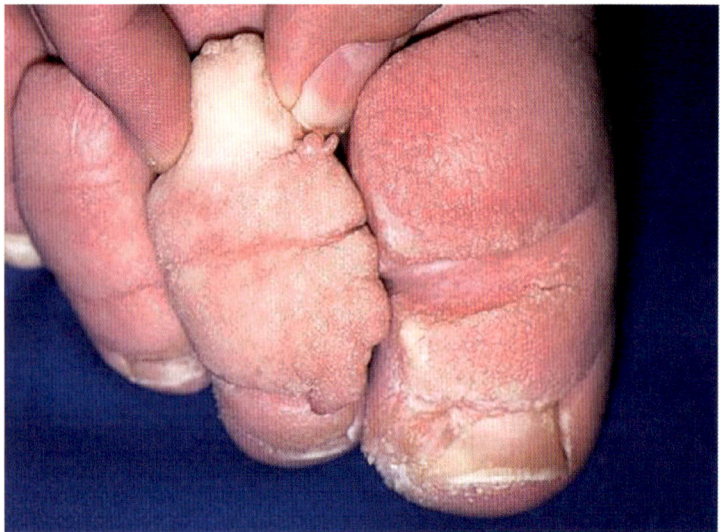

Figure 103.2 The Kaposi–Stemmer sign: an inability to pinch or pick up a fold of skin at the base of the second toe indicates lymphoedema.

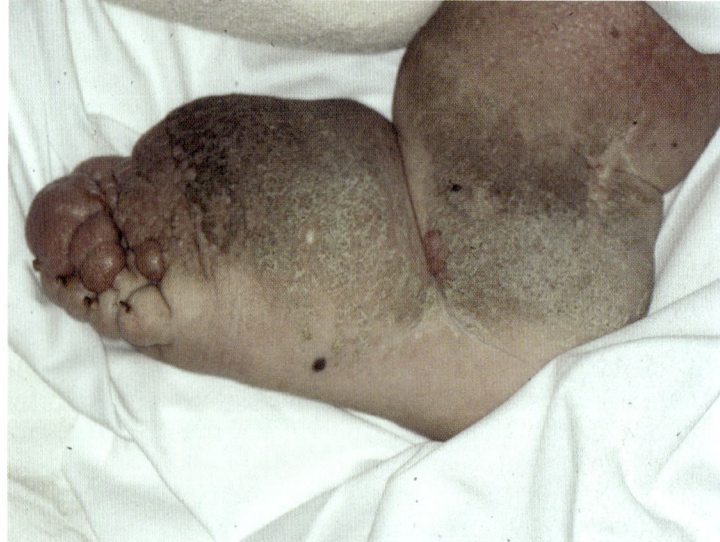

Figure 103.3 Elephantiasis nostras verrucosa showing marked hyperkeratosis and papillomatosis.

principles could have implications for the pathology of any skin disease where lymphatic dysfunction is involved [9].

Clinical features

Features that indicate primarily a lymphatic cause are (i) persistent swelling, which can be intermittent at first; (ii) oedema that does not resolve with overnight elevation; (iii) a poor response to diuretics; and (iv) recurrent cellulitis.

Inflammation, fibrosis and a component of fat all convey a more solid tissue texture to the lymphoedema. Nevertheless, fluid is invariably present giving rise to the brawny nature of the swelling. Lymphoedema is often alleged not to pit but this is only the case in very advanced elephantiasis. Conversely, in the early stages of lymphoedema pitting occurs easily. Therefore, the presence of pitting does not exclude lymphoedema.

With time, the skin doubles in thickness, a feature noticeable when trying to pick up a fold of skin between the fingertips. A failure to pinch a fold of skin at the base of the second toe is a positive Kaposi–Stemmer sign and is pathognomonic of lymphoedema (Figure 103.2). The skin also becomes warty due to hyperkeratosis.

Complications and co-morbidities

The major complications of lymphoedema and chronic oedema are swelling and infection.

Swelling. Limb swelling leads to discomfort, limb heaviness, reduced mobility and, on occasion, impaired function. The size and weight of affected limbs can result in secondary musculoskeletal complications such as back pain and joint problems, particularly in the case of asymmetrical lower limb swelling. Balance can be an issue with asymmetrical limb swelling affecting either the upper or lower limbs [10].

Skin changes. Elephantiasis refers to a big swollen limb but also to appearances resembling elephant skin. The epidermis becomes hyperkeratotic and warty and the dermis markedly thickened and fibrotic. Distended dermal lymphatics (lymphangiectasia) can

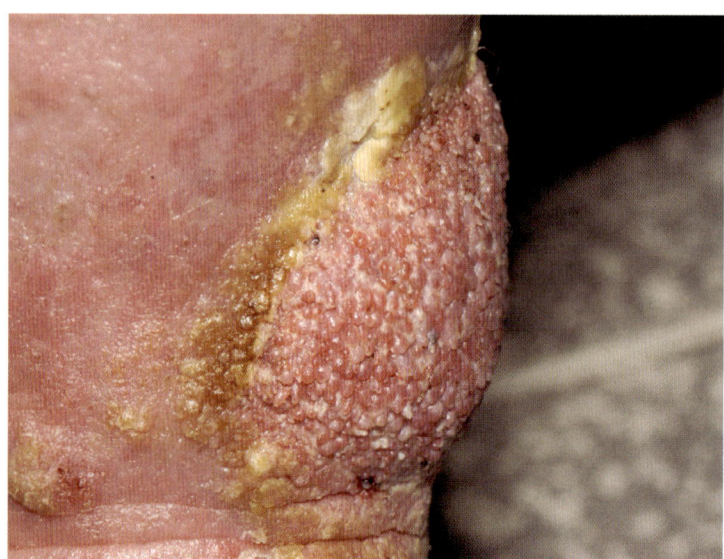

Figure 103.4 Acquired cutaneous lymphangiectasia leading to ulceration of the lower leg and lymphorrhoea.

bulge on the skin surface to create lymph blisters and, with time and tissue organisation, can produce a cobblestone appearance. Elephantiasis skin changes (elephantiasis verrucosa nostra) occur in established chronic lymphoedema, particularly in the lower limb or in circumstances of profound cutaneous lymph congestion (Figure 103.3). Thickening of the skin impairs joint mobility. Leakage of lymph through the skin (lymphorrhoea) may occur from lymphangiectasia (Figure 103.4).

Infection. Episodes of secondary infection, particularly cellulitis, are a characteristic feature of lymphoedema. Patients with lymphoedema irrespective of cause are liable to these attacks. Acute dermatolymphangioadenitis as seen in filariasis and podoconiosis represents the same process. It is likely that disturbances in immune cell trafficking compromise tissue immunosurveillance, but the exact mechanism is not known.

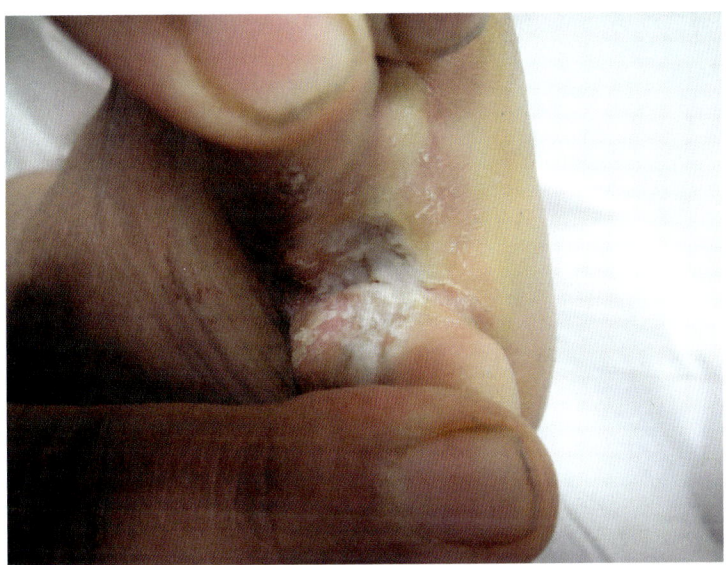

Figure 103.5 Macerated web-space skin leading to bacterial entry points and fungal infection.

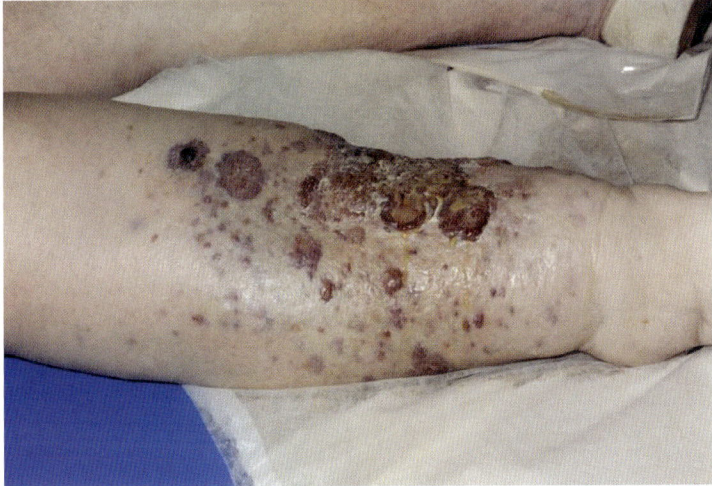

Figure 103.6 Lymphangiosarcoma arising in primary lymphoedema.

Constitutional symptoms such as fever, rigors, headache or vomiting can be profound and sudden in onset. Within 24 h, redness appears within the lymphoedematous area but without an advancing border. Pain and heat also feature. Recurrent episodes may be frequent and further impair lymph drainage, thereby exacerbating the lymphoedema. Thus, a vicious cycle is established. Haemolytic streptococci of groups A, B and particularly G have been demonstrated in the skin. Toxicity from infection can be extreme and even fatal [11].

It is not unusual for patients to comment that attacks of cellulitis can be induced by strenuous exercise or long car journeys. This suggests a mechanism not dissimilar to herpes simplex where the microorganism is always present but becomes reactivated.

Fungal infections, particularly tinea pedis, are difficult to avoid because of web-space skin maceration from swollen toes (Figure 103.5).

Opportunistic infections are also described in lymphoedema, lending further support to the localised immunodeficiency theory.

Psychosocial issues. In one study over 80% of patients (188/217) had taken time off work due to lymphoedema, with an estimated mean absenteeism of 10.5 days per year for medical appointments. Overall, 9% stated that the lymphoedema affected their employment status, with 4/209 (2%) respondents having to change jobs and 17/209 (8%) having to give up work because of it [3]. Relationships can also suffer.

The difficulty in finding clothes or shoes to fit creates social problems. Poor footwear will further compound the swelling by discouraging a normal gait or adequate exercise.

Patients with arm swelling in relation to breast cancer experienced functional impairment, psychosocial maladjustment and increased psychological morbidity.

Malignancy. Chronic lymphoedema has a permissive effect with certain types of malignancies, particularly angiosarcomas – the Stewart–Treves syndrome. The presumed mechanism is through immunodeficiency of the compromised drainage basin, in a similar way to malignancy complicating systemic immunodeficiency, such as in renal transplant recipients [12]. The Stewart–Treves syndrome describes lymphangiosarcoma developing from well-established postmastectomy oedema. However, lymphangiosarcoma is now described as occurring with lymphoedema of any cause (Figure 103.6) [13]. Other tumours that have been recorded to develop with lymphoedema include basal cell carcinoma, squamous cell carcinoma, lymphoma, melanoma, malignant fibrous histiocytoma, Merkel cell tumour and Kaposi sarcoma. Certain uncommon benign tumours are reported as being associated with lymphoedema [14].

Miscellaneous conditions. A range of cutaneous conditions has been reported as occurring preferentially at sites of lymphoedematous involvement. These include xanthomatous deposits, bullous pemphigoid, toxic epidermal necrolysis, atypical neutrophilic dermatosis and severe necrotising fasciitis.

Investigations

The gold standard investigation for lymphoedema is lymphoscintigraphy but indocyanine green lymphography and magnetic resonance lymphangiography are increasingly used. Biopsy generally does not reveal a cause for lymphoedema except in certain circumstances such as lymphoedema due to granulomatous diseases or malignancy.

Lymphoscintigraphy (isotope lymphography) involves the interstitial (dermis or subcutis) injection of a radiolabelled protein or colloid. Radioactivity, measured using a wide field-of-view gamma camera, is determined over the injection site depot and at regions of interest over vessels or nodes. The measurement of transit times and time activity curves permits a quantitative analysis of lymph drainage [15]. The measurement of tracer uptake within axillary or ilio-inguinal lymph nodes at a specified time will discriminate lymphoedema from oedema of non-lymphatic origin (Figure 103.7). Abnormalities on lymphoscintigraphy confirm lymphoedema but a negative scan does not exclude it.

Management

As yet there is no proven medical therapy nor any universally approved surgical procedure to improve lymph flow, although

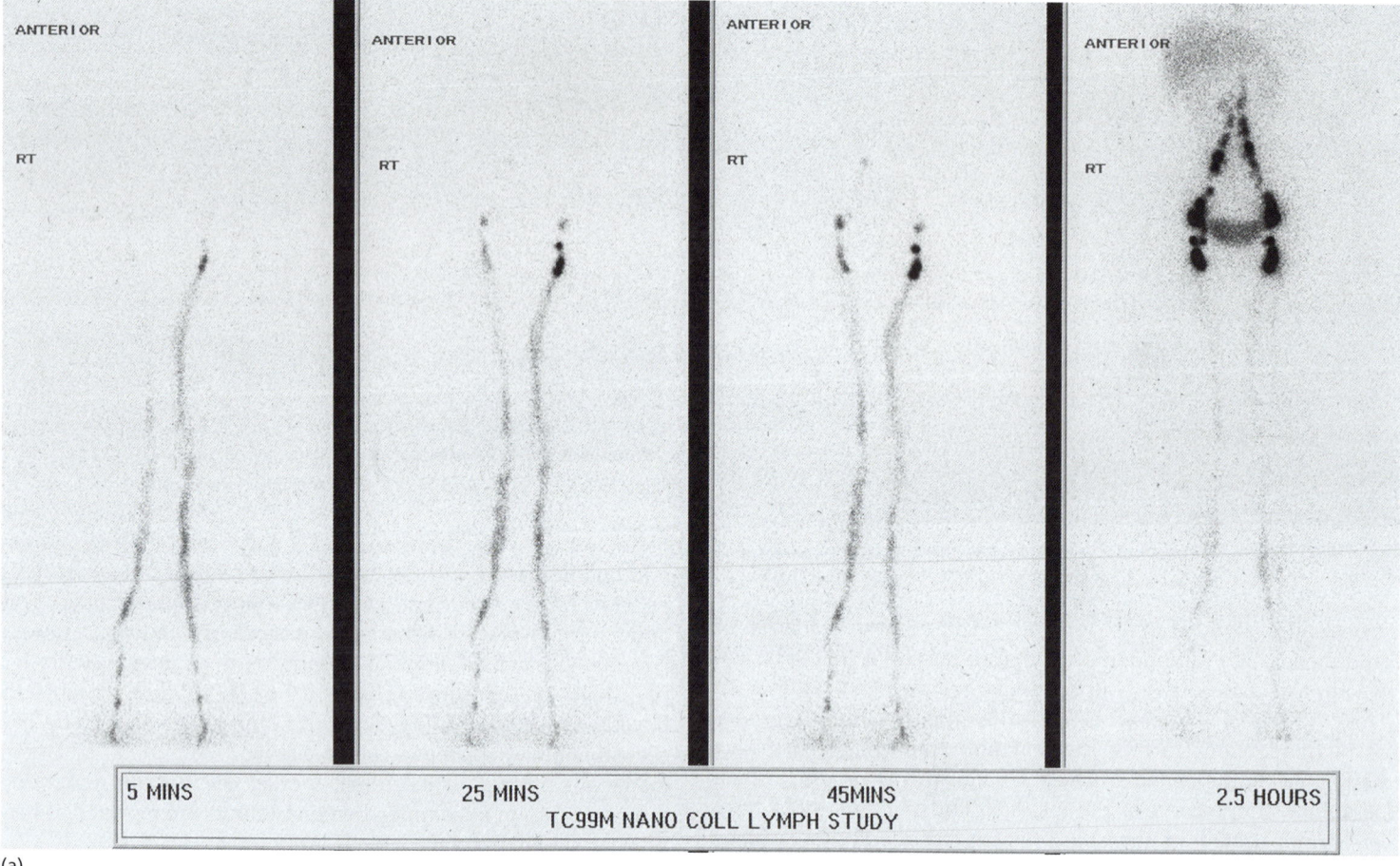

(a)

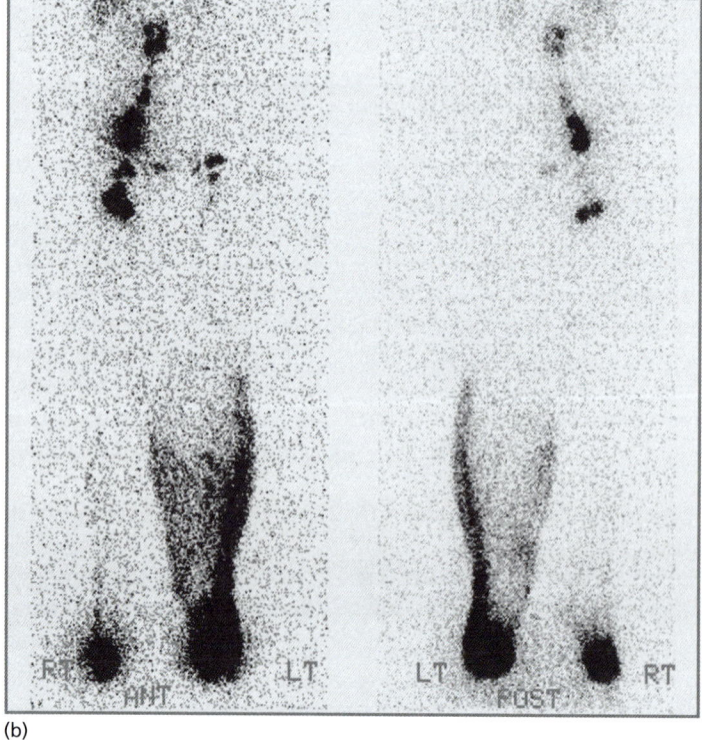

(b)

Figure 103.7 (a) Normal lymphoscintigraphy. Images show patent lymph routes draining tracer from the feet to the ilio-inguinal nodes. (b) Obstruction of lymph drainage at the groin leads to rerouting of tracer through the skin collaterals (dermal backflow). (a) Courtesy of Professor A. M. Peters.

Table 103.2 Causes of a swollen leg.

Genetic			Acquired				
Vascular	**Lymphatic**	**Other**	**Vascular**	**Lymphatic**	**Inflammatory**	**Musculoskeletal**	**Tumours**
Vascular malformation	Lymphoedema	Overgrowth spectrum:	DVT	Lymphoedema:	Cellulitis	Rheumatoid arthritis	Lymphoma
Diffuse phlebectasia	Lymphatic malformation	Fat hypertrophy	Post-thrombotic syndrome	Cancer surgery	Pretibial myxoedema	Ruptured Baker cyst	Sarcoma
Klippel–Trenaunay syndrome	Lymphangiomatosis	Lipomatosis	Chronic venous reflux	DXT	Varicose eczema	Joint effusion	Metastases
Parkes Weber syndrome		Lipoedema	Venous outflow obstruction	Filanosis	Psoriasis	Haematoma	
Maffucci syndrome		Proteus syndrome	Dependency syndrome	Podoconiosis	Pompholyx	Torn muscle	
		Muscle hamartoma/ overgrowth	Thrombophlebitis	Trauma	Sarcoidosis	Pathological fracture	
		Gigantism/ hemihypertrophy	Venous injury, e.g. IV drug abuse	Reconstructive surgery	Herpes simplex	Achilles tendonitis	
			Acute arterial ischaemia	Vein harvesting/vein stripping		Myositis ossificans	
			Idiopathic/cyclical oedema of women	Immobility/ armchair legs			
			Drugs, e.g. calcium channel antagonists	Factitial			
				Chronic regional pain syndrome			
				Obesity			

DVT, deep-vein thrombosis; DXT, radiotherapy; IV, intravenous.

there are new operations of value. First line treatment is physical therapy based on the physiological principles that movement and exercise stimulate lymph flow, and the addition of compression enhances that process. Massage in the form of a specific technique called manual lymphatic drainage is used to complement movement and compression for limb lymphoedema and is used as a primary treatment for midline lymphoedema (head and neck, trunk, breast and genital area).

The chronically swollen limb

Synonyms and inclusions
- Oedema
- Lymphoedema
- Overgrowth
- Vascular malformation
- Lipoedema

Introduction and general description
Swelling of a limb may be caused by fluid, in which case pitting should be evident to some degree, or it may be caused by an increase in volume of other tissue elements, for example bone, muscle or fat. Overgrowth syndromes, such as Klippel–Trenaunay syndrome, may have excessive growth of bone, fat or muscle (with or without additional fluid). Lymphatic and other vascular malformations can produce swelling but without pitting. Lipoedema is due to fat hypertrophy. A plexiform neurofibroma (neurofibromatosis) may cause tissue swelling from both the neural tumour and lymphoedema.

Epidemiology
Chronic leg swelling is common, but data are few. A point-prevalence study carried out during working day periods in

six general hospitals in four countries (Denmark, France, the UK and Australia) and one hospital oncology in-patient unit in Ireland showed that from a total of 1905 patients, swollen legs were present in 723 (38%) of the cohort [16]. In a separate report from Denmark, 595 hospitalisations of patients aged 75 years or over revealed 6.3% were due to suspected deep-vein thrombosis (DVT) or red swollen legs [17].

Pathophysiology
The cause of the swelling will depend on the tissue component that is increased. For fluid swelling the same principles of pathophysiology apply as they do for any chronic oedema. The cause of swollen legs is often multifactorial (Table 103.2). In the case of a swollen leg, differential diagnoses to consider are a ruptured Baker cyst, infection, trauma and malignancy. Inflammation of a joint or periarticular structure may cause oedema that is not primarily vascular.

Clinical features
Most cases of limb swelling will be due to fluid and will exhibit pitting to some degree but careful examination for causes of non-pitting swelling (e.g. fat hypertrophy, malformations, hamartomas, and benign and malignant tumours) is required. Therefore, the patient's individual history and an appropriate physical examination are important. A patient may perceive one leg to be swollen when in fact the other leg has become smaller, for example through atrophy of muscle or fat. Chronic, non-inflammatory, asymmetrical lower limb swelling should always suggest a cause within the hindquarter (e.g. chronic venous hypertension, lymphoedema and somatic mosaic disorders). Systemic causes of oedema including cardiac disease, renal disease or hypoproteinaemia should cause bilateral leg swelling.

Investigations
Blood tests are important to exclude hypoproteinaemia and heart failure, where measurement of plasma albumin and BNP (or

PART 9: VASCULAR DISORDERS

NT-proBNP) should be performed respectively. In cases of suspected venous and/or lymphatic obstruction, imaging such as ultrasound, CT or MRI of the root of the limb (e.g. the ilio-inguinal region) should be undertaken. CT or MRI of the limb can be helpful for determining the tissue component contributing to the swelling. Lymphoscintigraphy is the investigation of choice to confirm a lymphatic aetiology. Venous duplex ultrasound will identify whether venous reflux is contributory to the fluid swelling. A skin biopsy may be necessary if pathologies such as Kaposi sarcoma, pretibial myxoedema or malignancy are suspected.

Management

Treatment of a swollen leg is dependent on the cause. Fluid swelling should not be treated empirically with diuretics but should be managed through a reduction of any excess fluid filtration or improvement of lymph drainage or both.

Venous oedema, lymphovenous oedema and phlebolymphoedema

Definition and nomenclature

Venous oedema is oedema due to venous disease and specifically venous hypertension. Lymphovenous oedema means high lymph production from venous hypertension combined with lymphatic insufficiency. Phlebolymphoedema is lymphoedema arising from the effects of venous disease.

Synonyms and inclusions
- Venous oedema
- Venous hypertension
- Venous stasis
- Post-thrombotic syndrome
- Venous obstruction
- Chronic oedema
- Lymphovenous oedema
- Dependency oedema
- Orthostatic oedema
- Phlebolymphoedema

Introduction and general description

The veins and lymphatics are inextricably linked. Their endothelial parentage is identical as lymphatics and veins have a common embryological origin [18]. Consequently, genetic forms of lymphoedema are frequently associated with venous reflux.

Oedema is a common complication of venous disease. It is incorrectly assumed that venous oedema is the sole consequence of increased capillary filtration from venous hypertension. As lymph drainage is the main buffer against oedema, it is in fact the failure of local lymphatics to compensate for the increased lymph load from vascular filtration that leads to venous oedema. Lymphoedema associated with venous disease can give rise to significant swelling and skin changes owing to the combined effect of impaired lymph drainage and increased lymph load (Figure 103.8).

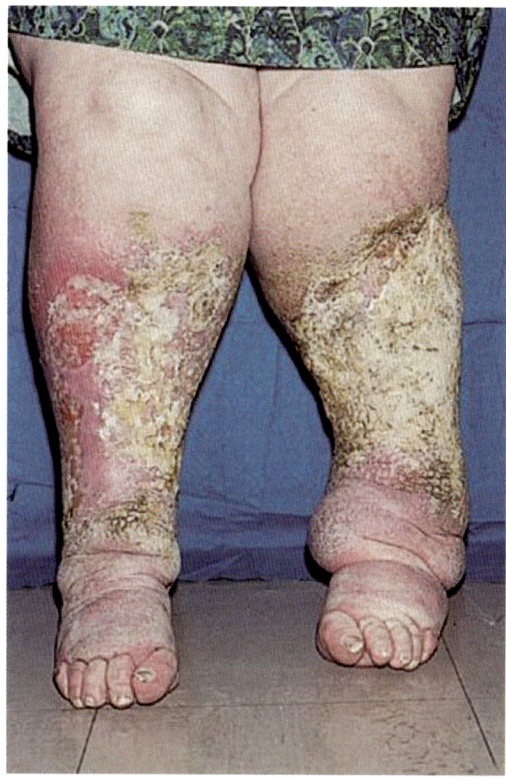

Figure 103.8 Lymphoedema associated with chronic venous disease.

Phlebolymphoedema results from high fluid filtration from venous hypertension overwhelming lymph drainage until eventually lymphatic routes become permanently damaged and lymphoedema ensues.

Epidemiology

Oedema is a common finding in chronic venous disease. The Bonn vein study identified 13.4% (11.6% men, 14.9% women) had pitting oedema of the lower limbs at the time of the investigation (oedema indicates a classification of C3 in chronic venous disease) [24].

Pathophysiology

Venous oedema is due to capillary filtration resulting from venous hypertension overwhelming the lymph drainage for a sufficient period of time. Contrary to popular belief, venous reabsorption of interstitial fluid cannot be maintained for any length of time in peripheral tissues. Interstitial fluid is reabsorbed almost entirely by the lymphatic vessels. Venous hypertension causes an increase in microvascular fluid filtration that requires greater lymph drainage if oedema is to be avoided. A reduction in venous pressure reduces capillary filtration sufficiently for lymph drainage to cope and thus the oedema resolves.

In the lower limbs, venous oedema may occur for many reasons including varicose veins, DVT or venous obstruction (Figure 103.9). In varicose veins and after a DVT there will often be venous valve failure (venous reflux).

Dependency oedema, like venous oedema, arises from venous hypertension increasing lymph production; the difference is that in dependency oedema the veins may be normal and the venous hypertension is solely due to gravitational forces. Because the calf muscle pump is important for venous return, immobility will

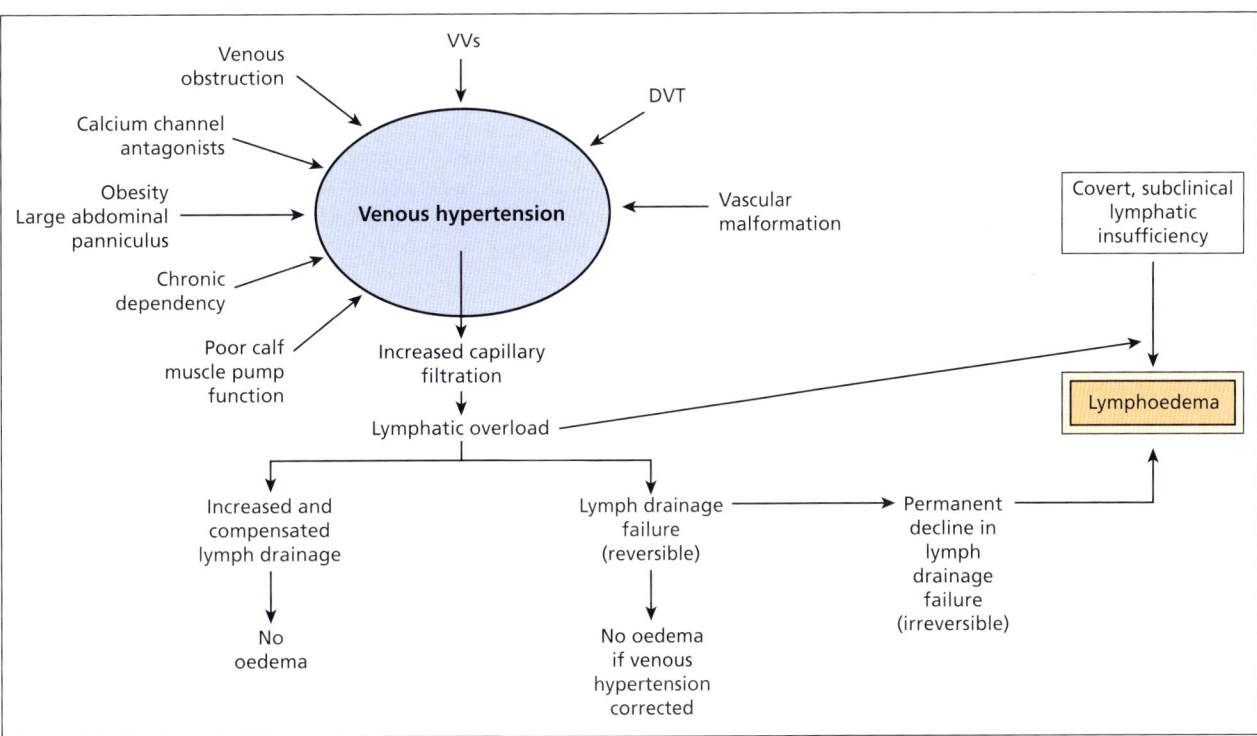

Figure 103.9 Causes of mixed lymphovenous disease and phlebolymphoedema. DVT, deep-vein thrombosis; VV, varicose veins.

encourage oedema. The lack of an effective calf muscle pump will cause venous hypertension and increased capillary fluid filtration (lymph production). Immobility will also cause a failure of lymph drainage so the combination of reduced venous return and poor lymph drainage can cause lymphovenous oedema. If immobility is combined with leg dependency where gravitational forces increase venous pressure, this is referred to as dependency or orthostatic oedema. A common scenario is 'armchair legs', where patients sit in a chair day and night with their legs dependent. Calcium channel antagonists inhibit contaction of lymphatic smooth muscle. This is a likely mechanism for the oedema seen with this class of drug [20].

Many primary lymphoedemas for which gene mutations are known also possess venous reflux because of a genetically determined venous valve failure. The best documented is lymphoedema distichiasis syndrome where the mutation is in the *FOXC2* gene All patients with the mutation appear to have superficial venous reflux [21].

Traditional surgical stripping of varicose veins or harvesting of the great saphenous vein for coronary artery bypass grafting can also damage leg lymphatics and lead to (lympho)venous oedema. Fortunately, both procedures are less commonly performed since the introduction of endovenous ablation therapy and stenting. Iliac vein obstruction can cause swelling of the left leg due to compression of the left iliac vein as it crosses the right iliac artery (May–Thurner syndrome).

Phlebolymphoedema arises when the effects of a high fluid load eventually lead to an irreversible lymphatic insufficiency. There may be numerous factors contributing such as overworked lymphatic vessels which fail in an analagous manner to the heart in high-output cardiac failure, and infection causing lymphangitis leading to permanent lymphangio-obliteration.

Intravenous drug abuse can produce thrombotic damage and sepsis, damaging veins and lymphatics leading to phlebolymphoedema in the upper and lower limbs.

Clinical features

Chronic venous disease may result in symptoms such as heaviness, aching, itching (from varicose dermatitis) and skin pigmentation (from purpura or haemosiderin). In the lower limb, symptoms worsen towards the end of the day, are relieved by overnight elevation and are usually exacerbated by heat and alcohol.

Venous oedema usually pits easily and resolves following overnight elevation. Signs of venous hypertension include varicose veins, haemosiderin deposition (particularly submalleolar), varicose eczema, atrophie blanche and ulceration. The greater the severity and duration of venous hypertension, the greater the damage to the skin. The CEAP classification (based on clinical manifestations (C), aetiological factors (E), anatomical distribution of disease (A) and underlying pathophysiological findings (P)) provides information on the staging of venous disease, with oedema featuring as stage III [22]. The reason why even severe venous disease may not exhibit oedema is where the lymph drainage is adequate.

Once venous oedema stops resolving with overnight elevation, it indicates a failing lymph drainage. Under such circumstances, clinical signs of lymphoedema begin to accompany the signs of venous hypertension, so-called phlebolymphoedema. Phlebolymphoedema most commonly occurs in the lower limb but can occur elsewhere in the body in circumstances of venous hypertension – for example a pendulous abdomen (hanging abdominal apron), large pendulous breast and upper limb venous outflow obstruction.

PART 9: VASCULAR DISORDERS

When lymphoedema dominates, the skin becomes harder. Advanced cases develop elephantiasis skin changes with hyperkeratosis and papillomatosis [23]. Recurrent cellulitis can occur due to disturbances in immune cell trafficking from the lymphatic insufficiency. Redness, pain and tenderness and warmth suggest lipodermatosclerosis and result from increased fluid congestion within the skin from the lymphovenous oedema. Poor wound healing can result in a chronic ulcer.

Investigations

Venous duplex ultrasound is the investigation of choice for chronic venous disease. It can detect venous reflux, thrombosis and venous obstruction. In cases of mixed vascular malformations and iliac vein obstruction, more specialist imaging with CT or MRI venography may be necessary.

Management

Compression and exercise treat both venous disease and lymphoedema. Compression may be achieved through bandaging or compression garments. Bandaging is helpful initially to produce a reduction in swelling and improve limb shape to enable a better fit for compression garments. Standard 'venous ulcer' compression bandaging will adequately treat most cases but if there is marked forefoot involvement (swollen or papillomatous toes) or if the swelling extends above the knee, then lymphoedema-style treatment in the form of decongestive lymphatic therapy (DLT) is preferred [**24**]. DLT involving toe and thigh bandaging can only be provided by trained therapists and is generally not available in the community. Wounds, dermatitis and infection need to be treated before, or at the same time as, compression is applied. Exercise is to be encouraged in preference to rest but when the patient is resting, the leg should be elevated to heart level. Patients should be discouraged from spending too long in a chair unless it is a reclining chair. In infirm patients, pneumatic compression therapy may be helpful [25]. Adjustable Velcro® compression devices can sometimes overcome the need for compression bandaging.

Superficial venous reflux may be amenable to endovenous therapy (EVT). Hopefully this will reduce the lymph load and so reduce oedema, but it is often still necessary to wear compression garments afterwards to encourage good lymph drainage and discourage recurrence of varicose veins [26]. If EVT fails to relieve oedema, then poor lymph drainage is likely to be the dominant physiological component.

Drug-induced oedema

Introduction and general description

A number of drugs can cause chronic oedema. Calcium channel antagonists are a common cause of peripheral oedema (up to 30% of cases), with amlodipine one of the worst offenders [27]. Discontinuing the drug will often resolve the oedema.

Epidemiology

A search of drug databases for drugs for which an unwanted side effect includes oedema revealed a large number of examples, some of which may include angioedema.

Pathophysiology

Drugs that induce fluid retention cause an increase in blood volume, which in turn leads to an increase in capillary pressure and an increase in capillary filtration. This will cause swelling if the lymph system cannot cope with the extra fluid. Drugs that may do this include corticosteroids, non-steroidal anti-inflammatory drugs (e.g. ibuprofen) and hormones (e.g. oestrogens). Other drugs may cause increased capillary filtration by increasing venous pressure as a result of arterial vasodilatation (e.g. calcium channel blockers such as amlodipine). Many chemotherapy agents cause oedema, particularly docetaxel; an increase in vascular permeability is probably to blame. Calcium channel blockers appear to cause oedema in those patients with reduced lymph drainage capacity. Mammalian target of rapamycin (mTOR) inhibitors (e.g sirolimus and everolimus) can cause lymphoedema probably by affecting lymphatic vessel repair.

Clinical features

The temporal relationship between the introduction of a drug and the onset of peripheral oedema suggests a cause and effect, particularly if withdrawal of the drug resolves the oedema, as is often the case with amlodipine. In most cases it is not so straightforward, particularly if a drug combination effect is involved. For example, rosiglitazone caused oedema in 4.8% of people in whom it was used as monotherapy for diabetes, but in combination with insulin the frequency increased to 14.7% [28]. Among the best-known drugs causing oedema are calcium channel antagonists, oral corticosteroids, sex hormones and related compounds (e.g. megestrol) (Box 103.1). Rates of oedema caused by sex hormones and related drugs are oestrogens (hormone replacement therapy) >1%, anastrozole 7–10%, tamoxifen 8–9% and megestrol 14%.

Box 103.1 Drugs causing oedema

- Calcium channel antagonists of dihydropyridine (DHP) class
- Cytotoxic chemotherapy, e.g. docetaxel (47–64%)
- Oral corticosteroids
- Sex hormones, e.g oestrogen, megestrol
- Anticonvulsants, e.g. pregabalin (5–12%)
- Antidepressants, e.g. trazodone (10%)
- Antidiabetics, e.g. rosiglitazone (5%)
- Antipsychotics, e.g. risperidone (16%)
- Bisphosphonates, e.g. zoledronic acid (21%)
- Mammalian target of rapamycin (mTOR) inhibitors, e.g sirolimus (>10%)
- Baclofen (1–10%)
- Others:
  - Dopamine receptor agonists: pramipexole, rotigoline and cabergoline
  - Lamotrigine (2% oedema)
  - Non-steroidal anti-inflammatory drugs (NSAIDs)
  - Morphine
  - Clonidine
  - Olanzapine
  - Thiazolidinediones
  - Quetiapine
  - Pemetrexed (eyelid oedema)

Management

In cases of drug-induced oedema (e.g. due to amlodipine), the drug should be replaced if possible or measures introduced to control swelling. The empirical use of diuretics is to be discouraged as they are often ineffective over time.

CELLULITIS

Recurrent cellulitis (erysipelas)

Definition and nomenclature

Cellulitis is an acute bacterial infection of the dermis and subcutaneous tissue, which can be recurrent. It is a common consequence of lymphatic dysfunction.

Synonyms and inclusions
- Erysipelas
- Lymphangitis
- Pseudo-erysipelas
- Pseudo-cellulitis
- Acute dermatolymphangioadenitis (ADLA)

Introduction and general description

Cellulitis (or erysipelas as it is more usually known in Europe) is one of the most common reasons for emergency admissions to hospital and up to half of patients have repeat episodes. Lymphoedema and leg ulcers provide the greatest risk for recurrent cellulitis. There is evidence that covert lymphatic insufficiency may predispose to first-time attacks of cellulitis [1]. Lymphangitis accompanies cellulitis but may not be clinically visible. Because an underlying microbiological cause is elusive in most cases of recurrent cellulitis occurring with lymphoedema, the terms pseudo-cellulitis and pseudo-erysipelas have been coined. In developed countries most patients with cellulitis are treated for the acute episode and discharged, yet the rate of recurrence is high, suggesting that underlying predisposing factors (e.g. lymphoedema) may not be sufficiently managed following the first episode.

Epidemiology

Recurrent cellulitis is common. In a recent study, 53% of subjects with a history of cellulitis had at least one recurrence during the 3-year trial [2]. In another study similar results were obtained: 22–49% of patients with cellulitis reported at least one prior episode; recurrences occurred in approximately 14% of cellulitis cases within 1 year and 45% of cases within 3 years, usually in the same location [3].

Pathophysiology

Beta-haemolytic streptococci cause nearly three-quarters of cases of cellulitis. *Staphylococcus aureus*, by comparison, tends to cause more purulent infections, such as abscesses [4]. Common predisposing conditions for recurrent cellulitis include wounds, venous disease, chronic oedema, obesity and diabetes [5,6]. Inflammatory destruction of lymphatic channels, followed by the development of lymphoedema, progresses with recurrent cellulitis. Equally, lymphoedema predisposes to cellulitis thereby leading to a vicious cycle.

Recurrent bacterial infections may also play a very important role in the pathogenesis of filarial lymphoedema, where it is called acute dermatolymphangioadenitis (ADLA), and may be responsible for its progression to elephantiasis and disability [7]. Web-space entry points appear very important for triggering ADLA [8]. ADLA also occurs in non-filarial elephantiasis, otherwise known as podoconiosis [9].

Causes of cellulitis and ADLA are likely to be similar. The afferent lymphatic vasculature provides the major exit route from the skin for soluble antigens and for immunologically active cells (e.g. lymphocytes, dendritic cells and macrophages) (Figure 103.10). It is likely that disturbances in immune cell trafficking compromise tissue immunosurveillance and predispose to infection, but the exact mechanism is not known [10].

Clinical features

The severity of recurrent episodes of cellulitis can vary. Some can be severe with marked systemic upset, high fever or rigors while others are milder, with minimal or no fever. Local signs always involve increased redness usually with pain, warmth and increased swelling of the affected area.

When associated with established lymphoedema, clinical features may differ from classic cellulitis. Onset may be in minutes (as opposed to hours as in classic cellulitis). Toxicity may be severe with flu-like symptoms, nausea and vomiting, headache and high fever. Systemic symptoms may occur well before local signs. The rash may be polymorphic with no defined border. In milder cases, inflammatory markers are not always raised. Episodes may be slow to resolve with oral antibiotics. Recurrence of infection is not unusual after only a week's course of antibiotics (Figure 103.11).

In some cases, associated with lymphoedema, symptoms and signs may grumble over a period of weeks, suggesting a surviving or extant infection. The patient may complain only of tiredness and feeling unwell but without fever. Local signs may be redness and swelling with 'flare-ups' of redness from time to time. Inflammatory markers are usually negative and only a prompt response to a prolonged course of antibiotics can confirm the diagnosis.

Episodes of ADLA are similar to cellulitis and characterised by malaise, fever, chills, diffuse inflammation, swelling of the limbs, lymphangitis, adenitis and, eventually, peeling skin.

The main differential diagnoses are DVT, necrotising fasciitis and lipodermatosclerosis. Other possibilities include gout, vasculitis, a ruptured Baker cyst and panniculitis.

Investigations

Cellulitis is a clinical diagnosis supported by a blood neutrophilia and raised CRP. Blood cultures should be performed but may be positive in only 10% of cases. Microbiology of any cuts or breaks in the skin or aspiration of blister fluid should be considered before antibiotics are started.

Management

Cellulitis is best managed by dermatologists because up to one-third of patients can be misdiagnosed and over a quarter of cases have

PART 9: VASCULAR DISORDERS

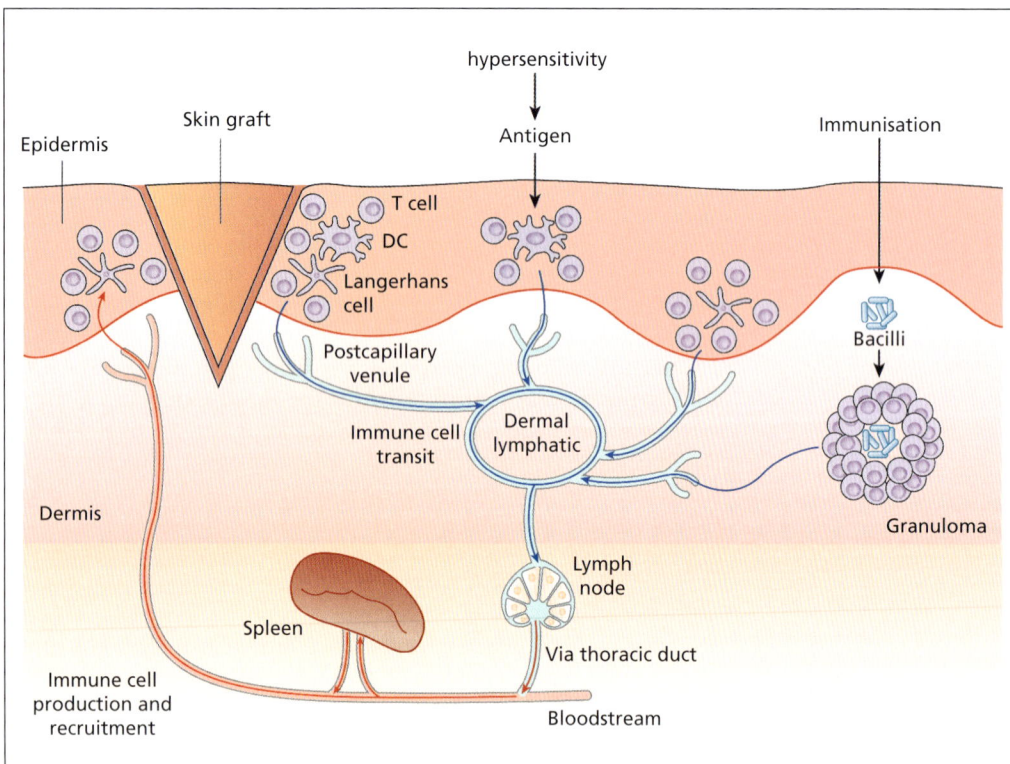

Figure 103.10 The lymphatic vessel sits centre stage for immune cell trafficking within the skin. DC, dendritic cell. Reproduced from Mortimer and Rockson 2014 [12] with permission of American Society for Clinical Investigation.

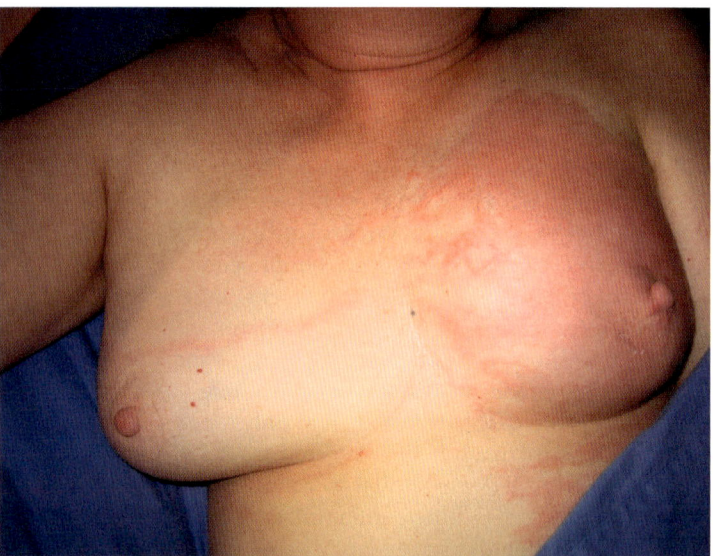

Figure 103.11 Recurrent cellulitis in lymphoedema following breast cancer treatment. Note lymphangitis crossing the watershed to the contralateral lymph node territory.

associated skin disease, treatment of which is likely to reduce the chances of cellulitis recurrence [11]. Wounds, breaks in skin integrity (particularly interdigital), dermatitis and fungal infections should be treated.

Low-dose prophylactic penicillin, phenoxymethylpenicillin 250 mg twice daily, given for a period of 12 months almost halves the risk of recurrence during the intervention period compared with placebo [2]. However, although some level of protection appears to be sustained for several months after the end of prophylactic therapy, this effect is lost by 36 months, a finding that suggests longer-

term prophylaxis may be required. Patients with a body mass index (BMI) of 33 or higher, multiple previous episodes of cellulitis or chronic oedema of the leg had a reduced likelihood of a response to prophylaxis [2]. A high BMI, multiple attacks and chronic oedema would all be associated with lymphatic dysfunction, supporting the view that lymphoedema is a very strong risk factor for cellulitis.

In patients allergic to penicillin, or in whom penicillin prophylaxis fails, alternative antibiotics such as clarithromycin or doxycycline should be considered although there are no data on efficacy or safety [12].

Lymphangitis

Definition

Lymphangitis is inflammation of the lymphatic vessels. It accompanies cellulitis but may exist in isolation and is most often caused by infection from bacteria, viruses or fungi or infiltration by cancer cells.

Introduction and general description

Lymphangitis represents inflammation of the lymphatic collector vessels and presents clinically as tender red streaks up the limb corresponding to the inflamed vessels. Oedema will often mask the red streaks. A more diffuse redness is seen extending up the medial side of the leg and thigh and thus distinction from an ascending cellulitis is difficult. In some circumstances the inflammatory response may be profound and painful inflammation of the regional lymph glands (lymphadenitis) may arise.

Pathophysiology

Lymphangitis may occur without any demonstrable inflammation or may be recurrent, for example following relapsing herpes simplex infection. Permanent obliteration of lymphatic collectors may follow severe or recurrent lymphangitis. In such cases, if reserve lymphatic capacity is limited, permanent swelling (lymphoedema) can result.

Lymphangitis occurring in filariasis is known as ADLA. Sporotrichoid spread (also known as nodular lymphangitis) describes a characteristic pattern of superficial cutaneous lesions that progress along the path of lymphatic drainage. Fungi, and classically sporotrichosis, exhibit this tendency but also nocardiosis, chromoblastomycosis and aspergillosis. Sporotrichoid spread through lymphangitis has been described with leishmaniasis and atypical mycobacterium (e.g. *Mycobacterium marinum*). Cutaneous squamous cell carcinoma can occasionally demonstrate sporotrichoid spread as can a hypersensitivity lymphangitis to an arthropod bite.

Snake toxin molecules are generally large and cannot directly enter the circulation but are readily taken up by the lymphatics. Snake bite venom will often cause lymphangitis. Pressure bandaging with immobilisation is the recommended first aid treatment with the intention of preventing lymph drainage.

Mondor disease is considered to be a form of superficial thrombophlebitis but it commonly complicates lymph node removal, thus a form of lymphangitis or lymphatic thrombosis may also be possible.

Lymphatic cording or axillary web syndrome following axillary lymph node intervention may be similar and is likely due to lymphatic thrombosis [13]. It is also described following a jellyfish sting. Lymph can clot and lymphangiothrombosis may occur more often than realised [14].

Sclerosing lymphangitis of the penis is a condition related to vigorous sexual activity, manifesting as an asymptomatic, firm, cord-like swelling around the coronal sulcus of the penis [15].

Carcinoma erysipeloides (lymphangitis carcinomatosa, carcinoma telangiectatica, carcinoma en cuirasse) occurs when cancer cells infiltrate the dermal lymphatics. It is a form of metastatic spread and occurs most commonly with breast cancer but can occur with melanoma and thyroid, lung, gastric, pancreatic, ovarian, prostate and colorectal cancer [16]. Carcinoma erysipeloides manifests clinically with a fixed red patch or plaque resembling cellulitis, but without fever. The inflamed area may show a distinct raised periphery and oedema secondary to lymphatic obstruction. A network or lattice pattern of telangiectatic vessels represents the infiltrated dermal lymphatics (Figure 103.12). Inflammatory breast cancer is a rare and very aggressive disease in which cancer cells block lymph vessels in the skin of the breast. This type of breast cancer is called 'inflammatory' or 'inflamed' because the breast often looks swollen and red.

Investigations

Lymphangitis is mainly a clinical diagnosis. Ultrasound examination may be helpful but non-specific. A definitive diagnosis requires biopsy particularly if malignancy is suspected.

Management

Treatment is dependent on cause. Lymphangitis from infection can settle spontaneously.

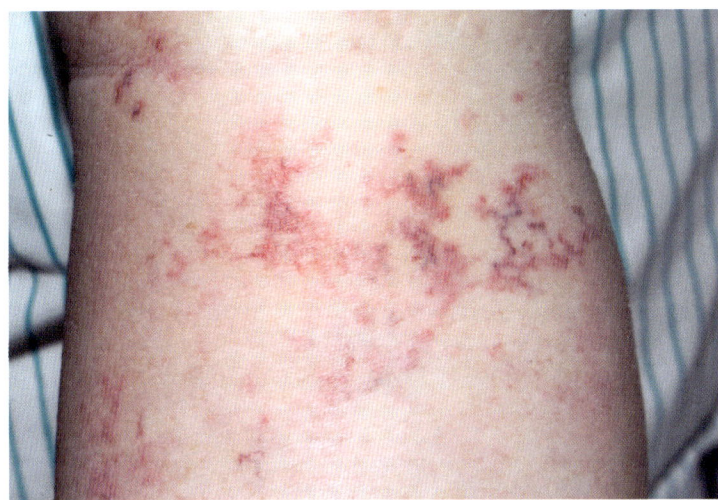

Figure 103.12 Carcinoma erysipeloides (carcinoma telangiectatica) on the ipsilateral arm of a breast cancer patient: the network of red vessels are dermal lymphatic vessels infiltrated with adenocarcinoma of the breast.

Lymphadenitis

Definition and nomenclature

Lymphadenitis means inflammation (*...itis*) of the *lymph* nodes (*...aden...*). Lymphadenitis means enlargement of one or more lymph glands due to inflammation, usually infection.

Synonyms and inclusions
- Swollen glands
- Lymphadenopathy

Pathophysiology

The swelling is due to the proliferation of lymphocytes but also recruitment of additional macrophages which plug the medullary sinuses, resulting in retention of lymph fluid. It is usually caused by the immune response to infection or vaccination but can occur in inflammatory conditions such as sarcoidosis, Kikuchi–Fujimoto disease, systemic lupus erythematosus or autoinflammatory disorders such as periodic fever.

Clinical features

Symptoms include tenderness and swelling of the lymph glands with or without redness of the overlying skin. Lymphadenitis may be confined to one lymph node group (e.g. axilla) or be generalised.

Investigations

Lymphadenitis is usually diagnosed clinically but ultrasound examination, with or without fine-needle aspirate, can be helpful.

Management

Treatment is dependent on the cause, but most cases will settle spontaneously.

Acute dermatolymphangioadenitis

Definition and nomenclature

According to the World Health Organization definition ADLA is 'acute onset fever and localised pain and warmth, with or without swelling or redness in the limb and/or genital area'. Two types of acute febrile attacks occur with filariasis: (i) caused by the death of adult filarial worms known as acute filarial lymphangitis (AFL); and (ii) due to secondary bacterial infections known as ADLA. ADLA is a common cause of elephantiasis both within and outside of filariasis endemic areas. Podoconiosis (non-filarial elephantiasis) also causes ADLA.

Synonyms and inclusions
- Cellulitis
- Lymphangitis

Epidemiology

Episodes of ADLA affect approximately one-third of patients with filarial lymphoedema [17]. Globally, podoconiosis affects an estimated 4 million people in 32 endemic countries, many of which are in the highlands of tropical sub-Saharan Africa, but also in parts of Central and South America and South-East Asia [18]. Patients with podoconiosis experience on average 5–23 episodes of ADLA per year and up to 90 days per year when they are incapacitated by it [19].

Pathophysiology

As with cellulitis in lymphoedema, the likely mechanism is disturbed access of antigen-presenting information to the lymph nodes and consequently a failure of the correct processing of the immune response to infection. In filarial lymphoedema, episodes of ADLA have been shown to accelerate damage to peripheral lymphatic vessels and to lead to fibrosis, resulting in a vicious cycle of impaired lymph drainage and more episodes of infection.

The causes of ADLA among patients with podoconiosis are likely to be similar to its causes among patients with other types of lymphoedema, such as filarial or postsurgical. In other words, disturbances in immune cell trafficking predispose to infection with frequent recurrences.

Clinical features

Episodes of ADLA are characterised by malaise, fever, chills, diffuse inflammation, swelling of the limbs, lymphangitis, adenitis and, eventually, peeling skin. Clinical descriptions of ADLA in filariasis endemic areas are remarkably similar to those of erysipelas and cellulitis.

Management

In a recent placebo-controlled clinical trial, while both amoxicillin (the standard antibiotic treatment for ADLA) and doxycycline reduced the frequency of ADLA, doxycycline also showed surprising efficacy in reversing the lymphoedema grade [20]. Participation in hygiene-based lymphoedema management was associated with a lower incidence of ADLA [21].

In podoconiosis endemic areas the cost of antibiotics, even simple penicillin, is prohibitive. A package containing instructions for foot hygiene, skin care, bandaging, exercises and the use of socks and shoes proved helpful. The incidence of ADLA was 19.4 episodes per person-year (95%CI 18.9–19.9) in the intervention group and 23.9 episodes per person-year (95%CI 23.4–24.4) in the control group [22].

Lipodermatosclerosis and chronic red leg

Definition and nomenclature

The chronically swollen red leg is a common sight in medical practice and is often due to lipodermatosclerosis (LDS). LDS is an inflammatory condition of the skin and subcutaneous tissues affecting the lower third of the leg, and is commonly, although incorrectly, called chronic cellulitis. It is often bundled together with stasis (or varicose) dermatitis and haemosiderin skin pigmentation as all can result from venous hypertension. However, LDS can exist independently with lymphoedema without venous disease.

Synonyms and inclusions
- Chronic cellulitis
- Red swollen legs
- Sclerosing panniculitis
- Hypodermatitis sclerodermiformis
- Stasis panniculitis

Epidemiology

There are few prevalence data on LDS alone. Often included with varicose eczema, LDS is considered common in the elderly and is reported to affect about 20% of people aged over 70 years [23]. Of 595 hospitalisations of patients aged 75 years or above in an emergency department in Denmark, 6.3% were due to suspected DVT or red swollen legs [24].

Pathophysiology

Lipodermatosclerosis is due to sustained 'congestion' – that is, high interstitial fluid and venous pressure. It is most usually described with chronic venous disease, but the common denominator is chronic oedema, frequently occurring in lymphoedema without venous reflux. The pathology of LDS is not well understood but is considered secondary to chronic venous hypertension. mRNA and protein expression of matrix metalloproteinase 1 (MMP-1), MMP-2 and tissue inhibitors of metalloproteinase 1 (TIMP-1) have been shown to be significantly increased, indicating that LDS is characterised by elevated matrix turnover [25]. LDS is always accompanied by tissue iron overload. It has been suggested that patients with LDS are unable to counteract venous-induced skin iron overload [26].

Clinical features

Lipodermatosclerosis mimics cellulitis but there are no systemic symptoms or signs of infection [27], and it is usually bilateral.

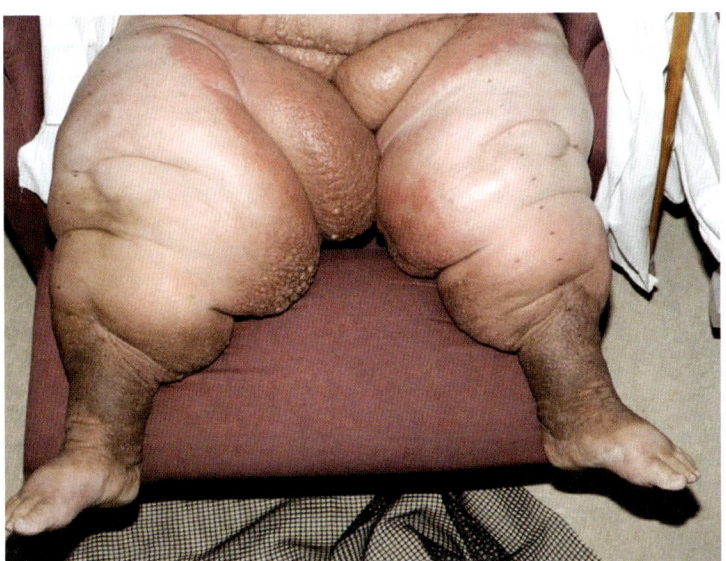

Figure 103.13 Acute and chronic lipodermatosclerosis; the bright red skin (acute) could be mistaken for bacterial cellulitis, but it is an inflammatory response to the skin blood and fluid congestion. The pigmented champagne bottle leg represents chronic lipodermatosclerosis. The treatment is decongestive lymphatic therapy with or without antibiotic cover.

Although redness and oedema are always present this is not always the case for warmth. Induration indicates that the underlying subcutaneous tissues are involved with the inflammatory process (sclerosing panniculitis). Pain and tenderness are always present but not itch; if itch does occur, varicose/stasis eczema probably coexists.

There are two forms of LDS: acute and chronic (Figure 103.13). Acute LDS mimics acute cellulitis with a flare of local redness, heat and pain. The differential diagnosis is acute cellulitis or DVT. With time, the chronic form supervenes. The skin becomes 'bound down' and retracted as the subcutaneous tissues become more fibrotic. Eventually redness gives rise to brown pigmentation and the leg contour takes on an 'inverted champagne bottle' shape. Pitting oedema will continue to exist both above and below the area of LDS and is a common feature (and common denominator) throughout. The skin surface remains smooth with no scaling as in eczema unless complications such as lymphorrhoea, infection or ulceration occur.

Investigations
Lipodermatosclerosis is a clinical diagnosis. Biopsy will reveal 'stasis dermatitis' changes together with a fibrotic panniculitis but there are no specific or diagnostic features. Furthermore, biopsy may induce ulceration if healing is poor.

Management
Compression therapy is the only proven therapy. Compression bandaging will achieve quicker results than compression hosiery but may not be tolerated if the affected tissues are very inflamed and tender. In such circumstances it may be necessary to start with bed rest or even topical steroids before introducing gentle compression. In more chronic cases, where there has been a change in shape of the leg, multilayer lymphoedema compression bandaging

works better [28]. Bandaging may have to be continued until a more normal contour is obtained. Only then will compression hosiery fit and work satisfactorily.

If superficial venous reflux is proven on duplex ultrasound then endovenous therapy (e.g. radiofrequency vein ablation, laser vein ablation or foam sclerotherapy) could be administered. If endovenous therapy is considered unsuitable then traditional ligation and stripping of superficial veins could be undertaken [29]. Bacterial infection (true cellulitis) can frequently complicate LDS but antibiotics alone do not resolve it and the only proven treatment is compression therapy to 'decongest' the tissues.

PRIMARY LYMPHOEDEMA

Primary lymphoedema

Definition and nomenclature
Primary lymphoedema (PL) is a build-up of lymph within tissues resulting from an inborn or intrinsic abnormality of lymph conducting pathways, that is, lymphatic vessels and nodes.

Synonyms and inclusions
- Lymphatic dysplasia
- Lymphatic anomalies
- Milroy disease
- Meige disease
- Lymphoedema congenita
- Lymphoedema praecox
- Lymphoedema tarda

Introduction and general description
Primary lymphoedema can be a presentation of complex genetic disease, with at least 20 identified pivotal causative genes identified. Recognition of clinical patterns is key to diagnosis, research and therapeutics. PL, or lymphoedema due to an underlying genetic abnormality, should always be suspected in a patient presenting with swelling and no obvious underlying medical cause. Suspicion of PL should be raised particularly if the presentation is during childhood or early adult years and when there is a family history.

Historically, PL was classified into three categories depending on the age of onset of swelling: congenita (lymphoedema present at birth), praecox (lymphoedema developing after birth but before the age of 35 years) and tarda (lymphoedema developing after the age of 35 years). It became apparent that this classification system, based purely on age of onset, was oversimplified and redundant in clinical practice as it failed to facilitate categorisation based on more specific phenotypes. Rigorous phenotyping of patients with PL has led to causal gene discovery and the possibility of a molecular diagnosis. This new approach to diagnosis is embodied in the St George's algorithm for clinical management [1].

The PL classification pathway is presented in the form of a colour-coded algorithm to illustrate the five main categories,

Table 103.3 Definition of terminology used in the classification pathway of primary lymphoedema.

Term	Definition
Congenital onset	Onset of lymphoedema before the age of 1 year
Cutaneous manifestations	Naevi/pigmentation variations (e.g. epidermal naevi/vascular malformations)
Distichiasis	Presence of aberrant eyelashes arising from the meibomian glands
Disturbed growth	Hypertrophy (overgrowth) and hypotrophy of bone or soft tissue resulting in altered length of a limb or body part
KT/KT-like	Klippel–Trenaunay/Klippel–Trenaunay-like syndrome
Late onset	Swelling presenting after 1 year of age
Prenatal onset	Detection of lymphatic abnormality in the prenatal period. Isolated pedal oedema is excluded from this definition as this may be a presentation of Milroy disease
Segment	A region of the body affected by lymphoedema (e.g. face, conjunctiva, genitalia, upper limbs, lower limbs – each constitutes one body part). Multisegmental refers to more than one segment affected by lymphoedema. Bilateral lower limb swelling is not considered to be multisegmental lymphoedema
Syndromic	A constellation of abnormalities, one of which is lymphoedema
Systemic involvement	Systemic lymphatic problems persisting beyond the newborn period or manifesting at any age thereafter. This includes hydrops fetalis, chylous ascites, intestinal lymphangiectasia, pleural and pericardial effusions and pulmonary lymphangiectasia
Vascular anomalies	Includes congenital vascular abnormalities

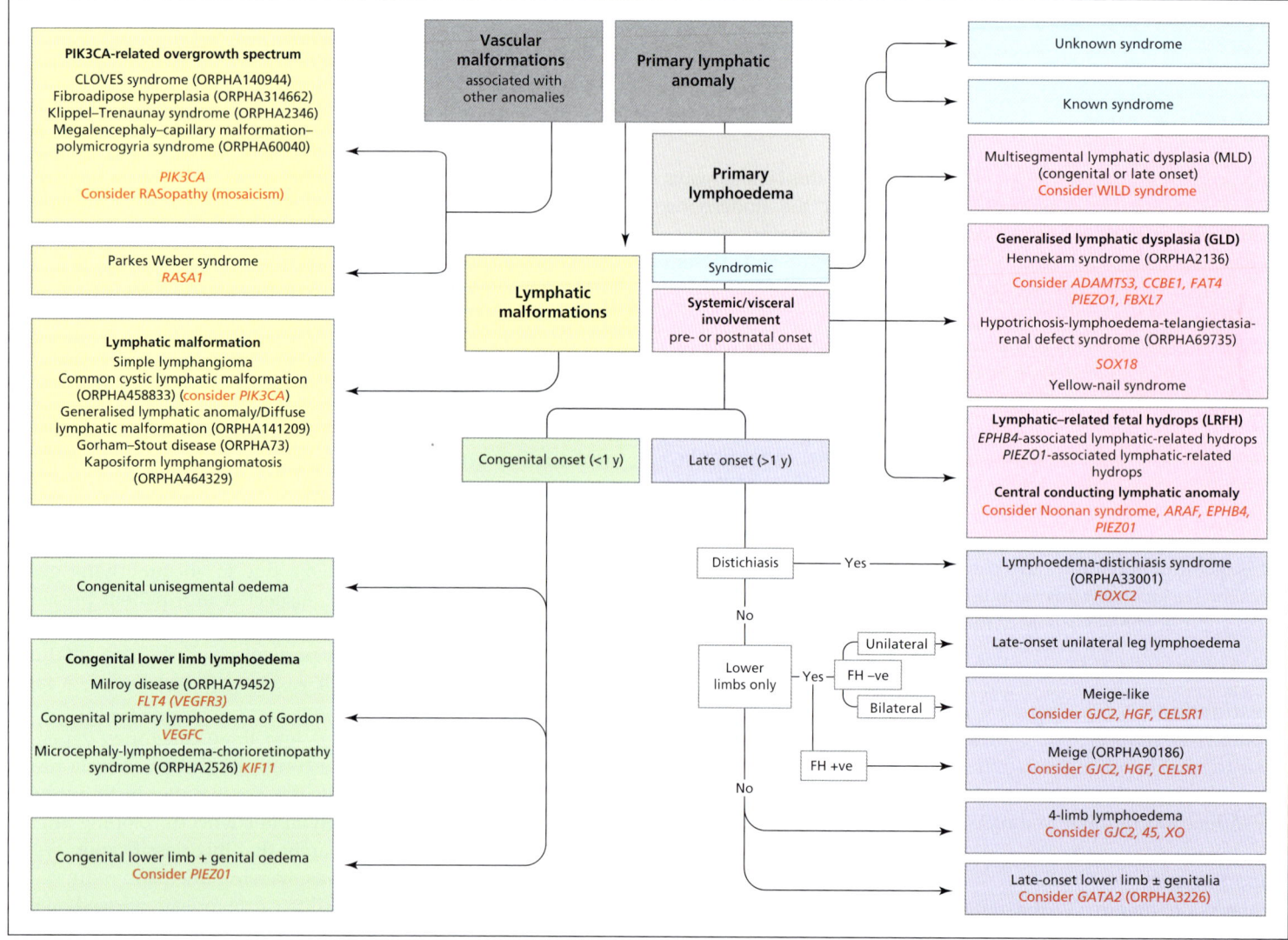

Figure 103.14 St George's classification algorithm for primary lymphatic anomalies showing the five main groupings (colour coded) with their various clinical subtypes of disease. Primary lymphoedema is the major clinical feature in the green, pink and purple sections. The text in red indicates the suggested genetic test and/or differential diagnosis for the subgroup, however the indicated genes do not explain the cause of disease in all patients in each grouping. For example, only 70% of patients with Milroy disease are explained by mutations in *FLT4/VEGFR3*. CLOVES, congenital lipomatous overgrowth, vascular malformations, epidermal naevi and scoliosis; FH, family history; +ve, positive; −ve, negative; WILD, warts, immunodeficiency, lymphoedema and ano-genital dysplasia. Courtesy of St George's Lymphovascular Research Group / Wikimedia Commons / CC BY-SA 4.0.

and the individual subtypes (including genotypes) within them (Table 103.3; Figure 103.14). The main categories are:

1 Syndromic associated with lymphoedema, but where lymphoedema is not the predominant feature) (blue).
2 Localised or generalised lymphoedema associated with systemic/visceral lymphatic abnormalities (pink).
3 Lymphoedema in association with disturbed growth and/or cutaneous/vascular anomalies (yellow).
4 Congenital-onset primary lymphoedema, that is, lymphoedema that is present at birth or develops within the first year of life (green).
5 Late-onset primary lymphoedema, that is, lymphoedema that develops after the first year of life (purple).

Epidemiology

Approximately 25% of causal genes for PL are now known although limited data exist on its prevalence. The prevalence of PL was estimated as 1 in 6000 based on one UK clinic but this is almost certainly an underestimate. In a case ascertainment study of chronic oedema, 12% were considered primary in type [2]. The prevalence of PL assessed from 8140 clinical records in nine lymphoedema services

in four countries was 17.5%. Italy and France had higher numbers of patients with PL (29.7% and 36.6%, respectively) compared with just 8.8% in Turkey [3]. This may be a disproportionately high number compared with the prevalence in the wider population as a number of specialist services specialise in managing patients with PL.

Pathophysiology

Primary lymphoedema may occur as a non-syndromic Mendelian condition, or less commonly as part of a complex syndromic disorder. Mutations in several genes are known as causative. Known causal genes are available for testing via the St George's lymphoedema gene panel [4]. Some, but not all, of these genes have been shown to play a role in the regulation of lymphangiogenesis (Table 103.4). The discovery of these genes has therefore informed their wider biological function. The first two genes to be identified as causative for human lymphoedema were *VEGFR3* (also known as *FLT4*) in Milroy disease [5] and *FOXC2* in lymphoedema distichiasis syndrome [6].

Developments in clinical phenotyping and identification of the genetic aetiology of a number of subtypes of PL demonstrate high

Table 103.4 A summary of genes causing primary lymphoedema and their phenotypes[a].

Gene name	Gene MIM number	Phenotype associated with a primary lymphatic anomaly	Phenotype ID number	Inheritance
GJA1/Cx43	121014	Oculo-dento-digital dysplasia (ODD) syndrome	ORPHA2710	AD
KIF11	148760	Microcephaly–lymphoedema–chorioretinopathy syndrome	ORPHA2526	AD
RAF1	164760	RASopathies (including Noonan syndrome)	ORPHA536391	AD
ADAMTS3	605011	Hennekam–lymphangiectasia–lymphoedema syndrome type 3	ORPHA2136	AR
CCBE1	612753	Hennekam–lymphangiectasia–lymphoedema syndrome type 1	ORPHA2136	AR
EPHB4	600011	*EPHB4*-related LRFH	ORPHA568065	AD
FAT4	612411	Hennekam–lymphangiectasia–lymphoedema syndrome type 2	ORPHA2136	AR
		Van Maldergem syndrome type 2	ORPHA314679	AR
PIEZO1	611184	*PIEZO1*-related GLD/LRFH	ORPHA568062	AR
SOX18	601618	Hypotrichosis–lymphoedema–telangiectasia–renal defect syndrome	ORPHA69735	AD, AR
FOXC2	602402	Lymphoedema distichiasis syndrome (LDS)	ORPHA33001	AD
GATA2	137295	GATA2-deficiency syndrome (Emberger syndrome)	ORPHA3226	AD
GJC2/Cx47	608803	Late-onset four-limb lymphoedema	OMIM613480	AD
VEGFC	601528	*VEGFC*-related congenital primary lymphoedema of Gordon	ORPHA79452	AD
VEGFR3/FLT4	136352	Milroy disease	ORPHA79452	AD
BRAF	164757	Mosaic RASopathies caused by postzygotic mutations		M
KRAS	190070			
MAP2K1	176872			
NRAS	164790			
PIK3CA	171834	*PIK3CA*-related overgrowth spectrum (PROS)	ORPHA530313	M
COUPTF-II	107773	Congenital heart defects, multiple types (but no primary lymphoedema association reported)	OMIM615779	AD
PROX1	601546	No reported phenotype		

Reproduced from Martin-Almedina *et al.* 2021 [**19**].

[a] Alterations in most of the genes listed cause different types of disease. These genes have been selected because primary lymphoedema is a major feature of the disease phenotype or because the role of the gene in lymphatic development is well documented. Some of the genes listed have no primary lymphoedema associated with them (*COUP-TFII*) or no phenotype at all (*PROX1*), but because their role in initiating the process of lymphangiogenesis is so crucial, they have been included in this review. The genes have been colour coded according to which of the categories of primary lymphoedema they are classified under in the St George's classification.

AD, autosomal dominant; AR, autosomal recessive; GLD, generalised lymphatic dysplasia; LRFH, lymphatic-related fetal hydrops; M, mosaic.

PART 9: VASCULAR DISORDERS

heterogeneity. A new classification system and diagnostic pathway have been developed in order to delineate specific phenotypes of PL and facilitate a molecular diagnosis as well as the discovery of new causative genes [1].

Infection in the form of cellulitis can manifest as PL [7]. In other words, cellulitis may be the presenting condition, but careful investigation will reveal an underlying pre-existing lymphatic insufficiency only evident on lymphoscintigraphy. Cellulitis may then be blamed as the cause of the lymphoedema, which is categorised as a secondary lymphoedema, but undetected primary lymphoedema was the true cause of both the cellulitis (because of altered immune cell trafficking) and the subsequent swelling.

Clinical features

Primary lymphoedema may not appear to be any different from any other form of lymphoedema except there will be no obvious cause. Swelling usually affects one or both legs but can be widespread, involving the upper limbs, face or genitalia. The more widespread the lymphoedema, the more likely there will be involvement of internal organs manifesting with pleural or pericardial effusions, ascites or chylous reflux. In such circumstances systemic immuno-deficiency may coexist as indicated by selective lymphopenia. Lymphatic or vascular malformations may often accompany PL.

The range of presentations for PL can be very varied with many different categories with different physical characteristics (phenotypes). The St George's classification suggests an approach that considers known syndromes (e.g. Turner syndrome or Noonan syndrome) first where lymphoedema may not be a dominant or common feature. Then one considers possible systemic involvement. Thereafter, time of onset is used to define phenotypes; for example congenital onset for Milroy disease caused by mutations

in *VEGFR3*, or late onset (there is no need to distinguish between pubertal and late adult onset) such as lymphoedema distichiasis syndrome caused by mutations in *FOXC2* or Emberger syndrome caused by mutations in *GATA2*. These phenotypes are called syndromes but are identified separately from the syndromic group because lymphoedema is a dominant and common feature. The final group to consider is the mosaic disorders where the gene fault is somatic and not germline. The identification of causal genes has permitted study of the exact phenotype for that gene.

Phenotyping and genotyping of patients with PL have led to a better understanding of the natural history and management of the specific categories and have guided genetic counselling.

Syndromic lymphoedema

Lymphoedema is a recognised feature of many syndromes where it is not the primary problem but is an associated feature. The genetic causes of many of these syndromes are known and testing is available. Table 103.5 provides a list of syndromes that include lymphoedema as part of the phenotype; these include Turner and Noonan syndromes.

Turner syndrome should always be suspected as the cause of congenital hand and/or foot swelling in female infants. It is a complex disorder caused by an absent or abnormal sex chromosome; karyotyping is necessary for diagnosis. It affects 1/2000 to 1/3000 live-born females. Congenital lymphoedema of the hands, feet and neck region is present in over 60% of patients. The majority of patients present at birth with four-limb lymphoedema, which often resolves in early childhood, but frequently recurs in later life.

Table 103.5 List of known syndromes associated with lymphoedema and the causative gene (or chromosomal abnormality) if known.

Known syndrome	Chromosome/gene
Aagenaes syndrome	Not known
Carbohydrate-deficient glycoprotein types 1a, 1b, 1h	*PMM2*, *PM1*, *ALG8*
Cardio-facio-cutaneous (CFC) syndrome	RAS-MAP kinase pathway including *KRAS*, *BRAF*, *MAP2K1*, *MAP2K2*
CHARGE syndrome	*CDH7*
Choanal atresia–lymphoedema	*PTPN14*
Ectodermal dysplasia, anhidrotic, immunodeficiency, osteopetrosis and lymphoedema (OLEDAID) syndrome	*IKBKG* (*NEMO*)
Fabry disease	*GLA*
Hennekam syndrome	*CCBE1*, *FAT4*
Hypotrichosis–lymphoedema–telangiectasia	*SOX18*
Irons–Bianchi syndrome	Not known
Lymphoedema–myelodysplasia (Emberger syndrome)	*GATA2*
Macrocephaly–capillary malformation (MCM)	*PIK3CA*
Microcephaly with or without chorioretinopathy, lymphoedema and mental retardation (MCLMR)	*KIF11*
Mucke syndrome	Not known
Noonan syndrome	RAS-MAPK pathway *PTPN11*, *KRAS*, *SOS1* and others
Oculo-dento-digital (ODD) syndrome	*GJA1*
Progressive encephalopathy, hypsarrhythmia and optic atrophy (PEHO) syndrome	Not known
Phelan–McDermid syndrome	22q terminal deletion or ring chromosome 22
Prader–Willi syndrome	15q11 microdeletion or maternal uniparental disomy 15
Thrombocytopenia with absent radius	1q21.1 microdeletion and *RBM8A*
Turner syndrome	45, X0
Velo-cardio-facial syndrome	22q11 microdeletion
Yellow-nail syndrome	Not known

CHARGE, coloboma, heart defects, atresia choanae, growth retardation, genital and ear abnormalities.

Systemic involvement (intestinal lymphangiectasia) can occur but is rare. Lymphoscintigraphy results suggest that the fault may be due to a failure of initial lymphatic (capillary) function [8].

The RASopathies, which include Noonan syndrome and cardio-facio-cutaneous syndrome (CFC) syndrome, are autosomal dominant disorders with genetic heterogeneity associated with germline mutations of genes in the RAS/mitogen-activated protein kinase (RAS–MAPK) pathway. Noonan syndrome and CFC syndrome in particular, are known to be associated with lymphatic problems.

Both conditions are characterised by facial dysmorphism, short stature and congenital heart disease. There is a characteristic lymphatic phenotype with bilateral lower limb lymphoedema, genital swelling and chylous reflux. There is frequent systemic involvement, including intestinal lymphangiectasia and chylothoraces, which may be progressive. Lymphoscintigraphy demonstrates reflux and/or rerouting of lymphatic drainage associated with incompetent veins on venous duplex scans [9].

Yellow-nail syndrome

Definition and nomenclature
Yellow-nail syndrome (YNS) comprises overcurved, smooth, translucent, slow-growing nails with a yellow discoloration along with respiratory ailments such as chronic sinusitis, bronchiectasis or pleural effusion and lymphoedema (Chapter 93). Although listed by McKusick as a genetic disease it more commonly develops late in adulthood as a sporadic condition (https://omim.org/, last accessed August 2022).

Synonyms and inclusions
- Lymphoedema and yellow nails

Introduction and general description
The first case series of 13 patients given a diagnosis of YNS was described by Samman and White [10]. Typically, the patient has (i) lymphoedema; (ii) a respiratory disease such as pleural effusion; and (iii) yellow dystrophic nails. Two of these features are required for the diagnosis, since the complete triad is only observed in about one-third of patients.

Epidemiology
A systematic review of 150 patients with YNS revealed that the median age was 60 years (range: newborn to 88 years) and occurred in all age groups but in 78.7% patients were aged between 41 and 80 years. The male : female ratio was 1.2 : 1. All cases had lymphoedema and 85.6% had yellow nails. Pleural effusions were bilateral in 68.3% of cases [11,12].

Pathophysiology
The pathogenesis is unknown. Lymphangiogram abnormalities have been described although a lymphoscintigraphic study demonstrated that a primary lymphatic abnormality is unlikely [13].

Pathology
The pleural effusion in YNS is an exudate in the vast majority of patients with lymphocytic predominance in 96% and a low count of nucleated cells. In 61 of 66 (92.4%) patients, pleural fluid protein values were >3 g/dL.

Genetics
Wells described a family with eight cases in four sibships of two generations. In the proband, who had yellow nails, lymphoedema began in the legs at the age of 51 years. At times oedema also affected the genitalia, hands, face and vocal cords. Lymphangiograms were interpreted as showing primary hypoplasia of the lymphatics [14].

Govaert *et al.* reported a girl who was born at 33 weeks' gestation with non-immune hydrops and a recurrent left chylothorax to a mother with YNS. The non-immune hydrops in this case was diagnosed on a 29-week ultrasound examination [15]. Slee *et al.* reported a case of a newborn infant who, at 23 weeks' gestation, was found to have hydrops on antenatal ultrasonography; bilateral chylothorax was found at delivery [16]. The mother had YNS with typical nail changes and bronchiectasis.

Clinical features
The average age of onset is during the sixth decade. Patients are usually first aware of not needing to cut their nails, of them becoming thicker and harder to cut. The nail may discolour yellow but also may lift up and become opaque (due to onycholysis) or turn green/black due to secondary haemorrhage or *Pseudomonas* infection. Manual dexterity may be affected due to tactile dysfunction. Nails may fracture or shed; nail units may become painful, particularly if affected by a paronychia. Cough is the commonest respiratory symptom and may be productive. Peripheral oedema usually starts in the ankles bilaterally but may become very widespread and involve the trunk, genitalia and upper limbs if severe.

Nail changes include slow growth, yellow-green discoloration, transverse and longitudinal overcurvature, onycholysis, shedding, cross-ridging and the loss of lunulae and cuticles. The nail plate remains translucent and smooth (Figure 103.15).

Although lymphoedema is the most consistent association with yellow nails, other associations include bronchiectasis, sinusitis, chronic cough and pleural effusions. Rarely a pericardial effusion can occur.

Recurrent chest infections are the commonest complication. Recurrent cellulitis frequently complicates lymphoedema. Acute

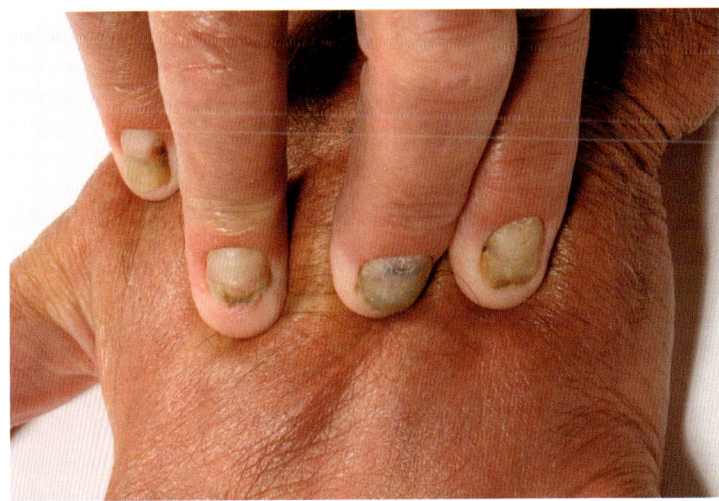

Figure 103.15 Yellow-nail syndrome showing slow-growing, overcurved, thickened nail plates and hand oedema.

paronychia can complicate the nail unit changes. In one study 4 of the 11 patients had complete recovery of their nails over a mean period of 4–5 years [17]. There are some suggestions that life expectancy is reduced.

Differential diagnosis

Onychomycosis in the setting of lymphoedema is an important differential diagnosis. A diagnosis of YNS is difficult without the characteristic nail changes.

Investigations

Yellow-nail syndrome is a clinical diagnosis. There is no confirmatory diagnostic test. Intranodal lymphangiography has revealed a slow contrast flow and narrowing of the thoracic duct, suggesting a pathogenic mechanism for the lymphatic phenotype in YNS [18].

Management

The most effective treatments for pleural effusions appear to be pleurodesis and decortication/pleurectomy. Diuretics do not improve lymph drainage, nevertheless diuretics such as spironolactone may be necessary if oedema is widespread and severe. Vitamin E is the most common treatment prescribed for the nail changes, but the evidence base for this is weak. Treatment of the chronic paronychia with fluconazole has been claimed to be beneficial in anecdotal reports.

Lymphoedema with systemic/visceral involvement

This is a widespread developmental abnormality of the lymphatic system that leads to systemic/visceral involvement and swelling that may not be confined to the limbs [**19**]. Lymphatic dysfunction may present prenatally with hydrothoraces or hydrops fetalis. The development of *in utero* oedema may cause dysmorphic facial features such as epicanthic folds, a broad nasal bridge and neck webbing with low-set ears. Systemic lymphatic abnormalities may present with pericardial and pleural effusions, chylous ascites and pulmonary and intestinal lymphangiectasia in the postnatal period. An individual with intestinal lymphangiectasia will complain of abdominal pain and diarrhoea following the ingestion of foods with a high fat content (as the intestinal lymphatics are responsible for fat absorption).

Management of systemic lymphatic impairment is not straightforward, and a multidisciplinary approach is key. Management includes the drainage of effusions and implementation of a medium-chain triglyceride diet to manage intestinal lymphangiectasia and chylous disorders.

Patients with systemic lymphatic abnormalities can be classified into one of two categories depending upon the clinical presentation: a multisegmental lymphatic dysplasia with systemic involvement (MLDSI) or a generalised lymphatic dysplasia (GLD).

Multisegmental lymphatic dysplasia with systemic involvement

Patients with MLDSI have a segmental pattern of lymphoedema. The swelling affects different body parts in association with a systemic lymphatic abnormality. For example, they may have lymphoedema of one or more limbs or body sites (including the face) in association with previous or current systemic lymphatic abnormalities (e.g. intestinal lymphangiectasia, recurrent chylous pleural effusions). The patient has no syndromic features and is of normal intelligence. The underlying mechanism is thought to be of somatic mosaicism, and no known causal genes have been identified to date. There is a low sibling and offspring recurrence risk.

WILD syndrome

This is a condition comprising clinical signs of *w*arts, *i*mmuno-deficiency, *l*ymphoedema and ano-genital *d*ysplasia (WILD) [20]. Lymphoedema affects regions of the body including the facial and conjunctival oedema and genital lymphoedema. Systemic involvement (intestinal lymphangiectasia/pleural or pericardial effusions) occurs in two-thirds of patients. Invariably there is a distinctive vascular malformation on the upper anterior chest wall and hyperpigmented lesions resembling epidermal naevi (but probably lymphatic in origin) can be found. Warts are common and often refractory [21]. In contrast to the previous single case report, ano-genital dysplasia is uncommon. Low CD4 counts and CD4/CD8 ratios typified the syndrome but monocyte counts were normal, unlike in GATA2 deficiency where warts may also be a presenting feature. WILD syndrome is a sporadic condition, suggesting probable somatic mosaicism. The underlying genetic cause has yet to be identified.

Generalised lymphatic dysplasia

Patients have a more global pattern of lymphoedema. Swelling typically affects all body parts and often presents *in utero* with hydrops fetalis. Patients with GLD may have a family history of lymphoedema suggestive of autosomal recessive inheritance, inferring a higher recurrence risk than in MLDSI.

Hennekam (lymphangiectasia–lymphoedema) syndrome. This is one type of autosomal recessive GLD and presents with lymphoedema of the lower limbs and genitalia although it can involve all four limbs. There is internal involvement with intestinal lymphangiectasia and a varible degree of pulmonary lymphatic dysplasia and learning difficulties. Characteristic facies include a flat face, flat and broad nasal bridge and hypertelorism. Associated problems include hypothyroidism, glaucoma, seizures, hearing loss and renal abnormalities. Lymphoscintigraphy has rarely been undertaken in this condition, but Bellini *et al.* demonstrated abnormal drainage in all four limbs and the thoracic duct in one patient [22].

The syndrome can be caused by biallelic variants in *CCBE1* (18q21.32) or *FAT4* (4q28.1) or *ADAMTS3* (4q13.3):
- Type 1 (mutations in *CCBE1*) [23].
- Type 2 (mutations in *FAT4*) [24].
- Type 3 (mutations in *ADAMTS3*) [25].

The diagnosis is based on the clinical phenotype. Intestinal lymphangiectasia may be suspected because of hypogammaglobulinaemia, hypoalbuminaemia and lymphopenia with a molecular diagnosis indicating type.

Hypotrichosis–lymphoedema–telangiectasia syndrome (HLTS). This is caused by mutations in *SOX18* (ORPHA69735; MIM: 607823). Dependent on the type of variant and which domain of the *SOX18* gene it resides in, HLTS can be described as either an autosomal recessive or an autosomal dominant disorder. No matter what the gene mutation, the phenotype is similar, and patients present with hypotrichosis (absence of hair including scalp, eyebrows and eyelashes) from infancy, primary non-congenital lymphoedema and telangiectasia (dilatation of cutaneous blood-filled capillaries). Thin transparent skin with widespread mottling (cutis marmorata) has also been described, although the expression of the disease features can be variable. Looking specifically at the primary lymphoedema phenotype, individuals with *SOX18* mutation(s) show variable ages of onset. The oedema is usually confined to the lower limbs, but most patients also have lymphoedema of the eyelids and periorbitally. Hydrocele, non-immune hydrops fetalis, progressive dilatation of the aorta and renal disease have been reported [26].

Lymphatic-related hydrops fetalis

Impaired lymphatic drainage causes lymphoedema in adults but in the fetus it can develop into a more severe and lethal condition known as hydrops fetalis. The term hyrops fetalis (HF) refers to excessive fluid accumulation in more than two fetal extravascular compartments and body cavities, and is characterised by generalised skin thickness of >5 mm, placental enlargement and oedema, pericardial or pleural effusion, or ascites. HF is further divided into immune HF related to Rhesus disease, or non-immune HF (NIHF). NIHF now accounts for 85–90% of all hydrops cases of which generalised lymphatic dysplasia is a major cause. Identified genetic causes of NIHF include all the Hennekam syndromes as well as muatations in *EPHB4*, *PIEZO-1* and *hCALCRL* [27]. Asking about hydrops when taking a history is important for the phenotyping of primary lymphoedema in children and adults.

Mosaic lymphoedema associated with disturbed growth and/or cutaneous/vascular anomalies

Genetic mosaicism is defined by the presence of at least two genetically distinct cell populations in the same organism. It results from postzygotic mutations. The clinical phenotype of mosaic disorders is determined by the cells affected, the timing of the mutation and the level of pathway activation. Generally, somatic mutations are not inherited.

Lymphatic abnormalities due to somatic mutations may develop in association with vascular abnormalities, disorders of growth and cutaneous abnormalities. Identifying the type of malformation and thereby the vessels involved is important for diagnosis and management. Several overgrowth syndromes, with overlapping phenotypic features, can all possess somatic mutations in the *PIK3CA* gene known as PIK3CA-related overgrowth syndrome or PROS. The best known of these syndromes is Klippel–Trenaunay syndrome, but others include megalencephaly–capillary malformation (MCAP) syndrome, CLOVES (congenital lipomatous overgrowth, vascular malformations, epidermal naevi and scoliosis)

syndrome as well as fibroadipose hyperplasia (FH) and hemihyperplasia multiple lipomatosis (HHML). Findings in PROS include adipose dysregulation, unilateral overgrowth that is predominantly left-sided, overgrowth that affects the lower extremities more than the upper extremities and progresses in a distal to proximal pattern, with often marked paucity of adipose tissue in unaffected areas [28].

An increased risk of thromboembolism has been recognised in individuals with mosaic overgrowth disorders, particularly Proteus syndrome and PROS, so surveillance for thrombosis is recommended in all cases [29].

These patients are challenging as there is considerable overlap in clinical findings and a clear-cut diagnosis based upon phenotype or genotype alone is not always possible. A molecular diagnosis can guide therapy. Sirolimus, an mTOR1 inhibitor, has shown promise in the management of vascular anomalies and now PROS [30]. The PIK3CA direct inhibitor, alpelisib (BYL719), was recently trialled with significant clinical benefit [31,32]. Miransertib, an AKT1 inhibitor, was found to decrease the size of the cerebriform connective tissue naevus and associated pain [33].

Conditions with gene abnormalities within the AKT/PIK3/mTOR pathway that are associated with lymphoedema

CLOVES syndrome. The spectrum of clinical signs includes congenital lipomatous overgrowth, vascular malformations, epidermal naevi and skeletal abnormalities. Somatic mosaicism of activating mutations within *PIK3CA* has been reported. The same gene and mechanism have also been implicated in several patients with Klippel–Trenaunay syndrome and fibroadipose hyperplasia [34]. Lymphatic malformations can arise as part of these conditions. Further molecular studies, together with careful phenotyping, will facilitate the understanding of this spectrum of diseases. It is likely that combined vascular malformations may arise as a result of somatic mosaicism.

Klippel–Trenaunay syndrome. This is a sporadic congenital vascular malformation which can possess somatic *PIK3CA* mutations as well as infrequent *KRAS* mutations. Patients present with a combination of several or all of the following within a single limb: limb length hypertrophy of muscle, fat or bone (e.g. presenting as increased limb length or girth), varicose veins, vascular malformation (e.g. capillary malformations) and lymphoedema. While Klippel–Trenaunay syndrome manifests with overgrowth and vascular malformations, the overgrowth is generally unilateral and overlapping with the vascular malformations. The typical vascular malformation is a lateral venous anomaly (lateral thigh varicose vein), and the skeletal overgrowth lacks the distortion and progressivity seen in people with Proteus syndrome. *PIK3CA* mutations are associated with scarring [35].

Proteus syndrome. Proteus syndrome is characterised by severe, progressive overgrowth that can affect nearly any region of the body [36]. Common syndromic manifestations include large superficial or deep lipomatous overgrowths, intellectual disability, seizures and other neurological problems and severe skeletal deformities with

PART 9: VASCULAR DISORDERS

skull overgrowth, kyphoscoliosis, asymmetrical macrodactyly and valgus or varus deformities of the knees. Lymphatic and capillary malformations are the most common vascular changes seen in this syndrome. The cerebriform connective tissue naevus of the soles found in many patients is a specific, but not a pathognomonic, finding. A somatic variant in the *AKT1* gene is the only reported cause of Proteus syndrome. AKT1 is a serine-threonine kinase that participates in the AKT/PI3K/mTOR pathway.

Somatic RASopathies associated with lymphatic abnormalities

Parkes Weber syndrome. When arteriovenous malformations coexist, Klippel–Trenaunay–Weber (or Parkes Weber) syndrome is often diagnosed. Capillary malformation–arteriovenous malformation is an autosomal dominant disorder, caused by heterozygous *RASA1* mutations, and manifesting with multifocal capillary malformations and a high risk for fast-flow lesions. *RASA1* mutations are responsible for aberrant lymphatic architecture and functional abnormalities in the Parkes Weber syndrome [37].

Mosaic RASopathies. These are developmental syndromes caused by germline mutations in genes that alter the RAS/MAPK pathway, and include neurofibromatosis type 1 and Noonan syndrome. Genes within this pathway that are only somatically mutated lead to a group of conditions which clinically overlap with PROS. These somatic RASopathies present mainly with vascular malformations but lymphatic malformations can coexist and if they interfere with lymph conducting pathways then lymphoedema can occur. Multiple mosaic-activating variants in four genes of the RAS/MAPK pathway, *KRAS*, *NRAS*, *BRAF* and *MAP2K1*, are responsible for the germline RASopathies. These variants are more frequent in high-flow than low-flow vascular malformations. MAPK inhibitors provide an opportunity for treatment [38].

Congenital-onset primary lymphoedema

Historically, all cases of congenital lymphoedema were classified as Milroy disease. However, several different types of congenital, lower limb, primary lymphoedema have been describd.

Milroy disease. This presents with congenital lymphoedema of the lower legs (usually symmetrical). The onset of swelling may occasionally be delayed but will occur within the first year of life, although may be missed if mild. Lymphoedema is typically confined to the feet and ankles but may progress to the knees. Up-slanting 'ski-jump' toenails are present as a result of disturbance of the nail bed by oedema. Prominent large-calibre veins are frequently present on the feet and pretibial regions. Varicose veins, with venous reflux in the great (long) saphenous veins, are a common finding in adults with Milroy disease, but do not appear to affect the paediatric population. A third of affected males have hydroceles [39]. Milroy disease can rarely present in the antenatal period with hydrops fetalis, but the outcome may be favourable (i.e. the swelling may regress and remain confined to the feet), or the hydrops may progress and result in intrauterine death.

Lymphoscintigraphy in Milroy disease confirms failure of the initial lymphatic vessels to absorb fluid. The term 'functional aplasia of lymphatic vessels' has been used to describe the characteristic lymphoscintigraphy results [40]. The initial lymphatic vessels (lymphatic capillaries) are present (confirmed on histological examination) but are unable to absorb interstitial fluid [41]. Abnormalities within the gene that encodes vascular endothelial growth factor receptor type 3 (VEGFR-3) on chromosome 5q35 are causal of Milroy disease [42]. Mutations in the tyrosine kinase domain of *VEGFR3* are found in 70% of patients with congenital-onset primary lymphoedema affecting both lower limbs. Inheritance is autosomal dominant but *de novo* cases may occur.

Gordon syndrome. Mutations in human *VEGFC* have been identified as the cause of congenital primary lymphoedema of Gordon (ORPHA79452) [43]. Vascular endothelial growth factor C (VEGF-C) is the ligand for VEGFR-3 and controls lymphatic sprouting during embryonic development. The lymphoedema usually is milder than in Milroy disease, but otherwise is very similar. In nearly all cases reported, swelling is confined to the lower limbs, often just the dorsa of the feet. One case had intermittent hand swelling. The lymphoedema usually presents at birth and there are no other major pathological features, apart from some patients who present with prominent varicose veins and hydrocele as in *VEGFR3* mutations of Milroy. Lymphoscintigraphy demonstrates poor uptake with tortuous lymphatics and rerouting.

Milroy-like lymphoedema. Individuals with congenital lower limb lymphoedema who do not have an underlying *VEGFR3* or *VEGFC* mutation are classified as having Milroy-like lymphoedema.

MCLID syndrome. *M*icrocephaly with or without *c*horioretinopathy, *l*ymphoedema or *i*ntellectual *d*isability (MCLID) syndrome is autosomal dominant, comprising congenital lower limb lymphoedema (mimicking Milroy disease) as well as microcephaly and variable degrees of learning difficulties that occur as a result of mutations in the *KIF11* gene on chromosome 10q24 [44]. The presence of chorioretinopathy is variable but should always be excluded by an expert ophthalmological opinion. Lymphoscintigraphy demonstrates the same pattern of lymphatic functional aplasia as that seen in Milroy disease. The KIF11 protein product is involved in spindle formation during mitosis but it is not clear how *KIF11* relates to the lymphangiogenesis pathway. MCLID should be considered in all patients with congenital bilateral lower limb lymphoedema and microcephaly.

Late-onset primary lymphoedema

The term late-onset lymphoedema is used to describe a primary lymphoedema that develops after the first year of life (i.e. non-congenital lymphoedema). This section contains a number of assorted conditions, some with life-threatening associated diseases (e.g. Emberger syndrome), but they share the common finding of non-congenital limb swelling.

Lymphoedema distichiasis syndrome. This condition presents with pubertal onset of bilateral lower limb lymphoedema. Distichiasis (aberrant eyelashes arising from the meibomian glands) is present in 95% of affected individuals and is frequently present at birth but rarely causes symptoms until childhood. While the distichiasis can be evident from birth, the lymphoedema of the lower limbs usually develops late in childhood or later in life and sometimes not until the fifth decade. Early-onset varicose veins (49%), ptosis (31%), cardiac defects (7%), cleft palate (4%), spinal cysts and structural kidney abnormalities are other associated complications. The majority of affected individuals have varicose veins [45]. Lymphoedema distichiasis syndrome occurs as a result of mutations in the *FOXC2* gene on chromosome 16q24 and is inherited in an autosomal dominant manner [46]. *FOXC2* encodes a transcription factor necessary for ensuring normal development of the lymphatic collecting vessels and valves. Lymphoscintigraphy of affected individuals demonstrates reflux of lymph within the lower limbs as a result of valve failure within the lymphatic vessels [47]. Similarly, abnormal venous valves lead to early-onset venous reflux in all patients with *FOXC2* mutations [48].

Emberger syndrome. This comprises late-onset (but in childhood), bilateral or unilateral lower limb with or without genital lymphoedema, together with myelodysplastic syndrome and/or acute myeloid leukaemia [49]. It may also be associated with a high-frequency, progressive, sensorineural deafness. Severe cutaneous warts occur as a result of the associated immune dysfunction.

Myelodysplasia may develop at any stage and will progress to acute myeloid leukaemia with a high mortality [50]. Lymphoedema often precedes the haematological abnormalities; it is recommended considering this syndrome when evaluating a patient with lymphoedema or extensive warts. Initially, the haematological abnormalities present as monocytopenia usually during the second decade and can develop into pancytopenia, myelodysplasia or acute myeloid leukaemia with high mortality. Therefore, this is a life-threatening condition that demands close monitoring. A high incidence of monosomy 7 or trisomy 8 in the bone marrow is frequently reported. Other features reported include mild hypertelorism, epicanthic folds and slender fingers. Mutations in the *GATA2* gene on chromosome 3q21 are causal and are inherited in an autosomal dominant manner [51]. *GATA2* is expressed in lymphatic, vascular and endocardial endothelial cells. Mouse studies suggest the lymphoedema occurs as a result of abnormal lymphatic valve development [52]. *GATA2* is also involved in the regulation of haematopoiesis, hence the association of lymphoedema with myelodysplasia in this rare, yet life-threatening, condition.

Meige disease. Meige disease is the most prevalent subtype of primary lymphoedema but as yet no causal gene has been identified [1]. It typically presents in females with bilateral lower limb lymphoedema that rarely extends above the knee. The onset of symptoms is in adolescence or adulthood. Family history is consistent with an autosomal dominant pattern of inheritance; there are no other associated features [53]. Lymphoscintigraphy frequently demonstrates abnormal, deep rerouting of lower limb lymph drainage as evidenced by an increased uptake of tracer within the popliteal lymph nodes and impaired main superficial lymphatic tract filling.

Late-onset four-limb lymphoedema. An autosomal dominant pattern of late-onset lymphoedema affecting either the lower limbs, or all four limbs, occurs as a result of mutations in the *GJC2* gene [54]. Apart from lower limb varicose veins, no other associated conditions have been reported. Lymphoscintigraphy demonstrates lymphatic tracts that appear normal but with significantly reduced quantification uptake of tracer, reflecting reduced absorption from tissues by peripheral lymphatics in all four limbs. The functional role of *GJC2* within the lymphatic system is unclear as it encodes for the connexin 47 protein located on chromosome 1q42 and is not known to be involved in the lymphangiogenesis pathway.

LYMPHATIC MALFORMATIONS

Definition and nomenclature

Vascular tumours are endothelial neoplasms characterised by increased cellular proliferation. Haemangioma is the most common and is almost exclusive to infants. Vascular malformations, including lymphatic malformations, on the other hand, are the result of abnormal development, and in particular overgrowth, of vascular elements during embryogenesis and fetal life. These may be single-vessel forms (capillary, arterial, lymphatic or venous) or a combination [1]. Once established, vascular malformations do not continue to express increased endothelial turnover. The same principles apply to lymphangioma which is proliferative and to lymphatic malformations which are non-proliferative and increase in size mainly from distension [2].

Synonyms and inclusions
- Lymphangioma circumscriptum
- Cavernous lymphangioma
- Microcystic lymphatic malformation
- Macrocystic lymphatic malformation
- Cystic hygroma
- Lymphangiodysplasia
- Mixed vascular anomaly

Lymphangioma circumscriptum

Introduction and general description

The term lymphangioma circumscriptum is in common usage to describe a lymphatic malformation. Strictly, a lymphangioma should be a 'growing lymphatic tumour' involving proliferating lymphatic endothelium. A lymphatic malformation (LM) once formed from an abnormal development of lymphatic vessels grows only by expansion/distension, not proliferation, and therefore lymphangioma is an inappropriate term for a malformation.

Localised congenital LMs can be divided into macrocystic (or deep) and microcystic (or superficial) lesions. LMs can have both microcystic and macrocystic components. Deeper, larger and cavernous LMs are macrocystic LMs [2]. Lymphangioma circumscriptum is a term best reserved for a LM that is localised to an area of skin, subcutaneous tissue and sometimes muscle [3].

LMs with few but large macrocystic swellings containing clear lymph are called *cystic hygromas* (hygroma = moist or watery tumour). The term cystic hygroma is usually reserved for those congenital LMs that present at birth or are diagnosed by prenatal ultrasound. Most occur in the neck, but they frequently extend into the upper mediastinum. In the neck they presumably arise from an embryonic jugular lymph sac. Individuals with Turner syndrome are particularly prone to both hydrops and cystic hygroma. Exceptionally, a cystic hygroma occurs in the groin, presumably from an embryonic iliac lymph sac. Fetal cystic hygroma can give rise to severe abnormalities, leading to fetal death.

Epidemiology

Lymphatic malformations account for 4% of all vascular malformations but comprise 25% of benign vascular growths in children [4]. Approximately 75% present at birth, while the remainder present by 2 years of age.

Pathophysiology

An LM is characterised by the size of the malformed channels: microcystic, macrocystic (often known as cystic hygroma if in the neck) or combined (microcystic/macrocystic). The contraction of thickened muscular linings may increase intramural pressure and cause cystic dilatation [5]. On light microscopy of biopsies, there are marked expanded channels in the dermis, which can extend into the subcutaneous and other deeper tissues. The channels are lined with flattened cells, which express CD31 and D2-40.

LMs can be isolated lesions disconnected from nearby normal lymphatic vessels (atruncular) or they can be connected (truncular) in which case lymphoedema will feature. In an LM, lymph fluid is trapped within the ectatic malformed lymph vessels, whereas in lymphoedema the lymph fluid is within the interstitial space of the tissues.

These malformations can be part of a syndrome such as Turner syndrome (due to monosomy X) or overgrowth syndromes, such as Proteus syndrome, Klippel–Trenaunay syndrome (capillary lymphaticovenous malformation) and CLOVES syndrome due to mutations in the AKT/PIK3 pathway [**1**].

Genetics

The lack of familial forms and the unifocality of the lesions suggest that the cause could be a postzygotic somatic mutation restricted to cells of the lesion. Such a mutation would be lethal if in the germline. Somatic activating mutations in the *PIK3CA* gene cause the majority of LMs. Both macrocystic and microcystic LM can be driven by an activating $PIK3CA^{H1047R}$ mutation, with the developmental timing of activation of the p110α PI3K signalling in lymphatic endothelia determining the LM subtype. The growth of $PIK3CA^{H1047R}$-driven microcystic LM in mice is dependent on the upstream lymphangiogenic VEGF-C/VEGFR-3 signalling. Combined inhibition of VEGF-C signalling and the PI3K downstream target mTOR using rapamycin, but neither treatment alone, promotes the regression of experimental LM in mice [6].

A recurrent somatic activating mutation has been discovered in the AKT1 pathway in patients with Proteus syndrome which can also cause malformations [7].

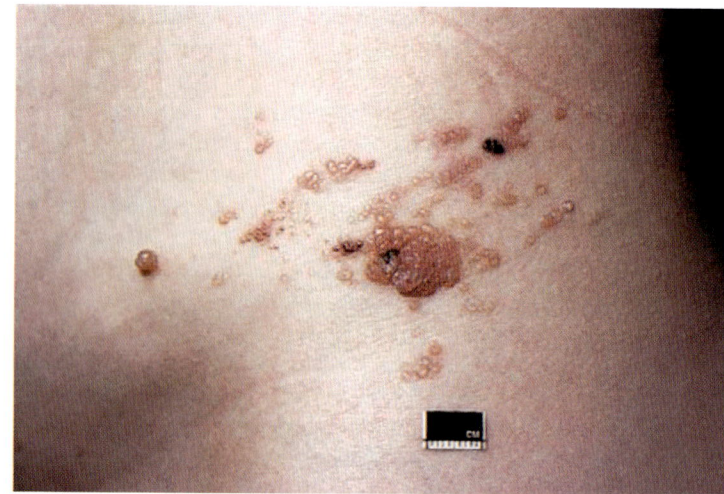

Figure 103.16 A lymphatic malformation otherwise called a lymphangioma circumscriptum showing fluid-filled vesicles resembling frogspawn. At times the vesicles can contain blood, weep clear fluid (lymphorrhoea) or become warty.

Clinical features

Lymphatic malformations (lymphangioma circumscriptum) manifest at birth or during infancy either as a localised subcutaneous swelling or as 'frogspawn' (groups of watery or haemorrhagic vesicles or lymph blisters) on the skin. Lymphangioma circumscriptum may present at any age but is usually noted at birth or appears during childhood. The commonest sites are the axillary folds, shoulders, flanks, proximal parts of the limbs and perineum. Clinically, the condition manifests with fluid-filled vesicles ('lymph blisters'), which bulge on the skin surface (Figure 103.16). They may be translucent when the overlying epidermis is very thin, or they may vary in colour from red to blue-black when they contain blood, which is a frequent occurrence. With time the surface of the lymphangiomas may appear extremely warty and the lesions may be mistaken for viral warts. The anatomical location of an LM is most frequently the head and neck (48%). LMs appear to involve the left side of the body more frequently.

LMs grow proportionally with the affected child. Some show marked progression especially during puberty and may not be noticeable until this time. Lymphatic malformations may occur at any site, although they often appear in the mouth, on the neck or jaw or around the axilla or groin. The most common symptom is recurrent oozing, usually of clear fluid (lymph), known as lymphorrhoea. If the malformation is disconnected from normally draining lymphatic pathways/trunks there will be no lymphoedema (atruncular) (Figure 103.17). If connections exist, then limb lymph drainage will be adversely affected and lymphoedema will be observed and may be the presenting feature (truncular) (Figure 103.18). Infection (e.g. cellulitis) can be a presenting feature because of the dysfunctional immune cell trafficking associated with an LM.

LMs of the neck region often lead to obstruction of the upper airways. The volume of the malformation increases with infection or trauma. Intracystic haemorrhage is also common. Frequent discharge of lymph fluid (lymphorrhoea), ulceration and infection are the most frequent complications. Pain can be a problem but it is difficult to know if the cause is infection, lymph thrombosis or lymphatic

Extensive LMs can have a blood vascular component. Consumption coagulopathy and in particular low platelets can complicate them. This may be because the correct separation of the lymphatic and blood vasculatures during embryonic development is dependent on CLEC-2-mediated platelet activation [8].

Differential diagnosis

Vascular birthmarks in the skin that look like blood capillary malformations may be mistaken for lymphatic capillary dermal malformations. Biopsy and staining with D2-40 may be necessary to make the distinction although the dermal vessels may be sufficiently undifferentiated to express both blood capillary and lymphatic phenotypes [9]. An LM can be mistaken for other vascular malformations, hamartomas or tumours. The surface lymph vesicles can be confused with human papillomavirus warts.

Investigations

Biopsy will reveal angulated channels, which stain for CD31 and D2-40. Ultrasound should demonstrate fluid-filled channels, which on duplex will be slow flow, making a distinction from a slow-flow venous malformation difficult. MRI can demonstrate the extent of the LM – that is, extension into muscle or bone. Overgrowth of tissue elements (fat, muscle or bone) may also be seen, as may any lymphoedema component. Lymphoscintigraphy should be normal in an atruncular lymphatic malformation but abnormal in a truncular lymphatic malformation.

Management

The majority of LMs are best managed conservatively [10]. Sclerotherapy is the mainstay of treatment of macrocystic LMs, but the response using traditional sclerosants is much less beneficial

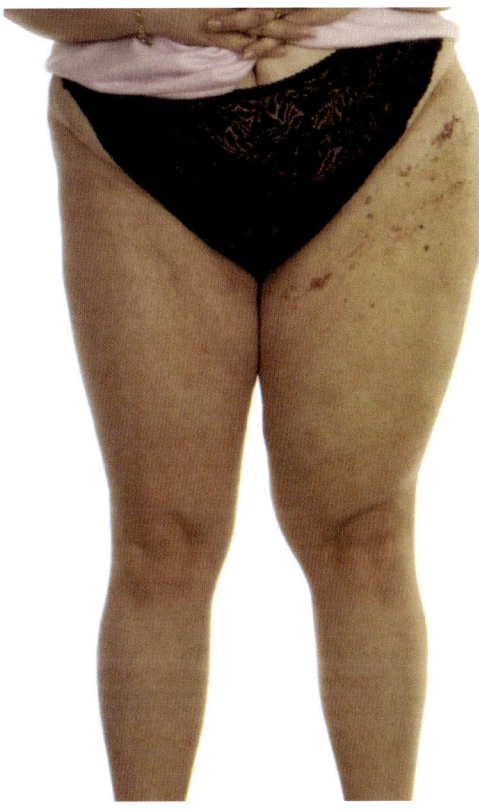

Figure 103.17 Atruncular lymphatic malformation without lymphoedema.

vessel distension from intralymphatic pressure. Squamous cell carcinoma is described arising within a lymphangioma. Prognosis is usually excellent, providing there is no lymphangiomatosis. Infection can rarely be severe and life threatening.

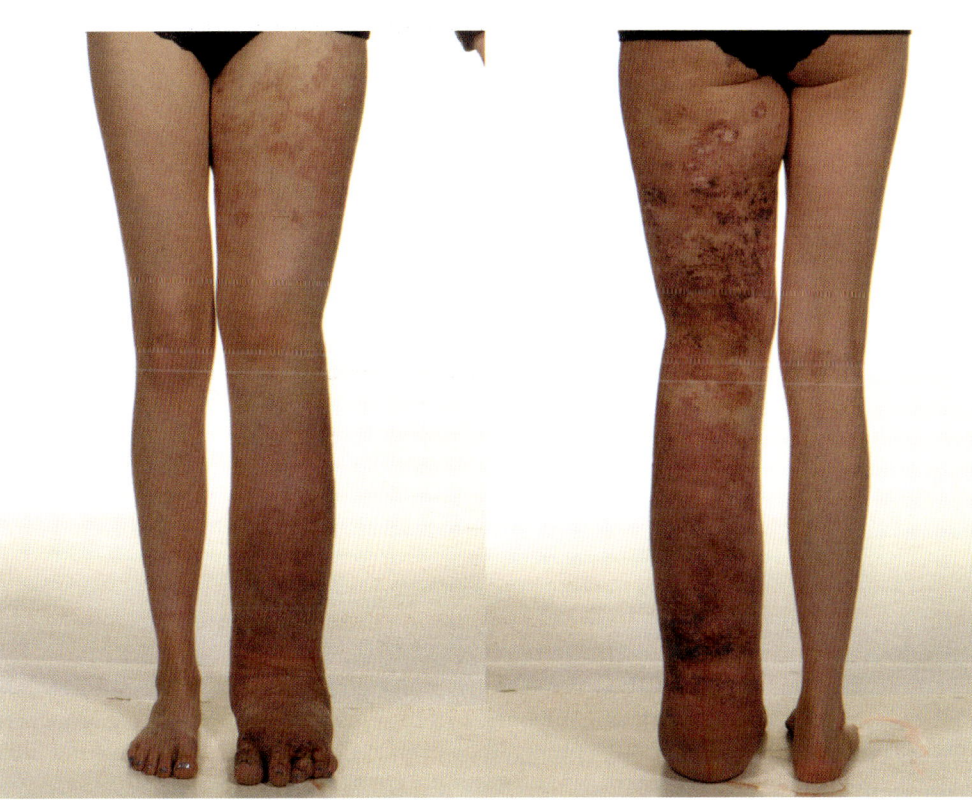

Figure 103.18 Truncular lymphatic malformation with blood-filled cutaneous lymphangiectasia and lymphoedema.

PART 9: VASCULAR DISORDERS

in microcystic lesions. Sclerotherapy of microcystic LMs using bleomycin is effective and safe, giving a complete response in 38% and a partial response in 58% ($n = 31$) in one series [10].

It is generally not possible to excise an LM because of its extent and ill-defined infiltration of surrounding tissues. Indeed, attempted excision may result in further growth of the remaining malformation. Debulking procedures may be necessary for very large malformations causing complications such as the obstruction of vital organs and their functions.

Surface vesicles that weep or bleed should be destroyed by diathermy or laser. Since the vesicles have a tendency to reform, such procedures can be repeated as often as necessary.

Infection should be treated promptly with antibiotics, as in lymphoedema. If recurrent attacks of infection occur then prophylactic antibiotics should be considered.

For truncular lymphatic malformations with lymphoedema, compression garments are recommended. In atruncular lymphatic malformations compression may prove fruitless, as the lymph fluid is trapped within the closed vessel system of the malformation.

Sildenafil can reduce LM volume and symptoms in some children [11].

A clearer understanding of the genetic underpinnings of LMs and mixed vascular anomalies has enabled the identification of therapeutic drug targets. The identified importance of PI3K/AKT/MAPK signalling led to treatment with sirolimus and then alpelisib (BYL719) with ARQ092 for AKT inhibition becoming available for PROS and Proteus syndrome [12].

Lymphangiomatosis, lymphangioleiomyomatosis and non-malignant lymphatic tumours

Definition and nomenclature

Lymphangiomatosis is a disorder of proliferative lymphatic vasculature. It is characterised by the progressive involvement of various body tissues and can involve the skeletal system, connective tissues and visceral organs. The process may vary from progressive overgrowth of an LM to a lymphatic tumour. A fundamental requirement is cellular proliferation of lymphatic endothelial cells.

Synonyms and inclusions
- Lymphangioma
- Kaposiform lymphangiomatosis
- Acquired progressive lymphangioma
- Benign lymphangioendothelioma
- Atypical vascular lesions
- Gorham–Stout disease
- Generalised lymphatic anomaly

Introduction and general description

There is no clear distinction between LMs, lymphangiomatosis and some non-malignant lymphatic tumours. Lymphangiomatosis implies there is progression through proliferation of aberrant lymph vessels, whereas in an LM there should be no progression other

than expansion though distension from intralymphatic pressure. Most LMs are stable and run a completely benign course. Conversely, some visceral thoracic and abdominal LMs can relentlessly progress, infiltrating vital organs with fatal outcome and making distinction from lymphangiomatosis and frank neoplasia difficult.

The identification of causal somatic mutations is helping to explain these findings. Mutations in *PIK3CA* and the somatic RASopathies have been described as causing LMs [13]. It would appear the same mutation (e.g. *PIK3CA*) can produce different phenotypes ranging from a limited benign lesion as in a simple lymphangioma circumscriptum to a progressive, infiltrating, multifocal disease such as lymphangiomatosis (generalised lymphatic anomaly). The process may vary from progressive overgrowth of an LM to a lymphatic tumour. The phenotype depends on the mutation, the cells affected and at what time in development the mutation has greatest effect.

Some non-malignant vascular tumours may exhibit a lymphangioma-like appearance with positive staining for lymphatic markers (e.g. tufted angioma, kaposiform haemangioendothelioma, multifocal lymphangioendotheliomatosis with thrombocytopenia, papillary intralymphatic angioendothelioma, retiform haemangioendothelioma and adult-type haemangioendotheliomas). However, it can be difficult to know if these are primarily lymphatic tumours. They can demonstrate locally aggressive behaviour and can be associated with life-threatening systemic complications such as Kasabach–Merritt syndrome.

Chylous reflux may complicate visceral lymphangiomatosis. Disseminated intravascular coagulation can occur and may give rise to thrombosis and haemorrhage [14].

Gorham–Stout disease (GSD). Gorham–Stout disease or disappearing/vanishing bone disease is characterised by massive osteolysis resulting from bone-replacing abnormal lymphatic capillary proliferation early in the disease or fibrous hyperplasia in the later stage. Lymphatic vessels are not present in normal bones, but they are present in the bones of patients with GSD and generalised lymphatic anomaly.

The major distinguishing characteristic is the progressive osteolysis seen in this disease. All bones could be affected, but the most common areas are the skull, shoulder girdle, pelvis and extremities. The osteolytic lesions in GSD are related to the local lymphatic vessel proliferation whereas no such vessels would usually be found in normal bones. ^{99m}Tc-antimony sulfide colloid lymphoscintigraphy and single photon-emission computed tomography (SPECT)/CT can detect GSD and other rare lymphatic disorders [15]. Treatment with a combination of drugs has been used such as bisphosphonates with sirolimus with or without surgery [16].

Generalised lymphatic anomaly (GLA). GLA, formerly known as lymphangiomatosis, is a sporadic disorder characterised by diffuse or multifocal LMs which are progressive and involve multiple tissue sites including bone. GLA frequently displays lymphatic abnormalities in the skin, soft tissues and abdominal and thoracic viscera as well as pericardial, pleural or peritoneal effusions, which can have lethal consequences. GLA can involve bone and is associated with the loss of medullary bone, pain and impaired mobility [17]. GSD typically presents with cortical and progressive osteolysis with adjacent soft tissue changes, and mainly axial skeletal involvement. GLA involves multiple bone and soft tissue sites and does not involve cortical bone; it typically presents at birth or in children and young adults. GLA can be caused by somatic activating mutations in *PIK3CA*. Mice that express an active form of PIK3CA in their lymphatic endothelial cells develop hyperplastic lymphatics and lymphatics in bone [18]. A mutation in *NRAS* was recently found in a patient diagnosed with GLA [19]. Rapamycin has been shown to reduce pain in patients with GLA [16].

Benign lymphangioendothelioma. Acquired progressive lymphangioma (benign lymphangioendothelioma) is a benign tumour that differs from simple 'acquired lymphangioma' or simple cutaneous lymphangiectasia by its clinical behaviour and histopathology [20]. It presents as reddish or bruise-like plaques, which are usually located on the abdominal wall, thigh or calf. Typically, the condition affects young adolescents but may also arise in adults. It is usually localised, flat and grows slowly. Acquired progressive lymphangioma is considered to originate from lymphatic endothelium. The histopathological appearance can mimic a low-grade sarcoma or Kaposi sarcoma. Anastomosing dilated channels, with a tendency to dissect the collagen bundles, are lined by swollen endothelial cells but without cellular atypia. It usually runs a long and benign course. D2-40 and Prox1 immunostains are positive [21].

Maffucci syndrome. This consists of diffuse haemolymphangiomatosis accompanied by severe, widespread deformities of bone and cartilage, notably enchondromas of the digits [22]. The lymphangiomas do not appear, on lymphography, to communicate with the main lymphatic pathways and often possess both blood vascular and lymphatic elements. Bony deformity may be gross; slowly uniting pathological fractures are common. The disease has high malignant potential including the development of lymphangiosarcoma [23]. Somatic mutations have been described [24].

Kaposiform lymphangiomatosis (KLA). Kaposiform lymphangiomatosis is a rare lymphatic anomaly affecting the lungs and mediastinum mainly in children, with a high mortality rate. Skin involvement resembles diffuse Kaposi sarcoma and can lead to lymphoedema. It is distinguished from GLA and diffuse pulmonary lymphangiomatosis in part by characteristic haematological abnormalities and haemorrhagic complications, including haemoptysis. Characteristic clusters or sheets of spindled lymphatic endothelial cells (human herpesvirus 8 negative) accompany malformed lymphatic channels histologically (Figure 103.19). Mutations in the RAS pathway, including NRAS and CBL, have been described with successful treatment with RAS pathway inhibition [25].

Lymphangioleiomyomatosis (LAM). Lymphangioleiomyomatosis is a slowly progressive, low-grade, metastasising neoplasm, associated with cellular invasion and cystic destruction of the pulmonary parenchyma. LAM is almost exclusively seen in women, especially during child-bearing age. LAM cells harbour mutations in the tuberous sclerosis genes. Lymphatic manifestations of LAM include thoracic duct wall invasion, lymphangioleiomyoma formation,

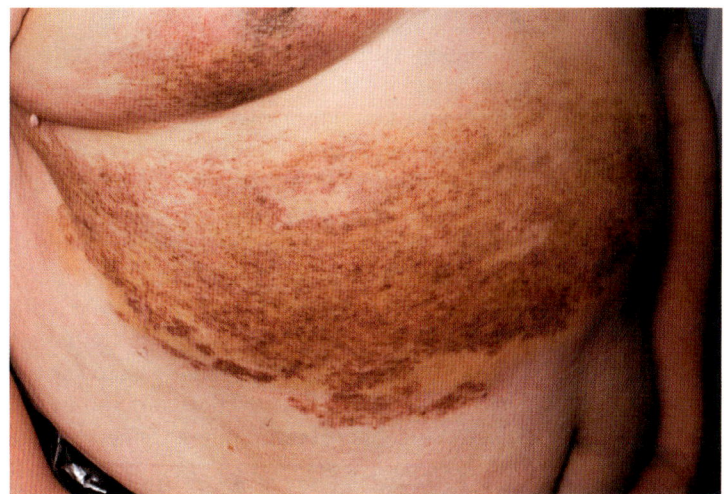

Figure 103.19 Kaposiform lymphangiomatosis showing a Kaposi sarcoma-like rash with localised lymphoedema of the breast and chest wall associated with haemoptysis.

chylous fluid collections in the peritoneal, pleural and pericardial spaces, chyloptysis, chyle leak from the vagina or umbilicus, chylous pulmonary congestion and lower extremity lymphoedema. Skin and kidney involvement is frequently found in tuberous sclerosis–LAM. Dermatological manifestations in tuberose sclerosis include angiofibromas, hypomelanotic macules, shagreen patch and ungal fibromas. Serum VEGF-D estimation and high-resolution CT can be helpful in diagnosis. mTOR inhibitors (e.g. sirolimus) are effective treatment [26]. The major histamine-derived metabolite methylimidazoleacetic acid (MIAA) is relatively more abundant in LAM plasma, and MIAA values are independent of VEGF-D. LAM tumorigenesis is reduced using approved drugs targeting monoamine oxidases A/B (clorgyline and rasagiline) or histamine H1 receptor (loratadine), and loratadine synergises with rapamycin [27].

Lymphoedema as a result of amniotic band constriction

Definition and nomenclature

Lymphoedema of a limb may be due to *in utero* circumferential entrapment of fetal parts by fibrous amniotic bands. These cause constriction and fibrosis, with subsequent impairment of regional lymphatic drainage, resulting in lymphoedema. Early surgical release may prove beneficial, but affected individuals typically suffer lifelong problems with lymphoedema.

Synonyms and inclusions
- Amniotic band syndrome
- Amniotic band sequence
- Amniotic deformity, adhesion and mutilation complex
- Pseudoainhum

Epidemiology

Incidence is less than 1 in 1 000 000.

PART 9: VASCULAR DISORDERS

Pathophysiology

It is a sporadic condition, with rare exceptions: a few affected families have been described. A study conducted by the National Center on Birth Defects and Developmental Disabilities (Atlanta, USA) observed that maternal cigarette smoking and aspirin use increased the risk of limb reduction deficiencies accompanied by amniotic bands [28].

Two theories for development have been suggested. Firstly, the amniotic band theory where bands occur due to a partial rupture of the amniotic sac. Fibrous bands of the ruptured amnion float within the amniotic fluid and encircle and constrict parts of the fetus. Subsequently, the fetus grows but the bands do not enlarge, causing constriction of the affected limb or digit. Constriction compromises the vascular supply, causing congenital abnormalities. Complete 'natural' amputation of an affected digit or limb may occur prior to birth. Secondly, the vascular disruption theory where an 'intrinsic' defect of the vascular circulation must be present, because the constricting mechanism of the amniotic band theory cannot fully explain the high incidence of cleft defects.

Clinical features

Amniotic bands rarely present on routine prenatal ultrasound imaging. Isolated amniotic bands are more likely to be detected at birth. Amniotic bands may affect digits or limbs. There is considerable variation in clinical presentation, depending upon the site of the amniotic band(s). Limb deformity and/or necrosis may be present.

Lymphoedema may develop in the antenatal period. The swelling will develop distal to the site of an amniotic band, enhancing the appearance of the narrow linear band around the affected limb (Figure 103.20). Milder cases (e.g. amniotic bands that are not fully circumferential) may not develop lymphoedema until later life, if at all. Aside from circumferential limb constrictions, pseudosyndactyly, intrauterine amputation and umbilical cord constrictions have been reported. The reduction in amniotic fluid and/or limb tethering by amniotic bands may result in reduced fetal movements, scoliosis, limb deformity, lung hypoplasia and hydrops. There is a strong association between amniotic bands and clubfoot (talipes). Other associated abnormalities include clubhand, haemangioma,

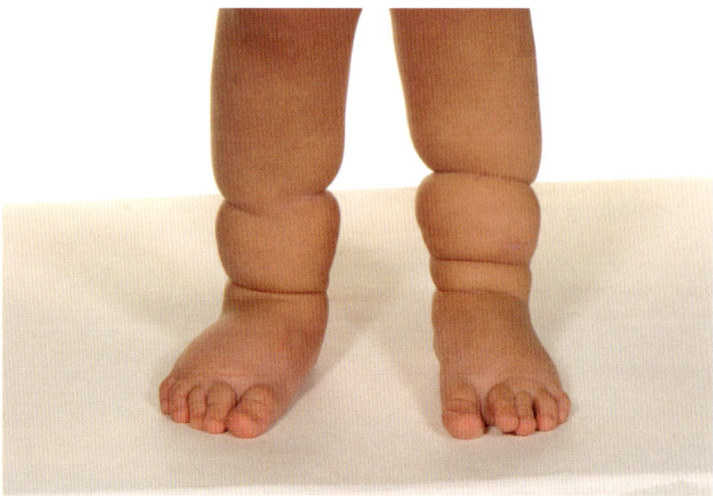

Figure 103.20 Amniotic bands and lymphoedema.

cleft lip and/or cleft palate. Affected individuals have an increased risk of infection (e.g. cellulitis) within the swollen limb due to impaired lymphatic drainage and subsequent reduced immune surveillance.

Differential diagnosis

The differentiation of amniotic bands from Adams–Oliver syndrome is usually straightforward. The latter condition is an autosomal dominant disorder characterised by transverse limb reduction defects, cutis marmorata and aplasia cutis congenita over the posterior parietal region with an underlying bone defect.

Investigations

Prenatal ultrasound scans may detect swelling of digits or limbs distal to the amniotic band constriction, but the band itself cannot be visualised. Three-dimensional ultrasound and MRI may be used for more detailed imaging when the index of suspicion is high.

Management

If amniotic bands occur with limb deformities, with or without necrosis, all attempts are made to salvage a necrotic limb, but amputation may be necessary. Treatment typically occurs after birth, but with the advancement of prenatal radiodiagnosis, fetal surgery *in utero* has been attempted. Children with circumferential or near-circumferential amniotic bands may undergo surgical release with a Z-plasty procedure. The aim of surgery is to release the fibrous tissue, thereby relieving constriction of both the vascular supply and draining lymphatic vessels of the limb. Surgery cannot completely reverse the constriction, so the child is often left with a degree of impaired lymphatic drainage within the affected limb. The child will benefit from the input of an experienced lymphoedema therapist to improve lymph drainage. Provision of made-to-measure compression hosiery can improve lymphatic drainage if worn on a daily basis. Fetoscopic release of the amniotic bands in the case of amniotic band syndrome is feasible with encouraging results [29].

LYMPHANGIECTASIA AND CHYLOUS DISEASE

Definition and nomenclature

Lymphangiectasia (or lymphangiectasis) means distension, expansion or dilatation of a lymph vessel. It is equivalent to telangiectasia of a blood vessel except lymphangiectasia can involve any size of lymphatic vessel whereas telangiectasia usually applies to skin capillaries. It could arise from dilatation of an otherwise normal lymphatic vessel due to raised intralymphatic pressure or it could arise from a structurally abnormal lymphatic vessel due to a fault in development.

Lymphangiectasia can affect any lymph vessel in any tissue (e.g. pulmonary lymphangiectasia, intestinal lymphangiectasia). Intestinal lymphangiectasia can be associated with a protein-losing enteropathy and cause peripheral oedema. Chylous disease can be due to lymphangiectasia and manifests with reflux of lymph draining from the gut. Because gut lymph is rich in fat it appears milky white (chyle) and can reflux into cutaneous lymphangiectasia in the genitalia and lower limbs.

Cutaneous lymphangiectasia

Introduction and general description

Cutaneous lymphangiectasia represents distended, but otherwise normal, dermal lymphatics engorged with lymph due to a failure of downstream drainage. The surface 'lymph blisters' or vesicles seen in cutaneous lymphangiectasia are not necessarily structurally or histologically different from those seen in an LM or lymphangioma. Acquired or secondary lymphangioma is an alternative term, but is confusing as there is neither a tumour nor a proliferative component.

Pathophysiology

Cutaneous lymphangiectasia arises following damage to previously normal, deep lymphatic vessels. The mechanism by which they form is identical to congenitally determined LMs [1]. Obstruction to drainage leads to back pressure and dermal backflow of lymph, with subsequent congestion and expansion of the upper dermal lymphatics. Lymphangiectases are neither true neoplasms nor hamartomas but represent simple expansion and engorgement (lymphangiectasia) of normal dermal initial lymphatic vessels due to raised intralymphatic pressure.

Histologically, the dermis exhibits expanded, angular, lymphatic vessels, which are CD31 and D2-40 positive. Endothelial cell atypia is usually absent.

Lower limb lesions usually arise in association with lymphoedema following either ilio-inguinal block dissection or pelvic surgery and radiotherapy for cancer, or when cancer relapses. Lymphangiectasias/acquired lymphangiomas have been described in association with scarring processes, including recurrent or chronic infections (such as the scrofuloderma variant of tuberculosis), hidradenitis suppurativa and genital involvement with Crohn disease or ano-genital granulomatosis (Table 103.6) [2]. They may also occur because of defective collagen or elastin, as documented in a report of penicillamine dermopathy.

Clinical features

For cutaneous lymphangiectasia, weeping and discharge of clear lymph or chyle is the commonest sign. Confusingly, the discharge may be blood-stained as blood readily enters lymph. The clinical appearance of cutaneous lymphangiectases/acquired lymphangiomas may vary greatly, ranging from clear, fluid-filled blisters to smooth, flesh-coloured papules or nodules. Typically, lymphangiectasia can be seen as translucent, almost flat, papules or vesicles in the skin, which may ooze lymph spontaneously or after trauma. Blood content may make them look black and like angiokeratomas.

Table 103.6 Causes of cutaneous lymphangiectasia.

Congenital causes	Acquired causes (acquired lymphangioma)
Lymphatic malformation (lymphangioma circumscriptum)	Post surgery
	Radiotherapy
Chylous reflux (intestinal lymphangiectasia)	Scarring: Accidental trauma
Noonan syndrome	Inflammatory:
Lymphoedema distichiasis	Filariasis
	Crohn/ano-genital granulomatosis
	Hidradenitis suppurativa
	Tuberculosis adenitis/scrofuloderma
	Chylous reflux, e.g. post radiation

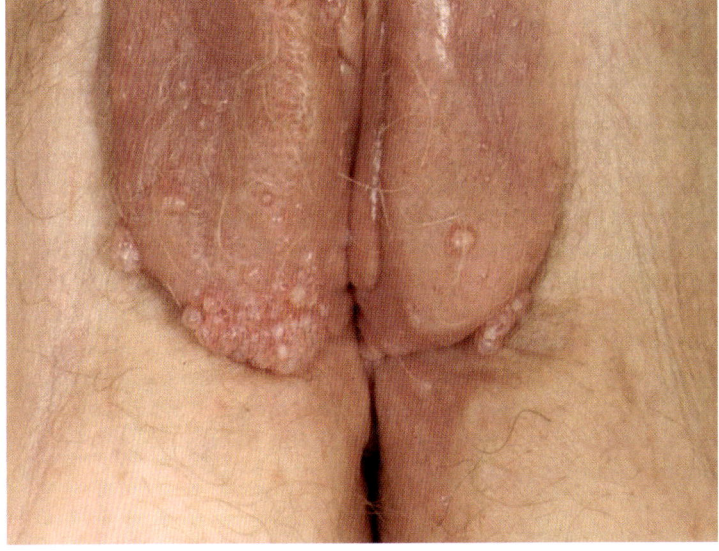

Figure 103.21 Vulval lymphangiectasia showing acquired lymphangiomas (lymphangiectasias) following cervical cancer treatment. The lymphangiomas were mistaken for genital warts.

Genital lesions may become hyperkeratotic on the surface and be mistaken for warts. Lesions may be solitary but scattered throughout a lymphoedematous limb, or they may be grouped, as seen in 'lymphangioma circumscriptum'. When involving the external genitalia, the scrotum or vulva is studded with multiple clusters of tiny, translucent vesicles (Figure 103.21).

The differential diagnosis includes human papillomavirus warts and molluscum contagiosum. Recognition and appropriate treatment of cutaneous lymphangiectasia are important because the lesions may act as portals of entry for infection. In addition, persistent leakage of lymphatic fluid may be mistaken for urinary incontinence in the case of vulval lymphangiectasia. In chylous reflux the lymph blisters/vesicles are white or cream coloured due to the milky chyle contained within.

Investigations

Skin biopsy with D2-40 stain is the definitive investigation.

Management

Treatment of cutaneous lymphangiectasia/acquired lymphangiomas is essentially the reduction of any underlying lymphoedema through compression plus the control of infection. Compression

PART 9: VASCULAR DISORDERS

may be relatively straightforward on the leg but is not so straightforward on the genitalia. Destruction of the 'lymph blisters' by laser or diathermy is helpful as palliative treatment [3]; recurrence is common.

Intestinal lymphangiectasia

Intestinal lymphangiectasia is an uncommon disorder and an important cause of protein-losing enteropathy [4]. It is relevant to dermatologists because it may manifest with peripheral oedema, cutaneous lymphangiectasia or chylous reflux (with milky lymph blisters appearing in the skin).

The major symptoms are peripheral oedema, and abdominal pain and diarrhoea following dietary fat challenge. Hypoproteinaemia and low serum albumin and immunoglobulin levels are found on investigation. A raised faecal alpha-1-antitrypsin enzyme supports the diagnosis. Biopsies of the small intestine show variable degrees of dilatation of lymph vessels in the mucosa and submucosa. Capsule endoscopy is the investigation of choice but has a high false negative rate [5]. Primary intestinal lymphangiectasia can be associated with the Turner, Noonan and Hennekam syndromes. In secondary intestinal lymphangiectasia, the dilatation of the lymphatics is caused by obstruction of the vessels or an elevated lymph pressure. Obstruction can be seen in patients with inflammatory bowel disease, sarcoidosis or lymphoma or in patients who have had pelvic radiotherapy. Secondary intestinal lymphangiectasia is observed in children with congenital heart disease who have undergone a Fontan operation [6].

Dietary avidance of fat with replacement by medium-chain triglycerides is recommended as these are absorbed and directed to the portal venous system rather than to the intestinal lacteals [7]. Diffuse intestinal lymphangiectasia and extensive lymphangiectasia require treatment with drugs (octreotide, sirolimus or everolimus) based on a comprehensive understanding of their mechanisms. Propranolol and tranexamic acid may be used in special conditions of primary intestinal lymphangiectasia [8].

Chylous disease

Fat is normally absorbed through the gut lymphatic vessels (lacteals) and drained through the cisterna chyli to the thoracic duct. Disturbances to this drainage route either within the gut wall (intestinal lymphangiectasia) or mesenteric lymphatics will result in a redistribution of chyle to other sites such as the pleural or pericardial cavities (chylous pleural or pericardial effusions) or peritoneal cavity (chylous ascites). An incompetence of valves within the main abdominal lymphatic trunks results in gross reflux of chyle to the lower limbs, perineum and genitalia [9]. The reverse flow to skin or 'dermal backflow' will result in chylous cutaneous lymphangiectasia. Chylous 'blisters' may occur on the toes. Chylous reflux can occur through a fault of lymphatic development such as in Noonan syndrome or be acquired from damage to lymph drainage routes through accidental or surgical trauma, filariasis or malignancy.

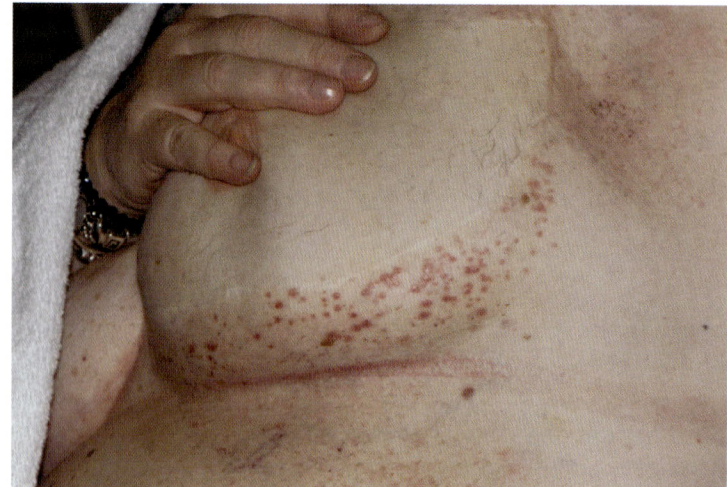

Figure 103.22 Benign lymphangiomatous papules (atypical vascular lesions) post radiotherapy.

Central conducting lymphatic anomaly (CCLA) is characterised by dilated lymphatic channels, lymphatic channel dysmotility and distal obstruction affecting internal lymphatic drainage and is classified as a channel-type LM [10]. *EPHB4* mutations cause CCLA and this suggests that extracellular signal-regulated kinase inhibitors may have therapeutic benefits in patients with complex lymphatic anomalies [11].

Atypical vascular lesions/benign lymphangiomatous papules

Cutaneous vascular proliferations occurring in the field of prior radiotherapy include angiosarcoma and small, cutaneous lesions with a pseudosarcomatous pattern that are reported as atypical vascular lesions or benign lymphangiomatous papules (Figure 103.22) [12]. Microscopically, the lesions are located mostly in the superficial/mid-dermis and are composed of expanded, irregularly jagged, vascular channels lined by a single layer of bland endothelial cells which are invariably D2-40 positive. Lesions can show additional cytological and/or architectural atypia but the prognosis is excellent [13].

Lymphocele, seroma and lymph fistula

Introduction and general description

Lymphoceles (lymphocysts) occur when afferent lymph vessels are disrupted, and lymph fluid accumulates in a potential space without a distinct endothelial lining. When copious lymph fluid drains externally it is referred to as a lymph fistula. A seroma is a pocket of clear serous fluid that also collects in a tissue space usually after surgery. Seromas may be difficult to distinguish from lymphoceles.

Lymphocele. Lymphoceles usually occur following surgery or accidental injury with disruption to lymphatic drainage channels. The wall of lymphoceles is 'false', in that no endothelial (or epithelial) lining exists and instead a dense network of fibrin with lymphocytes is present. Dermatologists might come across groin or axillary lymphoceles as they are superficial and frequently associated with infection and wound complications. In cases of groin lymphoceles, treatment options include observation, serial aspiration and compression, instillation of sclerosing agents, radiotherapy, negative pressure wound therapy and operative resection of the cavity with or without muscle flap coverage.

Lymphoceles following varicose vein surgery or vein harvesting have become much less common with changes in vascular surgical practice. With increasing levels of plastic surgery, particularly abdominoplasties and thigh lifts, lymphatic complications are likely to become more common.

Seroma. This is a localised swelling containing clear serous fluid which is indistinguishable from lymph. It may develop after lymphadenectomy where the fluid, referred to as a seroma, fills a tissue space [14]. Repeat aspiration is often necessary until collateral lymph drainage forms. A seroma, particularly if infected, may herald the onset of lymphoedema if alternative drainage routes are not established.

Lymph fistula. A lymph fistula occurs where a lymphatic vessel connects externally to the skin surface and weeps copious amounts of lymph. It usually occurs following trauma or surgery where lymph accesses the skin surface through a wound. It may be a feature of a lymphatic malformation. A chylous fistula drains fat.

SECONDARY LYMPHOEDEMA

Secondary lymphoedema occurs when an identifiable damage to lymph conducting pathways or a disease affects lymphatic function. Many examples of secondary lymphoedema can have more than one cause.

Lymphatic filariasis (filarial elephantiasis)

Definition and nomenclature
The single largest cause of lymphoedema worldwide is lymphatic filariasis (LF) [1]. It is a parasitic disease caused by microscopic worms that are transmitted by mosquitos. The adult worms live within the human lymphatic system and disrupt drainage, resulting in lymphoedema and hydroceles. Worldwide, 120 million people are infected and 40 million of these have lymphatic problems. Access to health care and lymphoedema treatment is often limited, resulting in a severe burden of disease in endemic countries.

Synonyms and inclusions
• Elephantiasis

Introduction and general description
Infection with one of three parasitic filarial worms causes LF: *Wuchereria bancrofti*, *Brugia malayi* and *B. timori*. *W. bancrofti* infection accounts for 90% of LF worldwide [2] (Chapter 33). The adult worms reside within the afferent lymphatic vessels (and/or the lymph nodes) while their larvae, the microfilariae, circulate within the peripheral blood and can infect mosquito vectors as they feed, facilitating transmission to other human hosts (Figure 103.23). The adult female worm may survive for more than a decade and is able to release thousands of fully formed microfilariae into the lymphatic circulation of the host each day. Infected patients may be asymptomatic or demonstrate acute or chronic manifestations. The clinical signs are related to the adult worms residing in the lymph vessels and are not due to the microfilariae. The filarial parasites specifically target the lymphatics and impair lymph flow, which is critical for the maintenance of fluid balance and physiological interstitial fluid transport [3,4].

Epidemiology
Lymphatic filariasis is endemic in 73 countries and 1.2 billion people are at risk of transmission and subsequent infection. An estimated 120 million individuals are currently infected. Approximately 40 million have chronic lymphatic pathology: 13 million with lymphoedema/elephantiasis and an additional 27 million males have hydroceles as a result of LF. Areas where LF is endemic include parts of Africa, South-East Asia, the western Pacific, the Americas and the Middle East. Transmission and morbidity are highest in South-East Asia and sub-Saharan Africa [2].

Pathophysiology
The pathogenesis of filarial disease remains poorly understood and has been the subject of great debate [5]. The clinical consequences of LF are believed to occur as a result of interaction between the pathogenic parasite, the immune response of the host and secondary bacterial and fungal infections that complicate the situation [6].

Lymphoedema may occur as a result of live adult worms within lymphatic vessels in the lower limbs and pelvic region. The live worms secrete irritant toxins that cause dilatation of the lymph vessels surrounding the worm. This causes a reduction in lymphatic flow. The subsequent oedema promotes fibrosis. Lymphoedema is further aggravated by secondary bacterial (ADLA) and fungal infections that arise as a result of impaired immune surveillance within the lymphoedematous region.

Lymphatic damage and subsequent lymphoedema may also occur as a direct result of dead adult worms within the lymphatic vessels (worm death due to old age or treatment). The presence of dead worms induces granuloma formation which leads to lymphatic outflow obstruction within the vessel and subsequent lymphoedema [4].

People residing for prolonged periods in tropical or subtropical areas where LF is endemic are at the greatest risk for infection. Repeated mosquito bites over several months are required in order to acquire LF. Visiting tourists have a very low risk of acquiring LF [7].

PART 9: VASCULAR DISORDERS

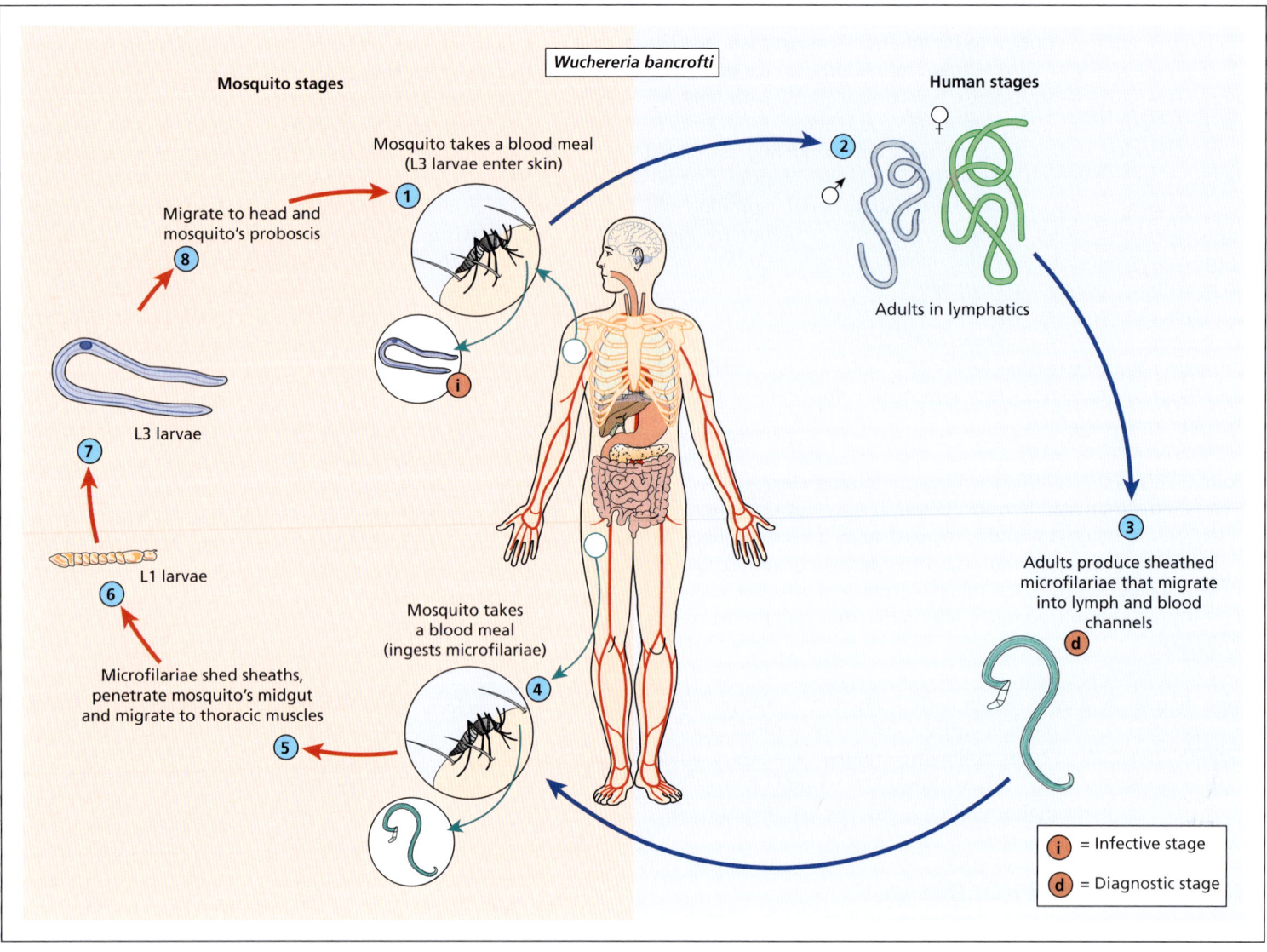

Figure 103.23 The life cycle of filarial nematodes in the human and mosquito hosts. *Wuchereria bancrofti*, *Brugia malayi* and *B. timori* have similar life cycles. The adult worms reside in the lymphatic system of humans and cause filarial disease. The female worm produces offspring (microfilariae), which leave the lymphatic system, enter the blood system of the human host and are taken up by mosquitoes during a blood meal. The microfilariae undergo development within the mosquito, become infective larvae and subsequently migrate to the mosquito's mouthparts. These larvae may be transmitted to humans when the mosquito takes its next blood meal. Once transmitted to humans, the larvae take approximately 6–12 months to mature into adult worms. From Centers for Disease Control and Prevention [1].

Causative organisms

Numerous parasitic filarial nematodes may infect humans but only *W. bancrofti*, *B. malayi* and *B. timori* species are responsible for LF. *W. bancrofti* is responsible for 90% of cases of LF worldwide.

Clinical features

Lymphatic filariasis has a range of clinical manifestations, varying from clinically asymptomatic microfilaria-positive individuals to those with disfiguring chronic filarial disease (elephantiasis). Overlap exists between the different symptom groups. While infections are contracted throughout life, most individuals remain asymptomatic until symptoms emerge during adolescence and adulthood. Males are more likely to be affected than females.

Clinical disease occurs in a minority of those infected with LF. The majority of infected individuals have few manifestations, despite the large number of circulating microfilariae in the peripheral blood. However, most will have some degree of subclinical disease, including microscopic haematuria and/or proteinuria, dilated and tortuous lymphatic vessels seen on lymphoscintigraphy, and scrotal lymphangiectasia in affected males.

One presentation of LF is with acute filarial lymphangitis in adolescence. This is caused by the death of adult worms, and is characterised by sudden-onset fever, skin heat, painful lymph nodes, lymphangitis and transient oedema. It is relatively uncommon in untreated persons, is usually asymptomatic or has a mild clinical course, and rarely causes residual lymphoedema. Involvement of the genitals appears to occur exclusively with *W. bancrofti* infection. Previously asymptomatic individuals may experience symptoms lasting 4–7 days, with a tendency to develop recurrent episodes.

The second syndrome, ADLA, is not caused by filarial worms *per se*, but probably results from secondary bacterial infections.

ADLA is a common cause of chronic lymphoedema and elephantiasis. Individuals with established LF and lymphoedema develop more severe and prolonged episodes of ADLA.

Chronic lymphatic obstruction as a result of filarial worms leads to the development of hydroceles, lymphoedema/elephantiasis skin changes (severe hyperkeratosis, papillomatosis and skin fissuring) and rarely chyluria. Hydroceles are the result of the accumulation of clear, straw-coloured lymphatic fluid within the tunica vaginalis because of obstruction of lymphatic vessels draining the retroperitoneal and subdiaphragmatic areas. The diameter of the hydroceles may be significant, reaching up to 30 cm.

Lymphoedema occurs as a result of the accumulation of lymphatic fluid within tissues following lymphatic vessel damage. The sites most affected are the lower limbs and scrotum. Other sites such as the upper limbs and trunk can be affected. Initially, the lymphoedema is intermittent and pitting in nature, but over time it becomes persistent and fibrotic. It is accompanied by gross skin changes referred to as elephantiasis – profoundly thickened and fibrotic skin with severe papillomatosis and secondary microbial infections.

Chyluria is a rare complication of LF and is the result of the presence of chyle (intestinal lymph) within the urinary tract. It occurs as a result of impaired drainage of retroperitoneal lymph below the cisterna chyli with subsequent reflux and flow of the lymph directly into the renal lymphatic vessels, which may rupture and permit flow of chyle into the urinary tract. The urine appears milky white in colour. Serious nutritional deficiencies may occur as a result of the loss of fat and protein within the urine.

Tropical pulmonary eosinophilia syndrome may rarely affect an individual with LF due to *W. bancrofti* or *B. malayi*. They develop respiratory wheeze and a paroxysmal nocturnal cough, similar to asthma. Chest radiographs demonstrate nodular or diffuse pulmonary lesions. Other features of this syndrome include elevated peripheral blood eosinophilia and high levels of serum IgE and specific antifilarial antibodies. Treatment with diethylcarbamazine is effective.

The clinical course of untreated LF is of progressive skin changes, worsening lymphoedema and increased incidence of secondary infection. A poor quality of life is associated with untreated disease. Elephantiasis and subsequent deformity lead to social stigma, financial hardship from loss of income and increased medical expenses. The socioeconomic burdens of isolation and poverty are immense.

Differential diagnosis

Filarial lymphoedema tends to be unilateral but frequently extends above the knee and can involve the groins and genitals causing hydrocele. The differential diagnosis includes podoconiosis and leprosy. In Ethiopia, where lower limb lymphoedema is common, leprotic lymphoedema is the second most common cause behind podoconiosis, accounting for more cases of lymphoedema than LF. Other causes of secondary lymphoedema include endemic Kaposi sarcoma, onchocerciasis (river blindness) and recurrent cellulitis/erysipelas [8].

Investigations

In endemic areas, adults with lower limb lymphoedema and/or male genital involvement are likely to have LF. A definitive diagnosis can be made by detection of the adult parasitic worm within the lymphatic vessels or accessible lymph nodes. Doppler ultrasound may detect motile adult worms within the scrotum. However, these diagnostic tests are not always suitable for use in developing countries.

Filarial parasites exhibit 'nocturnal periodicity' that restricts their appearance in the blood to the hours of 10 pm to 2 am. The diagnosis of LF has traditionally depended on the nocturnal laboratory examination for microfilaria in peripheral blood smears (stained with Giemsa or haematoxylin and eosin) between these hours to maximise the chances of detection.

In recent years, polymerase chain reaction and rapid antigenic assays have been developed. Antigen testing is a simple, sensitive and specific tool for the detection of the *W. bancrofti* antigen and is being used widely by lymphatic filariasis elimination programmes. The test detects infection within minutes and can be carried out at any time of day, unlike previous tests.

Lymphoedema, elephantiasis skin changes and hydroceles may persist in individuals with burned-out infections. Therefore, it is impossible to exclude a diagnosis of filarial-induced disease in the absence of circulating antigens or parasites. This situation may occur in patients who have received multiple courses of treatment or who no longer live in the endemic area.

Management

The World Health Organization (WHO) launched the Global Programme to Eliminate Lymphatic Filariasis (GPELF) to stop the spread of LF. Pharmaceutical companies have pledged to donate the required drugs. The strategy proposed by the WHO to achieve LF elimination comprises two components: (i) the interruption of transmission of filarial infection in all endemic countries by the drastic reduction of microfilariae prevalence levels; and (ii) the prevention and alleviation of disability and suffering in individuals already affected by LF. The interruption of transmission of infection is only possible if the entire at-risk population is treated by mass drug administration for a prolonged period of time to ensure a reduction in the blood levels of microfilariae to a level where transmission can no longer be sustained. The following drug regimens have been recommended by the WHO to be administered once a year for at least 5 years, with a coverage of at least 65% of the total at-risk population: (i) 6 mg/kg diethylcarbamazine citrate (DEC) in combination with 400 mg albendazole; or (ii) 150 µg/kg ivermectin in combination with 400 mg albendazole (in areas where onchocerciasis is prevalent) to avoid adverse drug reactions with DEC [7].

Lymphoedema, elephantiasis skin changes and acute inflammatory episodes are typically managed with simple measures of improved hygiene, skin care, exercise activities and elevation of affected limbs. The GPELF has pledged to provide access to a minimum package of care for every individual with chronic manifestations of LF in all areas where the disease is present.

Lifestyle measures can reduce the bacterial and fungal load that contributes to worsening lymphoedema. These include regular washing with soap and water, use of footwear and access to antibiotics and lymphoedema treatment [9]. Prevention of infection can be achieved by avoidance of mosquito bites. Lifestyle measures include sleeping under a mosquito net, using mosquito repellent on exposed skin and wearing long sleeves and trousers.

Podoconiosis (non-filarial lymphoedema)

Definition and nomenclature

Podoconiosis is a form of lymphoedema that occurs in tropical highland areas in genetically susceptible individuals who are exposed to irritant volcanic soils [8,10].

Synonyms and inclusions
- Mossy foot
- Verrucosis lymphatica
- Endemic non-filarial elephantiasis

Introduction and general description

Podoconiosis refers to the development of bilateral lower limb lymphoedema, thought to occur as a result of prolonged exposure to irritant mineral-rich soils present at high altitudes (Figure 103.24). These minerals appear to trigger an inflammatory response resulting in impaired lymphatic drainage and subsequent lymphoedema. Development of the condition is closely associated with barefoot living and working. A genetic susceptibility has also been postulated.

Podoconiosis is a leading cause of lower limb lymphoedema of young people in Africa, Central America and north India, yet it remains a neglected condition. It has been prevalent for centuries

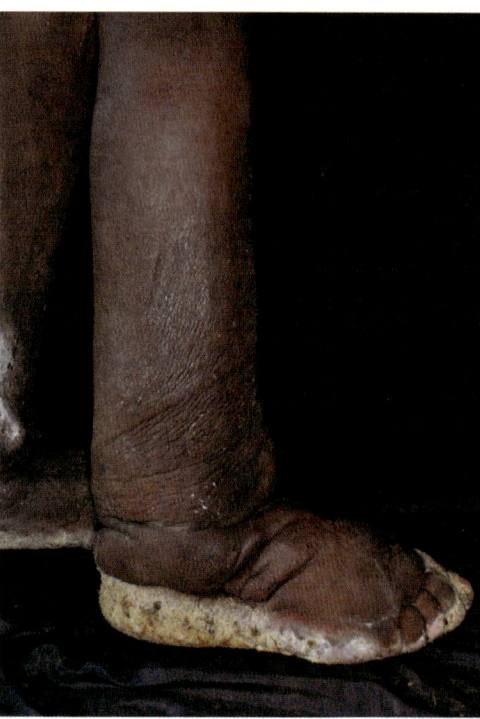

Figure 103.24 Lower limb lymphoedema due to podoconiosis. Note the presence of toe maceration and typical 'mossy' appearance of the foot. Reproduced with permission from D. Markos.

but was previously encompassed by the umbrella term 'elephantiasis' until the pathogenesis of filariasis was realised in the 19th century. All cases of elephantiasis were then assumed to be filarial in origin until the discrepancy between the widespread distribution of 'elephantiasis' cases and more focal distribution of filaria in North Africa, Central America and Europe prompted a review of this theory.

The term podoconiosis was proposed in the 1980s to describe non-filarial cases of elephantiasis skin changes and has since gained widespread acceptance. It is derived from the Greek for foot, *podos*, and dust, *konos* [11].

Epidemiology

It is estimated that 4 million people are affected by podoconiosis, mainly in tropical Africa, Central and South America and South-East Asia. Ethiopia is the country with the highest reported prevalence, with an estimated 1 million people living with the disease. Prevalence estimates are limited but have been made in Ethiopia (4%) [12], Cameroon (8%) and Uganda (4.5%). The variation in reported prevalence figures may be attributable to survey size and sampling methods. Onset is typically in the first or second decade of life but may occur later. Gender ratio results may be unreliable, especially in remote areas affected by podoconiosis. The recent Ethiopian survey reported that females are more likely to be affected than males.

People with certain occupations (i.e. those with prolonged contact with soil) are at higher risk of developing podoconiosis, especially farmers. Podoconiosis is associated with lower levels of income, poor education, being unmarried and the delayed introduction of footwear.

Pathophysiology

The pathogenesis of podoconiosis is not yet fully understood. Current evidence suggests a pivotal role of mineral particles within the soil, in a genetically susceptible individual [13]. One possible theory is that irritant particles cause an inflammatory response with subsequent impaired lymphatic drainage of the lower limbs, perhaps as a result of intraluminal lymphatic vessel obstruction by inflammatory cells. Supportive evidence for this theory includes the detection of elemental particles present in irritant clays (e.g. aluminium, silicon, magnesium or iron) within lower limb lymph node macrophages of affected individuals who live barefoot. The association between podoconiosis and exposure to irritant soil was established when maps of disease occurrence were superimposed onto geological survey maps, confirming a connection with clays derived from volcanic activity. Soil particles including smectite, mica and quartz are associated with podoconiosis prevalence and underpin the process.

An association has been reported between podoconiosis and variants in human leukocyte antigen (HLA) class II loci. Podoconiosis may be a T-cell-mediated inflammatory disease and could be a model for gene–environment interactions.

The climatic factors thought to be necessary for producing irritant clays are high altitude (greater than 1200 m above sea level) and high seasonal rainfall (over 1000 mm annually). These conditions contribute to the steady disintegration of volcanic ash and the reconstitution of the mineral components into irritant silicate clays.

Clinical features

The affected individual typically resides in a high-risk area and will have lived and worked barefoot. Podoconiosis presents with a prodromal phase of pruritus of the forefoot skin and a burning sensation of the feet and lower limbs prior to the onset of elephantiasis skin changes.

Early changes of podoconiosis are similar to those of any other cause of lower limb lymphoedema. The affected individual develops bilateral lymphoedema of the foot and ankle regions. Lymphorrhoea (leakage of lymph), hyperkeratosis, papillomatosis, fibrosis and gross disfigurement below the knee regions develop if the condition is untreated. The toes develop a characteristic macerated and 'mossy' appearance, hence the pseudonym 'mossy foot'. Recurrent lower limb cellulitis frequently complicates the clinical picture.

Clinical features of podoconiosis that differentiate it from filarial elephantiasis include the feet and ankles being the initial site of symptoms in podoconiosis rather than the groin or proximal lower limbs. Podoconiosis affects both lower limbs, albeit asymmetrically, whereas filariasis typically presents with unilateral lower limb swelling that extends above the knee. Groin involvement in podoconiosis is extremely rare, unlike in filariasis.

Progression is punctuated by episodes of ADLA, which occur as frequently as 23 times per year. The clinical presentation of ADLA resembles cellulitis, with diffuse swelling and redness of the limb, inflamed tender lymphatic vessels and lymph nodes and systemic symptoms including fever.

Without access to footwear and conventional lymphoedema treatment (skin care and compression), the condition is progressive and complicated by recurrent cellulitis.

Significant social stigma is attached to podoconiosis. Affected individuals are usually excluded from school, churches and mosques, and barred from marriage with unaffected individuals because of local beliefs that the condition is contagious. An affected individual is less likely to work, and this impacts financial status [14].

Differential diagnosis

Differential diagnoses include filariasis, endemic Kaposi sarcoma and leprotic lymphoedema. Podoconiosis may be distinguished from leprotic lower limb lymphoedema by the preservation of sensation within the lower limbs, and the absence of trophic ulceration, thickened palpable nerves or involvement of other body sites.

Investigations

Typically, affected individuals do not have access to lymphoscintigraphy or other investigative techniques. Filariasis, leprosy and endemic Kaposi sarcoma should be excluded if suspected by the clinician.

Management

Primary prevention of podoconiosis consists of avoiding prolonged contact between the skin of the feet and irritant soils by using good footwear. Prevention of disease progression and recurrent infections may be possible if affected individuals are instructed in the use of foot hygiene (e.g. daily washing of feet with soap and water and the use of antiseptics), and the use of shoes and socks for life. Emollients help to improve and maintain the integrity of the skin barrier. Simple compression bandaging is effective in reducing limb volumes if elephantiasis changes have not yet developed. A change in occupation or relocation may be beneficial but may not be feasible for the affected individual. Advanced cases of podoconiosis are managed with daily skin care, leg elevation and multilayer compression bandaging if the affected individual has access to health care providers. Debulking surgery has been employed with mixed success.

Resources

Footwork (The International Podoconiosis Initiative): www.podo.org (last accessed August 2022).

Cancer-related lymphoedema

Definition and nomenclature

Lymphoedema is rarely a presenting feature of cancer unless the cancer is already advanced but it is a common consequence of cancer treatment and relapsed cancer.

Synonyms and inclusions
- Breast cancer-related lymphoedema
- Postmastectomy lymphoedema
- Radiation-induced lymphoedema
- Malignant lymphoedema
- Carcinoma erysipeloides
- Carcinoma en cuirasse
- Lymphangitis carcinomatosa
- Telangiectatic carcinoma

Introduction and general description

Lymph flow is remarkably well maintained through malignant nodes; therefore, cancer does not usually present with swelling. The few exceptions to this general rule are lymphophilic tumours such as malignant eccrine poroma, Kaposi sarcoma, lymphangiosarcoma and inflammatory breast cancer (Table 103.7). Cancer-related lymphoedema usually results from cancer therapy: surgical lymphadenectomy, radiotherapy and chemotherapy.

Table 103.7 Cancers presenting with lymphoedema and causes of cancer-related lymphoedema.

Cancers where lymphoedema is a presenting sign	Cancer treatment causing lymphoedema
Inflammatory carcinoma	Lymphadenectomy
Lymphangiosarcoma	Radiotherapy
Kaposi sarcoma	Chemotherapy (taxanes)
Malignant eccrine poroma	Breast reconstruction
Advanced primary cancer, e.g. axillary or pelvic lymph node metastases	
Relapsed cancer:	
Lymph node metastases	
Carcinoma erysipeloides	
Lymphangitis carcinomatosa	
Carcinoma en cuirasse	

PART 9: VASCULAR DISORDERS

Advanced or relapsed cancer can present with lymphoedema. Extensive lymph node involvement can compromise lymph flow but other factors such as venous obstruction and hypoproteinaemia may also contribute to oedema formation. Recurrent cancer should always be considered as a cause of limb swelling, particularly if associated with pain. Full staging investigations should be undertaken in any cancer patient who develops new limb swelling.

Epidemiology

Breast cancer-related lymphoedema. More than one in five women who survive breast cancer will develop arm lymphoedema [15]. Taxane chemotherapy significantly contributes to this.

Lymphoedema related to cancers of the male and female uro-genital tract. The incidence of lower limb lymphoedema following radical hysterectomy alone was estimated at 5–10% but can be as high as 49% by 10 years of follow-up in patients who have also received adjuvant radiotreatment. The incidence after vulval cancer was reported at 28%. For prostate cancer, the rate was found to be 0–10% after extended pelvic lymphadenectomy. With extended-field irradiation for carcinoma of the prostate, an incidence of about 5% for genital and/or leg oedema has been noted and the oedema remained chronic in the majority of patients [16]. After penile cancer treatment the incidence of lymphoedema may be as high as 33% [17].

Melanoma-related lymphoedema. In a prospective study of lymphoedema after melanoma treatment, moderate lymphoedema (i.e. an increase in limb volume of >10%) occurred in 14.8% after sentinel lymph node biopsy but in 30.4% after therapeutic lymph node dissection [18].

Extremity soft-tissue sarcoma. The incidence of lymphoedema was 28.8% following limb salvage for extremity soft-tissue sarcomas. Nine percent of the cohort of 289 patients developed significant (grade ≥2) lymphoedema [19].

Pathophysiology

Extensive surgery (e.g. axillary lymph node dissection, greater number of lymph nodes dissected, mastectomy) and being overweight have been found to carry the highest risk for breast cancer-related lymphoedema. Recent evidence suggests axillary radiation may convey less risk than axillary clearance [20]. Cellulitis may be a trigger as may an insult to the limb such as a sterile or non-sterile skin puncture. Extreme resistance exercise such as carrying a heavy suitcase or shopping may trigger the swelling, as can a long-haul flight.

Breast cancer-related lymphoedema has been the most widely studied form of cancer-related lymphoedema. The pathology consists of an accumulation of fat as well as fluid, hence the justification for liposuction. While the cause was always assumed to be lymphatic obstruction in the axilla, evidence suggests the mechanism may be more complicated with constitutional, and pehaps genetic, predisposition [21].

Carcinoma erysipeloides is a form of metastatic spread and occurs most commonly with breast cancer but can occur with melanoma, thyroid, lung, gastric, pancreatic, ovarian, prostate and colorectal cancer [22].

Clinical features

Lymphoedema following cancer treatment may occur immediately after lymphadenectomy, particularly if complicated by wound infection or 'seroma', or may be delayed in onset for many years. Lymphoedema can ache but is predominantly painless unless associated with infection, thrombosis or active cancer.

Carcinoma erysipeloides (also called lymphangitis carcinomatosa, telangiectatic carcinoma or carcinoma en cuirasse) occurs when cancer cells infiltrate the dermal lymphatics. It represents metastatic disease. Bulk disease may be absent and therefore imaging may be normal. By obstructing collateral lymph drainage routes, dermal lymphatic infiltration by cancer is frequently associated with localised, or extensive limb, lymphoedema. It appears clinically with a fixed erythematous patch or plaque resembling cellulitis, but no fever. A network or lattice pattern of telangiectatic vessels represents the infiltrated dermal lymphatics (see Figure 103.12). Inflammatory breast cancer is a rare, aggressive disease where cancer cells block the lymph vessels in the skin of the breast. The breast often looks swollen and red, or 'inflamed'.

Investigations

If relapsed cancer is suspected, restaging investigations such as positron-emission tomography (PET)/CT are indicated. Skin biopsy is the investigation of choice for skin metastases. MRI can determine if the swelling is composed of fluid and therefore likely to be lymphoedema.

Management

If active cancer is diagnosed, then oncology treatment is the priority. If cancer is in remission or stable, then lymphoedema treatment (decongestive lymphatic therapy) can be implemented.

Obesity-related lymphoedema

Definition

Obesity leads to, and exacerbates, lymphoedema at all sites but particularly in the lower limbs.

Introduction and general description

Obesity is a significant risk factor for lymphoedema of the arms, legs and abdomen and for breast cancer-related lymphoedema after lymph nodes have been surgically removed [16]. Furthermore, dieting improves arm lymphoedema beyond that possible through the loss of subcutaneous fat alone (from weight loss irrespective of the diet used). The pathophysiology of lower limb lymphoedema can be complex, with increased fluid filtration from venous hypertension combined with impaired lymph drainage from an indirect effect of reduced mobility being the most important contributors (Box 103.2). The addition of obstructive sleep apnoea/sleep apnoea hypoventilation syndrome results in salt and water retention and heart failure.

Box 103.2 Contributing factors to obesity-related lower limb lymphoedema

- Poor mobility (to stimulate lymph drainage)
- Venous hypertension:
  - Dependency (armchair legs)
  - Abdominal girth/pendulous abdomen obstructing venous drainage in thighs
- Sleep apnoea syndrome
- Drug therapy, e.g. calcium-channel antagonists
- Co-morbidities, e.g. heart failure or post-thrombotic syndrome

Epidemiology

The prevalence of oedema in a UK bariatric service was 52.1% (25 of 48 participants had oedema), potentially linked to obesity, immobility and medications [23].

Pathophysiology

Fat and lymphatics appear to have a close relationship [24]. High-density lipoproteins require transport through the lymphatics to return to the bloodstream during reverse cholesterol transport, which requires lymph drainage [25]. In a model of hypercholesterolaemia, lymphatic function was severely compromised, including impaired dendritic cell migration. Mice with a heterozygous *Prox1*-inactivating mutation have leaky lymphatic vessels and develop obesity and inflammation [26].

Fat deposition is a striking feature of lymphoedema swelling and the justification for liposuction as a treatment for lymphoedema. Obesity impairs lymphatic transport capacity and impaired lymphatic function promotes adipose deposition. How obesity predisposes to lymphoedema is not clear. Lymph drainage requires movement and exercise to promote flow. In a cross-sectional study, 33% of severely obese participants had lymphoedema and those participants had worse physical function than those without lymphoedema. This association was independent of BMI [27].

It is the lower limb that is most closely linked with lymphoedema. In one study all 10 patients with a BMI between 30 and 53 had normal lower extremity lymphatic function, whereas the five patients with a BMI greater than 59 had abnormal lymphatic drainage consistent with lymphoedema [28]. Using an isotope clearance technique, lymph drainage was found to be significantly lower in obese human subjects when compared with lean controls [29].

A large abdominal apron resting on the thighs during sitting obstructs venous drainage and probably interferes with lymph drainage as well. The pressure in the ilio-femoral vein in morbidly obese patients is significantly higher than in non-obese subjects [30]. Abdominal adipose tissue potentially leads to elevated risk for both venous thromboembolism and chronic venous insufficiency.

Clinical features

Swelling is usually insidious in onset and progressive. Acute cellulitis may alert patient and carers to the swelling. More often a chronic redness with local pain and tenderness indicative of lipodermatosclerosis may develop. Trivial trauma may result in the weeping of fluid from the skin (lymphorrhoea). Persistent weeping will irritate the surrounding skin to promote dermatitis, extensive erosion and even ulceration. Odour may result from bacterial colonisation. The constant weeping can discourage the patient from going to bed (to avoid soiling the bed). Consequently, the patient sleeps in a chair, which further increases fluid filtration into the legs. The patient may choose to sleep in a chair anyway for reasons of comfort or sleep apnoea syndrome. As the legs swell more the extra weight further impairs mobility thereby reducing lymph drainage even more.

Skin changes of lipodermatosclerosis are invariably present in obesity-related lymphoedema. Distinction from bacterial cellulitis can be difficult with acute flares of pain and redness. Elephantiasis skin changes are common. Leg ulceration, heart failure and overwhelming sepsis are common complications. Co-morbidities such as diabetes, sleep apnoea syndrome and right-sided heart failure often coexist.

The prognosis is poor unless the patient loses weight and becomes more ambulant.

Differential diagnosis

Systemic causes of oedema (including cardiac disease, hypoproteinaemia and abdominal–pelvic malignancy) should always be considered, particularly if bilateral leg swelling is present. Calcium-channel blocking antagonists can cause peripheral oedema.

Investigations

Standard investigations such as venous duplex ultrasound and lymphoscintigraphy are probably unnecessary as they are unlikely to change management. More important are BNP to exclude heart failure, plasma protein estimation and D-dimers if thrombosis is considered likely.

Management

There are a number of management options to pursue:

1 Systemic conditions such as heart failure and sleep apnoea syndrome should be treated.
2 Compression therapy in the form of multilayer lymphoedema bandaging is the treatment of choice [31]. Standard venous ulcer bandaging will not address toe swelling with skin changes or oedema extending into the lower thighs. Pneumatic or adjustable Velcro compression devices can be useful adjunctive therapy. Compression garments should not be used until swelling is controlled and the skin is in good condition.
3 Exercise if logistically possible. This can be done through walking or static cycling, if safe. Active movements should always be encouraged but passive exercises are better than nothing.
4 Elevation of legs when resting. Encourage sleeping in a bed and not in a chair unless it is a reclining chair.
5 Treat active infection (e.g. cellulitis) [32].
6 Wound care should be undertaken where necessary.
7 Emollients such as 50/50 white soft and liquid paraffin should always be used. For the hyperkeratosis of elephantiasis, 10% salicylic acid is recommended.
8 Bariatric assessment and intervention.

PART 9: VASCULAR DISORDERS

Trauma-induced lymphoedema

Introduction and general description

Lymphoedema and other lymphatic complications, such as lymphocele or lymph fistula, can develop after therapeutic interventions or accidental damage to lymph drainage pathways. The failure of lymphatics to regenerate and re-anastomose satisfactorily through scarred or irradiated tissue is probably responsible for lymphoedema development.

Epidemiology

The incidence of lymphatic complications from 5407 surgical procedures for varicose veins was 118 cases (2.2%); a lymphocele on the limb occurred in 1.3%, an inguinal fistula or lymphocele in 0.7% and lymphoedema in 0.2% [33].

Pathophysiology

Trauma to lymphatics, either from elective surgery or by accident, usually needs to be extensive to induce lymphoedema. Indeed, the experimental production of lymphoedema is extremely difficult to achieve owing to the excellent regenerative powers of lymphatics.

It remains a puzzle as to why most women who have a full axillary lymph node clearance following breast cancer surgery do not develop lymphoedema, yet 6% of women who have a single sentinel lymph node biopsy develop arm swelling. Furthermore, it is not known why breast cancer-related lymphoedema can manifest immediately post surgery or be delayed for many years. A genetic predisposition may be relevant: mice with a heterozygous mutation in the adrenomedullin gene developed lymphoedema when subjected to surgery but wild-type mice did not [34]. Radiotherapy to lymph nodes can be as much a risk factor for lymphoedema as surgery. Wound infections increase the incidence of postsurgical and accidental lymphoedema.

Clinical features

Lymphoedema can develop after varicose vein treatment. Varicose vein surgery may be undertaken for reasons of 'venous oedema'. However, the chronic oedema may already reflect a compromised lymph drainage, in which case surgery may further undermine lymph drainage and make swelling worse. With the greater use of endovenous therapy using laser, radiofrequency or foam vein ablation (rather than traditional stripping and surgical ligation) the incidence of lymphoedema is likely to be reduced.

Lymphatics can be damaged and produce lymphoedema during saphenous vein harvesting for coronary artery bypass grafts. However, the increasing use of coronary stents has considerably reduced this risk. Similarly, great saphenous vein harvesting for critical limb ischaemia can result in lymphatic complications such as lymphocele.

Lymphoedema can develop at the donor site after reconstructive surgery such as a transverse upper gracilis free flap for breast reconstruction.

Resection of excess skin and soft tissue of the thighs after massive weight loss can also cause lymphoedema. The lymphatic collectors of the thigh sit superficial to the veins. Therefore, in a vertical medial thigh lift, choosing a dissection plane superficial to the great saphenous vein is unlikely to preserve the collectors of the ventromedial bundle [35]. Lymphoedema and other lymphatic complications (e.g. cellulitis, lymphocele) are a significant risk. An interruption of lymphatic pathways presumably results in a failure of adequate lymphangiogenesis and repair, resulting in lymphoedema.

Accidental trauma, such as a degloving injury to a limb, will produce lymphoedema distal to the injury if widespread circumferential scarring has occurred.

Self-inflicted injury, such as the repeated application of a tourniquet, will eventually cause permanent lymphatic damage and chronic swelling (Secrétan syndrome). The abrupt termination of the swelling often coincides with a skin contour change due to subcutaneous atrophy caused by a tight constricting band. Skin pigmentation may also coexist at the site. Factitious lymphoedema can be caused by tourniquets, blows to the arm or repeated skin irritation, usually in patients with known psychiatric conditions. Factitious lymphoedema results in symptoms and signs suggestive of chronic regional pain syndrome.

Intravenous drug abuse may cause lymphoedema due to a combination of infection and injected agents causing lymphangitis plus associated venous damage. Puffy hand syndrome is a long-term complication of intravenous drug abuse [36]. It can affect 7–16% of intravenous drug users [37].

Investigations

Lymphoscintigraphy is the investigation of choice to determine lymphatic insufficiency.

Management

Decongestive lymphatic therapy is first line treatment. Infection needs to be treated and prevented. The use of additional therapies such as pneumatic compression therapy and adjustable Velcro wraps can be considered.

Lymphoedema due to immobility

Introduction and general description

Lymph drainage, unlike blood flow, requires intermittent changes in local tissue pressure generated by movement and exercise in order to produce initial lymphatic transport. Main limb collector lymphatic vessels pump the lymph supplied from the initial lymphatics. Lymphatic collector vessels rely on innervation and effective smooth muscle contraction for pumping. Consequently, immobility, by reducing initial lymphatic absorption and transport, reduces lymph flow to the collectors. Less pumping promotes swelling, particularly if gravitational forces (dependency syndrome) encourage ongoing fluid filtration into the tissues but without sufficient compensatory lymph drainage.

Lymphoedema is well recognised with certain neurological conditions that restrict movement. Cerebrovascular accident, spina bifida and multiple sclerosis are those that are best described.

Postradiation brachial plexopathy following breast cancer treatment leads to severe lymphoedema, with paralysis being the major contributing factor.

Epidemiology

In a review of 240 electronic medical records from an adult spina bifida clinic, 22 patients (9.2%) had lymphoedema [38]. Lower limb oedema is common in multiple sclerosis patients, especially in those with reduced mobility. In one study, 93 patients (45%) of a total of 205 patients with definite multiple sclerosis had oedema with abnormal findings on lymphoscintigraphy [39].

Pathophysiology

Exercise and movement are essential for stimulating lymph drainage. Any reduction in movement lowers lymph drainage accordingly. Immobilising any body part in the face of sustained microvascular filtration will result in (lymph)oedema despite patent, and otherwise normal, lymphatic vessels. The lower limb is most affected because of the contribution from dependency/gravitational forces. Paralysis and neurological deficit cause lymphoedema for similar reasons.

Hand oedema after a stroke is not considered to be lymphoedema owing to normal lymphoscintigraphy. However, one would expect lymph drainage pathways to be patent but not functional owing to the lack of movement. Combine that fact with increased microvascular filtration (and high lymph load) due to dependency of the paralysed or spastic limb, and lymphoscintigraphy might be expected to be falsely normal. After all, if the lymphatics are working, oedema should be avoided irrespective of cause [40].

It is likely, but unproven, that with neurological deficit a failure of lymphatic pumping due to denervation contributes the most to oedema formation, but a lack of isotonic exercise (from muscle weakness or spasticity) will reduce initial lymph flow so making less lymph available for collector pumping.

With time, pathological changes within the failing, but hitherto normal, lymphatics occur. Lymphangiothrombosis [41] or luminal fibrosis [42] leads to an irreversible lymphoedema even if full mobility is restored.

Clinical features

Oedema associated with immobility will usually develop insidiously unless the immobility is sudden in onset (e.g. in a cerebrovascular accident hand or foot swelling is the norm because of the effect of gravity being maximal in the distal part of the limb). Peripheral oedema can cause pain and tissue tenderness. Extreme oedema may result in the weeping of fluid from the skin (lymphorrhoea).

A common scenario is 'armchair legs', a term coined by Sneddon and Church [43] where patients sit in a chair day and night with their legs dependent (otherwise known as elephantiasis nostras verrucosa because of the severe lymphoedema skin changes that ensue). No premorbid abnormalities of the lymphatics exist, but the immobility results in minimal lymph drainage and a functional lymphoedema due to a lack of movement or exercise to stimulate normal lymph drainage. Dependency of the limb compounds the problem by increasing capillary filtration. The syndrome is not confined to the legs, but can affect any chronically dependent and immobile part, as demonstrated in a pendulous abdomen [44].

Physical examination reveals swelling in which pitting is marked, due to a mixed aetiology of reduced lymph drainage and increased microvascular fluid filtration. Neuropathic limbs take on a particular appearance with a bluish hue and background livedo. As with all forms of lymphoedema, there is an increased risk of infection.

Differential diagnosis

Deep-vein thrombosis should be considered if onset is acute.

Investigations

In cases of possible DVT, D-dimers and compression ultrasonography should be considered. In breast cancer patients, PET/CT of the axilla should be undertaken to exclude axillary recurrence.

Management

Compression bandaging is the mainstay of treatment but needs to be undertaken with care if sensation is reduced. Oedema should reduce easily but refill occurs rapidly, therefore well-fitting compression garments are applied as soon as swelling is reduced. Pressure areas need to be carefully monitored. Skin care is of the utmost importance. The tendency of paralysed limbs to reswell means that bandaging may need to be continued or replaced with adjustable Velcro wraps (e.g. FarrowWrap®). When resting, elevation of the lower extremities is desirable, either while sitting in a wheelchair or lying in the bed, with the back of the knees and calves supported by pillows. The oedematous limb or limbs should be positioned higher than the hips, if possible.

Systems that encourage passive movements can prove helpful. Pneumatic compression pumps may be helpful as they simulate the muscle pump.

Pretibial myxoedema

Definition and nomenclature

Pretibial myxoedema (PTM) is a form of cutaneous mucinosis that typically occurs in association with Graves disease, hence the synonym thyroid dermopathy.

> **Synonyms and inclusions**
> - Localised myxoedema
> - Thyroid dermopathy
> - Infiltrative dermopathy

Introduction and general description

Pretibial myxoedema is a form of cutaneous mucinosis that occurs in association with Graves disease. Patients typically present with asymptomatic, pretibial nodules and plaques that may have a red-brown hue. Lower limb lymphoedema may develop in severe cases. The classic triad of Graves disease is (i) PTM; (ii) ophthalmopathy (e.g. exophthalmos and orbital myopathy); and (iii) thyroid acropachy (swelling of the digits and clubbing). It has been reported, on rare occasions, in association with Hashimoto thyroiditis and primary hypothyroidism and in euthyroid patients.

Epidemiology

Pretibial myxoedema affects up to 5% of patients with Graves disease, and affects up to 13% of patients with severe eye disease. It more commonly affects females, with a female : male ratio of 4 : 1 [45].

Pathophysiology

Deposition of hyaluronic acid within the dermis and subcutis causes the development of asymptomatic 'swelling', nodules and plaques, typically of the pretibal region of both lower limbs. The dermal accumulation of hyaluronic acid and other glycosaminoglycans is secreted by fibroblasts.

The hyperthyroidism of Graves disease occurs as a result of stimulation of the thyroid-stimulating hormone (TSH) receptor on thyroid follicular cells, by autoantibodies directed against it. However, the pathogenesis of Graves ophthalmopathy and PTM is less clear. The underlying mechanism of glycosaminoglycan (GAG) deposition is not clearly understood but is likely to occur as a result of several processes, including autoimmune, cellular and mechanical factors. For example, TSH receptor antibodies may bind to and stimulate dermal fibroblasts to increase the production of GAGs. Dermal GAG accumulation (i.e. mucin deposition) results in the separation of collagen fibres, the expansion of connective tissues and oedema formation. The obstruction of dermal lymphatic vessels by mucin results in lymphoedema [46]. The involvement of mechanical factors in the development of PTM may explain the lower limb predilection: dependency and trauma have been proposed.

Characteristic histopathological features of PTM consist of mucin deposition (i.e. GAGs including hyaluronic acid) within the reticular dermis. Alcian blue and periodic acid–Schiff stains demonstrate mucinous material between the collagen fibres. With extensive deposition of mucin, the collagen fibres become frayed and fragmented. Stellate fibroblasts may be observed, but the actual number of fibroblasts is not increased. There may be hyperkeratosis of the overlying epidermis.

Clinical features

Pretibial myxoedema occurs almost exclusively with Graves disease. The patient is likely to have a history of thyrotoxicosis (e.g. weight loss, palpitations and hyperhidrosis) and possible ophthalmopathy and acropachy. PTM may develop prior to, during or after the thyrotoxic state as it is not related to thyroid function. It usually occurs 12–24 months after the onset of Graves disease but may occur up to 12 years after its development.

PTM is typically confined to the lower limbs. The shins are the classic site, but the toes may be the only affected site. PTM may occur within surgical scars or sites of trauma. PTM may rarely affect other body sites, such as the head and neck region, torso and upper limbs, presumably triggered by trauma.

Patients typically present with firm, non-pitting, indurated nodules and plaques on the pretibial regions and feet. The lesions may be flesh coloured or have a reddish brown hue. A peau d'orange appearance may develop as a result of expansion of the interfollicular dermis. Cutaneous lesions may be asymptomatic, occasionally pruritic, or cause discomfort. Mild cases are usually asymptomatic and only of cosmetic concern. In severe cases of PTM, lesions may coalesce to give the entire extremity an enlarged, verruciform appearance (Figure 103.25). Functional impairment (inability to wear shoes as a result of toe disfiguration) and/or the development of secondary lymphoedema may occur.

PTM rarely causes significant morbidity. Local discomfort and difficulty in finding footwear may be experienced. Severe forms of the disease may cause lower limb lymphoedema and subsequent complications of increased incidence of infection.

Few studies exist on the evaluation of PTM outcomes. However, the prognosis for mild cases appears to be favourable. In mild cases,

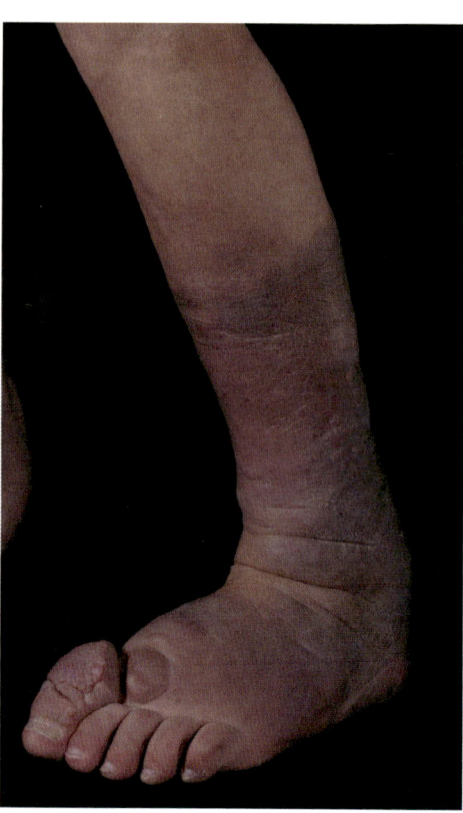
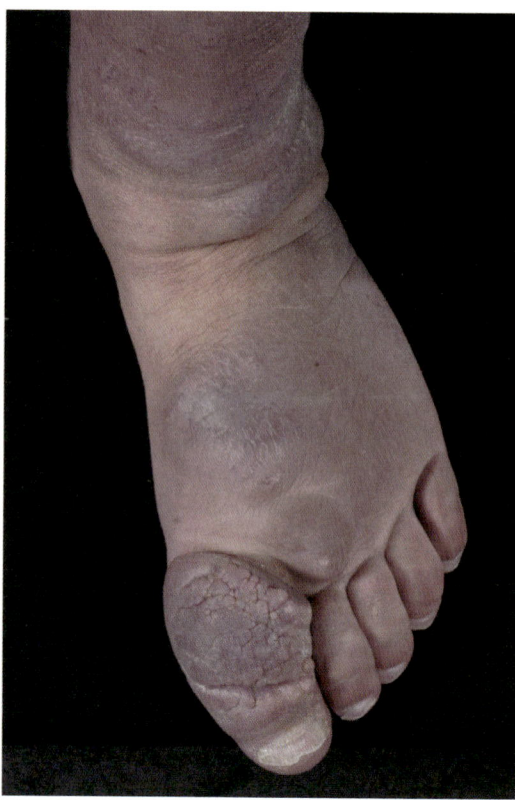

Figure 103.25 Pretibial myxoedema.

50% of patients achieve complete remission after several years. The largest series reports after 25 years of follow-up that 70% of mild untreated and 58% of treated severe cases achieved complete or partial remission. Very severe forms appear to be persistent.

Differential diagnosis

Differential diagnoses include lymphoedema, stasis dermatitis, obesity-associated lymphoedematous mucinosis and lichen amyloidosis. Mucin deposition restricted to an expanded papillary dermis, with nodular angioplasia, and haemosiderin deposition are more suggestive of stasis dermatitis rather than PTM.

Investigations

The diagnosis of PTM is possible from the patient's history and characteristic clinical findings. A positive blood TSH receptor antibody test is pathognomonic of Graves disease. It is rarely necessary to perform a skin biopsy, especially if there is a history of hyperthyroidism or Graves ophthalmopathy. If a biopsy is undertaken, the histopathological findings are characteristic.

The investigation of lymphatic function with lymphoscintigraphy is not routinely performed. However, lymphoscintigraphy and fluorescence microlymphography may confirm structural and functional alterations to the lymphatic drainage. Mucin deposition within the dermis may compress or occlude the initial lymphatic vessels, resulting in lymphoedema.

Management

Mild and asymptomatic cases of PTM may not require treatment. If symptomatic, treatment options include the use of potent topical corticosteroids under occlusion at night for several months. Prompt diagnosis and initiation of treatment appear to correlate with better outcomes. Compression hosiery or multilayer bandages may be used to manage the associated lymphatic impairment/secondary lymphoedema seen in more extensive and chronic cases.

A small number of case reports suggest surgical excision may be of benefit in select cases. However, surgery should be considered with caution as PTM may develop within areas of trauma.

Several therapeutic agents have been trialled in the treatment of PTM. Evidence of their efficacy is limited. These include intralesional steroids, systemic immunomodulators (e.g. prednisolone, plasmapheresis, intravenous immunoglobulin and rituximab) and octreotide.

REGIONAL SWELLING

Swollen breast and breast lymphoedema

Definition and nomenclature

Unilateral breast oedema is most often caused by breast cancer treatment but can also be caused by infection (e.g. cellulitis), malignancy (e.g. inflammatory breast cancer or angiosarcoma) and inflammatory mastitis. Rarely, it can occur with congestive cardiac failure, nephrotic syndrome and from treatment with mTOR

inhibitors such as rapamycin/sirolimus. It can also be due to overgrowth of breast tissue for genetic reasons.

> **Synonyms and inclusions**
> • Breast oedema
> • Swollen breast

Introduction and general description

As changes to breast cancer treatment have led to more breast-conserving surgery and increased use of therapeutic radiation to the breast, the incidence of lymphoedema localised to the breast has risen. The risk is higher in the obese and in women with larger breasts.

Epidemiology

Of 144 women enrolled into one study before cancer treatment, 38 developed breast lymphoedema (26%) [1].

Pathophysiology

Oedema is an excess of interstitial fluid. Any oedema, whatever the cause, is due to capillary filtration overwhelming the lymph drainage for a sufficient period of time. Interstitial fluid is reabsorbed almost entirely by the lymphatic vessels. Inflammation will increase blood flow and vascular permeability, both of which amplify microvascular fluid filtration. Inflammation can be caused by radiation and infection. Lymph drainage may be unable to respond to higher filtration because of the effects from axillary surgery in compromising lymph flow. Disturbances in the Starling principle of fluid exchange will be greatest in the most dependent regions of the breast.

Carcinoma erysipeloides refers to a red, swollen breast resulting from breast cancer infiltrating the dermal lymphatics overlying the breast. Removal of one or more axillary lymph nodes risks lymphoedema within the drainage basin, that is the ipsilateral upper limb and adjoining quadrant of the chest including the breast. Therapeutic radiation to the breast can also induce/exacerbate breast swelling. Obesity and size of breast increase risk, as may adjuvant taxane chemotherapy. In multivariate analysis from one study, factors associated with the development of breast lymphoedema in the axillary surgery subgroup included baseline BMI, surgical incision location and prior surgical biopsy [1].

Other systemic causes for breast lymphoedema include heart failure, low plasma proteins resulting from nephrotic syndrome or liver failure, axillary lymphadenopathy and central vein occlusion. There have been several reports of breast oedema associated with mTOR inhibitors [2].

Clinical features

Breast swelling can be observed immediately following axillary lymphadenectomy, particularly if a 'seroma' or wound infection has occurred (a seroma is a misnomer as it represents a collection of lymph not serum). The onset of swelling can be delayed for months or years, particularly when arising from radiation effects. Swelling may be triggered by an attack of cellulitis.

Symptoms are breast heaviness, swelling, indentations from a bra and sometimes pain and tenderness. Breast redness may feature,

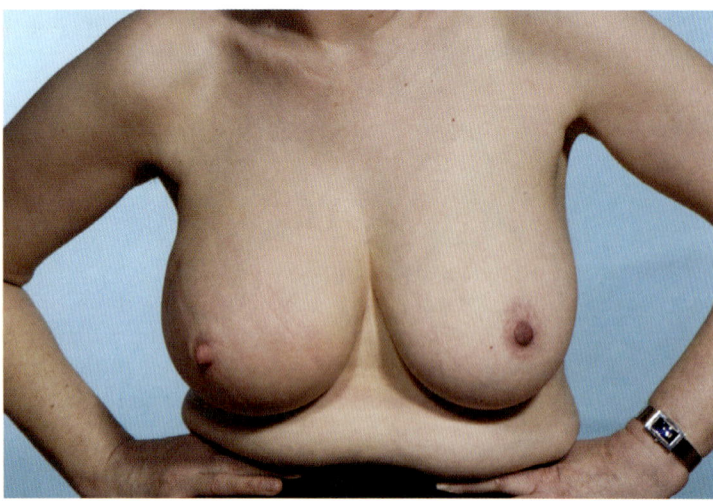

Figure 103.26 Breast lymphoedema following cancer treatment. Note pitting from bra indentations in the skin of the right breast.

indicating inflammation usually secondary to cellulitis, radiation effects or malignancy. Cellulitis can coexist and is difficult to distinguish from post-radiation changes (Figure 103.26). Pitting and peau d'orange skin changes are most noticeable on the undersurface of the breast.

Uncomplicated breast lymphoedema usually settles with treatment and resolves over time. Unexplained breast oedema should always be investigated in case of relapsed breast cancer or the development of (lymph)angiosarcoma.

Differential diagnosis

Oedema can be determined clinically from indentation due to pressure (pitting). Other differential diagnoses include swelling from hormonal effects and fat hypertrophy.

Investigations

Breast ultrasound is usually sufficient to confirm oedema and exclude malignancy; MRI is an alternative. A skin or breast biopsy may be necessary if malignancy is suspected.

Management

An infection, if present, should be treated and malignancy excluded. Obesity should be addressed, and weight reduced to as near normal as possible.

Lymphoedema treatment should involve a supportive bra (a sports bra is often best). It is recommended that the bra be worn both day and night to keep the breast uplifted, which overcomes gravitational factors. Massaging techniques are recommended, such as manual lymphatic drainage therapy, kinesiotaping and water immersion exercises (swimming aerobics), although the evidence base for their use is limited. Mastectomy is a last resort.

Swollen arm

Definition and nomenclature

Swelling of the upper limb is invariably due to oedema but overgrowth of tissue can occur. Oedema is likely to be caused either from lymphatic insufficiency (e.g. breast cancer treatment) or from venous obstruction.

> **Synonyms and inclusions**
> - Lymphoedema
> - Breast cancer-related lymphoedema
> - Postmastectomy lymphoedema
> - Thoracic outlet syndrome
> - Subclavian vein thrombosis

Introduction and general description

Swelling of an arm may be caused by oedema, in which case pitting should be evident to some degree, or it may be caused by an increase in the volume of other tissue elements, for example bone, muscle, fat or a tumour (Table 103.8). A swollen arm may be normal but perceived to be larger if the contralateral limb has shrunk. The commonest reason for upper limb swelling is lymphoedema following breast cancer treatment. Arm swelling can be a presentation of cancer with metastatic disease in the axilla.

Upper limb swelling may be due to primary lymphoedema (usually associated with lymphatic abnormalities elsewhere) or with a lymphatic malformation. Secondary lymphoedema can be caused by rheumatoid arthritis, psoriatic arthropathy, hand dermatitis, yellow-nail syndrome, chronic regional pain syndrome (reflex sympathetic dystrophy), PTM, sirolimus treatment and following repeated infections such as cellulitis and lymphangitis from herpes simplex.

Epidemiology

No data exist for upper limb swelling due to any cause, only for swelling caused by breast cancer.

Pathophysiology

Upper extremity swelling of vascular origin will be due to oedema or increased vascular volume (e.g. vascular malformation). A chronically swollen arm due to fluid indicates lymph drainage failure. This failure will be either due solely to lymphatic dysfunction (lymphoedema) or due to excessive microvascular fluid filtration overwhelming lymph drainage capacity. Increased filtration can be caused by high venous pressures or from enhanced vascular permeability from inflammation (e.g. dermatitis or infection).

Upper limb lymphoedema is most commonly caused by cancer treatment (i.e. axillary lymphadenectomy or radiation), but less commonly can be a presenting sign for advanced malignancy. Recurrent infections from herpes simplex can lead to upper limb lymphoedema [3]. Non-infective forms of inflammation due to chronic hand dermatitis [4], rheumatoid arthritis or psoriatic arthropathy can lead to lymphoedema [5]. Rarely lymphangiosarcoma can complicate any form of lymphoedema.

Venous outflow obstruction may be due to axillary/subclavian vein compression or stenosis (usually due to malignancy or radiation damage) or occlusion from thrombosis. Subclavian vein thrombosis is a rare condition that most often occurs in the context of central venous catheters, pacemakers, trauma, surgery immobilization, oral contraceptive pill use, pregnancy or malignancy. It occurs particularly in cancer patients receiving chemotherapy

Table 103.8 Causes of a swollen arm.

Congenital/genetic			Acquired			
Vascular	**Lymphatic**	**Other**	**Vascular**	**Lymphatic**	**Musculoskeletal**	**Tumours**
Vascular malformation	Lymphoedema	Overgrowth spectrum:	Subclavian vein thrombosis:	Lymphoedema:	Rheumatoid arthritis	Lymphoma
Diffuse phlebectasia	Lymphatic malformation	Proteus syndrome	Effort thrombosis	Axillary surgery	Haematoma	Sarcoma
Klippel–Trenaunay syndrome	Lymphangiomatosis	Fat hypertrophy	Venous catheterisation	DXT	Torn muscle	Metastases
Arteriovenous malformation		Muscle hamartoma	Chemotherapy ports	Cancer	Pathological fracture	
		Gigantism/hemihypertrophy	Chest radiotherapy	Neurological deficit	Myositis ossificans	
		Lipoedema	Thoracic outlet syndrome	Chronic regional pain syndrome	osteomyelitis	
		Dercum disease	Superior vena cava obstruction	Lymphangitis (bacterial infection, herpes simplex, psoriasis, rheumatoid arthritis)	Septic arthritis	
		Madelung disease (benign symmetrical lipomatosis)	IV drug abuse	Yellow-nail syndrome		

DXT, radiotherapy; IV, intravenous.

through central lines. It can also have primary causes such as anatomical anomalies, including thoracic outlet syndrome and Paget–Schröetter syndrome (so-called 'effort thrombosis'). Arteriovenous fistulae for haemodialysis will increase arm size from an increased blood flow but arm oedema will only occur with thrombosis or if lymph drainage is compromised.

Gene mutations causing tissue overgrowth have recently been identified [6]. *PIK3CA* mutations are frequently associated with a lymphatic anomaly and are usually mosaic/somatic in nature. Primary lymphoedema of the upper limb can be caused by a *CCBE1*, *FAT4* or *GJC2* mutation.

Clinical features

In its mildest form breast cancer-related lymphoedema may go unnoticed, even by the patient. Swelling of the hand or wrist may be observed. Alternatively, the patient may notice that their clothes are tight. Aching is frequently experienced.

Upper limb breast cancer-related lymphoedema should exhibit pitting oedema but in more advanced cases fat and fibrosis contribute more to the swelling, so the consistency of the swelling may be fatty or firm. The distribution of swelling along the arm varies between patients, and swelling may be confined to a specific region of the upper limb. In some patients the hand may be swollen, while in others the hand may be spared despite more proximal swelling of the forearm or upper arm. In cases of incipient or mild breast cancer-related lymphoedema, when the arm is not obviously increased in size, inspection may reveal decreased visibility of subcutaneous veins on the ventral forearm and dorsal hand ipsilaterally (the skin is thickened in lymphoedema and therefore more opaque) with smoothing or fullness of the medial elbow and distal upper arm contours. By pinching up the skin and subcutis of each arm between the finger and thumb, the thickened ipsilateral tissues can be palpated. Skin colour is normal except in the presence of venous outflow obstruction when it is red to blue; or with infection when it is pink to red; or with lipodermatosclerosis when it is deep to cherry red.

Differential diagnosis

Venous outflow obstruction due to axillary/subclavian vein compression or stenosis, or occlusion from thrombosis, will produce a discoloured (red/blue) painful swollen arm often with parasthesia.

A swollen arm due to overgrowth may be associated with lymphoedema or lymphatic malformation in which case there may be signs of a vascular birthmark often at the root of the limb. There may be overgrowth with fat either from lipohypertrophy, as in lipoedema, or with lipomatosis such as Madelung disease (Figure 103.27).

Other differentials to consider are musculoskeletal disorders (e.g. ruptured muscle, arthritis, myofascitis or polymyositis), infection, trauma, a neoplasm (including sarcoma and carcinoma), allergic reaction and factitious causes. Rarely, systemic causes such as heart failure, superior vena caval obstruction and hypoproteinaemia can produce arm swelling.

Investigations

Lymphoedema is usually a clinical diagnosis in the context of past cancer treatment. Imaging of the axilla is necessary to exclude a relapse of cancer (e.g. breast cancer or melanoma).

In cases of suspected non cancer lymphoedema, lymphoscintigraphy is the investigation of choice to confirm impaired lymph drainage. A venous duplex ultrasound examination is the first investigation of choice in suspected venous outflow obstruction, but CT or MRI venography may be necessary in neutral and stress postions to confirm a thoracic outlet obstruction. A thrombophilia screen is indicated in cases of thrombosis.

Where overgrowth is suspected, MRI comparing both upper limbs should identify enlarged muscle or fat. MRI can also help distinguish fat from fluid.

Management

Treatment of a swollen arm is dependent on the cause. In circumstances where systemic causes, for example cancer recurrence or heart failure, have led to, or coexist with, the lymphoedema, then

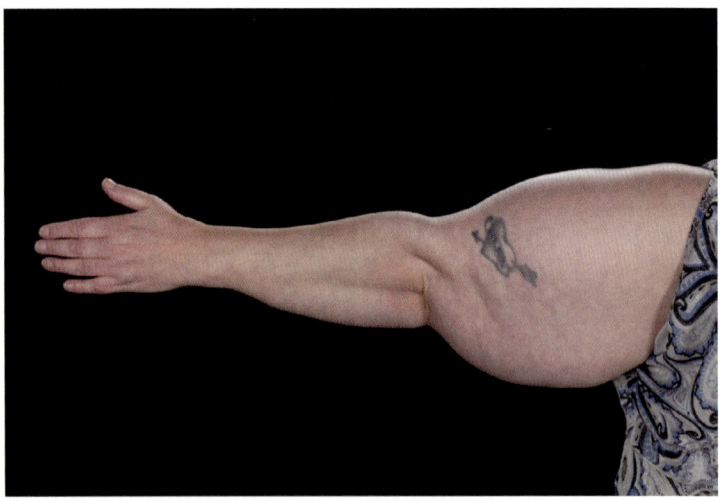

(a)

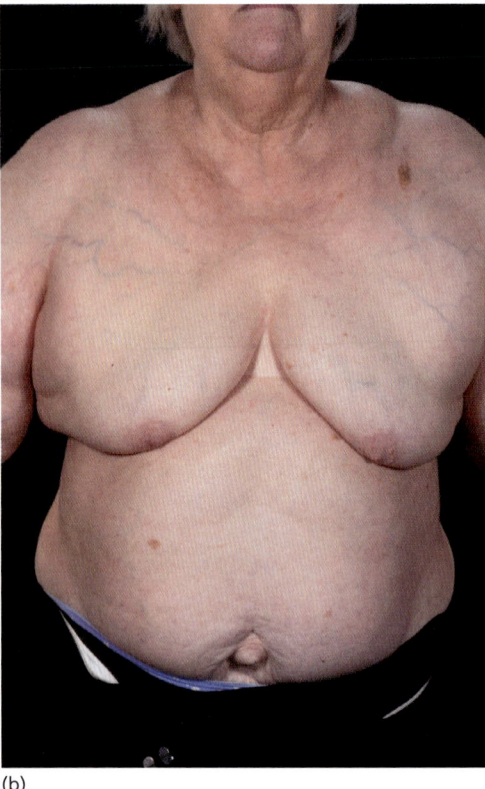

(b)

Figure 103.27 Madelung disorder. Benign symmetrical lipomatosis (also known as benign symmetrical lipomatosis of Launois–Bensaude, Madelung disease, multiple symmetrical lipomatosis and cephalothoracic lipodystrophy) is a cutaneous condition characterised by extensive symmetrical fat deposits in the head, neck and shoulder girdle area.

treatment of the medical condition must be undertaken before embarking on specific lymphoedema therapy. The general principle for treating a swollen limb is to limit increased microvascular filtration and enhance lymph drainage. Lymph drainage responds to exercise and movement done while wearing compression. Where cellulitis, particularly if recurrent, occurs then prophylactic antibiotics may be indicated.

Although surgical decompression and venous angioplasty may be considered for thoracic outlet obstruction, the typical treatment for primary subclavian vein thrombosis is oral anticoagulation only. Venous compression or stenosis may benefit from stenting.

Swollen face, head and neck

Definition and nomenclature
Facial swelling may be generalised or localised, for example to the eyelid(s), lips or one cheek. It may extend beyond the face to involve the head and neck. To be chronic it should persist for more than 3 months.

Synonyms and inclusions
• Puffy face
• Facial lymphoedema
• Rosaceous lymphoedema
• Morbihan disease
• Solid facial oedema
• Oro-facial granulomatosis
• Granulomatous cheilitis
• Melkersson–Rosenthal syndrome

Introduction and general description
Chronic swelling of the face is most often due to fluid oedema but can arise due to an increase in other tissue components, such as blood vessels in a port wine stain (capillary malformation), acromegaly, overgrowth spectrum (hemihypertrophy) or tumours (Table 103.9).

Oedema may extend beyond the face to involve the head and neck, which occurs after surgery and/or radiotherapy for head and neck cancer or with recurrent cancer. Lymphoedema is a frequent late effect of head and neck cancer. Head and neck lymphoedema may be categorised as involving external structures (e.g. the skin and soft tissue of the face and neck) and internal structures, such as the mucosa and underlying soft tissue of the upper aero-digestive tract (e.g. the pharynx and larynx). Other than the eyelids, the most common sites of external lymphoedema are the neck and submental area.

Oedema of the upper or lower lip (or both) may be from a vascular anomaly or result from recurrent angioedema, oro-facial granulomatosis, sarcoidosis, infective cheilitis or from the administration of lip fillers for cosmetic purposes.

Chronic oedema of the eyelids is common. Conditions that need to be considered include dermatomyositis, Graves disease and particularly rosacea/acne. Eyelid swelling may be quite simply due to acquired lax skin from photoageing and other processes that have undermined tissue compliance, such as blepharochalasis/dermatochalasis. In addition to an increase in the diameter and number of lymphatic vessels, a reduction in elastic fibres that are essential for the structure and function of the lymphatic system, a disarrangement in collagen fibres, stromal oedema and an increased number of macrophages play a role in the development of dermatochalasis [7].

Table 103.9 Causes of head and neck swelling.

Congenital/genetic			Acquired		
Vascular	**Lymphatic**	**Overgrowth**	**Tumours**	**Inflammatory**	**Miscellaneous**
Vascular malformation	Syndrome (neck webbing): Turner Noonan Generalised lymphatic dysplasia Mosaic with segmental lymphoedema Lymphangioma/ lymphatic malformation	Macrocephaly, e.g. macrocephaly capillary malformation syndrome	Metastatic head and neck cancer Angiosarcoma Radical neck lymphadenectomy Radiotherapy	Rosacea/acne Cellulitis/erysipelas Oro-facial granulomatosis Tuberculosis Sarcoidosis Dental abscess Sinusitis Dermatomyositis Dermatitis/eczema, psoriasis, contact allergy Dermatochalasis/ blepharochalasis Pediculosis Angioedema	Acromegaly Accidental trauma (cauliflower ear) Cushing syndrome Graves disease

Contact allergy or angioedema, if persistent or recurrent, may slowly compromise lymphatic function. Equally, one severe attack of facial cellulitis may damage the lymphatics sufficiently to cause lymphoedema.

Angiosarcoma or Kaposi sarcoma may infiltrate local lymph drainage, and manifest with eyelid oedema. Facial swelling can coexist with obvious primary lymphoedema of one or more limbs, suggesting that there is widespread congenitally determined lymphatic insufficiency.

Chronic inflammatory disorders (e.g. rosacea, psoriasis, eczema), bacterial cellulitis, pediculosis, trauma and primary (congenital) lymphoedema can all lead to localised, lymphoedematous enlargement of the ear. Rosaceous enlargement is called otophyma [8].

Epidemiology

There are no data for facial lymphoedema from inflammatory disorders. Chronic head and neck lymphoedema is highly prevalent following multimodal treatment for cancer. Most lymphoedema is internal (e.g. the floor of the mouth and pharynx) but 35% have combined internal and external (skin and subcutaneous tissues) [9].

Pathophysiology

Oedema is an excess of interstitial fluid. Any oedema, whatever the cause, is due to microvascular (capillary) filtration overwhelming the lymph drainage for a sufficient period of time. Interstitial fluid is reabsorbed almost entirely by the lymphatic vessels. Gravitational factors contributing to increased microvascular filtration do not play a part except overnight when the patient is lying down, hence facial swelling is often at its worst in the morning. However, sustained increased venous pressures (e.g. superior vena caval obstruction) can produce facial oedema.

If primary facial lymphoedema occurs it is invariably present at birth. It is usually asymmetrical and associated with lymphoedema elsewhere. Head and neck oedema occurring *in utero* may regress by birth but can leave signs such as prominent medial epicanthic folds or neck webbing postnatally, as seen in Turner and Noonan

syndromes. Congenital eyelid lymphoedema may be associated with conjunctival oedema.

A lymphatic malformation (lymphangioma) of the head and neck is more common than lymphoedema and gives rise to swelling from lymph fluid present within abnormally formed lymphatics (whereas lymphoedema is lymph fluid within the interstitial space). The mouth and particularly the tongue are common sites.

Facial lymphoedema may be secondary to other inflammatory pathologies of the skin such as rosacea or acne vulgaris. The skin or subcutaneous initial lymphatics fail rather than the main regional collecting trunks, but in addition telangiectasia and inflammation contribute to oedema through increased fluid filtration. Signalling neuropeptides, including pituitary adenylate cyclase-activating polypeptide (PACAP), a regulator of vasodilatation and oedema, are upregulated in rosacea skin. In a randomised, placebo-controlled trial sumatriptan was able to attenuate PACAP-38-induced rosacea flushing and oedema [10].

To what extent granulomatous rosacea, Morbihan disease and solid facial oedema (Figure 103.28) represent advanced versions of rosaceous lymphoedema remains unclear. Other inflammatory disorders considered to cause facial oedema include eczema, psoriasis, infection, pediculosis and trauma (cauliflower ears). Contact allergy or angioedema, if persistent or recurrent, may slowly compromise lymphatic function. One severe attack of facial erysipelas or cellulitis may damage the lymphatics sufficiently to cause lymphoedema.

Chronic oedema of the eyelids is common and may just be due to acquired lax skin from photoageing and other processes that have undermined tissue compliance.

Medical conditions associated with periocular oedema are dermatomyositis, Cushing syndrome (moon face) and thyroid disease particularly Graves disease. Renal disease, contrary to expectations, does not cause oedema unless associated with hypoproteinaemia (i.e. nephrotic syndrome) or when advanced. Inflammation within underlying structures may manifest with facial oedema (e.g. dental root infection, chronic sinusitis and salivary duct obstruction).

PART 9: VASCULAR DISORDERS

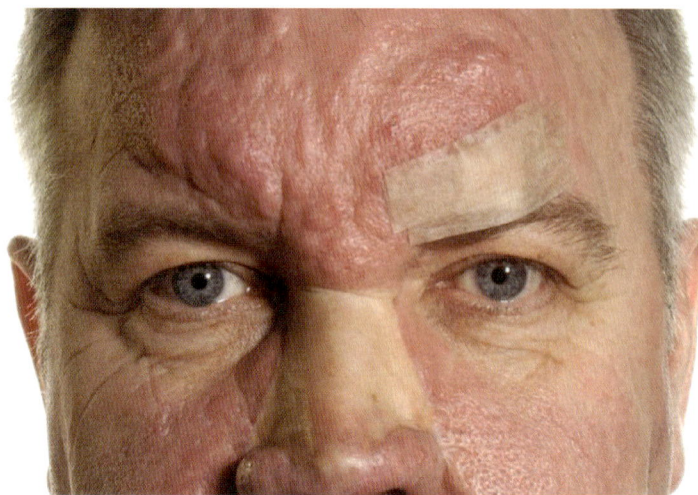

Figure 103.28 Solid facial oedema.

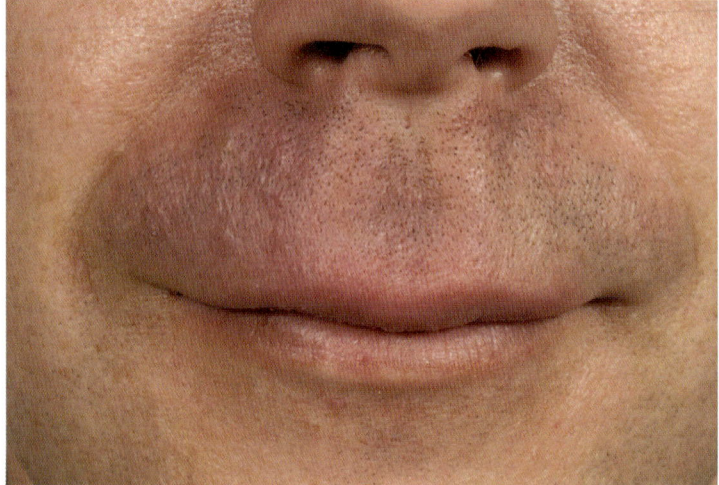

Figure 103.29 Oro-facial granulomatosis exhibiting redness and indurated swelling of the right upper lip.

Angiosarcoma or Kaposi sarcoma may infiltrate local lymph drainage routes and manifest with facial lymphoedema.

Oedema of the upper or lower lip (or both) may be congenital or result from chronic dermatitis, recurrent angioedema or oro-facial granulomatosis (OFG) (Figure 103.29). In OFG it may prove difficult to identify granulomas on biopsy therefore their absence does not necessarily exclude the diagnosis. If present, a diagnosis of OFG (also known as granulomatous cheilitis and Melkersson–Rosenthal syndrome) is made, but it remains unclear if the granulomas are cause or effect. Granulomatous inflammation may exist only locally but a thorough search for gastrointestinal Crohn disease or systemic sarcoidosis should be made. Crohn disease of the bowel can become apparent some time after presentation of OFG. Granulomatous inflammation from administration of lip fillers for cosmetic purposes can also cause chronic swelling [11].

Head and neck lymphoedema is becoming increasingly more common as more head and neck cancer is treated by lymph node neck dissection and radiotherapy. Fibrosis and secondary infection are frequent complications.

Clinical features

The clinical features of facial lymphoedema depend on the underlying aetiology. Swelling usually affects the central forehead, eyelids, cheeks and submental region. It may be surprisingly asymmetrical. Oedema may not diminish overnight when lying down. Redness is always present in rosacea, but inflammatory pustules and papules may be absent. OFG starts with intermittent bouts of swelling resembling angioedema affecting the lips or cheeks, but with time the condition may become persistent. An extension of the oedema within the mouth is common and is the reason for the rugose changes on the buccal mucosal and tongue (scrotal tongue).

Lymphoedema may be severe with head and neck cancer causing facial disfiguration and distress (Figure 103.30).

Investigations

Skin biopsy may be helpful if granulomatous disease, rosacea, dermatomyositis, angiosarcoma or Kaposi sarcoma is suspected. Lymphoscintigraphy can be performed on the head and neck but is difficult to interpret. MRI or CT imaging may be useful if an underlying pathology such as cancer, sinusitis or dental root infection is suspected. Such imaging may also help distinguish between swelling due to fluids and other tissue components such as fat.

Management

The treatment of facial lymphoedema will depend on the cause. Any inflammation will need to be treated to reduce the higher lymphatic load arising from increased vascular permeability and blood flow. Raising the head of the bed during overnight sleep helps to reduce venous pressure and therefore microvascular filtration. Otherwise, the standard principles of enhancing lymph flow through massage techniques and facial exercises apply. Modified decongestive lymphoedema therapy can be successful in treating head and neck lymphoedema following cancer treatment.

In rosaceous lymphoedema, antibiotic therapy appears disappointing in reducing swelling; low-dose isotretinoin has been advocated but may need to be sustained for 1–2 years. Laser ablation of the telangiectasia may reduce the fluid load on the lymphatics.

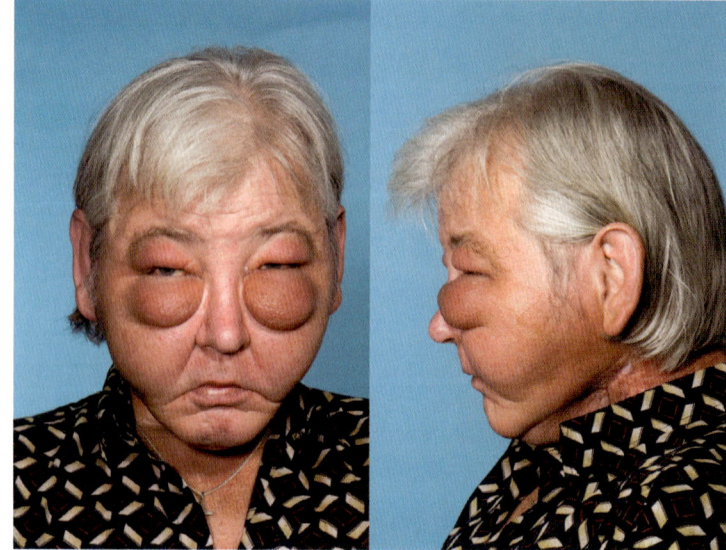

Figure 103.30 Severe facial lymphoedema following treatment for carcinoma of the tongue.

There are no data from clinical trials for the treatment of OFG. In one review of 45 patients who required treatment, 24 (53.3%) were treated with topical corticosteroids/immunosuppressants only, whereas 21 (46.7%) received a combined therapy (topical plus systemic corticosteroids/immunosuppressants and/or intralesional corticosteroids). The long-term outcome analysis showed complete or partial resolution of tissue swelling and oral ulceration in 78.8% and 70% of patients, respectively [12]. There are reports of therapeutic success with azathioprine, thalidomide, infliximab and mycophenylate mofetil.

Swollen genitalia and mons pubis

Definition and nomenclature
Genital lymphoedema may affect the shaft of the penis and/or scrotum plus the mons pubis.

Synonyms and inclusions
- Genital lymphoedema
- Peno-scrotal lymphoedema
- Vulval lymphoedema
- Elephantiasis
- Genital oedema
- Massive localised lymphoedema
- Acquired genital lymphangioma

Introduction and general description
Genital lymphoedema may be primary or secondary (Table 103.10). The genitalia have the option of bilateral lymph node drainage. For swelling to occur, drainage pathways to both inguinal regions must fail or local genital lymphatics must become occluded.

In primary genital lymphoedema gene mutations have been identified, including in *GATA2* and *FOXC2*.

Secondary lymphoedema may be caused by advanced or local infiltration of cancer, extensive scarring from accidental or surgical trauma, obesity, granulomatous disease such as Crohn disease

Table 103.10 Causes of lymphoedema of the genitalia and mons pubis.

Primary (congenital/genetic)	Secondary
Noonan syndrome	Cancer (advanced primary, inflammatory cancer, pelvic relapse, skin infiltration)
Hennekam syndrome (*CCBE1*, *FAT4*)	Lymphadenectomy (pelvic, bilateral, ilio-inguinal)
Generalised lymphatic dysplasia	Radiotherapy
Chylous reflux	Accidental trauma
Emberger syndrome (*GATA2*)	Obesity
Lymphoedema distichiasis (*FOXC2*)	Crohn disease/ano-genital granulomatosis
Yellow-nail syndrome	Hidradenitis suppurativa
	Infections:
	Filariasis
	Cellulitis
	Lymphogranuloma venereum
	Donovanosis
	Systemic causes (heart failure, nephrotic syndrome)

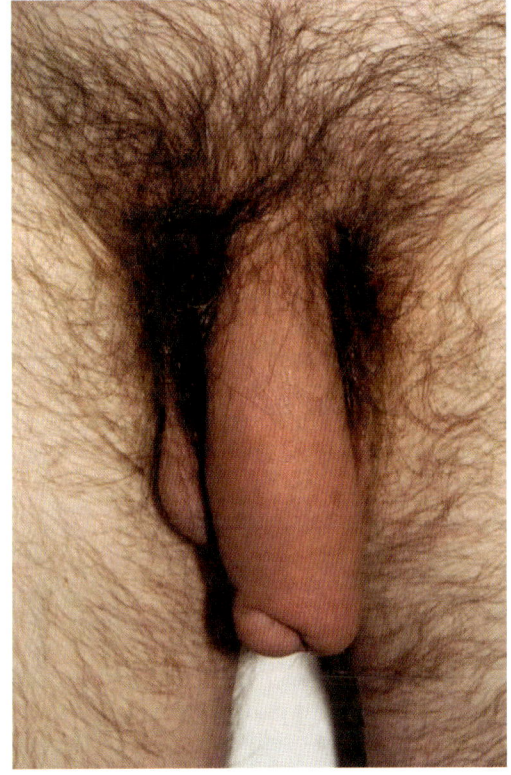

(a)

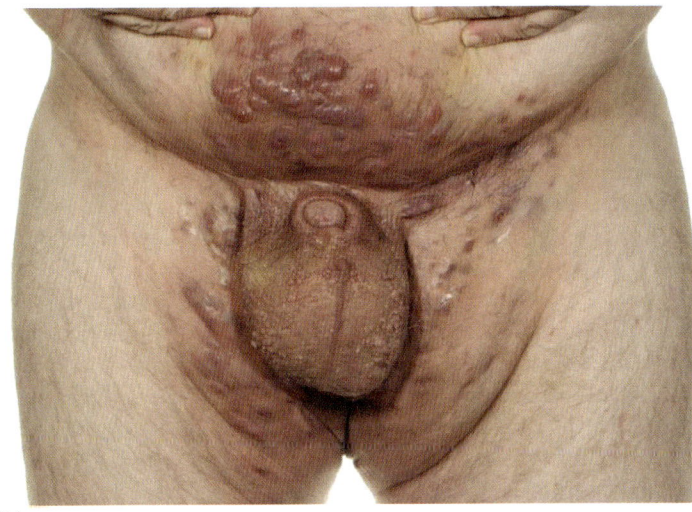

(b)

Figure 103.31 (a) Lymphoedema of the penis secondary to ano-genital granulomatosis. There may be no sign of inflammation. (b) Genital lymphoedema secondary to hidradenitis suppurativa. Note the cutaneous lymphangiectasia that predisposes to lymphorrhoea. (b) Reproduced from Thomas *et al.* 2014 [13].

or ano-genital granulomatosis (Figure 103.31a), hidradenitis suppurativa (Figure 103.31b) and infections such as filariasis, lymphogranuloma venereum and donovanosis.

Mons pubis swelling can develop in isolation but more often is associated with genital or lower limb lymphoedema.

Genital oedema occurring in isolation is usually a result of local inflammation, for instance due to infection, ano-genital granulomatosis (cutaneous Crohn disease), hidradenitis suppurativa or sarcoidosis. Genital oedema can be part of more widespread oedema from heart failure or nephrotic syndrome. Primary lymphoedema can affect the genitalia but not usually without lower limb involvement. Lymph or chylous reflux can produce genital oedema often with lymphangiectasia.

Pathophysiology
Pathology

In all forms of pure lymphoedema the pathology is the same, namely increased dermal and subcutaneous thickness through fluid, increased fat and fibrosis. A non-specific inflammatory infiltrate is invariably present. Lymphatic vessels may be increased in number and expanded due to increased lymphatic pressure, but they may also be reduced in number through genetically determined underdevelopment or if obliterated by fibrosis.

Causative factors

In primary lymphoedema a genetic cause is probable. To date there are at least four phenotypes for which mutations are known and which cause genital lymphoedema: Emberger syndrome, lymphoedema distichiasis syndrome, Hennekam syndrome and Noonan syndrome. Genital swelling may be a feature of congenital lymphoedema, particularly if part of a generalised lymphatic dysplasia. Chylous reflux into the scrotum may result from congenitally malformed retroperitoneal aortic and iliac lymphatics giving rise to megalymphatics or from intestinal lymphangiectasia.

Most cases (60%) of genital lymphoedema will be caused by obliteration of the upper thigh, inguinal and iliac lymph vessels for reasons which are not always apparent. One-quarter of cases will be caused by obliteration of outflow lymphatics from the scrotum and 15% caused by reflux [14].

The commonest cause of genital lymphoedema and hydrocele worldwide is filariasis. Other secondary causes of genital lymphoedema include active cancer and its treatment (e.g. bilateral inguinal lymphadenectomy or radiotherapy), granulomatous disease (e.g. Crohn disease and ano-genital granulomatosis) and extensive local inflammation and scarring (e.g. hidradenitis suppurativa). Genital swelling may occur as part of extensive oedema below the waist in heart failure, hypoalbuminaemia and inferior vena cava obstruction. Less common causes include tuberculous lymphadenitis, lymphogranuloma venereum and donovanosis [15].

Mons pubis lymphoedema is caused by local radiotherapy, obesity and local inflammatory disorders such as Crohn disease and hidradenitis suppurativa.

In both primary and secondary cases an infection or other forms of local inflammation (e.g dermatitis) may cause swelling. Compression of leg lymphoedema, through bandages or pneumatic compression pumps, can push fluid up to the trunk. This can result in genital oedema, especially if care is not taken to redirect the lymph through collateral drainage routes.

Genetics

Mutations in *GATA2* cause Emberger syndrome in which genital lymphoedema is one phenotypic feature [16]. Mutations in *FOXC2* cause lymphoedema distichiasis syndrome; uncommonly genital lymphoedema and lymphangiectasia can also feature [17]. Mutations in *CCBE1* and *FAT4* cause Hennekam syndrome

(lymphoedema–lymphangiectasia syndrome), a form of generalised lymphatic dysplasia; genital lymphoedema is variable as a feature [18]. In Noonan syndrome molecular genetic testing identifies a mutation in *PTPN11* in 50% of affected individuals, in *SOS1* in approximately 13%, in *RAF1* in 3–17% and in *KRAS* in fewer than 5%. Lymphatic dysplasia with a clinical lymphatic abnormality is one of the major features [19].

Clinical features

The development of swelling will be dependent on the underlying cause. The onset may be insidious or sudden with no obvious trigger. Infection (e.g. cellulitis) may be a provoking factor. A history of exposure to filariasis with travel to endemic areas must always be considered. Primary cases invariably have one or both lower limbs swollen at the time of onset of genital lymphoedema.

In primary lymphoedema swelling may be present at birth or develop later in life. Genital lymphoedema is much more common in men, probably because of anatomy and the dependent nature of male external genitalia. The various parts of the genitalia – the penis, scrotum and labia – are not always swollen equally.

Longstanding lymphoedema causes thickening and hyperkeratosis of the overlying skin with the production of papillomas. These probably arise from lymph congestion within the dermal lymphatics, which, in the early stages, can appear as 'lymph blisters' on the skin surface before the tissues become organised and fibrotic.

Episodes of cellulitis are common with genital lymphoedema. Each attack further undermines lymph drainage routes, leading to worse swelling and a higher risk of infections, so establishing a vicious cycle. Offending organisms may be many and difficult to identify. Gram-negative infections should always be considered. The inguinal lymph glands are often enlarged as a result of infection (filarial or bacterial).

Mons pubis lymphoedema presents as a dome-shaped swelling with peau d'orange skin changes. In the obese it can grow to epic proportions whereupon it resembles a pseudosarcoma and is called massive localised lymphoedema [20].

Genital lymphoedema can be complicated by infection (e.g. cellulitis) or the leakage of lymph or chyle with resulting contact dermatitis. Penile swelling may interefere with micturition and sexual function. Impotence may develop. A secondary balanoposthitis may occur.

Differential diagnosis

The characteristic skin changes make a diagnosis of lymphoedema relatively straightforward. However, systemic causes of oedema such as heart failure and nephrotic syndrome should be considered when accompanied by more widespread oedema. A hydrocele can be mistaken for oedema.

Investigations

Filariasis must be excluded by a complement fixation test, or night-time blood smears if active filarial infection is likely. A skin biopsy is essential to diagnose granulomatous disease or cancer infiltrating the dermal lymphatics.

Imaging with a CT or MRI scan is necessary to exclude lymphatic obstruction within the pelvis or ilio-inguinal glands from cancer or other pathologies (e.g. retroperitoneal fibrosis). Lymphoscintigraphy may be helpful in identifying lower limb lymphatic abnormalities. It may demonstrate tracer within the scrotal lymphatics in cases of reflux.

Management

Decongestive lymphatic therapy aims to reduce swelling through a combination of massage and compression [21]. This should only be undertaken if the underlying causes, such as cancer, granulomatous disease or infection, have been treated. Skin care should be scrupulous. Prophylactic antibiotics may be necessary to counter recurrent cellulitis. Compression is easier on the female genitalia than the male. Custom-made tights or shorts are recommended. Foam inserts can increase local pressure comfortably. A scrotal sling or harness may provide support and compression in the male.

Surgical reduction may be straightforward and effective [22]. Circumcision may resolve preputial swelling and any redundant foreskin. Hyfrecation or diathermy is best for lymphangiectasia. Antibiotic cover is recommended in all cases.

Abdominal wall lymphoedema

Definition and nomenclature

Abdominal wall lymphoedema is skin and subcutaneous oedema of the lower abdominal wall generated when ilio-inguinal lymph drainage is compromised bilaterally, or within a pendulous obese abdomen or in heart failure or nephrotic syndrome.

Synonyms and inclusions
- Pendulous abdomen
- Swollen abdominal panniculus
- Elephantiasis nostras verrucosa
- Secondary cancer-related lymphoedema
- Truncal lymphoedema

Introduction and general description

The abdominal wall is not considered a likely place for lymphoedema but is probably more common than generally realised. Diagnosis may be difficult because the soft tissues of the abdominal wall make pitting difficult to elicit. Furthermore, abdominal wall lymphoedema may manifest with more fat than fluid, making distinction from obesity demanding. Peau d'orange skin changes can be a helpful sign and palpation of fluid gives a more solid feel than fat.

Abdominal wall lymphoedema can develop following cancer treatment when ilio-inguinal lymph drainage is compromised. In such circumstances lower limb lymphoedema would likely coexist. Cancer relapse must be considered if swelling develops some time after curative cancer treatment. Cancer relapse may be in the pelvis or with infiltration of the abdominal wall skin (e.g. carcinoma erysipeloides).

Non-cancer-related lymphoedema of the abdominal wall is invariably related to obese abdominal panniculus, or in circumstances of extensive oedema such as heart failure, nephrotic syndrome or yellow-nail syndrome.

Pathophysiology

Causative factors include cancer treatment (e.g. bilateral inguinal or pelvic lymphadenectomy) or radiotherapy for gynaecological, penile, bladder or prostate cancer, as well as relapsed cancer and cellulitis. Obesity where the abdominal panniculus is pendulous is also a major risk factor.

Compromised ilio-inguinal lymph nodes affect all lymph drainage routes below the waist. This usually causes lower limb lymphoedema first, but in more severe cases the lower abdominal wall and genitalia are affected as well. External beam pelvic radiotherapy not only affects the lymph nodes but can also affect smaller collateral lymphatics within the skin and subcutaneous tissue of the mons pubis to cause lymphoedema within the radiation field.

Relapse of cancer with infiltration of the dermal and subcutaneous lymphatics of the lower abdomen can also produce lymphoedema. Advanced cancer can produce profound lymphoedema from the waist downwards, particularly if accompanied by iliac vein or inferior vena cava obstruction.

Obesity is known to cause lymphatic dysfunction and exacerbate lymphoedema. This is particularly so in abdominal panniculus when the abdomen becomes pendulous. This creates venous congestion so increasing fluid filtration into the abdominal wall. Intense oedema complicated by infection often leads to elephantiasis changes (elephantiasis nostras verrucosa). Obese patients often suffer sleep apnoea syndrome, which only further increases systemic salt and water retention.

Clinical features

The patient may not perceive mild abdominal wall oedema. With progression there may be a sensation of getting fatter, or tightness and discomfort within the affected area. There may be a history of past cancer treatment, obesity or cellulitis.

Pitting can usually be demonstrated only over the anterior superior iliac spine. Pinching a fold of lower abdominal skin will reveal thickening with a heavier, more solid feel than just fat. Peau d'orange skin changes may be observed. With time, and progressive accumulation of fat and fibrosis within the swollen area, the tissues will feel more indurated, particularly following an episode of cellulitis. More severe cases can develop marked hyperkeratosis, skin thickening and papillomatosis. These changes produce a warty, cobblestone appearance (Figure 103.32).

Cellulitis frequently occurs because of the compromised local tissue immunity. Recurrent attacks exacerbate the lymphoedema, leading to a vicious cycle. Lipodermatosclerosis may develop within the pendulous abdomen due to venous congestion and previous cellulitis. Progression of abdominal wall lymphoedema can result in a huge swelling, which may hang down as far as the patient's knees, thereby compromising mobility and risking overwhelming sepsis. There is a high morbidity and life-threatening sepsis in the very obese.

Differential diagnosis

Abdominal wall oedema may develop in heart failure, hypoalbuminaemia (nephrotic syndrome, liver disease and malnutrition) and inferior vena cava obstruction.

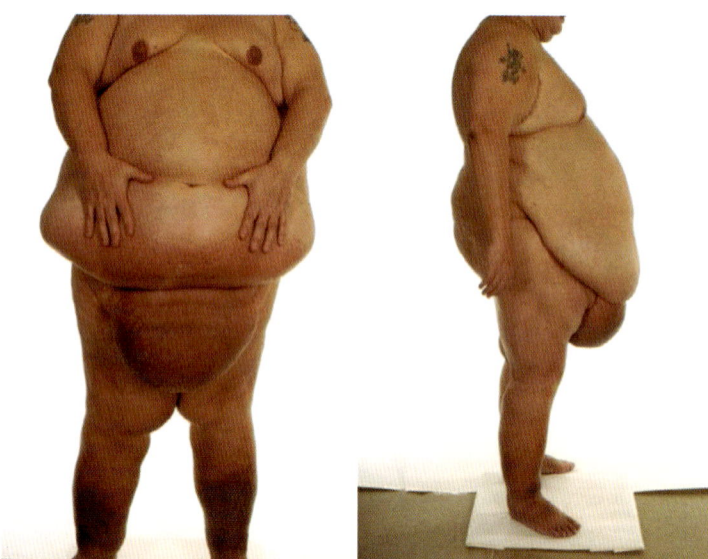

Figure 103.32 Lymphoedema of the pendulous abdomen and mons pubis due to obesity.

Investigations

In cancer patients, restaging using abdominal ultrasound or a PET/CT scan is recommended. Skin biopsy may be helpful if infiltrative cancer is a possibility. In the severely obese check for the following: (i) heart failure, using BNP estimation; (ii) low plasma albumin; and (iii) sleep apnoea syndrome, through sleep studies.

Management

Correction of any underlying causes is the first priority wherever possible. Diuretics are usually of little help in abdominal wall oedema except in heart failure, but may be tried for short periods where physiology involves increased microvascular filtration.

In severe morbid obesity (BMI >50) bariatric intervention should be considered.

Antibiotics should be given if infection is present. Prophylactic antibiotics may be given if there is recurrent infection.

Decongestive lymphatic therapy (manual lymphatic drainage and abdominal compression using binding or compression garments) should be administered.

A 'melon slice' surgical apronectomy may be considered but the risk of infection and wound dehiscence is high in obese patients.

Massive localised lymphoedema

Definition and nomenclature

Massive localised lymphoedema is a benign lymphoproliferative soft-tissue overgrowth in the morbidly obese patient. It represents gross lymphoedema usually confined to one area such as a thigh and appearing like a tumour.

Synonyms and inclusions

- Pseudosarcoma
- Elephantiasis nostras verrucosa

Introduction and general description

Lymphoedema typically affects a limb but uncommonly it can present as a localised mass resembling a tumour. It is not unusual for an area of lymphoedema on the lower inner thigh, leg, inguinal region or abdominal apron to hypertrophy into an enlarged fold and then, under the influence of gravity, progress into a pendulous swelling. Obesity and repeat attacks of infection locally increase risk.

Pathophysiology

Predisposing factors include obesity, filariasis and recurrent infection.

Solid or papillomatous plaques can mimic tumours but biopsy will reveal typical features of lymphoedema, namely oedema, dilated lymphatics, fibrosis, fat, epidermal acanthosis and hyperkeratosis, and inflammatory dermal infiltrate. In one series all 22 cases showed striking dermal fibrosis, expansion of the fibrous septa between fat lobules with increased numbers of stromal fibroblasts, lymphatic proliferation and lymphangiectasia. Multinucleated fibroblastic cells, marked vascular proliferation, moderate stromal cellularity and fascicular growth raised concern among referring pathologists for such conditions as atypical lipomatous tumour/well-differentiated liposarcoma, angiosarcoma and a fibroblastic neoplasm such as fibromatosis [23].

Clinical features

An area of lymphoedema becomes raised like a tumour, then under the effects of gravity may become polypoid. Lesions most resemble a benign tumour such as a pedunculated lipoma although a soft-tissue sarcoma could also be suspected. The overlying skin is markedly thickened with a 'cobblestone' appearance and elephantiasis (Figure 103.33). The structure often appears lobulated and can grow to a considerable size. Weeping of lymph fluid and ulceration are common. Infection with septicaemia frequently occurs. When very large the 'tumour' can interfere with mobility. A total of 65 cases of massive localised lymphoedema have been described in the literature, nine of which resulted in angiosarcoma (10.3% of all cases) [24]. The likelihood is that the lesion will continue to enlarge associated with chronic infection unless treated.

Differential diagnosis

Differential diagnoses include lipoma, lymphatic malformation, lymphocele and sarcoma.

Investigations

Magnetic resonance imaging typically demonstrates a sharply demarcated, pedunculated mass consisting of fat partitioned by fibrous septae surrounded by a thickened dermis. There is oedema both within the mass and tracking along the subcutaneous septae in a lace-like fashion outwards from the pedicle, outlining large lobules of fat [25].

Management

The only satisfactory treatment is surgical resection with reconstruction. However, this is not without hazard as wound dehiscence and overwhelming infection can present serious life-threatening risks. Intensive multilayer lymphoedema compression bandaging and IV antibiotics given first to shrink the mass might reduce the surgical complications and improve prognosis [26].

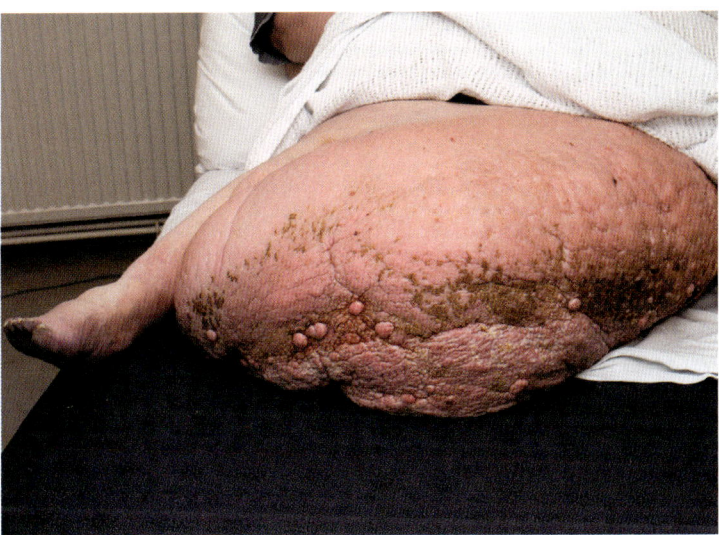

Figure 103.33 Massive localised lymphoedema of the right thigh showing marked 'cobblestone' skin changes.

LIPOEDEMA

Lipoedema

Definition and nomenclature
Lipoedema is a disorder of adipose tissue that occurs almost exclusively in women, usually at a time of hormonal change.

Synonyms and inclusions
- Adiposis dolorosa
- Painful fat syndrome
- Adipositas oedematosa
- Stovepipe legs

Introduction and general description
Lipoedema is a condition characterised by abnormal adipose deposition within the lower limbs. It occurs almost exclusively in females and is thought to be an inherited disorder. The onset of symptoms typically occurs at a time of hormonal change such as puberty or pregnancy. Patients complain of progressive fatty swelling of the lower limbs, with associated local easy bruising, skin tenderness and pain. Contrary to the name, fluid is not a dominant feature and the 'swelling' is caused predominantly by adipose tissue. Lipoedema was first described by Allen and Hines in 1940 as 'bilateral enlargement of the legs thought to be due to abnormal deposition of subcutaneous fat and accumulation of fluid in the lower legs' [1]. The lack of a clear definition of the disorder and no confirmatory test have led to significant confusion regarding diagnosis and management. In fact, some clinicians consider it a physiological variant of obesity rather than a disease [2]. However, lipoedema recently received acceptance as a medical condition and obtained an MIM number (614103) in 2011 [3].

Epidemiology
Limited prevalence data exist for lipoedema. Some clinicians believe it is a rare disorder, but many consider that it is more common than expected and is often misdiagnosed as simple obesity or lymphoedema.

Pathophysiology
The aetiology of lipoedema is still unknown. It has not yet been determined whether the cause of the 'fatty swelling' is due to adipocyte hypertrophy or hyperplasia, or a combination of the two. Histological examination of tissue biopsies and liposuction aspirates identifies oedema of the adipocytes and/or interstitium, but no other abnormalities are detected. One study postulated that activated adipogenesis occurs in lipoedema tissue leading to hypoxia and subsequent adipocyte necrosis and recruitment of macrophages, as occurs in obesity [4]. Child *et al.* proposed that a hormonal influence was likely to underlie the condition as lipoedema appeared to be expressed most commonly at puberty or other times of hormonal change.

Frequent observations of mother to daughter inheritance led to the hypothesis that lipoedema is a genetic disorder. Patterns of inheritance of the condition within families are consistent with either X-linked dominant inheritance or autosomal dominant inheritance with sex limitation [5].

Clinical features
Lipoedema occurs almost exclusively in females. No ethnic differences have been reported. Onset is typically at puberty or other times of hormonal change such as pregnancy or commencement of the oral contraceptive pill. Only six cases of lipoedema affecting males have been reported in the literature. All were thought to have developed lipoedema secondary to hormonal disturbances, with reduced testosterone levels being a common factor [6].

Affected individuals develop bilateral and symmetrical 'fatty' non-pitting swelling, usually confined to the legs and hips. The feet are spared, giving rise to an 'cuffing' or 'bracelet' effect at the ankles, sometimes called 'cankles' (Figure 103.34). Heavy deposition of fat on the thighs can result in knee hooding and loss of definition for the knee joint, saddlebags of fat on the hips, and excess buttock fat with a ledge between the buttocks and sacrum, so-called steatopygia. Patients frequently complain of tenderness and easy bruising of the affected areas. Over time, the patient may develop similar excess fat in their upper arms. Wold *et al.* have proposed a set of diagnostic criteria for lipoedema [6]:

1 Occurrence is almost exclusively in women.
2 It has a bilateral and symmetrical nature with minimal involvement of the feet, resulting in an 'inverse shouldering' or 'bracelet' effect at the ankle.
3 Minimal pitting oedema is seen.
4 There is pain, tenderness and easy bruising.
5 There is no reduction in limb size despite elevation of the extremities or weight loss.

In the teenager or young adult, the lipoedema phenotype is characteristic; the classic disproportionate distribution of fat below the waist, the coexisting features of tissue tenderness and easy bruising and the lack of response to weight-reducing diets all argue against a form of obesity. However, later in life, lipoedema can be complicated

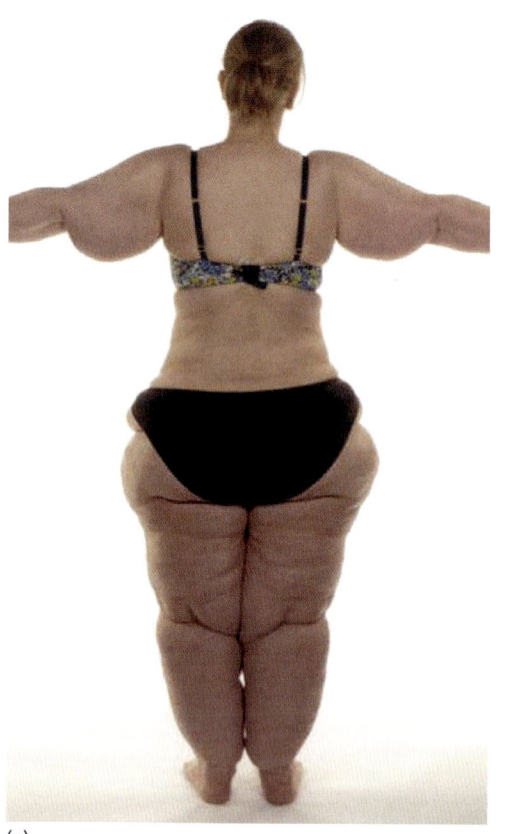

(a)

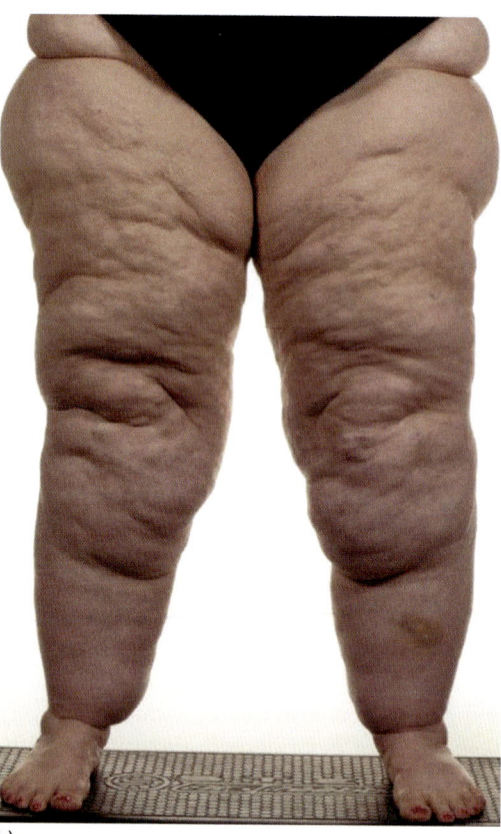

(b)

Figure 103.34 A patient with classic lipoedema. (a) Symmetrical fatty swelling of both lower limbs with sparing of the trunk. Increased adipose deposition of the upper arms is present. (b) Features include sparing of the feet with 'inverse shouldering' of the ankles. Fat pads are developing on the medial aspect of both knees.

by obesity and/or lymphoedema, rendering the diagnosis more difficult to make. In this case historical symptoms are key to the diagnosis. While lipoedema is confused with obesity by many clinicians, associated obesity has, nonetheless, been observed in most patients particularly when older.

Fluid oedema that develops during the day and resolves overnight can feature, and usually affects the legs below the knees. This oedema is called orthostatic oedema implying it is secondary to the effects of gravity in the upright posture. The feet usually remain unaffected. Allen and Hines proposed that this oedema formation in lipoedema was the result of poor resistance of accumulated fat against the hydrostatic passage of fluid from the capillaries into the interstitium [1].

Lipoedema is frequently complicated by the onset of a secondary lymphoedema, resulting in the clinical picture of lipo-lymphoedema. The clinical features of lipo-lymphoedema range from mild pitting oedema of the feet to severe asymmetrical swelling of the lower limbs because of impaired lymphatic drainage. Lymphoscintigraphy performed after the onset of lipo-lymphoedema will confirm impaired lymphatic drainage whereas in 'pure' lipoedema, lymphoscintigraphy is normal [7].

Hypermobility and disorders of gait, joint deformities (e.g. genu valgum) and pain may occur because of disproportionate adipose tissue of the legs. A number of women complain of knee pain prior to the onset of radiological changes, suggesting this is part of the lipoedema phenotype (possibly due to an associated disorder of connective tissue) or secondary to the strain put on the knee joint from increased limb volume. Venous telangiectasias are also common (but with no venous reflux on venous duplex examination).

Patients with lipoedema often develop psychological morbidity as a result of their chronic progressive disorder. Poorly managed lipoedema will undoubtedly progress and be complicated by obesity and lymphoedema. The unwieldy nature of the leg swelling, and the pain, can be disabling in older age particularly if obesity complicates the picture.

Differential diagnosis

Lipoedema must be differentiated from lymphoedema, a more well-known cause of bilateral lower limb enlargement. However, lymphoedema typically results in asymmetrical oedematous swelling due to the accumulation of lymph fluid within tissue spaces. Typical cutaneous findings of lymphoedema include brawny, hard and warty changes of the skin and subcutis. Pitting (where the skin remains indented for a few minutes after removal of firm finger pressure for 30 s) is usually present in lymphoedema, except in very advanced cases. In contrast, in pure lipoedema the skin remains characteristically soft and pitting is almost always absent. The experienced clinician will be able to differentiate the two conditions by the soft 'doughy' consistency of excess subcutaneous adipose deposition in lipoedema compared with the pitting, firmer tissue consistency of lymphoedema.

Dercum disease or adiposis dolorosa refers to a syndrome of painful fat disorder. Pain is the dominant feature and is considered to emanate from lipomas. Dercum disease can present with a phenotype similar to lipoedema. Lipomas can be a feature of lipoedema and Dercum disease where there are multiple, painful, diffuse or nodular lipomas (with chronic pain lasting more than 3 months) and generalised obesity. Men may be affected, but there is

Table 103.11 Stages of lipoedema.

Stage	Clinical signs
Stage I	The skin is smooth and the subcutaneous layer is thickened, soft and with an even structure. This stage can last for several years
Stage II	The skin might be cool in certain areas as a result of functional vascular imbalance. Over time, subcutaneous nodules develop and the skin surface becomes uneven
Stage III	After several decades, patients may develop large amounts of tender subcutaneous tissue and bulging protrusions of fat, mainly at the inner side of the thighs or knees, which lead to an impairment of gait

a female preponderance with a ratio of 5–30 : 1 [8]. Dercum disease is frequently misdiagnosed as fibromyalgia.

Table 103.11 contains the clinical stages of lipoedema as suggested by Schmeller and Meier-Vollrath [9].

Investigations

The diagnosis of lipoedema is currently clinical with no absolute phenotypic features or confirmatory test. Numerous investigations have been undertaken in patients with lipoedema, including lymphoscintigrams, venograms, arteriograms and magnetic resonance lymphangiography, all failing to demonstrate specific abnormalities but suggesting a subclinical reduction in lymphatic function in patients with lipoedema [10]. None of these investigations demonstrated specific diagnostic signs of lipoedema.

High-resolution cutaneous ultrasonography has been proposed as a method for differentiating lipoedema from lymphoedema. Naouri *et al*. reported a significant difference in dermal thickness between the two groups – no dermal thickening detected in lipoedema compared with marked dermal thickness in lymphoedema [11].

Management

No curative therapies are available for lipoedema. Management goals are aimed at the improvement of subjective symptoms (e.g. pain), prevention of progression and prevention of lipo-lymphoedema.

Conservative therapies including manual lymph drainage, intermittent pneumatic compression and multilayered short-stretch bandaging have been shown to reduce the perception of pain in patients with lipoedema. However, these treatments do not reduce limb volume unless there is coexistent lymphoedema. Compression therapy has been shown to prevent additional oedema formation.

The prevention of lipoedema progression is key. Physical activity should be encouraged as it will reduce the risk of obesity and may have a positive impact on the oedema component. Dietary advice for avoiding weight gain is a crucial part of the management plan. Patients should be made aware that obesity is a major exacerbating factor of lipoedema.

Liposuction has been accepted as a therapeutic option for lipoedema. Treatment is aimed at reducing limb volume/mass, and pain, and improving mobility. Treatment in the early stages

yields a better outcome than when liposuction is used in advanced cases or in lipo-lymphoedema. The long-term data on liposuction indicate good efficacy providing fitness is maintained [12]. Lipoedema legs have a delayed lymph transport. Tumescent liposuction does not diminish the lymphatic function in lipoedema patients, thus tumescent liposuction can be regarded as a safe treatment [13].

Patients must be aware that liposuction does not offer a cure. If the patient does not maintain their weight in the postoperative period then they will return to the original disease state.

Imaging of the lymphatic system

Introduction

Most patients with lymphoedema are diagnosed from the history and clinical findings. The use and value of imaging techniques are highly dependent on availability and expertise. Table 103.12 compares the different techniques available for imaging the lymphatic system. The techniques used to investigate the lymphatic system are discussed here, but some patients will benefit from additional imaging in order to understand the cause of their swelling. For example, MRI and CT scanning may be indicated to assess the presence of intra-abdominal or pelvic pathology or masses obstructing lymphatic drainage. MRI may also be requested to assess tissue hypertrophy or signs of overgrowth (e.g. in Klippel–Trenaunay syndrome). Venous duplex imaging may be requested to investigate the possibility that the lymphoedema is associated with venous incompetence.

Imaging techniques
Lymphography

X-ray contrast lymphography (lymphangiography) remains the gold standard mode of demonstrating lymphatic collectors and lymph nodes. However, it is rarely used as the technique requires the invasive procedure of direct cannulation of the lymphatics [1].

Lymphoscintigraphy

Lymphoscintigraphy (isotope lymphography) is currently the investigation of choice for determining if chronic oedema may be due predominantly to a failure of lymph drainage. It involves a simple intradermal/subcutaneous injection of a radiolabelled tracer protein, exclusively cleared by the lymphatics. Qualitative lymphoscintigraphy involves examination of images only. Measurement of tracer uptake and transit through the lymphatics that permits quantitative analyses of lymph drainage is referred to as quantitative lymphoscintigraphy and may discriminate lymphoedema from lipoedema [2]. Lymphoscintigraphy has the potential to distinguish between different types of primary lymphoedema and their mechanisms of lymph drainage failure. For example, initial lymphatic dysfunction in Milroy disease versus lymph collector reflux in lymphoedema distichiasis syndrome (Figure 103.35) [3]. However, lymphoscintigraphy suffers from poor spatial resolution with poor definition of the lymphatic vessels and limited functional measurements of actual lymph flow.

Table 103.12 Lymphatic imaging techniques and their properties.

Imaging technique	Contrast agent	Depth of imaging and comments	Invasiveness	Availability
Direct X-ray lymphography	Intralymphatic injection of a radio-opaque oil (e.g. lipiodol)	Anatomical imaging of lymphatic collectors and lymph nodes	Very invasive; requires the identification of a lymphatic collecting vessel by exploratory surgery	Rarely performed
Lymphoscintigraphy	Simple intradermal/subcutaneous injection of a radiolabelled tracer protein (e.g. technetium-99-labelled colloid)	Lymphatic collectors and lymph nodes Poor resolution compared with lymphography technique Limited functional data acquired Not anatomical	Minimal	Readily available in hospitals
Fluorescence microlymphangiog-raphy	Simple intradermal injection of fluorescent contrast agent (FITC-dextran)	Superficial dermal lymphatic vessels	Minimal	Research tool
Near infrared ICG lymphangiography	Simple intradermal/subcutaneous injection of ICG	Superficial dermal lymphatic vessels and superficial lymph nodes Contractility can be visualised but not quantified	Minimal	Increasing availability in departments offering lymphatic microsurgery
Magnetic resonance lymphangiography	Simple intradermal/subcutaneous injection of a gadolinium-based contrast agent	Lymphatic collectors and lymph nodes Subcutaneous fat and oedema also visualised	Minimal	Research tool
Intranodal MR lymphography	Injection of gadolinium-based contrast agent into the lymph nodes	Visualisation of internal lymphatic vessels and thoracic duct	Invasive	Specialised centres only

FITC, fluorescein isothiocanate; ICG, indocyanine green; MR, magnetic resonance.

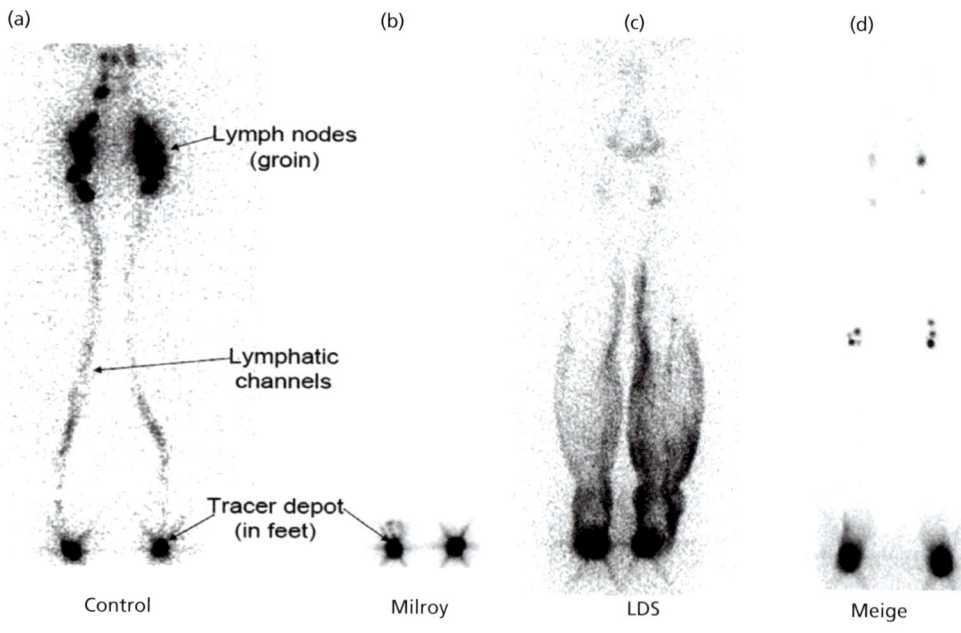

(a)   (b)   (c)   (d)

Lymph nodes (groin)

Lymphatic channels

Tracer depot (in feet)

Control   Milroy   LDS   Meige

Figure 103.35 Lymphoscintigraphs showing the uptake of technetium-99 in the inguinal lymph nodes (ILNs) at 2 h after injection in the normal lymphatic system and in patients with differing types of lower limb primary lymphoedema. (a) Healthy control. (b) Milroy disease, demonstrating functional aplasia of the lymphatics (i.e. no uptake into the ILNs). (c) Lymphoedema distichiasis syndrome (LDS) with reasonable uptake to the ILNs but evidence of marked reflux due to lymphatic valve incompetence. (d) Meige disease, with poor uptake and evidence of rerouting via the deep lymphatic channels resulting in uptake within the popliteal lymph nodes.

Fluorescence microlymphangiography

Fluorescence microlymphangiography (FML) is a research tool that uses a fluorescent contrast agent (fluorescein isothiocanate dextran) to provide information on superficial dermal lymphatic vessels. It has been used to improve understanding of lymphatic disease, including primary lymphoedema. For example, FML in conjunction with immunohistochemistry demonstrated that lymphatic dysfunction, and not aplasia, underlies Milroy disease [4].

Near infrared lymphangiography (ICG lymphography)

Near infrared (NIR) lymphangiography using indocyanine green (ICG) is a recently introduced and potentially useful technique used to demonstrate superficial lymphatic collecting vessels [5]. NIR imaging techniques use tracers that fluoresce under the excitation of NIR wavelengths (750–1000 nm) and external fluorescent detectors. ICG is a dye with properties of NIR absorption and fluorescence emission. ICG solution is injected intradermally or subcutaneously and enables real-time detection of the lymphatic vessels.

ICG is administered intradermally in order to map the lymphatic architecture. Fluorescent images have been collated to describe patterns of abnormal lymphatic structure in lymphoedema (e.g. dilated vessels with proximal obliteration) and diffuse constellation-like patches of dye accumulation (termed the 'Milky Way' feature). This method has also been used to quantify lymphatic function in the lower limb. NIR lymphangiography is now widely used to assess lymphatic vessel patency prior to lymphatico-venous or lymphatico-lymphatic anastomosis surgery [6].

Magnetic resonance lymphangiography

The use of contrast-enhanced magnetic resonance lymphangiography (MRL) has been reported in the investigation of patients with lymphoedema [7]. MRL has been used to demonstrate the presence of enlarged and tortuous lymphatic vessels in patients with unspecified lymphoedema. It is still mainly a research tool but could prove useful as it has the potential to provide high-quality images of anatomical abnormalities with high spatial resolution (Figure 103.36) and may be able to provide quantification of lymphatic function in the future.

Peripheral MRL has been successfully performed in the arms and legs of participants diagnosed with lymphoedema and in healthy participants. Intranodal MRL involves contrast agent injection into a lymph node, usually an inguinal lymph node, with needle positioning requiring ultrasound guidance. Imaging of intra-abdominal lymphatic vessels and the thoracic duct is possible. Central conducting anomalies can be diagnosed, and lymph leaks treated by embolisation [8].

Histopathological investigation of the lymphatic system

Skin biopsies may be useful when investigating a suspected lymphatic malformation. The distinction between lymphatic and blood vessels in skin biopsy sections has been made more straightforward by specific lymphatic markers. D2-40 (podoplanin) is considered the most robust as it stains the initial lymphatics, pre-collectors

and collecting vessels but not blood vessels. LYVE-1 stains the initial lymphatics but also macrophages and is downregulated by inflammation. Prox-1 and VEGFR-3 are also lymphatic-specific and stain larger vessels. A panel of markers is recommended, particularly in vascular malformations where differentiation between venous and lymphatic phenotypes may not be clear-cut [9]. CD31 and CD34 stain both lymphatic and blood vascular endothelium.

Lymphoedema management

Introduction

Failure of lymph drainage results in the accumulation of protein, fat and cells as well as water within the swollen tissues. Treatment is difficult because of the presence of the 'solid' component in the swelling. The management of lymphoedema varies greatly around the world. In developed countries, the emphasis is more on physical forms of therapy involving massage, exercise and compression designed to stimulate lymph drainage. In poorer, hotter countries where hosiery and appropriate bandages are too costly and uncomfortable, surgery may be the mainstay of treatment. Two particular problems need to be overcome with lymphoedema: swelling and predisposition to infection, particularly recurrent cellulitis.

There is limited research to inform evidence-based guidelines on the treatment of lymphoedema. Nevertheless, robust guidelines developed through consensus by experts do exist [1].

Unfortunately, there is no proven curative treatment for lymphoedema. Management is aimed at improving swelling through physical treatments designed to stimulate flow through existing or collateral drainage routes. Several surgical techniques have been implemented in recent years in a bid to improve lymphatic drainage or achieve limb volume reduction via liposuction. However, in the absence of robust data to support most surgical techniques, so-called 'conservative' physical therapies are relied on for the majority of patients.

Medical assessment

Medical assessment aims to identify, and treat, other causes of chronic peripheral oedema. In circumstances where systemic causes

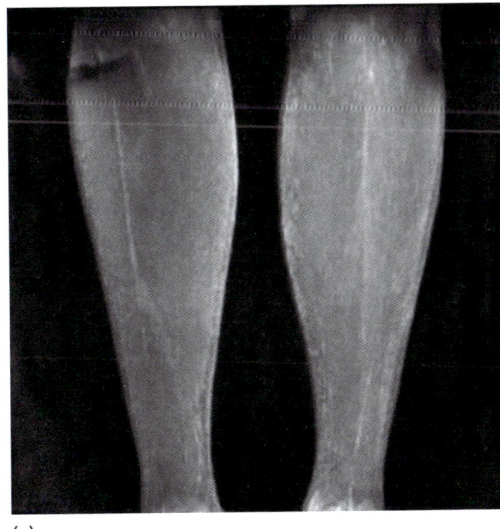
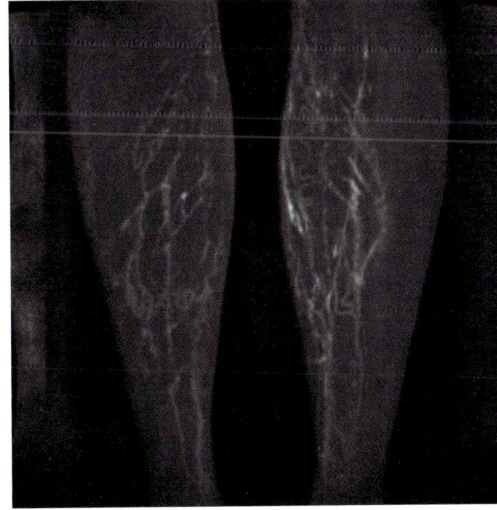

Figure 103.36 (a) Baseline magnetic resonance lymphangiography (MRL) images taken from a patient prior to contrast injection. His phenotype is of lymphoedema distichiasis syndrome (*FOXC2* positive). Two main vessels can be seen within the lower limbs. These could be venous or lymphatic in origin. (b) Post-contrast MRL images demonstrating multiple, dilated, tortuous lymphatic vessels seen in the below-knee regions.

(a)

(b)

for peripheral oedema, for example heart failure, have led to or coexist with the lymphoedema, then treatment of the medical condition must be undertaken before embarking on specific lymphoedema therapy. Where necessary, appropriate investigations should be performed to confirm lymphoedema and to identify treatable underlying causes (e.g. active cancer) or co-morbidities (e.g. superficial venous incompetence).

Physical therapies

All patients with a diagnosis of lymphoedema should be referred to a trained lymphoedema therapist. Management will focus on the needs of each individual patient. This may include (i) risk reduction, for example in breast cancer patients; (ii) swelling reduction and improvement of shape of a swollen limb; (iii) treatment and prevention of infection; (iv) treating skin problems such as elephantiasis, lymphorrhoea and wounds, as well as discouraging tissue fibrosis; (v) restoring functional independence and correcting posture imbalance; and (vi) pain and psychosocial management. Therapy assessment will include setting the benchmarks against which improvement can be judged, for example limb volume measurement, mobility and functional assessments. A treatment plan will depend on the site and severity of the lymphoedema and the need to engage other services, for example leg ulcer services, oncology or vascular surgeons.

Physical methods of treating lymphoedema have been practised in Europe for many years [2]. Therapy essentially aims to (i) control lymph formation (capillary filtration), including treatment of inflammatory causes and/or venous hypertension; and (ii) improve lymph drainage through existing lymphatics and collateral routes by applying normal physiological procedures that stimulate lymph flow. Physical treatment can, in most cases, improve quality of life considerably. Central to management is getting patients to understand their condition and know what they can do for themselves as self-management is an integral component of maintenance treatment. Only then can a high level of motivation and adherence to treatment be generated [3]. It is important to explain to patients that unlike blood, which is propelled by the heart, lymph drainage relies on local changes in tissue pressure generated by being active. Physical treatment exploits these principles, enhancing lymph flow as much as possible within the limits of a compromised drainage system. It should be appreciated that lymph flow still exists in lymphoedema, otherwise swelling would be a relentlessly progressive process.

The essential components of physical therapy include the following elements.

Care of the skin and prevention of infection

Elephantiasis skin changes are not only unsightly but lead to infection, odour, lymphorrhoea, restricted movement from fibrosis (pseudoscleroderma) and poor wound healing. Regular application of an emollient is important for hydrating the hardened skin, making it more supple and discouraging hyperkeratosis. Tinea pedis is almost invariable because of the closely apposed swollen toes – circumstances not improved by elastic hosiery. Modern antifungal creams macerate skin still further and therefore it is suggested that terbinafine cream is applied for 2 weeks to be replaced by an alcohol wipe in the longer term (assuming the skin is

not broken); in other words the alcohol wipes are to be introduced after 2 weeks of terbinafine cream application. For deep cracks and crevices that bacteria may readily colonise, regular toilet is necessary followed by an antiseptic soak, for example potassium permanganate. Hyperkeratosis can often be improved through the regular application of 5% salicylic acid ointment, but the best treatment to reverse elephantiasis skin changes is long-term compression. Areas that constantly seep lymph should also respond to sustained compression.

Prevention of infection, particularly lymphangitis/cellulitis, is crucial to the control of lymphoedema. Care of the skin, good hygiene, control of tinea pedis and good antisepsis following abrasions and minor wounds are important in reducing the risk of cellulitis, as maintenance of skin integrity and an effective barrier will reduce the entry of microorganisms.

Exercise

Exercise and movement are crucial to lymph drainage [4]. Dynamic muscle contractions (isotonic exercises) encourage both passive (movement of lymph along tissue planes or through non-contractile lymphatics) and active (increased contractility and therefore propulsion of lymph within contractile lymphatics) phases of lymph drainage. Overexertion and excessive static (isometric, e.g. gripping) exercise increase blood flow, which tends to increase oedema.

External compression

External compression (hosiery, bandage or pneumatic compression) complements the exercise programme. Such compression is not intended to 'squeeze' oedema but to act as a counterforce to striated muscle activity and so generate higher tissue pressures during contractions. This provides the most powerful stimulus to lymph drainage. Compression also limits capillary filtration by opposing capillary pressure. Compression is much less effective without exercise. Multilayer bandaging can be used for limb reduction, but also has the advantage of restoring limb shape so that subsequent use of compression garments (hosiery) is more effective at controlling swelling [5].

Bandaging may be the only method suitable for huge misshapen limbs and for controlling lymphorrhoea. Layers of strong, non-elastic (short stretch) bandages are applied to generate a high pressure during muscular contractions but low pressure at rest. The use of foam or soft padding helps to distribute pressure more evenly and to protect the skin. The digits are bandaged to control the swelling of the fingers and toes. The strategic positioning of rubber pads 'irons out' pockets of swelling and deep skin folds (Figure 103.37). Multilayer bandaging is a skill that takes time to learn and should not be undertaken without appropriate training. The compression administered may have to be modified in circumstances such as cancer requiring palliative treatment, moderate limb ischaemia or if there is any neurological deficit. Hosiery (below-knee or full-length stockings, half or full tights and sleeves) usually requires high compression and double layers may occasionally be required. Most garments last no more than 6 months. Two garments (or pairs) should be provided, one to wear and one for the wash. Washing is necessary to maintain the compression properties

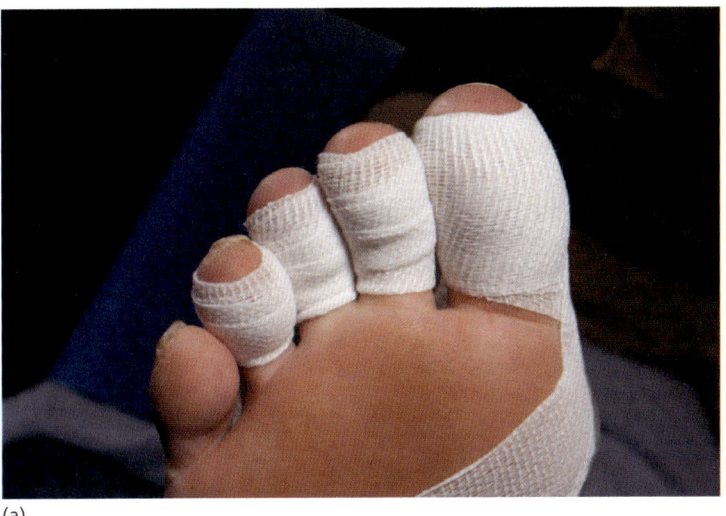

(a)

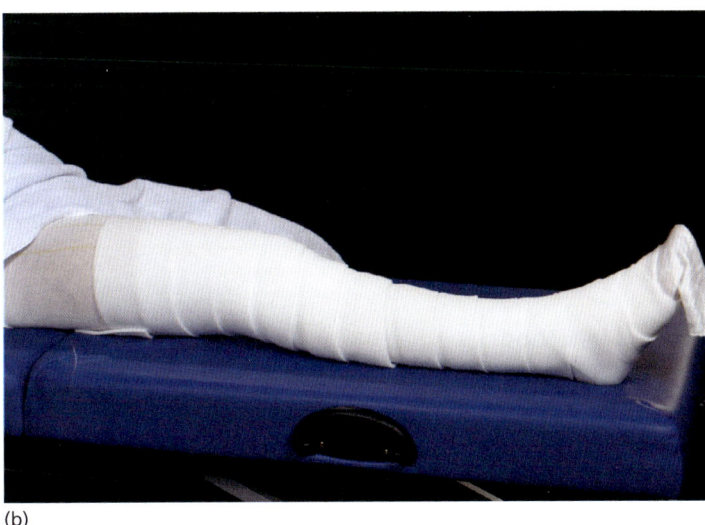

(b)

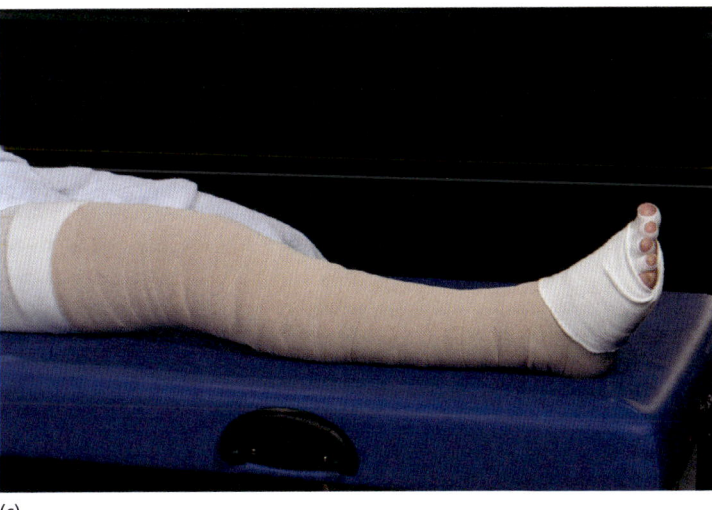

(c)

Figure 103.37 (a) Toe (or finger) bandaging with cotton crepe bandages. (b) Sub-bandage wadding over a tubular cotton bandage. (c) Short-stretch compression cotton bandages applied in layers in a figure of eight and/or spiral style.

of the garment. The patient's technique for the application, removal and care of garments is crucial for a successful outcome.

Pneumatic compression therapy (intermittent/sequential pneumatic compression) should not be used in preference to exercise and compression but can be useful in mixed lymphovenous oedema and in infirm patients [6]. An inflatable boot, legging or sleeve is connected to a motor-driven pump and lymph is displaced proximally towards the root of the limb. If hosiery is not fitted immediately following compression therapy, the swelling readily recurs. Pneumatic compression softens the tissues and reduces limb volume during treatment. Oscillatory pressure waves (OPW) generated by intermittent pneumatic compression therapy can entrain lymphatic contractility and modulate lymphatic function depending on the frequency and propagation speed of the OPW [7]. It is doubtful that any long-term benefit is gained over hosiery and exercise alone.

Massage (manual lymphatic drainage therapy)

Massage is an important component of treatment, particularly for midline lymphoedema where there are few alternatives. Manual lymphatic drainage is a massage technique performed by lymphoedema therapists with the aim of rerouting the accumulation of lymph from the swollen region via collateral lymphatic pathways to lymphatic basins that are able to drain normally. The initial step is to decongest central/proximal areas before massaging the oedematous region. This facilitates the drainage of lymph via lymphatic vessels/pathways that have been stimulated by the massage technique. Tissue movement must be gentle if it is to stimulate lymph flow without increasing blood flow [8].

A number of techniques are available but no single method appears to be superior. Manual lymphatic drainage is widely practised, and many patients, therapists and physicians advocate the benefits. Continuous manual lymphatic drainage delivered by a therapist is expensive and few health care providers will fund this long term. Simple lymphatic drainage is best delivered by a partner or carer trained in the technique and this can be a good maintenance option.

Breathing, postural exercise, elevation and rest

Breathing and postural exercises are important, particularly for clearance of lymph from the thorax and abdomen [9]. Without the dispersal of truncal lymph, there is no further drainage of peripheral limb oedema. Elevation *per se* does nothing to improve lymph drainage but lowering venous pressure (and therefore filtration) can help to reduce swelling. Rest and elevation alone, however, are not the correct treatment for lymphoedema.

Additional therapies that may be of benefit include:
- *Weight loss.* Many patients with lymphoedema are overweight because of obesity as well as fluid retention. Excessive weight gain is likely to impair lymph drainage in the same way as it impairs venous drainage, and obesity reduces mobility (and therefore exercise). Control of weight in combination with physical treatment may be sufficient to resolve oedema completely in some patients. Weight loss irrespective of type of diet has been shown to reduce arm volume over and above what would be expected from fat loss alone in breast cancer-related lymphoedema [10].
- *Hyperbaric oxygen (HBO), low-level laser therapy (LLLT) and kinesiotaping.* There are data recommending the use of HBO and LLLT

independently in breast cancer-related lymphoedema although a randomised controlled trial failed to demonstrate significant benefits from HBO treatment [11]. However, LLLT may reduce limb volumes and pain in patients with breast cancer-related lymphoedema [12]. Kinesiotaping has been shown to be effective in treating lymphoedema [13].

Intensive and maintenance treatment

Patients with mild limb lymphoedema, no fibrosis and no distortion of shape can be started on maintenance treatment with compression hosiery. Intensive therapy, comprising a 2–4-week course of daily skin care, manual lymphatic drainage, multilayer bandaging and exercises, is indicated for patients with moderate to severe limb swelling, poor limb shape or tissue changes such as fibrosis, elephantiasis or lymphorrhoea. Once intensive treatment is complete, maintenance treatment with hosiery is commenced immediately. While decongestive lymphatic therapy has become accepted first line therapy, the evidence for best treatment is weak.

Pharmacological therapies

There are many drugs available for treating disorders of the blood circulation, but there are none with proven efficacy for lymphoedema [14]. Diuretics alone demonstrate minimal improvement in lymphoedema, as their mode of action is to reduce capillary filtration by a reduction in circulating blood volume.

The chronic lymph accumulation in lymphoedema leads both to changes in the structure of the skin and also to impaired clearance of inflammatory cells and mediators, with dysregulated regional immune responses. Adipose tissue deposition and fibrosis lead to progressive anatomical distortion and eventually loss of function in the affected areas. Leukotriene B_4 (LTB_4) antagonism ameliorates experimental lymphoedema. LTB_4 was elevated in patient serum and was counterproductive to lymphatic repair in a mouse lymphatic surgery model, likely due to its various effects on lymphatic endothelial cell function and growth. Accordingly, blocking LTB_4 ameliorated clinical symptoms in the mice. This knowledge prompted the use of drugs known to inhibit the production of LTB_4, including ketoprofen and the leukotriene A_4 hydrolase inhibitor ubenimex. Ketoprofen did not reduce lower limb swelling but did produce improvements in skin histology, and a small trial evaluating ubenimex was negative [15].

Improvement in swelling can be obtained with antibiotics when subclinical infection is present. In a randomised controlled trial in a single setting (in Ghana) assessing the use of doxycycline for the treatment of filariasis, it was found that patients' lymphoedema stage improved regardless of the presence of active infection. This led the authors to suggest that a wider group of patients with lymphoedema might benefit from doxycycline [16].

Paroven (an oxerutin) and coumarin (a benzopyrone) have been trialled in lymphoedema and may produce a small reduction in limb volume by reducing vascular permeability and thus the amount of fluid forming in the subcutaneous tissues. However, this has been shown to be of little clinical benefit to the patient [17].

Animal studies involving vascular endothelial growth factors have stimulated excitement and hope among the lymphatic community that successful forms of drug therapy may be possible in the future. Introduction of VEGF-C into animal models of postsurgical lymphoedema (using mouse skin and rabbit ears) induced lymphatic vessel growth and a subsequent reduction in lymphoedema [18]. A similar study demonstrated regeneration of functional cutaneous lymphatics in the skin of *Chy* mice with primary lymphoedema by viral-mediated *VEGFC* gene transfer that caused overexpression of VEGF-C [19]. More recent animal studies have incorporated growth factors with lymph node transfer surgical methods. Studies using transplanted lymph nodes that were transfected with VEGF-C demonstrated that the lymphatic network in the defective area could be restored, with transplanted nodes and existing vessels becoming incorporated [20].

Research is currently being undertaken to optimise growth factor delivery with trials in patients with secondary lymphoedema. Lymfactin® is an adenovirus type 5-based gene therapy involving expression of human VEGF-C in the damaged tissue. It aims to correct deficient lymphatic flow by promoting the growth and repair of lymphatic vessels. Results from a phase II study investigating Lymfactin for the treatment of breast cancer-related lymphoedema in humans were inconclusive [21].

Surgical options

Surgery has a specific role in the management of lymphoedema [22]. It is of value in limb lymphoedema in a few patients in whom, even after conservative treatment, the size and weight of a limb inhibit its use or interfere with mobility. Surgery involves either removing excessive tissue or bypassing local lymphatic defects. Lifelong non-surgical measures such as hosiery must be continued postoperatively.

Excisional methods

Excisional surgical procedures for the management of lymphoedema, regardless of the underlying cause, have been employed for more than a century. They are now rarely utilised as the postoperative complications can be disastrous. Reduction (excisional) operations remove a longitudinal ellipse of skin and the underlying abnormal subcutaneous tissue down to the deep fascia in a 'melon slice' that permits primary closure of the skin edges (Sistrunk procedure). Undercutting of the skin allows the removal of additional tissue (Homans procedure). This procedure is preferred to circumferential excision and skin grafting (Charles procedure) or to the addition of in-rolling of a skin flap (Thompson buried dermis flap operation). Postoperative complications include skin transplant necrosis, poor cosmetic results and worsening lymphoedema distal to the surgical site. None of the excisional procedures has curative potential as all chances of restoring effective lymphatic transport have been surgically removed. Volume reduction may be achieved through tissue reduction, but not through lymphatic drainage improvement. The indications for this type of surgery should be restricted to rare cases lacking alternative conservative or surgical treatment options. The exceptions to this rule are cases of genital or eyelid lymphoedema, where reduction/debulking surgery is used sooner rather than later [23].

Liposuction (suction lipectomy)

Chronic lymphoedema may be associated with fatty tissue deposition in some patients, although the mechanisms are not fully understood. Excess adipose tissue will not respond to decongestive lymphoedema treatments, anastomosis surgery or lymph node transfer procedures. Liposuction creates significant volume reduction in therapy-resistant lymphoedema of the extremities, when combined with lifelong compression therapy [24]. This adjunctive therapy is used in compliant patients willing to wear lifelong compression garments. If patients disregard regular use of their garments, a relapse or worsening of lymphoedema is observed as liposuction may cause injury to the remaining subcutaneous lymphatics within the lymphoedematous extremities. However, liposuction has been shown to create a long-term volume reduction of 100% in compliant patients followed for up to 17 years. Liposuction techniques, although not curative, offer an effective symptomatic treatment.

Lymphovenous bypass (lymphatico-venous anastomosis)

Recently there has been much interest in lymphatico-venous anastomosis (LVA) surgery. LVA is a type of lymphovenous bypass, utilising a supermicrosurgical technique to anastomose distal subdermal lymphatic vessels with adjacent venules less than 0.8 mm in diameter in an attempt to improve regional lymph drainage and potentially remove the need for hosiery (an outcome that many patients are desperate to achieve). It is popular among surgeons as it is performed under local anaesthetic and the surgical incisions are small. Prior to LVA surgery patients undergo ICG fluorescent imaging to locate functional patent lymphatic vessels within the affected limb.

A review of the literature suggests that the efficacy of LVA surgery is limited. Postoperative results (within 1 year of surgery) vary greatly between centres, with limb volume reductions of 4–67% [25]. There is a lack of long-term data as the technique is relatively new. However, surgeons favour its use because of the low risk of complications. There is currently no method of determining its effect on lymphatic function. The development of imaging techniques could provide a tool to answer the question of its place in lymphatic treatment strategies.

Lymphatico-lymphatic anastomosis surgery

The rationale behind lymphatic grafting surgery is to avoid the inherent problems of LVA surgery caused by coagulation of blood within the lymphatics, by connecting the lymphatic system to itself. There is a lack of robust long-term data regarding efficacy.

Lymph node transfer surgery

Autologous transplantation of normal lymphatic tissue within a local or free flap to a site deficient of lymph nodes and vessels has been performed. The rationale is that the transplant of normal lymph nodes could encourage and improve lymphatic drainage in a previously oedematous region. Few surgeons perform this type of surgery but reported results appear encouraging, with one case series suggesting 40% of patients were cured of their lymphoedema [26]. However, no long-term data are available on its use. One important concern to raise with this type of surgery is that it relies on the transfer of normal lymph nodes to improve lymphatic drainage. This may be possible in a patient with secondary lymphoedema but may cause complications in patients with primary lymphoedema who may not have 'normal' lymph nodes, or 'normal' lymphatic vasculature, even at unaffected sites.

This concern is supported by reports of donor site lymphatic vessel dysfunction in patients undergoing microvascular lymph node transfer surgery for cancer-related lymphoedema [27].

Resources

Further information

Clinical Resource Efficiency Support Team (CREST). *Guidelines for the the Diagnosis, Assessment and Management of Lymphoedema*, 2008. https://www.lymphoedemasupportni.org/sites/default/files/crest_guidelines_on_the_diagnosis_assessment_and_management_of_lymphoedema.pdf.

Patient resources

A list of trained therapists can usually be accessed through national professional bodies for lymphoedema, for example:
Australasian Lymphology Association: www.lymphoedema.org.au.
Lymphoedema Support Network (UK): www.lymphoedema.org.
National Lymphedema Network (USA): www.lymphnet.org.
(All last accessed August 2022.)

Key references

The full list of references can be found in the online version at https://www.wiley.com/rooksdermatology10e

Introduction

1 Oliver G, Kipnis J, Randolph GJ, Harvey NL. The lymphatic vasculature in the 21st century: novel functional roles in homeostasis and disease. *Cell* 2020;182: 270–96.
9 Levick JR, Michel CC. Microvascular fluid exchange and the revised Starling principle. *Cardiovasc Res* 2010;87:198–210.

Diagnosis of lymphoedema

1 Levick JR, Michel CC. Microvascular fluid exchange and the revised Starling principle. *Cardiovasc Res* 2010;87:198–210.
3 Moffatt CJ, Franks PJ, Doherty DC *et al.* Lymphoedema: an underestimated health problem. *Q J Med* 2003;96:731–8.
12 Mortimer PS, Rockson SG. New developments in clinical aspects of lymphatic disease. *J Clin Invest* 2014;124:915–21.
24 Lymphoedema Framework. *Best Practice for the Management of Lymphoedema. International Consensus*. London: Medical Education, 2006. https://www.lympho.org/wp-content/uploads/2021/09/Best_practice.pdf (last accessed August 2022).

Cellulitis

2 Thomas KS, Crook AM, Nunn AJ *et al.* UK Dermatology Clinical Trials Network's PATCH I Trial Team. Penicillin to prevent recurrent leg cellulitis. *N Engl J Med* 2013;368:1695–703.
28 Lymphoedema Framework. *Best Practice for the Management of Lymphoedema. International Consensus*. London: Medical Education, 2006. https://www.lympho.org/wp-content/uploads/2021/09/Best_practice.pdf (last accessed August 2022).

Primary lymphoedema

1 Gordon K, Varney R, Keeley V *et al.* Update and audit of the St George's classification algorithm of primary lymphatic anomalies: a clinical and molecular approach to diagnosis. *J Med Genet* 2020;57:653–9.
19 Martin-Almedina S, Mortimer PS, Ostergaard P. Development and physiological functions of the lymphatic system: insights from human genetic studies of primary lymphedema. *Physiol Rev* 2021;101:1809–71.

Lymphatic malformations

1 Mäkinen T, Boon LM, Vikkula M, Alitalo K. Lymphatic malformations: genetics, mechanisms and therapeutic strategies. *Circ Res* 2021;129:136–54.

PART 9: VASCULAR DISORDERS

2 International Society for the Study of Vascular Anomalies (ISSVA). *ISSVA classification for vascular anomalies*. https://www.issva.org/UserFiles/file/ISSVA-Classification-2018.pdf (last accessed August 2022).

10 Chaudry G, Guevara CJ, Rialon KL *et al*. Safety and efficacy of bleomycin sclerotherapy for microcystic lymphatic malformation. *Cardiovasc Intervent Radiol* 2014;37:1476–81.

Lymphangiectasia and chylous disease

9 Browse NL. Management of lymph and chyle reflux. In: Browse NL, Burnand KG, Mortimer PS, eds. *Diseases of the Lymphatics*. London: Arnold, 2003:259–92.

Secondary lymphoedema

24 Escobedo N, Oliver G. The lymphatic vasculature: its role in adipose metabolism and obesity. *Cell Metab* 2017;26:598–609.

31 Lymphoedema Framework. *Best Practice for the Management of Lymphoedema. International Consensus*. London: Medical Education, 2006. https://www.lympho.org/wp-content/uploads/2021/09/Best_practice.pdf (last accessed August 2022).

32 British Lymphology Society; Lymphoedema Support Network. *Consensus document on the management of cellulitis in lymphoedema*. https://www.wwl.nhs.uk/media/community-pdfs/BLS-cellulitis-guidelines.pdf (last accessed August 2022).

Regional swelling

14 Browse NL. Management of lymph and chyle reflux. In: Browse NL, Burnand KG, Mortimer PS, eds. *Diseases of the Lymphatics*. London: Arnold, 2003:259–92.

21 Lymphoedema Framework. *Best Practice for the Management of Lymphoedema. International Consensus*. London: Medical Education, 2006. https://www.lympho.org/wp-content/uploads/2021/09/Best_practice.pdf (last accessed August 2022).

Lymphoedema management

1 Lymphoedema Framework. *Best Practice for the Management of Lymphoedema. International Consensus*. London: Medical Education, 2006. https://www.lympho.org/wp-content/uploads/2021/09/Best_practice.pdf (last accessed August 2022).

3 Mortimer P, Levine G. *Let's Talk Lymphoedema: The Essential Guide to Everything You Need to Know*. London: Elliott and Thompson, 2017.

22 Browse NL. Management of lymph and chyle reflux. In: Browse NL, Burnand KG, Mortimer PS, eds. *Diseases of the Lymphatics*. London: Arnold, 2003:259–92.

CHAPTER 104

Flushing and Blushing

Elizabeth Keeling and Síona Ní Raghallaigh

Beaumont Hospital, Dublin, Ireland

Flushing and blushing

Introduction

Flushing and blushing are the result of transient cutaneous vasodilatation that is usually physiological in nature. Although these terms are often used interchangeably, they are distinct processes. A blush signifies a psychosocial response to an experienced emotion, whereas a flush is a thermoregulatory response to increased body temperature. Patients who develop excessive or socially impeding flushing or blushing may present for medical consultation. Frequent blushing can be associated with anxiety states and, in some cases, social phobia. Excessive flushing may be associated with topical agents, food or alcohol intake, or rarely with underlying systemic disease. Clinical features useful in defining the diagnosis include the environmental setting in which the vascular reaction occurs, the extent and pattern of cutaneous involvement, and whether sweating or other systemic symptoms accompany the vasodilatation. Histological evaluation of skin is unhelpful but other investigations may be necessary in particular clinical circumstances. Understanding of the mechanisms by which these cutaneous reactions occur has increased, but treatment options remain limited.

Epidemiology

In the authors' experience, frequent blushing tends to be most problematic in younger individuals (i.e. early teens to mid-twenties) (Figure 104.1a,b) and diminishes with age. Flushing reactions can occur in all age groups. With the exception of menopausal flushing, excessive flushing does not appear to have any gender predilection. Flushing and blushing affect all ethnic groups. However, individuals with lighter skin types are generally most troubled by the social burden of frequent blushing, presumably because the contrast between erythema and unaffected skin is most marked in this group. Aldehyde dehydrogenase 2 deficiency, seen frequently in individuals of East Asian descent, results in alcohol-induced flushing due to the accumulation of acetaldehyde.

Physiology

Physiological transient vasodilatation plays an integral role in thermoregulation. This sympathetically mediated process is regulated by cutaneous arteriovenous anastomoses – the superficial venous plexus, located at the juncture of the papillary and reticular dermis, and the deep horizontal plexus, located at the juncture of the deep reticular dermis and panniculus [1]. Reflex cutaneous vasodilatation in response to an increase in core body temperature involves an initial abolition of the active vasoconstrictor tone that is dominant in normal circumstances. As body heating continues, active vasodilator neural activity to the cutaneous arterioles is enhanced, causing rapid increases in skin blood flow, which are often coincident with the onset of sweating. Overall, this active vasodilator system is responsible for 80–95% of the increase in skin blood flow that accompanies heat stress. During normothermic conditions, with the body at rest, total skin blood flow is approximately 200–500 mL/min. With full active vasodilatation, skin blood flow can increase to 8 L/min [2,3]. Neural control of cutaneous vasodilatation involves co-transmission by sympathetic cholinergic nerves, with the release of acetylcholine and one or more co-transmitters, such as substance P (and/or neurokinin-1 receptors), vasoactive intestinal peptide (VIP) and pituitary adenylate cyclase activating peptide (PACAP) [4,5,6]. This neurally mediated increase in blood flow in turn releases nitric oxide (NO) from endothelial cells, which, along with prostaglandins released from local keratinocytes, sustain these vasodilatory effects [7,8,9].

Pathophysiology of flushing

Abnormal, non-thermoregulatory flushing may result from circulating vasoactive mediators that act directly on the vascular smooth muscle or may be mediated by vasomotor autonomic innervation. Autonomic nerves also innervate eccrine sweat glands, therefore neurally activated vasodilatation tends to be associated with sweating, causing a 'wet flush'. Vasoactive substances typically cause a 'dry flush' [10]. A notable exception to this pattern of associated sweating is the carcinoid syndrome

Rook's Textbook of Dermatology, Tenth Edition. Edited by Christopher Griffiths, Jonathan Barker, Tanya Bleiker, Walayat Hussain and Rosalind Simpson.
© 2024 John Wiley & Sons Ltd. Published 2024 by John Wiley & Sons Ltd.

PART 9: VASCULAR DISORDERS

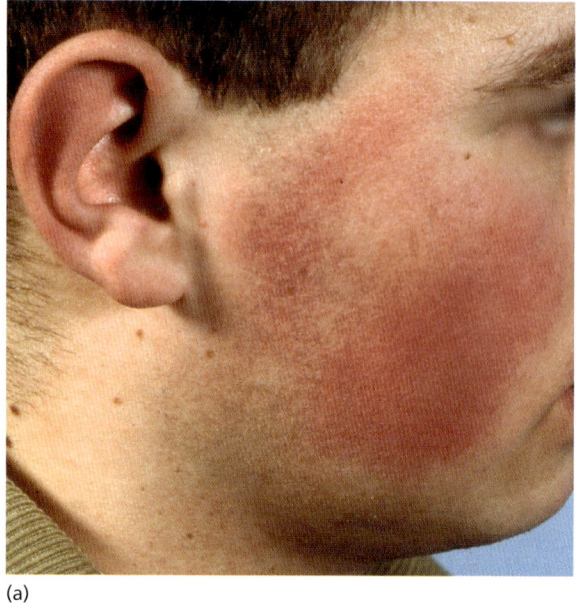

(a)

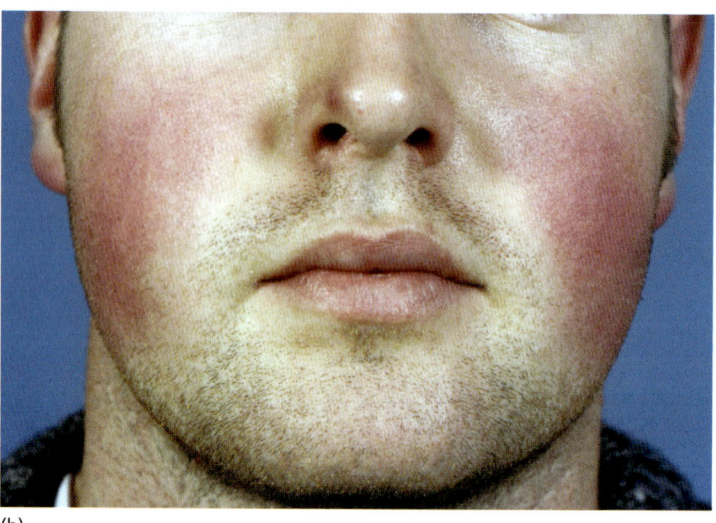

(b)

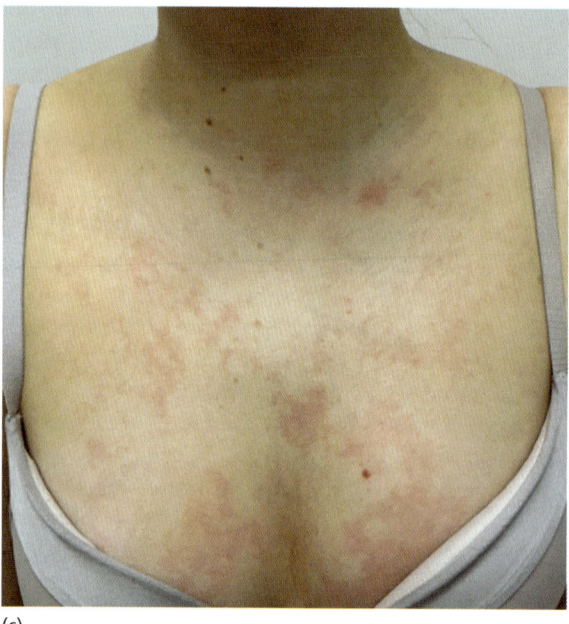

(c)

Figure 104.1 (a, b) Images demonstrating the typical distribution of the blush, as seen in two young men who presented for the management of frequent blushing. Note the 'skip areas' of pallor on the upper lateral cheek in (a). Sparing of the skin around the mouth suggestive of 'circumoral pallor' is evident in both cases. (c) Flush extending down onto the chest in a healthy 25-year-old woman.

Vasoactive mediators can be external or internal. External mediators include those found in food or drugs (Boxes 104.1 and 104.2). Specifically, foods containing tyramine, histamine, higher chain alcohols, monosodium glutamate, aldehyde, nitrites and sulphites may be associated with flushing [11]. Internal vasoactive mediators include neuropeptides (e.g. substance P, tachykinins, kallikrein, kinins, neurotensin, neuropeptide K, VIP, gastrin-related peptide, motilin), catecholamines (e.g. epinephrine, norepinephrine, dopamine), hormones (e.g. oestrogens, adrenocorticotrophic hormone, corticotrophin-releasing hormone, calcitonin), histamine and prostaglandins.

Disorders associated with flushing are listed in Box 104.3, with the clinical features of the flush associated with specific disorders described in Table 104.1. Causes of flushing in the paediatric population are listed in Table 104.2.

Psychosocial aspects of blushing

The blush reaction appears with the development of self-awareness in childhood, usually between the ages of 2 and 3 years [12]. This non-verbal signal of social discomfort has been shown to evoke affiliative, empathic responses in others [12]. Individuals who commonly blush often view it negatively and will try to conceal it. In

Box 104.1 Food that causes flushing

Alcohol (especially if alcohol dehydrogenase deficient)
Caffeine
Cheese (histamine rich – Roquefort)
Fish
- Scombroid poisoning (due to improper refrigeration, cooking does not prevent illness)
- Ciguatoxin (due to a toxin made by algae, notify public health if suspected)

Fruit (lemons, tomatoes)
Monosodium glutamate (food additive)
Sodium nitrite rich meats (e.g. salami)
Spicy food (especially chilli pepper)
Sulfite – common preservative and additive used in food and pharmaceuticals
Vegetables (spinach)

Box 104.2 Drugs that cause flushing

Anaesthesia combination with isoflurane and fentanyl
Angiotensin-converting enzyme (ACE) inhibitors: captopril, enalapril, lisinopril, perindopril, ramipril
Antimalarials
Bromocriptine
β3 adrenoceptor agonists: fluvoxamine, mirtazapine
Calcitonin
Calcium carbonate
Calcium-channel blockers: nifedipine, verapamil
Chemotherapeutics: tamoxifen, cyclosporine, doxorubicin, mithramycin, dacarbazine, cisplatin, interferon α-2, flutamide
Chlorpropamide
Contrast media with alcohol
Cyproterone acetate
Disulfiram with alcohol
Fumaric acid esters
Griseofulvin
Hormonal treatment for prostate/breast cancer (buserelin, triptorelin, goserelin, leuprorelin)
Hydralazine
Ketoconazole
Methylprednisolone: high-dose pulsed
Metrifonate
Metronidazole
Morphine and other opiates
Niacin
Nitrates: isosorbine mononitrate/dinitrate, glyceryl trinitrate
Non-steroidal anti-inflammatory agents including aspirin
Pilocarpine
Phentolamine
Phosphodiesterase inhibitors (sildenafil, tadalafil, vardenafil, mirodenafil)
Prostacyclin
Prostaglandin E
Raloxifene
Rifampicin
Tacrolimus ointment
Tamsulosin
Triamcinolone: oral, intrasynovial or intramuscular
Vancomycin
Venlafaxine
5-hydroxytryptamine (5-HT) 3 receptor antagonists: ondansetron, ramosetron, tropisetron

Box 104.3 Causes of flushing

Anaphylaxis
Autonomic epilepsy
Autonomic hyperreflexia
Auriculotemporal syndrome (Frey syndrome)
Basophilic granulocytic leukaemia
Brain tumours
Carcinoid syndrome
Cholinergic urticaria
Cluster headaches
Diabetic autonomic neuropathy
Dumping syndrome
Food, beverages, medication, alcohol (Boxes 104.1 and 104.2)
Harlequin syndrome
Horner syndrome
Malignant histiocytoma
Mastocytosis
Medullary carcinoma of the thyroid
Menopause
Migraine
Multiple sclerosis
Orthostatic hypotension
Pancreatic cell tumour
Parkinson disease
Phaeochromocytoma
POEMS (polyneuropathy, organomegaly, endocrinopathy, monoclonal gammopathy and skin changes) syndrome
Polycythaemia
Postsurgery (gastric/prostate/orchidectomy)
Psychiatric disorders
Red ear syndrome
Renal cell carcinoma
Rosacea
Rovsing syndrome
Spinal cord lesions
Trigeminal nerve damage
Thermoregulatory – heat exposure, exercise, fever

some cases this can progress to avoidance of situations they link to blushing and have a negative impact on quality of life [13]. This can progress in a small number to erythrophobia (i.e. an excessive fear of blushing resulting in social phobia and avoidance of social circumstances that might lead to blushing). Individuals with social anxiety frequently experience other autonomic and motor signs of anxiety during social encounters [14]. Psychologists can assess the degree and impact of blushing using validated questionnaires, such as the 'Blushing Propensity Scale' [15] and the 'Fear of Negative Evaluation Scale' [16]. The actual intensity of blushing (as measured by laser Doppler flowmetry or photoplethysmography) has been shown to be unrelated to the perceived intensity of, or the susceptibility to, blushing [17]. Similar findings have been shown in studies involving patients with rosacea who blush, and who perceive the blush to be more intense than it is [18]. Blushing appears to build up over repeated episodes in people who report that they blush frequently and frequent blushers have been shown to be more sensitive to vasodilating agents such as niacin [19]. It has been proposed that such individuals may have a physiological predisposition to delayed vascular recovery.

PART 9: VASCULAR DISORDERS

Table 104.1 Disorders associated with flushing.

Disease	Pathogenesis of flush	Characteristics of flush	Associated symptoms and signs	Investigations	Treatment	Notes
Menopause	The 'hot flush' of menopause is attributed to hypothalamic thermoregulatory dysfunction associated with fluctuations in oestrogen levels Flushing due to circadian cycling of core body temperature	Rising feeling of intense heat, profuse sweating and diffuse facial flushing; this may be followed by shivering; typical episodes last from 3 to 5 min and may occur up to 20 times/day	The flush may be associated with considerable discomfort and anxiety, affecting normal daily functioning and sleep patterns. Vasomotor symptoms typically appear in the late menopausal transition period, at which stage an interval of ≥60 days of amenorrhoea is likely to have occurred	FSH AMH Inhibin B	For postmenopausal women with moderate-to-severe vasomotor symptoms and no contraindications, consider HRT For women with moderate-to-severe hot flushes in whom oestrogen is contraindicated or not well tolerated, or for women who have stopped oestrogen and are experiencing recurrent symptoms but wish to avoid resuming oestrogen, therapy with gabapentin, SNRI or SSRI may be considered	Clonidine and opioid antagonism with naloxone have been used for climacteric-induced hot flushes. However, recent studies of clonidine have shown little or no benefit [22]
Rosacea	Neuroinflammatory mediators have been postulated to play a role in the flushing associated with rosacea Genes involved in vasoregulation and neurogenic inflammation are upregulated in rosacea patients Dysregulation of TRPV channels, which are expressed by both neuronal and non-neuronal cells, has enhanced gene expression in rosacea. Activation of nociceptive nerve fibres contributes to skin sensitivity in rosacea patients, and axon reflexes augment flushing in patients with the most severe symptoms [18]	Subgroup – longstanding predisposition to frequent flushing with specific triggers such as spicy food, moving from a cold to warm environment, etc. Not all patients with rosacea will flush	May be associated with telangiectasia, fixed facial redness, papules and pustules, phymatous and ocular rosacea, signs of photodamage, and with increased skin sensitivity	Occasionally a skin biopsy may be required to rule out other causes of facial redness	Avoidance of triggers Skin care regime Daily application of physical sunblock Topical brimonidine Topical oxymetazoline hydrochloride cream 1% Laser Intense pulsed light [23]	

Mastocytosis	Mast cell accumulation in at least one tissue with both chronic and episodic mast cell mediator release; mediators that may cause increased vasopermeability and vasodilation include histamine, cysteinyl leukotrienes (LTC4, LTD4, LTE4), prostaglandins (PGD$_2$) and platelet-activating factor	Sudden onset; features may be similar to that of an allergic or anaphylactic reaction; often with identifiable triggers such as narcotics, opioids, NSAIDs, systemic anaesthesia, exercise, massage, alcohol, infection, Hymenoptera stings	Skin findings: urticaria pigmentosa, diffuse cutaneous mastocytosis, isolated mastocytoma(s), or telangiectasias (TMEP). Associated pruritus, blister formation, Darier sign. Acute release of mediators: pruritus, hypotension, syncope, abdominal pain, nausea, vomiting, diarrhoea, fatigue, headache, collapse. Chronic mediator release: cachexia, chronic gastrointestinal symptoms, diffuse musculoskeletal pains, tissue remodelling and organ fibrosis; weight loss, neuropsychiatric symptoms; lymphadenopathy, splenomegaly, anaemia, eosinophilia; osteopenia, osteoporosis	Skin biopsy (inject local anaesthetic without epinephrine adjacent to the chosen lesion to avoid mast cell degranulation which makes histological examination difficult) with histopathological staining with Giemsa and/or immunohistochemical staining for tryptase and c-kit for cutaneous mastocytosis; this will not provide information about systemic involvement but may help to classify cutaneous disease. Complete blood count with differential. Liver function tests (including serum aminotransferases and alkaline phosphatase). Serum tryptase. Metabolites of mast cell activation (24-h urine for N-methyl histamine and 11-β-prostaglandin F2α) may be measured. Bone marrow biopsy and aspiration	Avoidance of triggers. Antihistamines: H$_1$ antihistamines (e.g. cetirizine, fexofenadine, hydroxyzine, doxepin) alone may be ineffective, combined blockade of H$_1$ and H$_2$ receptors prevents the vasodilatory effects of histamine. Ketotifen has been reported to have both mast cell stabilising and H$_1$ antihistamine properties, but is sedating. Aspirin (up to 650 mg twice daily) may be used to control flushing, but should be used with extreme caution and only in patients known to tolerate NSAIDs. Oral sodium cromoglycate. Steroids (oral and topical). Psoralen and ultraviolet A therapy for urticaria pigmentosa. Laser therapy for TMEP. Epinephrine autoinjector (e.g. Anapen) for patients with anaphylaxis. Patients with evidence of systemic mastocytosis, or those with unexplained anaphylaxis or hypotension, should be referred to the appropriate specialties for further investigation and management
Hyperthyroidism	Excess synthesis and secretion of thyroid hormones by the thyroid gland. Caused by Graves disease, toxic multinodular goitre or d toxic adenoma	Flushing. Skin may be warm and moist to touch	Tremor, anxiety, tachycardia, heat intolerance, perspiration, weakness and weight loss	Thyroid function tests. Thyroid auto-antibodies	Referral to specialist for definitive treatment. β-blockers can be used for symptom relief

(*Continued*)

Table 104.1 (continued)

Disease	Pathogenesis of flush	Characteristics of flush	Associated symptoms and signs	Investigations	Treatment	Notes
Carcinoid tumour/carcinoid syndrome (CS)	Carcinoid tumours arise from enterochromaffin cells; they can release many different polypeptides (e.g. kallikrein, bradykinin), biogenic amines (e.g. serotonin, histamine) and prostaglandins CS is typically caused by metastatic tumours of the midgut (jejunum, ileum, appendix, ascending colon). Hepatic metastases result in downstream release of tumour products, thereby bypassing the portal circulation and avoiding hepatic metabolism. CS due to foregut tumours (bronchial, gastric, duodenum, thymus) is less common. However, as their products are released directly into the systemic circulation, these tumours can result in CS in the absence of metastases. Hindgut tumours (distal colon, rectum, genitourinary) are usually hormonally inactive and therefore rarely cause CS. The main secretory products of carcinoid tumours are serotonin, histamine, tachykinins, kallikrein and prostaglandins. Serotonin does not cause flushing, but results in increased intestinal secretion and motility (diarrhoea) and increased fibroblast growth (cardiac valvular fibrosis) Histamine can be produced by primary gastric carcinoids and causes atypical flushing and pruritus Bradykinin (a product of kallikrein cleavage action) is a potent vasodilator and may result in flushing in some carcinoid patients. Prostaglandins E and F stimulate intestinal motility and fluid secretion in the normal gastrointestinal tract Some carcinoid tumours secrete tachykinins (substance P, neurokinin A, neuropeptide K) which may contribute to flushing and diarrhoea	The flush associated with classic CS (due to midgut carcinoids) begins suddenly and lasts from 30 seconds up to 30 minutes. The face, neck and upper chest may flush red to violaceous, with an associated mild burning sensation Severe flushes are accompanied by hypotension and tachycardia. As the disease progresses, the episodes may last longer and the flushing may be more diffuse and cyanotic The flushes associated with gastric carcinoid tumours are atypical and tend to be red-brown, patchy, sharply demarcated, with bizarre gyrate or serpiginous patterns that may resolve centrally, usually associated with an intense pruritus In patients with the bronchial carcinoid variant, the flushes can be very severe and prolonged, lasting hours to days. Atypical flushing may be associated with tremor, disorientation, lacrimation, salivation, oedema (including periorbitally) Most flushing episodes occur spontaneously, but they may be provoked by eating, drinking alcohol, defecation, emotional events, palpation of the liver and anaesthesia	Flushing is the most common symptom (occurring in 85% of patients with CS) Associated symptoms include secretory diarrhoea, hypotension, tachycardia, abdominal cramping, sweating and bronchospasm. As the disease progresses, valvular heart disease (right-sided fibrosis, tricuspid and pulmonary valves), venous telangiectasia, leonine facies and pellagra (diversion of dietary tryptophan for the increased production of serotonin) may occur	24-h urinary excretion of 5-HIAA (5-HIAA is the end product of serotonin metabolism; generally not useful in foregut and hindgut tumours, as these cannot convert 5-HT to serotonin) Urinary serotonin (may be of value in the rare patient with a foregut carcinoid in whom CS is suspected. DOPA decarboxylase in the renal parenchyma converts 5-HTP to serotonin) Chromogranin A (appropriate tumour marker for patients with an established diagnosis in order to assess disease progression, response to therapy or recurrence after surgical resection) Imaging studies of abdomen and pelvis; CT, MRI and SRS (octreoscans) are the primary imaging modalities used to identify carcinoid tumours Echocardiogram for patients with clinical evidence of carcinoid heart disease or if major surgery is being planned	Somatostatin analogues (e.g. octreotide) provide effective symptomatic control. Prophylactic preoperative subcutaneous or intravenous administration of octreotide is recommended for patients with CS undergoing surgery for metastatic disease Hepatic resection for patients with liver metastases; can provide long-term symptomatic relief of CS symptoms; useful in resectable disease, benefits need to be weighed in unresectable disease	Carcinoid crisis is a life-threatening form of CS that results from the release of an overwhelming amount of biologically active tumour products; it may be triggered by tumour manipulation (e.g. biopsy, surgery) or by anaesthesia. It is less commonly reported after chemotherapy, hepatic arterial embolisation or radionuclide therapy, mostly in patients with markedly elevated serum serotonin or urine 5-HIAA

Phaeo-chromocytoma	Catecholamine-secreting tumours that arise from chromaffin cells of the adrenal medulla; release of catecholamines (epinephrine, norepinephrine, dopamine) and other vasomediators (VIP, calcitonin gene-related peptide, adrenomedullin) episodically into the systemic circulation	Flushing of the face, neck, chest and trunk; paroxysmal attacks last 15 minutes to hours; usually occur spontaneously but may be triggered by deep abdominal palpation, diagnostic procedures (e.g. colonoscopy), induction of anaesthesia, surgery, with certain foods or beverages containing tyramine or with certain drugs (e.g. MAO inhibitors)	Hypertension (60% have sustained hypertension; 40% experience hypertension only during attacks); tachycardia; headaches, hyperhidrosis, piloerection; palpitations, a sense of impending doom, chest pain or abdominal pain associated with nausea and vomiting, pallor, weakness and collapse	24-h urine fractionated catecholamines and metanephrines Plasma fractionated metanephrines Biochemical confirmation of the diagnosis should be followed by radiological evaluation to locate the tumour. About 10% are extra-adrenal, but 95% are within the abdomen and pelvis CT/MRI MIBG scintigraphy. If abdominal and pelvic CT or MRI is negative in the presence of clinical and biochemical evidence of phaeochromocytoma, the diagnosis should be reconsidered. If it is still likely, then 123-I-MIBG scintigraphy may be done FDG-PET more sensitive than 123-I-MIBG and CT/MRI for detection of metastatic disease	Avoid precipitants (e.g. glucagon, histamine, metoclopramide) Combined α- and β-adrenergic blockade to control blood pressure and prevent intraoperative hypertensive crises Adrenalectomy	Check for cutaneous stigmata of neurofibromatosis
Medullary thyroid cancer (MTC)	Originates from the parafollicular cells (C cells), which produce the hormone calcitonin Also produces prostaglandins, histamine, substance P, ketacalcin, levodopa, ACTH and CRH	Can develop protracted flushing of the face and upper extremities	Most patients are asymptomatic If symptomatic, secretory diarrhea is the most prominent clinical finding Patients can also develop increased sweat production	US thyroid can detect nodule FNA from a thyroid nodule is usually diagnostic Serum calcitonin levels are usually elevated Carcinoembryonic antigen (CEA) may be elevated in advanced MTC	Total thyroidectomy with central lymph node dissection is the minimum recommended treatment. Genetic testing of the patient and all first-degree relatives should include RET mutation analysis	Caused by mutations in the RET proto-oncogene Sporadic or inherited in an autosomal dominant pattern as part of (MEN2A /MEN2B) or familial MTC
Pancreatic neuro-endocrine tumours (PNET)	Release numerous substances including: VIP Gastric inhibitory polypeptide Prostaglandin Insulin Gastrin Glucagon	Flushing can be seen in all forms of PNETs Flushing resembles gastric carcinoid syndrome Chronic flushing from PNETs may develop	Several subtypes including: VIPomas – watery diarrhea, hypokalemia, rarely flushing Gastrinomas – flushing rare Insulinomas – may produce flushing during hypoglycemic episodes Glucagonomas – present with hyperglycemia and a characteristic necrolytic migratory red rash	Biochemical work-up of the various secretory susbstances Imaging: ultrasound, CT	Surgical resection for localised disease and selected patients with metastatic disease Somatostatin analogues effective for symptoms of hormone overproduction	Majority benign, whilst some are malignant. When malignant can be known as islet cell carcinoma

(Continued)

PART 9: VASCULAR DISORDERS

Table 104.1 (continued)

Disease	Pathogenesis of flush	Characteristics of flush	Associated symptoms and signs	Investigations	Treatment	Notes
Renal cell carcinoma	Secretion of prostaglandins or via pituitary downregulation from release of gonadotropins can cause flushing	Flushing associated with sensation of warmth can be encountered	Classic triad of gross hematuria, flank pain and abdominal mass in fewer than 10% Often presents with hematuria alone Patients often experience fatigue, weight loss, and cachexia, anaemia and intermittent fever	Intravenous pyelography Renal ultrasound CT MRI	Radical nephrectomy for limited disease is treatment of choice In metastatic disease, chemotherapy, immunotherapy or hormonal therapy may be used	
Anaphylaxis	Mast cell and basophil vasoactive mediators release	Typically within minutes of exposure to trigger (if known); rarely presents with flushing alone	Urticaria, angioedema, hypotension, bronchospasm, rhinitis, chest pain, headache, tachycardia, collapse	Plasma mast cell tryptase Skin testing, in vitro IgE tests or both may be used to determine the stimulus causing the anaphylactic reaction – performed by specialist in immunology at a later date	During the anaphylactic episode, either IV or IM epinephrine (the latter via EpiPen (0.3 mg) or 0.3–0.5 mL of 1 : 1000 dilution) should be administered into either the anterolateral thigh muscles or the deltoid muscle every 5 min, as necessary, to control blood pressure and symptoms	
Acute alcohol sensitivity	ADH2, ALDH2 and CYP2E1 are important enzymes for the catalysis of the conversion of ethanol to acetaldehyde and to acetate in humans Genetic polymorphisms have been reported in these enzymes. Between 40 and 80% of several Asian groups have been found to be deficient in ALDH2. The accumulation of acetaldehyde following the ingestion of alcohol triggers catecholamine release from the adrenal medulla and sympathetic nerves	Unpleasant sensation following alcohol ingestion	Palpitations, headache, vomiting and sweating	An ethanol patch test may be a useful initial investigation	Alcohol avoidance	Up to 48% of the population of some East Asian countries, e.g. South Korea and Japan, have the ALDH2 polymorphism which produces flushing; this causes build-up of acetaldehydes, which after 2–3 standard alcoholic drinks are over 50 µM and mutagenic and hence tissues in contact with the alcohol in the nasopharynx and oesophagus have a much higher chance of malignancy [24–32]
Dumping syndrome	Rapid gastric emptying, occurring post gastrointestinal surgery including bariatric surgery Rapid hyperosmolar load transmitted from the stomach to the small intestines	Postprandial flushing	Tachycardia, sweating, dizziness, weakness and gastrointestinal disturbances	Glucose challenge test Gastric emptying scintigraphy	Small and frequent meals with fibre and protein Acarbose Octreotide Loperamide Surgery/enteral feeding if refractory	Early and late variants depending on time of symptom onset post meal

ACTH, adrenocorticotropic hormone; ADH2, alcohol dehydrogenase 2; ALDH2, aldehyde dehydrogenase 2 family; AMH, anti-mullerian hormone; CRH, corticotropin-releasing hormone; CT, computed tomography; CYP2E1, cytochrome P450 2E1; FDG-PET, fluorodeoxyglucose positron emission tomography; 5-HIAA, 5-hydroxyindoleacetic acid; 5-HT, 5-hydroxytryptamine; FNA, fine-needle aspirate; FSH, follicle-stimulating hormone; HRT, hormone replacement therapy; LTC4, leukotriene C4; LTD4, leukotriene D4; LTE4, leukotriene E4; MEN2A/MEN2B, multiple endocrine neoplasia 2A/2B; MAO inhibitors, monoamine oxidase inhibitors; MRI, magnetic resonance imaging; NSAID, non-steroidal anti-inflammatory drug; 123-I-MIBG, 123 I-metaiodobenzylguanidine; PGD2, prostaglandin D2; SNRI, serotonin and norepinephrine reuptake inhibitor; SSRI, selective serotonin reuptake inhibitor; SRS, somatostatin receptor scintigraphy; TMEP, telangiectasia macularis eruptive perstans; TRPV, transient receptor potential vanilloid; VIP, vasoactive intestinal peptide.

Table 104.2 Flushing in children. Many of the systemic diseases outlined in Box 104.3 may also apply to the paediatric population. However, this table outlines disorders that may be of particular relevance in children.

Pyrexia	–
Teething	Parents and professionals frequently attribute symptoms such as irritability, increased salivation and flushed cheeks to the eruption of primary teeth in infants. Little evidence exists to support these observations [33]
Mastocytosis	Table 104.1
Frey syndrome/ gustatory hyperhidrosis	Also known as auriculotemporal nerve syndrome, gustatory sweating results from a disruption of the auriculotemporal nerve pathways. Damage to the nerve may cause a misdirected regrowth that results in parasympathetic innervation of sympathetic receptors and, therefore, unilateral facial sweating and flushing with gustatory stimulation [34]
Raised intracranial pressure	Neurological deterioration associated with flushing involving either upper chest, face or arms in children has been reported. The flush typically lasts 5–15 min and dissipates quickly. The flushing reaction is postulated to be a centrally mediated response to sudden elevations in intracranial pressure [35]
Nephropathic cystinosis	Children with this lysosomal storage disorder display an inability to produce normal volumes of sweat. This deficiency results in heat intolerance and avoidance, flushing, hyperthermia and vomiting in small children [36]
Oesophageal atresia	Unilateral facial flushing has been reported following surgical repair of oesophageal atresia [37]
Harlequin colour change	A benign phenomenon, presenting as well-demarcated unilateral transient redness on the dependent side in a neonate. The flush lasts from 30 s to 20 min. It presents in the first 3 weeks of life, usually on days 2–5. It is believed to be caused by temporary imbalance in the tone of cutaneous blood vessels secondary to hypothalamic immaturity [38] (Figure 104.2)

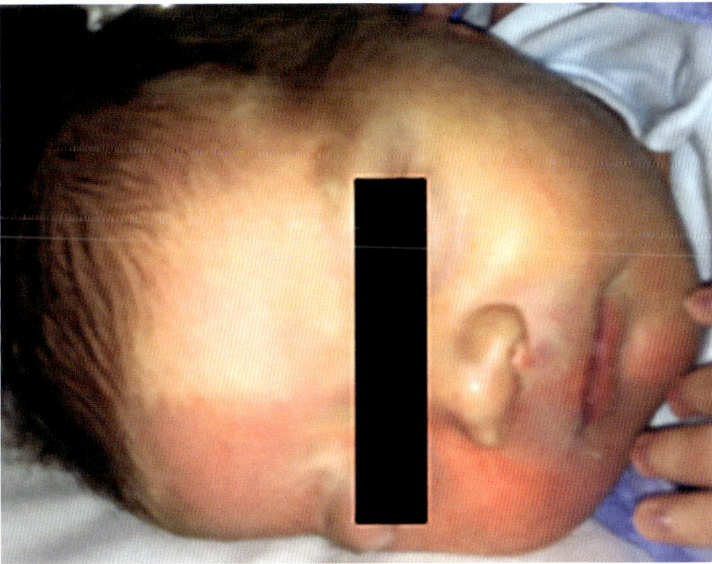

Figure 104.2 Harlequin colour change. Transient well-demarcated facial flush on the dependent right side of a healthy 2-day-old full-term male infant, which faded within minutes.

Clinical presentation of blushing

Patients with excessive blushing complain of an involuntary and prolonged reddening primarily of the facial skin, which is often precipitated by anxiety, emotion or psychological upset. Blushing usually starts on the lateral cheeks and spreads rapidly to involve the entire malar region. Frequently, 'skip' areas of pallor can be observed within the blush, with sparing of the area around the mouth, giving the impression of circumoral pallor. The blush may spread to the forehead and the sides of the neck. The ears characteristically develop an intense redness, involving primarily the helix and antihelix. Blushing is not usually associated with facial sweating, but there may be accompanying palmar hyperhidrosis and tremor. Because of the tendency to blush in certain social circumstances and their perception that the blush is more marked than it is, individuals may develop a degree of 'anticipatory anxiety' and blush even before they venture into these situations [20].

Clinical presentation of flushing

A flush may evolve in a similar manner to a blush, but often has a more widespread distribution extending to the anterior chest and sometimes the abdomen, particularly the epigastric region. Localised facial sweating may be a feature of flushing. Depending on the underlying aetiology, flushing can be episodic or constant. In patients with longstanding frequent flushing, fixed facial redness and telangiectases may develop [21].

Flushing must be distinguished from facial plethora, which is chronic, persistent redness that develops slowly over time. A menopausal flush can be sudden in onset and associated with a drenching sweat. Patients with rosacea who flush may describe associated symptoms such as heat intolerance and skin sensitivity.

Ingestion of alcohol can lead to dry flushing in those with aldehyde dehydrogenase gene polymorphisms. Ingestion of certain foods containing nitrites, sulfites and capsaicin can also lead to flushing. Rarely, scombroid fish poisoning, which results from bacterial conversion of histidine to histamine in inadequately preserved or refrigerated fish, can be associated with flushing along with other symptoms such as itch, vomiting and headache. Certain medications cause flushing (Box 104.2). Infusion reactions related to medications or blood products can also be associated with reactions in which flushing can occur.

In a minority of patients who experience flushing there may be associated systemic complaints, which warrant further investigation (Table 104.1). Patients with carcinoid syndrome can experience associated diarrhoea and wheezing. Flushing associated with itch can be seen in patients with mastocytosis. In most cases of malignancy, flushing is generally considered a symptom of late disease, with the exception of carcinoid syndrome. Superior vena caval obstruction can also be associated with facial flushing and congestion. In these cases, the Pemberton sign (facial plethora occurring secondary to bilateral arm elevation) will be seen.

Various neurological causes of flushing are well described (Box 104.3). Exertional flushing can sometimes be seen in patients with cholinergic urticaria. Flushing after a warm bath is occasionally reported in patients with polycythaemia. Flushing localised to the nose has been reported as a prodrome to migraine attacks. Men,

PART 9: VASCULAR DISORDERS

following surgery for prostate cancer, may experience flushing, particularly if they receive oestrogen therapy.

Investigations (Table 104.1 and Figure 104.3)

A thorough history, with particular emphasis on precipitating or exacerbating factors, drug and alcohol usage and food intake, and a detailed review of systemic symptoms including queries relating to anxiety and stress, is essential in the evaluation of an individual who presents with a complaint of excessive flushing. It may be useful for the patient to keep a record of flushing episodes, detailing possible triggers and associated symptoms such as headache, abdominal pain, wheeze, diarrhoea or chest pain. Patients who flush after alcohol intake can be tested by an ethanol patch test. In individuals deficient in the enzyme alcohol dehydrogenase, an area of redness develops in the tested skin. If an underlying systemic disorder is suspected, a detailed history and clinical examination should help to direct further workup. Initial investigations should include a full blood count,

renal and liver profiles, thyroid function tests, urinalysis, 24 h urine for 5-hydroxyindoleacetic acid (5-HIAA) (carcinoid syndrome), 24 h urinary fractionated catecholamines and metanephrines, plasma fractionated metanephrines (phaeochromocytoma), serum tryptase, 24 h urine histamine and calcitonin (medullary thyroid cancer). If the histamine is elevated or if there is mastocytosis such as urticaria pigmentosa, then referral to a haematologist for a potential bone marrow biopsy is indicated. Radiological imaging, when required, should be dictated by the underlying working diagnosis.

Management

The management of the flushing patient should be tailored to the individual and guided by the underlying cause (see Table 104.1 and Figure 104.4). However, most flushing patients will benefit from general guidance on managing the flush, such as identification of potential triggering factors (e.g. work environment, temperature, foods, alcohol, drugs) and their avoidance where feasible; information on histamine-releasing foods and medication;

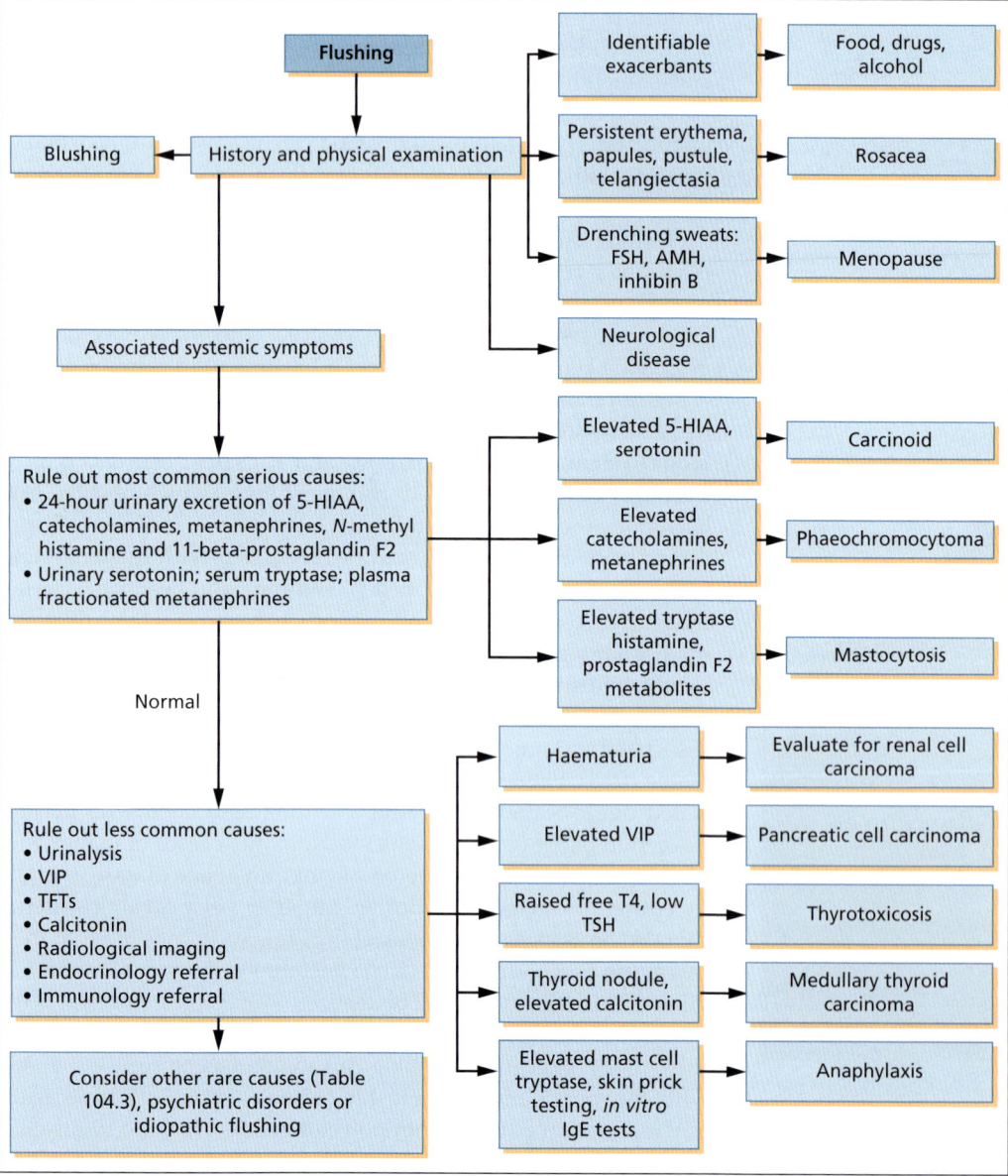

Figure 104.3 Algorithm for investigation of flushing and blushing.

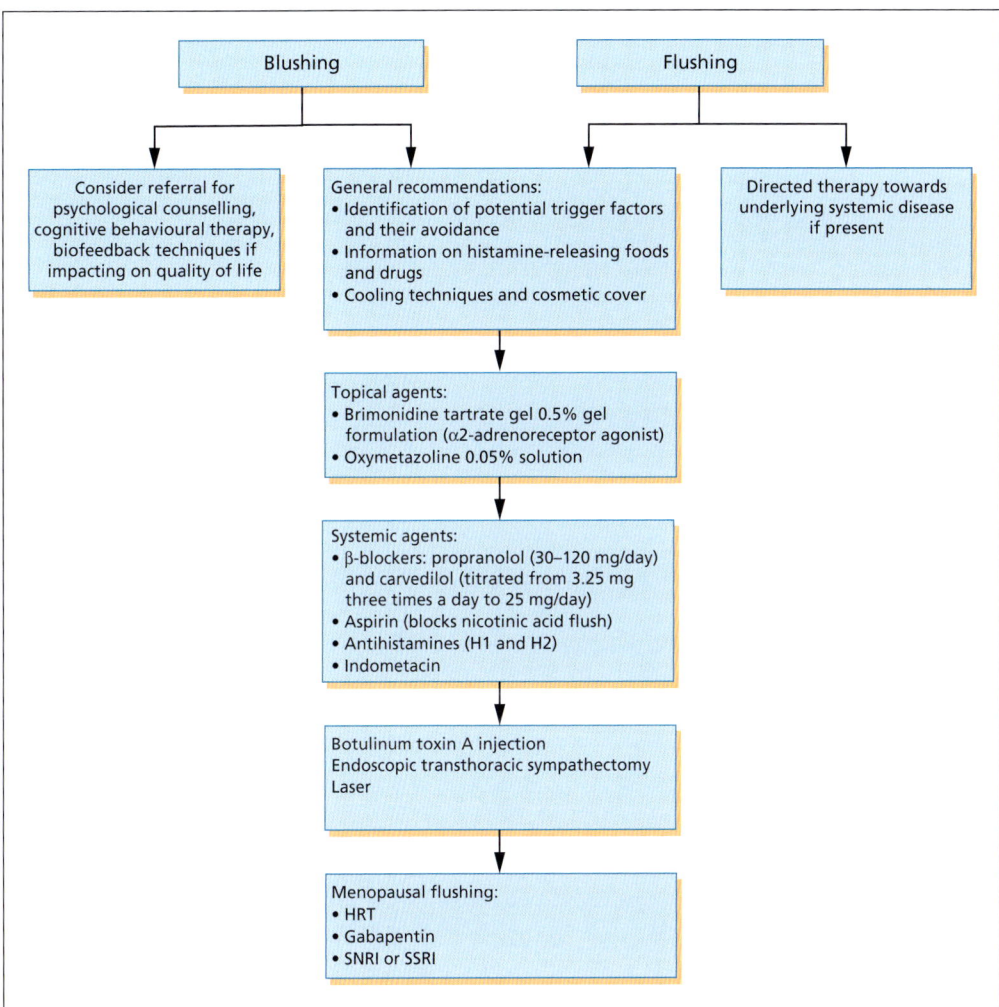

Figure 104.4 Algorithm for the management of flushing and blushing.

and advice on cooling techniques and temperature regulation (Figure 104.3). The management of blushing should encompass a comprehensive explanation of the psychosocial nature of the problem and its relationship to anxiety, as well as reassurance of the lack of disease association and the possibility of spontaneous improvement in younger patients with time. When blushing is associated with social withdrawal or excessive anxiety, consider referral for psychological counselling and cognitive behavioural therapy. Unfortunately, the studies examining its effectiveness are small in scale [39]. Biofeedback techniques may be useful in these patients.

Topical α-adrenoreceptor agonists, which produce cutaneous vasoconstriction, have shown efficacy in the treatment of flushing associated with rosacea. Brimonidine tartrate is a highly selective α2-adrenoreceptor agonist. Topical brimonidine tartrate gel 0.5% has been shown in controlled prospective randomised clinical trials to reduce facial redness after single and repeated once-daily applications [40]. Oxymetazoline hydrochloride cream, 1%, an alpha$_{A1}$ adrenoceptor agonist, has also been approved for treatment of persistent facial redness in rosacea [41]. Side effects of these agents include rebound erythema, burning sensation and irritant dermatitis. Patients should be counselled carefully on appropriate application of these agents, as well as the 'wear-off' timeframe.

Low-dose β-blocker therapy may be useful in some patients with either flushing or blushing. Non-selective β-blockers decrease sympathetic activity, thereby resulting in vasoconstriction. In addition, their anxiolytic effects may reduce the anxiety that may be associated with flushing. Serotonin reuptake inhibitors are a recognised treatment for social phobia. However, their effectiveness for facial blushing itself is not well documented [42].

Both propranolol (30–120 mg/day) and carvedilol (titrated from 3.25 mg three times a day to 25 mg/day) have been shown to reduce flushing episodes in patients with rosacea [43,44].

Other drugs reported to be helpful in certain subgroups include aspirin [45], antihistamines [46] and clonidine [47]. Evidence for the efficacy of these medications is lacking, and their potential toxicity should be considered before prescribing.

Laser techniques such as pulsed dye laser, intense pulsed light and potassium-titanyl-phosphate laser may be useful for the treatment of telangiectasia and erythema. Endoscopic transthoracic sympathectomy has been shown to be helpful in some patients with intractable flushing or blushing, but long-term side effects such as compensatory hyperhidrosis are common, and more serious complications may occasionally occur [48]. Botulinum toxin A, which acts presynaptically to abolish the release of all transmitters selectively from cholinergic nerves, has been used with success to treat neck and anterior chest wall flushing [49].

PART 9: VASCULAR DISORDERS

Key references

The full list of references can be found in the online version at https://www.wiley.com/rooksdermatology10e

1 Rowell LB. Reflex control of the cutaneous vasculature. *J Invest Dermatol* 1977;69:154–66.

2 Johnson JM, Kellogg DL Jr. Thermoregulatory and thermal control in the human cutaneous circulation. *Front Biosci* 2010;S2:825–53.

6 Kellogg DL Jr, Zhao JL, Wu Y, Johnson JM. VIP/PACAP receptor mediation of cutaneous active vasodilation during heat stress in humans. *J Appl Physiol* 2010;109: 95–100.

9 Charkoudian N. Mechanisms and modifiers of reflex induced cutaneous vasodilation and vasoconstriction in humans. *J Appl Physiol* 2010;109:1221–8.

10 Powell FC. *Rosacea: Diagnosis and Management.* Boca Raton, FL: CRC Press, 2009.

11 Izikson L, English JC 3rd, Zirwas MJ. The flushing patient: differential diagnosis, workup, and treatment. *J Am Acad Dermatol* 2006;55:193–208.

12 Crozier WR, de Jong PJ. *The Psychological Significance of the Blush.* Cambridge: Cambridge University Press, 2013.

14 Drummond PD, Lazaroo D. The effect of facial blood flow on ratings of blushing and negative affect during an embarrassing task: preliminary findings. *J Anxiety Disord* 2012;26:305–10.

18 Drummond PD, Su D. The relationship between blushing propensity, social anxiety and facial blood flow during embarrassment. *Cogn Emot* 2012;26:561–7.

40 Fowler J, Jackson M, Moore A. Efficacy and safety of once-daily topical brimonidine tartrate gel 0.5% for the treatment of moderate to severe facial erythema of rosacea: results of two randomized, double-blind, vehicle-controlled pivotal studies. *J Drugs Dermatol* 2013;12:650–6.

PART 10

Skin Disorders Associated with Specific Sites, Sex and Age

CHAPTER 105

Dermatoses of the Scalp

Paul Farrant[1], Megan Mowbray[2] and Anita Takwale[3]

[1]Department of Dermatology, Brighton General Hospital, University Hospitals Sussex, Brighton, UK
[2]Department of Dermatology, Queen Margaret Hospital, NHS Fife, Dunfermline, UK
[3]Department of Dermatology, Gloucestershire Royal Hospital, Gloucestershire Hospitals NHS Foundation Trust, Gloucester, UK

SCALING DISORDERS OF THE SCALP

Seborrhoeic dermatitis

Introduction and general description

Seborrhoeic dermatitis is an inflammatory condition of the skin that affects the scalp, face, groin and chest (Chapter 40). On the scalp there are a range of presentations from fine, dry flakes of skin or dandruff (previously referred to as pityriasis capitis) to thicker, greasy, yellow scales associated with an underlying inflammation of the scalp.

Epidemiology

Seborrhoeic dermatitis of infancy is probably a distinctive condition and may be a marker of the atopic state (discussed later). For others, the condition becomes more prevalent from puberty, probably driven by an increase in androgens and an increase in sebum production.

At the mild end of the spectrum, seborrheic dermatitis is a very common condition, with around 50% of 20-year-old white males having evidence of dandruff. Inflammatory seborrhoeic dermatitis affects 1–3% of immunocompetent adults [1]. Seborrhoeic dermatitis is more common in males, increases with age and is associated with a number of other skin conditions, with folliculitis being the most common (17%) [2]. There is a higher prevalence in patients with HIV infection, Parkinson's disease, epilepsy and following a stroke or spinal cord injury.

Pathophysiology

Seborrhoeic dermatitis results from *Malassezia* hydrolysation of free fatty acids with activation of the innate immune system. *Malassezia restricta* and *M. globosa* are the most virulent subspecies. *Malassezia* lipases hydrolyse sebaceous lipids, which generates increased amounts of irritating unsaturated fatty acids, such as oleic acids. It is believed that oleic acids are the main trigger for inflammation and there is likely to be individual sensitivity to these irritating chemicals [3]. Endogenous factors include increased sebaceous activity associated with androgen activity, altered immunity (HIV, lymphoma, bone marrow suppression) and neurological conditions, such as Parkinson disease and after a cerebrovascular accident. Facial immobility, sebum accumulation and increased sebum production are thought to play a role. Exogenous factors include stress, recent alcohol consumption [4], high humidity, epidermal growth factor receptor (EGFR) inhibitors and poor skin and hair care practices.

The role of diet remains controversial, but a high fruit diet may be protective and a typical Western diet may exacerbate the condition [5].

Clinical features

At one end of the spectrum, seborrhoeic dermatitis consists of fine, small, white or grey scales, which may be diffuse or localised in

PART 10: SPECIFIC SITES, SEX & AGE

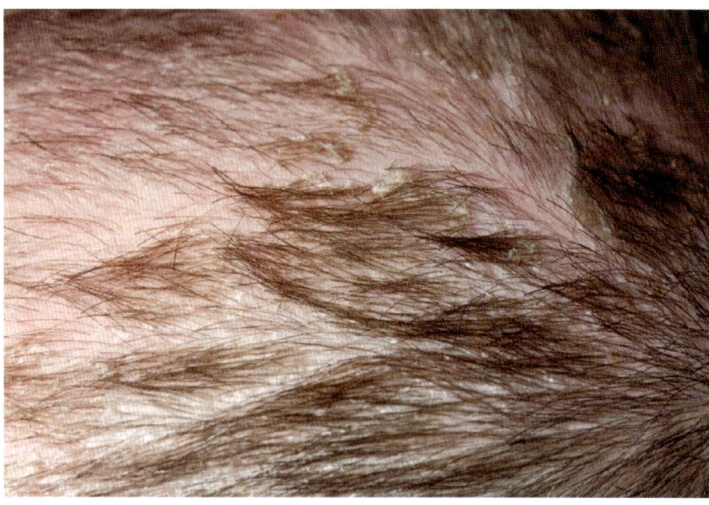

(a)

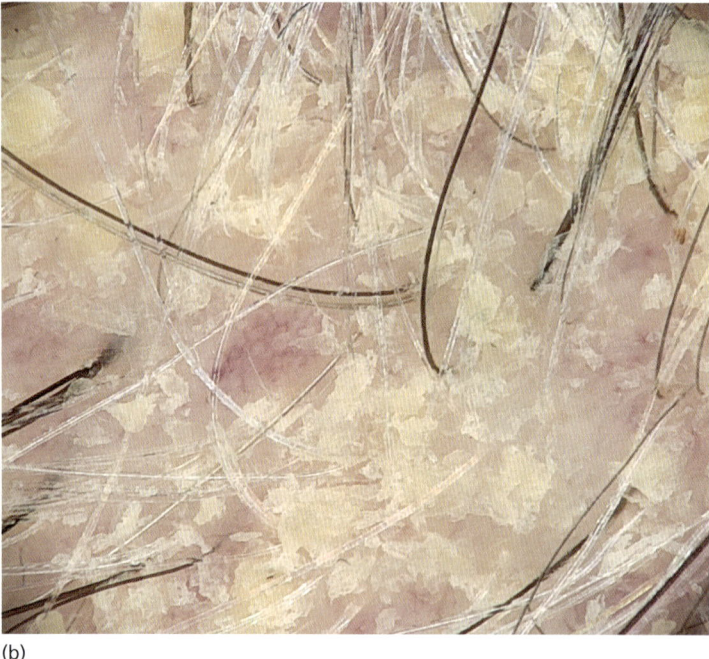

(b)

Figure 105.1 (a) Seborrhoeic dermatitis of the scalp and (b) showing a close-up of the thickened yellow adherent scales.

patches (Figure 105.1). Seborrhoea may bind the scale to produce more adherent mounds of yellowish, greasy scales. There may be associated perifollicular redness. As well as the scalp, seborrhoeic dermatitis commonly involves the eyebrows, naso-labial folds, chest and groins. In patients with darker skin, seborrhoeic dermatitis may present with hypopigmented scaly patches. Any underlying redness may be hard to appreciate. Arcuate and petaloid lesions may affect the hairline and face [6].

Differential diagnosis

The main differential diagnoses of seborrhoeic dermatitis are scalp psoriasis, tinea capitis and lichen simplex chronicus. Psoriasis is often characterised by a plaque of silvery scales with a well-demarcated edge and underlying redness of the skin, often involving the hair line. There may be some overlap of clinical features, which has led to the term 'sebo-psoriasis'. Dermoscopy has been reported as a diagnostic tool to help differentiate these two conditions, with arborising vessels being a feature of seborrhoeic dermatitis, and red dots, globules and twisted red loops being features of scalp psoriasis [7].

Tinea capitis may be confused with seborrhoeic dermatitis, especially tinea due to *Trichophyton* species, and one should have a low threshold for taking skin scrapings. Lichen simplex most typically involves the occiput and can be differentiated by itch, which is the characteristic feature of this condition.

Management

All treatments are aimed at control and not cure, and it is important that patients are made aware of this at the outset. Over-the-counter preparations include shampoos that are aimed at dandruff control; the active ingredients in these agents are zinc pyrithione, selenium sulphide, ciclopirox and ketoconazole. Coal tar shampoos can also be helpful in seborrheic dermatitis but are less cosmetically acceptable to patients. Medicated shampoos need to be used at least twice weekly for maintenance therapy to limit relapse. Both ketoconazole and ciclopirox have been shown to be superior to placebo at achieving early clearance and similar in efficacy to topical steroids but with fewer side effects [8].

The more inflammatory end of the seborrhoeic dermatitis spectrum requires the addition of an anti-inflammatory agent, typically a corticosteroid. Topical corticosteroids for scalp use are available in gels, lotions, mousses and shampoos. These should be used for a short period, on an intermittent basis, to avoid side effects.

Systemic oral antifungal agents such as ketoconazole, itraconazole and terbinafine should be reserved for severe unresponsive refractory cases. The evidence for efficacy of systemic antifungal agents is poor [9].

Future treatments may be aimed at altering the skin microbiome with topical and oral probiotics to increase bacterial diversity, with some initial studies showing decreased redness, scale and pruritus with topical *Vitreoscilla filiformis* and improvements of dandruff, redness and seborrhoea with oral *Lacticaseibacillus paracasei* [10].

Seborrhoeic dermatitis of infancy

Infantile seborrhoeic dermatitis or 'cradle cap' presents with greasy, yellow scales over the vertex of the newborn. It is often self-limiting and improves within the first year of life for the majority. It is regarded as a manifestation of the atopic state.

Psoriasis

Introduction and general description

Psoriasis is a common inflammatory skin disease that has a particular predilection for the scalp. It is not uncommon for the scalp to be the first site of involvement in psoriasis. The epidemiology, aetiology and pathology are all discussed in Chapter 35. The clinical features and treatment of scalp psoriasis are discussed here.

Epidemiology

Psoriasis affects 2–5% of the population and around 80% of psoriasis sufferers will have scalp involvement at some point.

Pathophysiology

In patients complaining of hair loss associated with psoriasis, scalp biopsies frequently show an increase in catagen and telogen hairs when viewed horizontally. Hair follicles often become miniaturised and there is atrophy of the sebaceous glands.

Clinical features

Psoriasis of the scalp is characterised by well-demarcated plaques covered in silvery thick scales (Figure 105.2). The scales may become matted together to form thickened plaques. Scalp psoriasis can be localised in patches or more diffuse throughout the scalp and occasionally covers the entire scalp. Psoriasis commonly involves the hair line, extending 1–2 cm beyond the hair line onto the forehead or neck. However, the earliest changes may be more subtle with diffuse scaling without specific features, and a diagnosis may only

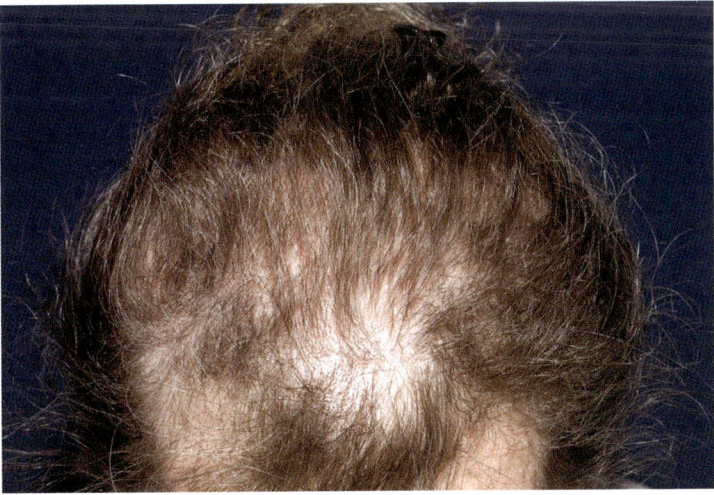

(a)

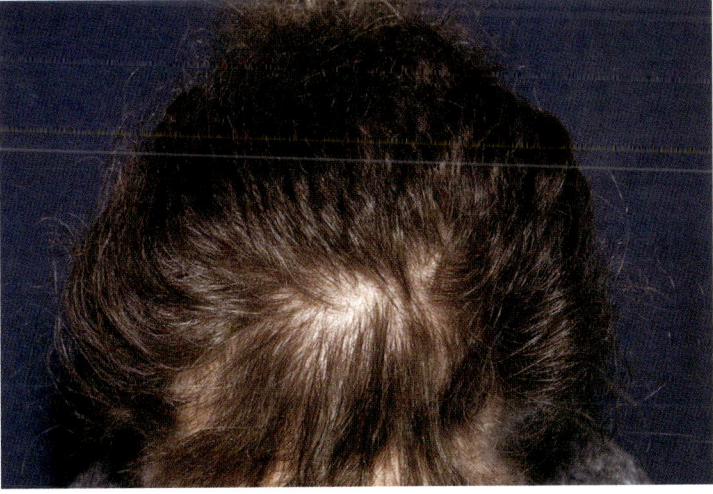

(b)

Figure 105.2 Scalp psoriasis with hair loss. (a) Psoriatic alopecia. (b) Hair regrowth after active management of scalp psoriasis.

be reached from the involvement of other sites or from a strong family history.

In erythrodermic psoriasis, scalp involvement may lead to marked hair loss. Scalp psoriasis is associated with an increase of hairs in the telogen phase and a degree of hair loss is not uncommon, but often under-recognised. Treatment of the psoriasis often leads to hair regrowth but scarring hair loss associated with psoriasis has been described [11].

Differential diagnosis

The main differential is seborrhoeic dermatitis, as discussed in the previous section. Examination of other body sites often provides clues to the true diagnosis but sometimes the conditions cannot be distinguished. Occasionally, discrete areas of discoid lupus can mimic psoriasis and a solitary scaly plaque on a bald scalp may represent Bowen disease.

Management

There are similarities with the management of scalp psoriasis and body psoriasis but important differences too. The main function of hair in today's society is largely cosmetic and treatments that impact on appearance are often considered unacceptable by patients. Creams and ointments that are messy, sticky and greasy need to be replaced with more suitable vehicles for hair-bearing skin such as gels, lotions, mousses or shampoo formulations. Counselling patients about long-term goals and the need for maintenance therapy is important, as the condition is controlled by treatment and not cured. Hair can provide a framework for scales to adhere to so that plaques become thickened and produce a barrier to the absorption of topical treatments. In severe cases of scalp psoriasis, removing these thickened plaques through physical means is an essential first step before the addition of any anti-inflammatory agent.

Medicated shampoos are commonly used in the management of scalp psoriasis and these often contain coal tar, which has mild anti-inflammatory properties and can be soothing for patients with itch. Other active ingredients may include cade oil, arachis oil, salicylic acid, coconut oil and urea. The addition of conditioners to scalp preparations may make them more acceptable to patients. Antidandruff shampoos may also be helpful as part of a regular routine.

In patients that have thickened plaques, efforts should be made to remove the scale. Scale can be softened with the use of oils (e.g. arachis or olive), petroleum-based emollients or pomades containing coal tar, salicylic acid or cade oils. These should be left on for several hours or overnight. Once the scale has been softened, it can be gently combed out, using a blunt tooth plastic comb, avoiding any trauma to the underlying scalp, which may exacerbate psoriasis due to koebnerisation. Assistance from a specialist nurse or friend or carer is often needed. If preparations are left on overnight, an ordinary shampoo should be applied to the scalp while the hair is still dry, rubbed in to produce an emulsion, and then the hair should be wetted and rinsed. For severe cases this procedure may need to be repeated for several days to make sufficient progress before proceeding to anti-inflammatory preparations.

In milder cases of psoriasis or in severe cases that have been de-scaled, treatment is then focused on the underlying psoriasis.

PART 10: SPECIFIC SITES, SEX & AGE

Vitamin D analogues, topical corticosteroids and combination products containing both, or topical steroid and additional ingredients such as salicylic acid, are the mainstay of treatment. Very potent or potent topical steroids are superior to vitamin D analogues, while vitamin D and steroid combinations are superior to potent steroid monotherapy [12,13]. The atrophic potential of corticosteroid treatments for scalp psoriasis remains unclear but has been described in trials investigating clobetasol propionate [14]. Topical corticosteroid or combination products often need to be used frequently at the outset, for example daily for up to a month, and then reduced to twice weekly or so for maintenance. It is important that patients are aware of the different formulations and efforts made to select the most appropriate vehicle. Newer formulations in the form of gels, foams and shampoos are targeted at addressing patient dissatisfaction at older treatments, with the aim of improving compliance [15].

In resistant cases of scalp psoriasis it may be necessary to use systemic agents to control the condition. Ciclosporin used short term can be particularly effective, especially if there is marked hair loss associated with the psoriasis. Ultraviolet therapy is less useful since the hair coverage acts as a barrier to UV light, but excimer laser therapy can be effective for hair line psoriasis in resistant cases [16].

Both the phosphodiesterese inhibitor apremilast [17] and the biological treatments etanercept, adalimumab, ixekizumab, brodalumab, guselkumab and secukinumab have shown specific benefit in treating scalp psoriasis and itch [**18**]. While most of these outcomes have been reported in subgroup analysis of patients being treated for body psoriasis, secukinumab was shown to have achieved a 90% improvement at week 12 in scalp psoriasis in 53% of participants in a dedicated trial investigating moderate to severe scalp psoriasis [19].

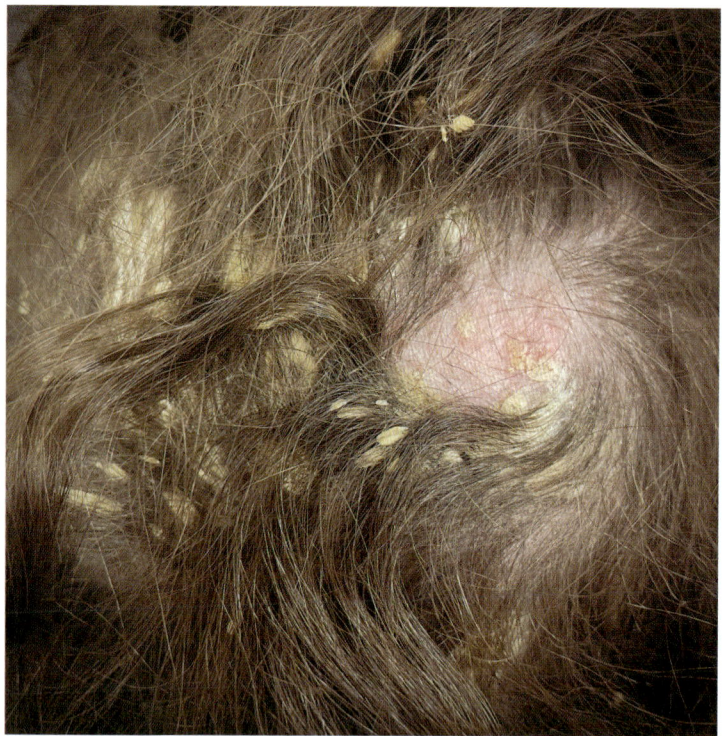

(a)

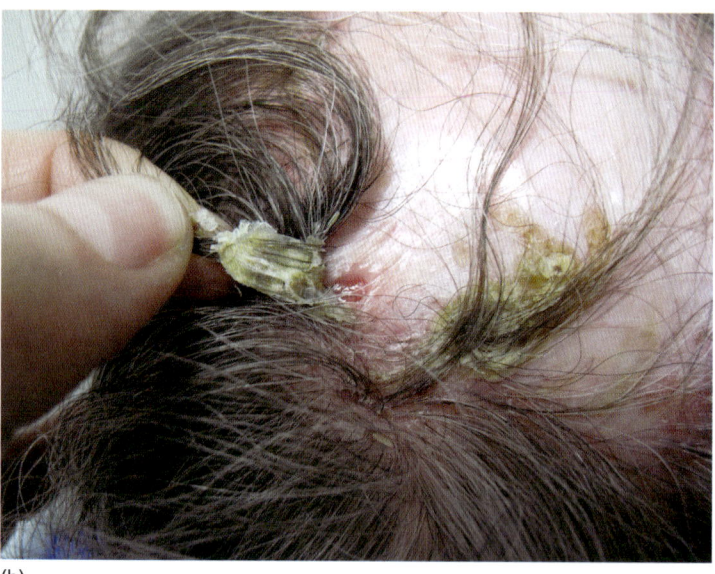

(b)

Figure 105.3 Pityriasis amiantacea, showing (a) localised build-up of thick adherent scale around the hair shafts with localised areas of hair loss and (b) close-up showing encasement of the hairs and surrounding scarring hair loss secondary to removal of the scale.

Pityriasis amiantacea

Introduction and general description

Pityriasis amiantacea refers to a scaling pattern on the scalp where the scales overlap like tiles on a roof. The matted scale is attached to the underlying hair shafts. The condition may be localised and confined to a small patch (Figure 105.3) or widespread involving the entire scalp, creating a skull cap-type appearance of scale and crust. Lifting up the scale often results in hairs coming away, revealing a moist red scalp. Hairs usually regrow if the underlying condition is treated. Some consider pityriasis amiantacea to be a form of severe psoriasis while others consider this a pattern that can be attributable to a range of causes such as seborrhoeic dermatitis, eczema, lichen simplex and psoriasis. It has been described after valproic acid therapy [20], vemurafenib [21] and bone marrow transplant [22].

Pathophysiology

Biopsies from 18 patients were examined by Knight [23]. The most consistent findings were spongiosis, parakeratosis, migration of lymphocytes into the epidermis and a variable degree of acanthosis. The essential features responsible for the scaling are diffuse hyperkeratosis and parakeratosis together with follicular keratosis, which surrounds each hair with a sheath of horn.

Management

Scale should be gently removed as described in the treatment of scalp psoriasis. Attention should then turn to treating the underlying condition, which typically involves the use of topical corticosteroids in an appropriate vehicle.

Contact dermatitis

Introduction and general description
Contact dermatitis of the scalp is an inflammatory condition resulting from an external agent and can be separated into irritant (non-immunogenic) or allergic (immunogenic, typically type IV). The scalp is surprisingly resistant to contact dermatitis and this may be due to either a thickened stratum corneum acting as a barrier or impaired antigen presentation from Langerhans cells. Most contact dermatitis from products used on the scalp present in the surrounding skin, such as the hair line, or on the hands of those that apply them, for example hand dermatitis in hairdressers.

Irritant contact dermatitis
The commonest causes of an irritant dermatitis are bleaches, thioglycolates (permanent waving solutions) and heat (blow drying) (Chapter 128). Shampoos may dry the scalp, but the majority of chemicals are washed off after a short contact period. Irritant dermatitis may present on the scalp with burning, soreness or tightness within a short period of time of the contact. There may be associated redness, oedema and exudation.

Allergic contact dermatitis
Causes include permanent hair dyes, bleaches, permanent waving solutions, hair straighteners and relaxers (Chapter 127). In a retrospective cross-sectional analysis of the North American Contact Dermatitis Group from 1996 to 2016, 4.8% of patients had scalp dermatitis and of those who had scalp and adjacent facial and neck involvement, 59.6% had a primary diagnosis of allergic contact dermatitis. The commonest allergens were p-phenlyenediamine, fragrance mix 1, nickel sulphate and balsam of Peru [24]. Contact allergic dermatitis may be iatrogenic and deliberate, such as with the use of diphencyprone in alopecia areata treatment.

Management
Contact dermatitis should be managed through identification and elimination of the offending contact irritant/allergen and the use of topical corticosteroids during the acute phase. Hair care practices may need to be altered.

Lichen simplex chronicus

Introduction and general description
Lichen simplex chronicus refers to a localised thickening of skin that results from chronic rubbing and scratching. The dermatoglyphics of the skin are often accentuated. The nape of the neck is frequently affected and can mimic psoriasis.

Epidemiology
Lichen simplex chronicus is rare before puberty and has a peak incidence between 30 and 50 years of age, with women being more commonly affected than men.

Pathophysiology
Typical histological features include hyperkeratosis and acanthosis with localised areas of both parakeratosis and spongiosis.

Clinical features
Lichen simplex chronicus can result from any underlying cause of itch that leads to scratching and rubbing. An underlying cause though may not be identified and it falls within the spectrum of neurodermatitis. The main symptom is itch and the most commonly associated diseases at this site are atopic eczema, seborrhoeic dermatitis and psoriasis.

Management
Management of lichen simplex chronicus requires education of the patient so that they have insight into the cause of the problem; any psychological aspect will need to be addressed. Efforts to break the itch–scratch cycle include treatment to manage the itch, which often involves potent or super-potent topical corticosteroids or intralesional corticosteroids. Occlusion of the affected area after the application of corticosteroid may be beneficial but is difficult to achieve on the scalp. Cognitive behavioural therapy, and in particular habit reversal, can be used in motivated subjects.

Radiodermatitis

Introduction and general description
After the discovery of X-rays in 1895 there were a number of applications for their use in the early 20th century in the management of hair-related problems. X-rays were advocated as a treatment for hirsutism and then subsequently as a treatment for scalp ringworm and this continued until the discovery of griseofulvin in 1958, with an estimated 300 000 children treated in this way. Unfortunately, X-rays later were found to induce skin cancers and now their use is limited to the management of malignancy.

Pathophysiology
In chronic radiodermatitis the epidermis becomes atrophic, with a loss of hair follicles and sebaceous glands. Superficial vessels are telangiectactic but deeper vessels may be partially or completed occluded by fibrosis.

Clinical features
Patients may still present many decades after scalp X-ray treatment. Common presentations include the development of a basal cell carcinoma or a localised area of alopecia or finer hairs at the site of treatment. It is not uncommon for patients to refer to previous 'light treatment' for ringworm rather than X-ray therapy. Patients treated with modern radiotherapy for malignancy present with a well-circumscribed patch of cicatricial alopecia. These may be red initially, fading to white in the chronic phase. In chronic radiodermatitis the skin is atrophic. Skin necrosis may occur and skin malignancies can develop years after treatment.

PART 10: SPECIFIC SITES, SEX & AGE

Table 105.1 Causes of secondary cicatricial alopecia.

Autoimmune		Cicatricial pemphigoid	
Inflammatory		Dissecting cellulitis of the scalp	
Degenerative		Follicular mucinosis	
Sclerosing		Morphoea	
		Scleroderma	
		Lichen sclerosus	
		Sclerodermoid porphyria cutanea tarda	
		Chronic graft-versus-host disease	
Granulomatous		Sarcoidosis	
		Necrobiosis lipoidica	
		Granuloma annulare	
Infectious	Bacterial	Folliculitis	
		Carbuncle/furuncle	
	Fungal	Kerion	
		Favus	
		Tinea capitis (rarely scarring)	
	Viral	Shingles	
		Varicella	
		HIV	
	Protozoal	Leishmaniasis	
	Treponemal	Syphilis	
	Mycobacterial	Tuberculosis	
Neoplastic	Benign	Cylindroma	
		Other adnexal tumours	
	Malignant	Primary	Basal cell carcinoma
			Squamous cell carcinoma
			Cutaneous T-cell lymphoma
		Secondary	Renal, breast, lung, gastrointestinal
			Lymphoma, leukaemia
Exogenous insults		Radiodermatitis	
		Mechanical trauma	
		Postoperative (e.g. flap necrosis)	
		Burns	
		Accidental alopecia	
		Dermatitis artefacta	
		Traction alopecia	
		Hot comb alopecia	
Developmental and hereditary		Aplasia cutis	
		Facial hemiatrophy (Romberg syndrome)	
		Epidermal naevi	
		Hair follicle hamartomas	
		Incontinentia pigmenti	
		Focal dermal hypoplasia of Goltz	
		Porokeratosis of Mibelli	
		Ichthyosis	
		Epidermolysis bullosa	
		Polyostotic fibrous dysplasia	
		Conradi–Hünermann syndrome (chondrodysplasia punctata)	

Management
There is no treatment, but localised areas of alopecia, malignancy or necrosis may be amenable to surgical excision.

SECONDARY CICATRICIAL ALOPECIA

In contrast to primary cicatricial alopecia (Chapter 87) where the hair follicle is the primary target of inflammation, secondary

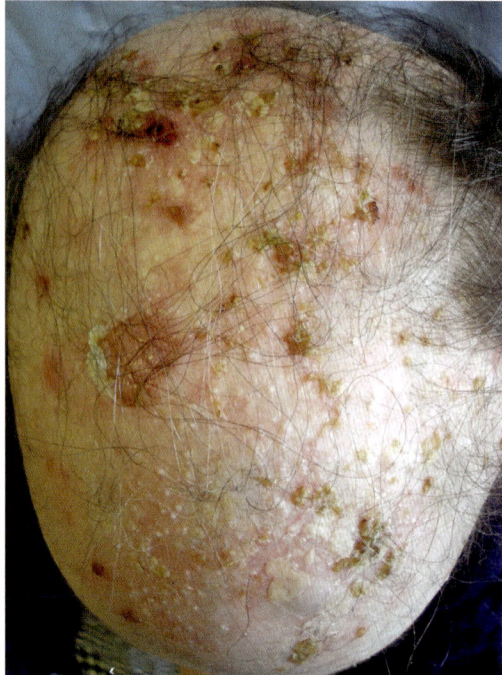

Figure 105.4 Cicatricial pemphigoid.

cicatricial alopecia occurs as a consequence of a separate primary insult. The causes for secondary cicatricial alopecia are listed in Table 105.1.

Cicatricial (mucous membrane) pemphigoid

Introduction and general description
Cicatricial pemphigoid is discussed in Chapter 50. The disease preferentially affects the ocular and/or genital mucous membranes with the skin being involved in 40–50% of cases and lesions may precede the mucosal lesions by months or years. The skin lesions repeatedly recur and leave scars. The favoured sites are the face and upper trunk; the scalp is involved in approximately 10% of cases. Lesions typically present as red plaques, with erosions, milia and cicatricial alopecia (Figure 105.4).

The Brunsting–Perry type originally described by Brunsting and Perry in 1957 is a rare variant of cicatricial pemphigoid, characterised by bullous lesions limited to the head, neck, scalp and upper trunk with mild or no mucosal involvement [25].

Management
Mild to moderate disease may be controlled with super-potent topical steroids. Systemic options may be needed, depending on disease severity, and may be required long term. Treatments include systemic corticosteroids, dapsone, mycophenolate mofetil, azathioprine, cyclophosphamide, rituximab, high-dose intravenous immunoglobulins and immunoadsorption [26].

Dissecting cellulitis of scalp

Synonyms and inclusions
- Dissecting folliculitis
- Perifolliculitis capitis abscedens

Introduction and general description

Dissecting cellulitis/folliculitis of the scalp is a chronic inflammatory condition associated with boggy swellings, superficial abscesses in the dermis, sinus tract formation and extensive secondary scarring hair loss.

The terminology dissecting cellulitis is misleading since this entity is not a cellulitis of infectious origin.

It can be associated with acne conglobata and hidradenitis suppurativa/acne inversa, often referred to as the follicular occlusion triad or tetrad if also associated with pilonidal sinus.

Epidemiology

Dissecting cellulitis of the scalp is rare and occurs predominantly in males aged between 18 and 40 years and is seen most commonly in those with Afro-textured hair. Familial cases are exceptional, as is childhood onset.

Pathophysiology

The aetiology of this inflammatory condition is unknown. Although staphylococci, streptococci and *Pseudomonas* may be cultured from various lesions, no specific causative organism has been isolated.

Pathology [27]

Histology shows a perifollicular inflammation with a heavy infiltrate of lymphocytes, histiocytes and polymorphonuclear cells. Abscess formation results, and leads to destruction of the pilosebaceous follicles initially, and eventually the other cutaneous appendages. Keratin fragments induce a granulomatous reaction, with foreign body giant cells, lymphoid and plasma cells. Special stains for bacteria, fungi and mycobacteria are negative.

Clinical features

Painful, firm, skin-coloured nodules develop near the vertex of the scalp and later become softer and fluctuant (Figure 105.5). Confluent nodules form tubular ridges with an irregular cerebriform pattern, on an inflamed, red and oedematous background. Thin, blood-stained pus exudes from crusted sinuses and pressure on one region of the scalp may cause discharge of pus from a neighbouring intercommunicating ridge. Cervical adenitis is present in some cases but is more remarkable for its absence in many others. Progressive scarring and permanent alopecia occur. Characteristically, hair is lost from the summits of these inflammatory lesions and retained in the valleys. The condition is chronic, with frequent acute exacerbations.

Differential diagnosis

While the clinical features are often distinctive and characteristic, differential diagnoses can include kerion, pyoderma gangrenosum and erosive pustular dermatosis of the scalp.

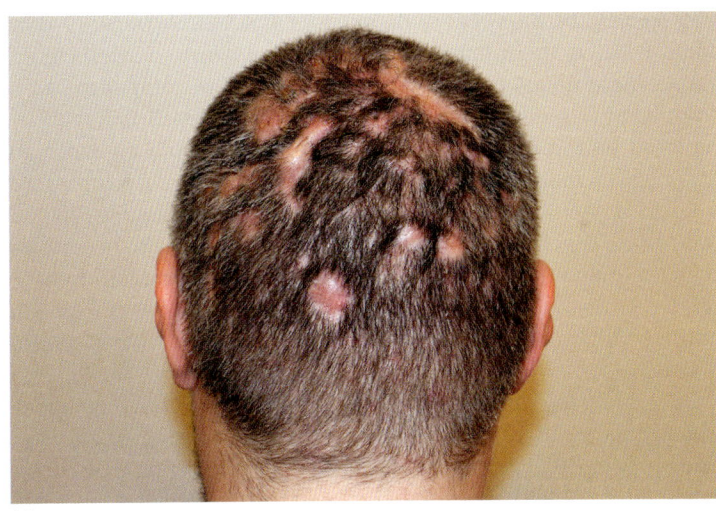

(a)

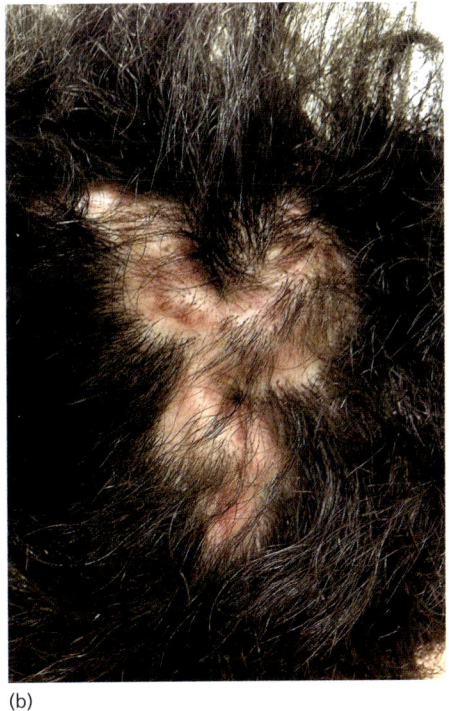

(b)

Figure 105.5 Dissecting cellulitis with diffuse occipital involvement (a) and more localised swellings over the crown (b). (a) Courtesy of Professor Bianca Maria Piraccini and Dr Michela Starace, Department of Experimental, Diagnostic and Specialty Medicine (DIMES), Alma Mater Studiorum University of Bologna, Italy. (b) Courtesy of Dr Leona Yip, Skin Partners Specialist Dermatologist, Brisbane, Australia.

Investigations

Culture from affected areas often grow bacterial organisms. Fungal cultures and a scalp biopsy for routine histology and direct immunofluorescences will exclude other causes of scarring alopecia.

Management

Although systemic antibiotics and topical or intralesional corticosteroids are sometimes helpful, relapses are frequent and the course is usually protracted. Isotretinoin (0.5–1 mg/kg daily), in combination with prednisolone (0.5–1 mg/kg daily) and erythromycin (500 mg four times daily), may induce a rapid remission and significant hair regrowth in areas not yet irreversibly damaged. Because the inflammation is predominantly perifollicular, a surprising amount of regrowth may occur. The antibiotics can be stopped after 4 weeks and the prednisolone gradually tailed off and replaced by topical steroids. The isotretinoin should be continued for at least 6 months and reintroduced if the condition relapses. For mild to moderate cases, alternative or adjuvant therapies include oral zinc. The benefit of isotretinoin in this condition contrasts with the frequent worsening seen with oral isotretinoin in folliculitis decalvans and suggests that these two conditions are distinct entities rather than different points along a spectrum of the same disease.

In recalcitrant cases, antitumour necrosis factor biologic agents, photodynamic therapy or laser therapy can be considered as second line options [28]. Widespread excision and grafting may be considered [29]. In older patients, superficial radiotherapy has been used with success. Intensity-modulated radiation therapy, which uses three-dimensional imaging guided mapping in conjunction with individual radiation beam modulation to tightly focus radiation, allows radiation to shape around the convexity of the scalp avoiding undertreated 'cold spots', overtreated 'hot spots', or excessive radiation exposure to adjacent structures [30].

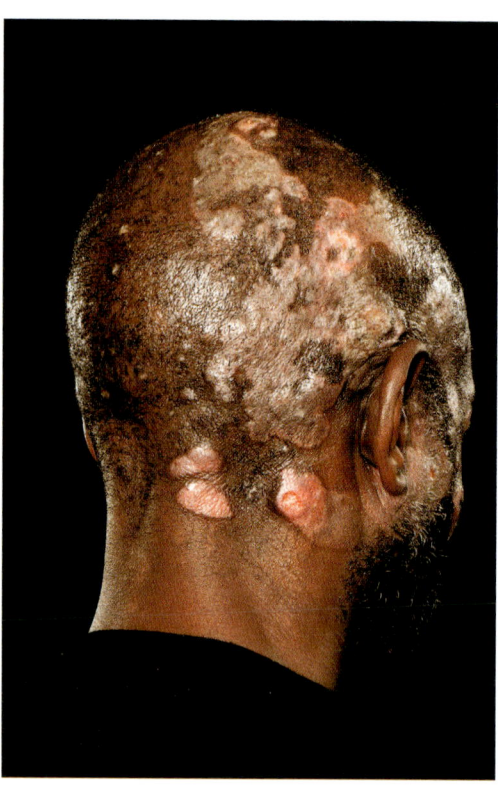

Figure 105.6 Lymphoma-associated follicular mucinosis, showing thickened plaques and associated alopecia.

Follicular mucinosis

Introduction and general description

Follicular mucinosis is a condition that often presents in the scalp with plaques and papules, usually associated with alopecia. While the primary form is idiopathic, the secondary form can be associated with mycosis fungoides [31].

Epidemiology

Follicular mucinosis is a rare condition. Two distinct forms are recognised: the primary form, idiopathic follicular mucinosis, is benign and occurs in children and young adults (10–40 years of age) with a self-limiting course, while the secondary form is lymphoma-associated and occurs in older adults.

Pathophysiology

The histopathological hallmarks of follicular mucinosis are the accumulation of mucin in the outer hair root sheath and sebaceous glands and a perifollicular and periadnexal inflammatory infiltrate, composed of lymphocytes, macrophages and eosinophils, with folliculotropism of the lymphocytes.

Clinical features

Follicular mucinosis is characterised by grouped follicular papules and scaly red plaques, usually located on the head and neck, resulting in alopecia showing patulous follicular openings (Figure 105.6). Sometimes the follicles are studded with horny plugs and some lesions may ulcerate. Hair loss does not always occur and for this reason the name follicular mucinosis is preferred to the original name 'alopecia mucinosis'. Linear lesions following Blaschko lines have been described.

Management

Many cases spontaneously improve. Topical or intralesional steroids are generally effective. Superficial radiotherapy and phototherapy are effective in treating follicular mucinosis secondary to mycosis fungoides. Hydroxychloroquine has been reported as a successful treatment inducing rapid remission and hair regrowth in idiopathic follicular mucinosis. Widespread pruritic lesions may benefit from low-dose systemic steroids or occasionally dapsone. Other anecdotal therapies include retinoids, minocycline, pimecrolimus and methotrexate.

Sclerosing conditions

Introduction and general description

Morphoea (Chapter 55) is a distinct autoimmune connective tissue disorder that can affect the scalp and produce localised areas of cicatricial alopecia. In early lesions of scalp morphoea, the centrifugally expanding lilac border is often obscured by hair. Well-established plaques of morphoea are white, smooth and hairless. Hair loss tends to be permanent. Lesional skin is thickened and indurated; as well as pallor there may be marginal hyperpigmentation. The lesions may be single or multiple.

Linear morphoea on the frontal scalp, also known as 'en coup de sabre', is the most frequent subtype in children. It is the most common clinical variant of scalp morphea. It is characterised by a

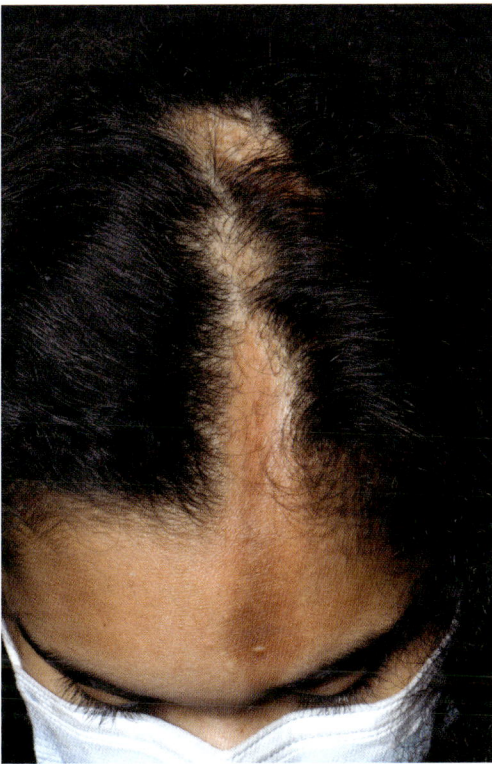

Figure 105.7 Linear morphoea (en coup de sabre).

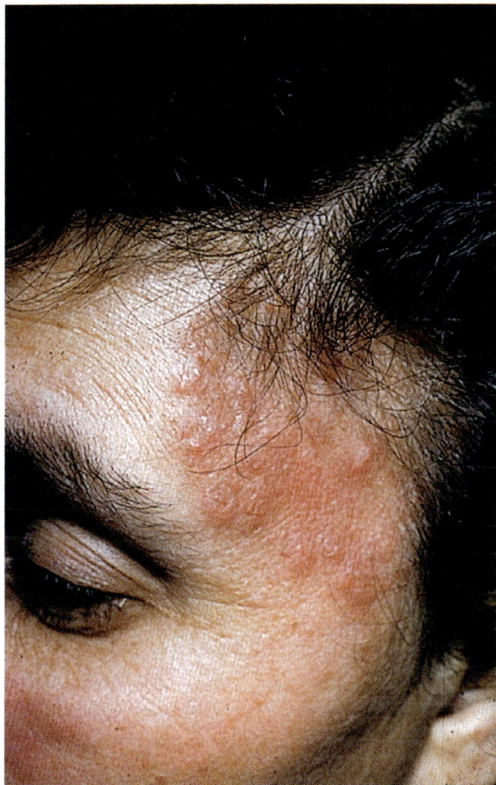

Figure 105.8 Sarcoidosis of the frontal hairline and forehead.

slowly progressive non-inflammatory linear alopecia (Figure 105.7). It has been suggested that lesions may follow the lines of Blaschko. The line of morphoea may extend inferiorly into the cheek, nose or upper lip. Rarely it may involve the mouth and tongue. A variety of neurological symptoms have been reported, which most commonly include seizures and headaches. In addition, computed tomography (CT) and magnetic resonance imaging (MRI) can reveal intracranial abnormalities, even in asymptomatic patients [32].

Histological examination shows chronic inflammation of the upper and mid-follicle and prominent fibrosis. Collagen bundles are densely packed in the reticular dermis, while eccrine glands appear atrophic [33]. A lymphocytic perineural infiltrate is a helpful histopathological feature [34].

The sclerodermatous phase of chronic graft-versus-host disease may involve the scalp to produce a cicatricial alopecia. Porphyria cutanea tarda may also produce scleroderma on the scalp.

Management
Potent topical steroids such as clobetasol propionate or intralesional triamcinolone may help, but systemic therapy incorporating methotrexate with or without oral corticosteroids is often required to stop progress. Mycophenolate mofetil, hydroxychloroquine and phototherapy have been used with varying success [35]. Surgical excision may provide definitive treatment, although recurrences occur, especially if the lesion is enlarging at the time of excision. Successful hair transplantation in linear morphoea has been described [36].

Granulomatous conditions

Introduction and general description
Distinguishing between necrobiosis lipoidica, granuloma annulare and sarcoidosis can be difficult on clinical grounds alone. Both granuloma annulare and necrobiosis lipoidica have been described affecting the scalp but are uncommon presentations of these diseases. Lesions typically present as annular, red or yellow plaques, with or without atrophy and telangiectasia, and often involve the forehead and frontal scalp.

Sarcoidosis is an idiopathic multisystem inflammatory non-necrotising granulomatous condition that has a highly variable presentation. It is more common in African and mixed-race individuals. The pattern of scalp involvement can range from annular plaques to infiltrated papules, nodules, scaly plaques and scarring alopecia (Figure 105.8). The age range of patients is between 30 and 60 years with males and females equally affected in the majority of cases. It is important to examine the rest of the skin since scalp involvement is commonly associated with cutaneous sarcoidosis [37].

Management
Treatment for sarcoidosis includes topical, intralesional or systemic corticosteroids, antimalarials, methotrexate and tetracycline antibiotics. Infliximab has been found to be beneficial in recalcitrant scalp sarcoidosis [38].

PART 10: SPECIFIC SITES, SEX & AGE

THICKENED SCALP DISORDERS

Cutis verticis gyrata

Introduction and general description

Cutis verticis gyrata (CVG) is a rare morphological syndrome characterised by hypertrophy and folding of the scalp skin, producing a gyrate or cerebriform appearance. In CVG there is overgrowth of the scalp in relation to the underlying skull. The diagnosis of CVG is based on clinical findings. CT and MRI scans may reveal a range of scalp lesions, as well as additional abnormalities in the head [39].

CVG is classified into primary and secondary forms. The primary forms are subdivided into primary essential CVG, where there are no associated features, and primary non-essential CVG, which is associated with a wide range of psychiatric, cerebral and ophthalmological abnormalities.

Primary CVG

Primary CVG is extremely rare and the aetiology remains unknown. Most cases appear to be sporadic, although familial forms have been reported in the context of complex syndromes. The skin changes typically develop after puberty and usually before 30 years of age. It is more common in men, with a male to female ratio of 5 : 1.

There is a strong association with learning difficulties [40]. Akesson found 47 cases (3.4%) of CVG in institutionalised subjects in Sweden, and CVG was observed in 22 out of 494 (4.5%) patients in an Italian psychiatric institution [41]. Cytogenetic analyses in the latter study showed chromosome fragile sites in nine subjects (chromosomes 9, 12 and X).

Secondary CVG

Secondary CVG is more common and often occurs as a response to multiple inflammatory or neoplastic processes. Congenital melanocytic naevi appear to be the most common but other naevoid abnormalities, such as naevus lipomatosus and connective tissue naevi, and acquired lesions such as neurofibroma may also cause CVG. CVG has been described in association with a variety of endocrine and genetic disorders, including acromegaly, myxedema, insulin resistance, Turner syndrome and eczema. The age of onset is more variable than in primary CVG and, in the naevoid forms, it may be present at birth.

Clinical features

CVG typically affects the vertex and occipital scalp but it may involve the entire scalp (Figure 105.9). The folds are usually arranged in an anteroposterior direction but may be transverse over the occiput. Hair density may be reduced over the convexities of the folds.

Differential diagnosis

The differential diagnosis includes pachydermoperiostosis (Chapter 155) and 'lumpy scalp syndrome'. The former is genetically determined and occurs mainly in men. It differs from CVG in several ways: (i) the scalp is folded but the skin of the face, hands and feet is also affected; (ii) the cutaneous changes are accompanied

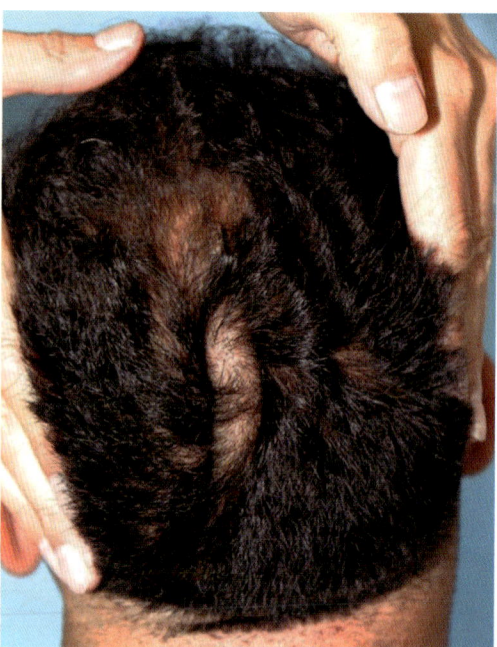

Figure 105.9 Cutis verticis gyrata. Courtesy of Mr Greg Williams FRCS (Plast), Hair Transplant Surgeon, Farjo Hair Institute.

by thickening of the phalanges and long bones of the limbs; and (iii) skin involvement progresses for 10–15 years, and then becomes static.

Management

Investigations are aimed at identifying the underlying causes. These may include neurological, endocrine, ophthalmological and cytogenetic studies. In early-onset CVG, a biopsy is advisable to identify those cases caused by a structural lesion, such as a melanocytic naevus. In the majority of cases, treatment is symptomatic. Patients should be educated in scalp hygiene to avoid accumulation of skin debris and secretions in the furrows. Surgical correction with skin expansion can be helpful in selected cases [42].

Lipoedematous alopecia

Introduction and general description

Lipoedematous alopecia is a rare, non-scarring symptomatic alopecia characterised by an increasing thickness of the subcutaneous layer of the scalp and inability to grow hair longer than 2 cm [43]. The condition more commonly occurs in women (Figure 105.10). The hormone leptin, which regulates the distribution of adipose tissue, has been postulated as playing a role in causing hyperplasia of the subcutaneous fat [44].

The pathogenesis remains unclear. The fundamental pathological finding consists of an approximate doubling in scalp thickness resulting from expansion of the subcutaneous fat layer. There is associated atrophy and fibrous replacement of many hair follicles. Light and electron microscopy suggests that the increase in scalp thickness is caused by localised oedema, with disruption and degeneration of adipose tissue. In addition to thickening of the adipose tissue layer, dermal oedema, lymphatic dilatation and

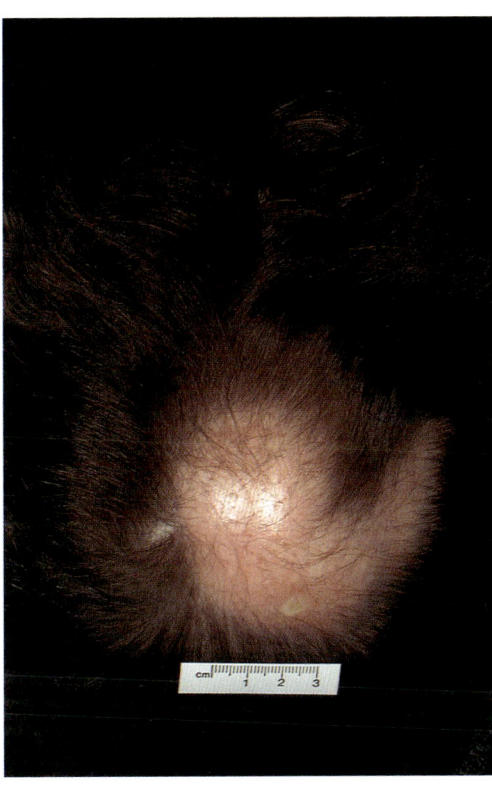

Figure 105.10 Lipoedematous alopecia. Courtesy of Dr Leona Yip, Skin Partners Specialist Dermatologist, Brisbane, Australia.

elastic fibre fragmentation are frequently seen which may suggest that the primary pathology is related to abnormal lymphatics [45] and lymphatic dilatation may be the mechanism of hair loss [46]. Mucin is not seen [47].

Management
Surgical debulking with scalp reduction has been described as a technique for managing a localised case [48]. Mycophenolate mofetil has also been described as a potential treatment, with a patient experiencing complete recovery of their hair [49].

TUMOURS OF THE SCALP

The scalp is a common location of tumours of the skin and these can be broadly categorised as benign, malignant or metastatic. Benign and malignant tumours can arise from the epidermis, the pilosebaceous unit or adnexal structures. Due to chronic sun exposure the scalp is a common site of squamous cell carcinoma, basal cell carcinoma, lentigo maligna, desmoplastic melanoma and angiosarcoma. Only tumours that have a particular predilection for the scalp are mentioned here.

Sebaceous naevus

Sebaceous naevus represents a common congenital hamartoma that presents as an orange-yellow hairless patch most commonly located on the scalp (Chapter 73). They may be present at birth or may become more obvious through childhood and adolescence. From puberty it is common for the patch to become thickened and more verrucous in nature. The development of basal cell carcinomas and other adnexal tumours has been described and for that reason some dermatologists advocate surgical removal of sebaceous naevi as a preventative measure. In a large retrospective study of 706 patients, the most common tumours found within a sebaceous naevus were trichoblastoma (7.4%) and syringocystadenoma papilliferum (5.2%). Malignant tumours were only found in 2.5% of cases (basal cell carcinomas 1.1% and squamous cell carcinomas 0.6%) and these did not occur in childhood, inferring that any removal can be planned for adolescence or adulthood [50]. Surgical techniques include primary excision with local tissue undermining and galeal scoring for small lesions, and rotation or transposition flaps, serial excisions and tissue expansion and excision for large lesions. However, over a third of patients experienced a poor outcome, even with small lesions [51].

Syringocystadenoma papilliferum

Syringocystadenoma papilliferum is a rare, benign, adnexal tumour of the apocrine or eccrine sweat ducts, which typically presents as a solitary, pink, dome-shaped nodule on the scalp (Chapter 137). It may occur in association with a sebaceous naevus. They are usually present from birth or infancy. Malignant change has been described, heralded by ulceration, bleeding and rapid enlargement. Surgical excision is recommended as a preventative measure.

Tumours of the pilosebaceous unit

Trichoepitheliomas
Trichoepitheliomas are firm, red nodules that commonly occur on the scalp (Chapter 136). Trichoepitheliomas can be solitary but typically multiple lesions coexist and can cover a large area of the scalp, which has led to the term 'turban tumour'. They are benign tumours, but they grow slowly and can cause considerable cosmetic issues. Trichoepitheliomas can be surgically excised.

Trichilemmal cysts
Trichilemmal cysts arise from the outer root sheath of the hair follicle (Chapter 132). Ninety per cent of trichilemmal cysts are located on the scalp due to the increased density of follicles. While lesions may be solitary, it is common for patients to have multiple lesions. Cysts can be surgically excised if treatment is required.

Scalp metastases

The scalp is a common site for cutaneous metastases, accounting for 12% of all skin metastases (Chapter 148). They usually present as a single, smooth, bald nodule in the scalp and are often initially

PART 10: SPECIFIC SITES, SEX & AGE

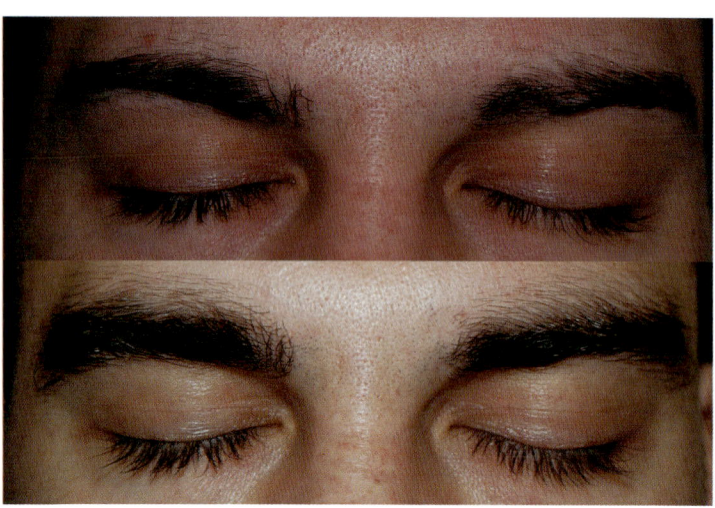

Figure 105.11 Typical patchy 'moth-eaten' appearance of syphilis of the eyebrows (a) and full regrowth after treatment (b). Courtesy of Dr Michela Starace and Professor Bianca Maria Piraccini, Department of Experimental, Diagnostic and Specialty Medicine (DIMES), Alma Mater Studiorum University of Bologna, Italy.

misdiagnosed as a benign cyst. Occasionally, they may be the first sign of an underlying malignancy. The primary tumour is commonly located in the lung, stomach, colon or kidney [52].

INFECTIONS OF THE SCALP

The scalp is a common site of skin infection and infestation. Hair loss can be a feature of this. Tinea capitis (Chapter 32), infestations (Chapter 34) and bacterial infections (Chapter 26) are discussed elsewhere.

Syphilis

Hair loss occurs in approximately 2.9–7% of cases of secondary syphilis and may be the presenting feature [53–55] (Chapter 29). The hair loss typically has a 'moth-eaten' appearance (Figure 105.11), but may be diffuse in nature [56]. Other features of secondary syphilis are present in most cases, particularly lymph node enlargement and hepatomegaly, but hair loss has been reported as the only sign of the disease [56]. Li *et al.* describe a rare case of nodular secondary syphilis that presented with multiple nodules on the scalp, resembling Rosai–Dorfman disease or cutaneous malignant metastasis [57].

Trichoscopy of 'moth-eaten' secondary syphilis shows that alopecia is mainly due to a reduction in the number of terminal hairs [58]. Trichoscopy of this presentation can also show black dots, focal atrichia, hypopigmentation of hair shaft and yellow dots [59].

Histological features include an increase in catagen and telogen hairs, and a peribulbar lymphocytic infiltrate, similar to the changes seen in alopecia areata [55]. Additional features in syphilis include lymphocytic infiltration of the isthmus region, parabulbar lymphoid aggregates and the presence of plasma cells within the infiltrate. Despite appropriate stains, *Treponema pallidum* is not usually seen. The alopecia is non-scarring and sometimes affects other hair-bearing areas [53,60]. The alopecia usually resolves within 3 months of appropriate treatment for syphilis [53].

The serpiginous nodulosquamous syphilide of tertiary syphilis may also affect the scalp. The syphilitic gumma is a cause of scarring alopecia.

Human immunodeficiency virus

A variety of alterations in hair growth have been described in patients with HIV infection (Chapter 31). Telogen effluvium is common; causes include chronic HIV-1 infection itself, secondary infections, nutritional deficiencies and drugs [61]. Hair loss on the body as well as the scalp has been reported with several antiretroviral drugs, particularly indinavir [62] and other protease inhibitors. In one case, a 62-year-old man with HIV infection experienced alopecia totalis 18 months after initiating antiretroviral treatment, which included iopinavir/ritonavir. The alopecia reversed completely 2 months after stopping iopinavir/ritonavir [63]. A review of the literature evaluating antiretroviral-related alopecia showed that the protease inhibitor class, in particular indinavir, was most commonly reported to cause hair loss, followed by the nucleoside reverse-transcriptase inhibitor, lamivudine. The majority of cases presented with alopecia of the scalp alone, with a median time of onset of 2.5 months. Management involved discontinuing the drug in most cases, with at least partial reversal in half the cases [64]. Case reports have implicated abacavir and tenofovir alafenamide in the development of alopecia [65,66].

There are also reports of alopecia areata occurring in patients with HIV infection [67–70]. Conversely, Ramot *et al.* describe the remission of longstanding alopecia universalis after HIV infection [71].

Tinea capitis, psoriasis and seborrhoeic dermatitis are all more common in patients with HIV infection. Straightening of the hair is a common feature of HIV infection in black patients [72]. Various forms of folliculitis are seen in HIV infection, including acneiform eruptions, staphylococcal folliculitis and eosinophilic pustular folliculitis.

PUSTULAR CONDITIONS OF THE SCALP

There are a large number of conditions that can present with pustules on the scalp. These vary from conditions where the pustules are isolated findings without hair loss, to those that are associated with localised cicatricial alopecia. Figure 105.12 shows a clinical diagnostic approach to pustules in the scalp.

Pustular conditions associated with cicatricial alopecia are discussed in Chapter 87.

Other conditions are also covered elsewhere in this book:
- Scalp folliculitis: Chapter 91.
- Pseudofolliculitis barbae: Chapter 91.
- Necrotising lymphocytic folliculitis of the scalp margin (acne varioliformis): Chapter 91.

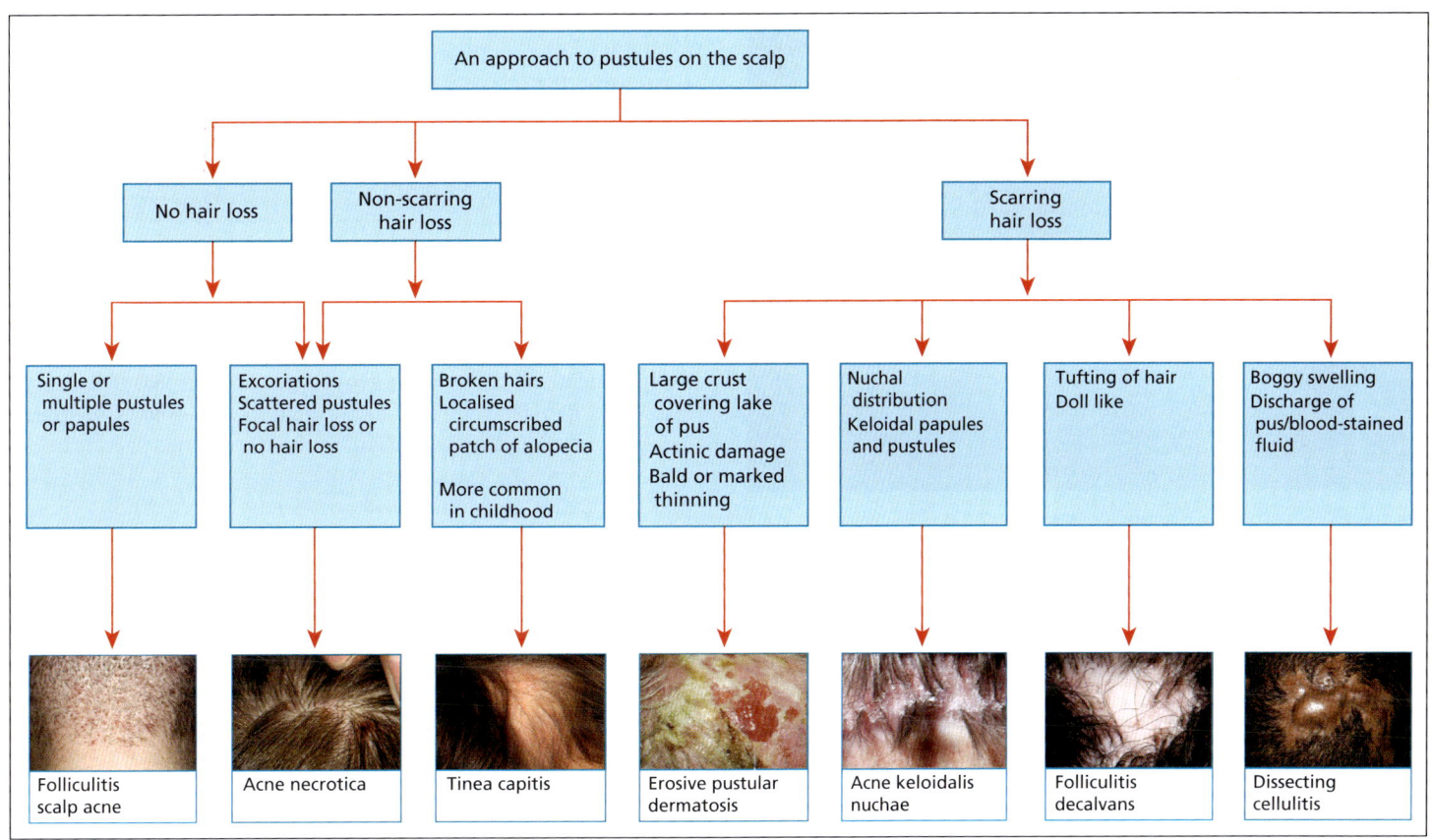

Figure 105.12 An approach to diagnosing pustules in the scalp.

- Dissecting cellulitis/perifolliculitis capitis abscedens et suffodiens: see under secondary cicatricial alopecias earlier in this chapter.
- Folliculitis keloidalis/acne keloidalis nuchae: Chapter 91.
- Folliculitis decalvans: Chapter 87.

Erosive pustular dermatosis of the scalp

Introduction and general description

Erosive pustular dermatosis of the scalp (EPDS) is an increasingly recognised type of scarring alopecia, predominantly affecting the elderly, that was first described by Pye *et al.* in 1979 [73]. While original reports detailed a female preponderance, more modern series have shown it to be more common in men [74].

It presents with a thick crust overlying erosions, granulation tissue and pus with associated scarring alopecia. It is commonly associated with androgenetic alopecia and actinic damage of the scalp. It has a chronic course, often spreading outwards.

Pathophysiology

The exact pathogenesis of EPDS remains unknown. It is commonly associated with androgenetic alopecia and actinic damage of the scalp and is usually preceded by trauma. Surgery, curettage, cryotherapy, photodynamic therapy, treatment of actinic damage

with imiquimod or ingenol mebutate, topical minoxidil and EGFR inhibitors have all been associated with triggering the condition. It has also followed herpes zoster infection. It is considered an aberrant wound healing response and has been associated with increased expression of matrix metalloproteinase 3 (MMP-3) in the non-healing skin. The lack of follicles, which normally have a wound healing role in the skin, altered immunity due to UV light or age, and atrophy and altered blood flow may all have a negative impact on the ability of the skin to heal itself [75]. It has also been postulated that autoimmunity could play a role, with the follicle being a target after initial trauma.

Pathology

The histological features of EPDS depend on the stage of the disease and whether there is hair or not. Early-stage disease is characterised by orthokeratosis, psoriasiform hyperplasia and a slight mixed inflammatory infiltrate, consisting of neutrophils, lymphocytes, plasma cells and mild fibrosis. More intermediate-stage disease shows greater fibrosis at the level of the isthmus and loss of sebaceous glands. Late disease shows an absence of follicles and diffuse and severe fibrosis. Miniaturised anagen follicles and shift to catagen are common, which is unsurprising given the association with androgenetic alopecia [76].

In patients who had biopsies from hair-bearing scalp, a dense neutrophilic and lymphocytic infiltrate was noted around the infundibula of terminal hair follicles, with prominent infundibular spongiosis and focal or total disruption of the follicle wall. Spongiform pustules were also present. These findings led authors to

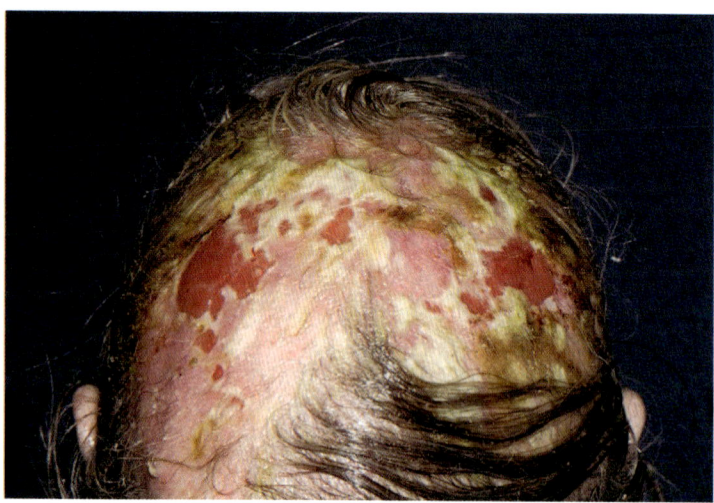

Figure 105.13 Erosive pustular dermatosis of the scalp.

postulate it should be considered a neutrophilic dermatosis with pathergy features similar to pustular pyoderma gangrenosum [74].

Clinical features

The characteristic clinical finding is crust overlying the scalp with underlying sterile pus sitting above a moist eroded scalp surface (Figure 105.13). It is commonly associated with androgenetic alopecia, miniaturised hairs and decreased hair density or baldness. Actinic damage of the scalp is very common and the condition may coexist with actinic keratoses. The vertex is the most common site, followed by the frontal, parietal and temporal regions. Scalp atrophy and scarring are often evident [76].

Due to marked skin atrophy, trichoscopic features include the absence of follicular ostia and the visualisation of both dermal vessels and hair bulbs [76].

Differential diagnosis

Pyogenic and yeast infection is excluded by bacteriological examination and the lack of response to antibacterial or antifungal agents. Biopsy may be necessary to exclude pustular psoriasis, cicatricial pemphigoid, 'irritated' solar keratosis or squamous cell carcinoma.

In one case series review of 30 patients, the most common clinical diagnosis at point of biopsy were squamous cell carcinoma (13), basal cell carcinoma (3), actinic keratosis (5) and autoimmune bullous disease (3). EPDS was only offered as a diagnosis in 3 patients. The final diagnosis was reached after careful exclusion based on histology, direct immunofluorescence and microbiological analysis [74].

Management

There is limited evidence from multiple case series to support the use of super-potent and potent topical steroids, with or without oral zinc, followed by maintenance with topical calcineurin inhibitors. Tacrolimus 0.1% has the advantage of not causing further atrophy of the scalp. There are studies that support the use of topical photodynamic therapy but this modality has also been associated with triggering the condition [77]. In cases induced by EGFR inhibitors, withdrawal or tapering of the drugs led to improvement [78]. In resistant cases, oral corticosteroids have been reported as

being efficacious and should be considered first line over other modalities like oral antibiotics. There are also positive reports supporting the use of systemic retinoids and ciclosporin [78].

OTHER CONDITIONS OF THE SCALP

Scalp pruritus

Introduction and general description of scalp pruritis

Scalp pruritus is a common symptom (Chapter 81). Pruritus, also known as itch, is an unpleasant sensation that evokes the desire to scratch [79]. An additional term, trichokinesis, has been introduced to describe itching sensations which increase by touching the hair [80]. It can be associated with a variety of conditions including dermatological, neurological and psychogenic diseases, as well as being a manifestation of a systemic problem, or being iatrogenically induced [81]. Scalp itch is distressing and causes significant morbidity. Often it can appear without any noticeable skin pathology. It can be both diagnostically and therapeutically challenging.

Epidemiology
Incidence and prevalence

Although scalp itch is recognised as common, there is a lack of information published on its incidence and prevalence [82]. In an epidemiological study conducted in a representative sample of the French population, 44% declared suffering from a 'sensitive scalp'. Of these subjects 25% complained of an itching sensation [83]. In 75 patients with generalised idiopathic pruritus without eruption, 14% described involvement of the scalp [84]. A large epidemiological study on the prevalence of chronic pruritus involving 2540 people found that 44.6% of subjects have scalp pruritus [85].

Age, sex and ethnicity

In a French study population who had a 'sensitive itchy scalp', differences were noted according to age: 31% were under 35 years old, 27% 35–50 years old and 42% over 50 years old. Women suffered more frequently from a sensitive scalp than men [83]. In 75 patients from Singapore with generalised idiopathic pruritus, there was no difference in sex or race affected. The mean age of those affected was 52 years. A cross-sectional study of 302 geriatric patients revealed a 28% prevalence of pruritus on the scalp area [86]. A cross-sectional study, designed to evaluate the prevalence of and risk factors for scalp pruritus in a general dermatology population, reports an overall prevalence of scalp pruritus of 25.3%. After adjustment for confounders, black participants had a more than twofold increased odds of scalp pruritus (odds ratio 2.13; 95% CI, 1.10–4.13) [87].

Associated diseases

Scalp pruritus can be associated with a variety of conditions. These include dermatological disease, systemic disease, neurological disease and psychiatric/psychosomatic diseases (Table 105.2) [79,84,88]. Vázquez-Herrera *et al.* propose a simple acronym (SCALLP) in order to easily recall the most common causes of scalp itch [89]:

Table 105.2 Diseases associated with scalp pruritus. Adapted from Ständer *et al.* [79], Goon *et al.* [84] and Rattanakaemakorn and Suchonwanit [**88**].

Type	Examples
Dermatological	Seborrhoeic dermatitis
	Psoriasis
	Urticaria
	Atopic eczema and lichen simplex chronicus
	Allergic contact dermatitis
	Alopecia areata
	Lichen planopilaris
	Central centrifugal cicatricial alopecia
	Discoid lupus erythematosus
	Dermatitis herpetiformis
	Acne necrotica
	Folliculitis decalvans
	Scalp folliculitis
	Infection and infestation
	Red scalp disease
	Bullous pemphigoid
	Dermatitis herpetiformis
Systemic	Chronic renal failure
	Cholestatic liver disease
	Haematological malignancy, e.g lymphoma or leukaemia
	Drug-induced pruritus
	Thyroid dysfunction
	Dermatomyositis
	Diabetes mellitus
Neurological (diseases or disorders of the central or peripheral nervous system)	Diabetic neuropathy
	Postherpetic neuralgia
	Migraine
	Atypical facial neuralgia
	Scalp dysaesthesia
	Brain and spinal cord injury
	Wallenberg syndrome
	Brain tumour
	Narrowing of the bony foramina from osteoarthritis
Psychogenic/psychosomatic	Anxiety disorders
	Delusional parasitosis
	Depression
	Obsessive compulsive disorders
	Schizophrenia
	Somatoform and dissociative disorders
	Tactile hallucinations

- Seborrhoeic dermatitis
- Contact dermatitis
- Anxiety
- Lichen planopilaris
- Lice
- Psoriasis

Pathophysiology

The scalp is unique in its innervation, vasculature and embryonic origin. The scalp is the most densely innervated peripheral organ in the body. Taken together with hair follicles, which are richly innervated, and a dense dermal scalp vasculature, these neuroanatomical features alone could account for the intensity of scalp itch [90]. However, numerous different cells and mediators in the scalp are thought to be involved in scalp itch. Figure 105.14 demonstrates the itch mediators that have been demonstrated in the scalp and where they have been found.

Mast cells release histamine, which induces pruritus via the H1 and H4 receptors on nerve fibres. Proteinase-activating receptor 2 (PAR-2) mediates chronic pruritus via calcitonin gene-related peptide (CGRP) and substance P. Exogenous activators of PAR-2 include serine proteases generated by bacteria, fungi and house dust mite. Transient receptor potential vanilloid type 1 receptor (TRPV1) can be activated by capsaicin, heat, acidosis and endogenous endovanilloids. Mas-related G-protein-coupled receptor (Mrgpr) can be activated directly by peptides with common C-terminal motifs. The endogenous opioid system includes three opioid receptors: mu (MOR), delta (DOR) and kappa (KOR), and the opioid peptides enkephalins, endorphins, dynorphins and endomorphins. KOR signalling suppresses itch while MOR signalling stimulates itch. Activation of cannabinoid receptors CB1 and CB2 leads to the inhibition of pruritus. Substance P binds with high affinity to the neurokinin-1 receptor (NK1R) on keratinocytes, endothelial cells and mast cells. Degranulation of mast cells releases pruritogenic pro-inflammatory cytokines. CGRP promotes itch on release after C-fibre activity. Four members of the neurotrophin (NT) family are involved in the pathogenesis of itch: NGF, BDNF, NT-3 and NT-4. Gastrin-related peptide receptor (GRPR) is activated by histamine-independent mechanisms. Endothelin-1 (ET-1) evokes pruritus in humans and animals. Interleukins (ILs) are implicated in the pathogenesis of pruritis including IL-2, IL-31 and IL-8 [**82**].

Mast cells are thought to be a key itch conductor in psoriatic scalp itch due to their ability to trigger neurogenic inflammation, activate the skin HPA-axis, process, integrate and orchestrate itch through mast cell interactions with hair follicles [90].

A study of patients with seborrheic dermatitis has shown an increase in cathepsin S levels in patients with dandruff/seborrheic dermatitis. Cathepsin S, pruritus and clinical severity were found to be well correlated. Cathepsin S is a cysteine protease which is selectively upregulated in human keratinocytes under stimulation by gamma interferon, suggesting a role in inflammatory skin diseases. The trigger of the increased expression of cathepsin S and the links between cathepsin S and itching remain to be determined [91].

Scalp pruritus can be a feature of dermatomyositis. A group from the University of Minnesota describe their discovery of a small-fibre neuropathy of the scalp in a patient with dermatomyositis and chronic, severe scalp pruritus. These findings may lead to new areas of research in the pathogenesis and therapy of scalp pruritus [92].

Bin Saif *et al.* propose that the non-itchy scalp demonstrates a significant insensitivity of small C nerve fibres of the scalp to thermal, heat pain, itch and neurogenic inflammation similar to that noted in significant neuropathies. They suggest that the scalp has an aberrant response of small C nerve fibres which makes the scalp a unique body site in somatosensation disorders [93].

Causative organisms

Malassezia species are found in high concentrations on the scalp. In normal conditions, *Malassezia* yeast reduces the production of pro-inflammatory cytokines by keratinocytes. This is related to the presence of a lipid-rich microfibrillar layer surrounding yeast cells. A high quantity of lipid may prevent the yeast cell from

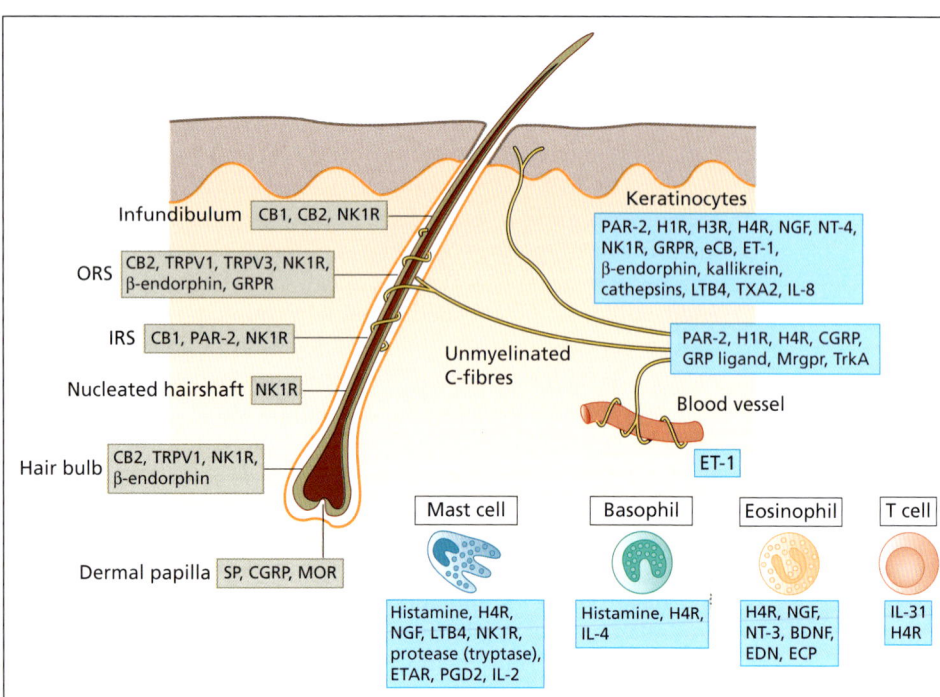

Figure 105.14 Cutaneous sensory receptors and mediators involved in the itchy scalp. BDNF, brain-derived neurotropic factor; CB, cannabinoid receptor; CGRP, calcitonin gene-related peptide; eCB, endogenous cannabinoids; ECP, eosinophil cationic protein; EDN, eosinophil-derived neurotoxin; ET-1, endothelin-1; ETAR, endothelin receptor A; GRP, gastrin-related peptide; GRPR, gastrin-related peptide receptor; H1R, histamine 1 receptor; H3R, histamine 3 receptor; H4R, histamine 4 receptor; IL, interleukin; IRS, inner root sheath; LTB4, leukotriene B4; MOR, mu opioid receptor; Mrgpr, Mas-related G-protein-coupled receptor; NGF, nerve growth factor; NK1R, neurokinin-1 receptor; NT, neurotrophin; ORS, outer root sheath; PAR-2, proteinase-activating receptor 2; PGD2, prostaglandin D2; SP, substance P; TrkA, high-affinity NGF receptor; TRPV, transient receptor potential vanilloid; TXA2, thromboxane A2. Adapted from Bin Saif *et al.* [82].

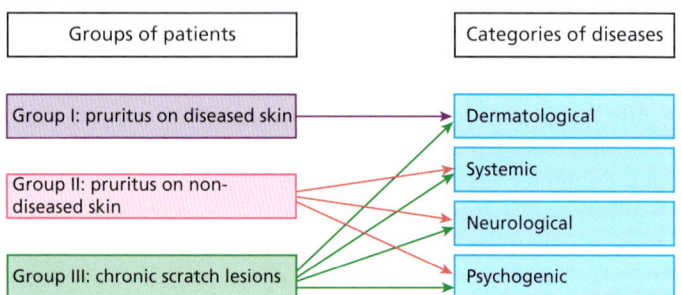

Figure 105.15 Clinical classification of scalp pruritus. Adapted from Ständer *et al.* [79].

Table 105.3 Investigation of scalp itch. Adapted from Ständer *et al.* [79] and Rattanakaemakorn and Suchonwanit [88].

Classification	Investigations
Pruritus on diseased skin	Microscopy and culture
	Skin biopsy for histology/immunofluorescence
Pruritus on non-diseased skin	Guided by medical history but may include:
	Full blood count
	Urea and electrolytes
	Thyroid function
	Liver function
	Ferritin
Pruritus with chronic scratch lesions	Often requires a combination of investigations for both pruritus on diseased skin and pruritus on non-diseased skin, e.g. biopsy and laboratory investigation

inducing inflammation, whereas low lipid content may induce inflammation [94,95]. This may explain the aetiology of seborrhoeic dermatitis itch.

Staphylococcus aureus may also induce itch. Staphylococcal endotoxins lead to IL-31 expression, a known mediator of itch. *Staphylococcus* can also mediate serine protease expression through PAR-2 receptor, which could explain why scalp folliculitis is itchy.

Clinical features

Pruritus is defined as an unpleasant sensation of the skin leading to the desire to scratch. This can be described as acute or chronic; the latter is defined as pruritus lasting 6 or more weeks.

Pruritus of the scalp can be classified as that occurring on apparently normal skin, on diseased skin or on scratch-evoked lesions (Figure 105.15).

Chronic pruritus can lead to scratching, rubbing and pinching. Scratching may induce skin damage such as excoriation, crusting, lichenification and excoriated papules and nodules. Lesions may coexist in different stages and secondary infection may occur. Lesions may resolve leaving atrophic, hyper- or hypopigmented scars.

The course and prognosis of scalp pruritus are dependent on the cause. Treatment of the underlying cause of pruritus should result in resolution. Chronic pruritus with no identifiable aetiology is more of a challenge and may persist for years, despite supportive treatment.

Investigations

Grouping pruritus as that occurring on apparently normal skin, on diseased skin or on scratch-evoked lesions can aid selection of the most appropriate investigation (Table 105.3).

Management

If there is evidence of a scalp dermatosis causing itch then that disorder should be treated. Principal topical medications used for the treatment of scalp pruritus include emollients (including oils, e.g.

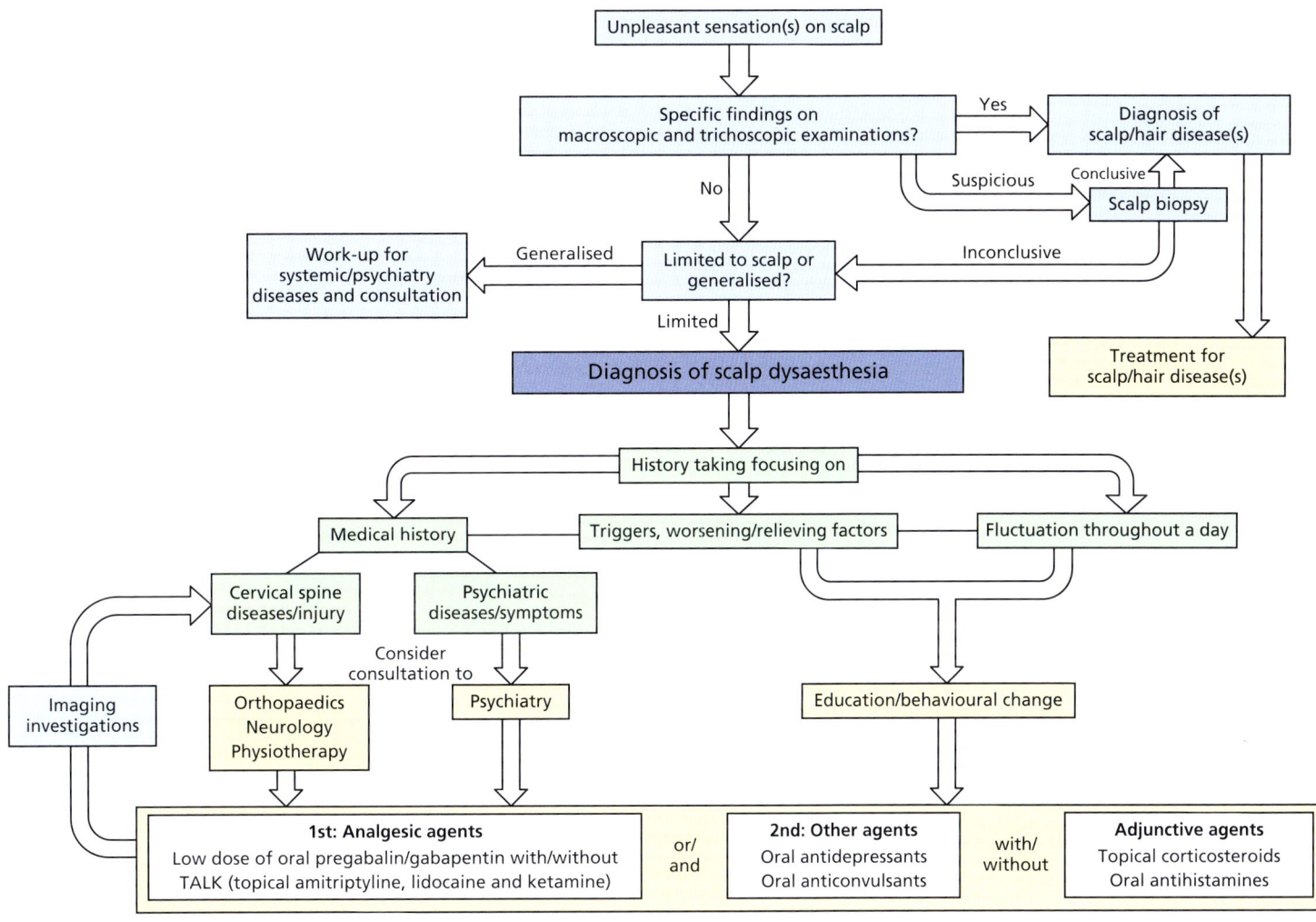

Figure 105.16 Proposal of diagnostic and therapeutic algorithm to manage scalp dysaesthesia. The process of investigations (blue boxes), history taking of associated factors (green boxes) and treatment approaches (yellow boxes) are demonstrated. Adapted from Lancer *et al.* [4].

coconut, olive or arachis), glucocorticoids, calcineurin inhibitors, menthol, capsaicin and shampoos with anti-inflammatory effects (coal tar, selenium sulphide, ketoconazole and shampoos containing zinc pyrithione).

Principal systemic medications utilised for scalp pruritus include antihistamines, anticonvulsants (gabapentin, pregabalin), opioids (naloxone, naltrexone, butorphanol), antidepressants (amitriptyline, paroxetine, mirtazapine), cyclosporin A and thalidomide [88].

Scalp dysaesthesia

Introduction and general description

Hoss and Segal first described scalp dysaesthesia as chronic severe pain, burning, stinging and/or pruritus of the scalp without objective findings [96]. The symptoms may be manifestations of an underlying psychiatric disorder or may represent a type of chronic pain syndrome (Chapter 82). Nerve trauma, either indirectly through muscle tension or directly through surgical trauma, has been indicated as a potential cause [97,98].

Epidemiology and aetiology

In a study looking at the epidemiology of scalp sensitivity from a representative sample of the French population, 44% reported having a sensitive scalp. Women suffered more frequently from a sensitive scalp than men and no relationship with age was found. Prickling, itch and burning were the most common symptoms in those with a sensitive scalp. No link was found between scalp sensitivity and any specific scalp disease. Triggering factors of scalp sensitivity were heat, cold, pollution, emotions, dry or wet air, water and shampoos [83].

Hoss and Segal considered whether alopecia could have caused or contributed to scalp dysaesthesia and found that 7 of 11 patients had mild androgenetic alopecia. It was concluded that this is not an increased incidence of androgenetic alopecia compared with the general population, therefore it was unlikely to be the sole cause of the scalp problems [96]. This study also considered the role of a psychiatric cause in scalp dysaesthesia. Five of the 11 patients studied had one or more physician-diagnosed psychiatric disorders; of these, 4 had problems that were present prior to the onset of scalp dysaesthesia. The symptoms in 7 of the 11 intensified with psychological stress [96]. Hoss and Segal remain uncertain as to whether their patients have pain secondary to an underlying psychiatric condition, or if the psychiatric problems are unrelated or caused by the scalp dysaesthesia.

Two additional aetiological theories consider neurological trauma as a cause. A retrospective review of 15 women with scalp dysaesthesia found that 14 patients had cervical spine disease confirmed by imaging [97]. The commonest finding on imaging was degenerative disc disease, with 10 out of 14 patients having changes at C5/C6. The authors postulated that chronic muscle tension placed on the pericranial muscles or scalp aponeurosis secondary to the underlying cervical spine disease may lead to the symptoms of scalp dysaesthesia [97]. Scalp dysaesthesia has been described as a postoperative complication of patients who have an endoscopic brow lift. It is thought to be caused by peripheral nerve damage during this procedure [98].

Management

Most treatment options are derived from case series/reports without comparisons with each other.

Nine of the 11 patients studied by Hoss and Segal experienced improvement or complete resolution of their scalp symptoms with low-dose antidepressants (doxepin, amitriptyline) [96]. Oral pregabalin and oral or topical gabapentin have been used effectively in the management of scalp dysaesthesia [97,99]. Naltrexone is an opioid receptor antagonist. Low-dose naltrexone, defined as daily doses ranging from 1 mg to 5 mg, has been shown to reduce pruritis in patients with lichen planopilaris [100]. Tortelly *et al.* recommend low-dose naltrexone as a therapeutic option for scalp dysaesthesia [101]. Laidler *et al.* studied 16 participants to evaluate the use of an exercise protocol consisting of cervical spine range of movement exercises, gentle mobilisation and muscle stretches: ten (62%) experienced a reduction in their symptoms, four (25%)

experienced complete resolution and two (13%) experienced no benefit [102]. Kinoshita-Ise and Shear describe two cases who responded to pregabalin 50 mg daily and two who responded to TALK (topical 5% amitriptyline, 5% lidocaine, 10% ketamine in lipobase; Leo Laboratories, Hurley, UK) [**103**]. This group present a useful initial version of a diagnostic and therapeutic algorithm for scalp dysaesthesia (Figure 105.16).

Key references

The full list of references can be found in the online version at https://www.wiley.com/rooksdermatology10e

3 Adalsteinsson J, Kausik S, Muzumdar S *et al.* An update on the microbiology, immunology and genetics of seborrheic dermatitis. *Expl Dermatol* 2020;29:481–9.

9 Gupta A, Richardson M, Paquet M. Systematic review of oral treatments for seborrhoeic dermatitis. *J Eur Acad Dermatol Venereol* 2014;28:16–26.

18 Alsenaid A, Ezmerli M, Srour J *et al.* Biologics and small molecules in patients with scalp psoriasis: a systematic review. *J Dermatol Treat* 2020;19:1–10.

28 Thomas J, Aguh C. Approach to treatment of refractory dissecting cellulitis of the scalp: a systematic review. *J Dermatolog Treat* 2021;32:144–9.

35 Mazori D, Wright N, Patel M *et al.* Characteristics and treatment of adult–onset linear morphea: a retrospective cohort study of 61 patients at 3 tertiary care centres. *J Am Acad Dermatol* 2016;74:577–9.

74 Tomasini C, Michelario A. Erosive pustular dermatosis of the scalp: a neutrophilic folliculitis within the spectrum of neutrophilic dermatoses. *J Am Acad Dermatol* 2019;81:527–33.

82 Bin Saif GA, Ericson ME, Yosipovitch G. The itchy scalp – scratching for an explanation. *Exp Dermatol* 2011;20:959–68.

88 Rattanakaemakorn P, Suchonwanit P. Scalp pruritus: review of the pathogenesis, diagnosis and management. *BioMed Res Int* 2019;1268430 eCollection 2019:1–11.

96 Hoss D, Segal S. Scalp dysesthesia. *Arch Dermatol* 1998;143:327–30.

103 Kinoshita-Ise M, Shear N. Diagnostic and therapeutic approach to scalp dysaesthesia: a case series and published work review. *J Dermatol* 2019;46:526–30.

CHAPTER 106

Dermatoses of the External Ear

Cameron Kennedy[1] *and Ashish Sharma*[2]

[1]Bristol Royal Infirmary and Bristol Royal Hospital for Children, Bristol, UK
[2]Nottingham University Hospital, Nottingham, UK

Introduction

Anatomy and physiology [1–3]

The outer ear, also known as the external ear or auris externa, is the external part of the ear and consists of the auricle (pinna) and the ear canal. The auricle, or pinna (Figure 106.1), is a convoluted, elastic and cartilaginous plate covered by skin which is continuous medially with the lining of the external auditory canal (EAC). The skin is bound firmly to the cartilage, except on the fibro-fatty lobe and at the back of the ear. The auricle is attached to the head by fibrous ligaments and three vestigial auricularis muscles.

The EAC is approximately 25–30 mm in length, extending backwards and upwards in an S-shaped curve. It is composed of a distal cartilaginous canal and proximal bony canal (Figure 106.2). The EAC's length gives it a fundamental tuning frequency of 3–4 kHz, which coincides with the spectrum of human speech [4].

The EAC begins at the external auditory meatus and ends at the tympanic membrane (eardrum). The lateral one-third of the EAC has a cartilaginous infrastructure covered by a layer of sebaceous and apocrine glands and hair. This fibroelastic cartilage contains two horizontal fissures of Santorini, which communicate with the parotid anteriorly and the soft tissue overlying the mastoid

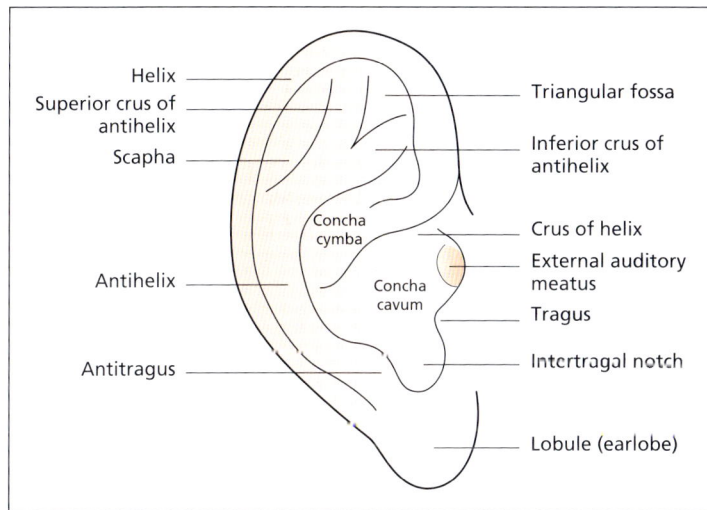

Figure 106.1 Anatomical landmarks of the auricle.

posteriorly. This may provide a portal for spread of infection or tumour. The skin overlying the lateral canal is approximately 1 mm thick and in direct contact with the perichondrium. The medial two-thirds of the EAC has osseous support from the tympanic

Rook's Textbook of Dermatology, Tenth Edition. Edited by Christopher Griffiths, Jonathan Barker, Tanya Bleiker, Walayat Hussain and Rosalind Simpson.

PART 10: SPECIFIC SITES, SEX & AGE

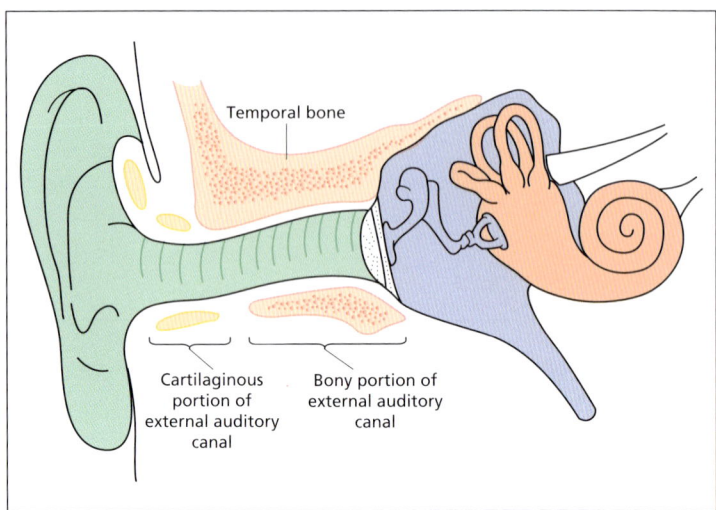

Figure 106.2 Anatomy of the external ear (green), consisting of the auricle, external auditory canal and the outer layer of the tympanic membrane. The middle ear (blue) and inner ear (light brown) are also shown.

portion of the temporal bone, with thinner skin that is devoid of adnexal structures.

The skin of the EAC is unique in that there is no frictional loss of stratum corneum; cerumen and epithelial debris have therefore to be removed by lateral epithelial migration towards the external os, a process that slows with age. The epidermis of the ear has a conspicuous stratum granulosum and a thick, compact stratum corneum. The dermis contains abundant elastic tissue. Eccrine sweat glands are not present in the auditory canal but modified apocrine (ceruminous) glands are numerous. Together with sebaceous glands, these contribute to the production of ear wax.

The blood supply to the auricle is provided by anastomosing branches of the superficial temporal and posterior auricular arteries, which are continuations of the external carotid artery (Figure 106.3a). Venous drainage is via posterior auricular and superficial temporal veins into the external jugular vein and via the superficial temporal, maxillary and facial veins into the internal jugular vein. Lymphatic drainage is to the superficial parotid,

retroauricular and superficial cervical lymph nodes. There is a complex nerve supply to the ear involving elements of the Vth, VIIth, IXth and Xth cranial nerves as well as cervical branches of the greater and lesser auricular nerves. The back of the ear is supplied by the greater auricular nerve (C2,3), the concha by the auricular branch of the vagus (Xth) and the anterior part of the pinna and the EAC by the auriculotemporal branch of the Vth cranial nerve (Figure 106.3b). Intercommunicating branches of the VIIth, IXth and Xth supply the deeper parts of the ear. With this complicated nerve supply, otalgia is more commonly due to referred pain than to disease in the ear itself [5].

The foramen of Huschke is a developmental defect in the bony EAC and may provide a route of communication to the parotid gland and infratemporal fossa. If disease breaches the EAC it can invade several areas including the stylomastoid foramen, carotid canal, jugular foramen, petrotympanic fissure and eustachian tube.

Hypertrichosis of the pinnae (MIM: 425500) was originally described as a Y-chromosome linked trait (Figure 106.4) [6]. An autosomal dominant genetic basis for hairy ears has also been noted in South Indian [7] and Maltese [8] people. Acquired hairy ears have been described in infants born of diabetic mothers [9,10] and in association with HIV infection [11].

Microbiology
The skin of the EAC in most healthy individuals supports the growth of multiple bacterial species, especially *Staphylococcus epidermidis*, *Corynebacterium* spp., *Bacillus* spp. and less often *Staphylococcus aureus*. *Pseudomonas aeruginosa*, often relevant to external otitis, and fungi are not normally found [2]. The normal flora can include organisms such as *Turicella otidis*, which can cause otitis media [12].

Cerumen (wax)
Cerumen is the combined product of sebaceous and apocrine glands, and its main function is to waterproof the EAC [13]. It contains both squalene and insoluble fatty acids and also diterpenoids [14]. Insufficient cerumen predisposes to infection, whereas thickened cerumen, which can be caused by genetics, metabolism, or age, fosters retention of water and debris. Extrusion is aided

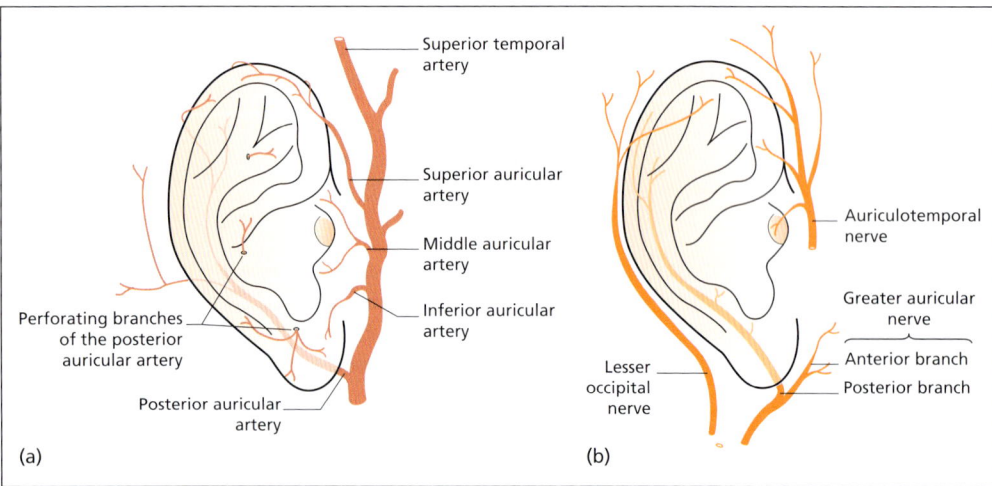

(a)   (b)

Figure 106.3 (a) Arterial and (b) nerve supply to external ear.

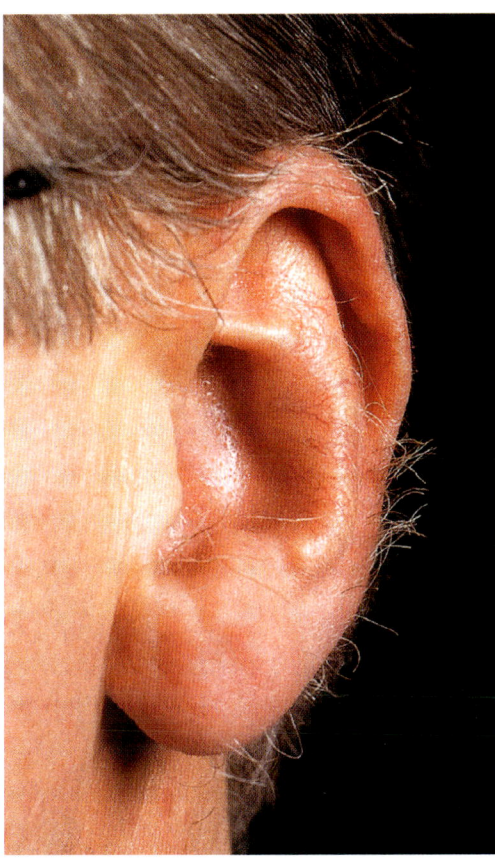

Figure 106.4 Coarse terminal hair on the auricle: a trait possibly associated with the Y chromosome.

by mastication. It is impeded if the ear canal is too narrow or tortuous, or when inflammation interferes with the normal migratory process.

There are genetically determined differences in cerumen composition and character: so-called 'dry' ear wax is light grey, dry and flaky; 'wet' ear wax is golden brown and sticky. The former is very common in Asian people. Wax phenotype is determined by a single gene pair, the wet wax allele being dominant [13]. Cerumen darkens with exposure to air.

Although not bactericidal, cerumen does not encourage bacterial or fungal growth. It is likely that antimicrobial peptides play a role

[15,16]; other possible reasons include the presence of lysozyme, immunoglobulins and polyunsaturated fatty acids. The surface pH of the EAC is around 6.9, which discourages microbial growth. It varies from 5.6 to 5.8 at the concha to 7.3 to 7.5 at 5–10 mm within the canal. With inflammation, the pH becomes slightly more acid.

Two populations have been shown to have excessive production and/or impaction of cerumen: individuals with learning difficulties and the elderly [13]. An increased secretion of cerumen occurs in patients treated with aromatic retinoids [17].

If wax becomes impacted or adherent, it can cause various symptoms such as hearing loss, tinnitus, vertigo, pain and itching, and can be a contributory factor to external otitis. It may be removed by irrigation techniques or by suction under direct vision [18,19]. Ear drops are based on water or oil, with and without active ingredients. A systematic review found that there is no good evidence to support one type of drop over another [20]. Regular use of an emollient liquid may have a role in prevention of impaction [21]. Inflammation interferes with normal epidermal migration and tends therefore both to induce and to encourage the retention of scale.

DEVELOPMENTAL DEFECTS AND CHANGES WITH AGEING

The auricle begins development in the fifth week of embryonic life. It arises from six auricular hillocks, described by His in 1885 [1]. These are mesenchymal proliferations located at the dorsal ends of the 1st (mandibular) and 2nd (hyoid) pharyngeal arches. The arches are also called branchial arches, derived from the Greek word for gill. These arches surround the first pharyngeal/branchial cleft, which will later become the external auditory meatus [2]. Together with the development of the face, these hillocks later fuse, deviate and gradually form the complex shape of the definitive auricle (Figure 106.5). The resulting fusion planes provide a potential path for the spread of skin cancer.

As the fusion of the auricular hillocks is complex, developmental abnormalities of the auricle are not uncommon. Cessation or retardation of the development at any stage will cause various

PART 10: SPECIFIC SITES, SEX & AGE

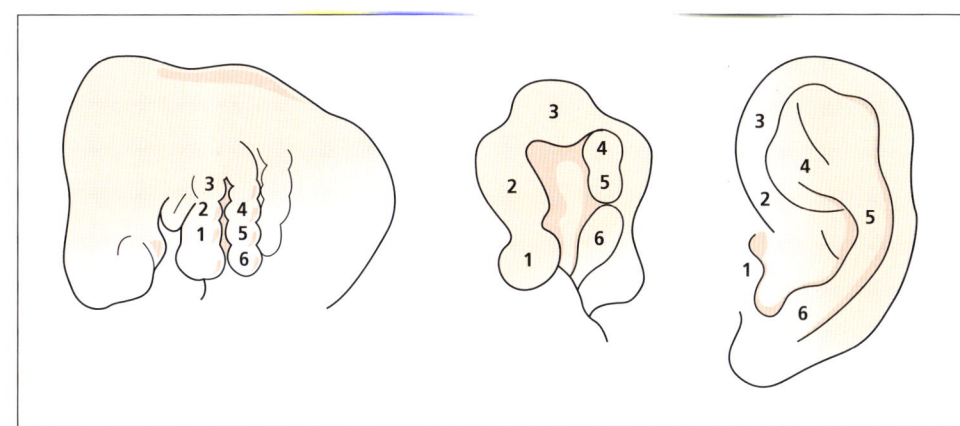

Figure 106.5 Developmental anatomy of the auricle. Numbers represent relative positions of fusion planes. Left, 6-week embryo; centre, 8-week embryo; right, adult.

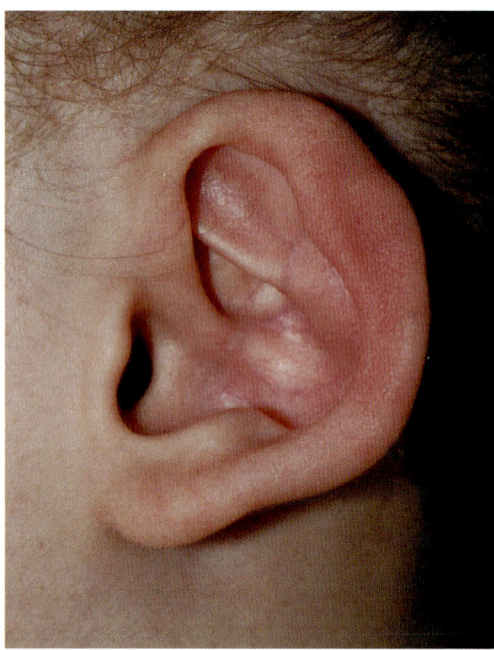

Figure 106.6 CHARGE syndrome: typical appearance of pinna with (i) almost triangular concha; (ii) discontinuity between the antihelix and antitragus; and (iii) 'snipped-off' appearance of the helical folds. Source: Dr Michael Saunders, Consultant Paediatric Otolaryngologist, Bristol Royal Hospital for Children, UK.

auricular anomalies, including a congenital auricular cleft, agenesis of the lobule, or a congenital bifid lobule [3]. Pinna abnormalities are associated sufficiently often with conductive hearing loss that screening tests should be carried out [4–8].

External ear malformations as part of a genetic syndrome account for fewer than 10% of all external ear abnormalities; isolated cases of ear malformation may either be non-genetic in origin or may have a genetic basis but with poor gene penetrance [9]. Some are associated with chromosomal abnormalities, such as Down syndrome, or inherited disorders such as CHARGE syndrome (Figure 106.6) or brachio-oto-renal syndrome (Figure 106.7).

Microtia (small ears)

Microtia designates a spectrum of underdevelopment of the pinna, from small ears to absence of an ear or ears (Figure 106.8) [10]. The prevalence varies between 1 and 17/17 000 in different populations [11]. Small ears are often associated with hearing deficit and may be a feature of many syndromes. In addition to being small, the pinna may be rudimentary, resembling the hillocks from which it is embryologically derived. The more primitive the appearance, the greater the likelihood of hearing abnormalities, in most cases due to defects or atresia of the ossicles. There may also be a narrowing or atresia of the auditory canal [10–13] and various abnormalities of the middle ear [14] and inner ear [15]. Small ears are a feature of many syndromes, including Down syndrome, Treacher Collins syndrome (Figure 106.9), Goldenhar syndrome, Apert syndrome, Mohr orofaciodigital syndrome, Duane retraction syndrome and thalidomide embryopathy.

Familial microtia inherited as an isolated autosomal dominant trait has been described [16]. Microtia is one of the birth defects that occurs more on the right than the left side [17].

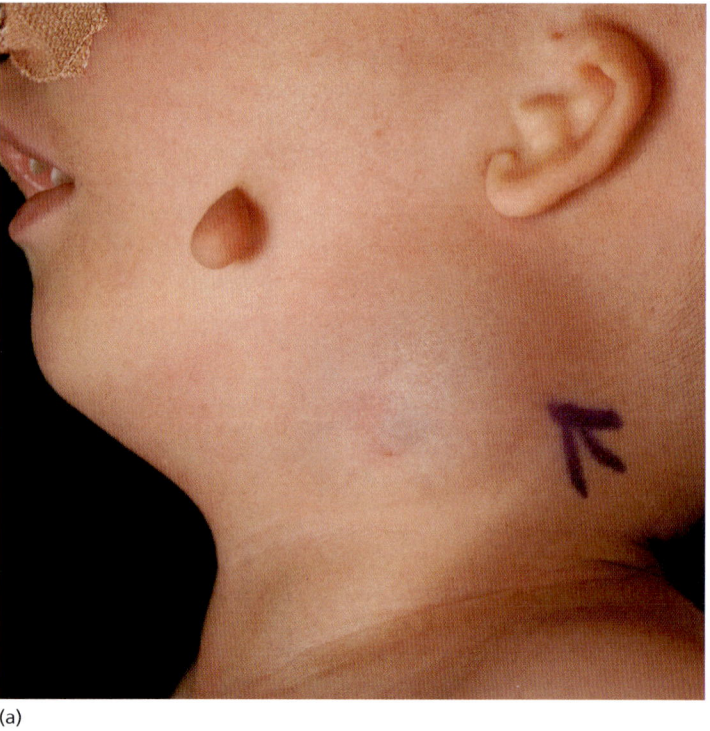

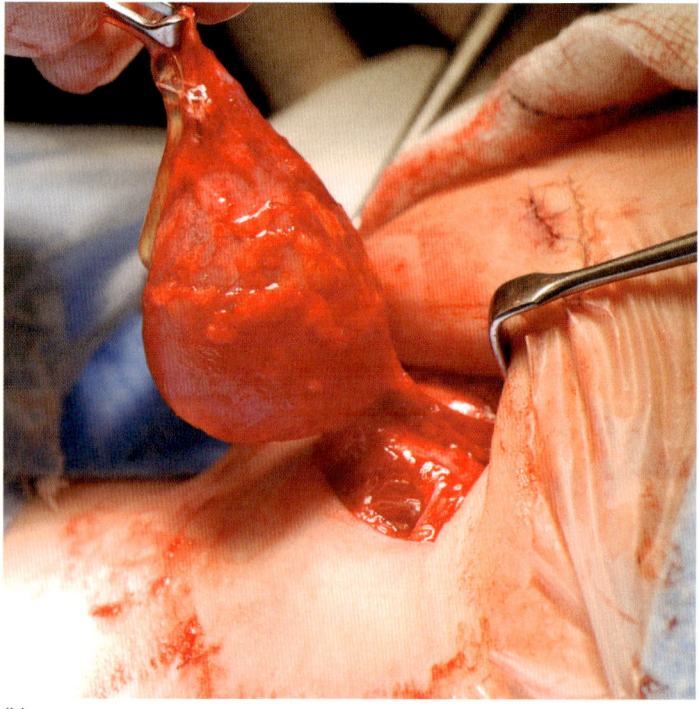

(a)   (b)

Figure 106.7 Branchio-oto-renal syndrome. (a) Second arch branchial cyst (arrowed), skin tag on lower cheek, pre-auricular sinus and microtia with absent ear canal. (b) Surgical excision of second arch branchial cyst. Source: Dr Michael Saunders, Consultant Paediatric Otolaryngologist, Bristol Royal Hospital for Children, UK.

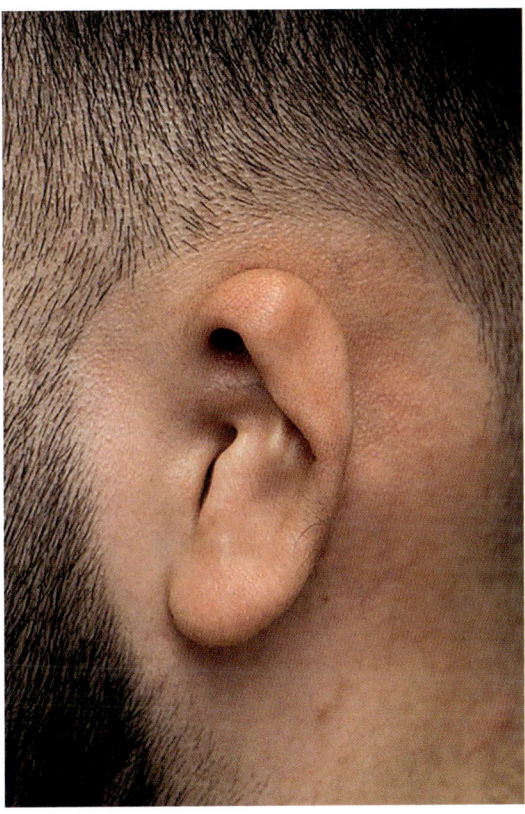

Figure 106.8 Microtia – reduction of auditory meatus, with partly formed pinna.

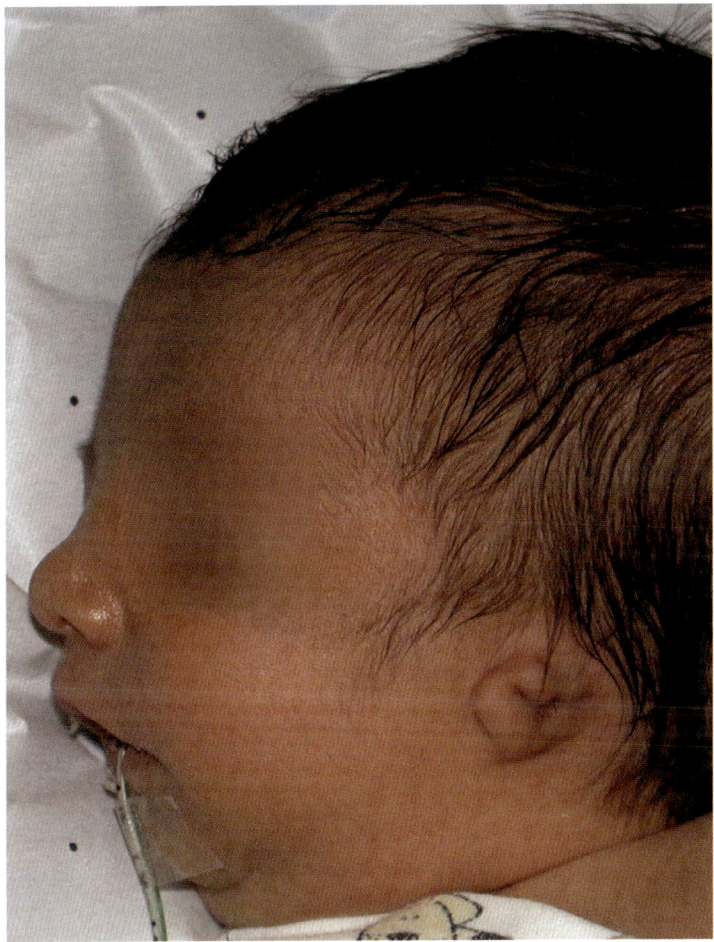

Figure 106.9 Treacher Collins syndrome – marked retrognathia, low set pinna with microtia. Source: Dr Michael Saunders, Consultant Paediatric Otolaryngologist, Bristol Royal Hospital for Children, UK.)

Macrotia (large ears)

Macrotia is a developmental variation in which the amount of tissue between the helix and antihelix is increased, causing the ears to wing out. The ear may also be diffusely enlarged or elongated. Such changes are common in Turner syndrome, and there may be associated sensorineural deafness. Large ears are well described in fragile X syndrome [18] and Kabuki syndrome, although in the latter they may also be smaller than normal [19]. Generally enlarged ears are sometimes seen in patients with the XXXXY chromosome defect. The cartilaginous parts of the ears are enlarged and soft in Zimmermann–Laband syndrome [20,21]. In this rare disorder the ears are large and floppy, in association with a bulbous soft nose.

Low-set ears

Normally, the top of the helix is at the same level as the eyebrow, the earlobe is above the angle of the mandible and the external auditory meatus is at the level of the ala nasi. Low-set ears may in addition be posteriorly rotated and are often small. The condition is usually bilateral. Although it may be isolated, it is often associated with major middle-ear or systemic malformations, appearing for example in Turner, Noonan, Patau and Crouzon syndromes.

Variations in the shape of the pinna

Minor variations in size and shape are common and not usually associated with any other abnormality. These include *bat ear* or protruding ear, in which the antihelix lacks the usual bulge; *lop ear*, in which there is an unrolled helix, a poorly developed antihelix and scapha, and a large concha resulting in a somewhat floppy ear; and *prominent auricular (Darwin) tubercle*. Variations in the contour of the helix and antihelix to produce a bulge of the anterosuperior part of the pinna account for so-called *Mozart ear*, and in *Wildemuth ear* the antihelix is prominent and the formation of the helix is poor. These minor ear anomalies can be a syndromic feature or can be associated with conductive and occasionally sensorineural hearing loss, but in most instances they are isolated. They may, however, be inherited, as in the Mozart family. A distinctive *railroad track abnormality* with marked prominence of the crus of the helix is said to occur in up to 30% of children with fetal alcohol syndrome [11,15] and a protruding auricle may, rarely, be a sign of neuromuscular disease [22]. Various abnormalities of the configuration of the pinna

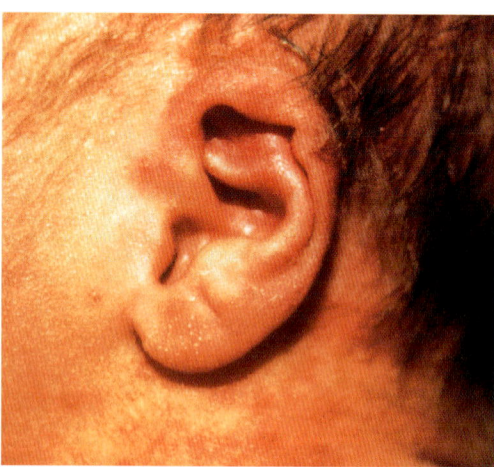

Figure 106.10 Diagonal earlobe crease in an infant with Beckwith–Wiedemann syndrome.

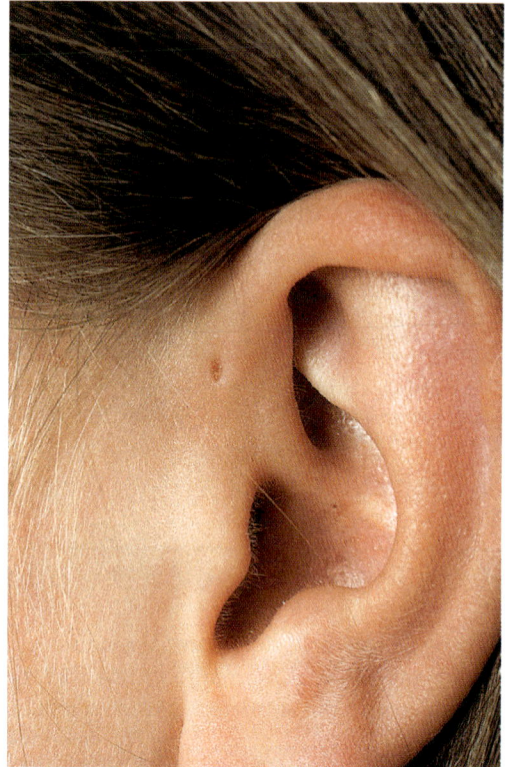

Figure 106.11 Pre-auricular sinus.

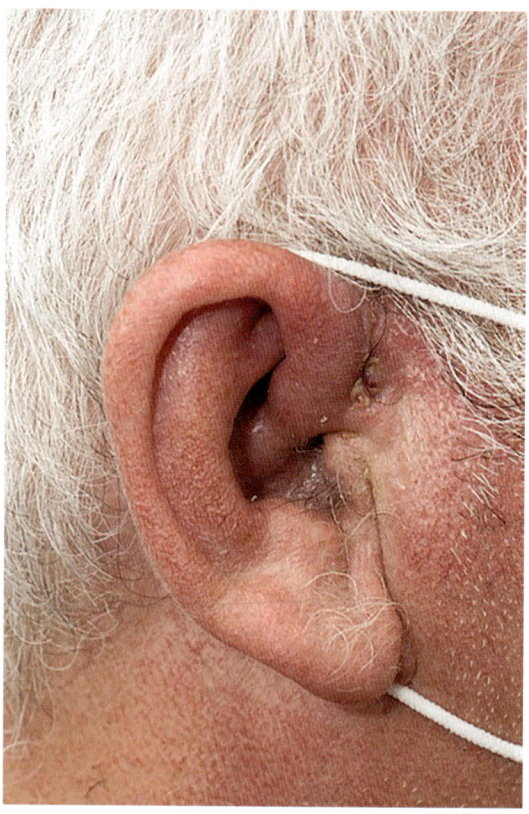

Figure 106.12 Pre-auricular sinus acting as a focus of infection, with acute otitis externa. An adult patient presenting with a new onset of discharge from a previously asymptomatic indentation in front of the right ear.

Peri-auricular anomalies

Pre-auricular sinus (PAS) (synonym: ear pit/fistula/tract) is a congenital malformation that manifests as a small opening in the external ear, usually near the anterior limb of the ascending helix (Figure 106.11). The term 'pre-auricular' is therefore a misnomer as the sinus opening is usually on the auricle, with occurrence reported along the superior helix margin, tragus and lobule [1].

The incidence varies between 0.47% and 2.5% [2–8], with bilateral lesions in 17–27% of cases [2,3,7]. The remaining unilateral lesions show no lateral preference, although one study found a left-sided predominance [7]. PAS is generally asymptomatic, with only one-quarter of subjects reporting an episode of symptomatic discharge, redness and pain [7] (Figure 106.12). If an abscess is present, it will likely need to be incised and drained. In the medical literature, some believe that even asymptomatic sinuses should be removed, others that surgery is only indicated if infection or other complications arise. Several surgical techniques are described for removal including use of methylene blue dye and probes [9]. Recurrence after surgery has been reported to be between 19% and 42% [10–12].

PAS may be sporadic or inherited, with bilateral lesions more likely in the latter. PAS may also be part of a multiple congenital abnormality syndrome, such as brachio-oto-renal syndrome

have been described in the distinctive *lumpy scalp syndrome* [23], in which other features include absent or rudimentary nipples and dermal nodules on the scalp [24]. The lobule can show isolated abnormalities, for example pits and clefts. Absence of the lobule is, however, usually associated with a syndrome of a more serious nature [4]. Diagonal linear creases in the lobule are seen in Beckwith–Wiedemann syndrome (Figure 106.10), and in adult life in association with some degenerative diseases, although they are also a common finding in normal individuals. Also see next section.

Table 106.1 Developmental disorders which display changes to the external ear.

Syndrome	Genetics	Clinical findings on ears	Other clinical features
Apert	*FGFR2* gene; autosomal dominant	Microtia (small or partially formed ears)	Acrocephalosyndactyly; hydrocephalus; fusion of fingers; exophthalmos; mid-face hypoplasia
Branchio-oto-renal	*EYA1*, *SIX5*, *SIX1* genes; autosomal dominant	Microtia with cupped appearance; overfolding of skin and cartilage of superior helix ('lop' ear); preauricular pits or tags	Branchial fistulas and cysts; kidney malformation or atresia
CHARGE	*CHD7* gene, in two-thirds of patients	Short, wide ear with little or no lobe; 'snipped off' helix; prominent antihelix which is discontinuous with tragus; triangular concha; decreased cartilage ('floppy' ear); may by asymmetric and stick out	Coloboma (notch in lower part of eye); heart defects; atresia of choanae; retardation of growth and development; ear abnormalities and deafness
Crouzon	*FGFR2* gene; autosomal dominant	Low-set ears; atresia of ear canal	Craniosynostosis (skull plates prematurely fuse); hydrocephalus
Down	Trisomy of chromosome 21	Overfolded helix; ear canal stenosis causing chronic wax impaction; chronic otitis media is common	Small chin; flat nasal bridge; single palmar crease; short stature; heart abnormalities
Duane retraction	*CHN1* gene	Microtia; preauricular tags	Strabismus
EEC	*TP63* gene in 90% of patients; autosomal dominant	Microtia, overfolded helix, low-set ears; attached earlobes; ear canal stenosis	Ectrodactyly, ectodermal dysplasia and cleft lip–palate
Fragile X	*FMR1* gene; X-linked dominant	Macrotia (large ears)	Intellectual impairment; large head; long face
Goldenhar	Gene not yet identified	Microtia or anotia (absence of ear)	'Oculo-auriculo-vertebral' spectrum; ocular dermoid cysts; scoliosis or kyphosis
Holoprosencephaly	Trisomy of chromosome 13	Low-set ears	Patau's syndrome; congenital heart defects
Kabuki	*MLL2* (autosomal dominant) and *KDM6A* (X-linked dominant) genes	Macrotia. Less commonly auricular atresia and preauricular fistula	Long palpebral fissures; everted lower eyelids; arched eyebrows; congenital heart defects
Nager	*SF3B4* gene	Microtia; blind-ending or absent ear canal	Acrofacial dystosis; micrognathia; cleft palate; clinodactyly or syndactyly
Noonan	*PTPN11 gene*; autosomal dominant	Low-set and posteriorly rotated ears	Hypertelorism; micrognathia; congenital heart defects
Orofaciodigital 1	*OFD1* gene; X-linked dominant	Milial cysts on ears	Accessory oral frenulum; cleft palate; hypertelorism; polycystic kidneys;
Orofaciodigital 2	Exact gene uncertain; autosomal recessive inheritance	Low-set and/or protruding ears	Mohr syndrome; accessory oral frenulum; cleft nasal tip; cleft tongue
Townes–Brocks	*SALL1* gene; autosomal dominant	Microtia; 'satyr' or 'lop' ear; preauricular skin tags	Imperforate anus; triphalangeal or duplicate thumbs; renal failure
Treacher Collins	*TCOF1* or *POLR1D* genes (autosomal dominant)	Microtia or anotia; atresia or stenosis of ear canal	Hypoplastic or absent malar, micrognathia, cleft palate, coloboma
Turner	Loss of X chromosome in females	Low-set ears; elongated or cup-shaped ears; thick earlobes	Short stature; premature ovarian failure; webbed neck; high arched palate
XXXXY	Presence of three extra X chromosomes in males	Macrotia; low-set and folded ears	Short stature; hypogonadism; hypertelorism; prognathism
Zimmermann–Laband	*KCNH1* gene	Macrotia; thick and floppy ears due to soft cartilage	Gingival fibromatosis; nail absence or hypoplasia

(Table 106.1). An association with renal structural abnormalities has been reported in 2.2–4.3% [13,14] of children with PAS. However, routine ultrasound scanning in the presence of PAS is not recommended, except in the presence of one of the following: another malformation or dysmorphic feature; a family history of deafness; auricular and/or renal malformations; a maternal history of gestational diabetes [15].

Pre-auricular tags are commonly described, although lesions on or near the tragus are probably best termed 'accessory tragus' [16] (Figure 106.13). The term 'accessory auricle' is sometimes used for this, and for similar firm elevations of skin and cartilage just near the ascending crus of the helix. They may be single or multiple and may occur anywhere in a line from the tragus to the angle of the mouth. Accessory auricles, congenital fistulae and other external ear manifestations may occur alone or may be associated with more widespread first and second branchial arch abnormalities, for example Treacher Collins and Goldenhar syndromes.

Ageing changes

Many changes seen on the skin of the pinna attributed to ageing are a result of its exposure to environmental factors, especially

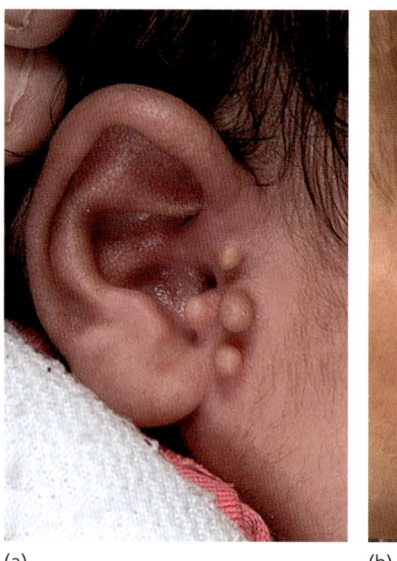
(a)

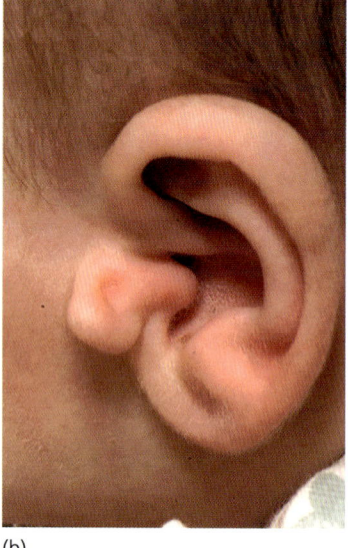
(b)

Figure 106.13 (a) Pre-auricular skin tags. (b) Accessory tragus.

UV radiation, cold (perniosis) and infrared radiation. The elderly exposed pinna often shows varying degrees of dermal and epidermal atrophy, solar/actinic keratoses and lentigines, solar elastosis, telangiectasia and venous lakes. If the pinna is at least partially light protected, as in many women, the skin may still appear somewhat thinned due to intrinsic ageing changes.

It has long been observed that the pinna grows progressively throughout life, more so in males than females, and this has been confirmed in a large study [17]. It is recognised in Chinese culture that length of the ear in men is a predictor for longevity [18]. Two studies would appear to confirm this: one from Kent, UK [19] and one from Japan [20]. The increase in length of the male ear from the age of 30 years onwards may have a 7-year periodicity [21].

Earlobe creases

An earlobe crease can be a marker for internal disease. The Frank sign appears as an earlobe crease extending 45 degrees diagonally from the tragus to the outer border of the lobe [22]. It has been proposed that this earlobe crease is a predictor of coronary artery disease. An explanation of this pathophysiology may be intimal thickening leading to microvascular ischaemia to earlobe end arterioles.

Nazzal *et al.* [23] examined 241 patients presenting to an acute stroke unit, with the Frank sign present in 73% of patients with a transient ischaemic attack and in 89% of patients with a cerebrovascular accident. Several other studies described the Frank sign as a predictor of future coronary heart disease [24–31], cerebrovascular disease [32–36] and peripheral vascular disease [37,38] although a systematic review [39] identified several studies disproving the association. Overall, the presence of the Frank sign with symptomatic cardiovascular disease should prompt physicians to evaluate for atherosclerotic disease, but it is not clear whether it is an independent risk factor.

Diagonal earlobe creases are seen in other contexts, for example Beckwith–Wiedemann syndrome [40] (Figure 106.10), and do not seem to be associated with coronary artery disease in Hawaiian [41], Native American [42] or Chinese [43] people. Earlobe creases have also been associated with primary open-angle glaucoma [44].

TRAUMATIC CONDITIONS

Contusion and haematoma

Bruises of the ear and perichondrial haematomas are usually due to blunt trauma and are common in contact sports, such as boxing, wrestling and rugby. In children, physical abuse may need to be excluded [1,2]. A distinctive condition known as *tin ear syndrome* has been considered pathognomonic of child abuse: a triad of isolated ear bruising, haemorrhagic retinopathy and a small, ipsilateral subdural haematoma [3]. In a study of 250 Indian schoolchildren, 18% reported physical abuse involving the ears, mostly related to poor performance in school. An overall mild or moderate hearing loss was detected in 50% of the affected children [4]. Following trauma, blood and serum collects in the plane between the perichondrium and cartilage resulting in ischaemia of cartilage. If the fluid is not removed early the cartilage will necrose and undergo fibrosis causing permanent swelling. Repeated trauma may result in the distorted nodular deformity known as *cauliflower ear*, which is due to varying degrees of cartilage necrosis, fibrosis and dystrophic calcification.

Management

Subperichondrial haematomas must be treated promptly, with full aseptic technique to avoid secondary perichondritis. Small collections of fluid can sometimes be aspirated by syringe, but usually need to be drained through a small incision and a laterally placed pressure dressing applied to prevent re-accumulation [5,6]. Another useful technique is to use a through-and-through suture technique to maintain bolsters over the area where the haematoma has been evacuated [7]. Other approaches include a posterior incision and suction drainage [8], or fenestrations in the cartilage to promote adhesion of the opposing perichondrial layers [9]. Prophylactic antibiotics are sometimes given. Improvement of cauliflower ear usually requires multiple corrective procedures.

Pseudocyst of the ear

Pseudocyst of the ear is an uncommon fluid-filled non-inflammatory swelling due to the appearance of a cavity within the cartilage. It is probably a result of trauma.

Epidemiology

It is most common in young men. It can occur over a wide age range [10] including infants [11]. There may be a predilection for Chinese people, although this could be due to reporting bias [12,13].

Pathophysiology

The exact pathophysiology is unknown. There is often minor repetitive trauma, such as rubbing and ear twisting. It has been reported in patients with neurological movement disorders [14]. Trauma may induce a break in the cartilage [15] or an underlying malformation of the cartilage may be present. A characteristic finding is elevation of isoforms 4 and 5 of lactate dehydrogenase (LDH) – these are released from chondrocytes [16]. A role for cytokines has been suggested [17].

Predisposing factors

Circumstances which cause trauma include rubbing due to atopic eczema [18], sporting injury, habit-related twisting of the ears, sleeping on hard pillows and wearing a motorcycle helmet and/or earphones.

Pathology

There is a cavity within the cartilage. The walls of the cavity are not lined by epithelium (hence the term *pseudo*cyst) and within the cartilage there is eosinophilic amorphous material. There may be focal fibrosis, especially in older lesions [19,20].

Clinical features

Patients present with a 1–5 cm painless swelling that is typically fluctuant and non-tender, developing over a 1–3 month period. It is usually on the upper outer aspect of the ear, involving the scaphoid, triangular fossa and antihelix (Figure 106.14). The condition is usually unilateral [21], although bilateral lesions have been reported [22–25]. If fluid is aspirated, it is clear or yellowish. Uncommonly, there may be some signs of inflammation and tenderness. Untreated,

the condition may lead to fibrosis causing deformity of the pinna. The differential diagnosis includes haematoma, cysts, tumours, perichondritis and relapsing polychondritis.

Management

Reassurance and observation is a reasonable management plan for small lesions, as the condition is benign.

First line

Needle aspiration of the contents is a relatively simple procedure that can be performed at the initial consultation. To reduce recurrence, chemical and mechanical obliteration of the residual 'dead' space can be performed. Injection with intralesional triamcinolone [26], fibrin [27], minocycline [28] or trichloracetic acid have been reported. A pressure dressing can then be applied for 3 weeks to prevent reaccumulation of fluid. This can be made from a thermoplastic material such as Aquaplast® [29], a plastic sheet [30] or a mastoid bandage.

Second line

Surgical deroofing of the cyst may be more successful than aspiration. Under sterile conditions, an incision is made along the antihelical line, through the anterior cartilaginous leaflet [31]. The use of a punch biopsy has been described [32], followed by a pressure bolster.

Chondrodermatitis nodularis

Chondrodermatitis nodularis (CN) is an idiopathic, benign, usually painful condition of the ear [1].

Synonyms and inclusions

- Chondrodermatitis nodularis chronica helicis and antihelicis (ante- is sometimes used as an alternative to anti-)

Epidemiology

Chondrodermatitis is most common in the middle aged and elderly, with an average age of 65 years [2] although it can occur in all age groups. In the older person, there is a ratio of 10 males to 1 female in most series [3]; it is relatively commoner in females in younger individuals.

When it occurs in the younger patient there is sometimes a structural abnormality and/or a pathological process in the cartilage. Only seven paediatric patients have been reported [4–7], the youngest being a 9-month-old infant [8]. Four of these patients had an underlying connective tissue disorder, including dermatomyositis, rheumatoid nodule, systemic lupus erythematosus and Beckwith–Weidemann syndrome. Simultaneous occurrence in monozygotic twins has been reported [9]. Magro *et al.* [10] observed an association between CNH and collagen vascular disease, scleroderma, hypertension, thyroid disease and heart disease, with a higher incidence of any of these medical problems in younger patients. Therefore, it is suggested to screen younger patients (below 40 years) for an underlying vasculopathy or autoimmune connective tissue disorder.

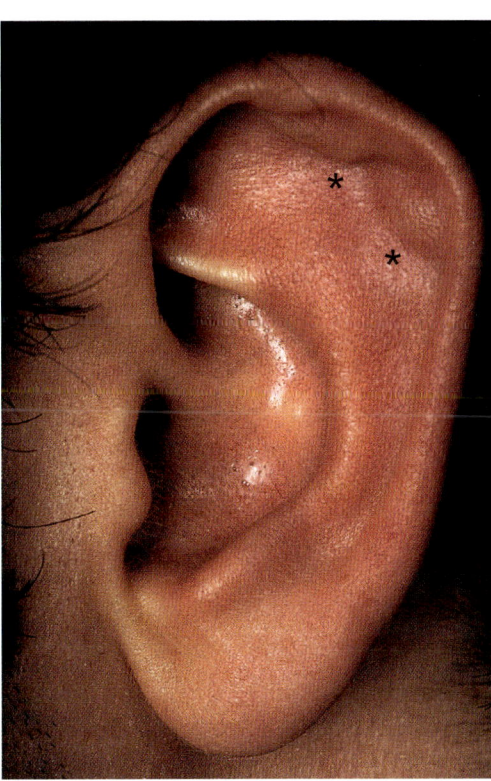

Figure 106.14 Pseudocyst. Bilobed fluctuant swelling (asterisks) on the upper pinna.

PART 10: SPECIFIC SITES, SEX & AGE

Predisposing factors

The small dermal blood vessels supplying the outer ear are vulnerable to compression, due to an external location, lack of bony support and thin subcutaneous tissue. Necrosis from trauma, cold or actinic damage can help initiate CN, and the disruption of blood perfusion can prevent adequate healing. Predisposing factors are therefore summarised as:

1 Prolonged and excessive pressure from, for example, sleeping on one side, headgear, mobile phone or headphones.
2 Solar radiation.
3 Exposure to cold and wind, with the formation of weathering nodules.
4 Connective tissue disorders associated with microvascular injury.
5 Abnormal structural variants of the pinna.

Pathology

A typical lesion of CN consists of a nodule of degenerate homogeneous collagen surrounded by vascular granulation tissue with an overlying acanthotic epidermis, and there may be a central ulcer through which the damaged collagen is extruded. In nearly all cases, there is inflammation and fibrosis of the underlying perichondrium, and degenerative changes may be seen in the cartilage (Figure 106.15). There is often transepidermal elimination of altered connective tissue [11]. Other findings of CNH reported in the literature include loss of elastic fibres in the central area of degenerated dermal collagen and nerve hyperplasia [12], which might account for pain.

Clinical features

The lesion usually begins as a globular or oval nodule, about 0.5–1 cm in diameter, raised above the often hyperaemic surrounding skin (Figure 106.16). It is commonly painful and exquisitely tender to touch which is virtually pathognomonic of the diagnosis. The surface may be scaly or crusted, concealing a small ulcer. Sometimes the condition is first noticed as an ulcer, requiring a biopsy to exclude a basal cell or squamous cell carcinoma. In men,

nearly 90% of nodules are situated on the helix, usually at the upper pole, but may occur on the antihelix, tragus, concha and antitragus, in order of decreasing frequency [13]. The posterior surface can be affected if the ear is folded during sleep [14]. Although bilateral cases have been reported [15], it is typically unilateral and the right side appears to be more commonly affected [16,17]. The conchal bowl can be affected by modern earphones [18].

The differential diagnosis includes: basal cell carcinoma, squamous cell carcinoma, actinic keratosis, benign tumours and weathering nodule of the ear.

Management

For symptomatic CN, measures should be taken to relieve pressure over the ear where this is a contributory factor. Initial success rates of 87% have been reported [19], but with a recurrence rate of 34%. Various interventions to provide relief of pressure during sleep include a doughnut-shaped pillow [20], protective hollowed-out foam [21], a moulded prosthesis and self-adhering foam [22].

Nitroglycerin causes local vasodilatation and restores adequate blood flow to the pinna. A 5 mg transdermal patch [23] or 2% ointment [24] is applied for 2 months, with a cure rate of 62–64%. This is much lower than surgery, but comparable to pressure relief, with which it can be combined. Diltiazem cream (2%) is reported to be effective [25]. Topical steroid is often used and can give some symptomatic relief [26]. Intralesional corticosteroid injection, e.g. triamcinolone 10 mg/mL can also help in the short term [27].

Surgical treatment can be curative in 85% of cases; removing the abnormal cartilage with or without the overlying skin is the best technique [28–30]. A modification of this using a sutureless closure has been described [31]. Many other surgical techniques have been used anecdotally, including curettage [32–34], shave excision, wedge excision, punch excision replacing the removed tissue with punch biopsy derived graft [35] and excision followed by flap repair [36]. However, surgical intervention may lead to the formation of adjacent cartilaginous nodules around the scar site and so care is needed to prevent a mismatch in height around the treated area.

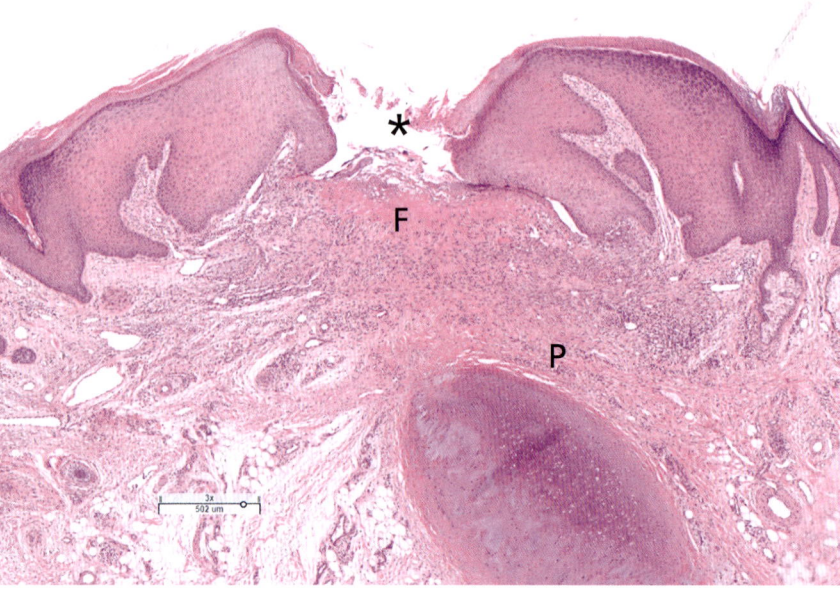

Figure 106.15 Chondrodermatitis nodularis helicis. Transverse section stained with H&E. There is an area of ulceration beneath a funnel-shaped defect (*) in the epidermis. Adjacent to the defect the epidermis is acanthotic. In the floor of the ulcer there is fibrin (F) and beneath this there is fibrinoid degeneration of the dermal collagen with a mixed inflammatory cell infiltrate. The perichondrium (P) is focally thickened. Courtesy of Dr J. Oxley, Southmead Hospital, Bristol, UK.

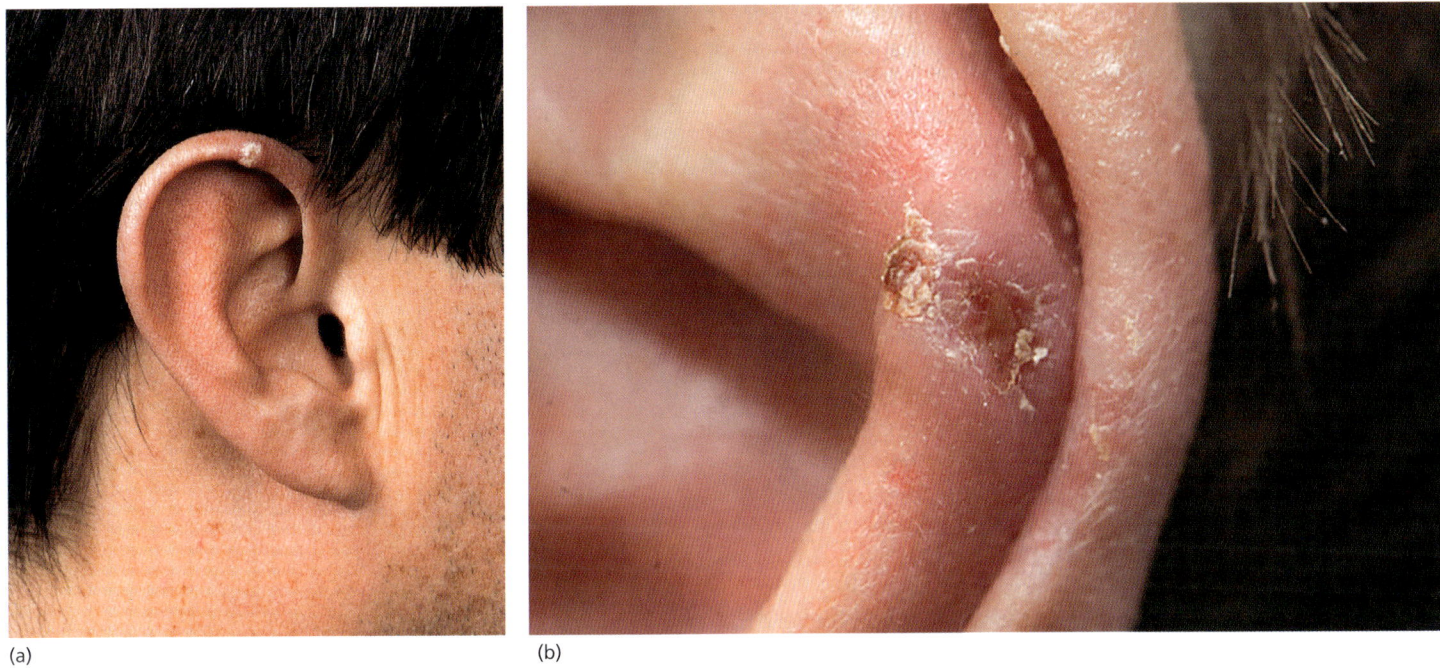

Figure 106.16 Chondrodermatitis nodularis of the helix. (a) A superficially ulcerated, exquisitely tender nodule on the superior helical rim. (b) Erythematous papule with superficial ulceration on the antihelix of a female patient.

Other options have minimal evidence and include cryotherapy, photodynamic therapy [37,38], cushioning from collagen injections [39] and carbon dioxide laser treatment [40].

Treatment ladder for chondrodermatitis nodularis

First line

Conservative treatment	Pressure avoidance and devices

Second line

Medical management	Topical treatment with nitroglycerin, diltiazem or corticosteroid; or

Third line

	intralesional steroid
Surgical intervention	Excision, curettage, shave, punch

Fourth line

Alternative modalities	Cryotherapy, PDT, laser

Ear piercing

Piercing of the earlobes has been performed among both sexes since ancient times for social, religious and cosmetic purposes [1], in both Eastern and Western societies. Body piercings other than earlobes represent a marker for risky behaviour [2–4]. While in most hands ear piercing is a rather low-risk procedure, it has its early and late complications [5,6]. Common local complications include: contact dermatitis, infection of the lobule, keloid formation beginning at the puncture site, lobular tissue loss from trauma through pulling the earring and splitting of the earlobe by the earring [7]. Embedding of the earring via a spring-loaded gun is a common problem in children [8]. The ear is also pierced in acupuncture as used in traditional medicine, and complications have been reported [9,10].

Complications
Bacterial infection
This is common and usually due to Gram-positive cocci. Predisposing factors include skin disease, such as atopic eczema or contact dermatitis. Life-threatening septicaemia has been described [11], and even in healthy individuals, infective endocarditis is a risk [12]. When cartilage is pierced the usual bacterial infection is with *Pseudomonas aeruginosa*, which causes perichondritis [13] or chondritis [14], and for which the best treatment is ciprofloxacin [15]. Any purulent material should be cultured, since other pathogens have been described (e.g. *Lactobacillus*) [16]. There is a report of pyogenic spondylitis [17]. Primary tuberculosis has been described [18].

Contact allergy
Earrings remain a major source of sensitisation to nickel, and ear piercing is one explanation for the higher incidence of nickel allergy in females [19,20]. Even stainless steel studs and clasps, which can produce irritant as well as allergic effects, may release sufficient nickel to elicit contact dermatitis [21]. When nickel in ear piercings was banned in Denmark in 1992, there was a substantial fall in nickel sensitisation [22].

Allergic contact dermatitis to pure gold is rare due to its stability and low tendency to ionisation [23], in contrast to that from nickel, copper or zinc. Earrings may be made of 24-carat pure gold. However, its malleability prevents screw threads being cut into the retaining bolt. Therefore, small quantities of copper, nickel, zinc or silver are added to the stem to retain strength. It is this part that is in direct and prolonged contact with the earlobe skin and may cause an allergic contact dermatitis. This allergic response may manifest as a weeping eczematous reaction of the skin, resulting in a gradual splitting of the earlobe or a keloid-like scar.

For gold to induce a contact dermatitis reaction, it must be converted into a soluble form and absorbed into the skin, probably by the action of amino acids in sweat [24]. Gold may ionise more in the dermis than in the epidermis [25]. The resulting cellular response in the dermis is distinct from that characterised by contact sensitivity on the epidermis. Fisher [26] describes a non-eczematous dermal contact dermatitis, where the epidermal changes are minimal and more marked dermal involvement is observed. This may be relevant in patients who develop split earlobes or keloid formation, where the initiating cause is a subclinical allergic reaction to gold earrings.

Patch testing is best carried out using gold sodium thiosulfate. Metallic (elemental) gold almost always tests negative and gold trichloride has been demonstrated to elicit more false-negative and false-positive reactions [27] (see Chapter 121 for reactions to gold and Chapter 127 for allergic contact dermatitis).

Contact dermatitis from other materials used in earrings, such as olive wood [28], copper [29], cobalt [30,31] and chromium [32], has been described, and may also occur from the use of topical antiseptics, antibiotics and dressings used to treat infection.

Granulomatous and lymphoid reactions

Reddish brown and purple papules and nodules at sites of ear piercing may denote a granulomatous response to gold [33] and lymphoma-like reactions have been described [34–37]. A foreign-body reaction following ear piercing presenting as a keloid-like nodule has been reported [38]. Similar reactions have been associated with palladium [39] and titanium [40]. Sarcoidosis and a sarcoidal tissue reaction have presented after ear piercing [41,42].

Other complications

Implantation epidermoid cysts due to ear piercing often present as tender, chronic, inflammatory swellings, sometimes with drainage. There is usually an epithelial lined track as well as cysts, and all epithelial tissue must be removed, for example with a skin punch [43].

Localised argyria presents as bluish macules, usually on the posterior surface of the earlobe [44,45].

Frostbite has followed the use of ethyl chloride topical anaesthesia [46].

A case of severe relapsing polychondritis following ear piercing has been reported [47].

Split earlobe

Split earlobes can be classified into two groups: congenital and traumatic [1]. The congenital group can be divided into three categories: anterior, posterior with doubled earlobe, and sagittal [2]. The traumatic group can be divided into two categories: complete and incomplete (Figure 106.17). Each can be unilateral or bilateral.

Complete clefts are often due to acute trauma, causing transection of the lobule. The wound edges usually heal without forming

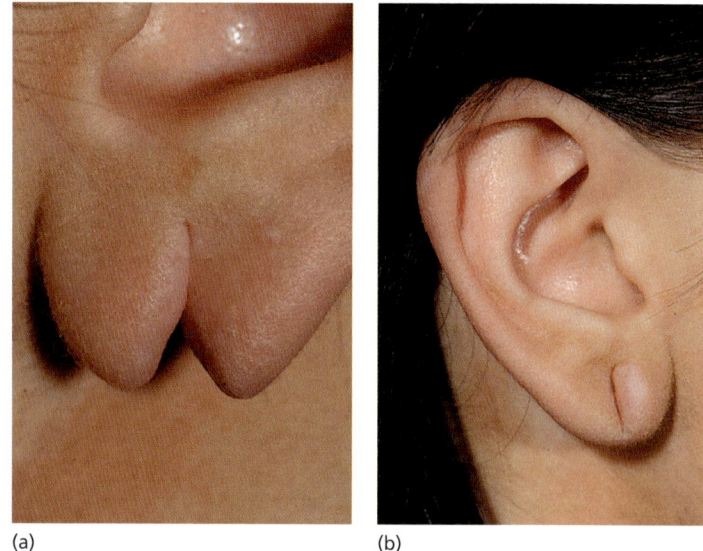

(a)   (b)

Figure 106.17 Traumatic cleft or split of the earlobe. (a) Complete. (b) Incomplete.

visible scar tissue, leaving a complete cleft of the earlobe. Prolonged traction from heavy or pendulous earrings can cause the piercing hole to gradually enlarge until it becomes a complete cleft. Other predisposing factors include chronic and repetitive tension from jogging or habitual fondling. Complete clefts can also be caused by pressure necrosis from clip-on earrings, causing progressive atrophy. Incomplete clefts may be seen in older women who have worn heavy earrings for several decades.

Incomplete clefts can be subclassified [3]:
1 Type 1: boundaries of the cleft hole extending less than half the distance from piercing site to inferior margin of the earlobe.
2 Type 2: boundaries of the cleft hole extending more than half the distance.
3 Type 3: cleft hole completely splitting the earlobe.

Type 1 clefts should be corrected by excising the borders and suturing them, without preserving the pierced hole. For Type 2 deformities, a complete cleft should be created by incising the bridge of remaining soft tissue.

In a study of the pathology of split earlobes in 21 patients wearing heavy gold earrings, an inflammatory reaction was seen in the majority of cases, with perivascular infiltration of lymphocytes, plasma cells and eosinophils [4]. Most of the patients reported that the split was preceded by a moist discharge or itching of variable intensity, indicating an inflammatory response. The authors proposed that an allergic reaction may often be involved, rather than pure trauma or prolonged traction.

Management

Reconstruction of a cleft earlobe can be divided into those involving direct suture and those using local flaps. All methods of earlobe repair concern the removal of the scar epithelium and some type of approximation of the fresh edges. Basic principles include primary straight-line closure with or without a V-shaped wedge excision or broken-line closures employing Z-plasty or L-plasty with full or partial-thickness flaps (Figure 106.18) [5–17].

Repairs can be performed with or without preservation of the earring hole. To create a new epithelialised earring hole, early

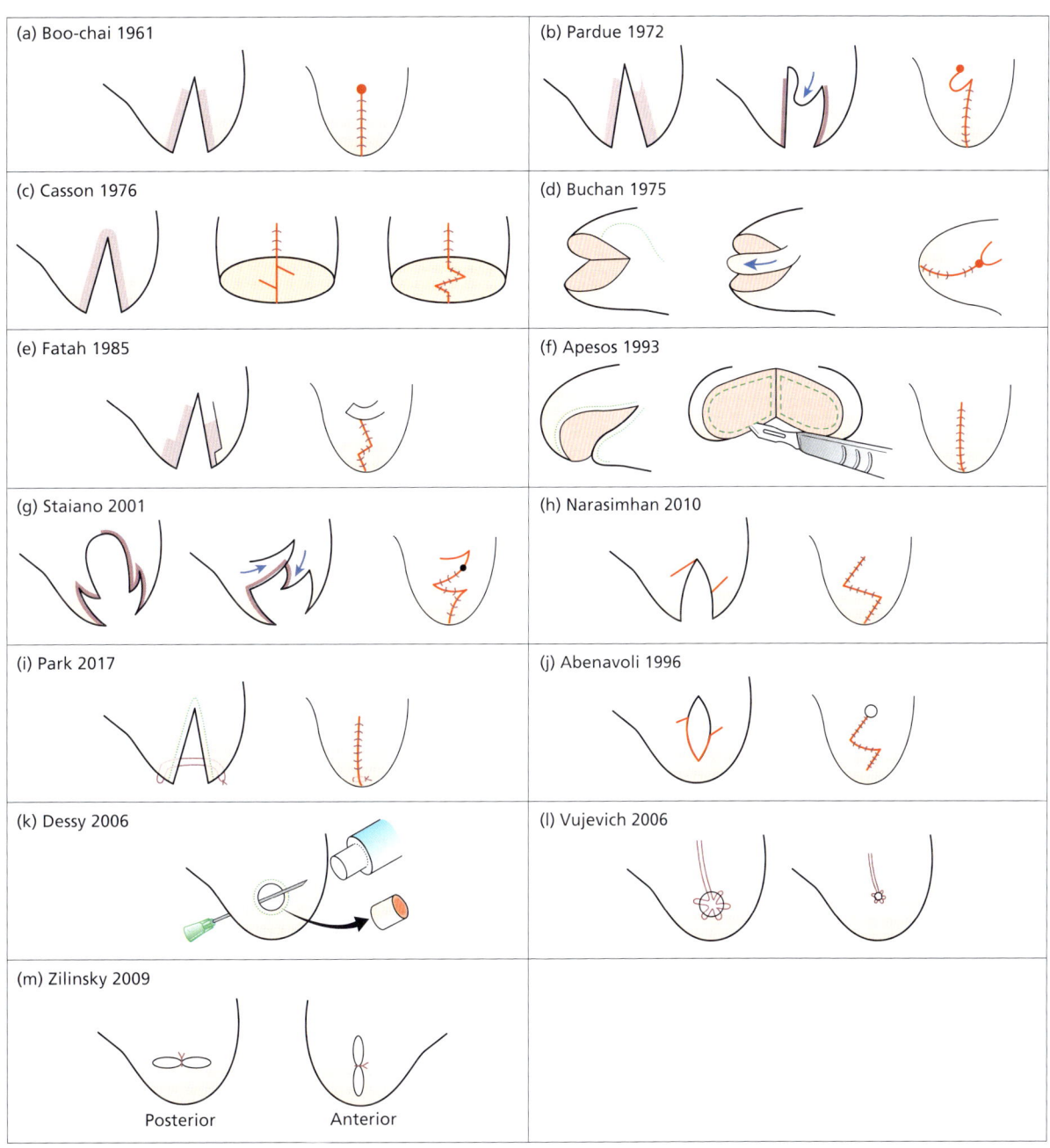

Figure 106.18 Repair techniques for complete clefts (a–i) and incomplete clefts (j–m) of the earlobe. (a) The edges of the cleft are excised and the margins opposed with sutures. (b) The edges of the cleft are excised, with a transposition flap at the superior aspect. (c) A Z-plasty at the inferior surface of the lobe, which prevents a notch developing from scar contracture. (d) A 2 mm flap of skin is raised, rotated 180 degrees, and drawn through the cleft repair to form the floor of the new earring canal. This may provide more strength to support the weight of a new earring, compared with techniques where the canal floor is lined with scar tissue. (e) An L-plasty is used to prevent notching from the contracture of a linear scar. A flap may or may not be included, to create an earring hole. (f) The cleft is excised and the edges are undermined for 1 mm. The skin edges are then everted and closed with simple sutures. (g) The cleft is excised and the wound divided into an upper and lower portion. An upper flap is created to form an epithelial-lined earring hole and the lower flap supports its position. (h) Excision of cleft followed by Z-plasty. (i) A vertical mattress suture is used to create eversion of the inferior lobe to reduce the risk of notching. (j) The earlobe is stretched and a Z-plasty performed to the lower half of the cleft, leaving the upper half to act as a new earring hole. (k) A needle is inserted through an incomplete cleft to act as a guide. A punch biopsy then removes the skin edges, which are then sutured. Adapted from Dessy 2006. (l) An incomplete cleft is excised and a 'purse-string' suture is placed in the periphery to partially close the defect. (m) A 'cross-stitching' technique where the anterior surface of the lobe is closed in a vertical orientation and the posterior surface closed in a horizontal orientation.

reports described a matchstick being left in the superior cleft for 2 weeks [5] or a nylon suture for 4–6 weeks [6]. Repair by direct closure leaves a vertical scar that renders the earring susceptible to being pulled through again. Flap repair options may prevent this, by supporting the scar with fresh tissue that resists the vertical tension of a new earring. Such flap repairs also prevent a notch forming, due to contraction of a direct closure scar. Rim modification techniques produce appropriate lobule contour, avoid excessive lengthening and prevent excessive grooves or notching along the inferior lobule [7].

Ideally the original position of the earring hole is preserved so that earrings remain symmetrical, especially in unilateral tears.

Photographs or a template from the opposite ear may help with positioning of the new earring hole.

Complicated flaps are difficult to handle on the fleshy and mobile tissues of the earlobe. Stability during reconstructive surgery can be achieved with the supportive use of chalazion clamps, skin hooks and sterile tongue depressors [18].

Keloids

Keloids occur due to aberrant wound healing, resulting in excessive and disorganised collagen deposition, forming nodules and plaques beyond the margin of the initiating trauma [1]. Factors involved in keloid formation include inflammation from infection, excessive wound tension and foreign material. Earlobe keloids are unique due to the low tension in this area, their tenancy to respond better to therapy and their lower recurrence rates after excision.

Earlobe keloids most often are the result of ear piercing (Figure 106.19). In a survey of 1200 pierced ears, Simplot and Hoffman [2] reported the incidence of keloid as 2.5%. Piercing before the age of 11 years is more likely to be followed by keloid than after that age [3]. The keloids seem to occur more on the back surface than the front of the earlobe [4], perhaps exacerbated by the presence of metal in the backs of earring [5]. A classification system for earlobe keloids has been proposed [6].

Management

The treatment of keloids is discussed in greater detail in Chapter 94.

Conservative treatment

Compression therapy has been used since 1860 [7], first described using elastic stockings in patients with keloids to burn scars. Recurrence rates can be low [8,9], but requires patient adherence to nearly continuous pressure application. This can be accomplished by means of acrylic splints [10], Oyster splints using dental plaster [11], silicone sheeting [12], a form pressure device [13] or special clip-on earrings. These devices are to be worn for 18–24 hours per day for between 4 and 6 months [14]. Early release of the device can lead to rebound hypertrophy, making it unsuitable for the non-compliant patient [15].

First Line

- For earlobe keloids, injection of corticosteroids can be used as monotherapy with a response rate of 5–100% and a recurrence rate 9–50% [16].
- Surgical excision as monotherapy has a high risk of recurrence, with a study of 43 patients reporting a recurrence in 51.2% after 1 year [8], similar to previous reports [17]. A preoperative photograph of the opposite lobule may help as a template for surgical reconstruction [18]. Combination therapy of excision followed by intralesional corticosteroids (using triamcinolone acetonide 10–40 mg/mL) can maximise treatment success. Recurrence rates are reported to be between 14% and 43% at 3–5 years [19–22].

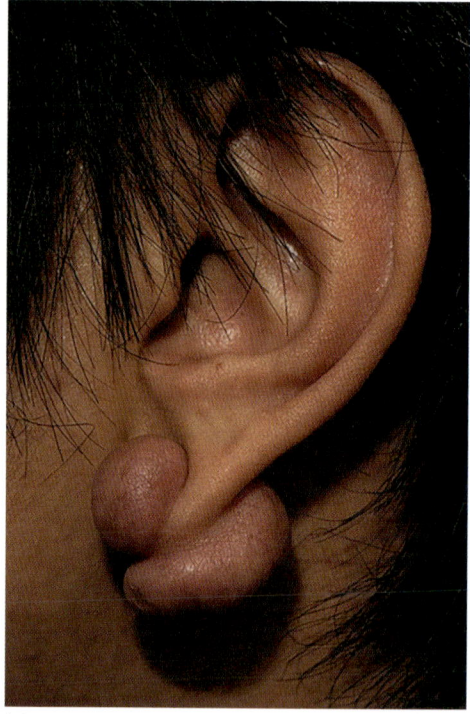

(a)

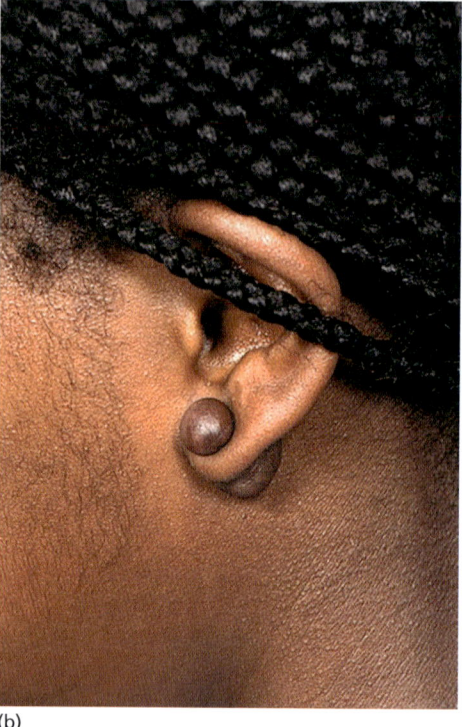

(b)

Figure 106.19 (a, b) Keloids secondary to ear piercing. A *barbell* keloid affecting, both the anterior and posterior aspects of the lobule.

Second line

Intralesional cryosurgery allows for a focused destruction of keloid scar tissue with minimal surface damage to the epidermis [23]. The keloid is pierced with a long, uninsulated, double-lumen cryoneedle, attached to a liquid nitrogen source. The cryogen gas is passed through the needle until the keloid is sufficiently frozen by visual inspection, typically taking 10–60 minutes depending on scar volume. A prospective study of 29 keloid scars, 11 on the ear, found a mean volume decrease of 63%, with recurrence in seven cases (24%) at one year [24].

Other

Radiation therapy has been used as monotherapy, with either external radiation or brachytherapy but is cautioned in young adults due to long-term carcinogenic potential. Adjuvant therapy following surgical excision can be useful, with a lower recurrence associated with shorter time intervals from excision to radiation [25,26]. This can be considered for recalcitrant keloids not responding to traditional therapies. For earlobe keloids in particular, the combination of adjuvant radiotherapy and surgical excision can result in low recurrence rates of 3–25% [27–29]. This technique is not widely practised. An uncontrolled study has suggested that imiquimod 5% may be a reasonably effective adjuvant therapeutic alternative for the prevention of recurrences in excised earlobe keloids [30].

Treatment ladder for keloid scars

First line
- Pressure, intralesional corticosteroid, surgical excision in conjunction with intralesional corticosteroid

Second line
- Intralesional cryosurgery

INFECTIONS

Otitis externa

Definition and nomenclature

Otitis externa (OE) is a diffuse inflammatory or infective condition of the skin of the auditory canal that can affect the adjacent pinna all the way to the tympanic membrane. It may cause varying degrees of pain, itch, deafness and discharge. It can be divided into acute and chronic forms (Figures 106.20 and 106.21).

Introduction and general description

The term OE may include a number of overlapping conditions:

Acute localised OE: this term is sometimes used for furunculosis of the ear canal.

Acute diffuse OE: this has a rapid onset and is generally due to infection, often precipitated by trauma and/or excessive exposure to water or high humidity. Although the infective agent is usually bacterial, viral infection, e.g. herpes zoster, can present as OE.

Chronic OE: this lasts for 2 months or more [1]. Factors that contribute to this include an inflammatory dermatosis, trauma, microbial flora, alterations in cerumen and anatomical variations.

Necrotising OE: this term is used for a more invasive and serious infection.

Otomycosis: this is a non-dermatophyte fungal infection of the EAC. Although included in the subclassification of OE, it is dealt with separately below.

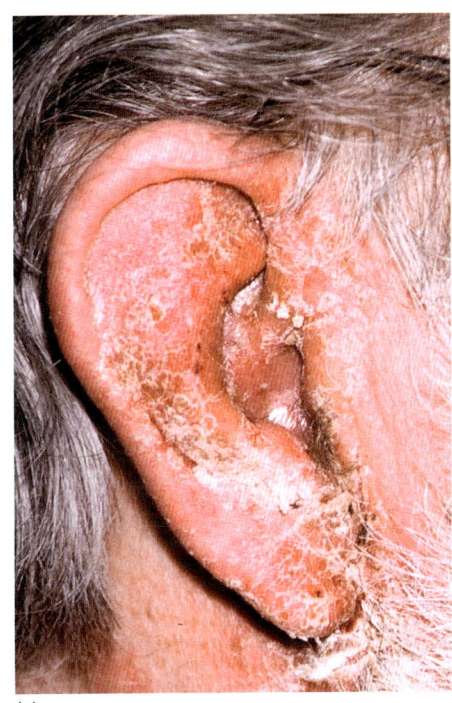

(a)

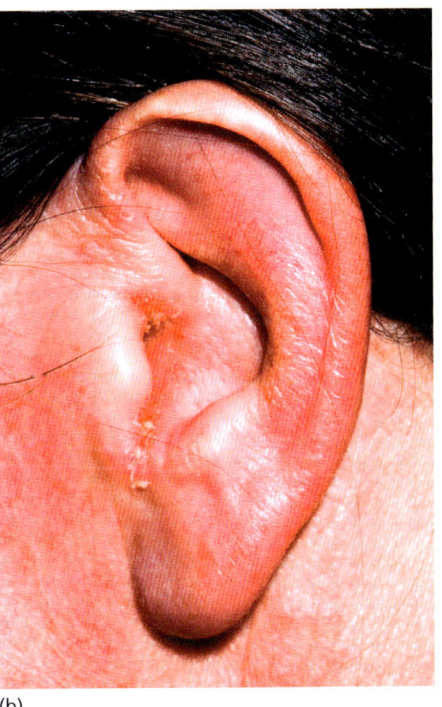

(b)

Figure 106.20 Acute otitis externa. (a) The pinna and adjacent skin are red with crusting and scaling, with narrowing of the auditory meatus. (b) Milder form with redness of the pinna and crusting at the meatus.

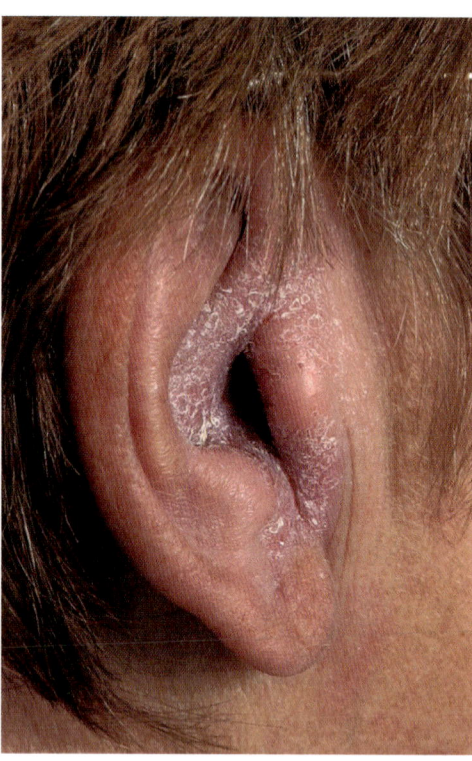

Figure 106.21 Chronic otitis externa. There is longstanding eczematous change, in part due to contact allergic reactions to ear drops, and induration causing narrowing of the canal.

Acute diffuse OE and chronic OE

Epidemiology

Incidence and prevalence

Most data relate to acute diffuse OE, which is common, some studies indicating an annual incidence of about 1 : 250 [2] and appears to be commoner in the summer months, probably because of higher temperatures, humidity and more people engaging in swimming and other water sports [3]. It is unilateral in 90% of cases.

Age

Some studies indicate that acute diffuse OE is more common in children, adolescents and young adults [4], peaking at age 7–12 years and declining after 50 years.

Sex

There is no sex predilection.

Ethnicity

There are significant racial and individual differences in susceptibility to OE. This may be due to anatomical differences in the curvature of the EAC or narrowing of the isthmus, e.g. natives of New Guinea with wide straight canals only rarely suffer from external otitis [5].

Associated diseases

Chronic OE is often associated with an inflammatory dermatosis, particularly atopic eczema, seborrhoeic dermatitis, contact dermatitis or psoriasis, but occasionally other skin diseases such as discoid lupus erythematosus (Figure 106.27).

Pathophysiology

Predisposing factors

1 Trauma is a common immediate precipitating factor. Examples include insertion of fingernails, paperclips, matches, hair grips and even hearing aid earpieces.
2 Water retention, e.g. from swimming, plugs of wax, a tortuous canal and abundant hair are also predisposing factors.
3 Absence of ear wax, e.g. from repeated water exposure or overzealous cleansing can contribute; some individuals may not produce enough cerumen.
4 Alkaline pH [6] may be associated with chronicity. Increased levels of proteases may also be associated with chronicity [7].
5 Variations in lectin binding may influence the likelihood of *Pseudomonas* infection – binding occurs more in individuals expressing blood group A on their epithelial cells [8].

Pathology

In most cases of OE, there is acanthosis, elongation of the rete ridges and an increase in orthokeratosis and parakeratosis. Spongiosis occurs in eczematous and seborrhoeic forms. The nature of the dermal infiltrate varies with both cause and chronicity. The histopathology is seldom diagnostic except when fungal mycelia are seen.

Causative organisms

Pseudomonas aeruginosa is the most common infection, particularly in swimmers and in hot humid environments, and the organism probably comes from resident flora in the ear canal. Some strains may be more pathogenic [9]. A recent study has shown evidence for increasing resistance to aminoglycosides but almost all isolates remain sensitive to fluoroquinolones [10]. In more temperate climates, *Staphylococcus aureus* is often isolated. This may be associated with evidence of skin disease elsewhere or with staphylococcal carriage. Methicillin-resistant *S. aureus* (MRSA) infections are becoming more common, especially when the patient has recently had hospital exposure [11].

In the tropics, mycotic infections of the external ear canal are relatively common. *Aspergillus*, *Candida*, *Penicillium* and *Mucor* spp. are the organisms most often incriminated. There is some debate, however, as to whether these fungi are pathogenic, opportunistic, saprophytic or simply commensal. Otomycosis is discussed later.

Environmental factors

Heat, humidity and moisture are undoubtedly important in hot-weather ear or swimmer's ear [12]. This condition is common, especially among white people in tropical and subtropical regions. High temperature, high relative humidity and swimming [13] all encourage maceration and secondary bacterial or fungal infections of the canal epithelium. Freshwater swimming appears to be a particular risk factor [14]. Failure to dry the ears completely after swimming, shampooing or showering may also be a factor in some cases [15].

Clinical features

Presentation: acute diffuse OE

Symptoms of acute diffuse OE typically include pain, itching and a sensation of fullness. There may be hearing loss and a clear or purulent discharge, which tends to be bluish-green when *Ps. aeruginosa* is the infective cause.

Examination of acute diffuse OE shows redness and swelling which may spread from the EAC to involve the concha or beyond. The EAC shows redness and oedema, and there is macerated debris and perhaps greenish pus present. In severe cases, inflammation can extend to involve the tympanic membrane. Hearing loss is due to oedema of the canal, and this may be sufficient to obscure vision of its full length. Traction on the pinna to examine the canal and pressure over the tragus characteristically elicit pain. There may be associated low-grade fever, malaise and regional lymphadenopathy. If there is a temperature of more than 38.5°C and/or obvious cellulitis, consider necrotising OE.

During examination, it is important to visualise the tympanic membrane; if it is not intact, the OE may be secondary to otitis media, and drops containing aminoglycosides are best avoided.

Presentation: chronic OE

In chronic OE, the main symptoms are itch, variable pain and discharge, which have persisted for more than 2 months. Signs will vary depending on the contributory pathologies.

Infection is very likely to be a factor. Microbiological assessment demonstrated a significant organism in 82% of cases in one series [16]: *S. aureus* in one-third, *Pseudomonas* in one-third and various other Gram-negative and Gram-positive organisms in the remainder; in addition, 17 of the 99 patients had fungal disease alone. There is often a dry canal due to lack of cerumen. In most cases of chronic OE, particularly when treatment has been used for the acute attack and symptoms have continued, concurrent dermatological disorders are usually present (Figure 106.21). For recalcitrant disease, clinicians should consider the possibility of an underlying systemic disease, such as HIV infection, malnutrition or uncontrolled diabetes; a poor therapeutic response is also seen in patients treated with high-dose steroids or chemotherapeutic agents [17].

Seborrhoeic dermatitis, atopic eczema and psoriasis usually occur only at the meatus but may sometimes extend further into the canal. Seborrhoeic OE is common and has been regarded by some dermatologists as the basis for many cases of chronic OE. The symptoms and signs are normally mild unless complicated by secondary factors, with only superficial scaling and a little discomfort or itching. Signs of pityriasis capitis or seborrhoeic dermatitis elsewhere are usually present. Psoriasis involving the canal (Figure 106.30) is likely to be present on the pinna and/or elsewhere.

Secondary bacterial infection is common. In this 'reactive' group the appearance is often that of a dermatitis spreading into the ear, in contrast with those cases with a primarily 'infective' aetiology where infection and/or inflammation often appears to be spreading out from the ear and where the entire length of the canal is commonly affected. The clinical appearance, however, is often non-diagnostic.

'Infective' eczema usually causes intense pruritus associated with exudate, and may complicate both otitis media and OE. Alternatively, it may develop from seborrhoeic dermatitis that has become secondarily infected. The condition may affect the meatus, concha, lobe and periauricular skin and often spreads widely. The post-auricular fold is commonly affected. The symptoms and signs are those of eczema with an accompanying or preceding aural discharge. Fissures and cellulitis are common complications.

Contact dermatitis is often occult and easily overlooked. It is both a complication (see later) and a contributory factor to chronicity. Sensitivity to topically applied medicaments is common in chronic external otitis. Neomycin and the related aminoglycosides are likely to be the commonest sensitisers [18–20], and medicated gauze should be considered [21]. Occlusion, the recurrent nature of the disease and frequent use of antibiotics on an already damaged skin probably account for the high incidence of contact dermatitis at this site. Other sensitivities include nickel from hair pins, metal implements, nail varnish, chromate and phosphorus sesquisulfide (from match heads introduced into the ears). One study of 37 patients [22] with chronic OE found a positive reaction in 59% of patients, with 63% of those having a reaction to two or more substances. Other studies have shown a 23–40% positive test in patients with OE [23–25]. It is characteristic that the degree of itching and burning is often markedly out of proportion to the amount of redness and oedema present. Contact dermatitis may also occur with ear moulds. In a study of 25 hearing aid users with persistent irritation, 56% of patients developed a positive patch test reaction to methyl methacrylate [26], also demonstrated in later studies [23,27]. In-the-ear moulds commonly feature in case reports [28], but behind-the-ear devices, bone-anchored hearing aids [29] and cochlear implants [30] have also been affected. Chemicals and resins of ear prostheses can also cause an allergic contact dermatitis.

Lichen simplex (neurodermatitis) may be localised to one area of the meatus or may occur more diffusely over the tragus, triangular fossa and adjoining skin. The condition is usually diagnosed by the history rather than the signs. Itching is intense, but often intermittent. The need to scratch or rub is compulsive, although often denied. Signs of inflammation are often minimal, but some degree of oedema and scaling is common. Complications from trauma, infection and sensitisation are frequent. Intermittent itching of the EAC (non-specific external otitis) can also occur, irregularly and over a long period, without any obvious cause and with minimal signs of disease. Clinically, it may be difficult to differentiate lichen simplex from contact dermatitis.

Whatever the primary aetiology, with the passage of time, chronic OE becomes an increasingly complex diagnostic and therapeutic problem.

Classification of severity

With acute diffuse OE there is a spectrum. Mild cases have earache and or itching, some hearing loss and little or no discharge. At the severe end, the symptoms are more intense with swelling involving not only the ear canal but also the pinna; there may be low-grade fever and lymphadenopathy. If there is a high fever, necrotising OE (see later) should be considered.

Complications and co-morbidities

Hypertrophic OE or localised elephantiasis nostra (lymphoedema) [31] of the ears may accompany recurrent OE, as a result of the effects of chronic lymphatic obstruction. Narrowing of the EAC coupled with the underlying lymphoedema makes recurrent and repeated infections more likely. Benign non-necrotising OE presents as chronic non-painful otorrhoea with an ulcer present in the floor of the EAC. Surgery may be a better alternative for this complication than long-term medical management [32]. Contact sensitisation, discussed above as a contributory factor to chronic OE, is a common complication. Causes include the aminoglycosides, neomycin, framycetin and gentamicin, quinolines, corticosteroids, nail varnish, nickel, chromate and phosphorus sesquisulfide

Disease course and prognosis

Acute diffuse OE usually responds well to topical therapy. Recurrence is likely if there are background factors such as heat, humidity, frequent swimming, an abnormal ear canal, eczema, etc.

Once OE becomes chronic, it is less likely that it can be eradicated.

Investigations

Investigations are probably not necessary for acute diffuse OE when there are no co-morbidities. Bacterial swabs are recommended if there has been no response to treatment after 7 days, if the patient is systematically unwell or if there is concern that the diagnosis is necrotising OE. For resistant disease, a swab should be cultured for bacterial sensitivities, and fungal investigations including microscopy and fungal culture may be appropriate. Patients with chronic OE should be patch tested.

Management [33,34]

Acute diffuse OE

For acute diffuse OE, topical treatment and appropriate analgesia is usually sufficient, with the condition resolving in a week or so. Ideally, the eardrum should be visualised before deciding on a topical therapy because of the potential ototoxicity of topical aminoglycosides although there is a consensus that aminoglycoside in ear drops is safe even if the drum is perforated, provided it is used for not more than 2 weeks [35].

When there is marked swelling of the ear canal, ear drops will be more effective if there is an ear wick in place. Wax and keratinous debris in the canal can be removed regularly by gentle suction, making treatment more effective. Alternatively, advise patients with a swollen ear canal to lie on one side with the affected ear up, holding position for 10 min after the introduction of ear drops.

Recent systematic reviews and commentaries [35,36–40] of treatments for acute diffuse OE have established that:

- A topical antibiotic plus steroid ear drop is effective and probably better than either alone.
- There is little to choose in efficacy between aminoglycosides such as neomycin, framycetin and gentamicin, polymyxin B, fluoroquinolones, i.e. ciprofloxacin (currently only available in the UK as eye drops), ofloxacin (not available currently in the UK) and the antiseptic clioquinol.
- Treatment should be for 7 days, but longer (up to a further 7 days) if necessary.
- Acetic acid drops are as effective as an antibiotic–steroid combination in the short term, but less effective if longer treatment is needed.
- Aluminium acetate ear drops are probably as effective as antibiotic–steroid drops.
- Treatment choice may be influenced by the possible risk of aminoglycoside toxicity, contact hypersensitivity (more likely

when there is a history of recurrent episodes), availability, cost, dosing schedule (acetic acid and aluminium acetate require frequent administration) and possible bacterial resistance.

Treatment ladder for acute diffuse OE

- When feasible use microsuction or dry swabbing to remove debris, allow visualisation of the drum and improve access of medication to the canal wall.
- Analgesia, e.g. paracetamol and ibuprofen.
- If the ear canal is swollen, to improve delivery of drops an ear wick should be used.
- The canal should be kept dry when bathing, etc.

First line
- Topical antibiotic/corticosteroid, e.g. ciprofloxacin with dexamethasone 4 drops BD for up to 14 days.

Second line
- As alternative to topical antibiotic/corticosteroid: flumetasone pivalate with clioquinol 3 drops BD for up to 14 days.

Third line
- As alternative to topical antibiotic/corticosteroid: aluminium acetate ear drops or spray.

If there is a failure of response by 14 days' topical treatment, the canal is completely stenosed or it remains full of debris, urgent referral to an otorhinolaryngology department should be considered.

Chronic OE

In cases of chronic OE it is important to review the likely cause(s) for chronicity. These include a dermatosis such as atopic eczema or psoriasis, an anatomical problem causing canal stenosis, contact dermatitis and fungal overgrowth. While awaiting the results of patch testing, aluminium acetate ear drops can be very useful. Topical 0.1% tacrolimus delivered via an ear wick is a useful alternative to topical steroids in chronic OE [41]. Pope wick and ichthammol wicks can be soothing.

Occasionally, chronic OE is due to narrowing of the external auditory meatus. Surgical enlargement of the meatus can then bring about resolution [42–44].

Treatment ladder for chronic OE

Chronicity is most likely due to one or more underlying skin diseases or abnormality of the ear canal. Contact dermatitis to medicaments is often a factor. Bacterial and/fungal infection may also be relevant. Initial investigations should include appropriate patch testing and microbial culture. If the ear canal is swollen, to improve delivery of drops an ear wick should be used. The canal should be kept dry when bathing etc.

First line

- If steroid +/- antibiotic have been used, particularly for a lengthy period, discontinue and use 2% aluminium acetate or 2% acetic acid drops 3–4 times daily

Second line

- Further treatment is likely to be guided by the assessment of underlying cause(s) and results of investigations. If severe oedema of the canal persists a short course of oral corticosteroid may be indicated.

Acute localised OE

This is a furunculosis of the hair-bearing part of the canal. It is usually due to infection with *Staphylococcus aureus*. In the ear canal, furunculosis typically causes pain, which can be aggravated by chewing when the anterior wall of the canal is involved. Furunculosis of the canal can usually be distinguished from acute diffuse OE by the normal appearance of the canal epithelium and the absence of a discharge; the two conditions can, however, coexist. Swelling may obstruct the entrance to the canal. There is often regional lymphadenopathy and sometimes fever. Usually this can be treated with analgesia and the application of warmth. If there are signs of severe infection, however, treat with an oral antibiotic and consider the need for incision and drainage.

Treatment ladder for acute localised OE

- Most cases are caused by *Staphylococcus aureus*.
- No fever or lymphadenopathy: antibiotic drops, e.g. ciprofloxacin.
- Fever and/or lymphadenopathy: flucloxacillin (if penicillin allergic, clarithromycin).
- If there is an abscess, drain and send sample for culture. Change treatment if necessary as determined by culture results.

Necrotising OE

Necrotising or malignant OE is a rare complication of OE, occurring in 0.5% of cases. Infection beginning in the EAC then spreads into the temporal bone causing osteomyelitis, then further into the base of the skull when cranial nerve palsies may occur. It is a serious and potentially fatal infection, typically affecting the elderly, immunosuppressed and diabetics [45]. Patients may report refractory purulent otorrhoea and severe otalgia that may worsen at night.

On examination, the EAC is always abnormal, with varying degrees of oedema and redness, and extensive granulation tissue formation is evident. This is particularly seen on the posterior and inferior aspect of the wall at the junction between the bony and cartilaginous segments of the canal. There may be exposed bone in the floor of the canal and swelling of the soft tissues of the pinna and beyond, leading to lymphadenopathy and trismus (pain on mouth opening). The tympanic membrane is frequently necrotic in children but is characteristically spared in adults [46]. Cranial neuropathies may be found in up to 40% of patients, most commonly a facial nerve palsy with extensive disease affecting cranial nerves IX, X and XI. There may be a high fever.

Management is a medical emergency requiring involvement of otorhinolaryngology colleagues. Prolonged antibiotic therapy of 6–8 weeks' duration and debridement surgery are among the treatment options. For a suspected mild case it is reasonable to initiate ciprofloxacin 750 mg PO twice daily. If there is no improvement, then refer as stated previously [47].

Infection of the pinna

The anatomy of the ear, with its many folds and the semi-occluded nature of the EAC, make it particularly susceptible to intertriginous infection, especially with Gram-negative organisms. The close anatomical relationship between the middle and external ear means that infections can pass relatively easily from one to the other, and the eardrum should always be examined. The cartilaginous and bony structures close to the skin are particularly vulnerable to infection.

Pyogenic infection

Staphylococcus aureus, alone or in association with group A β-haemolytic *Streptococcus*, may cause impetigo of the ear. This is a relatively common site for infection in infants and young children. *Staphylococcus aureus* is also the most common causative organism of furuncles (boils) and carbuncles, which are more common in the EAC (see previously, acute localised OE) than on the pinna. Cracks and fissures around the auricle are often the portal of entry for β-haemolytic streptococcal infection manifesting as erysipelas. This is more common in the elderly, the newborn and those suffering from malnutrition, disability, alcoholism, diabetes or immune deficiency states.

Erysipelas typically begins with high fever and constitutional upset, including malaise, vomiting and headache, and there is rapidly spreading redness and oedema from the pinna on to the face. There is often lymphadenopathy. Recurrent attacks of cellulitis of the face may have the same predisposing factors as at other body sites. Recurrent attacks of cellulitis lead to fibrosis and lymphoedema. Treatment of erysipelas and cellulitis is discussed in Chapter 26. Necrotising fasciitis has rarely been described arising from an initial infection of the pinna.

The term *infective eczematoid dermatitis* is still sometimes used for an oozing crusted eczematous condition occurring on and often below the pinna in association with chronic discharge from the ear. Coagulase-positive staphylococci are the most frequently isolated bacteria. The ear canal is oedematous and red, and purulent discharge may be seen coming from a perforated tympanic membrane. The condition should be differentiated from impetigo, secondarily infected contact dermatitis, seborrhoeic dermatitis and atopic eczema.

Other bacterial infections

Mycobacterial infection can rarely involve the external ear. Lupus vulgaris can produce extensive destruction and may mimic other conditions. Secondary involvement from underlying lymph node disease (scrofuloderma) can present with hearing loss, tinnitus and periauricular lymphadenopathy, with only minimal secretion in the ear canal.

Atypical mycobacteria that may involve the ear include *Mycobacterium marinum* acquired from swimming pool injuries. In leprosy, the ear is almost always involved in the lepromatous type, and there may be evident infiltration of the skin. The earlobe is often used for taking smears.

Syphilis may occasionally involve the ear, usually in the secondary stage.

Viral infections

Herpes simplex occasionally involves the ear, transmitted during contact sports such as rugby and wrestling. Herpes zoster may present as an isolated herpetiform eruption of the external ear or associated with ipsilateral facial palsy and auditory symptoms (Ramsay–Hunt syndrome; geniculate herpes). The condition usually begins with pain and may initially be mistaken for erysipelas. Vesicles usually appear on about the fifth day and involve the pinna, the EAM and, rarely, the tympanic membrane. There is usually malaise, pyrexia and lymphadenopathy. Facial palsy, when it occurs, is usually transient, but more severe and persistent cases do occur. Taste and lacrimation may also be affected. Compression damage to the VIIIth cranial nerve may lead to tinnitus, vertigo, nystagmus, nausea and deafness. Management of herpes zoster is discussed in Chapter 25.

Otomycosis

Definition and nomenclature

Otomycosis is an inflammatory condition of the ear canal in which yeast or fungal organisms play an essential part. It may occur as an isolated condition, as a complication of OE, or included as a subtype of OE.

Introduction and general description

Otomycosis is recognised clinically by visible growth of filamentous fungi on the skin of the ear canal. It is usually a chronic disorder. The use of topical corticosteroids and/or antibiotics in the treatment of OE predisposes to otomycosis; however, it can occur *de novo*. It is commoner in hot climates and when there is excessive exposure to water.

Epidemiology

There are little data on incidence or prevalence, but in tropical countries otomycosis constitutes about 10% of cases of OE. It can occur at all ages but is commoner in middle age. It is twice as common in males as in females. There is no ethnic, racial or genetic predilection recorded.

Associated diseases

Otomycosis is more common in patients with chronic OE treated with topical antibiotics and/or corticosteroids, and both diabetes and immunosuppression may make patients more susceptible.

Predisposing factors

Heat, humidity, trauma, frequent exposure to water, and prolonged use of antibiotics and/or steroid drops in the ear canal may all be important predisposing factors [1,2]. As such, it is probably commoner in hot and humid environments. Otomycosis can follow acute otitis media [3].

Pathology

The fungal hyphae are in the stratum corneum. There may be little or no inflammatory change. Particularly in the immunosuppressed, the fungi can penetrate into the dermis and beyond.

Causative organisms

Most cases are due to *Aspergillus* and *Candida* species. In tropical regions, *Aspergillus* predominate whereas in more temperate areas *Candida* isolates are more common [4]. *Candida* is also more common than *Aspergillus* in the immunocompromised [5]. Occasionally, other yeasts and fungi are found, including phycomycetes, *Rhizopus*, *Actinomyces* and *Penicillium*, and, rarely, dermatophytes. The fact that these organisms can be pathogenic as well as saprophytic has been confirmed in a number of studies [4,6,7]

Clinical features
History
The usual symptoms are itching, earache, discharge, hearing loss, a sense of fullness and pain. Pain may be relatively more common in the immunocompromised [8].

Presentation
On examination, the dominant feature is the presence of wispy filamentous masses, which may be isolated or diffusely present in the canal. These masses are white, grey or stippled black if *Aspergillus* is present. Inflammation of the canal epithelium is usually mild. There may be some epithelial debris, which may be either moist or dry. Otomycosis is usually unilateral, but commonly bilateral in the immunosuppressed [4].

Cellulitis of the surrounding soft tissues without bacterial infection represents more severe infection and is more likely in the immunocompromised. Perforation of the tympanic membrane can occur. Otomycosis can become an invasive disease with penetration into the temporal bone in the immunosuppressed. It is often a chronic disorder but can be cured if adequately treated and any predisposing factors corrected.

Management

Fungal microscopy and culture are needed to establish the diagnosis. The ear canal should be cleaned of debris and discharge, using gentle suction if available. Many treatments have been advocated, but there is little evidence for a particular agent. They include aluminium acetate, acetic acid, *m*-cresyl acetate, thiomersal, gentian violet, clioquinol, nystatin, amphotericin and the imidazoles.

Treatment ladder for otomycosis

First line
- 1% clotrimazole drops 2–3 times daily for at least 2 weeks.

Second line
- If there is tympanic membrane perforation or a likelihood of invasive disease, a systemic agent, e.g. itraconazole, should be used.

Third line
- If there is penetration into bone, voriconazole or posaconazole may be more effective systemic agents than itraconazole [9].

Superficial and deep mycoses

Dermatophyte fungi may rarely involve the ear, and when present can simulate granulomatous disease and chondritis. Pityriasis versicolor may involve the ears but is usually easy to diagnose. In cases of ulcerative granulomatous disease of the ear, deep fungal infections, for example sporotrichosis, should be considered. Biopsy, examination of smears, cultures and serological studies should enable accurate diagnosis. Deep fungal infection may prompt an enquiry for underlying immune deficiency.

EAR INVOLVEMENT IN SKIN DISEASE AND SYSTEMIC DISEASE

The external ear may be affected by a number of skin diseases and also can be a manifestation of a systemic disease presenting in the skin. Some of these cutaneous manifestations are shown in Table 106.2, with cross references to other chapters where the condition is covered in more detail.

Miscellaneous conditions

Petrified ear

This is a rare condition where the ear cartilage is replaced by ectopic calcification or ossification [1]. It can be easily highlighted in radiology images [2]. The clinical presentation is of a partially or wholly rigid auricle, which may be uncomfortable with pressure over it. One or both ears may be involved. Causes include frostbite, trauma, radiation therapy and systemic diseases, including Addison disease, diabetes, hypopituitarism, acromegaly and hypothyroidism. It has been reported in pseudopseudohypoparathyroidism [3].

Cholesteatoma

Cholesteatoma of the middle ear space is accumulation of keratinous debris within a sac-like squamous epithelial lining. A similar condition occurs rarely in the EAC, although its status as a true cholesteatoma is disputed [4,5]. The accumulation of stratum corneum occurs within a cyst-like penetration of the bony portion of the canal wall by the epithelial lining. There is localised ulceration of the skin of the floor of the canal, with underlying osteitis and sometimes necrosis of bone. Some cases are primary and several causes have been identified including previous trauma, operation and radiotherapy [6]. Examination may show a white cystic mass protruding into the canal. Treatment is by otorhinolaryngology colleagues.

Keratosis obturans

Due to a defect in the normal epithelial migration [7], there is a localised accumulation of desquamated keratin in the ear canal. It is usually bilateral and typically occurs in younger patients than those presenting with EAC cholesteatoma, which it can resemble. There is conductive hearing loss, sometimes with otalgia. It can be associated with paranasal sinus disease, bronchitis and the yellow nail syndrome [8]. Treatment consists of careful removal of the accumulated keratin. Irrigation with water should be avoided.

TUMOURS OF THE AURICLE

Despite accounting for 1% of the body surface area, approximately 6% of all cutaneous neoplasms are found in the auricular and periauricular skin [1]. The ear's external location and prominence may account for this disproportionate incidence. In addition, a survey of 269 skin cancer patients found 73% used sunscreen regularly but only 26% of these regularly applied it to their ears [2]. Over the whole body, around two-thirds are basal cell carcinoma (BCC) and one-third are squamous cell carcinoma (SCC). This BCC:SCC ratio has been reported as 3.5:1 in the UK [3] and 2.3:1 in Sweden [4], across all skin sites. For the cancers on the external ear, this ratio reduces to 1.4:1 in the UK [3] and 1:1 in California [2]. In a study of 426 patients in Birmingham, UK, Ahmad found a ratio of 1.3:1 on the ear and 4:1 on the head and neck [5], supporting the perception that for a suspicious nodule on the pinna, the risk of SCC is comparatively much higher.

These two keratinocyte skin cancers are the main focus of this section.

Basal cell carcinoma of the auricle

Aspects of basal cell carcinoma specific to the auricle and EAC are presented in this chapter. See Chapter 140 for a comprehensive account of BCC.

Epidemiology
Incidence
BCC is the most common cancer worldwide and its incidence is increasing in many countries. In the UK, Venables [3] identified a 5% increase between 2013 and 2015 using national data. This large study of over 200 000 tumours found that 6.5% of all BCCs in men, and 1.3% in women, were located on the ear. Subgroup analysis of facial BCCs shows that 17% of male and 3% of female BCCs on the

Table 106.2 Ear dermatoses that may indicate other skin disease or systemic disease.

Diagnosis	Clinical features	Chapter cross reference
Acne	Comedones frequently involve the concha and are occasionally found on the helix, tragus or earlobe. Inflammatory cysts may be found on the lobe, at the entrance to the external auditory canal, or in both the pre- and post-auricular areas	88
Acromegaly	There may be enlargement of the auricular cartilage and coarsening of the overlying skin	150
Addison disease	Pigmentary changes may involve the ear and ossification of the auricular cartilage (petrified ear) may occur in Addison disease [1]	150
Alkaptonuria	aka ochronosis This is typically associated with a bluish discoloration of the auricular cartilage due to oxidation of bound homogentisic acid (Figure 106.22). The cerumen in such patients may be very dark, a finding that can precede other clinical manifestations	
Amyloidosis, primary cutaneous	Asymptomatic papules on the helix and concha of the ear have been described as the sole manifestation of cutaneous amyloidosis [2,3], more generalised papular amyloid [4] and with macular amyloid of the back [5]	56
Angiolymphoid hyperplasia with eosinophilia	This commonly affects the pinna, external auditory meatus (Figure 106.23) and post-auricular area. The lesions are red–brown papules or nodules. Occasionally, they itch and can be painful or pulsatile [6]. The condition mainly affects young to middle-aged adults, and in some series there is a female preponderance	136
Asteatotic eczema	This common cause of a dry itchy ear is mainly seen in the elderly. Aggravating factors include overzealous cleansing, cold, windy weather, low humidity indoors and air-conditioned air during the summer. There may be little to see other than slight scaling. Similar changes can occur in the ear canal, where additional factors include drying vehicles used in ear drops, e.g. alcohol and acetone. Management will include avoidance of provocative factors and use of emollients	39
Atopic eczema	A crusted eczematous fissure at the junction of the earlobe and the face is a common finding in atopics and can be regarded as a reliable feature of atopy [7]. In addition to involvement of the infra-auricular crease, the tragal notch and sometimes the whole of the pinna may be commonly involved	41
Bazex syndrome	Bazex syndrome (acrokeratosis paraneoplastica) commonly affects the ears and is an important marker for internal malignancy [8]	148
Bullous diseases	Pemphigus, pemphigoid, dermatitis herpetiformis and epidermolysis bullosa aquisita may all involve the ear and occasionally the auditory canal. Blistering of the pinna and stenosis of the canal can occur in dystrophic epidermolysis bullosa [9]	50
Calcification, dystrophic	Calcium deposition may occur in many circumstances and occasionally the ear is involved. Usually, calcium deposits in the ear occur for local reasons, e.g. degenerative changes in the cartilage. In infants, congenital calcinosis cutis has been reported [10], although congenital nodular calcification of Winer should be considered [11]. A distinctive paediatric condition often found on the pinna is subepidermal calcifying nodule (Figure 106.24). Petrified ear (idiopathic auricular ossification) should be considered in the differential diagnosis [12–14]	59
Contact dermatitis	The external ear is commonly affected by both irritant and allergic contact dermatitis. As well as products and medicaments used on the scalp and around the ears, allergens may be transferred by fingers, e.g. nail varnish, plant resins. Unilateral involvement of the earlobe may indicate a facial allergic contact dermatitis [15]	127, 128
Crohn disease	Metastatic Crohn disease may rarely involve the ear [16]	153
Cutis laxa	Cutis laxa may result in distinctive pendulous earlobes [17]	94
Darier disease	Occasionally, Darier disease can present with involvement of the external ear as the principal affected site, with redness, oedema and crusting mimicking an eczematous reaction [18]	
Drug reaction	Purpura of the ears has been described in a series of children receiving levamisole for nephritic syndrome [19]. Both vasculitis and thrombotic changes occurred, and there was an association with circulating autoantibodies Hypertrophy of the retroauricular folds may be seen as a consequence of phenytoin therapy [20] Hypertrichosis of the ear canal due to minoxidil therapy can be a predisposing factor for external otitis [21] Pseudolymphoma of the ear can be induced by phenytoin [22] Fixed drug eruption can occur at the site of ear piercing [23]	64
Elephantiasis	Chronically red swollen ears may occur for a number of reasons, including longstanding eczema, psoriasis [24] and chronic streptococcal infection. Longstanding head louse infection has also been reported as a cause [25]	
Erythromelalgia	Typical erythromelalgia of hands and/or feet is occasionally accompanied by concurrent episodes of red swelling of one or both ears associated with a burning painful sensation [26]	
Gout	Gouty tophi frequently involve the pinna (Figure 106.25) and may predate the onset of joint disease or appear decades after the initial attack. The helix and antihelix are typical sites. Histology is distinctive	155
Granuloma annulare	Typical papular and annular dermal lesions of granuloma annulare may involve the pinna, sometimes in the absence of lesions elsewhere [27], and the perforating variant has been reported [28]	95
Granuloma faciale	The ear is an occasional site for the brownish red plaques of this distinctive disorder [29]	100
Granulomatosis with polyangiitis	Granulomatosis with polyangiitis (Wegener's granulomatosis) can present with serous or suppurative otitis and conductive or sensorineural deafness [30]	100
IgG4-related skin disease	This is a recently recognised syndrome characterised by mass-forming lesions with lymphoplasmacytic infiltration, with an increased number of IgG4 cells within the affected tissues. Presentation as nodules behind the ears has been reported [31]	
Jessner's lymphocytic infiltrate	This condition occasionally involves the ear and post-auricular region and sunlight may precipitate or worsen the eruption	133

Table 106.2 (*continued*)

Diagnosis	Clinical features	Chapter cross reference
Leprosy	Leprosy can present with swelling of the earlobe [32] and the earlobe is a valuable site for taking smears [33]	28
Leishmaniasis	Cutaneous leishmaniasis can present as a unilateral 'Dumbo' ear swelling, more common in Mexico [34]	
Lichen planus	Lichen planus typically causes discharge and hearing loss due to stenosis of the external auditory canal. Pruritus, pain and bleeding may also occur. The canal appears red and there may be Wickham's striae [35]	37
Lupus erythematosus	Discoid, subacute cutaneous and systemic lupus erythematosus can all involve the ears (Figure 106.26). The concha is a characteristic site for chronic discoid lupus erythematosus (Figure 106.27)	51
Lymphoma	Systemic lymphoma can occasionally present as an isolated lesion on the ear [36–38], as can other haematological malignancies.	138
Mudi-chood	This distinctive dermatosis, which typically affects the nape of the neck and upper shoulders of girls and young women in the state of Kerala in South India, can occur on the ears. It is thought to be the result of the frictional and occlusive effects of moist oily hair in a hot and humid environment. Individual lesions are hyperpigmented papules with a thin surrounding rim of scale, occurring on the posterolateral aspects of the pinnae [39,40]	
Otophyma	This is due to enlargement of the outer third of the external auditory canal and its entrance due to fibrosis, sebaceous hyperplasia and oedema. It can result in conductive hearing loss. It is usually associated with rosacea and other 'phymatous' enlargement of, for example, the nose, cheek, chin or eyelid. It can be managed by surgical reduction followed by low dose oral isotretinoin [41]	
Perforating disorders	The ear may occasionally be the site for lesions of Kyrle disease, elastosis perforans serpiginosa, perforating folliculitis and perforating papules of diabetic dialysis patients	
Photodermatoses	The ear is a common site for conditions provoked or aggravated by UV and/or visible radiation. A condition peculiar to the ear is juvenile spring eruption (Figure 106.28), a variant of polymorphic light eruption, typically found in young boys. A condition with a similar aetiology is seen in farmers, termed 'lambing ears' [42]	125
Porphyria	Porphyria cutanea tarda (Figure 106.29) may present with vesicles and bullae, often on a background of scarring, hyperpigmentation, milia, sclerodermoid plaques and hypertrichosis. Pseudocysts of the auricle and perichondritis may be simulated [43]	58
Psoriasis	Both guttate and plaque psoriasis involve the external ear. Sometimes this is by extension from the scalp, face or neck. Like seborrhoeic dermatitis, psoriasis often involves the concha and distal part of the external auditory canal, but usually its colour, the nature of the scaling (Figure 106.30) and the presence of psoriasis elsewhere allow it to be differentiated. Sometimes both conditions appear to coexist	35
Red ear syndrome	An episodic condition mainly described in children and young adults in which redness and swelling of one or both ears is associated with a burning sensation and headache, usually of the migrainous type [44]	
Relapsing polychondritis	Relapsing polychondritis is characterised by redness, tenderness and swelling of the entire ear, but with sparing of the lobe; however, it can affect only the tragus and conchal bowl [45]. A persistent ulcer may be the first clinical sign [46]. It has been associated with pseudocyst of the ear [47]. The differential diagnosis includes auricular erythromelalgia [48]	
Rheumatoid disease	Rheumatoid disease is characterised by nodules, which can occur on the ear, where they may ulcerate due to pressure from a pillow or spectacles	155
Sarcoidosis	Cutaneous sarcoidosis [49] can involve the ear, especially the lupus pernio variety	96
Seborrhoeic dermatitis	In its mildest form, seborrhoeic dermatitis simply causes a little scaling and inflammation at the entrance to the external auditory meatus, in the concha or in the auricular folds. When severe, the whole pinna may be affected and there may be infective eczematoid dermatitis both in and around the ear or post-auricularly	40
Systemic sclerosis	Scleroderma can produce pallor and telangiectasia of the auditory canal	54
Syphilis	This may occasionally involve the ear, usually in the secondary stage	
Tuberculosis	Mycobacterial infection can rarely involve the external ear [50]. Lupus vulgaris (cutaneous tuberculosis) can produce extensive destruction and presentation as a unilateral enlarged 'Turkey ear' has been reported [51]	
Viral infection	Herpes vegetans is a rare presentation of the herpes simplex virus, which presents as hyperkeratotic, verrucous eroded ulcerated plaques or nodules [52]. Orf can present on the ear as an isolated nodule [53]	
Verruciform xanthoma	This uncommon condition is typically found in the mouth but has been reported on the ear, where it can mimic squamous cell carcinoma [54]	60
Weathering nodules	These asymptomatic histologically distinct nodules are found on the free edge of the helix (Figure 106.31). They are quite common, increasingly so with age in older men [55], although can occur in women [56]	
Xanthogranuloma, adult	Symmetrical yellow–red nodular lesions with the same histology as juvenile xanthogranuloma have been described on the earlobes [57]	134
Xanthoma	Xanthomas occasionally occur on the ears, presenting as yellow nodules, and can occur without any associated lipid abnormality [58]	60

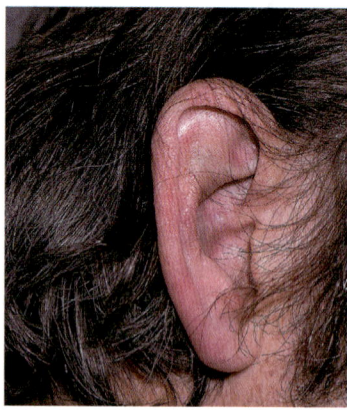

Figure 106.22 Alkaptonuria. The auricular cartilage has a distinctive blue colour. Courtesy of Dr P. Hollingworth, Southmead Hospital, Bristol, UK.

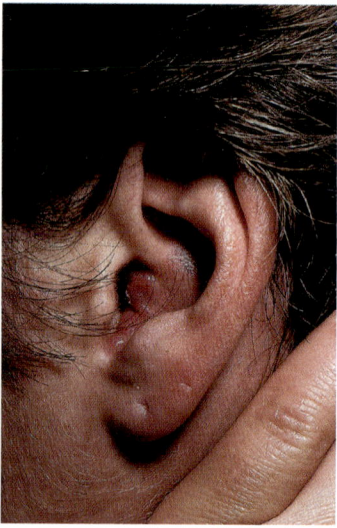

Figure 106.23 Angiolymphoid hyperplasia with eosinophilia. Firm red–brown nodules at the entrance to the external auditory canal.

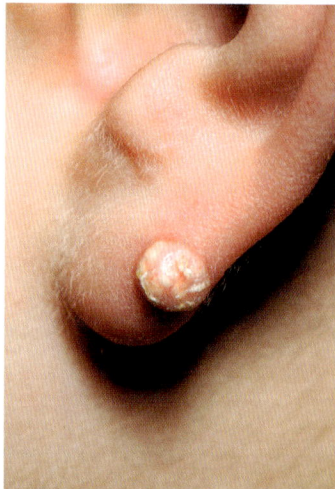

Figure 106.24 Subepidermal calcifying nodule. Hard whitish nodule with slight overlying scale.

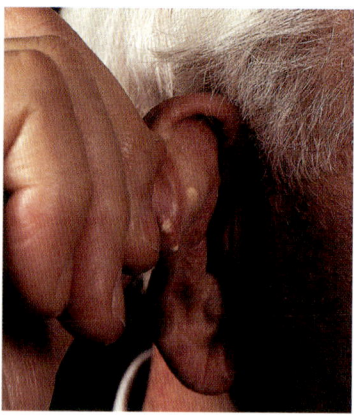

Figure 106.25 Gouty tophi. Yellowish dermal nodules

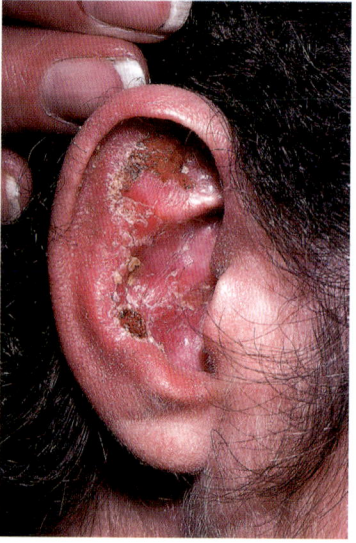

Figure 106.26 Cutaneous lupus erythematosus. Acute redness and erosions following sun exposure.

face are located on the ear. This supports studies from the USA [6] and Australia [7], which showed that 10% of head and neck BCCs were located on the ear, across both genders. Left and right-sided carcinomas are equally distributed [1,8].

Age

The average age of patients with BCC on the ear is reported as between 69 and 73 years [6], and 69 and 70 years [8]. This matches that seen for all BCC with a median age of 71 years [3].

Sex

Over the whole body, BCC has a slightly higher incidence in men than women. Studies relating to ears have shown a greater male preponderance. Mulvaney *et al.* [6] found that 86% of ear BCCs were in men, compared with 57% of non-ear locations. This is matched by Venables *et al.* [3] who showed an 86% male preponderance, compared with 54% of non-ear locations. In a study of 272 patients with BCC in the conchal bowl, this male bias increased to 92% [9]. Other reports shortened the majority to 79% male for the ear [8] and 71.4% male for both ear and nose BCCs [10].

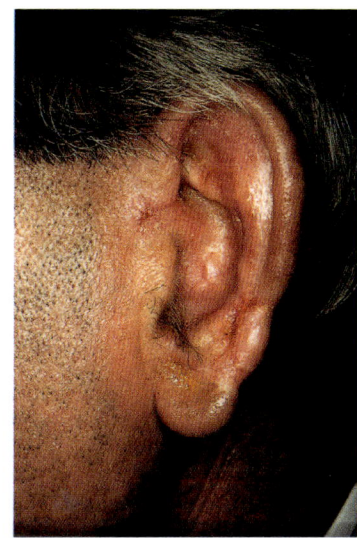

Figure 106.29 Porphyria cutanea tarda. Firm whitish sclerodermoid changes at the site of repeated blistering.

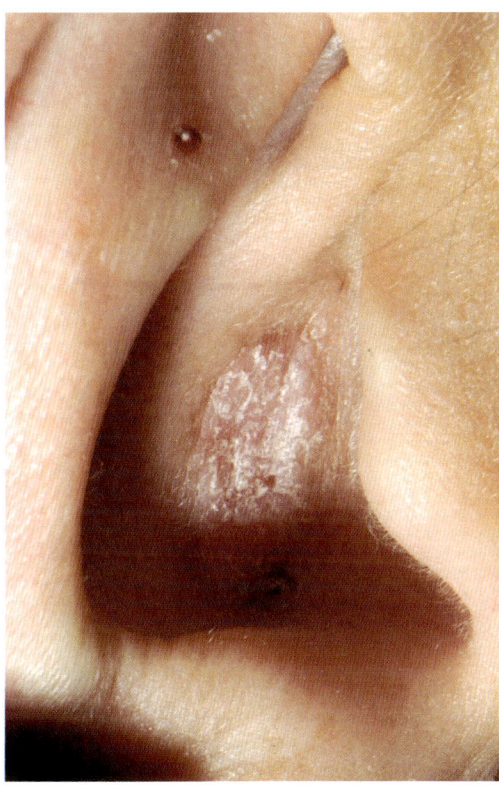

Figure 106.27 Discoid lupus erythematosus. Redness with adherent scaling extending into the ear canal.

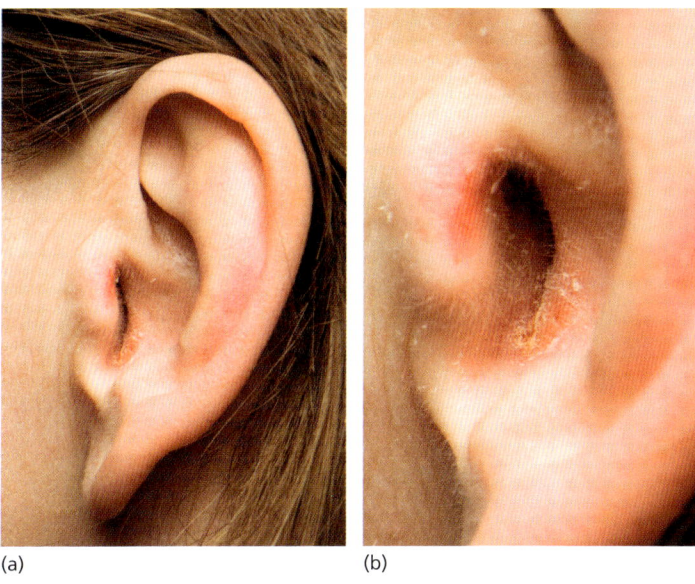

(a)   (b)

Figure 106.30 Psoriasis. (a) Well-defined redness with prominent scaling at entrance to ear canal – close-up in (b).

Pathophysiology

Embryology

BCCs are typically locally invasive and slowly spreading. Bailin *et al.* [11] describe the pattern of spread of auricular BCC, suggesting it is influenced by the convoluted embryologic fusion planes (Figure 106.5). Tumours of the preauricular skin tend to extend toward the ear to involve the superior helix and/or tragus, and, by further extension, the antihelix and lobule. Tumours of the helix spread along the helix and then extend toward the antihelix or posterior surface of the ear. Tumours of the antihelix spread in all directions concentrically. Tumours of the posterior surface of the auricle can extend laterally to the helix and medially to the postauricular sulcus.

BCC is more likely to occur in fusion planes of mid face [12]. Some infantile haemangiomas have also been shown to develop along

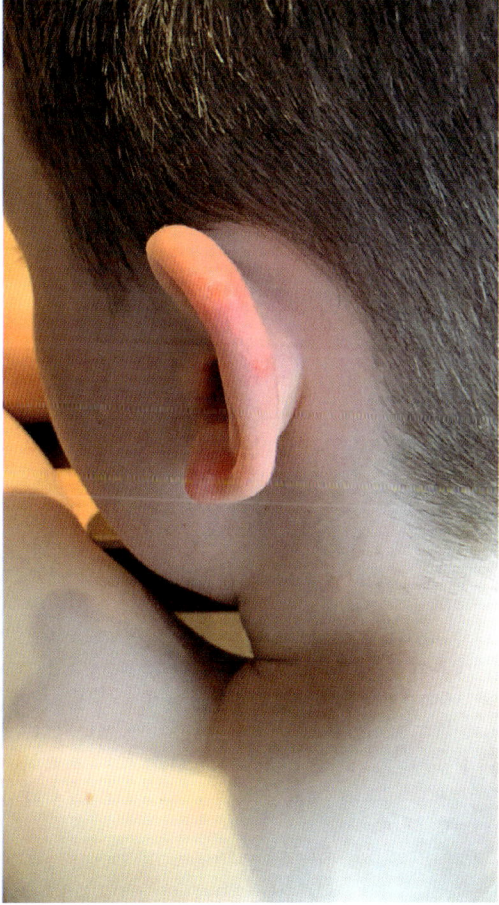

Figure 106.28 Juvenile springtime eruption: papules on the upper pinna of a boy following sunlight exposure during spring.

PART 10: SPECIFIC SITES, SEX & AGE

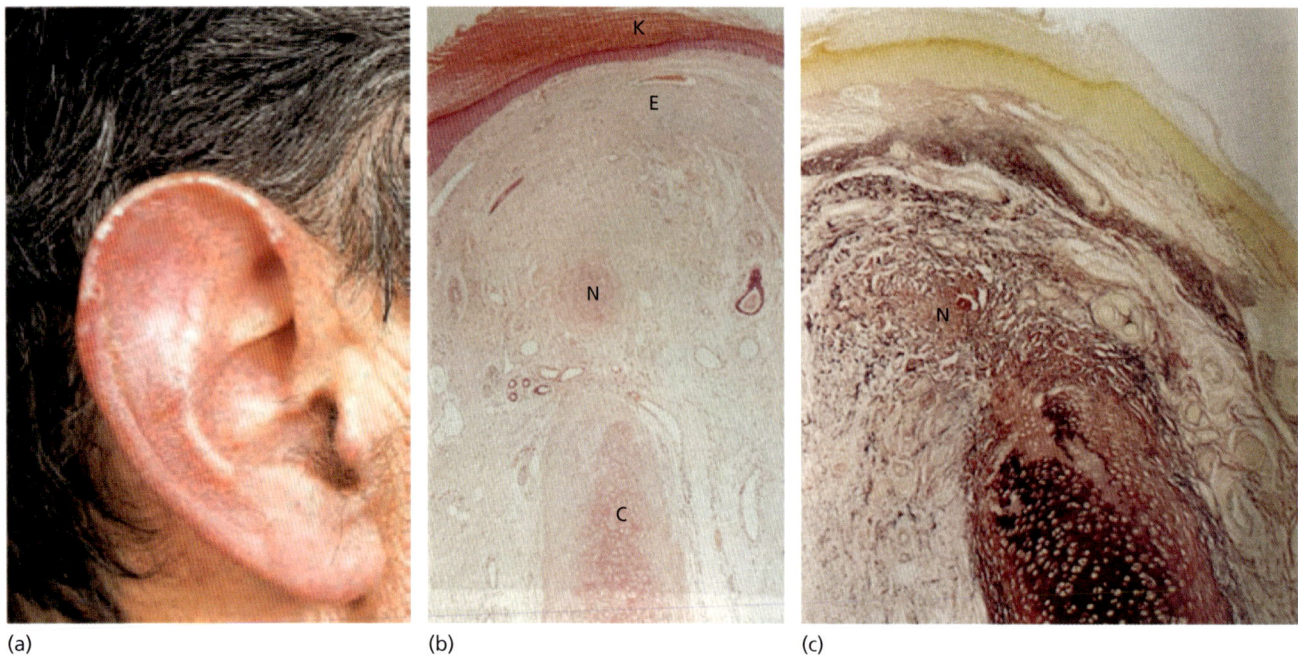

(a)   (b)   (c)

Figure 106.31 (a) Several firm white 'weathering' nodules on the helical rim. (b) Transverse section stained with H&E. N, a nodule comprising a focus of cartilage overlying the edge of the pinna cartilage; E, solar elastotic degeneration; K, an overlying flake of hyperkeratosis. (c) Transverse section stained with Millers and Van Gieson. Serial sectioning showed this was not a separate nodule (N) of cartilage but comprised cartilage metaplasia within a spur of fibrous tissue extending up from disrupted perichondrium of the underlying pinna cartilage (C). Reproduced from Kavanagh *et al.* 1996 [55] with permission of John Wiley & Sons.

these fusion lines [13]. Connecting these, it is postulated that embryonic fusion planes are areas especially hospitable to angiogenesis, with motility of cells and chemotaxis factors. A correlation is known to exist between degree of angiogenesis and BCC aggressiveness [14]. Similarly, the multiple embryonic fusion planes in the ear may provide a path of least resistance for unrestricted growth, within the undulations of the ear folds [15–18].

Pathology

There is an association between tumour site and histological subtype of BCC [19–23]. BCC on the ear is more likely to be of an aggressive subtype (including infiltrative, morphoeic and micronodular variants), with 57% of ear BCCs showing a high-risk phenotype compared with 38% on the cheek [8]. There is a high discordance rate between biopsy samples and Mohs histopathology, with 35% of ear BCCs being up-staged to a more aggressive phenotype during Mohs surgery compared with 9% of non-ear BCCs [24]. Small biopsy specimens from this architecturally complex site may therefore miss an aggressive subtype, supporting the recommendation for Mohs surgery on the ear. Cartilage invasion has been identified in 1.7% of auricular and nasal BCCs [25].

Location of BCC on the ear or midface is associated with a more aggressive clinical course and a significantly higher recurrence rate [26]. Location on the ears is one of the risk factors for extensive subclinical spread [27]. These tumours show greater subclinical extension, are more frequently associated with residual positive margins after excision and have a higher recurrence rate than at other sites. When analysing 758 BCCs on the ear, Mulvaney *et al.* [6] found they presented as larger lesions (1.28 cm^2 vs 0.98 cm^2) and produced a larger final defect following Mohs surgery (4.92 cm^2 vs 4.21 cm^2) than non-ear lesions. This indicates a clinically

aggressive behaviour, even when controlling for aggressive tumour subtypes.

Management

The complete management options for BCC are described in Chapter 140 and discussed further in national guidelines [28]. As a general rule, surgical excision is preferred (standard excision or Mohs surgery), although in individual cases there may be a role for other treatment modalities including cryotherapy, radiotherapy, 5% imiquimod cream and active non-intervention.

Small lesions may be treated by curettage or cryotherapy. Combination treatment with curettage–cryosurgery can be effective [29], with 5-year outcomes reported [30].

Surgical excision is often the treatment of choice for BCC. However, the multiple tissue planes and topography of the pinna can make histological interpretation difficult and confound total excision. Furthermore, the external ear is not a uniform visual unit. The helical rim, antihelix and conchal bowl are separate cosmetic units and will require different repair strategies if infiltrated by tumour. For these reasons, removal of BCC from the ear is best managed by total margin analysis of the surgical specimen. Mohs micrographic surgery (MMS) is indicated for BCC of the pinna for preservation of both function and appearance. Recurrence rates following MMS to the ear have been reported as 4.2% [31] and 6.9% [32]. In a case series of 69 patients, Bumsted and Ceilley [31] found that conventional surgical excision of auricular malignancies would have produced 180% and 347% larger defects in primary and recurrent lesions, respectively, than with MMS.

Where surgery is not appropriate, radiotherapy can be applied with good effect. This includes external beam radiation treatment and brachytherapy [33]. A study including 99 BCCs on the ear found a recurrence rate of 12% over an average 2-years' follow-up, with a good cosmetic result in 75% of patients [34]. Brachytherapy involves the creation of a wax mould, shaped to the contours of the ear, to deliver radiation directly to the skin surface. This may not be appropriate for lesions extending down the ear canal, as the deeper margin cannot be identified at the time of mould insertion. Photon therapy delivered with a planning CT scan may be more suitable in such cases.

Although cartilage necrosis is a recognised side-effect, the ear should be considered a suitable site for radiotherapy. However, cancer that is infiltrating the cartilage is best not treated by radiotherapy, as the post-tumour defects within the cartilage structure can lead to weakness and deformity. A similar problem is seen with hoarse voice due to a floppy larynx, after radiotherapy for invasive throat cancer.

Squamous cell carcinoma of the auricle

Aspects of squamous cell carcinoma specific to the auricle are presented in this chapter. Chapter 141 has a comprehensive account of SCC. Primary SCC arising within the EAC is rare, and usually managed by otolaryngology due to its proximity to the middle ear and temporal bone.

Introduction
Cutaneous SCC (cSCC) refers to malignancy developing from the keratinocytes of the epidermis. Overall, it is the second most common type of skin cancer, after BCC, accounting for one-fifth of all cutaneous malignancies [1,2]. A study of nearly 1500 lesions found that 12% of all cSCC were located on the ear [3]. Auricular cSCC most often develops on the helix and antihelix, followed by the retroauricular region and concha cavum [4,5,6]. The right ear is affected in 60% of cases, according to one study of 117 patients [5], supporting earlier observations demonstrating this figure [6,7].

Epidemiology
Age
The average age of patients with SCC on the ear is reported across studies as between 68 years and 81 years [4,5,8–10]. These figures are slightly lower than that seen for cSCC across all sites, which has a median age 79 years [11], but are generally higher than for BCC on the ear. As such, SCC occurs predominantly in elderly white men, although at a younger age in the immunosuppressed

Sex
The external ear, due to its location, is a site on the body that is exposed to sun on a regular basis. In females, however, the hairstyle determines the level of sun exposure. Several studies have noted a large male bias for auricular cSCC, with rates in females as low as 0.2–3% [9,12–14]. Recent UK data [11] showed that in men, 15.8% of all cSCC is located on the ear, but only in 1.3% women. The same study showed a higher incidence on the lower legs of women compared with men (25.1% vs 4.9%), further indicating that UV exposure is a major risk factor for cSCC.

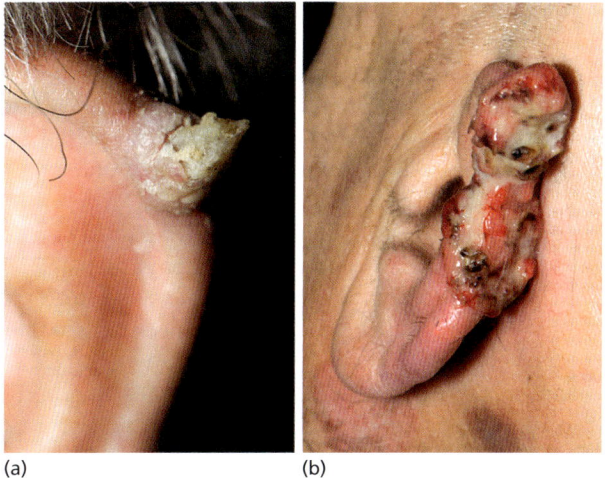

(a)   (b)

Figure 106.32 Squamous carcinoma. (a) Well-defined, symmetrical papule with a keratotic core and a raised pink base. (b) An ulcerated tumour on the superior helical rim, with an everted edge and destruction of the ear cartilage.

Tokez *et al.* [15] looked at the incidence of SCC-*in situ*, a premalignant condition of which 2–5% will progress to SCC if untreated. In this study of 88 754 patients in the Netherlands, the ears were a common location in men compared with women (10% vs 1%).

Clinical features
In most instances, SCC evolves from a premalignant lesion, usually a solar/actinic keratosis, but may appear *de novo* as a new growth or ulcer. Early SCC may be suspected when there is induration of the base of a scaly papule, nodule or cutaneous horn. There is often a keratinous core with well-differentiated SCCs, and keratoacanthoma can be closely mimicked. As an SCC grows, it typically becomes a nodular tumour, liable to be ulcerated and crusted. Poorly differentiated tumours tend to be friable and haemorrhagic, and do not show any evidence of keratinisation. With progression, SCC may invade the cartilage and can become grossly destructive (Figure 106.32). Symptoms are sometimes present and include pain and bleeding. Enlargement of the lesion is typically faster than that of a BCC.

Disease course and prognosis
Lymph node metastasis
Lewis in 1960 was one of the first to recognise that SCC of the pinna has a higher metastatic rate than cutaneous SCC that originates elsewhere [16]. His series of 150 auricular cancers included seven patients with locally invasive SCC, in whom two developed lymph node metastases (LNM). Since then, his findings have been supported by numerous studies, with metastatic rates at presentation ranging from 10% to 16% [9,10,14,17–21]. By comparison, Venables *et al.* [22] used English registry data to calculate the overall metastatic rate of cSCC as 1.1% for women and 2.4% for men, supporting earlier reported rates of 0.5–2.6% [23,24]. The reasons for the higher rate of metastatic cSCC of the ear remains unclear, but is perhaps related to the anatomy and lymph node drainage of this region.

A systematic review [18] found that 85% of metastases from auricular cSCC develop within 12 months and 98% within 24 months, although follow-up was limited to 12–36 months in most studies. This supports the current UK recommendations [25] for a follow-up period of 2 years for auricular cSCC, recognised as a 'high-risk' location. If other features are low risk then follow-up is not needed, e.g. thin depth, small diameter, well differentiated, no perineural invasion, no lymphovascular invasion and patient not immunocompromised.

Despite the gender bias in incidence, the likelihood of metastasis from auricular cSCC may be the same for both men and women. Venables *et al.* [22] showed the metastatic rates were greater for men for all body sites except the ears, scalp and neck, where rates were similar for both sexes.

The skin on the anterior part of the pinna is thin and tightly bound to the underlying cartilage. Therefore, epidermal tumours of the pinna need only grow a short vertical distance through the dermis before encountering larger dermal and subcutaneous lymphatic channels, and also cartilage. These anatomical features may explain the increased metastatic potential of auricular cSCC. The lymphatic drainage of the auricular region is plentiful and variable, with tumour location within the ear influencing the location of metastasis [26]. Spread to the parotid and upper deep cervical chain are most common and the postauricular nodes are also frequently involved (Figures 106.33 and 106.34, Table 106.3).

Five-year overall survival rates for patients with cSCC of the ear without lymph node metastases (LNM) are 73–98% [27,28], whereas with LNM this decreases to 20–46% [9,29]. Therefore,

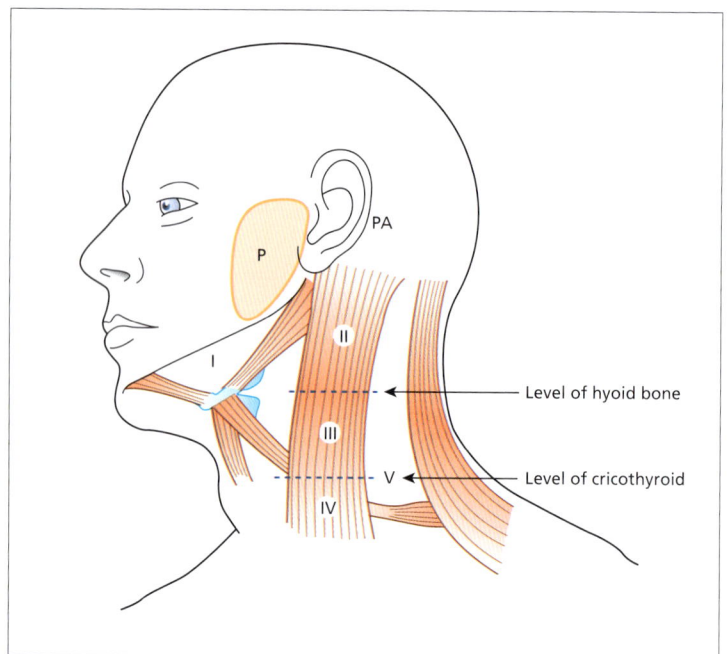

Figure 106.34 Lymph nodes and lymphatic drainage basins in the neck. P, parotid; PA, postauricular node.

Table 106.3 Frequency of positive nodal involvement following SCC of the ear. Data from Clarke *et al.* 2010 [10].

	Lymph nodes	Frequency of involvement
	Parotid	54%
	Postauricular	29%
Level I	Submandibular	4%
	Submental	
Level II	Superior spinal accessory	42%
	Superior jugular	
	Jugulo-digastric	
Level III	Midjugular	13%
Level IV	Jugular-omohyoid	8%
	Inferior jugular	
Level V	Inferior spinal accessory	13%
	Transverse cervical	

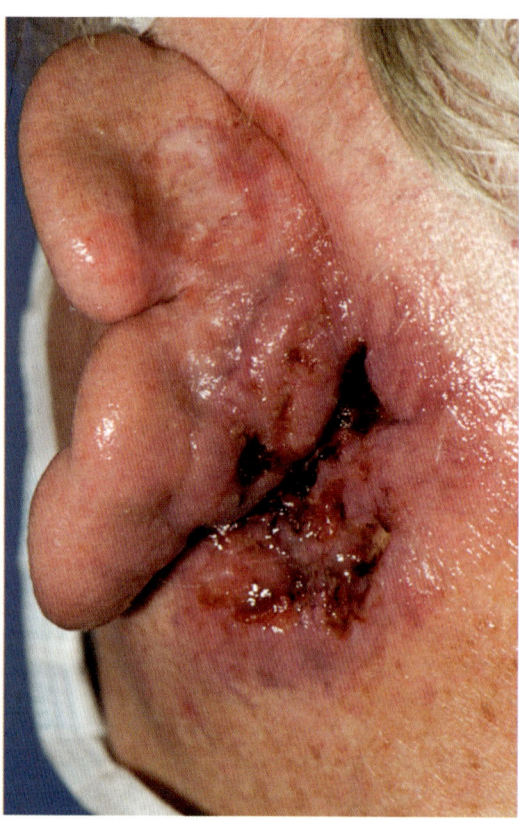

Figure 106.33 Recurrent squamous cell carcinoma on the posterior pinna, extending onto the left neck. A postauricular lymph node was clinically palpable with a CT scan identifying further nodes in Levels II, III, IV and V. A scar from the previous wedge excision is seen on the mid-helical rim.

identifying patients with cSCC of the ear who are at high risk of LNM may facilitate closer assessment and improve outcomes. Various prognostic factors for LNM in ear cancer have been reported [1,9,10,14,17,18,20,28–32]. However, the results are inconsistent and sometimes conflicting. For example, cartilage invasion has been identified as a predictor of LNM [10,17,18,28], not a predictor of LNM [31,33] and correlated but not predictive of LNM [14]. Studies have shown no correlation between histological features and LNM [4,9], indicating this is not a prognostic feature in isolation at this site.

Direct spread

SCC poses a higher risk of aggressive subclinical extension, both directly and via perineural invasion. Tumours at the tragus may spread deep along and under the anterior EAC wall toward the stylomastoid foramen. In such cases, there may be positive margins deep to the main trunk of the facial nerve necessitating a total parotidectomy. Spread along the EAC is well recognised; there is virtually no natural barrier to restrict tumour growth in any one direction within the cartilaginous canal [34]. Posterior extension through the cancellous portion of the EAC into the mastoid is rare. More commonly, there can be anterior extension through Santorini fissures (see anatomy section). Once into the bony canal, the compact tympanic bone restricts tumour extension. However, patency of Huschke foramen can permit anterior extension to the temporomandibular joint and into the parotid gland.

To assess for direct spread, patients should be evaluated for pain, otorrhoea, hearing loss, trismus (spasm of jaw muscles causing the mouth to remain tightly closed), facial weakness, hoarseness and dysphagia, with palpation for lymphadenopathy. Otoscopic evaluation is recommended to assess the bony EAC and tympanic membrane. Radiological imaging may be helpful, with either a high-resolution CT scan of the brain/parotid/neck or an MRI scan [35]. The EAC, neck, parotid, infratemporal fossa, glenoid fossa and temporal bone may be involved, despite the fact that they are not clinically suspected preoperatively.

Management

The complete management options for SCC are described in Chapter 141. It is helpful to discuss SCCs with high-risk features at a multidisciplinary meeting.

It is important to achieve control of the disease with the initial treatment for SCC. For small minimally invasive lesions, simple excision, cryotherapy or curettage with electrodesiccation may be adequate. Excellent results have been reported from the combination of curettage and cryotherapy for carefully selected cases [36], and the current UK guidelines [25] advocate curettage for small (under 1 cm), well-defined and low-risk SCC.

The highest incidence of SCC occurs on the helical rim and this anatomic location usually lends itself to wedge excision with primary closure [37] or excision with a skin graft [38]. If the tumour is very large or recurrent, partial or complete removal of the pinna may be required. Lesions arising in the concha bowl or tragus may extend down the EAC (see Basal cell carcinoma earlier) and a flap repair or skin graft may be required to prevent cicatricial narrowing of the canal. If the entire ear is removed, the area can be resurfaced with a skin graft and the defect covered with a highly cosmetically acceptable prosthesis. Two prostheses may be supplied to the patient, to match the skin colour in the summer and winter months. If there is spread beyond the auricle, resection of the parotid, temporal bone, temporomandibular joint or mandibular ramus may be required, with appropriate repair.

Several authors have recommended predetermined resection margins, for example: 1 cm [39], 6 mm with frozen section control [40], 8 mm for 1 cm diameter tumours and 1.5 cm for 3 cm diameter tumours [41], all with removal of the underlying cartilage. Historical data of 5-year recurrence rates shows an incidence of 18.7% for multiple modalities compared with 5.3% for MMS [20], with Mohs himself reporting 7.7% in 1988 [42]. A more recent study demonstrated a 5.7% recurrence rate over an average period of 3 years [5]. Overall, the evidence favours microscopic control of tumour margins to reduce long-term recurrence [34,43,44], although

no prospective comparison study has been performed for standard surgery versus MMS, unlike for BCC [45].

Squamous cell carcinomas in the tragal and pretragal location appear to have a greater tendency to spread along embryonic fusion planes and may only be curable by radical surgery, for example parotidectomy in association with removal of the tumour [33,34]. Various techniques can be employed to reconstruct the ear after curative surgery [43–55].

Sentinel lymph node biopsy (SLNB) may have a role in managing auricular SCC [56], by indicating those patients with possible occult metastatic spread. A systematic review of SLNB in head and neck SCC highlighted its feasibility and reliability [57]. However, SLNB for early detection of LNM currently lacks evidence to show improvement in SCC recurrence or survival rates and is not performed routinely. Prophylactic lymph node dissection has been proposed when certain high-risk features are present [10,19,28]. However, recent UK guidelines (2020) [25] do not recommend lymph node dissection in clinically node-negative patients.

Radiotherapy can be successful as a primary treatment for SCC of the auricle, megavoltage electron-beam therapy having therapeutic and cosmetic advantages over conventional superficial radiotherapy [58]. Although results can be as good as from surgery [59], there may be a higher recurrence rate compared with surgery for large tumours. Radiation therapy can be complicated by damage to the cartilage and associated chronic infection; deformity of the auricle is another long-term consequence. Adjuvant radiotherapy has a role in preventing local recurrence for tumours displaying perineural/perivascular invasion, or those excised with narrow histological margins.

In renal transplant recipients, reducing the degree of immunosuppression can improve survival in poor prognosis SCC without necessarily jeopardising the transplant [60].

For inoperable and metastatic tumours, local treatment will be palliative. There is a role for systemic treatment in the management of metastatic SCC. Chemotherapy and PD-1 inhibitors, such as cemiplimab, may be of value.

Management of tumours at the external auditory meatus

Keratinocyte skin cancers (BCC and SCC) close to, or surrounding, the external auditory meatus are difficult to treat (Figure 106.35). This includes tumours within the conchal bowl, a fossa that is bisected by the helicis crus into the cymba superiorly and cavum inferiorly (Figure 106.1). Accessing the peripheral margins at this location is difficult and further increased by the late presentation of many tumours. In a review of 407 auricular carcinomas by Niparko et al. [1], 41 (10%) occurred in the conchal bowl and 16 (4%) in the EAC. Duffy et al. [2] examined cancers on these non-visible parts of the ear, of which 73% were BCC. The surgical defect following excision of the tumour was 1.6–2.3 times larger as those on more visible portions of the ear, and 2.5–3.5 times larger than defects on the nose. This may reflect a degree of visual neglect, where patients only palpate those areas of the ear more amenable to touch, without

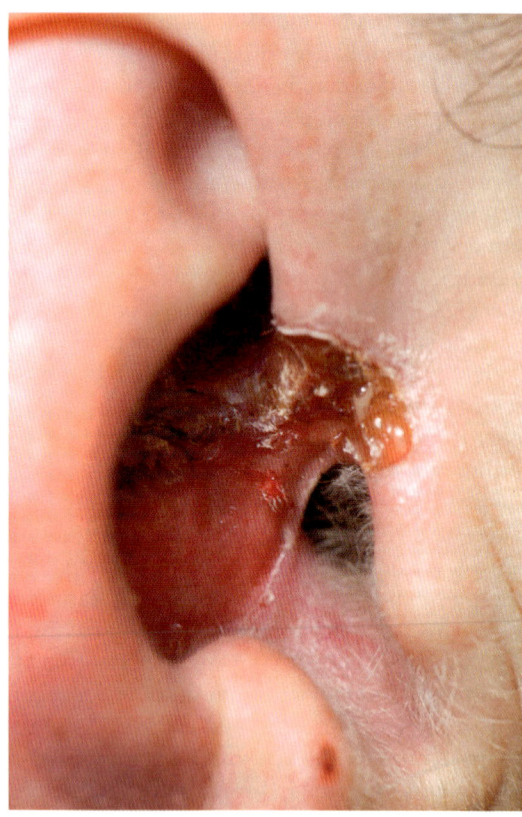

Figure 106.35 Basal cell carcinoma of the right conchal bowl, encircling the entrance to the external auditory canal.

direct visualisation of the entire ear. As a result, presentation is delayed until tumours are palpable.

Complete excision of tumours at the conchal bowl can be technically challenging under local anaesthetic, as medial extension into the EAC limits adequate surgical margins. Cartilage is often excised to maximise clearance at the deep margin. Substantial subclinical spread has been identified by tumours at these sites [3]. During Mohs surgery, the use of a tympanostomy blade [4] or a Beaver ophthalmic blade [5] may aid access to the medial aspects of the conchal bowl. A Dermablade [6] and Goulian knife [7] are better suited for flatter parts of the ear. A flap repair (such as the revolving door flap [8] may be preferable to a skin graft at the EAC, as the outward passage of migratory epithelium and cerumen may inhibit adequate uptake of the graft.

Several authors [9,10,**11**] have described their experience of managing conchal bowl tumours, the majority of which were BCC. Most could be managed by a single modality, either MMS or surgical resection of the deeper aspect under general anaesthetic. However, they found it useful to adopt a multidisciplinary approach for the rare cases where an extensive subclinical spread was encountered or complex reconstruction was required. If positive margins remain at completion of MMS, they suggest that positive areas are clearly identified with marking sutures, photography and a clinical drawing. This will assist the subsequent surgeon in reassessing the surgical field for wider excision. A proposed management algorithm is shown in Figure 106.36. In the UK, such cases are best discussed at a multidisciplinary team meeting. Complex surgical

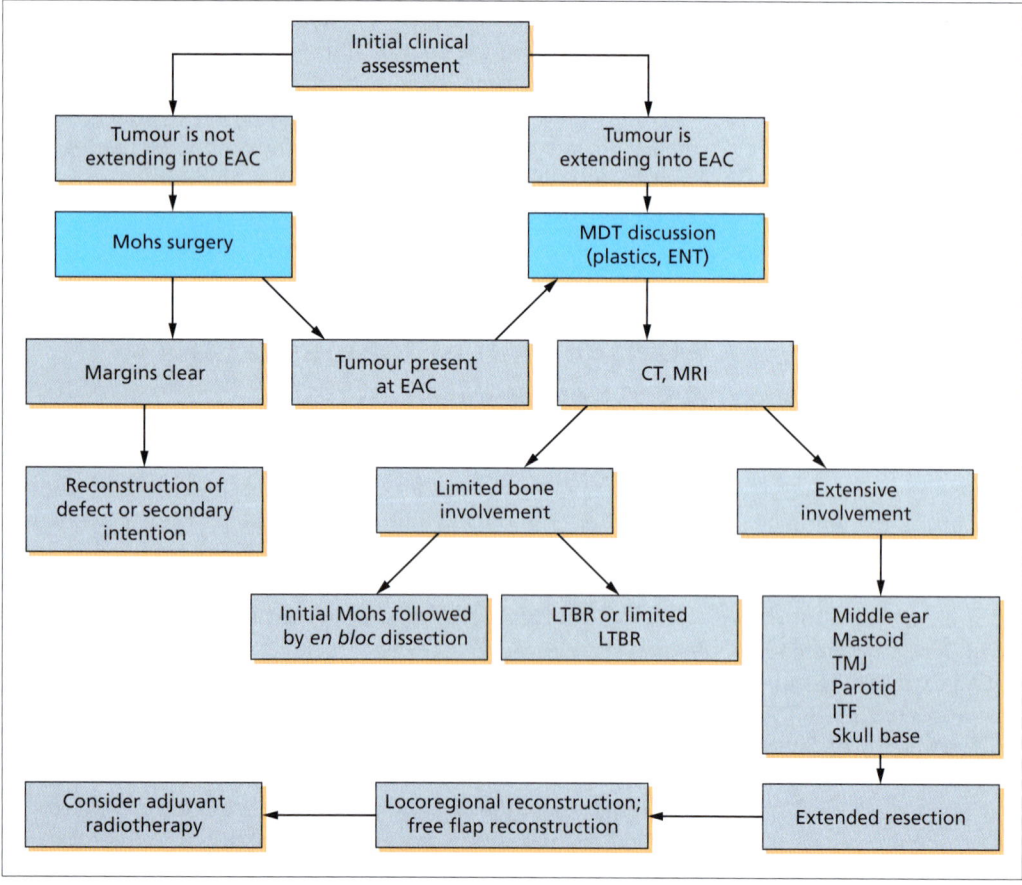

Figure 106.36 Management pathway for patients with a keratinocyte cancer close to the external auditory meatus. EAC, external auditory canal; LTBR, lateral temporal bone resection; TMJ, temporomandibular joint; ITF, infratemporal fossa.

procedures may proceed jointly with ENT and an oncologically trained plastic surgeon, for example sleeve resection of the skin lining the cartilaginous EAC, followed by flap repair of the resulting defect.

Melanoma of the auricle

Aspects of melanoma specific to the auricle are presented in this chapter. See Chapter 142 for a comprehensive account of melanoma.

Epidemiology

Incidence
Melanoma of the ear accounts for 10–20% of melanomas on the head and neck [1,2,3,4,5] and 1–4% of all cutaneous melanomas [3,6]. The incidence in the USA is 1.91 per 100 000 persons-per-year [7].

Sex
There is a male preponderance, perhaps due to the protective effect of long hair length in women. A systematic review found a male:female ratio of 3.5:1 [8].

Age
The mean age of patients is 59 years [8], although the incidence in young adults (aged 15–39 years) more than doubled between 1973 and 2012 [9].

Pathology
The commonest histological subtype is superficial spreading malignant melanoma, with the commonest location on the helix. The average Breslow thickness is 2.0 mm, which is non-significantly higher than for melanomas at other head and neck sites [1,4,8].

Clinical features
Melanoma can arise *de novo* or as a change in a pre-existing melanocytic naevus. Lesions on the ear can present with a variety of clinical appearances, from multicoloured macules to exophytic nodules [10]. The presence of pigment on dermoscopy is a characteristic feature.

Differential diagnosis
Given its rarity on the ear, the unwary clinician may omit melanoma from the differential diagnosis during a busy clinic, perhaps favouring a pigmented basal cell carcinoma (Figure 106.37). Benign melanocytic naevi are easily identified, but Spitz naevi can cause diagnostic confusion (Figure 106.38). Dermoscopy may show a homogeneous blue coloration, giving the false impression of a blue naevus [11].

Disease course and prognosis
The early literature suggested an aggressive biological behaviour of external ear melanoma [4,12–14]. This led to recommendations for extensive surgery including total amputation of the ear. Later studies failed to demonstrate a worse prognosis compared with other sites [1,2,15]. A prospective study of 162 patients showed a high

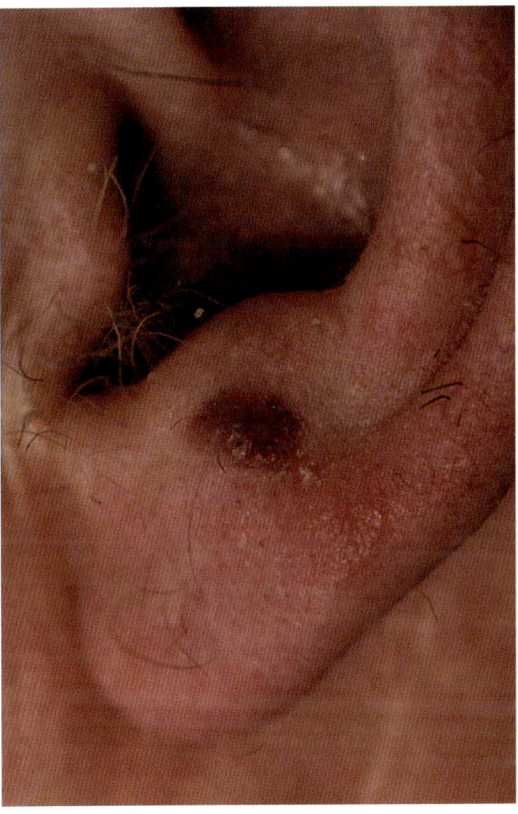

Figure 106.37 Desmoplastic melanoma – a pink cystic papule containing dots of pigmentation. The clinician had suspected a pigmented basal cell carcinoma.

survival rate for stage 1 and 2 melanomas of the ear, with a 3-year disease-specific survival rate of 98% [3]. The 5-year survival rate was also high at 96%, although in the literature this varies between 43% and 89% [6–8,16–19].

The location of a head and neck melanoma at the external ear is not an independent risk factor for overall and disease-free survival, or recurrence. As with other anatomic sites, increasing tumour thickness and ulceration are negative prognostic indicators.

Sub-group analysis of a large prospective trial [1] showed that loco-regional recurrence was non-significantly lower than for non-ear sites (8% vs 13%), although other reported rates vary between 13% and 37% [17,18,20]. Distant metastasis was also non-significantly lower than for non-ear sites (11% vs 14%), similar to other reported rates between 13% and 22% [17,18,20].

Management
As with all melanomas on head and neck, surgical resection is a balance between sufficient surgical aggressiveness and preservation of function and aesthetics of the ear [21]. There is no general agreement on the optimal surgical management, but a favourable prognosis tends to advocate a less invasive approach. There is no evidence to support the historical use of radical amputation, with several studies showing no relationship between surgical approach and survival. Furthermore, there is evidence that conservative resection margins, using wedge resection or cartilage-sparing wide local excision of the tumour, provide satisfactory outcomes with regard to survival and recurrence.

PART 10: SPECIFIC SITES, SEX & AGE

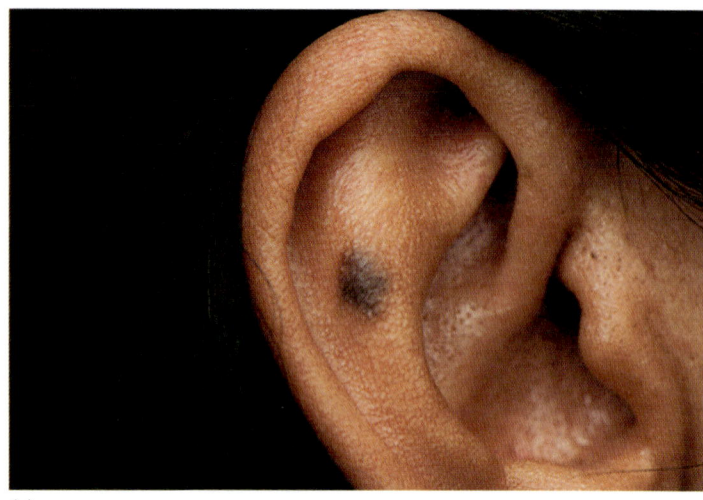

(a)

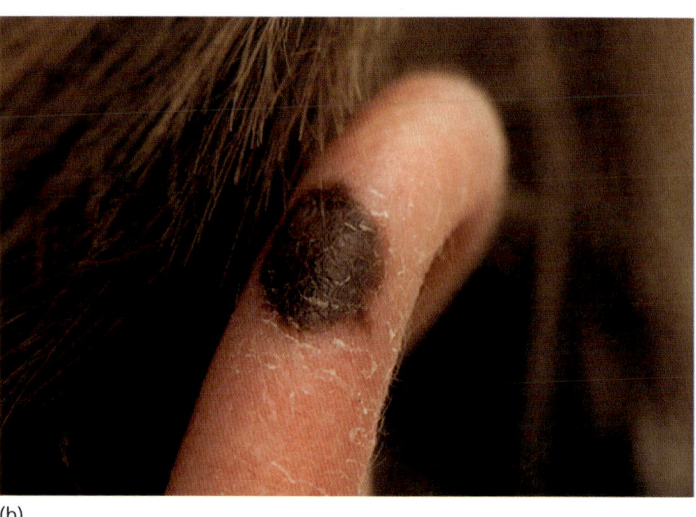

(b)

Figure 106.38 (a) Compound melanocytic naevus, a symmetrical pigmented papule with a dark but even coloration. (b) Spitz naevus, on the posterior border of the right helix. A broadly symmetrical, minimally raised, pigmented macule, with mild overlying scale. Despite the irregular edge and lateral pigment projection, histological analysis identified no atypical features.

Surgical margins

Resection margins for treatment of ear melanoma are often lower than the general recommendations, with the aim of preserving function and improving cosmetic outcome. This practice is seen elsewhere in the head and neck, including the eyelid [22]. Despite the average Breslow thickness being 2.0 mm, resection margins are often between 1 and 2 cm. Several authors report a minimum excision margin of 1 cm [15,16,20], with some proposing that this is adequate management for most ear melanomas [23,24]. Excision margins below 1 cm are correlated with a reduction in recurrence-free survival [3].

In a study of lentigo maligna melanoma [3], patients undergoing Mohs micrographic surgery had an average margin of 5 mm, with a 5-year recurrence-free survival rate of 90%. Those undergoing conventional surgery had an average margin of 10 mm, with a slightly lower survival rate. The melanomas were thicker in the Mohs cohort.

Overall, there is insufficient evidence to recommend deviation from established guidance. The methods detailed above are based on surgeons' preferred practice and only one study associated a 1 cm margin with a low risk of recurrence [20]. Indeed, some authors recommend following standard melanoma treatment guidelines to improve local tumour control [3,6], using excision margins as for other anatomical sites.

Cartilage excision

There is plenty of evidence to suggest that removal of cartilage is not necessary to improve survival and reduce recurrence in melanoma of the external ear. This permits a simpler reconstruction with better aesthetic and functional outcomes, without compromising prognosis.

In a histological review of 51 ear melanomas, the perichondrium was never violated by the tumour regardless of the Breslow thickness [25], supporting earlier observations [26]. Translating this into surgical practice, cartilage-sparing resections are not associated with a higher rate of local recurrence [15,20,27,28]. It is suggested that the perichondrium may serve as a barrier to the tumour and may not need to be removed for satisfactory surgical removal of ear melanomas.

Conversely, there is one report of cartilage invasion [29] and one author recommends cartilage excision for melanomas of >1.0 mm 'to avoid the risk of submicroscopic residual malignant cell in the perichondrium' [19].

There are several reports of melanoma in the EAC (Figure 106.39), where the tumour is always removed with a margin of surrounding cartilage and bone [30–33]. The authors justify this aggressive treatment because tumours at this specific location are often extensive, due to late diagnosis.

Sentinel node biopsy

The lymph node drainage of ear melanomas is unpredictable [16,34,35], as is true for many head and neck melanomas [36–41]. In a series of 111 patients undergoing lymphoscintigraphy for melanoma of the ear, lymphatic drainage occurred in a retrograde, antegrade or transaural pattern, although never contralaterally [42]. The SLNB procedure might therefore be less reliable on the ear. One retrospective study of 41 patients found a significantly lower rate of sentinel node positivity (10%) compared with other cutaneous sites (23%), despite similarity in other tumour prognostic features [43]. Some studies support this low positive SLNB rate of 7–8% [1,8,44], although others report a high rate of 22–23% [6,45]. A low rate might reflect a less aggressive behaviour, or a higher rate of false negativity related to the variability of lymphatic drainage patterns.

Despite the great variability, it has been demonstrated that SLNB is both feasible and useful in melanoma of the head and neck, including melanoma of the ear. Identification of the sentinel node is possible in >90% of cases [20,34,35], with predominance of drainage to level II.

Two prospective randomised trials have reported on the outcome of patients with a positive sentinel node. The MSLT-2 and DeCOG trials randomised patients to either elective completion lymph

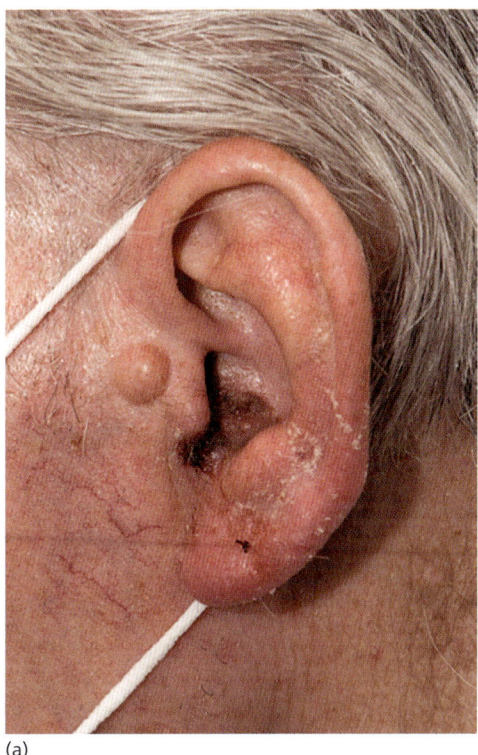

(a)

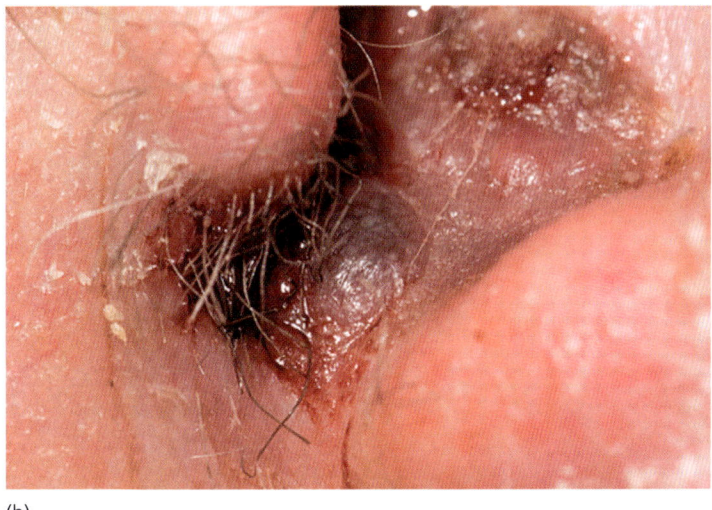

(b)

Figure 106.39 (a) Lentigo maligna melanoma of Breslow thickness 2.5 mm, with extension into the auditory canal. The patient had been treated in the community for recurrent otitis externa. (b) A pigmented plaque arising on a background of shiny redness, with a papular component and superficial erosions.

node dissection or nodal observation with radiological imaging [46,47]. The larger of these trials included 241 melanomas of the head and neck, although specific data for ear melanomas was not presented [46]. Neither trial demonstrated a survival benefit for having a completion lymph node dissection. This procedure is no longer routinely performed following a positive SLNB in patients with melanoma of the ear. However, adjuvant immunotherapy can provide a survival benefit and is the subject of ongoing research trials.

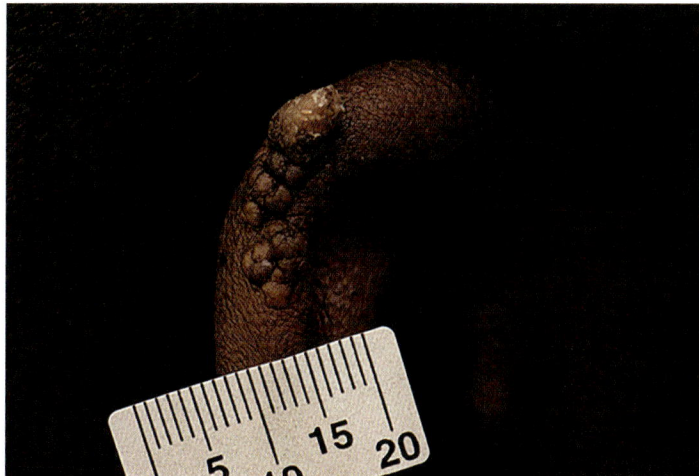

Figure 106.40 Sebaceous naevus. An elongated plaque present since birth, with a papillomatous surface that appears pale and slightly yellow in places.

Other lesions and tumours affecting the ear

Benign lesions

Benign mass lesions in the canal include exostosis and osteoma. Exostoses are usually bilateral, symmetrical, multiple, diffuse, broadly based growths of bone. Frequent exposure to cold water, such as from surfing, is an aetiological factor in nearly all cases. Somewhat similar are osteomas, although these can usually be differentiated by their solitary and unilateral distribution.

Other benign lesions that may present in the canal are fibrous dysplasia – both monostotic and polyostotic (Albright syndrome), eosinophilic granuloma, cholesteatoma and keratosis obturans, benign ceruminous gland tumours, cartilaginous choristomas and temporomandibular joint herniation. Papillomatosis of the canal presents with multiple rounded papules; it has been associated with human papillomavirus (HPV) 6. A sebaceous naevus may be suspected from its presence since birth, but in darker skin types may lack the classical orange–yellow coloration (Figure 106.40).

Premalignant lesions

Because of its high level of exposure to UV radiation, especially in men, the auricle is a common site for premalignant lesions of epidermal origin. Other predisposing factors include prior ionising radiation, a chronic dermatosis such as lupus vulgaris and genetic factors such as xeroderma pigmentosum and Gorlin syndrome.

The commonest premalignant lesion is the solar (or actinic) keratosis, which can occur on all sun-exposed aspects of the auricle, but is especially common on the upper surface of the helix. The clinical presentations include an red telangiectatic patch, a focal area of scaling or hyperkeratosis, or a cutaneous horn. Solar keratoses on the auricle are often multiple. Solar elastosis may be evident in the surrounding skin. With continued sun exposure, the dysplastic cells may involve the entire thickness of the epidermis. This is

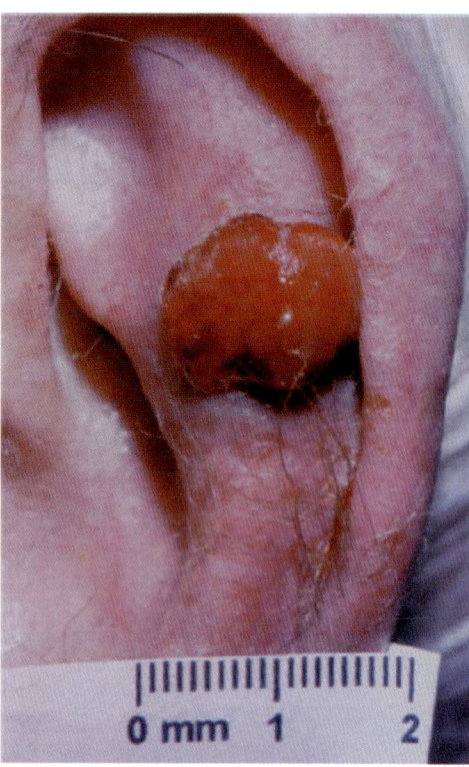

Figure 106.41 Atypical fibroxanthoma. A firm fleshy tumour of the pinna.

a squamous cell carcinoma *in situ* (or intraepidermal carcinoma or Bowen disease) and carries a higher risk of progression to SCC. A keratoacanthoma can closely resemble an SCC and should ideally be excised to ensure accurate diagnosis, unless it is clearly regressing.

Several forms of treatment can eradicate premalignant lesions from the auricle, but there are no high quality trials to compare them. Options include cryotherapy, 5-fluorouracil, imiquimod, curettage, photodynamic therapy and excision. The choice will depend on a number of factors, including the need for a tissue diagnosis, size and location of the lesion, likely cosmetic outcome and the available facilities. Although most patients can be discharged following education on skin surveillance, follow-up is recommended for immunosuppressed patients [1].

Other lesions

The dermatologist may also encounter sebaceous carcinoma, atypical fibroxanthoma (Figure 106.41), trichilemmal carcinoma, Merkel cell tumour, carcinosarcoma, Kaposi sarcoma, angiosarcoma and, mainly in children, rhabdomyosarcoma. Lymphomas and pseudolymphoma may occur on the external ear (Figure 106.42). The ear may be involved by direct extension from tumours nearby, for example the parotid, and also by metastases from distant sites.

Tumours of the ceruminous glands are rare. It is often difficult to distinguish between adenoma and carcinoma on histological grounds [2,3]. The tumours comprise benign and pleomorphic adenomas, adenocarcinomas, adenoid cystic carcinomas and perhaps others including mucoepidermoid carcinomas. The glandular tissue of a ceruminous adenoma has myoepithelial basal cells

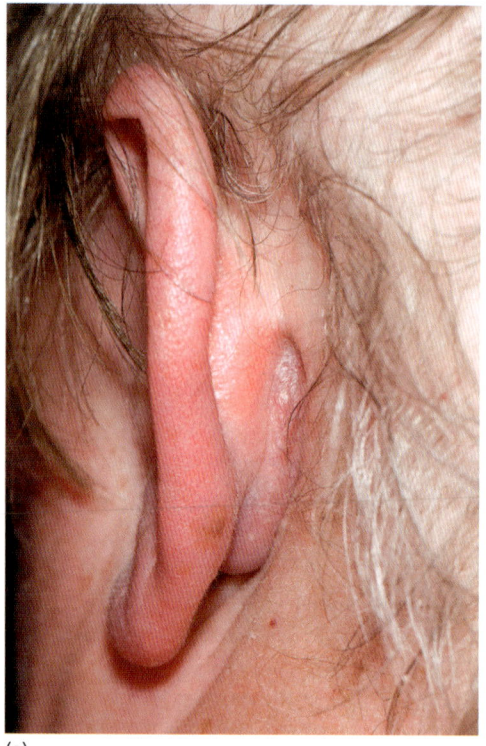

(a)

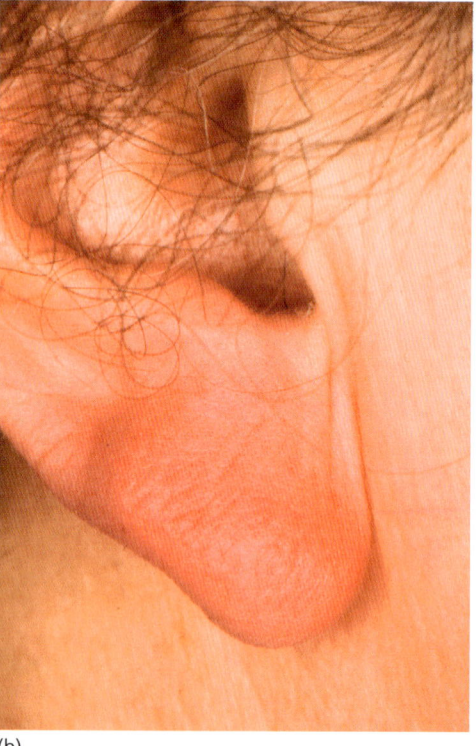

(b)

Figure 106.42 (a) B-cell lymphoma presenting as a purple nodular swelling in the retroauricular fold. (b) Erythematous swelling of the ear lobe due to infiltration by B-cell lymphoma.

which are positive for CK5/6, S100 and p63 and luminal cerumi-nous cells which stain for CK7 [4]. Tumours of the cerumen glands have been reported in association with other sweat gland tumours elsewhere [5].

Isolated cases of syringocystadenoma papilliferum, apocrine cys-tadenoma, benign eccrine cylindroma, hidradenoma papilliferum and carcinomas of eccrine and sebaceous origin have also been reported [6,7]. Extramammary Paget disease of the external ear and/or canal [8,9] resembles Bowen disease or an inflammatory dermatosis. Cutaneous schwannoma can occur, with pain present in around a third of cases [10]. Folliculosebaceous cystic hamartoma is a rare cutaneous hamartoma comprised of follicular, sebaceous and mesenchymal elements, and has been described on the ear and preauricular skin [11].

Key references

The full list of references can be found in the online version at https://www.wiley.com/rooksdermatology10e

Introduction
4 Manolidis S, Ratner D. External auditory canal defect management and reconstruction. Dermatol Surg 2014;40(Suppl. 9):S86–95.

Developmental defects and changes with ageing
1 Veugen CC, Dikkers FG, deBakker BS. The developmental origin of the auricula revisited. *Laryngoscope* 2020;130:2467–74.

Peri-auricular anomalies, ageing changes and earlobe creases
1 Scheinfeld NS, Silverberg NB, Weinberg JM, Nozad V. The preauricular sinus: a review of its clinical presentation, treatment, and associations. *Pediatr Dermatol* 2004;21:191–6.

Traumatic conditions
Contusion and haematoma pseudocyst, and pseudocyst of the ear
31 Patigaroo SA, Mehfooz N, Patigaroo FA *et al.* Clinical characteristics and comparative study of different modalities of treatment of pseudocyst pinna. *Eur Arch Otorhinolaryngol* 2012;269:1747–54.

Chondrodermatitis nodularis
1 Kechichian E, Jabbour S, Haber R, Abdelmassih Y, Tomb R. Management of chondrodermatitis nodularis helicis. *Dermatol Surg* 2016;42:1125–34.

Split earlobe
18 Niamtu J. Eleven pearls for cosmetic earlobe repair. *Dermatol Surg* 2002;28:180–5.

Keloids
16 Ogawa R. The most current algorithms for the treatment and prevention of hypertrophic scars and keloids. *Plast Reconstr Surg* 2010;125:557–68.

Infections
Otitis externa
35 Hajioff D, Mackeith S. Otitis externa. *BMJ Clin Evid* 2015;2015:0510.

Otomycosis
9 Vennewald I, Klemm E. Otomycosis: diagnosis and treatment. *Clin Dermatol* 2010;28:202–11.

Tumours of the auricle, basal cell carcinoma
24 Navrazhina K, Parra CE, Cressey BD, Xanthos C, Christos PJ, Minkis K. Basal cell carcinomas of the ear are more aggressive and have higher discordance rates between biopsy and Mohs histopathology. *J Am Acad Dermatol* 2020;83:1805–7.

Squamous cell carcinoma
5 Silapunt S, Peterson SR, Goldberg LH. Squamous cell carcinoma of the auricle and Mohs micrographic surgery. *Dermatol Surg* 2005;31:1423–7.

Management of tumours at the external auditory meatus
11 Fraser KM, Matthews TW, Kurwa HA. Epidermal carcinoma of the conchal bowl: creation of a multidisciplinary pathway approach. *J Cutan Med Surg* 2020;24:129–36.

Melanoma of the auricle
3 Jahn V, Breuninger H, Garbe C, Moehrle M. Melanoma of the ear: prognostic factors and surgical strategies. *Br J Dermatol* 2006;154:310–18.

CHAPTER 107

Dermatoses of the Eye, Eyelids and Eyebrows

Valerie P. J. Saw[1] *and Stuart N. Cohen*[2]

[1]Imperial College Healthcare NHS Trust, University College London Institute of Ophthalmology, London, UK
[2]Department of Dermatology, Liverpool University Hospitals NHS Foundation Trust; University of Liverpool School of Medicine, Liverpool, UK

PART 10: SPECIFIC SITES, SEX & AGE

Introduction

This chapter is not intended to be a comprehensive account of all diseases that affect the skin and eyes, for which there are several reviews [1–5,6,7]. The main focus is on those conditions that commonly occur in clinical practice and that present a problem with management. It is also intended to alert the dermatologist to conditions that might threaten visual acuity and require urgent referral to an ophthalmologist. Also, many systemic diseases affect both the skin and eyes, and ophthalmic assessment will be of help in making the correct diagnosis and in the long-term management of such patients.

Anatomy and physiology of the eye [1,2]

The eye and skin share a common embryological origin. The structure of the lid, conjunctiva, lacrimal gland and associated drainage apparatus are of surface ectodermal origin while the remainder of the eye arises from epithelium of the ectodermal neural plate.

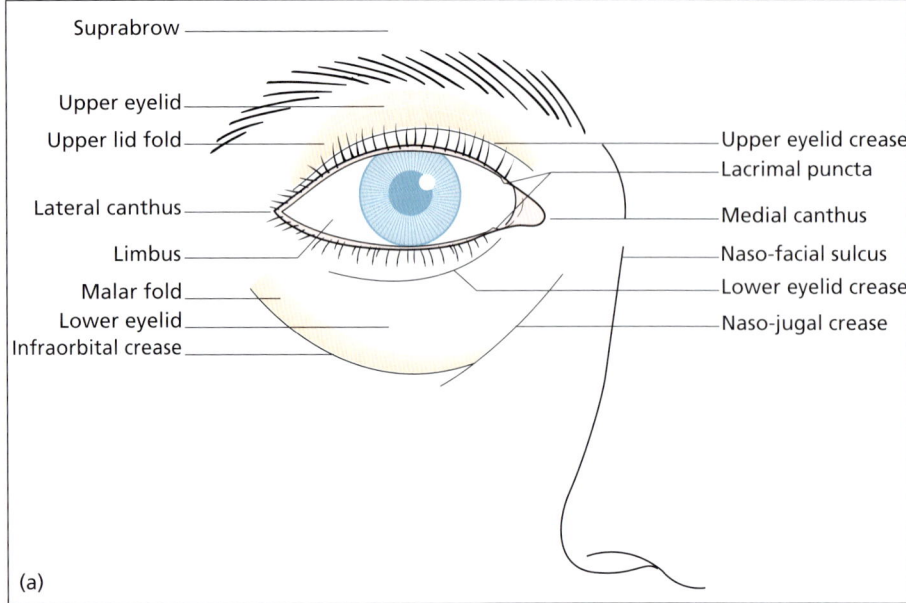

(a)

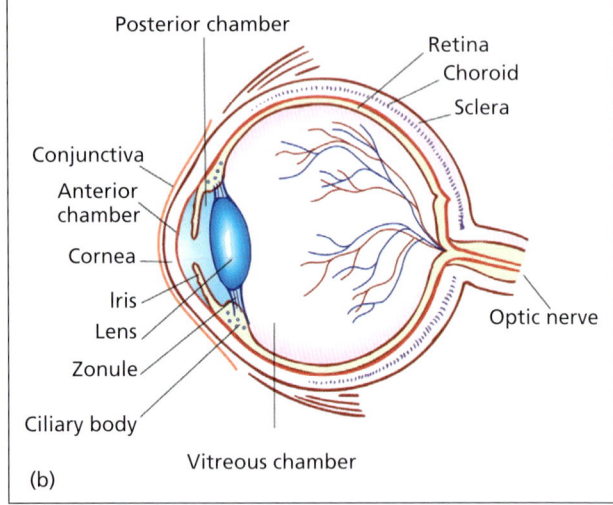

(b)

Figure 107.1 Anatomy of the normal eye. (a) The external appearance of the right eye. (b) Cross-section of the human eye.

The only mesodermal contribution to the eye is the myoblasts of the extraocular muscles. The anatomy of the eye is shown in Figure 107.1. The eye appendages are as follows.

Eyebrows

These hair-bearing areas rest on very mobile fat and muscle pads overlying the superior orbital ridge. Their mobility is important as a means of facial expression. The eyebrows help protect the eye from bright light and sweat.

Eyelids

The eyelids have distinct anatomical layers, comprising the skin with subcutaneous tissue and striated muscles that effect lid movement, the tarsal plate and conjunctiva (Figure 107.2). The grey line, an important anatomical landmark for surgical repair and pathological conditions of the lid margin such as blepharitis, divides the lid into an anterior lamella (skin and muscle) and a posterior lamella (tarsus and conjunctiva). The grey line represents the location of the marginal region of the orbicularis muscle (muscle of Riolan) seen through the lid skin.

The skin is thin and modified in several ways to protect the eyeball. It contains sebaceous glands associated with the fine hairs of the eyelashes (cilia) and both apocrine and eccrine sweat glands. There are about 300 eyelashes, arising in two rows along the eyelid margin, two-thirds of which are in the upper lid. They have no associated erector muscles, but rudimentary sebaceous glands (of Zeis) are present. Some lashes, particularly those of the lower lid, are associated with ancillary apocrine sweat glands (of Moll). The ducts of these glands open both into the lash follicles and directly onto the anterior lid margin between the lashes. The eyelashes help to protect against foreign bodies impinging on the eyeball. Each lash follicle has a rich nerve plexus, which is easily excited – even faint touch initiates reflex lid closure.

The tarsal plate of each eyelid gives the palpebral aperture shape and stability. They comprise dense, fibrous tissue surrounding modified sebaceous glands (meibomian glands). These secrete the outer lipid layer of the precorneal tear film through openings along the mucocutaneous junction of the eyelid margin. This lipid helps to stabilise the tear film and reduce evaporation. There are about 30 glands in the upper tarsal plate and 20 in the lower. Meibomian

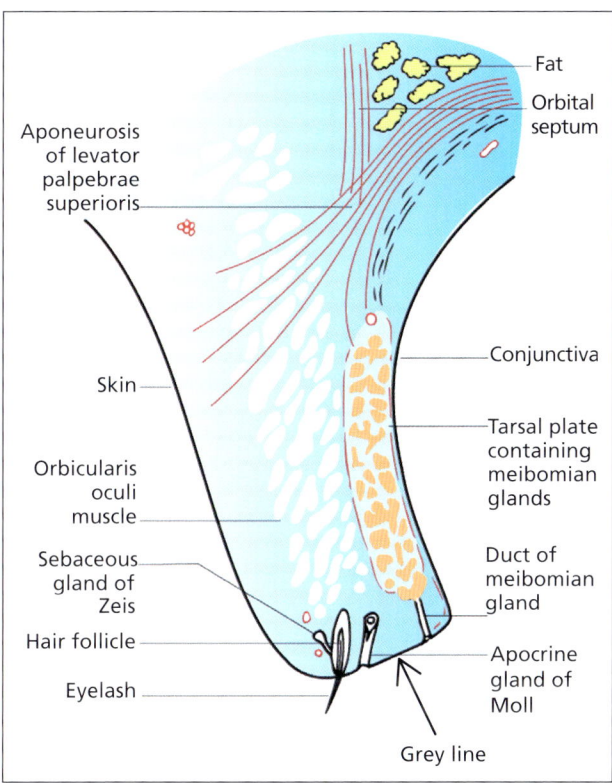

Figure 107.2 Cross-section of the upper eyelid.

glands have up to 20 acini surrounding a central vertical duct and are visible through the conjunctiva.

The eyelids are lined by a mucous membrane called the palpebral conjunctiva. It is reflected over the anterior portion of the eyeball up to the edge of the cornea as the bulbar conjunctiva. The folds formed by the reflection of the conjunctiva from the lids onto the eyeball are called the superior and inferior palpebral fornices. The conjunctiva contains numerous goblet cells secreting mucin into the tear film. It also contains about 50 accessory lacrimal glands and its substantia propria contains neural tissue, mast cells, lymphocytes and lymphoid follicles, which are important in mediating local immunological reactions.

The striated muscle of the levator palpebrae superioris opens the eye, and the striated orbicularis oculi muscle closes it. Both are innervated by the facial nerve. Two divisions of the trigeminal nerve supply sensation to the eyelids; the upper lid and medial (inner) canthus are supplied by the ophthalmic division, and the remainder of the lower lid by the maxillary division.

The eyelid has a rich blood supply, mainly through the medial and lateral palpebral arteries, which are branches of the ophthalmic artery. There is also a rich anastomosis between adjacent arteries arising from the internal and external carotid. The blood drains through a network of veins to the facial and orbital veins and the cavernous sinus. Lymphatics drain the conjunctiva and tarsal plate to the post-tarsal plexus, and the skin and orbicularis to the pretarsal plexus. The medial canthus and lower lid subsequently drain to the submandibular nodes while the lateral canthus and upper lid drain to the parotid and preauricular nodes.

Lacrimal glands

The main lacrimal gland is a modified sweat gland located in the lacrimal fossa, a bony depression just under the upper and outer margin of the orbit. It produces an aqueous secretion, which discharges through a network of ductules onto the surface of the palpebral conjunctiva. In addition, there is a variable number of accessory lacrimal glands in the upper and lower conjunctival fornices. The lacrimal gland and accessory lacrimal glands are both innervated, but the accessory lacrimal glands lack parasympathetic innervation [3].

Precorneal tear film

The eyelids make a vital contribution to the composition and stability of the precorneal tear film. The precorneal tear film is now believed, based on spectral domain optical coherence tomography techniques, to be about 4 μm thick [4]. It is a layered structure consisting of a thin 50–100 nm outermost lipid layer secreted primarily by the meibomian glands with a lesser contribution from the eyelid glands of Moll and Zeis (as discussed earlier) and a central aqueous–mucous layer secreted primarily by the main lacrimal gland and accessory lacrimal glands of Krause and Wolfring, with additional fluid and electrolytes secreted by ocular surface epithelial cells. The aqueous–mucin pool contains soluble gel-forming mucins secreted by conjunctival goblet cells. Anchored to the apical plasma membrane of the corneal and conjunctival epithelial cells are transmembrane mucins, which contribute to formation of a glycocalyx. Blinking consists of a lateral to medial movement of the eyelids, which enables resurfacing of the tear film of the cornea and propels the tears to the punctum of the tear duct; from here, they are actively removed by the lacrimal pump mechanism through the lacrimal canaliculi into the common canaliculus and lacrimal sac, and then via the naso-lacrimal duct into the nose (Figure 107.3).

The tear film has a number of functions:
1 To supply oxygen and other nutrients to the cornea.
2 To remove particulate matter from the surface of the eye.
3 To prevent drying of the eye.
4 To act as a lubricant and prevent adhesion of the palpebral to the bulbar conjunctiva.
5 To protect the eye surface through its antibacterial role; it contains white blood cells, various proteins, lysozyme and immunoglobulins.

Glossary of ophthalmological terms

A glossary is provided in Table 107.1.

Disorders affecting the eyebrows and eyelashes

There is a wide variation in the colour, distribution and density of the eyebrow hairs. The inheritance of the appearance of the eyebrows is polygenic. Some hereditary variations are of no known significance, but others are associated with other development defects or are part of a recognised syndrome.

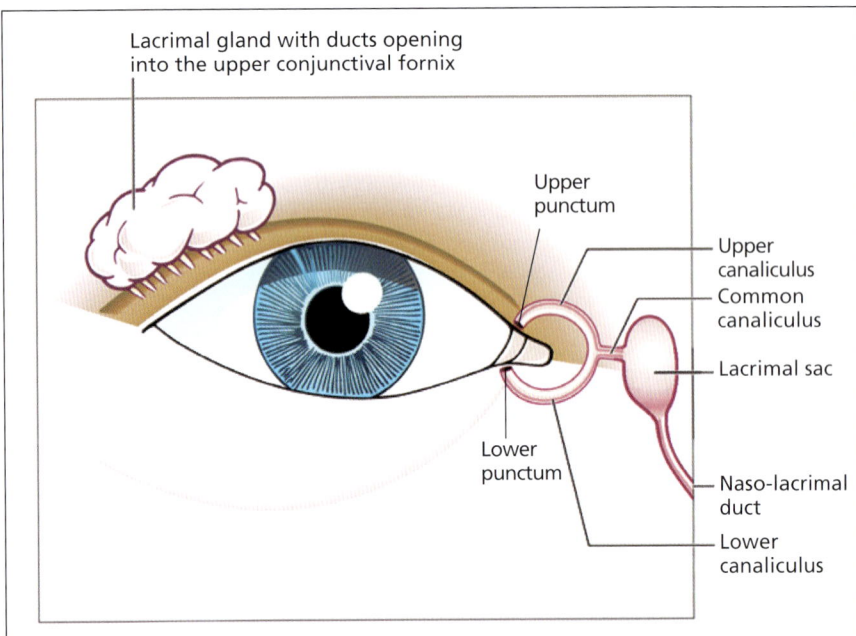

Figure 107.3 The lacrimal apparatus of the right eye.

Disorders of the eyebrows [1,2]

Synophrys

This term is applied when the eyebrows are profuse with a tendency to meet in the centre of the face. Synophrys is a feature of some genodermatoses. The eyebrows also tend to become more bushy in the ageing male for reasons that are unknown. Bushy eyebrows may also occur in other acquired forms of hypertrichosis, for example due to drugs such as diazoxide, and fusion of the eyebrows has been reported in kwashiorkor.

Reduction in eyebrow hair density

Some inherited diseases are characterised by hypoplasia of the eyebrows. Acquired conditions can cause sparsity or sometimes complete loss of the eyebrows. They may be the only site affected in alopecia areata. Thinning of the eyebrows occurs in hypothyroidism, follicular mucinosis and secondary syphilis. Lepromatous leprosy causes thinning of the outer third of the eyebrows in the early stages, often with depigmentation, progressing to total loss of the brows and lashes. These changes do not occur in tuberculoid leprosy. Plucking the eyebrows for cosmetic reasons is common, but true trichotillomania (hair-pulling disorder) of the eyebrows is sometimes seen in clinical practice. It may mimic alopecia areata but there is typically a history of hair-pulling [3]. Dermoscopic findings are reportedly the same as those seen in the condition when it affects the scalp [4]. Any cause of repetitive rubbing or scratching can lead to hair loss. This can occur in the eyebrow area in seborrhoeic dermatitis, atopic eczema and psoriasis, for example. Scarring alopecia may result from inflammation, such as in discoid lupus erythematosus, frontal fibrosing alopecia, lupus vulgaris or secondary or tertiary syphilis. Scarring may also follow chemical and thermal burns or radiation. Drugs and toxins are a further cause of alopecia including in this area, as may occur with chemotherapy. Loss of eyebrows can be camouflaged by the use of eyebrow pencils, permanent tattooing or by a hair prosthesis glued in place daily. Bimatoprost has been proposed as a treatment for eyebrow loss, although the use of such topical prostaglandin analogues is more established for alopecia of the eyelashes [5].

Disorders of the eyelashes

Trichomegaly [6–10]

This may be due to a genetic trait. Increased growth of the eyelashes has also been described in human immunodeficiency virus (HIV) infection and related to various drugs including ciclosporin, zidovudine, interferon, epidermal growth factor receptor inhibitors and topical prostaglandin analogues such as bimatoprost. The latter can be used for the treatment of hypotrichosis of the eyelashes and in alopecia areata [11]. However, chronic topical prostaglandin analogue use can be associated with worsening meibomian gland dysfunction leading to ocular surface inflammation and evaporative dry eye [12]. Long lashes also occur in some patients with phenylketonuria.

Madarosis

Madarosis is a decrease in the number of or complete loss of lashes [1]. Various causes have been recognised including alopecia areata, chronic anterior lid margin blepharitis (Figure 107.4),

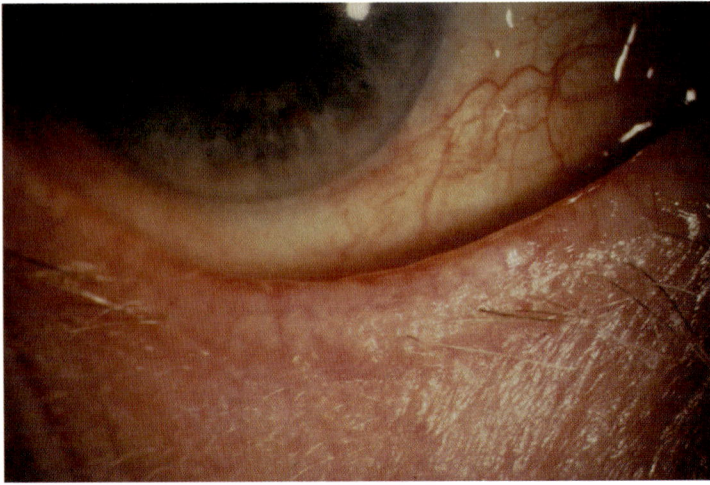

Figure 107.4 Madarosis due to staphylococcal blepharitis. Courtesy of Mr J. Dart, Moorfields Eye Hospital, London, UK.

PART 10: SPECIFIC SITES, SEX & AGE

Table 107.1 Glossary of ophthalmological terms

Term	Definition
Anophthalmia	Absence of eye
Astichiasis	Absence of lashes
Blepharitis	Inflammation of the eyelid margin
Blepharochalasis	A rare syndrome consisting of recurrent bouts of upper eyelid oedema associated with thinning, stretching and fine wrinkling of the involved skin
Bruch membrane	Retinal layer sandwiched between the retinal pigment epithelium and the vascular choroid
Chemosis	Swelling or oedema of the conjunctiva, due to exudation from capillaries
Coloboma	Congenital cleft created by failure of development of a portion of the eye or adnexal structures
Dermatochalasis	Loose and redundant skin of the eyelids, a common sign of periocular ageing
Distichiasis	Accessory row of eyelashes
Ectropion	Eversion of the eyelid
Entropion	Inversion of the eyelid
Epicanthal fold	Accessory fold of skin at the inner canthal region of the eye
Epicanthus inversus	Lower lid fold larger than upper lid fold
Epiphora	Excess tearing
Episcleritis	Inflammation of the superficial scleral tissues
Follicular inflammation	Inflammatory response of the conjunctiva characterised by discrete, round, elevated lesions of the conjunctiva with a vascular network around the follicle, diameter 0.5–5.0 mm. Composed of lymphocytes, macrophages and plasma cells; may form lymphoid follicles. Usually located in the inferior palpebral conjunctiva, sometimes superiorly
Grey line	An important anatomical landmark for surgical repair and pathological conditions of the lid margin such as blepharitis. The grey line divides the lid into an anterior lamella (skin and muscle) and a posterior lamella (tarsus and conjunctiva). It represents the location of the marginal region of the orbicularis muscle (muscle of Riolan) seen through the lid skin
Hypertelorism	Increased distance between the two eyes measured radiologically
Hypopyon	Presence of pus in the anterior chamber
Keratitis	Inflammation of the cornea. Various types are recognised, including: *filamentary keratitis* – the development of epithelialised mucous filaments on the corneal surface – and *interstitial keratitis* – inflammation of the corneal stromal layer
Keratoconjunctivitis sicca	Corneal and conjunctival inflammation associated with impaired tear secretion and ocular dryness
Keratoconus	Conical distortion of the central cornea as a result of a degenerative process in the stroma
Keratopathy	Corneal abnormalities including *exposure keratopathy* – from corneal exposure and drying of the cornea
Lagophthalmos	Persistent exposure of the eyeball despite closure of the eyelid
Limbus	Boundary between the cornea and sclera
Madarosis	Loss of the eyelashes and/or eyebrow hair
Pannus	Vascularised corneal scar
Papillary inflammation	Inflammatory response of the conjunctiva characterised by elevated polygonal hyperaemic areas each with a central fibrovascular core, separated by paler areas. Diameter of 0.3 mm (micropapillae) to 2.0 mm; 'giant' papillae if >1.0 mm. Composed of polymorphonuclear leukocytes and other acute inflammatory cells, with epithelial hypertrophy. Typically occur on the tarsal conjunctiva and at the limbus
Phlyctenule	Wedge-shaped, peripheral corneal or conjunctival nodule
Preseptal cellulitis	Cellulitis of the eyelids that has not penetrated through the orbital septum to involve the orbit
Symblepharon	Adhesions between the bulbar and palpebral conjunctiva resulting in complete or partial obliteration of the eyelid fornices
Telecanthus	Increased distance between the inner canthi
Trichiasis	Lashes that turn inward toward the cornea usually as a result of entropion
Uveitis	Inflammation of the uveal tract. It is subdivided into anterior uveitis (which is the most common), intermediate uveitis, posterior uveitis and panuveitis. *Anterior uveitis* is subdivided into iritis, in which the inflammation predominantly affects the iris, and iridocyclitis, in which both the iris and the anterior part of the ciliary body (pars plicata) are equally involved. *Intermediate uveitis* involves the posterior part of the ciliary body (pars plana) and the extreme periphery of the choroid and retina. *Posterior uveitis* is inflammation located behind the vitreous base. *Panuveitis* is involvement of the entire uveal tract

PART 10: SPECIFIC SITES, SEX & AGE

infiltrating tumours of the lid, burns, cryotherapy and radiotherapy, trichotillomania and discoid lupus erythematosus (see Figure 107.9e). Systemic diseases such as hypothyroidism and syphilis may also be responsible.

Abnormalities of the eyelids

These include dermatochalasis, blepharochalasis and lid laxity. Numerous developmental defects can affect the palpebral fissure or size and shape of the eyelids. A number of hereditary dermatoses affect the eyelids.

Blepharochalasis

Blepharochalasis is an eyelid condition that consists of chronic skin changes and episodic inflammation. This eyelid issue is bilateral and it tends to manifest in the upper eyelids.

Dermatochalasis

This is a condition in which the skin on the upper or lower eyelids loses its elasticity, causing it to sag and bulge. It is most commonly associated with old age, although certain inherited conditions, skin disorders, eye injuries and renal problems can also bring about dermatochalasis.

Ptosis

Drooping of the eyelids on one or both sides is a common genetic defect. Mild ptosis commonly develops in the elderly due to the laxity of the connective tissue. There are many important acquired causes, such as third nerve palsy, Horner syndrome and myasthenia gravis, which require neurological referral. Ptosis may be associated with other ocular abnormalities.

Skin diseases affecting the eyelids and periocular skin

While noting that skin disease confined to the periocular area can be challenging to differentiate, a large number of dermatological conditions can affect the eyelids as part of a more widespread process [1]. The diagnosis can then usually be made by examination and investigation of the rest of the skin. Psoriasis and lichen planus can both involve the lids and cause considerable irritation. These are chronic diseases and management can become a problem with the potential for use of potent topical corticosteroids on the eyelids over a prolonged period of time. The topical immunosuppressants tacrolimus and pimecrolimus are effective and can reduce topical corticosteroid exposure in facial psoriasis [2]. Unilateral inflammation of an eyelid raises the possibility of infective conditions, including dermatophytosis and mycobacterial infections.

Psoriasis [3,4]

Eye involvement can occur in 10–58% of patients with psoriasis, mostly in those with psoriatic arthritis. Men are more susceptible to ocular disease. Involvement of the eyelid gives rise to blepharitis, madarosis and the development of psoriatic plaques. Chronic non-specific conjunctivitis may occur over time and lead eventually to keratoconjunctivitis sicca with symblepharon formation and trichiasis. Conjunctivitis usually complicates eyelid margin involvement; white or yellow psoriatic plaques can spread from the lid on to the conjunctiva itself. Corneal changes are rare and are most commonly related to exposure and trichiasis. Anterior uveitis is rare but has been reported in patients with psoriatic arthritis and is similar to that seen in Reiter syndrome. Ocular psoriasis is treated with use of lubricants, topical corticosteroids and steroid-sparing topical calcineurin inhibitors where indicated. Patients with chronic eyelid involvement should be referred for ophthalmic assessment for possible impaired eyelid closure, and associated exposure keratopathy.

Contact dermatitis [5–11]

Contact dermatitis, whether irritant or allergic, is the responsible cause in approximately half of patients with periocular dermatitis. The remainder have manifestations of atopic or seborrhoeic eczema. The eyelid skin is very sensitive to primary irritants. These can cause dermatitis in their own right or can aggravate an underlying constitutional tendency in patients with either atopic or seborrhoeic eczema.

Allergic contact dermatitis can present after many years of exposure to the culpable allergen. Clinically, it is characterised by severe itching, redness and swelling of the eyelid, progressing to the formation of vesicles. A wide variety of allergens have been reported as causing allergic contact dermatitis of the lid and include preservatives (used in cosmetics, topical medications (Figure 107.5) and

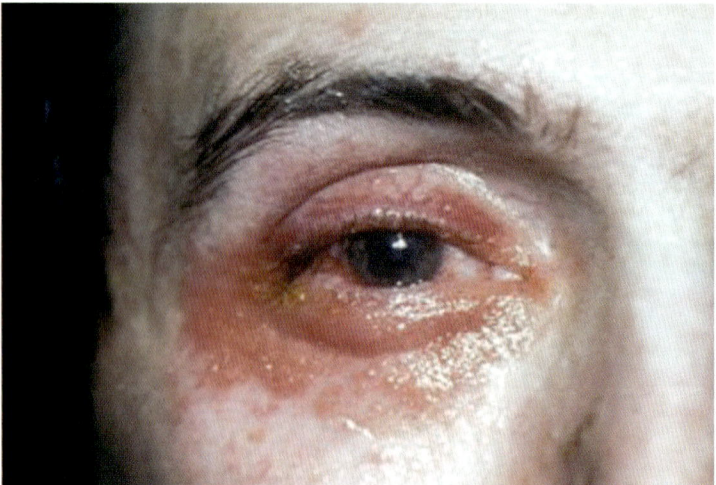

Figure 107.5 Allergic blepharoconjunctivitis due to topical medication. Allergic eyelid skin reaction. Courtesy of Mr J. Dart, Moorfields Eye Hospital, London, UK.

contact lens cleaning solutions), fragrances and various chemicals in cosmetic nail products. Patients with possible contact dermatitis of the eyelids should be patch tested. A careful history is of paramount importance to ensure that the relevant allergens are included in the test battery. The possibility of transferring antigen from the hands to the eyelids needs to be considered. Maibach described the upper eyelid dermatosis syndrome in which patients have discomfort of the eyelids with or without dermatitis; this is thought to be unrelated to the use of cosmetics.

Periorbital oedema [12,13]

The subcutaneous tissue of the eyelids is lax and prone to oedema. There are many systemic and dermatological causes of eyelid oedema that must be considered. Systemic causes include glomerulonephritis, hypoalbuminaemia (especially nephrotic syndrome), cardiac failure, superior veno-caval obstruction and thyroid disease. Some systemic infections, such as infectious mononucleosis and scarlatina, cause periorbital oedema. It may be the presenting feature of dermatomyositis and has been reported in systemic lupus erythematosus.

The most common dermatological causes of periorbital oedema are angioedema, lymphoedema, allergic contact dermatitis (Figure 107.6) and blepharochalasis; they are usually distinguished by

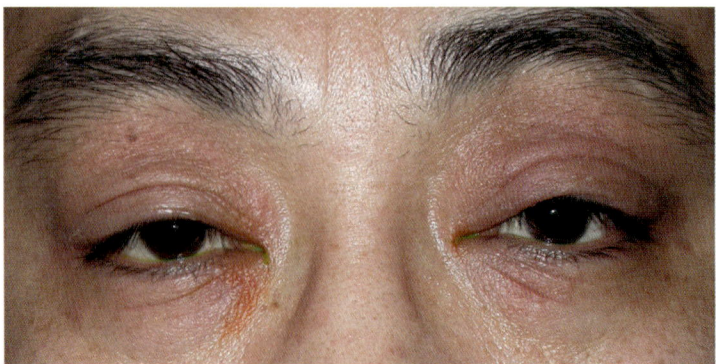

Figure 107.6 Periorbital oedema as a manifestation of allergic contact dermatitis.

the history. Angioedema is transient and often part of a more generalised urticarial eruption. Lymphoedema is persistent, tends to be worse first thing in the morning and improves during the day; it may be associated with underlying sinus disease or a chronic inflammatory condition such as granulomatous rosacea. Allergic contact dermatitis presents acutely with swelling, redness and itching. The typical eczematous scaling, which helps to differentiate this clinically from angioedema, may only become evident later. Blepharochalasis syndrome is an uncommon condition which may be inherited (autosomal dominant) or sporadic; it presents in the second decade with recurrent episodes of painless lid oedema, resulting in the development of excess skin and thickened subcutaneous tissue which may require treatment by blepharoplasty. Senile orbital fat prolapse through a deficient orbital septum may mimic periorbital oedema but is differentiated by the fact that there is minimal fluctuation in the associated swelling. Periorbital oedema may be the presenting feature of rosacea. Melkersson–Rosenthal syndrome is a rare cause of isolated eyelid oedema which can pose a diagnostic challenge [14].

Changes in pigmentation [15–19]

There are considerable racial and familial variations in the degree of pigmentation of the eyelids. Marked periorbital melanosis is seen as a genetic trait. Pigmentation of the periorbital skin can be post-traumatic, postinflammatory or can accompany melanocyte-stimulating hormone-induced melanosis of any cause. It can also be associated with metabolic syndrome and be a side effect of latanoprost eye drops. Infraorbital dark circles can be a significant aesthetic concern and are challenging to treat [20]. Chemical pigmentation can occur from prolonged use of a mercurial or silver preparation, producing a slate-blue or grey-brown discoloration. Mauve discoloration of the eyelids and periorbital area is an early part of chrysiasis from parenteral gold therapy. Grey discoloration can complicate long-term treatment with minocycline. Local hyperpigmentation may also be due to cosmetics containing phototoxic agents, usually psoralens. Postinflammatory hyperpigmentation commonly follows dermatoses such as eczema and especially lichen planus and its variants. Dyspigmentation is also a frequent consequence of discoid lupus erythematosus. The eyelids may be involved in vitiligo. Hypopigmentation can complicate the use of topical medications including thiotepa eye drops and mercurial ointments.

SKIN DISEASES AFFECTING THE EYE AND EYELIDS

Blepharitis, meibomian gland dysfunction, rosacea and seborrhoeic dermatitis [1–5]

Definition and nomenclature

An influential international workshop on meibomian gland dysfunction (MGD) formalised definitions and terminology [2].

Blepharitis is a general term describing inflammation of the lid as a whole. Anterior blepharitis describes inflammation of the lid margin anterior to the grey line and concentrated around the lashes. It may be accompanied by squamous debris or collarettes around the lashes, and inflammation may spill onto the posterior lid margin, resulting in posterior blepharitis. Posterior blepharitis describes inflammation of the posterior lid margin, which may have different causes, including MGD, conjunctival inflammation (allergic or infective) and/or other conditions, such as rosacea. MGD is a chronic, diffuse abnormality of the meibomian glands, commonly characterised by terminal duct obstruction and/or qualitative/quantitative changes in the glandular secretion. It may result in alterations of the tear film, symptoms of eye irritation, clinically apparent inflammation and ocular surface disease. MGD is further subcategorised into hyposecretory, obstructive and hypersecretory forms.

Introduction and general description

Table 107.2 classifies the five types of chronic blepharitis (including ocular rosacea) into those that principally affect the anterior lid margin structures (cutaneous margin with lash-bearing skin and associated glands) and those affecting the posterior lid margin (mucocutaneous junction, meibomian orifices). This classification corresponds with, and simplifies understanding of, the treatment of the different conditions, which differs between the anterior lid and posterior lid margin disorders but not between the individual conditions within each of these two groups. The commoner clinical signs of staphylococcal blepharitis are shown in Figure 107.7. Ocular rosacea is an important condition because of its severity and wide spectrum of clinical features (Table 107.3; Figure 107.8).

In addition to these very common types of blepharitis, there are other chronic causes in which the pathogenesis is clear. These are all uncommon and are often misdiagnosed as one of the types of chronic blepharitis described in Table 107.2. They include fungal infection (e.g. *Candida*), parasitic infection (e.g. phthiriasis), protozoal infection (e.g. leishmaniasis), some neoplasms and autoimmune conditions such as lupus erythematosus; some of these are illustrated in Figure 107.9. They should be considered when therapy for conventional blepharitis fails.

Acute blepharitis is a clearly defined group of conditions, for which the causes are summarised in Table 107.4.

Epidemiology

The epidemiology of blepharitis has been hampered by difficulties of disease definition, a lack of a standardised clinical assessment and the different perspectives of dermatologists and ophthalmologists [6,7,8].

Incidence and prevalence

Chronic blepharitis is very common and makes up about 70% of ophthalmic referrals. MGD is the commonest cause of blepharitis and affects 20–40% of all patients consulting ophthalmologists for routine eye examinations. The reported prevalence of MGD varies widely, with a suggested higher prevalence (>60%) in Asian populations compared with a prevalence of 3.5–20% in white people;

Table 107.2 Classification of types of chronic blepharitis (lid margin disorders) [1,3]

	Anterior lid margin[a]		Posterior lid margin[a]			Anterior and/or posterior lid margin
	Staphylococcal blepharitis	Seborrhoeic blepharitis	Meibomitis/ocular rosacea	Other meibomian gland dysfunction	Meibomian seborrhoea	Other blepharitis, e.g. atopic, psoriatic, fungal, protozoal, parasitic, neoplastic, lupus
Associations with other types of blepharitis	Secondary meibomitis; Demodex blepharitis (cylindrical dandruff or sleeves on eyelashes)	Staphylococcal blepharitis; Any posterior lid margin condition	Staphylococcal and seborrhoeic blepharitis	Seborrhoeic blepharitis	Seborrhoeic blepharitis	
Associated skin disease	Atopic eczema; Impetigo; Rosacea (rare)	Seborrhoeic dermatitis; Rosacea (rare)	Rosacea in up to 50% of cases	Rosacea in up to 50% of cases		Atopy; Psoriasis; Lupus
Associated eye disease	Dry eye; Atopic keratoconjunctivitis	Dry eye	Scleritis and episcleritis in ocular rosacea	Scleritis and episcleritis in ocular rosacea		Variable according to aetiology
Main features *Symptoms*	Burning; Itching; Photophobia	Minimal	Foreign body sensation; Burning; Discomfort; Photophobia with ocular rosacea	Variable: Foreign body sensation; Burning; Discomfort	Variable: Foreign body sensation; Burning; Discomfort	Lack of resolution with standard MGD treatment; Variable according to aetiology
Lid signs	Unilateral/patchy lid margin involvement (Figure 107.7d); Brittle fibrinous scales bleed when detached, form collarettes at lash base (Figure 107.7a); Dilated vessels, styes (external hordeolum, Figure 107.24a); Poliosis, madarosis, eyelash misdirection (Figure 107.7b); Eyelid ulceration and scarring when severe	Bilateral greasy scales (not fibrinous)	Chalazia (Figure 107.8b); Irregular lid margins; Distorted meibomian orifices and meibomian gland drop out; Inspissated secretions; Expression difficult; Surrounding inflammation; For lid signs in ocular rosacea see Table 107.3	Eyelash misdirection; Foamy discharge on eyelid margin; Poor-quality meibum; Expression difficult; Meibomian gland drop out; Chalazia; Irregular scarred lid margins in long-standing disease	Plugged and elevated orifices without inflammation	Variable according to aetiology
Conjunctival and corneal signs	Follicles, papillae and hyperaemia of lower tarsal conjunctiva and fornix (Figure 107.7c); Conjunctival and corneal phlyctenules may occur; Coarse punctate keratitis in lower third of cornea. Marginal keratitis (Figure 107.7e) typically at 10, 2, 4 or 8 o'clock and corneal vascularisation and thinning. Conjunctival scarring (Figure 107.8a)	Mild conjunctival injection; Coarse punctate keratitis in lower third of cornea	Early tear break up time; Foam/debris in tears; Punctate keratitis (dry eye); For conjunctival and corneal signs in ocular rosacea see Table 107.3	Early tear break up time; Foam/debris in tears; Punctate keratitis (dry eye); For conjunctival and corneal signs in ocular rosacea see Table 107.3	Minimal injection; Foamy tear film	Variable according to aetiology; Variable according to aetiology

[a] The anterior lid margin is the portion anterior to the meibomian gland orifices and the posterior lid margin is behind this, including the meibomian glands. Anterior and posterior lid margin disorders are commonly mixed, and there is often overlap in clinical features of these categories of blepharitis; frequent associations are shown in the table.
MGD, meibomian gland disease.

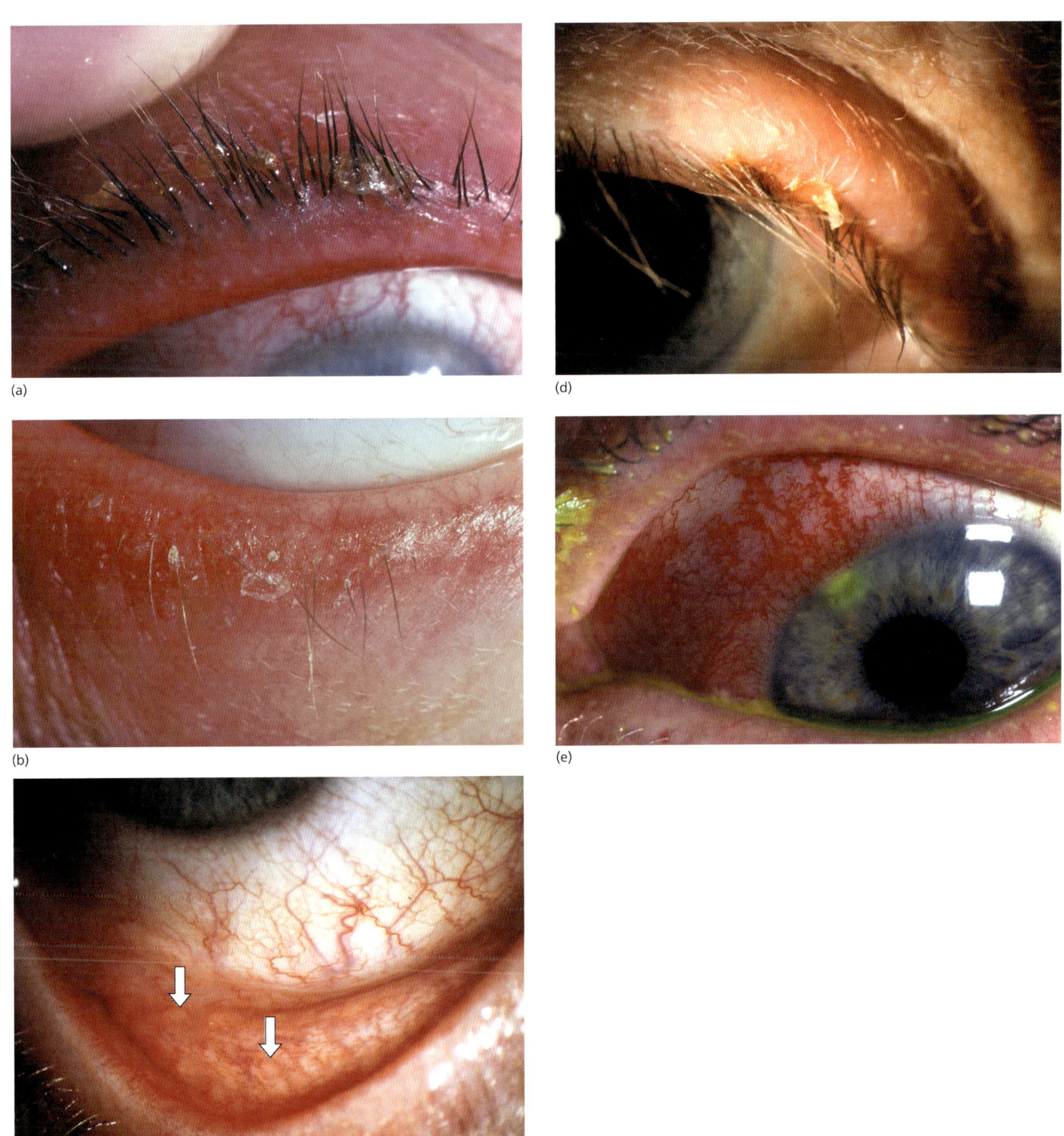

Figure 107.7 Staphylococcal blepharitis. (a) Fibrinous 'collarettes' lifting away from the skin as the lashes grow. (b) Fibrinous scales on the anterior lid margin with the madarosis (loss of lashes) and poliosis (white lashes) that accompanies chronic blepharitis. (c) Follicular conjunctivitis with arrows showing the white/yellow follicles. (d) Localised ulcerative blepharitis. Sectoral disease like this is quite common in staphylococcal blepharitis which can also be largely unilateral. (e) Marginal keratitis with ulceration, a common corneal complication of staphylococcal blepharitis (fluorescence occurs in the area where an ulcer is present. Courtesy of Mr J. Dart, Moorfields Eye Hospital, London, UK.

Table 107.3 Clinical signs of ocular rosacea

Signs	Common	Uncommon	Rare
Lid	Meibomitis (Figure 107.8a) Seborrhoeic blepharitis Lid margin telangiectasia Lid notching Retroplacement of the mucocutaneous junction Chalazia (Figure 107.8b,d) Hordeoleum	Entropion	
Conjunctiva	Conjunctival hyperaemia Papillary conjunctivitis	Reticular and linear tarsal scarring and fornix shortening (Figure 107.8a)	
Cornea	Phlyctenular keratoconjunctivitis Marginal corneal infiltration and ulceration (Figure 107.8c)	Pseudopterygium	Corneal perforation
Sclera and episclera		Episcleritis	Scleritis

however, there is significant variation in disease definition and the age of the study groups in these studies [6]. Between 3% and 58% of patients with rosacea have ocular involvement; this wide variation largely reflects differences in disease definition. Approximately half of patients with rosacea have signs of ocular rosacea, while one-quarter of patients with ocular rosacea has no dermatological disease. In participants with all types of blepharitis, the prevalence of rosacea ranged from 26.7% to 44%, and that of seborrhoeic dermatitis was 32.9% [9,10].

Age
In a case–control study conducted in San Francisco and Texas [1,11], the average age of onset of staphylococcal blepharitis was 42 years, the mean age of participants with seborrhoeic blepharitis was 50 years, and that of MGD blepharitis patients was 50 years. Rosacea may be found in early childhood as well as in the elderly, but it is most often diagnosed at aged 30–50 [12].

Sex
While staphylococcal blepharitis occurs more commonly in women (80%), the prevalence of seborrhoeic blepharitis, MGD and ocular rosacea is equal between men and women [1,13].

Ethnicity
Asian ethnicity has been suggested to be a risk factor for MGD [6]; however, MGD is also more common in fair-skinned individuals due to its association with rosacea, which is more prevalent in this population [12].

Associated diseases
See Table 107.2.

Pathophysiology
The pathogenesis of chronic blepharitis is, in general, poorly understood. There is some evidence to support hypotheses of pathogenesis in staphylococcal blepharitis and in meibomian dysfunction.

Predisposing factors
Ophthalmic factors associated with MGD include contact lens wear, *Demodex folliculorum* and dry eye disease. Systemic factors that may promote MGD include, among others, androgen deficiency, menopause, ageing, Sjögren syndrome, hypercholesterolaemia, psoriasis, atopy, rosacea, hypertension and benign prostatic hyperplasia (BPH). Medications associated with the pathogenesis of MGD include antiandrogens, medications used to treat BPH, postmenopausal hormone therapy (e.g. oestrogens and progestins), antihistamines, antidepressants and retinoids [6].

Pathology
Staphylococcal blepharitis. In staphylococcal blepharitis there is an association with *Staphylococcus aureus* and *S. epidermidis* colonisation of the lid margins, although colonisation by *S. aureus* is often transient and the numbers of either organism are often no greater than in normal controls [14] (Chapter 26). Although folliculitis, styes and lid margin ulcers may be due to infection by *S. aureus*, the persistence of lid inflammation after treatment and the sterile marginal ulcers are not explained by infection alone. The importance of cell-mediated immunity in the pathogenesis of the disease was shown by experimental studies in rabbits. When these were immunised with either whole *S. aureus* or with cell wall ribitol teichoic acid, ulcerative keratitis, phlyctenules and marginal corneal ulcers developed after secondary challenge, providing evidence for the hypothesis that these changes were due to the development of hypersensitivity to both viable and killed organisms [15,16]. These findings could not be reproduced for *S. epidermidis*. However, evidence for a similar pathogenesis in humans is lacking; the relationship between the clinical signs of staphylococcal blepharitis and hypersensitivity to subcutaneous injections of either whole *S. aureus* or of *S. aureus* cell wall protein A is poor. *S. epidermidis* is more often isolated than *S. aureus* from the lids of patients with staphylococcal blepharitis, but the role of a hypersensitivity response is assumed and not supported by any firm data [17]. The pathogenesis of the often severe follicular and papillary conjunctivitis that accompanies this condition is assumed to be due to a combination of transient infection and hypersensitivity. Some researchers have hypothesised that toxins produced by the bacteria may cause irritation, but no specific toxin has been identified [18,19].

***Demodex folliculorum* infestation.** *Demodex folliculorum* are small parasitic mites that live in hair follicles, sebaceous glands and meibomian glands. They are found in 30% of chronic blepharitis patients, but are also found with nearly the same prevalence in patients without blepharitis [20]. They may have a role in both anterior and posterior blepharitis. It is theorised that the infestation and wastage of mites cause blockage of the follicles and glands and/or an inflammatory response. Patients with recalcitrant blepharitis have responded to therapy directed at eradicating *Demodex* mite. Studies support its role in the activation of immune mechanisms in subtypes of rosacea (e.g. papulopustular rosacea [21]) and one study has found a correlation between serum immunoreactivity, ocular *Demodex* infestation, lid margin inflammation and facial rosacea [22].

Meibomian gland disease. The meibomian lipids (meibum) are a complex mixture of cholesterol esters and esterified unsaturated

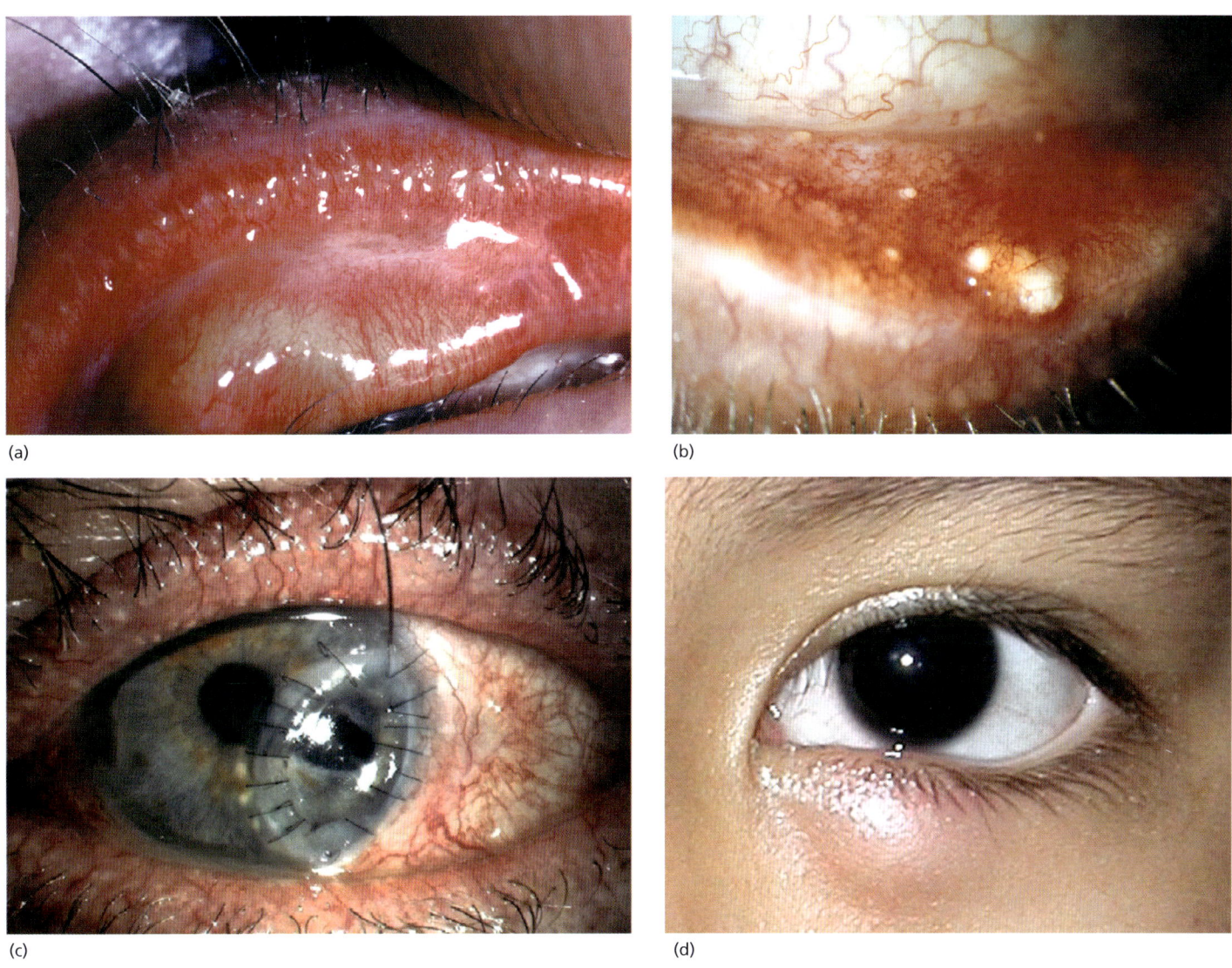

Figure 107.8 Ocular rosacea. (a) Scales on the anterior lid margin, meibomitis with posterior migration of the orifices associated with loss of the normal posterior lid margin architecture and scarring in the superior tarsal marginal sulcus. Entropion and trichiasis may result from this degree of scarring. (b) Meibomian dysfunction with blocked glands and small chalazia. (c) Corneal transplant following perforation of a marginal ulcer; also shows meibomitis. (d) Chalazion (meibomian gland cyst). (c) Courtesy of Mr J, Dart, Moorfields Eye Hospital, London, UK.

fatty acids. These lipids are responsible for maintaining a stable tear film, reducing tear film evaporation (and, therefore, preventing drying of the ocular surface) [23], preventing tear spill over the lid margins by lowering surface tension and reducing ocular surface contamination by sebum from the cutaneous surface of the lids, which otherwise forms dry spots. Three factors have been invoked as contributing to MGD: (i) keratinisation of the meibomian ductules; (ii) the effect of bacterial lipases on the meibum at the lid margin; and (iii) primary abnormalities in the production of meibum by individuals with MGD [24].

Normal meibomian gland ducts open just anterior to the mucocutaneous junction. As the duct lining is partially keratinised, abnormalities of keratinisation, analogous to those present in the sebaceous glands of patients with rosacea, may be important in the pathogenesis of MGD by altering gland function. Bacterial lipases are produced by all the bacteria that colonise the lid margin and have the potential to break down meibum into free fatty acids,

which destabilise the tear film [25]. These bacteria colonise the gland orifices, and expression of lipid from deeper within the glands can stabilise the tear film. Meibomian lipids differ between individuals and, as analytical methods increase in sensitivity, the relative roles of primary abnormalities of meibum and those secondary to the effects of bacterial lipases in the pathogenesis of MGD are likely to become clearer [26]. Neither the pathogenesis of the conjunctival inflammation that is common in meibomitis (and which is a feature of ocular rosacea), nor that of the keratitis in ocular rosacea, has been explained.

Ocular rosacea. The precise aetiology and pathophysiology of ocular rosacea remains unknown, although different theories have been proposed [27,28] (Chapter 89). Molecular studies propose that abnormal recognition of common environmental stimuli leads to activation of pro-inflammatory systems as well as innate immune responses. Factors that trigger the innate immune

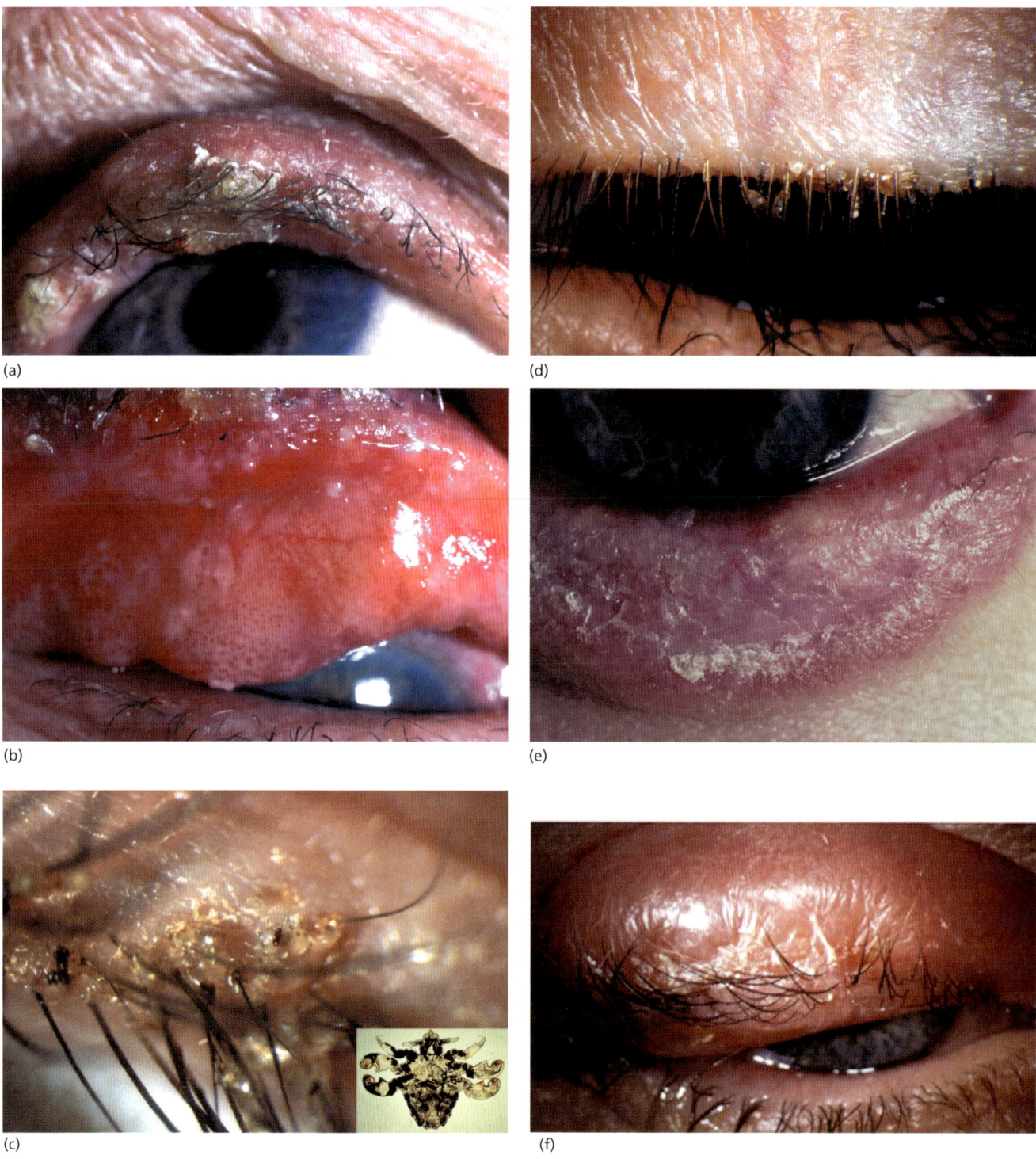

Figure 107.9 Rarer causes of chronic blepharitis. (a, b) Sebaceous carcinoma of the upper lid. (c, d) Blepharitis due to *Phthirus pubis*, showing the louse in (c) and the eggs ('nits') in (d). (e) Typical lid lesion of discoid lupus. (f) Cutaneous *Leishmania* infection of the upper eyelid. Diagnosis is by biopsy. (e) Courtesy of Mr J. Dart, Moorfields Eye Hospital, London, UK.

system lead to increased expression of certain cytokines and antimicrobial molecules such as cathelicidin, which is vasoactive and pro-inflammatory [29]. Overreaction to environmental stimuli is believed in part to be due to elevated expression of Toll-like receptor 2 in the epidermis of rosacea patients via a complex interplay between a variety of mediators including matrix metalloproteinase,

kallikrein 5, tumour necrosis factor α (TNF-α) and interleukins [27,28]. This leads to increased serine protease and cathelicidin production. Furthermore, tetracyclines, which improve the signs and symptoms of rosacea, inhibit the expression and activity of several matrix metalloproteinases, as well as a class of proteases that activate cathelicidin, thus supporting this theory.

Table 107.4 Causes of acute blepharitis

Location	Underlying diagnosis
Acute anterior lid margin	Folliculitis (infected lash follicles)
	External hordeoleum (stye) (Figure 107.24a)
	Angular blepharitis (at lateral canthus)
	Impetigo
	Herpes infection (Figure 107.22a)
Acute posterior lid margin	Chalazion (Figure 107.8b,d)
	Internal hordeoleum (Figure 107.24b)
Generalised anterior and posterior	Necrotising fasciitis

Causative organisms

Staphylococcal blepharitis is believed to be associated with staphylococcal bacteria on the ocular surface, but there are likely to be additional contributing factors, given that in some studies there is no difference in positive culture levels between controls and blepharitis patients.

Demodex mites have also been considered a causative factor in blepharitis and papulopustular rosacea. Another proposed mechanism is that *Demodex* mites may act as vectors for other organisms such as *Bacillus olenorius*, which may be responsible for initiating the inflammatory response via stimulation of Toll-like receptor 2 and the production of antigenic proteins [22].

Environmental factors

It has been postulated that staphylococcal blepharitis occurs more commonly in warmer climates, while MGD may be more common in cooler climates [30].

Clinical features

History

See Table 107.2.

Presentation

See Tables 107.2 and 107.3.

Clinical variants

See Tables 107.2 and 107.3.

Differential diagnosis

See Table 107.5.

Classification of severity

A severity grading for MGD, which can be used to guide treatment, has been described [31].

Complications and co-morbidities

See Tables 107.2 and 107.3.

In severe and longstanding staphylococcal blepharitis, trichiasis (misdirection of eyelashes towards the eye), poliosis (depigmentation of the eyelashes), madarosis (loss of eyelashes), eyelid ulceration and eyelid and corneal scarring may occur [3].

Blepharitis due to MGD can be complicated by:

1 Ocular surface damage with conjunctival and corneal involvement, including meibomian keratoconjunctivitis and phlyctenular keratitis [32,33].

Table 107.5 Differential diagnosis of blepharitis: other conditions associated with eyelid inflammation [3]

Condition	Entity
Bacterial infections	Impetigo (due primarily to *Staphylococcus aureus*)
	Erysipelas (due primarily to *Streptococcus pyogenes*)
Viral infections	Herpes simplex virus
	Molluscum contagiosum
	Varicella zoster virus
	Papillomavirus
	Vaccinia
Parasitic infection	Pediculosis palpebrarum (*Phthirus pubis*)
Immunological conditions	Atopic eczema
	Allergic contact dermatitis
	Erythema multiforme
	Pemphigus foliaceus
	Ocular mucous membrane pemphigoid
	Stevens–Johnson syndrome
	Connective tissue disorders
	Lichen planus
	Discoid lupus erythematosus
	Dermatomyositis
	Graft-versus-host disease
	Crohn disease
	Melkersson–Rosenthal syndrome
Other dermatoses	Psoriasis
	Ichthyosis
	Exfoliative dermatitis
	Irritant contact dermatitis
	Seborrhoeic dermatitis
	Other causes of erythroderma
Benign eyelid tumours	Pseudoepitheliomatous hyperplasia
	Actinic keratosis
	Squamous cell papilloma
	Sebaceous gland hyperplasia
	Haemangioma
	Pyogenic granuloma
Malignant eyelid tumours	Basal cell carcinoma
	Squamous cell carcinoma
	Sebaceous carcinoma
	Melanoma
	Kaposi sarcoma
	Mycosis fungoides
Trauma	Chemical
	Thermal
	Radiation
	Mechanical
	Surgical

2 Evaporative dry eye [33].
3 Other ocular disorders including contact lens intolerance and recurrent corneal erosion syndrome [34].

Disease course and prognosis

The natural history of MGD is not precisely known, but it is regarded as a progressive but treatable disease, in which therapy may prevent irreversible damage [33]. Therapy to prevent progression is most important when the sight-threatening complications of ocular rosacea and severe staphylococcal blepharitis including corneal vascularisation, corneal thinning, perforation, pseudopterygium and corneal phlyctenules are first detected. One of the most important aspects of caring for patients with blepharitis is educating them about the chronicity and recurrence of the disease process, and the likelihood that their symptoms can be improved but are rarely eliminated [3].

Investigations

There are no specific diagnostic tests for blepharitis, which depends on recognition of typical clinical signs and symptoms for diagnosis. However, cultures of the eyelid margins may be indicated for recurrent anterior blepharitis with severe inflammation, and for patients not responding to therapy. Microscopic examination of epilated lashes may reveal *Demodex* mites. A biopsy of the eyelid to exclude carcinoma should be considered in blepharitis unresponsive to therapy, especially if it is very asymmetrical, or in the context of unifocal recurrent chalazia which do not respond well to therapy.

Meibomian gland disease may be diagnosed in isolation, or more commonly in association with dry eye or ocular surface damage. A series of tests may be performed in the ophthalmology clinic, first to diagnose generic dry eye and then to differentiate between MGD-related evaporative dry eye versus aqueous deficient dry eye. These may include the administration of a validated symptom questionnaire such as the OSDI (ocular surface disease index), measurement of blink rate and blink interval, measurement of lower tear meniscus height, assessment of tear film break-up time and the Schirmer test. Characterisation of MGD is by quantification of morphological features, meibum expressibility and quality, and meibomian gland drop out [33].

If testing suggests the diagnosis of a generic dry eye and tests of tear flow and volume are normal, then evaporative dry eye is implied, and quantification of MGD will indicate the meibomian glands' contribution. This test sequence also allows a diagnosis of MGD, with or without ocular surface staining or dry eye, to be made. The grading scores for each test can be used to monitor the disease during treatment.

Management

The treatment of blepharitis is that of the underlying cause, if one can be identified. The blepharitis should initially be classified into either anterior or posterior lid disease or both (see Table 107.2). It is important to decide whether blepharitis is the cause of the symptoms; seborrhoea rarely causes symptoms and should not be used as a scapegoat to explain away symptoms possibly due to other, or undiagnosable, conditions. Other conditions that give rise to similar symptoms and signs (see Table 107.2) should be excluded or treated. Symptoms of dry eye, and associated skin disorders, should also be treated (Table 107.6).

Diffuse folliculitis is generally caused by *S. aureus* and requires a course of an appropriate systemic antibiotic. Laboratory investigations are of limited value – bacteriology samples can be taken from lid margins using swabs dipped in trypsin digest broth, but these are usually only performed for recurrent disease that has not responded to initial therapy.

Chalazia will resolve in time; approximately 60% of lesions will resolve in 6 months and the remainder will resolve spontaneously, given longer. Resolution of chalazia can be hastened by incision and curettage; the lid is incised, usually from the conjunctival surface, under local anaesthesia, and the necrotic granulomatous tissue in the centre of the lesion is removed with a curette. This leaves a linear conjunctival and tarsal scar. It is only recommended

Table 107.6 Treatment of chronic blepharitis

Aims of treatment	Therapeutic guidelines
For anterior lid margin disease	
Treat infection (may depend on local resistance patterns)	Staphylococcal and mixed staphylococcal/seborrhoeic groups
	Topical antibiotics (chloramphenicol or fusidic acid) 4 times daily to lid margins or topical azithromycin drops
	Oral tetracycline or macrolide (especially for women of childbearing age or children) for 10 days
	Tea tree oil lid scrubs for recalcitrant blepharitis due to *Demodex*
Clean lid margins	'Lid scrubs'[a]: 1–2 times daily with cotton pads dampened in boiled water or proprietary lid cleaning pads, to remove debris
Lid hyperaemia and exudate	Topical chloramphenicol and hydrocortisone 0.5–1.0% to lid margins 2–4 times daily for 2 weeks
For posterior lid margin disease	
Mechanically unblock meibomian glands	Apply hot compresses to eyelid margins[a] to liquefy meibomian secretions 1–2 times daily
Alter meibomian secretions	Oral tetracycline (e.g. doxycycline 100 mg daily or lymecycline 408 mg daily) or macrolide (e.g. erythromycin 250–500 mg twice daily) for 12 weeks minimum or azithromycin 500 mg daily for 3 days per week, for 3 weeks
For the tear film	
Restore tear film	Artificial tears drops 2–4 hourly or carbomer gel 3–4 times daily
For associated conjunctivitis (papillary or mixed follicular and papillary)	
Reduce inflammation	Fluorometholone 0.1% 4 times daily for 1 week, progressively reducing to once daily over a further 4 weeks
	Consider topical ciclosporin as a steroid-sparing agent
Treat associated skin disease	Treat coexisting seborrhoeic dermatitis conventionally with, for example, topical antiyeast agent
	Rosacea: oral lymecycline 408 mg or doxycycline 100 mg once daily, or erythromycin 250–500 mg twice daily for 12 weeks
For keratitis	
Coarse punctate keratitis and/or marginal keratoconjunctivitis and/or phlyctenules	Fluorometholone 0.1% 4 times daily for 1 week, progressively reducing to once daily over a further 4 weeks[b]
Corneal thinning and perforation	Exclude and treat any concomitant microbial keratitis and establish disease control by methods summarised above, apply tissue glue to perforations. Consider systemic immunosuppression (e.g. mycophenolate or azathioprine). Carry out tectonic corneal graft, if necessary, once the inflammation is controlled

[a] Lid scrubs, lid massage and low-dose systemic antibiotics take about 4–6 weeks to start to work. Do not assume that treatment has failed until at least 8 weeks on treatment has elapsed, and continue the regimen for a minimum of 2–3 months if benefit is shown. Then advise a maintenance regimen of lid scrubs (for anterior lid margin disease), hot compresses and tarsal massage (for posterior lid margin disease), ± artificial tears. In the case of relapse, repeat a 3-month course of oral antibiotic treatment.
[b] More prolonged courses of corticosteroid or more potent corticosteroids may be needed under specialist ophthalmological supervision. Topical ciclosporin has been shown to be effective for controlling inflammation in posterior blepharitis in small randomised trials and case series [36–39].

for cosmetic reasons or to improve vision in large lesions affecting the upper lid, which can cause temporary astigmatism.

Practice points for dermatologists are that the association between blepharitis and skin disease is variable, that treatment with tetracyclines may be beneficial for both the ocular and dermatological manifestations of these disorders, and that ocular rosacea and staphylococcal blepharitis may produce sight-threatening complications.

First line (Figure 107.10) [31]

Inform the patient about MGD and the potential impact of diet and environment on tear evaporation. Advise the patient on improving ambient humidity and increasing dietary omega-3 fatty acid intake.

Institute eyelid hygiene with eyelid warming (once or twice daily) followed by moderate to firm massage and expression of meibomian gland secretions.

Second line

First line management plus artificial lubricants (for frequent use, non-preserved is preferred). Consider topical azithromycin, topical emollient lubricant or liposomal lubricant.

Third line

Try oral tetracyclines and lubricant ointment at bedtime, and consider anti-inflammatory therapy (topical steroids, topical ciclosporin [35–40]) as indicated.

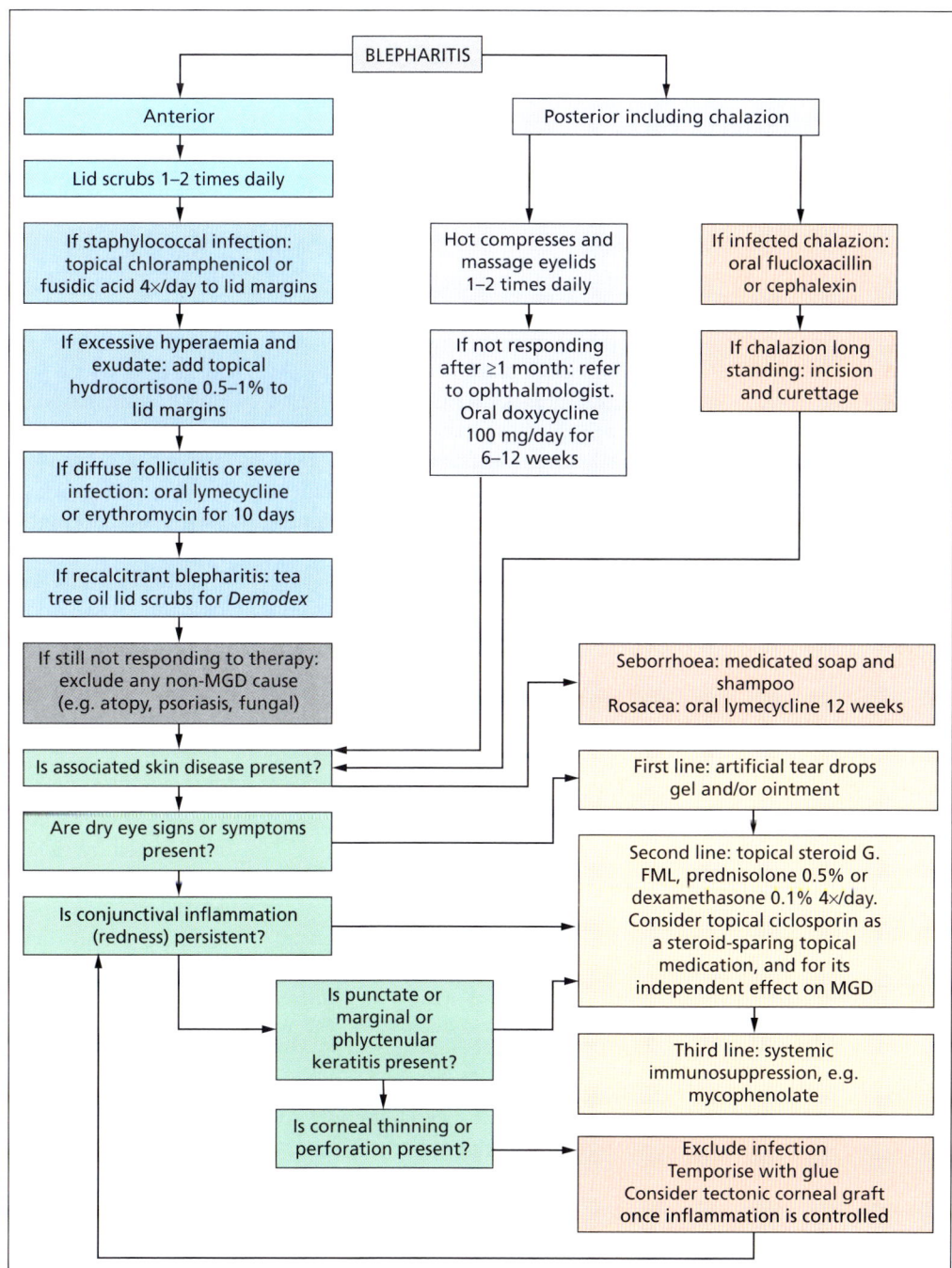

Figure 107.10 Management algorithm for blepharitis. MGD, meibomian gland dysfunction; FML, fluorometholone.

Atopy and atopic eye disease

Definition

The atopic eye diseases comprise a group of disorders that have in common a papillary conjunctivitis and evidence of a type I allergic mechanism (Chapter 41). They include the milder conditions of seasonal allergic conjunctivitis (SAC) and perennial allergic conjunctivitis (PAC) and the more severe atopic keratoconjunctivitis (AKC), atopic blepharoconjunctivitis (ABC) and vernal keratoconjunctivitis (VKC).

Atopic eczema is associated with these conditions. It commonly affects the eyelids but it is covered in Chapter 41 so will not be discussed in detail here.

Introduction and general description

The atopic eye diseases all involve immunoglobulin E (IgE) mediated hypersensitivity responses although each disease has specific immunogenic pathways. Ocular involvement in atopic patients ranges from 15% to 40% but is generally mild with features of SAC or PAC. Only a very small proportion of patients with atopic eczema have significant ocular disease. Table 107.7 summarises these disorders. Of these, only AKC and VKC can involve the cornea and threaten sight. They are often difficult to treat. The severity of symptoms is closely related to disease activity. Patients with minimal symptoms respond to simple topical measures and safe treatment with antihistamines and mast cell stabilisers. At the opposite extreme, acute exacerbations of AKC and VKC must be recognised and treated promptly as these may develop within hours and lead to blinding corneal complications within 1–2 days. ABC runs a similar course to AKC but has no corneal involvement and although infection with *Staphylococcus aureus* can be a significant complication, the disease in itself is not a potentially blinding condition.

Epidemiology [1]

Incidence and prevalence

The incidence of allergic conditions has increased significantly over the past 40 years. It has been estimated that 15–40% of atopic patients have some ocular involvement although this is usually mild. SAC is the commonest form of atopic eye disease (90%) followed by PAC (5%). The remaining 5% is accounted for by AKC, ABC and VKC.

Age

Seasonal allergic conjunctivitis and PAC can occur in any age group. AKC and ABC begin in the late teens or early twenties and persist often until the fifth decade of life. VKC occurs mainly in children and 90% of cases resolve by adult life.

Sex

These diseases affect the sexes equally with the exception of VKC which is more common in boys than girls before puberty.

Ethnicity

These conditions affect all ethnic groups although VKC is more common in patients of African and Asian origin.

Associated diseases

Atopic keratoconjunctivitis is associated with a predisposition to staphylococcal lid and eye infections, and also herpes simplex lid and eye infections, such that bilateral herpetic eye disease is more frequently observed (usually herpetic eye disease is a unilateral condition). It is thought that susceptibility to these infections is related to impaired T-cell immunity in AKC patients.

Pathophysiology [1–5]

Predisposing factors

There is usually a personal or family history of atopy.

Pathology

Recent advances in our understanding of the atopic eye diseases have come from investigation of the humoral mediators of inflammation in the tears and analysis of the cellular components by immunostaining and *in situ* hybridisation of conjunctival biopsies. These techniques have shown that SAC and PAC are primarily type I IgE-mediated hypersensitivity responses whereas the others show varying degrees of a coexisting type IV hypersensitivity response and also involve the production of cytokines by various effector cells.

SAC and PAC show mast cells and eosinophils in the conjunctival mucosa and submucosa with high levels of locally produced IgE to specific allergens being present in the tears. Symptoms are due to the release of histamine and other inflammatory agents by mast cells which lead to dilated blood vessels, irritated nerve endings and increased secretion of tears. The diseases can be mimicked by topical instillation of allergens and are blocked by drugs that are active against mast cells.

The pathogenesis of AKC and VKC involves both IgE-mediated type I and non-IgE-mediated type IV hypersensitivity responses, with the production of various cytokines by effector cells. These lead to the more severe inflammatory changes that cause corneal damage. AKC and VKC show the cellular components present in SAC and PAC but also increased fibroblast activity with connective tissue hyperplasia, CD4+ lymphocytes and plasma cells together with different subsets of mast cells. The T cells are probably important inducers of the cellular inflammatory response in these diseases. Differences in AKC and VKC phenotypes may be explained by differences in the predominance of T-helper subsets; the Th1 subset involved in delayed hypersensitivity responses and inactivated by ciclosporin is more predominant in AKC than VKC in which the Th2 subset predominates with a B-cell helper role. Mast cells and eosinophils are found in larger numbers in VKC than AKC and functional heterogeneity in their populations may also be determinants of disease phenotypes. Eosinophils play a central role in atopic eye diseases and it appears that the level of eosinophil activation rather than the absolute number is relevant to the development of corneal disease. Eosinophils elaborate a host of cytokines and release cationic proteins including major basic protein, which is epitheliotoxic and has been identified in the tears in VKC. It is probably a major factor responsible for the development of corneal epithelial erosions and macroerosions. The presence of the latter, with the mucus and debris present in acute exacerbations of keratopathy, accounts for the formation of plaque. Basophils have also been found to contribute to the atopic eye diseases through IgE-induced release of chemical mediators.

Environmental factors

These are most relevant in SAC and PAC where airborne allergens play a causal role. Symptoms for many patients are worse when the weather is warm and dry.

Clinical features [1–12]

History

From the dermatologist's perspective these patients will be under their care primarily for the management of atopic eczema but have or develop ocular symptoms. The dermatologist needs to be aware that any sudden deterioration of vision may herald one of the blinding complications of these diseases and should be treated as an emergency.

Presentation

The initial symptoms are similar for all the atopic eye diseases. Patients complain of itching, watering and the production of a sticky white mucus discharge. In the more severe variants of AKC, ABC and VKC exacerbations lead to rapid deterioration in symptoms. The itching may be superseded by extreme discomfort with soreness with a foreign body sensation and vision deteriorates. The lids may be difficult to open in the morning because of a combination of discomfort and discharge.

Clinical variants

Seasonal allergic conjunctivitis is the commonest form of atopic eye disease often presenting with other features of hay fever: nasal and pharyngeal symptoms. The onset of symptoms is seasonally related to specific circulating aeroallergens most commonly grass and tree pollens. Ocular involvement is usually bilateral. The conjunctival surfaces are mildly injected and oedematous, and lid oedema and papillary inflammation along tarsal conjunctival surfaces are features (Figure 107.11). PAC is a variant of SAC that persists throughout the year although 80% of patients have seasonal exacerbations. Dust mites, animal dander and feathers are the most common allergic associations. SAC and PAC are mild and never affect the cornea. They are reversible upon removal of the causal allergen.

   VKC is a severe, chronic, ocular inflammatory process affecting children, which typically manifests as cobblestone papillae in the upper tarsal conjunctiva (Figure 107.12a). The condition presents in children aged 5–15 years old who often have a history of seasonal allergy, asthma and eczema. Presenting symptoms include intense pruritus, eye watering and redness with mucus production. There is a marked seasonal incidence with the most frequent onset in spring. In VKC, involvement of one eye may be minimal while the other is severely affected. Lid margin signs are uncommon in VKC although an extra lower eyelid crease from oedema may be present (Dennie line). The lower tarsal conjunctiva is usually less involved than the upper lid, which can be seen to be thickened and velvety with papillary inflammation when the lid is everted. Persistent forms of VKC are associated with subepithelial fibrosis that appears as a white linear scar running parallel to the lid margin (Arlt line). Progressive fibrosis gives rise to giant upper tarsal papillae known as cobblestone papillae. This occurs more commonly in VKC than in AKC.

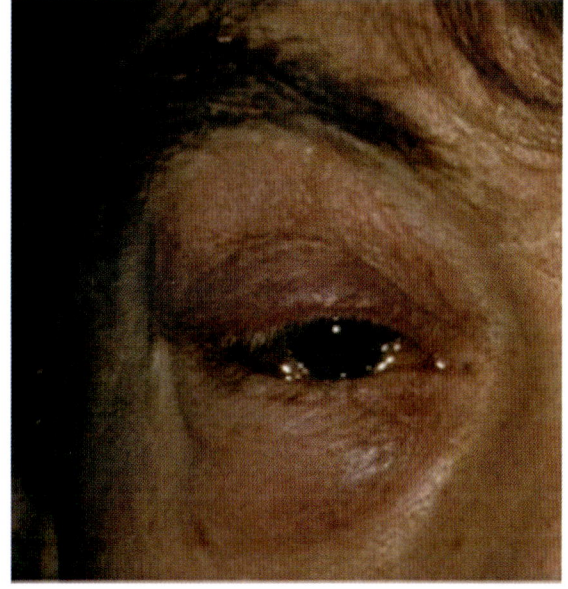

(a)

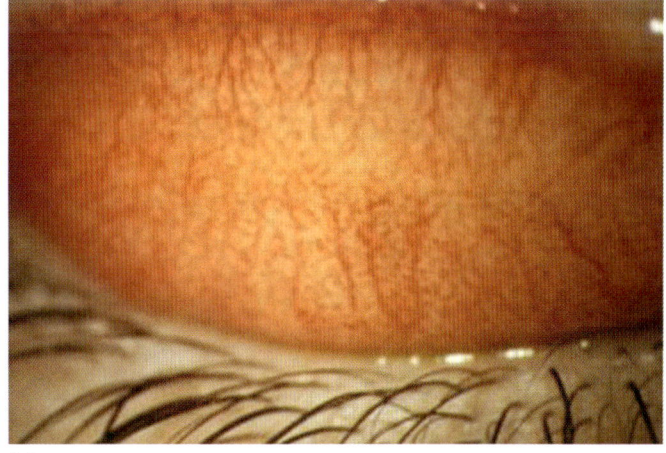

(b)

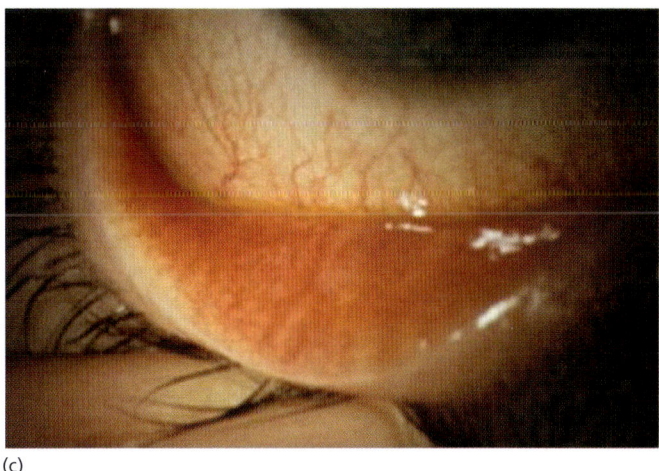

(c)

Figure 107.11 Seasonal and perennial allergic conjunctivitis (SAC and PAC) (a) Eyelid oedema and redness. (b) Upper tarsal papillary inflammation. (c) Lower tarsal papillary inflammation.

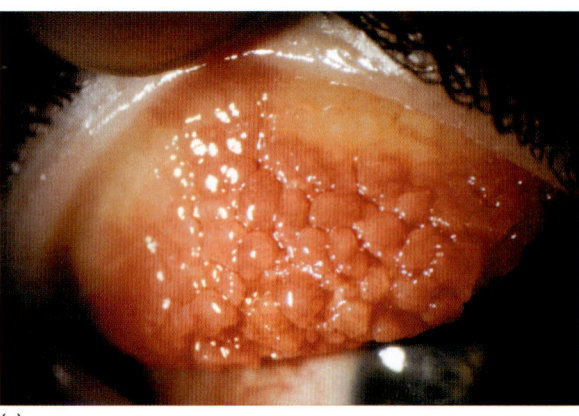

(a)

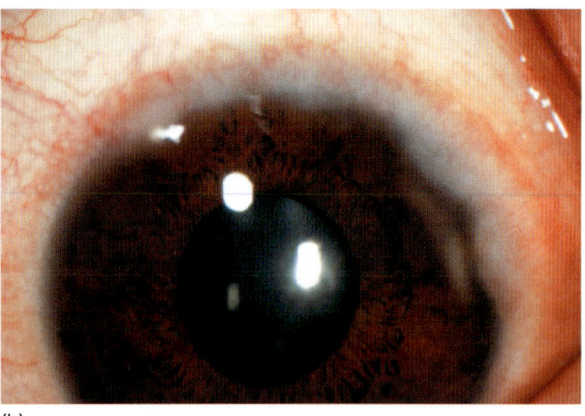

(b)

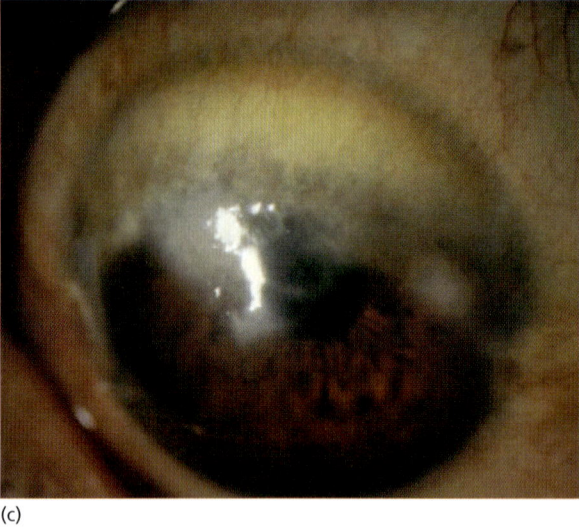

(c)

Figure 107.12 Vernal keratoconjunctivitis (VKC). (a) 'Giant' upper tarsal cobblestone papillae with mucous exudate in palpebral VKC. (b) Typical pale limbal papillae (Trantas dots) in limbal VKC. (c) Sclerosing variant of VKC.

VKC spontaneously resolves in 95% of children after 10 years. Those with VKC who continue to suffer actively inflamed atopic eye disease in adulthood have disease which is then termed AKC. In burnt-out quiescent VKC there may be sheet-like scarring of the upper conjunctiva as evidence of previous fibrotic–inflammatory episodes. There are two clinical patterns of VKC, limbal and palpebral, depending on which part of the conjunctiva is mainly

involved. Limbal VKC manifests with gelatinous macropapillae at the limbus (Trantas dots) (Figure 107.12b) and micropapillae on the upper tarsus. Palpebral VKC manifests with giant upper tarsal papillae (Figure 107.12a). Mixed forms show both limbal and palpebral disease. During exacerbations of VKC, the tarsal conjunctiva becomes very red and inflamed and covered with adherent mucus. In severe cases keratitis develops, most often in the upper cornea due to contact with cytokines released from the upper tarsal papillae. This initially manifests as punctate epitheliopathy and progresses to macroerosion, shield ulcer and then a vernal plaque. This results in severe discomfort to the patient with photophobia, tearing, pain and deterioration of vision. Central corneal scars may develop. VKC will threaten sight if it involves the cornea. A sclerosing variant of VKC has been observed, where the limbus is sclerosed and vascularised (Figure 107.12c), most likely a long-term fibrotic sequel of limbal VKC. In the majority of cases, VKC burns out by the age of 30 (<10 years after onset).

AKC affects patients in their early twenties to fifties. AKC usually presents with itching, burning and tearing which is more severe than with SAC and PAC. The disease is usually bilateral and symmetrical. AKC can recur at any time during the course of the associated atopic disease and is independent of its degree of severity. Patients with AKC may have prolonged exacerbations of the disease that are difficult to control, which are associated with redness, severe photophobia, pain and blurring of vision. Examination of patients with AKC shows severe eczema affecting the eyelids and periorbital skin often extending onto the cheeks. The associated blepharoconjunctivitis gives rise to thickened and inflamed lid margins (Figure 107.13e). Excessive tearing can result in maceration of the eyelid skin and secondary staphylococcal infection. AKC patients have an increased susceptibility to staphylococcal infections as well as herpes simplex infections, which can involve the cornea (Figure 107.13d) and eyelid. The cornea infections are sight threatening, sometimes bilaterally, which is uncommon in non-AKC patients with herpes simplex keratitis. There may be an absence of the lateral eyebrows from chronic rubbing. The conjunctivae are chronically inflamed. Papillary hypertrophy of both upper and lower tarsal conjunctiva is usual in the early years of the disease and giant (compound) upper tarsal papillae may occur in some patients (Figure 107.13c). The conjunctiva is often so thickened by infiltrate that the tarsal vessels are obscured (Figure 107.13b) – later in the disease the papillae may be obscured by sheet scarring. Shortening of the inferior fornix develops in some patients and less often the medial and lateral fornices may be obliterated by scar tissue (Figure 107.13f). The bulbar conjunctiva is inflamed during exacerbations but otherwise grossly normal except for the limbal region which may be thickened and nodular with the presence of pinpoint Trantas dots at the apices of the nodules (Figure 107.13g). One of the more common corneal changes is pseudogerotoxon (Figure 107.13h), in which there is a limbal pannus giving rise to an arcus senilis-like appearance.

ABC (Figure 107.14) runs a similar course to AKC but has no corneal involvement and is therefore not potentially blinding. It can, however, be associated with chronic staphylococcal infection with the associated risk of long-term complications.

Key clinical features distinguishing the different variants of atopic eye disease are summarised in Table 107.7.

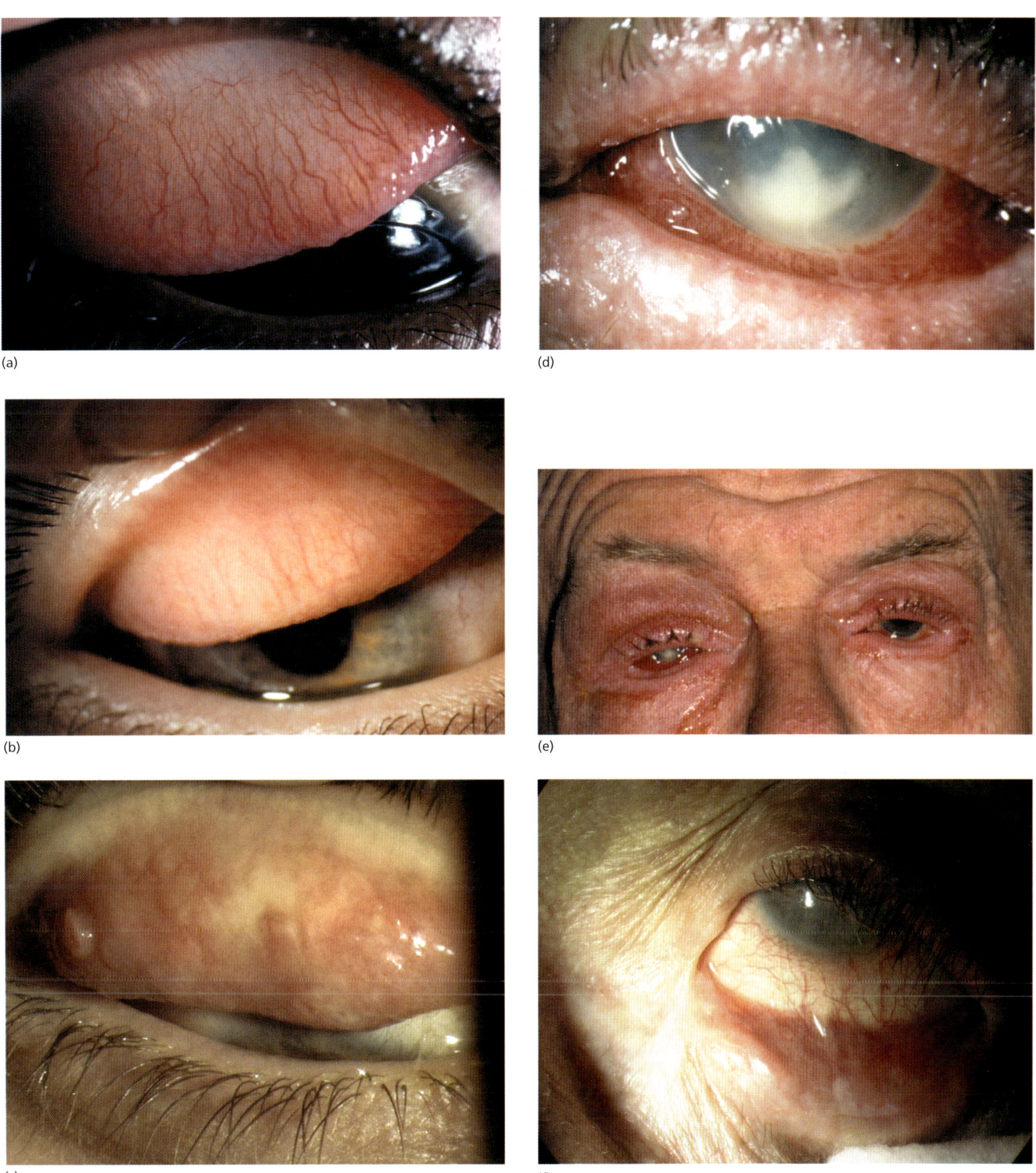

Figure 107.13 Atopic keratoconjunctivitis (AKC). (a) Normal upper tarsal conjunctiva; the tarsal vessels are clearly visible through the healthy conjunctival epithelium and substantia propria. (b) AKC with an infiltrated, papillary, upper tarsal conjunctiva. Compare with the normal tarsal conjunctiva in (a). (c) Giant upper tarsal papillae in AKC. (d) Bacterial keratitis complicating AKC showing a corneal infiltrate. The eyes of this patient are shown in (e), with atopic eczema localised to the eyelids; the eczema is often generalised. The right eye shows the infection in (d). (f) Inferior fornix and plical scarring. (g) Limbitis in AKC. (h) Pseudogerontoxon. (i) AKC anterior subcapsular 'polar bear rug' cataract.

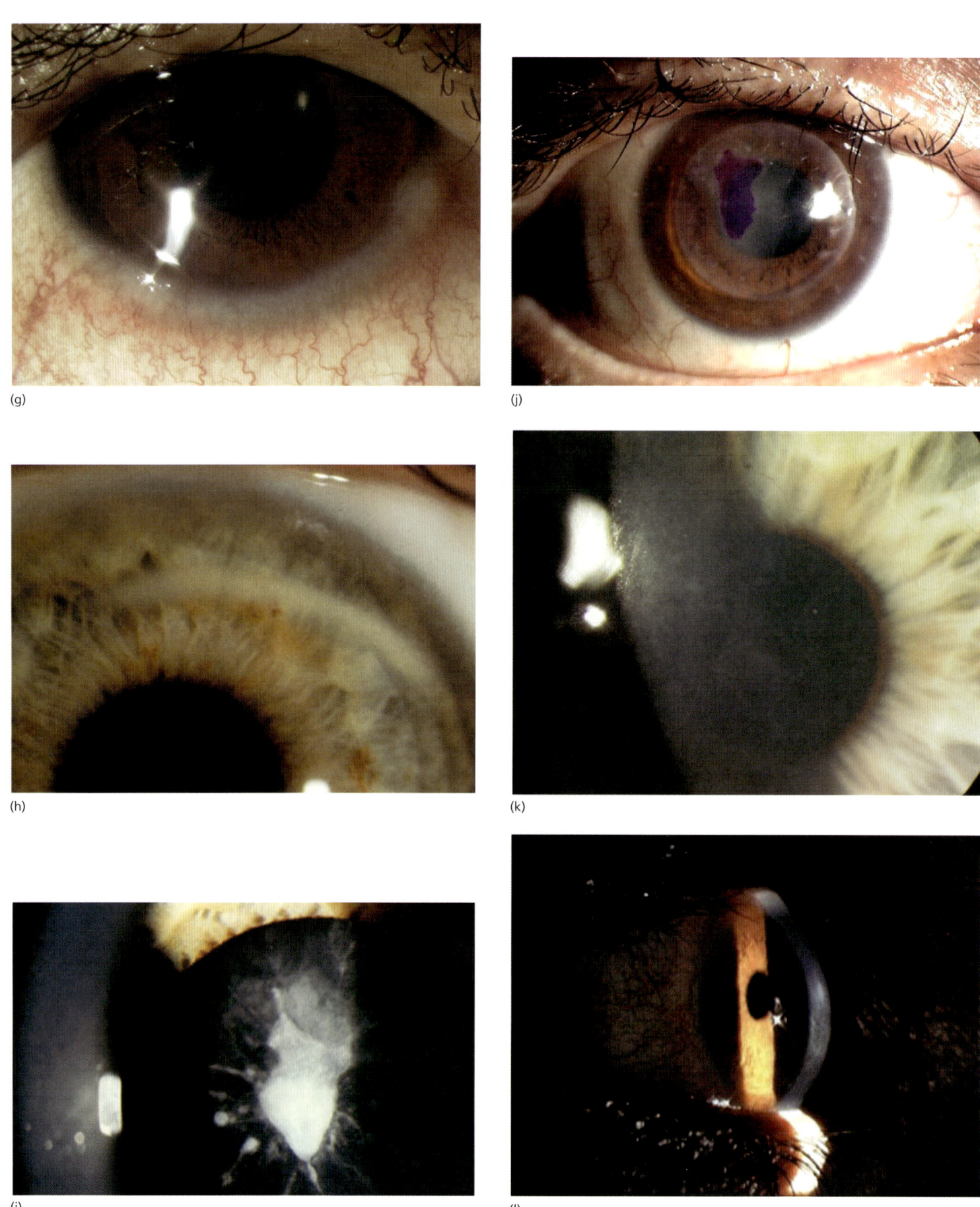

(g)

(j)

(h)

(k)

(i)

(l)

Figure 107.13 (*Continued*)

Table 107.7 Clinical characteristics and distinguishing features and diagnosis of the atopic eye diseases

Disease	Disease course	Conjunctival signs	Corneal signs	Disease associations	Diagnostic tests
Periocular atopic eczema	Onset variable but often in childhood Varies in severity over time	Typically none	None	Personal or family history of atopy	
Seasonal allergic conjunctivitis (SAC)	Onset 5–20 years Spontaneous remissions common Rare in old age Strikingly seasonal	Hyperaemia, stringy white discharge, oedema, micropapillae if severe	None	Personal or family history of atopy including atopic eczema	*Cytology*: usually normal. Serum and tear IgE often elevated but not diagnostic
Perennial allergic conjunctivitis (PAC)	As for SAC but symptoms all year round with seasonal exacerbations	Hyperaemia, stringy white discharge, micropapillae common	None	Personal or family history of atopy including atopic eczema	
Atopic keratoconjunctivitis (AKC)	Onset between 20 and 50 years Chronic course over many years (Figure 107.13e) Spontaneous resolution in old age Non-seasonal	Micropapillae with intense infiltrate (Figure 107.13b). Reticular and sheet scarring. Shortened fornices in some cases Trantas dots[a]	Punctate epithelial keratopathy, pannus, macroerosion[b] and plaque[c] Pseudogerontoxon[d] Herpes keratitis and bacterial keratitis (Figure 107.13d) common	*Systemic*: atopy and atopic eczema in all cases *Ocular*: staphylococcal lid disease, cataract, keratoconus, herpes simplex keratitis (often bilateral)	*Cytology*: shows eosinophils and mast cells. Serum immunoglobulin E (IgE) elevated. Skin prick tests positive to many allergens but not diagnostic *Upper tarsal conjunctival punch biopsy*: the gold standard for disease confirmation after a 2-week abstention from use of topical corticosteroids *Tear IgE*: useful unless the serum IgE is very high
Atopic blepharoconjunctivitis (ABC)	As for AKC	Micropapillae with intense infiltrate, reticular scarring	None	Personal or family history of atopy	
Vernal keratoconjunctivitis (VKC) – palpebral, limbal and mixed forms	Onset between 5 and 15 years. Spontaneous resolution in 95% after 10 years Seasonal exacerbations usual	*Palpebral form*: giant upper tarsal papillae (Figure 107.12a) often bilaterally asymmetrical *Limbal form*: micropapillae on upper tarsus but gelatinous macropapillae at limbus (Figure 107.12b) Trantas dots in both *Mixed form*: combines features of both diseases	*Palpebral form*: punctate epithelial keratopathy affecting upper half of cornea. Adherent mucus appearing as superficial syncytial opacity progressing to macroerosion, shield ulcer and then vernal plaque *Limbal form*: keratopathy extending in from limbus with associated epithelial dysplasia	*Ocular*: keratoconus and cataract (Figure 107.13i) *Systemic*: atopy in variable proportions from 0% to 100% depending on geographic location (atopy common in northern Europe but rare in Middle East)	

[a] Trantas dots: white, pinhead-sized dots consisting of eosinophils and necrotic epithelial cells usually at the limbus.
[b] Macroerosion: large epithelial erosions usually in the upper half of the cornea.
[c] Plaque (vernal plaque): laminated structure of protein and polysaccharide adherent to the anterior stroma with destruction of the Bowman layer.
[d] Pseudogerontoxon: arcus-like appearance in relation to limbal pannus; may disappear in remissions.

Differential diagnosis

The clinical features together with a personal or family history of atopy are usually sufficient for diagnosis. Diagnostic dilemmas usually occur in two settings: firstly, in those patients who do not respond to appropriate topical therapy as expected to control the disease process before starting systemic immunosuppression; secondly, in cases of conjunctival scarring to differentiate AKC from other causes of cicatrisation such as primary Sjögren disease, rosacea and mucous membrane pemphigoid (MMP) (see Table 107.10).

Classification of severity

There are no generally accepted or validated classifications of severity in these diseases; however, for the purposes of evaluating response to therapy in a treatment trial, severity grading scores have been used [13].

The more severely affected patients with AKC have associated blepharoconjunctivitis and corneal disease formation of an atopic cataract (Figure 107.13i) and are particularly vulnerable to infection with *Staphylococcus aureus* and herpes simplex virus. The corneal epithelium reveals punctate scarring with fluorescein and limbal inflammation with Trantas dots (Figure 107.13g). More severely affected patients can develop changes of a cicatrising conjunctivitis with subepithelial fibrosis, shallowing of the conjunctival fornix obliterated by scar tissue and symblepharon formation (Figure 107.13f). Corneal scarring and neovascularisation can lead to blindness.

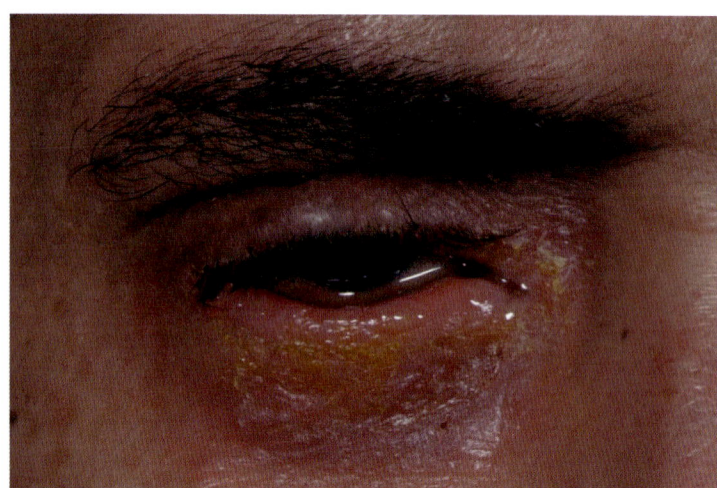

Figure 107.14 Atopic blepharoconjunctivitis (ABC).

Complications and co-morbidities

Cataracts occur in 8–12% of patients with severe atopic eczema, particularly young adults. They characteristically affect the anterior lens giving rise to a 'polar bear rug' appearance (Figure 107.13i). Posterior subcapsular cataracts are also present due to steroid usage. Keratoconus occurs in a small percentage of patients with AKC and VKC adding a further complexity to management – conversely, 16% of patients with keratoconus have atopic eczema. Patients with atopic eye disease are at risk of glaucoma because of the long-term use of topical steroid. It is difficult to treat, often requiring complex surgical procedures.

Disease course and prognosis

This is covered in the clinical variants section.

Investigations

Laboratory investigations may be required in patients who do not respond to therapy or who require topical or systemic immunosuppressive therapy for the relief of symptoms or when the diagnosis is uncertain. Raised serum IgE levels may be helpful in supporting a diagnosis of atopy, but skin prick testing is of limited value as the results do not necessarily identify the causal allergens. Ophthalmic investigations (upper tarsal conjunctival punch biopsy, tear IgE evaluation, impression cytology of the upper tarsal conjunctiva) are the province of the ophthalmologist and are summarised in Table 107.7.

Management [5,13–20,21]

Most cases of atopic eye disease are managed with topical ocular therapy which has no effect on the dermatological aspects of the disorder. Because of the potential sight-threatening complications more severe atopic eye disease (VKC, AKC) is best managed by a specialist ophthalmologist with an interest in these conditions. Treatment with courses of systemic agents when needed either for the dermatological or ophthalmological aspects of atopy is clearly going to be beneficial to the management of both. The risk of cataract and especially glaucoma with the use of potent topical steroids in the periocular skin demands that regular screening is carried out. Use of steroid-sparing topical calcineurin inhibitors (tacrolimus, pimecrolimus) is therefore preferable.

First line (Figure 107.15)

Simple measures of allergen avoidance, use of cold compresses and lubrication with preservative-free artificial tears are helpful first-line steps. An addition of a potent topical antihistamine or a systemic antihistamine may help relieve itch in some patients. Any long-term systemic antihistamine intake can lead to dry eye, the clinical features of which can complicate the ocular allergy features. Topical cromones are mast cell stabilisers (sodium cromoglycate 2–4% or the more recently introduced nedocromil or lodoxamide), and are helpful as first line treatments given once to four times daily depending on symptoms. Topical olopatadine and ketotifen fumarate combine the effects of a cromone with that of an antihistamine and are probably used more widely than cromones as a first line drug. These treatments are very safe and do not require ophthalmological supervision but are only effective for very mild disease. Cromones are often not tolerated until the inflammation is brought under control with high-dose topical steroids such as dexamethasone 0.1% or prednisolone 0.5%. Because of the attendant risk of glaucoma and steroid-induced cataract, topical ciclosporin and a less potent topical steroid (e.g. fluorometholone or hydrocortisone 0.335%) should be substituted as soon as the disease is brought under safe control. Topical calcineurin inhibitors (ciclosporin, tacrolimus) are used topically wherever possible as corticosteroid-sparing drugs. Novel agents, such as Janus kinase (JAK) inhibitors may be useful agents, on the horizon for these disorders [22].

Second line

The addition of topical calcineurin inhibitors is effective because T cells play a central role in the pathogenesis of the disease. Ciclosporin inactivates calcineurin which then inhibits T-cell activation and interleukin 2 (IL-2) production. It also inhibits histamine release from mast cells. Various preparations of topical ciclosporin are available for different regions, both for ocular allergy and for dry eye, including 0.05% and 0.1% concentrations, as well as an unlicensed 0.2% veterinary ointment formulation. Topical ciclosporin is more soluble in an oily vehicle, although this stings on application. Adverse effects apart from stinging are infrequent, so introduction of the drug for patients requiring high doses of topical corticosteroid has allowed the reduction or complete withdrawal of corticosteroid in many cases. Topical ciclosporin is best tolerated if introduced during remissions. Both the 1% and 2% concentrations have been reported to be safely used in children with VKC for up to 4 years, with no reports of malignancy or infection.

Topical tacrolimus (0.03% and 0.1%) ointment and pimecrolimus cream are both also useful as steroid-sparing agents when applied to the eyelids. There is also some benefit from spreading onto the conjunctival surface in treating other aspects of the disease.

Severe staphylococcal blepharitis often accompanies AKC and ABC and can be treated with a course of azithromycin followed by local therapy with an antibiotic ointment to which the skin flora are sensitive, usually chloramphenicol together with a topical ophthalmic corticosteroid ointment such as hydrocortisone 0.5% or 1% applied to the lids. Combined preparations often contain aminoglycosides which frequently cause toxicity or allergy and should be avoided.

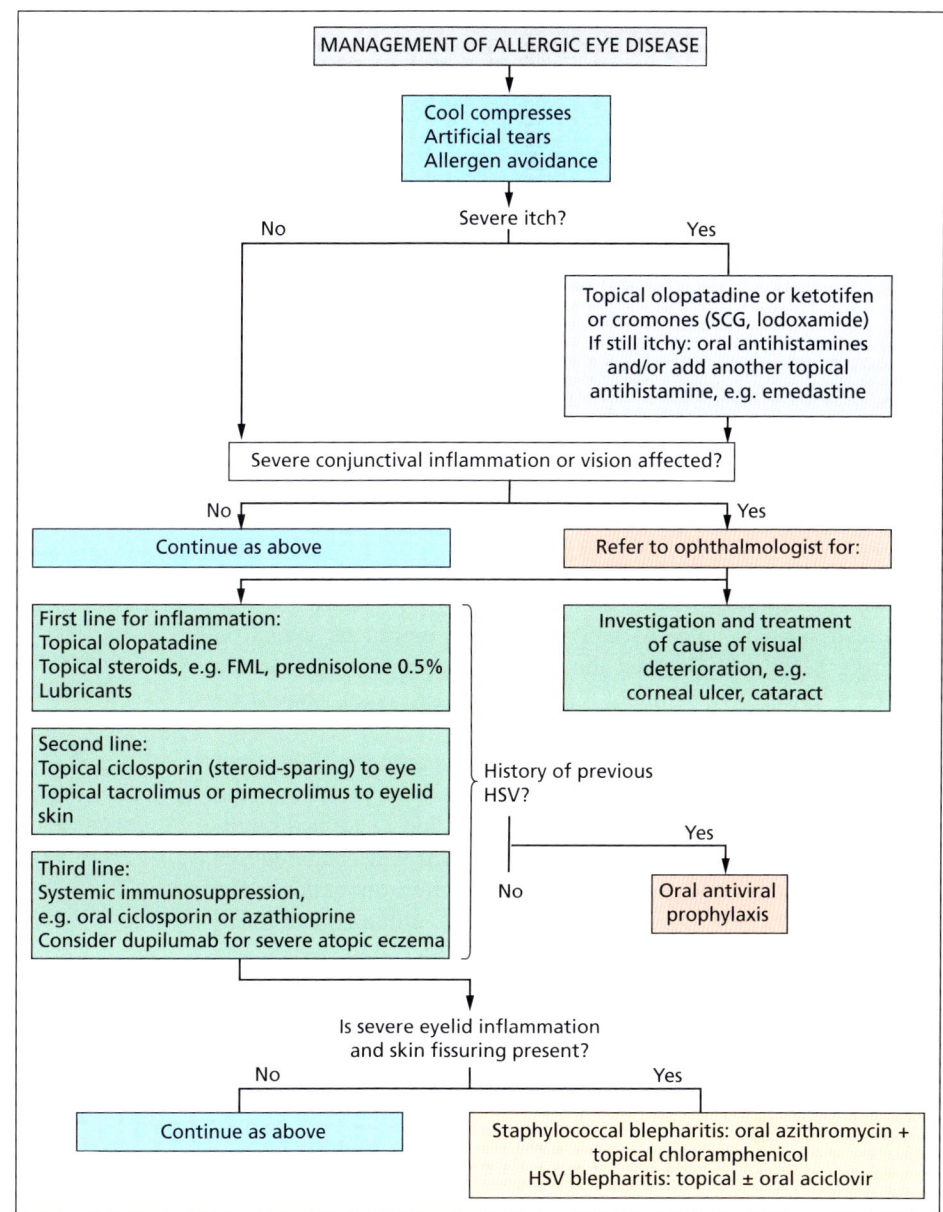

Figure 107.15 Management algorithm for allergic eye disease. FML, fluorometholone; HSV, herpes simplex virus; SCG, sodium cromoglycate.

Herpetic blepharitis may require treatment with local aciclovir ointment, and corneal involvement may require systemic aciclovir therapy combined with appropriate topical steroid (see the herpes infection sections later in this chapter).

Third line

Systemic immunosuppression is needed for severe exacerbations of disease; a 3–4-week course of systemic corticosteroids starting with prednisolone at a dose of 60 mg/day may be necessary to bring the disease under control while topical therapy is being introduced. Systemic steroids also carry a risk of glaucoma, but topical application of corticosteroid around the eyelids probably constitutes a higher risk.

Patients with a previous history of ocular herpes simplex virus or with serological evidence of previous exposure to herpes simplex virus, should be aware that they may develop herpes keratitis while on systemic or topical steroids. Patients who have had previous episodes of ocular herpes simplex should receive prophylaxis with oral aciclovir 400 mg BD (or valaciclovir 500 mg OD); topical prophylaxis is unnecessary and may complicate the clinical signs in patients with complex keratoconjunctivitis. Patients with AKC are predisposed to bilateral herpes keratitis and prophylactic antivirals are advisable when they are using corticosteroids.

Patients with severe or resistant AKC may benefit from oral immunosuppressive agents such as ciclosporin, azathioprine, mycophenolate mofetil and methotrexate. These are also likely to be beneficial for any associated eczema.

Future therapeutic agents

New biologics to modify T- and B-cell responses are all being trialled. Anecdotal reports suggest that omalizumab can be helpful in atopic eye disease.

PART 10: SPECIFIC SITES, SEX & AGE

Cicatrising conjunctivitis associated with immunobullous disorders

Definition and nomenclature

Cicatrising conjunctivitis is conjunctival inflammation with progressive scarring. The immunobullous disorder mucous membrane pemphigoid (MMP) is the commonest cause of progressive conjunctival cicatrisation [1] (Chapter 50).

Synonyms and inclusions
- Cicatricial pemphigoid (CP)
- Ocular cicatricial pemphigoid, benign mucous membrane pemphigoid
- Oral pemphigoid
- Desquamative gingivitis, and incorrectly ocular pemphigus

Introduction and general description

Mucous membrane pemphigoid was previously referred to as a number of synonyms, as well as ocular pemphigus, which is incorrect. MMP was deemed the most appropriate nomenclature in a 2002 consensus document [2]. The other synonyms should no longer be used for MMP.

Although uncommon, cicatrising conjunctivitis is one of the most difficult management problems in ophthalmology because of the widespread effects on the ocular surface, leading to corneal blindness in many patients. The classification of cicatrising conjunctivitis follows the dermatological classification of immunobullous and other autoimmune mucocutaneous disorders, although not all of the dermatological disorders are associated with conjunctivitis. The severity of the conjunctival involvement varies but is mild, without scarring, in pemphigus vulgaris, with variable degrees of scarring and severity in the remainder.

Early diagnosis and treatment of progressive conjunctival cicatrisation is important to try to prevent irreversible sequelae. Table 107.8 lists the different causes of progressive versus relatively static conjunctival cicatrisation. Henceforth, this section will focus on the commonest causes of autoimmune cicatrising conjunctivitis, first MMP, then erythema multiforme and graft-versus-host disease (GVHD).

Mucous membrane pemphigoid [2,3,4,5–7]

Introduction and general description

Mucous membrane pemphigoid is an immunologically heterogeneous group of systemic autoimmune disorders that share a cicatrising clinical phenotype, affecting mucous membranes and skin. Disease may be localised to one site or may affect multiple sites (Chapter 50). The proportion of patients with ocular involvement alone varies from 18% to 50%; these differences are likely to reflect differences in the referral base for each series. About 60% of patients presenting to a dermatology clinic will have conjunctival involvement, in addition to skin disease.

Table 107.8 Differential diagnosis of cicatrising conjunctivitis

Static or very slowly progressive conjunctival scarring	Progressive conjunctival scarring
1 Trauma – physical, chemical, thermal, radiation injury, artefacta	**1** Neoplasia – squamous cell carcinoma, sebaceous carcinoma, lymphoma
2 Infection: Trachoma Membranous streptococcal conjunctivitis Adenoviral conjunctivitis *Corynebacterium diphtheriae* Chronic mucocutaneous candidiasis	**2** Immunobullous disorders: Mucous membrane pemphigoid Paraneoplastic MMP (antilaminin-332 MMP) Drug-induced ocular MMP Linear IgA disease Epidermolysis bullosa acquisita Paraneoplastic pemphigus Dermatitis herpetiformis
3 Allergic eye disease: Atopic keratoconjunctivitis Vernal keratoconjunctivitis	**3** Other mucocutaneous disorders: Lichen planus SJS/TEN[a]
4 Drug-induced conjunctival cicatrisation (DICC)[a,b]	
5 Mucocutaneous disorders: SJS/TEN[a] Graft-versus-host disease Discoid and systemic lupus erythematosus[c]	
6 Immunobullous disorders: Linear IgA disease[a] Epidermolysis bullosa acquisita[a] Bullous pemphigoid Pemphigus vulgaris Dermatitis herpetiformis	
7 Systemic disease: Rosacea Sjögren syndrome Sarcoidosis[c] Scleroderma Granulomatosis with polyangiitis Inflammatory bowel disease Ectodermal dysplasia[a] Immune complex diseases Porphyria cutanea tarda Erythroderma ichthyosiform congenita	

Adapted from De Rojas *et al*. 2007 [**22**].

[a] A subset of patients with these diseases may develop autoantibody-positive *progressive* conjunctival scarring similar to ocular MMP.

[b] Associated with granulomatous conjunctival inflammation.

[c] Rare cases can develop *progressive* scarring.

IgA, immunogobulin A; MMP, mucous membrane pemphigoid; SJS, Stevens–Johnson syndrome; TEN, toxic epidermal necrolysis.

Epidemiology

Incidence and prevalence

Unambiguous data on the epidemiology of MMP are difficult to obtain because studies have been based on the site of involvement. A UK ophthalmic surveillance study found the incidence of ocular MMP to be 0.8 per million UK population, and the overall incidence of cicatrising conjunctivitis (including MMP, Stevens–Johnson syndrome (SJS) and other causes) to be 1.3 per million

UK population [1]. A French study of MMP patients presenting to dermatologists reported an incidence of 1.13 per million/year [8]. In ophthalmology centres, MMP affects between 1 : 8000 and 1 : 46 000 patients.

Age

The age range is 30–90 years with peak onset in the seventh decade, although patients may rarely present in childhood.

Sex

The male : female ratio is most commonly 1 : 3.

Ethnicity

No racial or geographic predilection to MMP is reported.

Associated diseases

Mucous membrane pemphigoid is associated with other autoimmune disorders including Sjögren syndrome, rheumatoid arthritis, systemic lupus erythematosus and polyarteritis nodosa. The antilaminin-332 (or antiepiligrin) subtype of MMP is associated with solid organ malignancies.

Pathophysiology

Predisposing factors

In the eye, drug-induced MMP (also known as pseudopemphigoid in the ophthalmic literature), SJS, toxic epidermal necrolysis (TEN) and ectodermal dysplasia [9–11] can also lead to the development of autoantibodies against basement membrane, and a clinical and immunopathological phenotype typical of ocular MMP. This suggests that chronic conjunctival damage can precipitate MMP in susceptible individuals, perhaps via epitope speading (the development of immune responses to endogenous epitopes secondary to the release of self-antigens during a chronic autoimmune or inflammatory response). Thus ocular MMP may be a final common pathway following various conjunctival insults.

Pathology

Current evidence suggests that MMP develops as a consequence of the loss of immunological tolerance to structural proteins in the basement membrane. This results in the production of circulating autoantibodies that bind the basement membrane and weaken adhesion of the overlying epidermis or mucosal epithelium, via inflammatory mechanisms in the case of autoantibodies to bullous pemphigoid antigen 2 (BPAG2) [12] or via non-inflammatory mechanisms in the case of autoantibodies to laminin-332 [13,14]. While the pathogenic activity of experimental or patient IgG versus the NC16A domain of BPAG2, and that of IgG versus laminin-332, have both been shown in passive transfer studies, the pathogenic activity of IgG versus integrin subunits α6 or β4 has not yet been shown. However, the latter IgGs against integrin subunits have been shown to induce basement membrane separation in skin organ culture models.

MMP is a heterogeneous group of disorders, with different subtypes identified according to the autoantigens recognised by circulating autoantibodies. Autoantigens identified include: the NC16 and C-terminal regions of BP180 in oral and other forms of MMP (ocular, nasal, hypopharyngeal); the integrin subunit β4 in some ocular MMP patients; the integrin subunit α6 in some oral MMP patients; laminin-332 in antiepiligrin MMP; and the NC1 domain of collagen VII [15].

In the eye, irreversible blinding consequences occur as a result of two main pathological processes: excessive inflammation (leading to limbal stem cell failure and/or corneal vascularisation) and fibrosis (trichiasis and entropion leading to corneal ulceration and microbial keratitis, and severe dry eye).

Inflammation. Immunohistology and cellular phenotyping studies have described the inflammatory cellular response in human ocular MMP, giving detailed phenotypic information but limited functional information [16]. In acute disease, subepithelial bulla formation is accompanied by inflammatory infiltration of the substantia propria by neutrophils, macrophages, dendritic antigen-presenting cells and some plasma cells, together with an increase in CD4 (helper) T cells, which probably reflects their role in recruiting other inflammatory cells. The cytokine profile observed in the acute phase of MMP indicates a mixed helper T-cell type 1 (Th1) IL-2, interferon γ (IFN-γ) and type 2 (Th2) IL-4, IL-5 and IL-13 response [17,18].

In chronic disease, macrophages and T cells are present, of which the Th1 subset is active, as demonstrated by the presence of the cytokines IL-2 and IFN-γ, as opposed to the Th2 subset that is involved in B-cell activation. This, coupled with the low numbers of B cells but increased number of plasma cells, suggests that B-cell activation must be occurring in the extraocular tissues with homing of mature plasma cells to the conjunctiva. Major histocompatibility complex (MHC) class II expression is increased, suggesting the potential for local antigen presentation to T-helper cells. There is a slight increase in activated T cells, which are involved in the recruitment of fibroblasts and macrophages.

Fibrosis. Growth factors including fibroblast growth factor (FGF), platelet-derived growth factor (PDGF) and transforming growth factor β (TGF-β) are all present in MMP. PGDF upregulates the extracellular matrix component (ECM) thrombospondin, which is itself important in activating latent TGF-β. PDGF is a powerful chemoattractant for macrophages and fibroblasts and is probably pivotal to the scarring response. However, only TGF-β is capable of stimulating fibroblasts to produce collagen and ECM components. It also blocks matrix degradation by decreasing protease synthesis and increasing protease inhibition. In acute disease, TGF-β is significantly increased and is produced by macrophages and fibroblasts in conjunctiva affected by ocular MMP. Once macrophages and fibroblasts are present in large numbers and activated they may become self-regulating; fibroblasts from ocular MMP conjunctiva display a profibrotic phenotype in cell culture [19].

Implications of immunopathological findings for therapy. Inflammation is important in acute disease; severe inflammation is associated clinically with rapid scarring and therefore demands urgent and effective immunosuppression. Inflammation may also play a role in chronic disease although scarring may continue even in the presence of minimal inflammation, suggesting that growth factor production by macrophages and fibroblasts may be relatively independent of the other inflammatory cells. Therefore, modulation of growth factor activity, collagen metabolism or fibroblast activity may be necessary to halt the disease process.

Genetics

A genetic predisposition to MMP has been found in an association with the HLA-DQB1*0301 haplotype [20].

Clinical features of ocular MMP [4]
History

In most patients the onset is insidious, with non-specific conjunctival symptoms including irritation, hyperaemia and discharge due to what is often thought to be recurrent conjunctivitis. In other patients the first symptoms are due to trichiasis, or less commonly ptosis as a result of cicatricial entropion affecting the upper lid. Dry eye and mucous deficiency are late signs. Acute disease occurs in about 20% of new patients with severe inflammation and conjunctival ulceration; this presentation may follow failed lid surgery for entropion on undiagnosed cases.

Presentation

Signs, in order of progression, often start at the medial canthus with loss of the plica and later of the caruncle (Figure 107.16f), subepithelial reticular fibrosis of the tarsal conjunctiva (Figure 107.16a), conjunctival infiltrate due to increased cellularity and collagen formation (Figure 107.16c, d), hyperaemia, shortening of the fornices (Figure 107.16a), symblepharon (Figure 107.16b), blepharitis, trichiasis and cicatricial entropion (Figure 107.16g), punctate keratopathy, limbitis (Figure 107.16d), conjunctival keratinisation (Figure 107.16e), corneal keratinisation and corneal surface failure (Figure 107.16e).

Clinical variants

Clinical variants of ocular MMP include:
1 Idiopathic autoimmune ocular MMP (most common).
2 Ocular MMP associated with other immunobullous disorders such as linear IgA disease, epidermolysis bullosa acquisita and antilaminin-332 MMP (Table 107.8) [21].
3 Ocular MMP arising as a result of drug-induced conjunctival damage (also known as drug-induced conjunctival cicatrisation (DICC) or drug-induced pseudopemphigoid).
4 Ocular MMP arising in association with SJS and other autoimmune conjunctival disorders.

Differential diagnosis

The conjunctival signs in MMP may be identical to those produced by the other immunobullous disorders that are summarised in Table 107.8. However, in the latter conditions, the skin disease precedes the ocular disease, so that there is rarely any confusion. In SJS/TEN, exacerbations of conjunctival inflammation can occur many years after the acute disease, leading to a condition indistinguishable from MMP both in terms of the clinical signs and immunopathology [22].

The principal problems in differential diagnosis relate to diseases other than the immunobullous disorders that may also cause cicatrising conjunctivitis (Table 107.8). Patients with conjunctival cicatrisation secondary to infective causes are sometimes referred for investigation of what has been longstanding conjunctival scarring, following a long-forgotten episode of infection, where the absence of a recent history of inflammation or of progressive symptoms usually indicates static disease. Patients with sarcoidosis or systemic sclerosis normally have a well-established diagnosis by the time conjunctival scarring develops. Sjögren syndrome may mimic early MMP, but can usually be differentiated by the presence of Sjögren-specific antibodies and/or a positive labial biopsy. AKC can occasionally be difficult to differentiate from slowly progressive MMP, but the history and clinical signs of severe eczema, and a tarsal conjunctival biopsy (performed after withdrawal of topical corticosteroids for 2 weeks) that shows excessive numbers of mast cells and eosinophils, can confirm the diagnosis. Iatrogenic conjunctivitis is non-progressive, except in the case of drug-induced MMP, which is indistinguishable from classic MMP. Awareness that conjunctival scarring can occur in ocular rosacea (see Figure 107.8a) and in staphylococcal blepharoconjunctivitis is usually enough to distinguish these conditions from MMP. Factitious conjunctival trauma is rare and usually more focal than classic MMP but can mimic MMP while the self-trauma is active.

Classification of severity

A validated scoring system, the Cicatrising Conjunctivitis Assessment Tool, incorporates three functional categories of inflammation, scarring and morbidity, and is recommended for severity assessment in ocular MMP [23].

Complications and co-morbidities

Late ocular MMP results in fusion of the lids and globe known as ankyloblepharon (Figure 107.16f), which may obscure the cornea completely. In these advanced cases the surface of the eye is extremely dry, keratinised, cicatrised and blind (Figure 107.16h). Persistent corneal epithelial defect, microbial keratitis and corneal perforation are common in ocular MMP, either occurring as a result of trichiasis abrading the cornea and/or severe cicatricial dry eye and/or exposure from scarred distorted eyelids. Corneal surface failure and these associated complications account for the management challenges posed by the disease.

Disease course and prognosis

Most patients with ocular MMP have progressive disease. Current aggressive treatment regimens with systemic immunosuppression have been shown to reduce the rate of progression. Because patients can occasionally progress to blindness within months from the onset, both early diagnosis and effective treatment are critical in improving the prognosis. At presentation, between 25% and 38% of patients with ocular disease have significant visual loss and about 30% become legally blind.

Investigations
Diagnostic problems in predominantly ocular MMP [1,2, 24–29]

The diagnosis of predominantly ocular MMP has been complicated by the definition of MMP used by the first International Consensus Statement on MMP [2] in which the disease was defined as 'a group of putative autoimmune, chronic inflammatory, subepithelial

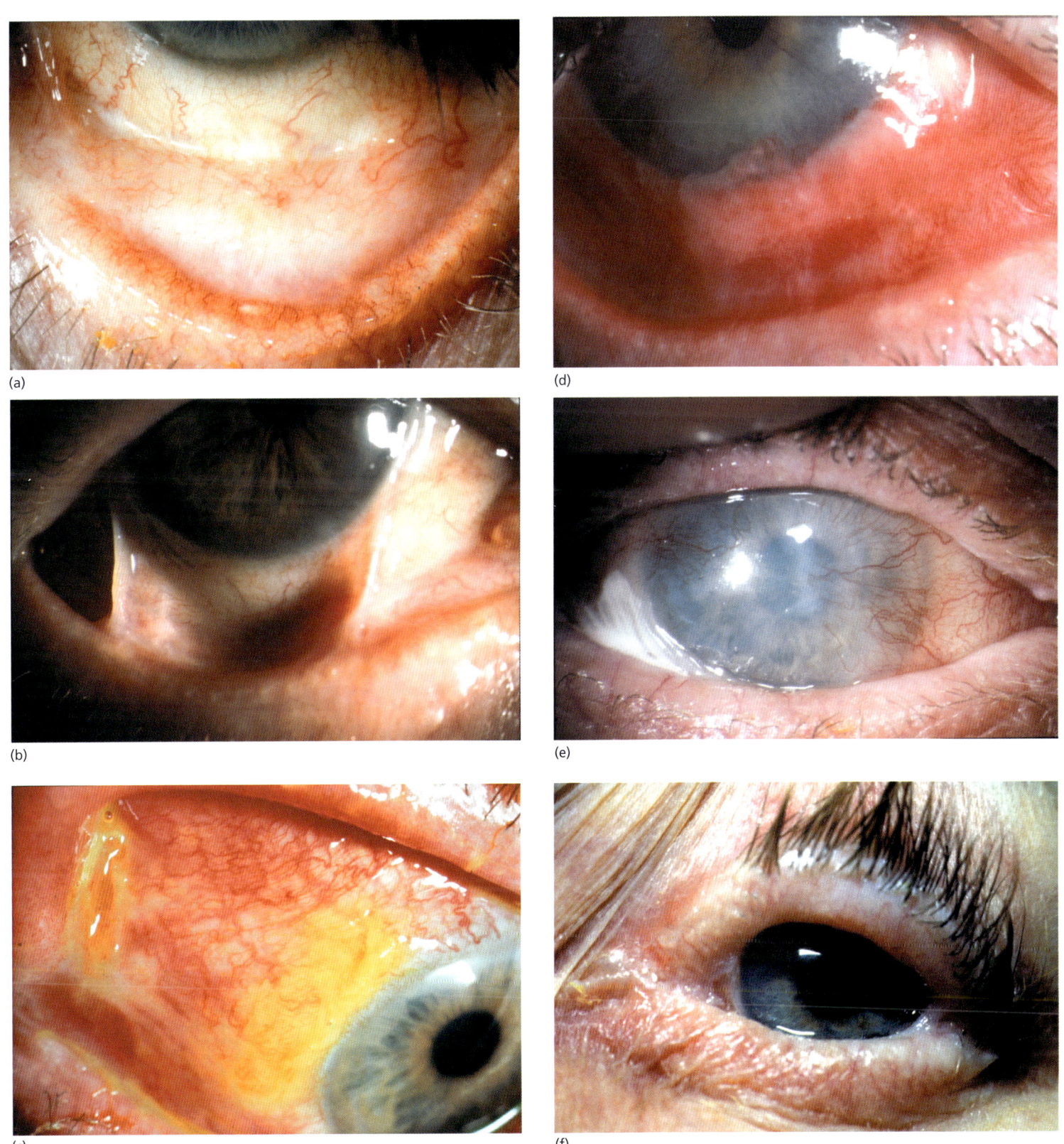

(a)

(b)

(c)

(d)

(e)

(f)

Figure 107.16 Ocular signs of mucous membrane pemphigoid (MMP). (a) Inferior fornix shortening and subconjunctival scarring. (b) Conjunctival symblepharon tethering the globe to the lower lid. (c) Acute exacerbation of conjunctival MMP showing conjunctival ulceration. This occurs in only 10% of patients presenting with MMP affecting the eye. (d) Severe conjunctival inflammation and limbitis. This leads rapidly to the ocular surface failure and corneal blindness shown in (e) unless it is promptly controlled with adequate immunosuppressive therapy. (e) Ocular surface failure and keratinisation (the white area) in advanced pemphigoid; this eye is blind. (f) Advanced ocular pemphigoid showing loss of the medial canthal structures (plica and caruncle) with a reduced interpalpebral aperture secondary to shortening of the fornices (as in (a)) and fusion of the tarsal and bulbar conjunctivae. (g) Upper and lower lid trichiasis due to cicatricial entropion. (h) Terminally dry keratinised blind eye with trichiasis and entropion. (f) Courtesy of Mr J. Dart, Moorfields Eye Hospital, London, UK.

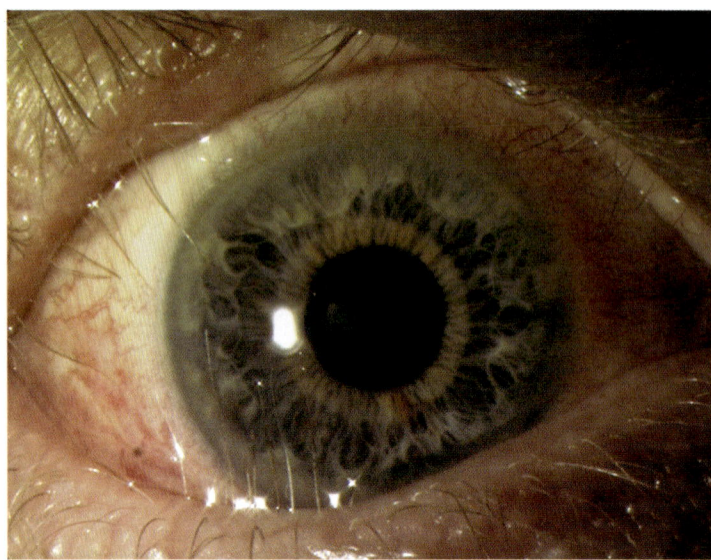

(g)

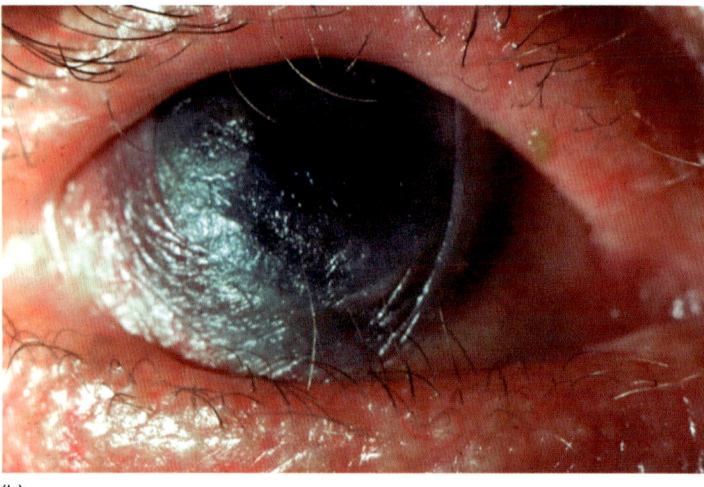

(h)

Figure 107.16 (*Continued*)

blistering diseases predominantly affecting mucous membranes that is characterized by linear deposition of IgG, IgA or C3 along the epithelial basement membrane zone'. While it has done much to harmonise the various definitions of MMP in terms of the clinical and diagnostic characteristics, and also to encourage both careful clinical phenotyping and the application of diagnostic immunopathology tests, the necessity of positive direct immunofluorescence (DIF) raises important issues for ocular MMP. It is well recognised that DIF is invariably positive from at least one site when MMP affects the oro-pharynx and skin as well as the eyes; compliance with a definition that requires positive DIF is therefore usually straightforward in such cases with multiple sites affected. However, from the perspective of clinicians caring for patients with MMP affecting the eyes alone, the 2002 Consensus Statement has resulted in a substantial proportion of patients (27.4–47.3% having negative DIF) failing to meet these immunopathological criteria for diagnosis. As a result, despite having a typical MMP phenotype and

response to treatment, they fall outside the Consensus Statement diagnostic criteria. Subsequent to the publication of the Consensus Statement, peer reviewers of studies on ocular MMP have suggested that this group of patients are omitted from studies on MMP. Extending this to clinical settings, the resulting uncertainty about the diagnosis has meant that immunosuppressive therapy has been delayed or deferred in some patients. Recently, S3 consensus-based European guidelines on the diagnosis and management of MMP have been established and these highlight the challenges in the diagnosis of ocular MMP [24].

Sensitivity and specificity of direct immunofluorescence for MMP

Direct immunofluorescence is not a specific test for MMP and a positive result does not exclude other immunobullous disorders, as is made clear in both consensus statements. In effect, a positive DIF test is used as a surrogate to provide evidence for an autoimmune pathogenesis. For DIF to be integral to a diagnosis of ocular MMP, the test should ideally be both highly sensitive and specific. Not only is DIF of low sensitivity in ocular MMP, it is also of low specificity. Conjunctival biopsies may have a positive DIF result typical of that found in MMP (linear IgG and/or IgA deposition along the basement membrane zone) in a range of disorders, including bullous pemphigoid, skin-dominated linear IgA bullous dermatosis, skin-dominated epidermolysis bullosa acquisita, drug-induced pemphigoid, SJS, rosacea and ulcerative colitis [2,27,28]. Most of these are immunobullous disorders with an autoimmune basis, but not all. Furthermore, some must be differentiated from each other by the clinical phenotype or may require more sophisticated tests to reliably distinguish them from each other, such as indirect immunofluorescence (IIF) studies on salt-split skin, immunoblotting and immunoelectron microscopy. In addition, DIF may not be consistently positive and may change with time [26,29]. With regard to the low sensitivity of DIF, studies have shown that there is a well-recognised DIF-negative subgroup comprising up to 27.4–47.3% of patients with ocular MMP, these subjects having scarring conjunctival inflammation that is phenotypically indistinguishable from MMP, and which responds identically to immunosuppressive therapy.

Indirect immunofluorescence in MMP

Indirect immunofluorescence positivity, detecting circulating autoantibodies in patient sera, occurs in 36–84% of MMP patients (using salt-split skin) [24]. Positive IIF provides evidence for an underlying autoimmune pathology, and may be positive in ocular MMP when DIF is negative.

European Consensus criteria for the diagnosis of predominantly ocular MMP

These are as follows [24].

Predominantly ocular MMP. This is a term used for those cases without any evidence of MMP affecting other systems. The term 'predominantly' is used to recognize the fact that, even with the most careful phenotyping, it is not possible to exclude asymptomatic involvement of, for example, the oesophagus.

Criteria for the diagnosis of ocular MMP.

1 Positive DIF on the conjunctiva and/or tissue from other sites. Patients with DIF showing IgG, IgA and/or C3, either in the conjunctiva or from another site, meet the currently widely adopted 2002 Consensus criteria. Biopsy of normal skin or oral mucosa may be positive when a conjunctival biopsy is DIF negative in ocular MMP.

- Where possible, bulbar conjunctival biopsies should be taken from uninflamed conjunctiva because of the reduced sensitivity in inflamed conjunctiva. When they are taken from inflamed conjunctiva, this should be recorded.
- Biopsies should be taken from another non-lesional site if the conjunctiva is inflamed, and because multiple biopsies improve the detection of a positive DIF. Non-lesional skin gives results similar to those of uninflamed conjunctiva, and buccal mucosal DIF may also be positive when the conjunctival DIF is negative. More data are needed regarding the numbers of biopsies that are optimal to provide good DIF sensitivity.
- Conjunctival DIF should also include staining for fibrinogen to identify lichen planus, which shows shaggy discontinuous fibrinogen deposits at the basement membrane zone.

2 Routine conjunctival histopathology is needed to exclude sarcoid and ocular surface tumours, both of which may present with inflammation and scarring. Ocular surface tumours are usually, but not always, unilateral.

3 Serology tests: patients with positive IIF, or the presence of antibodies to epithelial basement membrane zone proteins, can be diagnosed as having ocular MMP providing the clinical features are consistent. These tests are generally less often positive than DIF, and it is important to be aware that a variable proportion of age- and sex-matched healthy controls have positive serology findings.

4 When both DIF and serology are negative, and the other diseases that may cause cicatricial conjunctivitis have been excluded, this immunopathology negative subset of patients can be diagnosed as having ocular MMP. However, if the disease course or response to therapy is not as expected, all tests should be repeated.

Management

General principles of management [7,30–32]

The same strategies can be used to treat the ocular aspects of cicatrising conjunctivitis due to any cause, whether ocular MMP or SJS. The aim of treatment is the successful management of each of five principal components of these diseases.

1 Treating any ocular surface disease present (e.g. blepharitis, trichiasis, dry eye).
2 Excluding and treating any secondary infection.
3 Identifying any treatment toxicity.
4 Managing any underlying autoimmunity-driven inflammation.
5 Preventing and treating fibrosis.

These components of disease are present to variable degrees in different diseases. For example, in SJS, most patients have relatively little inflammation once the surface disease has been treated and any treatment toxicity eliminated, so it is the minority of these patients, with recurrent inflammation or progressive cicatrisation [22], who

require suppression of inflammation with systemic therapy. Conversely, most, but not all, MMP patients require management of all five components of disease, with 80% of patients requiring systemic immunosuppressive therapy to control the inflammation that persists once the surface disease, any infection or toxicity have been controlled. At present, there are few therapies widely used that specifically target fibrosis. The only demonstrated means of slowing the progression of scarring is good control of inflammation, usually with systemic therapy. However, even with conventional immunosuppressive regimens in ocular MMP, fibrosis of the eye can still progress in 11–53% of patients [7].

The following management strategy is depicted as an algorithm in Figure 107.17.

Manage any ocular surface disease. Ocular surface disease is secondary to previous or current lid and conjunctival scarring and inflammation. This surface disease causes much of the damage to the cornea and is responsible for additional inflammation. Trichiasis and entropion, blepharitis, dry eye and filamentary keratitis, keratinisation, persistent epithelial defect, microbial keratitis and corneal perforation may all result from a combination of a poor tear film, poor lid closure and corneal damage secondary to trichiasis. These are treated as follows.

- Trichiasis: epilate in the short term and use electrolysis or laser for odd lashes, cryotherapy for misdirected lashes and surgery for entropion (inferior retractor plication for lower lid and anterior lamellar reposition for upper lid, labial mucosal graft for conjunctival fornix reconstruction if indicated).
- Blepharitis: use oral tetracyclines and institute a lid hygiene regimen (see 'Blepharitis, meibomian gland dysfunction, rosacea and seborrhoeic dermatitis' earlier in this chapter).
- Dry eye and filaments: use non-preserved lubricants, topical acetylcysteine 5–10% as a mucolytic, punctal occlusion to conserve tears (once any blepharitis has been controlled), courses of topical steroids and topical ciclosporin.
- Keratinisation: topical retinoic acid is effective in 30% but is only available in specialised centres.
- Persistent corneal epithelial defect: exclude infection, treat ingrowing lashes, use non-preserved lubricants and therapeutic lenses (silicone hydrogel if the eyes are not too dry) and, if these measures are unsuccessful, close the eye with a botulinum toxin protective ptosis or with a temporary tarsorrhaphy. Other more specialised treatments may be needed.
- Corneal perforation: temporise with therapeutic contact lenses and/or corneal glue, followed by keratoplasty only if absolutely necessary.

Exclude and treat any secondary infection. The compromised environment of the cicatrised conjunctiva harbours more potentially pathogenic bacteria [33] and fungi such as yeasts. The index of suspicion for infection must be high, for example in the presence of any corneal epithelial defect, given that the typical clinical signs of a white cell-mediated corneal infiltrate may be suppressed in an immunosuppressed host, and topical steroids may also contribute to the lack of an infiltrate. Taking a swab or small scrape from the edge of the corneal epithelial defect and sending it for

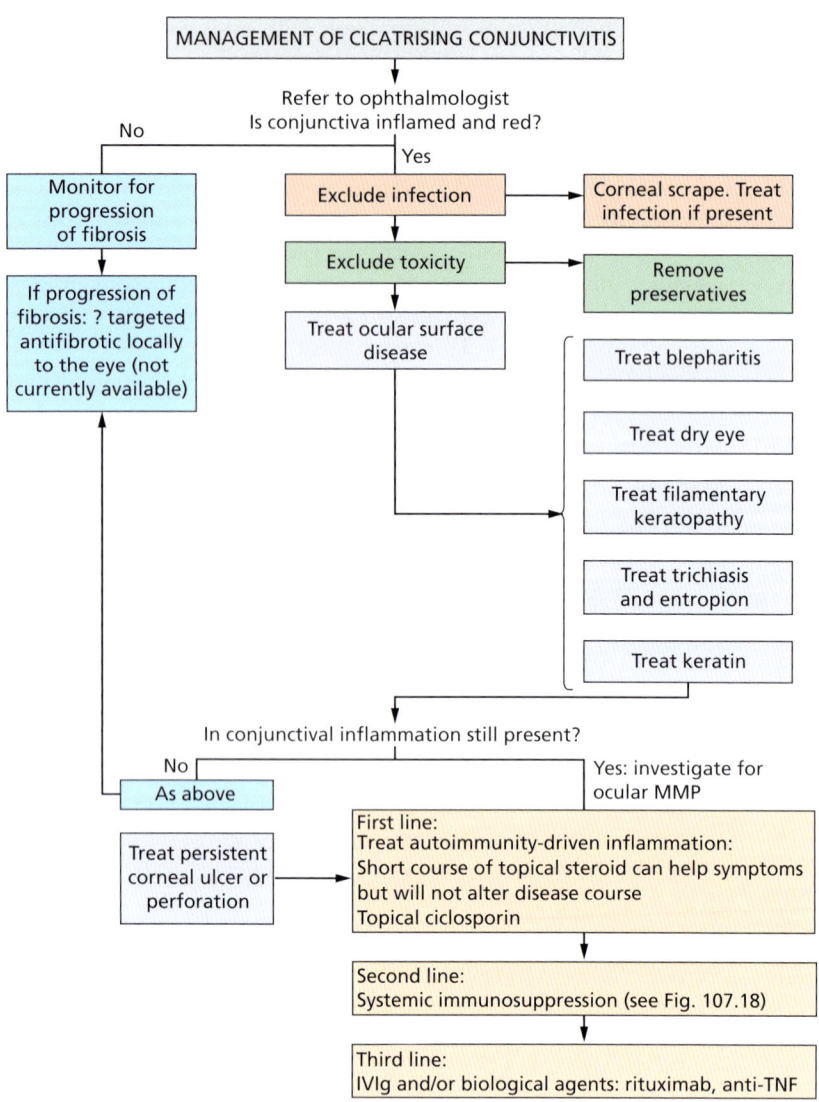

Figure 107.17 Management algorithm for the management of cicatrising conjunctivitis. IVIg, intravenous immunoglobulin; MMP, mucous membrane pemphigoid; TNF, tumour necrosis factor.

microbiology will help confirm that an infection is present and whether it is likely to respond to the empirical treatment instituted.

Eliminate or minimise treatment toxicity.
Treatment toxicity results principally from the preservative benzalkonium chloride, a component of most reusable bottles of eye drop preparations as well as of topical glaucoma medications and aminoglycoside eye drops. Unnecessary topical treatment should therefore be avoided and unpreserved drops or saline used as far as possible. The effects of topical treatment toxicity are hard to distinguish from those of the ocular surface disease. After withdrawal of toxic topical therapy, the mean recovery period is 2 weeks but may extend to 3 months.

Suppress inflammation/commence immunosuppressive therapy.
Any inflammation on the upper bulbar conjunctiva that persists once any ocular surface disease has been treated and any infection and treatment toxicity excluded is likely to be due to underlying autoimmune activity. The upper bulbar conjunctiva is a good location to assess underlying autoimmune disease activity

because it is less susceptible to the effects of blepharitis and dry eye, given the protection of the upper eyelid. In some cases, conjunctival autoimmune activity can, however, manifest as a patchy distribution of inflammation, and this may not necessarily involve the upper bulbar conjunctiva. In these cases, persistence of inflammation despite maximal treatment of ocular surface disease is an indication that systemic immunosuppression is needed (Figure 107.18).

It is worth pointing out that MMP disease activity at sites other than the eye may dictate how aggressively the condition should be treated. Guidelines recommend that all of ocular, naso-pharyngeal, laryngeal, oesophageal and genital involvement should be regarded as high risk for complications, but oral disease alone can be highly symptomatic and refractory cases may require treatment escalation [34].

First line
In *mild ocular disease* (hyperaemia and oedema), a low-dose topical corticosteroid for short durations may be helpful, particularly in

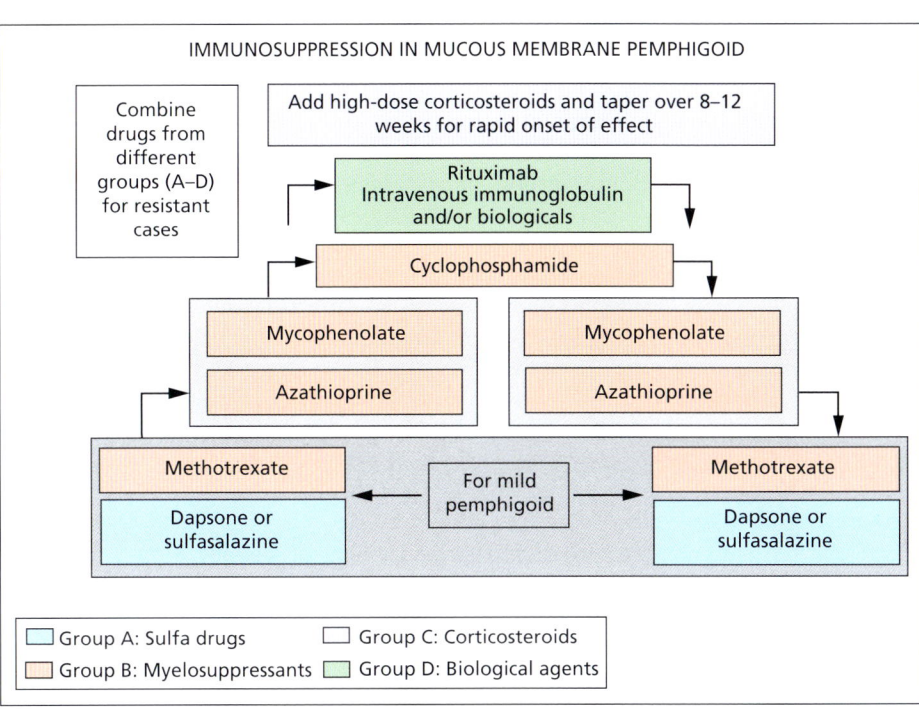

Figure 107.18 Systemic immunosuppression stepladder for ocular mucous membrane pemphigoid (MMP). Immunosuppression can be carried out using a 'stepladder' approach for the introduction of systemic drugs [7,39]. Mild disease may respond well to dapsone, sulfapyridine or sulfasalazine, or to methotrexate. If there is no response after 2–3 months, treatment is 'stepped up' to azathioprine or mycophenolate mofetil. If these drugs are not effective in another 2–3 months then rituximab (anti-CD20) or cyclophosphamide are the treatments of choice. Steroids, the sulfones (dapsone and sulfapyridine) and the bone marrow suppressive immunosuppressants (methotrexate, azathioprine and mycophenolate) can be combined although the neutrophil count, in particular, must be monitored. Rituximab can be combined with dapsone if needed. Rituximab may also be combined with bone marrow suppressants but there is an increased risk of life-threatening infection. Systemic ciclosporin has been little used in cicatrising conjunctivitis because of lack of evidence of efficacy and concern about potential fibrogenic side effects as well as likely renal toxicity in elderly patients.

the alleviation of the symptoms of very dry eye. However, prolonged topical corticosteroid use increases the risk of ocular surface infection in cicatrised eyes, which harbour more pathogenic flora (bacteria, fungi) compared with non-cicatrised eyes [4]. Topical ciclosporin preparations can be used as a steroid-sparing agent. This can similarly help with dry eye symptoms [31] but targets surface inflammation rather than the underlying autoimmune process [35].

Second line

For *moderate ocular disease* (hyperaemia, intense infiltration), immunosuppressants used initially include a sulfa agent such as dapsone or sulfasalazine [7], or the antimetabolite methotrexate. The dose of dapsone is 75 mg daily, increased each month by 25 mg daily to 125 mg, assuming that haemoglobin levels remain satisfactory; there is a 70% response in 1–2 months, reducing to 50% after 1 year. Methotrexate (5–25 mg once weekly) is sometimes used as a first line immunosuppressant in ocular MMP (effective in about 80% depending on the severity of the disease) [32]. Mycophenolate mofetil (1–2 g daily) has also been used as a first line systemic immunosuppressant in ocular MMP, with a greater efficacy (effective in about 80% depending on the severity of the disease) than sulfa agents yet less frequent side effects [36]. Azathioprine may also be considered (1–2 mg/kg/day; effective in about 60%), although it tends to be less well tolerated [7].

Third line

For *severe or refractory ocular disease* (hyperaemia, limbitis, conjunctival ulceration), start oral prednisolone 1 mg/kg/day, reducing the dose after 2 weeks and with the aim of tailing off after 2–4 months. This is ineffective at low doses in the long term and a steroid-sparing immunosuppressive agent is usually added for long-term disease control.

Cyclophosphamide. One of the most effective immunosuppressive agents for MMP is cyclophosphamide 1 mg/kg/day, but it is associated with significant toxicity (bladder toxicity, risk of pancytopenia). The dose of cyclophosphamide is adjusted to maintain a lymphocyte count between 0.5 and 1.0×10^9/L; other haematological parameters should remain normal. To minimise bladder toxicity, cyclophosphamide therapy is usually discontinued after 1 year and substituted by sulfonamides or alternative immunosuppressive agents.

Rituximab. Rituximab is an anti-CD20 chimeric monoclonal antibody [37,38]. It reduces circulating B cells and prevents their maturation into antibody-secreting plasma cells. There is significant level 3 evidence derived from systematic reviews and phase II studies, and as yet unpublished UK cost data, indicating that rituximab is more effective and safer than cyclophosphamide, and more cost effective and more convenient (and more rapidly effective) than intravenous immunoglobulin (IVIg) [38]. For this reason, rituximab is increasingly being considered for refractory ocular pemphigoid prior to using cyclophosphamide or IVIg.

Rituximab appears to induce complete remission rates ranging from ≥66% to 75% and up to 80%, often in response to a single cycle. There is also evidence of adjuvant (steroid and immunosuppressive agent) treatment-sparing effects. Relapse rates were of the order of 40–50%. Times to relapse were typically in the order of 12–18 months. In patients with relapse, rituximab retreatment induced previously observed disease control responses [38].

Rituximab is administered either as four infusions, each 375 mg/m^2, given at weekly intervals over 4 weeks (the 'lymphoma protocol') or two infusions of 1 g, 2 weeks apart (the 'rheumatoid arthritis protocol'). Current evidence supports the rheumatoid arthritis protocol in terms of higher response rates and greater steroid-sparing effect; however, it may also be associated with higher relapse rates [38].

Other agents. Intravenous immunoglobulin [39] and anti-TNF-α agents [40] may also be beneficial. Results of these therapies have been reported in non-randomised series or case reports.

Combination therapy. Most of this therapy is empirical. A sulfonamide (dapsone or sulfasalazine) can be used together with an alkylating agent (cyclophosphamide) or an antimetabolite (azathioprine, methotrexate or mycophenolate mofetil) to control inflammation. A sulfonamide can be combined with rituximab, and if necessary a bone marrow suppressive immunosuppressant can be combined with both of these, but the risk of infection is higher. This immunosuppressive strategy is summarised in Figure 107.18.

Preventing fibrosis

Currently, the only convincingly demonstrated means of slowing the progression of scarring is good control of inflammation with systemic immunosuppression. Therapy specifically targeted at fibrosis in MMP is limited. Mitomycin C has been delivered either subconjunctivally or applied intraoperatively following division of symblephara, but no controlled trials have been carried out. Adverse effects of mitomycin include tissue ischaemia, which may affect the success of mucous membrane graft reconstructive surgery, and potential limbal stem cell damage. Subconjunctival injection of 5-fluorouracil has also been used in view of its antifibrotic action and prior experience of its use in ophthalmology for other indications. Evidence is limited, although a recent report described positive effects on scarring and visual acuity in patients with ocular MMP and SJS/TEN in a retrospective, single-centre study [41].

Other subepithelial disorders and conjunctivitis

Other immunobullous disorders are much less frequently associated with conjunctival cicatrisation. As a result, little is known about the pathogenesis of the conjunctival disease as opposed to the events in the skin. Bullous pemphigoid generally results in mild conjunctivitis although severe cicatrisation has been reported. Epidermolysis bullosa aquisita, linear IgA disease [42], dermatitis herpetiformis and lichen planus may all be associated with progressive conjunctival scarring indistinguishable from that of MMP [2].

Stevens–Johnson syndrome/toxic epidermal necrolysis

The ocular complications of SJS/TEN are shown in Table 107.9 (Chapter 117) [43]. About 70–80% of patients admitted for treatment of these diseases will develop eye disease. This can result in profound, long-term morbidity in many such patients. In addition, the eye disease, unlike the lesions affecting the remaining mucosal surfaces, may progress years after the acute episode has resolved [**22**].

Acute ocular complications of SJS/TEN. These usually occur concurrently with the skin disease (Figure 107.19a) but may sometimes precede it by several days. The conjunctivitis varies from a papillary reaction with watery discharge (Figure 107.19b) to a membranous conjunctivitis with sloughing of the conjunctival epithelium. Corneal epithelial defects are common and may progress to corneal

Table 107.9 Ocular effects of Stevens–Johnson syndrome and toxic epidermal necrolysis (SJS/TEN)

Ocular effects	Resulting symptoms and signs
Loss of goblet cells	Disrupted tear film leading to poor vision and punctate keratopathy (Figure 107.19d)
Loss of accessory lacrimal glands	
Scarring of meibomian gland orifices	
Metaplasia of meibomian gland epithelium with development of metaplastic lashes	Trichiasis secondary to metaplastic lashes
Conjunctival scarring and obliteration of lacrimal gland ductules	Very dry eye with secondary conjunctival and corneal squamous metaplasia (Figure 107.19d)
Corneal and conjunctival keratinisation due to squamous metaplasia	Exacerbates drying and discomfort
Conjunctival scarring with fornix shortening and symblepharon formation leading to lid shortening	May cause lagophthalmos and corneal exposure
Retroplacement of meibomian gland orifices and irregularity of mucocutaneous junction	Disrupts tear film
Entropion of upper and lower lids with trichiasis of both metaplastic and normal lashes	Corneal punctate keratopathy and ulceration
Corneal epithelial failure secondary to limbal inflammation causing loss of palisades of Vogt, conjunctivalisation of the cornea, corneal neovascularisation and corneal opacification	Blindness

Reproduced from Jovanovic *et al.* 2021 [41] with permission of Wolters Kluwer Health, Inc.

ulceration with or without bacterial superinfection. The morbidity of the disease may be due to the acute corneal complications but is more usually due to conjunctival scarring.

Chronic ocular complications of SJS/TEN. These are numerous. The severe conjunctival inflammation leads to a loss of goblet cells and the accessory conjunctival lacrimal glands as well as disruption of the meibomian gland orifices leading to MGD. This results in a disrupted tear film and a secondary punctate keratopathy. In mildly affected patients, this causes chronic mild discomfort, photophobia and slightly reduced vision. In more severely affected patients, the conjunctival inflammation leads to cicatrisation of the lacrimal ductules, resulting in a severely dry eye accompanied by squamous metaplasia and keratinisation (Figure 107.19c) of both the conjunctival and corneal components of the ocular surface, thereby causing more severe discomfort and loss of vision (Figure 107.19d). In addition, the meibomian gland ductal epithelium undergoes metaplasia, resulting in the development of fine metaplastic lashes which are not a feature of MMP. The conjunctival shortening leads to entropion, resulting in ocular surface abrasion by normal as well as by metaplastic lashes, and may also cause lid shortening, leading to reduced eye closure (lagophthalmos), which is easily overlooked. Lash abrasion and trichiasis lead to the development of corneal epithelial defects which, as a result of the poor tear film, may persist. Persistent epithelial defect predisposes to corneal stromal melts and perforation, which are often precipitated by infection.

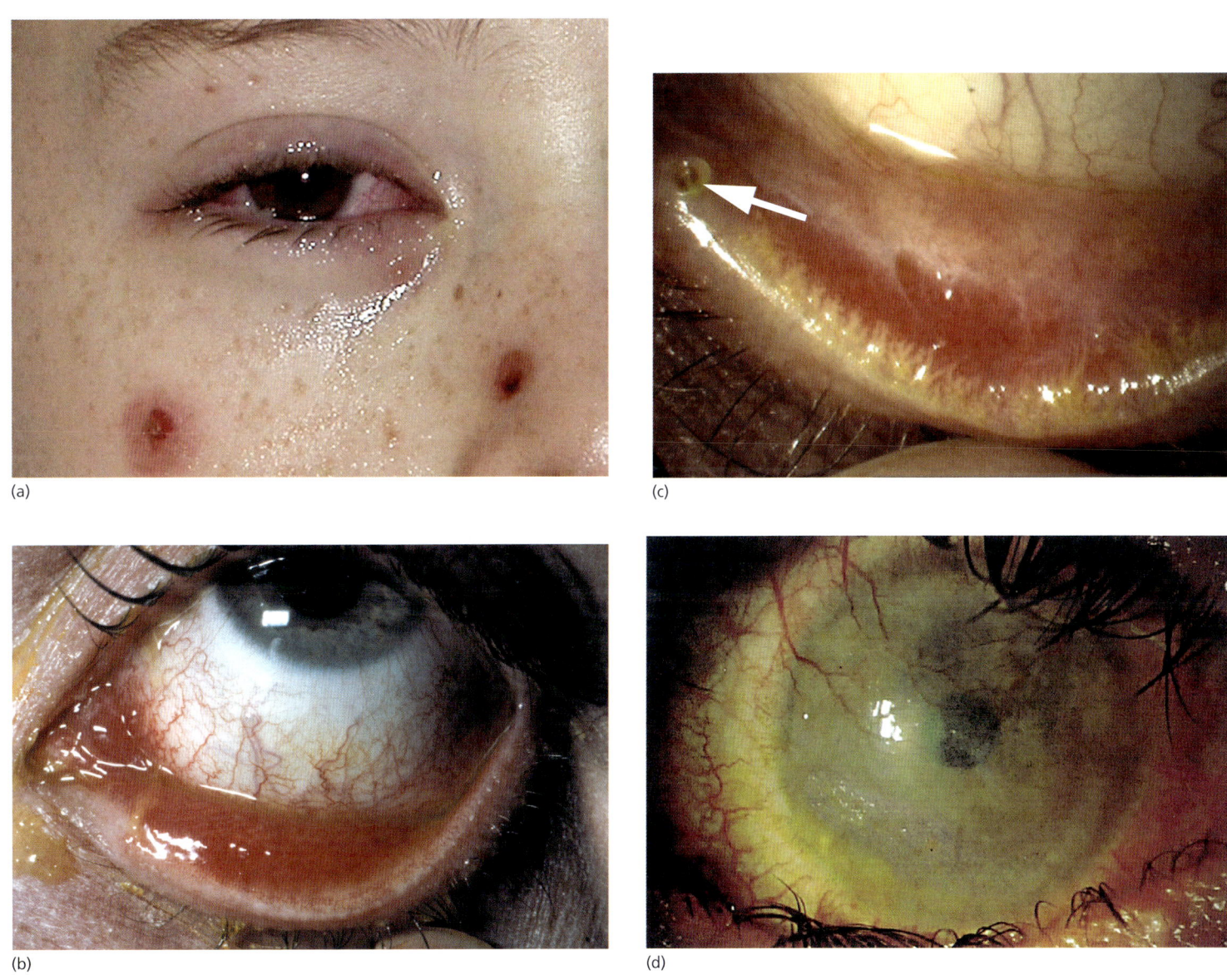

Figure 107.19 Ocular disease in Stevens–Johnson syndrome (SJS). (a) Acute conjunctivitis with mucus discharge occurring concurrently with erythema multiforme-like skin lesions. (b) Acute conjunctivitis in a patient with mild SJS. The conjunctiva is hyperaemic with a papillary reaction and mucopurulent discharge. (c) Lower tarsal conjunctival scarring with squamous metaplasia and keratinisation adjacent to the mucocutaneous junction of the lower lid. A punctal plug (arrow) is *in situ* to conserve tears in a dry eye. (d) The late ocular complications of SJS showing entropion, a dry eye with ocular surface failure (in this case an opaque keratinised epithelium). (b) Courtesy of Mr J. Dart, Moorfields Eye Hospital, London, UK.

PART 10: SPECIFIC SITES, SEX & AGE

This evolution of changes is not the direct consequence of the acute disease but is secondary to the effects on the tear film and lids. A grading system for the chronic ocular manifestations of SJS has been proposed [43].

The severe inflammation may also lead to blinding opacity of the corneal epithelium, not only as a result of squamous metaplasia but also by the loss of corneal epithelial progenitor cells (stem cells). Because of prolonged survival of transient amplifying cells, the progeny of stem cells, stem cell failure may not be manifest for 12–18 months after the onset of the disease.

An additional problem for patients with ocular complications of SJS is the development of severe conjunctival inflammation with or without progressive scarring that may be indistinguishable from MMP and may also be DIF positive. The latter can occur as

a continuation of the acute episode or may develop many years after the onset of disease. Necrotising sclerokeratitis may also follow SJS [22]. All of these severe inflammatory problems can precipitate stem cell failure and demand rapid control, usually requiring systemic immunosuppressive therapy. The cause of these late inflammatory complications is not understood.

Management
Management of acute ocular SJS/TEN includes topical steroids [44] (Chapter 117). Urgent amniotic membrane transplantation in acute disease with extensive ulceration can be helpful [45]. Management of chronic ocular SJS/TEN includes management of severe dry eye, trichiasis and entropion, limbal stem cell deficiency and inflammation. Systemic immunosuppression may be needed

if inflammatory complications of chronic disease (e.g. recurrent inflammation, secondary ocular MMP) do not respond to topical therapies. The immunosuppressive therapy strategy for ocular SJS/TEN is similar to that of cicatrising conjunctivitis in MMP, apart from the avoidance of sulfa agents which may precipitate SJS/TEN. A paradigm shift in ocular surface stabilisation in SJS with mucous membrane grafting for lid margin keratinisation and scleral contact lenses has been reported to maintain better visual acuity and prevent limbal stem cell damage [46].

Graft-versus-host disease

Ocular complications are common (60–90%) in patients with GVHD, and typically result from involvement of both the conjunctiva and the lacrimal gland (Chapter 38). The spectrum of chronic GVHD varies from dry eye to sight-threatening surface inflammation, scarring and, in rare cases, perforation, which may present many months after the bone marrow allograft. Notably, severe ocular disease can occur in the absence of systemic GVHD. Ocular GVHD can lead to loss of vision due to corneal involvement. In acute GVHD, conjunctivitis ranges from hyperaemia through chemosis to a pseudomembranous conjunctivitis, with or without corneal epithelial sloughing. Severe conjunctival involvement is a marker for the severity of acute GVHD, occurring in 12% of patients, and is a poor prognostic factor for mortality [47]. In chronic GVHD, conjunctival involvement has been observed in 11% of patients, for whom it was also associated with disease severity. Some of these patients develop a severe scarring response like that of MMP. Lacrimal gland involvement occurs in about 50% of patients with chronic GVHD who develop a Sjögren syndrome-type picture of dry eyes. The pathogenesis of the conjunctival disease has been examined in a few cases and appears to be similar to that in the skin. Involvement of panophthalmic structures can sometimes be evident in chronic GVHD. Although dry eye and cicatrising conjunctivitis are the commonest (90%) ocular findings in GVHD, choroiditis, retinitis and scleritis may also occur.

Anti-inflammatory treatments, particularly T-cell suppressants, can help manage GVHD. Topical anti-inflammatory therapy with steroids, and steroid-sparing calcineurin inhibitors such as ciclosporin and tacrolimus, should be instituted early in the course of the disease [48]. Autologous serum eye drops have beneficial effects. Antifibrotic agents such as tranilast may also help.

Systemic diseases with skin and eye involvement

Some multisystem diseases affect both the skin and eye [1,2–23]. It is not possible to catalogue every complication of all these diseases but the most frequent are summarised in Table 107.10.

INFECTIONS

A number of infections involve the eyelids, but the following are important to recognise because they are common, or require urgent therapy or referral to an ophthalmologist [1].

VIRAL INFECTIONS

Warts

Clinical features

These are common and found on the eyelid margins, often as a long thin (filiform) projection (Figure 107.20).

Management

Lesions in this site are most simply treated with careful cryotherapy with accurate application of liquid nitrogen to the base of the lesion using a cotton wool bud rather than cryospray. An alternative is surgical removal by snip or shave excision.

Molluscum contagiosum [2]

Clinical features

This condition mainly affects children and young adults (Chapter 25). It is also prevalent in patients with acquired immune deficiency syndrome (AIDS), who may develop multiple lesions around the eyelids. As elsewhere on the skin, typical lesions arise as dome-shaped papules with a central umbilication. Lesions may grow in the lash line as well as on the lid skin and, occasionally, on the mucocutaneous junction. Lesions can be easily overlooked or mistaken for an epidermoid cyst; this condition must always be considered in the differential diagnosis of patients with unilateral or bilateral follicular conjunctivitis. There is associated conjunctival discharge and a variable, often severe, follicular conjunctival response (Figure 107.21). A superficial epithelial keratitis may develop in longstanding cases which progresses to pannus formation across the cornea.

Management

In uncomplicated cases in immunocompetent individuals, treatment may not be required as the lesions will usually resolve spontaneously. Curettage or cryotherapy can be used.

Herpes simplex virus [3,4,5]

Clinical features

Primary herpes simplex virus infection is asymptomatic in many patients; in others it causes blepharoconjunctivitis (Chapter 25). However, most of the ocular manifestations of herpes simplex virus infection are due to reactivation of latent infection in the trigeminal ganglion. Both the primary infection, and reactivation of latent disease, may be particularly severe in patients with atopic eczema or with immunodeficiency. The blepharoconjunctivitis of herpes simplex virus usually results in crops of small vesicles, which may be associated with mild oedema of the lids with or without associated conjunctivitis (Figure 107.22a). As with herpes simplex virus elsewhere, the vesicles dry to a crust and heal within a few days. Neither the blepharitis nor conjunctivitis present a serious

Table 107.10 Systemic diseases with skin and eye involvement

Systemic disease	Eye disease
Sarcoidosis *Epidemiology*: ocular involvement the presenting feature in 10%; 20–30% of patients have eye disease at some stage [**1**,2–7]	*Lids and orbital findings*: clusters of granulomatous eyelid swellings. Proptosis from orbital granulomas. Dry eye from lacrimal gland involvement *Heerfordt syndrome* (uveoparotid fever): consists of uveitis and parotid gland enlargement, fever and facial nerve palsy. *Löfgren syndrome*: acute iritis, bilateral hilar lymphadenopathy, erythema nodosum and arthralgia. *Mikulicz syndrome*: bilateral swelling of lacrimal and salivary glands *Anterior segment findings*: *conjunctivitis*: occasionally a granulomatous conjunctivitis mimicking a follicular conjunctivitis. *Uveitis*: usually, but not always, bilateral granulomatous anterior uveitis in 80% of patients with eye manifestations with redness, pain, photophobia and blurred vision with floaters *Posterior segment findings*: rare
Systemic lupus erythematosus [8–10]	*Anterior segment findings*: dry eye, peripheral corneal ulcers. Scleritis is rare. Episcleritis occurs in 10% causing a red eye *Posterior segment findings*: retinal vasculitis common during exacerbations of systemic disease with flame-shaped haemorrhages and cotton wool spots. May be associated with severe central nervous system vasculitis or lupus nephritis
Sjögren syndrome [11]	*Lids and orbital findings*: lacrimal gland inflammation causing dry eye *Anterior segment findings*: symptoms: often severe with chronic discomfort, foreign body sensation, dryness and blurred vision. *Conjunctiva*: conjunctivitis and scarring in some cases. *Cornea*: punctate keratopathy, persistent corneal epithelial defects leading to corneal ulceration and perforation or corneal infection
Reactive arthritis (formerly Reiter syndrome) *Epidemiology*: ocular involvement in about 30% of patients [1]	*Anterior segment findings*: symptoms: red irritable eyes resolving spontaneously within 7–10 days. *Conjunctiva*: bilateral mucopurulent conjunctivitis is the most frequent manifestation affecting approximately 30% of patients; this usually follows a urethritis by about 2 weeks and precedes the onset of arthritis. *Cornea*: keratitis may occur in isolation and is rare. *Uveitis*: anterior uveitis (iritis) occurs in about 20% of patients either with the first attack of reactive arthritis or during a recurrence
Behçet syndrome *Epidemiology*: ocular involvement in 60–70% of patients [12,13]	*Anterior segment findings*: external eye diseases: conjunctivitis, keratitis and episcleritis may occur but are not specific for the condition. *Uveitis*: the commonest manifestation of the disease *Posterior segment findings*: visual impairment or blindness is a frequent complication of Behçet syndrome as a result of the retinal ischaemia
Inflammatory bowel disease *Epidemiology*: ocular manifestations in about 5% of patients [14,15]	*Anterior segment findings*: external eye diseases: conjunctivitis, limbitis, peripheral corneal infiltrates and episcleritis may occur. *Uveitis*: acute iritis in about 5% of patients which may occur at the same time as exacerbation of colitis
Acquired immune deficiency syndrome (AIDS) *Epidemiology*: ocular complications occur in about 75% of patients [16–20]	*Common features*: (i) opportunistic infections with viruses, mycobacteria and fungi; (ii) malignancies, e.g. Kaposi sarcoma; (iii) retinal microangiopathy; and (iv) neuro-ophthalmic lesions with intracranial infections and tumours *Anterior segment findings*: external eye diseases: *Molluscum contagiosum* is a common ocular finding in patients with AIDS, they tend to be large and when located on the lid margin can give rise to follicular conjunctivitis. The lesions can be complicated by epithelial keratitis with associated pannus formation. *Kaposi sarcoma* may involve the lids and conjunctiva. *Herpes simplex* keratitis tends to be severe with more frequent relapses. The peripheral cornea is more often involved in contrast to central disease in immunocompetent patients. *Herpes zoster ophthalmicus* is common and may be a presenting feature of human immunodeficiency virus (HIV) infection, especially if severe disease presents in young patients *Posterior segment findings*: retinal microangiopathy is common and characterised by retinal haemorrhages, microaneurysms and cotton wool spots. *Cytomegalovirus* retinitis and *Pneumocystis jirovecii* choroiditis are serious ophthalmic complications signifying severe systemic involvement
Porphyria [21,22]	*Common features*: ocular involvement results from either photosensitisation and/or neurological dysfunction. Photosensitisation can affect the eyelids, conjunctiva, cornea, sclera and possibly the retina *Lids and orbital findings*: inflammation can lead to vesicle and bulla formation, secondary infection to scarring with ectropion and hyperpigmentation *Neuro-ophthalmic complications*: these include optic neuritis, optic atrophy, ptosis and cranial nerve palsies
Granulomatosis with polyangiitis [23]	Episcleritis is very common in the active stages. Also retinal vasculitis, optic neuritis, orbital pseudotumour
Polyarteritis nodosa	Episcleritis, scleritis and keratitis
Dermatomyositis	Periorbital 'heliotrope rash'. Ocular signs may include conjunctival oedema, extraocular muscle dysfunction, nystagmus, iritis and retinopathy
Amyloidosis	Ocular amyloidosis can be highly variable: nephrotic syndrome can lead to periorbital oedema; mass or infiltration may affect the lacrimal glands or extraocular muscles, causing for example proptosis, ptosis, ophthalmoplegia or epiphora; amyloid deposits may also involve the conjunctiva, cornea and retina
Histiocytoses	Langerhans cell histiocytosis may present with a lytic lesion in the bones of the orbit; orbital and intraocular masses are reported in Rosai–Dorfman disease; Erdheim–Chester disease causes bilateral proptosis due to orbital masses in association with xanthelasmas; ocular lesions of juvenile xanthogranuloma occur, particularly affecting the iris

PART 10: SPECIFIC SITES, SEX & AGE

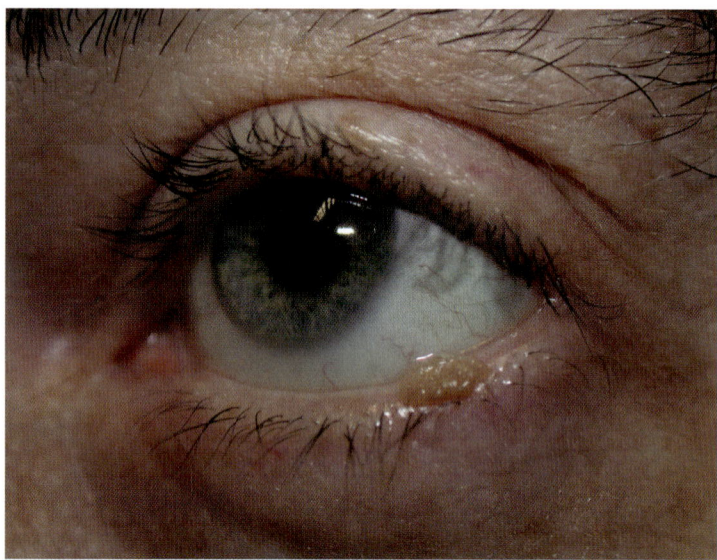

Figure 107.20 Wart on the eyelid.

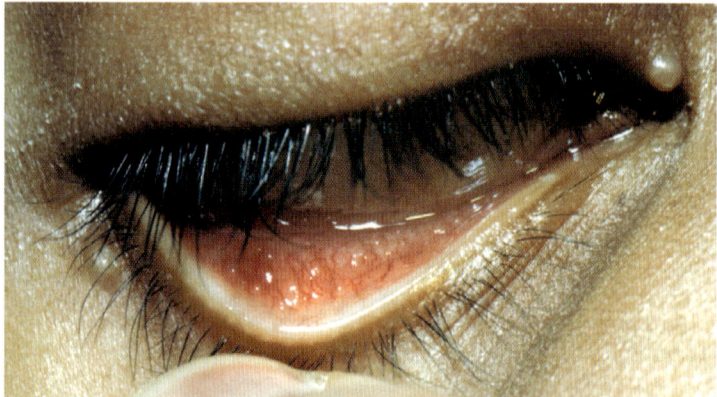

Figure 107.21 Molluscum contagiosum at the medial aspect of the upper lid margin with an associated follicular conjunctivitis. Courtesy of Mr J. Dart, Moorfields Eye Hospital, London, UK.

problem for most patients. The serious and sight-threatening ocular complications of herpes simplex virus infection of the eye are due to recurrent keratitis or keratouveitis. Herpetic keratitis may affect the epithelium alone (dendritic keratitis (Figure 107.22b)), the stroma (stromal herpetic keratitis (Figure 107.22c), geographic corneal ulceration or metaherpetic keratitis (Figure 107.22d)) or the endothelium (disciform keratitis or herpetic endotheliitis (Figure 107.22e)). Dendritic keratitis is in itself a benign disease unless treated with topical corticosteroids when the disease will rapidly spread, resulting in geographic keratitis, which may cause destructive corneal disease. Most cases of corneal disease represent reactivation of latent herpes simplex virus and patients may develop any of the corneal manifestations. Stromal and endothelial disease can progress to blinding corneal vascularisation, scarring (Figure 107.22f) and ulceration. Fortunately, the disease is normally unilateral, except in atopic individuals when it may be bilateral.

Management

Because of the difficulties of managing the ocular manifestations of this disease, patients with suspected herpes simplex virus involvement of the eye should be referred for urgent ophthalmic assessment. The conjunctivitis can be treated with ganciclovir gel or aciclovir ointment five times a day for 5 days or with oral aciclovir 400 mg five times per day for 5 days. Topical steroids alone will mask the symptoms and signs, leading to spread of the ulcer and corneal perforation with disastrous consequences for the patient's vision. Dendritic keratitis may ensue. The management of the stromal and endothelial keratitis is beyond the scope of this chapter except to state that it involves the judicious use of topical corticosteroids with systemic or topical antivirals. Keratouveitis involves the endothelium and stroma and may be associated with secondary glaucoma.

Herpes zoster [6–10]

Clinical features

Herpes zoster of the ophthalmic division of the trigeminal nerve (Figure 107.23a) is an important condition to recognise (Chapter 25). As occurs when it affects other sites, it often presents with a non-specific flu-like illness with fever and malaise, and symptoms of unilateral neuralgia. This develops over the distribution of the affected nerve and varies in severity from a mild tingling in the skin to a deep severe pain. The characteristic lesions of herpes zoster may appear up to a week after the initial symptoms. Red macules develop into clusters of papules and vesicles, becoming pustular and haemorrhagic after 3–4 days. The lesions then scab and are dry by 7–14 days, and sometimes result in pitted scars. Involvement of the naso-ciliary nerve, which supplies the skin on the side of the nose, occurs in about 35% of patients and vesicles at this site (Hutchinson sign) are associated with a high risk of ophthalmic complications. Ocular involvement may occur in the absence of naso-ciliary involvement but it is usually milder. Herpes zoster *sine eruptione* can cause ocular complications without the cutaneous eruption. It is rare but evidence of the infection can be found by polymerase chain reaction analysis of the aqueous fluid or sequential titres of varicella zoster virus antibodies. Patients whose eyes cannot be examined due to persistent lid oedema, or those with ocular signs and symptoms, should be referred for urgent ophthalmic assessment. The disease can affect any part of the eye, including the orbit, extraocular muscles, optic nerve and cornea, and may give rise to long-term complications including severe relapsing keratitis, glaucoma and cataract. The commonest ocular complications are dendritiform keratopathy (Figure 107.23b), stromal keratitis and uveitis.

Management

Antiviral drugs reduce the duration and severity of acute herpes zoster but must be given within the first 3 days of the onset of the rash to be effective. Oral aciclovir has been the standard therapy at doses of 800 mg five times a day for 7–10 days. Valaciclovir (1000 mg three times per day) or famciclovir (500 mg three times per day for 7 days) are now preferred because of simpler dosing

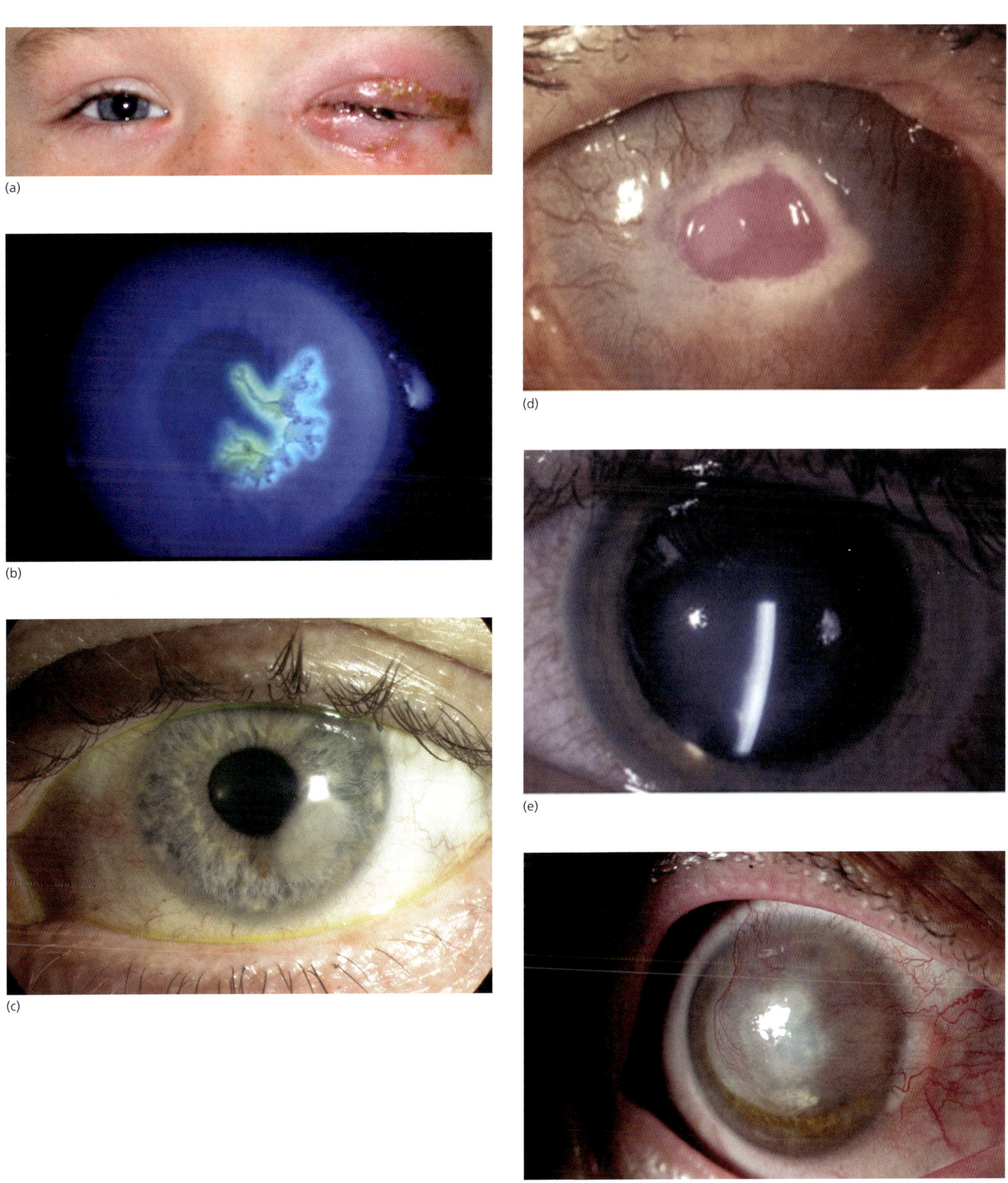

Figure 107.22 Herpes simplex virus. (a) Primary herpes simplex blepharoconjunctivitis in a child. (b) Dendritic epithelial keratitis. (c) Stromal herpetic keratitis. (d) Metaherpetic keratitis. (e) Herpetic endotheliitis. (f) Herpetic corneal vascularisation and scarring. (d) Courtesy of Mr J. Dart, Moorfields Eye Hospital, London, UK.

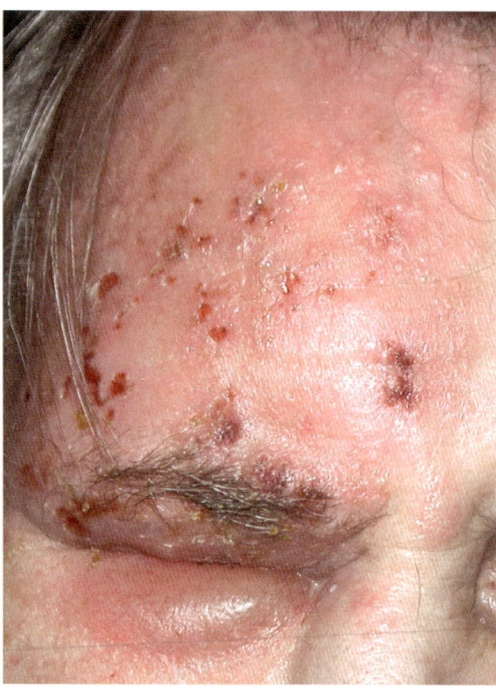

(a)

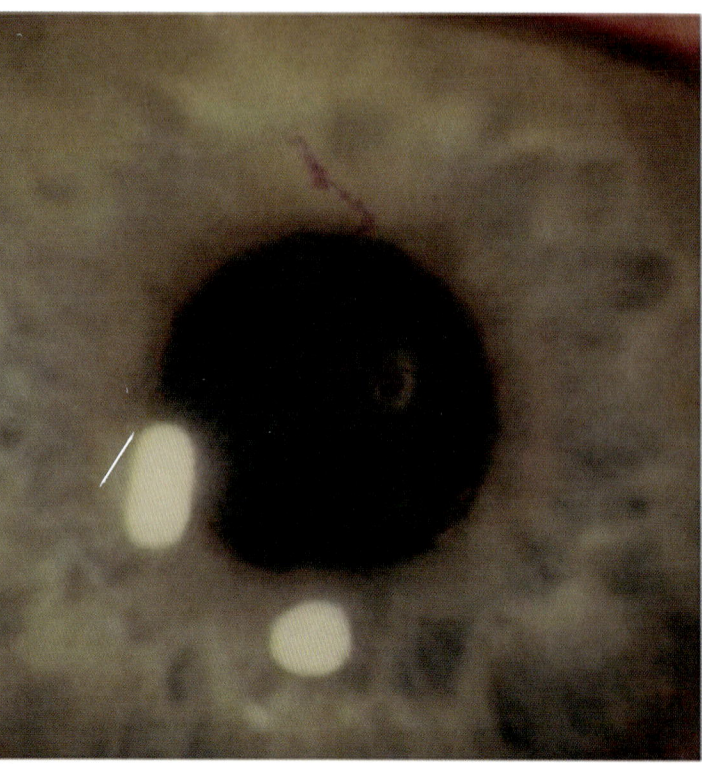

(b)

Figure 107.23 Herpes zoster. (a) Herpes zoster ophthalmicus. (b) Dendritiform keratopathy in herpes.

regimens and superior pharmacokinetics. Topical aciclovir is not indicated and unhelpful in almost all aspects of herpes zoster affecting the cornea, which respond to topical steroid treatment alone. One exception to this is late dendritiform lesions on the cornea in herpes zoster, which have been shown to be foci of productive varicella zoster virus [10], and thus require topical or

systemic antiviral treatment in addition to topical steroids. Topical corticosteroid therapy is necessary to control the numerous corneal manifestations of the disease and may need to be continued for several years. Some of these complications may be delayed and occur months after the initial skin eruption.

BACTERIAL INFECTIONS

Impetigo

Clinical features

Impetigo is a common staphylococcal or streptococcal skin infection that mainly affects children (Chapter 26). It can involve the eyelids, but usually as part of a general infection over the face. It presents as rapidly spreading red macules, developing into flaccid blistering, which become weepy before giving rise to surface crusting.

Management

The lesions need to be swabbed for bacteriology and appropriate topical or oral antibiotics given. Chloramphenicol drops or ointment are indicated if there is marked eyelid involvement.

Hordeolum

Clinical features

An external hordeolum (stye) is caused by staphylococcal infection of an eyelash follicle and its associated glands. It presents with a tender, red, inflamed swelling on the lid margin, which subsequently points anteriorly and discharges close to the lash roots (Figure 107.24a).

Management

No treatment is usually required beyond the application of local soothing compresses and removal of the affected lash. If there is local cellulitis then systemic antibiotics should be given. An internal hordeolum is a staphylococcal abscess of the meibomian glands (Figure 107.24b) and needs incision and drainage.

Erysipelas [11]

Clinical features

This represents subcutaneous spreading cellulitis, usually caused by β-haemolytic *Streptococcus* (Chapter 26). It usually presents with a rigor followed by a raised red plaque with a well-demarcated edge that spreads rapidly over the skin.

Management

Erysipelas is a serious skin infection that needs to be treated urgently with appropriate systemic antibiotics.

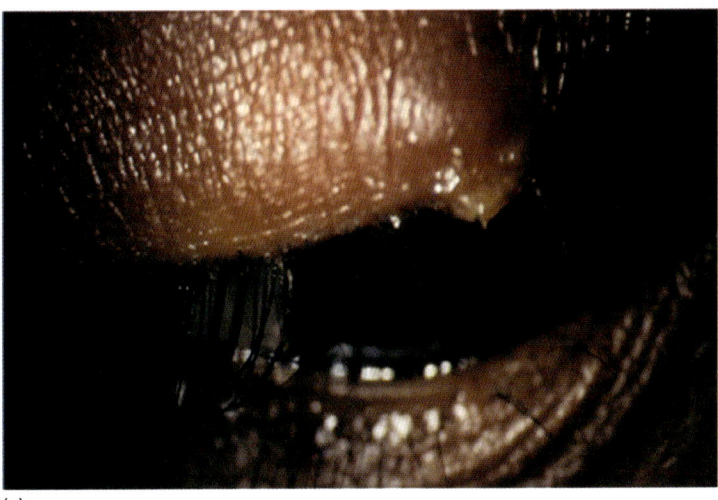

(a)

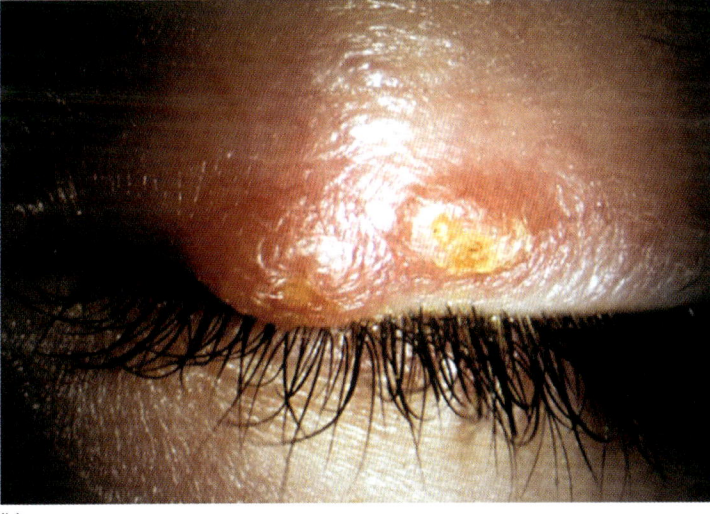

(b)

Figure 107.24 (a) External hordeolum (stye). (b) Internal hordeolum (infected chalazion) which has spontaneously discharged anteriorly through the skin (arrow), which is not uncommon. There is a large lesion on the left and a smaller lesion on the right.

Necrotising fasciitls [12]

Clinical features

This is very rare in the periorbital area, is typically polymicrobial and mainly affects elderly or debilitated patients (Chapter 26). A spreading purple discoloration of the eyelid rapidly progresses to gangrene.

Management

Early recognition, immediate institution of broad-spectrum intravenous antibiotics and referral to an ophthalmic plastic surgeon for emergency debridement of the necrotic tissue are mandatory as the condition carries a high mortality.

MYCOBACTERIAL INFECTIONS

Tuberculosis

Clinical features

There are no specific ocular findings in tuberculosis, and diagnosis is often based on indirect evidence such as intractable uveitis that is unresponsive to corticosteroid therapy, with negative findings for other causes of uveitis, and in the presence of tuberculosis at a distant body site (Chapter 27). Chronic iridocyclitis, which is usually granulomatous, is the commonest feature. Choroiditis and retinal vasculitis may occur.

Management

Appropriate antituberculous chemotherapy should be given.

Leprosy [13,14]

Clinical features

Ocular complications of leprosy are common, most frequently madarosis, conjunctivitis, episcleritis or scleritis (Chapter 28). Keratitis results from a combination of corneal anaesthesia, lagophthalmus, trichiasis and secondary infection. Iritis and its complications are the most common causes of blindness from leprosy. Lepromatous disease is more commonly associated with uveitis than is tuberculoid leprosy.

Management

Appropriate antilepromatous chemotherapy should be given.

TREPONEMAL INFECTIONS

Syphilis [15]

Clinical features

Ocular syphilis is very rare and there are no pathognomonic signs (Chapter 29). Eye involvement mainly occurs during the secondary and tertiary stages, although primary chancre of the conjunctiva may occur. External features include madarosis, scleritis and interstitial keratitis. Uveitis and chorioretinitis are rare but serious complications of syphilis and lead to blindness. Neuro-ophthalmic features include Argyll Robertson pupils, optic nerve lesions and palsies of the third and sixth cranial nerves. Gummatous involvement of the brain can cause visual field defects.

Management

Patients with suspected ocular syphilis should be referred to an infectious diseases or genito-urinary medicine specialist for assessment and therapy. Ophthalmic involvement should be assessed by an ophthalmologist, although definitive treatment is likely to be the same as for systemic infection.

Lyme disease [16,17]

Clinical features

Ocular manifestations of Lyme disease involve all parts of the eye (Chapter 26). As with syphilis, these vary according to the stage of the disease. In stage 1, a localised conjunctivitis with photophobia occurs in 10% of patients. This is mild and brief, and ophthalmologists are rarely consulted. In stage 2, various ophthalmic complications have been described including cranial nerve palsies; these may occur within 1 month of the appearance of erythema migrans. It is in the late stage 3 that most of the severe ocular complications are seen, including episcleritis, symblepharon, interstitial keratitis, uveitis, chorioretinitis and retinal vasculitis.

Management

Patients with suspected ocular involvement with Lyme disease should ideally be referred to an ophthalmologist with a specific interest in infection for assessment and management of the ocular complications.

PARASITIC INFECTIONS

Phthiriasis (lice) [18,19]

Clinical features

This is an infestation of the eyelashes by the pubic louse, *Phthirus pubis* (Chapter 34). It mainly affects children and causes chronic itching, irritation and rubbing of the lids. As with louse infection elsewhere, the adult lice can be difficult to see, although nits (eggs) and their shells are visible, adhering to the eyelashes (see Figure 107.9c, d). The skin nearest to the base of the lashes may show small bluish spots due to the louse bites (maculae caeruleae).

Management

A number of measures have been used to treat louse infestation of the eyelids, including mechanical removal with forceps, epilation and trimming of infested lashes, and the application of fluorescein, occlusive ointments (e.g. petrolatum) or aqueous malathion for 7–10 days.

Filariasis (onchocerciasis) [20]

Clinical features

Onchocerciasis or river blindness is caused by the filarial organism *Onchocerca volvulus* (Chapter 33). It is the second most common cause of preventable blindness in sub-Saharan Africa with an estimated prevalence of 500 000 cases with visual impairment and 270 000 with blindness. It appears that *Wolbachia endobacteria*, a bacterial symbiont, produces an endotoxin-like product which

constitutes a major pro-inflammatory stimulus in the eye, causing corneal inflammation and sclerosing keratitis.

Management

Patients with suspected ocular onchocerciasis should be referred to an ophthalmologist with a special interest in tropical diseases for assessment and management.

OTHER INFECTIONS

Protozoal infections

Clinical features

Ocular disease may complicate leishmaniasis. In *Leishmania donovani* infection, bilateral retinal haemorrhages may be a feature (Chapter 33). In *L. tropica* and *L. braziliensis* infection, eyelid lesions (see Figure 107.9f) and corneal lesions occur, and subsequent destruction may lead to loss of the eye. In trypanosomiasis, unilateral oedema of the lids may occur.

Management

Patients with suspected ocular complications of leishmaniasis should ideally be referred to an ophthalmologist with a special interest in the management of tropical diseases for assessment and management.

OTHER DISORDERS

INHERITED DISORDERS

A large number of inherited disorders affect the skin and eyes. Major reference texts are cited in [1–3]. The main ocular features are summarised in Table 107.11 [4–51].

OCULAR COMPLICATIONS OF DERMATOLOGICAL THERAPY

A number of drugs used by dermatologists have significant side effects on the eye and require careful monitoring.

Corticosteroids [1–15]

The use of corticosteroids can cause significant side effects on the eye. Both systemic and topical corticosteroids are responsible, although the greatest risk is to those receiving prednisolone at a dose of 10–15 mg/day for over a year. Continuous therapy is more likely to cause side effects than intermittent therapy.

Posterior subcapsular cataracts are induced by long-term systemic corticosteroids in as many as 30% of patients. They rarely occur at doses less than 10 mg/day and for less than 1 year. Children are particularly vulnerable. Reversibility of cataracts is not common and progression of cataracts may occur in spite of the reduction or discontinuation of corticosteroid therapy.

Table 107.11 Inherited disorders affecting the skin and eyes

Group	Condition	Inheritance	Ocular features
Nutritional deficiency	Acrodermatitis enteropathica [4]	AR (MIM 201100)	Loss of eyebrows and eyelashes, conjunctivitis, blepharitis, photophobia
Connective tissue disorder	Ehlers–Danlos syndrome [5]	Mainly AD (MIM 130000)	Lax eyelid skin with redundant folds, epicanthal folds, hypertelorism, strabismus, blue sclera, corneal abnormalities including keratoconus, angioid streaks (breaks in Bruch membrane), ectopic lens. Retinal detachments occasionally occur
	Marfan syndrome [6]	AD (MIM 154700)	Subluxation of lens – 60–80% of patients in early childhood. Amblyopia, myopia, cataract, corneal abnormalities, glaucoma. Retinal detachment is the most serious complication
	Pseudoxanthoma elasticum [7]	Types I and II AR (MIM 264800, 264810) Types III and IV AD (MIM 177850, 177860)	Angioid streaks in majority. Haemorrhagic maculopathy after trauma may cause visual loss
Dysplasias, hyperplasia, atrophies and aplasias	Ablepharon macrostomia syndrome [8]	Unknown (MIM 200110)	Absent eyelids and ectropion
	Aplasia cutis congenita [9]	AD (MIM 107600) AR (MIM 207700)	Congenital absence of skin leading to eyelid colobomas, corneal opacities, scleral dermoids and lamellar cataracts
	Blepharophimosis, ptosis, epicanthus inversus syndrome [10]	AD (MIM 110100)	Blepharophimosis, ptosis, epicanthus inversus, telecanthus. Amblyopia in 50% of patients
	Cockayne syndrome [11]	AR (MIM 216400)	Corneal opacities, cataracts in 30%, retinitis pigmentosa, optic atrophy, strabismus, photophobia
	Dyskeratosis congenita [12]	XR (MIM 305000)	Obliteration of the lacrimal puncta in 80% of cases, conjunctivitis, blepharitis, ectropion, loss of eyelashes and eyebrows
	Ectodermal dysplasias – a complex group of disorders with various inheritance patterns and a variety of ocular findings [13] Examples are:		
	(i) Christ–Siemens–Touraine syndrome	XR (MIM 305100)	Photophobia, dry eye
	(ii) Fischer–Jacobsen–Clouston syndrome	AD	Usually normal
	(iii) Ellis–van Creveld syndrome	AR (MIM 225500)	Coloboma of iris, microphthalmia, occasional cataract
	Focal dermal hypoplasia (Goltz syndrome) [14]	XD (MIM 305600)	40% have ocular abnormalities, the commonest being colobomas of iris, choroid, retina or optic nerve
	Fraser syndrome [15]	AR (MIM 219000)	Bilateral or unilateral absence of palpebral fissure with loss of eyebrows, anophthalmia, microphthalmia
	Frydman syndrome [16]	AR	Synophrys, blepharophimosis, weakness of extraocular and frontal muscles
	Hallermann–Streiff syndrome [17]	Unknown (MIM 264090)	Loss of hair of eyebrows and eyelashes, microphthalmos, cataracts, amblyopia, nystagmus
	MIDAS syndrome [18]	XD (MIM 309801)	Microphthalmia, sclerocornea
	Pachyonychia congenita (PC) [19]	AD; PC1 (MIM 167200) PC2 (MIM 167210)	Cataract and corneal dyskeratosis
Hair disorders	Brachmann–Lange syndrome [20]	AR	Synophrys, long thick eyelashes, narrow palpebral fissure, myopia, nystagmus, strabismus
	Monilethrix [21]	AD (MIM 158000)	Loss of eyebrows and lashes
	Pili torti [22]	AR (MIM 261900)	Loss of eyebrows and lashes
	Chondrodysplasia punctata [23]	AD (MIM 215105) XR (MIM 302950)	Cataracts Ocular albinism, cataracts, microphthalmia
Keratinisation disorders	The ichthyoses [24]:		
	(i) Ichthyosis congenita gravis	AR (MIM 242500)	Severe ectropion
	(ii) Ichthyosiform erythroderma	AD (MIM 242100)	Early development of ectropion is characteristic
	(iii) Lamellar ichthyosis	AR (various types)	Cicatricial ectropion with exposure keratitis Direct conjunctival involvement may occur
	(iv) X-linked ichthyosis	XL (MIM 308100)	Deep corneal opacities
	KID syndrome [25]	XD (MIM 148210)	Keratitis
	Refsum syndrome [26]	AR (MIM 266500)	Night blindness, posterior subcapsular cataracts develop in most cases
	Sjögren–Larsson syndrome [27]	AR (MIM 270200)	Blepharitis, conjunctivitis, punctate corneal erosions, pigmentary degeneration of the retina
	Ulerythema ophryogenes [28]	AD	Redness and perifollicular papules on eye to eyebrows, spreading medially and causing thinning of eyebrows (occurs in keratosis pilaris, Noonan syndrome, cardio-facio-cutaneous syndrome)

(continued)

PART 10: SPECIFIC SITES, SEX & AGE

Table 107.11 (*continued*)

Group	Condition	Inheritance	Ocular features
Metabolic disorders	Alkaptonuria [29]	AR (MIM 203500)	Scleral pigmentation is early sign, eyelid pigmentation
	Angiokeratoma corporis diffusum [30]	XL (MIM 301500)	Angiokeratomas of conjunctiva, corneal opacities, posterior capsular cataracts
	Homocystinuria [31]	AR (MIM 236200)	Myopia, cataracts, subluxation of lens, secondary glaucoma, retinal detachment
	Hurler syndrome [32]	AR (MIM 252800)	Early clouding of cornea
Neurocutaneous syndromes	Richner–Hanhart syndrome [33]	AR (MIM 276600)	Corneal lesions vary from erosions to deep ulcers Nystagmus and lens opacities
	Neurofibromatosis type I [34]	AD (MIM 162200)	Neurofibromas of eyelid, corneal clouding, Lisch nodules of iris, optic nerve glioma, palsies from cranial nerve involvement
	Neurofibromatosis type II [34]	AD (MIM 101000)	Cataract fundus lesions, extraocular motility abnormalities
	Tuberous sclerosis [35]	AD (MIM 191100)	Tumours of the lids or nodules on conjunctiva and retina
Photosensitive disorders	Basal cell naevus syndrome [36]	AD (MIM 109400)	Basal cell carcinoma of eyelid and periorbital area, hypertelorism, strabismus, colobomas of the choroid, cataracts, glaucoma in 5–10%
	Bloom syndrome [37]	AD (MIM 210900)	Telangiectasia on lower lids, blistering and scarring on lower eyelids
	Rothmund–Thomson syndrome [38]	AR (MIM 268400)	Sparse eyebrows and eyelashes, degenerative changes in cornea, 50% of patients have bilateral cataracts which develop in childhood, strabismus
	Xeroderma pigmentosum [39]	AR (various types)	Angiomas, keratoses, papillomas, carcinomas develop on eyelids, sometimes extending on to conjunctiva and cornea, scarring and atrophy of lids with exposure keratitis leading to corneal ulceration and symblepharon formation; ocular melanoma
Pigmentation disorders	Chediak–Higashi syndrome [40]	AR (MIM 214500)	Oculocutaneous albinism, corneal opacities
	Cross syndrome [41]	AR (MIM 257800)	Microphthalmia, small opaque cornea, coarse nystagmus
	Epidermal naevus syndrome [42]	Sporadic	Ocular melanocytic naevi, coloboma of the lids, iris and choroid; lipodermoid of conjunctiva or choroid
	Incontinentia pigmenti [43]	XD (MIM 308300)	35% of patients have eye abnormalities including strabismus, cataract and microphthalmia; retinal detachment may occur
	Hypomelanosis of Ito [44]	Sporadic (MIM 300337)	Hypertelorism, strabismus, myopia
	Oculocutaneous albinism [45]	AR (various types)	Total loss of pigment in eyes, nystagmus, absence of binocular vision
	Piebaldism [46]	AD (MIM 172800)	Absent pigmentation medially of eyebrows, eyelids and eyelashes, heterochromia of iris
	Waardenburg syndrome [47]	AD (MIM 193150)	Telecanthus, synophrys, partial albinism, heterochromia of iris
Vascular and haematological syndromes	Cutis marmorata telangiectatica congenita [48]	Unknown (MIM 219250)	Clouding of cornea, glaucoma
	Fanconi pancytopenia syndrome [49]	AR (MIM 227650)	Microphthalmia strabismus, nystagmus and colobomas
	Lymphoedema–distichiasis syndrome [50]	AD (MIM 153400)	Double row of eyelashes on upper and lower eyelids
	Sturge–Weber syndrome [51]	Sporadic (MIM 185300)	50% of patients have angiomatous changes of the ipsilateral choroid causing glaucoma

AD, autosomal dominant; AR, autosomal recessive; KID, keratitis, icthyosis and deafness; MIDAS, microphthalmia, dermal aplasia and sclerocornea; XD, X-linked dominant; XL, X-linked; XR, X-linked recessive.

Patients also risk developing open angle glaucoma, particularly if genetically predisposed. The precise mechanism is unknown, although it is thought to be due to decreased aqueous outflow. Particular risk factors include type 1 diabetes, high myopia, connective tissue disorders and a family history of glaucoma. Topical corticosteroids induce a rise in intraocular pressure more quickly than systemic corticosteroids. Topical corticosteroids applied to, or near, the eyelids may spread over the lid margin and are absorbed through the cornea; mid to high potency preparations can reach sufficient concentrations to elevate ocular pressures over long periods.

Topical corticosteroids also predispose patients to secondary surface infection. Injudicious use in herpes simplex virus infection masks the clinical signs of dendritic ulcer and risks perforation. Wearing contact lenses (including single-use lenses) increases the risk of infection when using topical ocular corticosteroid. The risk is higher with soft lenses than hard. Other ocular complications from corticosteroids include angioedema, papilloedema from raised intracranial pressure and toxic amblyopia. Systemic treatment with corticosteroids may cause serous chorioretinopathy or diffuse retinal pigment epitheliopathy.

The question arises of what constitutes 'safe' usage of topical corticosteroids in the context of dermatoses affecting the eyelids, the commonest scenario being that of atopic eczema. This is difficult to answer from the literature or major national guidelines. For example, neither those from the UK National Institute for Health and Care Excellence (NICE) [16] nor those of the American Academy of Dermatology [17] address the issue. A useful review by Beck *et al.* [18] published in 2019 stated the generally accepted view that lower potency corticosteroids are preferred on the eyelids. These authors noted a lack of prospective evidence. Anecdotal reports suggest that intraocular pressure (IOP) increases in some patients as a result of topical corticosteroid use; the results of retrospective studies have been inconsistent. The report noted that certain individuals are at higher risk of corticosteroid-induced elevation in IOP, including age <10 and >40 years, and those with diabetes, myopia, connective tissue disease, a history of refractive surgery or family or personal history of open angle glaucoma. Overall, however, which individuals will develop raised IOP from topical corticosteroid use cannot be predicted. It is thought that it takes a few weeks of use for IOP to occur and pressures usually return to normal 2–4 weeks after cessation. In relation to cataract formation, Beck *et al.* noted that this is associated with atopic eczema, but concluded that there is no evidence that long-term use of low-potency products or short-term use of higher potency products increases the risk.

The suggestion to treat in short bursts of a few days at a time with the lowest potency product that is effective seems sensible. In addition, it is advisable to monitor IOP closely – such as every 3 months – in individuals in whom long-term periocular use of topical corticosteroids cannot be avoided. Consideration should always be given to switching the topical corticosteroid to a calcineurin inhibitor if the indication is appropriate. The latter have not been associated with ocular adverse effects. Their use is limited in some patients by the sensation of burning or stinging, although this usually subsides after a few applications. It may be helpful to control acute inflammation initially using topical corticosteroids, before transitioning to the calcineurin inhibitor. In cases where the eyelid dermatosis does not respond sufficiently to topical treatment or where continuous or near-continuous potent corticosteroids are required, systemic therapies should be considered.

Patients on long-term systemic corticosteroids similarly require monitoring of IOP regularly (e.g. 1–6 monthly intervals) depending on their degree of risk. Long-term systemic corticosteroids (at any dose) can cause or worsen glaucoma, and patients and clinicians need to be aware of this risk and ensure appropriate regular monitoring is carried out.

Oral retinoids [19–21,22]

Isotretinoin, alitretinoin and acitretin can each cause ocular side effects. The most common is evaporative dry eye with associated conjunctivitis and blepharoconjunctivitis, giving rise to blurred vision. There may be associated staphylococcal infection. Exposure keratopathy and corneal ulceration rarely occur; asymptomatic corneal opacities may develop but resolve after 6–8 weeks. Patients should be warned that they may be unable to tolerate contact lenses while on retinoid therapy. Use of tear substitutes, humidification of the environment and lid hygiene measures help. Retinal abnormalities may also occur, with poor night vision and increased sensitivity to glare, and can be a significant problem in those who drive at night; pilots are not allowed to fly while taking isotretinoin due to the potential effects on night vision. The cause is unknown but may be due to competitive inhibition of ocular retinol dehydrogenase causing local vitamin A deficiency and reduction in rhodopsin formation. More serious side effects include papilloedema from raised intracranial pressure, optic atrophy and cataract. Although these are rare, a history of visual disturbance should be asked for when patients come for follow-up. Severe headache early in the course of treatment is significant. The ocular manifestations are dose dependent and usually reversible,

provided they are recognised and the treatment regimen adjusted. However, there have been reports of severe dry eye syndrome and night blindness persisting after retinoids have been discontinued. Laser eye surgery is contraindicated within 6 months of being on isotretinoin [23].

Antimalarials [24,25,26]

A key potential adverse effect of both hydroxychloroquine and chloroquine is irreversible retinopathy with resulting loss of vision. The mechanisms are not fully understood, but the drugs are thought to induce degeneration of the retinal pigment epithelium [24]. It is estimated that long-term exposure to hydroxychloroquine results in retinopathy in about 7.5% of patients. This can produce central visual loss and the characteristic 'bull's eye maculopathy'. Chloroquine appears to lead to similar problems, but more rapidly than hydroxychloroquine, whereas this problem has not been linked with mepacrine. Previous recommendations for prescribers of the two former drugs involved simple tests of visual acuity. With the development of more sensitive methods to detect retinopathy prior to the onset of symptoms or visual loss, UK guidelines for the surveillance of patients taking these drugs were released by the Royal College of Ophthalmologists. These were updated in 2020 [26] and recommend referral to ophthalmology for annual monitoring after taking hydroxychloroquine for 5 years or chloroquine for 1 year. Monitoring should preferably be with both spectral-domain optical coherence tomography (SD-OCT) and wide-field fundus autofluorescence imaging (FAF). Referral of patients prescribed hydroxychloroquine should take place sooner if there are additional risk factors, namely a dose greater than 5 mg/kg/day, concomitant tamoxifen or renal impairment (estimated glomerular filtration rate (eGFR) <60 mL/min/1.73 m^2). If retinal toxicity is identified, cessation of the causative drug will generally be recommended by the ophthalmologist as this is the only intervention likely to prevent progression. In some cases, retinopathy worsens despite stopping the drug, although this is more likely in the context of advanced disease.

Antibiotics for acne [27–31]

Oxytetracycline, minocycline and doxycycline can all cause raised intracranial pressure. The mechanism is unknown but is thought to be related to interference with the energy-dependent absorption mechanism of cerebrospinal fluid, which is mediated by cyclic adenosine monophosphate (cAMP) at the arachnoid granulations. Patients who complain of headache should be examined carefully with fundoscopy through dilated pupils to look for papilloedema, and should have formal testing of visual acuity and of visual fields. Permanent visual field loss can occur if the condition is not recognised early and the drug stopped. Sometimes treatment with acetazolamide is required to reduce the pressure. Erythromycin or trimethoprim may cause SJS/TEN or erythema multiforme with associated ocular changes. Pigmentation due to minocycline can occur in the skin and has also been reported in the sclera.

Psoralens [32–45]

Psoralens have been shown to bind to the lens proteins, and some animal studies have shown induction of anterior cortical opacities although others have not. 8-Methoxypsoralen can be detected in the human lens 12 h after oral ingestion. There has been a longstanding concern about the risk of cataract in patients having psoralen and long-wave ultraviolet A radiation (PUVA) therapy. Although PUVA has been used in the treatment of skin diseases for 30 years, and clinical studies have not yet shown any convincing evidence of an increase in cataracts as compared with the general population, it is still recommended that UVA-filtered spectacles are used for 12 h after ingestion of psoralens in case significant long-term sequelae eventually develop. Failure to do so may result in other signs of ocular toxicity such as conjunctival hyperaemia, decreased lacrimation and pinguecula formation, which represents elastotic degeneration of the cornea. Care must be taken to ensure that the spectacles are suitable for UV protection.

Botulinum toxin [46]

With the increased use of botulinum toxin for the treatment of facial wrinkling and eyebrow position, dermatologists need to be aware of the potential side effects. These include haematoma, ptosis, ectropion, diplopia and eyelid drooping, and are often related to poor injection technique.

Biologic agents

Dupilumab is the first biologic agent approved for eczema. It is a recombinant IgG4 monoclonal antibody that interrupts the pathways involved in type 2 inflammatory disease by inhibiting IL-4 and IL-13 [47]. While atopic eczema is known to be associated with a variety of eye disorders including dry eye syndrome, keratoconjunctivitis, conjunctivitis, blepharitis and several others [48], clinical trials of dupilumab found higher than expected rates of eye complications, usually described as conjunctivitis (8.6–22.1% in participants taking dupilumab versus 2.1–11.1% on placebo [47]). This appears only to occur in patients with eczema and not those with other indications such as asthma, chronic rhinosinusitis with nasal polyps or eosinophilic oesophagitis and is more common in individuals with more severe atopic eczema or a previous history of conjunctivitis [49]. It is thought that IL-13 has a role in the regulation of conjunctival goblet cells and its blockade results in impaired tear quality [50]. Most cases are mild to moderate in severity and discontinuation due to ocular adverse effects is rare [49,51].

Wollenberg *et al.* reported a good response to topical corticosteroid (fluorometholone 0.1% eye drops) or tacrolimus (0.03% eye ointment), whereas antihistamine drops and artificial tears were unhelpful [52]. On the other hand, Rial *et al.* reported good results in their small series of patients with severe atopic eczema from using prophylactic artificial tears from a week prior to initiation of dupilumab [50]. Hot compresses and topical ciclosporin may also be helpful.

The other IL-13 antagonists, tralokinumab and lebrikizumab, appear to be associated with similar ocular adverse effects of mild to moderate severity [53–55].

Potential ocular side effects of biologic agents used within oncology include (depending on the agent used) trichomegaly, blepharitis, conjunctivitis, cicatricial entropion, corneal erosion, reversible posterior leukoencephalic syndrome and possible optic neuritis. Further details can be found in Hager and Seitz [56].

BENIGN LESIONS OF THE EYELID

As would be expected of such complex tissue, the eyelid gives rise to a large number of skin tumours. Tumours can arise from the epidermis and dermis in addition to the adnexal structures, which include the meibomian and Zeis sebaceous glands, eccrine and Moll apocrine sweat glands, and the specialised hair follicles of the eyelashes. They may also originate from lymphoid neural and vascular tissue found in the preseptal tissues of the eyelid. Although optimal treatment of the tumours begins with accurate diagnosis, many are rather non-specific in their appearance and are only diagnosed with certainty by histology.

Seborrhoeic keratosis

Seborrhoeic keratoses occur on the eyelid and show similar clinical features to those at other sites. They can be treated if necessary with careful cryotherapy, or laser ablation or surgery under local anaesthesia.

Xanthelasma [1,2]

These present as yellowish cutaneous plaques, most commonly located on the medial part of the eyelids (Figure 107.25). They are usually bilateral and are much more common in elderly patients. About 60% of patients have associated hypercholesterolaemia and lipid levels should be measured. Patients often request treatment for cosmetic reasons. Although 90% trichloroacetic acid applied with a cotton wool bud is used there is a significant risk of spillage into the eye. More effective treatment is by surgical excision or ablation with carbon dioxide laser. Necrobiotic xanthogranuloma may look similar to xanthelasma but are thicker and more nodular. These lesions may involve the conjunctiva and sclera. On the rare occasions that they infiltrate the orbit, they may cause proptosis.

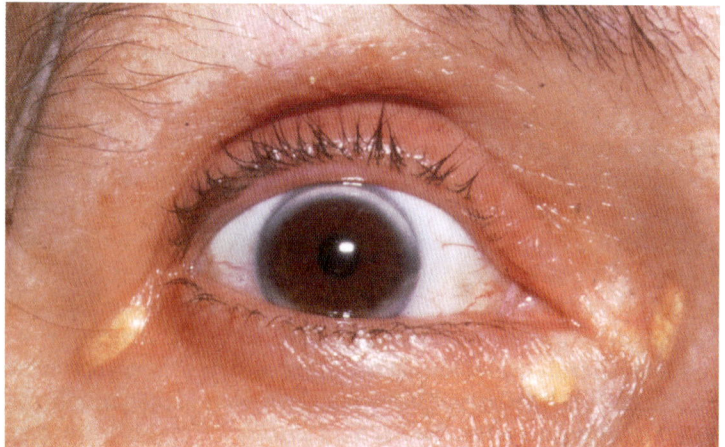

Figure 107.25 Xanthelasma. There are two lesions on the medial eyelid and one lesion on the temporal eyelid. The cornea shows arcus senilis, which is also associated with hypercholesterolaemia.

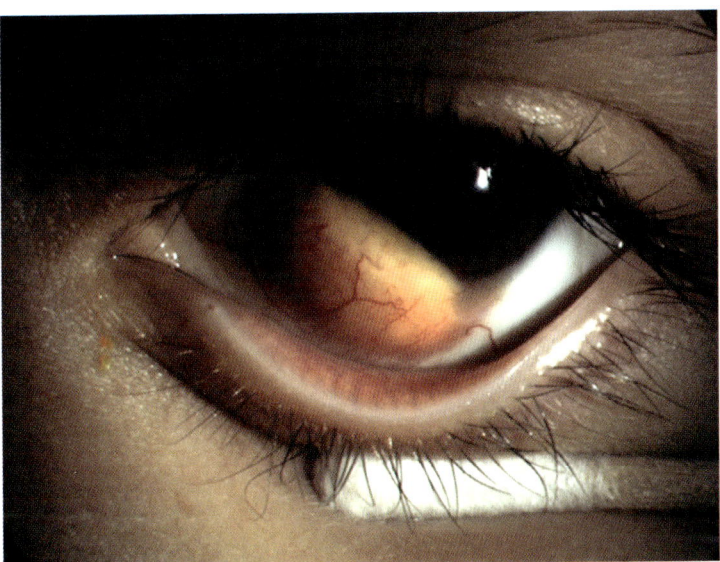

Figure 107.26 Juvenile xanthogranuloma.

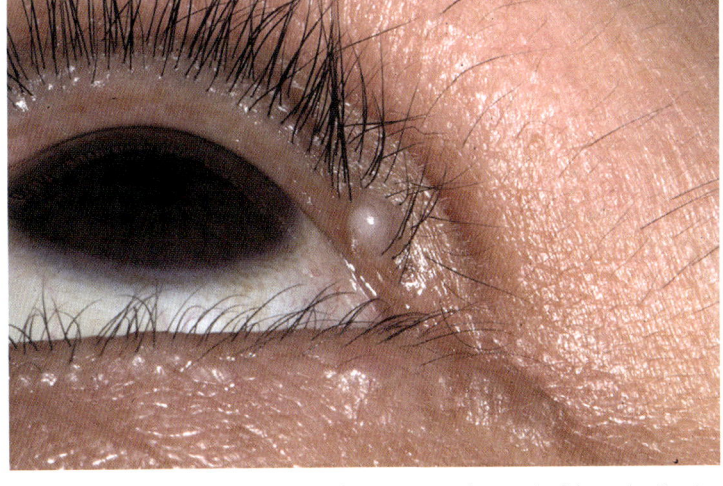

Figure 107.27 Cyst of Moll, a small translucent cyst on the anterior lid margin. Courtesy of Mr N. Joshi, Chelsea and Westminster Hospital/Medical Illustration UK, London, UK.

Juvenile xanthogranuloma [3]

These lesions occasionally involve the eyelid, conjunctiva or uveal tract. They may be associated with glaucoma and threaten sight. Patients need screening by an ophthalmologist (Figure 107.26).

Benign adnexal lesions [4]

Syringomas, milia, trichoepitheliomas and tricholemmomas present as small papules around the eyelids. They can be very difficult to distinguish from each other. Syringomas are the most common, but histology from a biopsy is the only way to make a definite diagnosis. Treatment is by local destruction of the lesions. Eccrine hidrocystomas can present in an eruptive fashion on the face and eyelids; they may respond to topical atropine.

Benign sebaceous lesions also occur in the periocular area. Histology is required for diagnosis and to differentiate them from sebaceous carcinoma, which is discussed later in this section. Confirmed diagnosis of a sebaceous lesion should prompt consideration of testing for mismatch repair genes, although sebaceous lesions occurring below the neck are much more strongly associated with Muir–Torré syndrome.

Benign cysts of the eyelid

Retention cysts may arise from either the glands of Moll or Zeis. A cyst of Moll usually presents as a small translucent lesion on the anterior lid margin close to the lacrimal punctum (Figure 107.27). Glands of Zeis are sebaceous glands and their retention cysts contain oily secretions and are more opaque than a cyst of Moll (Figure 107.28). An eccrine hidrocystoma is similar in appearance to a cyst of Moll but is not confined to the lid margin. These cysts

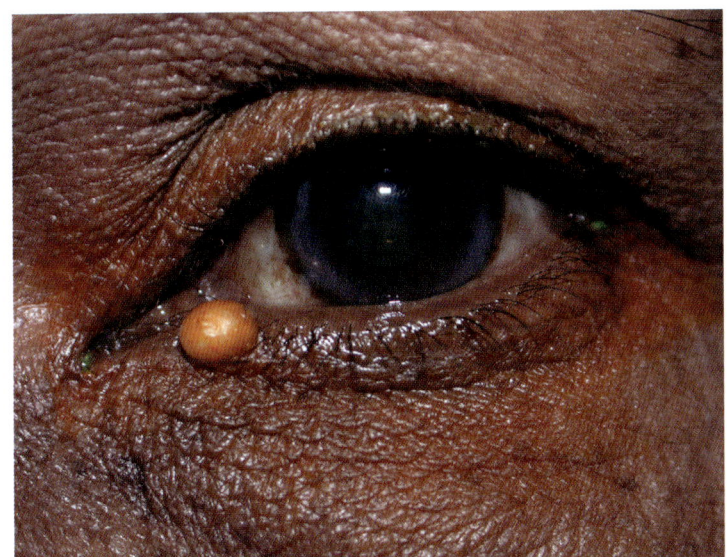

Figure 107.28 Cyst of Zeis. Opaque sebaceous cyst.

are easily confused with a basal cell carcinoma clinically and are treated by excision biopsy.

Chalazion [5]

This lesion represents a chronic granulomatous inflammatory reaction around a blocked sebaceous gland. Patients with seborrhoeic dermatitis and rosacea are at increased risk of chalazion formation. A chalazion presents as a firm lump in the eyelid (see Figure 107.8b, d), which is clearly visible when the lid is everted; an association with chronic posterior blepharitis is common. Chalazia will usually resolve spontaneously but large and troublesome lesions can be treated by everting the lid with a special clamp, incising the cyst and curetting the contents through the tarsal plate. Patients who develop recurrent chalazia associated with seborrhoeic dermatitis

PART 10: SPECIFIC SITES, SEX & AGE

and rosacea benefit from long-term antibiotic treatment using tetracyclines. Hot compresses reduce the inflammation.

Melanocytic naevi [6,7]

The skin on the eyelid can develop pigmented naevi. Their appearance, classification and potential malignant change is the same as elsewhere on the skin. Patients with dysplastic naevus syndrome should be referred to an ophthalmologist for ocular assessment (Chapter 131). Melanocytic lesions of the conjunctiva extending onto the cornea or pigmented lesions of the conjunctiva (Figure 107.29), which change in character, should also be referred with a view to excision biopsy.

Naevus of Ota [8]

This lesion affects the eyelids, conjunctiva and sclera (Chapter 73). Occasionally, the pigmentation is confined to the eye and uvea with no cutaneous involvement (Figure 107.30). Naevus of Ota carries an increased risk of ocular melanoma and glaucoma, and patients need to be referred for ophthalmic examination and long-term review.

Haemangioma [10–15]

Strawberry naevus (capillary haemangioma) can affect the eyelids (Chapter 116). It is more common on the upper lid and presents as a unilateral, red, raised lesion, which grows quickly during the first year of life (Figure 107.31). Spontaneous involution occurs usually by age 9 years. Amblyopia is the main potential complication of larger periorbital lesions and results either from physical closure of the eye and occlusion of the pupil, giving rise to stimulus deprivation, or from refractive errors caused by corneal distortion due to lid pressure. Lesions that threaten function such as sight or those

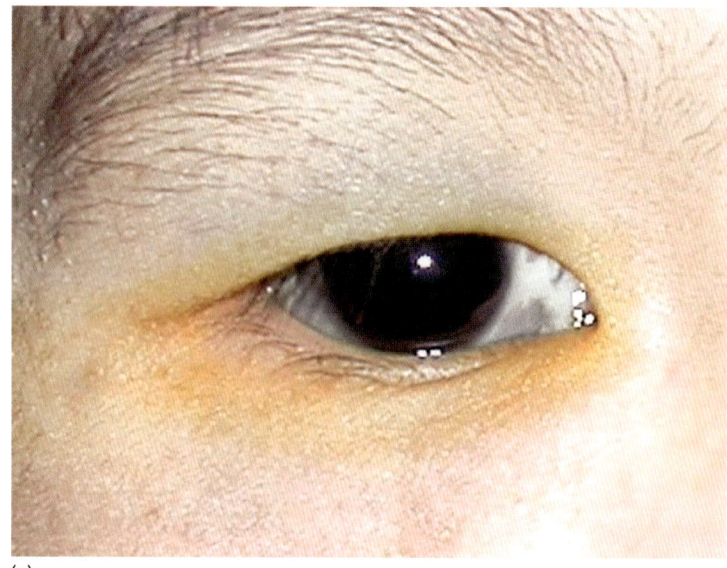

(a)

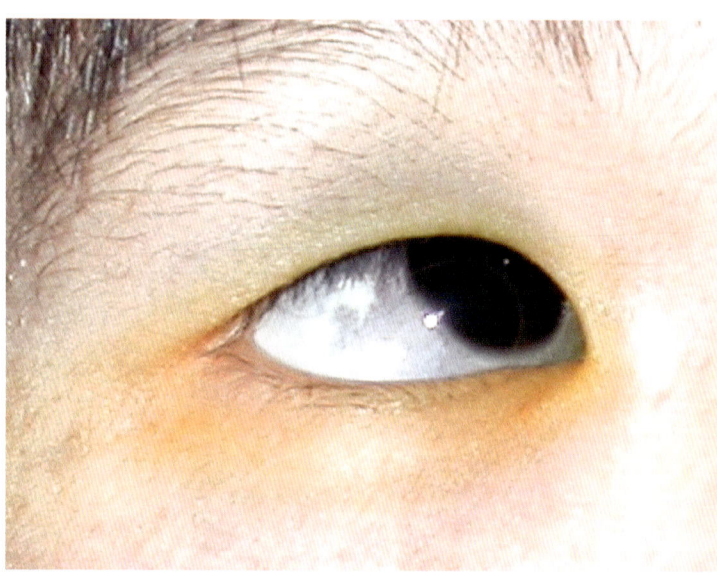

(b)

Figure 107.30 (a, b) Naevus of Ota. In this case the pigmentation is confined to the eye, with no cutaneous involvement. The yellow staining of the eyelid is due to fluorescein instillation into the eye to measure intraocular pressure.

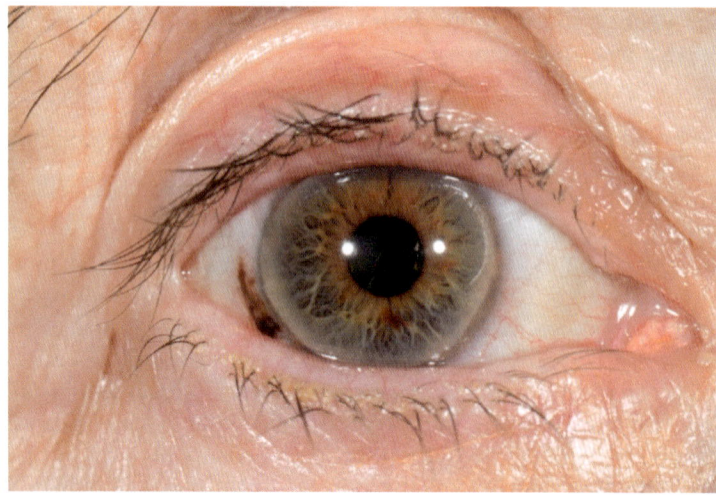

Figure 107.29 Primary acquired melanosis of the conjunctiva.

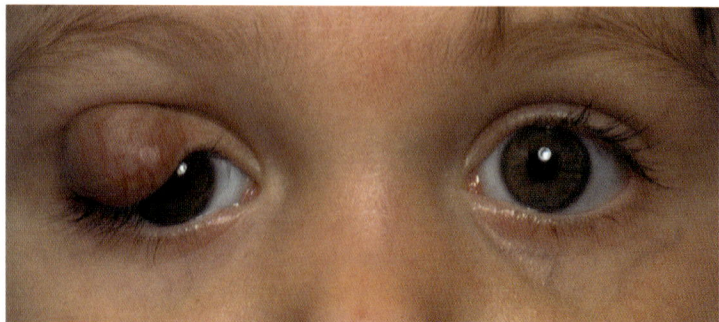

Figure 107.31 Capillary haemangioma. The enlarging lesion on the right upper lid is starting to occlude vision. Courtesy of Mr N. Joshi, Chelsea and Westminster Hospital/Medical Illustration UK, London, UK.

that are symptomatic are generally treated with systemic or topical β-blockers. Surgical resection or laser therapy is helpful in certain cases.

Port-wine stain [16,17]

This is an uncommon congenital vascular lesion, which may affect the eyelids (Chapter 71). It presents as a sharply demarcated, red, macular lesion, which becomes darker and thicker over time. Cases with upper eyelid and forehead involvement in particular may be associated with Sturge–Weber syndrome (SWS), which is characterised by a wide spectrum of neurological features including epilepsy and learning difficulties. Hennedige *et al.* found that SWS was present in only 3% of their series of 874 patients with facial port-wine stain [16]. There is also an association between facial port-wine stain and other ocular abnormalities. Rujimethapass *et al.*, for example, found that 18% of their patients with port-wine stain had glaucoma and recommended screening [17].

Keratoacanthoma

Keratoacanthoma may develop on the eyelid (Chapter 140). It presents as a rapidly enlarging papulonodule, which develops a characteristic keratin-filled crater and may reach up to 3 cm in diameter (Figure 107.32). The lesion then stops growing and remains static for weeks to months before spontaneously involuting. This can lead to unpredictable scarring of the eyelid so it is generally seen as preferable to excise lesions at this site at an early stage.

Squamous cell carcinoma in situ

Both actinic keratoses and Bowen disease can occur on the eyelid. They have similar clinical features to those elsewhere on the skin

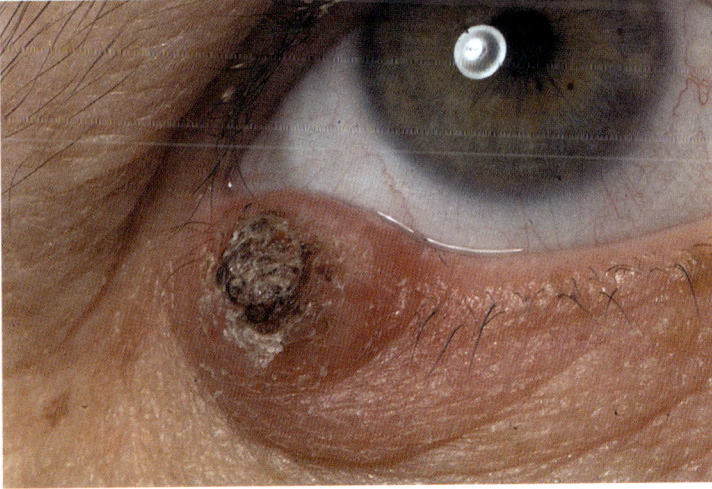

Figure 107.32 Keratoacanthoma. Keratin-filled crateriform nodule on the lid margin. Courtesy of Mr N. Joshi, Chelsea and Westminster Hospital/Medical Illustration UK, London, UK.

and can be treated similarly. Options include carefully applied cryotherapy, or laser ablation under local anaesthesia. Topical 5-fluorouracil cream can also be used with care in the periocular area [18] and is often the best option for larger lesions or in cases with more widespread actinic field change. Although surgical treatment may be required, curettage can be difficult in the periocular region: the skin is mobile and thin, making it difficult both to gain any purchase with the curette and also to control the depth of treatment. Recurrent actinic keratosis should be biopsied and sent for histological examination to make sure it is not a deceptive manifestation of skin cancer such as superficial basal cell carcinoma.

MALIGNANT LESIONS OF THE EYELID [1–4]

Basal cell carcinoma (BCC), squamous cell carcinoma (SCC) and malignant melanoma all occur on the eyelid as on other areas of the skin (Chapters 139 and 140). The same rules for management apply on the eyelid as at any site, but the eyelid poses specific problems in preserving good cosmesis and residual function. Clinical examination is an unreliable way of determining the extent of many of these lesions, particularly infiltrative BCC. For such lesions, margin-controlled excision, preferably Mohs micrographic surgery, should be considered as primary treatment, with reconstruction by an operator appropriately experienced and skilled in operating in this area.

Basal cell carcinoma [4–14]

This is the most common skin malignancy and in most series accounts for 90% of malignant tumours. Although it rarely metastasises, it can cause problems in the periocular area through local tissue destruction and invasion of periorbital tissue. This can lead to disruption of the delicate functioning of the eyelids and lacrimal system. Furthermore, infiltrative tumours may eventually extend behind the globe so that exenteration is the only potentially curative treatment. Over 70% of periocular BCCs arise on the lower eyelid, followed in order of frequency by the medial canthus, upper eyelid and lateral canthus. Tumours located near to the medial canthus can invade the orbit and sinuses. Treatment of these can be particularly problematic because of the high risk of damaging the tear duct. The majority of BCCs are solid or cystic and are fairly straightforward to recognise (Figure 107.33). The infiltrative or morphoeic subtype is more difficult to diagnose as it may lack some of the classic features of BCC and tends to present later. The paucity of reticular dermis and subcutaneous fat to resist deep invasion presents a particular problem around the eye. Once the orbital septum is penetrated the BCC can rapidly invade, threatening the orbit. At the medial canthus the lacrimal sac and the rich anastomosis of blood vessels offers little barrier.

Treatment of any periocular BCC is ideally by complete excision. Histological confirmation of an adequate excision margin is mandatory. Mohs micrographic surgery is often indicated in this area, both to be confident that ill-defined lesions are fully removed and also for tissue sparing in an area where it is vital to preserve function. This can minimise the complexity of the reconstruction and thus the likelihood of complications. Radiotherapy damages and scars the eyelid tissues and lacrimal system and should be reserved for situations when surgery is otherwise inappropriate. Cryotherapy should be avoided due to the risks of leaving residual tumour and excessive scarring. Hedgehog pathway inhibitors can be helpful in the management of patients with unresectable disease, such as large infiltrating eyelid BCC and in Gorlin syndrome where there may be numerous eyelid lesions; however, the drugs are poorly tolerated [7].

Squamous cell carcinoma [8,9]

This is much less common than BCC, accounting for between 5% and 10% of eyelid malignancies. SCCs usually occur on a background of marked actinic damage and are much more common in immunosuppressed individuals. They mainly affect the lower eyelid and lid margin, and may arise *de novo* or from pre-existing *in situ* disease. SCC of the eyelids may be nodular, plaque-like or ulcerated (Figure 107.34). Excision with adequate margins is the treatment of choice. Tumours greater than 2 cm in diameter and those with deep penetration have a higher risk of metastasis. Histological evidence of poor differentiation or of perineural invasion are also poor prognostic factors and require more aggressive treatment. Mohs micrographic surgery can be considered as a primary treatment in the periocular region where tissue sparing is likely to be a particular advantage, and especially if on conventional excision the margins are not free of tumour. Radiotherapy is a potentially curative alternative to surgery; it is usually used as an adjuvant treatment for high-risk lesions. Locally advanced tumours which are not suitable for these interventions may respond to immune checkpoint inhibitors or epidermal growth factor receptor inhibitors.

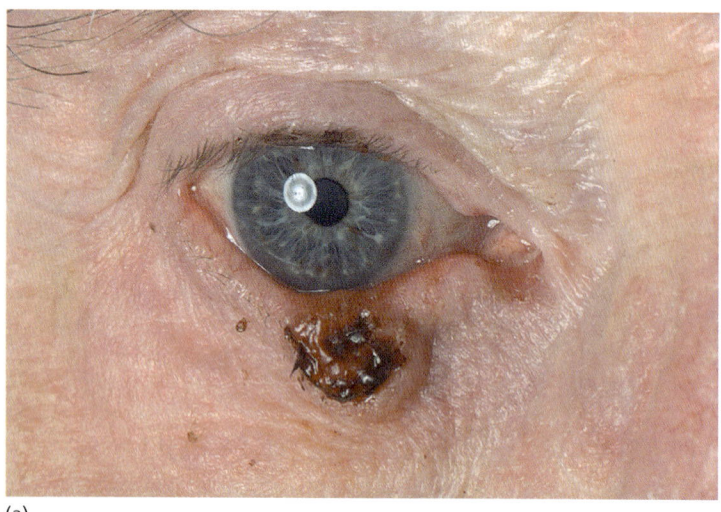

(a)

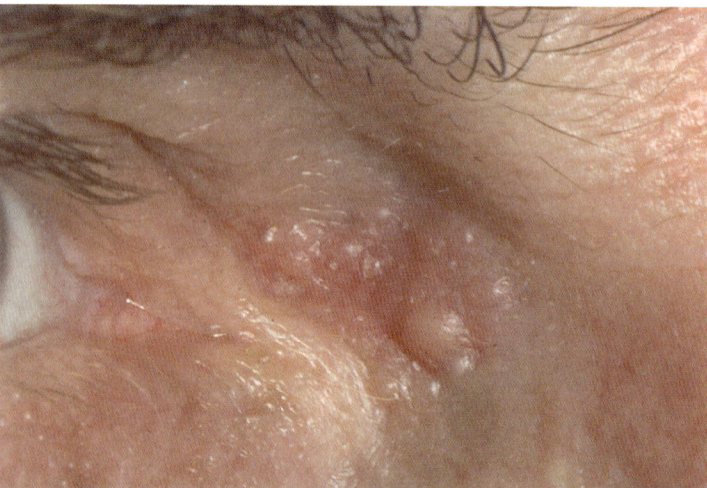

(b)

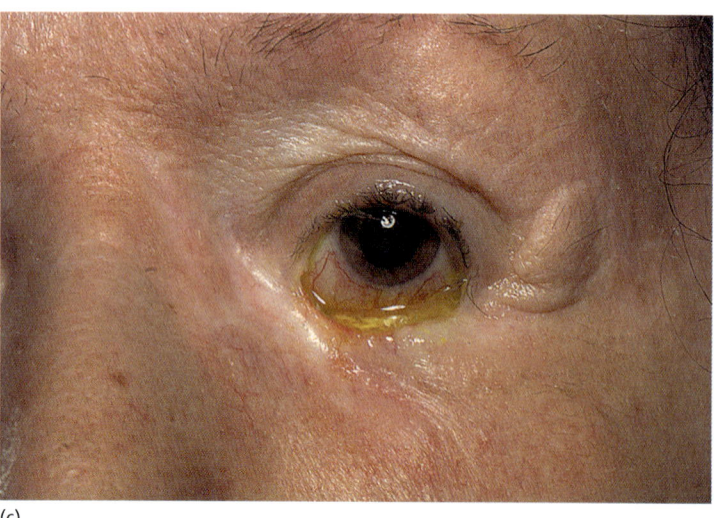

(c)

Figure 107.33 Basal cell carcinoma (BCC). (a) Ulcerated BCC on the lower lid. (b) Poorly defined BCC at the medial canthus. (c) Morphoeic BCC along the lower lid. Courtesy of Mr N. Joshi, Chelsea and Westminster Hospital/Medical Illustration UK, London, UK.

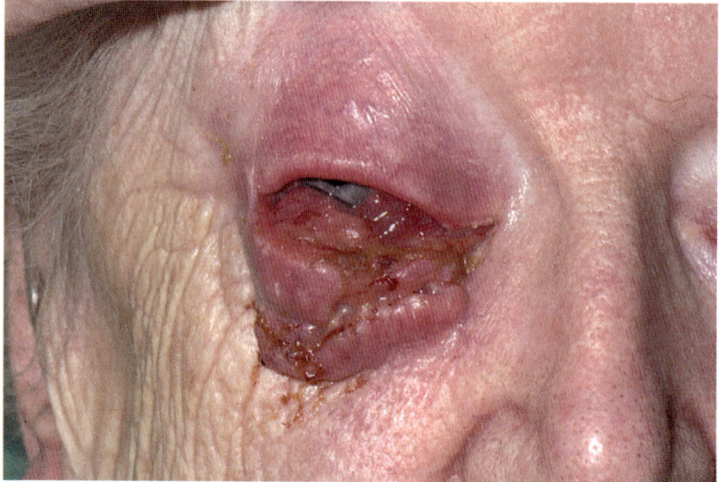

Figure 107.34 Squamous cell carcinoma (SCC). Infiltrating ulcerated SCC on the lower lid. Courtesy of Mr N. Joshi, Chelsea and Westminster Hospital/Medical Illustration UK, London, UK.

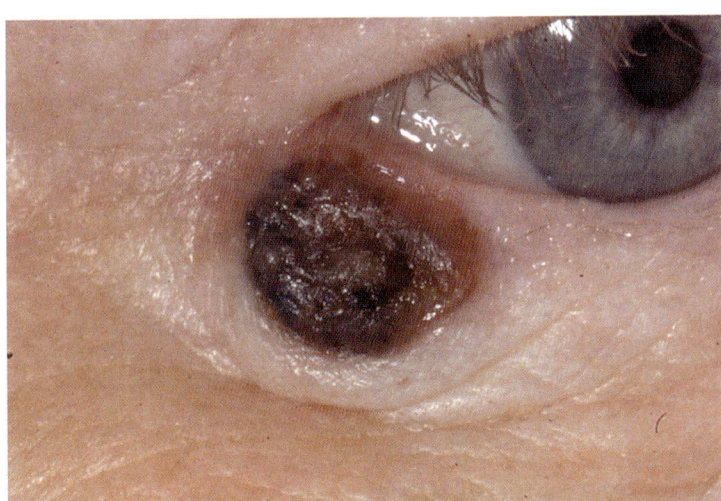

Figure 107.35 Malignant melanoma. Irregularly pigmented lesion on the lower lid. Courtesy of Mr N. Joshi, Chelsea and Westminster Hospital/Medical Illustration UK, London, UK.

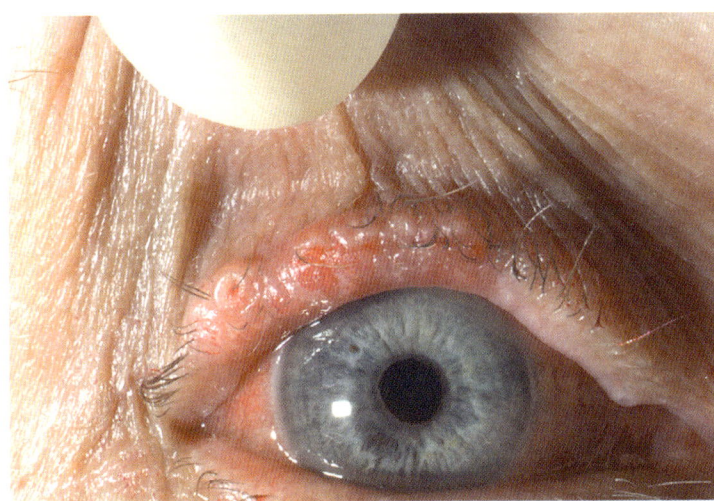

Figure 107.36 Sebaceous carcinoma. Infiltrating lesion on the upper lid. Courtesy of Mr N. Joshi, Chelsea and Westminster Hospital/Medical Illustration UK, London, UK.

Malignant melanoma [10]

This may occur on the eyelids or conjunctiva (Chapter 142) and will sometimes extend from one to the other. Its features are essentially the same as melanoma at other sites (Figure 107.35). However, a significant proportion of lid melanoma is amelanotic and this may give rise to difficulties with clinical diagnosis. Periocular melanoma most commonly affects the lower lid. The superficial spreading and lentiginous subtypes are most frequent. As with melanoma at other sites, treatment is generally by wide local excision. Difficulty can arise due to the proximity to the eye, as well as subclinical extension often seen in lentigo maligna. Such cases should be managed in conjunction with the skin cancer multidisciplinary team.

Sebaceous carcinoma [11,12]

This rare but aggressive cancer accounts for about 3–5% of malignant tumours of the eyelid, making it the third most common type of periocular cancer after BCC and SCC. It appears to be more common in Far Eastern populations. It usually arises from the meibomian glands although occasionally from the glands of Zeis. In contrast to BCC and SCC, the upper lid is the most common site for periocular lesions (Figure 107.36). Nodular lesions can be impossible to distinguish clinically from keratinocyte cancers, but sebaceous carcinoma is notorious for mimicking benign conditions, such as chalazia or blepharitis (see Figure 107.9a,b). The diagnosis is thus often delayed, with later presentation associated with poorer outcomes. A sebaceous tumour should be considered if a 'chalazion' lasts for more than 6 months, and one that recurs should be viewed with suspicion. Primary treatment is surgical, either by wide local excision or Mohs micrographic surgery.

Eccrine carcinoma [13]

This is a rare cancer of the eye and may present as an indurated thickening of the lid or with a signet-ring appearance. They are commonest in middle-aged or elderly men and may recur after excision.

Microcystic adnexal carcinoma [14]

This rare type of skin cancer most commonly presents on the head and neck in older white individuals. It tends to grow slowly and presents as a smooth papulonodule with features that may be indistinguishable from a variety of other benign and malignant lesions. Metastasis is rare but the tumour is infiltrating and locally aggressive. Wide local excision can be effective, but given the importance of tissue sparing in the periocular region, Mohs micrographic surgery is useful for such lesions.

Merkel cell carcinoma

This tumour very rarely occurs on the eyelid. It can also mimic a chalazion in its early stages, with a resulting delay in diagnosis (Chapter 146). It is highly malignant and has often metastasised by the time of excision.

Kaposi sarcoma

A vascular malignancy, Kaposi sarcoma presents as a reddish, purple or brown lesion on the eyelid or conjunctiva and can be mistaken for a benign haemangioma (Chapter 137). However, it will tend to enlarge, and may ulcerate and bleed. When it presents on the eyelid it is usually associated with HIV infection, of which it may be the sole manifestation at the time of presentation. If HIV-related, it may regress with retroviral therapy, although it is very radiosensitive, and this is otherwise the preferred mode of treatment once the diagnosis has been confirmed histologically.

Key references

The full list of references can be found in the online version at https://www.wiley.com/rooksdermatology10e

Introduction
6 Mannis MJ, Macsai MS, Huntley AC, eds. *Eye and Skin Disease*. New York: Lippincott-Raven, 1996.
7 Ostler HB, Maibach HI, Hoko AW, Swab IR, eds. *Diseases of the Eye and Skin: a Color Atlas*. Philadelphia: Lippincott, Williams & Wilkins, 2004.

Skin diseases affecting the eye and eyelids
Blepharitis, meibomian gland dysfunction, rosacea and seborrhoeic dermatitis
6 Nichols KK, Foulks GN, Bron AJ *et al*. The international workshop on meibomian gland dysfunction: executive summary. *Invest Ophthalmol Vis Sci* 2011;52(4):1922–9.

Atopy and atopic eye disease
21 Utine CA, Li G, Asbell P *et al*. Ocular surface disease associated with dupilumab treatment for atopic diseases. *Ocul Surf* 2021;19:151–6.

Cicatrising conjunctivitis associated with immunobullous disorders
4 Saw VP, Dart JK. Ocular mucous membrane pemphigoid: diagnosis and management strategies. *Ocul Surf* 2008;6:128–42.
22 De Rojas MV, Dart JK, Saw VP. The natural history of Stevens–Johnson syndrome: patterns of chronic ocular disease and the role of systemic immunosuppressive therapy. *Br J Ophthalmol* 2007;91:1048–53.

Systemic diseases with skin and eye involvement
1 Callen JP, Mahl CF. Oculocutaneous manifestation observed in multisystem disorders. *Dermatol Clin* 1992;10:709–16.

Infections
4 Herpetic Eye Disease Study Group. Oral acyclovir for herpes simplex virus eye disease. Effect on prevention of epithelial keratitis and stromal keratitis. *Arch Ophthalmol* 2000;118:1030–6.

Other disorders
Ocular complications of dermatological therapy
22 Ruiz-Lozano RE, Hernandez-Camarena JC, Garza-Garza LA *et al*. Isotretinoin and the eye: a review for the dermatologist. *Dermatol Ther* 2020;33:e14029.
26 Royal College of Ophthalmologists. *Hydroxychloroquine and Chloroquine Retinopathy: Recommendations on Monitoring*. 2020. https://www.rcophth.ac.uk/2020/12/hydroxychloroquine-and-chloroquine-retinopathy-recommendations-on-monitoring/ (last accessed November 2022).

CHAPTER 108

Dermatoses of the Oral Cavity and Lips

Barbara Carey[1] and Jane Setterfield[2]

[1]Department of Oral Medicine, Guy's and St Thomas' NHS Foundation Trust, London, UK
[2]Centre for Host-Microbiome Interactions, King's College London Faculty of Dentistry, Oral and Craniofacial Sciences, London, UK; Department of Oral Medicine and St John's Institute of Dermatology, Guy's and St Thomas' NHS Foundation Trust, London, UK

PART 10: SPECIFIC SITES, SEX & AGE

Introduction

Oral and labial lesions are usually the result of local disease but may be the early signs of systemic disease, including dermatological disorders. This chapter discusses disorders of the periodontal and mucosal tissues that may be related to skin disease and/or may present to a dermatology clinic.

It provides a brief overview of the biology of the mouth followed by review of the more common signs and symptoms affecting specific oral tissues and how to undertake an oral examination optimally. The remainder of the chapter is divided into sections based upon types of clinical presentations, e.g. lumps and bumps, pigmented, red or white lesions and oral ulceration. The chapter concludes with the oral manifestations of systemic diseases and oculo-cutaneous syndromes. Only the more classic oral lesions are illustrated. Approximately 20 of the colour illustrations are from *Oral and Maxillofacial Diseases*, 2010 (reproduced by kind permission of C. Scully, S. Flint, J.V. Bagan *et al.*, Informa, London). More detail of histology is available elsewhere [1]. Diseases affecting the teeth, salivary glands, jaws or temporomandibular joints are not discussed because problems in these sites should be referred directly to their dental surgeon, oral medicine or oral and maxillofacial surgery.

It is important to remember that diseases confined to the oral soft tissues may best be referred to oral medicine for diagnosis and management. Complex mucocutaneous disorders will, however, be optimally managed with a multidisciplinary team.

BIOLOGY OF THE MOUTH

The oral cavity is a unique anatomical structure, characterised by a combination of soft and hard tissues, which is continuously challenged by the external environment. It is a site where pathogens, antigens and allergens are often first encountered and thus it has significant protective and immunological roles. It is notable that the oral mucosa heals very effectively often with minimal scarring in

health, partly on account of the rapid turnover of epithelial cells. However, in disease it may be very slow to heal. Thus, it is vital to ensure that the clinician and patient are aware of this before changing doses or therapeutic interventions.

Lips

The opening of the oral cavity is surrounded by the lips. The lips mainly consist of bundles of striated muscle, particularly the *orbicularis oris* muscle. The labial mucosa on the inner lip is a wet surface within which there is a profusion of minor salivary glands. The outer lip, or vermilion, is the transitional zone between the glabrous skin and the mucous membrane, and is found only in humans. It contains no hair or sweat glands but does contain sebaceous glands (Fordyce spots). The epithelium of the vermilion is distinctive, with a prominent stratum lucidum and a very thin stratum corneum. The dermal papillae are numerous at this site, with a rich capillary supply, which produces the reddish-pink colour of the lips in white people. Melanocytes are abundant in the basal layer of the vermilion of pigmented skin, but are infrequent in white skin.

The *oral commissures* are the angles where the upper and lower lip meet. The upper lip includes the *philtrum*, a midline depression, extending from the columella of the nose to the superior edge of the vermilion zone.

Oral epithelium

The oral epithelium consists of a *functional compartment* – the progenitor cells (basal and parabasal cells) – which is the site of cell division; a *maturation compartment* (spinous and granular cells) where the cells become more terminally differentiated; and a superficial *cornified compartment* of squames and areas of keratinisation, either orthokeratotic or parakeratotic. In the non-keratinised regions such as the buccal mucosa (cheek) and floor-of-mouth, overt keratinisation and granular cells are absent and the surface cells are flattened, with elongated nuclei.

Oral mucosa

The mucosa is divided into masticatory, lining and specialised types. *Masticatory mucosa* (hard palate, attached gingiva) is adapted to the forces of pressure and friction and is keratinised, with numerous tall rete ridges and connective tissue papillae and little submucosa. *Lining mucosa* (buccal, labial and alveolar mucosa, floor of mouth, ventral surface of tongue, soft palate, lips) is non-keratinised, with broad rete ridges and connective tissue papillae and abundant elastic fibres in the lamina propria. The buccal mucosae are similar in structure to the lips with which they are continuous, but contain a fat pad in the subcutaneous tissue. The floor of the mouth is formed by mucosa overlying the mylohyoid muscle. In the midline lies the lingual frenum, on either side of which is the opening of the submandibular duct (Wharton's duct) from the associated submandibular gland. Similarly, in the upper arch midline is the labial frenulum that attaches the lip to the uppermost aspect of the attached gingiva.

Specialised mucosa on the dorsum of the tongue, adapted for taste and mastication, is keratinised, with numerous rete ridges and connective tissue papillae, abundant elastic and collagen fibres in the lamina propria and no submucosa. The tongue is divided by a V-shaped groove, the *sulcus terminalis*, into an anterior two-thirds and a posterior third (Figure 108.1). Various papillae on the dorsum include the *filiform papillae*, which cover the entire anterior surface and form an abrasive surface to control the food bolus as it is pressed against the palate, and the *fungiform papillae*. The latter are mushroom-shaped red structures covered by non-keratinised epithelium. They are scattered between the filiform papillae and have taste buds on their surface. Adjacent and anterior to the sulcus terminalis are eight to 12 large *circumvallate papillae*, each surrounded by a deep groove into which open the ducts of serous minor salivary glands. The lateral walls of these papillae contain taste buds.

The *foliate papillae* consist of four to 11 parallel ridges, alternating with deep grooves in the mucosa, on the lateral margins on the posterior part of the tongue. There are taste buds on their lateral walls. The *lingual tonsils* are round or oval prominences with intervening lingual crypts lined by non-keratinised epithelium. They are part of *Waldeyer's oropharyngeal ring* of lymphoid tissue. The lingual tonsil is a mass of lymphoid tissue in the posterior third of the tongue, between the epiglottis posteriorly and the circumvallate papillae anteriorly. It is usually divided in the midline by a ligament.

Teeth

The teeth are important in mastication. Each tooth consists of a crown, which varies in shape dependent on position in the mouth, with one or more roots. Teeth comprise a crown of insensitive enamel, surrounding sensitive dentine, and a root which has no enamel covering. Teeth contain a vital pulp (nerve and blood vessels) and are supported by the periodontal ligament which connects the root to the socket within the alveolar process of the jaws (maxilla and mandible). The fibres of the periodontal ligament attach through cementum on the root surface to the dentine surface. With erosion of the cementum and gingival recession, the root surfaces may become very sensitive. The alveolus is covered by the gingivae, or gums, which in health are pink, stippled and tightly bound down, and form a close-fitting cuff, with a small sulcus (gingival crevice) around the neck of each tooth.

The first or primary (deciduous or milk) dentition comprise 20 teeth. The secondary or permanent teeth begin to erupt at about the age of 6–7 years. The normal permanent (adult) dentition comprises two incisors, a canine, two premolars and three molars in each quadrant (32 teeth).

Junction of the mucosa with the teeth

The dentogingival junction represents a unique anatomical feature concerned with the attachment of the gingival (gum) mucosa to the tooth. Non-keratinised gingival epithelium forms a cuff surrounding the tooth, and at its lowest point on the tooth is adherent to the enamel or cementum. This 'junctional' epithelium is unique in being bounded both on its tooth and lamina propria aspects by basement membranes. Above this is a shallow sulcus or crevice (up to 2 mm deep), the gingival sulcus or crevice. Neutrophils continually migrate into the gingival crevice, and there is also a slow exudate of serum (crevicular fluid) into the saliva.

Saliva

Saliva is produced by the three paired major salivary glands (parotid, submandibular and sublingual), together with the many minor salivary glands throughout the oropharynx. A reasonable indication of salivary flow may be obtained by measuring the resting (unstimulated) salivary flow over a period of 10 minutes. In health, the rate will normally be around 0.35 mL/min, with a range of 0.2–0.5 mL/min. However, this will be reduced in patients with xerostomia secondary to xerostomic medications or underlying conditions such as Sjögren's syndrome. Saliva flow also reduces overnight and explains why patients often wake with a dry mouth.

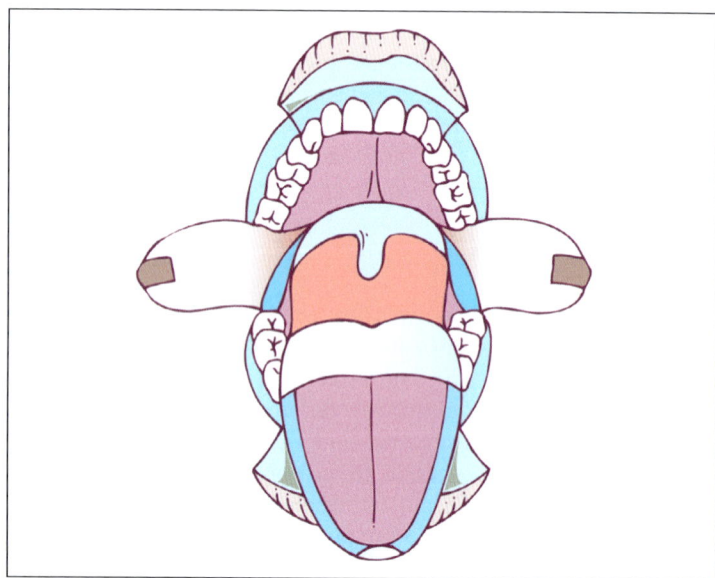

Figure 108.1 Diagram of the oral cavity.

Immunity in the oral cavity

The host defence in the oral cavity is complex and involves several components: saliva, the periodontium and the tonsilar lymphoid tissue. Additionally, movement of the soft tissues during speech and swallowing, and salivation, ensures that much foreign material is swallowed. The need for this cleaning mechanism is clearly apparent in patients with facial paralysis, or in those with xerostomia, in whom there is accumulation of oral debris and subsequent infection. Saliva aggregates bacteria and deters their attachment to surfaces. In xerostomia, patients have higher levels of dental plaque and an increased risk of periodontitis and candidiasis than otherwise healthy individuals. Additionally, saliva contains many molecular elements which restrict microbial growth. These include lysozyme which cleaves bacterial cell walls, lactoferrin which complexes iron ions and is an essential microbial nutrient, and antimicrobial peptides such as histatins that inhibit the growth of *Candida albicans* and *Streptococcus mutans*.

The gingival sulcus (the space between the tooth and the gum) is susceptible to inflammation caused by plaque bacteria. This region, however, has a high turnover of keratinocytes and a rich vasculature that enables leukocyte emigration, and both of which protect against bacterial invasion. Additionally, the sulcus is bathed with a serum exudate called gingival crevicular fluid, which carries complement components as well as antibodies, neutrophils and plasma cells.

The tonsils comprise the palatine, lingual and tubal tonsils as well as the adenoids (pharyngeal tonsils) and are collections of lymphoid tissue beneath the epithelium. The different tonsillar tissues form a ring of lymphoid tissue known as Waldeyer's ring. The tonsils are often a site of bacterial infection and are the main induction sites for mucosal immunity in the oropharynx. These are part of the common mucosal immune system leading to induction of secretory IgA antibodies locally and at distant mucosal sites as well as linking to the systemic immune system.

The mucosal immune system has evolved to provide protection against pathogens yet maintain a tolerance (termed 'oral tolerance') towards non-harmful commensal microbes and benign environmental substances. It is by far the largest component of the entire immune system with regard to the deployment of immune cells and the production of immunoglobulins [1]. Secretory IgA (SIgA) is produced in quantities far exceeding those of all other immunoglobulin isotypes combined [2]. Whereas bone marrow derived serum IgA is mostly monomeric, and consists predominantly of IgA1 subclass, SIgA is dimeric and consists of variable proportions of IgA1 and IgA2. Secretory IgA is produced in salivary gland tissue and derives its B cells from the gut-associated lymphoid tissue (GALT) system. Salivary acinar cells produce a secretory component (transport piece) needed for transport of immunoglobulin A (IgA) into the saliva and its stability in the presence of salivary or gastric proteolytic enzymes. Salivary IgA aggregates oral bacteria such as *Streptococcus mutans*, reducing the formation of dental plaque. Although the exact contribution to oral defence made by salivary IgA antibodies is difficult to assess, some patients who have IgA deficiency suffer from oral infections, and in animals it is possible to induce protective salivary IgA antibodies to caries-producing organisms such as *Streptococcus mutans*.

Neutrophils and other leukocytes are particularly essential for oral health as shown by the fact that patients with HIV infection, neutropenia, agranulocytopenia, leukaemia or chronic granulomatous disease are predisposed to severe gingivitis and rapid periodontal breakdown, as well as ulceration and infections.

Oral microbiome

The oral microbiome is defined as the collective genome of microorganisms that reside in the oral cavity. After the gut, it is the second largest microbial community in humans, comprising a core microbiome common to all individuals, and a variable microbiome which is unique to an individual but is determined by lifestyle and physiological differences. The teeth, tongue, cheeks, gingival sulcus, tonsils, hard palate and soft palate provide a rich environment in which microorganisms can flourish [3].

The role of the oral microbiome is an area undergoing extensive research and to date is poorly understood. However, it is recognised that both maintenance of health and conversely disease susceptibility, involves a complex interplay between host immunity, genetics and environmental factors including the host microbiome.

PRESENTATION OF ORAL LESIONS

Patients presenting to a dermatology clinic will generally complain of one of the following symptoms: pain (with or without visible changes in the mucous membranes), pain associated with epithelial thinning (atrophy), ulceration or blistering, a lump (persistent or fluctuating), a colour change (pigmentation, white or red lesion) or oral dryness. It is vital to take a detailed history of symptoms, comorbidities, concurrent medication and family history. This, combined with a detailed systematic examination, will determine the diagnosis in the majority of cases.

EXAMINATION OF THE MOUTH AND PERIORAL REGION

Examination includes inspection under a good light, and palpation of the cervical lymph nodes, salivary glands and oral cavity. The extraoral assessment includes inspection of the lips, face and neck, noting any obvious asymmetry, masses or changes to the skin. Malignant tumours in the face, head or neck may cause facial paralysis due to perineural tumour spread. Perineural invasion of the facial nerve result in facial palsy, while involvement of the trigeminal nerve may result in facial pain, facial numbness and/or weakness of muscles supplied by this nerve.

Assess any mass, swelling or lump by inspection and palpation. Note the shape of the lump and if the borders are regular or irregular. Check the consistency if it feels soft, hard (e.g. in malignancy) or rubbery (e.g. a lymph node). Assess if the lump feels mobile or is tethered to other local structures.

PART 10: SPECIFIC SITES, SEX & AGE

Table 108.1 Drainage areas of cervical lymph nodes.

Area	Draining lymph nodes
Central lower lip, the floor of the mouth and the tip of tongue	Submental
Cheeks, the lateral aspects of the nose, upper lip, lateral parts of the lower lip, gums and the anterior tongue. Also receive lymph from the submental and facial lymph nodes.	Submandibular
Scalp, face and neck	Superficial lymph nodes
Nose, the nasal cavity, the external acoustic meatus, the tympanic cavity and the lateral borders of the orbit	Superficial parotid
Nasal cavities and the nasopharynx	Deep parotid
Superficial areas of the face and temporal region	Pre-auricular
Posterior neck, upper ear and the back of the external auditory meatus	Post-auricular
Occipital area of scalp	Occipital
Superficial surfaces of the anterior neck	Anterior superficial cervical lymph nodes
Superficial surfaces of the neck	Posterior superficial cervical lymph nodes

Lymph nodes (Table 108.1)

Lymph from the superficial tissue of the head and neck generally drains first to groups of superficially placed lymph nodes, then to the deep cervical lymph nodes. Systematically, each region needs to be examined lightly with the pulps of the fingers, trying to roll the lymph nodes against harder underlying structures. With the patient seated upright, expose the neck from the jawbone to clavicles. Examine the patient from behind if possible. Ask the patient to tilt their chin slightly downwards to allow for muscle relaxation and allow easier palpation.

- Parotid, mastoid and occipital lymph nodes can be palpated simultaneously using both hands.
- Superficial cervical lymph nodes are examined with lighter palpation as they can only be compressed against the softer sternomastoid muscle.
- Submental lymph nodes are examined by tipping the patient's head forward and rolling the lymph nodes against the inner aspect of the mandible.
- Submandibular lymph nodes are examined in the same way with the patient's head tipped to the side being examined.
- The deep cervical lymph nodes, which project anterior or posterior to the sternomastoid muscle, can be palpated. The jugulodigastric lymph node should be specifically examined, as this is the most common lymph node involved in tonsillar infections.
- The supraclavicular region should be examined at the same time as the rest of the neck; lymph nodes here may extend up into the posterior triangle of the neck on the scalene muscles, behind sternomastoid.
- Any asymmetry in size, consistency, tenderness and swelling should be documented. Lymph nodes that are tender may be inflammatory (lymphadenitis). Nodes that are increasing in size and are hard or fixed to adjacent tissues may be malignant.
- Both anterior and posterior cervical nodes should be examined as well as other nodes, liver and spleen if systemic disease is a possibility.

Jaws

There is wide normal individual variation in morphology of the face. Most individuals have facial asymmetry but of a degree that cannot be regarded as abnormal. Maxillary, mandibular or zygomatic deformities or lumps may be more reliably confirmed by inspection from above (maxillae/zygomas) or behind (mandible). The jaws should be palpated to detect swelling or tenderness.

Salivary glands

The major salivary glands include the parotid and submandibular salivary glands [4]. Inspect and palpate for symmetry, enlargement, evidence of salivary flow from salivary ducts and the appearance of saliva. The parotid glands can be palpated by placing fingers over the pre-auricular region and angle of mandible. Early enlargement of the parotid gland is characterised by outward deflection of the lower part of the earlobe, which is best observed by looking at the patient from behind. This simple sign may allow distinction from simple obesity. The submandibular glands can be bimanually palpated using fingers inside the mouth and extraorally. The submandibular gland is best palpated with a finger of one hand in the floor of the mouth lingual to the lower molar teeth, and a finger of the other hand placed over the submandibular triangle. The submandibular duct (Wharton's duct) opens at the side of the lingual fraenum on the anterior floor of the mouth.

Intraoral examination

The examination should be conducted in a systematic fashion to ensure that all areas are included. If the patient wears any removable prostheses or appliances, these should be removed in the first instance. Use of a head light can be helpful for examining the oral cavity because it frees both hands for the examination. Dry the mucosa with gauze to improve visibility. White and red plaques and textural changes should be noted by careful palpation. Ulceration and lumps, their size, tenderness, and extension to adjacent anatomical sites should be recorded.

All mucosal surfaces should be examined, starting away from the location of any known lesions. The labial mucosa, buccal (cheek) mucosae, floor of mouth and ventrum of tongue, dorsal surface of the tongue, hard and soft palates, gingivae and teeth should then be examined in sequence and lesions noted on a diagram of the oral cavity (Figure 108.1).

Lips. The lips should be inspected first. Features such as cyanosis are seen mainly in the lips in cardiac or respiratory disease; angular cheilitis (stomatitis) is seen mainly in oral candidosis or in iron, vitamin or immune deficiencies. Examination is facilitated if the mouth is gently closed at this stage, so that the lips can then be everted to examine the labial mucosa.

Labial mucosa. Normally appears moist with a fairly prominent vascular arcade. In the lower lip, the many minor salivary glands are easily visible. Many adults have a few yellowish pinhead-sized papules in the vermilion border (particularly of the upper lip) and at the commissures; these are ectopic sebaceous glands (Fordyce spots), and may be numerous, especially as age advances.

Cheek (buccal) mucosa. This is readily inspected if the mouth is held half open. The vascular pattern and minor salivary glands are not obvious, but Fordyce spots may be conspicuous, particularly near the commissures and retromolar regions in adults. Place the surface of a dental mirror against the buccal mucosa. The mirror should lift off easily; if it adheres to the mucosa, then xerostomia is present.

Floor of mouth and ventrum of the tongue. These are best examined by asking the patient to push the tongue first into the palate then into each cheek in turn. This raises for inspection the floor of the mouth, an area where tumours may start. Its posterior part is the most difficult area to examine well and one where lesions are most easily missed. Lingual veins are prominent and, in the elderly, may be conspicuous (lingual varices). Bony lumps on the alveolar ridge lingual to the premolars are most often tori (torus mandibularis). The quantity and consistency of saliva should be assessed. Examine for normal pooling of saliva in the floor of the mouth.

Dorsum of the tongue. This is best inspected by protrusion, when it can be held with gauze. The anterior two-thirds of the tongue is embryologically and anatomically distinct from the posterior third and separated by large circumvallate papillae (Figure 108.2). The anterior two-thirds is coated with many filiform, but relatively few fungiform, papillae often located anteriorly (Figure 108.3). Behind the circumvallate papillae, the tongue contains several large lymphoid masses (lingual tonsil) and the foliate papillae lie on the lateral borders posteriorly. The tongue may be fissured but this is usually regarded as a developmental anomaly. A mild coating is not

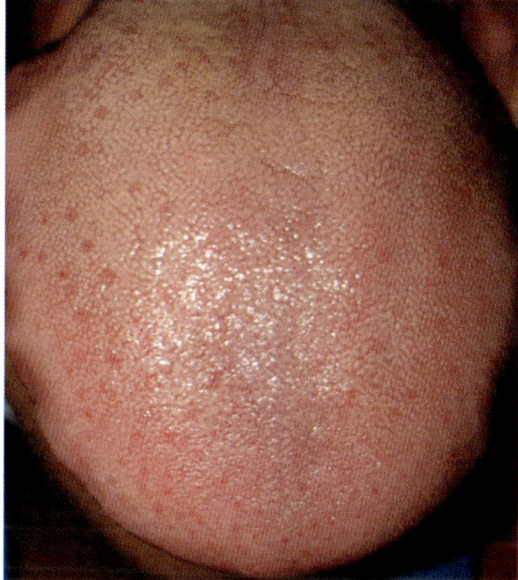

Figure 108.3 Anterior two-thirds of the tongue coated with many filiform and fewer fungiform papillae.

uncommon in healthy adults. Abnormalities of tongue movement (neurological or muscular disease) may be obvious from dysarthria or involuntary movements and any fibrillation or wasting noted. Hypoglossal palsy may lead to deviation of the tongue towards the affected side on protrusion.

Palate and fauces. These consist of an anterior hard and posterior soft palate, and the tonsillar area and oropharynx. The mucosa of the hard palate is firmly bound down and appears pink/grey as a mucoperiosteum (similar to the gingivae) and with no obvious vascular arcades. Rugae are present anteriorly on either side of the incisive papilla that overlies the incisive foramen. Bony lumps in the posterior centre of the vault of the hard palate are usually tori (torus palatinus). The palate should be inspected and movements examined when the patient says 'Aah'. The soft palate is delineated by two small palatal pits in the midline and is mobile. Using a mirror to depress the tongue, this permits inspection of the posterior tongue, tonsils, oropharynx, and can even offer a glimpse of the larynx. Glossopharyngeal palsy may lead to uvula deviation to the contralateral side.

Anatomical variants

Patients sometimes become concerned after noticing various anatomical variants in the mouth. These include tori and exostoses, which are developmental bony lumps [5,6]. Most common is torus palatinus, a slow-growing, asymptomatic, benign, bony lump in the midline of the palate (Figure 108.4). Tori mandibularis are bilateral, asymptomatic, benign, bony lumps lingual to the premolars (Figure 108.5).

The diagnosis is confirmed by radiography. These are excised or reduced only if causing severe difficulties with dentures. Rarely, there is a need to exclude other conditions such as Gardner syndrome and familial polyposis coli.

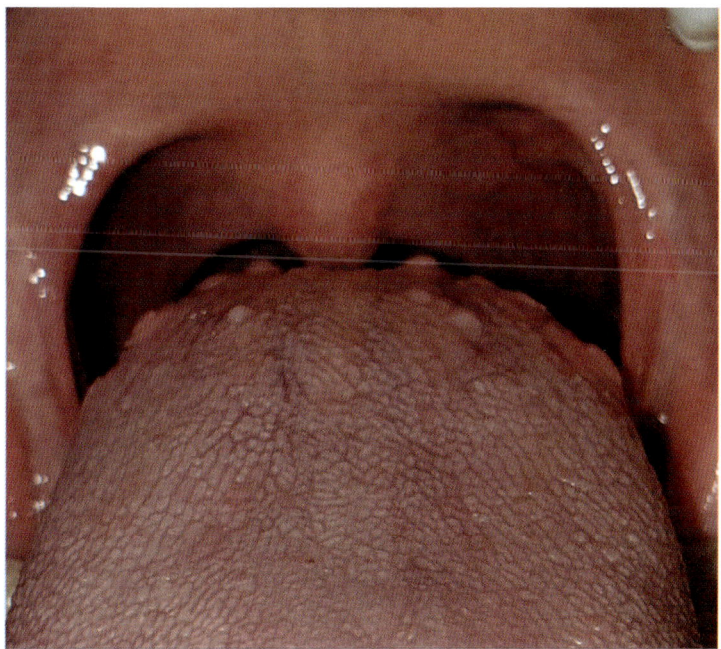

Figure 108.2 Circumvallate papillae involving the posterior dorsum tongue.

PART 10: SPECIFIC SITES, SEX & AGE

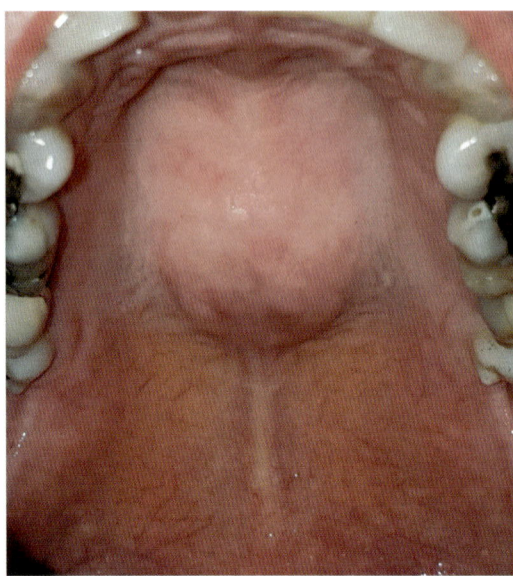

Figure 108.4 Torus platinus.

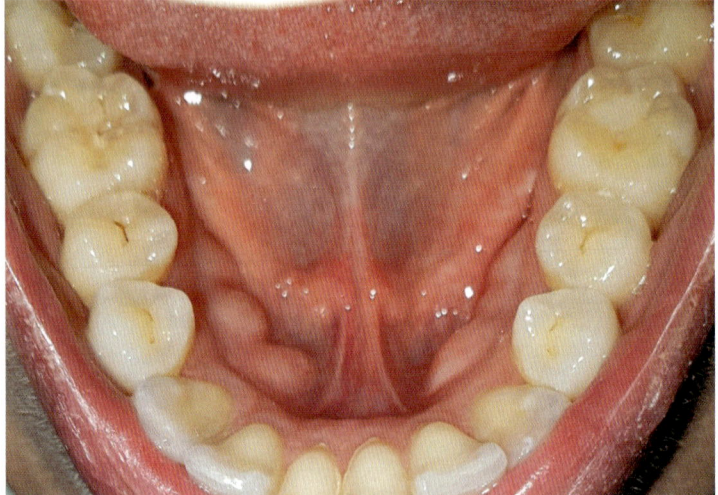

Figure 108.5 Tori mandibularis presenting as bilateral lumps lingual to the premolars.

Oral Disease Severity Score

The oral disease severity score (ODSS) (Figure 108.6) is a validated method of assessing oral disease scoring applicable to most oral mucosal diseases [7–9]. It has now been validated for use in pemphigus vulgaris (PV), oral lichen planus and mucous membrane pemphigoid. The ODSS records the presence of lesions and degree of activity at multiple oral sites. Additionally, it includes a subjective assessment of the patient's degree of oral pain over the preceding week. The ODSS divides the mouth into 17 sites weighted according to area of possible involvement and allocated a site score of 0–2. The sites include the outer/inner lips, left and right buccal mucosa, six gingival segments, hard palate (left/right or both), soft palate (left/right or both), dorsum tongue (left/right or both), left ventral tongue, right ventral tongue, floor of mouth (left/right or both), and oropharynx. Individual sites are allocated an activity score (0–3), reflecting mild inflammation (minimal erythema or a white 'healing' mucosa) = 1; moderate inflammation (marked erythema

Date:			Consultant:	
Name:			M / F:	
Hospital No.			Diagnosis:	
DoB:			Management:	

Site	Site	Activity		Pain
Upper lip (1)				0
Lower lip (1)				
R Buccal mucosa (1 or 2)				1
L Buccal mucosa (1 or 2)				
Gingivae (1 each segment)				2
Lower R				
Lower central				3
Lower L				
Upper R				4
Upper central				
Upper L				5
Dorsum of tongue (1 or 2)				
R Ventral tongue (1)				6
L Ventral tongue (1)				
Floor of mouth (1 or 2)				7
Hard palate (1 or 2)				
Soft palate (1 or 2)				8
Oropharynx (1 or 2)				
Total				9
				10

TOTAL SCORE	

Figure 108.6 Oral Disease Severity Score.

but no ulceration) = 2; and ulceration = 3. A subjective assessment of the patient's oral pain in the preceding week is included (based on a visual analogue scale 0–10). The theoretical maximum total score is 106. Combined with serological markers, the ODSS can confirm a clinical and immunological response to therapy.

The ODSS and Autoimmune Bullous Skin Disorder Intensity Score (ABSIS) have been validated for use in oral PV and mucous membrane pemphigoid. The disease-specific Pemphigus Disease Area Index (PDAI) and Mucous Membrane Pemphigoid Disease Area Index (MMPDAI) have been validated for use in oral PV and mucous membrane pemphigoid, respectively.

Measurement of quality of life provides a patient-based measure to assess disease burden and monitor activity. The Oral Health Impact Profile (OHIP) is the most common generic patient-based instrument used in oral medicine. The Chronic Oral Mucosal Disease Questionnaire (COMDQ) is a validated instrument to evaluate chronic conditions of the oral mucosa. The Autoimmune Bullous Disease Quality of Life (ABQOL) and Treatment of Autoimmune Bullous Disease Quality of Life (TABQOL) have been shown to be reliable and valid instruments for the assessment of quality of life in autoimmune bullous disease.

LUMPS AND SWELLINGS

Lumps and swellings in the mouth range from simple anatomical variants, which can cause the patient considerable concern, to

Box 108.1 Lesions that may cause lumps or swellings in the mouth

Normal anatomical features
- Pterygoid hamulus
- Parotid papillae
- Foliate or circumvallate papillae
- Unerupted teeth

Developmental
- Haemangioma
- Lymphangioma
- Palatal and mandibular tori
- Hereditary gingival fibromatosis
- Von Recklinghausen neurofibromatosis
- Cysts of developmental origin

Inflammatory
- Abscess
- Pyogenic granuloma
- Oral Crohn disease
- Orofacial granulomatosis
- Sarcoidosis
- Granulomatosis with polyangiitis

Traumatic
- Epulis
- Fibroepithelial polyp
- Denture-induced granuloma
- Mucocoele
- Herniation of buccal fat pad

Infective
- Various papillomatous lesions

Cystic
- Cysts of odontogenic origin (e.g. dental cysts)

Deposits
- Amyloidosis (oral manifestations of systemic diseases)

Drug therapy (gingival swelling only)
- Oral contraceptive (pill gingivitis)
- Phenytoin
- Calcium-channel blockers
- Ciclosporin

Hormonal
- Pubertal gingivitis
- Pregnancy epulis/gingivitis

Blood dyscrasias
- Leukaemia, lymphoma and myeloma

Benign neoplasms

Malignant neoplasms

Others
- Angioedema
- Fibro-osseous diseases
- Acanthosis nigricans (oral manifestations of systemic diseases)

pathological lumps caused by inflammatory, cystic, neoplastic and other disorders (Box 108.1).

Lip or facial swelling may be diffuse or localised. If it appears rapidly over a few minutes or up to an hour, it may be caused by an insect bite or sting, or angioedema. If the swelling appears over hours or days is often inflammatory in origin. Swelling that appears over days or weeks may be caused by granulomatous disorders (e.g. orofacial granulomatosis or sarcoidosis). Swelling that appears over weeks or months may be due to a neoplasm or deposits such as amyloidosis. Facial swelling that is persistent may be caused by fluid (e.g. vascular lesions or lymphangiomas), solids (e.g. neoplasms), deposits (e.g. amyloidosis) or foreign material (e.g. fillers).

SOFT TISSUE SWELLING

Abscesses

The two main types of dental abscess are periapical abscess (originates in the dental pulp) and periodontal abscess (originates in the supporting structures of the teeth) [1,2]. Periapical abscess formation is usually secondary to dental decay whereas periodontal abscess formation is associated with chronic periodontitis. Most intraoral abscesses are odontogenic in origin. Most discharge intraorally on the buccal gingiva but occasionally discharge palatally, lingually, on the chin or submental region (Figure 108.7). Very occasionally, abscesses follow trauma or a foreign body, or rarely are related to unusual oral infections such as actinomycosis or nocardiosis. The usual signs include swelling with cervical lymphadenopathy and gum swelling with a purulent exudate. Drainage and appropriate antimicrobials are indicated [3]. Dental attention is required; dental abscesses are drained by tooth extraction, incision and drainage, or through the root canal (endodontics).

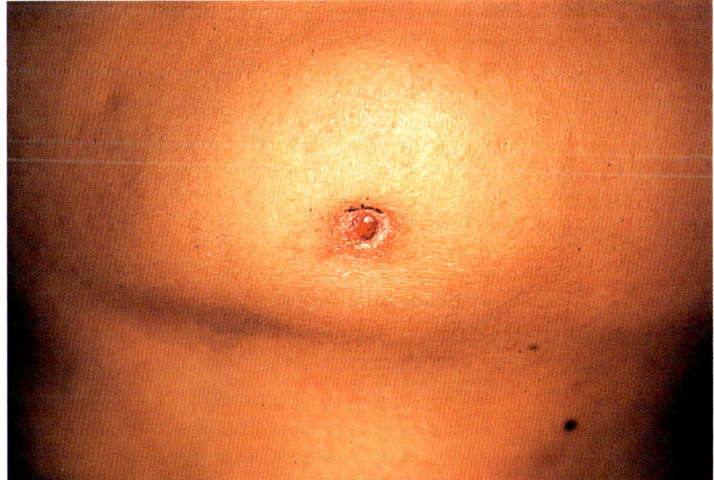

Figure 108.7 Sinus on the chin related to a dental abscess on a mandibular incisor tooth.

Angioedema

Angioedema manifests with rapid development of oedematous swelling of the lips, tongue and oral or facial swelling. It can be life-threatening as oedema may also involve the neck and compromise the airway. The swelling is usually relatively transient and the skin does not scale. Angioedema may be acquired or hereditary. Acquired forms may be of allergic origin (histaminergic angioedema) or non-allergic. Allergic angioedema is a type 1 hypersensitivity response seen predominantly in those with atopy. Hereditary angioedema is caused by a deficiency of the complement component C1 esterase inhibitor (C1-INH) [1–3]. Acquired angioedema may be drug-induced (mainly by angiotensin-converting enzyme inhibitors and non-steroidal anti-inflammatory drugs (NSAIDS)) or complement-mediated (due to an acquired deficiency of C1-inhibitor) [3]. Occasionally, the precipitating agent is not clearly identified. All types of angioedema may be aggravated by the oral contraceptive pill (OCP) or hormone replacement therapy.

- Allergic angioedema may be induced by foods (e.g. shellfish, eggs nuts), drugs (e.g. antibiotics, aspirin, exposure to latex or insect bites/stings). Allergic angioedema results from mast-cell and basophil activation, with release of histamine and bradykinin, causing vasodilatation and increased vascular permeability. The oedema appears within 60 minutes of antigen exposure and can cause pronounced itchy labial and periorbital swelling and involve any oral site.
- Non-allergic angioedema can manifest after many weeks of drug exposure. The swelling usually affects the lips, although it can be localised to the tongue or soft palate. Intramuscular adrenaline (epinephrine), and systemic corticosteroids and/or antihistamines, such as chlorphenamine may be indicated for allergic and non-allergic angioedema.
- Hereditary angioedema is a rare autosomal dominant disorder caused by C1-INH deficiency. It mimics allergic angioedema, although it produces a more severe reaction, with oedema affecting the lips, mouth, face and neck region, the extremities and gastrointestinal tract after minor trauma. It may not present until later childhood or adolescence, and nearly 20% of cases are caused by spontaneous genetic mutation. Type I hereditary angioedema exhibits low levels of functionally normal C1-INH, while in the type II variant, C1-INH is dysfunctional. In both types, plasma C4 levels fall but C3 levels are normal. Type III is X-linked and seen in women in relation to pregnancy or OCP use linked with F12 gene mutations. Blunt injury is the most consistent precipitating event. The trauma of dental treatment is a potent trigger, and some attacks follow emotional stress. It is characterised by acute onset of non-itchy or painful oedema affecting the lips, tongue, mouth, face and neck region, the extremities and the gastrointestinal tract – with abdominal pain and sometimes diarrhoea. Oedema may persist for many hours and even up to 4 days. Involvement of the airway is a constant threat. Management is with C1-INH replacement, plasminogen inhibitors such as tranexamic acid, the bradykinin-receptor antagonist icatibant, the plasma kallikrein inhibitor ecallantide, fresh frozen plasma, or androgenic steroids, such as danazol and stanozolol, which raise plasma C1-esterase inhibitor levels to normal [4,5].

Buccal fat-pad herniation

Trauma may rarely cause the buccal fat pad to herniate through the buccinator muscle, producing an intraoral swelling [1,2]. The condition is rare and usually occurs in males from 5 months to 12 years of age. Treatment options include excision or repositioning of the herniated fat.

Denture-induced hyperplasia

Denture-induced hyperplasia is a hyperplastic condition of the oral mucosa caused by chronic excessive mechanical pressure on the vestibular mucosa by ill-fitting dentures. Where a denture flange is overextended and irritates the vestibular mucosa, a linear reparative process may result, eventually producing an elongated fibroepithelial enlargement. Firm leaf-like painless swellings are seen, usually in the buccal or labial vestibule. It is usually asymptomatic but sometimes severe inflammation and ulceration can occur. The pathology is that of a fibrous lump. A denture-induced granuloma should be excised and examined histologically to exclude more serious pathology if modification of the denture does not induce regression.

Eruption cyst

This is a bluish, fluctuant cystic swelling over an erupting tooth. It is most frequently seen in babies overlying a primary tooth but may occur in childhood in association also with the permanent dentition. It is usually painless and spontaneously resolves in most cases (Figure 108.8).

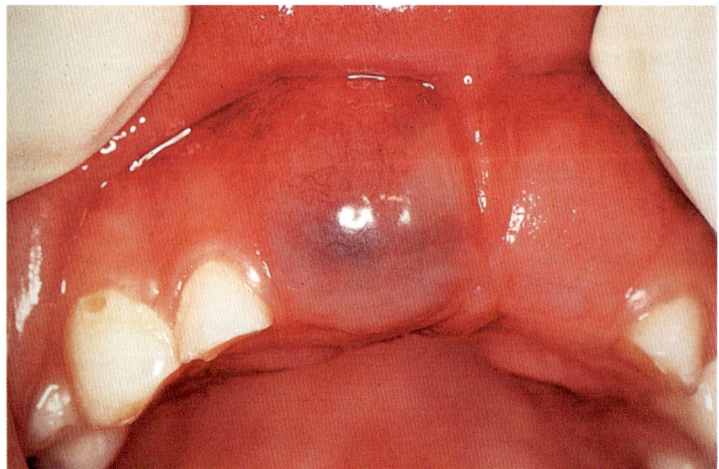

Figure 108.8 Bluish, fluctuant swelling of an oral cyst, in this case an eruption cyst over an erupting maxillary permanent incisor. (The lesion on the maxillary canine is early dental caries.)

Focal epithelial hyperplasia (multifocal epithelial hyperplasia)

Focal epithelial hyperplasia, also known as Heck's disease, is a rare benign familial disorder (through transmission of human papillomavirus (HPV)) with no sex predisposition, presenting with soft, nodular elevations of the oral mucosa [1–4]. Heck disease occurs particularly in American Indian people, in Inuit people in Greenland and in Chinese people but has been reported rarely from many other countries. The prevalence in Greenland and Venezuela approaches 35%.

The papillomaviruses HPV-13 and HPV-32 appear to be causal in patients with the genetic predisposition to focal epithelial hyperplasia [5]. Household transmission of HPV through saliva and the shared use of contaminated objects may be implicated.

The characteristics of focal epithelial hyperplasia are local epithelial hyperplasia, acanthosis and elongated 'Bronze Age axe' rete ridges, together with a ballooning type of nuclear degeneration. Koilocyte changes and mitosoid bodies are present in the superficial keratinocytes.

The condition is characterised by the occurrence of multiple circumscribed, sessile, soft, elevated papules or nodules in the oral cavity, especially on labial and buccal mucosa, lower lip and tongue, which sometimes form clusters [6].

Focal epithelial hyperplasia is a benign asymptomatic condition and requires no treatment, except in some cases of functional (e.g. lesions that are repeatedly traumatised on biting) or aesthetic impairment.

Foliate papillitis

The foliate lingual papillae may become inflamed and swell in response to oral or upper respiratory tract infection [1]. Because of their location on the posterolateral tongue this may give undue concern about malignancy. The condition resolves spontaneously.

Lingual tonsil

The lingual tonsil is a mass of lymphoid tissue in the posterior third of the tongue, between the epiglottis posteriorly and the circumvallate papillae anteriorly [1,2]. It is usually divided in the midline by a ligament (Figure 108.9). Although usually small and asymptomatic, it may become enlarged, especially in infections and atopy. It may be so prominent that it fills the vallecula and impinges against the epiglottis. If the lingual tonsil is large, it may cause a globus sensation, alteration of the voice, obstructive sleep apnoea or airway obstruction [3,4]. It tends to involute with increasing age.

Occasionally, there may be lingual tonsillitis with a red, swollen, painful tongue, fever and neutrophilia.

The condition should be distinguished from benign and malignant tumours of the tongue, including lingual thyroid, but the symmetry of the lingual tonsil and its midline division are helpful diagnostic pointers.

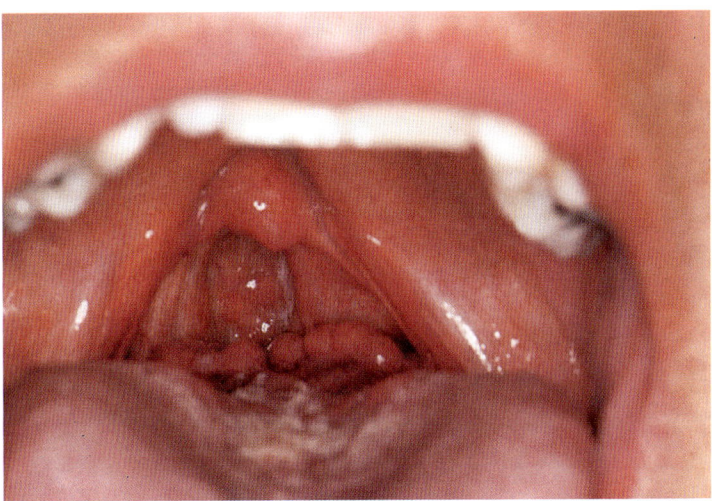

Figure 108.9 Lingual tonsil showing a well-demarcated midline groove. Courtesy of Dr C.T.C. Kennedy.

Treatment may be required if the enlarged tonsil causes symptoms. Surgery may be hazardous because of the copious blood supply to the tongue base. Electrocautery and cryotherapy are generally regarded as the safer procedures.

Gastro-oesophageal reflux and body mass index may be associated with lingual tonsil hypertrophy in adults with sleep-disordered breathing.

Lingual thyroid

Ectopic thyroid tissue may rarely present clinically in the mouth, although some 10% of cadaver tongues contain thyroid tissue. Typically, an asymptomatic, smooth-surfaced lump in the midline of the base of the tongue, between the sulcus terminalis and epiglottis at the site of the foramen caecum [1–3], a lingual thyroid may occasionally produce dysphagia, cough, pain or, rarely, airways obstruction [4].

Not all lingual thyroid tissue is functional, and function tends to decline with age. Where thyroid-stimulating hormone levels are high, thyroid hormone supplements are indicated. Malignant change is rare in lingual thyroid, although follicular carcinomas have been recorded. MRI and ^{99m}Tc pertechnetate scintiscanning is important to ensure the presence of normal thyroid tissue in the neck before considering treatment of a lingual thyroid by surgery or radioiodine. If removal is deemed appropriate a total lingual thyroidectomy transoral approach with use of either a microscope or a robotic endoscope for optical assistance is recommended [5].

Macroglossia

Macroglossia is enlargement of the tongue. True macroglossia (apparent enlargement of the tongue due to an underlying disease or condition) and relative macroglossia (normally sized tongue fills a small oral cavity) may be further subdivided into congenital and acquired disorders [1]. Congenital causes include

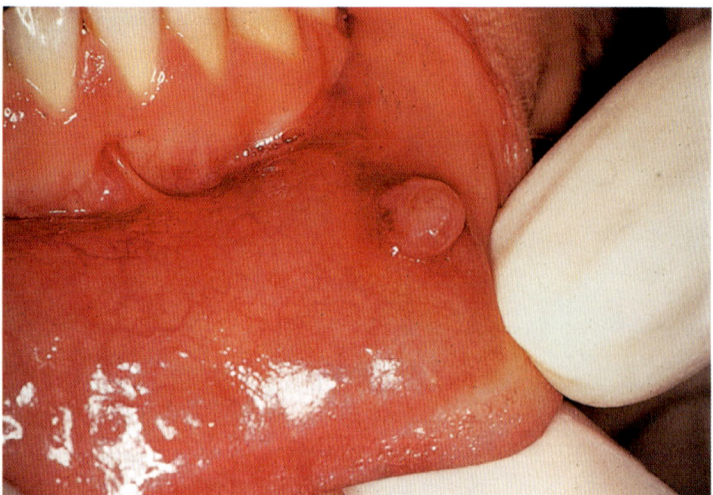

Figure 108.10 Mucocoele.

Down syndrome, Pierre Robin syndrome, Beckwith Wiedemann syndrome, mucopolysaccharidoses (Hunter syndrome and Hurler syndrome), Pompe disease, Robinow syndrome, Crouzon syndrome and idiopathic muscular hypertrophy. Focal enlargement is caused by congenital tumours such as haemangiomas and lymphangiomas. Acquired causes include allergic reactions, amyloidosis, neurofibromatosis, head and neck infections, trauma, polymyositis, inflammatory diseases, venous congestion, benign tumours (lymphangioma, haemangioma, lipoma), malignant tumours and endocrine disorders (hypothyroidism, acromegaly). Progressive macroglossia occurs in the mucopolysaccharidoses. Symptoms include drooling, difficulty speaking and eating, and airway obstruction.

Mucocele (mucous cyst)

Mucoceles are common and usually seen in the lower labial mucosa (Figure 108.10), resulting from the escape of mucus into the lamina propria from a damaged minor salivary gland duct (extravasation mucoceles). This type of mucocele is not, however, lined by epithelium, and therefore is not a true cyst. Mucoceles appear usually as solitary, painless, dome-shaped, fluctuant translucent, whitish blue papules or nodules [1–3]. Occasionally mucoceles are caused by saliva retention (retention mucoceles), especially in the floor of mouth and are termed 'ranula'. Care should be taken to ensure that the lesion is not a salivary gland tumour with cystic change, especially when dealing with an apparent mucocele in the upper lip. Mucoceles can be seen on the palate in graft-versus-host disease (GVHD) [4]. Superficial mucoceles may also be seen in lichen planus [5]. Mucoceles can be excised but they also respond well to cryosurgery [3,6].

Nodular fasciitis

Nodular (pseudosarcomatous) fasciitis affects the head and neck in 20% of cases but rarely involves the mouth [1–4]. In the mouth, most cases involve the lips and buccal mucosae. The spindle cells are positive for smooth muscle actin and muscle-specific actin (HHF-35) antibodies. Treatment typically involves conservative excision, but the lesion may regress spontaneously [1].

Oral allergy syndrome

Oral allergy syndrome (OAS), also known as 'pollen-fruit allergy syndrome', is a type of food allergy limited to the oral mucosa and caused by uncooked fruit, raw vegetables, flavours and nuts [1–3]. An IgE-mediated hypersensitivity to an environmental allergen triggers the food allergy. The most frequent symptoms are a combination of oral pruritus, irritation or swelling of the lips, tongue, palate and throat, sometimes associated with other allergic features such as rhinoconjunctivitis, asthma, urticaria, angioedema and anaphylactic shock. The adverse effects begin quickly after eating raw fruits or vegetables. OAS can happen at any time during the year.

In patients who are adversely affected by birch tree pollen, fruit such as apples, cherries, nectarines, peaches and pears may provoke a response. Likewise, in subjects with birch-pollen allergy, carrot, celery, almond and hazelnut may also cause oral pruritus. Individuals with grass allergy may have a response to kiwi, peach and tomatoes. Those with responses to ragweed may have OAS when eating melon, cucumber and banana. Latex-sensitive patients may be sensitive to bananas, avocado, kiwi and chestnuts. OAS may respond to antihistamines, corticosteroids and epinephrine (intramuscular). Cooking often destroys food allergens.

Papillary hyperplasia

Papillary hyperplasia is a benign lesion of the oral mucosa characterised by the growth of one or more nodular lesions, measuring about 2 mm or less. The lesion almost exclusively involves the vault of the palate. It is typically associated with the use of removable upper dentures and chronic denture-related stomatitis and may be related to *Candida* infection [1–3], although has also been found in patients with no history of a dental prosthesis. The lesion is mostly asymptomatic and the mucosa may vary from pink to red.

Papillary hyperplasia may require treatment with antifungals, excision, laser removal or cryotherapy.

SOFT TISSUE BENIGN TUMOURS

Dermoid cyst

Dermoid cyst is a hamartoma, a development lesion commonly arising in the midline of the neck, above the mylohyoid. It occasionally occurs elsewhere such as the tongue, antrum and rarely the parotid gland [1–6]. Dermoid cysts usually become clinically obvious in the second decade of life and cause elevation of the tongue. Occasionally, dermoid cysts become infected and then painful. Treatment is by surgical excision.

Leiomyoma

This benign tumour of smooth muscle is rarely encountered in the oral cavity. Leiomyomas present as a slow-growing, asymptomatic submucosal mass, usually in the tongue, hard palate or buccal mucosa [1–4]. They may be seen at any age. Sometimes it is an angioleiomyoma and rarely multiple. The diagnosis is mainly determined by histological studies and immunohistochemical stains confirm the smooth muscle origin. Excision is the usual management and recurrence is rare.

Lipoma

Lipomas are uncommon in the mouth, comprising fewer than 5% of oral benign tumours [1–3]. They present as asymptomatic slow-growing, spherical, smooth and soft semifluctuant lumps with a characteristic yellowish colour. Most involve the buccal mucosa or floor of the mouth. Occasionally, lipomas can develop within the tongue [1]. Although benign, they may rarely infiltrate. Histology shows adult fat cells gathered into lobules by vascular septa of fibrous connective tissue. Angiolipomas, spindle cell lipomas and liposarcomas are in the differential diagnosis. Surgery is the treatment of choice for lipomas interfering with speaking and mastication. Infiltrating lipomas are prone to recurrence.

Lymphangioma

Lymphangiomas are uncommon congenital hamartomas of the lymphatic system. They are usually diagnosed in infancy or early childhood. Many are of similar structure to haemangiomas and can clinically resemble them, with a 'frog-spawn' appearance, but they contain lymph rather than blood (Figure 108.11). Approximately 75% of lymphangiomas are located in the head and neck. The oral cavity is rarely affected. Although uncommon, the most frequent site of occurrence of lymphangioma in the mouth is on the tongue, followed by the palate, gingiva, lips, alveolar ridge and rarely buccal mucosa [1–5]. Lymphangiomas are usually solitary. They are occasionally associated with cystic hygroma.

Contrast-enhanced T1-weighted magnetic resonance imaging (MRI) can be used to differentiate between lymphangiomas and deep haemangiomas. Small lymphangiomas need no treatment. Larger lesions may require excision, although cryotherapy, laser therapy, sclerotherapy and radiofrequency ablation can be useful.

Multiple mucosal neuroma syndrome

The syndrome of multiple endocrine neoplasia (MEN) type 2b is inherited as an autosomal dominant condition, although new cases often arise sporadically. The gene locus is on chromosome 10 with germline mutations in the RET proto-oncogene.

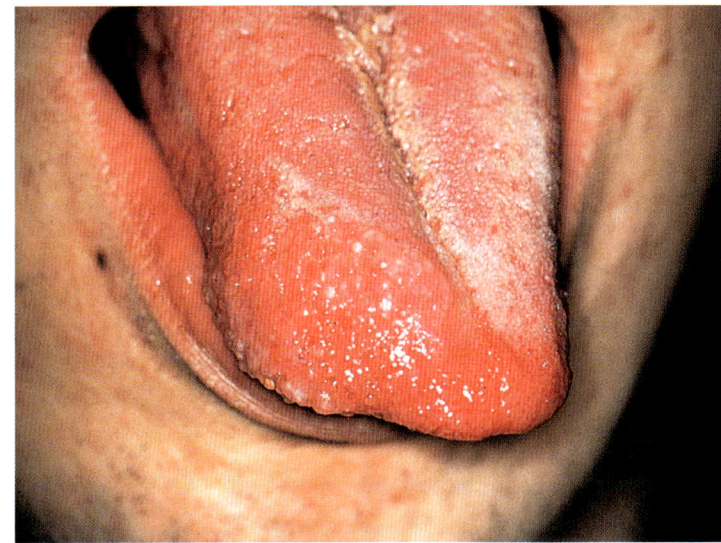

Figure 108.11 Lymphangioma of the tongue.

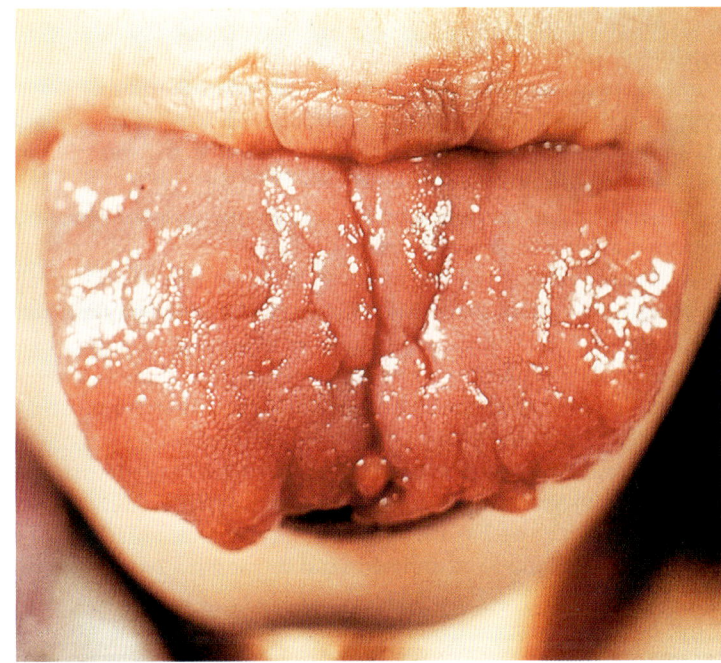

Figure 108.12 Multiple neuromas of the lips and tongue in a patient with multiple endocrine neoplasia syndrome (type 2). Courtesy of Dr M. Hartog.

Multiple endocrine neoplasia type 2b is characterised by medullary carcinoma of the thyroid and phaeochromocytoma, in association with multiple mucosal neuromas and an abnormal phenotype – a striking facial appearance, with thick slightly everted lips that usually have a slightly bumpy surface due to multiple neuromas [1–4]. These are mucosal and submucosal hamartomatous proliferations of nerve axons, Schwann cells and ganglion cells.

Lesions may also involve the tongue and commissures but are less frequent on the buccal mucosa, gingivae, palate, pharynx or larynx (Figure 108.12).

Most patients have a marfanoid habitus, with high arched palate, pectus excavatum, arachnodactyly and kyphoscoliosis, but the lens subluxation and cardiovascular abnormalities of Marfan syndrome are not present. Differential diagnosis includes multiple idiopathic mucosal neuromas and *PTEN* hamartoma–tumour (Cowden) syndrome.

Myxoma

Myxomas are rare in the oral cavity, mainly as odontogenic or soft tissue myxomas [1–4]. Neurothekeoma (nerve sheath myxoma) [5] may also affect the oral cavity. Myxomas arise in bone or soft tissue and, although benign, are aggressive and difficult to eradicate because of the tendency to infiltrate normal tissue.

Papilloma

Papilloma are benign epithelial neoplasms caused by HPV [1–3]. Papillomas can appear anywhere in the mouth, but are most common at the junction of the hard and soft palate. The papilloma is a white or pink, cauliflower-like lesion that may resemble a wart. Papillomas of normal colour may be confused with fibroepithelial polyps, although the latter are most common at sites of potential trauma. Papillomas are common in HIV-infected people and have increased with the introduction of HAART [4]. Unlike some papillomas of the larynx or bowel, oral papillomas are generally benign although some are dysplastic [5].

Oral papillomas should be removed and examined histologically to establish a correct diagnosis. Histology includes acanthotic and sometimes hyperkeratotic epithelium with occasional koilocytosis. Excision must be total, deep and wide enough to include any abnormal cells beyond the zone of the pedicle. Cryosurgery or pulse dye laser or carbon dioxide (CO_2) laser may also be used.

Both common warts (verrucae vulgaris) and sexually transmitted warts (condyloma acuminatum) are caused by HPV. They are rare in the mouth (Figure 108.13) but are more common in HIV disease, especially after long-term antiretroviral therapy [5]. None is known

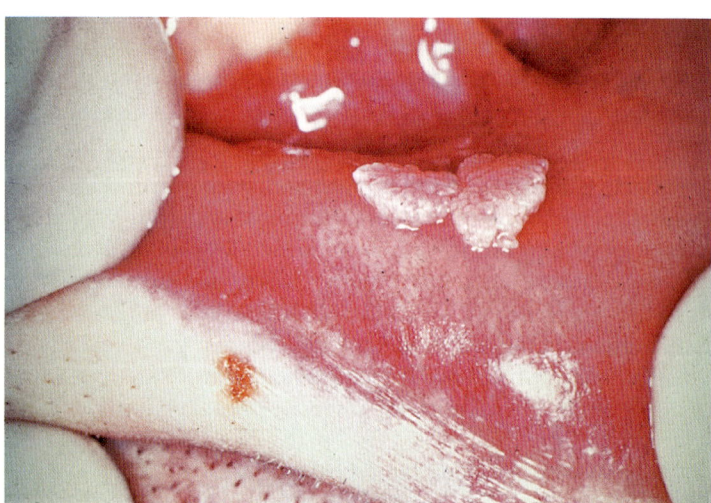

Figure 108.13 Warts on the lower lip in HIV infection.

to be premalignant. Most can be treated by excision, cryosurgery or laser.

Rhabdomyoma

Rhabdomyomas are rare but most extracardiac rhabdomyomas present in the mouth, typically as lumps in the floor of the mouth, tongue or soft palate [1–3]. Most are seen in the sixth decade, predominantly in males, most are solitary but cases with multiple lesions have been reported [3]. Surgery is effective provided total excision is achieved.

Verruciform xanthoma

Verruciform xanthoma is a very uncommon papillary growth seen chiefly in the oral mucosa but is also known occasionally to affect skin and non-oral mucosae [1,2]. The lesion is usually found in the fifth decade. The aetiology is unknown but may be a reaction to some irritant. The gingiva, alveolar mucosa and hard palate are the most common intraoral sites of involvement. It usually presents as an asymptomatic solitary, sessile or pedunculated lesion with a normal, pale, reddish or keratotic surface [1,2].

The lesions consist of parakeratotic verruciform epithelium, with large foamy xanthoma cells containing slightly periodic acid–Schiff-positive granules and abundant lipid in the lamina propria between the epithelial rete pegs.

Excision is rarely followed by recurrence. Verruciform xanthoma has been reported in GVHD [3].

HARD TISSUE BENIGN TUMOURS

Osteoma mucosae

There are rare cases of osteoma of the oral mucosa, usually in the tongue. Most have been in females in the third and fourth decades and have arisen as pedunculated hard painless lumps on the dorsum of the tongue immediately posterior to the foramen caecum [1–4]. They may arise from thyroid anlages. Simple excision suffices.

PIGMENTED LESIONS (BOX 108.2)

Most oral hyperpigmentation is physiological in origin and seen in patients with darker skin tones (Figure 108.14) but there are many other causes – especially various drugs – from antimalarials to imatinib. Seen mainly in people of African or Asian heritage, physiological pigmentation can also be noted in patients of Mediterranean descent, sometimes even in some fairly light-skinned people. It is most obvious in the anterior labial gingivae and palatal mucosa, and pigmentation is usually symmetrically distributed. Patches may be seen elsewhere. Pigmentation may be first noted by the patient in adult life and then incorrectly assumed to be acquired rather than congenital in origin. Generalised oral mucosal hyperpigmentation is usually racial in origin and only occasionally has a systemic cause, such as Addison disease.

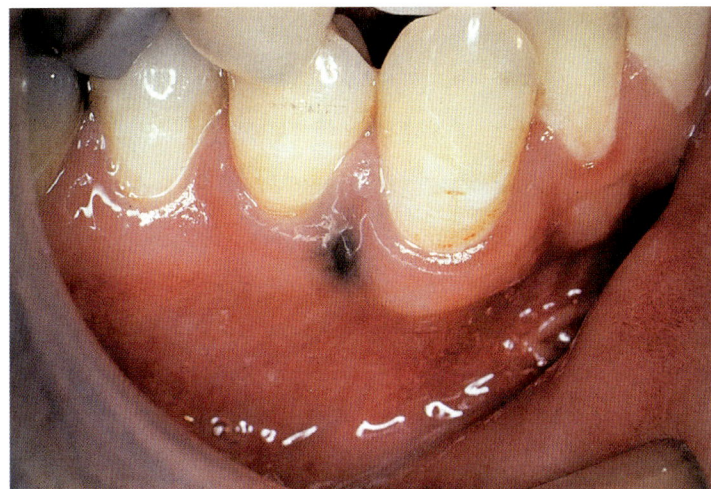

Figure 108.15 Amalgam tattoo.

Box 108.2 Causes of mucosal pigmentation

Localised
- Amalgam tattoo
- Ephelis (freckle)
- Naevus
- Malignant melanoma
- Kaposi sarcoma
- Peutz–Jeghers syndrome
- Laugier–Hunziker syndrome
- Melanotic macules

Generalised
- Physiological in darker skin tones
- Localised irritation, e.g. smoking
- Drugs, e.g. phenothiazines, antimalarials, minocycline, contraceptives
- Addison disease
- Nelson syndrome
- Ectopic adrenocorticotrophic hormone (e.g. bronchogenic carcinoma)
- Heavy metals
- Albright syndrome
- Other rare causes, e.g. haemochromatosis, generalised neurofibromatosis, incontinentia pigmenti
- Malignant acanthosis nigricans

The tongue is often discoloured due to superficial staining from foods, drinks or habits such as tobacco or betel use. Localised hyperpigmented lesions are usually due to pigmentary incontinence, amalgam tattoos, melanotic macule or naevi, although melanomas, Kaposi sarcoma and epithelioid angiomatosis must be excluded.

Wide variation in gingival colour is common clinically and may relate to physiological pigmentation and smoker's melanosis. Local causes, exogenous staining (e.g. due to betel, herbal preparations, beverages), systemic causes (including Peutz–Jeghers syndrome, acanthosis nigricans, Addison disease, chloasma, Albright

syndrome, neurofibromatosis), medications (quinacrine, phenolphthalein, minocycline, amiodarone) and heavy metal ingestion (lead, tin, mercury) may need to be considered depending on the pattern and distribution of gingival pigmentation.

Amalgam tattoos

Amalgam tattoos are a common cause of blue-black pigmentation, usually seen in the mandibular gingiva or at least close to the teeth (Figure 108.15), or in the scar of an apicectomy where there has been a retrograde root filling with amalgam used as root-end filling material [1–3]. The amalgam associates with elastin fibres. The lesion does not change significantly in size or colour and is painless. Opacities may or may not be seen on radiography. Similar lesions can result if, for some reason, pencil lead (graphite tattoo) or other similar foreign bodies become embedded in the oral tissues.

Biopsy may be indicated to exclude a melanoma but otherwise these innocuous lesions require no treatment.

Body art

Tattooing of the lower lip may occasionally be seen. A tattooed lower lip in a Sudanese woman, for example, signifies that she is married. The Wodaabe people of Nigeria and Cameroon may tattoo on the skin surface at the angle of the mouth, a practice which has its basis in the ritual of warding-off the 'evil eye'. The vermilion may be tattooed red in Western countries.

Intraoral tattooing is less common [1,2]. Traditional tattooing of the gingiva is common among some populations in Africa's Sahel region and is termed 'ethnobotanical tattooing' [3]. A number of different pigments and techniques are employed in gingival tattooing but most involve the use of soot coated thorns. Other reported tattooing agents include burnt seeds and herbs combined with lantern soot, lampblack mixed with unspecified herbs and applied with needles, lantern soot and resin from the plant *D. Stramonium* and soot.

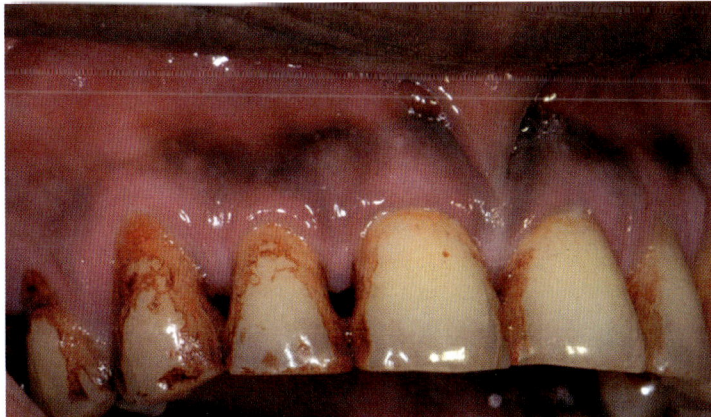

Figure 108.14 Betel staining of teeth with physiological pigmentation of the attached gingiva.

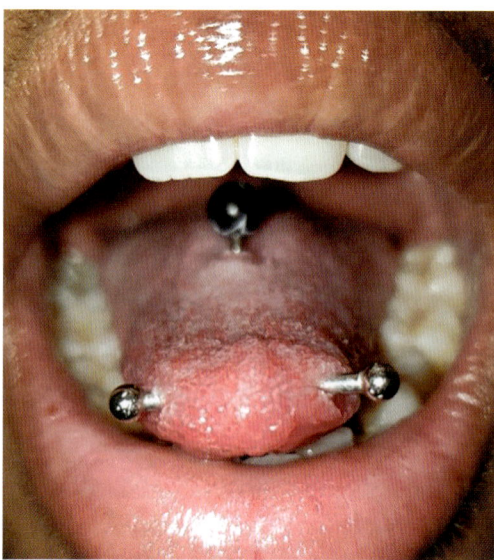

Figure 108.16 Tongue piercing.

The practice of piercing oral and facial soft tissues and then placing foreign objects/ornaments in the defects on a more or less permanent basis is one which has also been largely confined, historically, to certain tribal groups in continental Africa and isolated Amazon regions of South America. Piercing is now common in resource-rich countries. The most common sites are the tongue, followed by the lip (Figure 108.16).

Gingival recession is the most frequent complication of tongue and lip piercing [4]. Additional complications secondary to oral and facial piercings include pain, bleeding, dental fractures and gingival damage.

Carney complex

Carney complex is a rare multiple endocrine neoplasia syndrome characterised by distinctive pigmented lesions of the skin and mucosal surfaces, cardiac and non-cardiac myxomatous tumours, and multiple endocrine tumours. The Carney complex gene 1 is the regulatory subunit 1A of protein kinase A (PRKAR1A) located at 17q22-24. An inactivating heterozygous germ line mutation of PRKAR1A is observed in about two-thirds of Carney complex patients. Carney complex causes cardiac and cutaneous myxomas, with mammary myxoid fibroadenomas, spotty cutaneous hyperpigmentation, primary pigmented nodular adrenocortical disease, testicular Sertoli cell tumours and growth hormone-secreting pituitary adenoma. It may present with oral hyperpigmentation and myxomas [1–4].

The hyperpigmentation in Carney complex is facial and occurs on the vermilion of the lips in about 35%, although about 8% have pigmented lesions on the oral mucosa and about 2% have oral myxomas, usually on the palate or tongue [2,3]. Carney complex differs clinically from Peutz–Jeghers syndrome in that hyperpigmentation is less common intraorally but more common on the conjunctiva, and other manifestations are also present.

Carney complex has been previously called NAME (nevi, atrial myxoma, ephelides) and LAMB (lentigines, atrial myxoma, blue nevi) syndrome. In LEOPARD (lentigines, EKG (electrocardiogram) abnormalities, ocular hypertelorism, pulmonary stenosis, abnormal genitalia, retardation of growth, and sensorineural deafness) syndrome, lentigines tend to involve a large portion of the skin, including the face, neck and upper trunk, which is in contrast with the Carney complex.

Coated, furred, brown or black hairy tongue

Children rarely have a furred (coated) tongue in health but it may be coated with off-white debris in febrile and other illnesses. Adults, however, not infrequently have a coating on the tongue in health, particularly if they are edentulous, are on a soft non-abrasive diet, have poor oral hygiene or are fasting. The coating appears more obvious in ill patients or those with hyposalivation, especially those who cannot maintain oral hygiene.

The coating in most cases consists of epithelial, food and microbial debris; indeed, the tongue is the main oral reservoir of some microorganisms, such as *Candida albicans* and viridans streptococci. The filiform papillae become excessively long and stained by the accumulation of squames and chromogenic microorganisms.

Habits such as alcohol, tobacco and betel use, various medicaments such as chlorhexidine or iron, and confectionery or beverages can cause a black or brown superficial staining of the tongue (and teeth) [1–4].

Occasionally, a brown or black hairy tongue may be caused by drugs that induce hyposalivation, or antimicrobials, when it may be related to overgrowth of microorganisms such as *Candida* species.

Black hairy tongue usually involves the posterior and middle dorsal tongue (Figure 108.17).

Patients with black hairy tongue may find the condition improves if they avoid habits or drugs that stain the tongue, increase their standard of oral hygiene, brushing the tongue with a hard toothbrush, use sodium bicarbonate mouthwashes, chew gum, eating rougher foods such as raw fruits and vegetables, or suck a dry peach stone. Fresh pineapple (not tinned or pasteurised) contains a proteolytic enzyme called bromelaine that can break down the overgrown papillae.

Drug, food, habits and heavy metal induced hyperpigmentation

Causes (Box 108.2) can include [1–6]:
- Foods and beverages (such as beetroot, red wine, coffee and tea).
- Confectionery (such as liquorice).
- Smoking tobacco – a fairly common cause (smoker's melanosis) and this may produce extrinsic discoloration but also intrinsic pigmentary incontinence, with pigment cells increasing and appearing in the lamina propria. Nicotine may stimulate melanocytes located in the basal layer of the oral mucosa. It is

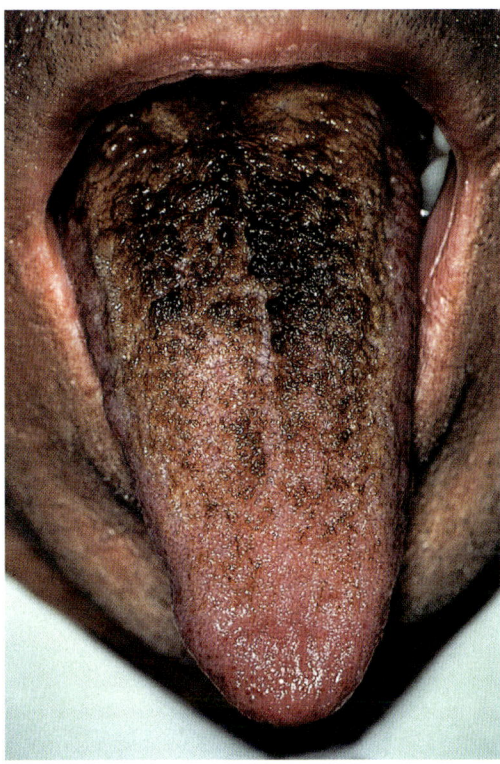

Figure 108.17 Black hairy tongue.

especially likely in persons who smoke with the lighted end of the cigarette within the mouth (reverse smoking), with pigmentation changes most common on the hard palate. Smoker's melanosis is characterised by irregular hyperpigmentation of the oral mucosa. Brown patches are most commonly located on the anterior labial gingiva in cigarette smokers and on the buccal mucosa in pipe smokers. Over months or years, smoker's melanosis gradually disappears after smoking cessation.

- Chewing betel may cause superficial brownish-red discoloration, mainly in the buccal mucosa (and on the teeth), with an irregular epithelial surface that has a tendency to desquamate, seen mainly in women from South and South-East Asia (see Figure 108.14). The epithelium in betel chewer's mucosa is often hyperplastic with material from the betel quid visible on the epithelial surface with ballooning of epithelial cells. Importantly betel use predisposes to submucous fibrosis and squamous cell carcinoma.
- Drugs and chemicals such as chlorhexidine, iron salts, griseofulvin, crack cocaine, minocycline, bismuth subsalicylate, lansoprazole and hormone replacement therapy. With these, hyperpigmentation may be due to deposition of the agent on oral mucosal surfaces, stimulation of melanin synthesis, drug or metabolite accumulation and bacterial metabolism.
- Drugs that cause intrinsic staining include:
  - Antimalarials produce a variety of colours in the mucosa, ranging from yellow with mepacrine to blue-black with amodiaquine.
  - Minocycline may cause grey/black discoloration of teeth, gingivae and bone, skin, sclera and even breast milk. Minocycline can, in a minority of patients, produce blue-grey gingival

pigmentation caused by staining of the underlying bone, and some intrinsic faint bluish-grey staining, mainly near the anterior teeth.
  - Busulphan, hydroxyurea, zidovudine and clofazimine oral contraceptives, phenothiazines, tetracycline, cyclophosphamide, bleomycin, fluorouracil and anticonvulsants may also occasionally produce, or increase, brown pigmentation.
  - Gold may produce purplish gingival discoloration. Many of the heavy metals formerly implicated in producing oral hyperpigmentation (such as mercury, lead and bismuth) are not used therapeutically now, although industrial or accidental exposure is still occasionally seen. Metallic sulphides deposited in the tissues were seen especially where oral hygiene was poor, with bacteria producing sulphides that resulted in pigmentation at the gingival margin (e.g. lead line).
- Some drug-induced hyperpigmentation resolves on cessation of exposure to the drug and improved oral hygiene, although resolution can take months or years.
- Endocrine causes: oral hyperpigmentation may be seen in adrenocorticotrophic hormone therapy, Addison disease, Nelson syndrome or ectopic adrenocorticotrophic hormone production (e.g. by bronchogenic carcinoma). The brown or black pigmentation is variable in distribution but is seen typically on the soft palate, buccal mucosa and at sites of trauma.

HIV infection

Oral hyperpigmentation may be seen in HIV infection, sometimes related to adrenal hypofunction or drug use [1,2].

Inherited patterned lentiginosis

This is an extremely rare, autosomal dominant condition reported in patients of **African descent**, especially those with mixed American Indian heritage. It is characterised by small discrete hyperpigmented macules on the face, lips, extremities, buttocks and palmoplantar areas [1]. No series of patients have been reported with oral mucosal lesions or internal organ system abnormalities.

This condition can resemble other lentiginosis syndromes, especially Peutz–Jeghers syndrome, centrofacial lentiginosis syndrome and Carney complex.

Lentiginoses

The lentiginoses (or lentigenoses) include Peutz–Jeghers syndrome, LEOPARD syndrome (lentigines, EKG (electrocardiogram) abnormalities, ocular hypertelorism, pulmonary stenosis, abnormal genitalia, retardation of growth, and sensorineural deafness), syndrome of arterial dissections with lentiginosis, Laugier–Hunziker–Baran syndrome, Cowden disease, Ruvalcaba–Myhre–Smith (Bannayan–Zonana) syndrome, and the centrofacial, benign patterned and segmental lentiginoses, all of which can be associated with a variety of developmental defects.

Laugier–Hunziker syndrome

Laugier–Hunziker syndrome is an acquired, benign disorder presenting in adults with labial, oral mucosal and nail hyperpigmentation [1–5]. A possible variant of this or Peutz–Jeghers syndrome has been termed *idiopathic lenticular pigmentation*, in which there are oral, labial, perianal and digital hyperpigmented lenticular macules. Treatment with cryosurgery, Q-switched alexandrite laser and Nd-Yag laser has been reported [6]. There are no underlying systemic abnormalities and no malignant predisposition.

Melanoma

Oral melanoma is rare and highly aggressive. Most patients are over 50 years of age and there is a male preponderance. Mucosal melanomas account for fewer than 1% of all melanoma. However, they account for approximately 10% of melanoma of the head and neck. The most common sites for mucosal melanoma are nasal, paranasal sinuses, oral cavity and nasopharynx. Malignant melanoma may arise in apparently normal oral mucosa or in a pre-existent pigmented naevus, most commonly (~80%) in the palate or maxillary alveolus [1–5]. The initial presentation is often swelling, which is usually with a brown, dark blue, or black macule. Satellite foci may surround the primary lesion. Advanced lesions may present as a raised, nodular or polypoid mass. Amelanotic oral melanomas are rare. Features suggestive of malignancy include a rapid increase in size, change in colour, ulceration, pain, bleeding, the occurrence of satellite pigmented spots, or regional lymph node enlargement. The prognosis is poor unless detected very early. Metastatic melanoma is rare. Surgery is the mainstay of treatment in oral melanoma. c-KIT (CD117) is overexpressed in more than 80% of mucosal melanoma [6]. BRAF protein mutations are uncommon in mucosal melanoma and found in fewer than 10%. Histology may show anaplastic spindle-shaped or squamoid cells. However, the histology is quite varied and staining with dopa or antibodies may be required to help the diagnosis. Most cases are positive for S-100, tyrosinase and Mart-1/melana-A. Lesions suspected to be melanoma should not be biopsied until the time of definitive surgical excision.

Melanocanthoma

Oral melanoacanthoma is a rare reactive melanocytic lesion with solitary or multifocal diffuse pigmentation, found mainly in children: most reported cases have been in individuals with highly pigmented skin. A hyperpigmented symptomless macule appears over a course of days or weeks. It is thought to be a reactive response to local trauma or chronic irritation. There is a female predominance among the patients with solitary oral melanoacanthoma,

whereas multifocal oral melanoacanthoma showed an equal gender distribution. Multifocal lesions tended to occur on the palate, and solitary lesions on the buccal mucosa. The sudden appearance and rapid radial growth often mimics melanoma. Biopsy is required to exclude mucosal melanoma and shows increased numbers of dendritic melanocytes in an acanthotic epithelium. The course is benign, and some cases resolve spontaneously within 6 months [1–5]. No specific treatment is required but argon plasma coagulation is a relatively safe and effective modality.

Melanotic macule

The melanotic macule is the most common mucosal pigmented lesion. It is an acquired, small, flat, brown to brown-black, asymptomatic, benign lesion, unchanging in character. Oral melanotic macule is similar to the ephelis and lentigo. Melanotic macules are usually solitary, discrete, pigmented brown collections of melanin-containing cells.

It can occur on the lips and intraorally, especially at the keratinised sites, such as gingiva and palate, and ranges in colour from brown to black (Figure 108.18). Most on the lips are seen near the midline, on the lower lip vermilion [1–4]. They are typically symmetric with sharp borders. Clinically, the melanotic macule may resemble other lesions such as early melanoma and ephelides, although the latter tend to fade in winter and darken in summer.

Histopathologically, the mucosal epithelium is normal apart from increased pigmentation of the basal layer, accentuated at the tips of rete ridges. There are no naevus cells or elongated rete ridges. There is melanin in the epithelial basal layer and/or upper lamina propria. Occasionally they are seen along with melanonychia striata (Laugier–Hunziker syndrome).

In contrast to melanoma, basal layer melanocytes are not increased. Melanotic macules occasionally appear suddenly as reactive lesions following trauma. Excision biopsy may be indicated to exclude melanoma or for cosmetic reasons.

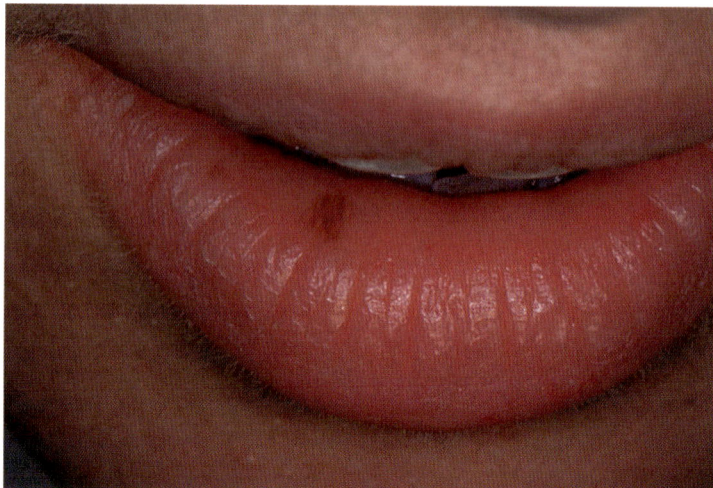

Figure 108.18 Melanotic macule of the lower lip.

Oral melanocytic naevi

Oral melanocytic naevi are much less common in the oral mucosa than in skin [1]. Approximately half of naevi are histologically of the intradermal (intramucosal) type; one-third are blue naevi; many others are compound naevi; and some are junctional naevi.

They are formed from increased melanin-containing cells, are flat or raised, do not change rapidly in size or colour, are painless and are seen particularly on the palate. The intramucosal type of naevus is most common (about 60%), while another 25% are blue naevi. Compound and junctional naevi and combined naevi are rare in the mouth. The intramucosal naevus consists of a collection of melanocytic cells in the lamina propria without involvement of the epithelium. The blue naevus consists of spindle cells at any level in the lamina propria. The junctional naevus consists of clusters of benign naevus cells at the epithelio–mesenchymal junction and the lamina propria is otherwise not involved. Naevi are seen particularly on the vermilion border of the lip and on the palate or buccal mucosa [2,3]. They usually present as a solitary, brown or blue, well-circumscribed nodule or macule, do not change rapidly in size or colour and are painless. There is no evidence that most pigmented naevi progress to melanoma [3]. However, pigmented naevi may resemble melanomas and if early detection of oral melanomas is to be achieved, all pigmented oral cavity lesions should be viewed with suspicion. Therefore, excisional biopsy is recommended to exclude malignancy and may also be performed for cosmetic reasons. This is particularly important if the lesions are raised or nodular.

Peutz–Jeghers syndrome

Peutz–Jeghers syndrome is an autosomal dominant trait most often due to germline mutations in the *STK11* (*LKB1*) gene encoding a serine threonine kinase mapped to chromosome 19p13.3 and is characterised by gastrointestinal hamartomatous polyps, mucocutaneous pigmentation, especially circumorally, and an increased risk of gastrointestinal and non-gastrointestinal cancer. Mucocutaneous pigmented macules are present in more than 95% of individuals with Peutz–Jeghers syndrome and are caused by pigment-laden macrophages in the dermis. Those affected have discrete flat brown to bluish black macules mainly around the oral, nasal and ocular orifices, 1–5 mm in size. The lips, especially the lower, have pigmented macules in about 98% of patients (Figure 108.19) [1–4]. The buccal mucosa in involved in 66% of Peutz–Jeghers syndrome individuals. Mucocutaneous pigmentation usually occurs during the first one to two years of life, increases in size and number over the ensuing years, and finally fades after puberty. Oral brown or black macules, unlike the circumoral lesions, do not fade after puberty. Malignant transformation is extremely rare.

Intestinal polyps are found mainly in the small intestine and rarely undergo malignant change but if they produce intussusception, surgical intervention is required. There is a slightly increased risk of gastrointestinal carcinoma and carcinomas of the pancreas, lung, breast, uterus and ovary.

Ruby and argon lasers have been used to treat the pigmentation of the lips and oral mucosa.

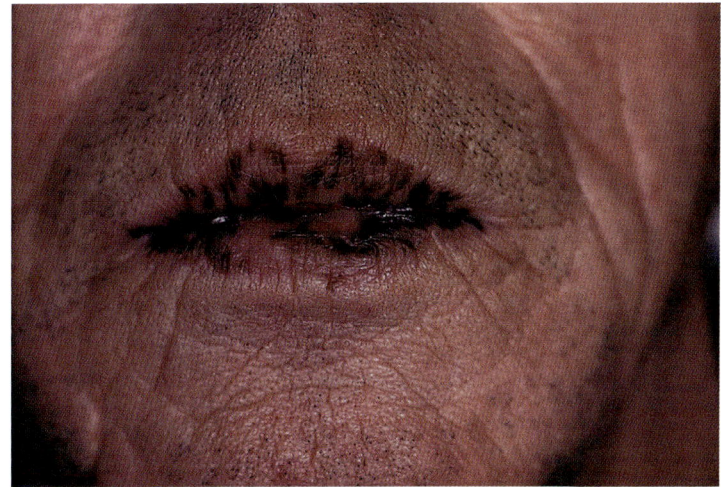

Figure 108.19 Peutz–Jeghers syndrome.

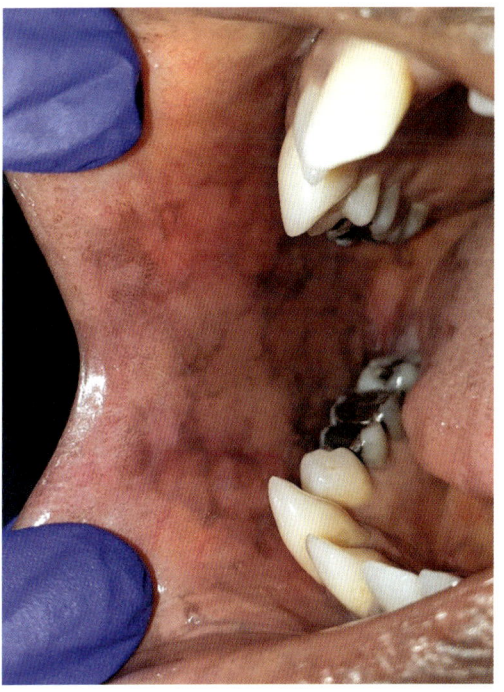

Figure 108.20 Postinflammatory hyperpigmentation in oral lichen planus.

Pigmentary incontinence

Melanin pigment ingested by macrophages in the upper lamina propria (pigmentary incontinence) may give rise to hyperpigmentation in lichen planus, especially in dark-skinned people (Figure 108.20) [1].

RED LESIONS

Some red lesions may be associated with localised inflammation (e.g. infections or traumatic injury), autoimmune conditions (e.g. mucous membrane pemphigoid) or may be additionally associated with epithelial thinning (atrophy) (e.g. geographic tongue or lichen planus) or desquamation (e.g. desquamative gingivitis). Lesions in pemphigus vulgaris are associated with epithelial thinning, will appear red and are very painful. Structural vascular changes are also often red (e.g. telangiectasia), with vascular proliferation (e.g. haemangiomas), increased vascular permeability (e.g. purpura) or malignant lesions (e.g. leukaemia or Kaposi sarcoma). This section will be grouped into:

1 Inflammatory lesions, e.g. infection or autoimmune, trauma or atrophic lesions.
2 Vascular lesions: structural anomalies or tumour-related.

INFLAMMATORY LESIONS

Acrodermatitis enteropathica

Acrodermatitis enteropathica is a rare autosomal recessive inborn error of metabolism resulting in zinc malabsorption and severe zinc deficiency. It is the result of mutations in the *SLC39A4* gene, which encodes a protein involved in zinc transport [1–4].

Clinical features

Diarrhoea, mood changes, anorexia and neurological disturbance are reported, most frequently in infancy. Growth retardation, alopecia, weight loss and recurrent infections are prevalent in affected toddlers and schoolchildren. A vesiculobullous dermatitis with perioral involvement may be seen, often sparing the vermilion [2]. Zinc deficiency during growth periods results in growth failure and lack of gonadal development in males. Other effects of zinc deficiency include skin changes, poor appetite, mental lethargy, delayed wound healing, neurosensory disorders and cell-mediated immune disorders. Skin lesions and poor wound healing are observed in severe forms and the disorder can be lethal.

Diagnosis

Assays of zinc in granulocytes and lymphocytes provide better diagnostic criteria for marginal zinc deficiency than plasma zinc assays.

Management

Patients with acrodermatitis enteropathica require high doses of zinc to overcome the defect in intestinal zinc absorption (approximately 3 mg/kg/day of elemental zinc).

Angina bullosa haemorrhagica

Angina bullosa haemorrhagica is an uncommon, acquired fragility of the non-keratinised mucosa resulting in haemorrhagic bullae that spontaneously rupture leaving a ragged ulcer that heals within 1–2 days. It usually affects individuals over the age of 50 and has no known structural or systemic underlying cause. Lesions frequently involve trauma prone sites, e.g the soft palate, buccal mucosa or ventrolateral tongue. Although the blister is subepidermal it heals rapidly and without scarring [1–6]. (Figure 108.21). Patients are otherwise well, with no detectable immunological or

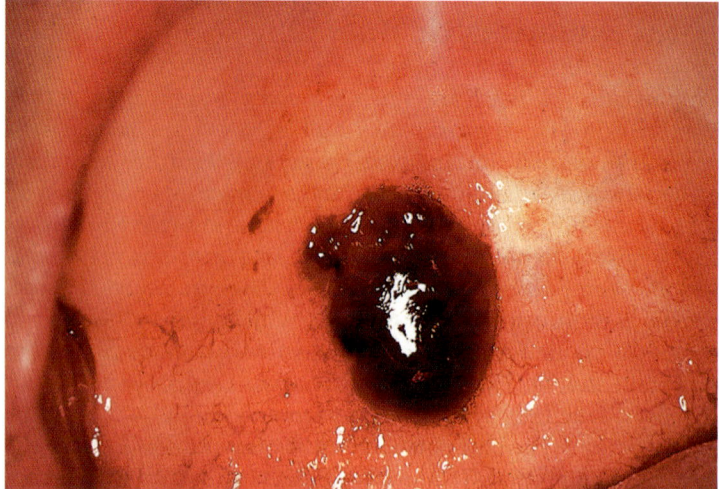

Figure 108.21 Angina bullosa haemorrhagica: a large blood blister in a typical site on the soft palate. The adjacent whitish lesions are from scarring after a previous biopsy.

bleeding disorder [1–6]. Occasional cases are related to the use of corticosteroid inhalers and trauma seems to be the major provoking factor. The diagnosis of angina bullosa haemorrhagica is mainly clinical. A clotting function test will exclude bleeding disorders that may present with intraoral blood-filled lesions. Only symptomatic care is available. The diagnosis is based upon the history and biopsy is not usually indicated.

Erythematous candidiasis

Candidiasis often presents with oral white lesions, but red variants are increasingly recognised. Erythematous or atrophic candidiasis may be seen in:

• Acute candidiasis
• Denture-related stomatitis
• Angular cheilitis
• Antibiotic- or steroid-induced stomatitis
• HIV infection

Acute candidiasis

Acute oral candidiasis may complicate corticosteroid or antibiotic therapy, particularly with long-term broad-spectrum antimicrobials. There is widespread erythema and soreness of the oral mucosa, particularly noticeable on the tongue, sometimes with associated thrush. Topical antifungals usually suffice.

Angular cheilitis

This presents as inflammation of the skin and contiguous labial mucosa located at the commissures of the mouth.

Denture-related stomatitis

This common form of mild, chronic, atrophic oral candidiasis occurs only beneath a denture, and is often asymptomatic [1–7]. It is a disease mainly of the middle-aged or older. Dentures worn

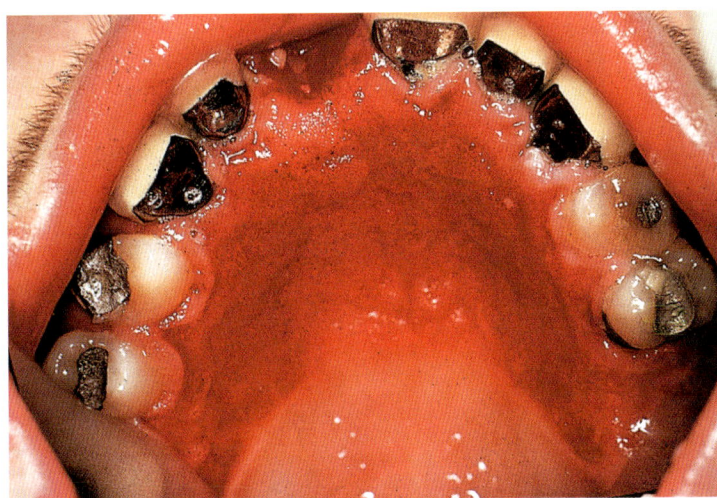

Figure 108.22 Denture-induced stomatitis showing diffuse erythema in the denture-bearing area.

throughout the night, or with a dry mouth, favour development of this infection with *Candida* species mainly. It is not caused by allergy to the denture material. It is more prevalent in women than men. Patients appear otherwise healthy. Denture-related stomatitis consists of mild inflammation and erythema of the mucosa beneath a denture (Figure 108.22).

Dentures can produce a number of ecological changes, including the following:
- Changes in the oral flora.
- Plaque accumulation between the mucosal surface of the denture and the palate.
- Saliva present between the maxillary denture and the mucosa may have a lower pH than usual.
- Accumulation of microbial plaque (bacteria and/or yeasts) on and in the fitting surface of the denture and the underlying mucosa.

Decreased salivary flow and a low pH under the denture probably results in a high *Candida* enzymatic activity, which can cause inflammation. Yeasts such as *Candida* are isolated from up to 90% of persons with denture-related stomatitis. The most frequently isolated species is *Candida albicans*. Of the *C. albicans* isolates, 75% are serotype A and 25% serotype B. *C. albicans* is the most frequently isolated species, followed by *C. tropicalis* and *C. glabrata*. Histological examination of the soft tissue beneath dentures has shown proliferative or degenerative responses with reduced keratinisation and thinner epithelium.

It is not clear why only some denture wearers develop denture-related stomatitis, since most patients appear otherwise healthy. Patients with denture-related stomatitis have no serious, cell-mediated immune defects but they may sometimes be deficient in migration inhibition factor and may have overactive suppressor T cells or other T-lymphocyte/phagocyte defects.

Predisposing factors
Dental appliances (mainly maxillary dentures), especially when worn throughout the night, or with a dry mouth, are the major predisposing factor. Diabetes, immunosuppressive therapy or a high-carbohydrate diet occasionally are predisposing factors. HIV

is a rare underlying factor. Factors that are usually *not* significant include allergy to the dental material, trauma, pharmacological agents and smoking.

Clinical features
The characteristic presenting features of denture-related stomatitis are:
- Chronic erythema and oedema of the mucosa that contacts the fitting surface of the denture.
- The mucosa below the lower dentures is rarely involved.
- Erythema is restricted to the denture-bearing area.
- Usually there are no symptoms.
- Uncommon complications include angular stomatitis and papillary hyperplasia in the vault of the palate.

Clinical variants
The lesions have been classified into three clinical types (Newton's types), increasing in severity:
- Type 1: a localised simple inflammation or a pinpoint hyperaemia.
- Type 2: an erythematous or generalised simple type presenting as more diffuse erythema involving a part of, or the entire, denture-covered mucosa.
- Type 3: a granular type (inflammatory papillary hyperplasia) commonly involving the central part of the hard palate and the alveolar ridge.

Investigations
Denture-related stomatitis is a clinical diagnosis. A full blood picture, haematinic assays and smears for fungal hyphae and culture may be warranted.

Management [8,9]
Any underlying systemic disease should be treated where possible. The oral biofilm must be removed regularly. The denture plaque and fitting surface is infested, usually with *C. albicans*, and dentures acts as a reservoir for microbial colonisation. To treat and prevent recurrence of denture-related stomatitis, dentures should be removed from the mouth at night, cleaned and disinfected, and stored in an antiseptic. Cleansing is crucial to therapeutic success. Sodium hypochlorite 0.5% can help disinfect denture liners and tissue conditioners. Hypochlorite is an effective anticandidal agent but can turn chrome cobalt dentures black. The incorporation of nystatin in those materials is also able to treat or prevent oral candidiasis. Many other cleansers are available (alkaline peroxides, alkaline hypochlorites, acids, yeast lytic enzymes).

The mucosal infection is eradicated by brushing the palate and using antifungals. Effective agents include nystatin pastilles or suspension, miconazole gel or fluconazole suspension or tablets, administered concurrently with an oral antiseptic such as chlorhexidine, which itself has antifungal activity.

HIV-associated candidiasis

It has been reported that up to 90% of HIV-infected patients develop oropharyngeal candidiasis at some time [1–8]. Low CD4 counts, denture-wearing, smoking, corticosteroid therapy, broad-spectrum

PART 10: SPECIFIC SITES, SEX & AGE

antibiotic therapy and hyposalivation predispose to candidiasis. The most dominant oral fungal species, in decreasing order of frequency, are:

- *C. albicans.*
- *C. glabrata.*
- *C. tropicalis.*
- *C. parapsilosis.*
- *C. krusei.*
- Other *Candida* species such as *C. dubliniensis, C. africanus* and *C. inconspicua.*

Erythematous or atrophic candidiasis may arise as a consequence of persistent acute pseudomembranous candidiasis when the pseudomembranes are shed, may develop *de novo*, or in HIV infection may precede pseudomembranous candidiasis. The clinical presentation is of erythematous areas generally on the dorsum of the tongue, palate or buccal mucosa. Lesions on the dorsum of the tongue present as depapillated areas. Lesions are often seen in the central palate. There can be an associated angular stomatitis.

Pseudomembranous candidiasis is a well-recognised feature of T-cell immunodeficiencies, particularly after the severe T-cell immunosuppression necessary for organ transplantation and in other secondary immunodeficiencies, such as leukaemia, diabetes or HIV/AIDS. It is a common and early feature of AIDS.

Furthermore, with increasing use of antimycotic therapy, especially in HIV disease, there is a shift towards not only resistant *C. albicans*, as well as the appearance of novel species, but also other species such as *C. glabrata* and *C. krusei*. Pseudomembranous candidiasis is characterised by white patches on the surface of the oral mucosa, tongue and elsewhere. The lesions develop to form confluent plaques that resemble milk curds, and can be wiped off to reveal a raw, erythematous and sometimes bleeding base. Complications of oropharyngeal candidiasis may sometimes present as lesions of the adjacent mucosa, particularly in the upper respiratory tract and the oesophagus. The combination of oral and oesophageal candidiasis is particularly prevalent in HIV-infected patients.

Antifungal therapy is indicated [9–12]. Tobacco habits should be stopped. Antiretroviral treatment reduces the frequency of candidiasis. The negative effects of antiretroviral treatment include: an increase in oral lesions from HPV, xerostomia, dysgeusia/ageusia, hyposmia, perioral paraesthesia, hyperpigmentation of oral mucosa, facial lipodystrophy and ulceration. Candidiasis in HIV disease may prove poorly responsive to polyene antifungal drugs, so systemic fluconazole is usually indicated.

Median rhomboid glossitis

Median rhomboid glossitis, or glossal central papillary atrophy, is a depapillated red rhomboidal area in the centre line of the dorsum of the tongue, just anterior to the sulcus terminalis [1–4]. It is uncommon and mainly found in older patients. There is a significant association between median rhomboid glossitis, *Candida* and diabetes, but the other possible risk factors, such as sex, smoking and denture wearing, may not be present. Occasionally, immune defects (including HIV) and diabetes predispose to this lesion.

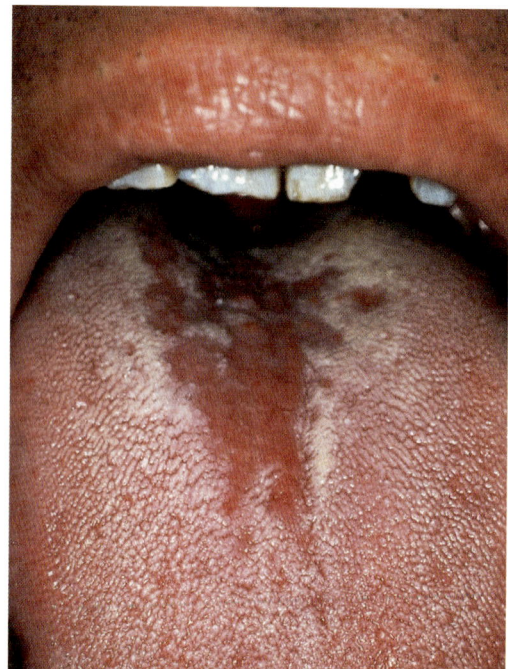

Figure 108.23 Median rhomboid glossitis.

Pathophysiology

The aetiology of the lesion is controversial. Formerly thought to be caused by persistence of the embryonic tuberculum impar, this lesion is now thought to be related to candidiasis. Culture frequently shows *Candida*. Histopathologically, candidal hyphae infiltrate the superficial layers of the parakeratotic epithelium and a neutrophil infiltrate occupies the epithelium, with elongated hyperplastic rete ridges (pseudoepitheliomatous hyperplasia) that may resemble a carcinoma (but it is not a malignant condition).

Clinical features

There is typically a red midline lesion, rhomboidal in shape, anterior to the sulcus terminalis on the dorsum of the tongue (Figure 108.23). It is usually asymptomatic. Occasionally it may have a hyperplastic or lobulated exophytic appearance. An opposing 'kissing' lesion may be seen in the palatal vault.

Investigations

Median rhomboid glossitis is usually diagnosed on clinical grounds. Long disease duration and no benefit from topical steroids are suggestive of this condition. The differential diagnosis may include haemangioma, pyogenic granuloma, amyloidosis, granular cell tumour, Kaposi sarcoma and neoplasms. Since some lesions are nodular and may simulate a neoplasm or other pathology, biopsy may be indicated.

Management

Median rhomboid glossitis may respond to cessation of smoking and to the use of antifungals. There is no good evidence that median rhomboid glossitis lesions completely resolve after topical antifungals.

Desquamative gingivitis

Desquamative gingivitis is a clinical descriptive term. It is usually the result of a disease process that causes separation of the epithelium from the underlying connective tissue. Desquamative gingivitis may be a manifestation of several mucocutaneous diseases, most commonly mucous membrane pemphigoid, pemphigus vulgaris and lichen planus [1–3]. Treatment consists of treating the underlying disease. Elimination of dental plaque and calculus can significantly improve the treatment outcome.

Epidermolysis bullosa

Epidermolysis bullosa is characterised by blisters, sometimes preceded by white patches, which develop rapidly, particularly where there is trauma. Blisters rupture to produce ulcers, often with eventual scarring, particularly in the recessive dystrophic types [1–5]. Oral manifestations differ in frequency and severity according to the disease subtype, but the most common are bullae, which leave painful ulcers on rupture, followed by scarring. Oral lesions are fairly common in dystrophic and lethal forms of epidermolysis bullosa but are rare in most simplex types except the superficial type, where they are found in 70% of patients. Overall, oral mucosal lesions are found in about 30% of patients with epidermolysis bullosa. There is a predisposition to oral squamous cell carcinoma (SCC), mainly in the Hallopeau–Siemens type.

Dental hypoplasia (and other defects) and delayed tooth eruption may also be a feature, especially in junctional epidermolysis bullosa (Table 108.2). Also, with the difficulty in maintaining adequate oral hygiene, there is a predisposition to caries.

Patients with recessive dystrophic epidermolysis bullosa suffer from severe growth inhibition due to reduced food intake as a result of severe oropharyngeal and oesophageal blistering or scarring, with smaller maxillae and smaller mandibles than normal.

Dental treatment is complicated by severe oral and perioral scarring, microstomia and ankyloglossia [6,7].

The oral manifestations in the various inherited forms of this condition are summarised in Table 108.2 and epidermolysis bullosa acquisita is discussed in Chapter 69.

Erythroplakia

Erythroplakia is defined as 'any lesion of the oral mucosa that presents as bright red velvety plaques which cannot be characterised clinically or pathologically as any other recognisable condition' [1–6]. It is uncommon and appears to occur mainly in the middle aged and elderly. Erythroplakia is usually solitary and involves the floor of the mouth, the ventrum of the tongue or the soft palate (Figure 108.24). Erythroplakia presents as a fiery red macule or patch with a soft velvety texture [1,2]. Lesions are usually irregular in outline, though well defined. There are usually no symptoms. Risk factors for erythroplakia are as for carcinoma, mainly tobacco, alcohol and betel quid chewing. Other possible aetiological factors include body mass index and nutritional status.

The overall risk of malignant transformation is 33.1% and the malignant transformation rate per year is 2.7% [5,6]. Many red lesions may present with carcinoma *in situ* or invasive disease at the time of diagnosis.

Surgical excision is the treatment of choice, either by scalpel or laser excision, and sent for histological examination. There is no reliable data about the prognosis or recurrence rate.

Table 108.2 Oral manifestations in epidermolysis bullosa (EB).

Type	EB subtype	Mucosal lesions	Dental hypoplasia
I: Epidermolytic (simplex); autosomal dominant	Generalised (Koebner)	±	–
	Localised (Weber–Cockayne)	–	–
	Localised (Kallin)	–	Anodontia
	With mottled pigmentation and punctate keratoderma	+	–
	With bruising (Ogna)		±
	Herpetiform (Dowling–Meara)	Blistering with scarring	–
	Superficial	+	–
II: Junctional; autosomal recessive	Generalised, severe (Herlitz)	+	++
	Generalised, mild	+	+
	Localised	±	+
	Inverse	±	+
	Progressive	+	–
III: Dermolytic (dystrophic)	Hyperplastic (Cockayne–Touraine)	±	–
Autosomal dominant	Albopapuloid (Pasini)	+	–
	Pretibial (Kuske–Portugal)	–	–
Autosomal recessive (Hallopeau–Siemens)	Localised	+	±
	Generalised	++	++
	Mutilating	+++	+++
	Inverse	+	–
VI: Acquired type	Adult form	±	–
	Child form	+	–

–, Absent; +, mild; ++, moderate; +++, severe.

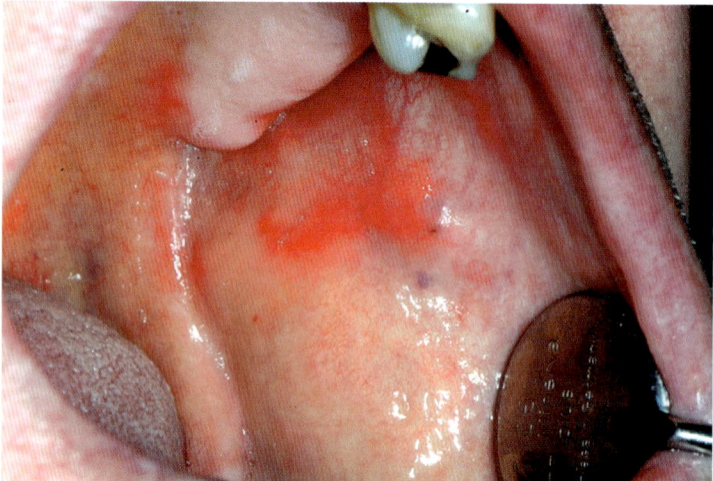

Figure 108.24 Erythroplakia involving the left buccal mucosa.

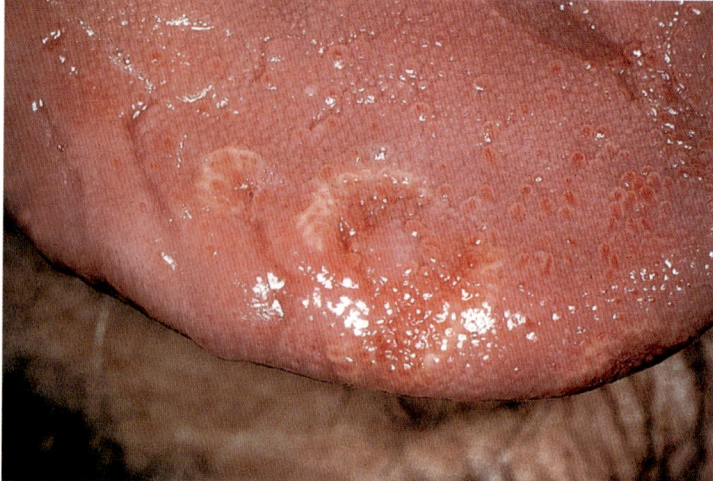

Figure 108.26 Somewhat less obvious signs of lingual erythema migrans.

Geographic tongue (benign migratory glossitis/erythema migrans)

A benign inflammatory condition of the tongue with map-like areas of erythema which are not constant in size, shape or location. The condition is unrelated to cutaneous erythema migrans.

Geographic tongue is characterised by map-like red areas with increased thickness of intervening filiform papillae. Alternatively, there are rounded, sometimes scalloped, reddish areas with a white margin (Figures 108.25 and 108.26). These patterns change from day to day and even within a few hours. It is a common condition, affecting about 1–2% of the population [1–6]. Patients of any age may be affected. There may be a positive family history.

Some patients with geographic tongue have atopic conditions such as hayfever and a few relate the oral lesions to a particular food [3].

Pathophysiology
There is epithelial thinning at the centre of the lesion with an inflammatory infiltrate mainly of polymorphonuclear leukocytes.

Clinical features
Geographic tongue may be asymptomatic or cause a sore tongue. Rarely, other sites, such as the labial or palatal mucosa, are affected (benign migratory stomatitis). The tongue is usually, but not invariably, affected simultaneously with the other sites. There are no complications.

Investigations
Clinical examination usually suffices to differentiate the condition. Many patients with a fissured tongue also have geographic tongue. Similar oral lesions may be seen in reactive arthritis (previously termed Reiter syndrome), generalised pustular psoriasis and acrodermatitis continua of Hallopeau [5].

Management
No effective treatment is available except reassurance, but benzydamine hydrochloride 0.15% spray or mouthwash may provide symptomatic relief.

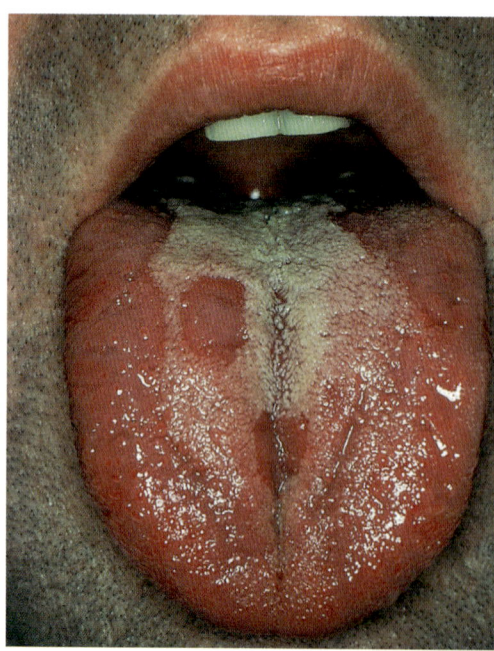

Figure 108.25 Classical geographic tongue (lingual erythema migrans).

Glossitis

Glossitis is characterised by atrophy of the filiform papillae of the tongue, giving the tongue a smooth, glossy, red appearance. Causes of glossitis include:
- Nutritional deficiencies (iron, vitamin B12, folic acid).
- Oral *Candida* infection.
- Coeliac disease.
- Lichen planus.
- Benign migratory glossitis.
- Protein–calorie malnutrition.
- Xerostomia.

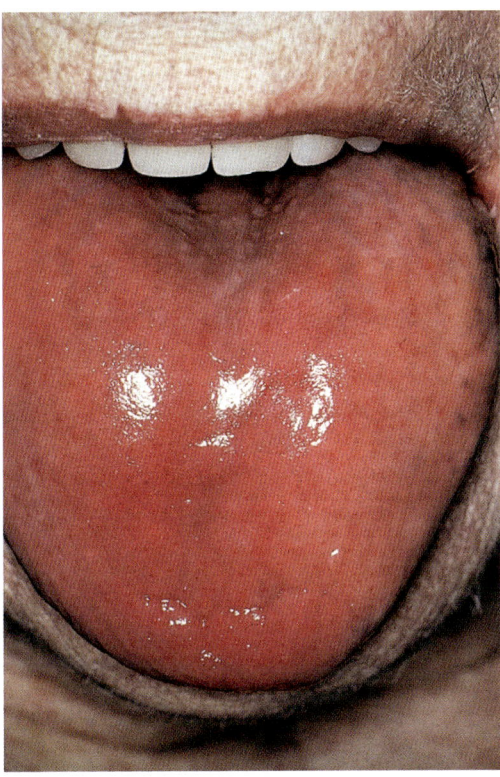

Figure 108.27 Atrophic glossitis in vitamin B$_{12}$ deficiency.

Deficiency glossitis may be related particularly to deficiency of iron, folate or vitamin B$_{12}$, and may then be associated with angular stomatitis and/or mouth ulcers. In anaemic glossitis the tongue is red, sore and smooth (Figure 108.27) [1–4]. Occasionally, pernicious anaemia can also produce red areas or patterns of red lines. Patients with glossitis often complain of a burning sensation and increased sensitivity when eating acidic or salty foods. Most causes of glossitis are self-limiting and require no treatment. Symptomatic relief is possible with good oral hygiene and mouthwash, e.g. benzydamine hydrochloride.

Immune defects

Mouth ulcers and early-onset periodontitis feature in congenital immune defects, including Chédiak–Higashi syndrome, Papillon–Lefèvre syndrome, familial neutropenia, cyclic neutropenia, Job syndrome, chronic granulomatous disease and glycogen storage disease type 1b [1–8].

Plasma cell gingivitis

Plasma cell gingivitis is a rare benign inflammatory condition characterised by extensive infiltration of plasma cells within the connective tissue of the oral mucosa [1]. The first cases were caused by hypersensitivity to a component of chewing gum. Flavouring agents such as cinnamaldehyde, mint candy, herbs and spices have also been recognised as causative factors [2–4]. Patients report

soreness and sensitivity, especially on eating acidic and spicy foods. The gingiva presents with diffuse erythema with swelling and loss of stippling, similar to desquamative gingivitis. Other oral sites such as the buccal and palatal mucosa may be affected. Biopsy shows sheets of polyclonal plasma cells. Identifying the causative agent is important and patch testing may be useful. Treatment includes topical and systemic corticosteroids. Lesions will persist if the patient is exposed to the antigen.

Strawberry tongue

A red denuded appearance of the dorsum tongue with persistent hypertrophic fungiform papillae may be seen in scarlet fever, Kawasaki disease [1] and Riley–Day syndrome (familial dysautonomia), giving rise to an appearance similar to a strawberry.

VASCULAR LESIONS

Blue rubber–bleb naevus syndrome

Oral haemangiomas may be seen [1–3].

Glomovenous malformations

Glomovenous malformations are disseminated variants of cutaneous glomus tumours. Some have been treated successfully with sequential pulsed dye Nd-Yag laser [1].

Haemangioma

Haemangiomas are usually deep red or blue-purple, blanch on pressure, are fluctuant to palpation, and are level with the mucosa or have a lobulated or raised surface. Most are small and of no consequence [1,2].

Most haemangiomas are seen in isolation, but a few may be multiple and/or part of a wider syndrome, such as Maffucci syndrome. Large facial haemangiomas, which can involve the lips, may be associated with Sturge–Weber syndrome or Dandy–Walker syndrome, or other posterior cranial fossa malformations.

Haemangiomas are at risk from trauma and prone to excessive bleeding if damaged (e.g. during tooth extraction). Occasionally, oral haemangiomas develop phlebolithiasis.

Oral lesions suspected of being haemangiomatous should not be routinely biopsied. Kaposi sarcoma and epithelioid angiomatosis should be excluded. After intravenous administration of contrast medium, enhancement is observed in haemangiomas in areas corresponding to those with high signal on T$_2$-weighted MRI.

Oral haemangiomas are left alone unless causing symptoms, when they are best treated with cryosurgery or laser if small, injection of 3% sodium tetra decyl sulphate locally or by ligation or embolisation of feeding vessels if large. Propranolol is an effective treatment of head and neck infantile haemangiomas.

Hereditary haemorrhagic telangiectasia (Osler–Rendu–Weber syndrome)

Hereditary haemorrhagic telangiectasia is an autosomal dominant disorder predominantly caused by mutations in *ENG* (encodes endoglin) and *ACVRL1* (encodes ALK1), which both belong to the transforming growth factor (TGF)-β signalling pathway [1].

The most common clinical findings are epistaxis, gastrointestinal bleeding and iron deficiency anaemia, along with characteristic mucocutaneous telangiectasia on the lips, perioral skin, oral and nasal mucosae as well as the gastrointestinal tract [1–4]. Mucocutaneous and gastrointestinal telangiectasia develop by the age of 30 years and increase in number over time [5]. Hereditary haemorrhagic telangiectasia manifests in the oral cavity as red spots approximately 1–3 mm in diameter that appear on the tongue, lips, buccal mucosa or palate. Visceral arteriovenous malformations of the liver, lung and central nervous system are common [6]. Complications include high-output heart failure, portal hypertension, liver failure, haemoptysis, polycythaemia, cerebral abscess and stroke.

Oral haemorrhage can be controlled by cryotherapy, cautery, infrared coagulation, Nd-Yag laser or intense pulsed light. Bevacizumab, a vascular endothelial growth factor (VEGF) inhibitor, may be efficacious in those with severe, intractable nosebleeds.

Kaposi sarcoma

Kaposi sarcoma (KS) accounts for 20–25% of sarcomas within the head and neck. Cases are most frequently associated with the human immunodeficiency virus. The pathogenesis of KS is poorly understood but it is known to be initiated by the human herpesvirus 8 (HHV-8) [1,2]. Clinical presentation of KS in the head and neck can vary from isolated blue/purple macules to exophytic or multifocal lesions. Intraorally, it commonly presents on keratinised surfaces, most frequently the gingiva and palate (Figure 108.28). Up to 95% of lesions are seen in the palate, 23% in the gingiva and others on the tongue or buccal mucosa [3–6]. A red–purple macule is the early lesion, progressing to a purple nodular swelling that may be extensive and ulcerated. Multiple lesions are common. Lesions are often asymptomatic, but more than 25% are painful and about 8% bleed.

Histologically, spindle cells proliferate along with irregular vessels which can appear slit-shaped. Mitoses are often abundant and central necrosis can occur. Immunohistochemistry to identify HHV-8 is useful to confirm the diagnosis.

Differential diagnoses should include benign and malignant lesions such as haemangioma, pyogenic granuloma, bacillary angiomatosis and melanoma.

Highly active antiretroviral treatment is effective in preventing and controlling HIV-related KS. Other treatment modalities can

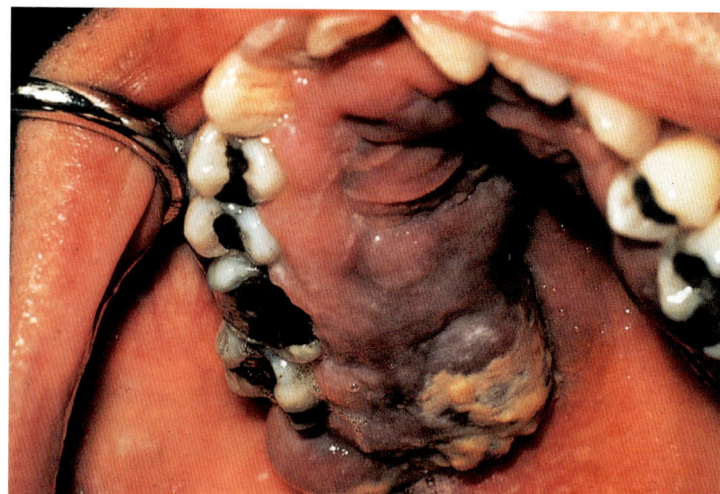

Figure 108.28 Kaposi sarcoma in a typical site with a characteristic purplish appearance. Courtesy of Dr J.B. Epstein.

include surgical excision and radiotherapy for localised lesions and chemotherapy (e.g. paclitaxel, doxorubicin) for widespread disease [7–10].

Klippel–Trenaunay–Weber syndrome

Haemangiomas of the buccal mucosa and tongue, macroglossia, maxillary hyperplasia and an anterior open bite have been recorded in this syndrome. Post-extraction bleeding can be a problem [1–3].

Maffucci syndrome

Oral haemangiomas may be seen [1–4].

Mucoepithelial dysplasia

Hereditary mucoepithelial dysplasia is an autosomal dominant dyskeratotic epithelial syndrome affecting oral, nasal, vaginal, urethral, anal, bladder and conjunctival mucosae, causing cataracts, follicular keratosis, non-scarring alopecia and terminal lung disease [1–3].

Pathology

The condition is probably a pan-epithelial cell defect of desmosomal and gap junction structure. Histochemically, there is a lack of cornification and keratinisation. Electron microscopy shows an abnormality in desmosomes and gap junctions, with a lack of keratohyalin granules, a paucity of desmosomes, intercellular accumulations, cytoplasmic vacuolisation and formation of bands and aggregates of filamentous fibres and structures in the cytoplasm resembling desmosomes and gap junctions. There is some acantholysis as well as benign dyskeratosis of individual cells.

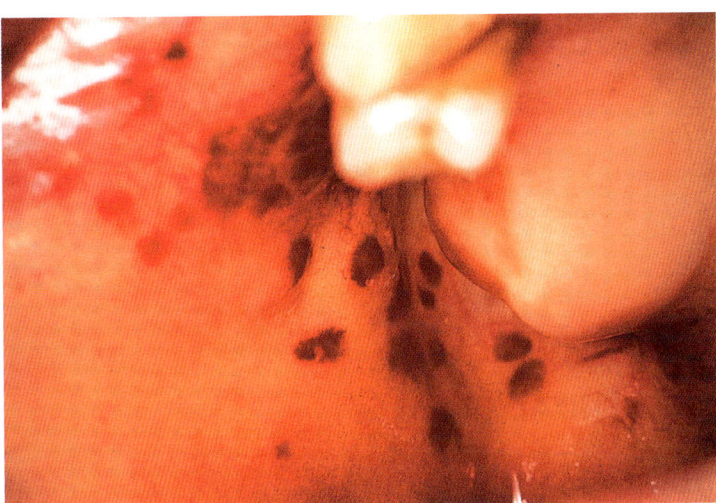

Figure 108.29 Oral purpura in thrombocytopenia.

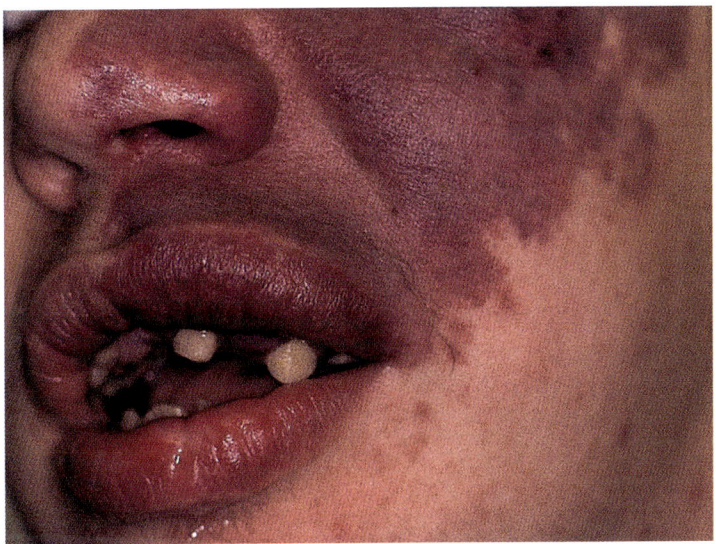

Figure 108.30 Haemangioma affecting the lip in Sturge–Weber syndrome.

Histologically, the mucosal epithelium shows dyshesion, thinning of the epithelial layer and dyskeratosis. Mucosal Papanicolaou smears show lack of epithelial maturation, cytoplasmic vacuoles and inclusions, and individual cell dyskeratosis.

Clinical features

Red periorificial mucosal lesions are typically noted during infancy and may persist throughout life. The oral lesions are painless red macules or maculopapules and are seen predominantly on the palate and gingiva. Angular cheilitis and fissured tongue are additional features. Severe photophobia, tearing and nystagmus in infancy herald the development of keratitis, corneal vascularisation and lens cataracts.

Purpura

Petechiae are usually caused by trauma, but senile purpura or a thrombocytopathy (as in chemotherapy, infectious mononucleosis, HIV infection or leukaemia) must be excluded (Figure 108.29) [1,2]. Thrombocytopenic lesions are usually on the soft tissues most susceptible to trauma, such as the buccal mucosa from cheek-biting, the junction between the hard and soft palate in denture-wearing individuals or the gingiva. Petechiae may be seen in parvovirus-related papular-purpuric 'gloves and socks' syndrome [3].

Blood-filled blisters may be seen in localised oral purpura (angina bullosa haemorrhagica) and pemphigoid, and occasionally in amyloidosis [4].

Sturge–Weber syndrome

The haemangioma in the trigeminal area in Sturge–Weber syndrome is usually unilateral, may involve the mouth but fortunately rarely involves bone (Figure 108.30). It may be associated with hypertrophy of affected tissues and, if the patient is treated with phenytoin, with gingival hyperplasia [1–3].

Telangiectasia

Oral telangiectases occur mainly in hereditary haemorrhagic telangiectasia, CREST (calcinosis, Raynaud, oesophageal, sclerodactyly, telangiectasia) syndrome, chronic liver disease, pregnancy and after irradiation.

Varicosities

Bluish oral varicosities may often be seen in elderly patients, particularly in the ventrum and lateral margin of the tongue. They are benign.

Vascular proliferative lesions

Benign atypical vascular lesions may exhibit cytological or architectural features that simulate angiosarcoma such that considerable caution is required in diagnosis [1]. The head and neck region is a common location, particularly for lobular capillary haemangioma (pyogenic granuloma), while the lip is an especially common site for lobular capillary haemangioma [2–5] and intravascular papillary endothelial hyperplasia (Masson haemangioma or pseudoangiosarcoma) [5,6]. Intravascular papillary endothelial hyperplasia is a benign non-neoplastic vascular lesion characterised histologically by papillary fronds lined by proliferating endothelium and probably represents an organising thrombus. Seen mainly in the lip or tongue in females, it may simulate angiosarcoma histologically. Excision suffices.

Vascular lesions such as epithelioid haemangioma, epithelioid haemangioendothelioma, spindle cell haemangioendothelioma, acquired progressive lymphangioma or angiosarcoma and Kaposi sarcoma may need to be excluded.

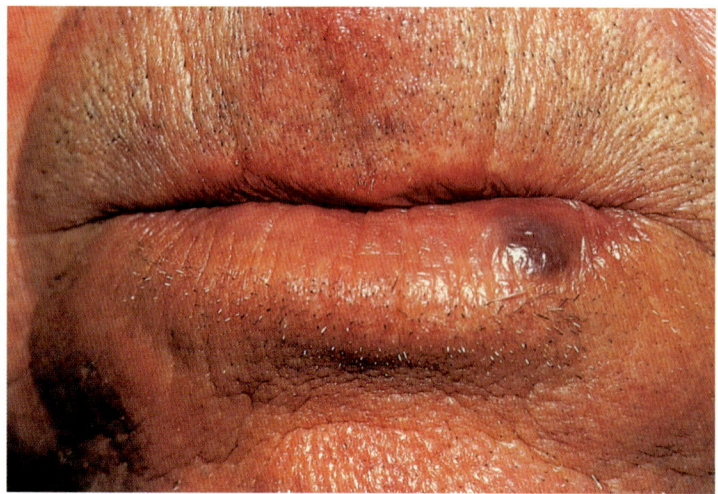

Figure 108.31 Venous lake of the lip. Courtesy of Addenbrooke's Hospital.

Venous lake

This is a bluish-purple soft swelling, 2–10 mm in diameter, usually seen on the lower lip of an elderly person, due to a venous dilatation (Figure 108.31). They are usually seen in people older than 50 and are more common in men than in women [1]. The lesion is lined by a single layer of flattened endothelial cells with a thick wall of fibrous tissue. The lesion empties on prolonged pressure. A venous lake (also referred to as phlebectasis or phlebectasia) may be only a trivial cosmetic problem or it can bleed after trauma. It can be excised but often leaves a permanent scar. Cryotherapy, electrocautery, infrared coagulation or treatment with an argon laser can also give good results. Cosmetic camouflage cream can make the lesion less noticeable [2–4].

Venous mucocutaneous malformation

The condition venous mucocutaneous malformation (VMCM) is characterised by the presence of small, multifocal bluish cutaneous and/or mucosal venous malformations [1]. They are usually present at birth and new lesions appear with time. Small lesions are usually asymptomatic, while larger lesions can invade subcutaneous muscle and cause pain. Venous mucocutaneous malformation are seen most commonly on mucous membranes, including the mouth, are lighter purple in colour than glomulovenous malformations, are compressible and not painful.

VMCM is a rare autosomal dominant condition with incomplete penetrance, reported in only about 20 families. VMCM are associated with amino acid substitutions in the tyrosine-protein kinase endothelial cell receptor (TEK/TIE2; 9p21). Approximately 90% of individuals with a *TEK* gene mutation develop the venous mucocutaneous malformation by age 20; and ~10% are clinically unaffected. More than 80% of individuals with multifocal VMCM have elevated D-dimer concentration. Treatment is with ethanol sclerotherapy. Surgery is effective for small lesions. Malignant transformation has not been described.

Wiskott–Aldrich syndrome

Oral petechiae and infections such as candidiasis may occur in Wiskott–Aldrich syndrome (associated with adaptive and innate immunodeficiency, thrombocytopenia, eczema, and an increased risk of autoimmune disorders and malignancy) [1–4].

WHITE LESIONS

CONGENITAL

Clouston syndrome

Hidrotic ectodermal dysplasia, Clouston type, is an autosomal dominant condition characterised by nail dystrophy, palmoplantar hyperkeratosis and abnormal hair. Individuals are able to sweat and generally have normal teeth but a tendency toward excess caries. HED2 is caused by variants in the gene encoding connexin-30, GJB6, on chromosome 13q11-q12.1. In the oral cavity, there may be diffuse white lesions in the buccal mucosa, palate, tongue and elsewhere [1–3].

Darier disease

Darier disease is a rare autosomal dominant genodermatosis. Oral lesions are seen in up to 50% of patients with skin lesions of Darier disease. They may also occur in the oesophagus and on the anogenital mucosa. The oral changes are typically flattish, coalescing, red plaques that eventually turn white and affect the keratinised mucosa of the dorsum of the tongue, palate and gingiva (Figure 108.32) [1–6]. Oral lesions may cause blockage of the salivary ducts, particularly of the parotid gland, and xerostomia [7,8].

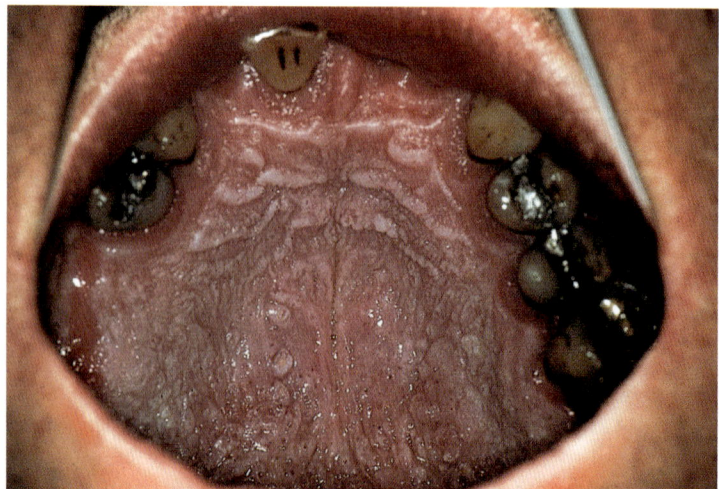

Figure 108.32 Darier disease: oral white lesions resemble those of nicotinic stomatitis.

Dyskeratosis congenita

Dyskeratosis congenita (DC) is an inherited disorder characterised by bone marrow failure, cancer predisposition and somatic abnormalities. DC is caused by mutations that interfere with normal maintenance of telomeres (specialised structures at the end of chromosomes that shorten with each cell division). It usually presents with oral lesions between the ages of 5 and 10 years, when the tongue and sometimes the buccal mucosa and palate develop leukoplakia [1–3]. Other rare oral features include taurodontism (an elongated crown affecting molar teeth with short roots) or hypocalcified teeth, mucosal hyperpigmentation and severe dental or periodontal disease. Head and neck SCC account for 40% of cancers reported in DC [4,5].

Focal palmoplantar and oral hyperkeratosis syndrome

This syndrome is an autosomal-dominant disorder characterised by hyperkeratosis of the attached gingiva and palmoplantar hyperkeratosis [1,2]. Biopsy of gingival lesions histologically show acanthosis and hyperkeratotic cornification of the epithelium.

Fordyce spots

Fordyce spots are sebaceous glands containing neutral lipids similar to those found in skin sebaceous glands [1] but are not associated with hair follicles. Fordyce spots are yellowish small grains seen beneath the buccal or labial mucosa. Fordyce spots are extremely common: probably 80% of the population have them. Fordyce spots are often not noticeable in children until after puberty (although they are present histologically), and they seem to be more obvious in male patients with greasy skin and the elderly. They are usually seen in the buccal mucosa, particularly inside the commissures (Figure 108.33), and sometimes in the retromolar regions and upper lip [1–4]. They may be associated with genital Fordyce spots. Fordyce spots are completely benign. No treatment is indicated, other than reassurance.

Hereditary benign intraepithelial dyskeratosis

Hereditary benign intraepithelial dyskeratosis is a rare autosomal-dominant disorder associated with chromosome 4 anomalies, first described and predominantly affecting descendants of Haliwa-Saponi American Indians. It is a disorder of the bulbar conjunctiva and oral mucosa, associated with epithelial hyperplasia and hyperkeratosis [1–4].

Oral milky white, smooth, somewhat translucent plaques appear in childhood and become more obvious by adolescence. These lesions affect predominantly the buccal mucosae, lips and ventrum of the tongue.

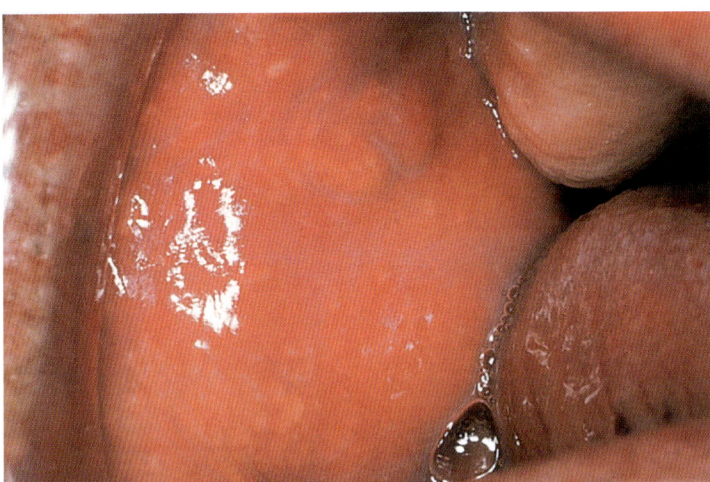

Figure 108.33 Fordyce spots: sebaceous glands in the buccal mucosa.

Ocular lesions include conjunctivitis with gelatinous conjunctival plaques, which become evident in infancy. Dilated superficial vessels in association with the conjunctival plaques give the eye a red appearance. Patients complain of symptoms of irritation, such as itching, excessive lacrimation and photophobia.

Oral biopsy is usually indicated for diagnosis. There is pronounced epithelial acanthosis, vacuolisation in the stratum spinosum and eosinophilic cells apparently engulfed by normal squamous cells ('tobacco cells').

No treatment is required. The plaques persist throughout life and sometimes progress, but may wax and wane.

Keratitis, ichthyosis and deafness syndrome

Keratitis, ichthyosis and deafness (KID) syndrome is a rare autosomal dominant disorder caused by heterozygous mutations in the *GJB2* gene. Dental dysplasia, persistent oral ulceration, chronic mucocutaneous candidiasis and occasional carcinoma may be seen in KID syndrome [1–3].

Leukoedema

Leukoedema is not a mucosal disease but simply the name given to the faint whitish lines seen in some normal buccal mucosae, often prominent in black people (Figure 108.34). It is the result of fluid accumulation within keratinocytes. The whitish lines are bilateral and disappear if the mucosa is stretched – a diagnostic test [1,2]. Confusion with lichen planus should thereby be avoided. A biopsy is rarely necessary. The condition is benign.

Linear naevus syndrome (naevus sebaceous of Jadassohn)

Linear naevus syndrome (naevus sebaceous of Jadassohn) is an epidermal naevus with predominant sebaceous glands on

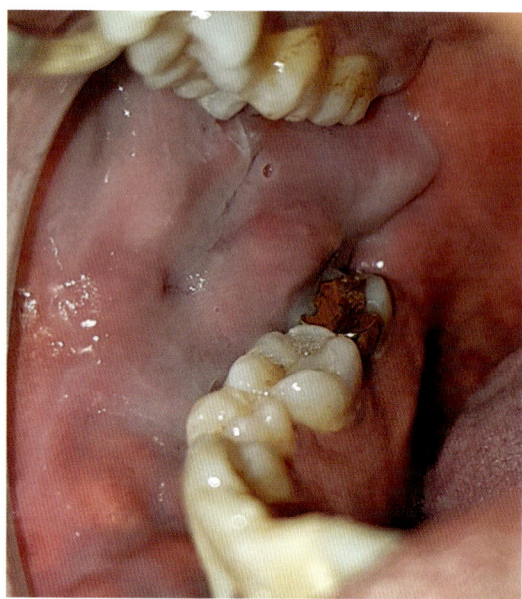

Figure 108.34 Leukoedema of the right buccal mucosa in a black individual.

histology. Oral involvement ranges from papillomatous growths on the tongue, gingiva and palate to dental abnormalities such as hypodontia, unerupted teeth, abnormal spacing of teeth and teeth of abnormal size [1–3].

Linear epidermal naevus

Linear epidermal naevus is a sporadic hamartomatous lesion of the skin caused by a proliferation of embryonic ectodermal cells distributed in a linear configuration along Blaschko's lines and composed primarily of surface epithelium. Lesions typically present as brown verrucous papules and plaques and tend to occur circumferentially on the trunk and longitudinally on the extremities. Most oral linear epidermal naevi are associated with cutaneous lesions [1,2].

Intraorally, lesions may present as unilateral or midline papules or nodules with a papillary or verrucous surface ranging in colour from that of normal mucosa to brown [1,2]. Lesions are unilateral and do not cross the midline. The lips, tongue and palate are the most frequently affected sites. Oral lesions require no treatment in the absence of symptoms or functional problems.

Olmsted syndrome (congenital palmoplantar and periorificial keratoderma with corneal epithelial dysplasia)

Olmsted syndrome is a rare palmoplantar keratinising disorder associated with diffuse alopecia, nail dystrophy, corneal dystrophy, recurrent infections and susceptibility to develop SCCs in keratotic areas. Keratotic plaques may be seen intraorally [1–5]. Most of reported Olmsted syndrome cases are sporadic, although familial

cases with different modes of inheritance have been described. Mutations in *TRPV3* (transient receptor potential vanilloid-3) gene have recently been identified as a cause of autosomal dominant (gain-of-function mutations) or recessive Olmsted syndrome. Mutations in *MBTPS2* (membrane-bound transcription factor protease, site 2) gene have been identified in a recessive X-linked form.

Pachyonychia congenita

Pachyonychia congenita is a rare autosomal dominant disorder of keratinisation affecting primarily the skin and nails [1–3]. It is caused by dominant negative variants in KRT6A, KRT6B, KRT6C, KRT16 or KRT17, which encode the keratins K6a, K6b, K6c, K16 and K17, respectively. The predominant clinical manifestations are a triad of hypertrophic nail dystrophy, plantar keratoderma and severe plantar pain. Other clinical findings reported include fingernail dystrophy, oral leukokeratosis, palmar keratoderma, follicular hyperkeratosis, hyperhidrosis, cysts, hoarseness due to laryngeal involvement and natal teeth. About 60% of patients have oral keratosis (white-greyish patches on the tongue and buccal mucosa), 16% have natal or neonatal teeth and 10% have angular stomatitis [3–6]. There is a higher likelihood of oral leukokeratosis in individuals with KRT6A mutations and a strong association of natal teeth and cysts in carriers of a KRT17 mutation.

The keratosis requires no treatment. Dental advice should be sought regarding natal or neonatal teeth.

Sebaceous adenoma

Sebaceous adenomas are exceedingly rare in the mouth, except in association with salivary glands but have been described in the buccal mucosa [1–4].

Tylosis

Tylosis is an autosomal dominant syndrome of palmoplantar hyperkeratosis that may predispose to oesophageal carcinoma. Oral leukoplakias have also been described [1–4]. The causative gene is *RHBDF2*, coding for a rhomboid protease involved in epidermal growth factor receptor.

Warty dyskeratoma (focal acantholytic dyskeratosis)

Warty dyskeratoma is a benign proliferative epidermal disorder, which originates from the pilosebaceous apparatus. It is rare in the oral cavity but typically presents as a whitish centrally umbilicated papule or nodule on keratinised mucosa, including maxillary and mandibular alveolar ridges and the hard palate [1–5]. Warty dyskeratoma is typically asymptomatic in both cutaneous and mucosal sites. The histology is similar to that of Darier disease and transient acantholytic dermatosis, with suprabasal epithelial splits and corps ronds.

White sponge naevus

White sponge naevus (also called white sponge naevus of Cannon) is a rare, autosomal dominant disorder caused by mutations in keratin 4 (KRT4) or keratin 13 (KRT13) genes [1–3]. It presents in childhood. The oral mucosa is almost invariably involved with non-painful white plaques primarily involving the buccal mucosae and floor of the mouth. Painless, shaggy or folded white lesions typically affect the buccal mucosa bilaterally, but may also involve other areas, although rarely the gingival margins [1,3]. Extra-oral lesions most often occur in the oesophagus or anogenital area, but almost invariably follow the development of typical oral lesions. There is hyperplastic acanthotic epithelium in which gross oedema causes a basket-weave appearance. The superficial epithelium has a 'washed-out' appearance as it stains only very lightly.

The family history and clinical examination are usually adequate to differentiate this from other more common causes of white lesions.

This is a benign condition with an excellent prognosis. Reassurance is all that is required, although some have suggested a beneficial effect with topical tetracyclines.

ACQUIRED

Acquired white lesions in the mouth are usually caused by materia alba (a soft whitish material formed from an accumulation or aggregation of microorganisms, desquamated epithelial cells, blood cells, and food debris loosely adherent to surfaces of teeth or soft tissue and is washed away with water) (Figure 108.35), cheek biting or chemical burns. However, keratoses, infections (mainly candidiasis), dermatoses (usually lichen planus), neoplastic disorders and other conditions must be excluded.

Actinic cheilitis

See later in this chapter.

Burns

Chemical burns (due, for example, to holding mouthwashes in the mouth or drugs against the buccal mucosa) or burns caused by heat, cold or irradiation can cause white sloughing lesions of the mucosa. Such lesions typically heal spontaneously within 1–3 weeks.

Candidiasis (see also 'Fungal infections' later in this chapter)

Of the several clinical presentations of oral candidiasis, only acute pseudomembranous candidiasis, candidal leukoplakia and chronic mucocutaneous candidiasis present as white lesions; the other types, acute and chronic atrophic candidiasis, are red.

Acute pseudomembranous candidiasis

Healthy neonates, who have yet to develop immunity to *Candida* species, may develop acute pseudomembranous candidiasis (thrush). In other patients, predisposing factors include antibiotic or corticosteroid use, xerostomia and severe T-cell immune defects associated with immunosuppression or immunodeficiencies such as leukaemia or HIV disease. Acute pseudomembranous candidiasis is a common and early feature of HIV infection.

Clinically, it presents as soft creamy patches of thrush, which resemble milk curds, and can be wiped off the oral mucosa with gauze, leaving an area of erythema (Figure 108.36) [1–3].

Chronic candidiasis

The aetiology of chronic oral candidosis is unclear and in only a few patients can either a local cause or underlying immune defect be identified [1–3]. HIV/AIDS and chronic mucocutaneous candidiasis syndromes are rare causes. Chronic hyperplastic candidiasis (candidal leukoplakia) is a persistent discrete lesion that varies from small, palpable, whitish areas to large, dense, opaque plaques, and are non-homogeneous 'speckled' leukoplakias in up to 50% [4–6]. They usually occur on the buccal mucosa on one or both sides, mainly just inside the commissure, and less often on the tongue dorsum.

The diagnosis of oral candidiasis is usually clinical, but it tends to be overdiagnosed by physicians. In contrast, erythematous candidiasis is probably underdiagnosed. In immunosuppressed patients, a Gram-stained smear should be taken to distinguish oral candidiasis from the plaques produced by opportunistic bacteria. Hyphae seem

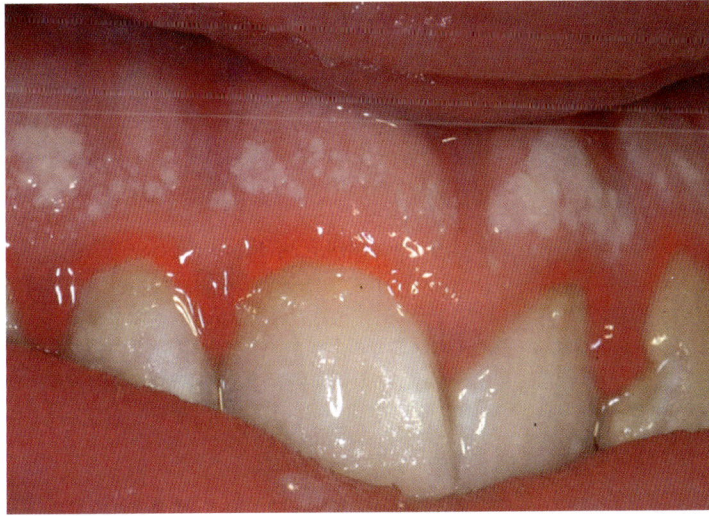

Figure 108.35 Materia alba.

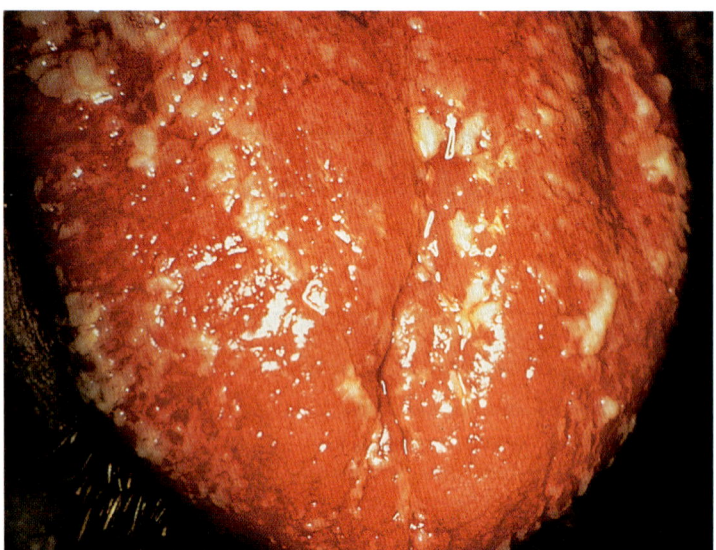

Figure 108.36 Thrush: scattered white lesions on an erythematous background.

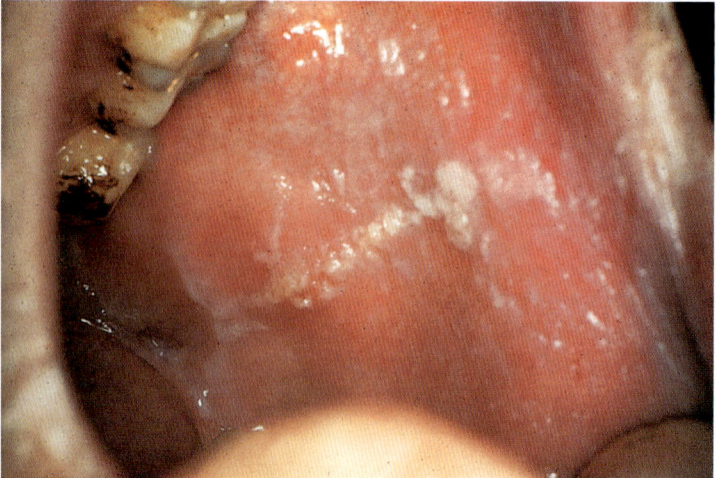

Figure 108.37 Frictional keratosis and cheek biting (morsicatio buccarum) at the occlusal line.

to indicate that the *Candida* organisms are acting as pathogens and not simple commensals.

Chronic hyperplastic candidiasis should be biopsied to distinguish it from other non-candidal lesions and to examine for dysplasia [6]. Although candidal hyphae and a neutrophil infiltrate may be seen on haematoxylin and eosin staining, periodic-acid Schiff will demonstrate the purple staining of the hyphae.

Management

Except in healthy neonates, possible predisposing causes should be looked for and treated. Topical polyenes such as nystatin or amphotericin, or imidazoles such as miconazole are often indicated [3]. Fluconazole may be required. The oral lesions of chronic hyperplastic candidiasis prove poorly responsive to polyene antifungal drugs and, in some cases, respond only to systemic fluconazole or itraconazole.

Chronic mucocutaneous candidiasis

Chronic mucocutaneous candidiasis (CMC) is the term given to a heterogeneous group of rare syndromes, sometimes familial, in which there is persistent mucocutaneous candidiasis of the skin, nails and mucous membranes that are usually resistant to topical treatment and there is an absence of invasive fungal infections. CMC is associated with a defect in T helper 17 (Th17) cell immunity or disruption to cytokines IL-17 and IL-22 [1–6]. CMC is associated with defects involved in *Candida* recognition (e.g. CARD9 and Dectin-1), Th17 differentiation (e.g. *STAT1* and *STAT3* mutations) and IL-17 signalling (e.g. anti-IL-17 autoantibodies). Persistent adherent white lesions are seen in the mouth, often with angular stomatitis. In autoimmune polyendocrinopathy-candidiasis-ectodermal dystrophy (APECED) (triad of mucocutaneous candidiasis, hypoparathyroidism and adrenal failure) there may also be enamel hypoplasia and, rarely, oral carcinoma. CMC is a prominent feature of a number of primary immune deficiencies including the hyperimmunoglobulin E syndromes (HIES) and autoimmune polyendocrine syndrome type I (APS-I). Patients with

autosomal dominant HIES have heterozygous loss-of-function (LOF) mutations in the *STAT3* gene. Patients with APS-I have LOF mutations in the *AIRE* gene. Autosomal dominant GOF mutation in *STAT1* is the most common cause of CMC and accounts for more than half of cases [7]. The genetic defect leads to an exaggerated Th1 cell response and a diminished Th17 response. The mainstay of treatment for patients with CMC is systemic and topical antifungals [3,7,8]. Long-term suppressive therapy is often required to prevent recurrence.

Cheek biting

A horizontal white line may be seen in the buccal mucosa of healthy people (linea alba) but can be exaggerated in individuals with a parafunctional habit. Cheek biting causes a whitish shredded appearance usually of the buccal or lower labial mucosa at the occlusal line (adjacent to where the teeth meet) (Figure 108.37) [1,2]. The lesion is benign but may simulate white sponge naevus, leukoplakia or lichen planus.

Hairy leukoplakia

Oral hairy leukoplakia is caused by the Epstein–Barr virus and is usually seen in immunocompromised individuals, such as those with HIV infection and systemic immunosuppression [1–8]. It is characterised by white painless corrugated non-removable plaques, usually involving the lingual squamous epithelium (Figure 108.38). There have been cases of oral hairy leukoplakia in those using immune-modulating medications, long-term corticosteroid inhaler use and diabetes. The diagnosis is largely clinical, supported by proof of Epstein–Barr virus and usually HIV testing [9]. Histological features include hyperparakeratosis, hyperplasia and ballooning of prickle cells, few or absent Langerhans cells, and only a sparse inflammatory cell infiltrate in the lamina propria. Treatment is not often required, but the condition often resolves

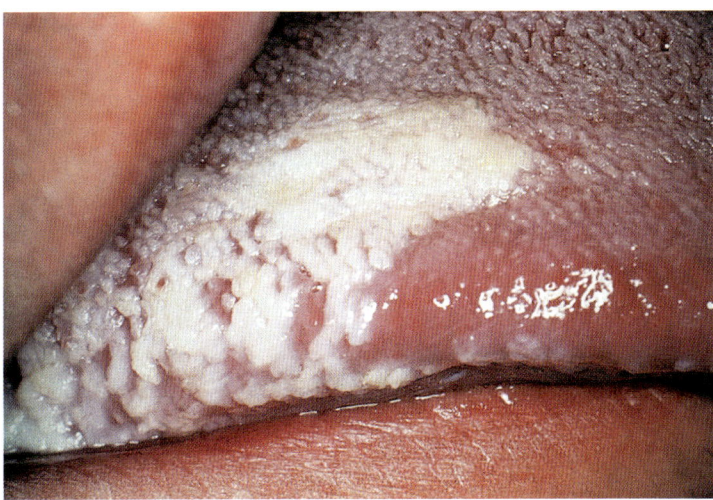

Figure 108.38 Hairy leukoplakia. Found mainly in HIV infection, vertical white ridges on the lateral margin of the tongue.

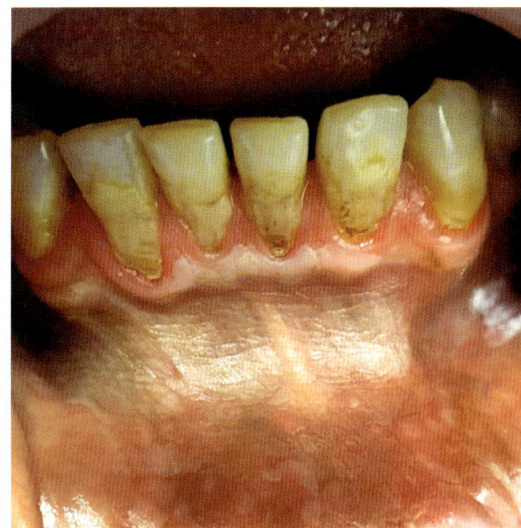

Figure 108.39 Homogeneous keratosis involving the labial gingiva and labial sulcus due to holding tobacco in the sulcus.

with aciclovir or other agents active against Epstein–Barr virus, or with antiretroviral agents. Oral hairy leukoplakia is not considered a premalignant lesion.

Keratoses

The cause of most keratoses is unknown (idiopathic keratoses) but some are caused by chronic irritation, particular lifestyle habits or infective agents.

- *Tobacco-induced keratoses.* Consumption of tobacco products has long been causally connected with oral cancer and is a common cause of keratosis. Tobacco use also predisposes to cancers elsewhere in the upper aerodigestive tract, bladder and other sites. Tobacco use should thus be discouraged.
- *Tobacco chewing.* Tobacco is chewed in many parts of the world and may induce keratosis. In many communities, tobacco is a component of betel quid, along with *Areca* nut and betel leaf, and sometimes slaked lime and spices. Sometimes betel is used without tobacco (pan or paan), though others use paan with tobacco. Oral carcinoma can result.
- *Reverse smoking (bidi).* In some communities, especially in Asia, cigarettes are smoked with the lit end within the mouth. Palatal or other oral carcinomas can result.
- *Cigarette-induced keratoses.* Mild keratosis may be seen especially on the palate, lip and at the commissures, along with nicotine-stained teeth. Malignant change is uncommon.
- *Pipe smoking.* Diffuse whiteness over the palate is termed 'smoker's keratosis' or 'stomatitis nicotina'. The palatal minor salivary gland orifices appear red against this white background.
- *Cigar smoking.* Cigar smokers may develop stomatitis nicotina and nicotine-stained teeth. Malignant change is uncommon.
- *Snuff dipper's keratosis and other smokeless tobacco lesions.* Snuff may produce keratosis – white hyperkeratotic lesions caused by snuff-dipping (holding flavoured tobacco powder in the oral sulcus or vestibule) (Figure 108.39).

Koplik spots

White specks may be seen in the buccal mucosa in early measles.

Leukoplakia

The World Health Organization defines leukoplakia as a predominantly white plaque of questionable risk having excluded (other) known diseases or disorders that carry no increased risk of cancer. By definition, the term excludes entities such as frictional keratosis or smoker's keratosis [1,2]. The main differential diagnoses include white sponge naevus, leukoedema, oral lichen planus and oral hairy leukoplakia.

Epidemiology
Leukoplakia occurs in about 0.1% of the population with a global prevalence of 2–4%. Most cases are seen in the 50–70 age group.

Risk factors
Risk factors for leukoplakia are as for carcinoma, mainly tobacco, alcohol and betel. Other factors may include personal or familial history of cancer or cancer therapy, chronic immunosuppression, age, syndromes such as dyskeratosis congenita, ultraviolet light damage for lesions of the vermilion and human papillomavirus in a small number of cases.

Pathology
Leukoplakias show, to a varying degree, three main microscopic features:
- Increased keratin production: increased keratin produces the white clinical appearance of keratosis.
- Change in epithelial thickness: thinning (hypoplasia) or thickening (hyperplasia) may be present. Malignant change is more likely in a hypoplastic epithelium.
- Disordered epithelial maturation.

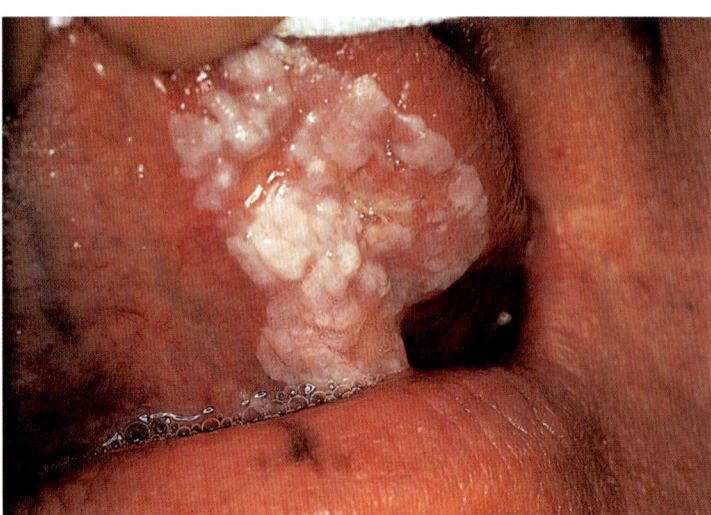

Figure 108.40 Sublingual keratosis.

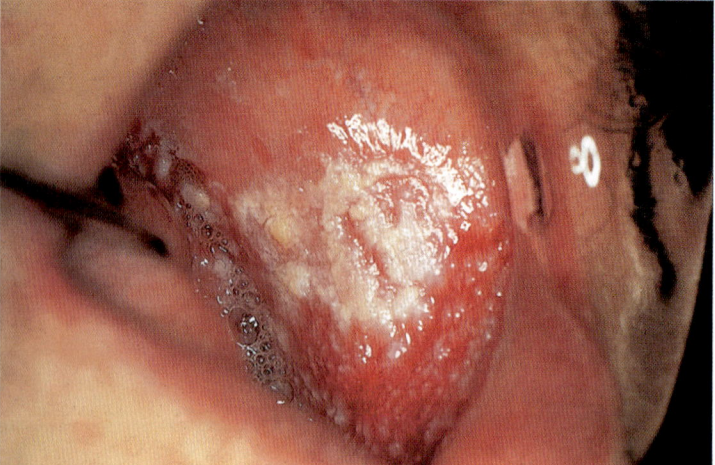

Figure 108.42 Speckled leukoplakia.

Clinical features

Leukoplakias vary in size: the majority are solitary, small and focal white plaques, others more widespread, occasionally involving very large areas of the oral mucosa. Leukoplakia has a wide range of clinical presentations, from homogeneous white plaques, which can be faintly white or very thick and opaque, to nodular white lesions, or lesions admixed with red lesions. It is generally asymptomatic. The tongue, gingiva, buccal mucosa and palatal mucosa are the most commonly affected sites. High-risk sites for malignant transformation include the soft palate complex, ventrolateral tongue and floor of the mouth (where sublingual keratosis has a particularly high risk of malignant change; Figure 108.40). Sublingual keratosis is more common in women than men, has a typical 'ebbing-tide' appearance clinically (Figure 108.40).

Leukoplakia is classified as:

- Homogeneous leukoplakia: most common type, well-demarcated, uniform white plaque, usually of *low* malignant potential (Figure 108.41).

- Non-homogeneous leukoplakia: *high* risk of malignant transformation.
  - Verrucous leukoplakia has a well-demarcated border, wrinkled or warty exophytic surface, often occurs on the gingiva.
  - Nodular leukoplakia surface has rounded exophytic lesions, well demarcated.
  - Erythroleukoplakia which has areas of erythema within the leukoplakia that may be patchy or speckled (speckled leukoplakia) (Figure 108.42).

Other leukoplakias

- Chronic hyperplastic candidiasis (candidal leukoplakia) may be associated with an increased risk of malignant change. The role of *Candida* in oral potentially malignant disorders remains contentious. Chronic hyperplastic candidiasis leukoplakias may respond to antifungals and cessation of smoking.
- Hairy leukoplakia is caused by Epstein–Barr virus. It usually has a corrugated surface and affects margins of the tongue. The condition is benign and self-limiting.
- Syphilitic leukoplakia, especially of the dorsum of the tongue, is a feature of tertiary syphilis and rarely seen now.

Prognosis

There is a higher risk of transformation for non-homogeneous leukoplakias. The malignant transformation rate has been reported as 3% for homogeneous lesions and 14.5% for non-homogeneous lesions [3,4,5,6].

Proliferative verrucous leukoplakia is a special subtype of verrucous leukoplakia, characterised by progressive involvement of the oral mucosa by white plaques, often verrucous, at multiple, non-contiguous sites, or it may present as a single large lesion with or without involvement of contiguous sites (Figure 108.43). The average age at diagnosis of proliferative verrucous leukoplakia is in the seventh decade. There is less association with smoking. The most common intraoral sites involved include the gingiva, alveolar mucosa and palatal mucosa. The malignant transformation rate is 49.5% [5]. It may be associated in some patients with preceding oral lichen planus.

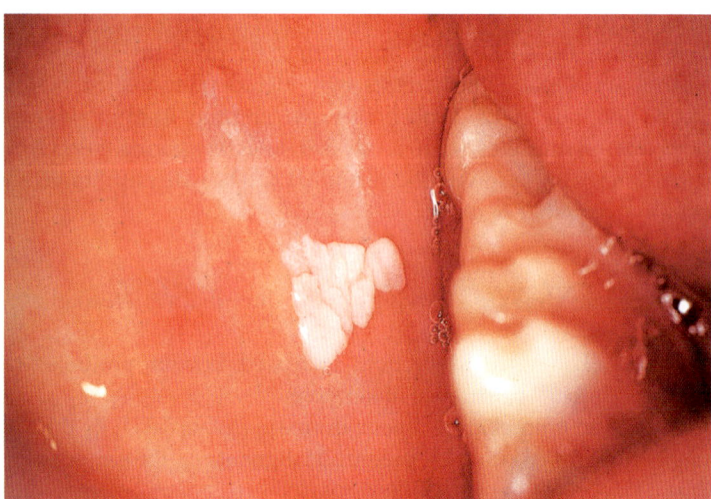

Figure 108.41 Homogeneous leukoplakia in the buccal mucosa.

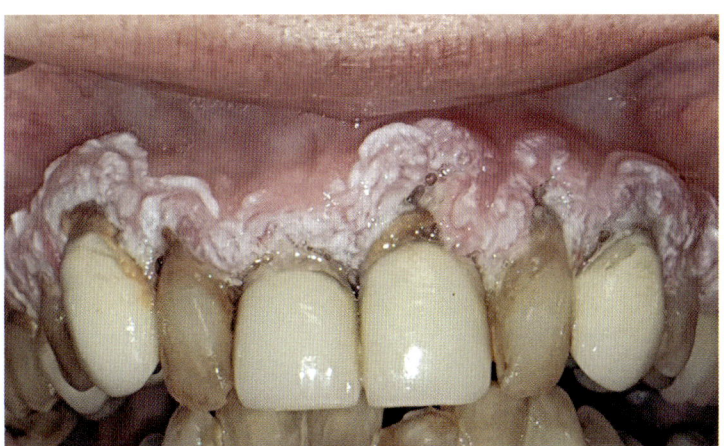

Figure 108.43 Proliferative verrucous leukoplakia involving the maxillary gingiva.

Leukoplakia has an annual malignant transformation rate of 1.56% and 9.3% for proliferative verrucous leukoplakia [5]. It is not possible to predict reliably which leukoplakias will progress to carcinoma, but currently, the most predictive markers of transformation in leukoplakias are (Box 108.3):
• speckled (erythroleukoplakia)
• verrucous
• from high-risk sites, including the soft palate/fauces, floor of the mouth/ventral tongue
• in a patient with previous cancer in the upper aerodigestive tract
• in non-smoking females
• dysplasia
• DNA polysomic (aneuploidy or tetraploidy)
• positive for genetic markers such as mutated tumour suppressor factor p53, or loss of heterozygosity on chromosomes 3p or 9p.

Box 108.3 Leukoplakias at increased risk of malignant transformation

• Non-homogeneous type
• Dysplasia
• In non-smokers
• In females
• High-risk sites – the soft palate/fauces, floor of the mouth/ventral tongue
• Size >200 mm^2
• Cancer history positive
• DNA aneuploidy
• Loss of chromosomal heterozygosity (LOH)
  • High risk – LOH for 9p, 17p and 4q
• p53 protein expression

No single molecular marker appears to be predictive of malignant transformation in leukoplakia. Malignant change to carcinoma is most frequent in women >50 years and in large lesions. Interestingly, leukoplakias developing in non-smokers have a higher rather than lower risk of malignant change. Some leukoplakias may regress clinically, not only when supposed aetiological factors have been removed but also sometimes spontaneously.

Diagnosis

There are no clinical signs or symptoms that reliably predict whether a leukoplakia will undergo malignant change. Biopsy can confirm the presence and degree of dysplasia. Dysplasia is characterised by cytological and architectural alterations reflecting the loss of normal maturation and stratification pattern of surface epithelium. Dysplasia is graded as mild, moderate or severe. The malignant transformation rate of dysplastic lesions is 1.7–15.0% for mild, 0.0–32.1% for moderate and up to 50.0% for severe. Biopsy is generally indicated for leukoplakias that are:
• in patients with previous or concurrent head and neck cancer
• non-homogeneous, i.e. have red areas, are verrucous or nodular
• in a high-risk site such as the floor of the mouth or tongue
• focal
• symptomatic
• without obvious aetiological factors.

In lesions that are large, multiple biopsies should be performed such as from a white area, from a red area, and from an indurated area.

Management

Lifestyle modification to eliminate risk factors is indicated. Up to 45% of leukoplakias may regress or totally disappear if tobacco use is stopped. Leukoplakias induced by smokeless tobacco may resolve if the habit is ceased. The current treatment for oral leukoplakia can range from careful observation to surgical intervention. 'Watchful waiting' may be considered in patients with mild dysplasia. Moderate-to-severe dysplasia are more likely to progress and should be excised with a scalpel with a clear margin or laser excision.

Current chemoprevention approaches to prevent malignant transformation include retinoids, epidermal growth factor receptor inhibitors/antagonists, cyclooxygenase-2 inhibitors, p53 modulators and topical agents such as bleomycin. Medical therapies are not reliably effective. Retinoids (13-*cis*-retinoic acid) can induce regression of leukoplakia. However, chemoprevention with retinoids is not a definitive treatment since there is a high lesion recurrence rate after stopping treatment [2,7].

Recurrence has been reported in approximately 7–38% of lesions. Follow-up is usually life-long with clinical photographs.

Oral lichen planus

See later in this chapter.

Psoriasis (Chapter 35)

The oral mucosa appears to be rarely involved in psoriasis, although there are occasionally lip lesions or white oral lesions, especially in the buccal mucosa, or lesions clinically indistinguishable from geographic tongue, particularly in generalised pustular psoriasis [1,2]. Oral lesions are more likely to develop in those with the more severe forms of psoriasis.

ULCERATION

Blisters

Box 108.4 lists the potential causes for oral blistering lesions. The commonest is trauma or mucocoeles. Most mucocoeles arise from damage to the duct which normally allows mucus to drain freely from minor salivary glands, e.g. within the lower lip to drain into the mouth. Minor trauma results in extravasation of mucus from the minor salivary glands forming a clear or bluish swelling. Superficial mucocoeles can also be seen on the soft palate in chronic GVHD.

Box 108.4 Causes of blisters

Trauma – friction, chemical burns
Mucocoeles
Infection – bacterial, viral (herpes simplex, coxsackie, varicella)
Angina bullosa haemorrhagica
Immunobullous disorders
Bullous lupus
Bullous lichen planus
Erythema multiforme
Stevens–Johnson syndrome/toxic epidermal necrolysis
Drugs
Amyloidosis

There are many other causes for oral blisters and these will be discussed in more detail. Many of these quickly burst and form erosions as in pemphigus or ulcers (full thickness loss of the epithelium). Many of these will be clear fluid filled or serosanguinous. Blood-filled blisters may be seen in angina bullosa haemorrhagica, pemphigus or in amyloidosis. Blisters in pemphigus are rarely seen as they break down rapidly to produce erosions. Epidermolysis bullosa acquisita and erythema multiforme may present with oral bullae or vesicles, although ulcers are more common. Vesicles may be seen in viral infections, especially in herpes simplex stomatitis, chickenpox, herpangina and hand, foot and mouth disease.

Erosions and ulcers

Erosions are typically erythematous areas of thinned epithelium where there has not been a breach in the basement membrane. They may be seen for example in pemphigus vulgaris or atrophic lichen planus.

Oral ulcers are often caused by trauma or recurrent aphthae. However, there are many potential causes that are listed in Box 108.5. Malignant neoplasms may present as ulcers. Various infections or systemic disorders, particularly those of the blood, gastrointestinal tract or skin, also produce mouth ulcers, as may drugs and irradiation. The causes of mouth ulcers are thus diverse. However, the history of the oral ulcer(s) will provide most of the clues for diagnosis. There are four main groups based upon clinical presentation (Box 108.5).

Box 108.5 Cause of oral ulcers

Single episode
- Local factors, e.g. trauma, dental appliances, sharp teeth, irradiation
- Infections
- Drugs, e.g. nicorandil
- Stevens–Johnson syndrome/toxic epidermal necrolysis

Recurrent episodic
- Aphthous ulcers
- Erythema multiforme

Persistent ulcers (see Oral manifestations of systemic diseases)
- Immunobullous disorders
- Lichen planus
- Lupus erythematosus
- Behçet syndrome/disease
- Vasculitis
- Ulcerative colitis/Crohn disease

Single persistent lesion (see Malignant lesions)
- Malignant neoplasms

SINGLE EPISODE OF ORAL ULCERATION

Mouth ulcers of local aetiology

Oral ulceration due to local factors tends to resolve spontaneously. Accidental cheek biting or facial trauma may cause ulceration; the history is usually quite clear and a single ulcer of short duration (5–10 days) is present. Ulceration due to biting an anaesthetised lower lip or tongue following a dental local analgesic injection is a fairly common problem in young children.

Orthodontic appliances or, more commonly, dentures are responsible for many traumatic oral ulcers. These ulcers are usually clearly related to the appliance. Chronic trauma may cause a well-defined ulcer with a whitish keratotic halo [1].

The possibility of some other aetiology for ulcers of apparently local cause should always be borne in mind. Riga–Fede disease consists of ulcers of the lingual frenum in neonates with natal lower incisors [2]. Child abuse may cause ulcers, especially over the upper labial fraena. Self-mutilation may be seen in some psychologically disturbed patients, patients with learning disability, individuals with sensory impairment and in Lesch–Nyhan syndrome [3]. Other local causes of ulceration include thermal burns, especially of the tongue and palate (e.g. 'pizza burn' – now more common with microwave oven use), chemical burns from the holding of medicaments or drugs (e.g. aspirin or cocaine) against the mucosa, and irradiation mucositis [4]. Most ulcers of local cause heal spontaneously within 7–14 days if the cause is removed.

Management

Maintenance of good oral hygiene and the use of hot saline mouth-baths and 0.2% aqueous chlorhexidine gluconate mouthwash aid healing. A 0.15% benzydamine mouthwash may help give relief. Occasionally, mechanical protection with a plastic guard may help. Patients should be reviewed within 3 weeks to ensure healing has occurred. Any patient with a single ulcer lasting more than 2–3 weeks should be regarded with suspicion and investigated further, usually by biopsy.

Traumatic ulcerative granuloma with stromal eosinophilia (eosinophilic ulcer)

Traumatic ulcerative granuloma with stromal eosinophilia (TUGSE) is a benign and self-limited lesion which typically affects the tongue [1–7]. It is rare and may be easily mistaken for a cancer or microbial infection.

Epidemiology
It affects older adults 50–80 years of age. There is a slight female predominance reported. The aetiology remains obscure but trauma has been found to be a contributing factor.

Pathophysiology
Pathological features show an extensive subepithelial inflammatory cell infiltration, with predominantly eosinophilic cells throughout the submucosa and histological similarities to CD30+ lympho-proliferative disorders [3]. It involves the superficial mucosa and extending deep into the submucosa involving the muscle and even salivary glands. The peripheral blood eosinophil count is normal.

Clinical features
TUGSE typically affects the lateral or dorsal surface of the tongue. It presents as a rapidly developing solitary ulcer with elevated or indurated margins. Lesions may vary in size from a few millimetres to several centimetres. In addition, submucosal masses, multifocal lesions and recurrences have also been described.

Investigations
A diagnostic biopsy is usually undertaken.

Management
A variety of approaches has been used including a conservative excisional biopsy and intralesional or topical corticosteroids.

RECURRENT (EPISODIC) ORAL ULCERATION

Ulcers are the most common lesions to affect the oral mucosa. Among the many causes, aphthae are the most frequent. There are three subtypes that need to be recognised: minor, major and herpetiform. Ulcers similar to aphthae (aphthous-like ulcers) may be seen in some multisystem disorders such as Behçet syndrome.

Recurrent episodes of ulceration may also be due to EM and infections such as recurrent herpes simplex (cold sores) or very rarely varicella-zoster.

Recurrent aphthous stomatitis

Recurrent aphthous stomatitis (RAS) is characterised by multiple recurrent, round or ovoid ulcers, which have circumscribed margins, erythematous haloes and a yellow or grey base. Lesions may be single or multiple and the three main subtypes are detailed in Table 108.3. Aphthae last only a limited period of time (from 1 to 6 weeks) depending upon the subtype, before healing spontaneously. Episodes are recurrent, unlike ulcers that persist without healing, such as malignant ulcers and those associated with vesiculobullous disorders. The natural history of RAS is one of eventual remission, but this may take many years.

Epidemiology
RAS is a common disease affecting 10–20% of the general population. RAS typically starts in childhood or adolescence. There is a slight female predisposition and it is often familial. There is no underlying systemic disease associated. However, there may be nutritional deficiencies aggravating the condition.

Pathophysiology
The aetiology of RAS is unclear [1–4]. There are identifiable predisposing factors in some patients (Table 108.3). There is no known association with systemic autoimmune disorders and it tends to resolve or decrease spontaneously with increasing age. It seems likely that a minor degree of immunological dysregulation underlies aphthae, and a genetic tendency to ulceration, and cross-reacting antigens between the oral mucosa and microorganisms may be involved. Immune mechanisms that appear to play a role in a people with a genetic predisposition to oral ulceration include [5–8]:
- A local cell-mediated immune response to Henoch–Schönlein purpura involving cytotoxic CD8+ T-cells, natural killer cells, macrophages and mast cells.
- T-helper cells (gamma-delta cells) predominate in early RAS lesions, along with some natural killer cells.
- Cytotoxic cells then appear in the lesions.
- IL-1β and IL-6 gene polymorphisms are associated with an increased risk for RAS.
- There is increased expression of TNF-α, IL-2, IL-4, IL-5 and interferon-γ in aphthous ulcers.

Immune dysregulation leads to an exaggerated proinflammatory process or a relatively weak anti-inflammatory response.

Infectious causes
Attempts to implicate a variety of viruses or bacteria in the aetiology of RAS have largely been unsuccessful.

Genetics
There is a genetic predisposition shown by a positive family history in about one-third of patients and by an increased frequency of human leukocyte antigen (HLA) types (HLA-A2, A11, B12 and DR2) [1–4]. There is an association between RAS and inheritance of a single-nucleotide polymorphism of the NOS2 gene (encoding inducible nitric oxide synthase) [9]. IL-1β and IL-6 gene polymorphisms are associated with an increased risk for RAS [10].

Table 108.3 Main features of recurrent aphthous stomatitis.

	Minor aphthae	Major aphthae	Herpetiform ulcers
Age of onset	Childhood or adolescence	Childhood or adolescence	Young adult
Ulcer size	2–4 mm	May be 10 mm or larger	Initially tiny but ulcers coalesce
Number of ulcers	Up to about 6	Up to about 6	10–100
Sites affected	Mainly vestibule, labial, buccal mucosa and floor of mouth; rarely dorsum of tongue, gingiva or palate	Any site	Any site but often on ventrum of tongue
Duration of each ulcer	Up to 10 days	Up to 1 month	Up to 1 month
Other comments	Most common type of aphthae	May heal with scarring	Affects females predominantly

Environmental factors

Stress underlies RAS in some cases. Trauma from biting the mucosa or from dental appliances may lead to aphthae. Cessation of smoking may precipitate or exacerbate RAS in some cases. In up to 20% of patients, deficiencies of iron, folic acid (folate) or vitamin B are found and sometimes the correction of this may relieve the ulceration. Endocrine factors are relevant in some women where RAS is related to the fall in progestogen level in the luteal phase of the menstrual cycle. RAS may regress temporarily in pregnancy.

Clinical features

Patients with RAS have no clinically detectable systemic symptoms or signs. There are three main clinical types of RAS (Table 108.3):
- Minor aphthous ulcers (~80% of all RAS).
- Major aphthous ulcers.
- Herpetiform ulcers.

Minor aphthous ulcers. This type of RAS occurs mainly in the 10–40 years age group. Ulcers are small, round or ovoid ulcers 2–4 mm in diameter and occur in crops of only a few ulcers (1–6) at a time, with initially yellowish floors surrounded by an erythematous halo and some oedema, but become greyish as epithelialisation proceeds (Figure 108.44). They affect mainly the non-keratinised mobile mucosae of the lips, cheeks, floor of the mouth, sulci or ventrum of the tongue and occasionally soft palate or fauces. Ulcers heal in 7–10 days and recur at intervals of 1–4 months. The ulcers heal without scarring.

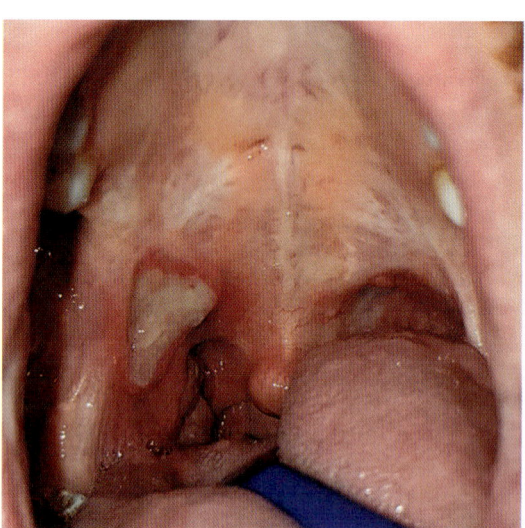

Figure 108.45 Major aphthous ulcer involving the right soft palate. There is evidence of scarring involving the left soft palate.

Major aphthous ulcers. The ulcers are round, ovoid or more angular as in Figure 108.45. They can be large, frequently about 1 cm in diameter. They are found on any area of the oral mucosa, including the keratinised dorsum of the tongue or palate. They occur in crops of only a few ulcers at one time and heal slowly over 10–40 days. They are extremely painful and may heal with scarring.

Herpetiform ulceration. This type of RAS are found in a slightly older age group than the other RAS and begin with vesiculation, which passes rapidly into multiple minute pinhead-sized discrete ulcers that increase in size and coalesce to leave large, round, ragged ulcers (Figure 108.46). They involve any oral site, including the keratinised mucosa, and heal in 10 days or longer. Herpetiform ulcers are often extremely painful and recur so frequently that ulceration may be virtually continuous. Their similarity to herpetic stomatitis gives herpetiform ulcers their name, but there is no evidence that herpes simplex virus (HSV) is involved.

Aphthous-like ulcers

The diagnosis of RAS is often misapplied to the similar ulcers (aphthous-like ulcers), which may be seen in a range of systemic conditions (Table 108.4). History and examination should be directed to eliciting any cutaneous, gastrointestinal, genital,

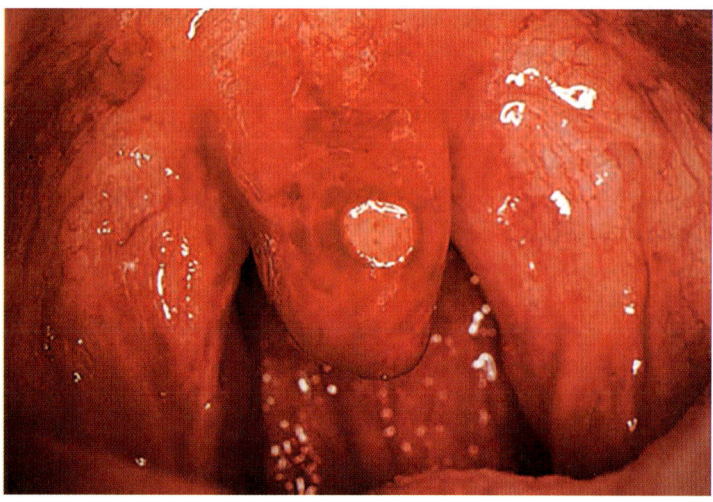

Figure 108.44 Recurrent aphthae.

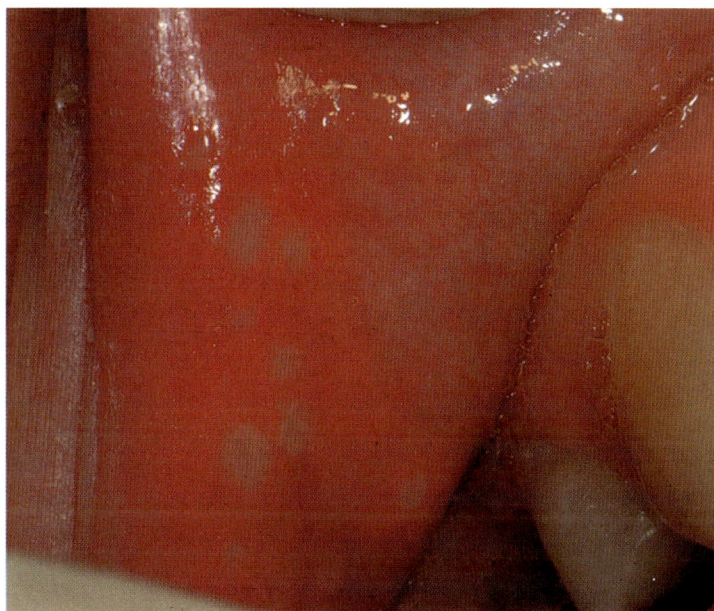

Figure 108.46 Herpetiform ulceration.

Table 108.4 Systemic factors that may occasionally underlie or be associated with aphthous-like ulcers.

	Comments
Autoinflammatory disorders	e.g periodic fever, aphthous stomatitis, pharyngitis and cervical adenitis (PFAPA) syndrome
Behçet disease	Association of recurrent mouth ulcers with ocular lesions, genital ulcers and multisystem disease
Gastrointestinal disease	Malabsorption states (coeliac disease and Crohn disease) may precipitate RAS in a small minority
Immunodeficiency	e.g. HIV, cyclical neutropenia
Sweet syndrome	See Chapter 49

ocular, joint problems or history of fever, which might point to these conditions. They include conditions such as:

- Immune deficiencies such as HIV, cyclical neutropenia and other immune defects.
- Behçet disease, where mouth ulcers are seen along with genital ulcers.
- Coeliac disease.
- Crohn disease.
- Autoinflammatory conditions such as periodic fever, aphthous stomatitis, pharyngitis and cervical adenitis (PFAPA) syndrome [11].
- Sweet syndrome.
- Drug use, especially NSAIDs and nicorandil.

Investigations

Diagnosis of RAS is based on history and clinical features; no specific tests are available. Biopsy is indicated only where some other cause of ulceration is suspected. To exclude a number of systemic disorders, it is often useful to undertake blood investigations:

- Full blood picture (haemoglobin, white cell count and differential, red cell indices.
- Red cell folate assay.

- Serum ferritin levels (or other iron studies).
- Vitamin B_{12} measurements.
- Calcium measurements (low in coeliac disease).
- Tissue transglutaminase and IgA anti-endomysial antibody assays (positive in coeliac disease).

The relevance of HLA studies for differentiating RAS from Behçet syndrome is discussed below.

Management

RAS in most patients resolves or abates spontaneously with age. An underlying, identifiable predisposing cause is particularly likely where ulceration commences or worsens in adult life [12–14].

Predisposing factors should be corrected:

- Trauma: patients should avoid hard or sharp foods.
- Any iron or vitamin deficiency should be corrected.

Relief of pain and reduction of ulcer duration:

- Good oral hygiene should be maintained; chlorhexidine mouthwash may help.
- Anti-inflammatory agents: topical agents, such as benzydamine, may help in the management of discomfort.
- Topical analgesics, e.g. 5% lidocaine gel or spray
- Topical corticosteroids can often control minor or major RAS. Topical corticosteroids are the primary therapeutic agents used to treat ulcerative mucosal lesions. A mild potency agent such as hydrocortisone hemisuccinate pellets (Corlan®) 2.5 mg or triamcinolone acetonide in carboxymethylcellulose paste (Adcortyl® in Orabase®) may be effective, but more typically a medium potency corticosteroid such as betamethasone (500 μg soluble tablets dissolved in 10 mL of water and used as a mouthwash) may be required [15–17]. Larger and recalcitrant ulcers can be treated by intralesional therapy such as triamcinolone injections. Topical tetracycline (a capsule of 100 mg doxycycline dissolved in 10 mL water) as a mouth rinse may provide relief and reduce ulcer duration [18]. Systemic immunomodulators may be required and include short courses of systemic corticosteroids (e.g. prednisolone) usually reserved for major aphthosis or other immunomodulatory agents (e.g. colchicine, azathioprine, pentoxifylline, ciclosporin, dapsone, interferon or anti-TNF agents) [19–28]. Colchicine is a useful second line agent. It is well tolerated if introduced slowly to mitigate the gastrointestinal adverse reactions that frequently occur. Treatment may be with 500 μg once daily, increasing after a week or two to twice daily. Occasionally three times daily is required in the more severe cases. Six-monthly full blood count is advisable. Azathioprine could be considered in those inadequately controlled with colchicine plus betamethasone mouth rinses.

Complex aphthosis

Complex aphthosis is a term usefully applied to patients with either: (i) more than three almost continual oral aphthae or (ii) recurrent oral and genital aphthae but with no other features to support a diagnosis of Behçet syndrome [1,2]. These patients very rarely progress to Behçet. It is important in these cases to undertake a full screening for underlying systemic causes (secondary complex aphthosis), especially for underlying inflammatory bowel disease. The majority, however, will be idiopathic, i.e. with no identifiable underlying cause.

Management

These patients are usually well-controlled with colchicine and betamethasone mouthwash or azathioprine. Combined colchicine and dapsone may also be used in these group [1,3].

Behçet syndrome (Chapter 48)

Behçet syndrome (BS)/Behçet disease is a systemic variable vessel vasculitis that involves the mucosa, skin, joints, eyes, arteries, veins, nervous system and the gastrointestinal system [1–4]. Turkey has the highest prevalence of BS at 420/100 000. The prevalence of BS is approximately 0.64/100 000 in the UK and up to 0.33/100 000 in the USA. Onset of the disease usually occurs in the third or fourth decade of life.

Aetiology

The aetiology of BS is unknown. There is a genetic predisposition to BS, which is strongly associated with HLA-B*51 (HLA-B*5101). The frequency of HLA-B51 along the Silk Route ranges between 50% and 80% among patients with BS (<25% in the population). In contrast, the frequency of HLA-B51 in Northern Europe and the USA is around 15% among patients with BS against 5% in the general population. HLA-DR/DQ haplotypes are important for the development of the mucocutaneous type of BS.

The aetiopathogenesis of BS is still unclear. The most widely accepted theory behind its pathogenesis is that an environmental stimulus elicits an abnormal immune response in a genetically susceptible host. A possible pathogenic role of certain bacterial antigens that have cross-reactivity with human peptides has been proposed. Heat shock proteins, streptococcal antigens, *Helicobacter pylori*, Herpes simplex virus, and parvovirus B19 have been implicated [5].

There are many immunological findings in BS similar to those seen in RAS, with various T lymphocyte abnormalities and increased polymorphonuclear leukocyte motility.

- There is increased T cell (Th-1) activity; cells infiltrating into lesions expressing interferon (IFN)-γ and reacting against heat shock proteins. Proinflammatory cytokines IL-12, IL-18 and tumour necrosis factor alpha (TNF-α) are increased. There may be a mix of Th1 and Th2 activity in BS and increased activity of Th17 cells.
- Circulating autoantibodies against a number of components, including oral mucosal antigens, endothelial cells, T cell costimulatory molecule CTLA-4, killer immunoglobulin-like receptors, oxidised low-density lipoprotein and kinectin.
- Hypercoagulability is also a feature. Von Willebrand factor, endothelin-1,2, thromboxane and thrombomodulin are increased and factor V Leiden and prothrombin mutations are associated with thromboses in BS.
- Endothelial dysfunction is a characteristic finding in BS.
- Polymorphonuclear leukocytes are activated.

Clinical features

BS is a chronic multisystem vasculitis characterised mainly by:

- Oral aphthous-like ulceration (90–100% cases) is usually the initial manifestation of BS. The minor form is by far the most common in BS, followed by the major and herpetiform variants.
- Recurrent painful genital ulcers that tend to heal with scarring (64–88% cases). In women, ulcers most commonly affect the labia and in men, the scrotum is regularly involved.
- Ocular lesions (30–70%) are more frequent and severe in men. Uveitis with conjunctivitis (early) and hypopyon (late), retinal vasculitis (posterior uveitis), iridocyclitis and optic atrophy can arise.
- Central nervous system lesions are predominantly subtentorial (affecting cerebellum, brainstem and spinal cord), with meningoencephalitis, cerebral infarction, psychosis, cranial nerve palsies, and hemi- and quadriparesis.
- Skin lesions (80%) include erythema nodosum-like lesions, papulopustular lesions and acneiform nodules. Pathergy phenomenon is not routinely tested for in UK or US patients.
- Cardiac or large vein thrombosis (of the inferior vena cava and cranial venous sinuses).
- Involvement of the joints, epididymis, heart, intestinal tract.
- Myalgia and migratory arthralgias without overt arthritis.

Diagnosis

BS is usually diagnosed on clinical grounds. Because BS is rare and the established features overlap those of many other diseases, the condition can be difficult to diagnose. The International Study Group for Behçet's Syndrome Criteria 1990 [6] suggests the diagnosis should be made on clinical grounds alone (Table 108.5). The International Criteria for Behçet's Disease (ICBD) (2013) criteria [7] use a points-based system whereby a score of 4 points or above is classified as BS (Table 108.6). This system is more useful for research studies in patients already confirmed as having BS. In clinical practice and to minimise overdiagnosis in what is a rare disease, the International Study Group criteria are generally used.

There are no specific tests for the diagnosis of BS. Findings of HLA-B51 (more frequently associated with ocular Behçet), raised serum IgD and antibodies to cardiolipin are supportive of a

Table 108.5 International Study Group for Behçet's Syndrome Criteria 1990.

Oral aphthous-like ulcers plus two or more of:
Recurrent genital ulceration
Typical eye lesions
Characteristic skin lesions
Pathergy reaction – venepuncture followed by pustulation.

Table 108.6 International Criteria for Behçet's Disease (ICBD) (2013).

Oral aphthous ulcers (2 points)
Genital ulceration (2 points)
Ocular lesions (2 points)
Skin lesions (1 point)
Vascular lesions (1 point)
Neurological manifestations, e.g. headache (1 point)

diagnosis of BS. Disease activity may be assessed by serum levels of acute-phase proteins (ESR, CRP).

The differential diagnosis for BS includes the following:

- Sweet syndrome: aphthae, conjunctivitis/episcleritis, inflamed tender papule or nodule
- Erythema multiforme: erosions, target lesions
- Pemphigoid: bullae, erosions
- Pemphigus: erosions, multiple flaccid bullae
- Reactive arthritis: ulcers, conjunctivitis, keratoderma blenorrhagica
- Ulcerative colitis
- Herpes simplex
- Syphilis
- Lupus erythematosus
- Mixed connective tissue disease.

Management

BS is not self-limiting. Central nervous system involvement, thromboses of major vessels and gastrointestinal perforation while rare, result in a poor prognosis.

The effects of BS may be cumulative, especially with neurological, vascular and ocular involvement; one main problem is ophthalmic involvement, which can result in blindness. Mortality, though low, may result from neurological involvement, vascular thromboses, bowel perforation or cardiopulmonary disease, or as a complication of immunosuppressive therapy. Few patients with Behçet syndrome have spontaneous remission and thus treatment is indicated. A multidisciplinary approach is essential and patients ideally managed in a tertiary referral centre [8,**9**,10–13].

Topical treatment for oral ulcers. Treatment for aphthous-like ulcers in BS includes tetracycline mouthwash and topical corticosteroids. Benzydamine hydrochloride and lidocaine are helpful for symptomatic relief.

Systemic treatment. Systemic therapy with colchicine (1500 µg daily) and dapsone is often useful for mucocutaneous lesions. In refractory cases, thalidomide, azathioprine or biological agents, such as tumour necrosis factor-α antagonists (infliximab, etanercept) may be necessary [8,**9**,10–13].

MAGIC syndrome

MAGIC syndrome is associated with mouth and genital ulcers and inflamed cartilage [1–4]. Other oculomucocutaneous syndromes (Table 108.7) may cause similar manifestations.

Ulcers in association with systemic disease

Aphthous-like ulcers may be associated with systemic disease especially haematological, gastrointestinal and dermatological disorders. Oral ulceration is also frequently caused by infections and can be caused by iatrogenic problems such as drugs or irradiation or GVHD (Table 108.4).

Table 108.7 Oculomucocutaneous syndromes.[a]

| Disease | Main lesions | | |
	Oral and genital	Ocular	Skin
Behçet syndrome	Aphthae	Uveitis	Erythema nodosum
Sweet syndrome	Aphthae	Conjunctivitis, episcleritis	Inflamed papule or nodule
Erythema multiforme	Erosions	Erosions	Target lesions
Cicatricial pemphigoid	Bullae	Erosions	Occasional dome-shaped bullae
	Erosions	Scarring	
Pemphigus	Erosions	Erosions (rare)	Multiple, flaccid bullae
Reactive arthritis	Ulcers	Conjunctivitis	Keratoderma blenorrhagica

[a] Ulcerative colitis, herpes simplex, lupus erythematosus, mixed connective tissue disease and other disorders may also cause oral, cutaneous and ocular lesions.

Acute febrile neutrophilic dermatosis (Sweet syndrome) (Chapter 49)

Aphthous-like ulcers particularly on the buccal mucosa, palate or tongue may be found in this condition. Additional reported oral findings include bullae, vesicles, gingival hyperplasia, necrotising ulcerative periodontitis, nodules, papules, pustules and tongue swelling [1–3].

Drugs

A wide range of drugs can occasionally induce mouth ulcers, by a variety of effects [1]. Oral local use of caustics or agents such as cocaine can cause erosions or ulcers. Oral ulcers are regularly produced by cytotoxic agents. Aphthous-like ulcers may follow the use of nicorandil or methotrexate [2]. The ulcers usually resolve in 10–14 days if the offending drug can be identified and withdrawn.

Drugs may also cause mucocutaneous lesions; ulcers of a lichenoid type may follow exposure to antimalarials, beta blockers, NSAIDs, phenothiazines and sulfonylureas [3]. The Stevens–Johnson syndrome/toxic epidermal necrolysis spectrum may be associated with many drugs including allopurinol, carbamazepine, lamotrigine, nevirapine, oxicam, NSAIDs, phenobarbital, phenytoin, sulfamethoxazole and other sulphur antibiotics, and sulfasalazine [4]. Rarely drugs may be implicated in erythema multiforme. Infection, however, is by far the most frequently identified trigger.

Miscellaneous causes

Glucagonoma. Glossitis, stomatitis, or cheilitis has been reported [1,2].

Mucha–Haberman disease. Oral, genital and conjunctival mucosal ulcerations have been reported in pityriasis lichenoides et varioliformis acuta (Mucha–Haberman disease) [1,2].

Kawasaki disease. Kawasaki disease is an acute self-limiting systemic vasculitis that affects medium-sized arteries. It is characterised by a fever lasting for 5 days or more, non-exudative conjunctivitis, oropharyngeal changes, and rash and cervical lymphadenopathy, lasting for an average of 12 days without therapy [1]. There is erythema of the lips and oral mucosa. It is common in childhood and occurs only rarely in adults. At least one oral feature should be present for the diagnosis to be made. The oral and pharyngeal mucosae become generally red and sore and the lips dry and fissured. There may be oral ulceration and a 'strawberry tongue' appearance [1–3].

Necrotising sialometaplasia. Necrotising sialometaplasia is an uncommon benign self-limiting condition seen predominantly in the posterior hard palate of young adult males, most of whom smoke tobacco [1–4] but has been reported at other oral sites, such as the tongue, floor of the mouth and salivary glands. Hypoxia-inducible factor (HIF)-1α, VEGF and epidermal growth factor receptor have been implicated in the pathogenesis. An association with bulimia has been reported [5,6].

A painless deep ulcer persists for several weeks before spontaneously healing. This benign lesion must be differentiated from malignancy. Biopsy is usually indicated and reveals necrosis and pseudoepitheliomatous changes probably resulting from squamous metaplasia following infarction of minor salivary glands [7].

Superficial mucocoeles. Superficial extravasation mucocoeles of the intraoral minor salivary glands in the palate, buccal mucosa or labial mucosa are not uncommon, especially associated with oral lichen planus in middle-aged or elderly women and with chronic GVHD [1]. This benign self-limiting condition may cause confusion with vesiculobullous disorders [2–4]. No treatment is available or required.

PREMALIGNANCY AND MALIGNANCY

PREMALIGNANT LESIONS

The WHO Collaborating Centre for Oral Cancer Workshop in 2020 defined oral potentially malignant disorders (OPMDs) as 'any oral mucosal abnormality that is associated with a statistically increased risk of developing oral cancer' [1]. The current classification of oral potentially malignant disorders include: leukoplakia, proliferative verrucous leukoplakia, erythroplakia, oral lichen planus, lichenoid lesions, oral submucous fibrosis, oral lupus erythematosus, actinic cheilitis, palatal lesions in reverse smokers, dyskeratosis congenita and oral graft versus host disease. Oral epidermolysis bullosa (OEB), chronic hyperplastic candidiasis (CHC) and exophytic verrucous hyperplasia were removed from the classification [1]. The prevalence of OPMDs varies and has been estimated to be 4.47%, ranging from 0.11% in North American populations to 10.54% in Asian populations [2].

Erythroplakia (see earlier in this chapter)

Leukoplakia (see earlier in this chapter)

Oral submucous fibrosis

Oral submucous fibrosis is a chronic, potentially malignant condition seen only in persons who chew betel (*Areca catechu*) nuts, pan masala or gutkha [1,2]. It is characterised by tightening of the buccal, and sometimes palatal and lingual mucosae, causing trismus [1]. Areca nut also causes or aggravates pre-existing conditions such as neuronal injury, myocardial infarction, cardiac arrhythmias, hepatotoxicity, asthma, central obesity, type II diabetes, hyperlipidaemia and metabolic syndrome. It affects the endocrine system, leading to hypothyroidism, prostate hyperplasia and infertility. It suppresses T-cell activity and decreases release of cytokines. It is associated with adverse birth outcomes when used during pregnancy. It is linked to cancers of the oral cavity, pharynx, oesophagus, liver and biliary tracts and uterus.

Epidemiology

It occurs at high frequency in Asian populations, especially in those from the Indian subcontinent. The prevalence of oral submucous fibrosis in India has been estimated to range from 0.2 to 2.3% in males and 1.2–4.6% in females. It usually affects persons between the ages of 30–65 years.

Predisposing factors

Chewing betel quid is available in various forms both in the countries of Asia and in peoples from those areas living in resource-rich countries:

- Betel quid without tobacco.
- Gutka (gutkha, guttkha or guthka): a manufactured version of betel quid with tobacco sold as a single-use sachet.
- Mainpuri tobacco: a mixture of *Areca* nut, tobacco, lime and various condiments. Sweeteners or spices (i.e. anise seed, cardamom, clove, mustard, saffron, turmeric) may also be added.
- Mawa (kharra): a combination of *Areca* nut, tobacco and lime.
- Pan: freshly prepared betel quid (with or without tobacco).
- Pan masala: a commercially manufactured powdered version of betel quid.

Commercially freeze-dried products such as pan masala, gutka and mawa have higher concentrations of *Areca* nut per chew and appear to cause oral submucous fibrosis more rapidly than self-prepared conventional betel quid.

Pathophysiology

Areca nut contains alkaloids (the most potent of which is arecoline), flavonoids and copper, all of which interfere with collagen metabolism [3–10]. Arecoline stimulates fibroblasts to increase collagen production. It induces production of interleukin 6, keratinocyte growth factor-1, insulin-like growth factor-1, cystatin C (a protein up-regulated in a variety of fibrotic diseases) and tissue inhibitor of matrix metalloproteinases (TIMP). Arecoline inhibits matrix metalloproteinases (MMPs, particularly MMP-2) and chewing areca quid may also activate NF-κB expression, thereby further stimulating collagen fibroblasts. Flavonoids, catechin, tannin and possibly copper in betel nuts stabilise collagen molecules causing collagen fibres to cross-link and inhibit collagenase. There is a subepithelial chronic inflammatory reaction with fibrosis extending to the submucosa and muscle. The carcinogenic properties of areca nut are attributed to polyphenols, alkaloids (most importantly, arecoline), metabolites of alkaloids (e.g. arecoline N-oxide), and areca nut-specific nitrosamines [9]. Chronic exposure to such molecules results in increased oxidative stress and subsequent DNA damage which, when unrepaired, may lead to carcinogenesis.

Genetics

Patients have an increased frequency of HLA-A10, HLA-B7 and HLA-DR3. Further, the HLA class I chain-related gene A (MICA), particularly the phenotype frequency of allele A6 of MICA, is increased in oral submucous fibrosis, expressed by keratinocytes and other epithelial cells and interacts with gamma/delta T cells in the submucosa. Increased levels of proinflammatory cytokines and reduced antifibrotic interferon gamma may be central to the pathogenesis.

Clinical features

The buccal mucosa is the most commonly involved site, but any part of the mouth can be involved, and the pharynx. Oral submucous fibrosis develops insidiously, often initially presenting with a burning sensation of the oral mucosa, ulceration, vesicle formation, petechiae, postinflammatory hypermelanosis and pain. This is followed by symmetrical fibrosis of the cheeks, lips, tongue or soft palate, which appears as vertical bands running through the mucosa, and oral opening becomes restricted. In advanced disease, the fibrosis can become so severe that the affected site appears mottled and marble-like, and severely restricts mouth opening and tongue and/or palate mobility resulting in difficulty in mastication, speech and swallowing [1,2].

There is epithelial atrophy and sometimes frank erythroplakia or leukoplakia. There may be oesophageal fibrosis and, if the palatal and paratubal muscles are involved, conductive hearing loss may appear because of functional stenosis of the Eustachian tube.

Prognosis

Oral submucous fibrosis may predispose to the development of leukoplakia and oral carcinoma, with 7–13% of cases exhibiting transformation to SCC (0.5–1.1% per year) [11,12].

Investigations

The diagnosis is usually clinical, based upon clinical features, history of betel chewing and often of slowly increasing trismus. Diagnosis can be confirmed by biopsy which shows collagen hyalinisation, blood vessel obliteration and extensive fibrosis. A biopsy should be undertaken when leukoplakia, erythroplakia or persistent ulceration is noted.

Management

Management is difficult [13–17]. Stopping consumption of betel products is the mainstay of management but the condition does not regress with cessation of the habit. Physiotherapy may be useful in the early stages. Surgery may be needed to relieve the fibrosis. Medical therapies range from topical medication (e.g. with COX-2 inhibitors) to intralesionally injected medicaments such as corticosteroids, collagenase or hyaluronidase, to systemic medication with lycopene or pentoxifylline [13–17].

MALIGNANT NEOPLASMS

Oral cancer accounts for a large proportion of cancers in the head and neck region. Cancer of the lip is the most common malignant tumour affecting the head and neck. More than 90% of cancers are oral squamous cell carcinomas (OSCC).

Basal cell carcinoma of the lip

Epidemiology

Ultraviolet light is a major aetiological factor in the development of basal cell carcinoma, with more than 85% occurring on the sun-exposed areas of the head and neck [1,2]. Fair-skinned individuals who burn and those whose occupations require excessive exposure to sunshine are at greatest risk; the tumour is rare in dark-skinned persons and 95% occur after the age of 40 years [3]. SCC is more common than basal cell carcinoma in the lower lip.

Other significant risk factors for the development of basal cell carcinoma include prior burns, vaccinations, irradiation, exposure to inorganic arsenic, genetic syndromes (e.g. xeroderma pigmentosum, naevoid basal cell carcinoma syndrome, albinism) and immunosuppression.

Clinical features

On the lip this manifests as a pearly, sometimes ulcerated, nodule or papule. Unlike SCCs, basal cell carcinomas only rarely originate on the vermilion but commonly occur periorally [4–6]. Basal cell carcinomas more commonly arise on the upper rather than the lower lip. The lesions can also arise *de novo* on the vermilion or occasionally the mucosa of the lip [7].

Basal cell carcinoma has multiple forms that can be divided as follows:
- Nodular: the most frequent type around the lips presents as a translucent nodule with fine telangiectasias and is often ulcerated.
- Morphoeic: an atrophic plaque resembling a scar, with an aggressive infiltrative growth pattern and high rate of recurrence after excision.
- Superficial: appears as an erythematous plaque with elevated borders and central atrophy or ulceration. It is rare around the lips.

Although the tumour rarely metastasises, it is responsible for considerable functional and cosmetic morbidity. Multiple lesions are commonly encountered and the various forms have overlapping clinical features.

Investigations

Basal cell carcinoma of the lips must be differentiated from other nodules, including SCC, keratoacanthoma and sebaceous adenoma. Since lesions that arise periorally are often aggressive, early detection and confirmation by biopsy will prevent infiltration and destruction of the underlying structures.

Management

Various treatment modalities for basal cell carcinoma include surgical excision, and laser surgery, radiation, and non-surgical topical interventions [8–10]. Selection of the treatment modality depends on the size, site and histological pattern of the tumour as well as the age of the patient. Mohs micrographic surgery offers the highest cure rate with the greatest preservation of tissue [11].

Keratoacanthoma of the lip

Keratoacanthoma is a rapidly growing lesion most likely derived from the follicular infundibulum. Keratoacanthomas are common self-limiting proliferative tumours that arise most frequently in men after the sixth decade of life [1,2]. The lesions mimic SCC both clinically and microscopically [3]. Keratoacanthomas rarely develop on mucosal surfaces [4,5]. The role of actinic damage is strongly supported by the fact that the majority of lesions occur on sun-exposed skin (90%), with up to 10% occurring periorally or on the vermilion border of the lips, often on the lower lip.

Clinical features

Keratoacanthomas often manifest at the vermilion border, as indurated dome-shaped nodules displaying a characteristic central, keratin-filled, crusted and frequently darkened crater. While cutaneous lesions are asymptomatic, labial and oral lesions are frequently painful [6–12]. They usually appear as an ulcer with a rolled margin, usually on the anterior or maxillary gingiva, clinically indistinguishable from SCC. Keratoacanthomas grow rapidly, attaining a size typically greater than 1 cm, may be locally invasive and result in significant tissue damage.

Diagnosis

Keratoacanthomas require differentiation from SCC [13]. When lesions develop intraorally or on the lips, they should immediately be subjected to biopsy for confirmation.

Management

Management is often by surgical excision. Spontaneous resolution of mucosal lesions usually does not occur.

Squamous cell carcinoma of the lip

SCC of the lip is the most common malignant tumour affecting the head and neck. SCC is the most common malignancy to affect the vermilion zone and, as with squamous carcinoma of the glabrous skin, usually due to actinic damage [1–3]. However, there are occasional cases of sebaceous carcinoma and other variants.

Like actinic cheilitis, SCC is most common on the lower lip of fair-skinned outdoor workers in sunny climates and is relatively rare in pigmented skin [4–6] (Figure 108.47). About 90% of tumours arise in the lower lip, 7% in the upper lip and 3% at the oral commissure. Lip cancer has a far better prognosis than intraoral cancers. SCC that arise in the upper lip and oral commissure have a worse prognosis than those originating in the lower lip. These tumours grow rapidly, ulcerate sooner, metastasise earlier and have the potential for invasion into the premaxilla and nasal cavity. Facts that support a relationship to actinic radiation include the following:

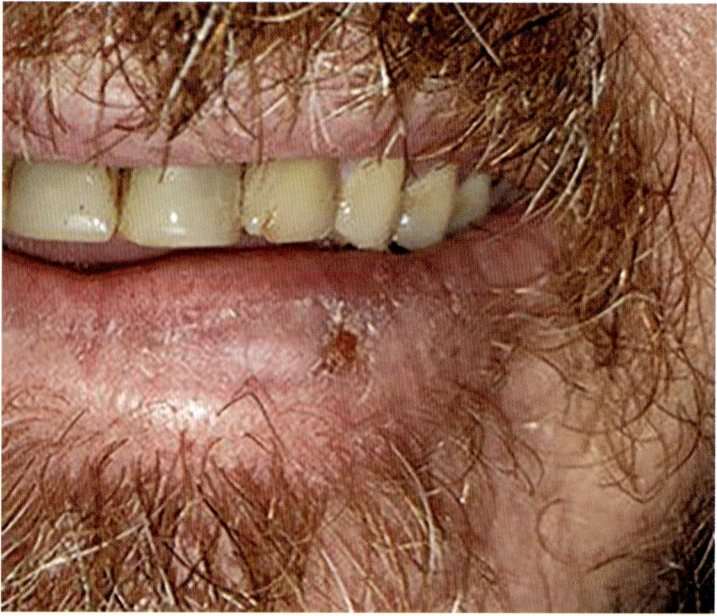

(a)

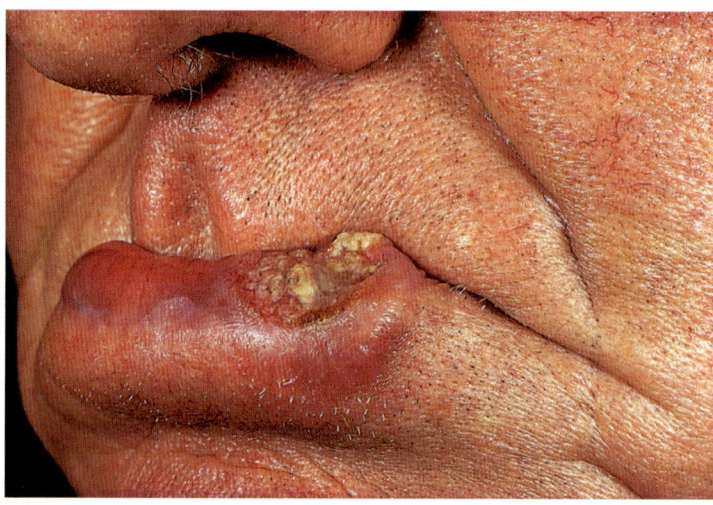

(b)

Figure 108.47 Squamous cell carcinoma of the lip. This may appear initially (a) as a subtle erosion on the lip with actinic cheilitis or (b) as an established ulcer on the lower lip.

- Lip cancer involves the more exposed lower lip, rather than the upper lip.
- There is a higher incidence of lip cancer in outdoor workers in occupations such as farming and fishing, and in rural populations.
- More fair-skinned than dark-skinned people tend to develop lip cancer (as well as skin cancer and melanoma) in sunny climates.

Other risk factors may include low social class, tobacco smoking and immunosuppression [1–5]. Several large cohort studies and a meta-analysis have shown that organ transplant patients (who of course are chronically immunosuppressed) have between 17 and 46 times an increased risk of lip cancer and 2–5 times an increased risk of mouth and pharyngeal cancers, compared with the general population. A US cohort study showed white people who were taking the photosensitising antihypertensive hydrochlorothiazide for 5 or more years had a fourfold increased risk of lip cancer.

The initial features are a keratinous growth or swelling of the lip (Figure 108.47), soreness and ulceration. Most lesions are amenable to surgical excision. Lymph node metastasis is not often seen, except in the presence of a large lesion. A margin ≥5 mm for resection is recommended [6,7]. Ten-year recurrence-free survival rate is 94% for stage I and 78% for stage II disease [8].

Florid oral papillomatosis

Florid oral papillomatosis is a rare but well-defined clinical entity [1–8]. Florid oral papillomatosis is a type of verrucous carcinoma. There is conflicting evidence for HPV involvement in oral florid papillomatosis. The papillomatous lesions are exuberant, warty or verrucous, and characterised by their benign appearance on histology. It destroys and extends into underlying tissue but is characterised by a low incidence of metastases to lymph nodes. Biopsy is required. Treatment in the early stage of the disease is usually successful. Surgical or laser excision is favoured.

Granular cell tumours

Congenital granular cell epulis is a rare lesion of unknown histogenesis with a predilection for the maxillary alveolar ridge of newborn girls. Microscopically, there are nests of polygonal cells with granular cytoplasm, a prominent capillary network and attenuated overlying squamous epithelium. The lesion lacks immunoreactivity for S-100, laminin, chromogranin and most other markers except neuron-specific enolase and vimentin [1–4]. This lesion should be distinguished from the more common adult granular cell tumour as well as other differential diagnoses.

Adult granular cell tumour (Abrikossoff tumour) develops between the second and sixth decades of life, more frequently among women and people of African heritage. The head and neck area is affected in 45–65% of cases and, of these, 70% are located intraorally (tongue, oral mucosa, hard palate) [5,6]. Both benign and malignant lesions have been reported, although malignancy is rare, comprising 2% of all granular cell tumours. The benign form shows polygonal cells with granular eosinophilic cytoplasm and small nuclei. The malignant form, however, is associated with a high mitotic index and pleomorphic cellular tissue. The clinical feature of either is a swelling covered by mucosa of normal clinical appearance. Histological examination is required. The treatment is surgery.

Metastatic oral neoplasms

Metastases to the oral cavity are rare, comprising only 1–3% of all malignant oral neoplasms [1]. In 25% of cases, oral metastases were found to be the first sign of the metastatic spread and in 23% it was the first indication of an undiscovered malignancy at a distant site. The jaw bones, particularly the mandible, were more frequently affected than the oral soft tissues (2:1). Most oral metastases originate from carcinomas of the breast, prostate, lungs, thyroid gland and kidneys [1–13]. The mandible is the most common location, with the molar area being the most frequently involved site [1]. In the soft tissues, the attached gingiva is the most frequently involved site (54%). In the early stages, gingival metastases resemble hyperplastic or reactive lesions.

Clinical features

Metastases usually present as a lesion in the jaw, sometimes only revealed coincidentally by imaging. Many metastases are asymptomatic but others manifest with:
- Pain
- Paraesthesia or hypoaesthesia
- Swelling
- Ulcer
- Tooth mobility
- Non-healing extraction sockets
- Pathological fracture
- Radiolucency or radio-opacity.

Early manifestation of metastases may resemble a hyperplastic or reactive lesion, such as pyogenic granuloma, peripheral giant cell granuloma or fibrous lump. Patients complaining of a numb chin should always raise the possibility of a metastatic disease in the mandible. Diagnosis is from history and clinical features supplemented by radiography and histopathology. In any case, where the clinical presentation is unusual, biopsy is mandatory. The prognosis of metastatic lesions to the oral cavity is very poor.

Oral squamous cell carcinoma

Carcinoma of the oral cavity may develop *de novo* or from a premalignant dysplastic lesion that appears clinically as leukoplakia, erythroplakia or an erythroleukoplakia. OSCC is among the 10 most common cancers worldwide. OSCC is seen predominantly in older patients (>65 years), but intraoral cancer is increasing, especially in younger adults (<45 years) and particularly in the oropharynx. OSCC is seen predominantly in males, but the male/female differential is decreasing. Mouth cancers include:
- Cancer of the lip is the most common malignant tumour affecting the head and neck. Lip cancer may follow chronic actinic cheilitis (Figure 108.47). About 90% of tumours arise in the lower lip, 7% in the upper lip and 3% at the oral commissure. Lip cancer has a far better prognosis than intraoral cancers. SCC that arises in the upper lip and oral commissure have a worse prognosis than those originating in the lower lip. These tumours grow rapidly, ulcerate sooner, metastasise earlier and have the potential for invasion into the premaxilla and nasal cavity.
- Most intraoral SCCs involve the lateral border of the tongue and/or the floor of the mouth (Figure 108.48) [1–5]. In the developing world, oral SCC is most common in the buccal mucosa and arises mainly from betel use.
- Oropharyngeal cancer arises in the fauces/posterior tongue.

Epidemiology

Worldwide, over 450 000 new cases of head and neck cancer are diagnosed each year. There is marked intercountry variation in

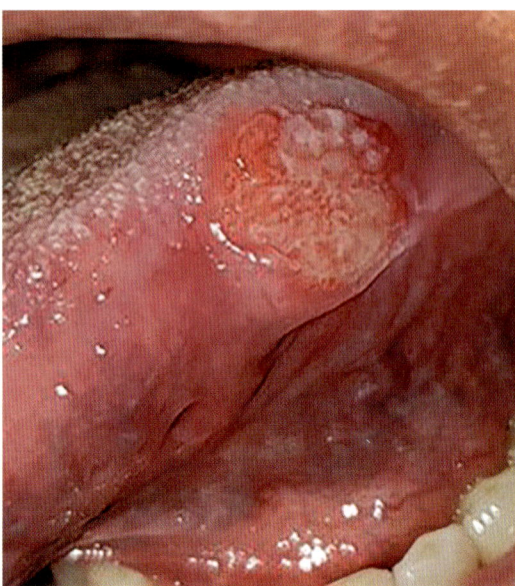

Figure 108.48 Squamous cell carcinoma on posterolateral border of the tongue with a raised rolled edge.

both the incidence of and mortality from OSCC. There is growing evidence of intracountry differences in OSCC, including ethnic differences in incidence and mortality. In South-East Asia and Brazil, the incidence of oral cancer is the highest in the world but varies widely in different areas. In the developed world, the incidence of OSCC varies between countries and between different regions of the same country. For example, OSCC is more than twice as common in Scotland than in England and Wales and, even within Scotland, there are regional differences. Oral cancer is the most common cancer for men and the third most common for women in India, Sri Lanka and Pakistan, whereas only 3% of new cases of cancer in the UK are oral cancer.

Predisposing factors

Factors important in mouth cancer include lifestyle modifiable risk factors and the following [5–11]:

- *Age*. Mouth cancer is more common in people over 45. Oropharyngeal cancer is increasing especially in younger adults (<45 years).
- *Gender*. Mouth cancer is generally more common in men than women, but the male/female differential is decreasing.
- *Social class*. Oral cancer is a problem particularly for people of resource-poor groups and ethnic minority groups. Many other explanations (e.g. habits, oral health, diet, nutrition) may be responsible.
- *Genetics*. There are a few familial cases, and people with certain syndromes have a high risk of mouth and throat cancer. Syndromes with a predisposition to mouth cancer include mainly:
  - Dyskeratosis congenita: a disease of defective telomere maintenance, characterised by mucocutaneous abnormalities, bone marrow failure and cancer predisposition. Leukoplakias occur in approximately 80% of patients and typically involve the buccal mucosa, tongue and oropharynx. Patients have an increased prevalence of SCC within sites of leukoplakia (especially the tongue), or of the skin, Hodgkin lymphoma, gastrointestinal adenocarcinoma, bronchial and laryngeal carcinoma, and leukaemia.
  - Fanconi anaemia: a recessively inherited disease, characterised by congenital anomalies and bone marrow failure, and a predisposition to develop cancer, particularly SCC in the head and neck and anogenital region, myelodysplastic syndrome, and acute myelocytic leukaemia.
  - Xeroderma pigmentosum: a rare disease of defective DNA repair mechanisms, predisposing to cancer in light-exposed areas such as skin and lips.

The main modifiable risk factors are as follows:

- *Tobacco use*. All forms of tobacco both smoked and smokeless are carcinogenic. There is a strong dose–response relationship. Smoking cessation leads to a fall in mouth cancer risk; by 20 years or more after cessation the risk is reduced to that of a never-smoker.
- *Alcohol*. The risk of developing oral cancer due to alcohol alone appears to be influenced by the type of alcoholic beverage and the frequency of consumption. Tobacco use, including smokeless tobacco, and excessive alcohol consumption are estimated to account for about 90% of oral cancers. Risk of a secondary primary tumour in the upper aerodigestive tract is also increased.
- *Betel use*. Some 20% of the world's population use betel. Betel may also cause oral submucous fibrosis (see earlier).
- *UV light*. Lip cancer, particularly on the lower lip, is an issue mainly in older men exposed over long periods to sunlight.
- *Human papillomavirus (HPV)*. Infection with oncogenic HPV, especially HPV-16 (>90%), are implicated mainly in oropharyngeal cancer (base of tongue, fauces) and does not appear as frequently in the oral cavity. The prevalence rates of HPV positivity were 41% in oropharyngeal cancer and 15% in oral cavity cancers. High-risk (oncogenic) HPV subtypes have been identified in a significant fraction of oropharyngeal tumours, including HPV-16, -18, -31 and -33.
- *Previous cancer*. There is an increased risk of mouth cancer following a previous cancer diagnosis. People with a previous head and neck cancer (including of the tongue, mouth, pharynx and larynx) have between a 12- and 16-fold increased risk of subsequent head and neck cancer. Survivors of oesophageal SCC have an almost sevenfold increase in risk of mouth and pharynx cancers. Previous irradiation for either malignant or benign disease has also been implicated.

History

Oral cancer in the initial clinically detectable stage is a red or red and white (erythroleukoplastic) area without symptoms. The initial lesions are usually solitary and asymptomatic. Lesions of oral cancer can range from a few millimetres to several centimetres in diameter in the more advanced cases (Box 108.6). In advanced cancers, there is often a red or red and white single lesion, ulcer or lump with irregular margins which are rigid to touch (indurated) and there may be pain especially in the tongue and floor of the mouth lesions. A typical malignant ulcer is hard with heaped-up and often everted or rolled edges and a granular floor. The *rule* is that a single lesion of three or more weeks' duration, especially a red and/or white lesion, an ulcer, a lump, or especially a combination of these, or if indurated (firm on palpation) should be regarded with suspicion, and a biopsy arranged.

Box 108.6 Features suggestive of oral squamous cell carcinoma

Red lesion	Erythroplakia may be associated
Mixed red/white lesion	Erythroleukoplakia may be associated
Irregular white lesion	Verrucous or nodular leukoplakia may be associated
Lump	Especially if enlarging and/or hard
Ulcer	Especially if persistent, or with fissuring or raised exophytic margins
Pain or numbness	May be a late feature
Abnormal blood vessels supplying a lump	
Tooth mobility	Destruction of the periodontium by malignant cells
Extraction socket not healing	
Induration beneath a lesion	Firm infiltration beneath the mucosa
Fixation of lesion	To deeper tissues or to overlying skin or mucosa
Lymph node enlargement	Especially if there is hardness in a lymph node or fixation
	Enlarged cervical nodes in a patient with OSCC may be caused by infection, reactive hyperplasia, secondary or metastatic disease
Dysphagia	
Weight loss	

Presentation

Some mouth cancers arise in clinically apparently normal mucosa, but some are preceded by a clinically obvious potentially malignant disorder. The risk of malignant transformation in the potentially malignant disorders is approximately as shown in Table 108.8. The presenting features of mouth cancer usually relate to the local effects of the primary tumour, occasionally to regional spread, metastatic disease or paraneoplastic phenomena. OSCC predominantly metastasises locally and to draining regional lymph nodes. Extraoral examination should therefore include cervical lymph node examination. A painless enlarged cervical lymph node may be the only presenting symptom.

Table 108.8 Potentially malignant disorders.

Entities	Approximate malignant potential over 10 years		
	Very high (70–85%)	**High (10–30%)**	**Low (1–5%)**
Main	Erythroplakia	Leukoplakia (non-homogeneous-nodular and speckled)	Leukoplakia (homogeneous)
	Proliferative verrucous leukoplakia		
			Lichenoid lesions
			Lichen planus
Less common		Actinic cheilitis	Discoid lupus erythematosus
		Dyskeratosis congenita	
		Submucous fibrosis	

Classification of severity

Grading is used as a prognostic indicator; well-differentiated or low-grade cancers have the better prognosis (Box 108.7). Low-grade tumours will usually grow more slowly and be less likely to spread than a high-grade tumour. High grade means the cells look more abnormal and the tumours metastasise more readily.

Box 108.7 Grades of carcinoma

Well differentiated
- Elongated rete pegs invading lamina propria, with keratin pearls

Moderately differentiated
- Irregular invading rete pegs; loss of cellular cohesion

Poorly differentiated
- Sheets of invading epithelium with no obvious architecture, but severe cellular abnormalities such as pleomorphism and hyperchromatism

OSCC should be staged according to the TNM (tumour, node, metastases) classification of the Union for International Cancer Control (UICC) – according to tumour size, nodal metastases and distant metastases (Tables 2 and 3) – since this classification relates well to overall survival rate (i.e. the earlier the stage of tumour, the better the prognosis and the less complicated and mutilating is the treatment). The current TNM staging system [12] (Table 108.9) now incorporates maximum depth of invasion. Patients with >5 mm depth of invasion have a minimum tumour stage of T2; patients with >10 mm depth of invasion have a minimum tumour stage of T3.

Disease course and prognosis

The quality of life during and after mouth cancer treatment has steadily improved over the years but survival rates have increased at a slower pace. The stage at which mouth cancer is diagnosed has a significant effect on overall survival and quality of life. For stage 1 and 2 oral cavity cancer, the 3-year survival is around 80%. For stage 3 and 4, the 3-year survival is almost 50%. Early diagnosis reduces mortality and also minimises morbidity, disfigurement, treatment duration and costs.

Investigations

Single ulcers, lumps, red patches or white patches, particularly if any of these persist for more than 3 weeks, may be manifestations of frank malignancy and thus biopsy is invariably indicated. Usually, examination under general anaesthesia may be indicated, particularly for patients with:
- Tumours in the posterior tongue.
- Tumours where the margins cannot be readily defined.
- An enlarged cervical node but no visible primary neoplasm.

Imaging and other studies which may help detect abnormalities missed during the clinical examination may include:
- An orthopantomogram (jaw), which might demonstrate bone invasion.
- A chest CT, which may demonstrate second primary tumours or metastases to lungs or hilar lymph nodes, ribs or vertebrae.

Table 108.9 TNM classification of cancer of the lip and oral cavity.

T - Primary tumour	
TX	Primary tumour cannot be assessed
T0	No evidence of primary tumour
Tis	Carcinoma *in situ*
T1	Tumour ≤2 cm with depth of invasion (DOI) ≤5 mm
T2	Tumour ≤2 cm, with DOI >5 mm and ≤10 mm; *or* tumour >2 cm and ≤4 cm, with DOI ≤10 mm
T3	Tumour >2 cm and ≤4 cm with DOI >10 mm; *or* tumour >4 cm with DOI ≤10 mm
T4a (lip)	Tumour invades through cortical bone, inferior alveolar nerve, floor of mouth or skin (chin or nose)
T4a (oral cavity)	Moderately advanced local disease. Tumour >4 cm with DOI >10 mm; *or* tumour invades adjacent structures only (e.g. through cortical bone of the mandible or maxilla, or involves the maxillary sinus or skin of the face)
T4b (lip and oral cavity)	Very advanced local disease. Tumour invades masticator space, pterygoid plates, or skull base and/or encases the internal carotid artery
N - Regional lymph nodes	
NX	Regional lymph nodes cannot be assessed
N0	No regional lymph node metastasis
N1	Metastasis in a single ipsilateral lymph node, ≤3 cm in greatest dimension
N2	Metastasis as specified in N2a, 2b, 2c below
N2a	Metastasis in a single ipsilateral lymph node, >3 cm but not >6 cm in greatest dimension
N2b	Metastasis in multiple ipsilateral lymph nodes, none >6 cm in greatest dimension
N2c	Metastasis in bilateral or contralateral lymph nodes, none >6 cm in greatest dimension
N3	Metastasis in a lymph node >6 cm in greatest dimension
M - Distant metastasis	
M0	No distant metastasis
M1	Distant metastasis

DOI, depth of invasion.

PART 10: SPECIFIC SITES, SEX & AGE

- MRI of the primary tumour site and of the neck to delineate the extent of cervical node metastases.
- Ultrasound and fine needle aspiration of neck lymph nodes that may contain metastases.

Management

Lip cancer is treated mainly surgically. Surgical resection is the mainstay of management for most oral cancers. Tumour resection should be performed with a clear margin of 1 cm (vital structures permitting). 'Close' margins (defined as a histopathological margin of <5 mm) mean further surgery or adjuvant radiotherapy. Neck dissection to clear the neck of cancer containing lymph nodes is often also needed in addition to the excision of the primary tumour. Reconstruction is crucially important to restore appearance and/or the function (e.g. the use of tissue flaps, bone grafts or prosthetic materials) and is best performed at the time of initial surgery. Adjuvant postoperative radiotherapy to the primary site and neck, with or without concurrent chemotherapy, is indicated for patients who have positive or close final resection margins, for those who have bone invasion, for patients with pathologically

positive lymph nodes or to treat the neck prophylactically without a neck dissection [13]. Concomitant chemoradiotherapy in cases of advanced neck disease, positive margins or extracapsular spread improves control rates [13]. Approximately, 80–90% of recurrences occur within the first 2–4 years.

Verrucous carcinoma

Verrucous carcinoma accounts for fewer than 5% of cases of SCC. Verrucous lesions clinically present as a velvety or warty exophytic mass [1–6]. It may develop from proliferative verrucous leukoplakia. Confirmation of the diagnosis by biopsy is particularly important because although they demonstrate progressive local growth, the prognosis is favourable. Complete surgical excision is the primary treatment.

Other oral malignant primary neoplasms

The following comprise up to 10% of all oral malignant tumours:
- Salivary gland tumours.
- Malignant melanoma (see earlier in this chapter).
- Lymphomas: non-Hodgkin lymphomas.
- Sarcomas.
- Kaposi sarcoma (see earlier in this chapter).
- Some odontogenic tumours.
- Maxillary antral carcinoma (or other neoplasms).
- Langerhans cell histiocytosis.
- Neoplasms of bone and connective tissue.

Complications of treatment

Bone marrow transplantation (haematopoietic stem cell transplantation)

Oral complications are common and can be a major cause of morbidity following bone marrow transplantation. Mucositis, infections, bleeding, xerostomia and loss of taste result from the effects of the underlying disease, chemotherapy or radiotherapy, and GVHD [1].

Graft-versus-host disease

The oral manifestations of acute GVHD are difficult or impossible to differentiate from chemotherapy-induced mucositis and consist of painful mucosal desquamation and ulceration. Erythema and ulceration are most pronounced at 7–11 days after human stem cell transplant (HSCT) and may be associated with obvious infection. The ventral surface of the tongue, buccal and labial mucosa and gingiva may be affected. Acute GVHD may also

Table 108.10 Scoring of oral chronic graft-versus-host disease lesions.

Erythema	None	0	Mild or moderate erythema (<25%)	1	Moderate (≥25%) or severe (≤25%) erythema	2	Severe erythema (≥25%)	3
Lichenoid	None	0	Lichen-like changes (<25%)	1	Lichen-like changes (25–50%)	2	Lichen-like changes (>50%)	3
Ulcers	None	0			Ulcers involving (≤20%)	3	Severe ulcerations (>20%)	6

Total score for all mucosal changes

manifest as cheilitis, hyposalivation, infections (candidiasis, HSV stomatitis (occasionally zoster), cytomegalovirus, protozoal and Gram-positive bacterial infections), purpura and bleeding.

The oral lesions of chronic GVHD (cGVHD) are painful and present as lichenoid lesions, hyperkeratotic plaques, generalised mucosal erythema, ulceration and mucoceles of minor salivary glands. Other problems include hyposalivation, taste abnormalities, infections, especially candidiasis, sclerodermatous changes manifesting as restricted mouth opening, loss of elasticity of the lips and restricted tongue movement [1–4]. The National Institute of Health (NIH) cGVHD Task Force developed a scoring system for cGVHD that includes three types of oral manifestations (erythema, lichenoid and ulcers) that can be graded in three activity levels (mild, moderate and severe) [5] (Table 108.10).

Management [6,7]

The aim of treatment is to alleviate symptoms to allow normal oral function. Pain relief with topical anaesthetic agents such as lidocaine or benzydamine hydrochloride mouthwash or spray and topical corticosteroids can be applied as solutions, gels, creams or ointments several times a day. Intralesional injections of corticosteroids (e.g. triamcinolone acetonide) for localised persistent ulcers is helpful. Calcineurin inhibitors may also be used for intraoral involvement.

Patients should be screened regularly as the risk for developing oral cancer is seven times higher in long-term survivors of allogeneic HSCT [8,9].

Mucositis

Mucositis, sometimes called *mucosal barrier injury*, is the term given to the widespread oral erythema, ulceration and soreness that is a common complication of a number of therapeutic procedures involving chemotherapy, radiotherapy or chemoradiotherapy, used largely in the treatment of cancer but also in the conditioning prior to bone marrow transplantation (i.e. haematopoietic stem cell transplantation) [1–5]. Mucositis appears 3–15 days after cancer treatment, earlier after chemotherapy than after radiotherapy.

Mucositis invariably follows external beam radiotherapy involving the orofacial tissues, and is also common in upper mantle head and neck radiation, and particularly in total body irradiation. Tissues such as the soft palate, and the lateral borders and ventral surface of the tongue and floor of the mouth, which have a good vascular supply or a higher cell turnover rate, are more susceptible to radiation mucositis. Risk factors for radiation mucositis include concurrent chemotherapy, younger age, alcohol, poor oral hygiene and dental disease.

Some two-thirds of patients on chemotherapy develop mucositis. Injury to mucosae tends to be acute but affects the whole gastrointestinal tract. Chemotherapy appears to cause injury to the mucosal barrier, with activation of the NF-κB pathway and release of cytokines such as TNF-α, IL-1 and IL-6. Most patients on high-dose chemotherapy develop severe oral mucositis that usually appears within 4–7 days after initiation of treatment and peaks within 2 weeks. The oral microflora is considered to play only a secondary role in the pathogenesis of mucositis. Risk factors for mucositis include age, body mass index, female gender, poor oral health, mucosal trauma and comorbidities (e.g. diabetes mellitus, impaired renal function). The impaired mucosal barrier in mucositis predisposes to life-threatening septic complications.

Clinical features

Mucositis typically presents with pain (which can be so intense as to interfere with eating and significantly affect the quality of life), widespread erythema, ulceration, swelling and sometimes bleeding.

Diagnosis

This is clinical and it is helpful to score the degree of mucositis in order to monitor progression and therapy [6].

Management

The basic strategies in the management of mucositis aim at pain relief, efforts to hasten healing and prevention of infectious complications. Interventions which have some proven success with some evidence base include [6–8]:

- Excellent oral care, including pre-treatment dental evaluation.
- Avoiding irritants (smoking, spirits or spicy foods).
  Topical analgesics used prior to meals to help combat pain and dysphagia, such as benzydamine hydrochloride and 2% lidocaine (lignocaine) gel.
- Oral cryotherapy using ice popsicles.
- Opioids, such as morphine and hydromorphone.
- Exposure to soft laser.
- Systemic administration of keratinocyte growth factor (palifermin), FDA-approved for use in patients with haematological malignancies receiving myelotoxic therapy requiring haematopoietic stem cell support.

Interventions that show some statistically significant evidence of a benefit also include aloe vera, amifostine, granulocyte-colony stimulating factor (G-CSF), intravenous glutamine, honey, sucralfate and polymixin/tobramycin/amphotericin (PTA) antibiotic pastille/paste. There are many other preparations used, often variants on the 'magic mouthwash' (viscous lidocaine, diphenhydramine, bismuth salicylate and a corticosteroid). Monitoring microbial colonisation and the institution of antiviral prophylaxis and antifungal prophylaxis, to avoid colonisation and superinfection, is particularly important in patients with low neutrophil counts.

INFECTIONS OF THE ORAL CAVITY

Infections frequently present with oral ulceration. It is a common presentation in some viral infections, typically in the herpesvirus or enterovirus infections seen in childhood. It can also be seen in HIV/AIDS and several bacterial diseases, notably acute necrotising gingivitis, but also in tuberculosis and syphilis. It is rare in fungal infections in resource-rich countries, although the deep mycoses may be responsible for infection in resource-poor countries or in the immunocompromised. Parasitic infections may occasionally cause ulceration. Infections may also present as blisters, e.g. Coxsackie, herpetic or varicella infections, or erythematous spots or macules, e.g. measles or candidal infection.

VIRAL INFECTIONS (CHAPTER 25)

Chikungunya

This togavirus (RNA), transmitted in areas around the Indian Ocean by the Asian tiger mosquito (*Aedes albopictus*) and now spread to Europe and the Americas, has an incubation period of 3–7 days. It presents with a high fever and joint pain. Similar to dengue fever and o'nyong'nyong virus, it features a maculopapular rash, headache, malaise and arthralgia [1,2]. The oral manifestations include oral ulceration, gingival bleeding, oral mucosal pain and burning, erythema, and pigmentation of the lips, tongue and hard palate [3]. Oral lesions occur 2–6 days after disease onset. Lesions mainly affected the gingiva, lips, tongue and buccal mucosa [4]. No cure or drug treatment is available.

Dengue

This is a mosquito-borne viral infection with an incubation period of 3–14 days. It characteristically presents with fever and headache, joint pains and morbilliform or maculopapular rash. Gingival and palatal bleeding, dry mouth and taste changes have been reported, but ulceration is not a prominent feature [1,2]. Osteonecrosis of the jaw associated with dengue fever was also reported.

Enteroviruses

Hand, foot and mouth disease (Chapter 25)

Aetiology
Hand, foot and mouth disease is caused by predominantly coxsackievirus A16 and enterovirus A71 [1,2]. Coxsackievirus A6

has increasingly been reported as a cause of outbreaks worldwide [3].

Clinical features
The incubation period is 3–10 days and, although young children are predominantly infected, there are occasional outbreaks in adults. Many infections are subclinical but features of the clinical syndrome include the following:
- General features: malaise, anorexia, irritability and fever may be present but usually only in severe cases.
- Anterior cervical lymph nodes may occasionally be slightly enlarged and tender. The oral lesions are most commonly on the tongue and buccal mucosa. The lesions begin as erythematous macules, which progress to vesicles, ranging from 1 to 5 mm. The vesicles rupture and form superficial ulcers with a greyish-yellow base and an erythematous rim [1].
- Rash: the exanthem may be macular, maculopapular or vesicular. The skin lesions are non-pruritic but may be painful when caused by certain serotypes (e.g. coxsackievirus A6). The lesions typically resolve in 3–4 days. The rash typically affects the hands, feet, buttocks, legs and arms.
   Hand, foot and mouth disease is self-limiting and only rarely complicated by systemic illness such as encephalitis. The condition tends to be more severe when it occurs in adults.

Diagnosis and management
As for herpangina later.

Herpangina

Aetiology
Herpangina is caused by 22 enterovirus serotypes, most commonly coxsackievirus A serotypes. The incubation period is 3–5 days and young children are predominantly affected.

Clinical features
Many infections are subclinical, but features of the clinical syndrome include malaise, anorexia, irritability, fever, sore throat, slightly enlarged and tender anterior cervical lymph nodes and mouth ulcers, predominantly on the soft palate [1,2]. Patients present with vesicles, ulceration, and diffuse erythema on the soft palate, fauces and tonsillar areas. The ulcers heal in 7–10 days.

Diagnosis
There may be a contact history. The main differential diagnosis is primary herpetic stomatitis, but in herpangina there is no acute gingivitis and ulceration is mainly restricted to the soft palate. A viral swab may be taken from the oropharynx for polymerase chain reaction.

Management
The condition is self-limiting and treatment is supportive only.

Herpesviruses

Herpesviruses are DNA viruses that can be transmitted in body fluids such as saliva, contracted in early life, characterised by latency and reactivated during immunosuppression [1].

There are eight subtypes of herpesviruses which span three subfamilies (α, β, γ).

- α herpesviruses include herpes simplex viruses (HSV-1 and HSV-2) and varicella-zoster virus. HSV causes primary herpetic stomatitis and recurrent herpes labialis or intraoral recurrences. Herpes varicella-zoster virus causes chickenpox and shingles.
- β herpesviruses include cytomegalovirus, which may cause some salivary infections.
- γ herpesviruses include EBV, which causes infectious mononucleosis, and may be associated with nasopharyngeal carcinoma, lymphomas and hairy leukoplakia. HHV-8 is associated with Kaposi sarcoma.

Chickenpox (Chapter 25)

Chickenpox (varicella) affects children predominantly and may present with intraoral vesicles that rupture to form ulcers on the tongue, buccal mucosa, gingival, palate and oropharynx. They are generally not very painful. Following the primary infection, the virus is transported via the sensory nerves to the dorsal spinal ganglia or trigeminal ganglion, where it remains latent. There is no gingivitis [1,2]. There may be a contact history. Following the primary infection, the varicella-zoster virus is transported via the sensory nerves to the dorsal spinal ganglia or trigeminal ganglion and remains latent and may be reactivated to produce shingles.

Cytomegalovirus infection

Cytomegalovirus may cause a glandular fever type of syndrome and rarely causes oral ulceration. Indolent cytomegalovirus-induced oral ulcers may be seen in immunosuppressed patients and in AIDS [1–3]. It has been termed the 'salivary gland inclusion virus' since there are inclusion bodies seen histopathologically in salivary glands of infected people [4]. These strikingly enlarged cells contain intranuclear inclusions that have the histopathological appearance of owl's eyes.

Epstein–Barr virus infections (Chapter 25)

Epstein–Barr virus is responsible for infectious mononucleosis and is found in pharyngeal epithelium and appears in the saliva of patients for several months after clinical recovery. Infection appears to be spread by close oral contact, especially kissing. It is typically a disease of the student population. It is also associated with oral hairy leukoplakia, a number of malignancies of the head and neck including oropharyngeal carcinoma and some lymphomas [1–3]. Infection is often subclinical [4]. Infectious mononucleosis is also protean in its clinical manifestations, which include particularly lymphadenopathy, sore throat, fever, malaise and rashes. In the anginose type (sore-throat type), the throat is sore with soft-palate petechiae and a whitish exudate on oedematous tonsils. There may be non-specific oral ulceration or pericoronitis and pharyngeal oedema may threaten the airway.

The glandular type of infectious mononucleosis is characterised by generalised lymph node enlargement and splenomegaly; the febrile type is characterised by fever.

Similar syndromes may be caused by cytomegalovirus, human herpesvirus (HHV)-6, toxoplasmosis and HIV. Characteristic of infectious mononucleosis are large numbers of atypical mononuclear cells in the blood and a wide variety of serological changes, particularly heterophil antibodies, which are detectable by the Paul–Bunnell or Monospot tests, usually during the first or second week of illness [5,6]. Several other antibodies against EBV appear during the course of infectious mononucleosis, but the most frequent is the antibody to viral capsid antigen, the titre of which reaches a peak at about 4 weeks [7]. Complications are rare but may include autoimmune haemolysis (and cold agglutinins), CNS involvement (meningitis, encephalitis, etc.), erythema multiforme, hepatomegaly or hepatitis, jaundice (from hepatic involvement or haemolysis), pericarditis or myocarditis, pneumonitis, splenic rupture and thrombocytopenia.

No specific treatment is available for infectious mononucleosis [1,2,6], but supportive care is important, not only because of the potential for airways obstruction but also because of the associated lassitude. Systemic corticosteroids are required if there is pharyngeal oedema severe enough to hazard the airway.

Herpes simplex gingivostomatitis

Oral infection is common with the herpesviruses. Inoculation of HSV-1 at mucosal surfaces permits entry of the virus into sensory and autonomic nerve endings, through which it is transported to the cell nuclei where it remains latent [1]. Reactivation results in recurrent HSV disease. Herpesviruses are often excreted in saliva, especially in immunocompromised persons.

Epidemiology

About 60% of the world population under the age of 50 has HSV-1 [2]. The prevalence is highest in low- and middle-income countries. It affects both sexes equally.

Primary infection affects predominantly children and adolescents. With improving socioeconomic circumstances and standards of hygiene, a larger number of children are not exposed to HSV and enter adult life without immunity. Cases of primary herpetic stomatitis are therefore now seen occasionally in adults. HSV transmission typically occurs via oral–oral, oral–genital, or genital–genital contact, as well as through skin abrasions with infected oral secretions. HSV transmission can occur if the source is asymptomatic or symptomatic [3–5].

Pathology

Transmission rate is higher when patients are symptomatic since the viral load is much greater [6]. Primary genital HSV-1 infection is thought to be transmitted most frequently through oral–genital contact. The incubation period for HSV infection ranges from 2 days to 2 weeks. Primary herpetic gingivostomatitis typically occurs in children but can occur in older children and adolescents.

Causative organisms

In general, HSV-1 causes primary herpetic gingivostomatitis and the secondary infection of recurrent herpes labialis. There are no precise distinctions now in the type of HSV causing oral herpes. Oral infection with HSV-2 is more frequently seen [7,8]:

- ~60% of adults are infected with HSV-1.
- ~12% of adults are infected with HSV-2.

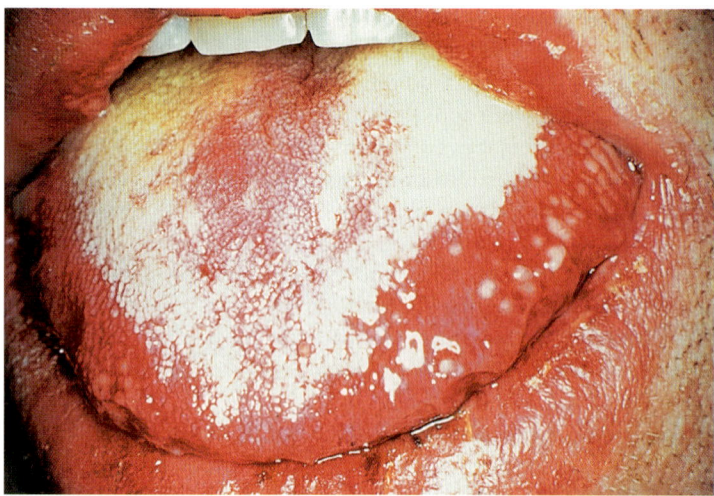

Figure 108.49 Scattered ulcers and a furred tongue in primary herpetic stomatitis.

It is possible to have genital outbreaks of HSV-1 and HSV-2 at different times. Acquiring HSV-1 in HSV-2-infected persons is unusual. In contrast, there is little protection against acquiring HSV-2 in those with a history of HSV-1 infection [8].

Clinical features

The incubation period is 2 days to 2 weeks, with a mean of 4 days. Many infections with HSV occur in childhood and are subclinical and, where there is disease, it varies greatly in severity. In many, it is trivial and misdiagnosed or passed off as 'teething'.

Primary herpetic gingivostomatitis typically presents with malaise, anorexia, irritability, fever, enlarged and tender anterior cervical lymph nodes, and a diffuse, purple, boggy gingivitis especially anteriorly. Multiple vesicles followed by round or ovoid ulcers 1–3 mm in diameter scatter across the oral mucosa and gingiva (Figure 108.49). They coalesce to form large, painful ulcers of the oral and perioral tissues. Lesions heal without scarring within 14 days. There are often perioral vesicular lesions (up to two-thirds of cases). In immunocompromised persons, herpes may manifest with chronic ulcers [9]. Halitosis may be an additional feature.

Differential diagnosis

The main differential diagnoses of herpetic gingivostomatitis in otherwise healthy persons are herpangina, hand, foot and mouth disease, aphthous ulcers and acute leukaemia. In immunocompromised persons, the differential is wider.

Disease course and prognosis

The resolution is spontaneous in otherwise healthy people but protracted in immunocompromised patients. Herpetic stomatitis resolves spontaneously in 7–14 days but HSV remains latent in the trigeminal ganglion. The most obvious sequel is that about one-third of patients are thereafter predisposed to recurrences. HSV is shed intermittently into the saliva [3–5]. HSV is implicated in many instances of erythema multiforme and may cause chronic ulcers in the immunocompromised (see later) or occasionally ulcers following trauma to the mouth. Complications of herpetic gingivostomatitis include dehydration, herpetic whitlow or herpetic keratitis from autoinoculation, eczema herpeticum, secondary

bacteraemia with upper respiratory bacteria *and* encephalitis. In immunocompromised patients, complications include severe local lesions, disseminated HSV infection (e.g. hepatitis), HSV pneumonitis and HSV encephalitis.

Investigations

Usually a clinical diagnosis. A full blood picture, white cell count and differential, and viral studies may be prudent [10]. The latter include the following:

- Nucleic acid studies. Polymerase chain reaction detection of HSV DNA: this is sensitive but expensive.
- Immunodetection: detection of HSV antigens is of some value. A rising titre of serum antibodies is confirmatory but only gives the diagnosis retrospectively.
- The Tzanck smear can be performed in patients with active lesions. It is only helpful if it is positive and does not distinguish between HSV-1, HSV-2 and varicella-zoster virus.

Management

Supportive care is the mainstay of therapy and includes antipyretic analgesics (e.g. acetaminophen/paracetamol), sponging with tepid water and a high fluid intake. An antihistamine such as promethazine may help sedate an irritable child.

- Encourage patient not to touch lesions.
- Avoid sharing eating utensils or toys.
- Wash utensils and hands frequently.
- Adequate pain control. Analgesics (as elixirs or syrups for children) and, in adults, lidocaine mouth-baths help ease discomfort and 0.2% aqueous chlorhexidine mouth-baths aid resolution.
- Blisters and sores should be kept dry.
- Antiviral medications can shorten outbreaks.
- For immunocompetent children with severely limited fluid intake and who present within 96 hours of onset, aciclovir may be given. In immunocompromised children with herpetic gingivostomatitis, IV or oral aciclovir *regardless of symptom duration before presentation* is recommended [11–14]. Topical antiviral agents are not helpful.

Recurrent labial HSV infection (RHL). Primary oral infection by HSV may produce perioral lesions (Figure 108.50). Approximately

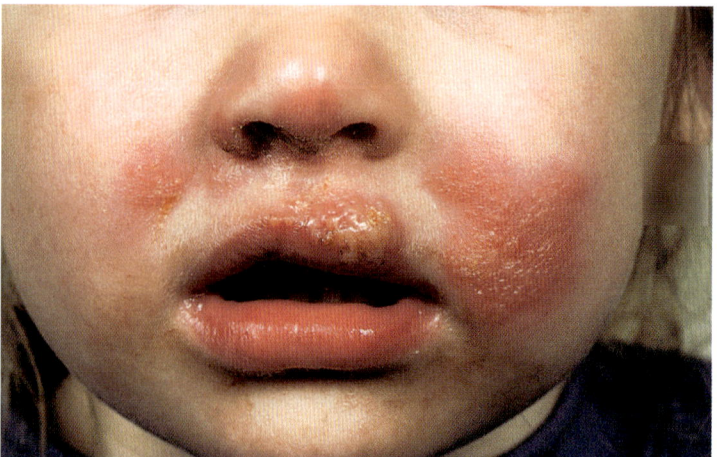

Figure 108.50 Primary herpetic stomatitis with extraoral lesions.

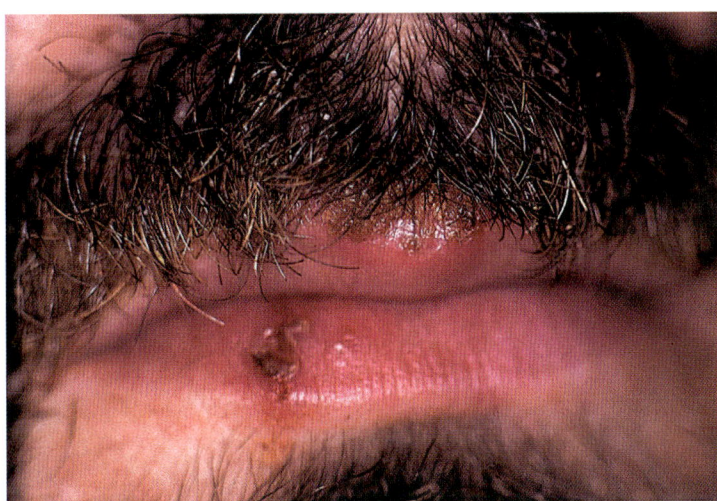

Figure 108.51 Herpes labialis.

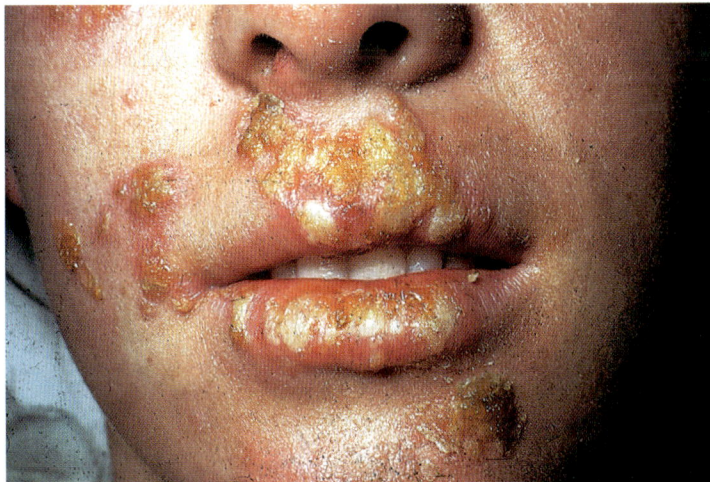

Figure 108.52 Impetigo.

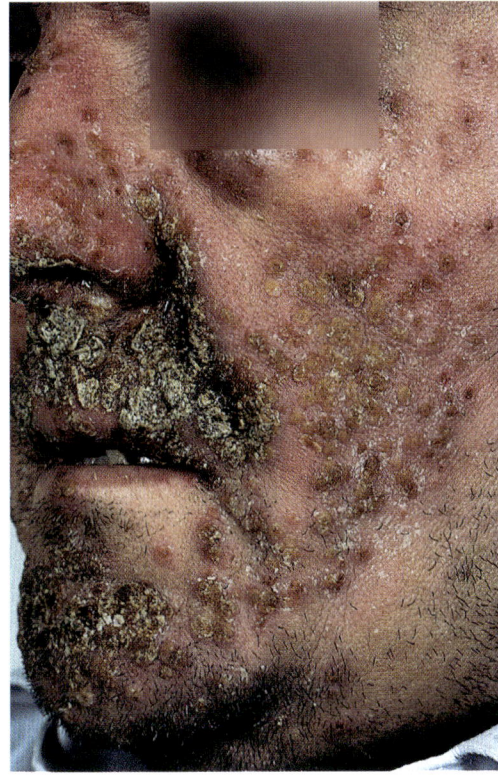

Figure 108.53 Eczema herpeticum.

Recurrent intraoral HSV infection. A small crop of ulcers, often with a raised white border and sometimes with a dendritic appearance, may occasionally affect apparently healthy individuals, especially at sites of trauma, for example following palatal infiltration of a local anaesthetic. Chronic indolent lesions, usually ulcerative or nodular, may be seen in patients with neutropenia or chronic leukaemia; in patients with more severe immunosuppression, such as acute leukaemia or HIV infection, more aggressive chronic, often dendritic, ulcers are seen frequently on the tongue dorsum. Aciclovir or other antivirals may be indicated systemically [17–21].

Herpesviruses 6, 7 and 8

Oral lesions have yet to be demonstrated in infections with HHV-6 or HHV-7. However, HHV-8 is implicated in oral Kaposi sarcoma [1]. Human herpesvirus 8 (HHV-8) is one of the human γ herpesviruses. Gamma herpesviruses play an important role in cellular proliferation and the development of malignancies. Host immunity plays an important role in the control of Kaposi sarcoma, as demonstrated by the increased incidence among transplant recipients and AIDS patients. Regression of Kaposi sarcoma has been shown with reduction of immunosuppressive treatment and in immune reconstitution following antiretroviral therapy [2]. Oral Kaposi sarcoma is discussed earlier in this chapter.

Herpes zoster (Chapter 25)

Recurrence of varicella-zoster virus causes zoster, or shingles. If shingles affects the maxillary or mandibular divisions of the trigeminal nerve, mouth ulcers are usually seen [1].

30% with primary HSV-1 will develop recurrent infection. It occurs mainly in adults and both sexes are affected. Recurrent HSV may recur at the site of initial inoculation or in the distribution of the associated nerves. Reactivating factors include sunlight, fever, trauma, immunosuppression, stress and hormonal changes. Recurrent herpes labialis involving the lip is the most common cause of blisters at the mucocutaneous junction (Figure 108.51). The lesions arise at the mucocutaneous junction as itching papules that progress to vesicles, pustules and then scab. They are unsightly and occasionally become infected with *Staphylococcus* or *Streptococcus*, resulting in impetigo (Figure 108.52). In immunocompromised persons, extensive and persistent lesions may result. In atopic persons, the lesions may spread to produce eczema herpeticum (Figure 108.53). Aciclovir has been the standard treatment used as a 5% cream and penciclovir 1% [15,16]. Hydrocolloid patches may be beneficial. Topical therapy must be administered multiple times per day and is less effective than oral antiviral therapy.

Prevention may be achieved with prophylactic antivirals; aciclovir (400 mg orally twice daily) or valaciclovir (500 mg orally once daily).

PART 10: SPECIFIC SITES, SEX & AGE

Clinical features

Thirty per cent of zoster is in the trigeminal region. The pain of trigeminal zoster may simulate toothache. Severe pain often precedes, accompanies and follows the rash, and postherpetic neuralgia may persist for months or years.

The rash is restricted to a dermatome and is unilateral, but sometimes a few chickenpox-type lesions can be found elsewhere. Oral ulcers appear in the distribution of the involved nerve division. There is ulceration of one side of the tongue, floor of the mouth and lower labial and buccal mucosa if the mandibular division of the trigeminal nerve is involved. One side of the palate, the upper gingiva and buccal sulcus are involved in maxillary zoster. Rarely, mandibular or maxillary zoster may disturb the formation of developing teeth [2] or cause jaw necrosis [3].

If the geniculate ganglion of the facial nerve is affected, there may be otitis externa, a unilateral lower motor neuron palsy of the facial nerve, ulceration of the soft palate and anterior two-thirds of the tongue unilaterally (Ramsay–Hunt syndrome) [4,5]. Herpes zoster keratitis or herpes zoster ophthalmicus can result from involvement of the ophthalmic branch of the trigeminal cranial nerve and can be sight-threatening [6].

Occasionally, there is misdiagnosis of toothache, leading to extraction, the true diagnosis becoming apparent only when the rash appears. Zoster resolves spontaneously. Postherpetic neuralgia (PHN) is defined as significant pain persisting for 90 days after the onset of rash. Numbness, dysaesthesias and allodynia may be noted in the affected dermatome.

Approximately 10–15% of patients with herpes zoster will develop PHN. Individuals older than 60 years and immunosuppressed patients have a higher incidence.

Management

An underlying immune defect, such as AIDS or malignancy, should be excluded in patients with zoster, although most zoster is related simply to lesser problems in advanced age. Treatment is mainly supportive but antivirals such as aciclovir can be useful [7–10]. Antiviral treatment is recommended for all immunocompetent patients over 50 years of age. Aciclovir tablets (400–800 mg) five times daily, or sugar-free oral suspension, for 7 days, or valaciclovir 1000 mg three times daily for 7 days, or famciclovir 500 mg three times daily for 7 days are useful. Addition of systemic corticosteroids may be beneficial in reducing PHN in patients over 50. In ophthalmic zoster, valaciclovir 1000 mg three times daily is indicated, and an ophthalmological opinion, since there can be corneal ulceration. Analgesics are indicated in zoster, although the pain may prove refractory to even potent analgesics, when antidepressants such as amitriptyline may have a place [9,11,12]. Treatment advances include lidocaine patches, opioid analgesics and gabapentin. Early recognition and treatment of high-risk herpes zoster patients with antiviral and analgesic therapies is mandatory.

HIV infection (Chapter 31)

Oral lesions include three types of oral and pharyngeal candidiasis (pseudomembranous, erythematous and angular cheilitis), hairy leukoplakia due to EBV infection, other herpes-group virus infections including herpes simplex and herpes zoster, papillomavirus warts, severe periodontal disease, salivary gland disease, Kaposi sarcoma and AIDS lymphoma [1–7]. Oral lesions of HIV infection can serve as early markers of the disease and indicators of disease progression in the untreated, and their presence correlates with HIV load and CD4 cell depletion.

Oral ulceration in patients infected with HIV may be due to any of the causes of mouth ulceration, and aphthous-like ulcers are also seen. Painful ulceration is one of the most distinctive manifestations of acute HIV infection and may be found on the oral mucosa [8]. However, it is important to exclude infections, mainly herpesviruses. There are also occasional examples of mouth ulcers due to mycobacteria, *Rochalimaea*, syphilis, *Histoplasma*, *Cryptococcus*, leishmaniasis and others. Malignant disease (mainly Kaposi sarcoma or non-Hodgkin lymphoma) may result in lumps that can ulcerate.

Aphthous-like ulcers in HIV may respond to local treatment or, failing that, thalidomide at a dose of 200 mg/day has been shown in randomised double-blind placebo-controlled trials to be effective in the treatment of HIV-related recurrent aphthous ulceration [9]. Other mouth ulcers should be treated as appropriate.

Use of long-term antiretroviral therapy may be associated with an increased risk of oral warts, hyposalivation, erythema multiforme, toxic epidermal necrolysis, lichenoid reactions and exfoliative cheilitis [10,11]. HPV-associated oral warts have a prevalence of 0.5% in the general population, up to 5% in persons living with HIV and in up to 23% of those on antiretroviral therapy.

BACTERIAL INFECTIONS (CHAPTER 26)

Acute necrotising (ulcerative) gingivitis and noma

Acute necrotising (ulcerative) gingivitis (ANUG), also called Vincent's angina or trench mouth, is typically an acute gingival ulceration, rarely complicated by gangrenous stomatitis (when it is called noma).

Epidemiology

ANUG is uncommon, typically seen in students, malnutrition or in conflict situations [1]. Noma is a serious destructive necrosis affecting the soft tissues and bones of the mouth and adjoining orofacial areas [2,3]. Noma is seen predominantly in sub-Saharan Africa, where the estimated frequency in some communities varies from 1 to 7 cases per 1000 population. ANUG is typically seen in children or adolescents and in young adults [4,5].

Predisposing factors

Viral respiratory infections, stress, smoking, malnutrition or immune defects may precede the onset of disease, suggesting depression of immunity as a predisposing cause. Necrotising ulcerative periodontitis may be a feature of HIV infection as well as patients with severe immunosuppression related to cancer chemotherapy or malnutrition. This manifests as severe loss of periodontal attachment and alveolar bone [5–7].

Causative organisms

Prevotella intermedia, *Fusobacterium* spp., *Tannerella forsythia*, *Treponema denticoli* and other oral spirochetes are associated with this infection [8,9].

Presentation

The mouth ulceration is usually initially restricted to the gingiva, specifically the interdental papillae, which appear blunted (Figures 108.54 and 108.55). The history is characteristic, with an acute onset of severe gingival soreness, bleeding and halitosis. Acute necrotising gingivitis occurs especially in the anterior part of the mouth where the affected gingiva are extremely tender to touch and an ulcerative necrotic slough forms on the gingiva. There is often anterior submandibular and submental lymphadenopathy and there may be pyrexia and malaise.

Failure to treat acute necrotising gingivitis adequately may predispose to recurrence and, in malnourished or immunocompromised individuals, may lead to noma (cancrum oris, orofacial gangrene).

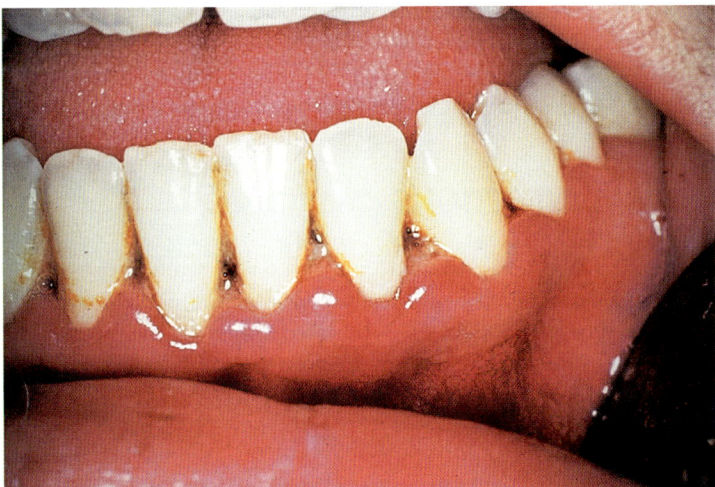

Figure 108.54 Acute necrotising gingivitis showing typical ulceration of interdental gingival papillae. This was in HIV infection.

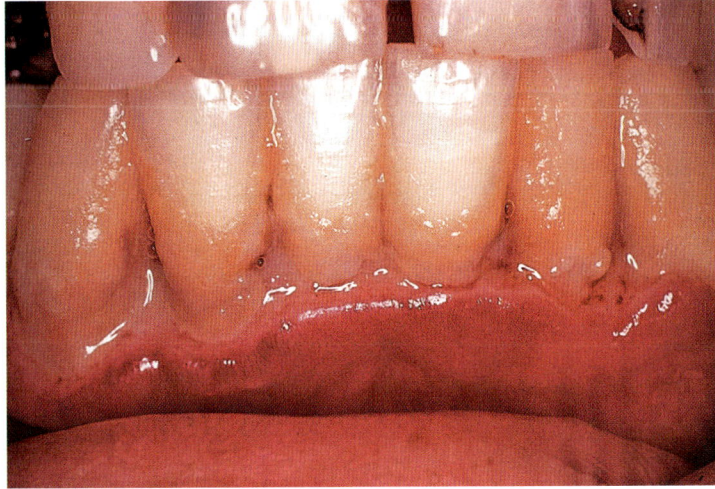

Figure 108.55 Untreated acute necrotising gingivitis can lead to extensive gingival ulceration and irreparable damage.

Management

Gentle cleansing with hydrogen peroxide or chlorhexidine gluconate mouthwash and a soft toothbrush is remarkably effective. Oral metronidazole 200 mg should be given three times daily for 3–7 days to limit the tissue destruction in ANUG. Penicillin is equally effective. The patient should also be referred for dental advice [1] and predisposing factors, including smoking, poor sleep hygiene and stress, should be addressed. Noma requires attention also to nutrition, antimicrobials and sometimes reconstructive surgery [3].

Epithelioid (bacillary) angiomatosis

(Chapter 26)

This condition is due to infection with *Bartonella henselae* or *Bartonella quintana*. It is uncommon but occurs in the immunocompromised, although it may also be seen in immunocompetent patients. It presents with skin papules and nodules. Oral lesions have been seen clinically in HIV disease [1–4], sometimes as the first manifestation of HIV infection [3]. Oral lesions can occur without skin involvement. Mucosal lesions appear as smooth purple papules or plaques on the gingiva, buccal mucosa, labial mucosa, hard palate and posterior pharynx [5].

Gonorrhoea

This is a sexually transmitted disease which may infect the oropharynx with the Gram-negative organism *Neisseria gonorrhoeae*. Oropharyngeal asymptomatic carriage of gonococci is found in around 4% of those attending clinics for sexually transmitted diseases [1–3]. Following contact with infected body fluid the incubation period is 7–21 days. Oral mucosal erythema, sometimes with oedema and ulceration, is occasionally seen in oropharyngeal gonorrhoea [1,2]. The majority are asymptomatic, although sore throat, pharyngeal exudates and cervical lymphadenopathy are present in some cases. Diagnosis is by a bacterial throat swab.

Leprosy

Mycobacterium leprae causes a bacterial infection presenting with skin, nerve, respiratory and ocular lesions. Oral involvement has been reported in up to 60% of leprosy cases. It is proportional to the duration of the disease. Intraoral manifestations are characterised as nodular lesions that tend to ulcerate leading to necrosis [1–4]. The incisive papilla and anterior maxillary gingiva, soft and hard palate, uvula and tonsils/glossopharyngeal arches are most commonly affected. Cranial nerve involvement, especially of the trigeminal and facial nerves, may occur leading to anaesthesia of the orofacial tissues and facial palsy, respectively [1–4]. It is an important differential for granulomatous oral diseases. Diagnosis is through oral biopsy [5].

Syphilis

Oral ulcers may be seen at any stage but particularly in secondary syphilis [1–6]. In primary syphilis, a primary chancre develops at the site of inoculation and may involve the lips, tongue or palate. A small, firm pink macule changes to a papule which ulcerates to form a painless round ulcer with a raised margin and indurated base [1,2]. Chancres heal spontaneously in 3–8 weeks but are highly infectious and are associated with painless regional lymphadenopathy.

Secondary syphilis follows after 4–6 weeks, with oral lesions in about one-third of patients. These are highly infectious and are usually fairly painless ulcers (mucous patches and snail-track ulcers) or raised nodules in the mouth, known as condyloma lata [2–4].

The most characteristic oral lesion of tertiary syphilis is a localised granuloma (gumma) that varies in size from a pinhead to several centimetres, affecting particularly the palate, or the tongue. Gummas break down to form deep chronic punched-out ulcers that are not infectious (Figure 108.56). There may be bone destruction with palatal perforation and oronasal fistula formation. Neurosyphilis can also give rise to trigeminal neuropathy and facial nerve palsy.

Oral manifestations of congenital syphilis are characterised by altered morphology of the anterior teeth (Hutchinson incisors), and the posterior dentition (mulberry molars), and perioral rhagades [2–4].

Diagnosis

The diagnosis of syphilis is usually based on a combination of clinical findings, serology and histopathological confirmation. Visualisation of *Treponema pallidum* bacterium via darkfield microscopy is rarely used. Treponemal tests looking specifically for *T. pallidum* or its components as antigens include *T. pallidum* haemagglutination assay (TPHA) and fluorescent treponemal antibody absorption assay (FTA-ABS). Importantly, the features of syphilis histologically are non-specific. A deep perivascular infiltrate containing plasma cells is suspicious of syphilis. Immunohistochemistry staining is essential to highlight and confirm *Treponema* antibody positive spirochetes [5].

Tuberculosis

Oral lesions can develop in pulmonary tuberculosis but are not common. A chronic ulcer with indurated, ill-defined margins, usually of the dorsum of the tongue, is the most common oral presentation but patches, papillomatous lesions and indurated soft tissue lesions have also been described. Tuberculous osteomyelitis involving the maxilla or mandible, or cervical lymphadenitis may be seen [1–4]. Rare tubercular involvement of the parotid gland has been reported [1]. Atypical mycobacteria are not uncommonly involved.

Mycobacterial oral ulcers, particularly caused by *Mycobacterium avium–intracellulare*, have been reported as a complication of AIDS and occasionally in apparently healthy individuals [5]. Cervicofacial infection is occasionally caused by *M. chelonei*, usually in the form of lymph node abscesses, or occasionally as intraoral swellings [6,7].

FUNGAL INFECTIONS (CHAPTER 32)

Oral fungal infections, apart from candidiasis, rarely causes mouth ulcers in resource-rich countries, where they are usually seen only in immunocompromised or debilitated patients, including those with AIDS. However, they may be seen occasionally in otherwise healthy persons from the tropics (Table 108.11).

Aspergillosis

Rhinocerebral aspergillosis may ulcerate through to the mouth. This is a rare event, except in the severely immunocompromised [1–3].

Table 108.11 Rare orofacial fungal infections.

Infection	Oral manifestations
Aspergillosis	Aspergilloma
	Rhinocerebral type causes palatal necrosis
	Disseminated in immunocompromised patients
Blastomycosis	
North American	Oral ulcers or suppurating granulomas
South American (paracoccidioidomycosis)	Oral ulcers and lymphadenopathy
Coccidioidomycosis	Rarely oral ulcers
Cryptococcosis	Oral ulcers
Histoplasmosis	Lumps or ulcers in mouth
Phycomycosis (mucormycosis, zygomycosis)	Antral involvement with palatal ulceration in immunocompromised patients, especially diabetics
Sporotrichosis	Oral lesions rare

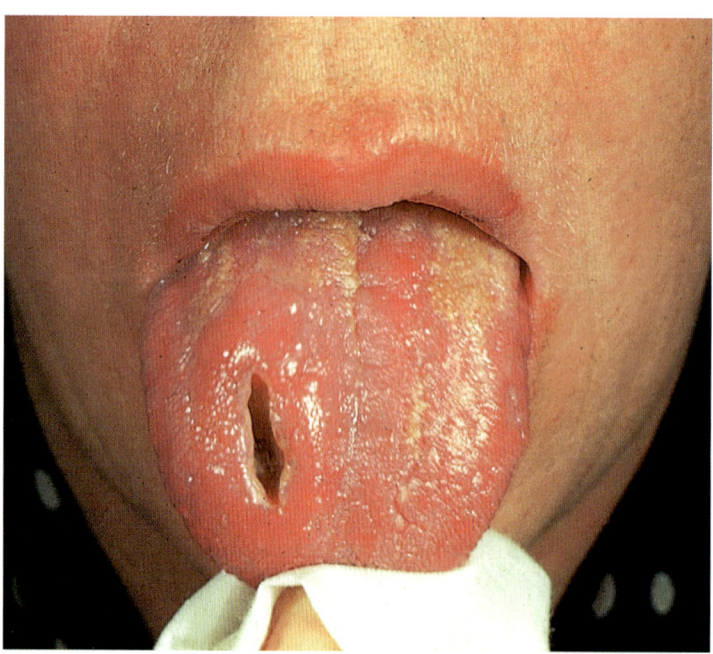

Figure 108.56 Gumma.

Mandibular aspergillosis has also been reported [4]. Occasionally, solitary aspergillosis arises as a consequence of endodontic treatment where root canal filling material enters the antrum [5], but this does not cause oral ulceration. Surgical debridement is usually indicated.

Blastomycoses

Blastomycoses may produce oral lesions which are typically mulberry-like ulcerated swellings especially seen on the gingiva and alveolus [1–3].

Candidiasis

At least 70% of the normal population carry the fungus *Candida albicans* as a normal oral commensal. Carriage is more common in cigarette smokers. *Candida* resides particularly on the posterior dorsum of the tongue. The commensal form is a unicellular budding yeast whereas the pathogenic form is a true hyphae with parallel-side wall. Infection with *Candida* (usually *Candida albicans*) known as candidiasis, or candidosis, is likely to result from xerostomia, local disturbances in salivary flora such as occurs during broad-spectrum antimicrobial treatment, or in people who are immunocompromised, e.g. HIV-infected patients, transplant recipients and chemotherapy patients. Acute pseudomembranous candidiasis, candidal leukoplakia and chronic mucocutaneous candidiasis present as white lesions (see earlier in this chapter); the other types, acute and chronic atrophic candidiasis, are red (see earlier in this chapter) (Table 108.12).

Table 108.12 Intraoral candidiasis.

Type of candidosis	Usual age at onset	Predisposing factors[a]
Acute pseudomembranous candidiasis (thrush)[b]	Any	Local: dry mouth, antimicrobials General: corticosteroids, leukaemia, HIV
Acute atrophic candidiasis (antibiotic sore mouth)	Any	Broad-spectrum antibiotics or corticosteroids
Erythematous candidiasis		Any, HIV especially
Chronic atrophic candidiasis (denture-related stomatitis)	Adults	Denture wearing, especially at night
Chronic hyperplastic candidiasis[b]	Usually middle-aged or elderly	Tobacco smoking, denture wearing, immune defect
Median rhomboid glossitis	Third or later decades	Tobacco smoking, denture wearing, HIV
Chronic mucocutaneous candidiasis[b]	Usually first decade	Often immune defect

[a] Immune defects can predispose to any form.
[b] White lesions.

Cryptococcosis

Cryptococcus neoformans may occasionally produce violaceous nodules of granulation tissue, swellings or ulcers in immunocompromised patients [1–4]. Oral lesions have been described on the gingiva, hard and soft palate, pharynx, oral mucosa, tonsillar pillar and after extraction [5–7].

Geotrichosis

Geotrichosis is a rare livid, sharply-defined enanthema of the oral mucosa with ulcerations seen in immunocompromised persons, such as those with leukaemia or HIV infection. *Geotrichum capitatum* is responsible and there may also be pneumonic lung infiltrates [1]. Treatment includes amphotericin, 5-fluorocytosine and itraconazole.

Histoplasmosis

Oral lesions of histoplasmosis are uncommon. They are typically seen in chronic disseminated histoplasmosis, usually as a fungating or ulcerative lesion on the tongue, palate, buccal mucosa or gingiva, sometimes in AIDS [1–5].

Mucormycosis

Rhinocerebral mucormycosis typically commences in the nasal cavity or paranasal sinuses and invades the palate to produce a black necrotic ulcer, although it might occasionally commence in the palate [1–4]. Although very rare, mandibular involvement can occur [5]. Cases are seen in diabetics or in immunocompromised patients such as those with AIDS [4,6]. Biopsy and radiography are required for diagnosis. Treatment is surgical debridement together with amphotericin intravenously and/or azoles.

PROTOZOAL INFESTATIONS

Leishmaniasis

Leishmaniasis is rare in northern Europe and the USA; it is not uncommon, however, in hotter climes and may cause ulcers in the mouth or more commonly on the lips [1] and is seen increasingly in HIV disease [2–4] or in other immunocompromised states.

LIP LESIONS

Lip lesions can be seen in many of the disorders described earlier in this chapter; this section covers conditions that manifest mainly or exclusively on the lips.

PART 10: SPECIFIC SITES, SEX & AGE

Actinic cheilitis (solar cheilosis)

Actinic cheilitis, also called solar cheilitis or solar cheilosis, is a premalignant disorder of the lip caused by chronic sun exposure [1–4].

Epidemiology

Most actinic cheilitis is seen on the lower lip of patients in their fifth to eighth decade of life. The frequency is higher in geographical areas with high ultraviolet (UV) radiation, in open-air workers and in people with fair skin.

Predisposing factors

The main factor is UV radiation. The vermilion of the lower lip in particular receives a high dose of UV irradiation and is poorly protected by keratin and melanocytes [5]. Tobacco smoking may aggravate the condition. Voriconazole therapy is a further risk factor [6]. Other forms of radiation such as arc-welding can occasionally cause similar damage. Actinic cheilitis rarely may be an early manifestation of a genetic susceptibility to light damage, as in xeroderma pigmentosum and oculocutaneous albinism. Immune defects, including immunosuppression in organ transplant recipients, also predispose to actinic damage and malignant transformation.

Pathology

Histology shows acanthosis, hyperkeratosis, focal areas of atrophy. An inflammatory infiltrate in which plasma cells may predominate can also be seen. Nuclear atypia and abnormal mitoses may be seen in the more severe cases, and some develop into invasive squamous carcinoma. The collagen generally shows basophilic (elastotic) degeneration [3,4].

Clinical features (Figure 108.57)

Actinic cheilitis tends to affect the lower lip with sparing of the oral commissures [1,2]. In the early stages there may be redness and oedema. Repeated exposure to UV radiation over long periods produces chronic tissue changes and the lip may become dry,

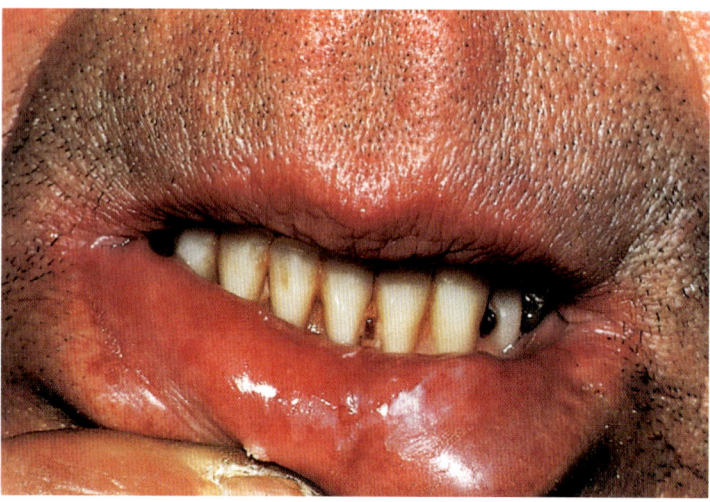

Figure 108.57 Chronic actinic cheilitis with leukoplakia. Courtesy of Addenbrooke's Hospital.

scaly and atrophic. The lip may become palpably thickened with small greyish white plaques. The border between the vermilion and the skin or mucosa becomes indistinct. Eventually, warty nodules may form, which may evolve into SCC. Suspicious features include: pain, chronic ulceration, a speckled area, generalised atrophy with focal areas of whitish thickening, persistent flaking and crusting.

Investigations

A biopsy should be taken from an area representative of the lesion's severity, as well as from areas with atrophy, ulceration or induration. The differential diagnosis includes lichen planus, lupus erythematosus, leukoplakia and SCC.

Management

Treatment of actinic cheilitis is required to relieve symptoms and to endeavour to prevent development of squamous carcinoma [7,8–10]. Wearing broad-brimmed hats, using broad-spectrum sunscreen (protection against both UVA and UVB rays) applied generously and frequently, and minimising sun exposure is advised. The highest success rates are reported with surgical approaches, laser therapy (mainly ablative CO_2 laser) or photodynamic therapy with aminolaevulinic acid. However, topical therapies are also very successful.

Topical chemotherapeutic approaches, e.g. topical applications of fluorouracil (5-FU) or 5% imiquimod have a good success rate of approximately 75% and are straightforward to prescribe and administer. Repeated courses over 2–3 weeks provide incremental success.

- 5% fluorouracil twice daily for 2–4 weeks. Imiquimod 5% cream may be applied to the involved area three times per week for 4–6 weeks. 50% trichloracetic acid or 3% diclofenac gel with 2.5% hyaluronic acid may also be effective.
- For patients with severe actinic cheilitis with evidence of high-grade dysplasia, vermilionectomy followed by defect repair by primary closure or mucosal advancement flap is the treatment of choice.
- Laser ablation may be an option for severe actinic cheilitis without evidence of high-grade dysplasia.
- Photodynamic therapy (PDT) with and without imiquimod is also a treatment option.

Following treatment, the regular use of a sunscreen lipsalve containing *p*-aminobenzoic acid probably gives the best protection. The estimated malignant transformation rate of actinic cheilitis into SCC approximately 3% [10,11]. Particular care should be taken to protect the vermilion of the lips with adequate sunscreens in patients with photosensitivity disorders such as xeroderma pigmentosum, in those whose exposure to UVB is high, and in those using photosensitising agents.

Actinic prurigo (Chapter 126)

Actinic prurigo is a photodermatosis often considered a variant of polymorphous light eruption, although actinic prurigo has distinct clinical features [1]. Actinic prurigo is characterised by symmetrical involvement of sun-exposed areas of the skin, lips and conjunctivae.

Epidemiology

Onset usually occurs in childhood, may spontaneously improve in adolescence, but can persist into adulthood. A family history is present in up to 50% of patients.

The condition predominates in women. It is seen mainly in native populations living at high altitudes especially in Latin America and in Asia, including in India, Thailand and China. The absence of mucosal involvement is a distinguishing feature between Asian and white populations.

Pathophysiology
Pathology

The diagnosis of actinic prurigo is often based upon clinical findings. Histological examination shows acanthosis, mild spongiosis, oedema of the lamina propria, moderate-to-dense in a band-like lymphocytic inflammatory infiltrate, eosinophils and, occasionally, lymphoid follicles [2].

Genetics

The specific locus, HLA-DRB1*0407, has been identified in 60–70% of patients [1,3–5]. In Singapore, there is a close association with HLA-DRB1*0301 [6].

Environmental factors

Lesions are induced by exposure to both UVA and UVB. UVA elicits the condition in most patients.

Clinical features

Facial skin and lips are involved in two-thirds of cases with an intensely itchy, excoriated papular and nodular skin eruption, and lip pruritus, oedema, scales, fissures, crusts and ulceration [7,8]. Polymorphic light eruption (PMLE) is usually present in the actinic prurigo of American Indians. It commonly presents in young women as a photosensitive facial rash with pruritic lower lip cheilitis, and it may be associated with conjunctivitis, pseudopterygium and eyebrow alopecia. Commonly, lesions are symmetrically distributed.

Investigations

On biopsy, actinic prurigo is distinguished from actinic cheilitis, which is due to prolonged and excessive exposure to UV irradiation, by the relative absence of epidermal dysplasia and solar elastosis. Serum immunoglobulin E (IgE) levels are elevated in nearly 50% and are associated with moderate or severe disease [9].

Management

Actinic prurigo treatment is with sunscreens, β-carotene and antihistamines. Topical corticosteroids can offer some relief. Topical application of tacrolimus may be effective in patients with milder disease. Phototherapy with psoralen plus ultraviolet A (PUVA) is an option in those with persistent symptoms [10]. Thalidomide has been successful in patients with resistant disease [11,12].

Pentoxifylline, cyclosporine and azathioprine are other options in resistant cases [13,14].

Angular cheilitis

Angular cheilitis is a chronic inflammatory lesion affecting usually both commissures. Most cases are seen in people with denture-related stomatitis and is related to *Candida* [1,2].

Epidemiology

Angular cheilitis is common. It occurs mostly in adults, particularly the older age group. It occurs in both males and females. There is no known geographic incidence.

Pathophysiology
Predisposing factors

Most cases are due to mechanical and/or infective causes or dry mouth, but nutritional or immune defects are also causes:
- *Infective agents* are the major cause.
- *Immune deficiency*, such as diabetes and HIV infection, may present with angular stomatitis [3–5]. Outbreaks of acute pustular and fissured cheilitis may occur in children, particularly if they are malnourished, and in some cases streptococci or staphylococci have appeared to be causative.
- *Mechanical factors* in edentulous patients who do not wear a denture or who have inadequate dentures, and also as a normal consequence of the ageing process, produce an oblique curved fold and keep the small area of skin constantly macerated.
- *Nutritional deficiencies*, particularly deficiencies of riboflavin, folate, iron and general protein malnutrition, may produce smooth shiny red lips associated with angular stomatitis, a combination called *cheilosis* [6].
- Disorders where the lip anatomical relationships are changed – such as when the vertical dimension of occlusion is reduced, or where lips are enlarged, such as in orofacial granulomatosis, Crohn's disease and Down syndrome [7,8] may cause angular cheilitis.
- *Hyposalivation*, such as after drug therapy, irradiation or in Sjögren syndrome may be a predisposing factor.

Causative organisms

Candida and/or staphylococci are isolated from most patients [9,10]. Permanent cure can be achieved only by eliminating the *Candida* beneath the upper denture [11,12]. Agents causing hyposalivation (e.g. irradiation, chemotherapy or anticholinergic drugs) can predispose to infections. *Candida albicans* or *Staphylococcus aureus* can be isolated in up to 54% of lesions.

Clinical features

The common complaints are of soreness, erythema and fissuring affecting the angles of the mouth. Typically, the condition persists or recurs. Atrophy, erythema, ulceration, crusting and scaling may be seen (Figure 108.58). Lesions occasionally extend beyond the vermilion border onto the skin in the form of linear furrows or

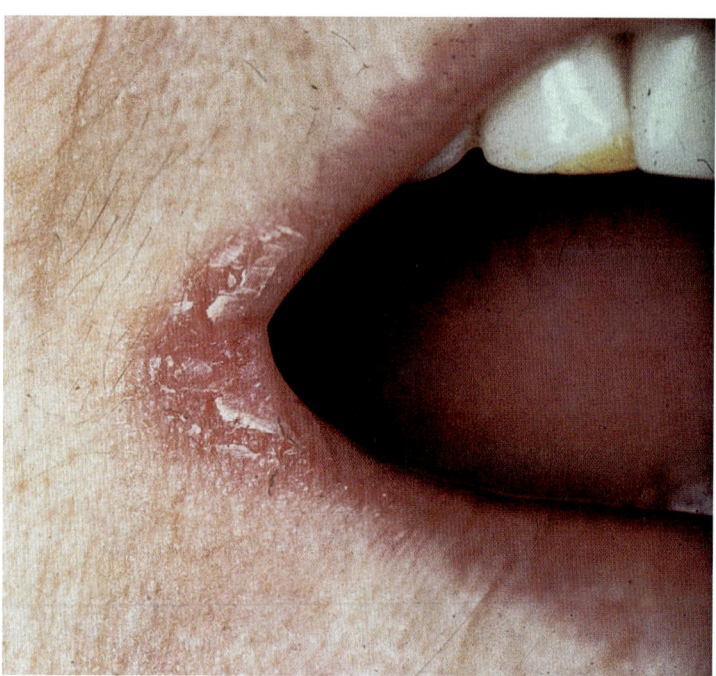

Figure 108.58 Angular cheilitis.

fissures radiating from the angle of the mouth (rhagades), mainly in the more severe forms, especially in denture wearers. An eczematous dermatitis may extend onto the cheek or chin as an infective eczematoid reaction.

Investigations

This is usually a clinical diagnosis, made by clinical examination. Intraoral inspection in angular cheilitis may reveal palatal erythema caused by associated denture-related stomatitis.

Management

Management of angular cheilitis is sometimes difficult and therapy may need to be prolonged. Dentures should be removed from the mouth at night and stored in a candidacidal solution such as hypochlorite. Denture-related stomatitis should be treated with an antifungal. Miconazole may be preferable treatment for candidiasis (cream applied locally, together with the oral gel) as it has some Gram-positive bacteriostatic action. New dentures that restore facial contour may help. The skin lesions should be swabbed and staphylococcal infection treated with fusidic acid ointment or cream at least four times daily. Miconazole plus hydrocortisone cream, fucidin plus hydrocortisone cream, clotrimazole plus hydrocortisone cream and nystatin plus hydrocortisone cream are other choices.

Blisters on the lips

Blistering is commonly due to recurrent herpes labialis but may be caused by various forms of cheilitis; trauma; burns from irradiation, heat or chemicals; solvent abuse; infections such as impetigo; mucoceles; allergies; lupus erythematosus; amyloidosis or vesiculobullous disorders [1–5].

'Chapping' of the lips

Chapping is a reaction to adverse environmental conditions usually caused by exposure to freezing cold or to hot dry winds. The keratin of the vermilion loses its plasticity, so that the lips become sore, cracked and scaly. The affected person tends to lick the lips, or to pick at the scales, which may aggravate the condition.

Treatment is by application of petroleum jelly and avoidance of the adverse environmental conditions.

Cheilitis

Cheilitis may arise as a primary disorder of the vermilion zone or the inflammation may extend from nearby skin or, less often, from the oral mucosa.

Contact cheilitis

Contact cheilitis is an inflammatory reaction provoked by an irritant (irritant contact cheilitis) or a sensitising compound leading to type 4 hypersensitivity (allergic contact cheilitis). Substances leading to allergic contact cheilitis include medicaments, cosmetics and toothpastes/mouthwashes but may also include other contact items, e.g. the mouthpiece of musical instruments [1–3]. Box 108.8 includes the most common as well as the rarer causes.

Box 108.8 Allergens associated with delayed contact cheilitis

Fragrances/flavour – fragrance mix, cinnamon, eugenol, oak moss, limonene, linalool, menthol, carvone, Balsam of Peru (*Myroxylon pereirae*), anethole
- Propolis (bee glue)
- Preservatives – gallates, benzoic acid
- Medicaments and ointment bases
- Metals – nickel, gold
- Shellac

Rarer causes
- Colourings/dyes
- Other metals, e.g. tin fluoride
- Sunscreens – benzophenones
- Nail varnish

It is essential to undertake patch testing that includes a standard European series plus cosmetics, flavourings and the patient's own products. Dental allergens for stomatitis with a history of restorative work should also be considered. Photopatch test for cheilitis caused by photocontact allergy to sunscreens, e.g. benzophenone-3. When considering irritancy with toothpaste, it is important to test diluted samples and undertake semi-open tests (Chapter 127).

Allergen groups may include drugs, vehicles, perfumes and flavourings, dental materials and photocontact products, e.g. sunscreens. Some of the specific allergens are detailed below:

- *Medicaments*. These may include: topical anaesthetics, corticosteroids, antimicrobials, e.g. antiviral, antibacterial, anti-yeast therapies plus their vehicles (lanolin, propylene glycol).
- *Cosmetics*. These include lip balms and lipsticks (Box 108.8). Components include: fragrances/flavourings, e.g. limonene, linalool, cinnamon, essential oils; propolis; preservatives/antioxidants; shellac; vehicle allergens such as lanolin and propylene glycol; sunscreens – consider potential photocontact allergy.
- *Toothpaste*: flavourings, e.g. mint/spearmint; allergens, e.g. limonene and linalool, carvone, surfactants, tin, other metals.
- *Mouthwashes* (borderline substances) contain flavourings and antiseptics (chlorhexidine, triclosan).
- *Dental materials*: acrylates, metals (nickel/chrome, gold), amalgam/mercury, topical anaesthetics, rubber, chlorhexidine.

Clinical features

Lipstick cheilitis is sometimes confined to the vermilion but more often extends beyond. There may be persistent irritation and scaling or a more acute reaction with oedema and vesiculation. Hyperpigmentation is an occasional complication.

Diagnosis

If acute eczematous changes are obviously present, the diagnosis of contact cheilitis is confirmed with patch testing. An irritant cheilitis will improve with avoidance of the contact factor. A history of eczema or atopy may otherwise indicate eczematous cheilitis.

Management

Avoidance of contact allergen and topical corticosteroids (fluticasone propionate, mometasone furoate) or tacrolimus.

Drug-induced cheilitis

Haemorrhagic crusting of the lips (Figure 108.59) is a feature Stevens–Johnson syndrome (Chapter 118).

Aromatic retinoids such as etretinate and isotretinoin frequently cause cheilitis, dryness and cracking of the lips [1,2]. Similar effects may follow use of voriconazole [3–5]. Many other drugs have been described as detailed in Table 108.13 [6].

Table 108.13 Drug-related cheilitis.

Drugs most commonly implicated	Drugs occasionally implicated
Isotretinoin	Atrovastatin
Acitretin	Busulfan
Protease inhibitors	Clofazimine
Vitamin A	Clomipramine
	Cyanocobalamin
	Methyldopa
	Psoralens
	Streptomycin
	Sulfasalazine
	Tetracycline

Eczematous cheilitis

The lips are often involved secondarily to atopic eczema (Chapter 41). The treatment is with emollients and topical corticosteroids. A potent steroid such as fludrocortisone may be required.

Exfoliative cheilitis

Exfoliative cheilitis is an uncommon inflammatory condition affecting the vermilion border of one or both lips that results in peeling, cracking, pain or burning and is a significant cause of morbidity (Figures 108.60 and 108.61) [1,2]. It is often ongoing with fluctuations in severity. Patients frequently search tirelessly for a solution and try numerous ointments and balms to ease symptoms. Making the diagnosis is essential as early as possible to break the habits that patients develop, explaining where possible the underlying cause and introducing optimal multidisciplinary approaches to management. The precise cause is unknown, but it is frequently associated with atopy or seborrheic dermatitis and is therefore often considered to be a localised form of eczema [3]. There is very little literature on this condition.

Epidemiology

Patients may present in adolescence or early adulthood although later presentation is also seen. Males and females may be affected. Age of onset varies.

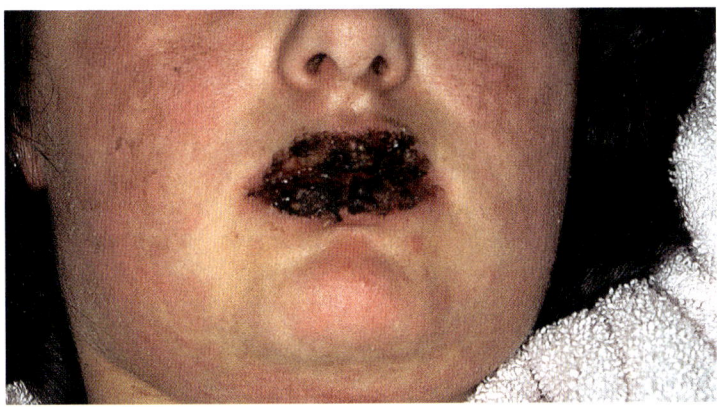

Figure 108.59 Haemorrhagic crusting of the lips in Stevens–Johnson syndrome.

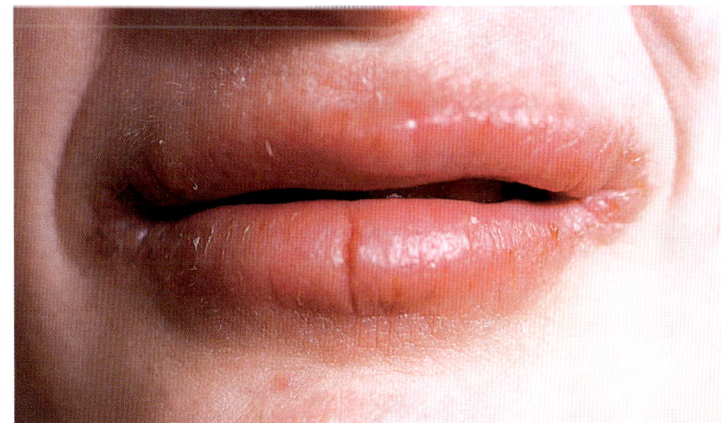

Figure 108.60 Factitious cheilitis due to repeated lip sucking.

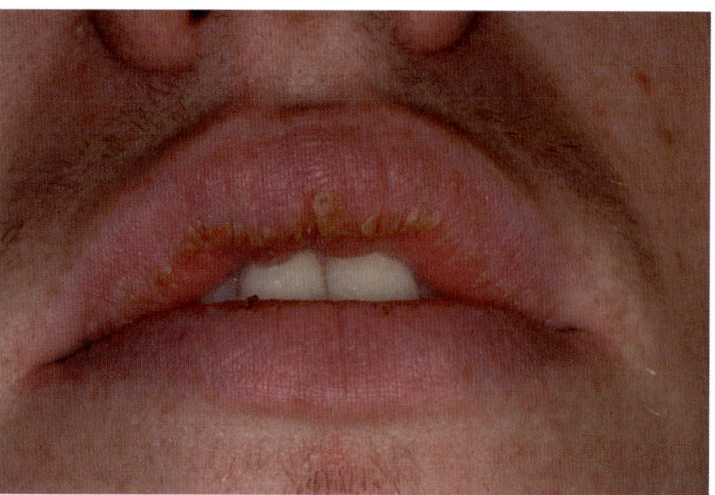

Figure 108.61 Exfoliative cheilitis.

Table 108.14 Some lip/facial fillers and implants.

Origin	Material	Usage
Natural fillers	Hyaluronic acid	Frequent
	Fat	Occasional
	Calcium hydroxylapatite	Occasional
Synthetic fillers	Poly-L-lactic acid	Occasional but more typically for volume restoration in other parts of the face
	Polyacrylamide and polymethylmethacrylate	Rare
Synthetic alloplastic implants	Silicone	Occasional use
		Rarely used
	Extended polytetrafluoroethylene	

Pathophysiology

An underlying tendency to eczema is present in about 40% of patients. Additionally, underlying mental health problems are also frequently present ranging from stress and anxiety to combined anxiety and depression, obsessive compulsive disorders and eating disorders. Contact dermatitis may be relevant in a significant proportion of patients. Secondary infection is also very frequent.

Clinical features

Patients slowly develop a tendency to dry, peeling lips at the onset. The process, which often starts in the middle of the lower lip and spreads to involve the whole of the lower or both lips, is more or less confined to the vermilion border, and persists in varying severity for months or years [1,2]. Patients find themselves picking and peeling the dry skin away and start to apply copious amounts of emollient. This harbours bacteria, most frequently *Staphylococcus aureus*, and yeasts. Patients complain of pain, burning and discomfort. There is a large psychological morbidity that further exacerbates a tendency to anxiety or depression. Patients start to avoid wetting their lips in the shower and guard their lips, trying to have as little contact with liquid or food as possible. Some drink through a straw and allow large amounts of keratin to sit on the lip surface.

Differential diagnosis

Contact and active cheilitis must be carefully excluded. Chronic exfoliative cheilitis is readily contaminated by *Candida*. Swabs of the nose and mouth for microscopy, culture and sensitivity are vital and need to be repeated frequently. Biopsy is not indicated. Patch testing is valuable.

Management

Some cases resolve spontaneously or with improved oral hygiene. Modification of unhelpful habits such as lip licking is important. Vaseline or lip balms should be limited to occasional use. Wiping away the loose keratin each morning after a shower is important, followed by a twice daily application of topical tacrolimus 0.1% for 6 weeks initially [4–6]. This can be continued as needed to control inflammation, but should be avoided if exposure to direct sunlight is likely during the day. Maintenance twice weekly is

essential. Treating infection in the nose and mouth with antibiotics and antifungals is important. Antiseptic mouthwashes should also be used daily. Finally, and most importantly, a psychological assessment is recommended in those with mental health problems [7]. Without this combined approach, treatment is unlikely to be successful.

Foreign body cheilitis

Injectable fillers used in cosmetic procedures are listed in Table 108.14. Hylauronic acid is the most frequently used, has a low side-effect profile and is dissolvable. These are temporary fillers lasting for 6 months, although some may have an effect for 2–3 years. Synthetic injectable materials are permanent and are now rarely used. They have been associated with a higher risk of complications.

Early complications of fillers may include oedema, erythema, paraesthesia, pain, bruising and haematoma [1]. Later complications include temporary lumps caused by volume effect, infection or a foreign body reaction [2–8]. Rarely, more serious complications have been described, such as delayed-onset nodules and vascular occlusion with resulting tissue necrosis [9].

MRI shows signs of intense inflammatory reactions in the affected areas. Histology reveals foreign body granulomas with multinucleated giant cells. The foreign material can be identified on histological examination.

Treatment of complications from hyaluronic acid fillers includes hyaluronidase to dissolve the filler and antibiotics for infection. Synthetic fillers are non-reversible; intralesional corticosteroid may be used for inflammatory reactions, use of a needle to break up clumps of material or surgical intervention.

Glandular cheilitis

Glandular cheilitis is characterised by inflammatory changes and swelling of salivary glands in the lips [1–4]. It is a clinical diagnosis based on the clinical finding of a swollen lip with dilated salivary gland ostia exuding a mucous substance and forms part of the spectrum of OFG. It is an uncommon idiopathic condition that in a few cases has apparently been familial. Although it was originally thought that the condition was due to inflammation of enlarged heterotopic salivary glands, the glands are often normal in size, depth and histology [3,4]. Several factors appear to play a role, including atopy, infection and tobacco use. Where swelling is persistent or has a fluctuating acute on chronic course, the diagnosis is now usually grouped into OFG and investigations for an underlying cause may be helpful. This is further discussed in the systemic disease section.

Infective cheilitis

Types of infective cheilitis are as follows:
- *Viral.* Lip infections with HSV are common, and varicella-zoster virus and HPV may also affect the lips. Rare viral infections such as orf [1–4] and vaccinia [5] can affect the lips.
- *Bacterial.* Dental infection or occasionally a furuncle or carbuncle may cause swelling of the lip. Impetigo may mimic herpes labialis (Chapter 25). Cancrum oris (fusospirochaetal infection) may cause labial and buccal necrosis [4].
  - The lip is the most common extragenital site for a primary syphilitic lesion. Most lip chancres in males tend to occur on the upper lip, in females on the lower lip. In secondary syphilis, moist flat papulonodular lesions (condylomata lata) often appear at the mucocutaneous junctions and on mucosal surfaces, especially at the commissures [5]. The tropical treponematoses may present similarly to syphilis.
  - Tuberculosis or leprosy may cause chronic lip swelling or ulceration [6].
  - Rhinoscleroma initially affects the nasal mucosa but may spread slowly to the upper lip, producing plaques or nodules with sunken centres. The extreme hardness of the infiltrations is characteristic. The lip can appear to fuse to the alveolar process, but the overlying skin and mucosa remain normal.
- *Protozoal.* Cutaneous or mucocutaneous leishmaniasis typically causes swellings on the upper lip with later enlargement and destruction of the lip [7], reflecting the three stages of oedema, granulomatous proliferation and then necrosis. Skin scraping or biopsy stained with Giemsa, culture and polymerase chain reaction are useful for diagnosis.
- *Fungal.* Blastomycosis and paracoccidioidomycosis are uncommon causes of chronic ulceration affecting the lip, producing very similar clinical lesions to leishmaniasis [8].
- *Others.* Red swollen lips with fissuring and exfoliation are prominent in mucocutaneous lymph node syndrome (Kawasaki disease).

Plasma cell cheilitis

Plasma cell cheilitis is an idiopathic benign inflammatory condition, presenting with a well-defined, indurated, or eroded erythematous plaque and characterised by dense plasma cell infiltrates in the lips and other mucosae close to body orifices [1,2]. The condition has been reported (under a wide variety of names) to affect the penis, vulva, lips, buccal mucosa, palate, gingiva, tongue, epiglottis and larynx.

Plasma cell cheilitis is the counterpart of Zoon plasma cell balanitis (Chapter 109). It presents as circumscribed flat or elevated patches of erythema, usually on the lower lip in an elderly person. Histology demonstrates a dense, band-like lichenoid infiltrate predominantly composed of mature plasma cells. The cause is unknown and treatment is difficult. It may respond to the

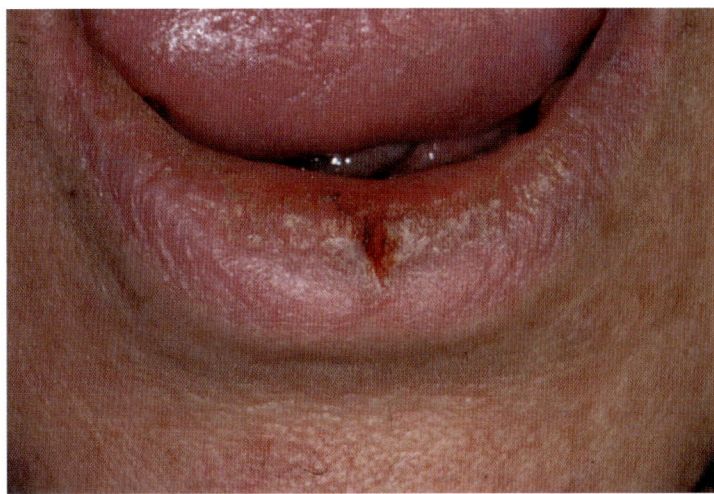

Figure 108.62 Lip fissure.

application of powerful topical corticosteroids such as clobetasol [3], or to the intradermal injection of triamcinolone [4,5], or to topical tacrolimus [6,7].

A similar lesion, which tends to form a tumorous mass with a hyperkeratotic surface and needs to be differentiated from extramedullary plasmacytoma [8], has been called *plasma-acanthoma* [9].

Other lesions of the lip

Calibre-persistent artery

A calibre-persistent artery is defined as an artery with a larger than normal diameter near a mucosal or external surface. When such arteries occur in the gut wall (Dieulafoy malformation) they may bleed, but in the lip they tend to cause chronic ulceration that can be mistaken for a mucocoele or a squamous cancer [1,2]. Intraoral examples have been reported [3]. The ulcer is attributed to continual pulsation from the large artery running parallel to the surface, although the exact mechanism is obscure. Ultrasound may assist diagnosis [4]. Ligation of the artery appears successful.

Lip fissure

A lip fissure may develop when a patient, typically a child, is mouth-breathing (Figure 108.62). Otherwise, the aetiology may be obscure, though sun, wind, cold weather and smoking are thought to predispose. A hereditary predisposition for weakness in the first branchial arch fusion seems to exist. Lip fissures are common in Down syndrome and the lips may also crack in this way if swollen, for example in cheilitis granulomatosa.

Clinical features

Most lip fissures are seen in males, typically median in the lower lip and chronic, causing discomfort and possibly bleeding from time to time [1]. Contrary to the clinical impression that fissures are seen only in the lower lip, there is also a high prevalence in the upper lip.

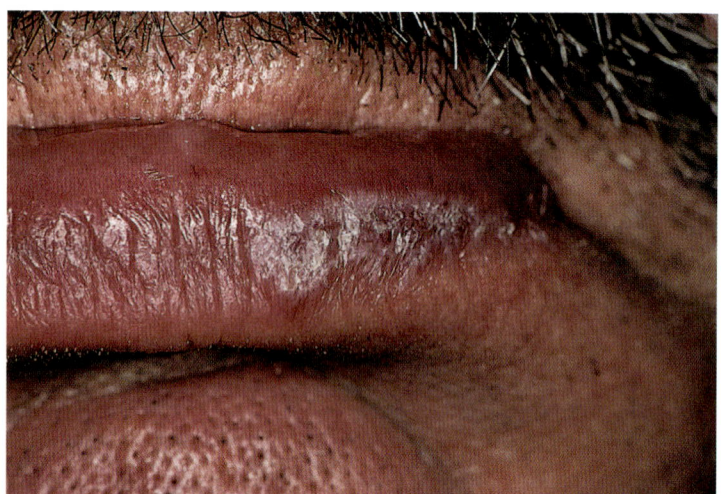

Figure 108.63 Discoid lupus erythematosus of the lower lip.

Diagnosis

The diagnosis is clinical.

Management

Predisposing factors should be managed. Bland creams may help the lesion heal spontaneously. Otherwise, local applications of 1–2% silver nitrate, 0.5% Balsam of Peru, salicylic acid and topical antimicrobials seem less effective than excision, preferably with a Z-plasty, cryosurgery [2] or carbon dioxide laser [3].

Lupus erythematosus (Chapter 51)

Involvement of the vermilion zone is quite common in both discoid erythematosus and systemic lupus erythematosus [1–4]. The cheilitis of systemic lupus erythematosus tends to be more severe, with erosions and haemorrhagic crusts. Lupus erythematosus can be very difficult to distinguish from lichen planus of the lips, both clinically and by histology (Figure 108.63). Discoid lupus can be premalignant [5–8] and should be treated with topical steroid ointments and sunscreens. Microinvasive squamous carcinoma arising in DLE lesions have been successfully treated with imiquimod 5% cream [9].

Reactive perforating collagenosis (Chapter 94)

Crateriform papules of the lower lip have been reported in reactive perforating collagenosis [1].

Sarcoidosis (Chapter 96)

Sarcoidosis may cause chronic violaceous lesions on, or swelling of, or in, the lips. See later in this chapter.

FACIAL PAIN SYNDROMES

Most oral pain is of local aetiology, usually resulting from odontogenic infections. Neurological, vascular and referred causes are less common, but must also be excluded.

Chronic oral soreness may be caused by ulceration, or by mucosal lesions in geographic tongue, lichen planus or deficiency states. Geographic tongue and burning mouth syndrome are common causes of a sore tongue. Lichen planus is the most common cause of chronic soreness in the buccal mucosae. Desquamative gingivitis is the common cause of persistently sore gingivae.

Burning mouth syndrome

Burning mouth syndrome (BMS), also known as oral dysaesthesia, is the term used when symptoms, usually described as a burning sensation, exist in the absence of clinically identifiable oral mucosal disease and when a medical or dental cause has been excluded. The International Headache Society defines BMS as an 'intra-oral burning or dysaesthetic sensation, recurring daily for more than 2 hours per day over more than 3 months, without clinically evident causative lesions'. A burning sensation may have defined causes. Haematinic deficiency states, erythema migrans (geographic tongue), ulcers, mucositis, lichen planus and candidiasis can cause oral soreness or burning sensation.

Epidemiology

BMS is seen especially in middle-aged or older patients. It is most frequent in postmenopausal women, with a general population prevalence of around 1% [1–3]. BMS is seen in women in a ratio of about 10:1.

Pathophysiology

Idiopathic BMS is considered 'primary' BMS, whereas 'secondary' BMS has an identifiable cause. Defined clinical conditions that must be excluded, since they can also present with a burning sensation, are shown in Box 108.9. There is consistent evidence for neuropathic alterations in primary BMS. Damage to peripheral small nerve fibres can produce a burning sensation and may result from deficiency, endocrine disorders, viral infection and Sjögren's

---

Box 108.9 Causes of burning mouth

Local
- Candidiasis
- Geographic tongue
- Lichen planus
- Oral submucous fibrosis
- Denture-induced allergy
- Ill-fitting dentures
- Parafunctional habits, e.g. tongue thrusting

Systemic
- Deficiency states
  - Pernicious anaemia and other vitamin B deficiencies
  - Folate deficiency
  - Iron deficiency
  - Zinc deficiency
- Diabetes
- Sjögren's syndrome
- Drugs (captopril, proton pump inhibitors, protease inhibitors)

syndrome [4]. Tongue biopsies have shown a lower density of small fibres in symptomatic areas suggesting damage of peripheral small fibres as a possible cause [5]. Nerve growth factor (NGF) peptide and tryptase activity appear significantly and persistently raised in saliva in BMS. It can also follow damage to the cauda tympani nerve [6].

In Parkinson disease, 40% of patients report burning mouth. The reduction in dopamine in the nigrostriatal neurons and the putamen in primary BMS patients found by positron emission tomography (PET) studies is similar to PET findings in early Parkinson disease [7].

The predisposition of BMS in peri-/postmenopausal females has suggested dysfunction of the hypothalamus–pituitary–gonadal (HPG) axis may play a role [8]. There is a high prevalence of psychiatric symptoms and/or disorders in BMS: anxiety, depression, somatisation, cancer phobia and insomnia are the most common diagnoses seen in this patient group [9,10].

Pathology

Burning mouth with a tongue of normal clinical appearance may be seen in deficiency states, drugs (e.g. angiotensin-converting enzyme inhibitors such as captopril, enalapril, lisinopril; protease inhibitors; cytotoxic agents; clonazepam) and diabetes. Uncommon causes that may need to be considered include hypothyroidism, lupus erythematosus, hypersensitivity (to sodium metabisulphite, nuts, dental materials and other substances) and galvanic reactions to metals in the mouth.

Clinical features

BMS most frequently affects the tongue, especially its tip and anterior two-thirds, but it can also affect the anterior palate or, less commonly, the lips or gingivae. Usually, symptoms are bilateral and symmetrical. Symptoms of BMS vary between occurring mildly with occasional symptom-free days, to unremitting constant burning. The pain tends to be worse as the day progresses. Dry mouth and dysgeusia (altered taste perception) are also frequently described, e.g. metallic or sour taste. Frequent comorbid conditions include depression and anxiety, chronic fatigue and gastrointestinal symptoms.

The symptoms are variable and may be.
- Moderately severe.
- Relieved by eating and drinking, in contrast to pain caused by organic lesions, which is typically aggravated by eating.
- Persistent though fluctuating in severity, but does not disturb sleep.
- Prolonged.

Investigations

BMS is the diagnosis when all organic causes have been excluded, investigations are all negative, and examination shows no clinically detectable signs of mucosal disease. Investigations indicated may include psychological screening using, for example, the hospital anxiety and depression scale (HADS). Hyposalivation should be excluded as this may predispose to candidiasis. Laboratory screening for anaemia, diabetes, a deficiency state or hypothyroidism should be undertaken.

Management

Few patients with BMS have spontaneous remission in the short term and thus an attempt at treatment is indicated [11–14]. Patient information is an important aspect in management and often reassurance is very helpful in alleviating anxiety from the outset. Active dental or oral surgical treatment, or attempts at 'hormone replacement', in the absence of any specific indication, should be avoided. Attention to factors such as haematinic deficiencies may occasionally be indicated [15,16]. Patients should avoid anything that aggravates symptoms. Cognitive behavioural therapy or a specialist referral may be indicated [17]. Some patients respond to medication:
- Topical medication: benzydamine rinse or spray [18]; capsaicin cream 0.025% (Zacin) or a clonazepam tablet 0.5 mg sucked for 2 minutes before discarding [19,20].
- Mouth wetting agents (for BMS patients with hyposalivation).
- α-lipoic acid systemically [21].
- Hormone replacement therapy (HRT).
- Anti-depressants in low doses [22–24].
  However, treatment is rarely completely successful [25].

Persistent idiopathic facial pain

Persistent idiopathic facial pain (PIFP) is described as a persistent facial and/or oral pain, with varying presentations but recurring daily for more than 2 hours per day over more than 3 months, in the absence of clinical neurological deficit. The pain cannot be attributed to any pathological process [1]. The diagnosis is difficult to make since it is reached only by the exclusion of organic disease. The current theory is that PIFP is a disproportionate reaction to a mild injury, but the exact pathophysiology is still unknown. There are often recent adverse life events, such as bereavement or family illness and/or dental or oral interventional procedures.

Epidemiology

PIFP is rare but may account for up to 20% of the patient population in orofacial pain clinics. Mean age of onset is in the mid-40s. Most patients are female.

Pathophysiology

PIFP is considered a neuropathic pain syndrome. Studies show increased neuronal excitability at the brainstem level, disturbed inhibitory function of the prefrontal cortex, and alterations in the dopamine systems associated with pain transmission and modulation [2–4]. Psychiatric and psychosocial disability have often been associated with PIFP, in particular anxiety and depression [5,6].

Clinical features

Onset is often associated with minor surgical or other invasive dental procedures [7]. The location of the pain is unrelated to the anatomical distribution of trigeminal nerve innervation, poorly localised, and sometimes crosses the midline to involve the other side or moves to another site [4]. It may be bilateral in up to 40% [8]. The pain is long-lasting (years) and often of a deep, dull, boring or burning type, persisting for much or all of the day, but does not wake the patient from sleep. There are few, if any, periods of remission. Objective signs are lacking. Investigations are normal. Response to treatment is poor.

Diagnosis

Making this diagnosis is not simple and follows a process of elimination of other potential causes of orofacial pain. Examination of at least the mouth, perioral structures and cranial nerves, and imaging (tooth/jaw/sinus/skull radiography, MRI/CT scan with particular attention to the skull base) to exclude organic disease are important. PIFP is a clinical diagnosis, only made after careful dental and otolaryngological evaluation, and other tests that rule out organic causes.

Management

A multidisciplinary approach is needed for the management of PIFP. Patient education on the condition is a very important aspect in management. Considering the chronicity and distress that result, behavioural interventions such as cognitive behavioural therapy may be indicated. Pharmacological treatment with antidepressants, antiepileptic or other drugs can also be tried. Amitriptyline is the primary choice starting at 10 mg at night, given as tablets or solution, increasing if needed by 10 mg each week to 50 mg [9]. Trials on duloxetine, venlafaxine and anticonvulsants have shown beneficial effects [10–13] High frequency repetitive transcranial magnetic stimulation (rTMS) is a promising new therapy in patients with neuropathic orofacial pain [14].

Post-herpetic neuralgia

Herpes zoster (shingles) is often preceded and accompanied by neuralgia. Neuralgia may also persist after the rash has resolved. Pain in the trigeminal region may follow an attack of zoster, especially in older patients. In half those patients the pain resolves within 2 months. Post-herpetic neuralgia is defined by the International Headache Society as pain developing during the acute phase of herpes zoster and persisting for more than 6 months thereafter. However, spontaneous improvement may follow after about 18–36 months in some patients.

Post-herpetic neuralgia causes continuous burning pain. Treatment is difficult, but there may be relief using gabapentin, antidepressants (amitriptyline), carbamazepine, topical capsaicin 0.025% or lidocaine, and transcutaneous electrical nerve stimulation [1–3].

Trigeminal neuralgia

Trigeminal neuralgia (TN) is a disorder of the trigeminal nerve that consists of episodes of unilateral intense, stabbing, electric shock-like pain that is abrupt in onset and termination in the areas of the face supplied by one or more divisions of the trigeminal nerve [1]. TN is not fatal, but it is universally considered to be one of the most painful afflictions known. TN may occur in tumours

of the trigeminal nerve (e.g. neuroma), with lesions affecting the trigeminal nerve at the cerebellopontine angle and in disseminated sclerosis or cerebral neoplasms, and these cases are termed secondary or symptomatic TN (STN), when there may be detectable physical signs – initially a reduced corneal reflex, progressing to trigeminal sensory loss. TN, however, much more frequently has no *clinically obvious* neurological cause (termed classic TN (CTN) or tic doloureux) and is then usually ascribed to pressure on the trigeminal nerve from an adjacent but atherosclerotic artery.

Epidemiology

CTN is uncommon; probably about four cases per 100 000 population [2,3]. The average age of onset is 53 years in CTN and 43 years in STN. It is slightly more common in women. There is no known geographic incidence.

Pathophysiology

CTN is caused by demyelination of primary sensory trigeminal afferents in the root entry zone. Demyelination results in neuronal discharge. In a significant proportion of patients, demyelination is caused by a neurovascular conflict (typically the superior cerebellar artery) resulting in morphological changes of the trigeminal nerve such as distortion, dislocation, distension and indentation.

Clinical features

In both CTN and STN, the pain is unilateral and follows the sensory distribution of cranial nerve V, typically radiating to the maxillary (V2) or mandibular (V3) area. TN has the following characteristics:

- Pain restricted to one or more divisions of the trigeminal nerve.
- Bilateral TN is very rare in CTN, and should raise suspicion of STN.
- Abrupt in onset and typically lasts only a few seconds (2 minutes at maximum).
- Pain may arise spontaneously but can be triggered by innocuous mechanical stimuli or movements such as eating, talking, washing the face, shaving or cleaning the teeth.
- Electric shock-like, shooting, stabbing or sharp in quality.
- No clinically evident neurological deficit.
- Usually entirely asymptomatic between paroxysms.
- There is no neurological deficit in CTN.
- TN patients may have autonomic symptoms.

Diagnosis

The diagnosis of TN is primarily based on patient history, as there is no definitive diagnostic test. Examination should include careful neurological assessment, especially of the cranial nerves – particularly the trigeminal nerve and those closely related to the trigeminal (i.e. cranial nerves VI, VII and VIII). Patients with CTN should have a completely unremarkable neurological examination. MRI of the brain should be undertaken early in the work-up to exclude tumours or multiple sclerosis.

Management

Patient information is an important aspect in management. Patients are best seen at an early stage by a specialist in order to confirm the diagnosis and initiate treatment [4].

Medical treatment. Successful for over 80% of patients. Carbamazepine or oxcarbazepine (better tolerability) are recommended as first-line treatments. Carbamazepine prevents attacks of neuralgia in 60% of patients [6–8]. Most patients respond to 200–400 mg carbamazepine three times daily. Combination treatment of carbamazepine with lamotrigine, pregabalin, gabapentin or baclofen may provide relief. These agents may also be used as monotherapy. Long-acting local analgesic injections as peripheral blocks (e.g. mepivacaine) may be of additional value. If these regimens fail to control TN, a neurosurgical opinion is necessary.

Neurosurgical treatment. Gasserian ganglion percutaneous techniques, gamma knife surgery and microvascular decompression [9] are the most promising options. Peripheral surgery involves deliberately interrupting nerve conduction in a division or branch of the trigeminal nerve and include: injections of long-acting analgesics such as ropivacaine, or alcohol or glycerol, local cryosurgery, chemical peripheral neurectomy or radiofrequency thermocoagulation. In medically refractory patients, with a neurovascular conflict, microvascular decompression is the first-choice treatment.

Trigeminal trophic syndrome

This is a rare dysaesthesia that follows damage to the trigeminal nerve [1–3]. The commonest causes are injuries or procedures such as trigeminal rhizotomy or injection of alcohol to the Gasserian ganglion for TN. While most frequently affecting the ala nasi, it can occasionally lead to oral lesions.

ORAL MANIFESTATIONS OF SYSTEMIC DISEASES

Acanthosis nigricans

Oral lesions may be a feature of familial [1] and malignant [2,3] acanthosis nigricans (AN). Malignant AN is most often associated with gastric adenocarcinoma. Between 30% and 50% of patients with malignant AN have oral lesions, which involve the tongue and lips predominantly as extensive papillomatous areas of normal mucosal colour and soft consistency. In malignant AN, successful treatment of the underlying cancer results in improvement of cutaneous or oral signs.

IgG4 disease

IgG4-related disease is a rare systemic fibroinflammatory disorder that was first described in 2003, and includes disorders formerly regarded as different entities such as Mikulicz disease, Küttner's tumour, Riedel thyroiditis and Ormond disease [1]. It is frequently associated with salivary gland swelling and xerostomia. It is characterised by high serum IgG4 levels and multiorgan inflammation that may target the salivary and lacrimal glands, periorbital structures, the pituitary gland, thyroid, pancreas, biliary tract, lungs, prostate gland and retroperitoneal cavity [2]. The classification criteria proposed by Umehara et al. in 2012 are based on the bioptic presence of IgG4$^+$ cells and high serum IgG4 level [3]. There are reports of mucosal manifestations of IgG4 related disease in the oral cavity. Most of these lesions have occurred on the mucosa of the gingiva, the alveolar mucosa, hard palate and floor of the mouth. Lesions characteristically show thickening and fibrosis of the tissues, nodules or ulcers [4].

Sarcoidosis

Head and neck manifestations can be seen in localised and systemic forms of sarcoidosis. Oral lesions are uncommon and may present as well-circumscribed brown-red papules, submucosal nodules, ulceration, gingival lesions, or facial or labial swelling [1–6]. Salivary gland involvement presents as painless swelling or salivary hypofunction. The buccal mucosa is the most frequently involved site, followed by gingiva, lips, tongue and palate. Intraosseous lesions are rare [7,8]. Oral involvement has been described in 33–58% of sarcoidosis cases and can be the first or only sign of systemic disease.

Histology demonstrates non-necrotising granulomatous inflammation. The granulomas may contain concentric calcifications (Schaumann bodies).

Stimulation or replacement of saliva may help in cases of salivary hypofunction. Surgery may be useful for single nodular lesions. Systemic treatments include corticosteroids, hydroxychloroquine, methotrexate and minocycline. Hydroxychloroquine is especially useful in the treatment of cutaneous and mucosal sarcoidosis. It is important to exclude systemic sarcoidosis in patients with isolated lesions involving the oral cavity.

RHEUMATOLOGICAL DISEASES

Rheumatological disorders relevant to the oral mucosa include dermatomyositis and other inflammatory myopathies, the vasculitides including lupus erythematosus, inflammatory arthritides, Sjögren's syndrome, Behçet syndrome and systemic sclerosis (Table 108.15). Oral lesions among these conditions are widely variable and include erythema, erosions, ulcers, sclerotic changes, xerostomia and dysaesthesia [1].

Dermatomyositis (Chapter 52)

Dermatomyositis and mixed connective tissue disease may be associated with non-specific mucosal erosions [1,2]. However, oral lesions in dermatomyositis are not infrequently reported to occur in 10–20% patients. The most frequently reported findings include mucosal oedema, erythema and telangiectasias. White plaques, vesicles, erosions and ulcers have also been noted. Among idiopathic

Table 108.15 Main oral features for rheumatological conditions.

Disease	Main oral features
Rheumatoid arthritis/juvenile chronic arthritis	Sjögren's syndrome
	Temporomandibular joint involvement (pain, crepitus, trismus, locking)
	Lichenoid lesions (e.g. drug-induced)
	Oral ulceration (e.g. secondary to anaemia)
	Amyloid deposits (rarely)
Systemic lupus erythematosus	Sjögren's syndrome
	Oral aphthous-like ulcers
	Oral mucosal white/red patches
	Lichenoid lesions (e.g. drug-induced)
	Trigeminal neuralgia or neuropathy
	Periodontitis
Discoid lupus erythematosus	Lichenoid lesions
	Characteristic chronic erosions/ulcers with sunray/brush border
Sjögren's syndrome	Xerostomia
	Candidiasis
	Salivary gland enlargement secondary to:
	Inflammation of the gland
	Acute suppurative sialadenitis
	Mucosa-associated lymphoid tissue (MALT) lymphoma
Systemic sclerosis	Sjögren's syndrome
	Microstomia
	Trismus
	Telangiectasia
	Widening of the periodontal space
	Trigeminal neuropathy
	Dysphagia
Immune-mediated myopathies including dermatomyositis	Erythema, oedema and telangiectasia
	Dysphagia
Behçet syndrome	Oral aphthous-like ulcers
Giant cell arthritis	Jaw claudication
Granulomatosis with polyangiitis	Strawberry-like gingivitis

inflammatory myopathies, additional oral associations included dysgeusia, dysphagia, burning mouth and xerostomia [3,4].

Inflammatory arthritides

Fibrosis or scarring of oral tissues

Fibrosis of oral tissues leads to restricted oral opening, and with loss of sulcal depth, difficulty in maintaining adequate oral hygiene. While the mouth in health heals rapidly, with chronic or severe inflammation scarring may occur. This may follow burns or irradiation. It may also be associated with habits such as the chewing of betel nut (*Areca*) (see earlier in this chapter), which predisposes to oral submucous fibrosis and may be caused by the connective tissue disorder, scleroderma. Rarely, it is occupational (polyvinylchloride workers). The autoimmune blistering disorders, mucous membrane pemphigoid and epidermolysis bullosa acquisita (see later) may result in scarring. Inherited dystrophic epidermolysis bullosa results in prominent scarring and microstomia. Additionally, subtypes of severe oral or mucocutaneous lichen planus, e.g. the vulvo-vaginal-gingival (VVG) variant may also lead to scarring.

Reactive arthritis (Reiter's syndrome)

Oral involvement in reactive arthritis is common (9–40%) and is often painless. Lesions may include red patches or superficial painless mucosal erosions that may resemble benign migratory glossitis (geographic tongue) both clinically and histologically [1]. Erosions or ulcers may also be present.

Rheumatoid arthritis

Rheumatoid arthritis (RA) is associated with increased periodontitis as well as potentially affecting the temporomandibular joint (TMJ). Similarly, juvenile chronic arthritis may also affect the TMJ. Both disorders may be associated with oral manifestations of immunosuppression including increased candidiasis. RA may also be associated with secondary Sjögren's syndrome and xerostomia (Table 108.15) [1].

It is now thought that RA is due to a combination of environmental factors such as smoking and microbiota, on a predisposed genetic background [2]. A number of observations support an association between periodontitis and RA [3]. These include a higher prevalence of periodontitis than controls. Both are chronic inflammatory conditions that share the overexpression of pro-inflammatory cytokines such as interleukin (IL)-1β, TNF-α, IL-6 and IL-8. *Porphyromonas gingivalis* (a component of the oral microbiota that is frequently associated with periodontitis) may promote aberrant citrullination (i.e. conversion of arginine to citrulline) via peptidyl arginine deiminase type IV, and eventually elicit the appearance of ACPAs [4]. Furthermore, the non-surgical treatment of periodontal disease is accompanied by a reduction in the severity of RA and periodontitis seems to negatively affect the response to RA treatment with biological agents such as TNF blockers.

Scleroderma (Chapter 54)

Oral features are common in systemic sclerosis (SSc) and are generally more obvious in those with diffuse rather than localised scleroderma. Rarely, however, the variant of localised scleroderma (en coup de Sabre) may involve the lip or intraoral soft and hard tissues.

Microstomia, which limits mouth opening in 70% of SSc patients, is the most frequent oral finding and is due to fibrosis of perioral soft tissue [1,2]. Decreased oral opening is correlated to oesophageal involvement. Subcutaneous collagen deposition in facial skin gives the face a characteristic smooth, mask-like appearance, and may be associated with perioral, labial or tongue telangiectasias. About 70% of patients have hyposalivation, most commonly in anticentromere antibody-positive cutaneous limited forms of SSc, and there is an increase in both caries and periodontal disease [2–4].

A characteristic finding is an increased width of the periodontal ligament space in all teeth on radiography, found in about 40% of SSc patients. It can be caused by a reduced number of periodontal capillaries, together with reduced levels of VEGF, as well as by increased collagen deposition, and may explain the high prevalence of tooth loss in SSc patients. There are mandibular erosions in the angle particularly, but also in the condyle, coronoid or digastric regions. Calcifications within the periodontal ligament space and pulp calcifications have been reported. Telangiectasia may be seen. The dropped head sign and tongue atrophy are rare manifestations in SSc associated myopathy. SSc patients are at increased risk of developing cancer, especially of the lung, oral cavity (particularly the tongue) and pharynx.

A multidisciplinary approach should be adopted to encourage oral hygiene and rehabilitation [5,6]. Specific mouth-opening rehabilitation programmes, connective tissue massage, Kabat's technique, kinesitherapy and home-based exercises may help oral opening. Autologous fat tissue grafting has been successfully used [7,8].

Vasculitides

Behçet disease/syndrome (see Chapter 48)

Giant cell arteritis (Chapter 100)

Giant cell arteritis, or temporal arteritis, is an autoimmune disease affecting the large blood vessels of the scalp, neck and arms. It typically involves the extracranial branches of the carotid artery such as the temporal artery, which may appear tortuous and be tender upon palpation. Inflammation leads to narrowing or ischaemia of the blood vessels that may result in blindness in up to 20%. The disease is commonly associated with polymyalgia rheumatica (40–60%) and is more frequent in white European females (F:M 3:1) over the age of 50. Patients may suffer ischaemic pain during mastication, intermittent claudication of the tongue or, rarely, facial palsy. Ulceration and necrosis of the tongue or occasionally the lip have also been observed [1–3]. Patients reporting jaw claudication should therefore be immediately evaluated by a rheumatologist.

Granulomatosis with polyangiitis

This rare (0.9/million) small- and medium-sized vessel necrotising vasculitis typically presents in 90% of patients with upper respiratory tract involvement. It is characterised by granulomatous sinusitis and if left untreated it may lead to the progressive destruction of maxillary and mandibular bone and nasal cartilage, nasal septum perforation, saddle nose deformity, damage to the walls of the sinus and orbit, and fistula formation. Additionally, it may have life-threatening complications such as lung and renal involvement.

The strawberry-like gingival lesions present with reddened, swollen and somewhat granular tissue that is often covered with petechiae and small punctate lesions. It is an almost pathognomonic clinical sign. Other oral manifestations include mucosal ulceration with non-specific histology findings, and lingual necrosis, which has also been reported as a rare presenting sign [1–6].

Lupus erythematosus (see Chapter 51)

Polyarteritis nodosa

Transient submucosal oral nodules may occur singly or in crops along the path of vessels and especially in the tongue. Other mucosal lesions include erythema, papules, haemorrhages, ulceration or necrosis [1].

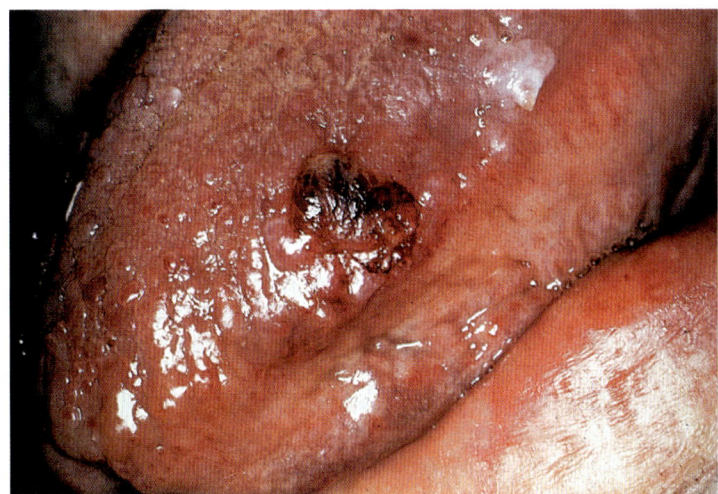

Figure 108.64 Macroglossia and oral petechiae in amyloidosis.

HAEMATOLOGICAL DISEASES

Amyloidosis

In primary amyloidosis the tongue is enlarged and firm or hard. There may also be yellowish submucosal nodules, lumps or petechiae (Figure 108.64). Rarely, there are similar deposits elsewhere (e.g. in the soft palate), and jaw claudication, salivary gland swelling or hyposalivation [1–10] and sometimes burning sensations.

Amyloidosis results from the abnormal folding of proteins forming insoluble amyloid fibrils with subsequent accumulation in various tissues and organs. It is classified as localised amyloidosis, acquired systemic amyloidosis, reactive systemic AA amyloidosis and hereditary systemic amyloidosis based on the specific protein deposited. Localised amyloidosis is the most common and results in the deposition of AL protein in an organ or tissue. Both localised and systemic amyloidosis may present with head and neck involvement with the tongue and the larynx being the most frequent sites of amyloid deposition. Amyloid deposition within the tongue manifests as macroglossia and results in restriction of tongue movement. Scalloping may be noted on the lateral borders of the tongue from impingement on the teeth. Discrete yellow papules and nodules affecting the tongue, palate, buccal and labial mucosa, haemorrhagic bullae, petechiae/ecchymosis (Figure 108.64) and ulceration are recognised presentations [1–10]. Infiltration in the salivary glands may manifest as decreased salivary flow and salivary gland swelling. Jaw claudication can occur in AL amyloidosis.

Secondary amyloidosis rarely involves the mouth except in the case of multiple myeloma or haemodialysis-associated amyloid. Amyloidosis of the tongue should be regarded as a marker of occult underlying plasma cell dyscrasia, in particular myeloma. Investigations should be undertaken focusing on the existence of gammopathies and underlying lymphoid and plasma cell malignancies.

Hereditary systemic amyloidosis is rare and results in the production of amyloid fibrils from inherited variant proteins such as transthyretin, gelsolin and apolipoprotein A-1 and fibrinogen. Hereditary gelsolin amyloidosis, a rare dominantly inherited systemic disease caused by a c.654G>A or c.654G>T gelsolin gene mutation, may cause oral dryness and cranial polyneuropathy.

A biopsy usually confirms the diagnosis. On light microscopy, amyloidosis appears as an eosinophilic amorphous substance, which on Congo red staining demonstrates green birefringence under polarised light [11].

Solitary intraoral amyloid is rare. Localised forms have an excellent prognosis and are not at increased risk of developing systemic involvement [12]. There is no cure for amyloidosis with current treatments focusing on the slowing amyloid accumulation and any subsequent organ dysfunction. For localised amyloidosis, therapeutic options include observation, surgery if functional or cosmetic disability is present, laser therapy, corticosteroids, radiotherapy and chemotherapy. Excision is usually curative in cases of localised amyloidosis in the head and neck. However, recurrence can occur.

Deficiency states

Low iron, folate or vitamin B12 levels may predispose to mouth ulcers. A few of these patients also have anaemia, sometimes with other oral features such as glossitis or angular stomatitis, but many have a deficiency state with no established anaemia [1]. Occasionally, patients with deficiency of B vitamins may develop other types of oral ulcer and sometimes epithelial dysplasia.

Extranodal NK/T-cell lymphoma, nasal type

Extranodal NK/T-cell lymphoma, nasal type (ENKTCL-NT) is a rare type of lymphoma that commonly involves the nasal cavity, oral cavity and/or pharynx but less commonly can also involve the eye, larynx, lung, gastrointestinal tract, skin and various other tissues. Patients presenting with highly localised midline facial disease fit the historical definition of lethal midline granuloma. These cases, unlike other cases of ENKTCL-NT with more widespread disease, often show no or relatively little progression of their disease over long periods of time [1].

Gamma heavy chain disease (Franklin disease)

This disease is characterised by an excessive production of heavy chains that are short and truncated. It is presumed to arise from a somatic mutation. It is associated with paraproteinaemia. Palatal oedema and oral ulceration have been described in a few patients with heavy-chain disease, but the former feature is not as invariable as initially described [1].

Graft-versus-host disease (see earlier in this chapter)

GVHD may follow as a complication of bone marrow transplantation. Oral lesions are usually lichenoid, often associated with hyperkeratotic plaques, mucosal ulceration and salivary gland dysfunction. Oral lesions can resemble reticular, atrophic, erosive and plaque-like oral lichen planus [1–3]. Palatal involvement is more frequent in GVHD than oral lichen planus. Regular monitoring of the oral mucosa is essential because patients are at increased risk of SCC of the oral cavity.

Granulocytic sarcoma (myeloid sarcoma)

Granulocytic sarcoma is a rare extramedullary tumour of immature granulocytic cells. It arises in myeloproliferative disorders especially in chronic myeloid leukemia and myelodysplastic syndromes. Granulocytic sarcomas are rare in the oral cavity. Most present with swelling or symptoms related to skeletal involvement [1,2]. The maxilla is particularly involved.

Hypereosinophilic syndrome

Oral erosions affecting buccal, gingival or labial mucosae may be a feature of the hypereosinophilic syndrome and may herald cardiac involvement [1,2].

Hypoplasminogenaemia

Also known as plasminogen deficiency type 1, this is a genetic disorder characterised by a lack of the protein plasminogen. Gingival swelling and ulceration are features of hypoplasminogenaemia [1].

Idiopathic thrombocytopenic purpura

This may present with oral purpura and/or spontaneous gingival haemorrhage. The differential diagnosis includes coagulation disorders, angina bullosa haemorrhagica, trauma and other causes of thrombocytopenia including bone marrow suppression, HIV, chemotherapy agents, etc. Full blood count and coagulation screen should be undertaken in patients presenting with blood blisters.

Langerhans cell histiocytosis

This condition typically produces lytic bone lesions, but gingival swelling, periodontal destruction with loosening of teeth,

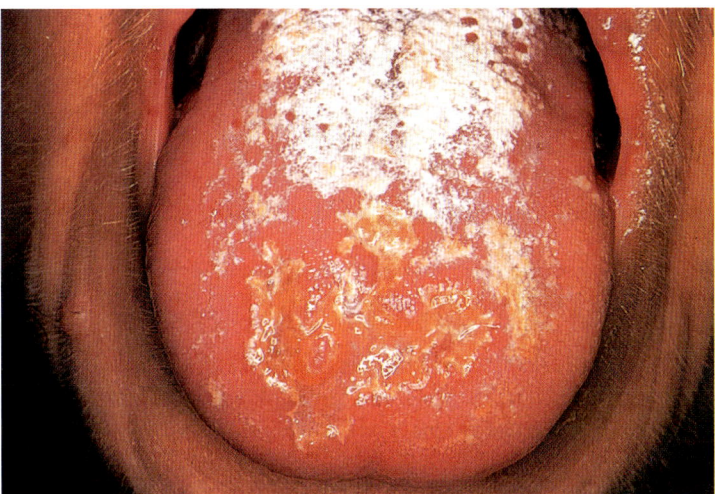

Figure 108.65 Herpes simplex lingual recurrence, and candidiasis in leukaemia: similar lesions may be seen in HIV infection.

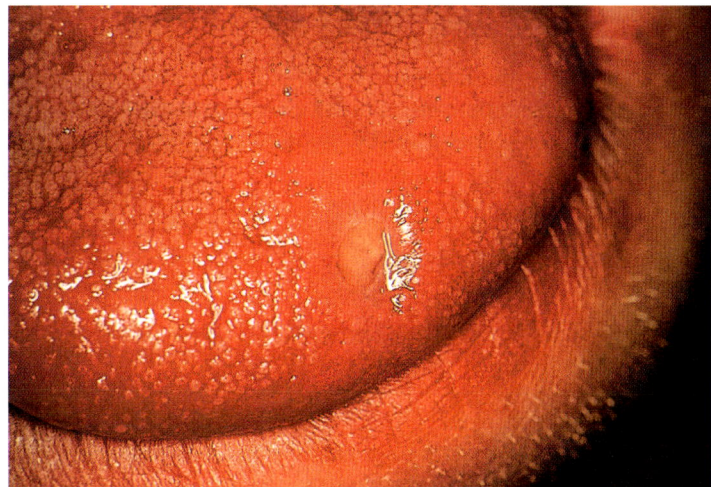

Figure 108.66 Aphthous-like ulceration in HIV disease.

non-healing extraction sockets and mouth ulceration may be seen [1–4]. FDG-PET/CT is useful alongside histology for diagnosis. Surgical treatment has been shown to be very effective in the treatment of localised oral manifestations of Langerhans cell histiocytosis and is usually regarded as being sufficient as a sole treatment, sometimes combined with steroid injections

Leukaemias

Oral ulceration may be a prominent feature, especially in the acute leukaemias. Other oral manifestations of leukaemia include mucosal pallor, gingival haemorrhage, gingival swelling, petechiae and ecchymoses [1,2]. Oral infections with *Candida albicans* and Gram-negative bacteria including *Pseudomonas* spp., *Escherichia coli*, *Proteus*, *Klebsiella* and *Serratia* spp. are common, especially in acute leukaemias, and may act as a portal for septicaemia. Herpes simplex or varicella-zoster virus ulcers are also common (Figure 108.65). Chemotherapy complicates the situation because it too can produce oral ulceration, as can bone marrow transplantation.

Other occasional findings include paraesthesia (particularly of the lower lip), facial palsy, extrusion of teeth or bone, painful swellings over the mandible and parotid swelling (Mikulicz syndrome).

Leukopenias and agranulocytosis

White cell dyscrasias and HIV infection are also often complicated by oral ulceration (Figure 108.66). Oral ulceration may be a major symptom in patients with leukopenias and the first manifestation of drug-induced agranulocytosis. Painful deep irregular ulcers, often with only a minimal inflammatory halo (in contrast to typical aphthous ulcers), involve the mouth and/or pharynx and tend to extend and penetrate slowly. In cyclic neutropenia, ulcers appear episodically at 21-day intervals in association with the neutropenic episodes. Severe periodontitis is often also a feature of leukocyte and

other immune defects and the patients may suffer from recurrent infections elsewhere [1–4]. Methotrexate can cause oral ulceration in the absence of leukopenia.

Lymphomas

Lymphomas make up 2.2% of all malignancies of the head and neck and are the second most frequent in that region surpassed only by epithelial malignancies [1–5]. Non-Hodgkin lymphoma is diagnosed in extranodal sites in 40% of cases, and the head and neck region is the second most affected, with an incidence of 11–33%, while Hodgkin lymphoma has a very low incidence in extranodal sites (1–4%).

Some 2–10% of lymphomas present first in the oral cavity. Of these, 80% are composed of follicular centre cells or post-follicular cells. Lymphomas usually occur on the pharynx or palate, but occasionally on the tongue, gingivae or lips; they may appear as oral swellings, which sometimes ulcerate and may cause pain or sensory disturbance. The manifestations of oral lymphomas are often difficult to diagnose because they present clinical features that mimic other diseases such as periodontal disease, osteomyelitis and other malignancies. This may delay the correct treatment thereby worsening the prognosis. Oral herpes zoster and herpes simplex infections are common in patients with lymphomas.

There is an increased incidence of oral lymphomas in HIV disease [6] including oral plasmablastic lymphomas. AIDS-related lymphomas have a rapid progression, poor response to treatment, high relapse rates and an overall poor prognosis.

Multicentric reticulohistiocytosis

Multicentric reticulohistiocytosis is a very rare multisystem arthropathic form of reticulocytosis [1]. It is a type of non-Langerhans cell histiocytosis characterised by skin and mucosal lesions, and arthritis.

Oral lesions are seen in up to 50% of patients with multicentric reticulohistiocytosis [2]. Lesions are collections of histiocytes that form nodular or granular lesions, particularly in the labial or buccal mucosa. The temporomandibular joint may also be involved as part of the polyarthropathy.

Mycosis fungoides

Oral mycosis fungoides is very rare and has been associated with advanced disease and a poor prognosis. Skin lesions are present for an average of more than 6 years before oral involvement occurs. The clinical appearance is highly variable with tongue, palate and gingiva most often affected. Oral lesions in mycosis fungoides typically are red or white areas on the tongue but may present as ulcers, erythematous plaques or tumours [1].

Myelodysplastic syndromes

Oral manifestations in myelodysplastic syndromes include particularly ulceration but also paraesthesiae, petechiae, burning mouth, gingival swelling, xerostomia and herpes labialis [1].

Myeloma and paraproteinaemias

Multiple myeloma very occasionally presents with an intraoral mass or oral bleeding. Osteolytic bone lesions are more common. Extramedullary plasmacytoma may also be seen; indeed, some 80% of these rare tumours are found in the head and neck region [1–4] but typically occur in the mucosa of the upper respiratory tract, especially in the supraglottic larynx, and only occasionally in the oral cavity. Extramedullary plasmacytoma is characterised by monoclonal restriction in immunoglobulin production identified using serum protein electrophoresis, immunofixation and serum-free light chains.

Patients with myeloma treated with intravenous bisphosphonates are at risk from medication-related osteonecrosis of the jaw (MRONJ).

Pseudolymphoma

Rare tumour-like lymphoproliferative infiltrates that lack the malignant potential of lymphomas may be seen intraorally, notably in the palate [1,2].

Waldenström macroglobulinaemia

Oral manifestations in Waldenström macroglobulinaemia include purpura, ulceration and occasional mental nerve anaesthesia [1–3].

GASTROINTESTINAL DISEASES

Gastrointestinal disorders may be associated with oral lesions and include Crohn disease, ulcerative colitis and coeliac disease. All may be associated with nutritional deficiencies and therefore a propensity to aphthous-like ulceration. However, there are additional oral manifestations that will be discussed below.

Coeliac disease

The two main oral manifestations of coeliac disease are related to nutritional deficiencies. These are recurrent aphthous ulceration and enamel defects in the permanent dentition [1,2].

Crohn disease

Oral lesions in Crohn disease form part of the spectrum of orofacial granulomatosis, though some aspects of the clinical presentation will suggest Crohn disease as the underlying cause. These include linear ulceration in the sulci, mucosal tags, cobblestoned appearance in the buccal mucosa and gingival hyperplasia. Patients with Crohn disease may also have signs of angular cheilitis, candidiasis and perioral erythema. A multidisciplinary approach is required for suspected patients with endoscopy, imaging and faecal calprotectin often indicated. Those with oral lesions tend to present in childhood or later in life. Treatment of the oral manifestations is for the underlying Crohn disease.

Orofacial granulomatosis

Orofacial granulomatosis (OFG) is a term applied to a spectrum of conditions associated with granuloma formation in the oral and perioral tissues [1]. Confusingly some patients may not be found to have clear granulomas on biopsy but are still classified from a management perspective in the same way. Underlying causes include Crohn disease, sarcoidosis, infections, allergy and the distinct Melkersson–Rosenthal syndrome [1]. It is now considered usual practice to try to identify any of the above causes. If an underlying cause such as Crohn disease is identified then 'oral Crohn' would be a more accurate name or 'orofacial sarcoidosis' [2]. For the remainder where the underlying cause is unclear then the term OFG is used. The majority of these cases will present with lip swelling as the main feature. Chronic lip swelling has also been termed granulomatous cheilitis. However, this is clinically and histologically indistinguishable from OFG.

Epidemiology
OFG is an uncommon condition. Onset is usually in children or young adults. There is no gender or geographic predilection.

Predisposing factors
- Dietary factors. There is an association with foods or additives including cinnamic aldehyde, benzoates, butylated hydroxyinosole or dodecyl gallate (in margarine), or menthol (in peppermint oil).

- There is a strong association with atopy.
- In adults, approximately 10% of cases over 10 years from diagnosis have or develop gastrointestinal Crohn disease (oral Crohn). In children, approximately 25% of cases over 10 years from diagnosis have or develop gastrointestinal Crohn disease.
- A small percentage may have sarcoidosis (orofacial sarcoidosis).
- A reaction to antigens (e.g. metals, such as cobalt), paratuberculosis or mycobacterial stress protein mSP65 has been suggested.

Pathophysiology

OFG is likely to represent a heterogeneous group of disease entities, each of which may arise from different combinations of genetic and environmental allergens. A delayed type of hypersensitivity reaction appears to be involved, although the exact antigen inducing the immunological reaction appears to vary in individual patients. The inflammatory response is a Th1-mediated immune response and is associated with non-caseating granulomas in the lamina propria, which appear to cause lymphatic obstruction and lymphoedema, resulting in the clinical swellings (Figure 108.67).

Genetics

The genetic background, any role of allergy and other diverse possible aetiological factors such as *Mycobacterium paratuberculosis* is unclear.

Clinical features

Intermittent acute or chronic swelling of one or both lips is present (Figure 108.67) and may be associated with perioral erythema and swelling of the surrounding skin. With repeated swelling the lips become firmer, developing a rubbery texture. Persistent lymphoedema and granulomatous changes may be associated with a more nodular texture with fissuring and peeling of the epidermis. Eventually the lips develop chronic oedema and angular cheilitis associated with infection, e.g. *Staphylococcus aureus* or *Candida* may be present. Intraorally, patients may have mucosal lesions including thickening and folding of the mucosa to produce a 'cobblestone' type of appearance and mucosal tags. Purple granulomatous enlargements may appear on the gingiva, along with full thickness gingivitis. Ulcers classically involve the buccal sulcus where they appear as linear ulcers, often with granulomatous masses flanking them [1,2].

In the rare Melkersson–Rosenthal syndrome, patients may present with facial palsy, facial swelling and a fissured tongue. Though intermittent at first, the palsy is lower motor neuron type and may become permanent. It may be unilateral or bilateral, and partial or complete. It has been reported in association with other conditions including taste disturbance and systemic diseases such as Crohn disease and sarcoidosis. Spontaneous remission occurs in 25% patients.

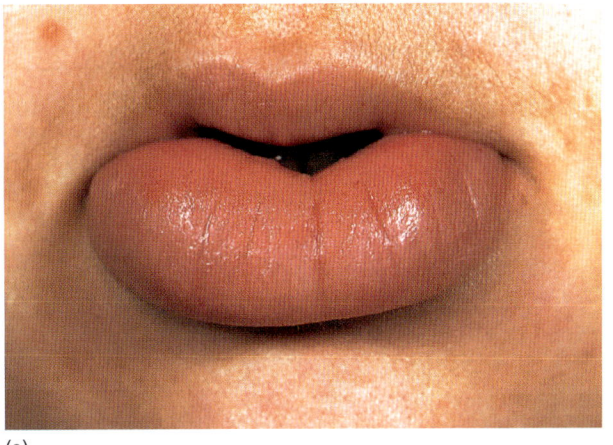

(a)

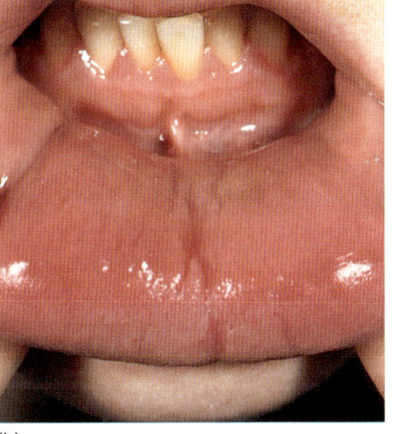

(h)

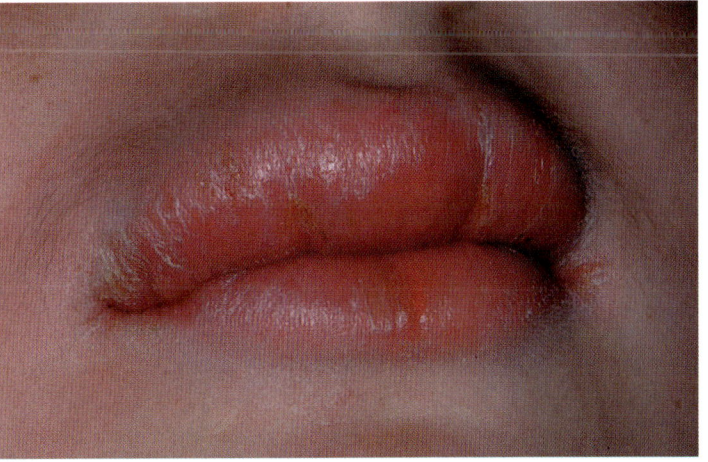

(c)

Figure 108.67 Granulomatous cheilitis may affect one or both lips. (a) Prominent swelling of the lower lip. (b) Midline fissuring is not infrequent and can be a nidus for infection. (c) Swelling of upper lip with secondary infection.

PART 10: SPECIFIC SITES, SEX & AGE

Investigations

The oral history is not specific and investigation of the gastro-intestinal tract is mandatory in patients with gastrointestinal symptoms. Investigations such as chest radiography, serum angiotensin-converting enzyme and a FDG-PET (fluorodeoxyglucose-positron emission tomography) CT scan may be required to exclude sarcoidosis. Patch tests and skin prick tests may be indicated to exclude reactions to various foodstuffs or additives [3]. A biopsy may be undertaken in more chronic cases to identify granulomas, avoiding the lip if possible. Salivary and skin microbiology is helpful to investigate possible *Candida* or *S. aureus* on the lips.

Management

The principal aims of treatment are to reduce lip swelling thereby improving the cosmetic appearance of the condition and reduce ulceration if present. Elimination diets such as a cinnamon and benzoate free diet should be introduced for a 3-month trial period and has been shown to improve 54–78% patients [3,4].

Topical corticosteroids or topical tacrolimus may be helpful for patients in the early stages of the condition or where there is an associated exfoliative cheilitis. Intralesional corticosteroids may be used for more chronic lip swelling and may effectively control the oral lesions [5]. Intralesional corticosteroid injections may also reduce the swelling. The injection of up to 10 mL triamcinolone (10 mg/L) into the lips after local analgesia may be effective. The injections may have to be repeated every 4–6 months once a response plateau has been reached.

Other therapies include short courses of prednisolone, and in patients with underlying Crohn disease treatment with azathioprine, methotrexate, mycophenolate mofetil or anti-TNF-α agents can be helpful. In patients with sarcoidosis, appropriate systemic therapy, e.g. hydroxychloroquine may be beneficial. Cheiloplasty is reserved for severely disfiguring cheilitis and only when the condition is quiescent and is often unsuccessful. Psychological support is important for patients and parents of children with the condition.

Table 108.16 lists potential causes of acute or chronic lip swelling. In early attacks of acute lip swelling, clinical differentiation of angio-oedema may be difficult. Persistence of the swelling between attacks would suggest an alternative diagnosis: sarcoidosis, tuberculosis or OFG/Crohn disease being the main differentials. In established cases, other causes of enlarged lips (Table 108.16) must be excluded. Lymphoma is a rare differential diagnosis. Ascher syndrome, associated with blepharochalasia, rarely causes confusion as the swelling of the lip is caused by redundant salivary tissue and is present from childhood. Cutaneous leishmaniasis and leprosy have also been reported to mimic OFG.

Pyostomatitis vegetans

The oral lesions termed pyostomatitis vegetans are deep fissures, pustules and papillary projections. Most patients have had inflammatory bowel disease, that is ulcerative colitis or Crohn disease [1–3]. The course of these lesions tends to follow that of the associated bowel disease. Although the oral lesions may respond

Table 108.16 Differential diagnoses of acute or chronic enlargement of one or both lips.

Acute	Chronic
Traumatic	Developmental
Infective	Familial
• Bacterial	• Double lip
• *Herpes simplex*	• Ascher syndrome
• Primary syphilis	• Lymphangioma
• Angio-oedema	• Haemangioma
	• Neurofibroma
Erythema multiforme	
	• Mucopolysaccharidoses
Actinic cheilitis (when secondarily infected)	
	Coffin–Siris syndrome
	Acquired
	• Post-traumatic
	• Lymphatic defect
	• Infective
	• Tuberculosis
	• Leprosy
	• Rhinoscleroma
	• Leishmaniasis
	Neoplastic
	Inflammatory
	• Meischer cheilitis (orofacial granulomatosis limited to the lip)
	• Melkersson–Rosenthal syndrome
	• Cheilitis glandularis
	• Sarcoidosis
	• Oral Crohn disease
	• Orofacial granulomatosis

at least partially to topical therapy (e.g. corticosteroids), systemic treatment is often needed.

Ulcerative colitis

Patients with ulcerative colitis may have oral aphthous-like ulcers, haemorrhaghic lesions, pyostomatitis vegetans or pyoderma gangrenosum [1,2].

Other gastrointestinal disease associations with the oral mucosa

Gastro-oesophageal reflux disease may be associated with oropharyngeal burning, erythematous lesions of the oropharyngeal region, hypersalivation, dysgeusia and dental erosion.

Hepatitis associated with jaundice may present with yellow oral mucosal pigmentation, oral mucosal atrophy, lichenoid lesions, hyposalivation and parotid gland swellings.

DERMATOLOGICAL DISEASES

Several conditions presenting to dermatologists may have oral and other mucosal presentations and it is essential that the dermatologist is able to recognise, assess and refer appropriately for multidisciplinary care. Some of these conditions are associated with oral ulcers or erosions while others may present as erythema, white patches or oral pain. The most common mucocutaneous disease is lichen planus which has a spectrum of oral presentations. The immunobullous diseases are less common but are generally more severe and again recognition of the oral features and an understanding of the chronicity of this site with its impact upon management is vital.

Erythema multiforme (Chapter 47)

Erythema multiforme (EM) is an uncommon inflammatory mucosal or mucocutaneous disease often presenting in young adults [1]. It is painful, but self-limiting, although episodes may be recurrent. Lesions may be oral, cutaneous or mucocutaneous with other sites, e.g. conjunctiva affected.

Epidemiology
The oral EM variant is an under-recognised form of EM. The peak age at presentation is between 20 and 40 years, although 20% of cases occur in children. Several reports suggest that males are affected more than females. However, in a large European series, 52% of patients were male and 48% were female, with a mean age of 38 years [2].

Pathophysiology
There may be a genetic predisposition, with associations of recurrent EM with HLA-B15 (B62), HLA-B35, HLA-A33, HLA-DR53 and HLA-DQB1*0301. HLA-DQ3 has been proven to be especially related to recurrent EM and may be a helpful marker for distinguishing this herpes-associated EM from other diseases with EM-like lesions. Patients with extensive mucosal involvement may have the rare HLA allele DQB1*0402.

The reaction is triggered by the following:
- *Infective agents*, particularly HSV (herpes-associated EM), which is implicated in 70% of recurrent EM. Bacteria (*Mycoplasma pneumoniae* and many others), other viruses, fungi or parasites are less commonly implicated [3,4].
- *Drugs* such as sulphonamides (e.g. co-trimoxazole), cephalosporins, aminopenicillins, quinolones, barbiturates, oxicam non-steroidal anti-inflammatory drugs, anticonvulsants, protease inhibitors, allopurinol and many others may trigger severe EM or toxic epidermal necrolysis in particular.
- *Food additives or chemicals* such as benzoates, nitrobenzene, perfumes, terpenes.
- *Immune conditions* such as bacille Calmette–Guérin (BCG) or hepatitis B immunisation, sarcoidosis, GVHD, inflammatory bowel disease, polyarteritis nodosa or systemic lupus erythematosus.

The aetiology of EM is unclear in most patients but appears to be an immunological hypersensitivity reaction with the appearance of cytotoxic effector cells (CD8+ T lymphocytes) in the epithelium, inducing apoptosis of scattered keratinocytes and leading to satellite cell necrosis.

EM has been classified into a number of variants – EM minor affecting one mucosa and EM major affecting two or more mucous membranes [5,6]. In Stevens–Johnson syndrome there is extensive skin involvement, multisite mucositis and an associated mortality rate of 10%.

Clinical features
Most patients with EM (70%), of either minor or major forms, have oral lesions. The oral mucosa may be involved alone or in association with skin lesions. Mucosal lesions begin as erythematous areas that blister and break down to irregular extensive painful erosions with extensive surrounding erythema. The labial mucosa is often involved, and a serosanguinous exudate leads to crusting of the swollen lips [1,5,6].

Mucosal erosions plus typical or raised atypical targets and epidermal detachment, involving less than 10% of the body surface and usually located on the extremities and/or the face, characterise herpes simplex-induced EM major. The gingivae are characteristically spared.

It may be a recurrent condition. In a large European study, the frequency of previous occurrences ranged from 0 to 10 [2].

Diagnosis
A diagnosis of EM can be difficult to establish easily, and there may be a need to differentiate from viral stomatitides, pemphigus, toxic epidermal necrolysis and the subepithelial immune blistering disorders (pemphigoid and others). There are no specific diagnostic tests. The diagnosis is mainly clinical. It may be helpful to undertake serology for *Mycoplasma pneumoniae* or HSV, or other microorganisms. Biopsy of perilesional tissue with immunostaining and histological examination may help to exclude other pathology, particularly PV.

Management
Spontaneous healing can be slow, up to 2–3 weeks in EM minor and up to 6 weeks in EM major. The use of oral corticosteroids is controversial [7]. In a series comprising eight EM major cases and four cases of Stevens–Johnson syndrome, patients were treated with fluocinolone, prednisolone or methylprednisolone in a variety of doses for 5–7 days during the acute illness. Oral assessment revealed a complete remission of buccal lesions in all patients 7–10 days after onset of systemic corticosteroid treatment.
- EM minor may respond to topical corticosteroids, although systemic corticosteroids may still be required and patients report faster healing with treatment.
- EM major should be treated with systemic corticosteroids (prednisolone 0.5–1 mg/kg/day tapered over 7–10 days) and/or azathioprine or other immunomodulatory drugs [7] if recurrences are frequent.
- Levamisole and thalidomide have occasionally been used to some effect. Plasmapheresis possibly has a place in the management of severe disease.
- Antimicrobials may be indicated:
  - Aciclovir in EM related to HSV 400 mg twice daily for 6 months is recommended [7]. Continuous therapy with valaciclovir 500 mg twice a day has also been reported to be effective.
  - Tetracycline is indicated in EM related to *Mycoplasma pneumoniae*.

Oral lichen planus (Chapter 37)

Oral lichen planus (OLP) is a chronic inflammatory condition that can involve the oral mucosa alone or in addition to other sites such as the skin, scalp, nails or genitalia. Less well recognised sites include the external auditory canal or the mucous membranes of the oesophagus, conjunctiva, vagina or urethra. These latter sites may be more frequently encountered in the *vulvovaginal–gingival syndrome*, which has a propensity for scarring with significant morbidity [1]. In the mouth, there is a dysregulation of epithelial turnover resulting in white striae, papules or plaques when there is reduced shedding. With increased shedding there is epithelial atrophy, and lesions are erythematous and often uncomfortable. With further thinning, ulceration may occur in any affected site and is painful.

Epidemiology

The prevalence of OLP has been estimated to be between 0.5% and 2.2% [2,3]. It presents most frequently after the fourth decade. It is twice as common in females and can affect more than one family member [4]. The reported incidence of cutaneous lesions in patients presenting with OLP ranges from 4% to 44% [5].

Pathophysiology

Most OLP is idiopathic. However, there are patients in whom a similar appearance both clinically and histologically may be associated with known triggers. These are termed 'lichenoid lesions' and may be associated with dental restorative materials, e.g. chromate, gold and thiomersal, chronic GVHD or hepatitis C virus (HCV) [6–10].

- *Genetics*: OLP is likely to result through combined genetic, environmental and gene–environment interactions. Genetic studies have focused on the major histocompatibility complex (MHC) region on chromosome 6p. In a phenome wide analysis performed in the USA, with 97 OLP cases and over 7000 population controls, a significant association between OLP and six single nucleotide polymorphisms (SNPs) in the region of HLA-DQB1*05:01 was reported. The VVG subtype of lichen planus has also shown association with the HLA-DQB1*0201 variant through candidate gene analysis, with 80% carriage rates of this allele (28/35) among individuals with vulvo-vaginal gingival lichen planus (VVG-LP) compared with 41.8% of healthy controls (74/177) [1,11,12].

- *Autoimmunity*: OLP demonstrates some features of an autoimmune condition, e.g. it more commonly affects women and has a tendency to cluster with other autoimmune conditions such as autoimmune thyroid disease, Sjögren's syndrome and systemic lupus erythematosus [13]. No autoantibodies have been identified for OLP, though through epitope spreading, low titre bullous pemphigoid antigens are sometimes detected. The antigens that trigger the immune activation of OLP are as yet unknown. However, a number of possible antigenic triggers have been suggested including local and systemic inducers of cell-mediated hypersensitivity, such as infection, drugs or dental materials [14].

- *Drugs*: lichenoid reactions may arise secondary to many classes of drugs, including non-steroidal anti-inflammatory drugs, antihypertensives (particularly ACE inhibitors), oral hypoglycaemics and antimalarials [15,16].

- *Infections*: a number of infectious triggers for OLP have been suggested, including bacterial and viral causes [17]. Proposed viral triggers include varicella-zoster virus, Epstein-Barr virus and cytomegalovirus. Many studies have demonstrated an association between chronic hepatitis C virus (HCV) infection and OLP, particularly in areas with higher prevalence of hepatitis C, such as Japan and the Mediterranean. However, while it is not believed to be a causal association there may be an increased risk of malignant transformation in those with hepatitis C.

- *Dental materials*: lichenoid reactions may be associated with contact allergic reactions to positive patch test reactions to chromate, gold and thiomersal [18]. Unilateral irritant contact reactions may also be observed with direct apposition of soft tissue to dental restorations, particularly amalgam.

Pathology

The pathology is similar to that of cutaneous lichen planus, although sawtooth rete ridges are rarely seen in oral biopsies, and other epithelial changes may be less distinct.

Clinical features

Oral lesions of lichen planus are bilateral and often symmetrical. There are a number of presentations which frequently overlap in any individual. These include reticular, papular or plaque-like lesions most frequently seen on the buccal mucosae or tongue (Figures 108.68–108.72). However, lesions may be atrophic, ulcerative and rarely bullous.

Reticular OLP

The reticular form is the most common oral presentation frequently involving the buccal mucosa, lips, tongue or gingivae. The majority of the patients are asymptomatic though some may complain of roughness or dryness of the affected areas. It presents as a white, linear or lacy pattern known as Wickham's striae (Figure 108.68).

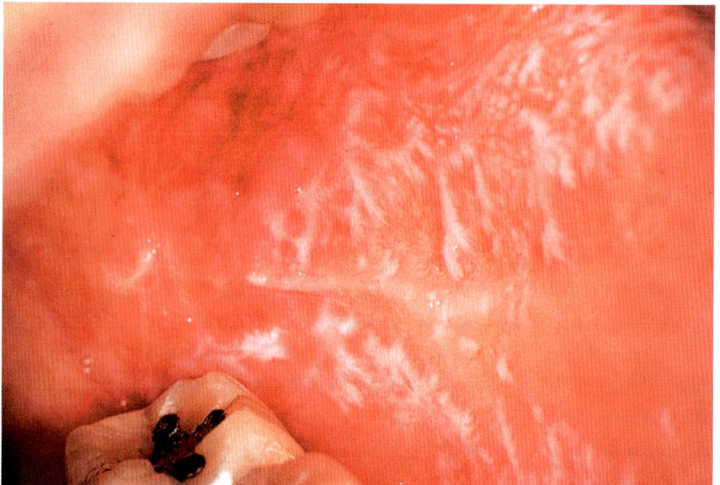

Figure 108.68 Lichen planus: reticulopapular lesions in the common oral site, the buccal mucosa.

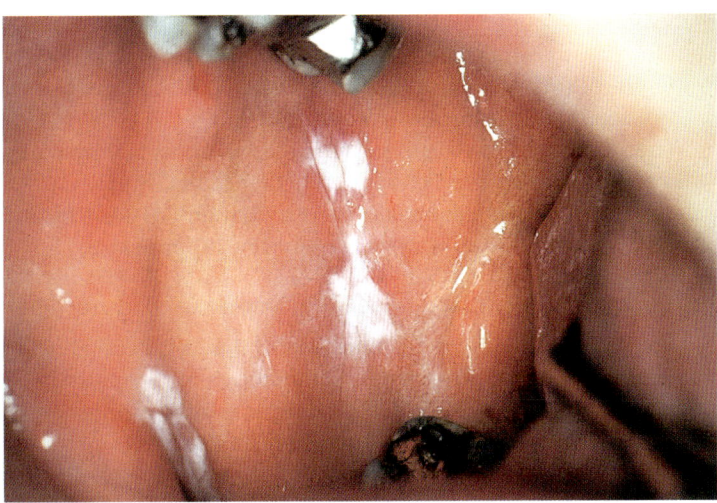

Figure 108.69 Lichen planus: plaque-like lesions resemble leukoplakia.

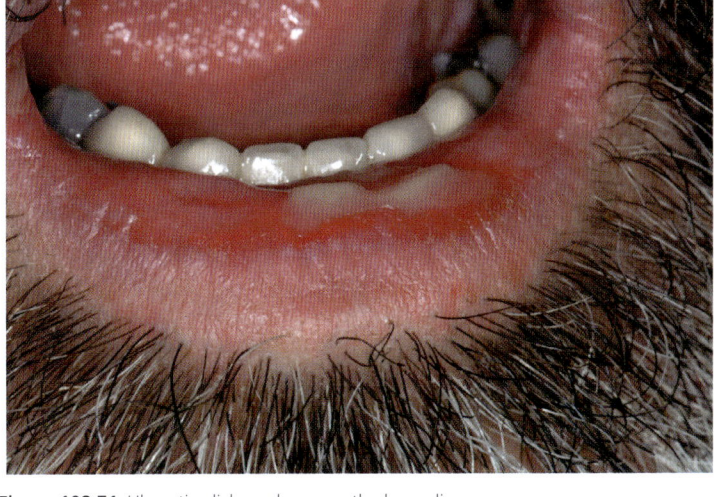

Figure 108.71 Ulcerative lichen planus on the lower lip.

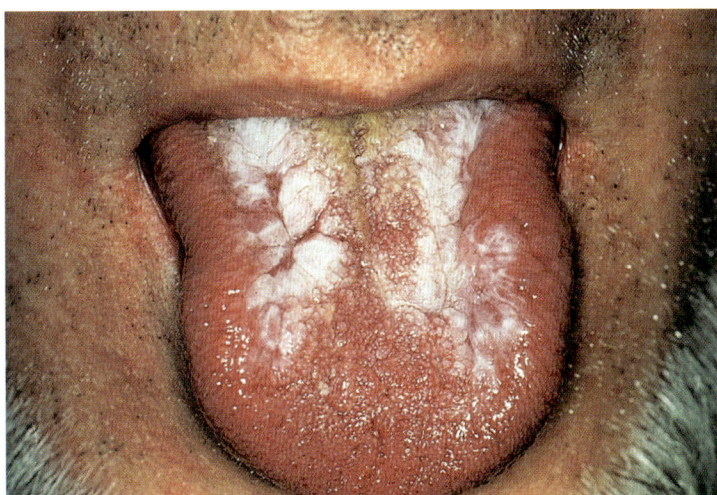

Figure 108.70 Plaque type lichen planus on the tongue with sparing of the lingual tip.

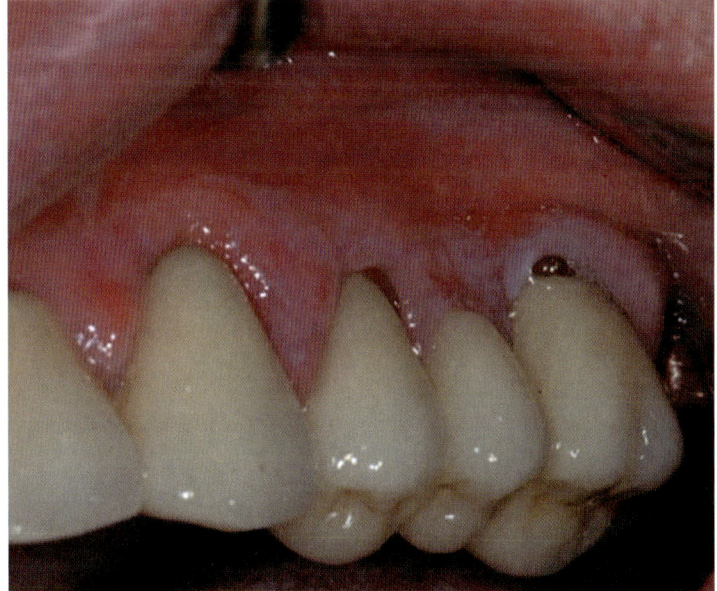

Figure 108.72 Lichen planus on the gingivae with a characteristic violaceous hue.

Papular or plaque OLP

Papular OLP is typically seen on the dorsal aspect of the tongue or buccal mucosa as slightly elevated areas which may eventually become more homogeneous (Figure 108.68). Plaque type lesions may present on any oral mucosal site. Most frequently they arise on the buccal mucosa or dorsum of tongue. Generally, a biopsy is advisable as the lesions are frequently asymmetrical and may represent an area of dysplasia arising within OLP. In some patients, plaques may become progressively thickened with a verrucous appearance as seen in Figure 108.70.

Atrophic and ulcerative OLP

Atrophic lesions are common (44%), appearing as symptomatic erythematous areas. When affecting the dorsum of the tongue, the lateral margins are affected initially, leading to a hemilunar depapillation often with sparing of the lingual tip. The depapillation may progress to involve the entire mid-dorsum. Once lost the papillae do not reappear, leaving a smooth atrophic surface. Within atrophic areas, progressive inflammation may lead to ulceration.

While these patients are very uncommon, they are the ones presenting to dermatology clinics and will often require systemic therapy.

Desquamative gingivitis

Gingival lichen planus may be mild with a violaceous hue or may appear as a glassy erythema with or without lichenoid striae, or may progress to form areas of desquamation or frank ulceration known as desquamative gingivitis (Figure 108.72). Patients with desquamative gingivitis may also be at risk of developing the VVG-LP subtype or rarely in males peno-gingival lichen planus. Gingival lichen planus may progress to a keratotic appearance and ultimately to verrucous changes called progressive verrucous leukoplakia which is a potentially malignant condition that needs to be closely monitored as it has a high transformation rate into OSCC.

PART 10: SPECIFIC SITES, SEX & AGE

Bullous OLP

Bullous OLP is rare and is characterised by the appearance of blisters, usually within an OLP lesion. It may be necessary to undertake direct immunofluorescence to distinguish from mucous membrane pemphigoid.

Prognosis

OLP is a chronic disease and may be present for many years. Long-term follow-up of patients with OLP reveals a malignant transformation rate of 1:200 patients/year with an approximate 1% lifetime risk [19,20]. The most frequently affected sites are the buccal mucosa and tongue with erosive, erythematous or atrophic lesions being more susceptible to malignant change. Modifiable risk factors such as smoking and alcohol consumption increase the patient's overall risk of developing SCC in the oral cavity.

Investigations

Biopsy with immunofluorescence may be undertaken if the diagnosis is unclear, when systemic therapy is being considered or where lesions are suspicious for dysplastic changes. An oral swab for *Candida* may be required if the degree of discomfort is disproportional to the clinical appearance or where the patient is at high risk of candidiasis.

Management

Treatment is aimed at improving symptoms. A stepwise approach is recommended according to symptoms and disease severity (Figure 108.73).
General advice:

- Assessment of disease severity using clinical outcome and patient reported outcome measures is essential. The oral disease severity score is ideal as it is validated for use in OLP [21].
- Improvement in oral hygiene is helpful. Additional antiseptic mouthwashes may reduce plaque.
- Avoiding foods that trigger discomfort is advisable, e.g. spicy or acidic food.
- Dental amalgams or gold crowns that are in direct contact with an area of localised OLP may have an irritant effect and may be replaced. However, there is no evidence that removing amalgams in the mouth is helpful and should not be advised.
- Identification of any lichenoid drug reaction is important so that the offending drug can be avoided.
- Identification of co-existing candidiasis is important and regular monthly antifungal therapy may be needed in patients with a propensity for infection (e.g. xerostomia, topical corticosteroid use, diabetes mellitus or systemic immunosuppression).

Mild symptomatic lichen planus

Topical corticosteroids are the mainstay of therapy. Betamethasone mouthrinses are typically used initially though higher potency corticosteroids such as clobetasol, fluocinonide or fluticasone may also be used. Suggested options are detailed in Table 108.17.

Moderately severe lichen planus

In addition to topical corticosteroids, intralesional triamcinolone for localised disease or systemic therapy may be required for uncontrolled symptoms. This might include reducing courses of oral prednisolone or a 3–6 month trial of hydroxychloroquine [22,23].

Severe lichen planus

In severe erosive (partial loss of epithelium) or ulcerative (full loss of epithelium) lichen planus, patients may require longer term systemic agents. There is very limited evidence for efficacy for these, derived mainly from small case series [24–28]. Options include hydroxychloroquine, systemic corticosteroids, mycophenolate mofetil, azathioprine or methotrexate. There is some evidence for retinoids and apremilast. There is emerging evidence to suggest that biologics may be of benefit particularly when targeting TNF. Adalimumab successfully cleared a patient with oral and cutaneous lichen planus in 6 weeks while in an OLP case there was improvement with etanercept. Preliminary evidence is emerging to support apremilast, the novel phosphodiesterase type IV inhibitor, in mucocutaneous lichen planus.

Differential diagnoses

Lichen planus pemphigoides. Oral lesions in lichen planus pemphigoides may be similar to those of lichen planus or pemphigoid [1–4], clinically and histologically, with direct immunofluorescence demonstrating linear deposits of immunoglobulin G and complement component C3 along the basement membrane.

Discoid lupus erythematosus. Oral involvement resembles atrophic, reticular or erosive lichen planus and may be unilateral rather than the typical bilateral presentation of OLP [1–3] (Figure 108.74). The typical oral lesion of discoid lupus erythematosus is a central erosion or erythema with a surrounding radial keratotic striae 'sun-ray' appearance and is often relatively painless.

Systemic lupus erythematosus. Up to 50% of patients with systemic lupus erythematosus may have oral lesions [1,2]. Typically, oral lesions include aphthous type ulcers or erythematous patches on the hard palate. However, lichenoid lesions may also be present and indistinguishable from OLP. Sjögren syndrome may also be present in systemic lupus erythematosus.

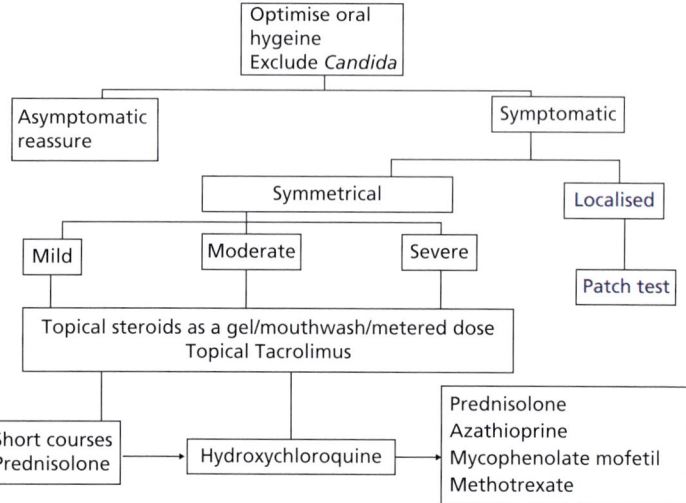

Figure 108.73 Algorithm for management of oral lichen planus.

Table 108.17 Topical therapeutic options for oral lichen planus.

Preparation	Treatment	Directions
Mouthrinse	Soluble prednisolone 5 mg tablets	5 mg dissolved in 15 mL of water as a mouthwash 3–4 times daily
	Flixonase nasules 400 μg with nystatin 100 000 units	1 mL of nystatin and 1 flixonase nasule added to 10 mL of water as a mouthwash twice daily
	Betamethasone sodium phosphate 500 μg tablets	500 μg tablet dissolved in 10 mL of water as a 3-minute mouthwash up to 4 times daily
Spray	Fluticasone propionate spray, 50 μg/puff	Applied to affected areas 3–4 times daily
	Beclomethasone spray, 100 μg/puff	Applied to affected areas 3–4 times daily
Ointment/cream	Clobetasol proprionate ointment (0.05%) ± orabase	Applied to painful areas 1–2 times daily
	Fluticasone cream (0.05%)	Applied to painful areas 3–4 times daily
	Tacrolimus 0.1% ointment	Applied to OLP of the lips twice daily for 6 weeks before as required use

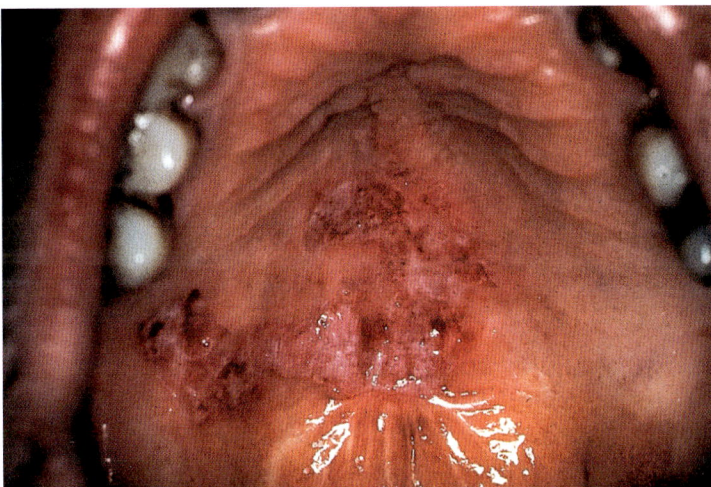

Figure 108.74 Oral lesions in discoid lupus erythematosus.

Chronic ulcerative stomatitis. Chronic ulcerative stomatitis may present as desquamative gingivitis with or without lesions on buccal or lingual mucosa and sometimes resembles lichen planus. It may be associated with lichenoid histology but is characterised by antinuclear antibodies directed against stratified squamous epithelia [1,2]. These autoantibodies are directed against a 70 kDa epithelial nuclear protein homologous to the p53 tumour suppressor and the p73 putative tumour suppressor, and shown to be a splicing variant of the *KET* gene. The lesions may respond to hydroxychloroquine [1,2].

Stevens–Johnson syndrome/toxic epidermal necrolysis (Chapter 118)

Stevens–Johnson syndrome/toxic epidermal necrolysis (SJS/TEN) are conditions that form part of a spectrum of disease severity with TEN having a high mortality proportional to the extent of skin involvement and patient comorbidities. It is characterised by extensive detachment of full-thickness epithelium. Most cases of SJS/TEN are drug induced [1]. A number of cases in patients with HIV/AIDS have been recorded.

Clinical features
Patients present with a cough, sore throat, burning eyes, malaise and low fever, followed after about 1–2 days by skin and mucous membrane lesions. Mucosal erosions plus widespread distribution of flat atypical targets or purpuric macules, and epithelial detachment involving 10–30% of body surface on the trunk, face and extremities are characteristic of drug-induced Stevens–Johnson syndrome.

In TEN, oral lesions can be seen in over 95% of patients. Gingival lesions are common and clinically are inflamed, with blister formation leading to painful widespread erosions. The blisters and erosions may precede the skin lesions by a day or so and may persist [1]. It is essential to have ophthalmology involvement alongside oral medicine assistance [1].

Diagnosis
Sheet-like loss of the epithelium and a positive Nikolsky sign are characteristic. Biopsy of perilesional tissue with immunostaining and histological examination are essential to the diagnosis. Histopathological examination is characteristic, showing necrosis of the whole epithelium detached from the lamina propria.

Management
Admission is required for SJS/TEN patients [1]:
- The mouth should be examined as a part of the initial assessment of a patient with SJS/TEN. Thereafter, daily oral review is necessary during the acute illness.
- Apply white soft paraffin ointment to the lips immediately, and then every 2 h throughout the acute illness. Protect ulcerated mucosal surfaces with a mucoprotectant mouthwash, used three times a day (e.g. Gelclair®). Clean the mouth daily with warm saline mouthwashes or an oral sponge, sweeping the sponge gently in the labial and buccal sulci to reduce the risk of fibrotic scars.
- Use an anti-inflammatory oral rinse or spray containing benzydamine hydrochloride every 3 hours, particularly before eating. If pain is inadequately controlled with benzydamine, then a topical anaesthetic preparation, e.g. viscous lidocaine 2%, 15 mL per application, may be used as an alternative. Cocaine mouthwashes 2–5% can be used for severe oral discomfort three times a day.
- Use an antiseptic oral rinse twice a day to reduce bacterial colonisation of the mucosa. Agents available include 1.5% hydrogen peroxide mouthwash (e.g. Peroxyl® mouthwash, 10 mL twice a day) or 0.2% chlorhexidine digluconate mouthwash (e.g. Corsodyl® mouthwash, 10 mL twice a day). Diluting 0.2% chlorhexidine mouthwash by up to 50% will reduce the soreness which can accompany this treatment.

PART 10: SPECIFIC SITES, SEX & AGE

- Oral and lip swabs should be taken regularly if bacterial or candidal secondary infection is suspected. Candidal infection should be treated with nystatin oral suspension 100 000 units four times a day for 1 week, or miconazole oral gel (e.g. Daktarin® oral gel) 5–10 mL held in the mouth after food four times a day for 1 week. Slow healing of the oral mucosa may reflect secondary infection by, or reactivation of, HSV.
- Consider using a topical corticosteroid four times a day (e.g. betamethasone sodium phosphate 0.5 mg in 10 mL water as a 3-min rinse-and-spit preparation). A more potent preparation, clobetasol propionate 0.05%, mixed in equal amounts with Orabase®, can be applied directly to the sulci, labial or buccal mucosae daily during the acute phase.

IMMUNOBULLOUS DISORDERS

Pemphigus (Chapter 50)

There are several variants of this group of intraepidermal blistering disorders. However, oral lesions are only present in pemphigus vulgaris (PV) and paraneoplastic pemphigus. PV is a rare mucocutaneous disorder presenting in over 90% of patients with oral lesions. These are very painful and can be recalcitrant to standard therapy. It is vital that the dermatologist understands the chronicity of oral PV, appreciates the need for objective disease severity assessment and how to manage patients optimally in a multidisciplinary team setting. Paraneoplastic pemphigus is a rare variant of pemphigus associated with an underlying neoplasm, e.g. lymphoproliferative disorders such as lymphoma, thymoma or the very rare Castleman disease. Extensive oral lesions are a major feature of this condition and require skilled management also in a multidisciplinary team setting.

Pemphigus vulgaris. The epidemiology and pathophysiology of pemphigus is discussed in Chapter 50.

Dsg3 is strongly expressed in oral epithelia and it is well recognised that increasing titres of Dsg3 IgG autoantibodies are associated with increasingly more severe oral disease [1,2]. Patients with both Dsg3 and Dsg1 may transform their clinical presentation over time, e.g. from PV to pemphigus foliaceous and vice versa.

Clinical features

The oral mucosa is almost invariably involved in PV and oral lesions are commonly the presenting feature (Figure 108.75) in over 60% of cases. At some point over the course of their disease, over 95% of patients will develop oral lesions. The most predominant site of involvement is the buccal mucosa, followed by palatal, lingual, labial mucosa and finally gingivae [1]. Oral lesions of PV are typically seen in adults, rarely in childhood.

Bullae appear on any part of the oral mucosa but are fragile and so are rarely seen. Typically, the patient presents with large, painful, irregular and persistent red lesions which can be difficult to differentiate clinically from those of other erosive conditions, such as mucous membrane pemphigoid, although intact bullae are more commonly seen in mucous membrane pemphigoid. The Nikolsky

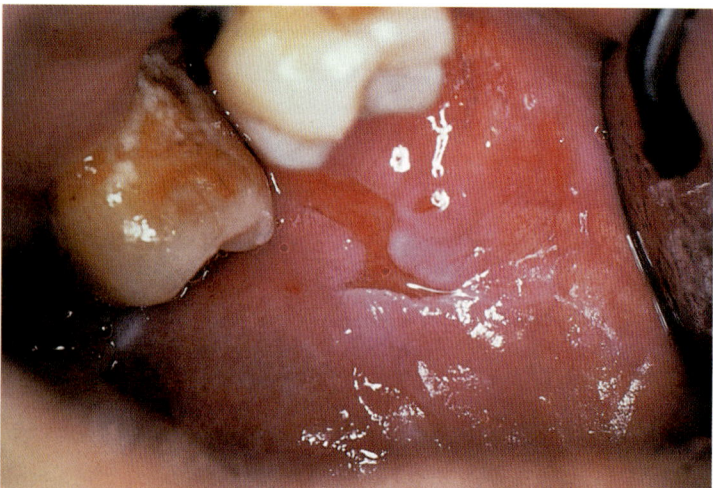

Figure 108.75 Pemphigus vulgaris: irregular persistent oral erosions.

sign, where application of lateral pressure to the edge of an erosion extends the lesion, is present in acute pemphigus but is painful and should be avoided. Furthermore, it can be seen in other immune blistering conditions.

Investigations

Diagnosis should be confirmed by biopsy and immunofluorescence studies. A biopsy of perilesional mucosa should be taken for haematoxylin and eosin stained sections and a normal adjacent area of tissue biopsied for direct immunofluorescence [3] (Table 108.18). Serum collected for autoantibody titres may be helpful for monitoring disease activity. Enzyme-linked immunosorbent assay (ELISA) are routinely undertaken.

Management

The management of PV is discussed in detail in Chapter 50 [4,5]. It is vital to use a validated clinical outcome measure and two main tools for multisite PV have been proposed: the pemphigus disease activity index (PDAI) [6] and the autoimmune bullous severity index score (ABSIS). For oral lesions, a more sensitive methodology has been devised and validated: the Oral Disease Severity Score (ODSS) [7]. Additionally, patient reported outcome measures are helpful. The Autoimmune Bullous Disease Quality of Life Questionnaire (ABQOL) has been devised for multisite disease, whereas for oral disease, the OHIP 14 and Chronic Oral Mucosal Disease Questionnaire (COMDQ) are recommended.

Treatment is largely based on systemic immunosuppression using corticosteroids, with mycophenolate mofetil, azathioprine, dapsone or methotrexate as adjuvants.

Specific management of oral lesions

Mucosal lesions are recalcitrant, often only healing long after skin lesions have resolved. Topical corticosteroids are helpful (Table 108.17). Tacrolimus topically may also be effective. However, patients will additionally require systemic immunosuppression for active oral disease. This needs to be maintained at a level that ensures healing before slowly reducing. It is vital to see the disease severity scores reduce before treatment is reduced.

Table 108.18 Immunostaining in oral mucosal vesiculobullous disorders.

Disease	DIF	Oral mucosal deposits mainly:	Pattern of IF	IIF	Autoantibodies against:
Pemphigus	+	IgG, C3	Epithelial intercellular	+	Dsg 1+3
Mucous membrane pemphigoid	+	IgG, C3, IgA	Linear epithelial BM	±	BP180, L332 (COL7)
Bullous pemphigoid	+	IgG, c3	Linear epithelial BM	+	BP180, BP230
Dermatitis herpetiformis	+	IgA +/– C3	Microgranular IgA dermal papillae and basement membrane	–	Transglutaminase 2 (TG2)
Linear IgA disease	+	IgA, C3	Linear epithelial BM	–	BP180 extracellular domain
Erythema multiforme	±	C3	Vessel walls in lamina propria	–	–
		IgM			
Lichen planus[a]	±	Fibrin[b]	Granular BM	–	–
Discoid lupus erythematosus[a]	+	IgG, IgA, IgM, C3	Granular epithelial BM	±	None, or antinuclear
Angina bullosa haemorrhagica	–	–	–	–	–

BM, basement membrane; DIF, direct immunofluorescence (biopsy); IF, immunofluorescence; IIF, indirect immunofluorescence (serology).
+, Present; –, absent; ±, sometimes.
[a] Rarely vesiculobullous; [b] non-specific deposits.

The anti-CD20 monoclonal antibody, rituximab, is a highly effective treatment for refractory PV. In the RITUX-3 study comparing rituximab plus a short course of prednisolone with high dose prednisolone alone there was an 89% sustained response over 2 years with a much lower total dose of prednisolone in a post-hoc analysis [8,9]. The earlier it is given the better the outcome. In the USA and parts of Europe it is available as first line therapy. However, in the UK it is only approved for third line use by NICE.

Paraneoplastic pemphigus. Paraneoplastic pemphigus is usually associated with lymphoproliferative diseases or thymoma [1–4]. Oral lesions may be the sole manifestation and have been seen in all reported cases of paraneoplastic pemphigus [1–4]. Patients present with painful hyperplastic ulcerative lesions often with a panstomatitis, painful paronychia and lichenoid papules may be seen, and histology may show lichenoid changes, acantholytic blister formation and apoptotic keratinocytes. Direct immunofluorescence is positive for IgG both in the epidermal intercellular spaces and along the basement membrane zone. Indirect immunofluorescence is similarly positive in a PV pattern.

There is often only a partial response to intravenous corticosteroids [5]. Recent therapeutic advances include the use of anti-CD20 monoclonal antibody (rituximab) and mycophenolate.

Pemphigus vegetans. Oral lesions in pemphigus vegetans are hyperplastic and are most frequently encountered at the commissures of the lips [1].

Other pemphigus variants. Oral lesions may be seen in less common pemphigus variants, especially in most cases with IgA pemphigus (intraepithelial IgA pustulosis or intraepidermal neutrophilic IgA dermatosis) [1–3], and in some cases of pemphigus associated with inflammatory bowel disease [4–10].

Pemphigoid (subepithelial immune bullous diseases)

A spectrum of immune-mediated subepithelial bullous diseases can present with oral blisters and/or erosions and/or desquamative gingivitis. These include bullous pemphigoid, mucous membrane pemphigoid, linear IgA disease and epidermolysis bullosa acquisita. P200 pemphigoid may also have oral lesions though diagnosis of this rare subtype is not routinely available in most laboratories.

Bullous pemphigoid (Chapter 50)

Oral lesions alongside skin lesions may be present but are usually transient and respond quickly to treatment. Lesions may present as blisters or ulcers but desquamative gingivitis would not be a feature. Where patients have troublesome or persistent oral lesions this suggests that the diagnosis is mucous membrane pemphigoid, linear IgA disease or epidermolysis bullosa acquisita [1].

Chronic bullous dermatosis of childhood (linear IgA disease of children) (Chapters 50 and 115)

Oral ulceration and desquamative gingivitis have been reported [1–5].

Dermatitis herpetiformis

Rarely, oral mucosal lesions may occur in dermatitis herpetiformis and if present may appear as erythema or ulcers. Dapsone and sulfapyridine are the most effective therapeutic agents along with a gluten-free diet [1].

Epidermolysis bullosa acquisita (Chapter 69)

Blisters or ulcers may be seen in the oral mucosa: typical sites include the tongue, lips and buccal mucosae. The gingivae are relatively spared. Scarring may be present and may result in ankyloglossia and microstomia. Perilesional biopsy for direct immunofluorescence shows dermal binding linear IgG and C3 with autoantibodies specifically targeting type 7 collagen [1,2]. Epidermolysis bullosa acquisita may be recalcitrant to treatment which includes dapsone, prednisolone and mycophenolate mofetil/azathioprine and/or rituximab.

PART 10: SPECIFIC SITES, SEX & AGE

Linear IgA disease of adults (Chapter 50)

Oral lesions are more frequently seen in linear IgA disease as vesicles, bullae and erosions or desquamative gingivitis [1,2].

Treatment is similar to that for MMP, with dapsone being first line.

Mucous membrane pemphigoid (Chapter 50)

Mucous membrane pemphigoid (MMP) is a mucocutaneous, immune-mediated, subepithelial blistering disease characterised by autoantibodies to a range of molecules in the basement membrane zone, although typically BP180 and/or L332 [1,2]. The mouth may be involved as part of a wider disease, although in many patients only oral lesions are seen [1].

Clinical features

MMP involves the oral mucosa in over 75% patients with or without conjunctival, nasopharyngeal, anogenital, cutaneous, oesophageal, laryngeal or rarely tracheobronchial lesions.

Oral MMP frequently presents with gingival lesions. Blisters may occasionally be visible on the gingivae but more typically patients will have gingival erythema with the appearance of a shiny smooth 'glassy' erythema with loss of stippling. More severe patients may have areas of ulceration, termed desquamative gingivitis. In contrast to PV, where desquamation sits around the neck of teeth as ragged gingival tip erosions, or marginal gingivitis associated with plaque, in MMP the inflammation affects much of the attached or bound-down gingivae and is visible as a band of erythema several millimetres in width. This inflammation is sometimes termed 'full thickness' desquamative gingivitis and is characterised by erythematous glazed often sore gingivae (Figure 108.76). Bullae when present may be seen in any affected sites but are not infrequently visible on the soft palate. They may be blood filled or are serosanguinous and rupture to form ulcers [1,3]. The buccal mucosa and hard or soft palate are also frequent 'extragingival' sites. Scarring is uncommon but when present is seen as whitish change in the buccal mucosae, loss of gingival sulci or flattening of the soft palate with distortion or loss of the uvula. Unusual sites in MMP include the tongue and lip. If these sites are affected, the patient may have an atypical subtype of L332 MMP or epidermolysis bullosa acquisita.

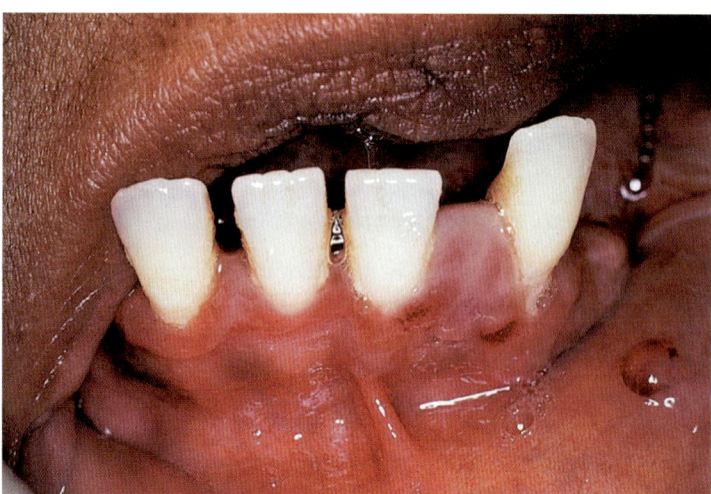

Figure 108.76 Pemphigoid: vesicles and desquamative gingivitis.

Investigations

A biopsy is required for diagnosis [3,4,5]. Direct immunofluorescence is positive for linear basement membrane zone IgG, IgA and/or C3. It is important to ensure that a representative sample is collected that maintains epithelium. Perilesional intact tissue is recommended [4]. Serum autoantibodies to epithelial basement membrane molecules may be detected in addition with salt-split skin substrate and may correlate with disease severity and sequentially with activity [6,7] (Table 108.18).

Management

Management of MMP is discussed in detail in Chapter 50.

Disease assessment

This is extremely important as the scarring sequelae of MMP may be severe and even life threatening. A multidisciplinary assessment is recommended for multisite involvement. However, an ophthalmology review is specifically recommended if any redness or dryness of the eyes is present, as is an ENT examination if there is nasal crusting, bleeding or hoarseness. Swallowing difficulties may also indicate oesophageal MMP. Clinical outcome measures are also useful for assessing baseline disease severity and sequentially to assess therapeutic efficacy. The Oral Disease Severity Score (ODSS) [8] has been compared with other proposed outcome measures and has been shown to be a more sensitive and reproducible technique compared with the Autoimmune Bullous Disease Severity Score (ABSIS) or the MMP Disease Activity Score (MMPDAI) [9,10]. Additionally, it is equally applicable to PV and OLP. When patients have an unusual clinical presentation or a more severe scarring phenotype it is important to consider atypical variants including L332 MMP because this is associated with an increased risk of malignancy [11–14].

Patient reported outcome measures are also vital and a variety of options are available including Dermatology Life Quality Index (DLQI), Oral Health Impact Profile (OHIP-14), a Chronic Oral Mucosal Diseases Questionnaire (COMDQ) and Autoimmune Bullous Disease Quality of Life questionnaire (ABQOL) [15–17].

Treatment

There is no high-quality evidence available upon which to base treatment recommendations [18,19]. Patients are typically treated with topical corticosteroids either alone where there is localised disease or, more typically, alongside systemic immunomodulating therapy. Systemic corticosteroids as a reducing short course may be used at initial presentation, but more typically an immunomodulating agent, such as dapsone or sulphapyridine, is introduced. These should be introduced slowly to minimise the risk of haemolysis and it is important to appreciate that response may be slow and progressive. Tetracyclines with or without nicotinamide may be used. Recalcitrant mucous membrane pemphigoid may respond to mycophenolate mofetil. A layered approach can be helpful in more complex cases with low dose prednisolone, dapsone and mycophenolate mofetil/azathioprine being combined. There is some evidence for use of intravenous immunoglobulins, rituximab or other biological agents [18]. The most recent European guidelines recommend that rituximab be considered a second-line agent in severe MMP and third-line in cases recalcitrant to standard therapies [18].

ENDOCRINE DISORDERS

- Addison's disease may be associated with oral and peri-oral melanotic pigmentation.
- Hyperparathyroidism can cause central and peripheral giant cell tumours, also known as 'Brown tumours'.
- Menopause has been associated with diminished salivation, mucosal atrophy, oral dysaesthesia and dysgeusia,
- Pregnancy may be associated with pyogenic granulomas, oral peripheral giant cell granuloma, angiogranuloma and periodontal disease.
- Autoimmune thyroid disease may be associated with lichen planus.
- Diabetes mellitus may be associated with mucosal atrophy and oral candidosis.

RENAL DISEASES

- Patients with acute kidney disease can present with oral ulcerative lesions or uraemic stomatitis. Chronic renal impairment may lead to oral candidosis, oral mucosal atrophy, hyposalivation and increased incidence of oral dysaesthesia.

NEUROLOGICAL DISEASES

- Multiple sclerosis can present with chronic orofacial pain, trigeminal neuralgia, oral paraesthesia and taste disturbances.
- Amyotrophic lateral sclerosis (motor neuron disease) may present with progressive paralysis of orofacial and pharyngeal function as well as an atrophied fasciculating tongue.
- Stroke patients may also present with chronic orofacial pain, oral dysaesthesia and taste disturbances.
- Patients with Parkinson's disease or dementia may have significant difficulty with sialorrhea.

PSYCHIATRIC DISORDERS

- Oral dysaesthesia and persistent idiopathic facial pain are often associated with a variety of psychiatric disorders, particularly anxiety and depression. Psychosocial factors, e.g. stress, are also known to aggravate and perpetuate chronic orofacial pain.
- Eating disorders can present with oral mucosal atrophy, oral candidiasis, salivary gland enlargement and dental enamel erosions that occur typically on the lingual/palatal surfaces of the anterior teeth.

OROCUTANEOUS SYNDROMES

Cleft lip/palate

Definition

The primary palate or premaxilla includes that portion of the alveolar ridge containing the four incisors. The secondary palate forms the remaining hard palate and all the soft palate. Cleft of the lip with or without cleft palate (CL/P) is one of the commonest congenital malformations in western countries. Based on their association with specific malformative patterns or their presence as isolated defects, CL/P can be classified as syndromic and non-syndromic, respectively. Both forms of CL/P are characterised by a strong genetic component. Syndromic forms are in many cases due to chromosomal aberrations or monogenic diseases. Non-syndromic CL/P is a multifactorial disease caused by the interaction between genetic and environmental factors.

Orofacial clefts result from an embryopathy in which there is failure of the frontonasal process and/or fusion of the palatal shelves. In the submucous cleft palate, the palatal shelves may fail to join, but the overlying mucous membranes are intact and the muscle attachments of the soft palate are abnormal, causing velopharyngeal insufficiency. Bifid uvula may signify a submucous cleft palate.

Epidemiology

The common clefts are cleft lip with or without cleft palate (CL/P) and cleft palate (CP) only. The total incidence of facial clefting is between two and three per 1000 live births. Cleft lip occurs in about 1/1000 white-skinned neonates. The prevalence is higher in Asian neonates (about 1.7/1000 births) and lower in black neonates (approximately 1/2500 births). CP has an incidence of 0.5/1000 births. The risk of recurrence in subsequent children is about 2% if one child has it, 6% if one parent has it, and 15% if one parent and one child have it. The male to female ratio of CL/P is 2:1, while the male to female ratio of CP is 1:2.

Associated diseases

Facial clefts are associated with a syndrome in up to 15–60% of cases and are then termed syndromic clefts. More than 100 syndromes may include a facial cleft as one manifestation and CL/P may be associated with many congenital syndromes.

However, the majority of cases are not syndromic and may be due to a combination of genetic and environmental factors. A number of teratogens (environmental agents that can cause birth defects) have been implicated, as well as defects in essential nutrients.

Pathophysiology

The development of the face and the upper lip takes place during the fifth to ninth week of pregnancy. CL/P and CP alone result from the failure of the first branchial arches to complete fusion processes and are the most common of all craniofacial anomalies. Failed fusion of the palatal shelves can be caused by different gene defects culminating in:

- A problem in the formation of the midline epithelial seam.
- Small size of the palatal processes.
- Unsynchronised timing of the elevation or growth of the palatal shelves with the growth of surrounding structures such as cranial base.
- A small mandible preventing the downwards relocation of the tongue which mechanically may prevent palatal fusion.

Predisposing factors [1–6]

CL/P is more prevalent in the lower socioeconomic classes. Environmental factors present during the first trimester of pregnancy and those which may generate CP include smoking or alcohol, obesity, diabetes and folate deficiency. Drugs recognised as teratogens with specificity for midfacial development include anticonvulsants (phenytoin, valproic acid, topimirate, carbamazepine), methotrexate, selective serotonin reuptake inhibitors (SSRIs), clomiphene, fluconazole, ondansetron and a number of other psychoactive drugs (e.g. cocaine, crack cocaine, heroin). A maternal age of 35 years or older has also been associated with an increased risk.

Genetics

Genetic factors have been identified for some syndromic conditions. Clefts can be seen in over 100 different syndromes (Box 108.10). The cause of non-syndromic CL/P is unclear but there is a strong genetic component. In monozygotic twins, there is nearly 40% concordance. A number of genes are involved, including cleft lip and palate transmembrane protein 1 and *GAD1* [7].

Box 108.10 Syndromes which may include cleft lip/palate

- Apert syndrome
- Basal cell carcinoma naevoid syndrome
- Carpenter syndrome
- Cleidocranial dysplasia
- Craniosynostosis
- Crouzon syndrome
- Freeman–Sheldon syndrome
- Goldenhar syndrome
- Hallerman–Streiff syndrome
- Hemifacial microsomia
- Hydrocephalus
- Microtia
- Miller syndrome
- Moebius syndrome
- Nager syndrome
- Nasal encephalocoeles
- Neurofibromatosis
- Orbital hypertelorism
- Parry–Romberg syndrome
- Pfeiffer syndrome
- Pierre Robin sequence
- Saethre–Chotzen syndrome
- Shprintzen syndrome
- Stickler syndrome
- Treacher Collins syndrome
- Van der Woude syndrome
- Velocardiofacial syndrome (DiGeorge syndrome or 22q11 deletion syndrome)
- Waardenberg syndrome

Clinical features

Presentation

A person may have a cleft lip, cleft palate or both cleft lip and palate. A unilateral cleft lip occurs on one side of the upper lip. A bilateral cleft lip occurs on both sides of the upper lip. In its most severe form, the cleft may extend through the nose base. Cleft lip is not always complete (i.e. extending into the nostril). A cleft may involve only the upper lip or may extend to involve the nostril and the hard and

soft palates. In about 9% of the cases, the cleft is associated with skin bridges or Simonart bands. Isolated cleft lip may be unilateral or bilateral (approximately 20%). When unilateral, the cleft is more common on the left side (about 70%).

Lips are more frequently cleft bilaterally (approximately 25%) when combined with cleft palate. CL/P is more common in men. CL/P comprises about 50% of cases, with cleft lip and isolated cleft palate each comprising about 25%. About 85% of bilateral cleft lips and 70% of unilateral cleft lips are associated with cleft palate. One subgroup have cleft lip and palate with median facial dysplasia and cerebrofacial malformations; others have laryngo-tracheal oesophageal clefts (Opitz–Firas or G syndrome) or cranial asymmetry (Opitz or B syndrome).

Clefts in the middle of the upper lip may be true or false. True median clefts have been described in association with bifid nose and ocular hypertelorism. Other cases of true median labial cleft are associated with polydactyly or other digital anomalies, constituting an autosomal recessive trait called *orofaciodigital syndrome II*.

Pseudocleft of the middle of the upper lip may occur in *orofaciodigital syndrome I*. A somewhat similar central defect, but of mild degree, is seen in chondroectodermal dysplasia (Ellis–van Creveld syndrome). Clefts in the lower lip are rare and usually median but may involve the mandible and sometimes the tongue. Management of cleft lip is discussed elsewhere.

Cleft palate may be incomplete involving only the uvula and the muscular soft palate. A complete cleft palate extends the entire length of the palate. Cleft palates can be unilateral or bilateral. Clefts are often accompanied by impaired facial growth, dental anomalies, speech disorders, poor hearing and psychosocial problems.

Clinical variants

Submucous cleft palate can be recognised by a notched posterior nasal spine, a translucent zone in the midline of the soft palate and a bifid uvula. However, not all these features are necessarily present and a bifid uvula may be seen in isolation. About 1/1200 births are affected and feeding difficulties, speech defects and middle-ear infections may develop in 90% of affected children. Adenoidectomy is contraindicated as it may reveal latent velopharyngeal insufficiency.

Complications and co-morbidities

A high percentage of patients with cleft palate develop otitis media with effusion. Up to 20% have additional abnormalities that can affect management in various ways. Systemic disorders are more frequent in patients with cleft palate than in those with cleft lip alone, and include especially skeletal, cardiac, renal and CNS defects.

Investigations

Health care providers that frequently participate in a multidisciplinary cleft palate team include: audiologists; maxillofacial, ear, nose and throat, and plastic surgeons; geneticists; neurosurgeons; nurses; dentists (paediatric dentist/orthodontist/prosthodontist); paediatricians; social workers/psychologists, and speech and language pathologists.

Management [8–10]

Treatment of the airway takes priority and may be managed with positioning but, in severe cases, may need tracheostomy. Aesthetics is a major issue for parents. One of the problems for the child is feeding: a Rosti bottle with Gummi teat often helps. The timing of the initial cleft lip and palate repair is controversial. In general, when the lip alone is cleft, initial cosmetic repair is carried out at about 3–6 months of age, although earlier operations are becoming popular. Many repair cleft lip and palate within the first few days of life because, after repair, the appearance is dramatically improved, feeding difficulties are significantly minimised and speech development is improved. If the palatal defect is too wide, it can be repaired 3 months later to allow for sufficient palatal growth. Cleft palate is now usually repaired before the child speaks, between 6 and 18 months, typically at 6–12 months of age.

Palatal ulcers seen in neonates with cleft lip and palate appear to result from trauma from the tongue and resolve if a palatal plate is fitted. Dental abnormalities include malocclusion (almost 100%), hypodontia (50%), hypoplasia (30%) and supernumerary teeth (20%). Children may have a higher prevalence of caries in both the primary and permanent dentitions, and significantly more gingivitis, especially in the maxillary anterior region.

Syndromic cleft palate

Syndromes account for approximately 30% of cases of CL/P and 50% of cases of CP. Van der Woude syndrome is the most common form of syndromic clefting, accounting for 1–2% of cases.

Other examples include:
- Stickler syndrome.
- Deletion of chromosome 22q11.
- Treacher Collins syndrome.
- SATB2 syndrome.

Cowden syndrome (Chapter 78)

Most cases of Cowden syndrome are caused by mutations in the *PTEN* tumour suppressor gene [1–3]. It is considered part of the *PTEN* hamartoma–tumour syndrome spectrum which also includes Bannayan–Riley–Ruvalcaba syndrome [4,5] and Proteus syndrome [6]. Characteristically, it starts in the third decade. There is an increased risk for breast, thyroid and endometrial cancer.

Clinical features
Patients present with multiple hamartomas, macrocephaly, trichilemmomas and papules in the mouth. Oral mucosal lesions may be found in the presence or absence of cutaneous stigma [6–11]. The oral lesions are typically 1–4 mm smooth, pink or whitish benign fibromas found especially on the palatal, gingival and labial mucosae. When they coalesce, they can form a distinctive cobblestone appearance.

De Lange syndrome

Classic Brachmann or Cornelia de Lange syndrome presents with a striking face, pronounced growth and learning disability, and variable limb deficiencies. Most cases are sporadic [1,2]. About 50% of patients have been found to have heterozygous mutations in the *NIPBL* gene with some cases being caused by mutations in *SMC1L1*, *HDAC8*, *RAD21* and *SMC3* genes [3]. A long philtrum and crescent-shaped mouth with down-turned corners is typical [4–6]. The characteristic face of classic de Lange syndrome is present at birth and changes little throughout life, although there is some lengthening of the face with age and the jaw becomes squared.

Double lip

Double lip is a developmental anomaly usually involving the upper lip. It is reported to be common among some groups of Africans [1]. Double lip may occur alone or in association with other anomalies. The association with blepharochalasis (laxity of the upper eyelid skin) and sometimes non-toxic thyroid enlargement is known as Ascher syndrome [2,3]. Non-syndromic double lip has been reported [4]. A fold of redundant tissue is found on the inner aspect of the involved lip [5,6]. Double lip requires no treatment unless except for cosmetic purposes.

Down syndrome

The incidence of clefts and of angular cheilitis is increased in people with Down syndrome, caused by an increased level of *Staphylococcus aureus* and *Candida albicans* [1,2]. Lip fissures may appear intermittently over a period of years or be intractable and longstanding. The tongue is often enlarged and may be fissured.

Erythropoietic protoporphyria
(Chapter 58)

Erythropoietic protoporphyria is thought to be caused by a compound loss-of-function mutation in the gene encoding ferrochelatase (FECH; 612386) found on chromosome 18q21. Typically, there is a mutation on one gene as well as a second, low-expression allele. Rarely, there is a gain in function mutation in ALA synthase (ALAS)-2 (X-linked dominant inheritance). Thus, inheritance can be autosomal recessive or autosomal dominant with incomplete penetrance (96% of patients in the UK). In very rare instances, erythropoietic protoporphyria has been reported to have been caused by myelodysplasia or myeloid leukaemia due to associated chromosomal instability, including knock-out loss of chromosome 18. The result is in inhibition of the conversion of protoporphyrin to haem.

Clinical features
Shallow elliptical or linear scars around the lips and linear perioral furrowing (pseudorhagades) are subtle changes that are pathognomonic when observed in children [1–3].

Focal mucinosis

Oral focal mucinosis is an uncommon clinicopathological entity considered to be the oral counterpart of cutaneous focal mucinosis and/or cutaneous myxoid cyst. The nature of the lesion is unknown. It occurs predominantly in adults during the fourth and fifth decade of life. It is most commonly found on the gingiva and presents as a painless, sessile or pedunculated mass of the same colour as the surrounding mucosa [1–3]. Histologically, it is characterised by localised areas of myxomatous connective tissue.

Gardner syndrome (Chapter 78)

Multiple jaw osteomas are a feature of Gardner syndrome of familial adenomatous polyposis coli. Some 80% of patients with familial adenomatosis polyposis coli have osteomas and 30% have dental anomalies such as unerupted teeth, supernumerary teeth, dentigerous cysts and odontomas [1–10].

Gorlin syndrome (Chapter 140)

Keratocystic odontogenic tumours (Kodontogenic keratocysts or primordial cysts) of the jaws are a prominent feature of Gorlin syndrome (naevoid basal cell carcinoma syndrome) [1–3]. The syndrome is caused by mutations in the Sonic Hedgehog *patched* gene, a tumour suppressor gene [4,5]. A single point mutation in one *patched* allele may be responsible for the various malformations found in the syndrome. Inactivation of both *patched* alleles results in the formation of tumours and cysts (basal cell carcinomas, odontogenic keratocysts and medulloblastomas). Three-quarters of odontogenic keratocysts present in the mandible [2,3,6]. The keratocysts should be surgically removed but have a tendency to recur [7].

There are also occasional reports of oral neoplasms, notably fibrosarcoma, ameloblastoma, squamous carcinoma, basal cell carcinoma and B-cell lymphoma [8–12].

Jacob disease

Jacob disease is a rare condition consisting of new joint formation between the coronoid process of the mandible and the inner aspect of the zygomatic arch [1,2].

Kindler syndrome

Kindler syndrome is a rare autosomal recessive type of epidermolysis bullosa due to a loss of function mutation in the *KIND1* gene encoding kindlin-1. It is characterised by skin blistering, photosensitivity, progressive poikiloderma and SCCs of skin and mucosal membranes [1–3]. Bulla formation starts at birth on areas of the skin that receive pressure and may lead to bilateral incomplete syndactylies involving all web spaces.

The oral mucosa is affected, with erosions and early and severe periodontitis leading to premature loss of teeth [4,5]. Trismus may also result.

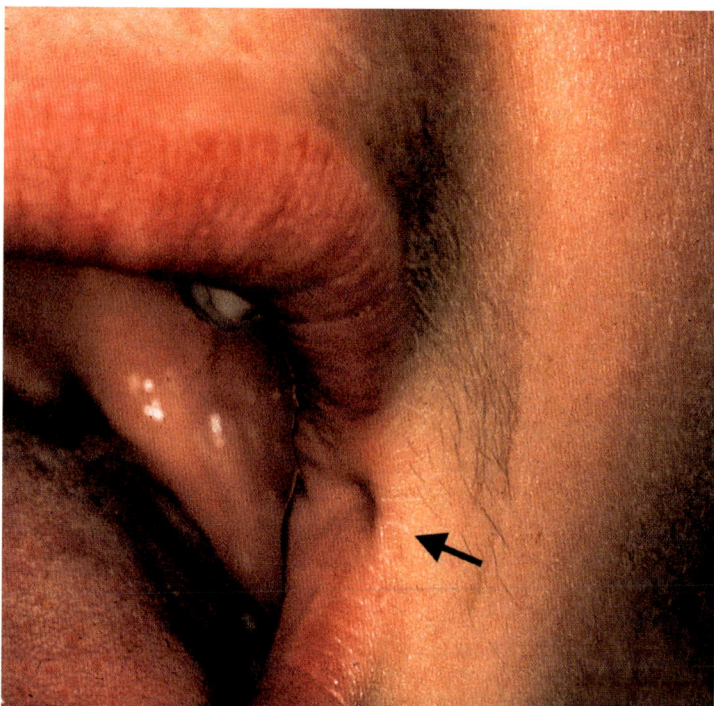

Figure 108.77 Angular sinus (lippit), a congenital anomaly.

Lip pits and sinuses

Congenital lip pits or sinuses are small blind fistulae on the vermilion border [1]. They are usually bilateral and symmetrical, often just to one side of the philtrum. The pits may be up to 3–4 mm in diameter and up to 2 cm deep. They may communicate with underlying minor salivary glands. They may appear as isolated findings but are often (67%) associated with cleft lip and/or palate (Van der Woude syndrome) [2–4] and caused by a DNA variation in *IRF6* [5].

Dimples are common at the commissures. They should be distinguished from *commissural pits*, which are distinct definite pits ranging from 1 to 4 mm in diameter and depth present from infancy [10,11], often showing a familial tendency and probably determined by a dominant gene (Figure 108.77). Commissural pits are sometimes associated with aural sinuses or pits. Rarely, they may be infected and present as recurrent or refractory angular cheilitis. Surgical removal may be indicated for cosmetic purposes.

Noonan syndrome

Noonan syndrome is an autosomal-dominant condition. It is caused by mutations in the RAS/mitogen-activated protein kinase (MAPK) pathway which is essential for cell cycle differentiation, growth and senescence. A number of mutations have been identified with the four most common being the *PTPN11* (50% of cases), *KRAS*, *SOS1* and *RAF1* genes [1,2].

The classic features include short stature and congenital heart disease. Central giant cell lesions or cherubism of the jaws may be present [3–8]. Dental anomalies such as malocclusion and abnormalities of tooth number or morphology are common.

Tuberous sclerosis

Oral manifestations in tuberous sclerosis include pit-shaped enamel defects in both dentitions, and gingival fibromatosis and intraoral fibromas [1–4].

Van der Woude syndrome

Van der Woude syndrome is a rare autosomal dominant syndrome [1] caused by mutations in the *IRF6* gene, located on chromosome 1q32-41 [2,3]. It is the most common syndromic form of cleft lip and palate, representing 1% of cases. It is characterised by pits and/or sinuses in the lower lip and cleft lip and/or cleft palate [2–5].

Velocardiofacial syndrome (22q11 deletion syndrome)

In approximately 90% of patients this arises as a sporadic mutation. In 10% of cases it is inherited from a parent with this syndrome. It is associated with many clinical features including cleft lip or palate, learning difficulties, congenital heart disease and hypoparathyroidism [1,2].

Von Recklinghausen neurofibromatosis

Neurofibromatosis consists of distinct variants due to *NF* gene mutations: type I (NF-I), often referred to as von Recklinghausen disease; and type II (NF-II), a much less common disorder of bilateral acoustic schwannomas. The incidence of head and neck manifestations in patients with NF varies between 14% and 37%. Multiple neurofibromas may occur as a feature of NF; cosmetic lesions include pigmentary changes (café-au-lait spots).

Neurofibromas may be seen mainly in NF-I. Neurofibromas may also be seen in NF-II, but bilateral acoustic neuromas are the hallmark of this disease and neurilemmomas and acoustic neuromas are the predominant neural tumours. Neurofibromas may also be part of the MEN syndrome (Chapter 148).

Oral lesions are not uncommon in von Recklinghausen generalised NF [1–5]. About two-thirds of patients have intraoral neurofibromas affecting predominantly the tongue, lips, buccal mucosa or palate [4,5]. Neurofibroma represents a benign overgrowth of all elements of a peripheral nerve (axon cylinder, Schwann cells and fibrous connective tissue), arranged in a variety of patterns. Enlarged fungiform papillae are found in about 50% of patients. About 60% of patients have radiographic evidence of disease, especially enlargement of the inferior alveolar canal or foramen, or branching of the canal. Neurofibromas may occur multiply as a feature of NF but only rarely undergo sarcomatous change [6]. Other rare, malignant tumours include nerve sheath tumour [7], triton tumour [8] and Merkel cell carcinoma [9].

Xeroderma pigmentosum

SCC of the lip may arise in patients with xeroderma pigmentosum and therefore it is crucial to institute sun protection [1–3]. Topical 5-fluorouracil or surgery may be used to treat potentially malignant lesions.

CONGENITAL ANOMALIES

Ankyloglossia

Ankyloglossia is an isolated anomaly that occurs when a short lingual frenulum or a tightly attached genioglossus muscle restricts tongue movement [1–3]. Most cases of ankyloglossia are sporadic. The association of cleft palate with ankyloglossia is inherited as a semidominant, X-linked disorder previously described in several large families of different ethnic origins and related to chromosome Xq21: the T-box transcription factor gene *TBX22* is mutated [4–6].

It results in impaired protrusion of the tongue and side-to-side movement of the tongue, and a heart shape to the tongue when it is protruded.

Speech is not affected in patients with ankyloglossia but difficulty breastfeeding, articulation problems and mechanical problems can result. No investigations are necessary. If necessary, surgery to the fraenum will relieve ankyloglossia [7].

Fissured tongue

Fissured tongue, a normal tongue variant seen in adults, presents with deep grooves located on the midline or evenly distributed on the tongue surface (Figure 108.78) [1]. It may be noted from childhood. Geographic tongue is commonly found in people with fissured tongues. Patients with Down syndrome often have a fissured tongue and it is a feature of the rare Melkersson–Rosenthal

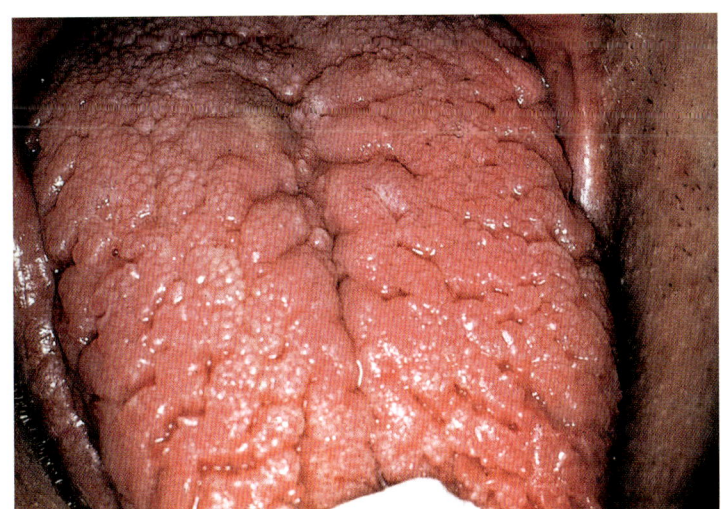

Figure 108.78 Fissured or scrotal tongue.

syndrome comprising recurrent orofacial swelling, facial palsy and plicated tongue. No investigations are required.

Patients are generally asymptomatic but may complain of halitosis. Reassurance only is required.

Key references

The full list of references can be found in the online version at https://www.wiley.com/rooksdermatology10e

Leukoplakia

1 Warnakulasuriya S, Kujan O, Aguirre-Urizar JM *et al*. Oral potentially malignant disorders: a consensus report from an international seminar on nomenclature and classification, convened by the WHO Collaborating Centre for Oral Cancer. *Oral Dis* 2021;27:1862–80.
5 Iocca O, Sollecito TP, Alawi F *et al*. Potentially malignant disorders of the oral cavity and oral dysplasia: a systematic review and meta-analysis of malignant transformation rate by subtype. *Head Neck* 2020;42:539–55.

Behçet syndrome

9 Hatemi G, Christensen R, Bang D *et al*. 2018 update of the EULAR recommendations for the management of Behçet's syndrome. *Ann Rheum Dis* 2018;77:808–18.

Oral squamous cell carcinoma

13 Kerawala C, Roques T, Jeannon JP, Bisase B. Oral cavity and lip cancer: United Kingdom National Multidisciplinary Guidelines. *J Laryngol Otol* 2016;130(Suppl. 2):S83–S89.

Actinic cheilitis (solar cheilosis)

7 Lai M, Pampena R, Cornacchia L, Pellacani G, Peris K, Longo C. Treatments of actinic cheilitis: a systematic review of the literature. *J Am Acad Dermatol* 2020;83:876–87.

Trigeminal neuralgia

5 Bendtsen L, Zakrzewska JM, Abbott J *et al*. European Academy of Neurology guideline on trigeminal neuralgia. *Eur J Neurol* 2019;26:831–49.

Stevens–Johnson syndrome/toxic epidermal necrolysis

1 Creamer D, Walsh SA, Dziewulski P *et al*. UK guidelines for the management of Stevens–Johnson syndrome/toxic epidermal necrolysis in adults 2015. *Br J Dermatol* 2016;174:1194–227.

Pemphigus vulgaris

3 Carey B, Joshi S, Abdelghani A, Mee J, Andiappan M, Setterfield J. The optimal oral biopsy site for diagnosis of mucous membrane pemphigoid and pemphigus vulgaris. *Br J Dermatol* 2020;182:747–53.
4 Antiga E, Bech R, Maglie R *et al*. S2K guidelines on the management of paraneoplastic pemphigus/paraneoplastic autoimmune multiorgan syndrome initiated by the European Academy of Dermatology and Venereology (EADV). *J Eur Acad Dermatol Venereol* 2023 Mar 25. doi: 10.1111/jdv.18931.
5 Harman KE, Brown D, Exton LS *et al*. British Association of Dermatologists' guidelines for the management of pemphigus vulgaris 2017. *Br J Dermatol* 2017;177:1170–201.

Mucous membrane pemphigoid

3 Rashid H, Lamberts A, Borradori L *et al*. European guidelines (S3) on diagnosis and management of mucous membrane pemphigoid, initiated by the European Academy of Dermatology and Venereology – Part I. *J Eur Acad Dermatol Venereol* 2021;35:1750–64.
8 Ormond M, McParland H, Thakrar P *et al*. An Oral Disease Severity Score validated for use in mucous membrane pemphigoid. *Br J Dermatol* 2020;183:78–85.
18 Schmidt E, Rashid H, Marzano AV *et al*. European Guidelines (S3) on diagnosis and management of mucous membrane pemphigoid, initiated by the European Academy of Dermatology and Venereology – Part II. *J Eur Acad Dermatol Venereol* 2021;35:1926–48.

CHAPTER 109

Dermatoses of the Male Genitalia

Christopher B. Bunker[1] *and Richard E. Watchorn*[1,2]

[1] University College London Hospitals and Chelsea & Westminster Hospitals, London, UK
[2] Beaumont Hospital, Dublin, Ireland

PART 10: SPECIFIC SITES, SEX & AGE

Rook's Textbook of Dermatology, Tenth Edition. Edited by Christopher Griffiths, Jonathan Barker, Tanya Bleiker, Walayat Hussain and Rosalind Simpson.
© 2024 John Wiley & Sons Ltd. Published 2024 by John Wiley & Sons Ltd.

Introduction

Male patients with non-sexually transmitted and non-urological skin problems commonly present to genito-urinary or urology clinics where the training and expertise are not orientated to adequate dermatological diagnosis and treatment [1].

Careful dermatological evaluation, including a full history and complete examination, usually allows confident clinical differential diagnosis. A biopsy and other investigations are sometimes indicated. It is important to consider the possibility of sexually transmitted disease or a urological disorder and refer accordingly.

Itching, rashes and tumours are the major components of general dermatology and the genito-crural area is not spared. The pruritic diseases that may affect the region are listed in Boxes 109.1, 109.2 and 109.3 and the causes of genito-crural intertrigo (any dermatosis affecting skin folds associated with occlusion and friction) are listed in Boxes 109.4 and 109.5. Itch occurring in the absence of specific diagnostic skin lesions is not usually confined to the genito-crural area, but if so it should not be labelled as psychogenic until all possible causes have been excluded. The intensity with which itch can be perceived in the ano-genital area may be a result of the vagaries of cortical representation afforded the region in the sensorium as well as anxiety about exposure to sexually transmitted disease and genital cleanliness.

While this chapter concerns male genitalia, it bears acknowledgement that patients with male genitalia may not identify as male; judicious use of gender terminology is particularly important in this context.

Box 109.1 Common causes of genital pruritus

- Eczema/dermatitis
  - Exogenous
    - Contact
      - Irritant
      - Allergic
  - Endogenous
    - Atopic
    - Seborrhoeic
    - Lichen simplex
- Psoriasis
- Lichen sclerosus
- Lichen planus
- Perianal streptococcal dermatitis (referred itch or involvement by direct extension to base of scrotum)
- Erythrasma
- Herpes simplex
- Candidosis
- Tinea
- Onchocerciasis (in developing countries)
- Phthiriasis
- Scabies

Reproduced from Bunker CB. *Male Genital Skin Disease*, 2nd edn. London: Bruce Shrink, 2019. © 2019, with permission from the author.

Box 109.2 Rare causes of genital pruritus

- Insect bites/papular urticaria
- Radiodermatitis
- Hirsutism (frictional irritation)
- Hyperhidrosis
- Fox–Fordyce disease
- Urticaria and dermographism
- Dermatitis herpetiformis
- Chlamydia
- Gonorrhoea
- Syphilis
- Other sexually transmitted diseases
- Trichosporosis
- Larva currens
- Cutaneous larva migrans
- Onchocerciasis (in western practice)
- Bowen disease
- Extramammary Paget disease
- Langerhans cell histiocytosis
- Drugs
- Foods
- Senescent pruritus
- Dysaesthesia syndromes

Reproduced from Bunker CB. *Male Genital Skin Disease*, 2nd edn. London: Bruce Shrink, 2019. © 2019, with permission from the author.

Box 109.3 Causes of genital itching in the absence of fixed clinical findings

- Symptomatic dermographism
- Contact urticaria
  - Non-immunological/allergic (e.g. mechanical friction of pubic hair, topical substances)
  - Immunological (latex, body fluids)
- Contact dermatitis
- Incognito disease
  - Psoriasis
  - Candidosis
  - Scabies
- Drugs and foods
- Senescent pruritus
- Delusional infestation
- Unexplained
- Dysaesthesia syndromes
- Psychosexual

Reproduced from Bunker CB. *Male Genital Skin Disease*, 2nd edn. London: Bruce Shrink, 2019. © 2019, with permission from the author.

Structure and function of the male genitalia

The penis is the male organ of urinary elimination and sexual function (for the insemination of the female). The prepuce

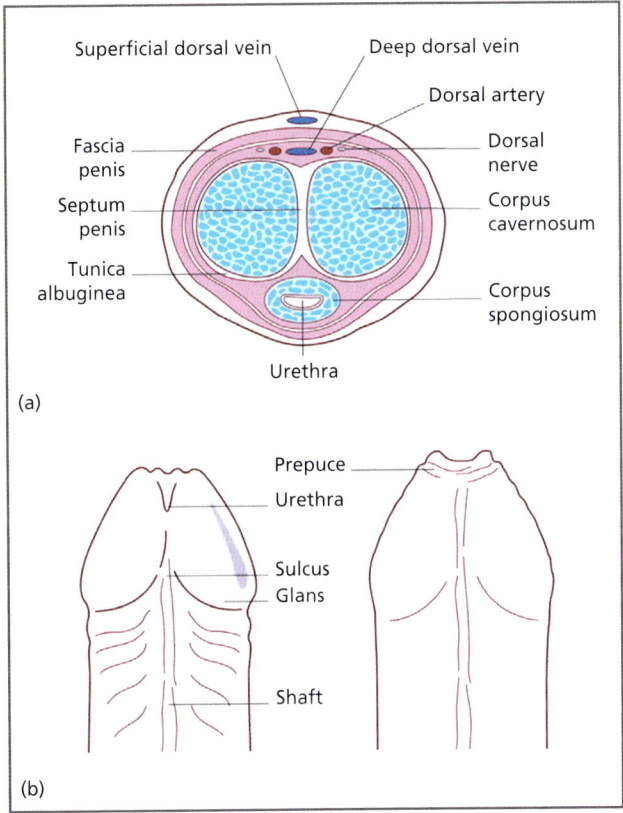

Figure 109.1 (a) Cross-section of the body of the penis. (b) Circumcised and uncircumcised glans penis. Adapted from *Last's Anatomy*, 9th edn. Reproduced from Bunker CB. *Male Genital Skin Disease*, 2nd edn. London: Bruce Shrink, 2019. © 2019, with permission from the author.

and its secretions provide physical and immunological protective functions, and it has erogenous properties (e.g. forms part of the penile dartos muscle and the corpuscular receptor-rich ridged band), but none of these is indispensable for erogenous function in copulation or other sexual activity [1]. The scrotum maintains the testes at the ideal temperature for spermatogenesis. The male genital structures are illustrated in Figure 109.1. The *anatomical position* is that of full penile erection.

The anatomy is explained by the embryology [2]. At about the third week of fetal development, mesenchymal tissue from the primitive streak forms cloacal folds around the cloacal membrane, joined anteriorly and cranially to form the genital tubercle, posteriorly and caudally to form an annulus. The cloacal membrane is thus divided into uro-genital and anal membranes craniocaudally, and lateral genital swellings appear as precursors of either the scrotum or labia majora.

Fetal and testicular androgens then induce lengthening of the genital tubercle to form first an urethral groove and then the urethral canal. The urethral epithelium of the penis is therefore derived from endoderm. Initially, it is incomplete cranially where the glans has developed from the genital tubercle. The glandular urethra and the meatus form from an invading canalising cord of ectoderm. The scrotal swellings fuse posteriorly at about 14 weeks but are empty until birth.

The prepuce [1] is formed by a midline fusion of ectoderm, neuroectoderm and mesenchyme, resulting in a pentalaminar structure consisting of (from the inner layer outwards) squamous mucosal epithelium, lamina propria, dartos muscle (also found in the penis and scrotum), dermis and glabrous skin. The preputial fold progressively extends, but there is also an ingrowth of a cellular lamella. It then fuses with the mucosa of the glans. The female analogue is the clitoral hood.

The ano-genital area is densely endowed with eccrine and apocrine sweat glands. Also in plentiful number are holocrine sebaceous glands, usually in association with hair follicles but also occurring

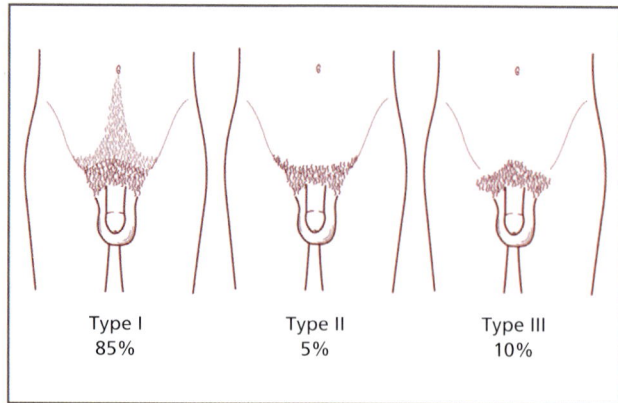

Figure 109.2 Normal distribution of pubic hair in men (three types). After McGregor [3]. Reproduced from Bunker CB. *Male Genital Skin Disease*, 2nd edn. London: Bruce Shrink, 2019. © 2019, with permission from the author.

as free glands at some sites such as the anal rim or around the coronal sulcus (Tyson glands). These secretions exist to lubricate hair, lubricate the mucocutaneous junctions to assist in the voiding of excreta and protect the epithelia from irritation, and to lubricate the penis for sexual activity (probably mainly the retraction of the foreskin rather than the penetration of the introitus and vagina).

Pubic hair appears in puberty as vellus hair that is focally replaced by terminal hair. The pattern of pubic hair in men is different from that in women, and its distribution varies widely between men. McGregor [3] defined three patterns (Figure 109.2). Generally, the abdominal wall, pubic mound, groins, scrotum and perineum are hairy but the natal cleft, perianal skin, distal penile shaft, prepuce and glans are hairless.

The pattern of keratinisation of the epithelium is different throughout the ano-genital area, particularly at the mucosal junctions, the prepuce and distal penile shaft and the glans in the circumcised male. The spectrum of differentiation of the male uro-genital tract is manifest in the expression of differing epithelial cytokeratins [4].

History and examination

The symptomatology of genital dermatology is more extensive than the standard symptomatic presentation of skin disease. This obliges the clinician to elicit symptoms resulting from sexual dysfunction (e.g. soreness, pain, bleeding or tearing on intercourse) [1] and the components of sexual function (erection, lubrication, libido, ejaculation, orgasm, fertility), urinary dysfunction (frequency, discharge, dysuria) or colorectal symptomatology (pain, bleeding, discharge).

Complete skin examination is mandatory to elicit important signs at extragenital sites. The physical examination of the male at any age is incomplete without examination of the penis and scrotum (but this is frequently not carried out in general clinical settings). Urologists teach that there are three primary reasons for careful examination of the scrotum: pain, swelling and absence of contents. The presence or absence of the prepuce (foreskin), phimosis or paraphimosis should be sought and the foreskin retracted gently (if present). The gluteal and crural folds should be parted to allow adequate inspection. Sometimes it is useful to elicit

dermographism of the inner thighs. Urinalysis is often done as part of the initial assessment (diabetes is an important cause of candidal balanoposthitis).

Findings specific to the male genitalia include phimosis, paraphimosis, balanitis and posthitis. Phimosis ('muzzling') refers to a non-retractable foreskin. The literature can be confusing; Rickwood *et al.* [2] have defined it as scarring of the tip of the foreskin. There are many possible causes of phimosis (Box 109.6). In adults, phimosis is often the consequence of lichen sclerosus (LSc), although erosive lichen planus, graft-versus-host disease or cicatricial pemphigoid may also be responsible. Diabetes may be present in up to 36% of adults with acquired phimosis [3,4], which may be due to obesity-induced LSc [5]. In boys, the histological findings may be normal in nearly half of those circumcised [6]. This finding does not exclude LSc or other dermatoses, since the prepuce may not be the seat of the disease, but might contribute to it.

Box 109.6 Causes of phimosis

- Non-specific balanoposthitis (e.g. in diabetes)
- Lichen sclerosus
- Lichen planus
- Hidradenitis suppurativa
- Crohn disease
- Cicatricial pemphigoid
- Chronic penile lymphoedema
- Penile intraepithelial neoplasia
- Cutaneous lymphoma
- Kaposi sarcoma

Reproduced from Bunker CB. *Male Genital Skin Disease*, 2nd edn. London: Bruce Shrink, 2019. © 2019, with permission from the author.

Paraphimosis refers to a foreskin fixed in retraction. Although some authors have used the term to describe a foreskin that is tight in retraction around the flaccid penile shaft, 'waisting' or 'constrictive posthitis' may be better terms [7]. Rickwood [8] has said that paraphimosis results from 'abuse' not disease of the foreskin, but some medical causes can be identified (Box 109.7).

Box 109.7 Causes of paraphimosis

- Acute contact urticaria
- Acute allergic contact dermatitis
- Lichen sclerosus
- Vigorous sexual activity or abuse
- Topical treatments (e.g. imiquimod, 5-fluorouracil)

Reproduced from Bunker CB. *Male Genital Skin Disease*, 2nd edn. London: Bruce Shrink, 2019. © 2019, with permission from the author.

Balanitis is inflammation of the glans penis; posthitis is inflammation of the prepuce [9]. Balanoposthitis means inflammation of the glans and prepuce and can be regarded as a special form of intertrigo (Boxes 109.8 and 109.9). By definition, therefore, balanoposthitis cannot normally occur in the circumcised male, but with age and obesity men may acquire a 'pseudo' foreskin, with attendant risks. Generally, dermatologists feel that balanitis, posthitis and balanoposthitis are probably more commonly caused by inflammatory and pre-cancerous dermatoses, in contrast to genito-urinary physicians, who teach that most cases are caused by infection, usually with *Candida* [10,11]. However, the evidence for *Candida* as a primary cause of balanoposthitis is not strong [12], although diabetes should always be excluded.

Box 109.8 Common causes of balanoposthitis

- Eczema
  - Exogenous
    - Allergic contact
    - Irritant contact
  - Endogenous
    - Seborrhoeic
- Psoriasis
- Reactive arthritis
- Lichen sclerosus
  - Zoon plasma cell balanitis
- Gonorrhoea
- Human papillomavirus
- Herpes simplex
- Candidosis (in the context of diabetes or secondary to another primary penile dermatosis, e.g. lichen sclerosis)

Reproduced from Bunker CB. *Male Genital Skin Disease*, 2nd edn. London: Bruce Shrink, 2019. © 2019, with permission from the author.

Box 109.9 Rare causes of balanoposthitis

- Crohn disease
- Streptococcal dermatitis
- Staphylococcal cellulitis
- Gonorrhoea
- Syphilis
  - Chancre with balanitis of Follmann
  - Mucous patch
- *Mycoplasma*
- *Trichomonas vaginalis*
- Lymphogranuloma venereum
- Non-syphilitic spirochaetal ulcerative balanoposthitis
- Tinea
- Amoebiasis
- Myiasis
- Scabies
- Eccrine syringofibroadenomatosis
- Erythroplasia of Queyrat
- Kaposi sarcoma
- Chronic lymphatic leukaemia
- Fixed drug eruption

Reproduced from Bunker CB. *Male Genital Skin Disease*, 2nd edn. London: Bruce Shrink, 2019. © 2019, with permission from the author.

The principal causes of male genital ulceration are sexually transmitted and non-sexually transmitted infection, cancer and artefact [13]. Several causes can co-present, especially in HIV/AIDS. Dorsal perforation of the prepuce is a recently highlighted complication of several ulcerative penile diseases, sexually and non-sexually acquired, as listed in Box 109.10 [14,15]. Penile necrosis is a rare but devastating presentation with an important differential diagnosis.

Box 109.10 Causes of dorsal perforation of the prepuce

- Hidradenitis suppurativa
- Pyoderma gangrenosum
- Florid condylomata
- Podophyllin
- Chancroid
- Herpes simplex

Investigations

In genito-urinary clinics, application of 3–5% acetic acid to the penis has been used as an aid to the clinical diagnosis of viral warts and is held to reveal subclinical infection [16] but is not felt to be clinically useful in dermatological practice so is not in routine use. Human papillomavirus (HPV) polymerase chain reaction (PCR) screening suggests that the acetowhite test is not very specific [16–18]. Penoscopy (i.e. the use of a colposcope and acetowhite testing) is not practised by dermatologists. There is an increasing literature on the utility of dermoscopy in the differential diagnosis of genital dermatoses. A penis biopsy is not often necessary but can be informative in carefully selected cases of suspected neoplasia rather than the differential diagnosis of the inflammatory dermatoses [19,20]. It is safe to use small amounts of epinephrine (adrenaline) with the local anaesthetic. In practice, 1–3 mL of lidocaine + 1 in 200 000 adrenaline is adequate for most diagnostic biopsies. A penile ring block is useful for bigger excisions. Beware of the distal ventral midline area where the urethra is very close to the skin surface. It is often not necessary to suture a punch biopsy site but two 5/0 Vicryl Rapide surface sutures can be inserted to help haemostasis and shorten the healing time.

Normal variants

Normal male genital variants include pigmentary variation, hair variation (as discussed earlier), skin tags, pearly penile papules, sebaceous prominence, melanocytic naevi, prominent veins, angiomas and angiokeratomas, common congenital abnormalities and circumcision.

Skin tags are common in the groins, especially of obese men. They may catch on clothing, bleed and become infected. Treatment is by electrodessication or scissor amputation and cautery. Fibrosed haemorrhoids result in perianal skin tags. Larger, fleshier, more oedematous skin tags should arouse the suspicion of Crohn

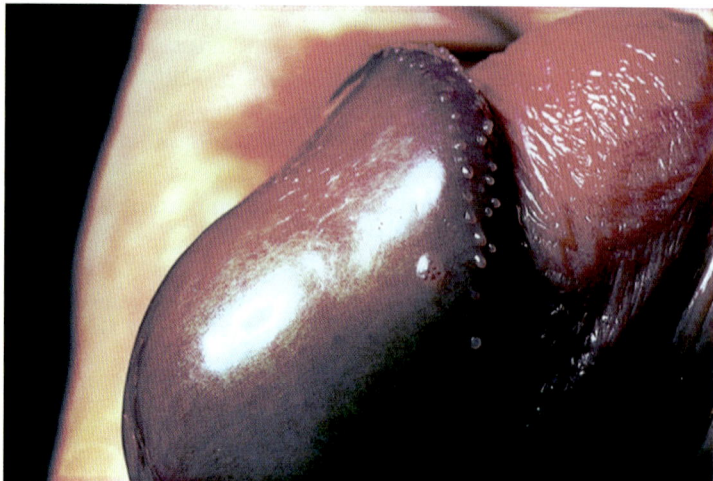

Figure 109.3 Pearly penile papules. Courtesy of Dr D.A. Burns, Leicester, UK.

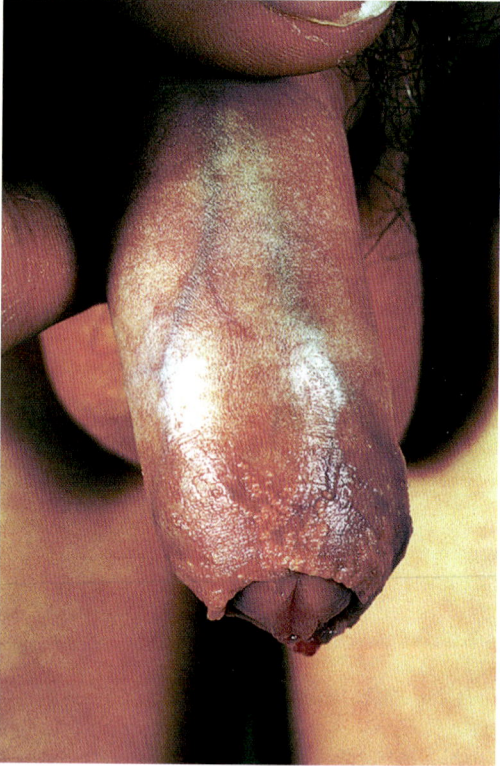

Figure 109.4 Prominent sebaceous glands on the penis. Courtesy of Dr F.A. Ive, Durham, UK.

disease and can predate gastrointestinal disease by several years. Sigmoidoscopy and biopsy should be considered [1].

Pearly penile papules are common; they may be found in up to 50% of men [2,3]. They present as flesh-coloured, pink, smooth, rounded, 1–3 mm papules, occurring predominantly around the coronal margin of the glans, rarely on the glans, in rows or rings (Figure 109.3). Ectopic lesions on the penile shaft have been reported [4]. They are frequently mistaken for warts and misdiagnosed as Tyson glands or ectopic sebaceous glands of Fordyce. The patient is often an anxious adolescent. Disproportionate concern and impact on life suggest the possibility of body dysmorphic disorder (BDD). The histology is that of angiofibroma. The lesion is analogous to other acral angiofibromas such as adenoma sebaceum, subungual and periungual fibromas, fibrous papule of the nose, acquired acral angiofibroma and oral fibroma [5]. Reassurance is usually sufficient but cryotherapy and laser treatment can be effective [6,7].

Sebaceous gland prominence, Tyson glands, sebaceous hyperplasia and ectopic sebaceous glands of Fordyce are all virtually synonymous, common, normal variants of the skin of the scrotal sac and penile shaft, but they may cause concern to the patient (Figure 109.4). They have been held to be very rare or their presence doubted at all [8]. Fordyce's condition also commonly affects the vermilion border of the lips. Naevoid linear lesions on the penile shaft have been seen [9–11]. The glans can be affected [12]. Reassurance is usually all that is required, but BDD can occur.

Congenital and acquired melanocytic naevi are not uncommon in the male genital region. It is possible that naevi on the penis occur more frequently in patients with the atypical naevus syndrome, but this has not been formally documented. Genital epithelioid blue naevus is very rare [13]. A man who developed multiple blue naevi on the glans penis has been described [14]. Spitz naevus has been described [15]. Divided or 'kissing' naevus (analogous to the entity recognised on the eyelids) has been reported, with one component located on the glans and the other on the distal penile shaft or prepuce, separated by uninvolved skin across the coronal sulcus [16,17,18]; melanoma developed in one case [19]. Large 'bathing trunk' naevi frequently involve the ano-genital area and pose significant management problems, including the risk of melanoma.

Prominent veins are common, if not universal, and occasionally give rise to concern. Vascular white spots are sometimes seen on the glans, and are possibly analogous to Bier spots seen on the palms and forearms.

Cherry Campbell de Morgan angiomas may, unusually, be confined to the genitalia. Angiokeratomas on the genitalia have also confusingly been given the Fordyce eponym (Figure 109.5). They

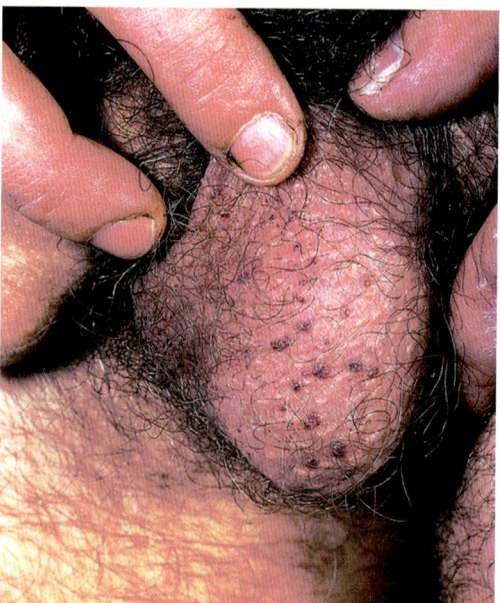

Figure 109.5 Scrotal angiokeratoma of Fordyce. Courtesy of Dr D.A. Burns, Leicester, UK.

are usually multiple, blue to purple, smooth, 2–5 mm papules on the scrotum; angiokeratomas occur rarely on the penile shaft [20] and glans [10,21]. The role of local venous hypertension in the causation of these lesions is controversial [22]. Angiomas and angiokeratomas may bleed following trauma. The differential diagnosis includes angiokeratoma corporis diffusum, acquired capillary and cavernous haemangiomas, Masson tumour, glomus tumour, epithelioid haemangioma, bacillary angiomatosis, Kaposi sarcoma and epithelioid haemangioendothelioma. One case of florid genital angiokeratomatosis has been associated, perhaps coincidentally, with corporeal papular xanthomatosis [23]. Most patients are content with reassurance, and a biopsy is not usually necessary. Hyfrecation, electrocautery or laser ablation [24] can be offered, but lesions recur. Appearing in some contexts, such as HIV infection or follow-up for genital cancer, they can cause alarm [25]. Diffuse angiokeratomas should alert the physician to the possibility of Fabry disease, a rare X-linked lysosomal storage disorder.

The foreskin

The prepuce has been present in primates for 65–100 million years and its function is controversial [1–4]. It is usual for it to be adherent to the glans at birth. Four per cent of boys have a retractable foreskin at birth, 15% at 6 months, 50% at 1 year and 80–90% at 3 years; the process should be complete by 17 years [5]. The foreskin varies in length and retractability: 'short' and 'long' variants are seen.

Circumcision

Circumcision, surgical removal of the prepuce, has been performed for religious, cultural or medical reasons throughout history [1] and a variety of techniques or alternative surgical procedures are now employed [2,3]. Worldwide, it has been estimated that approximately 25% of men have been circumcised [4].

There is some controversy around routine neonatal circumcision [5,6–8]. The UK General Medical Council (GMC) undertook a review of infantile circumcision in 1997, which 'demonstrated widely conflicting views in society that neither doctors nor the GMC can resolve' [9]. The debate still rages although some policy makers now endorse the procedure for derived health benefits [10]. The effects of circumcision on male sexual function and sensitivity are also disputed [11,12].

During infancy, circumcised boys have a higher incidence of penile problems than the uncircumcised, but after infancy the situation is significantly reversed [13,14]. Circumcision decreases the total bacterial load of the penis (coronal sulcus) and in particular decreases the abundance of putative anaerobic bacterial families, and reduces microbiota biodiversity [15,16]. Circumcision is protective against HPV infection, cancer of the penis and urinary tract, and sexually transmitted infections including HSV-2 and HIV [15–17,18–21]. Also, the effects of circumcision on the other outcomes may be small [22] (e.g. urethritis may be more common in the circumcised, whereas ulcerative disease is more common in the uncircumcised).

Circumcision is important in the management of disorders of the penis and the foreskin, including dermatological disease.

Circumcision protects men from certain inflammatory genital dermatoses including seborrhoeic dermatitis and LSc, while variable results have been identified in lichen planus and psoriasis [23–25]. Variability exists between clinicians in the indications for circumcision, especially in children. They include true phimosis, recurrent balanoposthitis, LSc, penile lymphoedema, intraepithelial neoplasia and carcinoma.

The consensus is that circumcision has insignificant adverse effects on health, but it is not risk-free or complication-free. Postoperatively, almost all patients have swelling, and altered sensation (long-term reduced sensation or short-term hyperaesthesia) [26]. The complication rate for therapeutic circumcision (e.g. those performed due to preputial disease such as phimosis or balanoposthitis) is 7.47% with adhesions, meatal stenosis and infections the most frequent complications [27]. Rarely bleeding, necrosis, bridges, chronic penile lymphoedema, fistula, keloid, concealed or buried penis, amputation, necrosis, excessive excision of penile skin, meatitis and meatal ulcer, cysts, chordee, hypospadias and epispadias, amputation neuromas, abnormal sexual behaviour, psychological distress, and dissatisfaction with appearance including penile dysmorphic disorder occur [28–39]. There does not appear to be a risk of sexual dysfunction with circumcision [40,41]. In some developing world settings, the complication rate can be very high [38], implying that better training is required if circumcision is going to become more commonly adopted as part of HIV-prevention strategies [18]. 'Uncircumcision' describes preputial restoration performed throughout history for various reasons [42,43].

As circumcised men age and become obese the penis may retract into the pubic mound – the 'vanishing penis syndrome'. This phenomenon can create a 'pseudoforeskin', especially if the initial circumcision was inadequate or incomplete, and this is likely to explain the observation of dermatoses found characteristically only in uncircumcised men, such as LSc [44].

Congenital and developmental abnormalities

Congenital and developmental anomalies are common, reflecting the complicated embryogenesis and subsequent sexual differentiation of the ano genital region. The dermatologist may not be called upon to make a primary diagnosis but needs to be aware of syndromic associations as well as anatomical and functional abnormalities because these additionally predispose the area to dermatoses and infections. Naevi are discussed earlier. Other common abnormalities include meatal pit, sacral pit, hypospadias, median raphe cysts, canals and sinuses, and ambiguous genitalia [1–3].

Rarer anomalies include hypospadias variants, epispadias, penile hypoplasia, mucoid or urethral cysts, dermoid cyst, juvenile xanthogranuloma, buried penis, urethral atresia, penoscrotal transposition, congenital lymphoedema, lymphangiectasia, lymphangioma, giant preputial sac, megaprepuce, accessory scrotum, haemangiomas, strawberry naevus, white sponge naevus, os penis, congenital megaprepuce, true aposthia, faun tail, aphallia, diphallia, chordee, penoscrotal webbing and micropenis [2,4–7].

Examples of syndromes that may be associated with one or other of these common or rarer anomalies include ano-genital haemangiomas in the PELVIS syndrome (Perineal haemangioma, External genitalia malformations, Lipomyelomeningocele, Vesicorenal abnormalities, Imperforate anus and Skin tag) [8], ano-genital lymphoedema in Hennekam syndrome [9], the micropenis of the MORM syndrome (Mental retardation, truncal Obesity, Retinal dystrophy and Micropenis) and Kabuki make-up syndrome [10,11], the cribriform scrotal atrophy associated with an unusual form of ectodermal dysplasia [12] and genital leukoplakia associated with dyskeratosis congenita [13].

TRAUMA AND ARTEFACT

Definition

Exogenous causes of penile trauma.

Introduction and general description

This is a rarely encountered phenomenon in male genital dermatology clinics.

Penile haematoma and rupture

The genitals may be readily traumatised, including by sexual activity. The penis is very vascular but haematoma formation and 'fracture' (penile rupture) are quite rare [1,2]. Pain, swelling and deformity associated with the history of a cracking noise during strenuous or contorted intercourse characterise the diagnosis. Splitting of the tunica albuginea of the corpus cavernosum can result in urethral damage, haematoma and retention. The prognosis is generally good but Peyronie disease can occur [3]. Injection of drugs for erectile dysfunction can be complicated by haematoma.

Sclerosing lymphangitis

Non-sexually transmitted sclerosing lymphangitis/penile sexually transmitted oedema/Mondor phlebitis/localised penile (sexually transmitted) lymphoedema/penile lymphocele presents with a serpiginous mass in the coronal sulcus. The lesion usually arises after prolonged or frequent sexual intercourse with a passive or unenthusiastic partner; subsequent sexual activity may result in tenderness and enlargement. The circumferential scar left by circumcision may be a predisposing factor. There may be spontaneous resolution or surgical excision may be needed [4]. It is not known whether lymphangitis or phlebitis is the cause [5]. True phlebitis of penile and scrotal veins has been reported in three patients, of whom one had been injured by a golf ball, but the other cases were idiopathic [6]. Its occurrence after taking tadalafil for erectile dysfunction has been used to argue for an anatomical variation in the distal draining subcoronal venous emissary arcade [7]. Thrombophlebitis of superficial penile and scrotal veins is analogous to

Mondor phlebitis of the chest wall, but it may be associated with polyarteritis nodosa and thromboangiitis obliterans [8]. Penile thrombophlebitis has been misdiagnosed as Peyronie disease and has also been the initial manifestation of a paraneoplastic migratory thrombophlebitis resulting from pancreatic cancer [9]. Given the circumstances that usually create the problem, patients should be screened for underlying sexually transmitted infection, despite the appellation [10].

Strangulation of the penis

The penis may be strangulated by ring devices [11,12], including vacuum erection equipment [13], condom rings [14], rubber bands, string, rings (washers), nuts, bushes and sprockets, which are placed deliberately on the penis by the patient for masturbation or to prolong erection [15,16]. In boys, strangulation can occur following experimental use of rubber bands, string or thread to control enuresis, or can result from encoiled hair after circumcision [17]. Penile strangulation – the tourniquet syndrome – causes pain, swelling, urethral fistula, pseudoainhum, gangrene, amputation and even death [18].

Foreign body

Self-instrumentation of the external genitalia may have an auto-erotic, psychiatric, therapeutic (relief of itch [19], aiding voiding, cleaning) or accidental aetiology [20]. Complications include frequency, haematuria, abscess, retention, fistulae and calculi. The diagnosis is made by palpation and radiography. Endoscopic removal is usually possible for foreign bodies below the uro-genital diaphragm.

Glass beads, spheres of plastic or small round smooth stones (even pearls) may be introduced under the skin of the penis for erotic reasons, causing clinical and radiographical confusion. In the Philippines this practice is called 'bulleetus', in Sumatra 'persimbraon', in Korea 'chagan ball' and in Thailand 'mukhsa' or 'tancho' [21,22,23]. Extrusion of a testicular prosthesis has been reported as a cause of scrotal ulceration [24].

If oil, petroleum jelly or silicone is used then a paraffinoma, silicone granuloma or (sclerosing) lipogranuloma can result.

Lipogranuloma

Patients may take it upon themselves to inject various substances with the aim of maintaining erection or enlarging the penis. The consequences may not be desirable. Infection is an obvious risk [25]. Mineral oil, petroleum jelly and silicone introduced into the genital skin can elicit lipogranuloma or paraffinoma. Most cases are self-induced, either to increase penile size or enhance sexual pleasure, but some may be accidental [26,27]. One patient injected his penis with an industrial high-pressure pneumatic grease gun [28]. Idiopathic cases attributed to endogenous fat liberation have been reported, predominantly from Japan [29]. The psychological consequences may be debilitating [30].

Dermatitis artefacta and mutilation

Dermatitis artefacta of the genitalia is rare but does occur. Lesions are typically geometrical, angulated and rectilinear. External trauma can be induced by needles, knives or cigarette burns, and extraneous foreign material may be introduced into the skin (lipogranuloma and silicone granuloma are discussed earlier).

Self-mutilation of genitalia may be performed by those who do not identify as their assigned sex [30]. It may also be undertaken by psychotic individuals [30]. It may be performed as a cultural practice: Australian aborigines create a slit in the penis by opening the urethra ventrally, thereby creating hypospadias; this is called subincision [31,32,33]. Biopsy and other investigations may be necessary to exclude penile cancer. It is important also to consider pyoderma gangrenosum, which is rare but frequently omitted from the differential diagnosis of penile ulceration by non-dermatologists.

Child abuse

Physical and sexual child abuse should be considered in the differential diagnosis of cutaneous disease of the ano-genital area in children (Box 109.11), but signs should be interpreted with caution and re-examination should be avoided [34,35–38]. Child abuse may be erroneously suspected (Box 109.12) when the ano-genital area is involved by a dermatosis or a diarrhoeal illness [39].

Box 109.11 Ano-genital signs of child abuse

- Overall context
- Emotional disturbance
- Passivity on ano-genital examination
- Anal relaxation/dilatation
- Purpura, bruising, tearing
- Signs of sexually transmitted disease

Reproduced from Bunker CB. *Male Genital Skin Disease*, 2nd edn. London: Bruce Shrink, 2019. © 2019, with permission from the author.

Box 109.12 Ano-genital mimics of child abuse

- Nappy rash
- Innocent skin tags and fissures
- Threadworms
- Eczema
- Phytophotodermatitis
- Lichen sclerosus
- Henoch–Schönlein purpura
- Acute haemorrhagic oedema of childhood

- Ano-genital streptococcal dermatitis
- Causes of diarrhoea
  - Haemolytic–uraemic syndrome
  - Crohn disease
- Causes of constipation
  - Hirschsprung disease

Reproduced from Bunker CB. *Male Genital Skin Disease*, 2nd edn. London: Bruce Shrink, 2019. © 2019, with permission from the author.

The significance of ano-genital warts in suggesting possible child sexual abuse is controversial. However, early recognition as a marker for child sexual abuse is in the child's long-term best interest [40].

Other traumatic and artefactual conditions

Sometimes the penis is bitten by another individual or an animal [41]. Purpura and ecchymoses may develop after oral sex ('love bites') or the use of vacuum erection devices [13]. Post-traumatic neuromas may be encountered and be mistaken for genital warts or pearly penile papules [42]. Degloving injuries can occur in accidents with industrial or agricultural equipment [43]. Electrical burns are rare [44]. Sex aids can result in abrasions, eczema and ulceration. Self-circumcision might be attempted, with adverse consequences [45]. Ano-genital tattoos are commonplace [46].

Localised gangrene of the scrotum and penis resulting from arterial embolisation with particulate matter complicating accidental femoral self-injection of heroin in an addict has been reported [47]. Scrotal gangrene from a snake bite has been described [48].

INFLAMMATORY DERMATOSES

Psoriasis

Introduction and general description
This is a common condition that can affect the genital region in isolation or as part of widely distributed disease. Psoriasis of the glans may exhibit circinate morphology (circinate balanitis) and may be severe.

Epidemiology
Approximately 2–3% of the population are said to have psoriasis [1] but it is possible that many more than 2% of men may have or have had ano-genital psoriasis at some time; it is certainly a common ano-genital diagnosis in isolation. Genital psoriasis is found in 30–40% of patients with psoriasis [2–4], but 63% of patients with psoriasis have experienced genital involvement [5]. Men are affected more often than women [4]. In 2–5% of psoriasis patients, the genital area may be the only affected area [6].

Pathophysiology

Psoriasis and its clinical manifestations and the relationship of psoriasis to HIV/AIDS are discussed in other chapters (Chapters 35 and 31).

Clinical features

Presentation

Ano-genital presentations of psoriasis may be vague in symptomatology and non-specific on examination. Itch is very common, but is not universal [5]. Pain, burning and dyspareunia are observed in approximately 50%, and exacerbation following intercourse occurs in a substantial minority [5,7]. Sexual function may also be impacted by the presence of scale, embarrassment or fear of rejection [7–9,10,11].

Clinical features are those of symmetrical sharply demarcated redness, with or without scale; fissuring is also seen [3,4]. Genital appearances may be challenging to interpret, especially on the glans or inner foreskin of the uncircumcised patient. The diagnosis is usually easier in the circumcised male where the tissue is keratinised and morphology is similar to extragenital lesions. A comprehensive examination, with particular focus on typically affected sites, should be undertaken for signs of the disease.

Although the prevalence of genital involvement is increased in patients with inverse psoriasis [12], genital psoriasis is distinct from inverse psoriasis, as only 22% of patients with genital psoriasis also have inverse psoriasis [13]. Non-specific presentation and patient embarrassment may both lead to delayed diagnosis. Failure by physicians to examine may also lead to non-detection of genital involvement in patients with extragenital psoriasis [4].

Risk factors for genital involvement include male sex, overall severity of psoriasis, flexural psoriasis, and involvement of scalp, nails or external auditory canal [2,4,5].

There does not appear to be an association between genital involvement and psoriatic arthritis [2,4,5].

Differential diagnosis

Eczema, fixed drug eruption, lichen planus, carcinoma *in situ*, extramammary Paget disease and dermatitis (atopic, seborrhoeic, allergic contact) are the differential diagnoses.

Investigations

Usually, the diagnosis of psoriasis is clinical, but a biopsy may be necessary (e.g. of a solitary mucosal lesion in an uncircumcised individual) to distinguish psoriasis from Zoon balanitis, lichen planus, carcinoma *in situ* (Bowen disease, erythroplasia of Queyrat) or Kaposi sarcoma. Carcinoma *in situ* and extramammary Paget disease may be misdiagnosed as psoriasis when there are single or several foci on the penile shaft and/or in the groins.

Management

Standard clinical tools such as the Psoriasis Area Severity Index (PASI) and Physician's Global Assessment (PGA) may lead to underestimation of the impact of genital psoriasis as they do not include a specific measurement of these areas [14]. The static Physician's Global Assessment of Genitalia (sPGA-G) is a more helpful tool in determining the clinical severity of psoriasis [9].

Determination of the impact on quality of life may be helpful in informing treatment choices; Genital Psoriasis Sexual Frequency Questionnaire (GenPs-SFQ) and Genital Psoriasis Symptoms Scale (GPSS) are validated scores for assessment of the severity of disease symptoms in genital psoriasis and their impact on a patient's quality of life. The psychological impact of the condition may be more significant than physical symptoms and this must be taken into account when determining treatment options.

Circumcision does not play a role in the treatment of psoriasis; it appears to neither improve nor aggravate psoriasis [5].

Supportive measures play an important role in the management of genital psoriasis [15]. These include reducing of friction with emollients, use of lubricant during sexual activity to minimise symptoms and koebnerisation, omission of soap in favour of emollient soap substitutes, and loose-fitting clothing.

Of patients with genital psoriasis, 45% have never applied treatment to their genital psoriasis [16]. Topical corticosteroids of mild to moderate potency represent first line treatment in genital psoriasis [15]. The literature provides little information on adverse effects of topical corticosteroids in the context of psoriasis [15]. Topical calcineurin inhibitors (tacrolimus, ciclosporin, pimecrolimus) and vitamin D analogues particularly calcitriol are well tolerated and are effective [17–23], although satisfaction with topical treatments in general appears to be low overall [5]. Phototherapy is not recommended for genital psoriasis, due to the risk of genital cancer [24,25], although studies indicate the risk of photocarcinogenesis of NB-UVB is low [26].

A stepwise algorithm for topical therapies has been suggested for patients with genital psoriasis, with varying potencies of topical steroids and/or non-steroidal agents such as tacrolimus of vitamin D analogues, with reported success in an open-label study [27].

Weak tar solutions represent another treatment option. Strong crude tar preparations should be avoided at this site given that ano-genital skin has a propensity to increased absorption of topical agents and because of the risk of genital cancer. Dithranol and tazarotene are usually avoided in this region.

Crisaborole ointment (2%), a topical phosphodiesterase E4 inhibitor approved by the Food and Drug Administration (USA) to treat mild to moderate atopic eczema, has been shown to be effective in ano-genital psoriasis in a small randomised controlled trial [28]. Topical JAK inhibitors are an emerging therapy in dermatology but are not currently routinely available. However, they may prove useful for the treatment of genital psoriasis in the future [29].

Severe or recalcitrant ano-genital involvement in psoriasis may be an indication for systemic treatment, even if the genital region is used in isolation. The evidence base for the efficacy of systemic treatments in genital psoriasis is limited [15]; one study indicates that approximately 25% of patients on conventional systemic agents and biologics have persistent genital involvement [4].

Among biologics that have been studied specifically in genital psoriasis, ixekizumab has been found to be effective, with the majority of patients experiencing either clearance or minimal disease with treatment [30–33]. A randomised controlled trial has also indicated efficacy of secukinumab for genital psoriasis [34]. A small observational study of psoriasis in difficult to treat sites has suggested that adalimumab is effective in genital psoriasis [35]. Apremilast is currently undergoing clinical trials in genital psoriasis [36].

Eczema

Introduction and general description

Eczema and a history of atopy are common in the general population and may be a risk factor for developing male genital skin disease. In a retrospective study of 331 new patients attending a specialist clinic, the most common primary diagnosis was irritant contact dermatitis in 67 patients. Of uncircumscribed patients in the whole cohort, 69% had a history of eczema [1,2]. Eczema is covered in more detail in other chapters (Chapters 39, 40 and 41). Eczema has several clinical manifestations and causes, and may present with genital involvement in isolation.

Clinical variants and presentation

Eczematous dermatoses

Itching and lichenification, particularly around the scrotum, are common presenting problems [2]. Contributory factors include pre-existing dermatoses such as xerosis, atopy, sedentary occupations, long-distance travel, and tight underclothing and trousers.

Irritation is a key adverse exogenous influence to which anogenital sites are vulnerable, and sweat, sebum, desquamated corneocytes, dirt, excreta, sexual secretions, clothing, detergents, toiletries, cosmetics, barrier contraceptives and some therapeutic topical treatments are all potential irritants.

Frequently underrated are the effects of overwashing and the excessive use of soap and toiletries, especially in the presence of skin symptoms or urinary or bowel problems, and particularly if patients feel that they might have been exposed to a sexually transmitted disease.

Lichen simplex

Lichen simplex is not uncommon around the male genitalia and may eventuate from different forms of dermatitis and other dermatoses. It is not usually a flexural condition but can be seen on the penile shaft and scrotum (Figure 109.6). Giant forms (of Pautrier) occur, giving an appearance like the outside of a pineapple [3]. The skin may be broken by excoriations and become secondarily impetiginised or colonised by *Candida*.

Irritant contact dermatitis

Irritant contact dermatitis is relatively common and is caused by non-immunological physical or chemical damage to the genital tissue; nappy (diaper) rash is a common example. Contact allergy requires exclusion with comprehensive assessment and patch testing. It may become superinfected with staphylococci or *Candida*, or both. An erythematous weeping or crusted eruption develops in the area of contact with irritants [4]. Irritant contact dermatitis is typically less florid than allergic contact dermatitis [1]. However, erosion or ulceration may be observed [5]. With chronicity, lichenfication and hyperkeratosis are observed. Ano-genital irritants are discussed earlier and listed in Box 109.13. Friction [6], maceration, overwashing and concomitant ano-rectal or urological disease are the chief influences. Irritant sources may be surfactants, e.g. sodium lauryl sulphate in soaps and other cleansers, preservatives, fragrances, ammonia or adhesives. Men also may be overusing soaps after sex or masturbation, or do so as a reflex response to

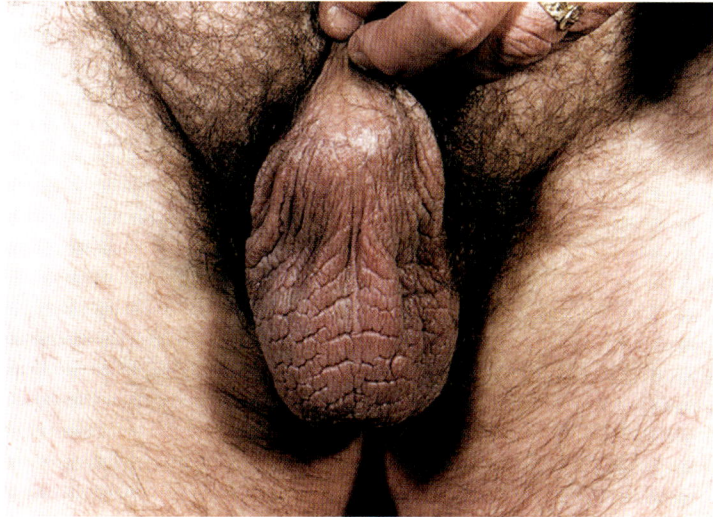

Figure 109.6 Scrotal lichen simplex. Courtesy of Dr F.A. Ive, Durham, UK.

developing redness or itching in their genital region [7]. It may develop due to antiseptic agents in emollient soap substitutes [8]. There may be an association with atopy; Birley *et al.* [9] diagnosed irritant dermatitis in 72% of patients presenting to a genito-urinary clinic with 'balanitis' (probably meaning balanoposthitis) of whom a possible 67% had a history of atopy, but none of these patients was patch tested. Topical 5-fluorouracil used to treat keratoses at extragenital sites has caused genital irritant dermatitis [10]. Topical retinoids for the treatment of genital warts may also cause irritant dermatitis [11]. The scrotum is particularly vulnerable to irritants [12]. Erosive dermatosis of Jacquet, classically described in infants in association with irritancy by urine, may also be observed in adults with urinary incontinence [13,14,15].

Box 109.13 Ano-genital irritants

- Sweat
- Sebum
- Desquamated corneocytes
- Dirt
- Excreta
- Sexual secretions
- Wart treatments (topical retinoids)
- Clothing
- Soap and detergents
- Antiseptic agents
- Topical antibiotics
- Toiletries
- Toilet paper
- Cosmetics
- Solvents
- Contraceptives
- Therapeutic agents
- Friction
- Maceration

Reproduced from Bunker CB. *Male Genital Skin Disease*, 2nd edn. London: Bruce Shrink, 2019. © 2019, with permission from the author.

Allergic contact dermatitis

Patch testing may reveal a diagnosis of allergic contact dermatitis (ACD) in a substantial proportion of patients with ano-genital skin problems [16]. In the genital region, as in other areas, ACD may manifest with redness, oedema, blistering, erosions and ulceration. Other skin conditions affecting the genital area, particularly irritant contact dermatitis, are likely to predispose individuals to ACD [17,18]. The patient may also present with phimosis or paraphimosis, due to oedema [19]. Eczematous symptomatology can appear approximately 1 week after first contact with the allergen if previously unsensitised, or within a few hours if already allergic. More immediate symptomatology and acute redness and angio-oedema suggest a contact urticaria, which can occur with some of the rubber constituents of condoms and gloves [16,20–22]. Allergens may be transferred from another part of the body, such as the hand, to the genital area (e.g. urushiol as in poison oak, poison ivy and poison sumac dermatitis).

Among the most common allergens leading to genital involvement are preservatives, fragrances (in personal care products and medicaments), dyes, rubber vulcanisation accelerators, medications, emulsifiers, corticosteroids, nickel sulphate, surfactants and lubricants [23,24]. Other triggers include tattoos (p-phenylenediamine) and metal piercings (nickel). Allergy to methylisothiozolinone, a ubiquitous preservative, has become an often reported phenomenon [25,26], although legislation in the European Union permits this in limited concentrations and only in wash-off products. Contact allergy to corticosteroids may also develop [27]. Contact with allergens may be indirect, such as fragrances on a partner's face, hands or genitalia [28], known as ACD by proxy dermatitis (synonym 'connubial' dermatitis as relating to the relationship between a couple).

While genital presentations of rubber and rubber accelerator contact allergies are usually observed in sexually active male condom users and their partners, they may also be observed in men suffering incontinence that use external urinary collection devices [29–35]. Patients may become sensitised to the spermicide [36]. Contact allergy to topical anaesthetics, e.g. benzocaine and lidocaine in condoms to delay ejaculation, has also been reported [37]. Contact allergy to benzyl alcohol, a preservative and solvent, has also been reported [23,26,38,39,40]. Lubricants may be either silicone-based or oil-based and may contain formaldehyde, parabens, benzoic acid, propylene glycol as a humectant, flavourings such as strawberry, mint or piña colada, fragrances, colourings, aloe vera and thermoactive substances – all of which may result in contact allergy [23].

Clothing dye dermatitis of the penis and scrotum [17,41,42] is common. Dietary nickel appears to be relevant in ano-genital ACD, but its exact role is not understood [17]. Other reported allergens include coal tar allergy. Amputees who have a prosthetic limb appear to be at high risk of developing a number of contact allergies which may result in penile ACD potentially [43]. Allergens may also come from occupational exposures [44].

Atopic eczema

Genital involvement may occur in up to 45% of patients with atopic eczema (AE), and causes itch, stinging, burning and pain [46,47].

Genital involvement may be associated with poor health-related quality of life, and a proportion of patients indicate impairment of sexual function [46,47,48] and emotional distress. It is not known how genital AE responds to circumcision, or its relationship to sexually transmitted disease. Based on the experience of AE patients, genital involvement appears to receive inadequate attention, with a majority indicating that their dermatologist had not paid any attention to this aspect of their condition [46].

Unlike other common chronic dermatoses such as seborrhoeic dermatitis and psoriasis, AE rarely affects the genital region in isolation. Isolated involvement of the genital region should prompt consideration of differential diagnoses such as contact dermatitis (irritant or allergic), lichen simplex chronicus, Hailey–Hailey disease, tinea cruris and extramammary Paget disease, or rarely secondary syphilis [49–52].

Radiodermatitis

Radiodermatitis is not usually a diagnostic challenge or a therapeutic problem in the acute stage after radiotherapy to the ano-genital skin for skin cancer or internal cancer, e.g. anal. In the chronic state, there may be pruritus together with the typical poikiloderma. Radiotherapy was historically used for the treatment of numerous ano-genital dermatoses over the years, including Bowen disease, erythroplasia of Queyrat, squamous cell carcinoma, psoriasis, Peyronie disease and pruritus ani [53]. Chronic worsening atrophy can lead to fragile skin and erosions especially when the scrotum has been treated. Radiotherapy also confers a long-term increased risk of skin cancer.

Seborrhoeic dermatitis

Genital involvement appears to be highly variable with this common dermatosis [2,54]. Careful examination of other sites typically affected may support the diagnosis, although the groins and penis may be the only sites involved. On the scalp, the face, in the flexures and at ano-genital sites, seborrhoeic dermatitis and psoriasis may be indistinguishable.

Investigations

The diagnosis is usually clinical. Investigations such as patch testing or biopsy are indicated in recalcitrant, persistent or atypical cases, and scrapings for mycology where scale is present.

Management

Management of all forms of dermatitis follows common principles. Irritants should be identified and eliminated or reduced. Where patients are attempting to self-treat the issue with zealous bathing, disinfectants or shower gels, this must be identified and counselling should be undertaken to address this. Soaps should be replaced with emollient soap substitutes.

Patients should be advised to apply emollients frequently and educated in emollient application technique. Patients must also be advised to avoid sources of friction (e.g. vigorous rubbing with towels and toilet paper). Topical corticosteroid ointments of moderate potency are recommended to control the dermatitis. Where secondary infection is present, swabs must be taken and antibiotics prescribed. Topical local anaesthetics should be avoided because of the risk of sensitisation. For specific scenarios, additional treatment may be needed.

Treatment of male genital lichen simplex may require a potent or super-potent topical corticosteroid and/or occlusion. Counselling regarding the itch–scratch cycle is crucial. Systemic treatment such as dupilumab may be required for recalcitrant cases [55]. Surgery is not usually considered as a treatment modality in this condition. However, two cases of extensive giant lichen simplex of the scrotum resistant to medical therapy have been successfully treated by hemiscrotectomy [3,56].

Recalcitrant or florid cases of eczema may merit patch testing to detect ACD. The broad principle of managing ACD on genital skin is elimination of the allergen(s) (Box 109.14), although the condition may persist even after withdrawal of the trigger allergen.

Box 109.14 Allergens of particular relevance to genital contact dermatitis [17,45]

Fragrances	Balsam of Peru
	Hydroxycitronellal
	Geraniol
	Isoeugenol
	Eugenol
	Cinnamic aldehyde
	Cinnamic alcohol
	α-amyl cinnamic alcohol
	Majantole
Food	Nickel (dietary)
Antimicrobial/ antiseptics	Neomycin
	Chlorhexidine
	Benzyl alcohol
	Benzylalkonium chloride
	Fusidic acid
	Polymyxin
	Clotrimazole
	Clindamycin
	Nystatin
	Iodopropynyl butylcarbamate (IPBC)
	Aciclovir
Personal care/ medicaments	Propylene glycol
	Cocamidopropyl betaine
	Wool alcohols/lanolin
	Ethylenediamine
	Methyldibromo glutaronitrile (MDBGN)
	Amidoamine
	Oleamidopropyl dimethylamine
	Oleamidopropyl betaine
	Propolis
	Dimethylaminopropylamine (DMAPA)
	Cocamide diethanolamine
	Lavender oil
	Bufexamac
	Sorbisan sesquioleate
Preservatives	Methylisothiazolinone
	Methylchloroisothiazolinone (MCI)/ methylisothiazolinone (MI)
	Parabens
	Formaldehyde
	Formaldehyde releasing preservatives (bronopol, diazolidinyl urea, DMDM hydantoin, imidazolidinyl urea, Quaternium 15)
	Methyldibromoglutaronitrile
	Ethylenediaminetetraacetic acid disodium salt (EDTA)
Rubber products	Vulcanisation accelerators (thiurams, dithiocarbamates, thiazoles)
	Antioxidants (N-isopropyl-N-phenyl-p-phenylenediamine (IPPD), N-cyclohexyl-N-phenyl-p-phenylenediamine (CPPD) and N,N-diphenyl-p-phenylenediamine (NPPD))
	4-Tert-butylphenol formaldehyde resin
	Ethylenediamine
	Carba mix
	Black rubber mix
Corticosteroids	Hydrocortisone
	Hydrocortisone-17-butyrate
	Tixocortol-21-pivalate
	Triamcinolone
	Budesonide
	Desoximetasone
Local anaesthetics	Benzocaine
	Lidocaine (lignocaine)
	Dibucaine
	Cinchocaine
Textile dyes	Disperse blue 106
	Disperse blue 124
	Disperse orange 3
Additional components in condoms	Local anaesthetic (benzocaine)
	Spermicides (nonoxynol-9)
	Fragrances
	Dyes
	Flavours
	Lubricants
Lubricants	Formaldehyde
	Parabens
	Benzoic acid
	Propylene glycol
	Ethylenediamine
Miscellaneous	Compositae
	Bisphenol A epoxy resin
	Calendula
	Roman chamomile
	Testosterone

In florid or acute cases of genital dermatitis, treatment with potassium permanganate soaks, systemic corticosteroids and antibiotics may be required.

Where seborrhoeic dermatitis is asymptomatic, reassurance may suffice. When treatment is desired, topical antifungals (such as clioquinol, nystatin and imidazoles) as ointments, creams, lotions or shampoos, and mixtures of the same agents with mild and moderately potent topical corticosteroids, can be effective. Topical calcineurin inhibitors are also effective in seborrheic dermatitis [57]. In severe cases, patients with concomitant seborrhoeic folliculitis, or in patients with HIV/AIDS, treatment with an oral imidazole and/or an oral tetracycline may be suitable.

Zoon balanoposthitis

Introduction and general description

An asymptomatic, inflammatory and irritant condition of the glans and mucosal prepuce. Zoon balanoposthitis is probably overdiagnosed.

Epidemiology

Zoon plasma cell balanoposthitis is a disorder of the middle-aged and older uncircumcised male [1,2], although an analogous condition has been reported to afflict the vulva, mouth, lips [3] and epiglottis [3,4].

Pathophysiology

Since the original report in 1952 by Zoon, a Dutch dermatologist, there have been many accounts in the literature, but the aetiopathogenesis remains poorly defined. There is no evidence of an infectious cause and immunohistochemical findings suggest that Zoon balanoposthitis represents a non-specific polyclonal tissue reaction [5,6], consistent with an irritant process. The presence of the foreskin is pivotal; the potential curative effect of circumcision raises the possibility that retention of urine and squames between two tightly apposed and infrequently and inadequately separated and/or inappropriately bathed, commensally hypercolonised, desquamative, secretory epithelial surfaces leads to a disturbed 'preputial ecology' and excessive frictional trauma (Zoon balanoposthitis is often located on the dorsal aspect of the glans and/or the adjacent 'kissing' prepuce, sites of maximal friction on foreskin retraction), and irritation by urine [7,8,9,10].

The evidence suggests that Zoon balanoposthitis is a chronic, reactive, principally irritant pattern brought about by a dysfunctional prepuce.

The existence of Zoon balanoposthitis as a distinct entity has been questioned [8,11–13] and the literature contains many examples of purported cases of the entity that describe or exhibit clinically pathognomonic features of LSc [8,14,15,16,17]. Cases of premalignant and malignant transformation in the context of Zoon balanoposthitis have been reported [18,19,20,21]. Phimosis has been described in Zoon balanitis [8] and proposed by some authors to predispose to the condition [14,22].

Pathology

The classic histology is of epidermal attenuation with absent granular and horny layers, and diamond- or lozenge-shaped basal cell keratinocytes with sparse dyskeratosis and spongiosis. Epidermal erosion may be present [5,6,8]. There is a band of dermal infiltration with plasma cells of variable density. Extravasated erythrocytes, haemosiderin and vascular proliferation are also seen. Although Zoon stressed the presence of the plasma cell infiltrate in this condition, the plasma cell numbers can be very variable [9,10,23]. In biopsies reported as Zoon balanoposthitis, these histological features are inconsistently present and findings are often non-specific [12]. In some cases, such non-specific features mask other inflammatory patterns. The histological diagnosis of 'Zoon balanitis' is thus ill-defined and appears to be loosely applied to a number of variable pathological features. It has been proposed that these

histological features should be considered a reactive pattern rather than a histological diagnosis [12]. Zoonoid histological features may be present in LSc [24] and other dermatoses.

Clinical features

The presentation is classically indolent and asymptomatic, although staining of the underclothes with blood has been reported [25]. Well-demarcated, glistening, moist, bright red or autumn brown patches involve the glans and visceral prepuce, with sparing of the keratinised penile shaft and foreskin (Figure 109.7). Erosions may be present [5,6,8]. The navicular fossa may be involved. Other signs include dark red stippling – 'cayenne pepper spots' – and purpura with haemosiderin deposition, solitary or multiple lesions of differing sizes (guttate or nummular), characteristically symmetrical about the axis of the coronal sulcus and 'kissing'. Although vegetative and nodular presentations have been recorded, atypical or unusual morphology should be viewed with great suspicion and biopsied [9,10].

Differential diagnosis

The differential diagnosis includes LSc, erosive lichen planus, psoriasis, seborrhoeic dermatitis, contact dermatitis, fixed drug eruption, secondary syphilis, histoplasmosis [26], erythroplasia of Queyrat [27] and Kaposi sarcoma. A confident clinical diagnosis is not always possible or safe [8,10,28], so a biopsy is advisable if there is any diagnostic uncertainty and the pathologist should be asked to look for concomitant disease. Frank cases of LSc, lichen planus, Bowenoid papulosis (BP) and penile cancer often appear

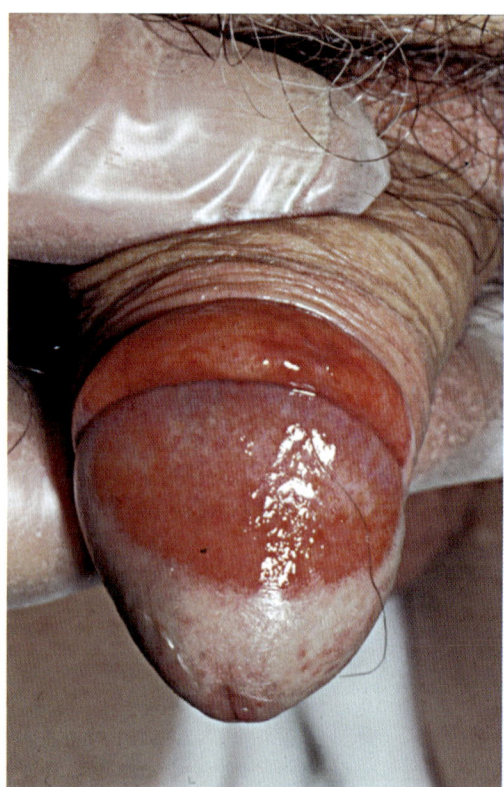

Figure 109.7 Zoon balanitis. Symmetrical moist redness of the glans and prepuce. Courtesy of Professor C.B. Bunker and with permission from Medical Illustration UK, Chelsea & Westminster Hospital, London, UK.

PART 10: SPECIFIC SITES, SEX & AGE

to have Zoon balanitis-like changes on clinical examination and on histology [10,28]. In other words, the signs of Zoon balanitis may be secondary to underlying preputial disease [10]. It is likely that some of the clinical and histological variants that have been reported [29–31] are a consequence of this phenomenon. Zoon balanitis indicates a dysfunctional foreskin and a more common or more sinister dermatosis may be concealed [10]. Most patients diagnosed with Zoon balanoposthitis probably have clinically subtler underlying LSc.

Investigations

The diagnosis of Zoon balanoposthitis is usually clinical. Biopsy is subject to 'sampling error'; Zoonoid inflammation may be present in LSc, therefore Zoonoid histological features may erroneously 'confirm' a diagnosis of Zoon balanitis if a biopsy is taken from areas of clinically Zoonoid inflammation, whereas if taken from a different area of the same genital dermatosis, it may illustrate histological features of LSc.

Zoonoid inflammation and balanoposthitis may resemble erythroplasia of Queyrat [5], and biopsy is indicated in clinically equivocal cases.

Management

Zoon balanitis may be treated with topical corticosteroid (potent or super-potent strength is usually needed, testifying to the likelihood of the underlying condition *actually* being LSc) and improved washing practices, although it usually persists or relapses [9,10], ultimately requiring circumcision in such cases [9,10]. In uncircumcised patients, follow-up may allow detection of fibrosis suggestive of LSc, or cancerous transformation. Case reports concerning the use of topical calcineurin inhibitors have appeared [17,32–34] but given the frequency of underlying LSc already highlighted they are not recommended [35]. Various other treatments have been reported to be effective, including topical imiquimod 5% and erbium:YAG or carbon dioxide laser [10,36–41].

Lichen sclerosus

Definition and nomenclature

LSc is a common inflammatory dermatosis with a predilection for ano genital skin.

Synonyms and inclusions
- Lichen sclerosus et atrophicus
- Balanitis xerotica obliterans
- Posthitis xerotica obliterans

Introduction and general description

LSc is a chronic inflammatory scarring dermatosis with a genital predilection that incurs a risk for penile carcinoma. It is a common cause of dermatological problems in the genital region.

Epidemiology

The prevalence of LSc is unknown. It is perceived that symptoms are underreported by patients and even when reported, the condition is often unrecognised and/or misdiagnosed by clinicians [1]. A further impediment to establishing accurate epidemiological statistics is the presentation of the condition to and management by multiple separate specialties including dermatology, genitourinary medicine and urology [1]. Genital LSc (GLSc) is more common than extragenital or oral disease, but there may (rarely) be concomitant involvement of these sites. In adults, ano-genital LSc is said to be about 10 times more common in women than men. Perianal disease is very rare in the male. The age of presentation is bimodal [2], although peak incidence occurs in the sixth and seventh decades of life [3,4]. The first report of male genital LSc (MGLSc) in children appeared only in 1977 [5]. MGLSc may be much more frequent than is generally supposed in early childhood, being diagnosed histologically in 14–95% of prepuces removed for phimosis [6,7].

Pathophysiology

The inflammatory process in LSc appears to be driven by $CD4^+$ and $CD8^+$ T-lymphocytes; $CD1a^+/HLA-DR^+$ dendritic cells and the expression of several cytokines including tumour necrosis factor α (TNF-α), interferon γ (IFN-γ) and interleukin 1 (IL-1) is increased [8,9–12].

The aetiology of male and female GLSc remains contentious and the current consensus is that it is multifactorial [13]. Among proposed aetiological factors are genetic predisposition, autoimmunity, immune dysregulation, aberrant fibrogenesis, occluded exposure to urine, infection, site-specific dysbiosis and epithelial susceptibility. There is an inconsistent association with organ-specific autoimmune disease [10,14–16,17,18,19,20,21,22,23–25,26] and atopy [27], and a variable association with *ECM1* autoreactivity (probably an epiphenomenon) [21,28,29]. HLA distributions in GLSc do not support an autoimmune association [18,25,30,31–33].

MGLSc is extremely rare in those circumcised at birth and circumcision is usually curative, indicating a pivotal role for occlusion and the foreskin in its aetiopathogenesis [2,34]; occlusion is also likely to underlie the relationship with obesity [35]. The presence of the histopathological features of LSc in a percentage of acrochordons (skin tags) suggests that occlusion of flaccid skin is a pathogenic factor [36]. Evidence points to the crucial role of chronic occluded exposure of susceptible epithelium to urine [2,37–40].

In contrast with women, the male perineum or perianal skin, which is not subject to chronic urinary irritation, is spared in MGLSc [2]. A high incidence of MGLSc is seen in patients with hypospadias, including those who have been circumcised [1,41]. MGLSc is also commonly encountered in patients with failed hypospadias repair [42].

There is increasing evidence to support the role of urine; these include clinical observations of LSc following fistulating genital piercing, and occurrence around ureterostomies and urethrostomies [43,44–46], including in the perineal area, which is usually unaffected in male patients. Recently, a prospective cross-sectional study of female patients demonstrated an association between urinary incontinence and LSc [47]. Patients also frequently report postmicturising dribbling or 'micro-incontinence' [48]. Nuclear magnetic resonance spectroscopy of urine has not identified a single culpable chemical constituent of urine [49].

The potential role of infectious agents has been subject to much investigation. HPV has been extensively studied but does not appear to play a causative role [30,50–59,60,61–75]. Borreliosis

[17,76,77,78–85,86,87–89] and hepatitis C [90] have been implicated and refuted. The epidemiology and clinical tenor of LSc are not those of an infectious or sexually transmitted disease: it is rarely seen in sexual partners [91]. Microbes have received renewed investigative attention; however, rather than frank infection, recent studies have focused on the potential role of dysbiosis. Differences in microbiota composition have been demonstrated between MGLSc and controls, in both the balanopreputial sac and urinary tract [92,93], with increased relative abundance of *Fusobacterium* spp. in the balanopreputial sac of MGLSc patients compared with healthy controls, and its abundance in the balanopreputial sac is closely associated with that of the urine. *Fusobacterium* spp. exhibit properties and associations that could be relevant to the defining characteristics of MGLSc, specifically pro-inflammatory and pro-carcinogenic properties [94]. *Fusobacterium* spp. mediate carcinogenesis via Wnt/β-catenin signalling, which plays a role in penile carcinoma [95]. Circumcision significantly reduces the abundance of *Fusobacterium* spp. [96,97], which could explain the curative effect of circumcision in LSc.

Pathology

The epidermis is atrophic with flattening of the rete ridges and basal cell hydropic degeneration. Variable hyperkeratosis may be seen. The superficial dermis is oedematous and hyalinised [98–100]. Deep to the hyalinised zone is a band-like lymphohistiocytic infiltrate. In early cases, the inflammatory infiltrate may be found superficially. Plasma cells are seen in addition to lymphocytes and histiocytes. Inflammation may be minimal or absent in late stages. Telangiectatic vessels are common, as is purpura. Perivascular lymphocytic infiltrates and lymphocytic vasculitis are sometimes seen [101]; the occasional association of endarteritis led originally to the usage of the term 'obliterans' [102]. Sometimes, LSc may be difficult to differentiate from lichen planus, and criteria to assist, in the vulva, have been proposed by Fung and LeBoit [103]. The histological features may simulate mycosis fungoides [104].

Clinical features

LSc of the penis may be asymptomatic, but diverse, sometimes vague, symptomatology is usually encountered at rest or during or after sexual congress. Patients may describe itching, burning, bleeding, tearing, splitting, rash, haemorrhagic blisters, discomfort with urination and narrowing of the urinary stream, and/or they may be concerned about the changing anatomy of their genitalia. Discomfort or pain occurs during or following sexual intercourse (male dyspareunia) in a majority of patients. In a substantial minority it is asymptomatic [23,105]. The development of secondary phimosis in school-age boys is highly suggestive of LSc [106]. In the older male, persistent primary phimosis or the secondary development of phimosis in a previously retractable foreskin may be related to LSc [107].

The clinical features of MGLSc are highly variable. It may present initially as a non-specific balanoposthitis [107]. The skin may exhibit whitened atrophic skin (leukoderma) on the glans or prepuce (Figure 109.8), or a more subtle appearance of etiolation. There may be telangiectasia and sparse purpura. Shiny-red 'moist' erythema of the glans and/or the inner prepuce may be evident, resembling the classic description of Zoon balanitis. Predominant

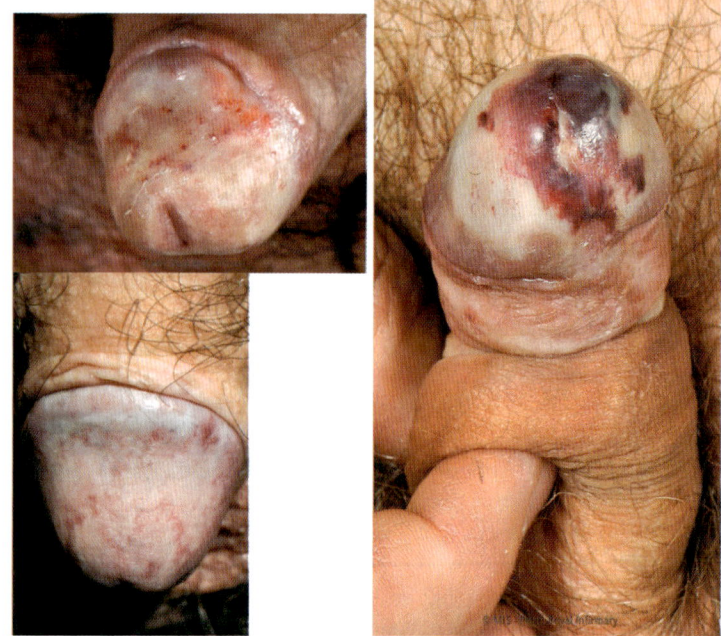

Figure 109.8 Chronic lichen sclerosis of the glans with pallor, fibrosis and area of telangiectasia. Courtesy of Dr A. Affleck, Dundee, UK.

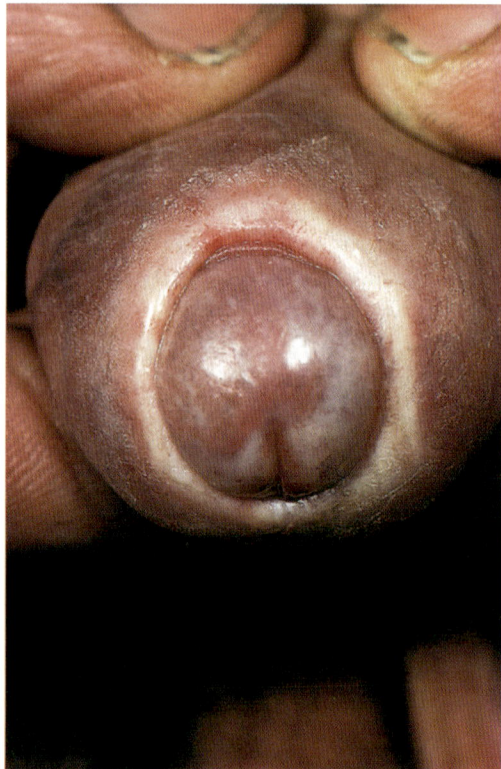

Figure 109.9 Lichen sclerosus causing phimosis. Courtesy of Dr D.A. Burns, Leicester, UK.

purpura, angiokeratomas, bullae, erosions and ulceration may be encountered. Postinflammatory hyper- and hypopigmentation are often seen.

Phimosis or paraphimosis may be evident (Figure 109.9); there may also be incomplete phimosis or paraphimosis caused by a constrictive posthitis, whereby constriction of the prepuce

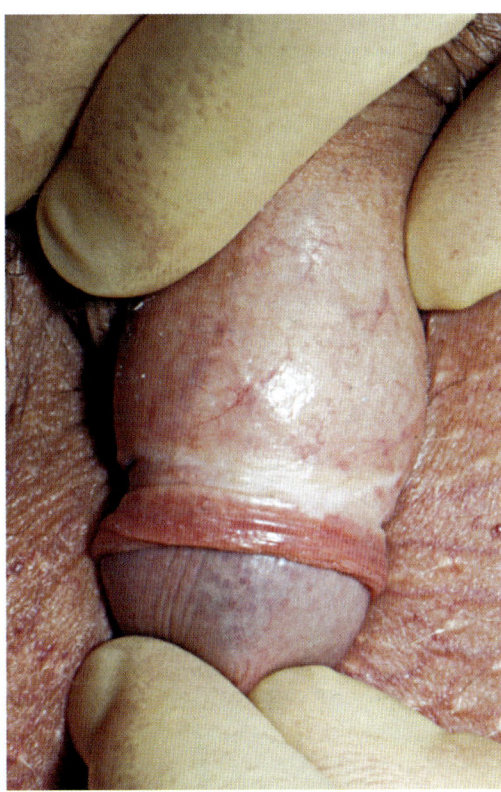

Figure 109.10 Lichen sclerosus. Sclerotic band of the prepuce causing a constrictive posthitis 'waisting'. Courtesy of Professor C.B. Bunker and with permission from Medical Illustration UK, Chelsea & Westminster Hospital, London, UK.

creates an 'hourglass' appearance when the prepuce is retracted (Figure 109.10). This sign has also been called 'waisting' [107]. Signs may, however, may be more subtle, with meatal 'pin hole' narrowing. Chordee (congenital or acquired due to frenular disease) may be evident to varying degrees.

Adhesions are common. Detection of small subcoronal adhesions may require retraction of the corona, whereas transcoronal adhesions are more easily visualised. Loss of anatomical definition may manifest in dissolution or effacement of the normally sharply defined architectural features. For example, extensive transcoronal adhesions may cause complete loss of the coronal sulcus but milder expressions of the disease may lead to a more subtle effacement of the coronal sulcal architecture. Similarly, the frenulum may be effaced. Adhesions may also be observed in the inguinal folds. Pearly penile papules may be destroyed. The arrangement of the naviculo-meatal fossa and meatus may be abnormal, as described earlier. Involvement of the meatus occurs in approximately 16% of cases and it may lead to stenosis in 12% of affected individuals manifesting in a 'pin hole' appearance [21,23,107,108].

LSc in men may extend into the navicular fossa, the penile urethra or rarely the bulbar urethra resulting in urinary symptoms, including impaired urinary stream and dysuria [109,110]; LSc is the commonest cause of penile urethral strictures in young and middle-aged adults [109]. The involvement of the anterior urethra can be serious; in some cases, urethral strictures may cause obstructive nephropathy and renal failure [109].

MGLSc may rarely be hyperkeratotic [107]. Pseudo-epitheliomatous micaceous and keratotic balanitis (PEMKB) is

a rare entity believed to represent a form of chronic, untreated MGLSc with a high risk of transformation to verrucous carcinoma [6,111,112]. It manifests as irregular, thin or thick scaly patches on the glans [113,114].

MGLSc may also develop in association with chronic penile oedema [115]. There may be evident signs of dysplasia, carcinoma *in situ* (usually erythroplasia of Queyrat clinically, whereas the histological type of penile intraepithelial neoplasia (PeIN) usually associated with both male and female GLSc is the differentiated pattern) or of an invasive cancer.

Lichen planus, non-specific balanoposthitis and very rarely mucous membrane pemphigoid are in the differential diagnosis. A biopsy is not usually required for the diagnosis of MGLSc, as it is a clinical diagnosis [116,117,118]. Moreover, histology in LSc may be non-specific, particularly in early cases, or lead to misdiagnosis of the underlying condition [1]. Reliance on histological diagnosis may also lead to progression of the disease when typical histological features of LSc are not demonstrated [108,118]. However, biopsies should be performed if there is clinical doubt or if the result might impact on management decisions, e.g. PeIN, particularly in the context of lesions that are eroded, ulcerated or verrucous.

Investigations

A biopsy is required in cases of suspected malignant transformation or when PeIN cannot be excluded clinically.

Management

Guidelines for the management of LSc have been published by the British Association of Dermatologists [13].

The aims of treatment are (i) early diagnosis and effective treatment to obtain normalisation of sexual function; (ii) to minimise dermatological and urinary morbidity; (iii) to prevent transformation to penile cancer or pre-cancer (or detect such transformation early where it has already occurred); and (iv) preservation of the foreskin if possible [107,119]. Contact with soap, pubic hair and urine should be avoided; a barrier emollient and a soap substitute are advocated and pubic hair should be trimmed. A super-potent topical corticosteroid (usually 0.05% clobetasol propionate) used under supervision for a finite course (twice daily for 1 month is the authors' practice) is effective [107,120–122]. Super-potent topical steroids can be useful for urethral and meatal disease [123,124]. The use of super-potent topical corticosteroids is usually safe, but herpes simplex and wart reactivation do occur [13,61], and counselling must take this into account. Prophylactic aciclovir merits consideration in those with a history of genital herpes simplex virus (HSV).

The plasticity of the male genital epithelium seems to allow significant remodelling, with the relief of phimosis, improvement of incomplete phimosis or constrictive posthitis, improvement in the histological changes and avoidance of circumcision [107,121,125]. Approximately 50% of patients will achieve a durable remission with medical treatment [126]. Topical clobetasol propionate has been shown to relieve undifferentiated 'phimosis' in many boys and so obviate the need for circumcision [122]. Treatment may prove difficult to apply in cases of severe phimosis [13]. Although currently evidence is lacking for the use of systemic retinoids in LSc generally, they may be of some benefit, particularly in hyperkeratotic LSc [13,127]. The use of topical calcineurin inhibitors is to be deprecated because of the theoretical risk of accelerated carcinogenesis [1,128,**129**,130].

Reasons for failure to respond to medical treatment may include ongoing urinary contact or occlusion (often due to anatomical abnormalities), a coincident second diagnosis such as psoriasis or ACD, or poor adherence to treatment [13]. In cases of genuine treatment failure, circumcision is indicated. Additional surgical options may be offered depending upon the clinical presentation, including division of adhesions in those with extensive coronal adhesions, frenuloplasty in cases of chordee, meatotomy in cases of meatal stenosis or distal urethral strictures, or glans resurfacing in cases of pseudoepitheliomatous keratotic and micaceous balanitis [131,132]. In boys, complete circumcision is the treatment of choice because all affected tissue is removed. Any secondary involvement of the glans probably regresses or resolves. This phenomenon may also occur in adult patients.

Fundamental to planning of penile surgery for LSc is the recognition of the pernicious role in the initiation and progression of MGLSc played by the chronic occluded exposure of genital skin to urine [133]. Causes of failure to respond to circumcision include distortion of meatal anatomy by instrumentation (e.g. during cystoscopy), genital piercing (which may cause fistula formation between the urethra and the skin) and congenital anatomical abnormalities, including hypospadias [1]. A so-called 'neo-foreskin' may develop in obese or elderly patients; this may also cause resistance to treatment by circumcision, or recurrence in those who initially responded to circumcision [1,35].

The vast majority of patients respond to either medical treatment or circumcision; ongoing symptoms were reported by a small minority of fewer than 3% [126]. Superimposed penile dysaesthesia or penodynia may account for some patients with ongoing symptoms that have no clinical evidence of inflammatory activity [13].

Persistent disease requires individualised follow-up and management. Residual burnt-out fibrosed disease on the glans may improve with long-term topical retinoid treatment. Subdermal injection of polydeoxyribonucleotide (a mitogen for fibroblasts, endothelial cells and adipocytes) has been reported [134]. Squamous carcinoma of the penis is the most serious potential complication of LSc [1,13,107]. Carcinoma *in situ* and early microinvasive disease can be difficult to diagnose clinically against a background of LSc [1,107,135]. Squamous hyperplasia and the basal and parabasal dysplasia of the differentiated PeIN seen histologically in association with LSc-associated squamous carcinoma can be subtle and underappreciated by histopathologists and clinicians [136]. The risk of squamous carcinoma complicating MGLSc suggested by the literature is 0–12.5%, depending on the size of study, length of follow-up and approach to management; the latent period may be one to three decades [1,135–143]. Involvement of the glans penis confers a greater risk [137]. The types of squamous carcinoma associated with LSc are the 'usual' and verrucous subtypes [136,144]. One-third to one-half of all established penile cancer is associated with LSc [142,145,146]. The effect of medical and surgical treatment on the subsequent incidence of penile cancer is not precisely known [147,148]. Liatsikos *et al.* [141] report squamous carcinoma of the glans developing in one of eight patients followed up after circumcision for LSc. However, evidence from the large cohorts of patients

reported by Edmonds *et al.* and Kravvas *et al.* suggest that accurate diagnosis and effective medical and surgical management abolish or significantly attenuate the risk of squamous cell carcinoma [23,126]. A subset of patients requires long-term follow-up, including those in whom circumcision has not been performed or disease activity persists despite treatment.

Resources

Further information
British Association of Dermatologists Guidelines
http://www.bad.org.uk/

Patient resources
https://www.bad.org.uk/pils/lichen-sclerosus-in-males/
(Both last accessed November 2022.)

Lichen planus

Introduction and general description
It is a common inflammatory dermatosis with a particular predilection for the oro-genital epithelium [1] (Chapter 37).

Pathophysiology
The aetiopathogenesis of lichen planus is poorly understood. The cytokine profile indicates a Th1 IFN-γ-induced immune response [2]. Drugs can cause a generalised lichenoid eruption; a case of a lichenoid drug eruption confined to the penis resulting from propranolol has been reported [3]. Lichen planus involving the genital region has also been reported as a paraneoplastic phenomenon [4].

The pathophysiology is described in more detail in Chapter 37.

Clinical features
Lichen planus can present in, and remain localised to, the anogenital area, including the groins and perianal skin. Like the classical disease at other sites, it presents as itchy red-purple papules, patches or plaques (Figure 109.11). Lesions may be hyperkeratotic, polygonal or annular morphology, or a combination; the male genitalia represent the commonest site for the annular subtype of lichen planus [5,6]. Wickham's striae, fine white reticular lines, may be prominent. It may rarely exhibit erosive morphology; this subtype is usually painful and is associated with adhesions and scarring. There is a male equivalent of the vulvovaginal syndrome of Hewitt – the genitogingival syndrome – with chronic erosive gingival and genital lesions [7]. Lichen nitidus is a condition that may represent a variant of lichen planus, or an independent entity. It manifests in very small, smooth, translucent and glistening 'micropapules' with an affinity for the penis, specifically the glans penis and prepuce [5]. It is sometimes seen on penile skin in isolation in young Asian males. Lichen nitidus can be difficult to diagnose because the signs may be subtle, even when the lesions are widespread. Hypertrophic penile lichen planus has also been described [8,9].

It may rarely present as phimosis [5,10], more frequently an erosive subtype. The Koebner phenomenon may partly explain the oro-genital predilection [11]. In most cases, ano-genital lichen

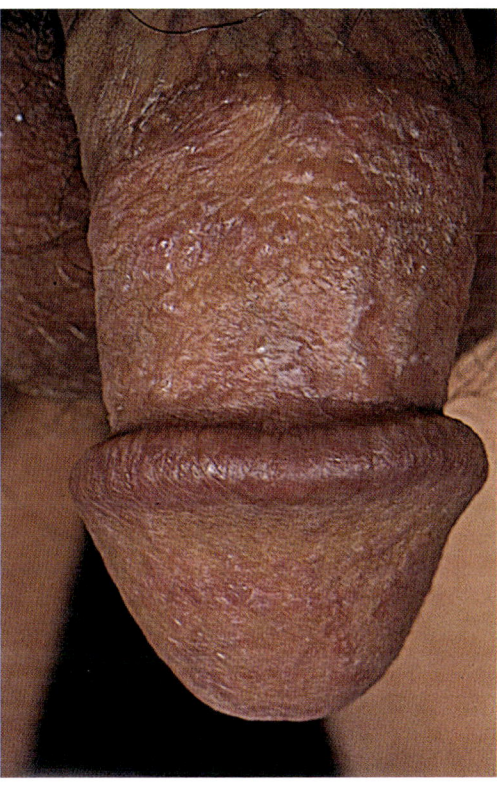

Figure 109.11 Lichen planus. Papules and annular lesions with striae of Wickham on the glans and shaft. Courtesy of Professor C.B. Bunker and with permission from Medical Illustration UK, Chelsea & Westminster Hospital, London, UK.

planus is self-limiting, although some patients remit and relapse. Postinflammatory hyperpigmentation can persist for months or years.

The link between lichen planus and squamous cell carcinoma is unclear. Chronic mucosal erosive lichen planus is associated with a risk of progression to squamous carcinoma, but most reports of this concern oral lichen planus. There are rare reports of squamous carcinoma eventuating from chronic penile dermatoses thought to be lichen planus [8,9,12–17]. Such reports appear to be very rare.

Overlap syndromes in which both LSc and lichen planus are present may occur [18].

Differential diagnosis

The differential diagnosis includes psoriasis, Zoon balanitis, LSc, viral warts, BP and porokeratosis. The differential diagnosis of ano-genital lichen planus is influenced by the morphology; for example, annular lichen planus may resemble porokeratosis, while lichen nitidus may resemble penile pearly papules. Similarly, erosive lichen planus requires specific consideration of infective and neoplastic differential diagnoses.

Complications and co-morbidities

In the follow-up of cases of chronic ano-genital lichen planus, erosive, ulcerative or verrucous features arouse concern about the development of squamous carcinoma.

Investigations

A biopsy is frequently necessary for diagnostic purposes.

Management

The current evidence base for treatment of genital lichen planus is limited. Potent and super-potent topical corticosteroids usually suffice for treatment. Patients are told to continue with the treatment until the lesions are non-itchy and flat; they are warned about postinflammatory hyperpigmentation. Reactivation of genital warts may occur [19]. Calcineurin inhibitors including tacrolimus and ciclosporin have been used in topical and oral forms but are not favoured due to the potential risk of squamous cell carcinogenesis [20–24]. Although evidence varies on the impact of circumcision [25,26], circumcision may be helpful particularly in the context of phimosis [27] or refractory erosive disease [28]. Photodynamic therapy has been reported as effective [29]. Pulsed dexamethasone therapy has been used for erosive disease [30]. Acitretin and secukinumab have been reported as being effective in erosive penile lichen planus [**31,32**].

Chronic penile oedema

Chronic penile lymphoedema is a relatively rare, disfiguring condition that causes sexual dysfunction and phimosis (Chapter 103) [**1**]. It is often chronic, leading to substantial psychosocial and physical morbidity. It has been called tumorous lymphoedema or elephantiasis verrucosa nostra [**2**]. It may be congenital or acquired [**3**].

Pathophysiology

Numerous causes have been described (Boxes 109.15–17).

Box 109.15 Causes of genital lymphoedema

- Idiopathic congenital lymphoedema (Milroy disease)
- Lipogranuloma and silicone granuloma
- Strangulation of the penis
- Iatrogenic
- Radical abdomino-pelvic surgery
- Radiotherapy
- Granulomatous lymphangitis
  - Crohn disease
  - Sarcoid
- Postinfectious
  - Cellulitis and erysipelas
  - Chronic penile lymphoedema
  - Chancroid
  - Lymphogranuloma venereum
  - Tuberculosis
  - Leprosy
  - Syphilis
  - Filariasis/onchocerciasis
- Carcinomatosis
  - Lymphatic involvement
  - Lymphatic blockage
- Lymphoma

Reproduced from Bunker CB. *Male Genital Skin Disease*, 2nd edn. London: Bruce Shrink, 2019. © 2019, with permission from the author.

Rigorous clinical evaluation is important [3]. Causes of ano-genital lymphoedema and penoscrotal swelling are listed in Boxes 109.15, 109.16 and 109.17.

Box 109.16 Commoner causes of penoscrotal swelling

- Paraphimosis
- Foreign body
- Strangulation of the penis
- Iatrogenic
  - Contact dermatitis
  - Continuous ambulatory peritoneal dialysis
  - Genital oedema resulting from raised right heart filling pressure in ITU
  - Postoperative
  - Postradiotherapy
- Varicocele
- Hydrocele
- Strangulated hernia
- Priapism
- Peyronie disease
- Epididymitis and orchitis
- Cellulitis
- Idiopathic chronic penile lymphoedema
- Testicular tumours

Reproduced from Bunker CB. *Male Genital Skin Disease*, 2nd edn. London: Bruce Shrink, 2019. © 2019, with permission from the author.

Box 109.17 Rarer causes of penoscrotal swelling

- Lymphangiectasia (with chylous reflux) [7]
- Giant haemangioma
- Urethral diverticulum
- Segmental urethral hypospadias
- Accessory scrotum [8,9]
- Herniation of scrotal contents into penile shaft
- Foreign body
- Haematocele
- Lipogranuloma and silicone granuloma
- Aortic aneurysm [10]
- Scrotal fat necrosis
- Henoch–Schönlein purpura
- Familial Mediterranean fever
- Acute haemorrhagic oedema of childhood
- Pancreatitis
- Infected cyst
- Abscess of corpus cavernosum [11]
- Fournier gangrene
- Tuberculosis
- Paracoccidioidomycosis
- Amputation of septic limbs in diabetics
- Giant scrotal tumours (e.g. neurilemmoma)
- Epithelioid haemangioma
- Kaposi sarcoma
- Epithelioid haemangioendiothelioma
- Lymphoma
- Sarcoma
- Drugs (e.g. angio-oedema caused by lisinopril)

Reproduced from Bunker CB. *Male Genital Skin Disease*, 2nd edn. London: Bruce Shrink, 2019. © 2019, with permission from the author.

Several factors may be involved in any individual case, and the aetiopathogenesis of penile lymphoedema requires careful consideration in each patient. Once the process of lymphatic damage has been initiated, each episode of acute or acute-on-chronic infection leads to loss of elastic fibres, hyperplasia of the collagenous connective tissue and scarring, resulting in permanent swelling with progressive loss of function and worsening appearances [4]. It is therefore likely that the worse the oedema becomes, the lower the chances of full recoverability.

Acquired lymphoedema can be the result of neoplasia, surgery or radiation to the pelvis [4]. Radical cancer surgery and/or radiotherapy to the ano-genital area and the lymphatics can cause swelling because of lymphoedema, early or delayed [5,6]. Infections may also be culpable [7,8] and may complicate or aggravate cases due to other causes. Bacteria appear to be the most common cause, in particular *Streptococcus*, which is known to be lymphatolytic [9,10]. Penile sexually transmitted oedema has been associated with gonococcal and herpes infection, and scabies infestation, and resolves after treatment of the underlying disease [11].

Inflammatory disorders that distort lymphatics may be culpable, including granulomatous disorders such as sarcoidosis or Crohn disease (CD), and non-granulomatous disorders such as hidradenitis suppuritiva [12,13,14,15]. Of note, genital (metastatic) CD may develop before bowel involvement, or in the context of occult and asymptomatic CD; CD may be present in up to one-third of patients with genital lymphoedema [13,16,17,18,19,20].

Many cases are viewed as idiopathic; idiopathic cases may be due to primary lymphatic hypoplasia but comprehensive work-up may reveal an underlying cause.

Reactive causes include trauma (including compulsive masturbation, chronic strangulation and circumcision) [21–23], venous thrombosis and angio-oedema. Localised genital lymphoedema can be associated with obesity (due to neolymphovascularisation of the scrotal region below the tunica dartos muscle and its associated hypertrophy) [18,24] However, scrotal lymphoedema after weight loss (resulting from lymphatic stasis in the redundant skin) has also been reported [25]. Acute idiopathic oedema of childhood is self-limiting; adult cases are very rare [26]. Congenital defects of the inguinal canal and other non-inguinal peritoneal leaks can lead to scrotal and penile swelling as a manifestation of dialysate oedema in patients with end-stage renal failure treated by continuous ambulatory peritoneal dialysis [27]. Contact allergies may also cause genital lymphoedema [28].

Peno-scrotal oedema has also been attributed to continuous ambulatory peritoneal dialysis [29], amputation of septic limbs in diabetes [30] and acute necrotising pancreatitis [31]. It may also be caused by disorders of fluid balance.

Clinical features

Patients with chronic penile oedema present with chronic swelling of the penis, foreskin, scrotum, pubic mound, buttocks and thighs, which may be warm and red [16]. The penis may resemble a saxophone. Some cases of penile lymphoedema are transient and self-limiting. In others, there may be intercurrent attacks of cellulitis and/or erysipelas with systemic symptoms and partial or complete remission of the oedema.

Investigations

Investigations should be directed at elucidating possible underlying causes and predisposing factors, as discussed earlier (Boxes 109.15, 109.16 and 109.17). Investigations required in the work-up include imaging, and serological and faecal screening diagnostics, and may include biopsy (Box 109.18). Computed tomography or magnetic resonance imaging of abdomen and pelvis may be performed [32] to delineate the subcutaneous lymphatic oedema and exclude other causes of lymphatic obstruction; it may illustrate features of occult inflammatory bowel disease. Imaging of lymphatic channels is not particularly helpful [21]. Other tests include screening for sexually transmitted diseases and filariasis (in cases of previous travel history to endemic areas), antistreptolysin antibody titre (ASOT) and faecal calprotectin [33] to screen for CD. Genital biopsy may be performed if specific diagnoses such as CD or sarcoid are being considered; the risk of delayed healing must be considered, and diagnostic tissue may be difficult to obtain, leading to a false negative.

Box 109.18 Evaluation of penile lymphoedema

- Consider in all patients:
  - History (focused on onset, associated symptoms, travel, constitutional, urethral, gastrointestinal and respiratory symptoms)
  - Physical examination (focused on identifying extent of oedema, associated cellulitis and possible bacterial portals of entry)
  - Imaging of abdomen/pelvis (ideally magnetic resonance imaging)
  - Surgical opinion (for suspected acute surgical causes)
- Based on these findings, consider:
  - Investigations including:
    - Screening for sexually transmitted infection
    - Screening for filarial infections
    - Serum angiotensin converting enzyme
    - Antistreptolysin O titre
    - Faecal calprotectin
    - Chest radiography
    - Genital skin biopsy
    - Patch testing
    - Multidisciplinary discussion led by initial results

Management

Treatment may comprise a multifaceted approach, tailored to the individual case and its aetiology. Management options are informed by the cases and series of chronic penile oedema that have been reported [1,16,18,34], and the principles include early aggressive treatment with antibiotics, prevention of recurrent episodes of cellulitis with antibiotic prophylaxis, aggressive treatment of relapses,

surgical debulking and removal of the grossly dysfunctional pre-puce, and long-term follow-up.

As outlined earlier, all cases of peno-scrotal oedema require aggressive treatment at first presentation to optimise outcome, as inadequate treatment can increase the risk of lymphatic scarring and subsequent recalcitrant oedema [16,35]. Glucocorticoids are most appropriate in patients with acute and rapid presentation of oedema.

Long-term treatment with lymecycline, erythromycin, clarithro-mycin, clindamycin, clindamycin plus rifampicin, amoxicillin–clavulanic acid, trimethoprim, sulphamethoxazole plus trimetho-prim or ciprofloxacin appears to ameliorate and stabilise the process. Antibiotics may be alternated or rotated in relapsing and remit-ting disease. Patients should be evaluated, treated and counselled regarding prevention for dermatoses, particularly tinea pedis, that cause fissures or erosions in the skin because these can serve as a portal of entry for bacteria.

Treatment directed to CD, sarcoid or hidradenitis suppurativa should be instituted as appropriate; a multidisciplinary approach with gastroenterology or respiratory input may be appropriate in the case of CD or sarcoid.

The aim of medical treatment is to minimise sufficiently preputial and penile oedema to allow therapeutic debulking circumcision [18,35]. Plastic repair or skin grafting using full- and split-thickness skin grafts may be necessary after excision of affected tissue [16,35–37] and may lead to improvement in quality of life [16,38]. Prophylactic antibiotics may need to be continued long term after surgery.

MISCELLANEOUS INFLAMMATORY DERMATOSES

Non-specific balanoposthitis

Balanoposthitis presents a wide differential diagnosis. Sexually transmitted disease, eczematous dermatoses, psoriasis, lichen planus, LSc, Zoon balanitis, cicatrising pemphigoid and penile carcinoma *in situ* need to be considered. However, in practice, clin-ical signs may be non-specific and diagnostic investigations may not contribute to a specific diagnosis. Where specific causes have been excluded, the term non-specific balanoposthitis is assigned [1,2]. Non-specific balanoposthitis is a relatively common diag-nosis in male genital dermatology [3,4], runs a chronic relapsing course and is likely to reflect a dysfunctional foreskin. Symptoms of dyspareunia are common. Microbiological investigations yield higher rates of positive results in balanoposthitis patients than controls, including *Staphylococcus aureus*, group A and group B streptococci, *Candida albicans*, *Mycoplasma genitalium* and *Malassezia* spp. [5,6,7,8], although identification of these organisms does not necessarily signify causation. Syphilis may present as balanitis, termed 'syphilitic balanitis of Follman', which typically presents with clear erosions [9]; however, subtle forms of syphilitic balanitis have been reported [10].

The principles of management include supportive therapy of emollients, avoidance of soap and other irritants, and potent or super-potent topical corticosteroids. Treatment for candidosis may be considered. Diagnostic investigations include swabs, patch testing and biopsy.

Non-specific balanoposthitis often proves recalcitrant to medical treatments [11], and in these cases circumcision must be considered. Circumcision may yield a specific diagnosis in some cases.

Ulcerative disease and penile necrosis

The causes of genital ulceration are listed in Boxes 109.19 and 109.20, and the causes of penile necrosis in Box 109.21. Many of the causes are discussed in this or other sections.

Box 109.19 Common causes of genital ulcers

- Trauma
- Behçet disease
- Pressure sores
- Aphthae
- Pilonidal sinus
- Anal fistula
- Anal fissure
- Erythema multiforme/Stevens–Johnson syndrome
- Hidradenitis suppurativa
- Crohn disease
- Chancroid
- Donovanosis/granuloma inguinale
- Lymphogranuloma venereum
- Syphilis: primary chancre
- Squamous cell carcinoma

Reproduced from Bunker CB. *Male Genital Skin Disease*, 2nd edn. London: Bruce Shrink, 2019. © 2019, with permission from the author.

Box 109.20 Rare causes of genital ulcers

- Extrusion of testicular prosthesis
- Embolisation
- Dermatitis artefacta
- Penile necrosis
- Spontaneous scrotal ulceration
- Degos malignant atrophic papulosis
- Calciphylaxis
- Haematological
  - Hypereosinophilic syndrome
  - Langerhans cell histiocytosis
- Drug reaction
- Inflammation
- Autoimmune bullous diseases
  - Bullous pemphigoid
  - Cicatricial pemphigoid
  - Linear IgA disease
- Necrobiosis lipoidica
- Dermatomyositis

- Pyoderma gangrenosum
- Sarcoid
- Erythema elevatum diutinum
- Necrotising vasculitis
  - Granulomatosis with polyangiitis
  - Polyarteritis nodosa
  - Systemic lupus erythematosus
  - Idiopathic systemic vasculitis
  - Hereditary spherocytosis with vascular necrosis
- Infections
  - Staphylococcus
  - *Pseudomonas*
  - Ecthyma gangrenosum
  - Necrotising ano-rectal ulcer in leukaemia
  - Gonorrhoea
  - Chancroid
  - Donovanosis (granuloma inguinale)
  - Lymphogranuloma venereum
  - Fournier gangrene
  - Tuberculosis and tuberculides
  - Atypical mycobacteria, e.g. *Mycobacterium ulcerans*
  - Syphilis: snail track ulcers
  - Yaws
  - Non-syphilitic spirochaetal ulcerative balanoposthitis
  - Herpes simplex
  - Herpes zoster
  - Cytomegalovirus (CMV)
  - HIV
  - Chikongunya
  - Deep fungal infections
    - Histoplasmosis
    - Blastomycosis
    - Cryptococcosis
  - Actinomycosis
  - Paracoccidioidomycosis
  - Leishmaniasis
  - Amoebiasis
  - Filariasis
- Neoplasia
  - Extramammary Paget disease
  - Basal cell carcinoma
  - Squamous carcinoma
  - Verrucous carcinoma
  - Sweat gland carcinoma
  - Melanoma
  - Kaposi sarcoma
  - Leukaemia
  - Lymphoma

Reproduced from Bunker CB. *Male Genital Skin Disease*, 2nd edn. London: Bruce Shrink, 2019. © 2019, with permission from the author.

Box 109.21 Causes of penile necrosis

- Decubitus ulcer
- Injection of foreign material
- Spider bite
- Priapism

- Embolism
- Strangulation and tourniquet syndromes
- Vacuum erection device
- Systemic vasculitis [46]
  - Lupus erythematosus
  - Polyarteritis nodosa [47]
- Granulomatosis with polyangiitis
- Diabetes [48,49]
- Chronic renal failure [50]
- Thrombocytopenia
- Polycythaemia
- Cryoglobulinaemia
- Coagulopathy [51]
- Pyoderma gangrenosum
- Calciphylaxis
- Ecthyma gangrenosum
- Fournier gangrene
- Herpes simplex
- Leukaemia
- Mucormycosis (in acute myeloblastic leukaemia) [52]
- Warfarin
- Fixed drug eruption

Reproduced from Bunker CB. *Male Genital Skin Disease*, 2nd edn. London: Bruce Shrink, 2019. © 2019, with permission from the author.

Aphthous ulceration of the penis and scrotum can occur, including in HIV/AIDS, but specific exclusion of sexually transmitted diseases and consideration of other causes of genital ulceration, especially Behçet syndrome, is necessary. The causes are obscure and the histology is non-specific.

Rare cases of spontaneous scrotal ulceration in young, previously fit men have been described – juvenile gangrenous vasculitis of the scrotum [1]. Histology shows non-specific vasculitis and spontaneous resolution can occur. This entity may be related to idiopathic scrotal panniculitis and fat necrosis. Both are distinct from other causes of the acute scrotum in prepubertal boys, presenting as acute, tender, sometimes painful swelling (classically, but not always, after swimming in cold water). Masses may be palpable in the scrotal wall. Otherwise, the patient is well, with no fever or leukocytosis. Idiopathic scrotal necrosis in a 2-month-old boy has been documented by Sarihan [2], where trauma, extreme cold and Fournier gangrene were excluded. Management is expectant and conservative [3,4]. In adults, one case of idiopathic scrotal panniculitis has been reported [5] and another associated with pancreatitis [6].

Subtle or severe oro-genital ulceration can occur in erythema multiforme or Stevens–Johnson syndrome.

Adamantiades–Behçet disease is discussed in another chapter (Chapter 48). Recurrent genital ulceration is not mandatory for the diagnosis; if patients do not have genital ulceration then they must have ophthalmic and dermatological involvement or a positive pathergy test [7]. In practice, there are many patients who have an incomplete syndrome. Other ano-genital manifestations include epididymitis and urethritis [8], spontaneous haematocele from venous rupture resulting from lymphocytic venulitis [9] and erectile dysfunction [10]. The genital ulcers of Behçet disease in men can be very painful and occur anywhere in the ano-genital area, including the perianal skin. Generally, they are larger, deeper, fewer and less recurrent than those in the mouth. Patients with relapsing polychondritis and Behçet disease have been reported, and the acronym MAGIC (mouth and genital ulcers with inflamed cartilage) syndrome has been proposed [11,12]. The histology of Behçet disease is non-specific and does not enable it to be distinguished from idiopathic aphthae, although sometimes necrotising vasculitis can be present.

Scrotal involvement can occur in Hailey–Hailey disease [13].

Degos malignant atrophic papulosis can cause painful penile ulceration that may precede the development of the eruption elsewhere and be associated with fatal involvement of other organs, despite aggressive treatment [14,15].

The hypereosinophilic syndrome involves the skin in up to 50% of cases, with oro-genital ulceration, erythroderma and urticaria. It may occur in HIV infection [16].

Granulomatosis with polyangiitis may present with glans penis ulceration and necrosis; repeated antineutrophil cytoplasmic antibodies (ANCA) estimation may be needed and it may be some time before systemic manifestations declare themselves [17–20,21].

There has been one case report of a patient with erythema elevatum diutinum causing penile ulceration [22]. Three cases of necrobiosis lipoidica have been reported presenting as erythematous ulcerated lesions of the glans penis. One patient was diabetic and also had lesions on the legs [23]; the others had penile lesions only, and were treated with oral pentoxifylline [24,25].

There are a number of case reports of pyoderma gangrenosum, including the variant superficial granulomatous pyoderma [26], involving the penis and scrotum in adults and children (where the ano-genital area is a site of predilection as well as the head and neck) (Figure 109.12) [27,28]. Genital pyoderma gangrenosum may occur following local trauma such as urological surgery [29,30] or treatment for cancer [31], or complicate ulcerative colitis [32] or chronic lymphocytic leukaemia, or it may be idiopathic [33–36].

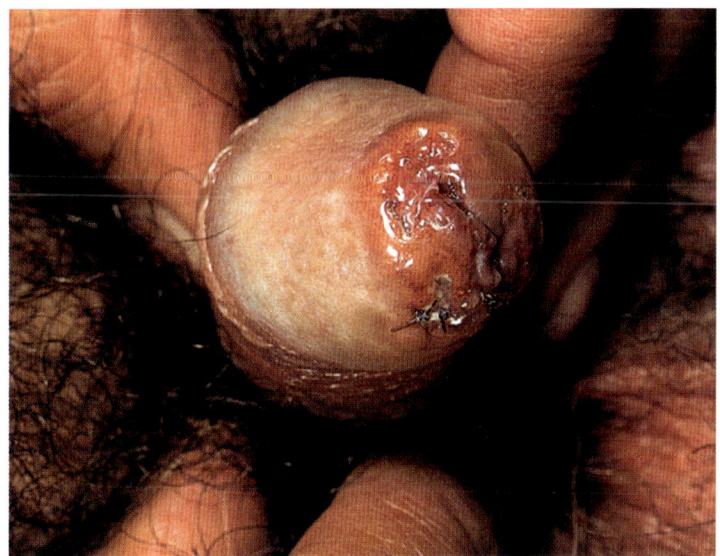

Figure 109.12 Pyoderma gangrenosum in a patient with severe seronegative arthropathy. Courtesy of Dr F.A. Ive, Durham, UK.

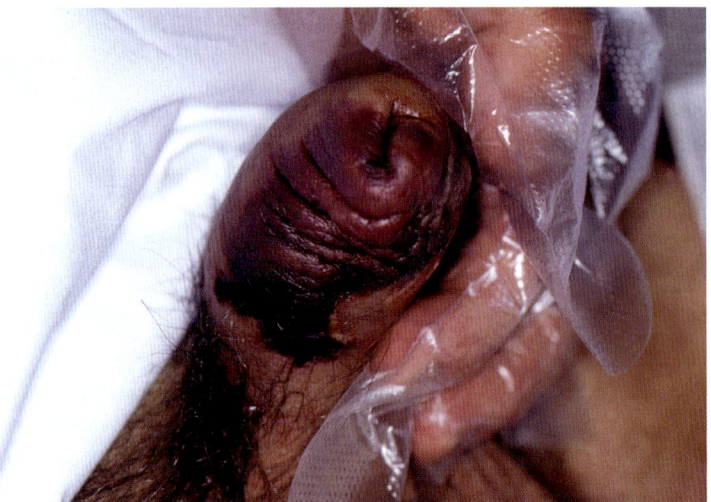

Figure 109.13 Calciphylaxis involving the penis in a patient with end-stage renal disease.

Pyoderma gangrenosum is a diagnosis made when other causes of purulent ulceration, such as infection (sexually acquired and exotic or rare, including Fournier gangrene), malignancy and artefact have been excluded. Systemic treatment is usually required but one case has responded to topical tacrolimus [**37**].

Calciphylaxis is a rare and serious complication of chronic renal failure in which extending ischaemic gangrenous necrosis affects acral tissues and sometimes the thighs, buttocks and genitals (Figure 109.13) [38,39,**40,41**,42,43].

Ulcers in the peno-scrotal region have been reported to appear 2–4 weeks after chikungunya, a novel togavirus arboviral infection that causes fever, headache and arthralgia [44].

There has been one case report of primary cutaneous T-cell lymphoma of the penis presenting with a 2-year history of 'recurrent balanitis', a preputial ulcer and phimosis [**45**]. Other reports include genital ulceration due to amoebiasis, methicillin-resistant *Staphylococcus aureus* (MRSA) infection, tuberculosis and in association with leukaemias [46–50].

Penile necrosis is rare but has been reported with polyartertitis nodosa, systemic lupus, hyperparathyroidism, calciphylaxis, diabetes, vena caval thrombosis and opportunistic fungal infection [51–60].

Pilonidal sinus

Pilonidal sinus very rarely affects the penis [**1**], but when it does it usually occurs in the coronal sulcus [2,3]. Some of the reported cases have been complicated by actinomycosis [2,4], and one has been associated with a dermoid cyst [5].

Penile acne

There is no literature on this condition but it is occasionally encountered. Patients have comedones, papules, pustules and inflammatory nodules of the proximal shaft of the penis. The differential diagnosis should include chloracne. Patients respond to conventional treatment for acne.

Peyronie disease

Peyronie disease [1,2], which affects middle-aged and older men, is a localised fibrotic disorder involving tissue immediately adjacent to the erectile tissues. It presents with pain and curvature on erection, a sensation of a cord within the penis, palpation of a lump or knot, decreased erection distal to the plaque, interference with intercourse and progressive impotence. It may be subclinical in many men, given that 23% of autopsies have shown histological evidence of the condition [1]. Psychological complications and marital difficulties occur. The penis curves towards the lesion, with dorsal curvature being most common. Peyronie (a physician to Louis XV) described nodules as 'rosary beads' but plaques vary in size. It has been associated with systemic sclerosis [**3,4**], and such patients may have penile Raynaud phenomenon [5]. It has occurred as a complication of the use of a vacuum erection device [6], but in most men the cause is unknown. Some evidence has been advanced for an autoimmune pathogenesis [7]. A case complicating chronic graft-versus-host disease has been reported [8].

The differential diagnosis includes congenital curvature, fibrosis secondary to trauma or urethritis and abscess, syphilitic gumma, lymphogranuloma venereum and infiltrative tumours (e.g. lipogranuloma). Penile thrombophlebitis as the initial presentation of a paraneoplastic migratory thrombophlebitis resulting from pancreatic cancer has been misdiagnosed as Peyronie disease [9].

In some men, there may be spontaneous regression. Treatment tends to be by a urologist and includes intralesional corticosteroid injection [**10**], including delivery by Dermojet® [**11**]. Surgery is avoided, but some specialised techniques are available [12]. Symptomatic relief has been claimed following iontophoresis of drugs such as dexamethasone, lidocaine (lignocaine), *para*-aminobenzoic acid and verapamil [**13,14**].

Drug reactions

The penis is a site of predilection for fixed drug eruption. Symptoms are itch or burning. The eruption is acute, with a red plaque, sometimes with central blister formation, erosion and ulceration. Cases have occurred in men after congress with sexual partners who have taken the drug to which they were known to be sensitive: co-trimoxazole, diclofenac, isosorbide and aspirin are the drugs cited [**1,2**]. The differential diagnosis of penile fixed drug eruption includes herpes simplex and localised erythema multiforme.

Ulceration has been reported following the inadvertent subcutaneous injection of papaverine for the treatment of erectile impotence [3]. All-*trans* retinoic acid has been reported to induce scrotal ulceration in a patient with acute promyelocytic leukaemia [4]. Foscarnet is a recognised cause of genital ulceration in HIV-infected patients [**5,6,7,8**]. Nicorandil is a recognised cause of ano-genital and peristomal ulceration and has been reported to have been triggered by circumcision [9,10,11]. Isolated penile ulceration following nivolumab treatment has also been reported [12]. Erosion following the use of topical steroids has been seen. Penile argyria due to chronic application of silver sulfadiazine has been reported [13], as has necrosis following warfarin administration [14,15].

Other inflammatory dermatoses

Bottomley and Cotterill [1] have described an acutely tender erythematous scrotum associated with zinc deficiency in a patient with Crohn disease. Necrolytic migratory redness can be localised to the genitalia [2]. Skin fragility and ulceration in the ano-genital area are features of prolidase deficiency [3].

Autoimmune bullous diseases such as pemphigus can involve the penis (the glans is the usual site) (Figure 109.14), but very rarely in isolation [4]. Pemphigus vegetans presenting with a 4-year history of indolent tender balanitis has been reported [5]. In this case, the glans penis was involved with a moist vegetative plaque with beefy red erosions separating irregular hyperkeratotic mounds [5]. Linear IgA disease commonly involves the mucosae. Mucosal lesions of bullous pemphigoid are uncommon; their presence suggests another diagnosis or an underlying neoplasm.

Cicatricial pemphigoid or mucous membrane pemphigoid is a rare variant of bullous pemphigoid in which blisters affect the skin and the mucous membranes. Skin lesions are usually less widespread than in bullous pemphigoid and they may heal with scarring. Oral lesions predominantly involve the palate and

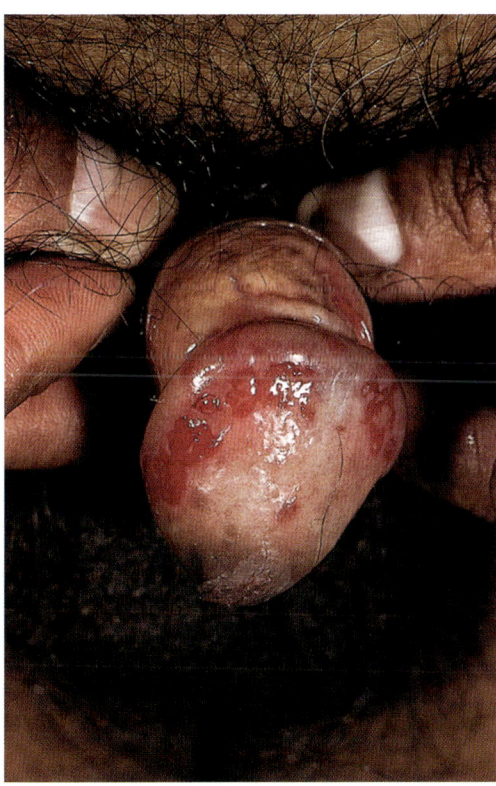

Figure 109.14 Pemphigus of the penis. Courtesy of Dr F.A. Ive, Durham, UK.

gingivae, but there may be oesophageal involvement with dysphagia, and conjunctival disease can lead to blindness. Involvement of the penis may be with blisters, erosions, ulcers, transcoronal adhesions, scarring and phimosis [6,7,8]. Although direct immunofluorescence is usually positive, circulating antibodies to the basement membrane zone are rarely found. The disease often proves difficult to treat, but options include oral corticosteroids, dapsone, cyclophosphamide, azathioprine, mycophenolate mofetil, thalidomide, intravenous immunoglobulin and rituximab.

One patient with Darier disease developed an HPV-16 associated squamous carcinoma of the scrotum during oral isotretinoin treatment; he had not previously had radiotherapy to the genito-crural area [9]. Genito-crural papular acantholytic dermatosis can involve the penis, as can granuloma annulare. Erythematous smooth, round and linear nodules are described in the latter. Most patients are uncircumcised. Extragenital granuloma annulare is uncommon in these patients.

Occasionally, patients with generalised cutaneous sarcoid present with genital lesions [10]. Tender erythematous induration of the distal shaft of the penis and yellowish subcutaneous nodules on the glans have been described [11]. A case presenting with penile ulceration has been reported [12]. Importantly, sarcoid can masquerade as testicular malignancy [12,13–15].

A granulomatous lymphangitis may be found histologically in the investigation of penile lymphoedema [16]. It can be a rare feature of the Melkersson–Rosenthal syndrome. Crohn disease can involve the penis and scrotum, presenting as peno-scrotal lymphoedema or erosions and ulcers [17–20,21,22,23].

Primary cutaneous amyloidosis of the penis is a rare entity. Nodular cutaneous amyloid is associated with systemic disease and up to 10% of cases with associated paraproteinaemia progress to systemic disease [24]. A soft-tissue mass in the penis associated with systemic amyloid has been reported [25]. True penile-limited cutaneous amyloidosis is highly associated with nodular amyloidosis. Primary amyloid of the urethra is very rare indeed, but accurate diagnosis is essential, as its presentation simulates carcinoma, with dysuria, bloody discharge and tender induration of the penis [26], or as an obstructive voiding syndrome, with tender periurethral masses and irregular urethral strictures [27].

One case each of eccrine syringofibroadenomatosis with penile involvement manifesting as a balanoposthitis [28], benign mucinous metaplasia with a preputial 0.6 cm papule replacing the superficial epidermis [29], and mucinous syringometaplasia with an ulcerated papule on the shaft of the penis [30] have been reported.

Acute scrotum is a clinical syndrome defined as acute painful swelling of the scrotum or its contents, usually in boys, accompanied by local signs and general symptoms [31]. It is a urological emergency. The critical differential diagnosis is torsion of the testis or spermatic cord. Other causes include idiopathic scrotal oedema, epididymitis, orchitis, hernia and haematocele. Thromboangiitis obliterans has been found in two cases [32]. Acute scrotal swelling may be a physical sign of primary peritonitis in children and infants [33] or secondary peritonitis resulting from appendicitis, healed meconium peritonitis in the neonate, haemoperitonitis (ruptured spleen) and pseudotorsion resulting from ventriculoperitoneal shunts inserted for hydrocephalus that have migrated into the scrotum from the peritoneum. Acute idiopathic scrotal oedema usually affects children aged 4–12 years. Allergy, infection (umbilical sepsis), trauma, insect bites, urinary extravasation and Henoch–Schönlein purpura have all been considered as causes. It is rare in adults, but cases in association with septic diabetic foot have been reported [34].

Henoch–Schönlein purpura/anaphylactoid purpura/allergic vasculitis may affect the genitalia. Ureteritis, renal pelvic haemorrhage and pain and swelling of the spermatic cord have been reported. The incidence of scrotal involvement ranges from 2% to 38%. Penile shaft involvement is less common and involvement of the glans very rare [35]. In some cases, the presentation has masqueraded as testicular torsion, resulting in unnecessary surgical exploration. Ultrasonography can help to distinguish between them [36]. However, testicular torsion can also be a real and serious complication of Henoch–Schönlein purpura [36].

Acute haemorrhagic oedema of childhood may present as tenderness, redness and swelling of the penis and scrotum with the development of more widespread haemorrhagic lesions [37]. The differential diagnosis includes acute febrile neutrophilic dermatosis, erythema multiforme, Henoch–Schönlein purpura and child abuse. The prognosis for complete recovery is excellent. Acute inflammation of the scrotum in patients with familial Mediterranean fever can occur [38]. It is manifested by pain, redness and swelling, fever, leukocytosis and elevated erythrocyte sedimentation rate (ESR). It may occur in isolation or accompanying peritonitis. The differential diagnosis includes torsion, orchitis and epididymitis in boys.

Polyarteritis nodosa may be associated with testicular and epididymal involvement, with scrotal pain and swelling. In one case these were the sole presenting features and testicular biopsy provided the diagnosis [39–41].

There has been one patient who presented with 'inaugural' painless erythematous papules on the penis that histologically showed granulomatous vasculitis, leading to the diagnosis of Churg–Strauss syndrome (eosinophilic granulomatosis with polyangiitis) [42].

NON-SEXUALLY TRANSMITTED INFECTIONS

Staphylococcal cellulitis

Cellulitis may affect the penis. Piercing and genital jewellery predispose to infection. Cellulitis and abscess formation can complicate cysts, sinuses and fistulae, and sexually transmitted infections.

Ano-genital infection is a serious complication in patients with malignant disease, and potentially life-threatening necrotising fasciitis and Fournier gangrene may occur.

Perineal streptococcal dermatitis/perianal cellulitis

This syndrome occurs in children and also occurs in adults [1], but it is much more common in boys in whom, if the penis is involved, there may be dysuria, redness and swelling of the penis and balanoposthitis. Bullous necrotic erysipelas of the penis due to *Streptococcus pyogenes* has been reported [2].

Ecthyma gangrenosum

Ecthyma gangrenosum has a predilection for the acral and anogenital regions, and may affect the penis in isolation, leading to gangrene [1]. The prognosis is poor. A case has been reported that was probably caused by direct arterial septic embolisation of the penis from femoral heroin injection [2].

Fournier gangrene

Fournier gangrene is analogous to necrotising fasciitis and Meleney gangrene. In 1883, the Parisian dermatologist Jean Alfred Fournier described five cases of spontaneous genital gangrene and ulceration, but Baurienne (1764) probably first reported this condition [3]. The disease begins with urethral or appendageal polybacterial infection. Most of the organisms isolated are resident urethral or lower gastrointestinal flora, and most patients have mixed infections. In children, staphylococci and streptococci are most commonly isolated [4]. A necrotising vasculitis ensues, possibly exotoxin mediated, with devastating consequences for involved skin, subcutis, fascia and muscle. It is held to be the human counterpart of the local Shwartzman phenomenon [5,6]. A typical presentation is characterised by painful, red, non-suppurative swelling of the genital skin (particularly the scrotum [7], where a dark red or a black spot may appear [8]), or the perianal zone or lower abdominal skin, accompanied by crepitus [9], marked systemic toxicity (may be absent in children [4]) and urinary retention. Necrosis of skin and deeper tissues can occur rapidly, and there is a very high mortality unless the diagnosis is made promptly and radical management undertaken. The diagnosis is clinical, but imaging including plain X-rays (that may show soft-tissue gas [10]), ultrasound, computed tomography and magnetic resonance imaging may assist with the diagnosis in established cases and determine the extent of disease. Predisposing factors are listed in Box 109.22. Preceding surgery, including vasectomy and instrumentation, including genital piercing [11], especially in patients with the listed risk factors, is particularly important. The differential diagnosis is given in Box 109.23.

Box 109.22 Risk factors for Fournier gangrene

- Diabetes
- Alcoholism
- Ano-genital infection
- Chemotherapy
- HIV
- Postinstrumentation (especially in the immunocompromised)
- Postoperative (urological and colorectal)
- Heroin addiction
- Trauma
- Unconventional sexual practices

Box 109.23 Differential diagnosis of Fournier gangrene

- Trauma
- Herpes simplex
- Cellulitis (streptococcal, staphylococcal)
- Streptococcal necrotising fasciitis
- Gonococcal balanitis and oedema
- Ecthyma gangrenosum
- Allergic vasculitis
- Polyarteritis nodosa
- Necrolytic migratory erythema
- Vascular occlusion syndromes
- Warfarin necrosis

Reproduced from Bunker CB. *Male Genital Skin Disease*, 2nd edn. London: Bruce Shrink, 2019. © 2019, with permission from the author.

If a diagnosis of Fournier gangrene is made, radical surgical debridement of all affected tissue is undertaken and broad spectrum systemic antibiotic therapy initiated. Plastic repair can be undertaken if the patient survives [7]. Hyperbaric oxygen, high-dose systemic steroids and unprocessed honey treatment have been used [6,12,13,14,15]. In adults, the mortality is approximately 25%. Children can be treated with more conservative surgery and their mortality rate is lower [4,16].

Trichomycosis pubis

Trichomycosis pubis causes asymptomatic yellow, red or black micronodules around hair shafts [1]. Pubic and axillary hair may be involved. The skin is normal but the sweat may be discoloured. Trichomycosis pubis is rare in western dermatological practice but is common in the Middle East [2] and may occur concomitantly with trichosporosis in India [3]. It is caused by *Corynebacterium* spp. The differential diagnosis includes true mycoses such as white or black piedra. Treatment is with topical benzoic acid, salicylic acid, clindamycin or naftifine [1].

Tuberculosis

Tuberculosis of the penis is rare [4] but important given the resurgence of the disease. Primary penile ulceration (solitary and multiple), with or without inguinal lymphadenopathy, caused by sexual infection or contact with infected clothing may occur [5], or the ulceration may be secondary to tuberculosis elsewhere (e.g. the lung) [6]. A cold abscess (presenting as erectile impotence) has been reported [7]. Tuberculides have involved the penis, including in isolation [8]. Penile manifestations have also followed immunotherapy [9,10].

Non-syphilitic spirochaetal ulcerative balanoposthitis

This condition is recognised in the Tropics and South Africa, presenting as large serpiginous foul-smelling ulcers in uncircumcised men, associated in some with non-tender inguinal lymphadenopathy. Treatment is with penicillin or metronidazole [11].

Yaws

An ulcerated, crusted and papillomatous lesion has been reported on the prepuce as part of disseminated early yaws (with other skin lesions elsewhere) in a patient in an endemic region. Several family members were also infected. The genital lesion probably arose from autoinnoculation [12].

Candidosis

Genito-urinary physicians maintain that *Candida* can be the cause of urethritis and balanoposthitis [13] and cause erosive disease of the glans and prepuce. *Candida* of the penis (with a prevalence of approximately 10% of that of vaginal candidosis) has attracted very little research interest [14]. However, *Candida* may be more often a secondary pathogen than a sexually acquired infection. Observing the signs of candidosis, or demonstrating the presence of the organism, does not prove that it is the cause of all the symptoms and signs. An underlying dermatological or medical cause should be excluded. The symptoms and signs of *Candida* may be more florid than the underlying predisposing cause. Medical causes include diabetes, iatrogenic immunosuppression and systemic antibiotic treatment. Although oropharyngeal candidosis is almost invariably found in HIV infection, candidal balanoposthitis is not generally associated, perhaps because it is overlooked or because many patients take long-term imidazole antifungals orally.

Candida albicans is such a ready opportunist organism because it is a part of the resident flora of the gastrointestinal tract and may be retrieved from intertriginous areas, including the preputial folds, in the absence of symptoms and signs. Candidal balanoposthitis could be a sexually transmitted disease that may have an affinity for the anatomically or physiologically abnormal penis, or in individuals predisposed by other factors or disease, and where there is chronic vaginal or anal carriage in a partner. Screening should be performed for other sexually transmitted diseases.

Underlying disease should be identified and treated, and predisposing factors rectified. Treatment includes topical nystatin, clioquinol or an imidazole, often usefully combined with hydrocortisone or a moderately potent corticosteroid. In severe disease, an oral imidazole may be indicated.

Tinea

Tinea of the penis or scrotum is uncommon and when it occurs it is usually associated with crural disease. Rarely encountered is the occurrence of tinea on the glans penis as a seat of itch or pain and producing a red patch or a crop of scaly papules [15–19,**20**]. Penile tinea in India has been associated with occlusion resulting from the wearing of a langota – a T-shaped piece of cloth tied over the genitalia [17].

Deep fungal infections

Although histoplasmosis is a common cause of disseminated fungal infection in the USA, urological and ano-genital disease (usually ulceration and adenopathy in an ill patient) is rare [21,**22**]. An otherwise well man with a small warty nodule on the glans penis has been reported [23]. One patient with a penile ulcer transmitted the disease sexually to his wife [24]. Another report documents a phimosis at presentation [25]. In blastomycosis, although the genito-urinary tract (prostate and epididymis) is involved in 20–30% of cases [26], involvement of the genital skin is rare. However, lesions of the prepuce and perianal skin have been recorded [27,**28**]. Paracoccidioidomycosis can be the cause of scrotal swelling and genital nodules and erosions [29]. Zygomycosis is usually regarded as a rhinocerebral infection but a diabetic with purulent lesions of the penis has been described [**30**].

Other non-sexually transmitted infections

Bacillary angiomatosis is important in the differential diagnosis of AIDS-related Kaposi sarcoma. A case in which the presenting tender red nodules affected the scrotum and groins has been published [1].

Buruli ulcer of the penis and scrotum due to *Mycobacterium ulcerans* is a rare disease. Medical treatment is disappointing, and lesions need excision and grafting [2].

Male genital involvement with leprosy is uncommon, but there are reports, and it may occur in isolation [3,**4**,5].

The penis is rarely affected by pityriasis versicolor and probably almost never in isolation [6,7]. However, *Malassezia* yeasts may colonise both the circumcised and uncircumcised penis [8]. Occasionally, the anterior pelvic girdle is the site involved.

Only one case of superficial phaeohyphomycosis manifesting as multiple, 1–3 mm pigmented papules, resembling seborrhoeic keratoses, on the scrotum of an HIV-positive patient has been described. Microscopy showed a mass of mycelia and two dematiaceous fungi were cultured [9].

Genital herpes simplex may be acquired non-sexually (e.g. during contact sports such as rugby [10]). A phenomenon of chronic erosive and verrucous herpes as part of immunoreconstitution disease has been described in HIV infection [**11**].

Sacral herpes zoster lesions may be found on the scrotum and penis [**12**], and urinary retention and constipation can occur.

It is not unusual for the herald patch of pityriasis rosea (thought now to be due to human herpesvirus (HHV)-6/7) to appear on suprapubic skin or in the groin. Incomplete or limited presentations (e.g. affecting the pelvic girdle) are not rare, although careful examination may elicit another patch on the neck or in the axilla.

A distinctive sequel of chikungunya may be ulcers in the penoscrotal region [13]. Amoebiasis can rarely present as a painful ulcerative balanitis, with swelling, frequency, dysuria and retention [**14**]. Self-inoculation from concomitant intestinal infection, by heterosexual intercourse where the female partner has amoebic vaginitis, or by anal intercourse are the putative mechanisms. Amoebiasis as the cause of genital ulceration should lead to the suspicion of underlying HIV infection [**15**].

Cutaneous leishmaniasis can affect the genitalia [**16**,17]. A red scaly plaque [**18**] and a giant hyperkeratotic nodule on the glans [**19**], as well as a sporotrichoid distribution on the shaft of the penis [**20**], have been reported. Post-kala-azar dermal leishmaniasis of the penis and scrotum has been described. Rarely, genital skin lesions may lead to the diagnosis of schistosomiasis. They occur because ova shed by worms enter the perineal vessels [21]. The papules and nodules may be skin coloured, pink or brown, scattered or grouped, affecting the penis and scrotum. They can spread onto the perineum and around the anus, and may develop into soft, warty, vegetating lesions. Ulceration is rare and, even more rarely, concomitant carcinoma has been reported [21].

The ano-genital consequences of onchocerciasis are 'leopard skin' hypopigmentation (the scrotum is commonly involved), ileal crest and scrotal nodules, 'hanging groin' and scrotal enlargement [**22**,23]. The differential diagnosis of the scrotal enlargement includes bancroftian filariasis [24]. Other filarial infections can lead to mild hydrocele or gross elephantiasis. Filariasis can cause secondary lymphangiectasis. Excision, grafting and genital reconstruction can be undertaken [25].

Primary penile cryptococcal infection has been reported [**26**,27] and treated successfully with oral azoles and amphotericin.

DERMATOLOGICAL ASPECTS OF SEXUALLY TRANSMITTED DISEASE

MRSA

MRSA presents increasing challenges in general dermatology. There is evidence that community-associated MRSA can be a sexually transmitted disease [1].

Syphilis

Syphilis is endemic throughout the world. After a period of reduced incidence, it has undergone a resurgence [**2**]. All manifestations of syphilis can affect the genital region [3]. Balanoposthitis can complicate and obscure penile chancre. The granulomatous gumma may affect the genital area as an ulcer, a white plaque or an atrophic scar. Pseudochancre redux describes gummatous (tertiary stage) recurrence at the site of the primary chancre [4]; it is very rare.

Viral warts

The burden of genital infection with HPV is enormous (Chapter 25) [5]. Circumcised men are more likely to have genital warts than the uncircumcised, but when warts are present in uncircumcised men they are more likely to be distally situated [6]. The risk of acquiring genital warts is significantly reduced by using condoms [7]. Clinically inapparent disease may present as balanoposthitis [8]. Subclinical or latent genital HPV infection may be 100 times more common than classical condylomas [9]. The prevalence of HPV in the genital tract of men is similar to that in women, and is between 3% and 45% depending on the age and population [10]. The estimated lifetime risk of acquiring HPV sexually is greater than 50% and may be 80% [9]. Only 25% of the population of the USA were thought to have no prior or current genital HPV infection in 1997 [11]. The 5% acetic acid test is not a very specific aid to the identification of warts or dysplastic lesions [12]. Accurate diagnosis of HPV infection can probably only be achieved by molecular methods [13]. Congenital and acquired immunosuppression increases the susceptibility of the ano-genital region to HPV infection and reactivation and progression to dysplasia and frank malignancy [14]. Topical steroid treatment of genital dermatoses may reactivate genital warts [15].

The clinical diagnosis of genital warts caused by HPV infection is usually certain, but condylomata lata (secondary syphilis), lichen planus, molluscum contagiosum, BP and pearly penile papules enter the differential diagnosis. Solitary lesions have a wider differential diagnosis, including giant condyloma, squamous carcinoma and transitional cell carcinoma of the distal urethra, which can present as a warty lesion at the urethral meatus [16]. Biopsy should be performed if there is diagnostic doubt. Patients with ano-genital warts and their partners may require full sexually transmitted disease and sometimes colorectal assessment. Treatment can be challenging, due to the Koebner phenomenon, and is not generally the preserve of the dermatologist [3,5]. Treatment options include salicylic acid, podophyllotoxin, cryotherapy, imiquimod and curettage; combination therapy with 5-fluorouracil/salicylic acid is an unlicensed option [17–20]. There have been case reports of treatment response to cidofovir and postexposure Gardasil vaccination [19,21,22].

Molluscum contagiosum

Young men are commonly seen with penile and pubic lesions and it is assumed that this is a sexually transmitted infection, but this may not always be the case.

HIV infection

Ulcerative genital disease is a risk factor for HIV [23,24], but ano-genital ulceration may be a consequence of HIV infection [25]. Box 109.24 lists the main causes. Biopsy, with special stains and culture, is mandatory. Other genital problems in HIV, such as psoriasis,

warts, intraepithelial neoplasia, squamous carcinoma and Kaposi sarcoma, are discussed elsewhere in this chapter and in Chapter 31 - HIV and the Skin.

Box 109.24 Causes of penile and scrotal ulcers in HIV infection

- Syphilis
- Chancroid
- Herpes simplex
- Squamous cell carcinoma
- Drugs (e.g. foscarnet)*
- *Pseudomonas*[a]
- Penicilliosis[a]
- Amoebiasis[a]
- Kaposi sarcoma[a]

[a] Denotes causes that are typically observed in the context of AIDS.

Phthiriasis

Phthiriasis (crab louse) can present with marked genital and pubic itching with few overt physical signs, or as an infected genito-crural and pubic eczema that conceals the underlying primary signs. In hirsute men, the abdomen, chest, axillae and thighs may also be involved. Screening for other sexually transmitted diseases should be offered to the patient and partner(s).

Scabies

Scabies may present with ano-genital itch, 'folliculitis' (including of the buttocks) and penile, scrotal and pubic nodules (Figure 109.15). An AIDS patient with a single non-pruritic, 'crusted' lesion on the glans penis has been described [26]. Topical pimecrolimus has been used with benefit in the treatment of steroid-resistant post-scabies nodules [27].

Other infections

Human bite injuries acquired during oro-genital contact usually heal well but a penile ulcer infected with the oral flora organism *Eikenelia corrodens* has been reported [28].

BENIGN TUMOURS

The following entities are all encountered in the male genital area: pearly penile papules (angiofibromas); angiomas and angiokeratomas, and angiokeratoma corporis diffusum; basal cell papillomas (may be mistaken for viral warts [1] or BP); melanocytic naevi; inguinogenital epidermoid or (much rarer) pilar (including giant

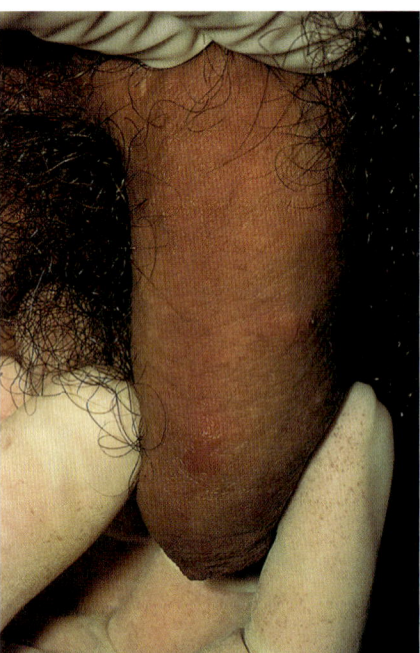

Figure 109.15 Papules on the penis in scabies. Courtesy of Dr C. White, University Hospital of North Durham, Durham, UK.

forms) cysts; these may become infected, and lesions containing molluscum contagiosum have been described [2,3].

Median raphe cysts

Congenital cystic median raphe anomalies may remain unobtrusive until adulthood. Cystic or nodular and linear swellings of the ventral penis occur near the glans. In adolescence or adulthood they may become traumatised or infected with staphylococci, gonococci or *Trichomonas* and present as tender, red, purulent nodules [4]. Histologically, they are either dermoid or mucoid, depending on their embryology or epithelial lining [5]. Very rarely, the basal epithelial lining of the cysts may contain melanocytes, imparting a brown-black pigment to the lesion [6].

Mucoid cysts

These are rare lesions that are present at birth or develop in childhood as small, flesh-coloured, mobile cystic papules or nodules with no punctum, commonly on the ventral glans or foreskin, rarely in the perineum. They can be asymptomatic, become infected or interfere with intercourse. The histological features suggest that they arise from ectopic urethral tissue during embryological development [7].

Scrotal calcinosis

Scrotal calcinosis is a relatively common, benign, idiopathic disorder presenting as solitary or multiple, hard, smooth, white papules or nodules on the scrotum, rarely the penis (Figure 109.16).

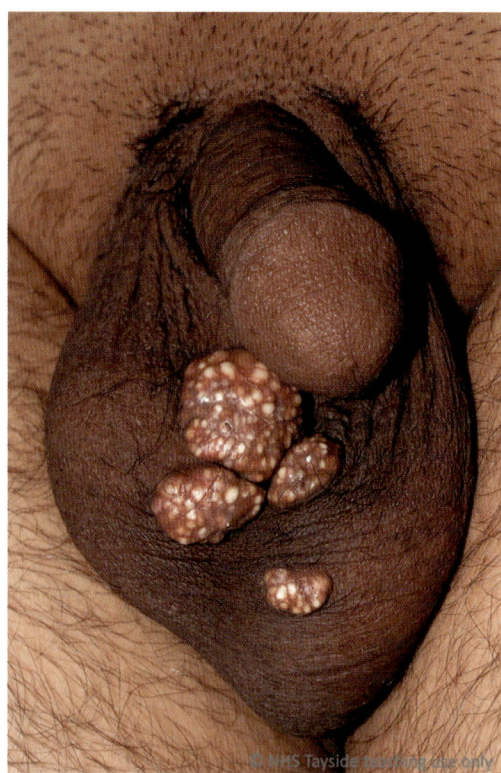

Figure 109.16 Benign, idiopathic scrotal calcinosis. Courtesy of Dr A. Affleck, Dundee, UK.

Interestingly, these lesions are much rarer on the vulva [8]. Occasionally, they may become secondarily inflamed or infected following trauma. Their occurrence was first described by Hutchinson [9]. Their origin has been debated: they have been said to arise from epidermoid cysts, eccrine duct milia, eccrine epithelial cysts, dystrophy of the dartos muscle, trauma and the presence of foreign bodies [10–20]. Scrotal calcinosis may occur after meconium peritonitis, with leakage of meconium through the processus vaginalis, and in testicular tumours such as teratomas, gonadoblastomas and Leydig cell tumours [**17**]. In endemic areas of onchocerciasis, calcified scrotal cysts may be caused by the living or dead nematodes, and patients have evidence of the disease elsewhere [21,**22**]. Onchocercal nodules are more common on the iliac crests and the rib cage. The unsightly and embarrassing lesions can be treated by incision and eventration under local anaesthesia. Idiopathic calcinosis of the penis is very rare [23,24]. A man who presented with a dome-shaped nodule on his glans has been described; the dystrophic calcinosis here was thought to derive from syringoma [25]. Other associations are trauma, self-injection with papaverine, Peyronie disease and cytotoxic chemotherapy [23]. Metastatic cutaneous calcinosis may affect the scrotum and is due to renal failure and secondary hyperparathyroidism.

Verruciform xanthoma

Verruciform xanthoma mainly affects the mouth. The genital skin is the next most frequently involved area, where it presents as a painless, yellow-brown or red, verrucous, sessile or papillary plaque. The histological findings are hyperkeratosis, focal parakeratosis, acanthosis and fat-filled foam cells in the papillary dermis. Verruciform xanthoma is thought to represent epidermal degeneration, with keratinocyte lipid then taken up by dermal macrophages [26] or fibroblasts to form the foam cells. Treatment is by surgical excision.

Other benign tumours

Naevus comedonicus of the glans penis, generally devoid of pilosebaceous structures, has been reported [27]. Keloid is rare, but can complicate circumcision [28,29,30] and other surgery and trauma [31,32]. Keloid has been simulated on the dorsum of the penis by chronic oedema caused by a condom catheter [33]. Dermoid cyst affecting the penis, presenting with pain, swelling and suppuration from abscess formation, has been reported [34]. Acanthosis nigricans almost always affects the groins. In pseudoacanthosis nigricans, the associated obesity is almost always responsible for intertrigo and skin tags. Penile colloid degeneration has been described, presenting as a dermal plaque of the dorsal shaft [35]. Some cases of multiple syringomata localised to the penis have been described, mimicking genital warts or lichen planus [36–39]. Other benign tumours that have been reported rarely to affect the genital area include apocrine cystadenoma [40,41], syringocystadenoma papilliferum [42], mixed syringocystadenoma papilliferum and papillary eccrine adenoma occurring in a scrotal condyloma [43], composite adnexal tumour [44], dermatofibroma [45], reticulohistiocytoma [46], giant cell fibroblastoma [47], connective tissue naevi (scrotum) [48], fibrous hamartoma of infancy [49], leiomyoma [45,50], genital smooth muscle hamartoma (scrotum) [51,52], traumatic neuroma [53], neurofibroma, neurilemoma, granular cell myoblastoma [45,54–56], varicosities/venous lakes, acquired capillary and cavernous haemangioma [45] (other angiomatous lesions are very much rarer, and controversy exists as to whether they represent a true neoplasm, herniation of the corpus spongiosum or vascularisation of a haematoma or thrombus [57]), Masson vegetant intravascular haemangioendothelioma [58], angiokeratoma circumscriptum of Mibelli [59], glomus tumour [48,60], port-wine stain, strawberry naevus [61–63], haemangiomas and PELVIS syndrome [64], epithelioid haemangioma [65], epithelioid haemangioendothelioma [45,66], pyogenic granuloma [67], angiolymphoid hyperplasia with eosinophilia/Kimura disease (penis and spermatic cord) [68,69,70] and lymphangioma circumscriptum [71,72].

PRE-CANCEROUS DERMATOSES AND CARCINOMA *IN SITU*

Erythroplasia of Queyrat, Bowen disease of the penis and bowenoid papulosis

Definition

PeIN is a histological term for the precursor state of invasive penile squamous cell carcinoma (PSCC).

Introduction and general description

There is a heterogeneous spectrum of clinical and histological presentations of carcinoma *in situ* of the penis: erythroplasia of Queyrat, Bowen disease of the penis (BDP) and BP. Nomenclature used for its clinical classification is distinct from that used for its histological classification. Clinical nomenclature categorised the entity by clinical morphology: BP, erythroplasia of Queyrat and BDP [1,2,3,4]. Histologically, PeIN is classified into undifferentiated (HPV-related) and differentiated (LSc-related, unrelated to HPV) that in turn are associated with specific PSCC subtypes [5–9]. PeIN is characterised histologically by dysplasia with an intact basement membrane. Differentiated PeIN is associated with squamous hyperplasia and LSc and the 'usual' and verrucous keratinising subtypes of squamous carcinoma of the penis. Undifferentiated PeIN is associated with HPV and the warty, condylomatous, basaloid and 'mixed' subtypes of penile squamous carcinoma [7,10].

Aetiology and pathophysiology

The two principal aetiological factors for PeIN are LSc (differentiated PeIN) and HPV (undifferentiated PeIN). Other contributory aetiological factors include smoking, the presence of the foreskin, poor hygiene, ultraviolet light exposure, immunological dysfunction and, potentially, other chronic dermatoses such as lichen planus [1,4,7,11,12]. Iatrogenic or acquired immunosuppression is also a risk factor for PeIN [13].

Undifferentiated PeIN results from integration of HPV genome into the DNA of the host epithelial cell, leading to oncogene expression [14,15,16,17,18,19,20]. Evidence of HPV infection is found in 70–100% of all cases of PeIN. HPV 16 is the most prevalent type encountered; this and other implicated types (18, 31, 33, 35, 39, 45, 51, 52, 54, 56, 58, 59, 66, 68 and 69) have been incriminated in 22–45% of PSCC and in over 70% of PSCC *in situ* [7,11,12,21]. It is possible that the various clinical phenotypes of HPV-related PeIN may have distinct molecular HPV signatures. One study has shown that in BP, 90% of HPV types are genital types, of which 35% are HPV 16, with the next most prevalent being HPV 6, whereas in erythroplasia of Queyrat, 90% are also genital types of which approximately 50% are HPV 16, followed by HPV 45 and 68. In BDP, 80% are genital types of which 50% are HPV 16, followed by HPV 33 and 18 [22].

The prevalence of PeIN appears to be high among male sexual partners of women with cervical intraepithelial neoplasia [23,24], but the exact risk of transmission is not known; the prevalence of HPV among male partners of women with cervical intraepithelial neoplasia varies between 12.95% and 86% [25]. Immunosuppression is an important risk; in one study, 50% of HIV patients with ano-genital warts had carcinoma *in situ* on histology in one study [26].

LSc is present in 10–42% of all cases of PeIN and in up to 100% of cases of differentiated PeIN [6,10,13,27,28,29]. The association with LSc is likely to explain the fact that neonatal circumcision protects against penile carcinoma [12,30,31]. Circumcision in later life may reduce the risk but does not abolish it, especially if the circumcision was performed for penile disease [1,12,32–34].

Upregulation of Wnt/β-catenin signalling is observed in penile carcinoma [35] and this signalling pathway is up-regulated by *Fusobacterium* spp., the relative abundance of which is increased in patients with MGLSc; this genus is also implicated in oral squamous cell carcinoma and colorectal carcinoma [36–40], raising the possibility that this genus is also implicated in LSc-associated penile carcinoma.

Spontaneous regression can occur [12] including with restitution of immunocompetence in the treatment of HIV [41].

Epidemiology

Erythroplasia of Queyrat and BDP are typically seen in older patients than BP; in one study the difference in the mean age between the two groups was around 16 years (mean ages: BDP 58.1; erythroplasia of Queyrat 56; BP 41) [13].

BP is the most common clinical subtype of PeIN, with BDP the next most common and erythroplasia of Queyrat the least common, being approximately three times less common than both BP and BDP [13].

Using data from the Office for National Statistics, it has been calculated that the UK age standardised incidence in 2011 was 0.66 per 100 000; the estimated 10-year prevalence is 3.089 per 100 000 [13,42,43,44]

In the UK, undifferentiated PeIN is more than eight times as common as differentiated PeIN [13], although this ratio is likely to be substantially higher in societies in which circumcision is a more prevalent practice.

Clinical features

In contrast to the relatively distinct histological definitions of PeIN subtypes, the clinical spectrum of PeIN is heterogeneous. There are three principal morphological variants: erythroplasia of Queyrat, BDP and BP [1,4]. These clinical entities possess differences in epidemiology and malignant potential [45]. BP appears as multiple, grouped brown or red papules that are smoother topped, more polymorphic and more coalescent than common genital viral condylomata acuminata (Figure 109.17), while erythroplasia of Queyrat is characterised by red, moist, shiny patches or minimally elevated plaques of the glabrous glans and inner ('mucosal') aspect of the prepuce in the uncircumcised [45]. BDP manifests as paucifocal, scaly plaques affecting hair-bearing, keratinised epithelium [2,12,46]. Clinical features of PeIN lie along a continuum and features of different clinical variants of PeIN can be present concomitantly.

Even with experience and appreciation of the morphological subtleties, a high index of suspicion and a low threshold for biopsy are required for the diagnosis of PeIN [13]. Biopsies can be both non-specific and false-negative [6,8,13,47,48].

The non-specificity of the clinical appearances makes for an important differential diagnosis, which includes psoriasis, LSc (especially with Zoonoid manifestations), lichen planus and extramammary Paget disease. The differential diagnosis of BP includes lichen planus, common warts, seborrhoeic warts, naevi and condylomata lata. Reflectance confocal microscopy may prove useful for diagnosis [49], although this diagnostic modality is not widely available.

In most reports, PeIN is preferentially distributed on the glans and prepuce [27,50] and one series indicates that the shaft is also a predominantly affected site [2,51].

Dermoscopic features of PeIN include structureless areas, vascular structures, particularly dotted vessels, scale and scar-like areas [52]. Other features include erosions and pigmentation consisting of brown-grey dots and globules.

The risks of transformation to PSCC in PeIN have been estimated as 1% for BP, 5% for BDP and 10–33% for erythroplasia of Queyrat [12,13,27,46,53–58,59]. Reports of overall progression rates vary from 0% to 7% (mean 6.7, median 6.0 years) [13]. Progression to PSCC may have occurred in 8.7–1-% of cases at the time of biopsy or circumcision [13].

Investigations

Biopsy is required to confirm a diagnosis of PeIN. Where there is clinical suspicion and biopsies are negative or equivocal, repeat biopsies are required.

Histology

PeIN – differentiated or undifferentiated – constitutes the latest nomenclature, having been adopted in the World Health Organization classification of urological malignant tumours, and is endorsed by the International Society of Urological Pathology [5,7,8,47].

In undifferentiated PeIN (Figure 109.17b), atypia are present in at least two-thirds of the epidermis, with dyskeratosis, parakeratosis and disorganised epithelial architecture; nuclei are enlarged, hyperchromatic and pleomorphic with atypical mitoses; koilocytes are also observed. Warty, basaloid and mixed warty-basaloid subtypes are described.

In differentiated PeIN (Figure 109.17c), dyskeratosis, acanthosis and elongated rete ridges are observed. In the superficial epithelium, keratinocytes lack atypia and maturation is preserved; koilocytes are not a feature. Atypical basal and parabasal keratinocytes are observed, with hyperchromatic irregular nuclei, with some mitotic figures and abundant cytoplasm. Squamous pearls may occasionally be visualised at the tip of the rete ridges. Differentiated PeIN may be discontiguous. Differentiated PeIN is frequently associated with squamous hyperplasia [14,60,61] (see later).

Nevertheless, the histological distinction diagnosis can be difficult, especially with small biopsies [6,8]. The triple panel of p16, p53 and Ki-67 may prove useful to help distinguish between the two forms of PeIN as follows: differentiated PeIN (p16 [-ve], Ki-67 [+ve], p53 [±ve]), squamous hyperplasia (p16 [-ve], Ki-67 [±ve], p53 [-ve]); undifferentiated (HPV-associated) PeIN (p16 [+ve], Ki-67 [+ve], p53 [±ve]) [62,63]. However, sensitivity and specificity are as yet poorly defined.

Differentiated PeIN is associated with 'usual', papillary, pseudohyperplastic, verrucous and sarcomatoid carcinomas, whereas undifferentiated PeIN is associated with warty, basaloid and mixed warty-basaloid carcinomas [7,28].

Management

The goals in managing PeIN are cure with tissue conservation, concomitant restoration and preservation of sexual and urinary function, and, crucially, prevention of PSCC [13,64].

Multidisciplinary management is ideal, as at least half of patients will require more than one treatment modality [13].

Treatment modalities for PeIN include topical chemotherapy (5-fluorouracil) [1,3,4,65], topical imiquimod [46,66–68], surgical procedures including curettage and electrocautery, excisional surgery, circumcision, glans resurfacing, Mohs micrographic

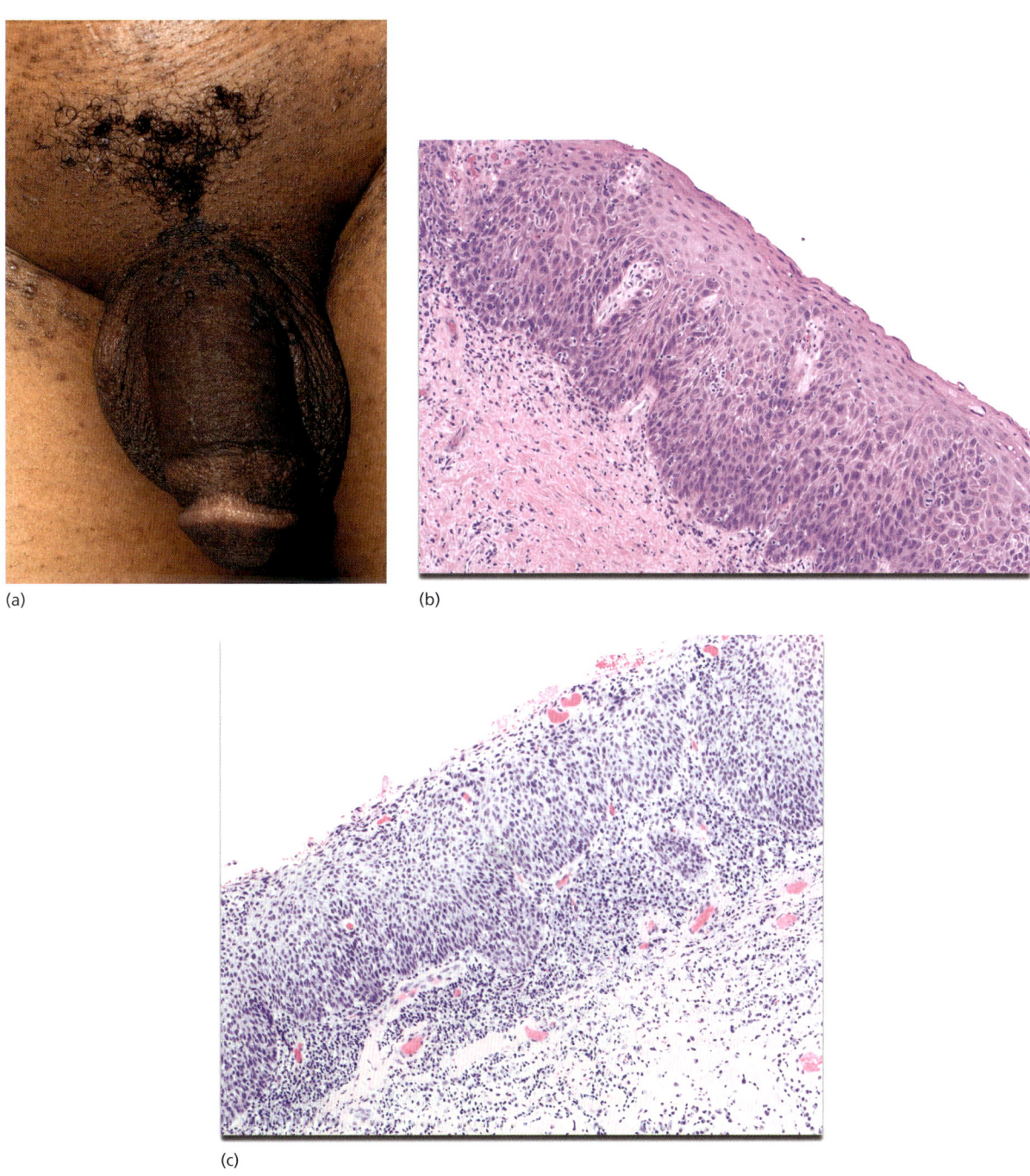

(a)

(b)

(c)

Figure 109.17 (a) Bowenoid papulosis affecting penile shaft and groins. Courtesy of Dr A. Affleck, Dundee, UK. (b) Haematoxylin and eosin stain. Magnification ×10. Undifferentiated PeIN basaloid type. Full-thickness atypia of the surface squamous epithelium with a monotonous population of basophilic cells. Courtesy of Dr A. Haider, University College Hospital, London, UK. (c) Haematoxylin and eosin stain. Magnification ×10. Differentiated PeIN (pleomorphic variant): marked pleomorphism of the basal and parabasal keratinocytes. There is surface maturation. Courtesy of Dr A. Haider, University College Hospital, London, UK.

surgery, and other procedures including cryotherapy, laser and photodynamic therapy [1,3,4,12,69,70]. Topical cidofovir has been used [71–73].

Treatment choice depends on many factors [3,4,12], including anatomical site of genitalia affected, histological subtype and patient's overall health status. The available guidelines lack structured management protocols and are limited by the poor quality of the evidence available [65,74,75]. Although many treatment modalities (particularly topical treatments and cryotherapy) are associated with high failure rates, incomplete response to treatment necessitates re-evaluation and consideration of repeat biopsy, as this could reflect subclinical progression to invasive disease.

Circumcision has a crucial role in the management of PeIN, as it (i) removes the occlusive environment that is crucial for development of LSc, which serves as a major risk factor for PeIN and PSCC; (ii) removes a substantial proportion of susceptible tissue; (iii) provides extensive tissue for histological analysis; (iv) triggers 'eukeratinisation' of the residual, largely glanular, epithelium; and

(v) facilitates clinical follow-up [4,76]. However, circumcision is not universally required, specifically in cases of BP and in cases of BPD of the shaft without involvement of balanopreputial epithelium. PeIN on the glans may respond to circumcision alone [77].

Topical treatments and cryotherapy play a role in the management of the majority of cases of PeIN, albeit alongside other modalities, as they are only successful alone in a small minority (14%) of cases [13].

Imiquimod yields a response rate of 40–100%, with a recurrence rate of 20%, while 5-fluorouracil yields a 48–74% response rate with an 11% rate of recurrence. Adverse effects occur in 5–12% of cases with these agents, with severe irritation and associated pain among the most common examples. Discontinuation of treatment by patients treated with imiquimod and 5-fluorouracil occurs in 10% and 11% of cases, respectively. A discontinuation rate of topical agents due to side effects has been reported as 12% [77].

Risks of cryotherapy include meatal stenosis, severe inflammation, spontaneous bleeding, pain and infection [13]. Perimeatal disease represents a particular challenge for cryotherapy and topical treatments, with risks of penetration, oedema, infection and scarring [13,70].

Scarring can incur morbidity and functional impairment, but also can render monitoring and surveillance by gross inspection more challenging [70]. Glans resurfacing represents an important advance, as it can overcome many of the shortcomings of other treatments. Glans resurfacing restores normal anatomy and the risk of local recurrence is reduced by the replacement of diseased epithelium and subepithelial tissues with healthy extragenital skin. There is an additional advantage in the removal of diseased epithelium, in turn allowing accurate histopathological staging. Penile form and function and length are preserved, while optimising cosmesis and oncological control [78]. A substantial proportion (28%) requires subsequent further surgery for positive surgical margins or understaging of their primary disease, although the need for further surgery does not compromise oncological control.

Laser treatment (CO_2 and Nd:YAG), photodynamic therapy, Mohs micrographic surgery and radiotherapy are also among treatments described [46,79–81,**82**,83,84,**85**,86–89,**90**]. Radiotherapy should be avoided.

Response rates for laser therapies were 52–100%, with recurrence in 7–48%; laser therapy precludes the opportunity to examine the tissue that is removed [77]. Excision (including undefined 'wide local excision') leads to a recurrence rate of 25%, compared with 4% for Mohs surgery, 5% for total glans resurfacing and 10% for glansectomy [77].

HPV vaccines against oncogenes E6, E7 and others hold promise for future treatment of HPV-driven intraepithelial neoplasia [**91**], but they are not currently commercially available. In their absence, adjunctive postexposure HPV vaccination with available options (e.g. Gardasil) has been advocated in the management of undifferentiated PeIN [**92**]. These target the L1 capsid protein, although trials against established HPV-driven neoplasia have not shown clear efficacy [**91**].

Smoking is a risk factor for penile carcinoma and smoking cessation is therefore an important component of management. Patients should be screened for sexually transmitted diseases, including HIV infection. Sexual partners should be advised to seek assessment.

Follow-up forms an essential component of management, as the overall recurrence rates lie between 3% and 10% [3,4,**13**,93,**94**] and the risk of progression to invasive penile cancer is significantly increased with estimates at between 5% and 33% [**13**,58,59]. BP that does not involve the balanopreputial sac may represent an exception, given the low risk of invasion.

Miscellaneous pre-cancerous conditions

Squamous hyperplasia and squamous intraepithelial lesion(s)

Squamous hyperplasia manifests clinically as small, red or white patches (Box 109.25) that are either thin and atrophic or hypertrophic and verrucous [1]. It is associated with differentiated PeIN, underlying LSc and penile carcinoma of the 'usual' and verrucous subtypes. Although squamous hyperplasia is the most common epithelial abnormality found in association with invasive squamous carcinoma of the penis, histologically there is *no* cytological atypia. The other histological features of squamous hyperplasia are those of hyperkeratosis with orthokeratosis or parakeratosis, acanthosis, elongated rete ridges, absence of koilocytosis; maturation of the squamous cells is normal with hypergranulosis [2]. The hyperplasia may sometimes be verrucous; the French term 'hyperplasie épithéliale verruqueuse' overlaps with this entity, and also encompasses PEMKB [1].

Box 109.25 Causes of male genital white patches and plaques

- Post-traumatic or surgical scar
- Lichen simplex
- Lichen sclerosus
- Vitiligo
- Mucous membrane (cicatricial) pemphigoid
- Peyronie disease
- Syphilis
  - Leukoderma: postsecondary syphilide
  - Gumma
  - Postgummatous atrophic scar
- Viral warts
- Pityriasis versicolor
- Pseudoepitheliomatous micaceous and keratotic balanitis
- Intraepithelial neoplasia
- Squamous hyperplasia
- Squamous cell carcinoma

Reproduced from Bunker CB. *Male Genital Skin Disease*, 2nd edn. London: Bruce Shrink, 2019. © 2019, with permission from the author.

Squamous intraepithelial lesions present clinically as redder or more pigmented papules and plaques; they are classified histologically into squamous, basaloid or warty, high- or low-grade subtypes; they are associated with undifferentiated (or 'usual' type) bowenoid PeIN, HPV and the warty, condylomatous, basaloid and 'mixed' subtypes of penile squamous carcinoma [2,3].

Penile horn

Penile horn refers to dramatic protruding hyperkeratosis. It is rare for cutaneous horn to affect the penis [4]. The underlying causes include PEMKB [5], verrucous carcinoma [6–9], squamous carcinoma [10] or condyloma acuminatum [11]. Chronic inflammation and recent circumcision for longstanding phimosis are said to be important predisposing factors [11–13]. Penile horn may be associated with PeIN or frank carcinoma in a substantial proportion of cases; the limited literature available suggests that over a third are associated with squamous cell carcinoma at the time of presentation [14]. The exact risk of malignant transformation is not known, but in the authors' experience the development of penile horn is likely to signify a high risk of transformation even in many cases where such histological features fall short of PeIN or squamous cell carcinoma. Treatment should be dictated by precise diagnosis, achieved by adequate excision and histology of the underlying epithelium. Given the association with premalignant and frank malignant change, circumcision is recommended by experts in the field. Follow-up is mandatory because recurrence may occur.

Porokeratosis of Mibelli

Porokeratosis of Mibelli has been reported on the penis and scrotum in rare cases. It may be commoner in Asian populations [15]. Pruritus and ulceration may occur [16].

It classically manifests as a slightly atrophic lesion with an annular, raised border and may have overlying scale [17,18]. It may be inherited; other potential causes include irradiation, infection, trauma, immunosuppression and other drugs. Porokeratosis may be confused with psoriasis, Bowen disease, granuloma annulare or lichen planus; biopsy differentiates these conditions [19]. Porokeratosis is due to clonal expansion of keratinocytes that exhibit varying degrees of dysplasia and consequently are thought to be premalignant; the risk of malignant transformation varies between 7.5% and 11.6% [20,21]. Topical 5-fluorouracil and imiquimod have been used for treatment [22,23].

Porokeratosis ptychotropica

Porokeratosis ptychotropica, also known as verrucous porokeratosis, is a rare variant of porokeratosis, only relatively recently described [24]. The term 'ptychotropica' derives from the Greek words 'ptyche' and 'trope,' meaning 'fold' and 'turning' respectively. Its aetiology is unknown. It manifests clinically as symmetrical, scaly red papules and plaques, typically located on the natal cleft and buttocks but they may also occur in the genital area [25,26,27]. The dermatosis has been described as having a 'butterfly' pattern, symmetrically affecting both buttocks but sparing the anal mucosa. The rash is slowly progressive over many years, expanding through the formation of peripheral satellite lesions that coalesce, and it can be associated with pruritus. Porokeratosis ptychotropica has been reported with other classical forms of porokeratosis [28] and there has been a single reported case with progression to squamous cell carcinoma [29].

Porokeratosis ptychotropica can be confused clinically with inflammatory dermatoses such as psoriasis, fungal infection or condyloma accuminatum. Diagnosis relies on clinicopathological correlation, with its distinctive features being its distribution, recalcitrance to treatment and the presence of multiple cornoid lamellae throughout the lesions on histology. The diagnosis is often missed because, although well described in the literature, it is underrecognised by dermatologists, and prominent secondary changes such as lichenification are often present, which obscures the cornoid lamellae both clinically and histologically [30]. A further impediment to diagnosis is inadequacy of biopsies, as these often do not capture cornoid lamellae that are appreciated clinically. Treatment represents a challenge [31]. Various therapies, including topical corticosteroids, tacrolimus, calcipotriol, psoralen ultraviolet A, 5-fluorouracil, podophyllin, topical retinoids, intralesional bleomycin, cryotherapy and CO_2 laser, often yield negligible benefit. Treatment success has been reported with oral acitretin, 5% imiquimod, photodynamic therapy and surgical excision [32].

Pseudoepitheliomatous micaceous and keratotic balanitis

PEMKB is a rare condition that represents chronic, unstable, inadequately treated or treatment-refractory (even after circumcision), LSc. PEMKB is a clinicopathological diagnosis, with clinical features of thick scaly micaceous patches on the glans of an uncircumcised penis [5,33] and histological features of acanthosis, hyperkeratosis and pseudoepitheliomatous hyperplasia [34]. Basal atypia is also seen in the majority of patients [35], and other features include prolongation of the rete ridges.

Its association with LSc [36–38] has been outlined in the literature by direct observation, analysis of published clinical photographs demonstrating pathognomonic features of LSc, and via an observed association with acquired phimosis [35]. HPV has not been demonstrated to play an aetiological role in PEMKB [35].

PEMKB is associated with differentiated PeIN [35] and may also progress to verrucous squamous cell carcinoma [36,37,39]. Metastatic spread has not occurred except where there was a penile horn [40], and in one patient who developed an aggressive soft tissue sarcoma of the penis [41].

Glans resurfacing appears to lead to the best outcomes with complete remission and favourable patient reported outcomes [35]. Limited excision may prove effective. Topical agents are ineffective in most cases [35]; cryotherapy and photodynamic therapy have also been reported. Radiotherapy is described in the historical literature [5] but does not play a role in current practice.

SQUAMOUS CARCINOMA AND OTHER MALIGNANT NEOPLASMS

Carcinoma of the penis

Introduction and general description

The earliest stages of penis cancer and pre-cancer form a heterogeneous spectrum of disease as discussed in detail earlier [1,2].

Although some penile cancers arise *de novo*, others develop from premalignant situations, which may be misdiagnosed or may be difficult to diagnose, and there are the issues of multifocality, field change and the temporal dynamic to acknowledge. The precise aetiologies of the types of PeIN and squamous carcinoma of the penis are unknown, but as outlined previously, there is a dichotomous pathway, HPV-related or LSc-related, as in the vulva. Verrucous carcinoma is verruciform in morphology, unrelated to HPV and with better survival compared with other forms of squamous cell carcinoma due to a low rate of metastasis.

Epidemiology

The incidence of penile carcinoma in Europe is 0.9–2.1/100 000 per annum [3]. Of the approximately 500 new cases per year, carcinoma of the penis causes about 100 deaths per annum in the UK and accounts for fewer than 1% of deaths from cancer in the USA. It constitutes 10–20% of tumours seen in males in either developing countries or in areas where early circumcision is not commonly practised; overall, the highest incidence is in Africa, South America and Asia (2–4/100 000 inhabitants) and lowest in the USA and Europe (0.3–1/100 000) [1,4].

Pathophysiology

Risk factors for penis cancer are listed in Box 109.26. The pathophysiology is discussed in detail earlier in this chapter.

Box 109.26 Risk factors for squamous carcinoma of the penis

- Uncircumcised
- Phimosis
- Long foreskin
- Poor hygiene
- Chronic irritation, inflammation, scarring
- Smoking
- Many sexual partners
- Lichen sclerosus
- Lichen planus
- Human papillomavirus
- HIV
- Squamous hyperplasia/squamous intraepithelial lesion
- Bowen disease
- Erythroplasia of Queyrat
- Bowenoid papulosis
- Pseudoepitheliomatous micaceous and keratotic balanitis
- Giant condyloma/verrucous carcinoma
- Photochemotherapy
- Iatrogenic immunosuppression
  - Renal transplantation
  - Systemic lupus erythematosus
- Radiotherapy

Phimosis and balanitis are known risk factors for penile cancer [5,6]. The possession of a 'long' foreskin may be important. Poor personal and sexual hygiene [6] and phimosis are risk factors. It is not widely appreciated that phimosis is a physical sign and not a diagnosis.

LSc is a common cause of phimosis in males and it predisposes to penile carcinoma [1,7–10]. Powell *et al.* [11] found that half of patients with penis cancer had a clinical history and/or histological evidence of LSc.

Verrucous carcinoma is unrelated to HPV but associated with LSc [12], and cases in association with hidradenitis suppurativa and very rarely lichen planus have occurred [13–15].

Regarding other chronic dermatoses, chronic erosive and hypertrophic lichen planus are premalignant conditions, and lichen planus is a cause of phimosis [5]. Chronic irritation and inflammation or scarring are all risk factors for squamous carcinoma of the skin generally and the penis is no exception; penis cancer complicating a burn scar and a chronic sinus tract have been reported [5].

Smoking is a risk factor, independent of phimosis, for penile carcinoma [5,16], and is also a recognised risk factor for anal and cervical cancer. Smoking may cause squamoepithelial cancer, not only in parts of the body in contact with smoke but also at distant sites by dissemination of carcinogens in the circulation or in secretions. The presence of tobacco-specific nitrosamines in the preputial secretions of rats has been demonstrated [5].

Penile carcinoma is a complication of psoralen and UVA therapy (PUVA) [5,17], and possibly other treatments for psoriasis.

Penis cancer complicates immunosuppression in solid organ transplantation [5,18] and HIV infection [5] (risk increased five- to sixfold). It is also seen in men with psoriasis treated with immunosuppressive drugs [5,19,20]. Topical immunosuppressive agents such as the calcineurin inhibitors should be used with extreme caution for genital dermatoses, especially in the uncircumcised, because of the risk of squamous carcinoma [21,22,23]. There is no evidence for a risk attributable to topical steroids [24].

The HPV-dependent pathway leads predominantly to basaloid and warty subtypes and the LSc–related pathway leads mainly to usual and verrucous subtypes [1,4,25].

Pathology

There is a spectrum of histological subtypes of PSCC [1,4,26,27]. Histological signs of squamous hyperplasia, squamous intraepithelial lesion (SIL), carcinoma *in situ* (CIS), PeIN, LSc and HPV are commonly found. HPV typing and immunohistochemistry, for example for p16INK 4a (as a co-factor for HPV), are emerging as adjunctive diagnostic tools [4,27]. Chaux and Cubilla [4] have classified PSCC as detailed in Table 109.1.

Verrucous carcinoma represents a distinct subtype of squamous cell carcinoma that is well-differentiated with histological features that include papillomatososis, acanthosis, hyperkeratosis, fibrovascular cores, broad pushing tumour base and stromal reaction. If tumours are non-invasive and well-differentiated, metastases do not occur [4]. Where invasion in lamina propria is present focally (microinvasive verrucous carcinomas), prognosis is not affected. Verrucous carcinomas may undergo dedifferentiation; if dedifferentiation is extensive, the tumour classification changes to 'mixed verrucous carcinoma (hybrid)' and the risk of metastasis increases to 25% [4].

Carcinoma cuniculatum represents a variant of verrucous carcinoma, named for a characteristic labyrinthine growth pattern that resembles rabbits' burrows [4].

Table 109.1 Classification of squamous cell carcinomas of the penis [**4**,**28**].

	Subtype
HPV-related	Papillary basaloid carcinoma
	Basaloid carcinoma
	Warty carcinoma
	Warty–basaloid carcinoma
	Clear cell carcinoma
	Lympho-epithelioma-like carcinoma
Non-HPV-related	Usual squamous cell carcinoma/NOS
	Verrucous carcinoma
	Adenosquamous carcinoma
	Pseudohyperplastic carcinoma
	Carcinoma cuniculatum
	Pseudoglandular carcinoma
	Sarcomatoid carcinoma
	Papillary carcinoma/NOS

Clinical features

Itch, irritation, pain, bleeding, discharge, ulceration or the discovery of a mass are the presenting symptoms of squamous carcinoma. There is often a long history of preceding problems with the penis and foreskin, which may manifest as dyspareunia, balanoposthitis or phimosis and dysuria. Irregular nodular and ulcerative morphology is found on examination (Figures 109.18 and 109.19) and there may be background BDP, erythroplasia of Queyrat and BP, LSc or lichen planus. Undiagnosed, untreated disease is destructive and mutilating. Phimosis should be regarded as a sinister situation, not least because it impedes complete inspection and palpation of the glans and coronal sulcus. The inguinal lymph glands must be palpated, although in penile cancer only 50% of enlarged glands will be found to contain tumour [29].

Verrucous carcinoma is a verruciform tumour with an exophytic and papillomatous pattern of growth.

The differential diagnosis includes the manifestations of intraepithelial neoplasia (and the differential diagnosis of these), erosive or ulcerative sexually transmitted disease, basal cell carcinoma, Kaposi sarcoma, pyoderma gangrenosum and artefact. Genito-urinary and urological assessment should be sought.

Investigations

Diagnosis is confirmed histologically by incisional or excisional biopsy. An incisional biopsy should be of adequate size and depth, and it may be necessary to sample several sites. Particular care is needed in verrucous carcinoma to obtain a biopsy of adequate depth, as the histological differential diagnosis can be challenging.

The biopsy(ies) *may* need to be performed by a urologist under general anaesthesia. Patients who have negative or equivocal biopsies, but who have risk factors or in whom there is a high index of suspicion, should be followed up closely and undergo repeat biopsy if indicated. Staging should not be based on incisional biopsies.

Management

Staging of all PSCC is as per TNM detailed in Table 109.2. The treatment of genital squamous carcinoma is not the province of the dermatologist. Nonetheless, dermatologists have a crucial role in diagnosis and treatment of its precursor conditions, LSc, HPV and PeIN, and are thus particularly well placed to detect and/or prevent progression from intraepithelial disease to invasive disease.

Table 109.2 TNM clinical and pathological classification of penile cancer.

Clinical classification

T – Primary tumour

TX	Primary tumour cannot be assessed
T0	No evidence of primary tumour
Ta	Carcinoma *in situ*
	Non-invasive verrucous carcinoma
T1	Tumour invades subepithelial connective tissue

	T1a	Tumour invades subepithelial connective tissue without lymphovascular invasion and is not poorly differentiated
	T1b	Tumour invades subepithelial connective tissue with lymphovascular invasion or is poorly differentiated
		If either of the following are present, it is T1b rather than T1a: sarcomatoid change, perineural invasion

T2	Tumour invades corpus spongiosum with or without invasion of the urethra
T3	Tumour invades corpus cavernosum with or without invasion of the urethra
T4	Tumour invades other adjacent structures

N – Regional lymph nodes

NX	Regional lymph nodes cannot be assessed
N0	No palpable or visibly enlarged inguinal lymph nodes
N1	Increased to >2 unilateral inguinal lymph node (LN) metastases without extranodal extension
N2	Increased to >2 unilateral or bilateral inguinal LN metastases without extranodal extension
N3	Fixed inguinal nodal mass *or* pelvic lymphadenopathy, unilateral or bilateral

M – Distant metastasis

M0	No distant metastasis
M1	Distant metastasis

Pathological classification
The pT categories correspond to the clinical T categories
The pN categories are based upon biopsy or surgical excision

pN – Regional lymph nodes

pNX	Regional lymph nodes cannot be assessed
pN0	No regional lymph node metastasis
pN1	Metastasis in one or two inguinal lymph nodes
pN2	Metastasis in more than two unilateral inguinal nodes or bilateral inguinal lymph nodes
pN3	Metastasis in pelvic lymph node(s), unilateral or bilateral extranodal *or* extension of regional lymph node metastasis

pM – Distant metastasis

pM1	Distant metastasis microscopically confirmed

G – Histopathological grading

GX	Grade of differentiation cannot be assessed
G1	Well differentiated
G2	Moderately differentiated
G3	Poorly differentiated
G4	Undifferentiated

Adapted from Hakenberg *et al.*, EAU Guidelines on Penile Cancer, and Paner *et al.*, Updates in the Eighth Edition of the Tumor-Node-Metastasis Staging Classification for Urologic Cancers [**3**,**30**].

The overriding general principles of treatment are to obtain complete disease control, conserving tissue where possible in order to minimise residual sexual dysfunction [31].

The penile surgery may need to be radical, total or partial, depending on location and extent.

To conserve tissue and minimise residual sexual dysfunction, conservative techniques are increasingly used, with narrow excisional

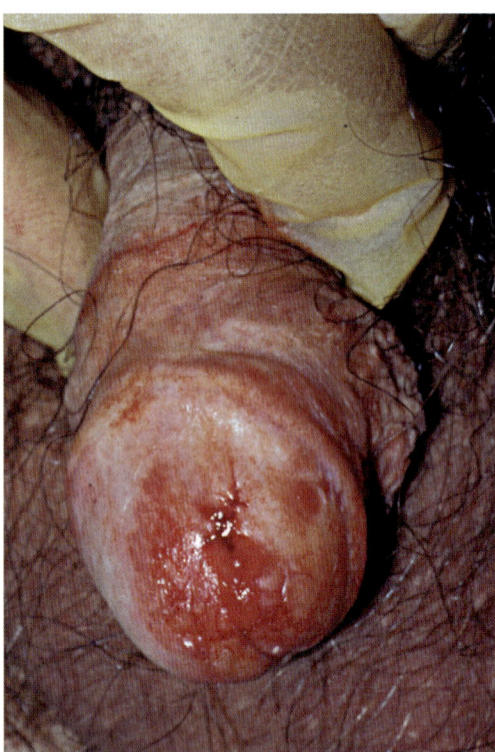

Figure 109.18 High-grade dysplasia and invasive squamous carcinoma. Courtesy of Professor C.B. Bunker and with permission from Medical Illustration UK, Chelsea & Westminster Hospital, London, UK.

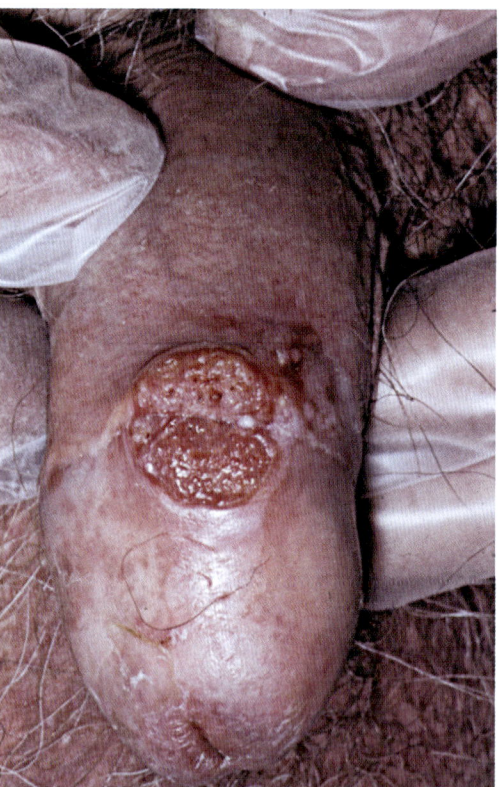

Figure 109.19 Squamous carcinoma. Severe background lichen sclerosus. Reproduced with permission from Elsevier.

margins and innovative plastic repair, as is Mohs micrographic surgery for squamous carcinoma of the penis.

The concepts of field change, multifocality and the temporal dynamic and implications of infection by HPV must also be considered.

Fundamental to the planning of penile surgery for penile carcinoma associated with LSc is the recognition of the pernicious role in the initiation and progression of LSc played by the chronic occluded exposure of genital skin to urine [32]; the laudable goals of organ-saving surgery in penis cancer should include the avoidance of new or, more likely, recurrent LSc, because of the ensuing morbidity and risk of second squamous cancers. For this reason, patients with a diagnosis of penile carcinoma should undergo circumcision, even if the carcinoma is on the glans.

A diagnosis of penile carcinoma dictates individualised expert multidisciplinary treatment, in the UK, by a multidisciplinary team.

PSCC limited to the prepuce may be treated by circumcision. Verrucous carcinoma of the glans, if non-invasive (pTa), may be treated with glans-sparing techniques, including local excision or glans resurfacing; other options described include focal chemotherapy or immunotherapy, laser ablation, radiation therapy or surgery [3].

Treatments for PeIN (carcinoma *in situ*/pTis) are discussed earlier in this chapter.

Complete excision of the tumour with a clear histopathological margin is needed; there is no clear evidence on the optimal surgical margins, but a 3.5 mm margin is considered likely to be satisfactory [3,33]. The use of Mohs micrographic surgery has been described [34].

Invasion of the corpus spongiosum (pT2) or the corpora cavernosa (pT3) necessitates glansectomy, and extensive tumours (pT4), in some cases including removal of the tips of the corpora. In these cases, plastic reconstruction should also be attempted. Extensive tumours (pT4) require either partial or radical penectomy [3].

Radiotherapy in the form of external beam radiotherapy or focal brachytherapy may be performed in stages T1 and T2 for tumours ≤4 cm, but local control rates are less favourable compared with the surgical options of glansectomy or glans resurfacing [3]. Potential complications of radiotherapy include urethral stenosis, glans necrosis and late fibrosis of the corpora cavernosa [3].

PSCC exhibits a tendency for early metastasis to regional (inguinal and pelvic) lymph nodes. One in seven patients has lymph node metastasis at the time of diagnosis [35]. Given the limitations in non-invasive imaging in detecting lymph node metastases in those without palpable lymphadenopathy, invasive diagnostic investigations are undertaken in stage pT1 and grade G2–3 and beyond, including dynamic sentinel lymph node biopsy (DSNB).

In those with confirmed lymph node metastasis, radical inguinal lymphadenectomy is indicated. Ipsilateral pelvic lymphadenectomy is required if additional inguinal lymph node metastases are detected at completion of lymphadenectomy.

If metastases are only detected in one lymph node, and capsular penetration or extranodal extension is detected, the disease is classified as pN3, and adjuvant chemotherapy can be offered.

The most common sites for distant metastases of penile carcinoma are the lungs, liver and brain [3]. Palliative chemotherapy, usually a triple regimen including both cisplatin and paclitaxel, can achieve a limited improvement in survival [3].

Data for targeted therapies remain limited [3], although a number of trials are ongoing [36]. Dacomitinib, a pan-HER tyrosine kinase inhibitor, has undergone an open-label phase 2 study and showed an overall response rate of 32.1% in patients with either lymph node or systemic metastases [37], lower than standard chemotherapy regimens. There are case reports indicating treatment response to PD-1 inhibitors [38,39] and epidermal growth factor receptor (EGFR) inhibitors [40–42]. In a case series of six patients with advanced penile carcinoma treated with sunitinib or sorafenib, a response (partial) was observed in just one patient [43].

The overall 5-year relative survival rate for localised disease is 80%, while regional metastasis reduces 5-year relative survival to 50% [44]. Distant metastasis portends a poor prognosis, with only 9% of patients surviving 5 years.

Carcinoma of the scrotum

Squamous cell carcinoma of the scrotum is rare, with an incidence of approximately 0.34/100 000 per year in a European population [1]. It has historically been recognised in chimney sweeps (exposed to carcinogens in soot) [2], mule spinners (exposed to carcinogens in lubricating oils for the spinning jenny in the cloth industry), Persian nomads (who travelled with pots of burning charcoal between their legs) and Indian jute oil processors [3–7]. Oil-mist exposure in industry continues to be widespread and, apart from scrotal cancer, has been associated with other cutaneous problems (such as contact dermatitis and oil acne) and respiratory diseases, including cancer [8].

Other individuals at risk of scrotal squamous carcinoma include those with a history of psoriasis treated with arsenic, coal tar, UVB and PUVA, radiotherapy [9–11,12,13,14], scrotal HPV infection, hidradenitis suppurativa, Bowen disease and multiple cutaneous keratoses and epitheliomas [15–19]. The 5-year survival for squamous cell carcinoma of the scrotum is 77% [1]. The incidence of scrotal squamous cell carcinoma has remained stable, despite increased recognition and mitigation of industrial exposures [1].

The clinical presentation of scrotal carcinoma may include symptoms of itch, irritation, pain, bleeding, discharge, ulceration or the discovery of a macule, ulcer or lump. The differential diagnosis includes the manifestations of intraepithelial neoplasia (and the respective differential diagnoses of each manifestation of this), erosive or ulcerative sexually transmitted disease, basal cell carcinoma, Kaposi sarcoma, metastasis, extramammary Paget disease, pyoderma gangrenosum and artefact. The diagnosis is confirmed by biopsy [20].

Buschke–Löwenstein tumour/giant condyloma

Introduction and general description

Buschke–Löwenstein tumour is a large HPV-related ano-genital tumour that can affect the penis and the ano-rectal region.

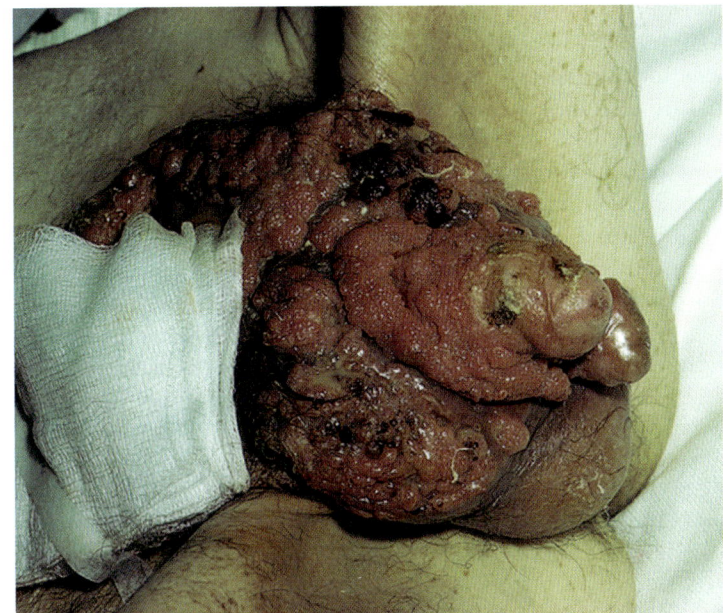

Figure 109.20 Gross condylomas of Buschke–Löwenstein of the penis. Courtesy of Professor R.M. MacKie, Glasgow University, Glasgow, UK.

Literature on the entity is problematic; it is composed almost entirely of case reports and case series, and the characteristics of lesions described as Buschke–Löwenstein tumours vary substantially [1]. A definition has therefore been recently proposed in which Buschke–Löwenstein tumour refers to an HPV-related ano-genital verrucous mass larger than 5 cm in total diameter, occupying greater than one-third of the circumference of an ano-genital organ (e.g. the penis, anus or vaginal introitus), with histological features of papillomatosis, hyperkeratosis, parakeratosis, acanthosis and mild koilocytosis [1].

Clinical features

Buschke–Löwenstein tumour exhibits a characteristically verruciform appearance [1,2]. It may appear dramatically polypoid or cauliflower-like (Figure 109.20). The term 'giant condyloma' has been variously used as a synonym for Buschke–Löwenstein tumour, or a precursor lesion that lacks downward growth (towards deeper tissue).

Buschke–Löwenstein tumours may be associated with symptoms of malodour, discomfort and bleeding [1]. They may also be associated with sinus tract formation [1]. Patients are frequently, but not always, immunocompromised. The tumours are often described as slow growing, but rapid growth has also been described [1].

Buschke and Löwenstein classified the entity as a non-carcinoma in their original description [3]. Löwenstein later elaborated on the basis for this classification, referring to the absence of metastasis or invasion of blood vessels, and the fact that apparent infiltration was 'not active' but rather reflected downward displacement of tissue by the prolific growth of the overlying condyloma [3].

However, subsequent literature has been characterised by inconsistencies and controversies regarding its clinical behaviour, and the classification of the entity varies between sources, with some classifying it as premalignant [4], others as 'semimalignant' [5,6] and others leaving the issue of classification open or undefined. Malignant transformation has been reported, but due to publication bias, the true risk of malignant transformation is difficult to estimate. A further impediment to determining the malignant potential of the entity is the pervasive confusion between Buschke–Löwenstein tumour and verrucous carcinoma in the literature; the terms are frequently used as synonyms, and it is frequently erroneously proffered that Buschke–Löwenstein tumour is classified as a form of verrucous carcinoma [1]. In addition, given the obscure definition of Buschke–Löwenstein tumour, it is possible that lesions reported as such may in fact have been misdiagnosed squamous cell carcinomas from the outset [1]. Analysis of reported cases indicates that death related to malignant transformation is extremely rare [1]. Instead, where mortality occurs related to the condition, infectious complications are the predominant cause. These observations suggest that the risk of malignant transformation, as implied in literature, is probably exaggerated [1].

Pathology

Histological features include papillomatosis, hyperkeratosis, parakeratosis, acanthosis and mild koilocytosis [1]. An exoendophytic growth pattern is observed, in which the tumour 'pushes' into adjacent tissue [3,5,7]. The basement membrane is intact [6,7], although it may be obscured by a lymphocytic infiltrate [3].

Pathophysiology

Buschke–Löwenstein tumour is most frequently associated with low-risk HPV types 6 and 11, but high-risk types 33, 52, 56 have also been detected [1]; and it is highly likely that HPV type influences the malignant potential of each tumour.

Investigation and management

In terms of management, true invasion must be excluded, with biopsy of any areas of induration or ulceration, although invasion may prove difficult to exclude conclusively without complete excision [1]. Cross-sectional imaging may be indicated to assess for invasion and for operative planning [7].

The predominant modality of treatment in the literature is surgical excision; given the low risk of malignant transformation, organ-preserving techniques are favoured [1,7].

Other procedural modalities described include electroresection, shave excision and cautery [8], ablative laser [9] and angioembolisation of supplying vasculature [10].

Medical treatment has also been reported to be effective, including agents such as topical imiquimod [11–13], photodynamic therapy [8], topical cidofovir, podophyllotoxin, liquid nitrogen cryotherapy [14], oral acitretin [15] and antiretroviral therapy [16]. Injectable treatments including mycobacterial vaccination and interferon alfa-2a [5] have also been reported.

Chemoradiation is also documented relatively frequently [17–20] and immunotherapy (pembrolizumab) has also been reported [21], but treatment response was not discussed.

Local recurrence following surgery is common, reportedly occurring in up to two-thirds of patients [22], possibly reflecting the Koebner phenomenon.

Extramammary Paget disease

Definition

Extramammary Paget disease (EMPD) is a malignant skin condition in which there is intraepidermal infiltration by neoplastic cells showing glandular differentiation.

Introduction and general description

Clinically, EMPD typically presents as unilateral well-demarcated, persistent and red eczematous patches or plaques in the ano-genital region.

It tends to progress slowly over a number of years so that a delay in diagnosis is not uncommon. EMPD is often associated with an underlying malignancy [1]. The condition has been classified into primary EMPD, in which it is not associated with an underlying carcinoma, and secondary EMPD, in which it is associated with an underlying carcinoma of a dermal adnexal gland or underlying viscera [2].

Although properly regarded as a type of carcinoma *in situ*, EMPD may itself become invasive and metastatic. There may be subjacent carcinoma (e.g. in periurethral glands) or distant carcinoma (e.g. prostate or bladder) or both (e.g. in periurethral glands and bladder). Pagetoid epidermal invasion of inguinal cutaneous metastatic mesothelioma of the tunica vaginalis of the testis has been reported. The prognosis for *in situ* or minimally invasive disease appears to be generally favourable [2].

Epidemiology

EMPD typically presents between the ages of 60 and 70. The incidence is six per million person-years [3].

Pathophysiology

Immunohistochemical evidence points to sweat gland epithelium or primitive epidermal cells as the source of Paget cells in primary EMPD [2]. The distribution along the 'milk line' has led to the suggestion that the 'clear cells of Toker' are the histogenic precursors of both clear cell papulosis and mammary and EMPD, respectively [4,5]. HPV is not present [6], but the c-erbB-2 oncoprotein may have a role in the pathogenesis of EMPD. It has been proposed that EMPD may be triggered by a central oncogenic stimulus that causes multicentric intraepidermal, adnexal and distant adenocarcinomas [7].

Pathology

Histological examination shows nests of large vacuolated cells with circular nuclei and foamy pale cytoplasm in the epidermis (Paget cells). Dermal involvement signifies a poor prognosis. CK7 is a sensitive marker for EMPD. Immunohistochemistry may also be helpful in determining the probability of an underlying visceral malignancy; expression of GCFDP-15 and lack of expression of CK20 indicate that an underlying malignancy is relatively less likely [2].

Clinical features

EMPD appears as unilateral well-demarcated, persistent and red eczematous patches or plaques that may exhibit crusting, scaling, lichenifcation, ulceration or bleeding on a unilateral red patch or plaque affecting the ano-genital skin, or other sites rich in apocrine glands; they may be solitary or multifocal [8]. In skin types IV–VI, EMPD may present as a hypopigmented macule or patch [9]. There may be papillomatous components or deep ulceration that may be suggestive of invasion [10]. Lesions are usually itchy; pain may also occur [11]. These are associated with symptoms of irritation and burning.

EMPD can occur anywhere in the ano-genital area, including the glans penis [1,6,12]. Localisation outside the 'milk line' has also been described and is termed 'ectopic EMPD' [13]. EMPD may appear concurrently in two different areas, termed 'synchronous EMPD' [13]. Penile EMPD is frequently misdiagnosed as psoriasis, eczema, tinea or Bowen disease [6,12]. An 'underpants' pattern of redness has been reported in a number of patients. Subclinical EMPD has been documented, where the skin looks normal macroscopically but is involved microscopically. EMPD behaves indolently, spreading by local extension and metastasis [1].

The concurrence of genital and extragenital EMPD is extremely rare, but overt and latent axillary EMPD can coexist and change daily in association with penile and pubic EMPD. Also very rare is depigmented EMPD of the genitalia, evoking the differential diagnosis of vitiligo, hypopigmented mycosis fungoides and LSc. A focus of cutaneous squamous carcinoma has been reported complicating genital EMPD [14].

Estimates of associated adnexal neoplasms are 7% [11] to 35% [2], while associated internal malignancies affect 12–40% [11,15]. The exact risk of underlying malignancy is difficult to determine due to limitations in the literature such as reporting bias, disparate definitions of terminology such as 'underlying malignancy', variability in methods used to investigate for underlying malignancy, and reporting bias [2]. The risk of internal malignancy appears to be lower in penoscrotal EMPD than in other anatomical locations [2].

Investigations

Diagnosis is by biopsy. Age-appropriate cancer screening should be undertaken, including urinalysis cytology, cystoscopy, chest X-ray, cross-sectional imaging of the thorax, abdomen and pelvis (to investigate for secondary malignancy and also to investigate for metastasis), colonoscopy and a prostate-specific antigen test [2,16,17]. Serum carcinoembryonic antigen may be helpful in invasive disease [2]. Associated cancers may be metachronous, however, and there are currently no guidelines regarding the frequency of cancer screening.

Management

While the condition presents challenges for surgical management, including its multifocal nature and poorly defined margins, wide excisional surgery has generally been the treatment of choice; margins of 2 cm or 5 cm have been recommended [13,18]. A 'clockface' mapping biopsy technique has been proposed to reduce the risk of incomplete excision; this involves marking the skin radially from the positions of 1 o'clock to 12 o'clock, with punch biopsies taken at 1 cm intervals to 5 cm from the visible edge of the lesion [8]. Mohs micrographic surgery for primary EMPD appears to lead to reduced

rates of recurrence (8–23%) compared with conventional surgical excision (33–44%) [11,18,19–22].

Sentinel lymph node biopsy may be useful in prognostic prediction in invasive disease [13,23,24]. An approach has been proposed in which sentinel lymph node biopsy is routinely performed where invasion is more than 1 mm and only performed in other cases where clinical suspicion is present [2].

Other treatments used for EMPD [6] include topical therapy, laser therapy (CO_2 and Nd:YAG), radiotherapy, photodynamic therapy and cryotherapy. Topical imiquimod has been found to be effective in patients with both primary and recurrent EMPD with complete response in 52–100% and recurrence rates of 6–60% [2,13,25,26]. Aminolevulinic acid-photodynamic therapy (ALA-PDT) has been reported as effective with a complete response rate of 33% and a recurrence rate of 50% [27]. Cryotherapy and topical 5-fluorouracil have been described in case reports and series, and efficacy appears to be poor [11,23,28]. Radiation therapy has also been utilised, with a reported complete response rate of 55% with a recurrence rate of 39% [29]. A combination of treatments is often required.

Regression of EMPD has been observed to occur following excision of an underlying neoplasm [30].

For metastatic EMPD, there is no standardised chemotherapeutic regimen, although many reported regimens include cisplatin and 5-fluorouracil [2].

Long-term follow-up is required, as recurrences have been reported 15 years following diagnosis [13]. There is no consensus regarding when repeat cancer screening for metachronous secondary malignancy should be undertaken [16].

Malignant melanoma

This is a rare condition of the penis. It is estimated to account for 1–1.5% of all malignancies of the penis [1,2] and fewer than 0.15% of all melanomas [3]. Melanoma is even rarer on the scrotum, with only 20 cases appearing in a recent literature review [4–6].

Genital melanoma presents as a pigmented macule or as a pigmented or amelanotic papule or nodule, possibly developing from a pre-existing dysplastic naevus that may ulcerate or bleed [1,2,7–10]. One case has been reported of a melanoma arising in a divided or 'kissing' naevus (naevi that became divided during embryogenesis) of the penis [10]. Multifocal melanoma of the glans penis has been reported [11]. Patients are usually middle-aged or older, although it has been reported in a boy [12]. It is exceedingly rare in Asian people and has not been reported in Afro-Caribbean people (although a case of melanoma of the urethra has been seen) [13]. The diagnosis is often delayed [2].

Between 60% and 70% of lesions occur on the glans. There may be a family history of melanoma and other atypical or 'dysplastic' naevi on examination. The inguinal and other nodes, as well as the abdomen, should be palpated. Between 40% and 50% of patients have lymphatic or other metastatic dissemination at the time of presentation. Clinically, atypical lesions should be biopsied and the histology critically reviewed [14,15]. Malignant melanoma of any histological subtype may be encountered [16].

Treatment is by primary excision.

PART 10: SPECIFIC SITES, SEX & AGE

Kaposi sarcoma

Solitary Kaposi sarcoma of the penis was very rarely seen before the HIV epidemic and cases are still occasionally seen in HIV-negative patients [1–4], but genital Kaposi sarcoma is essentially an HIV-associated disorder. It presents on the penis or scrotum, perineum or perianal skin in one of its classic forms: purple, slightly scaly patches or plaques, nodules or ulcerative lesions [5]. More atypical presentations that have been seen include engorgement with hypervascularity [6], penile lymphoedema [7] and phimosis. The differential diagnosis includes cellular naevus, histiocytoma, angioma, angiokeratoma, pseudo-Kaposi sarcoma [8], bacillary angiomatosis and melanoma.

Other malignant neoplasms

Although basal cell carcinoma is the most common type of skin cancer, it is rare in the ano-genital area [1,2]. Most reported cases have been located on the shaft, appearing clinically as plaques or nodules, and the majority are either nodular or superficial types on histology, with one case report of fibroepithelioma of Pinkus affecting the base of the penis [2,3]. A case of multiple erosive scrotal basal cell carcinomas with metastasis has been described [4].

Fibrosarcoma, haemangiopericytoma, leiomyosarcoma, malignant fibrous histiocytoma, epithelioid sarcoma, dermatofibrosarcoma protuberans and spindle cell sarcoma may occur, presenting as painful or painless nodules, masses or swelling with dysuria and erectile difficulties (e.g. masquerading as Peyronie disease) [5–7]. Other rarities include Merkel cell carcinoma [8], malignant eccrine poroma [9], malignant schwannoma [5,10] and solitary reticulohistiocytic granuloma of the scrotum [11]. Scrotal angiosarcoma complicating oedema following surgery and radiotherapy for carcinoma of the rectum has been described [12].

Involvement of the penis with Langerhans cell histiocytosis is very rare; fleshy papules on the dorsal penis, a painful nodule of the prepuce and penile ulceration have been reported [13,14].

Mycosis fungoides can be confined to, or concentrated in, the genital region. Localised perianal involvement [15], a solitary plaque on the penis [16] and response to treatment with imiquimod have been described [16,17].

Although lymphoma is the most frequent secondary tumour of the testis, it is rare in other parts of the male uro-genital tract [5]. Penile lymphoma can present as painless subcutaneous nodules, erythematous swelling, phimosis and ulceration [18–23]. There may be no evidence of systemic lymphoma. Ulcerating scrotal lymphoma has been reported [24], as have scrotal and penile ulceration resulting from leukaemic infiltration [25,26].

Metastases to the penis are rare, but several hundred cases have been reported [27,28]. They are usually secondary to cancer of the uro-genital tract [29] or gastrointestinal system, or other common cancers such as of the lung [30], and present with pain, swelling, priapism, urinary symptoms or haematuria. A very rare cause is secondary melanoma [27,31] and primary cholangiocarcinoma [32].

MISCELLANEOUS CUTANEOUS MALE GENITAL CONDITIONS

Penile melanosis

Causes of ano-genital hypo- and hyperpigmentation are listed in Boxes 109.27 and 109.28.

Box 109.27 Causes of genital postinflammatory hypopigmentation

- Following cryotherapy
  - Electrotherapy
  - Chemocautery
  - Laser surgery
- Contact dermatitis
- Lichen sclerosus
- Systemic sclerosis
- Lichen planus
- Cicatricial pemphigoid
- Gonococcal dermatitis
- Syphilis
  - Leukoderma: postsecondary syphilide
  - Gumma
  - Postgummatous atrophic scar
- Herpes simplex
- Pityriasis versicolor
- Onchocerciasis 'leopard skin'
- Peyronie disease
- Pseudoepitheliomatous micaceous and keratotic balanitis

Reproduced from Bunker CB. *Male Genital Skin Disease*, 2nd edn. London: Bruce Shrink, 2019. © 2019, with permission from the author.

Box 109.28 Causes of genital postinflammatory hyperpigmentation

- Post-traumatic
- Lichen planus
- Herpes simplex
- Fixed drug eruption

Reproduced from Bunker CB. *Male Genital Skin Disease*, 2nd edn. London: Bruce Shrink, 2019. © 2019, with permission from the author.

Pigmented macules are not uncommon on the glans and shaft of the penis [1,2]. They are benign but, because they may be large or enlarging, with irregular edges and multifocal and variegated pigmentary patterns, they arouse concern about atypical melanocytic proliferation and acral lentiginous melanoma. Such clinical concerns should lead to biopsy [3]; it is important to decolourise slides from deeply pigmented lesions because large quantities of melanin can obscure cytological detail [2]. Postinflammatory hyperpigmentation (e.g. LSc, lichen planus) may be the cause in many patients. Some cases have been associated with previous treatment with dithranol, PUVA therapy or diabetes [4,5]. The eruptive appearance of melanotic macules and papules in the ano-genital region may be associated with advanced metastatic adenocarcinoma [6].

The term penile melanosis has been used to describe pigmented lesions without lentiginous hyperplasia [5,7], but the field is confusing and this definition may be problematic. Revuz and Clerici [7] proposed the grouping of penile melanosis, vulvovaginal melanosis and the predominantly oral mucosal hyperpigmentation of the Laugier–Hunziker syndrome under the umbrella of essential melanotic hyperpigmentation of the mucosa. Lenane *et al.* [8] used the term genital melanotic macules. On histological examination there may be increased basal epidermal pigmentation, with or without benign lentiginous melanocytic hyperplasia (despite some definitions), or an increase in basal melanocyte number. Breathnach *et al.* [9] have proposed that depigmentation is an essential element of penile melanosis and demonstrated melanocytic hyperplasia in areas of hyperpigmentation. Harmelin *et al.* have reported vitiligo-like macules in penile melanosis, speculatively due to local antimelanocyte autoimmunity [10].

Patients ask for treatment of penile melanosis as it is unsightly and embarrassing, but options are limited [2]. Laser treatment or topical depigmenting agents may help [11]. Follow-up decisions are by necessity individualised.

Acral lentiginous melanoma is very rare but important [12,13].

Hypopigmentation

Striae as a consequence of growth or weight surges are common around the pelvic girdle, or represent a complication of topical corticosteroid application [14]. Initially, they are often purple-red in colour. Vitiligo is a commonly observed affliction of the male genitalia, although patients may be unaware of it and clinicians might not always observe it [15]. Penile vitiligo attributed to the use of topical imiquimod for the treatment of genital warts has been described [16].

Idiopathic lipogranuloma

Cases of characteristic, spontaneously resolving, painless, Y-shaped swelling of the scrotum embracing the penile root, with sclerosing eosinophilic lipogranuloma on histology and electron microscopy (but no exogenous lipids) and associated with blood eosinophilia (one patient had arthralgia), have been reported from Japan [1].

Dysaesthesia and chronic pain syndromes

It is not uncommon to encounter florid symptomatology affecting the genital skin with a paucity or absence of primary dermatological signs. These symptoms may include itching, excessive redness, burning and discomfort – in some cases so severe that it prevents the patient from sitting down. The skin may be completely normal or there may be redness. These presentations are grouped under the umbrella term of genital dysaesthesia, and related chronic uro-genital and rectal pain syndromes include orchialgia, prostatodynia, coccygodynia, proctalgia fugax, perineal pain, and the descending perineum syndrome [1–3]. It has been proposed that persistent genital arousal disorder, also known as restless genital syndrome, should also be classified among these disorders [4].

Redness may be present or absent in such disorders, although no other primary pathological morphology should be observed that could provide an alternative explanation for the symptoms. Localised dermographism should be sought by stroking the inside of the thigh with a chaperone present, because such patients may be helped by oral antihistamine treatment. The possibilities of zinc deficiency and necrolytic migratory erythema should also be considered. A history of infection with herpes zoster may explain the symptoms in some cases, as this can lead to damage or dysfunction of peripheral and skin nerve fibres and chronic pain and/or pruritus can develop as a consequence [5]; localised pain without cutaneous signs may also indicate a new infection or recurrent episode of herpes simplex.

In addition to the presence or absence of redness, the presentation of genital dysaesthesia is also heterogeneous in terms of the specific anatomical area(s) involved and the symptoms experienced (e.g. itch or pain or both). A well-described form of genital dysaesthesia is the red burning scrotum syndrome as defined by Fisher [6]. It manifests as 'persistent redness of the anterior half of the scrotum that may involve the base of the penis usually accompanied by a persistent itching or burning sensation and hyperalgesia'. It is a chronic condition that is resistant to treatment and its cause is unknown [6,7], although it has been proposed that it may represent a localised form of erythromelalgia [8,9].

The neurophysiological basis for chronic genital dysaesthesia is likely to be heterogeneous, reflecting the variability observed in clinical manifestations. Among the possible causes are small fibre neuropathy, nerve injury, inflammation or entrapment [5,10,11,12,13]; the role of somatisation is debated [14]. Small fibre polyneuropathy, affecting small unmyelinated C-fibres and thinly myelinated A-delta fibres, is prevalent in complex chronic pain syndromes, in which genital pain syndromes are observed as a co-morbidity [12]. There is some evidence to suggest increased expression of transient receptor potential vanilloid type 1 (TRPV1) ion channels by nociceptors in patients with vulvodynia [13]; these play a role in modulating itch and pain signals. There may be additional neural components that contribute to amplification or perpetuation of pain and these may be peripheral or central, and the immune system may also contribute [10]. Magnetic resonance imaging, which may include specialised techniques such as magnetic resonance neurography, may prove helpful in the diagnosis [10].

Pudendal nerve entrapment syndrome can result in cutaneous symptoms anywhere from the anus to the penis (or clitoris) [15]. In this syndrome, pain is predominantly experienced while sitting and pruritus may accompany pain, but does not occur in the absence of pain [15]. Normal electrophysiological studies do not exclude pudendal nerve entrapment syndrome, and pudendal nerve block is both diagnostic and therapeutic [14].

Treatment in these situations can be challenging and multidisciplinary management is often necessary [16], with input from dermatologists, pain specialists, psychologists, physiotherapists and radiologists. A diagnosis of a chronic pain syndrome implies the prospect of considerable psychological morbidity [14]. Body dysmorphic disorder, depression and psychosis may be present, and the risk of suicide must be considered [17,18].

Cognitive–behavioural therapy and physiotherapy may prove beneficial in genital dysaesthesia, as observed in female patients with vestibulodynia [19]. Patients should be counselled on avoidance of scratching to prevent lichenification and perpetuation of the itch–scratch cycle [20]. Topical lidocaine and oral doxepin, dosulepin, amitriptyline and paroxetine can afford some relief [6,20]. Topical capsaicin has also been reported to be successful [21]. Intradermal botulinum toxin has also been described as showing benefit in a case of genital (scrotal) dysaesthesia without redness [22].

Treatment success in the red burning scrotum syndrome has been reported with several agents including doxycycline [23–25], pregabalin [26,27], ivermectin [28], carvedilol [29], timolol [30] and indometacin [31].

Involvement of a pain specialist is crucial if nerve entrapment is suspected. If lumbosacral radiculopathy is confirmed, then paravertebral blockade can be offered [11]. Neuromodulation including techniques such as spinal cord stimulation, pudendal nerve stimulation and sacral neuromodulation may also prove a useful therapeutic option for patients [10].

Miscellaneous

Penile dysmorphic disorders may lead to patients seeking plastic surgery to the penis [1] for psychosexual reasons (e.g. body dysmorphic disorder).

The koro syndrome is a psychiatric disorder characterised by fear of genital retraction (i.e. the penis shrinking, retracting or disappearing into the abdomen), acute anxiety, and fear of death and genital pain. There is rarely real associated genital pathology. Although originally thought to be a culture-specific condition in South-East Asia and China, it has been observed in the West, without fear of death [2].

Key references

The full list of references can be found in the online version at https://www.wiley.com/rooksdermatology10e

Structure and function of the male genitalia

1 Cold CJ, Taylor JR. The prepuce. *BJU Int* 1999;83(Suppl. 1):34–44.
2 Ammini AC, Sabherwal U, Mukhopadhyay C *et al*. Morphogenesis of the human external male genitalia. *Pediatr Surg Int* 1997;12:401–6.
4 Achtstätter T, Moll R, Moore B, Franke WW. Cytokeratin polypeptide patterns of different epithelia of the human male urogenital tract: immunofluorescence and gel electrophoretic studies. *J Histochem Cytochem* 1985;33:415–26.

History and examination

7 Bunker CB. *Male Genital Skin Disease*. London: Saunders, 2004.
9 Waugh MA. Balanitis. *Dermatol Clin* 1998;16:757–62.
10 Edwards S. Balanitis and balanoposthitis: a review. *Genitourin Med* 1996;72:155–9.
11 English JC, III, Laws RA, Keough GC *et al*. Dermatoses of the glans penis and prepuce. *J Am Acad Dermatol* 1997;37:1–24.
13 Rosen T, Brown TJ. Genital ulcers: evaluation and treatment. *Dermatol Clin* 1998;16:673–85.
19 Mallon E, Ross JS, Hawkins DA *et al*. Biopsy of male genital dermatosis. *Genitourin Med* 1997;73:421.
20 Rao A, Bunker CB. Male genital skin biopsy. *Int J STD AIDS* 2011;22:418–19.

Normal variants

3 Sonnex C, Dockerty WG. Pearly penile papules: a common cause of concern. *Int J STD AIDS* 1999;10:726–7.
4 Neri I, Bardazzi F, Raone B *et al*. Ectopic pearly penile papules: a paediatric case. *Genitourin Med* 1997;73:136.
5 Ackerman AD, Kornberg R. Pearly penile papules. *Arch Dermatol* 1973;108:673–5.
6 Porter W, Bunker CB. Treatment of pearly penile papules with cryotherapy. *Br J Dermatol* 2000;142:847–8.
13 Izquierdo MJ, Pastor MA, Carrasco L *et al*. Epithelioid blue naevus of the genital mucosa: report of four cases. *Br J Dermatol* 2001;145:496–501.
14 de Giorgi V, Massi D, Brunasso G *et al*. Eruptive multiple blue nevi of the penis: a clinical dermoscopic pathologic case study. *J Cutan Pathol* 2004;31:185–8.
15 Aoyagi S, Sato-Matsumura KS, Akiyama M *et al*. Spitz naevus of the glans penis: an unusual location. *Acta Derm Venereol* 2004;84:324–5.
18 Phan PT, Francis N, Madden N, Bunker CB. Kissing naevus of the penis. *Clin Exp Dermatol* 2004;29:471–2.
22 Erkek E, Basar MM, Bagci Y *et al*. Fordyce angiokeratomas as clues to local venous hypertension. *Arch Dermatol* 2005;141:1325–6.
23 Caputo R, Passoni E, Cavicchini S. Papular xanthoma associated with angiokeratoma of Fordyce: considerations on the nosography of this rare non-Langerhans cell histiocytoxanthomatosis. *Dermatology* 2003;206:165–8.

The foreskin

1 Whitfield H. Circumcision. *BJU Int* 1999;83(Suppl. 1):1–113.
2 Porter WM, Bunker CB. The dysfunctional foreskin. *Int J STD AIDS* 2001;12:216–20.
3 Taves DR. The intromission function of the foreskin. *Med Hypotheses* 2002;59:180–2.
4 Bunker CB. *Male Genital Skin Disease*. London: Saunders, 2004.
5 Cold CJ, Taylor JR. The prepuce. *BJU Int* 1999;83(Suppl. 1):34–44.

Circumcision

5 Whitfield H. Circumcision. *BJU Int* 1999;83(Suppl. 1):1–113.
9 Anonymous. *Guidance for Doctors Who Are Asked to Circumcise Male Children*. London: General Medical Council, 1997.
10 American Academy of Pediatrics Task Force on Circumcision. Circumcision policy statement. *Pediatrics* 2012;130:585–86.
11 Morris B, Krieger J. Does male circumcision affect sexual function, sensitivity or satisfaction? A systematic review. *J Sex Med* 2013;10:2644–57.
13 Fergusson DM, Lawton JM, Shannon FT. Neonatal circumcision and penile problems: an 8 year longitudinal study. *Pediatrics* 1988;81:537–41.
15 Liu CM, Hungate BA, Tobian AAR *et al*. Male circumcision significantly reduces prevalence and load of genital anaerobic bacteria. *mBio* 2013;4:e00076.
16 Price LB, Liu CM, Johnson KE *et al*. The effects of circumcision on the penis microbiome. *PLoS One* 2010;5:e8442.
17 O'Farrell N, Egger M. Circumcision in men and the prevention of HIV infection: a 'meta-analysis' revisited. *Int J STD AIDS* 2000;11:137–42.
22 Laumann EO, Masi CM, Zuckerman EW. Circumcision in the United States: prevalence, prophylactic effects and sexual practice. *JAMA* 1997;277:1052–7.
23 Mallon E, Hawkins D, Dinneen M *et al*. Circumcision and genital dermatoses. *Arch Dermatol* 2000;136:350–4.
24 Chang HC, Sung CW, Lin MH. Association of circumcision status with genital lichen planus: a systematic review and meta-analysis. *Acta Derm Venereol* 2019;99:1049–50.
25 Ryan C, Sadlier M, De Vol E *et al*. Genital psoriasis is associated with significant impairment in quality of life and sexual functioning. *J Am Acad Dermatol* 2015;72:978–83.

44 Doiron PR, Bunker CB. Obesity-related male genital lichen sclerosus. *J Eur Acad Dermatol Venereol* 2017;31:876–9.

Congenital and developmental abnormalities

1 Baskin LS, Ebbers MB. Hypospadias: anatomy, etiology and technique. *J Pediatr Surg* 2006;41:463–72.

2 Bunker CB. *Male Genital Skin Disease*. London: Saunders, 2004.

3 Park CO, Chun EY, Lee JH. Median raphe cyst on the scrotum and perineum. *J Am Acad Dermatol* 2005;55:S114–15.

4 Browne WG, Izatt MM, Renwick JH. White sponge naevus of the mucosa: clinical and linkage data. *Ann Hum Genet* 1969;32:271–81.

5 Jorgenson RJ, Levin LS. White sponge nevus. *Arch Dermatol* 1981;117:73–6.

6 Shah A, Meacock L, More B, Chandran H. Lymphangioma of the penis: a rare anomaly. *Pediatr Surg Int* 2005;21:329–30.

7 Stadler HS, Peters CA, Sturm RM *et al*. Meeting report on the NIDDK/AUA Workshop on Congenital Anomalies of External Genitalia: challenges and opportunities for translational research. *J Pediatr Urol* 2020;16:791–804.

8 Girard C, Bigorre M, Guillot B, Bessis D. Pelvis syndrome. *Arch Dermatol* 2006;142:884–8.

9 Musumeci ML, Nasca MR, De Pasquale R *et al*. Cutaneous manifestations and massive genital involvement in Hennekam syndrome. *Pediatr Dermatol* 2006; 23:239–42.

10 Hampshire DJ, Ayub M, Springell K *et al*. MORM syndrome (mental retardation, truncal obesity, retinal dystrophy and micropenis), a new autosomal recessive disorder, links to 9q34. *Eur J Hum Genet* 2006;14:543–8.

11 Vaccaro M, Salpietro DC, Briuglia S *et al*. Cutis laxa in Kabuki make-up syndrome. *J Am Acad Dermatol* 2005;53:S247–51.

Trauma and artefact

1 Nouri M, Koutani A, Tazi K *et al*. Fractures of the penis: apropos of 56 cases. *Prog Urol* 1998;8:542–7.

21 George WM. Papular pearly penile pearls. *J Am Acad Dermatol* 1989;20:852.

25 Al-Mutairi N, Sharma AK, Zaki A *et al*. Penile self-injections: an unusual act. *Int J Dermatol* 2004;43:680–2.

29 Matsuda T, Shichiri Y, Hida S *et al*. Eosinophilic sclerosing lipogranuloma of the male genitalia not caused by exogenous lipids. *J Urol* 1988;140:1021.

31 Greilsheimer H, Groves JE. Male genital self-mutilation. *Arch Gen Psychiatry* 1979;36:441–6.

34 McCann J, Voris J. Perianal injuries resulting from sexual abuse: a longitudinal study. *Pediatrics* 1993;91:390–3.

39 Vickers D, Morris K, Coulthard MG, Eastham EJ. Anal signs in haemolytic uraemic syndrome. *Lancet* 1998;1:998.

40 Hobbs CJ, Wynne JM. How to manage warts. *Arch Dis Child* 1999;81:460.

43 Hrbaty J, Molitor M. Traumatic skin loss from the male genitalia. *Acta Chir Plast* 2001;43:17–20.

45 Sagar J, Sagar B, Shah DK. Penile skin necrosis – complication following selfcircumcision. *Ann R Coll Surg Engl* 2005;87:W5–7.

Inflammatory dermatoses

Psoriasis

2 Meeuwis KA, de Hullu JA, de Jager ME, Massuger LF, van de Kerkhof PC, van Rossum MM. Genital psoriasis: a questionnaire-based survey on a concealed skin disease in the Netherlands. *J Eur Acad Dermatol Venereol* 2010; 24:1425–30.

3 Meeuwis KA, de Hullu JA, Massuger LF, van de Kerkhof PC, van Rossum MM. Genital psoriasis: a systematic literature review on this hidden skin disease. *Acta Derm Venereol* 2011;91:5–11.

4 Larsabal M, Ly S, Sbidian E *et al*. GENIPSO: a French prospective study assessing instantaneous prevalence, clinical features and impact on quality of life of genital psoriasis among patients consulting for psoriasis. *Br J Dermatol* 2019; 180:647–56.

5 Ryan C, Sadlier M, De Vol E *et al*. Genital psoriasis is associated with significant impairment in quality of life and sexual functioning. *J Am Acad Dermatol* 2015;72:978–83.

10 Meeuwis KA, de Hullu JA, van de Nieuwenhof HP *et al*. Quality of life and sexual health in patients with genital psoriasis. *Br J Dermatol* 2011;164:1247–55.

Eczema

1 Shah M. Clinical outcomes in a specialist male genital skin clinic: prospective follow-up of 600 patients. *Clin Exp Dermatol* 2017;42:723–7.

2 Elakis JA, Hall AP. Skin disease of penis and male genitalia is linked to atopy and circumcision: caseload in a male genital dermatology clinic. *Australas J Dermatol* 2017;58:e68–72.

3 Porter WM, Bewley A, Dinneen M *et al*. Nodular lichen simplex of the scrotum treated by surgical excision. *Br J Dermatol* 2001;144:915–16.

14 Van L, Harting M, Rosen T. Jacquet erosive diaper dermatitis: a complication of adult urinary incontinence. *Cutis* 2008;82:72–4.

17 Warshaw EM, Kimyon RS, Silverberg JI *et al*. Evaluation of patch test findings in patients with anogenital dermatitis. *JAMA Dermatol* 2020;156:85–91.

23 Eubel J, Diepgen TL, Weisshaar E. Allergien im Genitalbereich. *Hautarzt* 2015;66:45–52.

40 van Ulsen J, Stolz E, van Joost T, Geursen-Reitsma AM. Allergy to spermicidal lubricant in a contraceptive. *Contact Dermatitis* 1987;17:115–16.

45 Gilissen L, Schollaert I, Huygens S, Goossens A. Iatrogenic allergic contact dermatitis in the (peri)anal and genital area. *Contact Dermatitis* 2021;84:431–8.

46 Woo YR, Han Y, Lee JH *et al*. Real-world prevalence and burden of genital eczema in atopic dermatitis: a multicenter questionnaire-based study. *J Dermatol* 2021;48:625–32.

47 Misery L, Seneschal J, Reguiai Z *et al*. The impact of atopic dermatitis on sexual health. *J Eur Acad Dermatol Venereol* 2019;33:428–32.

Zoon balanoposthitis

1 Zoon JJ. Vereningingsverslagen. *Ned Tijdschr Geneeskd* 1950;94:1528–30.

2 Zoon JJ. Balanoposthite chronique circonscrite bénigne à plasmocytes. *Dermatologica* 1952;105:1–7.

6 Farrell AM, Francis N, Bunker CB. Zoon's balanitis: an immunohistochemical study. *Br J Dermatol* 1996;135(Suppl. 47):57.

8 Altmeyer P, Kastner U, Luther H. Die Balanitis/Balanoposthitis chronica circumscripta benigna plasmacellularis – Entität oder Fiktion? *Hautarzt* 1998;49:552–5.

11 Bunker CB. Zoon balanitis – does it exist? *J Eur Acad Dermatol Venereol* 2020;34:e116–17.

12 Shah M, Maleki N, Edward S. Zoon's balanitis is a nonspecific reactive pattern and not a clinical diagnosis. *J Am Acad Dermatol* 2015;72(S1):AB87.

13 Weyers W, Ende Y, Schalla W, Diaz-Cascajo C. Balanitis of Zoon: a clinicopathologic study of 45 cases. *Am J Dermatopathol* 2002;24:459–67.

16 Bari O, Cohen PR. Successful management of Zoon's balanitis with topical mupirocin ointment: a case report and literature review of mupirocin-responsive balanitis circumscripta plasmacelluaris. *Dermatol Ther* 2017;7:203–10. Erratum in *Dermatol Ther* 2017;7:211.

17 Giorgio CMR, Briatico G, Licata G *et al*. Topical cyclosporine 5% cream in Zoon's balanitis resistant to other therapies: a case report. *Dermatol Ther* 2021;34:e14807.

18 Davis-Daneshfar A, Trüeb RM. Bowen's disease of the glans penis (erythroplasia of Queyrat) in plasma cell balanitis. *Cutis* 2000;65:395–8.

19 Balato N, Scalvenzi M, La Bella S, Di Costanzo L. Zoon's balanitis: benign or premalignant lesion? *Case Rep Dermatol* 2009;1:7–10.

24 Kravvas G, Shim TN, Doiron PR *et al*. The diagnosis and management of male genital lichen sclerosus: a retrospective review of 301 patients. *J Eur Acad Dermatol Venereol* 2018;32:91–5.

35 Bunker CB, Neill S, Staughton RCD. Topical tacrolimus, genital lichen sclerosus and risk of squamous cell carcinoma. *Arch Dermatol* 2004;140:1169.

Lichen sclerosus

1 Bunker CB, Shim TN. Male genital lichen sclerosus. *Indian J Dermatol* 2015; 60:111–17.

6 Ridley CM. Lichen sclerosus et atrophicus. *BMJ* 1987;295:1295–6.

7 Meffert JJ, Davis BM, Grimwood RE. Lichen sclerosus. *J Am Acad Dermatol* 1995;32:393–416.

9 Gambichler T, Skrygan M, Tigges C, Kobus S, Gläser R, Kreuter A. Significant upregulation of antimicrobial peptides and proteins in lichen sclerosus. *Br J Dermatol* 2009;161:1136–42.

10 Terlou A, Santegoets LA, van der Meijden WI *et al*. An autoimmune phenotype in vulvar lichen sclerosus and lichen planus: a Th1 response and high levels of microRNA-155. *J Invest Dermatol* 2012;132:658–66.

11 Farrell AM, Dean D, Millard PR, Charnock FM, Wojnarowska F. Cytokine alterations in lichen sclerosus: an immunohistochemical study. *Br J Dermatol* 2006;155:931–40.

PART 10: SPECIFIC SITES, SEX & AGE

12 Russo T, Currò M, Barbera A *et al*. Expression of transglutaminase in foreskin of children with balanitis xerotica obliterans. *Int J Mol Sci* 2016;17:E1551.

13 Lewis FM, Tatnall FM, Velangi SS *et al*. British Association of Dermatologists guidelines for the management of lichen sclerosus, 2018. *Br J Dermatol* 2018;178:839–53.

17 Lipscombe TK, Wayte J, Wojnarowska F, Marren P, Luzzi G. A study of clinical and aetiological factors and possible associations of lichen sclerosus in males. *Australas J Dermatol* 1997;8:132–6.

19 Cooper SM, Ali I, Baldo M, Wojnarowska F. The association of lichen sclerosus and erosive lichen planus of the vulva with autoimmune disease: a case-control study. *Arch Dermatol* 2008;144:1432–5.

21 Kantere D, Alvergren G, Gillstedt M, Pujol-Calderon F, Tunbäck P. Clinical features, complications and autoimmunity in male lichen sclerosus. *Acta Derm Venereol* 2017;97:365–9.

23 Edmonds EVJ, Hunt S, Hawkins D, Dinneen M, Francis N, Bunker CB. Clinical parameters in male genital lichen sclerosus: a case series of 329 patients. *J Eur Acad Dermatol Venereol* 2011;26:730–7.

24 Kreuter A, Kryvosheyeva Y, Terras S *et al*. Association of autoimmune diseases with lichen sclerosus in 532 male and female patients. *Acta Derm Venereol* 2013;93:238–41.

25 Marren P, Yell J, Charnock FM, Bunce M, Welsh K, Wojnarowska F. The association between lichen sclerosus and antigens of the HLA system. *Br J Dermatol* 1995;132:197–203.

28 Oyama N, Chan I, Neill SM *et al*. Autoantibodies to extracellular matrix protein 1 in lichen sclerosus. *Lancet* 2003;362(9378):118–23.

29 Edmonds EVJ, Oyama N, Chan I, Francis N, McGrath JA, Bunker CB. Extracellular matrix protein 1 autoantibodies in male genital lichen sclerosus. *Br J Dermatol* 2011;165:218–19.

30 Shim TN, Harwood CA, Marsh SG *et al*. Immunogenetics and human papillomavirus (HPV) in male genital lichen sclerosus (MGLSc). *International Journal of STD AIDS* 2020;31:1334–9.

34 Pugliese JM, Morey AF, Peterson AC. Lichen sclerosus: review of the literature and current recommendations for management. *J Urol* 2007;178:2268–76.

35 Doiron PR, Bunker CB. Obesity-related male genital lichen sclerosus. *J Eur Acad Dermatol Venereol* 2017;31:876–9.

44 Farrar CW, Dowling P, Mendelsohn SD. Peristomal lichen sclerosus developing posturostomy. *Clin Exp Dermatol* 2003;28:223–4.

45 Al-Niaimi F, Lyon C. Peristomal lichen sclerosus: the role of occlusion and urine exposure? *Br J Dermatol* 2013;168:643–6.

46 Shim TN, Andrich DE, Mundy AR, Bunker CB. Lichen sclerosus associated with perineal urethrostomy. *Br J Dermatol* 2014;170:222–3.

47 Kirby L, Gran S, Orekoya F, Owen C, Simpson R. Is urinary incontinence associated with vulval lichen sclerosus in women? A cross-sectional study. *Br J Dermatol* 2021;185:1063–5.

48 Bunker CB, Patel N, Shim TN. Urinary voiding symptomatology (micro-incontinence) in male genital lichen sclerosus. *Acta Derm Venereol* 2013;93:246–8.

60 Regauer S, Reich O, Beham-Schmid C. Monoclonal gamma-T-cell receptor rearrangement in vulvar lichen sclerosus and squamous cell carcinomas. *Am J Pathol* 2002;160:1035–45.

76 Edmonds E, Mavin S, Francis N, Ho-Yen D, Bvunker C. Borrelia burgdorferi is not associated with genital lichen sclerosus in men. *Br J Dermatol* 2009;160:459–60.

77 Eisendle K, Grabner T, Kutzner H, Zelger B. Possible role of Borrelia burgdorferi sensu lato infection in lichen sclerosus. *Arch Dermatol* 2008;144:591–8.

86 Farrell AM, Millard PR, Schomberg KH, Wojnarowska F. An infective aetiology for lichen sclerosus re-addressed. *Clin Exp Dermatol* 1999;24:479–83.

90 Shim TN, Bunker CB. Male genital lichen sclerosus (MGLSc) and hepatitis C. *Br J Dermatol* 2012;167:1398–9.

92 Watchorn RE, van den Munckhof EHA, Quint KD *et al*. Balanopreputial sac and urine microbiota in patients with male genital lichen sclerosus. *Int J Dermatol* 2021;60:201–7.

93 Cohen AJ, Gaither TW, Srirangapatanam S *et al*. Synchronous genitourinary lichen sclerosus signals a distinct urinary microbiome profile in men with urethral stricture disease. *World J Urol* 2021;39:605–11.

94 Han YW. Fusobacterium nucleatum: a commensal-turned pathogen. *Curr Opin Microbiol* 2015;23:141–7.

95 Arya M, Thrasivoulou C, Henrique R *et al*. Targets of Wnt/ß-catenin transcription in penile carcinoma. *PLOS One* 2015;1:e0124395.

96 Liu CM, Hungate BA, Tobian AAR *et al*. Male circumcision significantly reduces prevalence and load of genital anaerobic bacteria. *mBio* 2013;4(2):e00076.

97 Price LB, Liu CM, Johnson KE *et al*. The effects of circumcision on the penis microbiome. *PLoS One* 2010;5:e8422.

101 Regauer S. Immune dysregulation in lichen sclerosus. *Eur J Cell Biol* 2005; 84(2–3):273–7.

105 Shah M. Sexual function is adversely affected in the majority of men presenting with penile lichen sclerosus. *Clin Exp Dermatol* 2021;46:723–6.

111 Ridley CM. Pseudoepitheliomatous micaceous and keratotic balanitis. *Br J Dermatol* 1988;118:856–7.

112 Bunker CB, Francis N. Pseudoepitheliomatous keratotic and micaceous balanitis: comment. *Clin Exp Dermatol* 2012;37:434–5.

115 Shim TN, Doiron PR, Francis N *et al*. Penile lymphoedema: approach to investigation and management. *Clin Exp Dermatol* 2019;44:20–31.

118 McCarthy S, MacEoin N, O'Driscoll M *et al*. Should we always biopsy in clinically evident lichen sclerosus? *J Low Genit Tract Dis* 2019;23:182–3.

126 Kravvas G, Shim TN, Doiron PR *et al*. The diagnosis and management of male genital lichen sclerosus: a retrospective review of 301 patients. *J Eur Acad Dermatol Venereol* 2018;32:91–5.

129 Bunker CB. Male genital lichen sclerosus and topical tacrolimus. *Br J Dermatol* 2007;157:1079–80.

Lichen planus

2 Terlou A, Santegoets LA, van der Meijden WI *et al*. An autoimmune phenotype in vulvar lichen sclerosus and lichen planus: a Th1 response and high levels of microRNA-155. *J Invest Dermatol* 2012;132:658–66.

5 Bunker CB. *Male Genital Skin Disease*, 2nd edn. London: Bruce Shrink, 2019.

8 Worheide J, Bonsmann G, Kolde G, Hamm H. Plattenepithyelkarzinom auf dem Boden eines Lichen ruber hypertrophicus an der Glans penis. *Hautarzt* 1991;42:112–15.

31 Rezzag-Mahcene C, Cardot-Leccia N, Lacour JP, Montaudié H, Passeron T. Successful treatment of recalcitrant genital lichen planus with secukinumab. *J Eur Acad Dermatol Venereol* 2021;35:e321–3.

32 Poon F, De Cruz R, Hall A. Acitretin in erosive penile lichen planus. *Australas J Dermatol* 2017;58:e87–90.

Chronic penile oedema

1 Porter WM, Dinneen M, Bunker C. Chronic penile lymphoedema. *Arch Dermatol* 2001;137:1108–10.

3 Weinberger LN, Zirwas MJ, English JC, III. A diagnostic algorithm for male genital oedema. *J Eur Acad Dermatol Venereol* 2007;21:156–62.

6 Horinaga M, Masuda T, Jitsukawa S. A case of scrotal elephantiasis 30 years after treatment of penile carcinoma. *Hinyokika Kiyo* 1998;44:839–41.

9 Mendelson J, Miller M. Streptococcal venereal edema of the penis. *Clin Infect Dis* 1997;24:516–17.

10 Cunningham MW. Pathogenesis of group A streptococcal infections. *Clin Microbiol Rev* 2000;31:470–511.

13 Saha M, Edmonds E, Martin J *et al*. Penile lymphoedema in association with asymptomatic Crohn's disease. *Clin Exp Dermatol* 2009;34:88–90.

16 Bunker CB, Shim TN. Male genital edema in Crohn's disease. *J Am Acad Dermatol* 2014;70:385.

18 Shim TN, Doiron PR, Francis N *et al*. Penile lymphoedema: approach to investigation and management. *Clin Exp Dermatol* 2019;44:20–31.

19 Palamaras I, El-Jabbour J, Pietropaolo N *et al*. Metastatic Crohn's disease: a review. *J Eur Acad Dermatol Venereol* 2008;22:1033–43.

27 Kopecky RT, Funk MM, Kreitzer PR. Localized genital oedema in patients undergoing continuous ambulatory peritoneal dialysis. *J Eur Acad Dermatol Venereol* 2007;21:156–62.

33 Alibrahim B, Aljasser MI, Salh B. Fecal calprotectin use in inflammatory bowel disease and beyond: a mini-review. *Can J Gastroenterol Hepatol* 2015;29:157–63.

38 Modolin M, Mitre A, da Silva J *et al*. Surgical treatment of lymphedema of the penis and scrotum. *Clinics (Sao Paulo)* 2006;61:289–94.

Miscellaneous inflammatory dermatoses
Non-specific balanoposthitis

1 Bunker CB. *Male Genital Skin Disease*, 2nd edn. London: Bruce Shrink, 2019.

2 Alessi E, Coggi A, Gianotti R. Review of 120 biopsies performed on the balanopreputial sac. *Dermatology* 2004;208:120–4.

4 Shah M. Clinical outcomes in a specialist male genital skin clinic: prospective follow-up of 600 patients. *Clin Exp Dermatol* 2017;42:723–7.

6 Hasegawa T, Hata N, Matsui H, Isaka M, Tatsuno I. Characterisation of clinically isolated Streptococcus pyogenes from balanoposthitis patients, with special emphasis on emm89 isolates. *J Med Microbiol* 2017;66:511–16.

8 Norimatsu Y, Ohno Y. Streptococcus pyogenes balanoposthitis. *IDCases* 2020; 21:e00832.

10 Babu CS, Vitharana S, Higgins SP. Primary syphilis presenting as balanitis. *Int J STD AIDS* 2007;18:497–8.

11 Edwards SK, Bunker CB, Ziller F, van der Meijden WI. 2013 European guideline for the management of balanoposthitis. *Int J STD AIDS* 2014;25:615–26.

Ulcerative disease and penile necrosis

2 Sarihan H. Idiopathic scrotal necrosis. *Br J Urol* 1994;74:259.

12 Orme RL, Nordlund JJ, Barich L, Brown T. The magic syndrome (mouth and genital ulcers with inflamed cartilage). *Arch Dermatol* 1990;126:940–4.

13 Chan C-C, Thyong H-Y, Chan Y-C, Liao Y-H. Human papillomavirus type 5 infection in a patient with Hailey–Hailey disease successfully treated with imiquimod. *Br J Dermatol* 2007;156:579–81.

14 Thomson KF, Highet AS. Penile ulceration in fatal malignant atrophic papulosis (Degos' disease). *Br J Dermatol* 2000;143:1320–2.

21 Bories N, Becuwe C, Marcilly MC *et al.* Glans penis ulceration revealing Wegener's granulomatosis. *Dermatology* 2007;214:187–9.

29 Farrell AM, Black MM, Bracka A, Bunker CB. Pyoderma gangrenosum of the penis. *Br J Dermatol* 1998;138:337–40.

37 Lally A, Hollowood K, Bunker CB, Turner R. Penile pyoderma gangrenosum treated with topical tacrolimus. *Arch Dermatol* 2005;141:1175–6.

40 Boccaletti VP, Ricci R, Sebastio N *et al.* Penile necrosis. *Arch Dermatol* 2000; 136:261–4.

41 Woods M, Pattee SF, Levine N. Penile calciphylaxis. *J Am Acad Dermatol* 2006; 54:736–7.

45 Thorns C, Urban H, Remmler K *et al.* Primary cutaneous T-cell lymphoma of the penis. *Histopathology* 2003;42:513–14.

Pilonidal sinus

1 Al-Qassim Z, Reddy K, Khan Z, Reddy I. Pilonidal sinus cyst of the penis. *BMJ* 2013;2013:bcr2013009718.

2 Val-Bernal JF, Azcarretazabal T, Garijo MF. Pilonidal sinus of the penis: a report of two cases, one of them associated with actinomycosis. *J Cutan Pathol* 1999;26:155–8.

3 O'Kane HF, Duggan B, Mulholland C, Crosbie J. Pilonidal sinus of the penis. *Sci World J* 2004;4(Suppl. 1):258–9.

4 Rashid AMH, Menai Williams R, Parry D, Malone PR. Actinomycosis associated with pilonidal sinus of the penis. *J Urol* 1992;148:405–6.

5 Tomasini C, Aloi F, Puiatti P, Caliendo V. Dermoid cyst of the penis. *Dermatology* 1997;194:188–90.

Peyronie disease

2 Billig R, Baker R, Immergut M, Maxted W. Peyronie's disease. *Urology* 1975;6:409–18.

3 Simeon CP, Fonollosa V, Vilardell M *et al.* Impotence and Peyronie's disease in systemic sclerosis. *Clin Exp Rheumatol* 1994;12:464.

5 Mooradian AD, Viosca SP, Kaiser FE *et al.* Penile Raynaud's phenomenon: a possible cause of erectile failure. *Am J Med* 1988;85:748–50.

8 Grigg AP, Underhill C, Russell J, Sale G. Peyronie's disease as a complication of chronic graft versus host disease. *Hematology* 2002;7:165–8.

9 Horn AS, Pecora A, Chiesa JC, Alloy A. Penile thrombophlebitis as a presenting manifestation of pancreatic carcinoma. *Am J Gastroenterol* 1985;80:463–5.

10 Desanctis PN, Furey CA, Jr. Steroid injection therapy for Peyronie's disease: a 10-year summary and review of 38 cases. *J Urol* 1967;97:114–16.

11 Winter CC, Khanna R. Peyronie's disease: results with dermo-jet injection of dexamethasone. *J Urol* 1975;114:898–900.

12 Chun JL, McGregor A, Krishnan R, Carson CC. A comparison of dermal and cadaveric pericardial grafts in the modified Horton–Devine procedure for Peyronie's disease. *J Urol* 2001;166:185–8.

13 Riedl CR, Plas E, Engelhardt P *et al.* Iontophoresis for treatment of Peyronie's disease. *J Urol* 2000;163:95–9.

14 Paullis G, Cavallini G, Brancato T, Alvaro R. Peironimev-Plus in the treatment of chronic inflammation of tunica albuginea. Results of a controlled study. *Inflamm Allergy Drug Targets* 2013;12:61–7.

Drug reactions

1 Gruber F, Stasic A, Lenkovic M, Brajac I. Postcoital fixed drug eruption in a man sensitive to trimethoprim-sulphamethoxazole. *Clin Exp Dermatol* 1997;22:144–5.

2 Zawar V, Kirloskar M, Chuh A. Fixed drug eruption – a sexually inducible reaction? *Int J STD AIDS* 2004;15:560–3.

3 Borgstrom E. Penile ulcer as complication in self-induced papaverine erections. *Urology* 1988;32:416–17.

4 Esser AC, Nossa R, Shoji T, Sapadin AN. All-trans-retinoic acid-induced scrotal ulcerations in a patient with acute promyelocytic leukaemia. *J Am Acad Dermatol* 2000;43:316–17.

5 Evans LM, Grossman ME. Foscarnet-induced penile ulcer. *J Am Acad Dermatol* 1992;27:124–6.

6 Gross AS, Dretler RH. Foscarnet-induced penile ulcer in an uncircumcised patient with AIDS. *Clin Infect Dis* 1993;17:1076–7.

10 Ogden S, Mukasa Y, Lyon CC, Coulson IH. Nicorandil-induced peristomal ulcers: is nicorandil also associated with gastrointestinal fistula formation? *Br J Dermatol* 2007;156:575–612.

11 Chuah SY, Byrne DJ, Edwards S, Affleck A. Nicorandil-associated penile and anal ulceration triggered by circumcision. *Br J Med Surg Urol* 2010;3:175–7.

12 Baaklini GT, Thompson MJ, Krauland KJ, Walker DR, Hudak SJ. Isolated penile ulceration after Nivolumab therapy for non-small cell lung carcinoma. *Urol Case Rep* 2020;33:101339.

13 Griffiths MR, Milne JT, Porter WM. Penile argyria. *Br J Dermatol* 2006;154:1074–5.

14 Harmanyeri Y, Taskapan O, Dogan B *et al.* A case of coumarin necrosis with penile and pedal involvement. *J Eur Acad Dermatol Venereol* 1998;10:248–52.

15 Chang I, Ha M, Chi B *et al.* Warfarin-induced penile necrosis in a patient with heparin-induced thrombocytopenia. *J Kor Med Sci* 2010;25:1390–3.

Other inflammatory dermatoses

2 Bewley AP, Ross JS, Bunker CB, Staughton RC. Successful treatment of a patient with octreotide-resistant necrolytic migratory erythema. *Br J Dermatol* 1996;134:1101–4.

4 Sami N, Ahmed AR. Penile pemphigus. *Arch Dermatol* 2001;137:756–8.

8 Fueston JC, Adams BB, Mutasim DF. Cicatricial pemphigoid-induced phimosis. *J Am Acad Dermatol* 2001;46:S128–9.

12 Mahmood N, Afzal N, Joyce A. Sarcoidosis of the penis. *Br J Urol* 1997;80:155.

21 Slaney G, Muller S, Clay J *et al.* Crohn's disease involving the penis. *Gut* 1986;27:329–33.

24 Merika EE, Darling MI, Craig P *et al.* Primary cutaneous amyloidosis of the glans penis. Two case reports and a review of the literature. *Br J Dermatol* 2014;170:730–4 (review).

31 Melekos MD, Asbach HW, Markou SA. Aetiology of acute scrotum in 100 boys with regard to age distribution. *J Urol* 1988;139:1023.

33 Udall DA, Drake DJ, Rosenberg RS. Acute scrotal swelling: a physical sign of primary peritonitis. *J Urol* 1981;125:750–1.

35 David S, Schiff JD, Poppas DP. Henoch–Schönlein purpura involving the glans penis. *Urology* 2003;61:1035.

42 Rivollier C, Martin L, Machet L *et al.* Genital papules revealing a Churg–Strauss syndrome. *Ann Dermatol Venereol* 2002;129:1049–52.

Non-sexually transmitted infections
Perineal streptococcal dermatitis/perianal cellulitis

1 Zhang C, Haber RM. The ABCs of perineal streptococcal dermatitis. *J Cutan Med Surg* 2017;21:102–7.

2 Akkilic M, Weger W, Kränke B, Komericki P. Bullous necrotic lesion of the penis. *J Eur Acad Dermatol Venereol* 2006;20:1024–6.

Ecthyma gangrenosum and Fournier gangrene

1 Rabinowitz R, Lewin EB. Gangrene of the genitalia in children with Pseudomonas sepsis. *J Urol* 1980;124:431–2.

3 Smith GL, Bunker CB, Dineen MD. Fournier's gangrene. *Br J Urol* 1998;81:347–55.

4 Adams JR, Jr, Mata JA, Venable DD *et al.* Fournier's gangrene in children. *Urology* 1990;35:439–41.

6 Schultz ES, Diepgen TL, von den Driesch P, Hornstein OP. Systemic corticosteroids are important in the treatment of Fournier's gangrene: a case report. *J Dermatol* 1995;133:633–5.

7 Ferreira PC, Reis JC, Amarante JM *et al.* Fournier's gangrene: a review of 43 reconstructive cases. *Plast Reconstr Surg* 2007;119:175–84.

8 Bubrick MP, Hitchcock CR. Necrotizing anorectal and perineal infection. *Surgery* 1979;86:655–62.

9 Chang I-J, Lee C-C, Chen S-Y. Fulminant gangrenous and crepitating scrotum. *Arch Dermatol* 2006;142:797–8.

10 Fisher JR, Conway ML, Takeshita RT *et al*. Necrotizing fasciitis: importance of roentgenographic studies for soft-tissue gas. *JAMA* 1979;241:803–6.

14 Tahmaz L, Erdemir F, Kibar Y *et al*. Fournier's gangrene: report of thirty-three cases and a review of the literature. *Int J Urol* 2006;13:960–7.

16 Bunker CB. *Male Genital Skin Disease*, 2nd edn. London: Bruce Shrink, 2019.

Trichomycosis pubis, tuberculosis, non-syphilitic spirochaetal ulcerative balanoposthitis, yaws, candidosis, tinea and deep fungal infections

3 Kamalam A, Senthamilselvi G, Ajithadas K, Thambiah AS. Cutaneous trichosporosis. *Mycopathologia* 1988;101:167–75.

4 Minkin W, Frank SB, Cohen HJ. Penile granuloma. *Arch Dermatol* 1972;106:756.

5 Rossi R, Urbano F, Tortoli E *et al*. Primary tuberculosis of the penis. *J Eur Acad Dermatol Venereol* 1999;12:174–6.

11 Piot P, Duncan M, van Dyck E *et al*. Ulcerative balanoposthitis associated with non-syphilitic spirochaetal infection. *Genitourin Med* 1986;62:44–6.

12 Engelkens HJ, Judanarso J, van der Sluis JJ *et al*. Disseminated early yaws: report of a child with a remarkable genital lesion mimicking venereal syphilis. *Pediatr Dermatol* 1990;7:60–2.

14 Odds FC. Genital candidiasis. *Clin Exp Dermatol* 1982;7:345–54.

20 Pielop J, Rosen T. Penile dermatophytosis. *J Am Acad Dermatol* 2001;44:864–7.

22 Preminger B, Gerard PS, Lutwick L *et al*. Histoplasmosis of the penis. *J Urol* 1993;149:848–50.

28 English JC, III, Laws RA, Keough GC *et al*. Dermatoses of the glans penis and prepuce. *J Am Acad Dermatol* 1997;37:1–24; quiz 25–6.

30 Cohen-Ludmann C, Kerob D, Feuilhade M *et al*. Zygomycosis of the penis due to *Rhizopus oryzae* successfully treated with surgical debridement and a combination of high dose liposomal and topical amphotericin B. *Arch Dermatol* 2006;142:1657–8.

Other non-sexually transmitted infections

4 Mukhopadhyay AK. Primary involvement of penile skin in lepromatous leprosy. *Indian J Lepr* 2005;77:317–21.

11 Fox PA, Barton SE, Francis N *et al*. Chronic erosive herpes simplex virus infection of the penis: a possible immune reconstitution disease. *HIV Med* 1999;1:10–18.

12 Spray A, Glaser DA. Herpes zoster of the penis: an unusual location for a common eruption. *J Am Acad Dermatol* 2002;47:S177–9.

14 Cooke RA, Rodriguez RB. Amoebic balanitis. *Med J Aust* 1964;5:114–17.

15 Gbery IP, Dheja D, Kacou DE *et al*. Chronic genital ulcerations and HIV infection: 29 cases. *Med Trop* 1999;59:279–82.

16 Cain C, Seabury-Stone M, Thieburg M, Wilson ME. Non-healing genital ulcers. *Arch Dermatol* 1994;130:1311–16.

18 Grunwald MH, Amichai B, Trau H. Cutaneous leishmaniasis on an unusual site: the glans penis. *Br J Urol* 1998;82:928.

20 Masmoudi A, Boudaya S, Bouzid L *et al*. Penile sporotrichoid cutaneous leishmaniasis. *Bull Soc Pathol Exot* 2005;98:380–1.

22 Zawahry ME. Cutaneous amoebiasis. *Indian J Dermatol* 1966;11:77–8.

26 Narvaez-Moreno B, Bernabeu-Wittel J, Zulueta-Dorado T *et al*. Primary cutaneous crytococcosis of the penis. *Sex Transm Dis* 2012;39:792–3.

Dermatological aspects of sexually transmitted disease

2 Angus J, Langan SM, Stanway A *et al*. The many faces of secondary syphilis: a re-emergence of an old disease. *Clin Exp Dermatol* 2006;31:741–5.

5 Fox PA, Tung M-Y. Human papillomavirus: burden of illness and treatment cost considerations. *Am J Clin Dermatol* 2005;6:365–81.

7 Wen LM, Estcourt CS, Simpson JM, Mindel A. Risk factors for the acquisition of genital warts: are condoms protective? *Sex Transm Infect* 1999;75:312–16.

11 Koutsky L. Epidemiology of genital human papilloma virus infection. *Am J Med* 1997;102(5A):3–8.

12 Voog E, Ricksten A, Olofsson S *et al*. Demonstration of Epstein–Barr virus DNA and human papillomavirus DNA in acetowhite lesions of the penile skin and the oral mucosa. *Int J STD AIDS* 1997;8:772–5.

14 Daneshpouy M, Socic G, Clavel C *et al*. Human papillomavirus infection and anogenital condyloma in bone marrow transplant recipients. *Transplantation* 2001;71:167–9.

15 Von Krogh G, Dahlman-Ghozlan K, Syrjänen S. Potential human papillomavirus reactivation following topical corticosteroid therapy of genital lichen sclerosus and erosive lichen planus. *J Eur Acad Dermatol Venereol* 2002;16:130–3.

17 Jung JM, Jung CJ, Lee WJ *et al*. Topically applied treatments for external genital warts in nonimmunocompromised patients: a systematic review and network meta-analysis. *Br J Dermatol* 2020;183:24–36.

18 Batista CS, Atallah AN, Saconato H, da Silva EM. 5-FU for genital warts in non-immunocompromised individuals. *Cochrane Database Syst Rev* 2010; Issue 4:CD006562.

19 Lipke MM. An armamentarium of wart treatments. *Clin Med Res* 2006;4:273–93.

20 Lacey CJ, Goodall RL, Tennvall GR *et al*. Perstop Pharma Genital Warts Clinical Trial Group. Randomised controlled trial and economic evaluation of podophyllotoxin solution, podophyllotoxin cream, and podophyllin in the treatment of genital warts. *Sex Transm Infect* 2003;79:270–5.

21 Venugopal SS, Murrell DF. Recalcitrant cutaneous warts treated with recombinant quadrivalent human papillomavirus vaccine (types 6, 11, 16, and 18) in a developmentally delayed, 31-year-old white man. *Arch Dermatol* 2010; 146:475–7.

22 Silling S, Wieland U, Werner M, Pfister H, Potthoff A, Kreuter A. Resolution of novel human papillomavirus-induced warts after HPV vaccination. *Emerg Infect Dis* 2014;20:142–5.

24 Sardana K, Sehgal VN. Genital ulcer disease and human immunodeficiency virus: a focus. *J Dermatol* 2005;44:391–405.

Benign tumours

7 Cole LA, Helwig EB. Mucoid cysts of the penile skin. *J Urol* 1976;115:397–400.

17 Swinehart JM, Golitz LE. Scrotal calcinosis. *Arch Dermatol* 1982;118:985–8.

22 Akogun OB, Akoh JI, Hellandendu H. Non-ocular clinical onchocerciasis in relation to skin microfilaria in the Taraba River Valley, Nigeria. *J Hyg Epidemiol Microbiol Immunol* 1992;36:368–83.

27 Abdel-Aal H, Abdel-Aziz AM. Naevus comedonicus: report of three cases localized on glans penis. *Acta Derm Venereol* 1975;55:78–80.

29 Gürünlüoglu R, Bayramicli M, Dogan T, Numanoglu A. Unusual complications of circumcision. *Plast Reconstr Surg* 1999;104:1938–9.

45 Dehner LP, Smith BH. Soft tissue tumours of the penis. *Cancer* 1970;25:1431–47.

60 Macaluso JN, Sullivan JW, Tomberlin S. Glomus tumor of the glans penis. *Urology* 1985;25:409–10.

65 Srigley JR, Ayala AG, Ordóñez NG, van Nostrand AW. Epithelioid hemangioma of the penis: a rare and distinctive vascular lesion. *Arch Pathol Lab Med* 1985; 109:51–4.

70 Sezer E, Erbil H, Koseoglu D *et al*. Angiolymphoid hyperplasia with eosinophilia mimicking Bowenoid papulosis. *Clin Exp Dermatol* 2007;32:281–3.

71 Osborne GE, Chinn RJ, Francis ND, Bunker CB. Magnetic resonance imaging in the investigation of penile lymphangioma circumscriptum. *Br J Dermatol* 2000;143:467–8.

Pre-cancerous dermatoses and carcinoma *in situ*

Erythroplasia of Queyrat, Bowen disease of the penis and bowenoid papulosis

1 Bunker CB. *Male Genital Skin Disease*, 2nd edn. London: Bruce Shrink, 2019.

2 Wikström A, Hedblad M-A, Syrjänen S. Penile intraepithelial neoplasia: histopathological evaluation, HPV typing, clinical presentation and treatment. *J Eur Acad Dermatol Venereol* 2012;26:325–30.

5 Canete-Portillo S, Sanchez DF, Cubilla AL. Pathology of invasive and intraepithelial penile neoplasia. *Eur Urol Focus* 2019;5:713–17.

6 Chaux A, Velazquez EF, Amin A *et al*. Distribution and characterization of subtypes of penile intraepithelial neoplasia and their association with invasive carcinomas: a pathological study of 139 lesions in 121 patients. *Hum Pathol* 2012;43:1020–7.

7 Chaux A, Cubilla AL. Advances in the pathology of penile carcinomas. *Hum Pathol* 2012;43:771–89.

8 Calonje E, Lewis FM, Bunker CB *et al*. Diseases of the anogenital skin. In: Calonje E, Brenn T, Lazar AJ, Billings SD, eds. *Mckee's Pathology of the Skin: With Clinical Correlations*, 5th edn. Edinburgh: Elsevier, 2020:470–558.

9 Cubilla AL, Velazquez EF, Young RH. Epithelial lesions associated with invasive penile squamous cell carcinoma: a pathologic study of 288 cases. *Int J Surg Pathol* 2004;12:351–64.

10 Renaud-Vilmer C, Cavelier-Balloy B, Verola O et al. Analysis of alterations adjacent to invasive squamous cell carcinoma of the penis and their relationship with associated carcinoma. *J Am Acad Dermatol* 2010;62:284–90.

13 Kravvas G, Ge L, Ng J et al. The management of penile intraepithelial neoplasia (PeIN): clinical and histological features and treatment of 345 patients and a review of the literature. *J Dermatolog Treat* 2022;33:1047–62.

16 Mannweiler S, Sygulla S, Winter E et al. Two major pathways of penile carcinogenesis: HPV-induced penile cancers overexpress p16ink4a, HPV-negative cancers associated with dermatoses express p53, but lack p16ink4a overexpression. *J Am Acad Dermatol* 2013;69:73–81.

18 Dauendorffer JN, Cavelier Balloy B, Bagot M, Renaud-Vilmer C. HPV-induced penile intra-epithelial neoplasia: Bowenoid papulosis. *Ann Dermatol Venereol* 2017;144:220–4.

21 Fernàndez-Nestosa MJ, Guimerà N, Sanchez DF et al. Human papillomavirus (HPV) genotypes in condylomas, intraepithelial neoplasia, and invasive carcinoma of the penis using laser capture microdissection (LCM)-PCR: a study of 191 lesions in 43 patients. *Am J Surg Pathol* 2017;41:820–32.

22 Shim TN, Harwood CA, Marsh SG et al. The prevalence of human leucocyte antigen and human papillomavirus DNA in penile intraepithelial neoplasia in England 2011–2012. *Int J STD AIDS* 2021;32:388–95.

23 Barrasso R, De Brux J, Croissant O, Orth G. High prevalence of papillomavirus associated penile intraepithelial neoplasia in partners of women with cervical intraepithelial neoplasia. *N Engl J Med* 1987;317:916–23.

24 Kennedy L, Buntine DW, O'Connor D, Frazer IH. Human papillomavirus: a study of male sexual partners. *Med J Aust* 1988;149:309–11.

26 Voltz JM, Drobacheff C, Derancourt C et al. Papillomavirus-induced anogenital lesions in 121 HIV seropositive men: clinical, histological, viral study, and evolution. *Ann Dermatol Vénéréol* 1999;126:424–9.

28 Velazquez EF, Chaux A, Cubilla AL. Histologic classification of penile intraepithelial neoplasia. *Semin Diagn Pathol* 2012;29:96–102.

29 Kristiansen S, Svensson A, Drevin L et al. Risk factors for penile intraepithelial neoplasia: a population-based register study in Sweden, 2000–2012. *Acta Derm Venereol* 2019;99:315–20.

30 Wolbarst AL. Circumcision and penile cancer. *Lancet* 1932;1:150–3.

31 Schoen EJ, Oehrli M, Colby CJ, Machin G. The highly protective effect of newborn circumcision against invasive penile cancer. *Pediatrics* 2000;105:E36.

35 Arya M, Thrasivoulou C, Henrique R et al. Targets of Wnt/ßcatenin transcription in penile carcinoma. *PLoS One* 2015;10:e0124395.

36 Al-Hebshi NN, Nasher AT, Maryoud MY et al. Inflammatory bacteriome featuring *Fusobacterium nucleatum* and *Pseudomonas aeruginosa* identified in association with oral squamous cell carcinoma. *Sci Rep* 2017;7:1834.

37 Zhao H, Chu M, Huang Z et al. Variations in oral microbiota associated with oral cancer. *Sci Rep* 2017;7:11773.

38 Castellarin M, Warren RL, Freeman JD et al. *Fusobacterium nucleatum* infection is prevalent in human colorectal carcinoma. *Genome Res* 2012;22:299–306.

39 Kostic AD, Chun E, Robertson L et al. *Fusobacterium nucleatum* potentiates intestinal tumorigenesis and modulates the tumor-immune microenvironment. *Cell Host Microbe* 2013;14:207–15.

40 Binder Gallimidi A, Fischman S, Revach B et al. Periodontal pathogens *Porphyromonas gingivalis* and *Fusobacterium nucleatum* promote tumor progression in an oral-specific chemical carcinogenesis model. *Oncotarget* 2015;6:22613–23.

42 Rodney S, Arya M, Muneer A. Is the incidence of penile carcinoma in situ increasing in England and the rest of Europe? *Eur Urol Suppl* 2017;16:e1224–5.

43 Rippentrop JM, Joslyn SA, Konety BR. Squamous cell carcinoma of the penis: evaluation of data from the surveillance, epidemiology, and end results program. *Cancer* 2004;101:1357–63.

47 Moch H, Cubilla AL, Humphrey PA et al. The 2016 WHO Classification of tumours of the urinary system and male genital organs – Part A: renal, penile, and testicular tumours. *Eur Urol* 2016;70:93–105.

48 Rao A, Bunker CB. Male genital skin biopsy. *Int J STD Aids* 2011;22:418–19.

52 Chan SL, Watchorn RE, Panagou E et al. Dermatoscopic findings of penile intraepithelial neoplasia: Bowenoid papulosis, Bowen disease and erythroplasia of Queyrat. *Australas J Dermatol* 2019;60:e201–7.

59 Epstein JI, Cubilla AL, Humphrey PA. *Tumors of the prostate gland, seminal vesicles, penis and scrotum.* Washington, DC: American Registry of Pathology, Armed Forces Institute of Pathology, 2011.

60 Velazquez EF, Cubilla AL. Lichen sclerosus in 68 patients with squamous cell carcinoma of the penis: frequent atypias and correlation with special carcinoma variants suggests a precancerous role. *Am J Surg Pathol* 2003;27:1448–53.

61 Dauendorffer JN, Cavelier Balloy B, Bagot M et al. Penile squamous hyperplasia. *Ann Dermatol Venereol* 2018;145:72–5.

62 Chaux A, Velazquez EF, Cubilla AL. Distinctive immunohistochemical profile of penile intraepithelial lesions: a study of 74 cases. *Am J Surg Pathol* 2011;35:10.

63 Dauendorffer JN, Renaud-Vilmer C, Cavelier Balloy B et al. [Penile intra-epithelial neoplasia.] *Prog Urol* 2018;28:466–74.

65 Morton CA, Birnie AJ, Eedy DJ. British Association of Dermatologists' guidelines for the management of squamous cell carcinoma in situ (Bowen's disease) 2014. *Br J Dermatol* 2014;170:245–60.

70 Hadway P, Corbishley CM, Watkin NA. Total glans resurfacing for premalignant lesions of the penis: initial outcome data. *BJU Int* 2006;98:532–6.

74 Edwards S, Bunker CB, Ziller F et al. 2013 European guideline for the management of balanoposthitis. *Int J STD Aids* 2014;25:615–26.

75 Hakenberg OW, Compérat EM, Minhas S et al. EAU guidelines on penile cancer: 2014 update. *Eur Urol* 2015;67:142–50.

76 Arya M, Kalsi J, Kelly J et al. Malignant and premalignant lesions of the penis. *BMJ* 2013;346:f1149.

77 Issa A, Sebro K, Kwok A et al. Treatment options and outcomes for men with penile intraepithelial neoplasia: a systematic review. *Eur Urol Focus* 2022;8:829–32.

78 Shabbir M, Muneer A, Kalsi J et al. Glans resurfacing for the treatment of carcinoma in situ of the penis: surgical technique and outcomes. *Eur Urol* 2011;59:142–7.

82 Harth Y, Hirshovitz B. Topical photodynamic therapy in basal and squamous cell carcinoma and penile Bowen's disease with 20% aminolevulinic acid, and exposure to red light and infrared light. *Harefuah* 1998;134:602–5.

85 Mohs FE, Snow SN, Messing EM et al. Microscopically controlled surgery in the treatment of carcinoma of the penis. *J Urol* 1985;133:961–6.

90 Lukowiak TM, Perz AM, Aizman L et al. Mohs micrographic surgery for male genital tumors: local recurrence rates and patient-reported outcomes. *J Am Acad Dermatol* 2021;84:1030–6.

91 Pham CT, Juhasz M, Sung CT et al. The human papillomavirus vaccine as a treatment for human papillomavirus-related dysplastic and neoplastic conditions: a literature review. *J Am Acad Dermatol* 2020;82:202–12.

92 Doiron PR, Bunker CB. Expanding the benefits of HPV vaccination to boys and men. *Lancet* 2016;388(10045):659.

94 Zreik A, Ismail M, Nigam R. Penile intraepithelial neoplasia: management and outcomes. *Hum Androl* 2013;3:6–9.

Miscellaneous pre-cancerous conditions

1 Dauendorffer JN, Cavelier Balloy B, Bagot M et al. Penile squamous hyperplasia. *Ann Dermatol Venereol* 2018;145:72–5.

2 Calonje E, Neill S, Bunker CB, Francis N, Chaux A, Cubilla A. Diseases of the anogenital skin. In: Calonje E, Brenn T, Lazar A, McKee PH, eds. *McKee's Pathology of the Skin*, 4th edn. London: Elsevier Saunders, 2012:437–519.

3 Renaud-Vilmer C, Cavelier-Balloy B, Verola O et al. Analysis of alterations adjacent to invasive squamous cell carcinoma of the penis and their relationship with associated carcinoma. *J Am Acad Dermatol* 2010;62:284–90.

4 García Paños JM, Buendia Gonzalez E, Jimenez Leiro F et al. Penile cutaneous horn: report of a case and review of the literature. *Arch Esp Urol* 1999;52:173–4.

5 Bart RS, Kopf AW. Tumor conference No. 14: on a dilemma of penile horns – pseudoepitheliomatous, hyperkeratotic and micaceous balanitis. *J Dermatol Surg Oncol* 1977;3:580.

14 Solivan GA, Smith KJ, James WD. Cutaneous horn of the penis: its association with squamous cell carcinoma and HPV-16 infection. *J Am Acad Dermatol* 1990;23:969–72.

15 Chen T-J, Chou Y-C, Chen C-H et al. Genital porokeratosis: a series of 10 patients and review of the literature. *Br J Dermatol* 2006;155:325–9.

19 Levell NJ, Bewley AP, Levene GM. Porokeratosis of Mibelli on the penis, scrotum and natal cleft. *Clin Exp Dermatol* 1994;19:77–8.

21 Sasson M, Krain AD. Porokeratosis and cutaneous malignancy. A review. *Dermatol Surg* 1996;22:339–42.

22 Porter WM, Du P, Menagé H, Philip G, Bunker CB. Porokeratosis of the penis. *Br J Dermatol* 2001;144:643–4.

24 Lucker GP, Happle R, Steijlen PM. An unusual case of porokeratosis involving the natal cleft: porokeratosis ptychotropica. *Br J Dermatol* 1995;132:150–1.

25 Ong ELH, Calonje E, Bakkour W, Muneer A, Barker J, Bunker CB. An intractable under-recognized anogenitogluteal rash. *Clin Exp Dermatol* 2021;46:769–72.

26 Kogut M, Schiller M, Hadaschik E, Enk A, Haenssle HA. Porokeratosis ptychotropica involving the glans penis: a unique case of this rare condition. *JDDG* 2016;14:181–3.

35 Spencer AH, Watchorn RE, Kravvas G *et al*. Pseudoepitheliomatous keratotic and micaceous balanitis: a series of eight cases. *J Eur Acad Dermatol Venereol* 2022;3:1851–6.

36 Ridley CM. Lichen sclerosus et atrophicus. *BMJ* 1987;295:1295–6.

37 Bunker CB, Francis N. Pseudoepitheliomatous keratotic and micaceous balanitis: comment. *Clin Exp Dermatol* 2012;37:434–5.

38 Ridley CM. Pseudoepitheliomatous micaceous and keratotic balanitis. *Br J Dermatol* 1988;118:856–7.

Squamous carcinoma and other malignant neoplasms
Carcinoma of the penis

1 Brady KL, Mercurio MG, Brown MD. Malignant tumors of the penis. *Dermatol Surg* 2013;39:527–47.

2 Porter WM, Francis N, Hawkins D *et al*. Penile intraepithelial neoplasia: clinical spectrum and treatment of 35 cases. *Br J Dermatol* 2002;147:1159–65.

3 Hakenberg OW, Compérat E, Minhas S *et al*. EAU guidelines on penile cancer. Updated 2018. https://uroweb.org/guideline/penile-cancer/ (last accessed November 2022).

4 Chaux A, Cubilla AL. Advances in the pathology of penile carcinomas. *Hum Pathol* 2012;43:771–89.

5 Bunker CB. *Male Genital Skin Disease*, 2nd edn. London: Bruce Shrink, 2019.

12 Weber P, Rabinovitz H, Garland L. Verrucous carcinoma in penile lichen sclerosus et atrophicus. *J Dermatol Surg Oncol* 1987;13:529.

21 Bunker CB, Neill S, Staughton RCD. Topical tacrolimus, genital lichen sclerosus and risk of squamous cell carcinoma. *Arch Dermatol* 2004;140:1169.

22 Bunker CB. Male genital lichen sclerosus and topical tacrolimus. *Br J Dermatol* 2007;157:1079–80.

24 Edmonds EVJ, Hunt S, Hawkins D *et al*. Clinical parameters in male genital lichen sclerosus: a case series of 329 patients. *J Eur Acad Dermatol Venereol* 2011; 26:730–7.

25 Renaud-Vilmer C, Cavelier-Balloy B, Verola O *et al*. Analysis of alterations adjacent to invasive squamous cell carcinoma of the penis and their relationship with associated carcinoma. *J Am Acad Dermatol* 2010;62:284–90.

26 Chaux A, Velazquez EF, Amin A *et al*. Distribution and characterization of subtypes of penile intraepithelial neoplasia and their association with invasive carcinomas: a pathological study of 139 lesions in 121 patients. *Hum Pathol* 2012;43:1020–7.

27 Calonje E, Neill S, Bunker CB *et al*. Diseases of the anogenital skin. In: Calonje E, Brenn T, Lazaar A, McKee PH, eds. *McKee's Pathology of the Skin*, 4th edn. Amsterdam: Elsevier Saunders, 2012:437–519.

28 Sanchez DF. What is new in the pathologic staging of penile carcinoma in the 8th Edition of AJCC TNM Model: rationale for changes with practical stage-by-stage category diagnostic considerations. *Adv Anat Pathol* 2021;28:209–27.

30 Paner GP, Stadler WM, Hansel DE, Montironi R, Lin DW, Amin MB. Updates in the Eighth Edition of the Tumor-Node-Metastasis Staging Classification for Urologic Cancers. *Eur Urol* 2018;73:560–9.

31 Muneer A, Arya N, Horenblas S, eds. *Textbook of Penile Cancer*. Berlin: Springer, 2012.

32 Bunker CB, Shim TN. Male genital lichen sclerosus. *Indian J Dermatol* 2015; 60:111–17.

33 Minhas S, Kayes O, Hegarty P, Kumar P, Freeman A, Ralph D. What surgical resection margins are required to achieve oncological control in men with primary penile cancer? *BJU Int* 2005;96:1040–3.

35 Kirrander P, Sherif A, Friedrich B, Lambe M, Håkansson U; Steering Committee of the Swedish National Penile Cancer Register. Swedish National Penile Cancer Register: incidence, tumour characteristics, management and survival. *BJU Int* 2016;117:287–92.

44 Howlader N, Noone AM, Krapcho M *et al*., eds. SEER Cancer Statistics Review, 1975–2017. Bethesda, MD: National Cancer Institute. https://seer.cancer.gov/csr/1975_2017/, based on November 2019 SEER data submission, posted to the SEER website April 2020.

Carcinoma of the scrotum

1 Verhoeven RH, Louwman WJ, Koldewijn EL, Demeyere TB, Coebergh JW. Scrotal cancer: incidence, survival and second primary tumours in the Netherlands since 1989. *Br J Cancer* 2010;103:1462–6.

12 Archier E, Devaux S, Castela E *et al*. Carcinogenic risks of psoralen UV-A therapy and narrowband UV-B therapy in chronic plaque psoriasis: a systematic literature review. *J Eur Acad Dermatol Venereol* 2012;26(Suppl. 3):22–31.

20 Azike JE. A review of the history, epidemiology and treatment of squamous cell carcinoma of the scrotum. *Rare Tumors* 2009;1:e17.

Buschke–Löwenstein tumour/giant condyloma

1 Davis KG, Barton JS, Bivin W, Krane S, Orangio G. Buschke-Lowenstein tumors: a review and proposed classification system. *Sex Transm Dis* 2021;48:e263–8.

3 Steffen C. The men behind the eponym – Abraham Buschke and Ludwig Lowenstein: giant condyloma (Buschke-Loewenstein). *Am J Dermatopathol* 2006; 28:526–36.

4 Hakenberg OW, Compérat E, Minhas S *et al*. EAU guidelines on penile cancer. Updated 2018. https://uroweb.org/guideline/penile-cancer/ (last accessed November 2022).

7 Sporkert M, Rübben A. Buschke-Löwenstein-Tumor. *Hautarzt* 2017;68:199–203.

22 Chu QD, Vezeridis MP, Libbey NP, Wanebo HJ. Giant condyloma acuminatum (Buschke-Lowenstein tumor) of the anorectal and perianal regions. Analysis of 42 cases. *Dis Colon Rectum* 1994;37:950–7.

Extramammary Paget disease

1 Helwig EB, Graham JH. Anogenital (extramammary) Paget's disease: a clinicopathological study. *Cancer* 1963;16:387–403.

2 Lam C, Funaro D. Extramammary Paget's disease: summary of current knowledge. *Dermatol Clin* 2010;28:807–26.

3 Master VA, Herrel L, Johnson TV, Delman KA. Extramammary Paget's disease of the penis and anogenital area: seer analysis. *J Clin Oncol* 2011;29(s7):abstr 220.

4 Willman JH, Golitz LE, Fitzpatrick JE. Vulvar clear cells of Toker: precursors of extramammary Paget's disease. *Am J Dermatopathol* 2005;27:185–8.

5 Lloyd J, Flanagan AM. Mammary and extramammary Paget's disease. *J Clin Pathol* 2000;53:742–9.

8 Adashek JJ, Leonard A, Nealon SW *et al*. Extramammary Paget's disease: what do we know and how do we treat? *Can J Urol* 2019;26:10012–21.

11 Zollo JD, Zeitouni NC. The Roswell Park Cancer Institute experience with extramammary Paget's disease. *Br J Dermatol* 2000;142:59–65.

13 Simonds RM, Segal RJ, Sharma A. Extramammary Paget's disease: a review of the literature. *Int J Dermatol* 2019;58:871–9.

14 Chen YH, Wong TW, Lee JY. Depigmented genital extramammary Paget's disease: a possible histogenetic link to Toker's clear cells and clear cell papulosis. *J Cutan Pathol* 2001;28:105–8.

16 Christodoulidou MM, Alnajjar MHM, Parnham MA *et al*. Multidisciplinary approach for the management of penoscrotal extramammary Paget's disease – an eUROGEN study. *Urol Oncol* 2021;39:501.e1–10.

17 Schmitt AR, Long BJ, Weaver AL *et al*. Evidence-based screening recommendations for occult cancers in the setting of newly diagnosed extramammary Paget Disease. *Mayo Clin Proc* 2018;93:877–83.

18 Bae JM, Choi YY, Kim H *et al*. Mohs micrographic surgery for extramammary Paget disease: a pooled analysis of individual patient data. *J Am Acad Dermatol* 2013;68:632–7.

24 Ogata D, Kiyohara Y, Yoshikawa S, Tsuchida T. Usefulness of sentinel lymph node biopsy for prognostic prediction in extramammary Paget's disease. *Eur J Dermatol* 2016;26:254–9.

25 Machida H, Moeini A, Roman LD, Matsuo K. Effects of imiquimod on vulvar Paget's disease: a systematic review of literature. *Gynecol Oncol* 2015;139:165–71.

30 Bowling JCR, Powles A, Searle A, Nasiri N, Bunker CB. Spontaneous regression of extramammary Paget's disease after excision of primary apocrine carcinoma in an immunosuppressed patient. *Br J Dermatol* 2005;153:676–7.

Malignant melanoma

2 Brady KL, Mercurio MG, Brown MD. Malignant tumors of the penis. *Dermatol Surg* 2013;39:527–47.

16 Lucia MS, Miller GJ. Histopathology of malignant lesions of the penis. *Urol Clin North Am* 1992;19:227–46.

Other malignant neoplasms

1 Brady KL, Mercurio MG, Brown MD. Malignant tumors of the penis. *Dermatol Surg* 2013;39:527–47.

2 Nguyen H, Saadat P, Bennett RG. Penile basal cell carcinoma: two cases treated with Mohs micrographic surgery and remarks on pathogenesis. *Dermatol Surg* 2006;32:135–44.

28 Chaux A, Amin M, Cubilla A, Young R. Metastatic tumours to the penis: a report of 17 cases and review of the literature. *Int J Surg Path* 2010;19:597–606.

Miscellaneous cutaneous male genital conditions
Penile melanosis and hypopigmentation

1 Kaporis A, Lynfield Y. Penile lentiginosis. *J Am Acad Dermatol* 1998;38:781.

4 Rhodes AR, Harrist TJ, Momtaz TK. The PUVA-induced pigmented macule: a lentiginous proliferation of large, sometimes cytologically atypical, melanocytes. *J Am Acad Dermatol* 1983;9:47–58.

5 Barnhill RL, Albert LS, Sharma SK *et al.* Genital lentiginosis: a clinical and histopathologic study. *J Am Acad Dermatol* 1990;22:453–60.

Dysaesthesia and chronic pain syndromes

5 Stumpf A, Ständer S. Neuropathic itch: diagnosis and management. *Dermatol Ther* 2013;26:104–9.

6 Fisher BK. The red scrotum syndrome. *Cutis* 1997;60:139–41.

7 Markos AR. The male genital skin burning syndrome (dysaesthetic peno/scroto-dynia). *Int J STD AIDS* 2002;13:271–2.

8 Prevost N, English JC, 3rd. Case reports: red scrotal syndrome: a localized phenotypical expression of erythromelalgia. *J Drugs Dermatol* 2007;6:935–6.

12 Chen A, De E, Argoff C. Small fiber polyneuropathy is prevalent in patients experiencing complex chronic pelvic pain. *Pain Med* 2019;20:521–7.

13 Tympanidis P, Casula MA, Yiangou Y, Terenghi G, Dowd P, Anand P. Increased vanilloid receptor VR1 innervation in vulvodynia. *Eur J Pain* 2004;8:129–33.

14 Anyasodor MC, Taylor RE, Bewley A, Goulding JM. Dysaesthetic penoscrotodynia may be a somatoform disorder: results from a two-centre retrospective case series. *Clin Exp Dermatol* 2016;41:474–9.

15 Labat JJ, Riant T, Robert R, Amarenco G, Lefaucheur JP, Rigaud J. Diagnostic criteria for pudendal neuralgia by pudendal nerve entrapment (Nantes criteria). *Neurourol Urodyn* 2008;27:306–10.

20 Raef HS, Elmariah SB. Vulvar pruritus: a review of clinical associations, pathophysiology and therapeutic management. *Front Med* 2021;8:649402.

Miscellaneous

2 Cabellero JM, Avila A, Cardona X *et al.* Genital pain without urogenital pathology: the koro-like syndrome. *J Urol* 2000;163:243.

CHAPTER 110

Dermatoses of the Female Genitalia

Fiona Lewis

St John's Institute of Dermatology, Guy's and St Thomas' NHS Foundation Trust, London, UK

Introduction

Common dermatoses that are easily recognised elsewhere may have a modified appearance on the vulva, where the typical clinical features are often altered significantly. The ano-genital skin is vulnerable, with the local environmental influences of heat, moisture and friction all acting as irritants; changes in the normal bacterial flora are also important.

There has been some confusion regarding the terminology used for vulval disease. The classification of vulval disorders has been clarified and older terms such as vulval dystrophy, leukoplakia and kraurosis vulvae should no longer be used [1].

The development of vulval clinics has helped to improve the management of women with vulval disease. A multidisciplinary approach is needed as the management of many vulval disorders will require the expertise of different specialties including dermatology, gynaecology and genito-urinary medicine. Clinicopathological correlation involving discussion with a histopathologist is vital [2]. A study showed that consensus reporting between surgical and dermatopathologists can increase diagnostic confidence and

Rook's Textbook of Dermatology, Tenth Edition. Edited by Christopher Griffiths, Jonathan Barker, Tanya Bleiker, Walayat Hussain and Rosalind Simpson.
© 2024 John Wiley & Sons Ltd. Published 2024 by John Wiley & Sons Ltd.

improve overall reporting, particularly in select cases [3]. Clear pathways of care and links with other specialties including plastic surgery, urology, paediatrics, psychology and psychosexual medicine are important in the management of specific conditions. Standards of care for vulval clinics are now published [4].

History and examination

An accurate diagnosis depends on a thorough history, examination of the genital and extragenital skin, and relevant investigations. The history must include the nature and duration of the presenting complaint, how the problem changes (e.g. variation with menstrual cycle) and the type, regimen and effectiveness of any prescribed or over-the-counter treatment used. The complaint of 'irritation' should be defined, since the patient may use the term to describe the sensation of itch, dryness, pain or burning. This is important as a patient with itch will scratch or rub the skin, and the response will be lichen simplex or lichenification, whereas with discomfort or pain there will be no such change as the patient avoids touching the area.

A personal and family history of autoimmune disease, atopy or psoriasis should be established, together with any known skin sensitivities. The patient should also be asked about vaginal discharge, urinary symptoms and bowel function. It is helpful to know if there have been any abnormalities with cervical cytology, whether the human papillomavirus (HPV) vaccine has been administered and also whether the patient smokes cigarettes, as this is a major risk factor for intraepithelial neoplasia. As the vulva is important for normal sexual function, questions relating to dyspareunia and any psychosexual difficulties should be included.

The patient often finds the examination embarrassing and so it must be carried out sympathetically, with all the equipment that may be required such as swabs and speculums readily available. Good lighting and a means of magnification are needed. A methodical approach will ensure that all areas of the vulva and perianal skin are examined fully. It is important to know the normal anatomy of the vulva as some dermatoses result in scarring and therefore architectural changes can give diagnostic clues. The examination must also include inspection of other flexural sites and mucosae, the scalp and nails. It is also useful to determine if the patient exhibits dermographism [5], as this may be relevant for dyspareunia caused by pressure urticaria. The vagina and cervix should be examined in patients who have dermatoses that affect the mucosal surfaces and in any patient with symptoms of dyspareunia, vaginal discharge or postcoital bleeding. This may require referral to a gynaecologist for hysteroscopy or transvaginal ultrasound as significant vaginal bleeding is rarely related to skin disease.

Investigations

Investigations are determined by the specific problem. If an unusual or sexually transmitted infection is high on the list of differential diagnoses, it is important to involve a genito-urinary physician in the investigation and work-up of these patients and their sexual partners.

Vulval biopsy is often required and is very useful in the diagnosis of ano-genital dermatoses. However, careful clinicopathological correlation and discussion with a dermatopathologist are vital.

It is very important to include a clinical differential diagnosis when submitting biopsies for histological examination.

Some investigations are not the usual remit of the dermatologist but are necessary in patients with ano-genital dermatoses, for example cervical smear and proctoscopy in patients with high-grade squamous epithelial lesions.

Structure and function of the female genitalia

The vulva is the collective term used for the structures that comprise the female external genitalia. Anatomically, it is the region known as the uro-genital triangle, bounded anteriorly by the symphysis pubis, the pubic rami laterally and the transverse perineal body posteriorly. The vulval structures included within this area are the mons pubis, labia majora and labia minora, clitoris, vulval vestibule and hymen (Figure 110.1a). It is now recognised that there can be a wide variety in the size and appearance of these components [1,2]. The epithelia that cover the vulva change from skin on the outer aspects to mucosa on the inner aspects of the labia minora.

The mons pubis lies in front of and above the upper part of the symphysis pubis. The densely hair-bearing epithelium covers a thick cushion of subcutaneous fat.

The labia majora are paired, rounded folds of skin and are the homologue of the scrotum. They extend downwards and backwards from the mons pubis and meet posteriorly in the midline to form the posterior commissure, which lies approximately 2 cm anterior to the anus. The structure is similar to that of the mons pubis in that there is a thick layer of adipose tissue and a dense distribution of hair on the outer surfaces of the labia. Hair is absent from the inner surfaces but numerous sebaceous glands remain. The inner aspects of the labia majora fuse into the outer aspects of the labia minora laterally, forming the interlabial sulci.

The labia minora are the equivalent of the male prepuce, and are paired pendulous folds, which lie between the labia majora and the vulval vestibule. Anteriorly they split into two folds on each side, which fuse in the midline. The superior folds form the clitoral hood, and the lower folds fuse on the inferior aspect of the clitoris, forming the clitoral frenulum. Posteriorly, the labia minora fuse to form the fourchette, and sometimes form a depression in the midline – the fossa navicularis. The labia minora possess little subcutaneous fat. Their epithelium lacks hair but there are numerous sebaceous glands and sweat glands. The epithelium is cornified but its barrier function is not as effective as skin elsewhere.

The clitoris is the homologue of the penis and contains all the vascular and muscular structures found in its male counterpart. The end of the clitoris is surmounted by a small rounded tubercle, the glans clitoris (Figure 110.1b).

The vestibule is the area that lies between the labia minora and contains the openings of the urethra and vagina. The vaginal opening is partially closed by the hymen. When the hymen is ruptured, its remnants form rounded crenulations, the hymenal caruncle. Sometimes a line of demarcation between the keratinised epithelium of the labia minora and the non-keratinised mucosa of the vestibule can be clearly seen (the Hart line). The vestibule is a

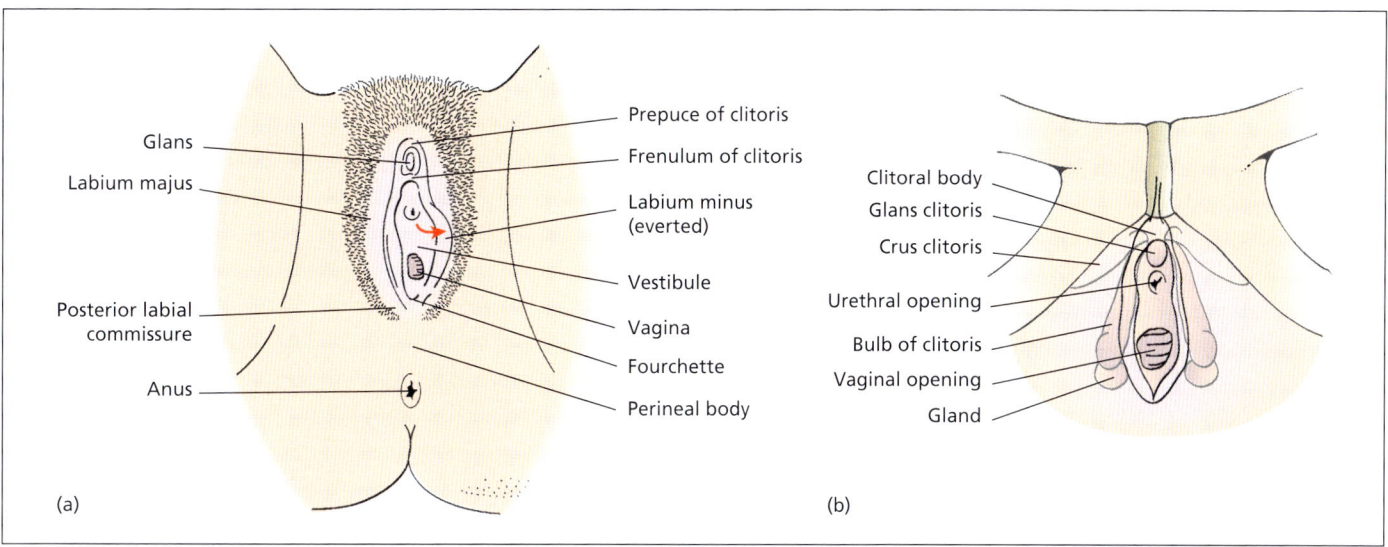

Figure 110.1 (a) The vulva. (b) The clitoris. Reproduced from Neill and Lewis 2009 [13] with permission of John Wiley & Sons.

mucosal epithelium and lacks hairs and sebaceous glands. On each side, the duct of the Bartholin glands can be seen sited between the hymenal ring and posterior part of the labium minus. The ducts of the minor vestibular glands, the Skene glands, open on either side of the urethral orifice.

Labial and clitoral variations

There is a wide variety of normal appearances of all structures on the vulva and it is important to recognise these to reassure the patient and to avoid unnecessary surgical modification. The labia minora are often asymmetrical and the rims may be pigmented [1].

Labial adhesions are common in children and are probably due to minor irritation and inflammation occurring in a low oestrogen state, but they can be inherited as a familial trait [3] or occur in association with disorders of sexual differentiation. In general, most occur in the neonatal period and early infancy, and usually divide spontaneously by the time the child is 6 years old. No intervention is necessary unless there is a problem with urination with pooling of urine and frequent urinary tract infections [4]. Some cases of labial adhesions in older children and adults result from lichen sclerosus.

Accessory labio-scrotal folds are well described in males, usually in association with a perineal lipoma. The equivalent in women, accessory labial folds, are extremely rare with only two cases having been reported [5].

The clitoris may be absent because of a failure of the genital tubercle to fuse, it may remain hypoplastic [6] or it may be enlarged because of congenital adrenal hyperplasia. The Lawrence–Seip syndrome, which is a congenital generalised lipodystrophy with the onset of insulin-resistant diabetes around the time of puberty, may also result in clitoral hypertrophy. Clitoral tumours may mimic disorders of sexual differentiation [7–9]. A pseudocyst of the clitoris, caused by a build-up of keratinous debris under clitoral hood adhesions, can occur in lichen sclerosus.

Virilisation of the external genitalia may also occur with maternal ingestion of testosterone or synthetic progestogens in the first trimester, and if taken later in pregnancy there may be clitoral hypertrophy alone.

An imperforate hymen is usually discovered at puberty and is caused either by failure of the epithelial cells of the hymen to degenerate or by scarring after an inflammatory reaction in the hymen at birth.

Normal flora

The skin of the perineal area has a higher pH, temperature and degree of humidity than skin elsewhere and, because of its proximity to the vagina and rectum, harbours many of the flora from these sites. The main resident organisms are micrococci, diphtheroids and lactobacilli. Lactobacilli are probably the most common organisms, particularly on the mucosal surfaces, as the glycogenated epithelium of the vagina, under the influence of oestrogen, encourages colonisation by them. The lactobacilli in turn metabolise the glycogen to lactic acid, which keeps the vaginal pH at approximately 4.5, restricting the growth of many organisms. Study of the vulval microbiome is an emerging field [10].

Normal variants
Angiokeratomas

Angiokeratomas are small (1–4 mm) vascular papules found on the labia majora. They vary in colour from red to blue-black and are normally asymptomatic, but can become quite large and bleed if traumatised, particularly in pregnancy (Figure 110.2).

Fordyce spots

These are sebaceous glands seen on the inner aspects of the labia majora and labia minora where the glands do not usually have an associated hair unit. They open directly onto the surface and may be very prominent and numerous. The yellow, uniform papules are often best seen when the skin is stretched (Figure 110.3). Rarely, they become very large and can be mistaken for a sebaceous gland adenoma [11]. They can disappear in lichen sclerosus.

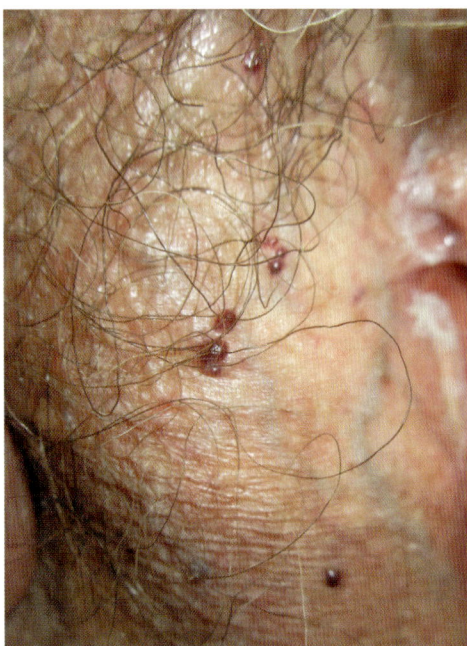

Figure 110.2 Angiokeratomas

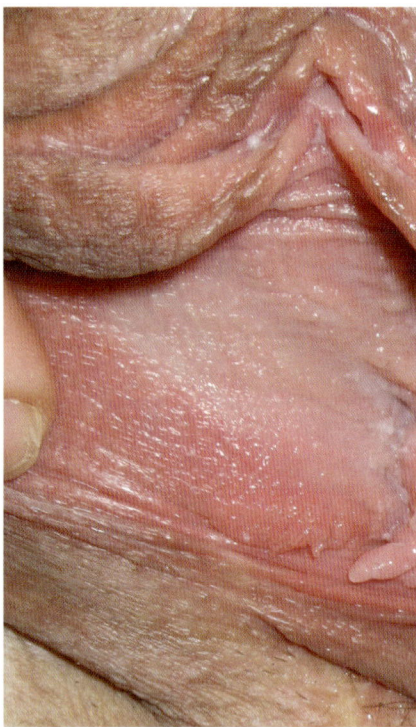

Figure 110.4 Vestibular papillomatosis.

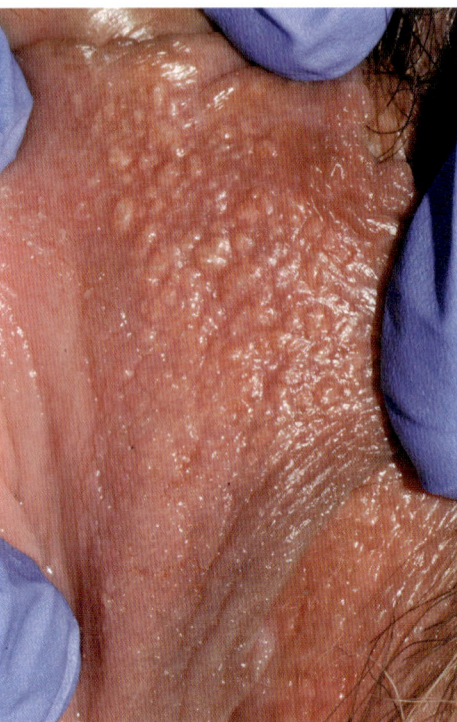

Figure 110.3 Fordyce spots (prominent sebaceous glands) of the inner labia.

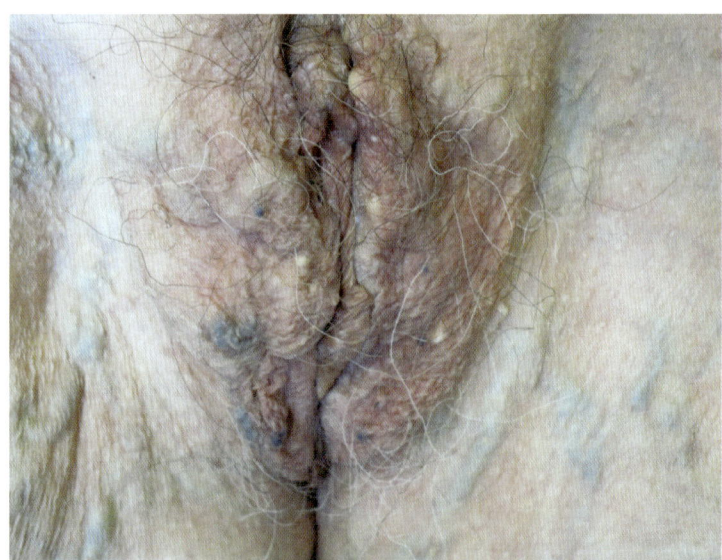

Figure 110.5 Vulval varicosities.

Vestibular papillomatosis

Vestibular papillomatosis is the term used to describe the occasional normal finding of multiple, tiny, filiform or soft, frond-like projections on the vestibular epithelium and inner aspects of the labia minora. Vestibular papillae are symmetrically distributed and each papilla has a solitary base. Previously, there was some confusion as the vestibule has heavily glycogenated epithelial cells that become vacuolated on processing and may resemble koilocytes. It is now known that HPV infection is not associated with these papillae [12] and that they are a normal entity and possibly the female equivalent of pearly penile papules (Figure 110.4).

Varicosities

Varicosities of the labial veins (Figure 110.5) may occur unilaterally in association with limb varicosities, or appear in pregnancy. Other changes in pregnancy include a fall in the pH and increased pigmentation. At the menopause, vascularity decreases and the sebaceous glands become less active.

Table 110.1 Classification of disorders of sexual development (DSDs).

Chromosome abnormality	Example disorder
Sex chromosome DSD	Klinefelter syndrome (XXY)
	Turner syndrome (XO)
46XY DSD	
46XX DSD	
Disorders of gonadal development	Gonadal dysgenesis
	Ovo-testicular DSD
Androgen excess	Testicular DSD
Others	

CONGENITAL ABNORMALITIES

Disorders of sexual development

Definition and nomenclature

This group of disorders relates to those where there is an abnormality in gonadal development or sexual differentiation.

Synonyms and inclusions
- Ambiguous external genitalia
- Intersex disorders

Introduction and general description

In a newborn, the external genitalia may not be phenotypical of either a male or female. Evaluation and management of these infants require an expert multidisciplinary team (MDT). The disorders of sexual development (DSDs) have been reclassified [1] as shown in Table 110.1.

The 46XX is the most common type of DSD encountered and 60% will be due to congenital adrenal hyperplasia. The ovaries are normal but the masculinisation of the external genitalia results from androgen exposure *in utero*.

GENODERMATOSES

Epidermolysis bullosa

Definition

Epidermolysis bullosa (EB) is a group of disorders characterised by skin fragility and blister formation.

Introduction and general description

The forms of EB that specifically involve the vulva are junctional EB inversa and recessive dystrophic EB inversa (Chapter 69).

Clinical features
Presentation

Extensive erosion and ulceration can affect the ano-genital area and may heal with scarring [1]. In junctional EB inversa, blistering and erosions occur in the flexures, vulva and vagina and oesophagus. There may be nail dystrophy and atrophic scarring elsewhere.

In recessive dystrophic EB inversa, oral lesions are always present and oesophageal involvement may be severe. Vaginal strictures have been reported [2].

Complications and co-morbidities

Vulval squamous cell carcinoma (SCC) has been reported [3].

Management

The management depends on expert nursing care and follows the principles used for other sites.

Hailey–Hailey disease

Definition and nomenclature

Hailey–Hailey disease (HHD) is an autosomal dominant inherited disorder of keratinisation with incomplete penetrance (Chapter 64).

Synonyms and inclusions
- Benign familial chronic pemphigus

Epidemiology
Age

The clinical features usually start in the teenage years but may present at any time up to the fourth decade.

Pathophysiology
Pathology

Acantholysis is seen throughout the epidermis, giving rise to the 'delapidated brick wall' appearance. Direct immunofluorescence will be negative.

Clinical features
History

Patients complain of painful erosions in flexural sites, particularly the axillae and inguinal folds. The use of the adjective 'benign' is a misnomer.

Presentation

Moist red plaques are seen in the flexures and these may be eroded and crusted. The vulva and perineum are frequently involved. Heat, friction and pregnancy may exacerbate the symptoms.

Differential diagnosis

Hailey–Hailey disease is often misdiagnosed as intertrigo initially. Flexural psoriasis, Darier disease, pemphigus erythematosus and extramammary Paget disease can have similar clinical features.

Complications and co-morbidities

Secondary infection with bacteria (most commonly *Staphylococcus aureus*), viruses (herpes simplex) and *Candida* is a common

PART 10: SPECIFIC SITES, SEX & AGE

complication and needs appropriate management. SCC has also been described [1,2].

Investigations
A skin biopsy will confirm the diagnosis.

Management
First line
First line management is a reduction in friction, with the use of emollients and a moderately potent topical steroid.

Second line
Topical tacrolimus may be of benefit [3] but a case of SCC developing after treatment has been reported [4]. Long-term antibiotics may be required for those where secondary infection is a major issue.

Third line
There is one case report of a patient with perineal disease responding to alefacept which inhibits T-cell activation and proliferation [5]. Photodynamic therapy [6] and CO_2 laser [7] have been used. Botulinum toxin has been used in axillary, submammary and inguinal HHD but is rarely reported on the vulva [8].

Resources

Patient resources
Hailey–Hailey Disease Society: www.haileyhailey.com (last accessed April 2022).

Darier disease

Definition
Darier disease is an acantholytic disorder of keratinisation, usually with autosomal dominant inheritance (Chapter 64).

Epidemiology
Age
Lesions develop in childhood and adolescence and tend to fluctuate in severity.

Clinical features
History
Patients complain of uncomfortable lesions on the vulva and in the inguinal folds. The lesions can weep and become macerated.

Presentation
All areas of the vulva can be affected, and rarely it may be the only site affected [1,2].

Differential diagnosis
There can be considerable overlap with HHD and genital papular dyskeratosis.

Complications and co-morbidities
Secondary bacterial and viral infections are common on ano-genital lesions. There is one case report of an SCC developing in vulval Darier disease [3].

Management
The management of vulval Darier disease is the same as for other sites but topical preparations may be more irritant in the ano-genital area. Prompt treatment of any infection is important.

INFLAMMATORY DERMATOSES OF THE VULVA

Lichen sclerosus

Definition and nomenclature
Lichen sclerosus (LS) is a common inflammatory dermatosis with a predilection for ano-genital skin (Chapter 55).

Synonyms and inclusions
- Lichen sclerosus et atrophicus

Introduction and general description
Lichen sclerosus is one of the most common dermatoses to affect the ano-genital skin [1]. The aetiology is still unknown but there is some evidence in women that LS is a genetically determined autoimmune disorder, and antibodies to extracellular matrix protein 1 have been identified in about 75% of women with the disease [2].

Epidemiology
Incidence and prevalence
Lichen sclerosus is estimated to occur in 1 in 30 postmenopausal women [3]. The prevalence in children is not clear but was suggested to occur in 1 in 900 girls in one study [4].

Age
Lichen sclerosus can affect females of any age, but there are two peaks of incidence, in prepubertal girls and postmenopausal women.

Sex
Lichen sclerosus is 6–10 times more common in females than males.

Associated diseases
There is a link with other autoimmune disorders in 21% of patients [5], with thyroid disease being the commonest association. However, this link is not as great in males [6]. It is also observed that there is often concomitant psoriasis in patients with LS [7,8].

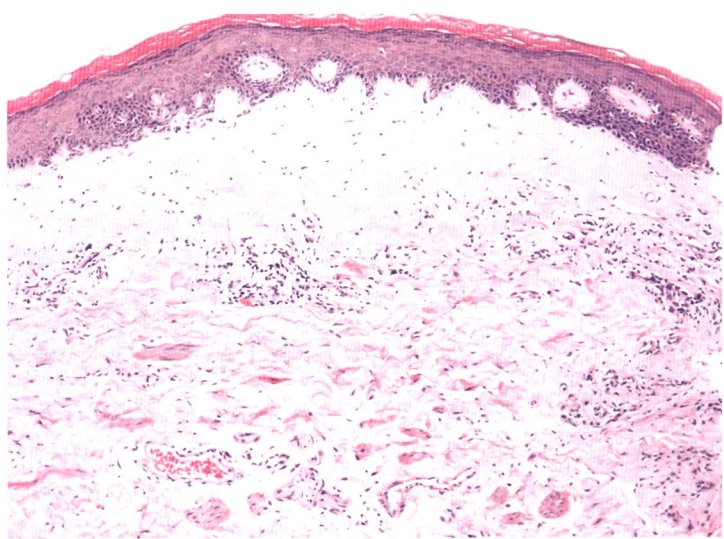

Figure 110.6 Histological features of lichen sclerosus.

Pathophysiology

Predisposing factors

Lichen sclerosus is known to exhibit the Koebner phenomenon and is sometimes seen in episiotomy scars. The Koebner phenomenon has also been reported at sites of radiotherapy [9], scar tissue [10], vaccination [11] and congenital haemangioma [12].

Pathology

The classic histological features are of a thinned epidermis with flattening of the rete pegs. The underlying dermis is pale and hyalinised and there are often extravasated red cells. Below the hyalinised area is a band-like zone of chronic inflammatory cells, mainly composed of CD4+ T lymphocytes (Figure 110.6). There is an absence of elastic fibres in the upper dermis. Attempts have been made to grade the histological appearances but there is probably little correlation between the timing of a lesion and its histological appearance [13]. In some cases the epidermis is thickened, and this is found in approximately 30% of cases of LS in association with vulval SCC [14].

There are abnormalities of the basement membrane, but it is uncertain whether these are a primary or secondary event [15]. Immunofluorescence studies are usually negative or demonstrate non-specific fibrin deposition at the dermal–epidermal junction. There is also an alteration of the elastin and fibrillin in the affected dermis [16]. Studies of cell kinetics show active regeneration of collagen [17] and there is altered p53 expression and epidermal cell proliferation [18]. Increased numbers of CD1+ Langerhans cells are found at all stages of disease [19]. There may be epigenetic phenomena in addition [20].

Causative organisms

Borrelia burgdorferi has been implicated in LS but there is no consistent evidence that it is causative.

Genetics

A positive family history is recognised in 12% of patients [21] and the disorder has been described in twins, both identical [22] and

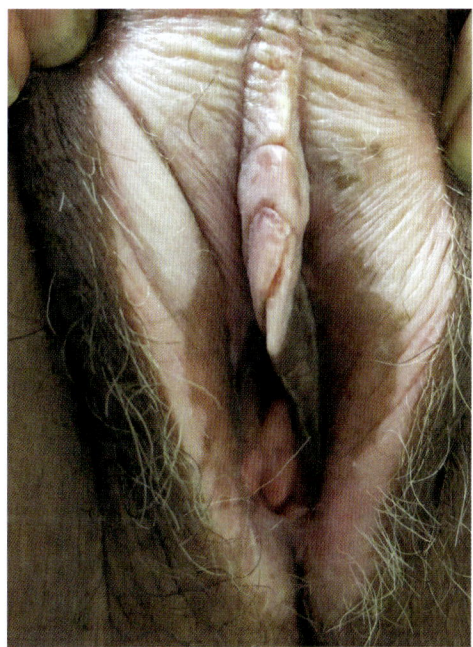

Figure 110.7 Lichen sclerosus showing white sclerotic plaques and architectural change.

non-identical [23]. There is an increased incidence of DQ7 in both adults [24] and girls [25].

Clinical features

History

The presenting symptom is usually itching, which is often severe and distressing. Patients may also complain of discomfort and dyspareunia if there is introital narrowing or fissuring. Constipation is a common feature of LS when it occurs in prepubertal girls.

Presentation

Ano-genital disease tends to be characterised by flat, atrophic, whitened epithelium (Figure 110.7), which may become confluent, extending around the vulval and perianal skin in a figure-of-eight configuration. There may also be oedema, purpura or ecchymosis (Figure 110.8), bullae, erosions, fissures (Figure 110.9) and ulceration. Sometimes the epithelium can become thickened (Figure 110.10). The sites most commonly affected are the inguinal folds, the inner aspects of the labia majora, labia minora and clitoral hood. Vestibular involvement is rare and vaginal lesions do not occur as LS seems to spare the mucosal epithelium. The one exception to this is when significant prolapse causes the skin to keratinise, which may then become affected by lichen sclerosus [26,27]. Perianal lesions occur in approximately 30% of female patients. The classic lesions seen on the extragenital skin are ivory-white papules and plaques with follicular delling. These occur in 10% of women with vulval disease. The extragenital areas may be truncal, at sites of pressure, or on the upper back, wrists, buttocks and thighs. Facial [28], lip [29], scalp [30] and nail [31] involvement have all been recorded.

Lesions of LS in the oral cavity are extremely rare but are reported on the tongue [32]. Many of the reports of oral involvement in the literature have often not been confirmed histologically [33] and may have been examples of lichen planus. It is not uncommon for patients with vulval LS to have coexistent oral lichen planus [34].

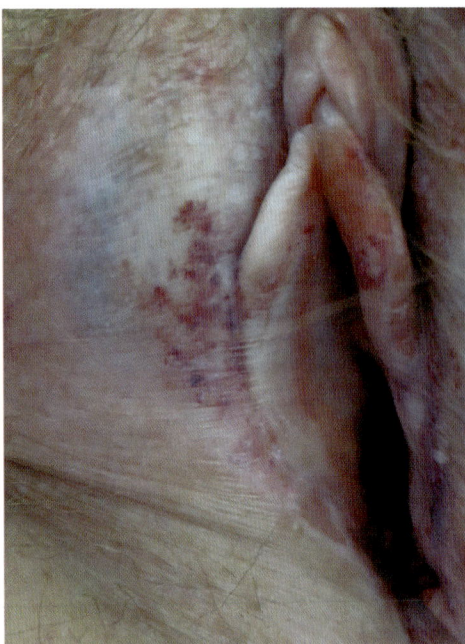

Figure 110.8 Ecchymosis (purpura) in lichen sclerosus

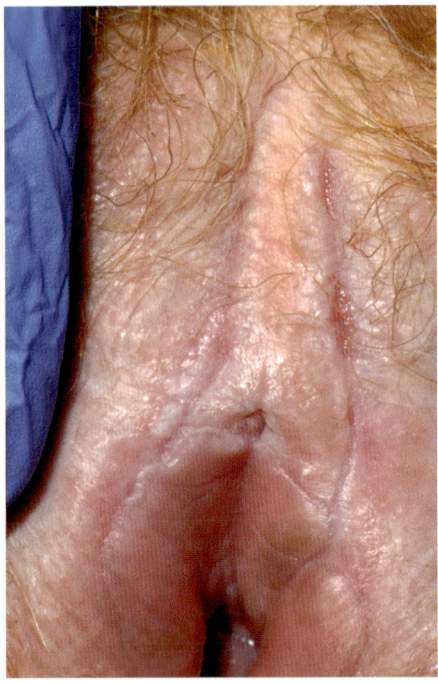

Figure 110.9 Fissuring in lichen sclerosus.

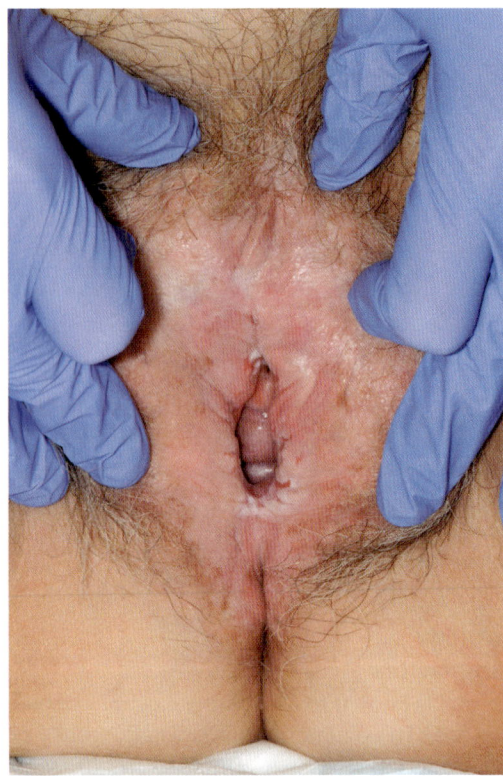

Figure 110.10 Thickened epithelium in acanthotic lichen sclerosus.

and LS, and they may represent a spectrum of disease rather than three distinct conditions [35]. The two conditions may coexist on the vulva [36].

LS and other dermatoses can be mistaken for sexual abuse [37–40], but sometimes the sexual abuse may be the initiating or exacerbating factor of the dermatological condition [41]. Thus it is important to consider sexual abuse if there are any concerns as the two can exist together.

Complications and co-morbidities

There is undoubtedly an association between vulval SCC and LS (Figure 110.12) but the incidence is less than 4% [42]. However, in retrospective reviews of pathological specimens of vulval carcinoma, histological evidence of LS is found in approximately half of the cases [43,44,45], and may be underrepresented [46]. These series included patients presenting with SCC as well as those on long-term follow-up for LS. A longitudinal cohort study of 211 patients showed that the number of invasive SCCs significantly exceeded that in an age-matched group [47]. The oncogenic HPV types do not appear to be implicated in the development of SCC on LS [48,49].

The histological patterns associated with SCC arising on LS include epithelial hyperplasia and differentiated intraepithelial neoplasia (dysplastic changes that are confined to the basal layers). Several studies have looked at markers to predict possible progression to SCC [50], but none is confirmatory or used in routine practice.

LS has been reported in association with verrucous carcinoma [51,52], basal cell carcinoma [53] and melanoma [54–56]. However, malignant melanoma and atypical genital naevi are known to be

LS is a scarring dermatosis and the changes that can occur on the vulva include loss of the labia minora and sealing over of the clitoral hood, burying the clitoris (Figure 110.11). Introital narrowing resulting from anterior and posterior labial fusion sometimes results in a tiny opening into the vestibule. Milia may occur.

Differential diagnosis

Vitiligo, mucous membrane pemphigoid, lichen planus and morphoea may present with a similar clinical appearance. There can be clinical and histological overlap between morphoea, lichen planus

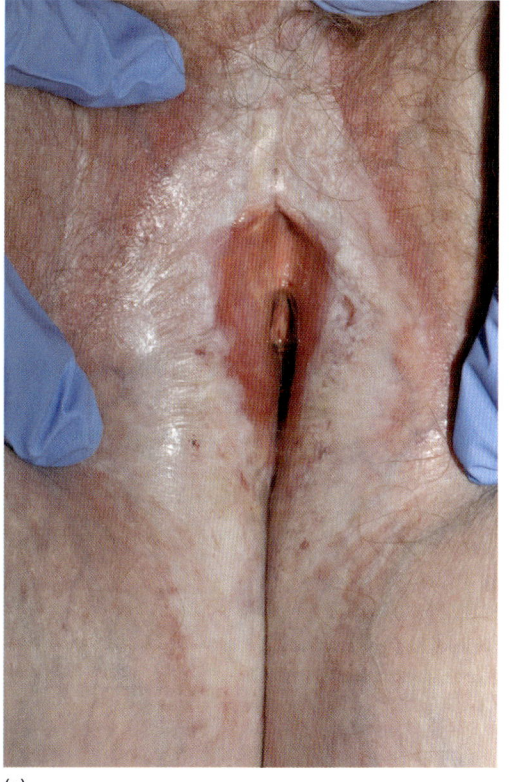

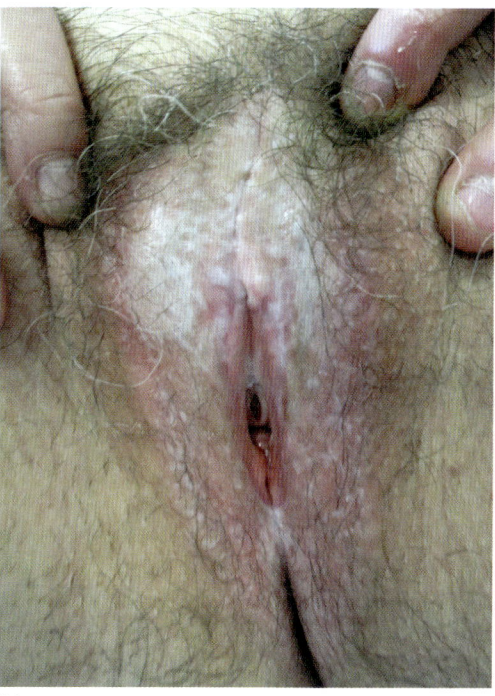

Figure 110.11 (a) Scarring in lichen sclerosus with mild ecchymosis. (b) Scarring in lichen sclerosus with loss of the labia minora and sealing of the clitoral hood.

(a)

(b)

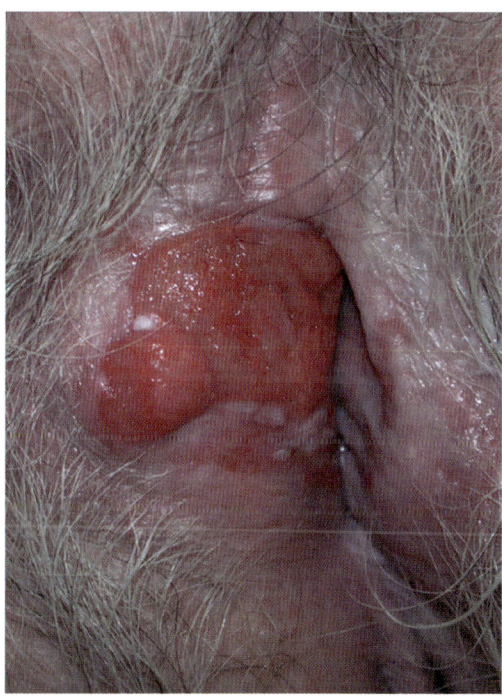

Figure 110.12 Squamous cell carcinoma arising on a background of lichen sclerosus.

difficult to diagnose in the presence of LS [57,58] and are generally reported in children with LS. It is thought that the inflammatory process may activate melanocytes.

Other complications of LS include urinary and sexual dysfunction. The role of urinary incontinence as an aetiological factor in women is not proven.

Disease course and prognosis

There is usually a good response to a super-potent topical steroid [59] but some patients have a relapse of symptoms, requiring repeated treatment. Most patients will require intermittent treatment to maintain control of symptoms and signs [60]. This has been shown to reduce scarring and risk of malignancy. Many girls with LS who are treated early and whose disease responds well before puberty do well and it often remits at that point. However, it can persist and require ongoing treatment and follow-up [61,62].

Investigations

A biopsy can confirm the diagnosis and is essential in atypical disease or if there is a failure to respond to treatment.

Management

First line

Super-potent topical steroid, clobetasol propionate 0.05%, is the first line treatment [63,64]. This has been shown to be superior to topical tacrolimus in a randomised controlled trial. The regimen currently recommended for a newly diagnosed case is initially clobetasol propionate ointment once nightly for 4 weeks, then alternate nights for 4 weeks, and twice a week for a further 4 weeks [64]. This tapering regimen is as effective as once-daily treatment. A 30 g tube of clobetasol propionate should last 12 weeks, and the patient is then reviewed. The treatment is then individualised to control symptoms and signs. Most patients seem to require 30–60 g annually. Although some patients do go into remission and do not require further treatment with no signs of active disease, most continue to have flares and remissions and they are advised to use clobetasol propionate ointment to maintain control. A soap substitute is also recommended such as emulsifying ointment. Barrier preparations may be helpful in those with urinary incontinence.

Second line
It is rare for LS not to respond to a potent topical steroid and it is important to exclude other causes for the symptoms such as infection, contact allergy or vulvodynia. An alternative topical steroid can be tried [**64**].

Other treatments
Topical testosterone has no role in the management of LS. It is expensive and is not as effective as clobetasol propionate [65]. Recent reports have suggested the use of the calcineurin inhibitors tacrolimus [66] or pimecrolimus [67] as steroid-sparing alternatives. The use of these topical immunosuppressants should be limited to the treatment of the rare cases of LS that prove unresponsive to a potent topical steroid. The treatment should be a short course and it should not be used long term as the safety of these immunosuppressants is still unknown, particularly as the condition carries a risk of neoplastic change. Ciclosporin [68] and UVA1 [69] have also been used to treat recalcitrant disease.

Surgery is only indicated for the management of functional problems caused by postinflammatory scarring, premalignant lesions and malignancy [70]. There is no evidence for the use of laser [71] or platelet-rich plasma to treat LS [72].

Resources

Further information
British Association of Dermatologists guidelines: https://onlinelibrary.wiley.com/doi/full/10.1111/bjd.16241.

Patient resources
Association for Lichen Sclerosus: www.lichensclerosus.org/.
International Society for the Study of Vulvovaginal Disease information sheets: https://www.issvd.org/resources/vulvar-lichen-sclerosus.
(All last accessed April 2022.)

Lichen planus

Synonyms and inclusions
- Syndrome of Hewitt and Pelisse
- Desquamative vaginitis

Introduction and general description
Lichen planus (LP) is an inflammatory dermatosis that can affect the skin and mucous membranes. It may affect the ano-genital skin and mucosa without involvement elsewhere but can also present at multiple sites, requiring multidisciplinary management [**1**] (Chapter 37).

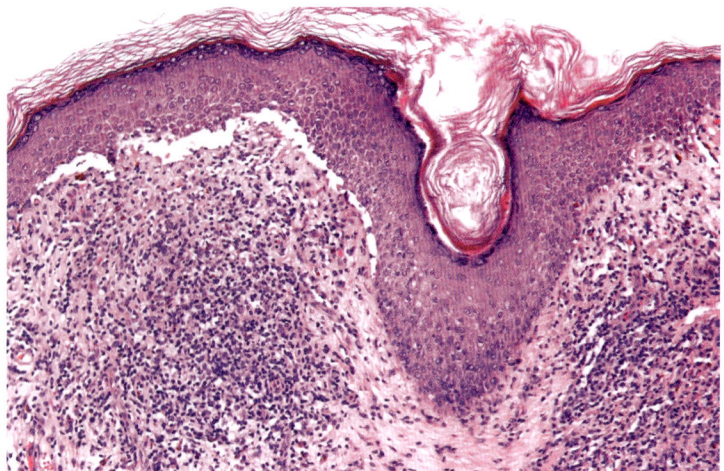

Figure 110.13 Histological features of lichen planus.

Epidemiology
Incidence and prevalence
The incidence in the general population is unknown but in one study of 3350 women attending a vulval clinic, 3.7% had vulval lichen planus [2]. Vulval LP was also found in 57% of patients with oral LP [3] and in 51% of those presenting with cutaneous lesions. Many were asymptomatic [**4**].

Age
The symptoms usually start in the fifth and sixth decades of life [5].

Associated diseases
There is an association of LP with autoimmune diseases including alopecia areata, vitiligo and thyroid disease. An association with hepatitis C infection has been reported in some Mediterranean and Japanese populations but not in northern Europe [6].

Pathophysiology
Lichen planus is probably a T-cell-mediated inflammatory disorder but no causative antigen that may trigger the T-lymphocyte response has been found. Antibasement membrane antibodies have been reported [7].

Pathology
On a cornified epithelium there is hyperkeratosis, irregular acanthosis with a typical saw-tooth appearance of the rete pegs, an increased granular layer and disruption of the basal layer with a closely apposed, dermal band-like lymphocytic infiltrate (Figure 110.13). The acanthosis and hyperkeratosis are marked in the hypertrophic form, and the characteristic band-like infiltrate may be focal. Eosinophilic colloid bodies may be seen. The classic histological features in the epidermis may not be seen in erosive disease, and mucosal lesions may show many plasma cells, which is where the diagnosis of Zoon vulvitis is often made incorrectly. Immunofluorescence studies reveal uneven staining of the basement membrane zone for fibrinogen and immunoglobulin M (IgM), cytoid bodies and, on occasion, IgG or IgA.

Genetics

Familial cases have been described and although human leukocyte antigen (HLA) findings are conflicting, an association with HLA-DR1 is postulated [8]. The DQB*0201 allele is associated with the vulvo-vaginal–gingival syndrome form of erosive LP [9].

Clinical features

History

The symptoms will depend on the clinical type of LP. Itching may be predominant in the classic and hypertrophic variants, whereas soreness, pain and dyspareunia are the common complaints in erosive LP. If vaginal disease is present, a serosanguinous discharge and postcoital bleeding may occur.

Presentation

The clinical features vary with clinical type.

Clinical variants

Three clinical forms are recognised but there may sometimes be overlap features.

1 *Classic/papular lichen planus*. This type can occur with cutaneous lesions. The typical violaceous papules are seen on the outer labia majora, interlabial sulci and clitoral hood. These may coalesce into small plaques or annular lesions (Figure 110.14a). The hallmark Wickham striae may be present (Figure 110.14b). Hyperpigmentation is common and may affect other flexural sites including the inguinal and inframammary folds and axillae. Lichen plano-pilaris has also been described on the vulva [10].

2 *Hypertrophic lichen planus*. This is the least common form of LP seen on the genital skin. Thickened, intensely pruritic plaques, sometimes with a violaceous edge, are seen on the labia majora, perineum and perianal skin. Vaginal lesions do not occur in classic or hypertrophic LP.

3 *Erosive lichen planus*. Erosive LP is the commonest type to affect the female genital area. On the vulva, symmetrical erosions are most commonly seen at the fourchette and vestibule. These may have an irregular lacy edge with Wickham striae. Diagnostic criteria have been put forward for the diagnosis of erosive LP [11], with the suggestion that three supportive criteria should be present to make the diagnosis. Clinicopathological correlation yields the most reliable diagnosis of vulval lichen planus [12].

4 *Vulvo-vaginal–gingival (VVG) syndrome*. This distinctive erosive subtype of LP principally affects the inner aspects of the labia minora, vestibule and vagina (Figure 110.15), together with a characteristic gingival erythema (Figure 110.16), which may be asymptomatic [13,14,15]. In the past, many cases labelled desquamative vaginitis were probably this entity [16]. The mucosa is eroded and there may be marked loss of architecture (Figure 110.17). The anal margin, external urethral meatus and cervix may also be involved.

The vaginal lesions are velvety red erosions or bright red, glazed erythema, which is friable and bleeds when touched. Vaginal synechiae and adhesions develop, which may rapidly lead to vaginal stenosis and unfortunately many patients present at this stage. Vaginal examination is therefore mandatory in these patients.

This is increasingly recognised as a multisite disease with lesions described on the conjunctiva [17], lacrimal duct (Figure 110.18) [18], oesophagus [19,20] and external auditory canal [21]. The manifestations of this syndrome do not necessarily all occur synchronously.

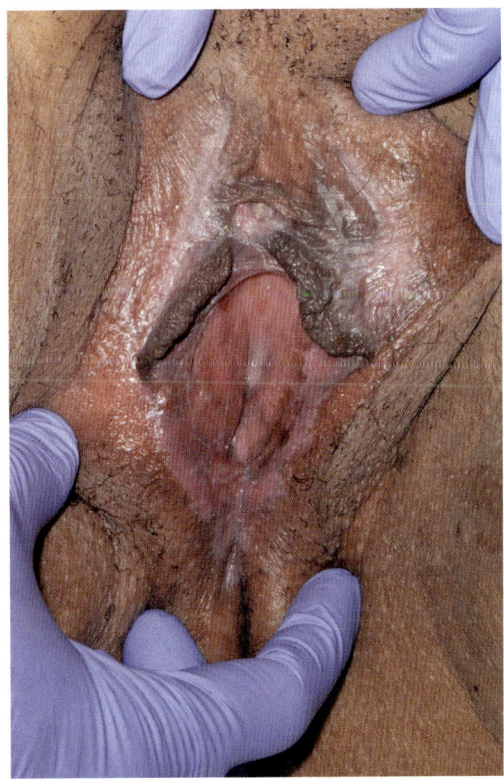
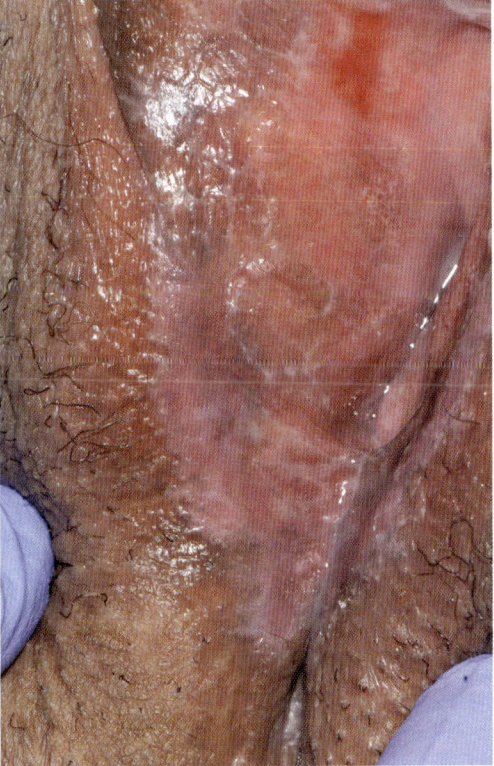

Figure 110.14 (a) Classic vulval lichen planus showing plaques in the interlabial sulci. (b) Classic vulval lichen planus with Wickham striae.

(a)

(b)

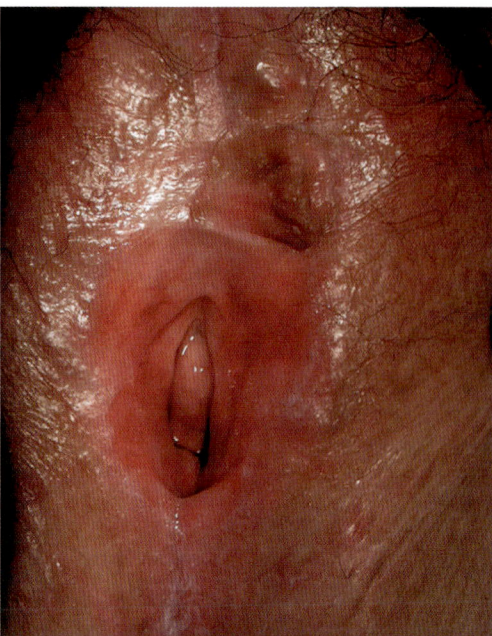

Figure 110.15 Lichen planus: vulval aspect showing glazed erythema and distortion of the architecture, with a remnant of the left labium minus and buried clitoris above it.

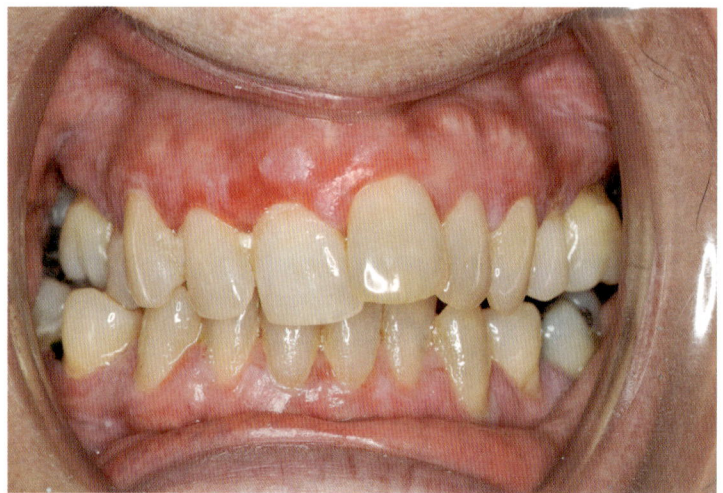

Figure 110.16 Gingival erythema in vulvo-vaginal–gingival syndrome.

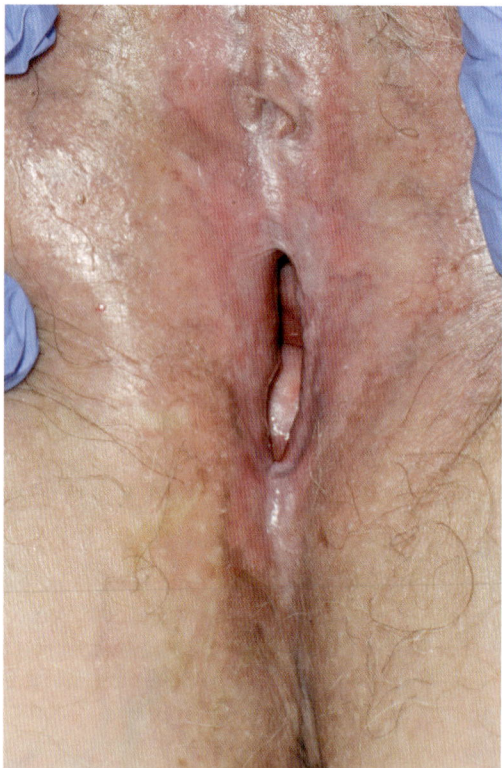

Figure 110.17 Scarring in erosive vulval lichen planus.

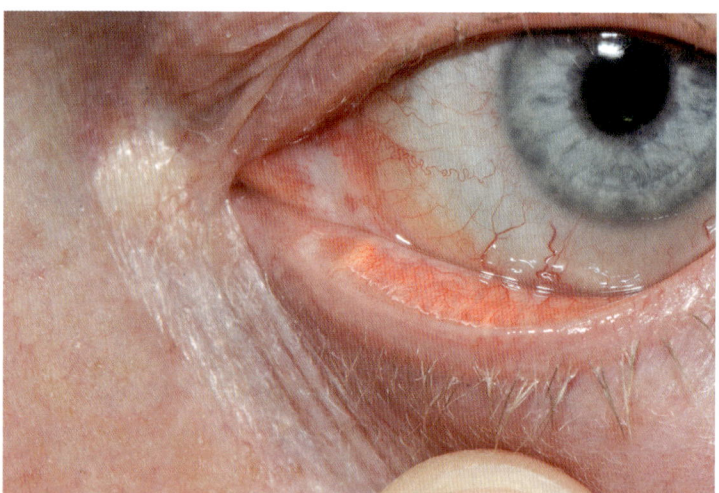

Figure 110.18 Lacrimal duct scarring in erosive lichen planus in vulvo-vaginal–gingival syndrome.

Differential diagnosis

The main differential diagnosis is usually LS, but mucous membrane pemphigoid, morphoea and lichenoid drug eruptions should also be included. In some cases, the differentiation between LS and LP can be extremely difficult as the two diseases have so many features in common [22,23]. The lichenoid form of graft-versus-host disease has clinical features that may be indistinguishable from erosive LP but this diagnosis should be clear from the history. Frequently, there are cases of LP misdiagnosed as Zoon vulvitis. Some hypertrophic lesions can mimic malignancy and histology is vital.

Complications and co-morbidities

Scarring is a major issue, particularly in erosive LP, and early diagnosis and appropriate management are important.

Malignancy is not thought to occur in erosive LP but SCC and SCC *in situ* have been reported in other forms of the disease [24–26]. Studies of patients with vulval SCC have shown that LP is present in the surrounding tissue in about 15% of patients [**27,28**].

In addition to the sites mentioned earlier which may be involved in the VVG syndrome, oral manifestations may be seen in all forms of genital LP on the buccal mucosa, tongue and palate. Nail changes are sometimes seen and scarring alopecia may occur in any form of genital LP. Frontal fibrosing alopecia was the commonest association in one series [29].

Disease course and prognosis

Classic LP often clears completely with little or no scarring. Hyperpigmentation may take months to resolve. Erosive and hypertrophic disease tends to pursue a chronic course with flares of disease. It can have a significant impact on quality of life [30].

Investigations

The clinical diagnosis can be confirmed on biopsy. The use of topical anaesthesia may obscure the true histological diagnosis [31].

Management

There are no definitive randomised controlled trials of treatment in genital LP and most therapy is based on small case series and single case reports [32]. A Cochrane review of treatments for mucosal erosive LP did not identify any studies of genital disease [33].

First line

Use super-potent topical steroid ointment for the vulva and intravaginal foam preparations for vaginal disease [34,35]. Emollients are also used as an adjunct to first line active treatment.

Second line

There are reports about the use of calcineurin inhibitors [36–38] but these must be used with caution, as in LS, as there have been concerns about malignant change after their use [39,40].

Third line

Oral retinoids, dapsone and ciclosporin have been used anecdotally but there is little evidence for their use [41]. Low-dose methotrexate, either alone or in combination with topical steroids and tacrolimus, has been reported to be useful [42–44]. Hydroxychloroquine was reported to be of benefit in one series [45].

Surgery to release vulval and vaginal adhesions may be required [46] but the use of super-potent topical steroids in the early postoperative phase is vital to prevent restenosis [47].

Photodynamic therapy has been trialled [48]. There are single case reports of the use of biologics to treat widespread erosive LP [49,50], but lichenoid eruptions may be a side effect [51,52] so they should be used with caution.

Resources

Patient resources

International Society for the Study of Vulvovaginal Disease information sheet: https://www.issvd.org/resources/vulvar-lichen-planus.
UK Lichen Planus: www.uklp.org.uk/.
(Both last accessed April 2022.)

Zoon vulvitis

Synonyms and inclusions

- Vulvitis circumscripta
- Plasma cell vulvitis

Introduction and general description

Although Zoon balanitis is well described, true Zoon vulvitis is rare. The criteria needed to make the diagnosis have varied in the literature, and there is some doubt whether plasma cell vulvitis is a distinct clinicopathological entity, as many of the reports of vestibular Zoon are probably LP [1]. It is likely that it represents a reaction pattern to another inflammatory condition. A plasma cell-rich infiltrate in a vestibular biopsy may be a misleading finding, because plasma cells are commonly found in inflammatory conditions of the vestibule. Many of the cases are examples of unrecognised dermatoses such as LP, or a chronic postinflammatory phenomenon.

Pathophysiology
Pathology

The essential features are epidermal thinning, absent horny and granular layers and distinctive lozenge-shaped keratinocytes with widened intercellular spaces. In the dermis there is a dense, inflammatory infiltrate composed largely of plasma cells, with dilated blood vessels and usually a lot of haemosiderin. Russell bodies and dermal–epidermal splitting have also been described [2].

Clinical features
History

Patients may complain of pruritus or discomfort, but it can be asymptomatic [3].

Presentation

The original description was of red, glazed patches, usually on the labia minora or vestibule [4]. The clitoris is rarely, if ever, affected.

Clinical variants

It is not uncommon to find patients with purpuric patches, often at the vestibule (Figure 110.19), in which haemosiderin and plasma cells are found without any specific epidermal change, and the term *chronic vulval purpura* may be a more accurate description [5]. An association with lichen aureus has been suggested, as pressure factors are thought to be relevant in the extravasation of blood [6].

Differential diagnosis

Lichen planus, postinflammatory pigmentation and vulval adenosis have similar features.

Disease course and prognosis

It follows a chronic but benign course.

Investigations

A vulval biopsy will show the features described.

Management
First line

First line management is with emollients and a potent topical steroid [7,8].

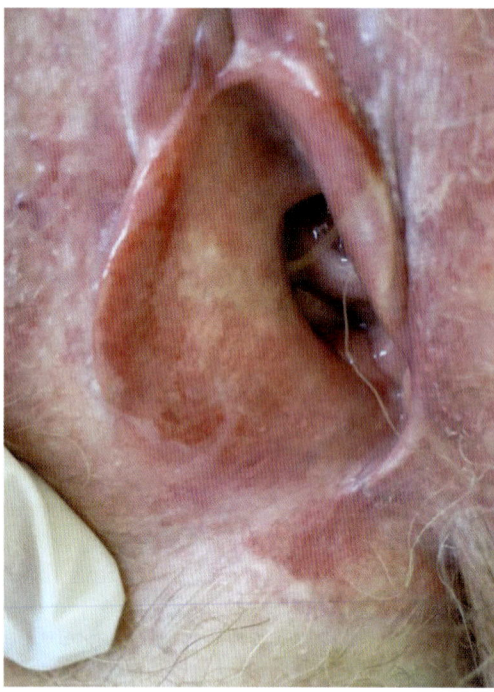

Figure 110.19 Chronic vulval purpura.

Second line

There are case reports of the use of misoprostol [9] and intralesional interferon α [10]. Topical tacrolimus has not been found to be useful [11].

Seborrhoeic eczema

Introduction and general description

This is a common type of eczema in younger people and may affect the vulva (Chapter 40).

Pathophysiology
Pathology

Histological examination is not always helpful as there may be features of both eczema and psoriasis. There is moderate acanthosis with slight spongiosis and a mild dermal inflammatory infiltrate.

Clinical features
History

Patients describe intermittent itching and soreness if fissures occur.

Presentation

The signs may be subtle, but scaling and redness are seen on the inguinal folds, labia majora, perineum and perianal skin. Keratin debris may build up in the interlabial sulci and sometimes under the clitoral hood.

Vulval involvement may be associated with skin changes on the scalp and changes at other flexural sites.

Differential diagnosis

This condition has both eczematous and psoriasiform features, sometimes making differentiation between it and psoriasis difficult.

In psoriasis, the lesions are usually better defined and thickened. The keratin debris can be mistaken for candidiasis but the discharge with this latter condition is seen in the vestibule and lower vulva.

Disease course and prognosis

Vulval lesions may recur and require intermittent treatment until resolution.

Investigations

The diagnosis is usually clinical.

Management

Treatment ladder for seborrhoeic eczema

First line
- Emollients
- Mild topical steroid once daily as needed

Second line
- Topical calcineurin inhibitors may be used but are not always well tolerated on the vulva

---

Irritant eczema

Synonyms and inclusions
- Irritant contact eczema
- Irritant contact dermatitis

Introduction and general description

If the barrier function of the vulval skin is impaired, as measured by transepidermal water loss, there is an increased susceptibility to irritant contact eczema [1,2] (Chapter 128).

Epidemiology
Age

An irritant contact eczema is common in children and in older women, particularly those who are incontinent.

Pathophysiology
Predisposing factors

The problem may occur because of the dampness and maceration secondary to a heavy vaginal discharge, or increased contact with urine in the incontinent patient. Contact with irritant chemicals in topical agents, particularly cleansers, bubble baths, lubricants, perfumed products, deodorants and medicaments, may all be responsible for an irritant dermatitis.

Clinical features

History

Soreness is often more common than pruritus in an irritant contact eczema. If severe, it can be painful, especially with micturition.

Presentation

Redness is most pronounced on the convex areas – the outer labia majora, perianal skin and buttocks – which are the sites most in contact with external irritants.

Differential diagnosis

There are some features in common with seborrhoeic eczema but extravulval involvement is unlikely. There is less scaling in irritant dermatitis compared with seborrheoic eczema.

Complications and co-morbidities

In severe cases of irritant dermatitis, most commonly in older women with urinary incontinence, ulcerative lesions similar to those seen in infantile gluteal granuloma may occur. These are often on the outer labia majora [3]. Jacquet erosive dermatitis and papulonodular verrucous plaques are likely to be a spectrum of the same disease [4].

Investigations

The diagnosis is clinical.

Management

Treatment ladder for irritant dermatitis

First line
- Removal of irritants
- Referral to a uro-gynaecologist can be helpful to improve urinary incontinence
- Emollients as soap substitute
- Barrier preparations

Second line
- Mild topical steroid, with antibacterial/antifungal if appropriate

---

Allergic contact dermatitis

Introduction and general description

Allergic contact dermatitis is a type IV delayed hypersensitivity reaction. It is rare as a primary cause of vulval symptoms but can complicate other dermatoses (Chapter 127).

Epidemiology

Incidence and prevalence

A high incidence of vulval contact dermatitis has been described [1,2,3,4] but this may be explained by many patients who also have perianal involvement. One study has shown a higher incidence of positive patch tests in patients with ano-genital dermatoses if both the genital and perianal areas are involved, compared with dermatoses affecting the genital skin alone [5].

Pathophysiology

Predisposing factors

There are reports of allergy to vaginal preparations and an intrauterine device [6–8], sanitary wear [9] and condoms [10]. Oestradiol may rarely cause a localised allergic contact dermatitis at a transdermal patch site, or generalised contact dermatitis with oral therapy [11]. Many other allergens can cause a vulval allergic contact problem [12,13].

Clinical features

Presentation

An allergic contact dermatitis most commonly presents with pruritus but, if acute, an erosive eruption may be seen which frequently extends down the thighs. An eczematous eruption can be seen which can extend to the perianal skin.

Differential diagnosis

Other forms of eczema and ano-genital psoriasis may have similar features.

Disease course and prognosis

Once the causative allergen is established and then avoided, the problem should resolve.

Investigations

A detailed history is vital; patch testing is needed in patients where an allergic contact dermatitis is suspected. It is important to include allergens that may be important in the genital area, and vulval/perianal allergen series are widely available. It may also be helpful to include the patient's own products.

Management

Treatment ladder for allergic contact dermatitis

First line
- Remove relevant allergens
- Emollients
- Moderately potent topical steroid ± an antibacterial or antifungal

Second line
- Potassium permanganate soaks (1 . 10 000 dilution applied on gauze) if weeping and eroded
- Antibiotics if secondary infection

Resources

Patient resources

British Society for Cutaneous Allergy patient information: https://cutaneousallergy.org/resources/patient-information-leaflets-pils/.

International Society for the Study of Vulvovaginal Disease information sheet: https://www.issvd.org/resources/contact-dermatitis-of-the-vulva.

(Both last accessed April 2022.)

PART 10: SPECIFIC SITES, SEX & AGE

Allergic contact urticaria

Introduction and general description

This is a type I immediate hypersensitivity reaction; the two most common causes of contact urticaria in the vulvo-vaginal area are latex and semen (Chapter 42). Seminal fluid usually induces an urticarial immediate type I reaction and rarely produces a type IV contact allergy. There are reports of mixed sensitivities; one patient was allergic to semen and latex and another to her husband's semen and sweat [1,2]. However, semen itself may not be the responsible allergen, the problem being caused by a medication or other allergen carried in the seminal fluid [3–5].

Epidemiology

Associated diseases

There is often a history of atopy.

Clinical features

History

The history is helpful diagnostically since immediate swelling of the vulva will occur. A condom will abolish the symptoms if the patient is allergic to semen but will cause the problem if latex is the relevant allergen.

Presentation

Immediate swelling occurs during or just after intercourse.

Differential diagnosis

Pressure urticaria can cause identical clinical features but occurs with or without a condom and dermographism elsewhere is usually seen.

Investigations

Intradermal testing with appropriate precautions can be done for semen allergy. Serological tests for latex can be used.

Management

Remove the cause – for instance, use non-latex condoms if the patient is latex allergic. Antigenic treatment of semen before artificial insemination has resulted in successful pregnancy if there is semen allergy [6]. Patients need referral to a specialised allergy or immunology centre.

Lichen simplex

Synonyms and inclusions

- Lichen simplex chronicus
- Lichenification
- Neurodermatitis

Introduction and general description

Lichen simplex is used to describe the changes seen on apparently normal skin secondary to rubbing the skin in response to itch, although the provoking symptom of itch may be initiated by a low-grade dermatosis. The term lichenification is used for similar changes arising on a background of a visible dermatosis (Chapter 81).

Epidemiology

Associated diseases

Lichen simplex occurs more commonly in patients who have a background of psoriasis or eczema.

Pathophysiology

Pathology

There is hyperkeratosis, acanthosis, a prominent granular layer, lengthened rete ridges and a chronic inflammatory dermal infiltrate. In addition, lamellar thickening of the papillary dermis and perineural fibrosis can be seen. Twelve cases of what was termed multinucleated atypia of the vulva have been reported [1], but this is thought to be a non-specific change found in lichenified skin [2,3].

Clinical features

History

The patient describes intense itching which may keep them awake at night. This often starts on the vulva but frequently spreads to involve the perineum and perianal skin.

Presentation

There are localised, thickened plaques, most commonly affecting the outer labia majora (Figure 110.20). The perianal skin is frequently involved. The epidermis becomes ridged and the trauma of continued rubbing can lead to hair loss in hair-bearing skin.

Differential diagnosis

It is always important to exclude an underlying dermatosis or naevoid lesion where the lichenification may be a secondary phenomenon [4,5].

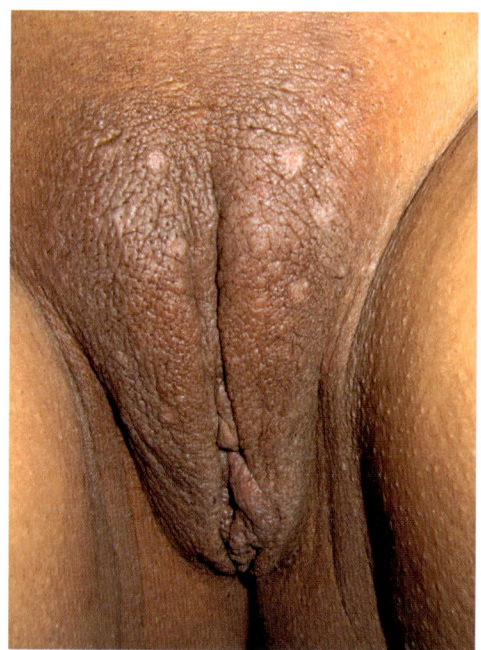

Figure 110.20 Lichen simplex.

Disease course and prognosis

In many cases, patients respond well to appropriate treatment but some enter a chronic itch–scratch–itch cycle that is more challenging to treat. Dysaesthesia may develop when the lichenification has resolved.

Investigations

The diagnosis is usually made on clinical grounds but if there are atypical features or a failure to respond to treatment, a biopsy will be helpful.

In cases where an allergic contact dermatitis trigger is suspected, patch testing is useful, but is not done routinely.

Management

> **Treatment ladder for lichen simplex**
>
> **First line**
> - Emollients and a potent topical steroid on a reducing regimen over 2–3 months. The symptoms may improve quickly but there is often relapse if the treatment is stopped before the lichenification has resolved
>
> **Second line**
> - Sedative antihistamines at night, e.g. hydroxyzine 25–50 mg
>
> **Third line**
> - Doxepin, low-dose tricylics in increasing doses, e.g. 10 mg nocte and increasing by 10 mg increments every 3–4 weeks. Low-dose naltrexone can also be considered

Psoriasis

> **Synonyms and inclusions**
> - Flexural psoriasis
> - Inverse psoriasis
> - Intertriginous psoriasis

Introduction and general description

Psoriasis may affect the ano-genital area as part of generalised disease but can occur in isolation (Chapter 35).

Epidemiology

Incidence and prevalence

Vulval psoriasis accounts for up to 5% of patients who present with persistent vulval symptoms [1]. Over 60% of patients with psoriasis will have genital involvement at some time [2,3]. Patients often find the problem embarrassing and do not consult readily about the issues [4].

Associated diseases

Many patients with lichen sclerosus are also noted to have psoriasis [5,6].

Pathophysiology

Pathology

Flexural psoriasis does not always have the typical histological features of psoriasis seen elsewhere and there may be marked spongiosis and papillary oedema.

Environmental factors

Friction and occlusion are important aggravating factors in vulval psoriasis.

Clinical features

History

Most patients complain of itching, but soreness and pain can occur, particularly if the lesions become fissured. Dyspareunia may also be a feature, which can have an impact on sexual function [7] and quality of life [8].

Presentation

Well-demarcated erythematous plaques are seen on the labia majora, and extension on to the mons pubis, inguinal folds, perianal skin and gluteal cleft is common (Figure 110.21). The typical silvery scale seen elsewhere is lost but may be seen on the mons. Rarely, there may be some scarring associated with vulval psoriasis, with loss of the labia minora [9]. However, it is possible that some of these patients may have had previous lichen sclerosus.

Differential diagnosis

Seborrhoeic eczema and intertrigo can have very similar clinical features. Extramammary Paget disease occasionally has psoriasiform features.

Disease course and prognosis

Ano-genital psoriasis generally runs a chronic course. It is reported that over 90% of adults and children respond to treatment but this may need to be used intermittently to control the disease [3].

Investigations

Psoriasis is usually diagnosed clinically and a biopsy is rarely needed. Swabs may be required if there is extensive fissuring and evidence of secondary infection.

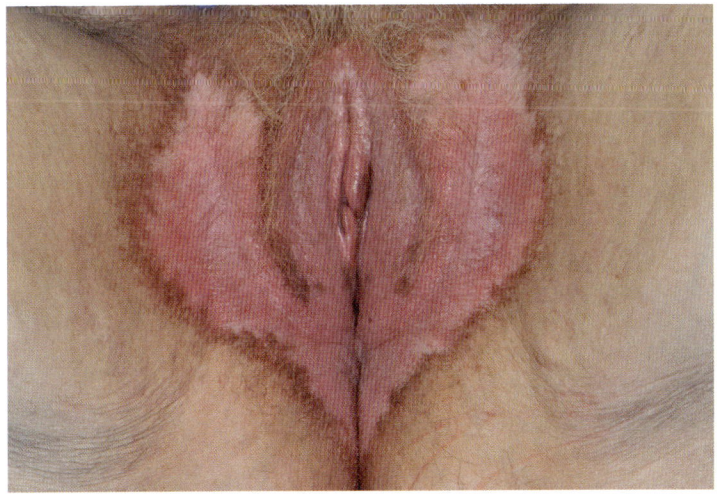

Figure 110.21 Vulval psoriasis.

Management

Resources

Patient resources

International Society for the Study of Vulvovaginal Disease information sheet: https://www.issvd.org/resources/vulvar-psoriasis.

Psoriasis Association: www.psoriasis-association.org.uk.

(Both last accessed April 2022.)

Reactive arthritis

Definition and nomenclature

Reactive arthritis is the triad of polyarthritis (of over a month's duration following gastrointestinal or lower genital tract infection), urethritis and non-gonococcal conjunctivitis. A scaly and erosive dermatosis of the vulva may accompany these features.

Synonyms and inclusions
- Circinate vulvo-vaginitis
- Reiter syndrome

Epidemiology
Sex
Genital lesions are rare in women.

Pathophysiology
Pathology
Histology shows hyperkeratosis and parakeratosis, an absent granular layer and prominent neutrophil epidermal microabscesses.

Causative organisms
Shigella dysentery (*Shigella flexneri* and *S. dysenteriae*) were the first infections to be associated with reactive arthritis, but species of *Salmonella*, *Yersinia*, *Campylobacter*, *Streptococcus* and *Mycoplasma* have all been associated with the disease. Sexually transmitted infections with *Chlamydia trachomatis* may also lead to reactive arthritis.

Genetics
It is more likely to occur in HLA-B27-positive individuals and also those with HLA-B51 positivity.

Clinical features
Presentation
Scaling, crusting and erosions are seen and the whole vulva may be involved including the mucosa [1]. A rash on the hands and feet that is indistinguishable from psoriasis is often present.

Differential diagnosis
The vulval lesions in reactive arthritis may resemble psoriasis and candidiasis.

Complications and co-morbidities
Cervicitis may develop.

Disease course and prognosis
The disease may follow a relapsing course. It is more difficult to control in patients with human immunodeficiency virus (HIV) infection.

Investigations
Associated infection must be sought. A biopsy may also be informative.

Management
Management should be shared with rheumatology, especially in complex cases. Any infection should be treated and this may require the input of a genito-urinary specialist.

ULCERATIVE AND BULLOUS DISORDERS

The differential diagnosis of genital ulceration is wide and an accurate diagnosis involves careful history taking, clinical examination and appropriate microbiological and histological investigation.

Table 110.2 Causes of vulval ulcers.

Genetic
Epidermolysis bullosa
Acantholytic dermatoses

Infective

Non-sexually transmitted
Herpes simplex/zoster
Epstein–Barr virus, HIV
Tuberculosis, actinomycosis, amoebiasis
Leishmaniasis, schistosomiasis

Sexually transmitted
Chancroid
Lymphogranuloma venereum
Granuloma inguinale
Syphilis

Inflammatory

Bullous
Autoimmune bullous disorders
Erythema multiforme
Stevens–Johnson syndrome/toxic epidermal
    necrolysis

Non-bullous
Aphthae
Lichen sclerosus/lichen planus
Crohn disease
Behçet disease
Lupus erythematosus
Graft-versus-host disease
Pyoderma gangrenosum
Hidradenitis suppurativa
Drug reactions, fixed drug
    eruptions, foscarnet, nicorandil
Rheumatoid nodule
Reactive arthritis

Tumours

Malignant
Squamous cell carcinoma/vulval intraepithelial
    neoplasia
Extramammary Paget disease
Basal cell carcinoma
Cutaneous lymphoma/leukaemia
Langerhans cell histiocytosis
Melanoma

Benign
Capillary haemangioma

Trauma
Blunt/sharp accidental/non-accidental trauma
Chemical – irritant contact dermatitis
Dermatitis artefacta
Radiation damage
Mechanical hymenal fissures

The major causes of vulval ulceration are listed in Table 110.2 and many are discussed fully elsewhere in this book.

Aphthous ulcers

Introduction and general description
Aphthous ulcers are recurrent, often multiple, small ulcers affecting the oral and genital mucosa.

Epidemiology
Age
The age of onset is in childhood, and there may be a family history.

Clinical features
History
There is acute onset of painful ulcers, and oral ulcers may be concurrent. Sometimes there are premenstrual exacerbations once the menarche is reached.

Presentation
The lesions are usually multiple, small (2–10 mm), superficial and painful. They are sited most frequently on the labia minora. They have a yellow base surrounded by a red rim and tend to heal quickly. Less commonly aphthous ulcers are solitary or few in number. Larger ulcers are referred to as giant aphthae.

Differential diagnosis
Herpes simplex and ulcers caused by Behçet disease are similar.

Disease course and prognosis
Lesions frequently recur in some patients.

Investigations
The diagnosis is clinical.

Management
Topical steroids and local anaesthetic preparations are helpful.

Non-sexually acquired reactive genital ulcers

Synonyms and inclusions
- Ulcus vulvae acutum
- Lipschutz ulcers

Introduction and general description
These are acute vulval ulcers presenting in young girls, usually as a reactive phenomenon to infection. They were first described by Lipschutz in 1913 [1].

Epidemiology
Age
These ulcers typically occur in teenagers and young adults [2].

Pathophysiology
Causative organisms
They have been most commonly linked with Epstein–Barr virus infection, which has been isolated from the ulcers in some cases [3,4]. Typhoid, paratyphoid fever, mumps and several other infections have also been associated [5,6]. They are also reported in association with Covid-19 infection [7].

Clinical features
History
The onset is acute with rapidly expanding, and very painful, vulval ulcers. There may be a history of preceding systemic illness or sore throat.

Presentation
The lesions start as haemorrhagic blisters and then enlarge and ulcerate. The base is covered by thick slough. They are usually located on the lower inner labia majora and may be bilateral ('kissing' ulcers).

Differential diagnosis
Major aphthae and Behçet ulcers can have similar features. One case mimicked a lymphoma [8].

Disease course and prognosis
The ulcers heal spontaneously over a few weeks. Recurrence is uncommon. Despite the deep nature of the ulcers, scarring is rare.

Investigations
Viral serology may be helpful. The diagnosis is usually clinical.

Management
Small ulcers can be treated with a moderately potent topical steroid; 5% lidocaine ointment and oral analgesia are helpful in relieving symptoms. Larger lesions may require a short course of oral prednisolone (e.g. 15–20 mg/day for 10 days) or doxycycline [9].

Behçet disease

Introduction and general description
Behçet disease is a multisystem disease with ulceration affecting the mucous membranes and is associated with systemic features (Chapter 48).

Clinical features
Presentation
The vulval ulcers seen in Behçet disease are recurrent, deep and heal with scarring after a few weeks. They can occur on the labia minora and majora and may be accompanied by some oedema. Vaginal ulcers have been reported [1].

Differential diagnosis
Initially, the genital ulcers can have similar features to simple aphthae and herpes simplex, but are larger and more persistent.

Investigations
Patients need full investigation for manifestations at other sites.

Management
Topical steroids are helpful initially for the genital ulcers. Management requires a multidisciplinary approach and is discussed elsewhere (Chapter 48).

Immunobullous disease

Synonyms and inclusions
- Mucous membrane pemphigoid
- Cicatricial pemphigoid
- Linear IgA disease of children
- Chronic bullous disease of childhood

Introduction and general description
The features of those diseases that commonly affect the genital area in females will be covered here – bullous pemphigoid (BP), mucous membrane pemphigoid (MMP), pemphigus vulgaris (PV), epidermolysis bullosa acquisita (EBA) and linear immunoglobulin A (IgA) disease.

Epidemiology
Incidence and prevalence
Genital involvement is common in BP and MMP, where 50% of adults with these conditions will have vulval involvement [1]. In those with linear IgA disease, 50% of adults and 80% of children will have vulval lesions.

Clinical features
Presentation
See Table 110.3 for the clinical presentations of immunobullous diseases on the vulva.

Differential diagnosis
Erosive lichen planus and lichen sclerosus can show similar scarring to MMP. It is also important to exclude herpes simplex in the early stages.

Complications and co-morbidities
Scarring of the vulva and vagina can occur in MMP.

Investigations
Investigations are the same as for autoimmune bullous disease on extragenital skin.

Management
Topical steroids and potassium permanganate soaks for open, eroded areas are helpful, but most patients will require systemic therapy as for diseases at other sites.

PIGMENTARY DISORDERS

Vitiligo

Introduction and general description
This is an acquired disorder characterised by loss of pigmentation in the skin and hair (Chapter 86).

Clinical features
History
Asymptomatic areas of hypopigmentation are noticed.

Presentation
There is complete depigmentation of the skin, which is otherwise normal. The edge is well defined and the outer labia majora are usually affected. There may be extension into the inguinal folds and perianal skin (Figure 110.22). In hair-bearing skin, the hair may also lose its colour (poliosis).

Table 110.3 Clinical presentation of immunobullous disease on the vulva.

	Bullous pemphigoid	Mucous membrane pemphigoid	Pemphigus vulgaris	Linear IgA	Epidermolysis bullosa acquisita
Age	Elderly; a localised form is described in children but is rare [2]	Adults; uncommon in children	Usually middle-aged	Children and adults	Rare; adults and children
Clinical features	Tense fluid-filled bullae	Vaginal lesions common with scarring	Flaccid bullae, painful erosions Vaginal disease can cause a discharge [3]	Tense bullae, may be clustered in children	Tense bullae

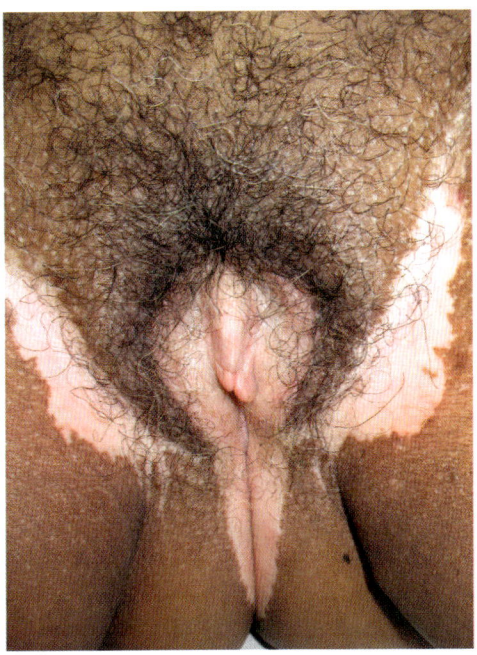

Figure 110.22 Vulval vitiligo with extension into the inguinal folds.

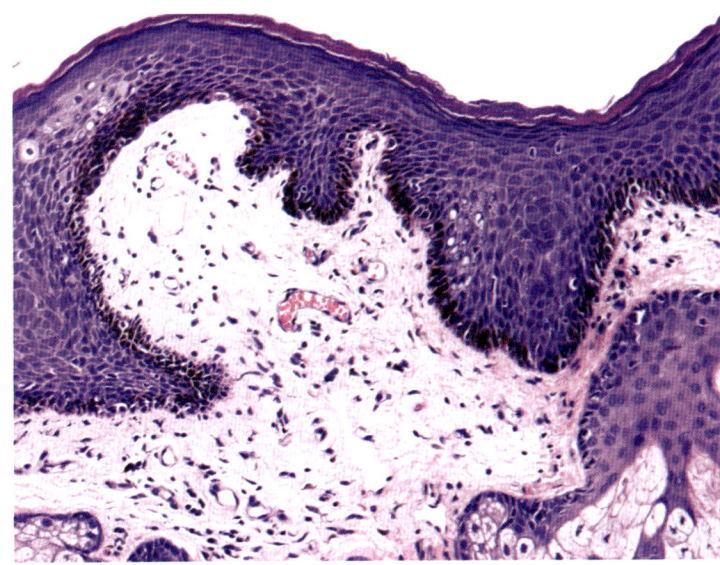

Figure 110.23 Histological features of vulval melanosis.

Differential diagnosis

The major differential diagnosis is lichen sclerosus but there is no architectural change in vitiligo and the texture of the skin is normal. The pallor sometimes seen in lichenification can also mimic vitiligo.

Complications and co-morbidities

Vitiligo and lichen sclerosus can coexist.

Management

No treatment is needed and treatment modalities used at other sites (e.g. psoralen and ultraviolet A (PUVA)) are inappropriate on the genital skin.

Vulval melanosis

Definition and nomenclature

Vulval melanosis is characterised by hyperpigmented lesions in the absence of any previous cause. There is no increase in melanocytes [1,2].

Synonyms and inclusions
• Idiopathic lenticular mucocutaneous pigmentation

Epidemiology
Age
Vulval melanosis is seen more commonly in young women.

Pathophysiology
Pathology
There is basal cell layer hyperpigmentation but no increase in the number of melanocytes. Pigmentary incontinence and pigment-rich macrophages may be seen in the dermis (Figure 110.23).

Clinical features
History
Melanosis is asymptomatic and usually an incidental finding.

Presentation
The lesions are usually multifocal (a single lesion would be termed a genital melanotic macule) and often irregular and asymmetrical. The colour may vary. They are most common on the inner labia

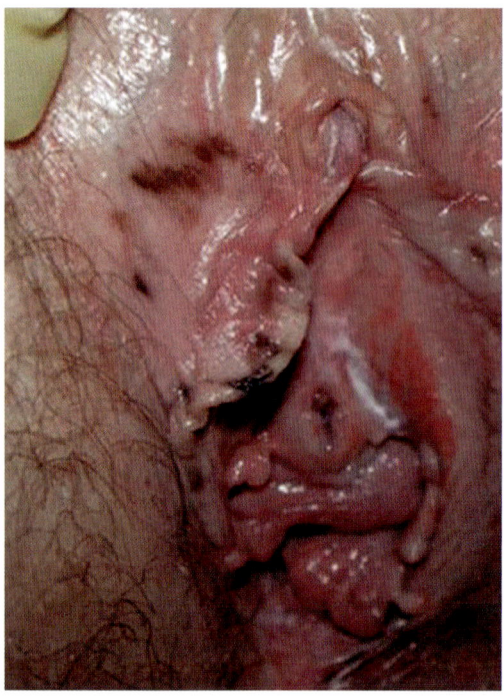

(a)

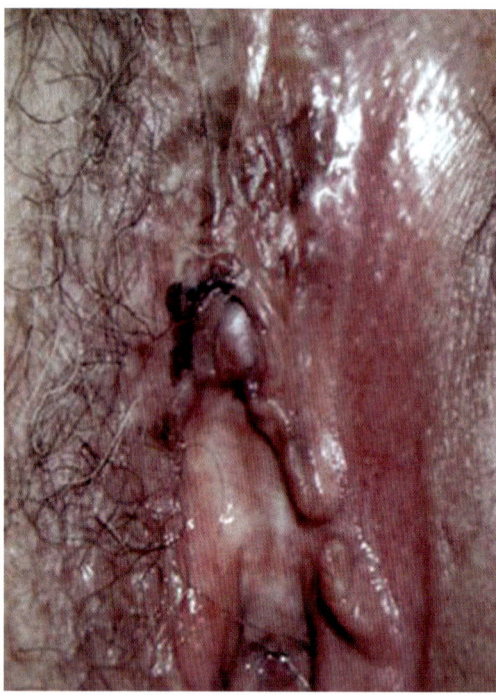

(b)

Figure 110.24 (a) *In situ* melanoma. (b) Vulval melanosis. Clinical appearances are almost indistinguishable and pigmented vulval areas such as this require biopsy for diagnosis.

minora and vestibule but the vagina and cervix may also be involved [3,4]. There may be similar lesions on the oral mucosa.

Differential diagnosis

The main differential diagnosis is from genital lentigines, but this term is used when there are increased numbers of melanocytes. The clinical appearance can mimic melanoma (Figure 110.24) and hence biopsy is always recommended. Melanosis is often darker than postinflammatory hyperpigmentation.

Disease course and prognosis

Melanoma has not been reported in vulva melanosis and the accepted view is that vulval melanosis is a benign condition, but there are no long-term follow-up studies.

Investigations

Dermoscopy can be helpful but if there is any uncertainty then the diagnosis is easily confirmed on vulval biopsy.

Management

There are no guidelines on follow-up but simple observation by the patient using photographs or diagrams as an aid is usually sufficient.

Acanthosis nigricans

Definition

Acanthosis nigricans is characterised by hyperpigmentation and thickening of the skin, particularly in the flexures.

Epidemiology

Associated diseases

Acanthosis nigricans is associated with insulin resistance in almost all cases. In adults, it can be a cutaneous sign of an underlying malignancy, usually an adenocarcinoma. If linked with malignancy, the onset and progression are rapid and unusual sites such as the eyelids, lips and palms (tripe palms) may be involved.

Clinical features

Presentation

The genital area is almost always involved [1] and velvety, dark plaques are seen on the labia majora, extending into the inguinal folds. These then develop a warty texture and skin tags are common on the plaques.

Differential diagnosis

Pseudoacanthosis nigricans may be seen in obese patients and is related to moisture, friction and subsequent maceration. Epidermal naevi may have similar clinical and histological features but are unlikely to occur at several sites.

Investigations

The diagnosis can be made clinically and confirmed on biopsy. A fasting blood glucose is indicated to check for type 2 diabetes. Referral for endocrine investigation is important to investigate insulin resistance. If there is a rapid onset or unusual features in an adult, then a potential associated malignancy should be sought.

Management

Keratolytics, retinoids and laser treatment have all been tried. These may be irritant in the genital skin.

Dowling–Degos disease

Definition and nomenclature

This condition is characterised by reticulate pigmentation in the flexures.

Synonyms and inclusions
- Reticulated pigmented anomaly of the flexures

Epidemiology
Age

Lesions typically appear in the third or fourth decade of life.

Pathophysiology
Pathology

Irregular elongation of the rete ridges is seen with melanin at the tips. The number of melanocytes is not increased.

Genetics

It is probably inherited in an autosomal dominant pattern with loss of function in the keratin 5 gene [1].

Clinical features
History

Dowling–Degos disease is asymptomatic.

Presentation

Reticulate pigmentation is seen on the vulva, which may be involved in isolation rarely [2] or as part of more widespread disease [3].

Clinical variants

Galli–Galli disease has acantholysis as a feature.

Differential diagnosis

Simple lentigines and the postinflammatory pigmentation seen with lichen planus have similar clinical features. Multiple genital lentigines are occasionally features of Laugier–Hunziker disease, Carney complex or LAMB syndrome (lentigines, atrial myxomas, mucocutaneous myxomas and blue naevi).

Investigations

A skin biopsy will show typical histological features.

Management

Depigmenting agents, adapalene and laser treatment have been reported to be successful in individual cases [4].

VULVAL OEDEMA

The causes of vulval oedema are generally classified into acute and chronic (Table 110.4) and most cases are due to leakage through the capillaries. The skin of the vulva is lax and fluid easily accumulates.

Table 110.4 Causes of vulval oedema.

Acute causes	Chronic causes
Inflammatory dermatoses, e.g. acute eczema	Primary lymphoedema secondary to congenital lymphatic hypoplasia
Infections, e.g. candidiasis	Crohn disease
Urticaria – pressure urticaria after intercourse	Hidradenitis suppurativa
Type 1 allergy (see allergic contact urticaria)	Infections, e.g. filariasis
Ovarian hyperstimulation syndrome	Lymphangioma – lymphangioma circumscriptum [1] and cavernous lymphangioma [2]
Pre-eclampsia	Malignancy
	Post-radiotherapy or lymphadenectomy
	Cyclist's vulva [3,4]

Crohn disease

Definition

Crohn disease is an inflammatory disease of the gastrointestinal tract.

Introduction and general description

Vulval disease may present many years before intestinal involvement, and in some cases there is vulval oedema only, with no other features of inflammation [1–3].

Epidemiology
Incidence and prevalence

Ano-genital lesions may occur in about 30% of patients with gastrointestinal Crohn disease. This may either be by direct extension or by so-called 'metastatic' disease. However, it can occur in patients without any bowel involvement and the cutaneous lesions may precede it.

Age

The average age of presentation is in the fourth decade but it has been reported in children [4].

Associated diseases

Crohn disease may be associated with pyoderma gangrenosum, erythema nodosum and a leukocytoclastic vasculitis.

Pathophysiology
Pathology

Initially, only dermal oedema and lymphangiectasia may be seen. Non-caseating granulomas occur later with features of ulceration in more severe disease. Granulomatous histology is seen in about 80% of cases so absence does not exclude the diagnosis.

Clinical features
History

The patient may simply complain of vulval oedema initially but soreness, pain and discharge occur in more severe disease.

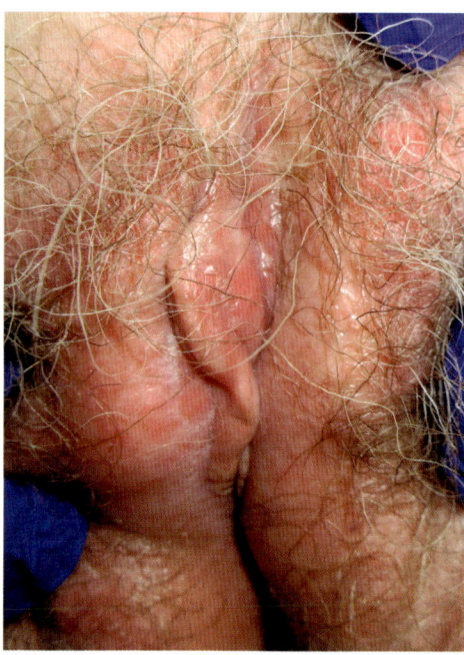

Figure 110.25 Vulval Crohn disease with swelling, erosion and early fissuring.

Presentation
Oedema may be the initial finding, which may be unilateral and generally affects the labia majora first [5]. Ulceration, erosions, abscesses, sinuses and fistulae can form and the classic feature is that of deep linear fissures (knife cut sign) along the skin creases (Figure 110.25). This is common in the gluteal cleft but can also occur in the abdominal folds.

Clinical variants
A separate form of vulval granuloma akin to the oro-facial lesions seen in Melkersson–Rosenthal syndrome has been described [6,7]. The term 'ano-genital granulomatosis' is sometimes used when there are granulomatous skin changes but no evidence of gastrointestinal Crohn disease [8,9]. However, most of these cases are likely to be related to Crohn disease that may present later.

Differential diagnosis
Hidradenitis suppurativa is the main differential diagnosis and there are some patients with features of both conditions.

Complications and co-morbidities
Bowen disease has been reported to occur in Crohn disease [10] and rarely squamous cell carcinoma [11].

Disease course and prognosis
The disease follows a chronic course with secondary infection being a common feature. The oedema may become firm and fixed and is the most challenging feature to influence with treatment.

Investigations
A biopsy may be helpful, but may show only oedema.

Management
If genital Crohn disease is the presenting problem it is important to involve a gastroenterologist in management as these patients need a full work-up to assess if there is intestinal disease as well.

First line
In patients who have no systemic disease, topical measures may be sufficient to control the cutaneous lesions in mild cases, that is the use of a super-potent topical steroid or topical tacrolimus [12]. An oral tetracycline or metronidazole can also be helpful [13].

Second line
In ulcerative disease it is essential to exclude any fistulous tracts with magnetic resonance imaging (MRI) scans, especially if anti-tumour necrosis factor (anti-TNF) agents are being considered. More severe disease may respond to oral steroids but recalcitrant ulcerative ano-genital lesions and fistulous tracts may require systemic immunosuppressants and/or biologic agents [13,14]. The cutaneous involvement can be more resistant to treatment than the gastrointestinal involvement [13,15].

NON-SEXUALLY TRANSMITTED INFECTIONS

The majority of infections in the ano-genital area are sexually acquired and these are dealt with elsewhere. Non-sexually acquired routes of infection include transfer by touch, fomites or contact with contaminated water. Threadworms and *Candida* species may spread from the anus.

DIAGNOSIS OF VAGINAL DISCHARGE

The diagnosis usually falls into one of the categories seen in Table 110.5. If an infective cause is suspected, the patient should

Table 110.5 Causes of vaginal discharge.

Cause	Example	Clinical features
Physiological	Excess physiological secretion of mucus, usually resulting from cervical erosion or an increase in the amount of vaginal transudate	The discharge is thick, with a grey-white appearance, and is odourless and non-irritant. Vaginal pH is normal
Iatrogenic	Tamoxifen, oral contraceptive pills, danthron [1]	
Infective	Bacterial vaginosis	pH usually >6. Grey, watery discharge with fishy odour
	Infective cervicitis (gonorrhoea, *Chlamydia*, herpes simplex, trichomonas)	Associated with deep pelvic pain
	Threadworms [2]	
Inflammatory	Erosive lichen planus, pemphigus	Chronic odourless discharge, which may be blood-tinged. Postcoital bleeding may occur
Neoplastic	Tumours of the fallopian tubes, uterus, cervix and vagina	

be referred to a genito-urinary clinic for full evaluation and management.

Resources

Patient resources

International Society for the Study of Vulvovaginal Disease information sheet: https://www.issvd.org/resources/vaginal-discharge (last accessed April 2022).

BACTERIAL INFECTIONS

Staphylococcal infections

Introduction and general description

Staphylococcus aureus is usually the causative agent in infective folliculitis, boils and abscesses of the vulva (Chapter 26). Panton–Valentine leukocidin *S. aureus infection* [1] can cause infection in the ano-genital skin.

Epidemiology
Associated diseases

Staphylococcal infection is often associated with diabetes and immunosuppression.

Pathophysiology
Predisposing factors

Shaving and waxing to remove hair can predispose to folliculitis.

Pathology

The impetiginous lesion shows subcorneal pustules filled with neutrophils and some spongiosis, with a moderate inflammatory response in the papillary dermis. Acute folliculitis may be superficial, with a subcorneal pustule present at the follicular opening, or be deep and associated with a perifollicular abscess and destruction of the follicle wall and sebaceous gland. Chronic deep intrafollicular abscesses may have the additional features of fibrosis and foreign body giant cells.

Causative organisms

Staphylococcus aureus is the most common bacteria causing folliculitis and furunculosis.

Clinical features
Clinical variants

A staphylococcal folliculitis on the buttocks may occur secondary to the pruritus induced by intestinal infestation with pinworm.

Menstrual toxic shock syndrome is caused by *S. aureus* superantigenic toxins and is associated with fever, hypotension and macular erythema. In the 1980s, retained tampons were a common focus of infection but this is now rare.

Staphylococcal scalded skin syndrome is a toxin-mediated infection and the flexural areas may often be the first to be involved.

An abscess of the Bartholin gland caused by acute infection of the duct may be caused by *S. aureus*.

Differential diagnosis

Pseudofolliculitis is a sterile folliculitis that may follow shaving or waxing and is caused by the newly regrowing hairs inducing an inflammatory reaction. It is a foreign body reaction and results in changes from mild inflammation to the formation of abscesses and sinuses.

Investigations

Microscopy and culture of lesional swabs will confirm the diagnosis. If recurrent, exclude staphylococcal carriage at other body sites.

Management

Topical antibiotics may be sufficient for mild folliculitis with antibacterial washes. Oral or intravenous antibiotics are required for more severe or widespread infection.

Streptococcal infections

Introduction and general description

Group B haemolytic streptococcal species are commonly found as commensals in the vulva and vagina, and do not cause symptoms [1]. However, if the patient is pregnant, this must be treated to prevent infection in the neonate. Group A species can cause cellulitis and more severe infections such as necrotising fasciitis (Chapter 26). These organisms may also cause secondary infection in patients with psoriasis [2].

Pathophysiology
Causative organisms

Streptococcus pyogenes and other β-haemolytic Lancefield group A bacteria are the usual cause of vulval cellulitis. *Streptococcus faecalis* may cause Bartholin abscesses.

Clinical features
Clinical variants

- *Vulval cellulitis*. The redness and oedema may be extreme, and vesicles and bullae may develop. There are usually associated systemic features. The infection arises at sites of trauma and is most commonly seen following a vulvectomy with lymphadenectomy. If there is residual lymphoedema then further attacks of cellulitis are more common.
- *Streptococcal dermatitis*. This usually affects the ano-genital area of children.
- Necrotising fasciitis (synergistic bacterial gangrene). This severe, rapidly extending and life-threatening disease is caused by the synergistic effect of a microaerophilic *Streptococcus* and *Staphylococcus aureus*. Anaerobes and Gram-negative bacilli may also be involved.

Differential diagnosis

It is important to distinguish more severe infection from pyoderma gangrenosum, as the management is completely different for these conditions and high-dose steroids would be required for pyoderma gangrenosum.

PART 10: SPECIFIC SITES, SEX & AGE

Investigations

Microscopy and culture of the lesion confirm the diagnosis. In severe infection, blood cultures may be positive.

Management

Appropriate antibiotic therapy and supportive care are needed in severe infections. Immediate surgical debridement is needed in necrotising fasciitis.

Mycobacterial infections

Synonyms and inclusions
- Genital tuberculosis
- Leprosy

Introduction and general description

Tuberculosis of the female genital tract is common in endemic areas (Chapter 27). Vulval lesions are rare and the upper genital tract is most commonly affected [1].

Pathophysiology

Predisposing factors

Genital tuberculosis is more common in HIV-positive patients and has been reported in a renal transplant patient [2].

Causative organisms

Mycobacterium tuberculosis is the cause of tuberculosis and occurs by haematogenous spread from foci outside the genital tract, by distal spread from the upper genital tract or as a primary exogenous infection contracted from sputum or sexual intercourse.

Mycobacterium leprae causes leprosy.

Clinical features

Presentation

In a primary infection the initial lesion may be inconspicuous, the main feature being a caseating lymphadenopathy. In other cases the lesions are masses or nodules that may ulcerate and lead to lymphoedema. The Bartholin gland may be involved.

Vulval lesions are rare in leprosy [3] and may present with loss of pubic hair.

Investigations

Investigation is similar to that at other sites.

Management

Management of both tuberculosis and leprosy requires specialist input from infectious disease specialists.

Malakoplakia

Introduction and general description

Malakoplakia is a rare inflammatory lesion that usually occurs in the urinary bladder. There are reports of it affecting skin sites and the tongue. It results from an atypical inflammatory response to *Escherichia coli* or other pathogens.

Epidemiology

Associated diseases

There is often underlying immunosuppression, the aetiology of which may include malignancy, dermatomyositis [1], lupus erythematosus, rheumatoid arthritis and organ transplantation [2].

Pathophysiology

Predisposing factors

Malakoplakia is due to macrophage dysfunction, and primary or acquired immunodeficiency is common [3].

Pathology

There are confluent sheets of histiocytes with eosinophilic granular cytoplasm and small eccentric nuclei. Round, sometimes laminated, structures are found with these cells and are known as Michaelis–Gutmann bodies. The histiocytic infiltrate may be mixed with neutrophils, lymphocytes and plasma cells, with associated granulation tissue. Electron microscopy of malakoplakia shows that the histiocytes contain numerous phagolysosomes within which there may be occasional intact and partly digested bacteria.

Causative organisms

It is not usually caused by one specific agent but the organisms involved include *E. coli*, *Pseudomonas* and *Staphylococcus aureus*.

Clinical features

Presentation

Malakoplakia most often affects the urinary or gastrointestinal tract but cutaneous lesions may occur on the vagina, vulva and perineum [4]. Involvement of Bartholin gland has been described [5]. The lesions are non-specific and include persistent pink/red plaques, ulcers, nodules and sinuses with pin-point bleeding. They are often multiple.

Differential diagnosis

Crohn disease, hidradenitis suppurativa and malignancy may have similar features.

Investigations

A culture of lesions and histology will confirm the diagnosis.

Management

Long-term antibiotics are needed and surgery may be required if sinuses are present.

Other bacterial infections

Synonyms and inclusions
- Actinomycosis
- *Mycoplasma* infection

Introduction and general description

Some other bacteria will cause genital infections, primarily actinomycosis species and *Mycoplasma* organisms.

Pathophysiology
Predisposing factors

Genital infection usually arises from bowel disease [1], but isolated lesions of the vulva have been reported.

Causative organisms

The Gram-positive acid-fast organisms responsible for actinomycosis are predominantly *Actinomyces israelii* and *A. gerencseriae*.

Mycoplasma hominis and *Ureaplasma urealyticum* are found in the vagina and rarely cause vulval disease.

Clinical features
Presentation

Actinomycosis organisms may colonise intrauterine devices and are usually asymptomatic, but invasion of the genital tract can occur [2,3].

Investigations

Cultures of lesional skin and histology are needed.

Management

Penicillin is the treatment of choice, and treatment may need to be prolonged. Tetracyclines, clindamycin and erythromycin are alternative agents.

FUNGAL INFECTIONS

Candidal vulvo-vaginitis

Synonyms and inclusions
- Thrush infection
- Yeast infection

Introduction and general description

Candida albicans causes vulvo-vaginitis and 75% of women will experience at least one episode (Chapter 32).

Epidemiology
Incidence and prevalence

Vulvo-vaginal candidiasis is the second most common genital infection (bacterial vaginosis being the commonest) in the western world [1].

Age

It is rare before menarche as the vaginal microbiota are different and the number of lactobacilli are reduced. It is most prevalent in the third and fourth decades.

Pathophysiology
Predisposing factors

Pregnancy, diabetes, possibly oral antibiotics, high-dose oestrogen oral contraceptive pills and immunosuppression may all be predisposing factors.

Causative organisms

Candida and *Torulopsis* are both yeasts that can infect the vulva and vagina. *Torulopsis* accounts for very few infections, whereas *Candida albicans* is the most frequently isolated and accounts for 90% of symptomatic episodes. It is a non-pathogenic commensal in the gastrointestinal tract in 30% of the normal population.

Changes in host factors and cell-mediated immunity are important in the transition to pathogenicity.

Clinical features
History

The major symptom is pruritus. Some patients may report vulval swelling.

Presentation

The primary infection arises in the vagina, causing inflammation and a heavy, white, curdy discharge, which then leads to a secondary vulvitis with well-demarcated sheets of erythema on the outer aspects of the vulva, sometimes extending on occasions into the genito-crural folds and perianally. There may be a scaly or vesiculopustular edge. Beyond this edge lie grouped or isolated superficial small pustules, which rupture rapidly, leaving a slightly scaly periphery.

Differential diagnosis

Eczema and flexural psoriasis may have similar appearances.

Complications and co-morbidities

In some cases of vulval eczema and psoriasis, *Candida* is cultured from skin swabs but the candidal overgrowth is a secondary problem arising on a background of an inflamed epithelium. Treating the dermatosis alone with a topical steroid will usually resolve the problem, without the addition of anticandidal agents.

Investigations

The diagnosis is confirmed by direct microscopy and culture. In resistant and recurrent infection, swabs for species and sensitivities are indicated.

Management

Treatment of vulvo-vaginal candidiasis requires vaginal pessaries or creams and/or oral imidazoles. In those patients with recurrent infection, that is, four or more proven infections in one year, it is always important to consider diabetes. In those with recalcitrant symptoms, referral to a genito-urinary physician is helpful as species and sensitivities may need to be known if they require alternative treatment regimens.

Resources

Further information

British Association for Sexual Health and HIV guidelines on the management of vulvo-vaginal candidiasis 2019: https://www.bashhguidelines.org/media/1249/vvc-ijsa-pdf.pdf.

Patient resources

International Society for the Study of Vulvovaginal Disease information sheet: https://www.issvd.org/resources/candidiasisyeast-infection.
(Both last accessed April 2022.)

Tinea cruris

Introduction and general description

Tinea cruris is a dermatophyte infection affecting the inguinal folds, which may extend to the vulva and perianal area (Chapter 32).

Epidemiology

Sex

Fungal infection in the genital area is more common in men.

Pathophysiology

Predisposing factors

Heat, occlusion and humidity predispose to this infection.

Causative organisms

The causative agents are *Trichophyton rubrum* and *Epidermophyton floccosum*.

Clinical features

History

The rash is usually itchy.

Presentation

The lesions are red and scaly, with a spreading serpiginous edge (Figure 110.26). Folliculitis is also seen, particularly in the perianal

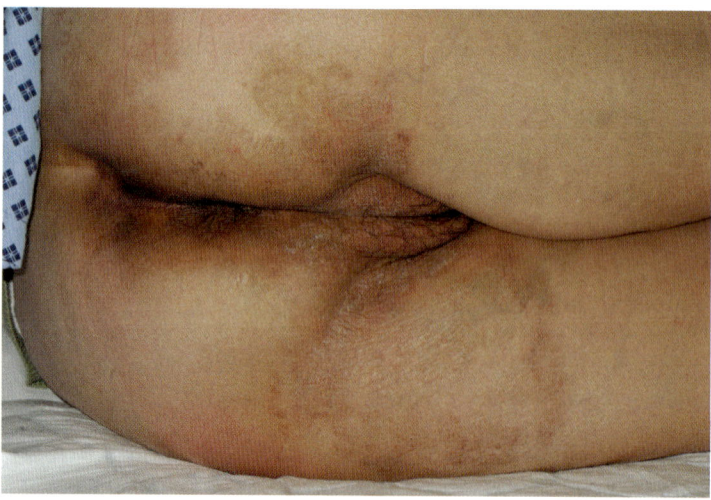

Figure 110.26 Tinea incognito, extension to the perianal area and thighs.

area. Tinea incognito may also occur perianally following the inappropriate use of a topical steroid in the presence of an unrecognised dermatophyte infection.

Differential diagnosis

Flexural psoriasis, eczema, erythrasma and candidiasis are the major differential diagnoses.

Pityriasis versicolor classically occurs on the trunk, but in severe widespread infection there may be vulval involvement [1,2].

Complications and co-morbidities

Deep fungal infections are rare but have been reported with *Microsporum canis* infection [3] and a kerion will usually affect the mons pubis [4]. Vulval phycomycosis has been described [5]. Subcutaneous infections occur in children and young adults. Histologically, the epidermis is unremarkable, but subcutaneously there are deep granulomatous masses containing hyphae. There is one case report of chromomycosis (chromoblastomycosis) affecting the vulva [6]. *Cryptococcus neoformans* can induce painless ulceration of the vulva in the immunosuppressed patient [7].

Investigations

The diagnosis is usually made by direct microscopy and the culture of skin scrapings.

Management

> **Treatment ladder for tinea cruris**
>
> **First line**
> - Topical azoles if non-hair-bearing skin
>
> **Second line**
> - Oral terbinafine 250 mg/day for 4 weeks or itraconazole 200 mg BD for 2 weeks

VIRAL INFECTIONS

Three groups of viruses are important causes of infection in the genital area: the poxviruses, papillomaviruses and herpesviruses (Chapter 25). Other viruses seldom give rise to distinctive clinical pictures, although vulval lesions may occur as part of a generalised viral infection.

Poxvirus infections

Synonyms and inclusions
- Molluscum contagiosum
- Orf
- Cowpox

Introduction and general description

The most common poxvirus infection of the vulva is molluscum contagiosum but isolated reports of orf [1] and cowpox [2] infection exist (Chapter 25).

Epidemiology
Age
Molluscum infection can occur in adults and children.

Pathophysiology
Predisposing factors
Atopic eczema, immunodeficiency, HIV infection and Darier disease can all predispose to mollusum contagiosum.

Causative organisms
Molluscum contagiosum virus (MCV) has four subtypes. MCV I usually causes childhood infection, whereas MCV II is a common cause in adults and is the major type seen in HIV-positive individuals.

Clinical features
Presentation
Lesions are often found on the mons pubis and labia majora, and the typical lesions are small, pearly papules with an umbilicated centre. Lesions of molluscum contagiosum can be profuse and large in immunosuppressed women.

Clinical variants
Giant molluscum lesions may occur and these can be mistaken for large genital warts.

Differential diagnosis
They may resemble genital warts and other infections and, if inflamed, mimic folliculitis.

Complications and co-morbidities
Adults with gential molluscum should be offered screening for other sexually transmitted infections.

Disease course and prognosis
The lesions regress spontaneously but may take many months to do so.

Investigations
The diagnosis is usually made clinically. If there is any doubt, then a biopsy will show characteristic cytoplasmic inclusions (molluscum bodies). The inflammatory response can vary from total absence to an intense lymphohistiocytic dermal inflammation.

Management
No treatment is needed as lesions will resolve. However, podophyllotoxin [3] and imiquimod [4] have shown cure rates of over 90% in controlled trials. Cryotherapy, curettage and extirpation of the core are other treatments used.

Resources

Further information
British Association for Sexual Health and HIV guidelines on the management of molluscum contagiosum: https://www.bashhguidelines.org/media/1055/mc_2014-ijstda.pdf (last accessed April 2022).

Herpes simplex virus infections

Epidemiology
Incidence and prevalence
Sexual transmission is responsible for 95% of herpes simplex virus (HSV) infections. The remainder are cases of autoinoculation or non-sexual contact (Chapter 25).

Pathophysiology
Causative organisms
Once this sexually transmitted DNA virus is acquired it lies dormant in the dorsal root ganglia and can give rise to recurrent symptomatic lesions. It exists in two types: I and II. Type I usually affects non-genital sites and type II is responsible for 50–80% of genital infections.

Clinical features
History
There may be prodromal symptoms of tingling or tender, enlarged inguinal nodes. Paraesthesiae may occur, affecting S2–S4, which may lead to urinary retention. Pain and oedema may also lead to retention, particularly in primary infections.

Presentation
The lesions are typically painful vesicles or ulcers, which are often multiple in primary infection but are fewer and usually localised to one side with recurrences. Cervical ulceration may be seen.

Clinical variants
Hypertrophic HSV infection in immunosuppressed patients can mimic tumours [1].

Differential diagnosis
Varicella-zoster virus may also affect the vulva if the third sacral dermatome is involved. It may be accompanied by bowel and bladder dysfunction [2].

Cytomegalovirus infection can sometimes resemble herpes simplex. This has been reported in an infant with congenital HIV disease who presented with pustular and ulcerative lesions on the perineum [3].

Complications and co-morbidities
Herpes simplex virus infection is an important co-factor in the transmission of HIV. Autonomic dysfunction can lead to constipation and hyperaesthesia of the perineal and sacral region. Aseptic meningitis is reported in up to 36% of women [4].

PART 10: SPECIFIC SITES, SEX & AGE

Investigations

It is important to obtain a definite diagnosis with a positive culture of HSV, and it is necessary to perform the test as soon as the blisters arise as the virus is harder to culture from older lesions. Polymerase chain reaction (PCR) techniques are increasingly used in diagnosis [5].

Patients should also be screened for other sexually transmitted infections.

Management

The treatment is either oral aciclovir 200 mg five times daily for 5 days, valaciclovir 500 mg twice daily for 5 days or famciclovir 250 mg three times daily for 5 days. Suppressant therapy is sometimes required for patients with frequent recurrences (six or more in a year). It is especially important to manage HSV infection in pregnancy and there are obstetric guidelines for this.

Resources

Further information

British Association for Sexual Health and HIV guidelines on the management of ano-genital herpes: https://www.bashhguidelines.org/media/1019/hsv_2014-ijstda.pdf.

British Association for Sexual Health and HIV guidelines on the management of genital herpes in pregnancy: https://www.bashhguidelines.org/media/1060/management-genital-herpes.pdf.

Patient resources

International Society for the Study of Vulvovaginal Disease information sheet: https://www.issvd.org/resources/genital-herpes.

(All last accessed April 2022.)

Human papillomavirus infections

Introduction and general description

Human papillomavirus is a small DNA virus, and the types that most commonly infect the vulval skin are HPV-6, -11, -16 and -18 (Chapter 25).

Epidemiology

Incidence and prevalence

Human papillomavirus is the commonest sexually transmitted infection and up to 85% of people will be infected with at least one type in their lifetime.

Age

Warts are more common in the younger age groups after sexual activity starts. If seen in children, this must always raise the possibility of sexual abuse [1].

Associated diseases

Immunosuppressed patients often have more florid infection with lesions that are difficult to treat. They are also at greater risk of developing HPV-related ano-genital cancers.

Pathophysiology

Predisposing factors

There is an increased risk of acquiring genital warts with a higher number of sexual partners, the presence of other sexually transmitted infections and a history of smoking.

Pathology

The histology of genital warts is characterised by the koilocyte, a vacuolated squamous cell with a basophilic and pyknotic nucleus in the upper part of the epidermis. It is important not to confuse it with the heavily glycogenated clear cells of vestibular epithelium. Other histological features are elongated dermal papillae, acanthosis, a prominent granular layer often containing koilocytes, and a stratum corneum of variable thickness.

Clinical features

Presentation

The warty lesions are known as condylomata acuminate (Figure 110.27). Extensive vegetating masses can cover the vulva and perianal area, particularly in diabetes, pregnancy and immunocompromised patients.

Differential diagnosis

Secondary syphilis may also present with extensive papulosquamous lesions.

Complications and co-morbidities

Human papillomavirus types 16, 18 and sometimes 33 are associated with ano-genital intraepithelial neoplasia and SCC.

Disease course and prognosis

Warts may resolve spontaneously, but may persist and be resistant especially in the immunosuppressed.

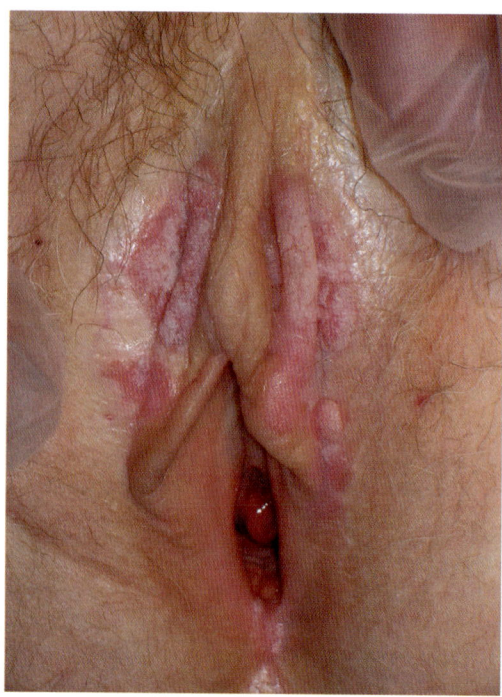

Figure 110.27 Vulval warts with plaques in the interlabial sulci.

Investigations

The diagnosis is usually clinical, but if there are atypical features it is important to exclude vulval intraepithelial neoplasia with histological examination. Patients with genital warts should also be screened for other sexually transmitted infections.

Management

The treatment of genital warts is usually undertaken in the setting of a genito-urinary clinic. Podophyllotoxin, cryotherapy, topical imiquimod and destructive treatments are used [2]. Imiquimod has to be used with care as it induces an inflammatory response in patients who have latent or active dermatitis. It should be used with extreme care in any patient with any inflammatory vulval dermatosis or vulval aphthous ulcers, as these can flare significantly.

In pregnancy, only cryotherapy or destructive techniques with cautery or hyfrecation can be used safely.

Prophylactic vaccination prior to exposure is now available for HPV types 6, 11, 16 and 18 and has been shown to reduce the incidence of warts and genital intraepithelial neoplasia [3,4].

Resources

Further information

British Association for Sexual Health and HIV guidelines on the management of ano-genital warts: https://www.bashhguidelines.org/media/1075/uk-national-guideline-on-warts-2015-final.pdf (last accessed April 2022).

BENIGN TUMOURS

The main benign tumours are discussed in this section, with Table 110.6 giving details of some others [1,2,3,4]. Nodular fasciitis [5] and glomus tumours [6,7] are rarely reported.

Mucinous cysts

Introduction and general description

Mucinous cysts occur at the site if there is obstruction of the duct of a minor vestibular gland.

Epidemiology

Age

These occur in adult women and rarely in adolescence.

Pathophysiology

The cysts are of uro-genital sinus origin and not, as was once thought, of Müllerian origin [1,2].

Pathology

The cysts are lined by a layer of mucinous epithelium.

Clinical features

Presentation

The lesions present as single or multiple lesions in the vestibule.

Management

Simple excision is curative.

Bartholin cyst

Introduction and general description

Bartholin cysts are common and arise as a result of obstruction of the main duct of the Bartholin gland.

Epidemiology

Age

These are most common in women of child-bearing age.

Pathophysiology

Pathology

The cyst is lined with transitional epithelium which may exhibit squamous metaplasia.

Clinical features

History

Simple cysts are asymptomatic and the patient may simply notice a lump.

Presentation

The lesions present as swellings 1–3 cm in size on the lower third of the inner labium majus.

Differential diagnosis

Benign or malignant tumours can present in a similar way.

Complications and co-morbidities

If the cysts become infected, then this abscess leads to painful swelling. There is a case report of an SCC arising within a cyst [1].

Management

The treatment is enucleation of the cyst but if incompletely removed they can recur. Several methods are used to treat these cysts but there is no evidence base to recommend one method over another [2].

Papillary hidradenoma

Definition and nomenclature

This sweat gland adenoma with apocrine differentiation occurs almost exclusively in the ano-genital region of middle-aged white women [1].

Synonyms and inclusions
• Hidradenoma papilliferum

Table 110.6 Other benign tumours of the vulva.

	Fibroma	Fibroepithelial polyps	Epidermal cyst	Lipomas	Verruciform xanthoma [1]	Granular cell myoblastoma [2,3]	Urethral caruncle	Neurofibroma	Leiomyoma	Syringoma [4]
Origin	Deeper connective tissue structures, e.g. introitus, perineal body		Epithelial implants after surgery or at fusion sites during embryogenesis	Fatty tissue of labia majora			Inflamed eversion of urethral mucosa	Solitary or part of generalised neurofibromatosis	Smooth muscle of erectile tissue, round ligament or myoepithelial cells of the Bartholin duct. Not associated with uterine lesions	Adenoma of eccrine sweat glands
Sites	Labia majora		Labia majora		Labia majora usually		Urethral meatus	Labia majora	Labia, clitoris	Labia majora
Clinical features	Penduculated	Soft polypoidal nodules	Single or multiple		Solitary plaque or warty lesion	Flesh coloured, sometimes pedunculated or ulcerated solitary lesion		Painless nodules, can mimic intersex problems	Painless nodules. Can enlarge during pregnancy	Multiple, may be pruritic
Pathology	Fibrovascular core covered by epithelium. Cellular atypia occasionally seen				Acanthosis, papillomatosis and foamy macrophages in papillary dermis		Vascular connective tissue with glandular structures or islands of urethral mucosa in inflamed stroma			Small ducts with comma-like tails

Epidemiology
Age
These occur in middle-aged women.

Pathophysiology
Pathology
A well-demarcated nodule is seen that is composed of papillary processes that extend into cystic spaces. Periodic acid–Schiff (PAS) stain-positive cytoplasmic granules are common.

Clinical features
History
The lesions are often asymptomatic but may be painful.

Presentation
The lesions are 1–2 cm nodules and occur most commonly on the labia majora, interlabial sulcus, lateral surfaces of the labia minora or perineal region [2]. Although usually single, there are occasionally multiple lesions. Curiously, when they are multiple, all the lesions tend to develop on one side of the vulva. In most patients, the covering epidermis remains intact, but in a proportion the elevated epithelium may become ulcerated. Larger lesions are described [3]. They are rarely described on the nipple, eyelid and external auditory meatus.

Complications and co-morbidities
Malignant change within a papillary hidradenoma has been reported, producing apocrine carcinoma [4] and adenosquamous carcinoma [5].

Management
Simple excision is curative.

Cutaneous endometriosis

Introduction and general description
Endometrial deposits on the vulva are rare [1].

Pathophysiology
Pathology
Endometrial glands and stroma are seen.

Clinical features
History
The lesions may be painful and patients may report a variation in size with the menstrual cycle. They may bleed at the same time as menstruation.

Presentation
The lesions present as small, bluish nodules and common sites are the perineum or episiotomy scars and the umbilicus.

Management
Surgical excision is usually curative.

Atypical genital naevi

Synonyms and inclusions
- Atypical melanocytic naevi of genital type

Introduction and general description
All types of naevi can occur on the genital skin but they may show atypical and concerning features, and it is important to be aware of the entity to avoid aggressive treatment (Chapter 131).

Epidemiology
Incidence and prevalence
The prevalence of vulval naevi has been estimated as 2.3% in one series [1].

Age
These are most commonly seen in young women, but children and teenagers can be affected as well.

Pathophysiology
Pathology
The histological features of these lesions can be difficult to interpret [2]. They may be asymmetrical with the junctional component often involving the adnexae and exhibiting large nests of cells. The naevoid cells are atypical with this cytological atypia visible in both junctional and dermal parts. Dermal mitoses may be evident.

Clinical features
History
The naevi are asymptomatic and often an incidental finding.

Presentation
The most common sites where naevi develop are the inner aspects of the labia majora, the labia minora and the clitoris.

Differential diagnosis
Melanoma is usually seen in elderly women.

Disease course and prognosis
There are no long-term follow-up studies but these naevi are thought to be benign [3].

Investigations
Histological examination reveals the findings discussed.

Management
Complete excision is recommended.

PREMALIGNANT CONDITIONS

High-grade squamous intraepithelial lesions

Synonyms and inclusions
- Vulval intraepithelial neoplasia (VIN)
- Bowen disease
- Bowenoid papulosis
- Carcinoma *in situ*
- Carcinoma simplex

Introduction and general description

High-grade squamous intraepithelial lesions (HSIL) are non-invasive, premalignant disease that may progress to vulval SCC. This is HPV related. The other premalignant change is that of differentiated vulval intraepithelial neoplasia (VIN), which occurs on a background of lichen sclerosus (Table 110.7).

The previous three-tier grading of VIN was misleading as there is interobserver variation in the grading, and in clinical practice many cases of VIN 1 with basal atypia are not truly premalignant but reparative (e.g. LP), or proliferative as in a benign condyloma. Therefore, in 2004, the International Society for the Study of Vulvo-vaginal Disease (ISSVD) proposed replacing the three-tier grading system with two types of VIN, undifferentiated and differentiated. This classification eliminates the term VIN 1 and replaces the terms VIN 2 and 3 with 'undifferentiated VIN'. 'Differentiated VIN' remains as the term reserved for the severe atypia confined to the basal layers, most often seen on a background of a chronic scarring dermatosis. This classification did not include extramammary Paget disease or melanoma *in situ* [1]. The most recent change is to align the terminology with that of cervical disease and so the current classification is of low-grade (i.e. condylomata) and high-grade (previously undifferentiated VIN) squamous intraepithelial lesions. Differentiated VIN remains as a precursor of invasive malignancy on a background of inflammatory disease [2].

Table 110.7 Differences between types of premalignant lesions.

	HSIL	Differentiated VIN
Age	Younger women	Older women
HPV infection	Types 16 and 18 strongly associated	Very rare
Lichen sclerosus	Not generally associated	Usually associated
Lesions	Often multifocal	Usually unifocal
Risk factors	Smoking, immunosuppression	None known
Progression to SCC	Low risk (9% within 1–8 years)	High risk
Treatment	Responds to medical treatment	Surgical excision is treatment of choice

HPV, human papillomavirus; HSIL, high-grade squamous intraepithelial lesions; SCC, squamous cell carcinoma; VIN, vulval intraepithelial neoplasia.

Epidemiology
Incidence and prevalence
The incidence of HSIL has been increasing, with an estimated doubling of incidence to 2.1 per 100 000 population in 2005 [3]. However, the incidence of invasive SCC is not increasing at the same rate.

Pathophysiology
Predisposing factors
Smoking is a known risk factor in HSIL. HIV-positive women have an increased incidence and prevalence of both HSIL and vulval cancer [4].

Pathology
There is two-thirds to full-thickness loss of cellular stratification throughout the epidermis, with large hyperchromatic cells, dyskeratosis, multinucleated cells and numerous typical and atypical mitoses (Figure 110.28). In warty lesions, the appearance may be condylomatous, whereas basaloid lesions have a thickened epithelium with a non-papillomatous surface.

In differentiated VIN (dVIN), the histology may be mistaken for a benign dermatosis as there may be subtle abnormalities in the basal layers with normal keratinocyte differentiation above this (Figure 110.29). In addition to the basal changes, the rete ridges may be long and forked with keratin pearls. This change on a background of LS/LP either represents very early invasive disease or heralds its imminent onset.

Causative organisms
Multifocal ano-genital HSIL is strongly associated with the oncogenic papillomaviruses, particularly HPV types 16 and 18 [5,6].

Clinical features
History
The main symptom is pruritus, but some patients are asymptomatic.

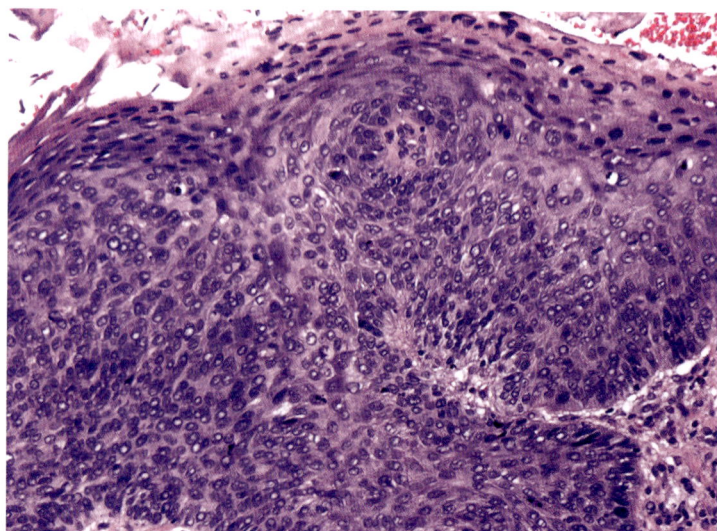

Figure 110.28 Histological features of a high-grade squamous intraepithelial lesion.

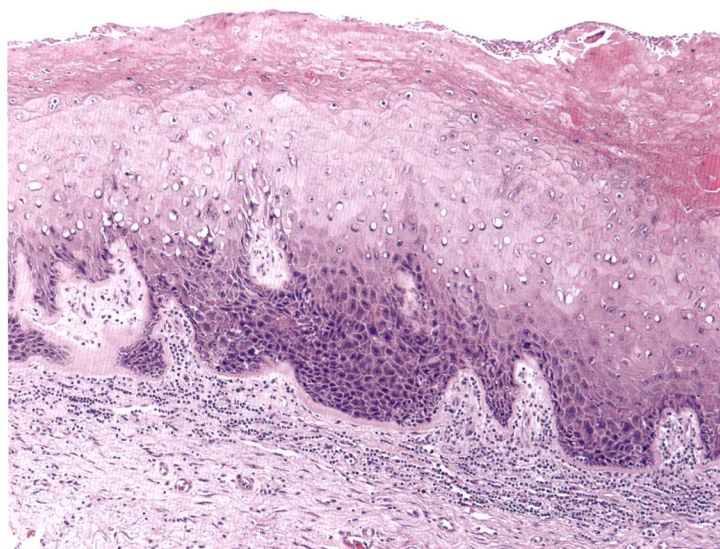

Figure 110.29 Histological features of differentiated vulval intraepithelial neoplasia.

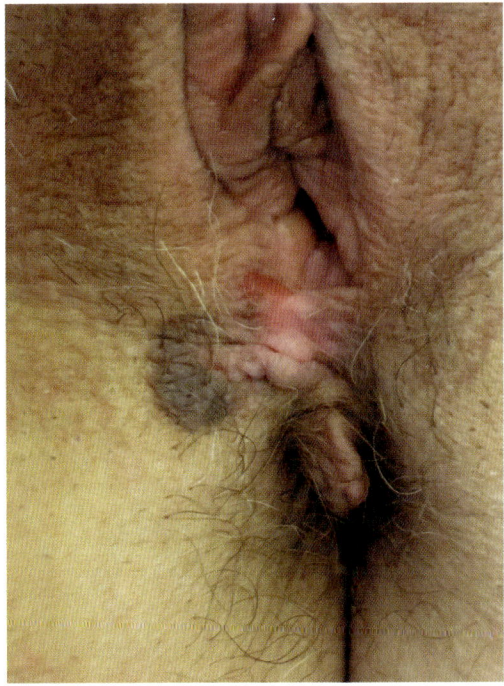

Figure 110.30 High-grade squamous intraepithelial lesions.

Presentation

The lesions of HSIL can be solitary or multiple. The morphology of the lesions is also diverse, with lesions that resemble viral warts, plaques that may be shiny and smooth, skin-coloured, red or white, or others that are warty and pigmented and resemble seborrhoeic keratoses (Figure 110.30). Less commonly, the lesions may be large and papillomatous, particularly perianally, where they may be polypoid. Vaginal involvement can be associated and should be checked by colposcopy.

Differentiated VIN is often subtle but red, hyperkeratotic or irregular lesions on a background or lichen sclerosus should be biopsied early and subjected to good clinicopathological correlation to confirm the diagnosis.

Differential diagnosis

The warty lesions of HSIL need to be distinguished from simple condylomata. The reddened lesions can resemble dermatoses and extramammary Paget disease.

Complications and co-morbidities

High-grade squamous intraepithelial lesions occur almost exclusively in smokers. The condition is caused by a failure of the host to mount an immune response to HPV. Patients who are immunocompromised have a higher incidence of this problem, but the majority of young women with this problem do not have an identifiable immunodeficiency. In addition to being multifocal, HSIL may be associated with multicentric disease, with lesions of intraepithelial neoplasia involving the cervix, vagina and perianal skin. Up to two-thirds of patients with HSIL have a current or past history of cervical intraepithelial neoplasia.

Disease course and prognosis

The risk of progression to invasive disease is estimated as 10% or less in multifocal HSIL, but this risk is likely to be higher in immunocompromised patients, those with perianal disease and in the older woman with a solitary plaque. Patients with dVIN are much more likely to develop an invasive tumour and in fact dVIN is rarely diagnosed prior to the development of SCC [7].

Investigations

High-grade squamous intraepithelial lesions are a multicentric problem, and other sites that need to be monitored are the cervix, vagina and perianal area. If there is perianal disease, anoscopy should be performed to exclude involvement of the anal canal.

Management

This is tailored to the individual but the patient should be managed in a specialised vulval clinic. In the case of a solitary lesion that is amenable to simple excision, this is the treatment of choice; surgical excision is always needed for areas of dVIN. In the woman with extensive HSIL, surgery would be mutilating physically and distressing psychologically, and does not guarantee a cure as the risk of recurrence is significant, due to the presence of oncogenic HPV. Such patients require regular and long-term follow-up, with biopsies of suspicious areas. Thick or polypoid lesions should be excised, as early invasive changes are difficult to detect in these areas [8].

Cryotherapy is not effective, but 5-fluorouracil can be used successfully for lesions of the labia minora, vestibule and clitoral area. It is not effective on the hair-bearing parts of the vulva, probably because of the deep adnexal structures, which can all be involved. Laser vaporisation has a high recurrence rate, particularly if the hair-bearing parts of the vulva are involved, and there is the additional danger that early invasive disease may be missed and therefore inappropriately treated. It is also extremely painful postoperatively.

Imiquimod has proved very effective in the treatment of multifocal HSIL in younger patients and recurrent disease after surgical

PART 10: SPECIFIC SITES, SEX & AGE

excision [**9,10**]. Lower recurrence rates compared with surgery have also been confirmed.

The development of HPV vaccines, which became licensed in Europe for preventative management in 2006, have already had an impact on the incidence of HSIL and should continue to do so.

Resources

Patient resources

International Society for the Study of Vulvovaginal Disease information sheet: https://www.issvd.org/resources/vulvar-squamous-intraepithelial-lesions.

Macmillan Cancer Support information sheet: https://www.macmillan.org.uk/cancer-information-and-support/worried-about-cancer/pre-cancerous-and-genetic-conditions/vulval-intraepithelial-neoplasia.

(Both last accessed April 2022.)

MALIGNANT NEOPLASMS

Squamous cell carcinoma

Introduction and general description

Squamous cell carcinoma is the most common malignancy occurring on the female genitalia (Chapter 141).

Epidemiology

Incidence and prevalence

Squamous cell carcinoma accounts for 90% of all vulval malignancies. The incidence of vulval SCC is 1–2 per 100 000.

Pathophysiology

Predisposing factors

Aetiologically, there appear to be two types of vulval SCC [**1,2**]. The first and largest group occurs in elderly women on a background of a chronic dermatosis such as LS or LP. The second type, which accounts for approximately 40% of cases, occurs in younger women and is associated with intraepithelial neoplasia associated with oncogenic-type HPV infection. There is, however, some overlap, and SCC arising in lichen sclerosus may be HPV positive [**3**].

Pathology

In the older age group, the tumours are usually well to moderately differentiated and keratinising, whereas in the younger HPV-associated group, they are poorly differentiated and often non-keratinising.

There is also an adenoid variant of SCC with acantholysis in the centres of some of the infiltrating nests, producing cystic spaces lined by cubocolumnar nests. These pseudocysts do not contain mucin, which differentiates them from adenosquamous cell carcinoma.

Causative organisms

High-risk oncogenic HPV types 16 and 18 are associated with VIN and the development of SCC in the younger age group.

Clinical features

History

The common symptoms are soreness and pruritus. The patient may present because of the presence of a nodule or plaque that causes few symptoms. Bleeding can occur if the tumour has ulcerated.

Presentation

Tumours can occur on any area of the vulva but common sites are the labia majora, clitoris, perineal body and fourchette.

Differential diagnosis

Some forms of ulcerated exophytic infection can mimic SCC. Hypertrophic infection with herpes simplex in immunosuppressed individuals can present as a tumour-like growth.

Classification of severity

There are combined TNM (tumour size, lymph nodes, distant metastasis) and FIGO (Federation of Gynaecology and Obstetrics) staging systems based on clinical examination and histological criteria. The depth of stromal invasion is measured from the epithelial–stromal junction of the adjacent dermal papilla to the deepest point of invasion by the tumour [**4**].

Disease course and prognosis

The overall 5-year survival is approximately 75%, which rises to 90% or greater in those with no nodal metastases. The main reason for failure of treatment is the inability to control lymphatic and distant metastases, lymphatic spread being the most important factor.

Investigations

A biopsy can confirm the diagnosis, and multiple mapping biopsies may be needed in multifocal disease. The patient must also be assessed for other sites of disease with cervical cytology, colposcopy and anoscopy if appropriate. Imaging will be needed to look for nodal involvement and distant spread.

Management

Surgery remains the primary treatment modality of locally resectable vulval cancer. In view of the rarity, the procedure should ideally be performed in dedicated cancer centers to achieve optimal disease control and maintain continence and sexual function whenever possible [**5,6**].

Surgical excision is tailored to the individual and is determined by the size and site of the tumour. Less radical surgery has not reduced survival rates but has significantly improved morbidity [**7**]. These patients are managed in a multidisciplinary setting with gynaecology oncologists, plastic surgeons and clinical and medical oncologists.

The vulval lymphatics drain to the inguinal and femoral nodes and from there to the pelvic nodes. Central lesions (those placed near the clitoris, urethra, vagina, fourchette and perianal area) have a bilateral lymphatic drainage, and it is important in these cases that the inguino-femoral nodes on both sides are excised. Radiotherapy is used as an adjuvant in patients with positive nodes and in those with inoperable tumours. It is also sometimes used as a primary treatment, together with chemotherapy, in tumours of the anus and urethra, to reduce their size before surgery and to try to preserve sphincter function.

Sentinel lymph node biopsy techniques are now being used in the management of these patients.

Resources

Patient resources

International Society for the Study of Vulvovaginal Disease information sheet: https://www.issvd.org/resources/vulvar-cancer.

Macmillan Cancer Support information sheet: https://www.macmillan.org.uk/cancer-information-and-support/vulval-cancer.

(Both last accessed April 2022.)

Verrucous carcinoma

Definition and nomenclature

A verrucous carcinoma is a low-grade and slowly growing form of SCC (Chapter 141).

Synonyms and inclusions
- Well-differentiated epidermoid squamous cell carcinoma
- Epithelioma cuniculatum
- Carcinoma cuniculatum
- Buschke–Löwenstein tumour
- Giant condyloma of Buschke–Löwenstein

Epidemiology

Age

These tumours occur in older women.

Associated diseases

Verrucous carcinomas can arise on a background of lichen sclerosus [1].

Pathophysiology

Pathology

The histological changes include epidermal acanthosis, with large bulbous rete ridges which compress and push down the underlying stroma. There is very little cellular atypia and the few, if any, mitoses are confined to the basal layers. The upper keratinocytes are often paler and there is a loss of the granular layer. Lymph node and distant metastases occur rarely.

Causative organisms

A proportion of cases may harbour HPV [2,3].

Clinical features

Presentation

Clinically, the lesions appear as a warty plaque or cauliflower-like tumour (Figure 110.31) which can ulcerate and become extremely large.

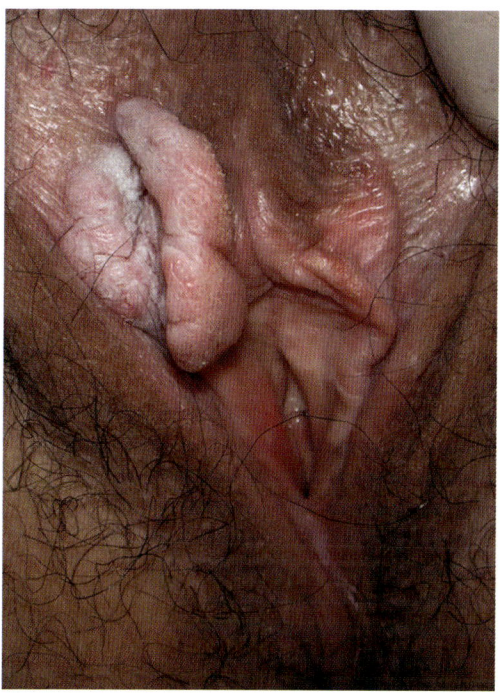

Figure 110.31 Verrucous carcinoma arising on a background of lichen sclerosus.

Differential diagnosis

Verrucous carcinomas are often misdiagnosed as squamous papillomas or condylomata because of the benign histological features.

Investigations

Multiple biopsies are often required to reach a firm diagnosis.

Management

Treatment is wide, local excision. Oral retinoids may also be helpful [4].

Extramammary Paget disease

Definition

Primary extramammary Paget disease (EMPD) is an intraepithelial adenocarcinoma arising in the epidermis or skin appendages. Secondary EMPD is epidermal involvement from an internal neoplasm, either by direct extension or metastasis.

Introduction and general description

The proposed classification for EMPD is shown in Table 110.8 [1]. In contrast to Paget disease of the nipple, the association with malignancy is only about 30%.

The differentiation between primary and secondary disease is not always straightforward clinically and sometimes relies on immunohistological investigations (Table 110.9) [2,3–5].

Table 110.8 Classification of extramammary Paget disease (EMPD).

Primary EMPD	Secondary EMPD
Primary intraepithelial neoplasm	Secondary to anal or rectal carcinoma
Intraepithelial neoplasm with invasion	Secondary to urothelial neoplasia
Manifestation of primary adenocarcinoma of a skin appendage or subcutaneous gland	Secondary to adenocarcinoma or related tumours of other sites

Adapted from Wilkinson and Brown 2002 [1].

Table 110.9 Immunocytochemical markers in extramammary Paget disease (EMPD).

Marker	Primary EMP	Secondary EMP	Bowen	Malignant melanoma
PAS	+	+	−	−
CK7	+	+	−	−
CK20	Usually −	Usually +	−	−
CEA	+	+	−	−
CAM5.2	+	+	−	−
GCDFP-15	+	+	−	−
S100	−	−	−	+
Melan A	−	−	−	+
Uroplakin III	+ if urothelial Ca			

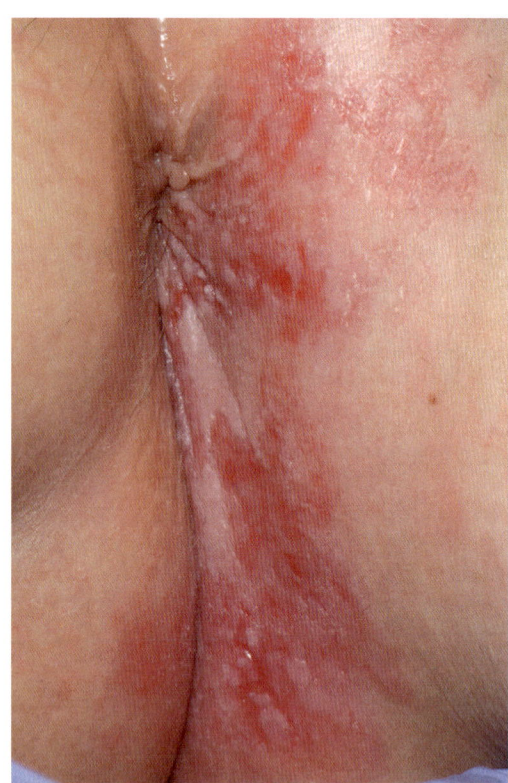

Figure 110.32 Extramammary Paget disease.

Epidemiology
Incidence and prevalence
The true prevalence is unknown but it accounts for 1–2% of all vulval malignancies.

Age
It generally affects women over 50 years [6,7].

Pathophysiology
Pathology
There is frequently epidermal hyperplasia. The epidermis is infiltrated with pale-staining Paget cells. The Paget cells are PAS positive and diastase resistant, and stain with Alcian blue and markers for the simple keratins.

Clinical features
History
The lesions may be asymptomatic initially and patients may report a longstanding eruption. Itching and burning are common symptoms.

Presentation
The lesions are typically moist, red plaques (Figure 110.32). The site of the lesions is important, as disease involving the urethra and perianal skin is more likely to be associated with an underlying malignancy of the urinary or gastrointestinal tract, respectively.

Differential diagnosis
The clinical differential diagnosis includes psoriasis and eczema. HSIL can have similar features. The important histological differential diagnoses are HSIL, melanoma and Bowen disease.

Complications and co-morbidities
The two most common tumours associated with secondary vulval EMPD are ano-rectal adenocarcinoma and urothelial carcinoma of the bladder or urethra. Other associated tumours reported include the cervix, endometrium and ovary [2,6].

Disease course and prognosis
Recurrence is common with all currently available treatment modalities. Regular monitoring and evaluation for invasion are important. The prognosis for primary intraepithelial disease is excellent. Invasive disease has an estimated 5-year survival of 72% [8].

Investigations
The diagnosis is confirmed histologically. Patients should have a full clinical examination and cervical cytology and mammography should be up to date. Further urological and bowel investigation should be undertaken if appropriate for secondary EMPD. There is no evidence for a routine screening programme for these malignancies in patients diagnosed with primary non-invasive VPD [2,9].

Management
In primary EMPD, excision of visible disease is often recommended for treatment and to exclude underlying appendageal adenocarcinoma. Sometimes in the very elderly, with extensive disease or recurrence after vulvectomy, this is not always an option. Patients should be regularly monitored, and topical steroids can be used if there is troublesome pruritus. Recurrence rates of over 40%

are reported after surgery, and even with Mohs micrographic surgery, the disease can recur in up to 27% and large margins are required [10].

Topical 5-fluorouracil, bleomycin and oral retinoids have been used, with some success. The recurrence rates are high after carbon dioxide laser and radiotherapy. Photodynamic therapy is reported to be of some benefit [11] but long-term results have not been evaluated.

There has been interest in the use of 5% imiquimod and although it is not licensed to treat EMPD, it can be useful in widespread disease and in recurrence after surgery [2,6,12].

Overexpression of the HER-2/neu protein is found in about 30% of cases, and in recurrent disease there are reports of the use of trastuzumab as targeted therapy [13].

In secondary disease, the treatment is directed predominantly at the associated carcinoma.

Resources

Patient resources

International Society for the Study of Vulvovaginal Disease information sheet: https://www.issvd.org/resources/extra-mammary-pagets-disease (accessed April 2022).

Basal cell carcinoma

Introduction and general description

Basal cell carcinomas account for 2–5% of all vulval malignancies (Chapter 140).

Epidemiology
Age
These tumours generally occur in the elderly but can be seen in younger women.

Clinical features
Presentation
Vulval basal cell carcinomas present as an eroded plaque, which may be pigmented. Less commonly, the tumour may form a nodule or ulcer. They occur most frequently on the labia majora or mons pubis [1–3].

Disease course and prognosis
Inadequate excision accounts for a high recurrence rate and vulval BCC has been reported to metastasise to regional lymph nodes [4].

Management
Due to their uncommon nature, consider discussing cases of vulval BCC at an MDT meeting. Complete histological excision should be achieved, be it wide local excision or margin-controlled surgery (Mohs micrographic surgery) in large or ill-defined lesions, or in cases where tissue preservation may have functional impact [5,6].

Vulval melanoma

Introduction and general description
Vulval melanoma is rare. All types of melanoma may occur on the vulva [1] (Chapter 142).

Epidemiology
Incidence and prevalence
Vulval melanoma accounts for about 2–10% of vulval malignancy. About 3% of all melanomas are found on the genital tract and the estimated annual incidence is about 1 per 1 million women.

Age
It is more usually found in the sixth and seventh decades of life. It has been reported in children but is extremely rare [2].

Pathophysiology
Genetics
Mutations in the KIT pathway are more common in vulval melanomas than in other mucosal lesions [3].

Clinical features
History
Vulval melanoma is often asymptomatic until it ulcerates, or becomes nodular. Bleeding may occur.

Presentation
The labia majora and clitoris are most common sites involved (Figure 110.33). The vagina is rarely involved and the cervix even less so. The clinical features are similar to melanoma elsewhere but

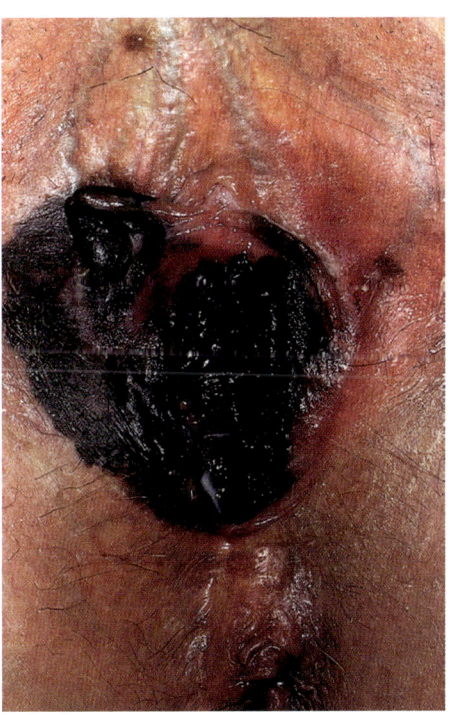

Figure 110.33 Melanoma of the vulva. Courtesy of Dr F. A. Ive, Durham, UK.

in one study of 219 patients, 27% were amelanotic [4]. Dermoscopy can aid in diagnosis and prompt early detection of thin melanomas [5] but is not always easy to do on the vulva.

Differential diagnosis
Amelanotic variants can mimic SCC and other tumours. Melanosis can have similar features to early lentigo maligna melanoma.

Disease course and prognosis
There is often a delay in diagnosis and a poorer prognosis for vulval and vaginal melanoma in particular. A 5-year survival rate of 11.4% has been estimated for female genital tract melanoma [6].

Investigations
The diagnosis is made histologically.

Management
The primary management is wide, local excision, with input from a specialist MDT. Adjuvant treatment with immunotherapy may be needed [7,8].

Resources

Further information
Gore M, Bagwan I, Board R *et al. Ano-uro-genital Mucosal Melanoma. Full Guideline.* Melanoma Focus 2018. https://melanomafocus.com/wp-content/uploads/2018/05/2_Full-Guideline-V.7.4-FINAL-29.5.18.pdf (last accessed April 2022).

Langerhans cell histiocytosis

Definition
Langerhans cell histiocytosis is a systemic disease with growth and proliferation of the Langerhans cells (Chapter 135). It can affect many organs and its presentation is variable.

Epidemiology
Age
Vulval Langerhans cell histiocytosis can present from childhood to old age. Primary or isolated involvement of the genitalia is uncommon [1,2].

Pathophysiology
Pathology
Large histiocytic cells with coffee bean nuclei are seen. Langerhans cells stain positively with S100 and characteristic Birkbeck granules are seen on electron microscopy.

Clinical features
Presentation
In infants, it may present as a resistant napkin eruption with yellowish and sometimes purpuric lesions. In adults, the lesions are papular, and scarring and ulceration may be prominent.

Differential diagnosis
The differential diagnosis is wide as it can mimic dermatoses and malignancy.

Management
Small localised lesions can be excised, but for more extensive disease this is impractical and radiotherapy, chemotherapy and thalidomide have been used [3].

Other malignant vulval neoplasms

There are some other tumours that are seen on the vulva but these are uncommon. They are detailed in Box 110.1.

Box 110.1 Other vulval neoplasms

Adenocarcinoma	Presents as painless subcutaneous nodules that can invade deeply. The mucinous carcinomas may be of cloacal origin [1]
Lymphoma	Non-Hodgkin lymphoma is more common than Hodgkin lymphoma [2] and has been reported post-transplantation [3] and in HIV-positive individuals [4]
Bartholin duct tumours	These may be better regarded as hyperplasia or hamartomas [5,6]
Bartholin gland carcinoma [7]	
Dermatofibrosarcoma protuberans [8]	
Liposarcoma [9]	
Epithelioid sarcoma [10]	
Merkel cell carcinoma [11]	
Myofibroblastic tumours	Angiomyofibroblastoma, cellular angiofibroma and aggressive angiomyxoma have a predilection for vulval soft tissues [12]
Metastatic tumours	These are uncommon and may be from malignancies of the cervix, endometrium, vagina, ovary, urethra, kidney, breast and lung [13]

PAIN DISORDERS

Vulval pain

Definition and nomenclature
Vulvodynia is defined as vulval discomfort, most often described as burning pain, occurring in the absence of relevant visible findings or a specific, clinically identifiable neurological disorder [1] (Chapter 82).

Introduction and general description

There has been much confusion in the literature about the terminology used for vulval pain and a system has been established by the ISSVD which replaces the 2003 classification (Box 110.2). A diagnosis of vulvodynia should be strictly reserved for those patients who have symptoms of pain or in the absence of any visible abnormality or explanation that would account for their symptoms. If any active dermatosis or dermographism is found that could account for the symptoms, then that condition is the diagnosis rather than vulvodynia. However, it is possible to have a dermatosis or other problem that is completely treated with no signs of activity, and vulvodynia as the condition that accounts for the symptoms of burning and discomfort.

Box 110.2 International Society for the Study of Vulvovaginal Disease (ISSVD) terminology and classification of vulval pain 2015

A. **Vulvar pain caused by a specific disorder**
   - Infectious (e.g. recurrent candidiasis, herpes)
   - Inflammatory (e.g. lichen sclerosus, lichen planus, immunobullous disorders)
   - Neoplastic (e.g. Paget disease, squamous cell carcinoma)
   - Neurological (e.g. postherpetic neuralgia, nerve compression or injury, neuroma)
   - Trauma (e.g. female genital cutting, obstetric)
   - Iatrogenic (e.g. postoperative, chemotherapy, radiation)
   - Hormonal deficiencies (e.g. genito-urinary syndrome of menopause (vulvo-vaginal atrophy), lactational amenorrhoea)
B. **Vulvodynia**
   - Localised (e.g. vestibulodynia, clitorodynia) or generalised or mixed (localised and generalised)
   - Provoked (e.g. insertional, contact) or spontaneous or mixed (provoked and spontaneous)
   - Onset (primary or secondary)
   - Temporal pattern (intermittent, persistent, constant, immediate, delayed)

Adapted from Bomstein et al. [1].

The two common types seen are provoked vulvodynia and generalised spontaneous vulvodynia. There is frequently overlap between the two types.

It is also important to remember that a form of dysaesthesia, probably more accurately labelled postinflammatory vulval hyperaesthesia, is a problem following inflammatory conditions of the vulva, particularly those involving the vestibule. It is seen most frequently following LP, when the patient still has symptoms despite the fact that the dermatosis has responded to treatment.

Epidemiology
Incidence and prevalence
The exact prevalence is not known but 16% of women in one study reported vulval pain lasting more than 3 months [2].

Age
Vestibulodynia occurs in young women, whereas the generalised form is more common in older postmenopausal women.

Associated diseases
There is frequently a history of other pain issues such as fibromyalgia, migraine and back pain [3]. Irritable bladder symptoms are particularly common in patients with vulvodynia.

Depression is a common feature in chronic pain but it is difficult to determine if this is a primary cause or a secondary effect of the symptoms.

Pathophysiology
The pathophysiology of vulvodynia is unknown but the existence of complex regional pain syndromes is now well recognised. Chronic pain syndromes are rarely caused by primary psychiatric disorders as originally thought, but are the result of peripheral and/or central neuronal sensitisation.

Predisposing factors
The majority of patients affected by vestibulodynia are psychologically normal but they do have higher anxiety and somatisation scores [4].

Pathology
There is now good evidence that inflammation is not a feature in vulvodynia [5].

Causative organisms
There is no evidence to support an association with chronic infection with either *Candida* or HPV, although there is sometimes a history of this prior to onset of symptoms.

Clinical features
History
In provoked vulvodynia, the classic history is of pain with penetration at intercourse. This can also occur with the use of tampons or speculum examination. Patients will sometimes relate the onset of symptoms to a particular event such as a severe episode of candidiasis or urinary tract infection. They frequently complain of increased sensitivity at other sites.

In the generalised form, the history is of constant pain with no obvious trigger factors. The pain may vary in intensity and patients may complain of shooting pain into the pelvis, thighs or anal area. Dyspareunia is not generally a feature.

Presentation
The vulva looks completely normal on examination. In provoked vulvodynia, there will be touch-provoked tenderness over the

vestibule when pressure is applied with a cotton-tipped swab (the touch test). This is usually at a maximum between 5 and 7 o'clock, but can affect the anterior vestibule also. In some patients, the pain is localised to the clitoris and this is then termed clitorodynia.

Differential diagnosis
Dermatoses, infections and malignancy can cause pain but the signs are evident. Dermographism, mechanical hymenal tears and vestibular fissures can cause pain with intercourse and sometimes it is helpful to examine the patient soon after intercourse to assess these. Pudendal neuralgia can be confused with generalised vulvodynia but here the pain is alleviated by standing.

Disease course and prognosis
Spontaneous resolution may occur but is unusual. As with any chronic pain problem, most patients show a steady but slow response to treatment and sometimes combination therapies are needed. Treatment outcomes are summarised in guidelines [6,7].

Investigations
The diagnosis is clinical and investigation is unhelpful.

Management
First line
Lidocaine 5% ointment can be applied regularly to the maximum points of tenderness. This is particularly helpful for provoked pain. Sensitisation is very rarely a problem with the use of the 5% lidocaine ointment. If alternative preparations are used, allergic or irritant dermatitis may occur.

Second line
Low-dose tricyclics (e.g. amitriptyline 10 mg nocte increasing by 10 mg increments to a maximum of 100 mg/day) may be used, however side effects can be troublesome and newer agents are increasingly favoured including pregabalin, gabapentin and duloxetine. Physiotherapy is particularly useful for associated vaginismus [8].

Third line
Referral to a pain clinic and expert psychosexual counselling are helpful. Vestibulectomy has been used for provoked vulvodynia but is only suitable for a small minority and there are few long-term results of efficacy. Psychological issues must be dealt with as these have an impact on outcome. Vestibulectomy is not advocated as a routine procedure and surgery is rarely used for other neuropathic pain problems.

There is often a need for combination therapies [9].

Resources

Patient resources
British Vulval Pain Society: www.vulvalpainsociety.org.
International Society for the Study of Vulvovaginal Disease information sheets: https://www.issvd.org/resources/vulvodynia.
National Vulvodynia Association: www.nva.org.
(All last accessed April 2022.)

TRAUMATIC LESIONS

There are various causes of vulval trauma, including accidental injury, obstetric tears and self-induced lesion [1,2]. Sclerosing lipogranuloma [3] is a granulomatous response induced artefactually.

Mechanical hymenal fissures

Synonyms and inclusions
- Postcoital fissures
- Hymenel fissures
- Nympho-hymenal tears

Introduction and general description
Mechanical hymenal fissures are a cause of dyspareunia and occur in nulliparous women on each intercourse.

Clinical features
History
Postcoital bleeding and pain at the site of the tear are the main symptoms. Abstinence, even for long periods of time, does not prevent recurrence.

Presentation
Fissures occur radially at 3 and 9 o'clock (Figure 110.34). They can be bilateral and extend from the hymenal ring into the vagina. Similar lesions can occur in the midline at the fourchette.

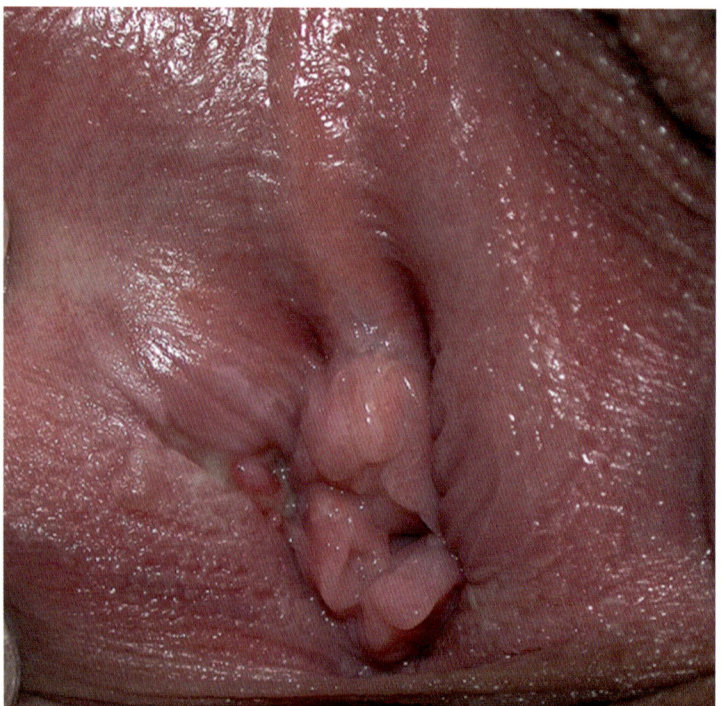

Figure 110.34 Tear of the right inferior aspect of the nympho-hymenal sulcus.

Differential diagnosis

The symptoms of provoked vulvodynia may be similar, but these usually improve very quickly after the pressure of intercourse stops. With mechanical hymenal fissures, the symptoms can last for over 48 h after intercourse.

Disease course and prognosis

They heal rapidly within a few days but recur at the same site with each intercourse. They may leave a pale scar.

Investigations

The diagnosis is clinical. It is important to examine the patient within 24 h of intercourse and to stretch the hymenal ring or the signs may be missed.

Management

Excision of the radial fissure with resuturing usually resolves the problem. For the midline fissures, good emollients and topical oestrogens applied directly to the area twice weekly can help, but surgery may be required to remove the area of recurrent fissuring. This should be done in the context of a specialised clinic.

Female genital mutilation

Synonyms and inclusions
- Female circumcision
- Cutting

Introduction and general description

Female genital mutilation (FGM), although banned in most European countries, is still forced on many women worldwide. Many cases are now being seen in the UK because of the rise in immigration of women who have had previous FGM. It involves a variety of procedures to remove parts of the female genitalia for non-medical reasons [1].

Epidemiology
Incidence and prevalence
It may affect up to 140 million women worldwide.

Age
Most FGM occurs before the age of 1, but in Egypt girls are likely to be circumcised between 5 and 15 years old.

Clinical features
Presentation
There are four types of operation performed, which vary according to the country and culture:
1 Clitoridectomy: removal of the clitoris and/or the clitoral hood (Sunna circumcision).
2 Excision: removal of the clitoris and part or all of the labia minora.

3 Narrowing of the introitus by cutting and apposing the labia minora and/or the labia majora, with or without excision of the clitoris (infibulation), leaving a tiny opening for urination and menstruation.
4 All other practices, which might involve cauterisation, applying corrosive material, and piercing or cutting of the clitoris, surrounding skin or vagina.

Complications and co-morbidities

There may be immediate damage to the urethra and vagina but the later complications are often only seen during delivery in those who have had infibulation. Many of the women who have had FGM experience difficulties with sexual intercourse, urination and pregnancy [2].

Management

Referral to a specialist clinic for further management is recommended.

Resources

Further information
Royal College of Obstetricians and Gynaecologists 2015 guidelines: https://www.rcog.org.uk/globalassets/documents/guidelines/gtg-53-fgm.pdf.
World Health Organization information: https://www.who.int/health-topics/female-genital-mutilation#tab=tab_1.

Patient resources
Foundation for Women's Health Research and Development: www.forwarduk.org.uk. (All last accessed April 2022.)

MISCELLANEOUS DERMATOSES

Graft-versus-host disease

Definition

Graft-versus-host disease (GVHD) occurs with acute followed by chronic features after allogeneic stem cell transplant, and is due to the donor cells reacting against host tissue (Chapter 38).

Epidemiology
Incidence and prevalence
Genital GVHD can occur in up to 49% of patients after transplant [1].

Clinical features

Presentation
Vulval and vaginal redness and erosions are seen [2].

Differential diagnosis

The clinical features are indistinguishable from erosive lichen planus. This is sometimes difficult to differentiate histologically as there may be a lichenoid infiltrate present.

Complications and co-morbidities

Vaginal involvement leads to the development of synechiae and complete stenosis, hence early recognition is vital [3]. It may be associated with cutaneous and oral GVHD.

Management

Treatment ladder for graft-versus-host disease

First line
- Super-potent topical steroids [4]

Second line
- Systemic steroids or immunosuppressive agents as guided by transplant physicians [5]. Patients also respond to ciclosporin [6]

Third line
- Extracorporeal photophoresis. Those with vaginal stenosis need expert surgical intervention to open the adhesions. Potent topical steroids must be used immediately postoperatively to maintain patency of the vagina

Vulvo-vaginal adenosis

Definition
Vulvo-vaginal adenosis is the presence of metaplastic cervical or endometrial epithelium.

Epidemiology
Associated diseases
Vulval adenosis may follow a severe erosive disease such as toxic epidermal necrolysis [1].

Pathophysiology
The pathogenesis is unknown but it is postulated that it develops from remnant tissue of paramesonephric origin.

Predisposing factors
Prolonged use of the oral contraceptive pill and trauma can predispose to adenosis. Upper vaginal disease is well recognised to occur after *in utero* exposure to diethyl stilboestrol taken during pregnancy.

Clinical features
Presentation
The lesions are red and very friable.

Complications and co-morbidities
Vaginal adenosis has been associated with vaginal adenocarcinoma [2].

Investigations
Histology shows mucous or endometrial glands are seen within the epithelium.

Management

Laser treatment has been used successfully.

Necrolytic migratory erythema

Synonyms and inclusions
- Glucagonoma syndrome

Introduction and general description
This dermatosis is usually seen in patients with the glucagonoma syndrome, but it is possible for it to occur in the absence of a glucagonoma or increased levels of glucagon [1] (Chapter 47).

Pathophysiology
The aetiology is unknown and even though there is a vey strong link with high levels of glucagon in the glucagonoma syndrome, this does not appear to cause it. The eruption is not reproduced by application or injection of glucagon and does not occur in other conditions where increased levels of glucagon are found, such as diabetes and renal failure.

Pathology
The keratinocytes are vacuolated and pale; necrosis leads to intraepidermal clefting. Subcorneal pustules may be a feature.

Environmental factors
Moisture, friction and trauma may precipitate fresh lesions.

Clinical features
History
The lesions are pruritic, and flaccid bullae occur which then rupture and crust over. This may occur in cycles.

Presentation
The lesions occur on the vulva, perineum and perianal skin and extend onto the thighs and lower abdomen. The central face and limbs may rarely be involved. Extensive eroded erythema with crusting and a desquamative, serpiginous edge, which spreads out centrifugally, give rise to the characteristic annular lesions.

Differential diagnosis
A similar clinical picture is seen with zinc and protein deficiency and there are now a number of reports of necrolytic migratory erythema occurring with liver diseases in the absence of a glucagonoma [2]. Acrodermatitis and pellagra have similar histological features.

Disease course and prognosis
The eruption may relapse and remit and postinflammatory hyperpigmentation can last for a few weeks. The eruption resolves rapidly after surgery or medical treatment of the glucagonoma.

Investigations

A skin biopsy will show the features described, and further endocrinological and imaging investigations are required to confirm any associated glucagonoma.

Management

Expert advice from an endocrinologist is needed for management. Topical steroids are helpful.

Genital papular acantholytic dyskeratosis

Introduction and general description

This was first described in 1984 [1], and is characterised by the presence of multiple papules or, less frequently, a single papule or plaque-like lesion on genital skin [2–5].

Epidemiology

Age

Middle-aged females are most affected.

Pathophysiology

Pathology

Histology shows hyperkeratosis and acantholysis.

Clinical features

History

The main symptom is pruritus.

Presentation

Multiple, small papules up to a few millimetres in size appear in the inguinal folds and may extend to the thighs and perineum. They may coalesce into nodules and small plaques.

Clinical variants

Cases with disseminated lesions have been described [6]. A case with positive immunofluorescence has been reported [7].

Differential diagnosis

The histological changes are similar to those seen in Darier disease or Hailey–Hailey disease, but there is no family history or evidence of these diseases at other sites.

Investigations

The diagnosis is made on histology.

Management

Laser treatment has been reported to be useful in those who are unresponsive to topical steroids or retinoids [8].

Vulval acne

Introduction and general description

This condition has recently been described [1].

Epidemiology

Age

Younger women below the age of 40 are generally affected.

Pathophysiology

Pathology

Histology shows folliculocentric inflammatory change.

Clinical features

History

Patients develop painful papules and nodules usually premenstrually. They can discharge or just spontaneously resolve.

Presentation

Small papules and pustules are seen on the inner labia majora or minora.

Differential diagnosis

Early hidradenitis suppurative can have similar features.

Investigations

The diagnosis is made on the clinical features and histology.

Management

Treatment is with oral antibiotics, the oral contraceptive pill or low-dose isotretinoin in persistent cases.

Key references

The full list of references can be found in the online version at https://www.wiley.com/rooksdermatology10e

Introduction

1 Lynch PJ, Moyal-Barracco M, Scurry J, Stockdale C. 2011 ISSVD terminology and classification of vulvar dermatological disorders; an approach to clinical diagnosis. *J Lower Gen Tract Dis* 2012;16:339–44.
4 British Association of Dermatologists. *Standards of Care for Women with Vulval Conditions*. https://cdn.bad.org.uk/uploads/2021/12/29200128/Standards-of-Care_Vulval-Conditions-Report.pdf (last accessed April 2022).

Structure and function of the female genitalia

1 Lloyd J, Crouch NS, Minto CL, Liao L, Creighton SM. Female genital appearance: 'normality' unfolds. *Br J Obstet Gynaecol* 2005;112:643–6.
2 Kreklau A, Vâz I, Oehme F et al. Measurements of a 'normal vulva' in women aged 15–84: a cross-sectional prospective single-centre study. *BJOG* 2018;125:1656–61.
4 Bacon JL, Romano ME, Quint EH. Clinical recommendation: labial adhesions. *J Pediatr Adolesc Gynecol* 2015;28:405–9.

Congenital abnormalities
Disorders of sexual development

1 Hughes IA. Disorders of sexual development: new definition and classification. *Best Pract Res Clin Endocrinol Metab* 2008;22:119–34.

Genodermatoses
Epidermolysis bullosa

1 Almaani N, Mellerio JE. Genitourinary tract involvement in epidermolysis bullosa. *Dermatol Clin* 2010;28:343–6.

Inflammatory dermatoses
Lichen sclerosus

1 Meffert JJ, Davis BM, Grimwood RE. Lichen sclerosus. *J Am Acad Dermatol* 1995;32:393–416.

6 Kreuter A, Kryvosheyeva Y, Terras S *et al*. Association of autoimmune diseases with lichen sclerosus in 532 male and female patients. *Acta Derm Venereol* 2013;93:238–41.

7 Simpkin S, Oakley A. Clinical review of 202 patients with vulval lichen sclerosus: a possible association with psoriasis. *Austral J Dermatol* 2007;48:28–31.

43 Zaki I, Dalziel KL, Solomons FA *et al*. The under-reporting of skin disease in association with squamous cell carcinoma of the vulva. *Clin Exp Dermatol* 1997;21:334–7.

59 Cooper S, Gao X-H, Powell JJ, Wojnarowska F. Does treatment of lichen sclerosus influence its prognosis? *Arch Dermatol* 2004;140:702–6.

60 Lee A, Bradford J, Fischer G. Long-term management of adult vulvar lichen sclerosus: a prospective cohort study of 507 women. *JAMA Dermatol* 2015;151:1061–7.

62 Morrel B, van Eersel R, Burger CW *et al*. The long-term clinical consequences of juvenile vulvar lichen sclerosus: a systematic review. *J Am Acad Dermatol* 2020;82:469–77.

63 Chi CC, Kitschig G, Baldo M, Brackenbury F, Lewis F, Wojnarowska F. Topical interventions of genital lichen sclerosus [Review]. *Cochrane Database Syst Rev* 2011;Issue 7:CD008240.

64 Lewis FM, Tatnall FM, Velangi SS *et al*. British Association of Dermatologists guidelines for the management of lichen sclerosus, 2018. *Br J Dermatol* 2018;178:839–53.

Lichen planus

1 Ebrahimi M, Lundqvist L, Wahlin YB, Nylander E. Mucosal lichen planus, a systemic disease requiring multidisciplinary care: a cross-sectional clinical review from a multi-disciplinary perspective. *J Lower Gen Tract Dis* 2012;16:377–80.

4 Lewis FM, Shah M, Harrington CI. Vulval involvement in lichen planus: a study of 37 women. *Br J Dermatol* 1996;135:89–91.

9 Setterfield JF, Neill SM, Shirlaw PJ *et al*. The vulvovaginal gingival syndrome: a severe subgroup of lichen planus with characteristic clinical features and a novel association with the class II HLA DQB1*0201 allele. *J Am Acad Dermatol* 2006;55:98–113.

13 Pelisse M, Leibowitch M, Sedel D, Hewitt J. Un nouveau syndrome vulvo-vagino-gingival. Lichen plan erosive plurimuqueux. *Ann Dermatol Vénéréol* 1982;109:797–8.

27 Zaki I, Dalziel KL, Solomons FA *et al*. The under-reporting of skin disease in association with squamous cell carcinoma of the vulva. *Clin Exp Dermatol* 1997;21:334–7.

28 Derrick EK, Ridley CM, Kobza-Black A *et al*. A clinical study of 23 cases of female anogenital carcinoma. *Br J Dermatol* 2000;143:1217–23.

32 Cooper SM, Haefner H, Abrahams-Gessel S, Margesson LJ. Vulvovaginal lichen planus treatment: a survey of current practices. *Arch Dermatol* 2008;144:1520–1.

34 Cooper SM, Wojnarowska F. Influence of treatment of erosive lichen planus of the vulva on its prognosis. *Arch Dermatol* 2006;142:289–94.

41 Panagiotopoulou N, Wong CSM, Winter-Roach B. Vulvovaginal-gingival syndrome. *J Obstet Gynaecol* 2010;30:226–30.

47 Rajkumar S, Lewis F, Nath R. The importance of topical steroids after adhesiolysis in erosive lichen planus and graft versus host disease. *J Obstet Gynaecol* 2019;39:82–5.

Zoon vulvitis

1 Scurry J, Dennerstein G, Brennan J. Vulvitis circumscripta plasmacellularis. A clinicopathologic entity? *J Reprod Med* 1993;38:14–18.

3 Virgili A, Corazza M, Minghetti S, Borghi A. Symptoms in plasma cell vulvitis: first observational cohort study on type, frequency and severity. *Dermatology* 2015;230:113–18.

7 Virgili A, Borghi A, Minghetti S, Corazza M. Comparative study on topical immunomodulatory and anti-inflammatory treatments for plasma cell vulvitis: long-term efficacy and safety. *J Eur Acad Dermatol Venereol* 2015;29:507–14.

Allergic contact dermatitis

1 O'Gorman SM, Torgerson RR. Allergic contact dermatitis of the vulva. *Dermatitis* 2013;24:64–72.

4 Haverhoek E, Reid C, Gordon L *et al*. Prospective study of patch tests in patients with vulval pruritus. *Australas J Dermatol* 2008;49:80–5.

12 Woodruff CM, Trivedi MK, Botto N, Kornik R. Allergic contact dermatitis of the vulva. *Dermatitis* 2018;29:233–43.

13 Warshaw EM, Furda LM, Maibach HI *et al*. Anogenital dermatitis in patients referred for patch testing: retrospective analysis of cross-sectional data from the North American Contact Dermatitis Group, 1994–2004. *Arch Dermatol* 2008;144:749–55.

Allergic contact urticaria

6 Lee-Wong M, Collins JS, Nozad C, Resnick DJ. Diagnosis and treatment of human seminal plasma hypersensitivity. *Obstet Gynecol* 2008;111:538–9.

Psoriasis

2 Meeuwis KAP, Potts Bleakman A, van de Kerkhof PCM *et al*. Prevalence of genital psoriasis in patients with psoriasis. *J Dermatol Treat* 2018;29:754–60.

3 Kapila S, Bradford J, Fischer G. Vulvar psoriasis in adults and children: a clinical audit of 194 cases and review of the literature. *J Lower Gen Tract Dis* 2012;16:108.

10 Meeuwis K, de Hullu J, Massuger L *et al*. Genital psoriasis: a systematic literature review on this hidden skin disease. *Acta Derm Venereol* 2011;91:5–11.

11 Larsabal M, Ly S, Sbidian E *et al*. GENIPSO: a French prospective study assessing instantaneous prevalence, clinical features and impact on quality of life of genital psoriasis among patients consulting for psoriasis. *Br J Dermatol* 2019;180:647–56.

Ulcerative and bullous disorders
Non-sexually acquired reactive genital ulcers

3 Portnoy J, Arontheim GA, Ghibu F *et al*. Recovery of Epstein–Barr virus from genital ulcers. *N Engl J Med* 1984;311:966–8.

4 Halvorsen JA, Brevig T, Aas T *et al*. Genital ulcers as initial manifestation of Epstein–Barr virus infection: two new cases and review of the literature. *Acta Derm Venereol* 2006;86:439–42.

6 Vismara SA, Lava SAG, Kottanattu L *et al*. Lipschütz's acute vulvar ulcer: a systematic review. *Eur J Pediatr* 2020;179:1559–67.

9 Dixit S, Bradford J, Fischer G. Management of nonsexually acquired genital ulceration using oral and topical corticosteroids followed by doxycycline prophylaxis. *J Am Acad Dermatol* 2013;68:797–802.

Immunobullous disease

1 Marren P, Wojnarowska F, Venning V, Wilson C, Nayar M. Vulvar involvement in auto-immune bullous diseases. *J Reprod Med* 1993;38:101–7.

3 Batta K, Munday PE, Tatnall FM. Pemphigus vulgaris localized to the vagina and presenting as a chronic vaginal discharge. *Br J Dermatol* 1999;140:945–7.

Pigmentary disorders
Vulval melanosis

1 Barnhill RI, Alber LS, Shama SK *et al*. Genital lentiginosis: a clinical and histopathological study. *J Am Acad Dermatol* 1990;22:453–60.

2 Haugh AM, Merkel EA, Zhang B *et al*. A clinical, histologic, and follow-up study of genital melanosis in men and women. *J Am Acad Dermatol* 2017;76:836–40.

4 De Giorgi V, Gori A, Salvati L *et al*. Clinical and dermoscopic features of vulvar melanosis over the last 20 years. *JAMA Dermatol* 2020;156:1185–91.

Dowling–Degos disease

4 Ong Kang H, Hur J, Woo Lee J *et al*. A case of Dowling–Degos disease on the vulva. *Ann Dermatol* 2011;23:205–8.

Vulval oedema
Crohn disease

1 Barret M, de Parades V, Battistella M *et al*. Crohn's disease of the vulva. *J Crohns Colitis* 2014;8:563–70.

2 Foo WC, Papalas JA, Robboy SJ, Selim MA. Vulvar manifestations of Crohn's disease. *Am J Dermatopathol* 2011;33:588–93.

3 Martin J, Holdstock G. Isolated vulval oedema as a feature of Crohn's disease. *J Obstet Gynecol* 1997;17:92–3.

13 Laftah Z, Bailey C, Zaheri S *et al.* Vulval Crohn's disease: a clinical study of 22 patients. *J Crohns Colitis* 2015;9:318–25.

Non-sexually transmitted infections
Streptococcal infections
2 Liegeon AL, Berville S, Wendling-Héraud J, Moyal-Barracco M. Group A streptococcal vulvitis in adult women: clinical features and association with psoriasis. *J Low Genit Tract Dis* 2019;23:287–9.

Candidal vulvo-vaginitis
1 Sobel JD. Recurrent vulvovaginal candidiasis. *Am J Obstet Gynecol* 2016;214:15–21.

Herpes simplex virus infections
4 Lautenschlager S, Eichmann A. The heterogenous clinical spectrum of genital herpes. *Dermatology* 2001;202:211–19.
5 Garland SM, Steben M. Genital herpes. *Best Pract Res Clin Obstet Gynaecol* 2014;28:1098–110.

Human papillomavirus infections
2 Scheinfeld N. Update on the treatment of genital warts. *Dermatol Online J* 2013;19:18559.

Benign tumours
1 Fite C, Plantier F, Dupin N, Anil MF, Moyal-Barracco M. Vulvar verruciform xanthoma: ten cases associated with lichen sclerosus, lichen planus or other conditions. *Arch Dermatol* 2011;147:1087–92.
4 Juang YH, Chuang YH, Kuo TT *et al.* Vulvar syringoma: a clinicopathologic and immunohistologic syudy of 18 patients and results of treatment. *J Am Acad Dermatol* 2003;48:735–9.

Papillary hidradenoma
2 El-Khoury J, Renald MH, Plantier F, Avril MF, Moyal-Barracco M. Vulvar hidradenoma papilliferum (HP) is located on the sites of mammary-like anogenital glands (MLAGs): analysis of the photographs of 52 tumors. *J Am Acad Dermatol* 2016;75:380–4.

Cutaneous endometriosis
1 Agarwal A, Fong YF. Cutaneous endometriosis. *Singapore Med J* 2008;49:704–9.

Atypical genital naevi
1 Rock B, Hood AF, Rock JA. Prospective study of vulvar nevi. *J Am Acad Dermatol* 1990;22:104–6.
2 Brenn T. Atypical genital naevus. *Arch Pathol Lab Med* 2011;135:317–20.
3 Ribé A. Melanocytic lesions of the genital area with attention given to atypical genital nevi. *J Cutan Pathol* 2008;35(Suppl. 2):24–7.

Premalignant conditions
High-grade squamous intraepithelial lesions
1 Sideri M, Jones RW, Wilkinson EJ *et al.* Squamous vulvar intraepithelial neoplasia: 2004 modified terminology, ISSVD Vulvaroncology Subcommittee. *J Reprod Med* 2005;50:807–10.
2 Darragh TM, Colgan TJ, Cox JT *et al.* The Lower Anogenital Squamous Terminology Standardization Project for HPV-Associated Lesions: background and consensus recommendations from the College of American Pathologists and the American Society for Colposcopy and Cervical Pathology. *J Low Genit Tract Dis* 2012;16:205–42.
3 Terlou A, Blok LJ, Helmerhorst TJM, van Beurden M. Premalignant epithelial disorders of the vulva: squamous vulvar intra-epithelial neoplasia, vulvar Paget's and melanoma in situ. *Acta Obstet Gynecol* 2010;89:741–8.
9 Van Seters M, van Beurden M, Ten Kate FJW *et al.* Treatment of vulvar intraepithelial neoplasia with topical imiquimod. *N Engl J Med* 2008;358:1465–73.
10 De Witte CJ, van de Sande AJ, van Beekhuizen HJ *et al.* Imiquimod in cervical, vaginal and vulvar intraepithelial neoplasia: a review. *Gynecol Oncol* 2015;139:377–84.

Malignant neoplasms
Squamous cell carcinoma
1 Singh N, Gilks CB. Vulval squamous cell carcinoma and its precursors. *Histopathology* 2020;76:128–38.
4 Benedet JL, Hacker NF, Ngan HYS *et al.* Staging classifications and clinical practice guidelines of gynaecologic cancers. *Int J Gynecol Obstet* 2000;70:209–62.
7 Rogers LJ, Cuello MA. Cancer of the vulva. *Int J Gynaecol Obstet* 2018;143(Suppl. 2):4–13.

Extramammary Paget disease
1 Wilkinson EJ, Brown HM. Vulvar Paget disease of urothelial origin: a report of three cases and a proposed classification of vulval Paget disease. *Hum Pathol* 2002;33:549–54.
2 Van der Linden M, Meeuwis KA, Bulten J *et al.* Paget disease of the vulva. *Crit Rev Oncol Hematol* 2016;101:60–74.
6 Delport ES. Extramammary Paget's disease of the vulva: an annotated review of the current literature. *Aust J Dermatol* 2013;54:9–21.

Basal cell carcinoma
4 Renati S, Henderson C, Aluko A, Burgin S. Basal cell carcinoma of the vulva: a case report and systematic review of the literature. *Int J Dermatol* 2019;58:892–902.
6 Sinha K, Abdul-Wahab A, Calonje E, Craythorne E, Lewis FM. Basal cell carcinoma of the vulva: treatment with Mohs micrographic surgery. *Clin Exp Dermatol* 2019;44:651–3.

Vulval melanoma
1 Postow MA, Hamid O, Carvajal RD. Mucosal melanoma: pathogenesis, clinical behaviour and management. *Curr Oncol Rep* 2012;14:441–8.
2 Egan CA, Bradley RR, Logsdon VK *et al.* Vulvar melanoma in children. *Arch Dermatol* 1997;133:345–8.
3 Omholt K, Grafstrom E, Kanter-Lewensohn L *et al.* KIT pathway alterations in mucosal melanomas of the vulva and other sites. *Clin Cancer Res* 2011;15:3933–42.
8 Wohlmuth C, Wohlmuth-Wieser I, May T *et al.* Malignant melanoma of the vulva and vagina: a US population-based study of 1863 patients. *Am J Clin Dermatol* 2020;21:285–95.

Langerhans cell histiocytosis
2 Jiang W, Li L, He Y, Yang K. Langerhans cell histiocytosis of the female genital tract: a literature review with additional three case studies in China. *Arch Gynecol Obstet* 2012;285:99–103.
3 El-Safadi S, Dreyer T, Oehmke F, Muenstedt K. Management of adult primary vulvae Langerhans cell histiocytosis: review of the literature and a case history. *Eur J Obstet Gynecol Reprod Biol* 2012;163:123–8.

Pain disorders
Vulval pain
1 Bornstein J, Goldstein AT, Stockdale CK *et al.* Consensus Vulvar Pain Terminology Committee of the International Society for the Study of Vulvovaginal Disease (ISSVD), the International Society for the Study of Women's Sexual Health (ISSWSH), and the International Pelvic Pain Society (IPPS). 2015 ISSVD, ISSWSH and IPPS consensus terminology and classification of persistent vulvar pain and vulvodynia. *Obstet Gynecol* 2016;127:745–51.
6 Mandal D, Nunns D, Byrne M *et al.* Guidelines for the management of vulvodynia. *Br J Dermatol* 2010;162:1180–5.
7 Haefner HK, Collins ME, David GD *et al.* The vulvodynia guideline. *J Lower Gen Tract Dis* 2005;9:40–51.

Traumatic lesions
2 Jones IS, O'Connor A. Non-obstetric vulval trauma. *Emerg Med Australas* 2013;25:36–9.

Female genital mutilation
1 Simpson J, Robinson K, Creighton SM, Hodes D. Female genital mutilation: the role of health professionals in prevention assessment and management. *BMJ* 2012;344:37–41.

PART 10: SPECIFIC SITES, SEX & AGE

2 Rushwan H. Female genital mutilation (FGM) management during pregnancy, childbirth and the postpartum period. *Int J Gynaecol Obstet* 2000;70:99–104.

Miscellaneous dermatoses
Graft-versus-host disease
1 Zantomio D, Grigg AP, MacGregor L *et al*. Female genital tract graft-versus-host disease: incidence, risk factors and recommendations for management. *Bone Marrow Transplant* 2006;38:567–72.
2 Smith Knutsson E, Björk Y, Broman AK *et al*. A prospective study of female genital chronic graft-versus-host disease symptoms, signs, diagnosis and treatment. *Acta Obstet Gynecol Scand* 2018;97:1122–9.

3 Hirsch P, Leclerc M, Rybojad M *et al*. Female genital chronic graft-versus-host disease: importance of early diagnosis to avoid severe complications. *Transplantation* 2012;93:1265–9.
4 Stratton P, Turner ML, Childs R *et al*. Vulvovaginal graft versus host disease with allogeneic haemopoetic stem cell transplantation. *Obstet Gynecol* 2007;110:1041–9.

Vulval acne
1 Foo S, Lewis F, Velangi S, Walsh S, Calonje JE. Vulval acne: a case series describing clinical features and management. *Clin Exp Dermatol* 2021;46:319–23.

CHAPTER 111

Dermatoses of Perineal and Perianal Skin

Eleanor Mallon

Department of Dermatology, St Mary's Hospital, Imperial College Healthcare NHS Trust, London, UK

Introduction

History and examination

The correct diagnosis of skin disease affecting the perineum and perianal skin depends on detailed history taking, thorough methodical examination including of extragenital skin and relevant investigations. The history should include a history of topical treatments that have been used including over-the-counter remedies and wet wipes. Examination using a Wood light can be helpful in the diagnosis of conditions including erythrasma and vitiligo.

Investigations in perineal and perianal dermatology

Investigations are determined by history and clinical findings. Clinicopathological correlation is essential through discussion with a dermatopathologist. Clinicians should have a low threshold to take bacterial and viral swabs, or scrapings for fungal culture. Diagnostic imaging techniques such as pelvic magnetic resonance imaging (MRI) and endoanal ultrasound are utilised in the investigation of conditions such as anal fistula and anal malignancy.

Structure and function of the ano-genital region

The perineum is a diamond-shaped region that lies below the pelvic floor and corresponds to the outlet of the pelvis (Figure 111.1).

The anterior boundary is formed by the symphysis pubis, the posterior boundary by the coccyx, the anterolateral boundary by the ischio-pubic rami and ischial tuberosities, and the postero-lateral boundary by the sacrotuberous ligaments. The deep limit of the perineum is the inferior surface of muscles forming the pelvic diaphragm and the superficial limit is the skin, which is continuous with the skin of the groins and lower abdomen. An imaginary line drawn transversely joining the ischial tuberosities divides the perineum into an anterior uro-genital triangle and a posterior anal triangle. The perineal body is the central point between the uro-genital and anal triangles. The anal triangle contains the anal canal and its sphincters and the ischio-anal fossae, a horseshoe-shaped region filling the majority of the anal triangle. The uro-genital triangle contains the male or female genitalia.

The anal orifice lies in the midline approximately 2–3 cm in front of and slightly below the tip of the coccyx. The anus is principally for the evacuation of faeces, but may also be an organ of sexual utility. The anal canal is the terminal portion of the large intestine and is anatomically defined as extending from the dentate line to the anal verge (Figure 111.2) [1]. The anal verge is a narrow band of tissue that separates the anal canal from perianal skin. It extends from the intersphincteric groove onto the skin surrounding the anus. It is covered by thin squamous epithelium that can be identified by the lack of hair follicles. It is marked by a sharp turn where the squamous epithelium lining the lower end of the anal canal becomes

Rook's Textbook of Dermatology, Tenth Edition. Edited by Christopher Griffiths, Jonathan Barker, Tanya Bleiker, Walayat Hussain and Rosalind Simpson.
© 2024 John Wiley & Sons Ltd. Published 2024 by John Wiley & Sons Ltd.

PART 10: SPECIFIC SITES, SEX & AGE

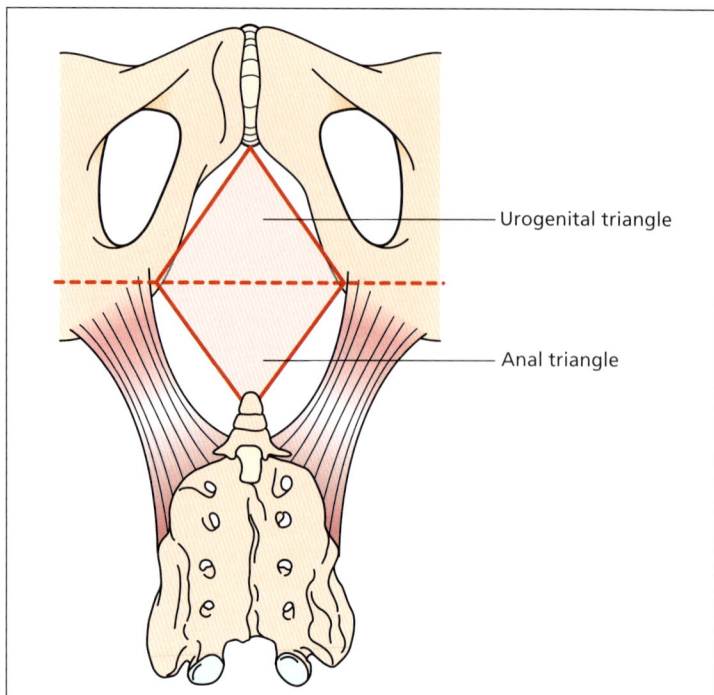

Figure 111.1 The perineum is a diamond-shaped region that lies below the pelvic floor. A transverse imaginary line drawn between the ischial tuberosities divides the perineum into an anterior urogenital triangle and posterior anal triangle. Adapted from Snell 2012 [10]. Reproduced with permission of Lippincott Williams & Wilkins/Wolters Kluwer.

Labels: Urogenital triangle; Anal triangle

somatic origin. The anal glands originate within either the internal anal sphincter or the intersphincteric plane between the internal and external anal sphincter (Figure 111.2) and open into small depressions, anal crypts, in the anal valves [2]. The ducts carry mucous from the glands to the valves. The glands are branched and lined by stratified columnar epithelium. Cystic dilatation of the glands may extend through the internal sphincter and further into the external sphincter. Infection of the anal glands is the main cause of anal sepsis, including anal abscesses.

The upper portion of the anal canal is lined by columnar epithelium similar to that of the rectum and contains secretory and absorptive cells. The columnar epithelium in the mid anal canal is thrown into 6–10 vertical folds, the anal columns. Each column contains a terminal radicle of the superior rectal artery and vein. The columns are expanded in three areas in the anal canal to form the anal cushions. The lower end of the columns form semilunar folds, called the anal valves, between which lie small recesses referred to as anal sinuses. The anal valves and sinuses together form the dentate line. The dentate line represents an important landmark because the blood supply and innervation of the anal canal transition at this point. Proximal to the dentate line, the anus is innervated by parasympathetic and sympathetic nerves with an absence of pain fibres. Distal to the dentate line, the anal canal has numerous somatic nerve endings derived from the inferior rectal nerve and is sensitive to pain, temperature, touch and pressure.

The columnar epithelial cells of the upper anal canal transition to non-keratinised squamous epithelial cells approximately 1–1.5 cm proximal to the dentate line in an area referred to as the anal transition zone. Mucosa below the dentate line lacks sweat and sebaceous glands and hair follicles. It extends to the intersphincteric groove, a depression at the lower border of the internal sphincter. The canal below the intersphincteric groove is lined by hair-bearing, keratinising, stratified epithelium that is continuous with perianal skin.

The smooth muscle of the internal anal sphincter is innervated by sympathetic and parasympathetic nerves and is in a state of tonic contraction. The striated muscle of the external anal sphincter is innervated by the inferior rectal nerve. The external anal sphincter is also in a state of tonic contraction but has a component of

continuous with the skin of the perineum (Figure 111.2). The skin of the anal verge is pigmented and is puckered due to the contraction of fibres of the conjoint longitudinal layer. Identification of the anal verge may be difficult, particularly in males in whom the perineum may funnel upwards towards the lower anal canal. The distinct border between the anal verge and perianal skin, as identified by the appearance of hair follicles and keratinising epithelium, is called the anal margin. The anal margin extends for 5 cm in circumference distal to the anal verge.

The anal canal measures approximately 2.5–5 cm in length and consists of an epithelial lining, vascular subepithelium and anal sphincters, and has a dense neuronal network of autonomic and

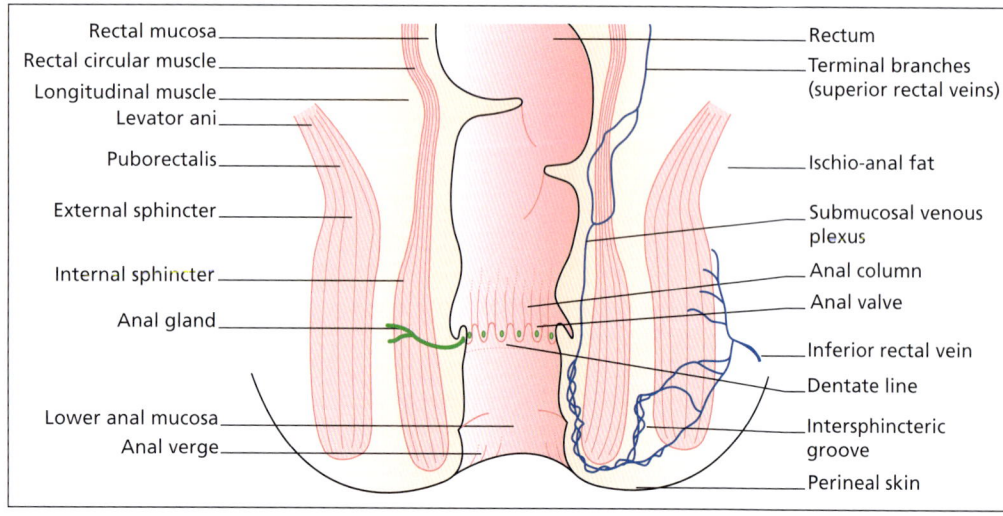

Labels: Rectal mucosa; Rectal circular muscle; Longitudinal muscle; Levator ani; Puborectalis; External sphincter; Internal sphincter; Anal gland; Lower anal mucosa; Anal verge; Rectum; Terminal branches (superior rectal veins); Ischio-anal fat; Submucosal venous plexus; Anal column; Anal valve; Inferior rectal vein; Dentate line; Intersphincteric groove; Perineal skin

Figure 111.2 Coronal section through the anal canal. From Standring 2008 [1]. Reproduced with permission of Elsevier.

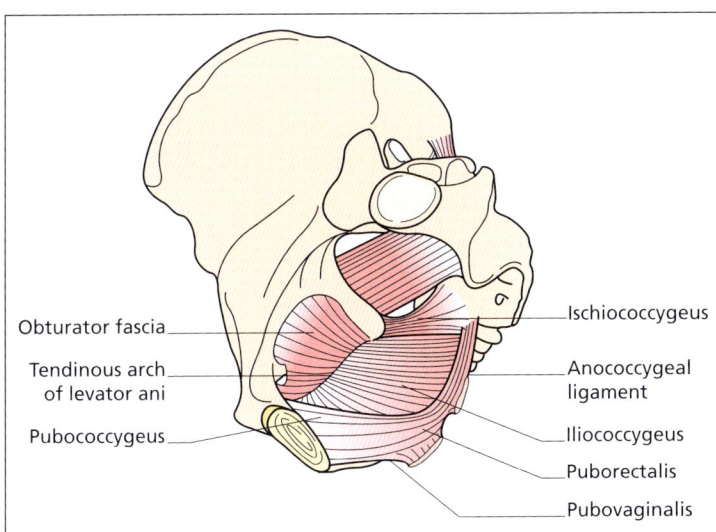

Figure 111.3 Muscles of the pelvic floor in a female. The levator ani muscle complex is composed of the ischiococcygeus, iliococcygeus and pubococcygeus muscles. The levator ani forms a large part of the pelvic floor, dividing the abdominal cavity from the perineum. From Standring 2008 [1]. Reproduced with permission of Elsevier.

voluntary control. The anal canal remains closed at rest as a result of tonic circumferential contraction of the sphincters and the presence of the anal cushions.

The ischio-anal fossa is a wedge-shaped space on each side of the anal canal filled with loose adipose tissue. The base of the wedge is formed by perianal and buttock skin. Infections, tumours and fluid collections may spread relatively freely within the ischio-anal space to the side of the anal canal and across the midline to the opposite side. The inferior rectal nerve supplies the perianal skin.

The lymphatic vessels of the perianal skin and the lower anal canal (below the dentate line) drain into inguinal lymph nodes. Lymphatic drainage above the dentate line is to the mesorectal, lateral pelvic and inferior mesenteric nodes. Lymphatic spread of malignant disease from the lower half of the anal canal is to the inguinal lymph nodes.

The deep natal cleft (gluteal cleft), the inguinal (crural) folds and the infragluteal folds are intertriginous sites because they are areas where two layers of skin come into close apposition. The natal cleft is deep and firmly fixed to the underlying fibrous and fascial tissues, and its sides are steep and closely apposed. Mucous discharges, excreta and moisture are retained easily within this cleft.

The levator ani muscle complex forms the pelvic diaphragm and divides the abdominal cavity from the perineum (Figure 111.3).

Embryogenesis of the ano-genital region

In the early embryo, the blind ending diverticulum called the allantois and the hindgut open into a common cavity called the cloaca [3]. The cloaca is partitioned into the uro-genital sinus anteriorly and the ano-rectal canal posteriorly (Figure 111.4). The anal membrane disintegrates at about 9 weeks to open into an ectodermal anal pit formed in the posterior cloacal folds. The mucosa of the upper half of the anal canal is derived from hindgut endoderm and is lined by columnar epithelium, it is innervated by autonomic nerves and the lymphatics and veins drain towards the portal system in the abdomen. The lower half of the anal canal is derived

from ectoderm, is lined by stratified squamous epithelium, has a somatic nerve supply and venous drainage is towards the external iliac system while the lymphatics drain to the inguinal lymph nodes.

Congenital and developmental abnormalities

Complete or partial failure of the anal membrane to resorb during embryogenesis can result in anal stenosis. Other congenital abnormalities resulting from defective embryogenesis of the cloacal region include imperforate anus, anal agenesis, anal duplication, perineal groove and perineal fistulae.

Dermoid cysts are ectodermal growths that occur at embryonic fusion lines. They can occur on or adjacent to the perineal raphe and sacral area.

Congenital hypertrichosis over the midline in the lumbosacral area (the faun tail) is a sign of underlying spinal dysraphism (e.g. spina bifida). Other skin lesions presenting in the sacral region that can be associated with spinal dysraphism include congenital melanocytic naevi and hamartomas.

Infantile haemangiomas may involve the perianal skin (Figure 111.5). Large perineal infantile haemangiomas may be associated with structural abnormalities including lipomyelomeningocele and imperforate anus [4].

Chordomas arise from the embryonic precursor of the axial skeleton, the notochord. They can involve the skin of the perineum, sacral area and buttocks by direct extension, recurrence or metastasis [5]. They present as single or multiple, smooth, skin-coloured, non-tender nodules. Persistent sacrococcygeal pain including coccygodynia may precede the diagnosis by many years.

Perianal keratotic plaques may occur in Olmsted syndrome [6]. Inflammatory linear verrucous epidermal naevi can affect the ano-genital region [7]. Hereditary mucoepithelial dysplasia is associated with perineal intertriginous plaques [8].

Infantile perianal pyramidal protrusion
Definition

Infantile perianal pyramidal protrusion is a rare benign perineal lesion characterised by a solitary flesh-coloured or pink-red nodular protrusion in the midline anterior to the anus. It may be present at birth or develop later in childhood, usually in association with constipation or lichen sclerosus. It is commoner in girls [9]. Differential diagnoses include haemorrhoids, skin tags, viral warts, Crohn disease, haemangiomas and sexual abuse. Lesions tend to resolve spontaneously.

PERIANAL SENSORY DISTURBANCES

Pruritus ani

Definition

This is the symptom of perianal itch or burning. Pruritus ani can be primary (idiopathic) or secondary and is not a diagnosis unless qualified as constitutional or idiopathic.

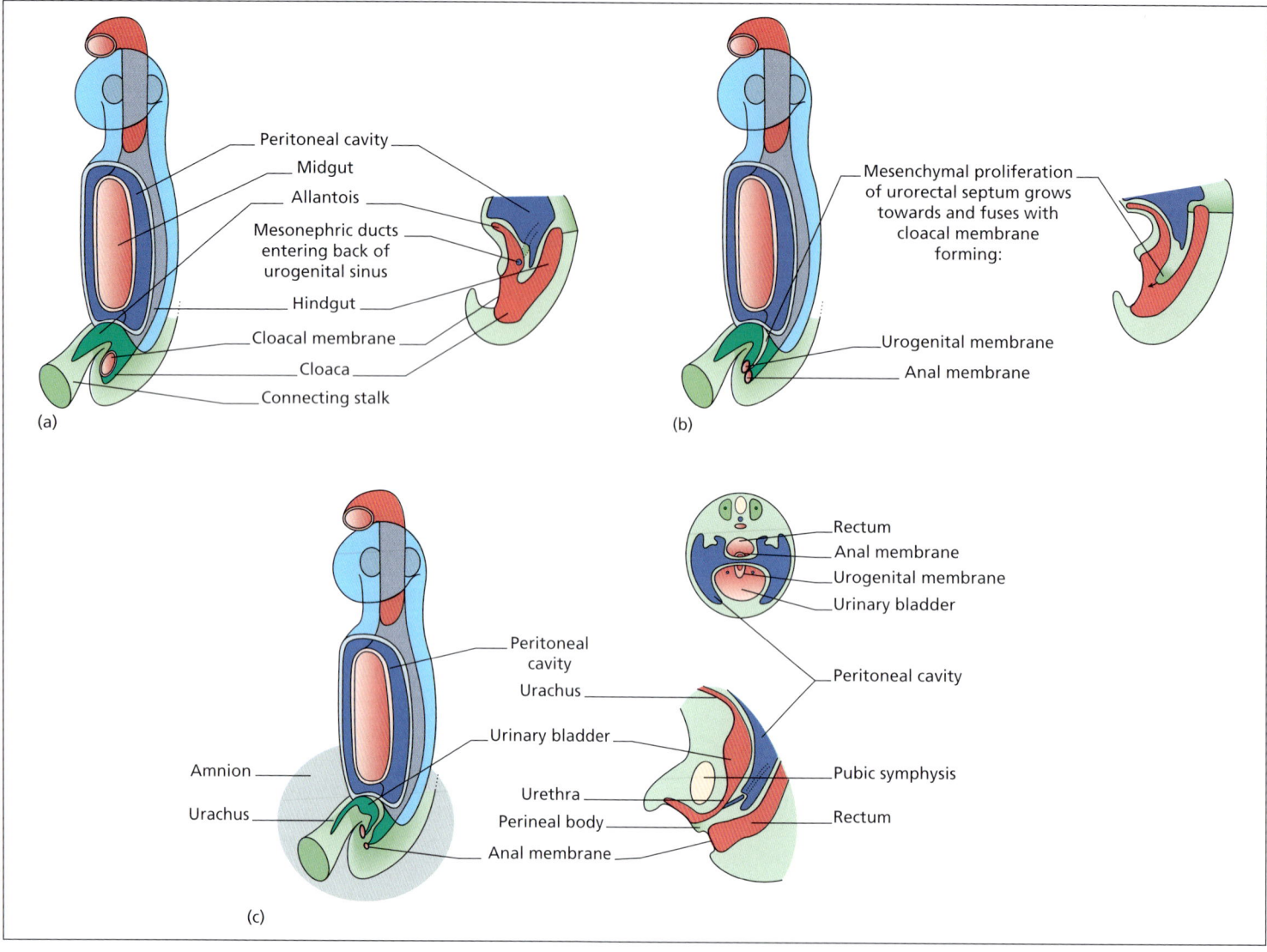

Figure 111.4 Partitioning of the cloacal membrane into the uro-genital membrane and anal membrane with the formation of the perineum occurs at 5–7 weeks' gestation. It is brought about by the separation of the cloacal portion of the hindgut by the uro-rectal septum growing caudally between the allantois anteriorly and the hindgut posteriorly to fuse with the cloacal membrane. The area of fusion becomes the perineal body and separates the dorsal anal membrane from the larger ventral uro-genital membrane. (a) Early cloaca. (b) Proliferation of the urorectal septum. (c) Separation of the urethra and the anal canal. From Standring 2008 **[1]**. Reproduced with permission of Elsevier.

Introduction and general description

The symptom of pruritus ani has many causes. Management requires detailed assessment to determine whether there is an underlying cause. Pruritus ani can be associated with most forms of ano-rectal disease or perianal skin disease. Typically, an itch–scratch cycle develops irrespective of the underlying cause. Management strategy involves breaking the itch–scratch cycle.

Pruritus ani is considered idiopathic when no dermatological or ano-rectal cause can be found. Idiopathic pruritus ani is responsible for 50–90% of all cases of pruritus ani [1]. The pathogenesis of idiopathic pruritus ani is thought to be primarily the consequence of faecal contamination or possibly the intake of certain food or drinks. The discussion here primarily deals with idiopathic pruritus ani. See Box 111.1 for secondary causes.

Box 111.1 Secondary causes of pruritus ani

Inflammatory skin disease
- Endogenous eczema including seborrhoeic and atopic
- Allergic or irritant contact dermatitis
- Psoriasis
- Lichen planus
- Urticaria
- Lichen sclerosus (almost always females)
- Hidradenitis suppurativa

Infections
- Candidiasis and dermatophytes
- Erythrasma (*Corynebacterium minutissimum*)
- *Staphylococcus aureus*, β-haemolytic streptococci
- Gonorrhoea, syphilis

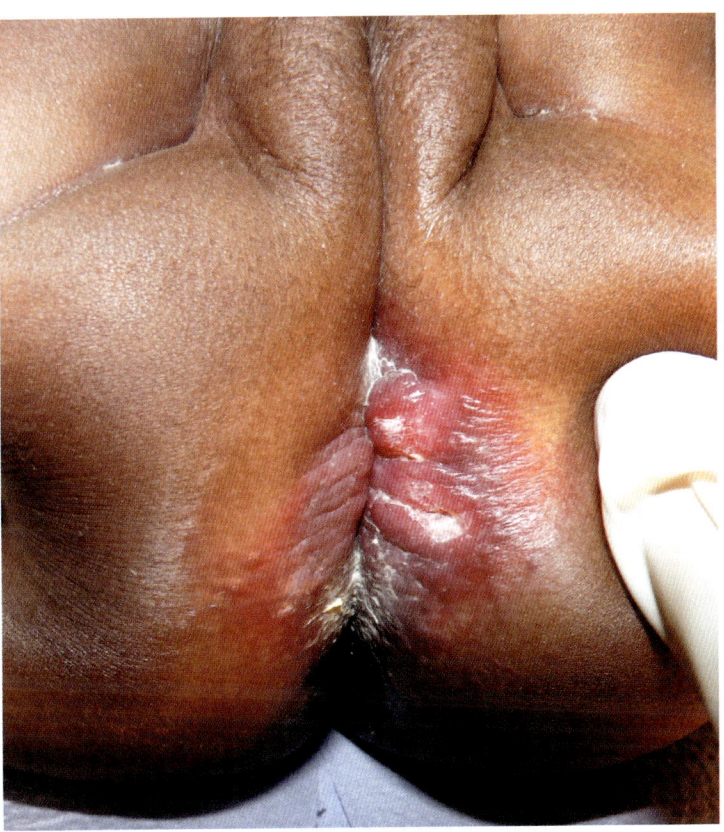

Figure 111.5 A 4-month-old female child with a perianal infantile haemangioma.

- Human papillomavirus, herpes simplex virus
- Human immunodeficiency virus

Infestations
- Threadworms (*Enterobius vermicularis*)
- Pubic lice (*Phthiriasis pubis*)

Perianal premalignant or malignant disease
- Anal intraepithelial neoplasia, anal carcinoma
- Extramammary Paget disease

Ano-rectal disease
- Haemorrhoids, anal fissure
- Perianal fistula, perianal abscess
- Inflammatory bowel disease

Systemic disease
- Metabolic including diabetes, renal, thyroid and liver disease
- Iron deficiency anaemia
- Malignancy including leukaemia and lymphoma
- May be psychoneurogenic/secondary to a psychiatric disorder

Epidemiology
Incidence and prevalence
It affects 1–5% of the general population [2].

Age
It most commonly presents in the fourth to sixth decade.

Sex
It is four times commoner in men than women.

Ethnicity
It is commoner in middle-aged white males [2].

Pathophysiology
Predisposing factors
The common factor linking most cases of idiopathic pruritus ani is faecal contamination. Faeces contain potential irritants and allergens, demonstrated by positive skin patch tests to autologous faeces and enzymes of bacterial origin that are capable of inducing itch and inflammation. Patients with idiopathic pruritus ani have a high incidence of loose stools and are rarely constipated. Patients with a colostomy do not suffer from pruritus ani. Any factor that increases faecal contamination exposes perianal skin to irritants. A sedentary lifestyle has been implicated.

Causes of faecal contamination include the following (more than one factor may be operative):
1 Difficulty cleaning the perianal area:
  - Obesity leads to poor ventilation and maceration.
  - Anatomical factors including deeply placed 'funnel anus' and hirsutism can cause mechanical problems in the maintenance of hygiene.
2 Anal leakage:
  - Local causes that alter anal morphology or function such as haemorrhoids, perianal tags or fissures can lead to anal incontinence.
  - Primary anal sphincter dysfunction. Exaggerated recto-anal inhibitory reflex and anal sphincter dysfunction may result in faecal soiling. Caffeine can lower anal resting pressure.
3 Loose frequent stools. These will cause faecal soiling and an increase in perianal trauma from frequent wiping of the skin. Underlying conditions include irritable bowel syndrome.
4 Flatulence. Leads to aerosolised delivery of faecal irritant material to perianal skin.

Other contributing factors include the following:
1 Food and drink. The role of food and drinks is uncertain but coffee, tea, cola, alcohol, chocolate, tomatoes, spices and citrus fruits are implicated. The mechanisms proposed include effects on anal sphincter tone, production of loose stools and undigested food components irritating or sensitising the perianal skin.
2 Psychological factors. Idiopathic pruritus ani has been attributed to stress and anxiety. Patients may be tense individuals in whom everyday problems induce a profound colonic reflex, with diarrhoea subtype irritable bowel syndrome, which may result in defecation and soiling.

Clinical features
History
The complaint is of itching, stinging or soreness that may be chronic and recurrent. Symptoms may be triggered by a bowel movement or wiping with toilet paper, but may occur at night when the patient is asleep.

Presentation
Physical signs include redness, excoriations, abrasions and lichenification which result from the effects of rubbing and scratching (Figure 111.6), secondary infection or contact dermatitis. There may be no visible abnormality at the time of examination.

PART 10: SPECIFIC SITES, SEX & AGE

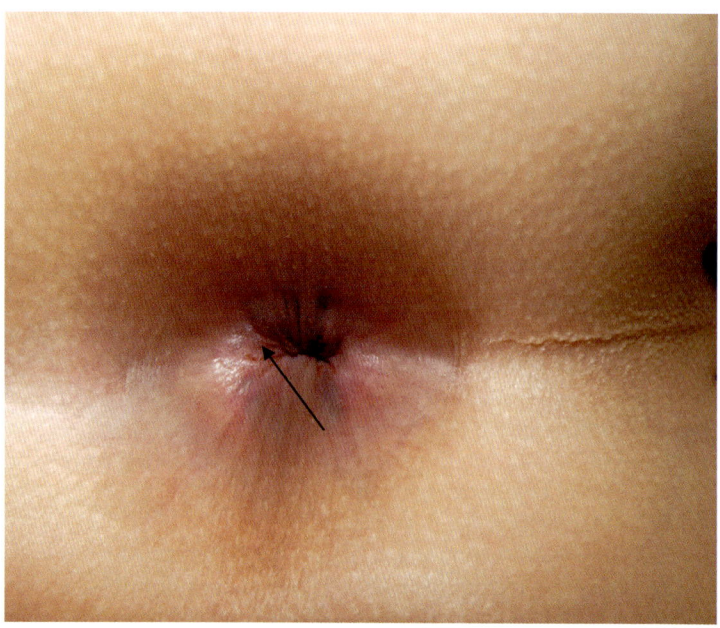

Figure 111.6 Excoriations and lichenification (arrow) secondary to idiopathic pruritus ani in a 6-year-old boy. It is important to exclude threadworms at this age.

Differential diagnosis

Fungal infection often causes intense pruritus, and diabetes must be excluded in all severe or persistent candidal infection. See Box 111.1 for other secondary causes.

Complications and co-morbidities

Lichenification, excoriations and secondary infection can occur. A contact irritant or allergic dermatitis can result from overwashing and treatment. Patients with pruritus ani are at high risk of sensitisation from topical medicaments, toiletries and wet tissue wipes. Chronic pruritus ani can lead to disruption in quality of life, irritability and depression [3].

Disease course and prognosis

Generic measures usually improve symptoms in 90% of patients [2]. Many patients who undergo surgery for potentially implicated causes such as haemorrhoids continue to have symptoms.

Investigations

In the young, threadworms should be sought with the Sellotape test or by stool examination. Skin patch testing should be considered at an early stage to assess for contact allergy. Common allergens include fragrance, topical anaesthetics, topical antifungals (e.g. neomycin), topical antibiotics, methylisothiazolinone [4] and rarely topical steroids [5].

Management

Specific secondary causes should be addressed. Clear explanation is helpful. The aim of management should be to break the itch–scratch cycle. Management includes attention to the patient's washing habits. It is important to maintain cleanliness and to ensure that the perianal area is dried after washing. Soap substitutes should be used and shampoo residues washed off. An emollient should be applied after each wash. A barrier preparation can be preapplied to the perianal skin before the bowels are opened. Washing perianal skin after defecation is preferable to wiping with toilet paper. Rubbing with toilet paper should be discouraged and dabbing recommended. Premoistened toilet paper or wet wipes should be avoided. Underwear should be loose and preferably made of cotton. Topical anaesthetic preparations should be avoided as sensitisation commonly occurs. Fingernails should be kept short.

A reduction of coffee consumption or elimination of food or drinks implicated may help. A high-fibre diet should be encouraged if there is any history of constipation or haemorrhoids and, conversely, a lower-fibre diet if diarrhoea is a feature.

Referral to a colorectal specialist is indicated if ano-rectal disease is suspected. Haemorrhoidectomy or excision of prominent skin tags may enable better perianal hygiene and lead to improvement in symptoms.

First line

The aim of treatment is to break the compulsive itch–scratch cycle. Habit reversal behavioural techniques are desirable. Local applications should be soothing and as mild as possible. Use of a twice daily liquid cleanser can be as effective as twice daily potent topical steroid application [6]. Mild steroid ointments (1% hydrocortisone) can be helpful [7] and these can be combined with antibacterials or antifungals. Caution should be exercised with topical steroids because perianal skin is occluded and atrophy may occur, although in practice, short courses of potent topical steroids are often helpful.

Second line

Other treatments that have been advocated include zinc paste with 1–2% phenol, 0.006% capsaicin ointment [8], 0.1% tacrolimus ointment [9], oral antihistamines, intralesional corticosteroids and corticosteroid suppositories.

Third line

Successful treatment of refractory idiopathic pruritus ani with intradermal injection of 1% methylene blue in combination with 1% lidocaine has been reported. Samalavicius *et al.* reported a high symptom improvement rate with low recurrence rate in patients with idiopathic pruritus ani [10]. The intradermal injections were administered after saddle block anaesthesia. Cryotherapy has also been used.

Perineal and perianal pain

Functional ano-rectal pain occurs in the absence of any underlying discernable organic disease. Functional disorders of the perineum causing pain include proctalgia fugax, levator ani syndrome and idiopathic coccygodynia [1], and may be part of the pelvic pain syndrome (Chapter 82).

Proctalgia fugax is characterised by severe, self-limiting, fleeting, episodic ano-rectal pain. Attacks tend to be infrequent, averaging once monthly [2]. Sudden-onset cramp-like pain occurs and lasts from a few seconds up to 20 min. Patients usually cannot identify any triggers. The prevalence is 4–18% and it is commoner in females [3]. The pathogenesis is unknown but may be due to spasm of the internal anal sphincter or compression of the pudendal nerve.

Chronic proctalgia (chronic idiopathic anal pain) can be defined as chronic or recurrent episodes of ano-rectal pain lasting more than 20 min in the absence of organic cause. Levator ani syndrome causes recurrent or persistent pain, pressure or discomfort in the perineal region and is commoner in females [4]. It is thought to be due to spasm of the levator ani muscles. Digital rectal examination distinguishes between levator ani syndrome and unspecified functional ano-rectal pain. Tenderness occurs on palpation of the puborectalis muscle in levator ani syndrome but not in patients with unspecified functional ano-rectal pain.

Coccygodynia is the symptom of pain in and around the coccyx. It is usually precipitated by prolonged sitting and rising from the seated position. Idiopathic coccygodynia is commoner in females and is associated with obesity. Secondary causes of coccygodynia include trauma, arthritis or rare tumours such as chordoma, intradural schwannoma, perineural cyst or intraosseous lipoma [5].

Descending perineum syndrome is commoner in females and is associated with multiparity. Clinical features include poorly localised deep perineal discomfort, faecal incontinence, constipation, rectal prolapse and perineal descent [6].

Precipitating factors of pain in chronic pain syndromes include sitting, defecation and psychological stress. Treatment is usually unnecessary for the transient symptoms of proctalgia fugax. Treatment options for chronic pain include analgesia, biofeedback, sitz baths, tricyclic antidepressants, botulinum toxin injections and sacral nerve stimulation (Chapter 82). Coccygectomy has been advocated for refractory coccygodynia [7].

Perianal trauma and pressure sores

Definition

Trauma includes accidental, self-induced or iatrogenic injury, as well as sexual abuse.

Introduction and general description

Anal, perianal and perineal trauma is not uncommon. Trauma can lead to anal stenosis.

Clinical variants

Pressure sores (synonym decubitus sores) due to tissue damage caused by sustained pressure are common and in most cases are preventable [1]. Reported prevalence rates range from 4.7% to 32% in hospital populations, and 22% in nursing homes [2]. The most common locations in adults are over the bony prominences of the sacral or hip region [1]. Sustained pressure over a bony prominence leads to tissue ischaemia and necrosis. Risk factors include neurological or cognitive impairment, diabetes and congestive cardiac failure. A persistent patch of non-blanchable red skin on the sacral or ischial region is a sign of impending ulceration. Oedema, induration or pain may also be present. Progression to ulceration can be prevented if this early stage is identified promptly [3]. Risk assessment tools have been developed to identify individuals at risk.

Dermatologists should be able to recognise early changes that occur before skin breakdown and to identify the different stages of ulceration to prevent delay in appropriate care [3]. Management of pressure ulcers includes pressure relief, assessment of nutritional status, wound care including managing infection and consideration of surgical techniques including debridement [4]. Squamous cell carcinoma (SCC) is a rare complication of pressure ulcers occurring in 0.5% of cases.

Clinical signs of perianal and anal trauma following sexual abuse in children include gaping of the anus and anal fissures [5]. Perianal skin diseases can be mistaken for sexual abuse, including lichen sclerosus and perianal *Streptococcus* infection. The presence of definitive skin disease does not exclude sexual abuse.

Obstetric perineal trauma is sustained in more than 85% of women during vaginal delivery in the UK and up to 69% will require sutures [6]. Injury may occur spontaneously or be iatrogenic (Figure 111.7). Prevalence is dependent on variations in obstetric practice. Prospective studies using endoanal ultrasound scanning

PART 10: SPECIFIC SITES, SEX & AGE

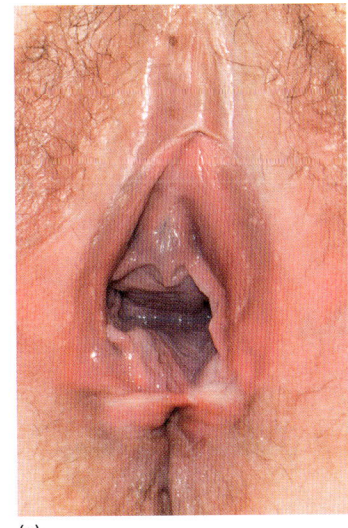
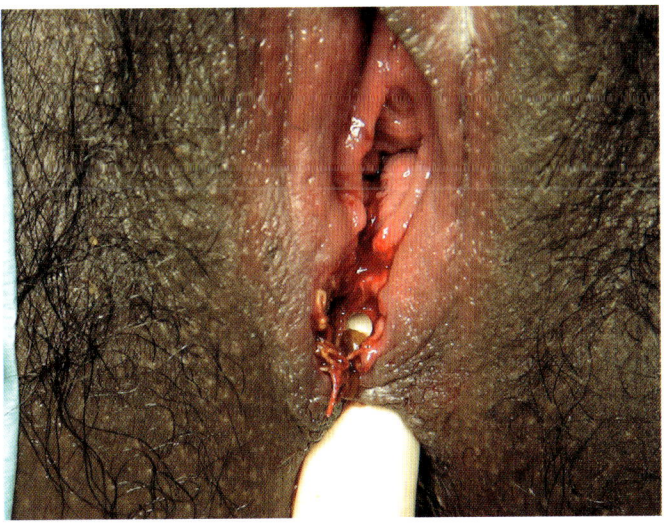

Figure 111.7 Obstetric perineal trauma. (a) Cloacal-like defect following a missed third-degree tear. The perineal body is absent and there is minimal tissue separating the anus from the vagina. (b) Breakdown of a wound following the repair of a fourth-degree tear has occurred, leading to a recto-vaginal fistula. Suture threads from the perineal tear closure are visible. Courtesy of Mr A. Sultan, Department of Obstetrics and Gynaecology, Croydon University Hospital, UK.   (a)   (b)

Table 111.1 Classification of obstetric perineal trauma.

Degree of trauma	Definition
First degree	Laceration of vaginal mucosa or perineal skin only
Second degree	Involvement of perineal muscles but not anal sphincter
Third degree	Disruption of anal sphincter muscles:
	3a: <50% of external anal sphincter torn
	3b: >50% of external anal sphincter torn
	3c: internal anal sphincter also torn
Fourth degree	Third-degree tear with disruption of anal epithelium

Adapted from [5].

have identified that occult anal sphincter injury is common [6]. See Table 111.1 for a classification of obstetric trauma [7].

INFLAMMATORY DERMATOSES

SUPERFICIAL INFLAMMATORY DERMATOSES

The microenvironment of the ano-genital and genito-crural region may alter the usual morphology of skin conditions easily recognised elsewhere. Skin disease may take on a vegetating appearance, especially in hot humid climates and in the presence of infection (Figure 111.8). Specific inflammatory dermatoses that commonly affect the perineum and perianal region are briefly described. The reader is referred to detailed description of specific diseases in relevant chapters.

In adults, inflammation may result from the coexistence of several factors such as haemorrhoids, anal discharge and the effects of scratching. In all cases of perianal and perineal inflammation, the urine should be tested for glucose, and swabs and scrapings tested for organisms. Inflammatory skin conditions can cause diagnostic difficulties because clinical features may be altered by the perianal microenvironment. Macerations and erosions can be a feature as demonstrated by the case of pemphigus foliaceus (Figure 111.8) and flexural psoriasis (Figure 111.9).

Seborrhoeic dermatitis. This causes a brownish-red inflammation with large greasy scales towards the edge, extending beyond and outside the natal cleft (Figure 111.10). Other areas may be involved including the scalp and other flexures.

Psoriasis. Psoriasis has a smooth glazed surface, dull red hue and is often fissured (Figure 111.9). Other signs of the disease are usually present including scalp and nail changes.

Lichen simplex. This simulates psoriasis but is usually unilateral, except when it involves the perianal area. It may occur as a small, intensely irritable area, localised to the edge of the anus.

Fungal infection. This should be suspected, particularly if there has been prior use of topical corticosteroids.

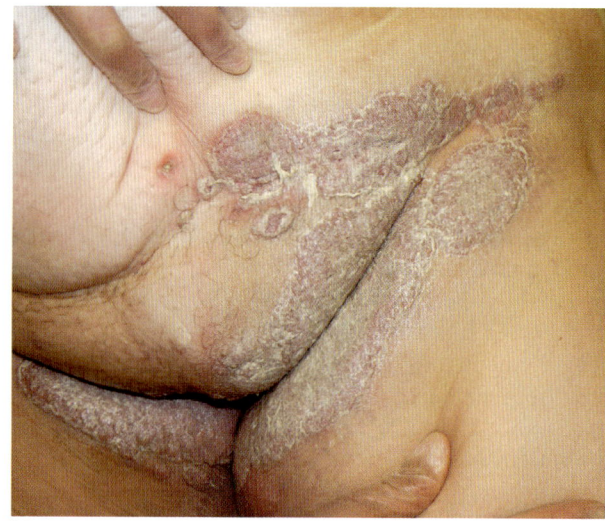

(a)

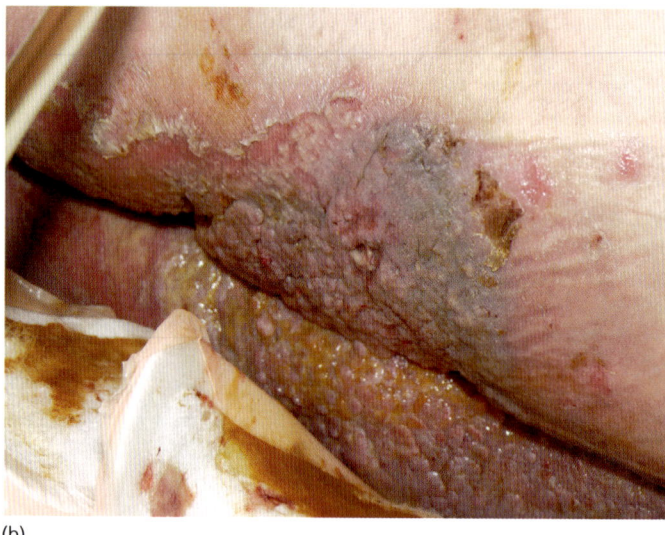

(b)

Figure 111.8 Vegetative pemphigus foliaceous. (a) Affecting the genito-crural region and lower abdomen. (b) Affecting the perianal region and buttocks in the same patient.

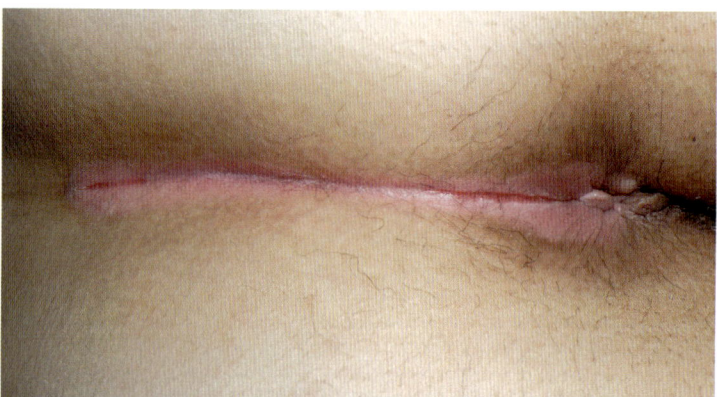

Figure 111.9 Perianal and natal cleft psoriasis causing fissures in a 42-year-old woman.

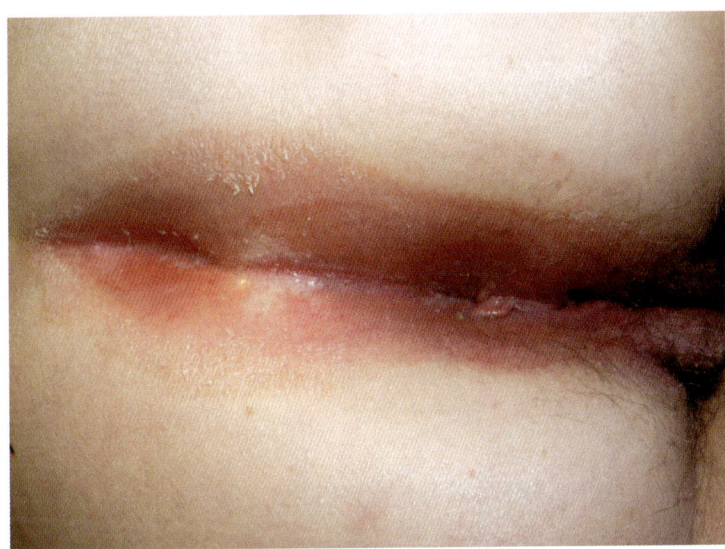

Figure 111.10 Seborrhoeic dermatitis affecting the natal cleft and perianal skin.

Irritant contact dermatitis. Perineal dermatitis can commonly arise as a result of contact with urine or faeces. Common chemical irritants include alcohol and detergents. Danthron redness is a form of irritant contact dermatitis caused by the use of laxatives containing danthron.

Lichen sclerosus. This extends from the vulval skin to the perianal skin in 30% of women, producing a typical figure-of-eight distribution (Figure 111.12). Perianal lichen sclerosus occurs in 30% of women with genital lichen sclerosus and its occurrence has been associated with urinary incontinence [3]. This pattern reflects the areas of ano-genital skin that come into contact with urine. Men rarely if ever have perianal lichen sclerosus, probably because the male perineum is rarely exposed to urine [4]. The development of perineal lichen sclerosus on previously healthy perineal skin has been described in men following perineal urethrostomy for anterior urethral stricture [5]. It is possible that chronic occluded contact of urine with susceptible epithelium is involved in the pathogenesis

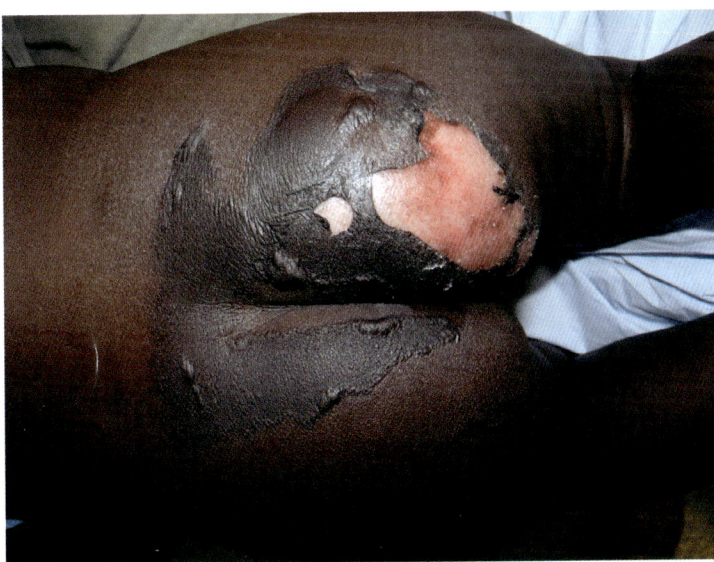

Figure 111.11 Contact dermatitis causing blistering in an infant due to the use of wet wipes containing methylisothiazolinone.

Allergic contact dermatitis. Allergic contact dermatitis is caused by a type IV immune response to specific allergens. It can lead to markedly inflamed perianal skin and may have an ill-defined spreading border. Blistering may occur (Figure 111.11). Patients with chronic perianal dermatoses are at a higher risk of developing sensitisation to topical medicaments than patients with genital dermatoses [1]. Skin patch testing is required to determine what specific allergens are implicated. Common contact allergens in the ano-genital region include neomycin, fragrance and Balsam of Peru. Methylisothiazolinone, a preservative that can be present in household items including wet wipes, cosmetics, toiletries and detergents, is a common cause of allergy in patients presenting with perineal eczema [2]. Carers may present with a hand dermatitis. Condom or spermicide allergy may develop in those practising anoreceptive sex.

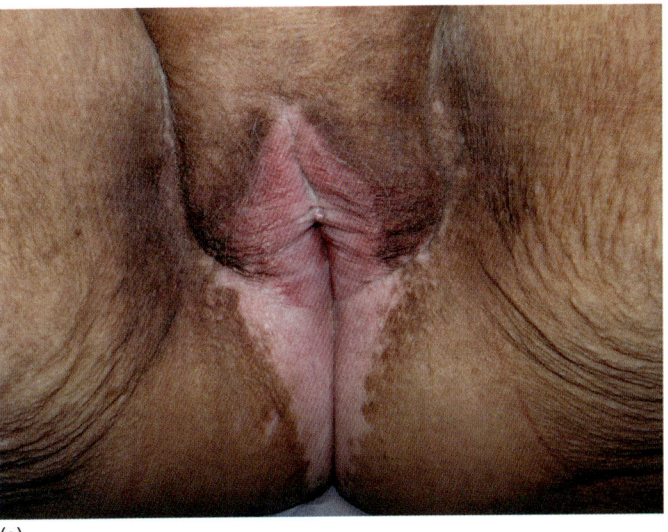

(a)

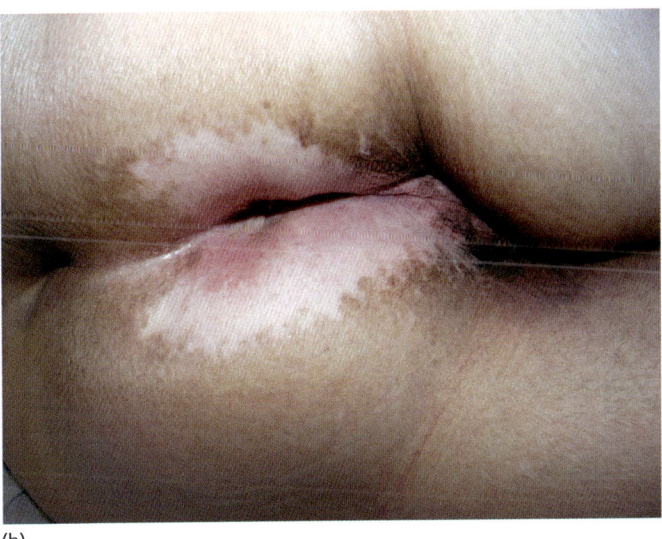

(b)

Figure 111.12 Lichen sclerosus. (a) Ano-genital lichen sclerosus in a female in a typical figure-of-eight configuration. (b) Perianal lichen sclerosus.

of ano-genital lichen sclerosus. The barrier function of wet skin is diminished and it is more permeable to irritants. In addition, wet skin has an increased frictional coefficient and higher microbial content [5].

Lichen planus. Lichen planus affecting the perianal region is typically very pruritic and may become excoriated or hypertrophic. Solitary involvement of the perianal region may occur (Figure 111.13).

Hailey–Hailey disease (Chapter 64). Heat, friction, infection and contact dermatitis can predispose to exacerbations in the ano-genital region (Figure 111.14). It is frequently misdiagnosed as other skin diseases such as seborrhoeic dermatitis. Histology and negative direct immunofluorescence are required to confirm the diagnosis.

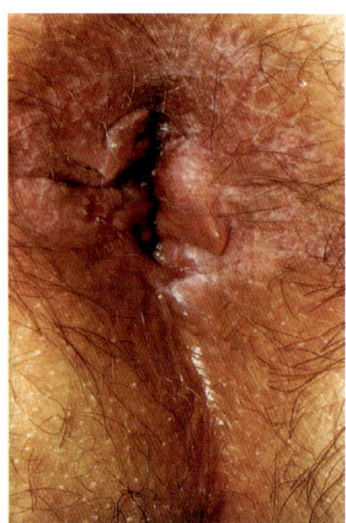

Figure 111.13 Perianal lichen planus showing Wickham's striae. Courtesy of Dr F. Ive, Durham, UK.

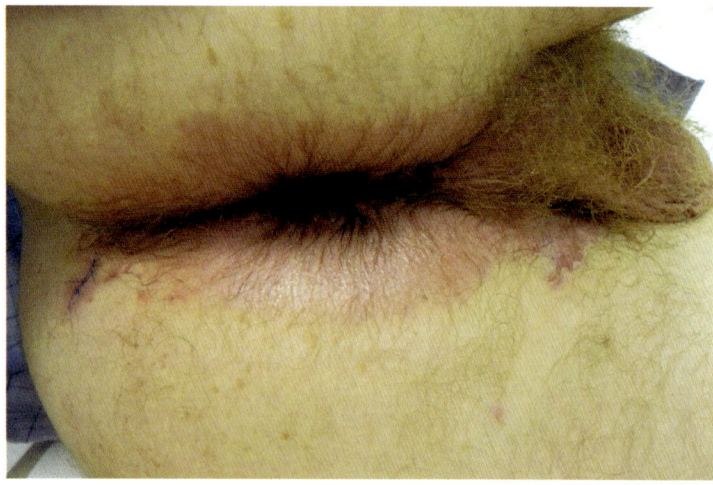

Figure 111.14 Hailey–Hailey disease affecting the ano-genital region and causing inflammation and superficial blistering. A skin biopsy has been taken for histology and direct immunofluorescence.

Acrodermatitis enteropathica (Chapter 61). This should be considered in the differential diagnosis of perianal inflammation in children or adults resulting from malnutrition or malabsorption.

Cicatricial pemphigoid and Stevens–Johnson syndrome (Chapters 12 and 50). These may cause perianal inflammation, ulceration and scarring and lead to anal stenosis.

Behçet disease (Chapter 48). Behçet disease can present with multiple shallow ulcers and fissures of the anal margin.

Radiodermatitis (Chapter 109). This may be encountered following treatment for anal carcinoma.

DEEP INFLAMMATORY DERMATOSES

Hidradenitis suppurativa

Definition and nomenclature
Hidradenitis suppurativa is a chronic, follicular, occlusive, inflammatory skin disease that affects the hair follicles in apocrine gland-bearing skin of the axillae, ano-genital and perianal region, buttocks, groin and inframammary region. It is characterised by recurrent abscesses, sinuses and scarring (Chapter 90).

Synonyms and inclusions
- Acne inversa
- Verneuil disease
- Chronic perianal proderma

Introduction and general description
It is characterised by recurrent, painful, deep-seated nodules and abscesses that progress to the development of bridged comedomes, sinus tracts and scars. It typically affects the ano-genital region in men and the axillae in women. Follicular occlusion is the primary event followed by inflammation of the apocrine gland.

Epidemiology
Incidence and prevalence
Prevalence is up to 4% [1].

Age
The average age of onset is the early twenties. Peak prevalence is in the fourth decade and declines with age [2].

Sex
There is a female to male ratio of 3 : 1.

Ethnicity
It is commoner in Afro-Caribbean people [3].

Associated diseases
These include other follicular occlusive disorders that form the follicular occlusion tetrad, namely acne conglobata, dissecting

cellulitis of the scalp and sacrococcygeal pilonidal sinus disease. Other disease associations include inflammatory bowel disease, pyoderma gangrenosum, spondyloarthropathies and non-melanoma skin carcinoma.

Pathophysiology
Predisposing factors
These include obesity, smoking, friction and pressure.

Pathology
Features include infundibular plugging, follicular hyperplasia, ductal hyperkeratosis, chronic inflammation, abscess formation, sinus tract formation, fibrosis and scarring.

Genetics
There may be a positive family history in 30–40% of cases. It is associated with an autosomal dominant pattern of inheritance with variable penetrance.

Clinical features
History
There is usually a history of painful recurring lumps with a discharge that is often malodourous and blood stained. Quality of life can be severely affected; activities such as sitting, walking and defecation can be impaired.

Presentation
There is a clinical spectrum overlapping with chronic furunculosis (Figure 111.15) through to severe disease. Mild or localised forms are frequently misdiagnosed as furunculosis or infected cysts. Recurrent deep-seated nodules occur at the same site.

Groin disease is common (Figure 111.16a). Women are more likely to have upper torso and axillary involvement (Figure 111.16b), while men are more likely to have perineal or perianal disease (Figure 111.17). In established hidradenitis suppurativa, fluctuant abscesses, bridged comedomes and deep, burrowing, discharging sinuses occur as well as scarring, including keloid scars

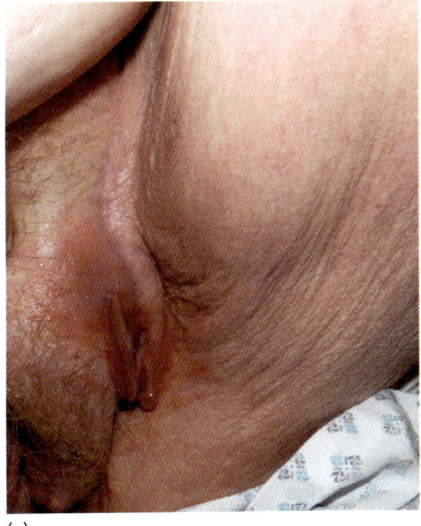

(a)

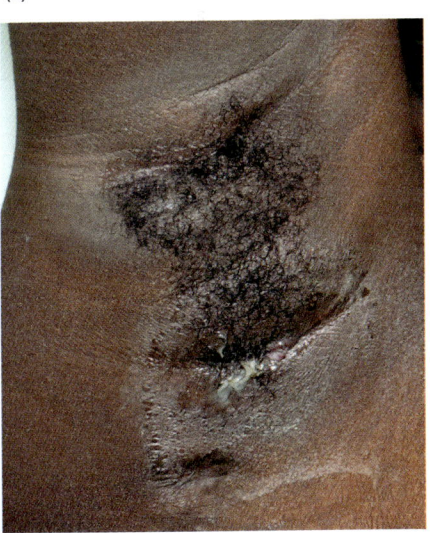

(b)

Figure 111.16 Hurley stage II hidradenitis suppurativa. (a) Affecting the groin of a female causing sinus track formation and scarring. (b) Affecting the axilla of a female causing sinus track formation and scarring.

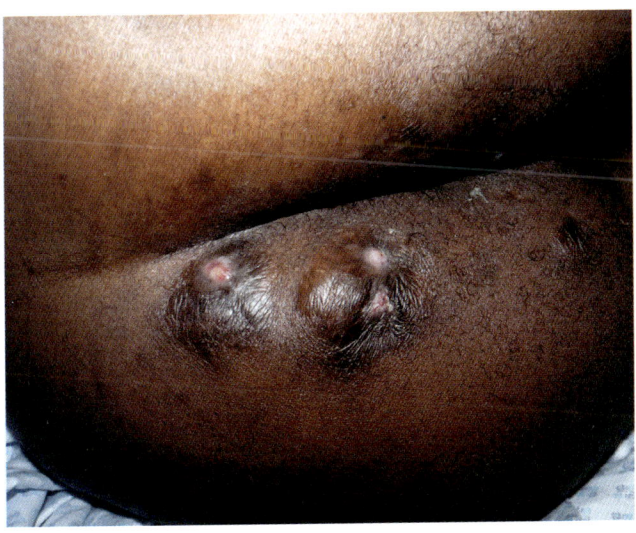

Figure 111.15 Hurley stage I hidradenitis suppurativa presenting as chronic furunculosis on the buttocks.

(Figure 111.17a). Men tend to have more severe disease and a history of severe acne [4]. Inflammation can invade fat and extend widely over the buttocks and thighs (Figure 111.17b). Persistent perineal sinuses are frequent and deep-seated lesions may lead to anal fistulae.

Differential diagnosis
Crohn disease can coexist with and may simulate hidradenitis suppurativa. Acne conglobata, pyoderma gangrenosum, lymphogranuloma venereum, developmental fistulae and chloracne should all be considered.

Classification of severity
The Hurley staging system can be used (Table 111.2) [5]. Males and smokers are more likely to have higher stage disease severity [2,4].

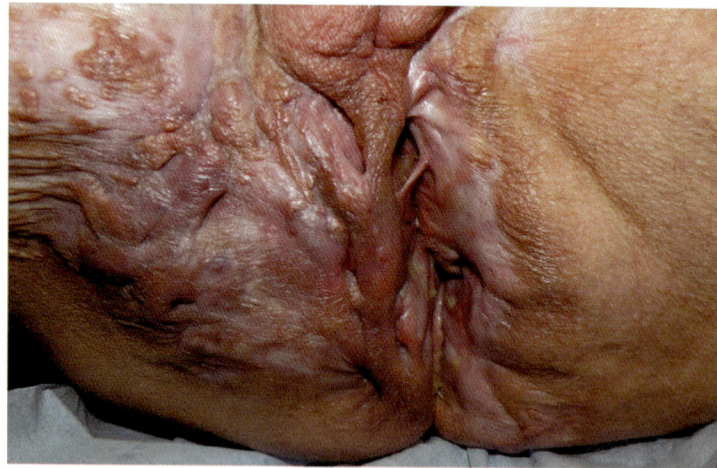

(a)

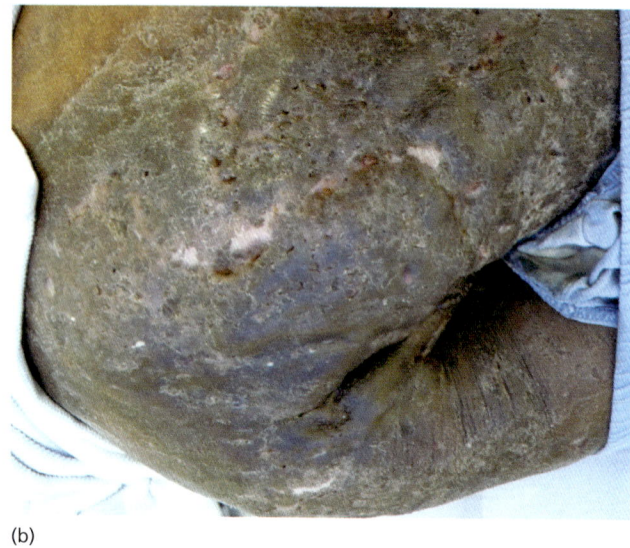

(b)

Figure 111.17 Hurley stage III severe hidradenitis suppurativa. (a) Affecting the perineum and causing extensive keloid scar formation in a 75-year-old male patient. (b) Affecting the buttocks and thighs causing extensive sinus formation and scarring.

Complications and co-morbidities

Secondary bacterial infection including with streptococci or staphylococci may occur. Complications of severe disease include anaemia, development of malignancy such as SCC, genital lymphoedema, contractures and reactive arthritis. Other conditions that are also part of the follicular occlusion tetrad are acne conglobata, pilonidal cyst and dissecting cellulitis of the scalp, which may co-exist with hidradenitis suppurativa.

Disease course and prognosis

The disease course is chronic and recurrent. Prevalence decreases with age.

Investigations

Swabs should be taken for bacterial culture.

Management

Hidradenitis suppurativa can be a difficult and recalcitrant condition to treat. A combination of different treatment modalities is often required.

Table 111.2 Hurley severity stages.

Stage	Definition
Stage I	Solitary or multiple abscesses occurring without formation of sinus tracks or scarring
Stage II	Recurrent abscesses with sinus track formation and scarring occurring within an anatomical region but separated by areas of normal skin
Stage III	Confluent involvement of an entire anatomical region with multiple interconnected abscesses, nodules, sinus tracks and scarring

Adapted from [5].

First line

Topical antibiotics and long-term combination oral antibiotic therapy should be used. The combination of rifampicin and clindamycin can be an effective treatment. The mode of action of antibiotics is likely to be mainly anti-inflammatory rather than bactericidal in nature. Oral antibiotic therapy is seldom of lasting value, although the elimination of specific secondary infection organisms such as *Streptococcus milleri* may be effective.

Small localised sinuses may be phenolised successfully, and early lesions may respond to intralesional corticosteroids. Surgical and laser therapy are useful adjuncts for early disease. Marsupialisation and diathermy of the affected tissue have been successful in some cases. Wide local excision for severe disease has been advocated [6]. Disease recurrence rates are high.

Second line

Oral retinoids have been used with mixed results [7].

Third line

Biologic drugs such as infliximab and adalimumab have been shown to be effective [7].

Resources

Further information

Hidradenitis Suppurativa Foundation: https://www.hs-foundation.org (last accessed June 2022).

DRUG REACTIONS

Fixed drug eruption. Fixed drug eruptions may produce striking pigmentation.

Cutaneous atrophy. Prolonged use of potent or superpotent topical steroids can cause dusky redness, telangiectasiae, atrophy and induration. Acneiform lesions and comedones may occur.

Perianal contact dermatitis. Topical treatments such as imiquimod or 5-fluorouracil cream may cause a contact dermatitis that can be irritant or allergic in nature (Figure 111.18).

Perianal ulceration. Painful perianal ulceration is a well-recognised complication of nicorandil (Figure 111.19). Complications include

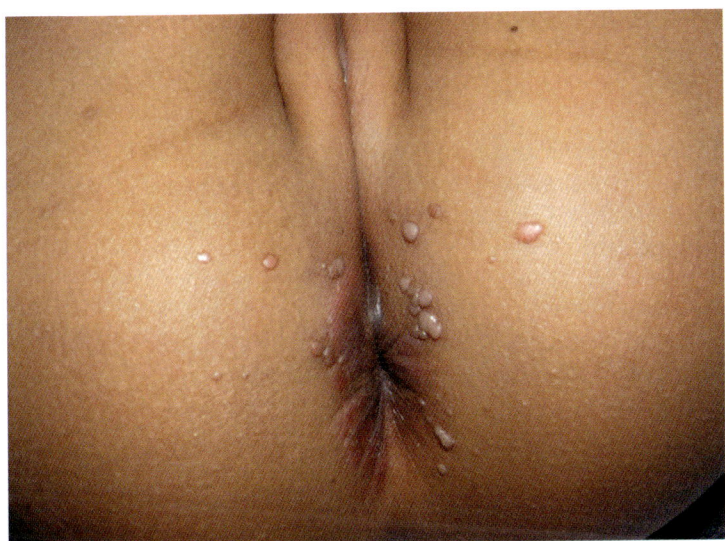

Figure 111.18 Perianal contact dermatitis caused by imiquimod cream used to treat perianal molluscum contagiosum.

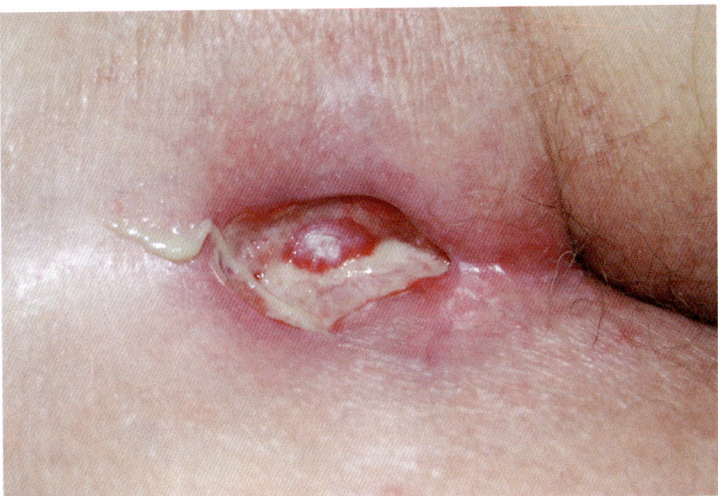

Figure 111.19 Perianal ulceration due to nicorandil. Courtesy of Dr S. Baron and Dr E. Kulakov, Kent, UK.

infection and fistula formation. Ulceration may commence shortly after starting treatment or years after treatment is commenced. The pathogenesis is unknown. The drug should be withdrawn. Oral isotretinoin can lead to vulnerability to mucocutaneous injury due to frictional forces including in genital and perianal skin [1].

INFECTIONS

BACTERIAL INFECTIONS

Folliculitis and furunculosis

Definition and nomenclature

Folliculitis is a superficial inflammatory or infective process occurring in the hair follicle. Furunculosis is a deep infection of the hair follicle and can lead to abscess formation and is usually caused by *Staphylococcus aureus*.

> **Synonyms and inclusions**
> • Boils

Introduction and general description

The ano-genital area, particularly the buttocks and thighs of men, can be susceptible to infection particularly with *S. aureus*. Severe involvement with furunculosis and abscesses suggests an overlap with hidradenitis suppurativa.

Epidemiology

Incidence and prevalence

These infections are common.

Age

All age groups are affected.

Sex

Both sexes are affected equally.

Associated diseases

Diabetes, immunodeficiency, anaemia and atopic eczema are all associated. Eosinophic folliculitis is associated with immunosuppression, including HIV infection [1].

Pathophysiology

Predisposing factors

The high temperature and humidity of the ano-genital area, combined with pressure and friction, encourage colonisation with *S. aureus*. Poor personal hygiene, hyperhidrosis, obesity, anaemia, family history and skin conditions such as atopic eczema are also predisposing factors. Nasal carriage of *S. aureus* is the primary risk factor for recurrent furunculosis and occurs in 60% of individuals [2]. Recurrent furunculosis may be a manifestation of underlying immunodeficiency including HIV infection, diabetes and malnutrition. Neutrophil dysfunction may contribute to recurrent furunculosis including iron deficiency-associated reduction in myeloperoxidase activity [3].

Folliculitis is a side effect of drugs including epidermal growth factor receptor inhibitors (e.g. cetuximab).

Pathology

An inflammatory infiltrate occurs within the follicle and may rupture through the follicular epithelium. Organisms may be identified within the follicle.

Causative organisms

Staphylococcus aureus is the commonest pathogen. Methicillin-resistant *S. aureus* (MRSA) and *S. aureus* possessing the Panton–Valentine leukocidin (PVL) virulence factor are common causes of recurrent furunculosis (Figure 111.20) [2]. PVL consists of two proteins that cause lysis and cell death of neutrophils, leading to tissue necrosis and abscess formation. Other organisms include

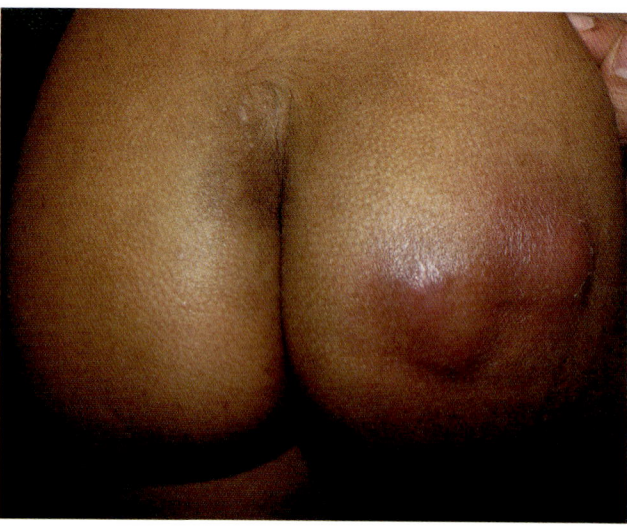

Figure 111.20 Panton–Valentine leukocidin *Staphylococcus aureus* infection affecting the buttock of a 3-year-old female.

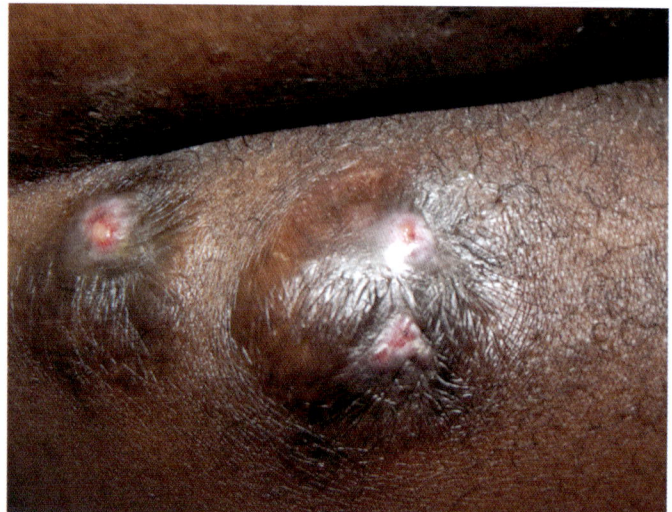

Figure 111.21 Furunculosis affecting the buttocks of a 22-year-old female.

Pseudomonas species (hot tub or wet suit folliculitis), *Malassezia furfur* (*Pityrosporum* folliculitis), *Klebsiella* (Gram-negative folliculitis) and herpes simplex virus.

Clinical features
History
Symptoms include pruritus, painful nodules and purulent discharge.

Presentation
Papules, pustules and suppurative nodules are seen (Figure 111.21). Scarring and hair loss may occur. PVL infection is associated with larger, redder, painful furuncles and may affect other family members [2].

Differential diagnosis
This includes hidradenitis suppurativa, pyoderma gangrenosum, pilonidal sinus and Crohn disease.

Complications and co-morbidities
These include bacteraemia, infective endocarditis and necrotising pneumonia.

Disease course and prognosis
Most patients present with a few boils that resolve with first line treatment. Colonisation with *S. aureus* may lead to recurrent furunculosis.

Investigations
Bacterial, fungal or viral swabs or scrapings should be taken. Swabs of nasal and other carrier sites including of close contacts should be considered.

Management
Antibacterial soaps and good personal, interpersonal and environmental hygiene should be advised. Incision and drainage may be required. A topical decolonisation regimen should be considered in recurrent furunculosis and where MRSA or PVL *S. aureus* infection has been identified.

First line
Topical antibiotics may be helpful in superficial folliculitis. Systemic antibacterial therapy is usually required for furunculosis based, if possible, on the results of culture.

OTHER BACTERIAL INFECTIONS

Streptococcal dermatitis/perianal cellulitis. Group A β-haemolytic streptococcal perianal dermatitis is most common in children between the ages of 6 and 10 months [1] but may occur in adults [2]. The child may present with pruritus, perianal soreness and painful defecation. Examination reveals a sharply demarcated, boggy redness. Satellite pustulosis may be present on the buttocks. It is commoner in boys. β-haemolytic streptococci are frequently cultured from the pharynx [1] and streptococcal perianal dermatitis may trigger guttate psoriasis [3]. Treatment includes systemic antibiotics.

Ano-genital cellulitis. Cellulitis and abscess formation can complicate cysts, sinuses and fistulae. The differential diagnosis is given in Box 111.2.

Box 111.2 Differential diagnosis of ano-genital cellulitis

- Staphylococcal cellulitis
- Streptococcal cellulitis
- Hidradenitis suppurativa
- Crohn disease
- Gonococcal cellulitis
- Necrotising soft-tissue infections, e.g. necrotising fasciitis, Fournier gangrene
- Malakoplakia
- Extramammary Paget disease
- Carcinoma erysipeloides (bladder, prostate, colon)

Adapted from Bunker 2004 [4]. Reproduced with permission of Elsevier.

Perianal tuberculosis. Perianal tuberculosis can cause indolent, irregular, painful ulcers, fistulae and abscesses and may be difficult to distinguish from Crohn disease. Lupus vulgaris may spread widely over the buttocks and perianal region or assume a fungating, vegetating appearance. Perineal scrofuloderma (secondary skin involvement from underlying lymph node disease) may cause diagnostic difficulty.

Necrotising soft-tissue infections. A number of overlapping, severe, gangrenous, necrotising conditions may affect the ano-rectal and perineal skin and subcutaneous tissues including muscle. Previously known by names such as clostridial and non-clostridial gangrene, gas gangrene and Fournier gangrene, they are now referred to by the generic term of necrotising soft-tissue infection [5]. Pathogens such as *Streptococcus* and *Clostridium* species are usually involved. Early recognition and intervention are crucial as delay in diagnosis increases mortality. Necrotising fasciitis is one of these infections.

Necrotising fasciitis most often affects middle-aged and elderly people but all ages can be affected. Risk factors include diabetes, intravenous drug use, trauma and haematological malignancy. Pain (often severe and out of proportion to physical signs), fever and cellulitic skin changes usually develop first. A distinct, dusky red to black spot may appear on affected skin. Tenderness and dusky red redness extend with extreme rapidity to involve wide areas of the perineum. Crepitus is an important feature, as is the presence of a dark brown, turbid fluid without pus. Deterioration and septicaemia may occur rapidly. Swift surgical intervention with exploration and debridement of affected tissue is essential to improve outcome.

Ecthyma gangrenosum. Ecthyma gangrenosum is usually caused by *Pseudomonas aeruginosa* and occurs in the critically ill or immunosuppressed. It has a predilection for the ano-genital region and may cause severe, painful, necrotising, ano-rectal ulceration and septicaemia. The mortality is high.

Perianal malakoplakia. Malakoplakia is a rare inflammatory condition associated with infections, malignancy and immunosuppression [6]. It has been reported in many different organs including the bladder, kidney, lung, pancreas and rarely the skin. The most common reported skin site affected is perianal skin. The pathogenesis is not understood but it is thought to result from a defect in macrophage function. Management depends on the extent of disease and the underlying condition. Antibiotic therapy in combination with surgical excision achieves the best results.

FUNGAL INFECTIONS

The possibility of fungal infection should be considered in all unusual forms of perianal dermatitis. The presence of superficial longitudinal fissures is typically seen. Microscopy and culture should be performed.

Candidiasis. This causes a bright red, glazed area, often with outlying small pustules, and may spread to the groins or natal cleft.

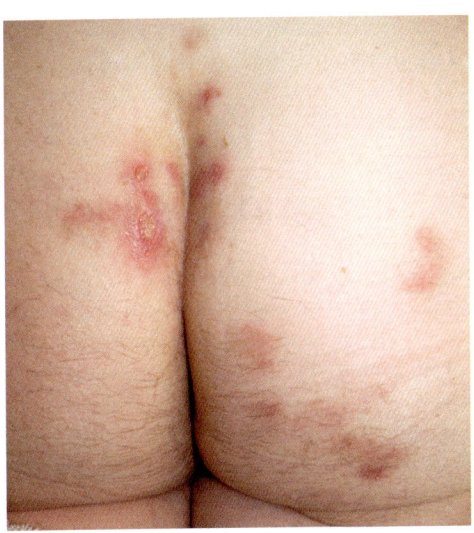

Figure 111.22 Ulcerated and inflamed skin affecting the natal cleft and buttock secondary to herpes simplex type II virus infection.

Dermatophyte infection. Dermatophyte infection (e.g. with *Trichophyton rubrum*) produces a well-defined, scaly patch with a circinate edge. Prior treatment with corticosteroids may disguise the appearance.

Histoplasmosis and blastomycosis. These can produce perianal lesions.

VIRAL INFECTIONS

Herpes simplex virus infection. This commonly affects the buttocks and perianal skin (Figure 111.22). Most ano-genital infections are sexually transmitted and are caused by herpes simplex virus (HSV) type 2. HSV type 1 infection can be transmitted to the ano-genital region by oral sex. Symptoms include ano-rectal pain, discharge and fever. Clinical features include perianal vesicles, ulceration and discharge. The diagnosis should be confirmed, e.g. by viral HSV DNA polymerase chain reaction (PCR). HSV becomes latent in the sacral ganglion after primary infection and may become reactivated to cause recurrent symptoms.

Human papillomavirus infection. See the section on human papillomavirus later in this chapter.

Molluscum contagiosum infection. Molluscum contagiosum infection is caused by a virus from the Pox family and is common in children. It may be secondary to eczema and spread by scratching. Typically, the lesions are pale waxy papules with an umbilicated centre (Figure 111.18). Molluscum contagiosum is often sexually transmitted in adults but can be transmitted from clothes or towels. Molluscum contagiosum infection can be a manifestation of HIV infection in adults. Testing for underlying HIV infection should always be considered.

Cytomegalovirus infection. This may cause perianal ulceration. It is rare in the immunocompetent but may occur in HIV infection.

Kawasaki disease. The cause is unknown but of possible viral aetiology. A red, desquamating, perineal eruption occurring in the first week of the disease may be the first cutaneous feature in up to two-thirds of children [1].

HELMINTH INFESTATIONS

Strongyloides stercoralis. Strongyloides stercoralis usually presents with cutaneous or gastrointestinal symptoms but may be asymptomatic in over 60% of cases and indicated only by a raised blood eosinophil count [1]. In chronic infection, filariform larvae passed in the stool can attach to the perianal skin and lead to autoinfection by migrating through the skin at this site (exoauto-invasion). Rapid intradermal migration of these infectious larvae causes the rash of larva currens and usually presents with very itchy red papules and serpiginous tracts on perianal, buttock and upper thigh skin. Larva currens is pathognomonic for strongyloidiasis [2].

Cutaneous larva migrans. This results from migration of infective larvae from the dog or cat hookworms *Ancylostoma brasiliense* or *A. caninum* after percutaneous invasion and may occur on perineal skin.

Schistosomiasis (bilharziasis). Perineal granulomatous lesions are a rare manifestation presenting as pruritic papules in the ano-genital region in endemic countries.

OTHER INFESTATIONS

Scabies infection. Infection with *Sarcoptes scabiei* var *hominis* can cause nodules on the buttocks and perineum.

Amoebiasis. This is caused by the protozoan *Entamoeba histolytica*. The spectrum of disease includes proctocolitis, liver and perianal abscess, and perianal ulceration. Transmission usually occurs by the faecal–oral route but direct inoculation of abraded perianal skin may occur. The highest prevalence is in developing countries. Ulcers typically extend slowly, but may progress rapidly until a phagedenic ulcer completely destroys the perianal and sacral tissue [1].

OTHER DISEASES AND INFECTIONS

Sexually transmitted diseases

Introduction and general description
Clinical descriptions pertinent to perineal/perianal skin only are discussed. The reader is directed to detailed description of specific sexually transmitted infections elsewhere.

In female patients, perianal symptoms may be caused by the posterior spread of genital infections such as candidiasis or trichomoniasis. An irritant perianal dermatitis may occur due to vaginal or anal discharge.

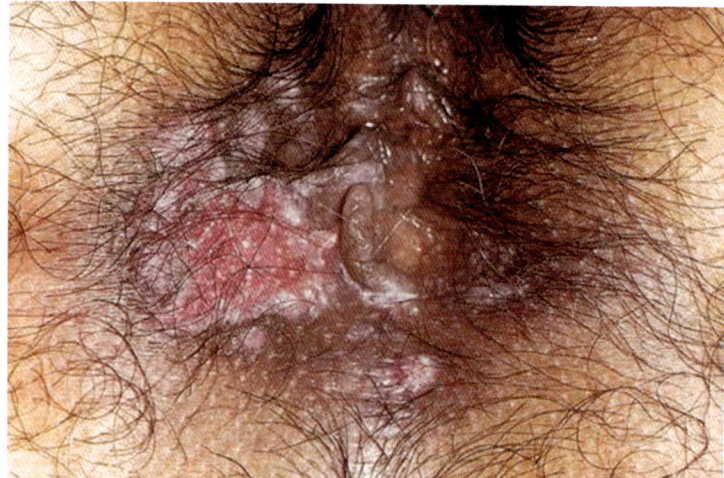

Figure 111.23 Condylomata lata. Courtesy of Dr S. Gold, London, UK.

Clinical features
Gonorrhoea. This may cause anal inflammation and discharge or an oedematous perianal dermatitis with multiple fissures and erosions.

Syphilis. This should always be considered as a cause of perianal and anal ulceration, especially in men who have sex with men (MSM). Primary chancres can be mistaken for anal fissures. In secondary syphilis, papular lesions may coalesce in moist areas such as the perianal region to form highly contagious condylomata lata (Figure 111.23). These can be mistaken for genital warts (condylomata acuminata). A granulomatous gumma of tertiary syphilis may affect the perianal area and present as an ulcer, white plaque or atrophic scar. Congenital syphilis may cause perianal rhagades.

Lymphogranuloma venereum (LGV). LGV is a sexually transmitted infection endemic in tropical areas including West Africa. It is caused by one of three invasive serovars (L1, L2 or L3) of *Chlamydia trachomatis* and usually presents with an inguinal syndrome. Infection has become endemic in the UK since 2004 in MSM, particularly HIV-positive men [1]. Similar outbreaks have been reported across Europe and the USA [2]. An ano-rectal LGV syndrome is the usual presentation in industrialised countries with the development of ulcerative haemorrhagic proctitis that can mimic Crohn colitis. Perianal ulcers and fissures may occur [1]. If untreated, LGV may progress to cause widespread vegetating and scarring lesions of the genito-perineal area.

Human papillomavirus (HPV) infection. HPV infection is the commonest viral sexually transmitted disease. Anal warts are common in young adults but are not always sexually transmitted.

Herpes simplex virus infection. HSV type 2 infection is a common cause of acute painful perianal and anal ulceration and proctitis in MSM. Proctitis can occur often without visible perianal ulceration [3].

Granuloma inguinale (Donovanosis). This is an infection caused by *Klebsiella granulomatis*. It is most frequently seen in tropical countries and is rare in temperate climates. It usually affects perineal skin, causing relatively painless papules and nodules that ulcerate. Ulcers may be phagedenic. Nodules may be mistaken for lymph nodes (pseudobubo). Perianal lesions can scar leading to anal stenosis and SCC can occur.

Chancroid. Chancroid is an infection caused by *Haemophilus ducreyi* and is characterised by painful ano-genital or perianal ulceration and inguinal lymphadenopathy. The prevalence of chancroid has decreased worldwide.

Infestations. Infestations including *Phthiriasis pubis* (pubic lice) should be considered.

Management
Patients should be managed by a genito-urinary medicine specialist.

Human immunodeficiency virus infection

Introduction and general description
Many skin conditions can affect perianal skin, including seborrhoeic dermatitis and flexural psoriasis, and are associated with HIV infection. The reader is referred to Chapter 31. Ano-rectal disease is common in HIV infection. Up to 66% of patients may have more than one condition [1]. Anal warts are the commonest disorder. There is a higher risk of progression to anal intraepithelial neoplasia and frank malignancy in HIV-positive men and women [2].

Painful perianal and intra-anal ulcers are also common, occurring in 32% of patients in a cohort of 180 HIV-positive men and women with ano-rectal symptoms [3]. Most of the ulcers were idiopathic; 12% were due to HSV infection and 7% due to cytomegalovirus reactivation.

Ano-genital ulceration can increase the risk of HIV acquisition per sexual exposure by a factor of 10–50 for male to female transmission and of 50–300 for female to male transmission [4].

Severe, painful recrudescence of ulcerated herpes simplex infection type 2 may occur, including as a manifestation of immune reconstitution after initiation of antiretroviral therapy [5].

Box 111.3 lists the main causes of anal ulceration associated with HIV infection.

Box 111.3 Causes of anal/perianal ulceration in HIV infection

- Herpes simplex virus infection
- Syphilis (primary chancre)
- Lymphogranuloma venereum
- Idiopathic (aphthous)
- Anal fissures
- Anal sepsis (perianal abscess, perianal fistula)
- Haemorrhoids
- Cytomegalovirus infection
- Kaposi sarcoma
- Non-Hodgkin lymphoma
- Squamous cell carcinoma
- Pruritus ani
- Trauma
- Amoebiasis

Human papillomavirus infection

Definition and nomenclature
Human papillomaviruses are DNA viruses that infect squamous epithelia or cells with the potential for squamous maturation, including the skin and mucosae of the ano-genital region.

Synonyms and inclusions
- Condylomata acuminata
- External genital warts

Introduction and general description
Infection with HPV of the ano-genital region is the commonest viral sexually transmitted disease. Perianal and intra-anal HPV infection is common. Approximately 40 out of the 180 known HPV genotypes have been associated with ano-genital lesions. The majority of HPV-associated diseases are caused by HPV types 6, 11, 16 and 18. HPV genotypes are divided into low-risk types such as HPV-6 and -11 that predominantly cause benign ano-genital warts and high-risk types such as HPV-16 and -18 that may cause neoplasia, including anal intraepithelial neoplasia (AIN) and anal cancer. At least 13 of the known HPV genotypes have oncogenic potential.

Epidemiology
Incidence and prevalence
The annual incidence of clinically visible ano-genital HPV infection has been estimated to be 1–2% in sexually active individuals. Many other patients may have subclinical or latent infection. The estimated lifetime risk of ano-genital wart infection is 10% [1].

Age
The peak prevalence of genital HPV infection occurs in females in their late teens and twenties and prevalence declines in subsequent decades. Men acquire infection in their late teens but prevalence does not decline with age [2]. The rate of acquiring a new genital HPV infection decreases with age in women but does not vary by age in men.

Sex
Genital HPV prevalence is higher in men than women. Anal HPV infection has been studied more frequently in men than women. Anal HPV prevalence among MSM is twice that of women and anal HPV prevalence in women is twice that of men who have sex with women [2]. The prevalence of anal HPV in men who have sex with women has been shown to be 12% [2] and up to 70% in MSM [3]. Anal HPV prevalence is higher in women with HPV-related cervical disease and women at risk of HPV infection [2].

Pathophysiology

Predisposing factors

Warts in the anal canal are associated with anoreceptive sex. An increased number of lifetime sexual partners and immunosuppression are risk factors for HPV infection.

Pathology

Histology is characterised by papillomatosis, acanthosis, hyperkeratosis and parakeratosis (Figure 111.24a). Koilocytes in the granular cell layer as well as coarse keratohyaline granules are characteristic (Figure 111.24b,c).

Causative organisms

Viral gene expression is confined to the keratinocytes. HPV infects and replicates in differentiating squamous epithelium only and is effective at evading host recognition and immunity [4]. HPV-6 and -11 are low-risk HPVs and are responsible for over 90% of ano-genital warts [5]. The presence of low-risk HPV infection may be a marker for the carriage of high-risk genotypes such as HPV-16.

Clinical features

History

Symptoms include pruritus ani, discomfort, bleeding and palpable lesions.

Presentation

Warty papules, plaques and nodules are seen and may be profuse and extend into the anal canal.

Clinical variants

Perianal viral warts may occur in infants and young children (Figure 111.25). Sexual abuse needs to be considered in all cases, particularly in children older than 2 years where vertical transmission is less likely. The upper age limit for vertical transmission is uncertain as latent infection may occur. Furthermore, HPV genotypes do not seem to show the same degree of tropism for either mucosal or cutaneous sites as occurs in adults [6]. The presence of warts or HPV DNA alone is not sufficient to make a diagnosis of sexual abuse and social, behavioural and other supporting clinical information is required.

Differential diagnosis

Molluscum contagiosum, condylomata lata, lichen planus, AIN and anal carcinoma should all be considered as possible diagnoses.

Complications and co-morbidities

Diagnosis of ano-genital warts is associated with a long-term risk of ano-genital neoplasia and other malignancies including oropharyngeal carcinoma. There is a higher risk of progression to AIN and anal carcinoma in the immunosuppressed.

MSM with ano-genital HPV infection have a significantly higher risk of acquiring HIV infection [7].

Disease course and prognosis

The average incubation period from sexual exposure to HPV and development of ano-genital warts in young adults is 3 months.

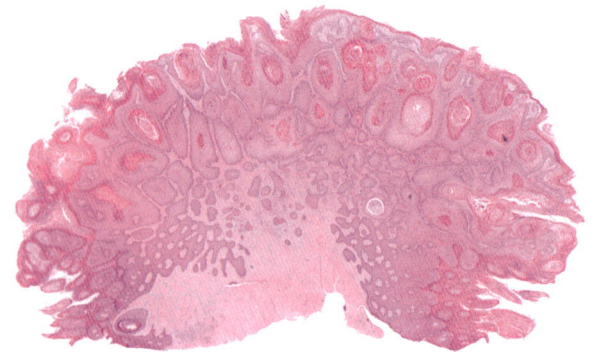

(a)

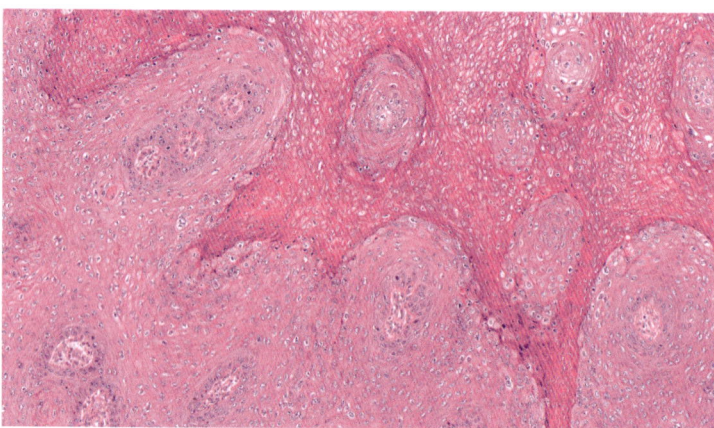

(b)

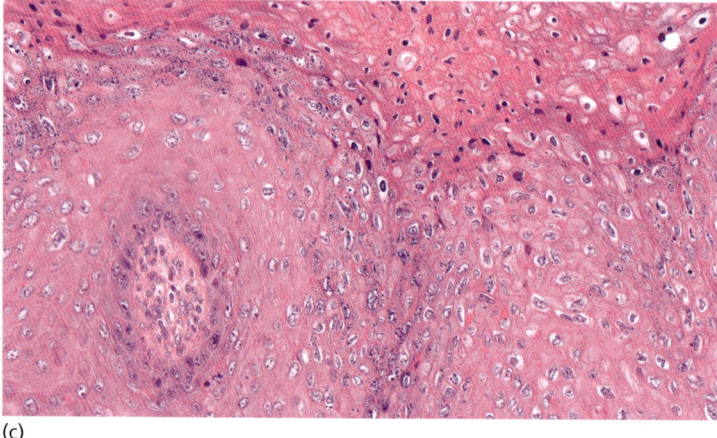

(c)

Figure 111.24 Perianal wart. (a) Low-power histological features of a perianal wart showing hyperkeratosis, acanthosis and papillomatosis. Magnification 40x. (b) Higher-power view of a perianal wart showing papillomatosis, hyperkeratosis, coarse keratohyaline granules and koilocytosis. Magnification 200x. (c) High-power view of a perianal viral wart showing keratohyaline granules and koilocytes. Magnification 400x. Courtesy of Dr Eduardo Calonje, London, UK.

Approximately 80–90% of ano-genital HPV infections regress due to a successful cell-mediated immune response. Persistent HPV infection with high-risk oncogenic genotypes able to evade host immunity can lead to the expression of potent oncogenes E6 and E7, with subsequent neoplastic transformation and progression to high-grade AIN or anal carcinoma [4].

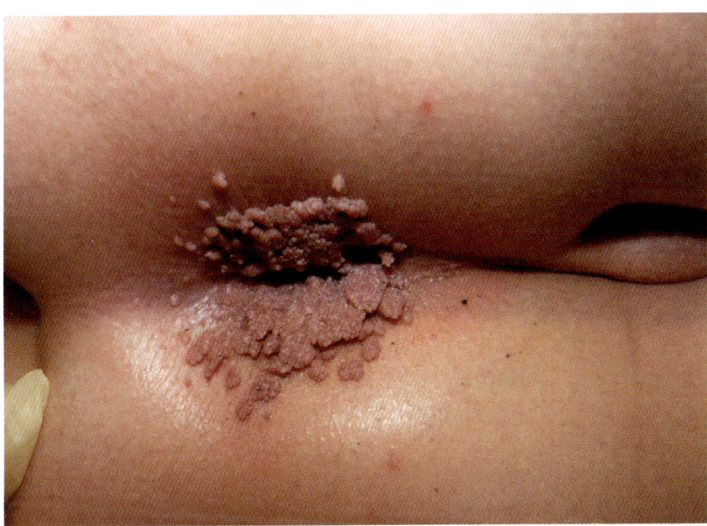

Figure 111.25 Florid perianal warts in a 5-year-old male.

Investigations

Infection with HPV can be investigated using molecular hybridisation to detect HPV DNA in biopsy specimens, swabs or scrapings obtained from the mucosa or skin.

Management

Patients should be managed by a genitourinary medicine specialist. A full sexual health screen is required and colorectal assessment if intra-anal disease is suspected. A biopsy should be performed if diagnosis is in doubt or dysplasia suspected. The treatment choice depends on the morphology, number of lesions and patient preference. Relapse is common.

HPV vaccination

The quadrivalent HPV vaccine consists of virus-like particles assembled from major capsid proteins (L1) of HPV-16, -18, -6 and -11. It has been shown to reduce ano-genital HPV infection prevalence in young females by more than 90%, as well as reducing high-grade cervical intraepithelial neoplasia in the same population [8]. Randomised controlled trials with the quadrivalent HPV vaccine have also demonstrated high efficacy against the development of ano-genital warts in men who have sex with women and MSM [9]. A gender-neutral vaccination programme has been advocated to induce true herd immunity and prevent all HPV-associated disease including anal cancer and oropharyngeal cancer in men and women [10]. Currently a quadrivalent vaccine is offered to boys and girls in the UK at age 12 and 13.

First line

Options include imiquimod cream 5%, podophyllin, podophyllotoxin or trichloroacetic acid solution and cryotherapy.

Second line

Options include ablative therapy with cryotherapy or electrocautery, curettage, surgical excision or laser therapy.

Third line

Topical, intralesional or systemic interferon treatment has been described. Interferons are not recommended for routine management of ano-genital warts. Various regimens have been described using interferons α, β and γ as creams and as intralesional or systemic injection [11].

Resources

Further information

British Association for Sexual Health and HIV: www.bashh.org/guidelines (last accessed May 2022).

Anal intraepithelial neoplasia

Definition and nomenclature

This is an intraepidermal, non-invasive, squamous neoplasia that can affect the anal canal and perianal skin. It is the precursor for anal SCC.

Synonyms and inclusions
- Anal intraepithelial dysplasia
- Carcinoma *in situ*
- Anal squamous intraepithelial lesion
- Bowen disease
- Bowenoid papulosis

Introduction and general description

The clinical presentation of AIN is variable. Perianal lesions are often referred to as Bowen disease. The high-risk HPV genotypes HPV-16 and -18 are strongly associated with the development of AIN and anal carcinoma. It is thought that early diagnosis and management of AIN are important to prevent progression to invasive SCC, although there is no current clear evidence that this is the case. There are several different classifications for AIN. Classification into low- or high-grade squamous intraepithelial lesion (LSIL and HSIL) has been adopted by many centres [1].

Epidemiology

Incidence and prevalence

The incidence of high-grade AIN is estimated to be 0.45 per 100 000 of the general population. The prevalence is higher in high-risk groups and is estimated to occur in 52% of HIV-positive MSM and 5% of renal transplant recipients [2].

Age

It is commoner in older women and younger men.

Sex

Anal intraepithelial neoplasia is commoner in women and in MSM.

PART 10: SPECIFIC SITES, SEX & AGE

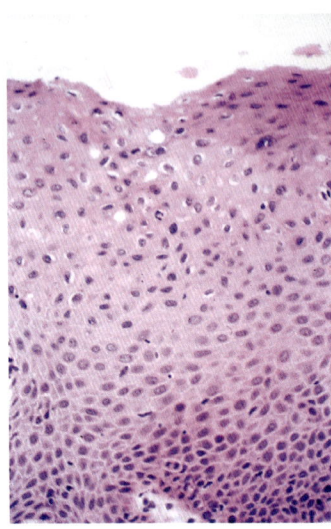

Figure 111.26 Histopathology of low-grade anal intraepithelial neoplasia. Koilocytes are present high in the upper half of the epidermis. Magnification 200×. Courtesy of Dr Nick Francis, London, UK.

Associated diseases

Anal intraepithelial neoplasia can be part of multicentric disease affecting other genital sites including the vulva, cervix and penis. There is a higher risk of malignancy including AIN and colorectal cancer in patients with hidradenitis suppurativa.

Pathophysiology

Predisposing factors

Predisposing factors include receptive anal sex, a history of ano-genital warts, smoking, lifetime number of sexual partners and immunosuppression including renal transplant recipients. The highest risk group for AIN is HIV-positive MSM.

Pathology

Cytological atypia is confined to the epidermal layer. AIN is characterised by varying degrees of loss of stratification and nuclear polarity, dyskeratosis, nuclear pleomorphism and hyperchromatism, and increased mitotic activity with the presence of mitoses high in the epithelium. Koilocytes may be present. Atypia can be graded into low grade (Figure 111.26) or high grade (Figure 111.27) depending on severity. Expression of proliferative biomarkers such as p16 can be a useful diagnostic tool to confirm the grade of disease.

Causative organisms

There are approximately 15 recognised high-risk oncogenic ano-genital HPV genotypes. HPV-16 and -18 are predominantly associated with AIN in men and women [1].

Clinical features

History

Anal intraepithelial neoplasia is often asymptomatic. Symptoms include pruritus ani and bleeding.

Presentation

Lesions can be solitary or multifocal. Intra-anal AIN when visible macroscopically may present as papillomatous papules or plaques that can appear red, white, pigmented or fissured. Induration or ulceration may indicate invasion. Intra-anal AIN can be identified after the application of 3% acetic acid during high-resolution anoscopy. AIN is often an incidental finding on surgical specimens.

Clinical variants

Perianal Bowen disease presents as relatively asymptomatic red, shiny or scaly plaques (Figure 111.28). There may be continuity with dysplastic lesions in the anal canal. HPV-16 has been identified in 60–80% of cases [1]. Perianal Bowen disease is estimated to progress to invasive SCC in 2–6% of cases [2].

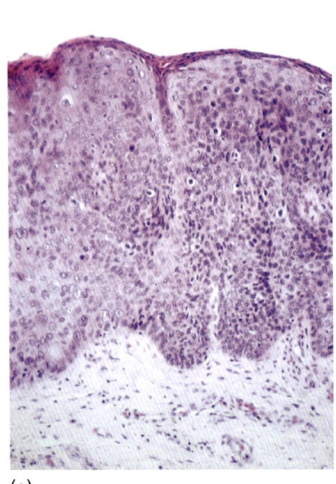
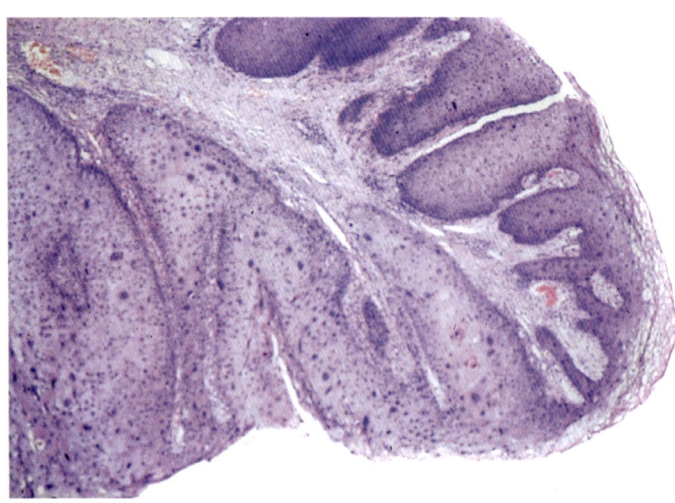
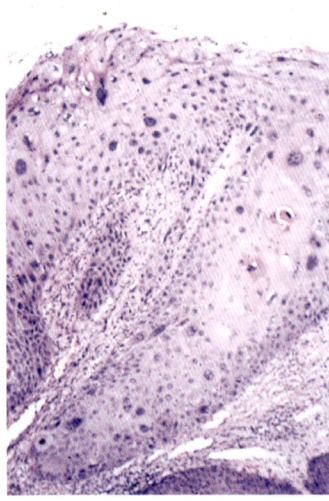

(a)   (b)   (c)

Figure 111.27 Histopathology of high-grade anal intraepithelial neoplasia (AIN). (a) High-grade, full-thickness AIN. Magnification 100×. (b) High-grade AIN occurring within a perianal wart. There is marked nuclear atypia, dyskeratosis and basal crowding of the nuclei. Magnification 40×. (c) High-grade AIN occurring within a perianal wart. Magnification 100×. Courtesy of Dr Nick Francis, London, UK.

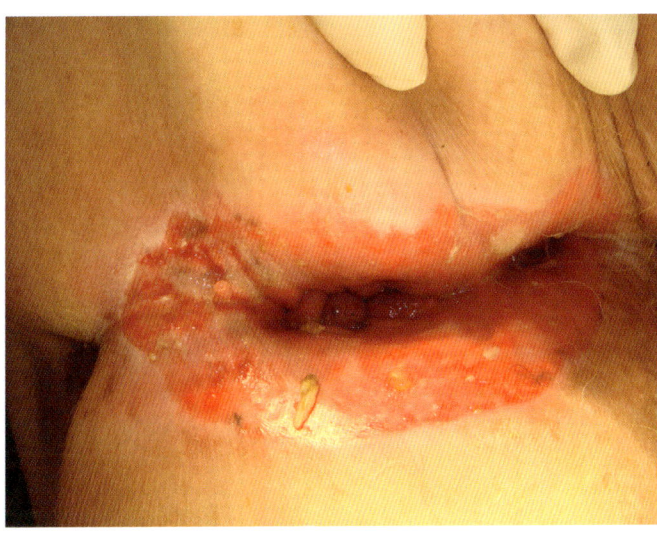

Figure 111.28 Extensive eroded plaque of perianal high-grade intraepithelial neoplasia (Bowen disease) in a 75-year-old female.

Bowenoid papulosis is a distinct clinical entity presenting as solitary or multiple, reddish-brown, pigmented or flesh-coloured papules with a flat or verrucous surface that can merge into plaques. It typically occurs in the ano-genital region or groin of young, sexually active individuals. Histology is of full-thickness epithelial dysplasia. HPV-16 is usually implicated. The risk of progression to invasive carcinoma is unknown.

Differential diagnosis
Anal carcinoma, HPV infection, psoriasis and lichen planus should be considered.

Classification of severity
Anal intraepithelial neoplasia is commonly defined as low or high grade based on the degree of cytological atypia.

Disease course and prognosis
The risk of progression to anal or perianal SCC is poorly understood, partly because there are relatively few trained experts in anoscopy and few and limited published data. The risk of progression of high-grade AIN to invasive anal carcinoma in immunocompetent patients over 5 years is approximately 10% [2]. The risk of progression to anal carcinoma in HIV-positive patients is currently unknown but invasive disease can develop quickly [2].

Investigations
Histological assessment of the suspected area of AIN is required to confirm the diagnosis and investigate whether there is evidence of invasive disease. Screening for AIN includes anal cytology and high-resolution anoscopy with mapping biopsies of suspicious areas.

Management
Multidisciplinary specialist management is essential. Digital rectal examination and anoscopy are required to determine if there is intra-anal disease. Genital skin should be examined for evidence of associated diseases. All females with AIN require gynaecological assessment in view of the high prevalence of concomitant cervical intraepithelial neoplasia.

The aims of management are to alleviate symptoms and prevent progression to anal cancer. Management of AIN is not standardised. There is no consensus on which modality of AIN treatment is optimal and whether treatment of AIN prevents development of anal SCC [3,4]. Some advocate close follow-up for low-grade intra-anal disease. Recurrence is common following intervention, especially in the immunosuppressed.

First line
Topical 5% imiquimod and 5-fluorouracil cream are therapeutic options for perianal or intra-anal disease and can be self-applied [5]. Targeted ablation options include CO_2 laser, electrocautery or infrared coagulation. Solitary, small perianal lesions may be amenable to surgical excision [6]. Risks of surgery include anal stenosis and faecal incontinence.

Second line
Photodynamic therapy or radiofrequency ablation can be considered.

Screening and prevention
The utility of screening for AIN using anal cytology and high-resolution anoscopy is currently controversial in terms of cost-effectiveness and there are no national screening programmes in place, but it has been recommended for high-risk populations including MSM and HIV-positive patients [7].

HPV vaccination has been shown to reduce the prevalence of AIN in MSM [8]. HPV vaccination is also being explored as a therapeutic option to prevent recurrence of AIN. Authors in a recent review of the efficacy of treatment options for AIN have concluded that HPV vaccination is unlikely to be an effective treatment for high-grade AIN [9].

Anal and perianal malignancy

Synonyms and inclusions
- Anal cancer
- Squamous cell carcinoma
- Epidermoid carcinoma

Introduction and general description
Malignancies of the anal region are relatively uncommon, comprising 2–4% of all ano-rectal malignancies. Tumours of the anal region include tumours of the anal canal and anal margin. Distinction between tumour location at the anal margin or anal canal is important as there are differences in management and prognosis. Unfortunately, the literature has often grouped these two anatomical sites together, leading to difficulties in interpreting the results of interventions.

SCC is the most common type of anal cancer, comprising approximately 80% of cases [1]. Anal adenocarcinoma accounts for fewer than 10% of all anal cancers [2]. Other rarer malignancies affecting the anal region include melanoma, lymphoma and Kaposi sarcoma. Ano-genital Kaposi sarcoma is essentially HIV related.

SCC of the anal region is usually preceded by AIN. Most cases are a result of sexually acquired infection with oncogenic HPV subtypes, predominantly HPV-16 and -18. Prevention may be possible through the use of HPV vaccination.

The following discussion will be limited to SCC.

Epidemiology
Incidence and prevalence
Anal SCC is rare, but the incidence is increasing worldwide in men and women. The rise in incidence in women is thought to be due to more women having anoreceptive sex with a resultant increased risk of exposure to high-risk HPV types. The rise in incidence in men is attributed to prolonged survival of patients with HIV infection, enabling progression of persistent high-risk HPV infection to AIN and subsequent invasive malignancy. The incidence of SCC of the anal canal is approximately 1.5 cases per 100 000 per year globally [3]. Anal cancer is not an AIDS-defining diagnosis but the incidence is 40–70 times higher in HIV-positive patients, and highest in MSM who practise anoreceptive sex [4].

Age
Women older than 50 years have a higher incidence rate. Men have a higher incidence rate in the 20–49-year age group [5].

Sex
It is commoner in women and HIV-positive men.

Associated diseases
Associated diseases include ano-genital HPV infection and other sexually transmitted diseases, vulval, penile and cervical intraepithelial neoplasia and carcinoma. Chronic inflammation and ulceration from severe hidradenitis suppurativa is also a risk factor.

Pathophysiology
Predisposing factors
Factors that increase the risk of ano-genital HPV infection or modulate the host immune response to HPV are associated with anal SCC. These include anoreceptive sex, lifetime number of sexual partners, immunosuppression (including organ transplant recipients) and smoking. Anal SCC is also increased in autoimmune disease including psoriasis and granulomatosis with polyangiitis [6]. The highest-risk group is HIV-positive MSM. HIV control as measured by the per cent of time with undetectable HIV viral load has been reported to decrease the risk of anal SCC [7]. Optimising antiretroviral therapy and control of HIV viral load may decrease the risk of anal SCC.

Perianal SCC can also develop on a background of chronic dermatoses including lichen planus, lichen sclerosus and hidradenitis suppurativa.

Pathology
Anal intraepithelial neoplasia is thought to be the precursor of invasive SCC (Figure 111.29). Histological features of anal

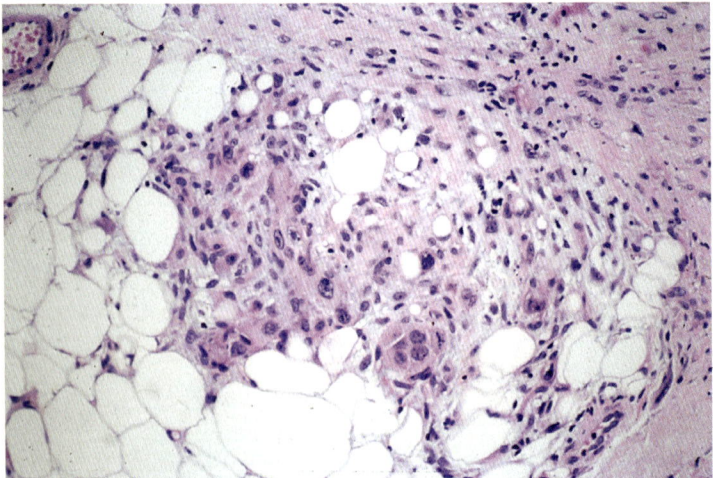

Figure 111.29 Squamous cell carcinoma infiltrating adipose tissue that has developed from adjacent high-grade anal intraepithelial neoplasia. Magnification 400x. Courtesy of Dr Nick Francis, London, UK.

SCC include hyperkeratosis, acanthosis, ectopic keratinisation, nuclear pleomorphism and mitoses. Cells can vary from large, pale eosinophilic cells to small, basaloid or spindle-shaped cells. Tongues of atypical keratinocytes invade the dermis. The invasive margin can vary from well circumscribed to irregular. A lymphocytic infiltrate of varying degrees may be present. No significant association between histological subtype and prognosis has been established.

Causative organisms
Anal SCC is associated with high-risk HPV infection, including HPV-16, in more than 96% of cases [8].

Clinical features
History
Symptoms include pruritus ani, bleeding, pain, tenesmus, faecal incontinence, discharge, change in bowel habit, ulceration and presence of a mass. History may include ano-genital HPV infection, HIV infection, anoreceptive sex or smoking.

Presentation
Presentation includes an ulcer or a hard mass that can be flat, raised or polypoid (Figures 111.30 and 111.31). SCC of the anal margin is at least fivefold less common than of the anal canal [9], but is the commonest tumour of the anal margin. Anal margin SCC is commoner in men [10]. It can be difficult to determine from the outset whether the tumour originated in the anal canal or anal margin as often both areas are involved at the time of diagnosis.

Locally advanced disease may present with perianal infection, fistula formation and inguinal lymphadenopathy. Lymph node involvement at diagnosis occurs in 30–40% of cases with distant extrapelvic metastases recorded in 5–8% at diagnosis. Rates of metastatic progression after primary treatment vary between 10% and 20% [10]. Tumours distal to the dentate line drain to the inguinal and femoral nodal chains.

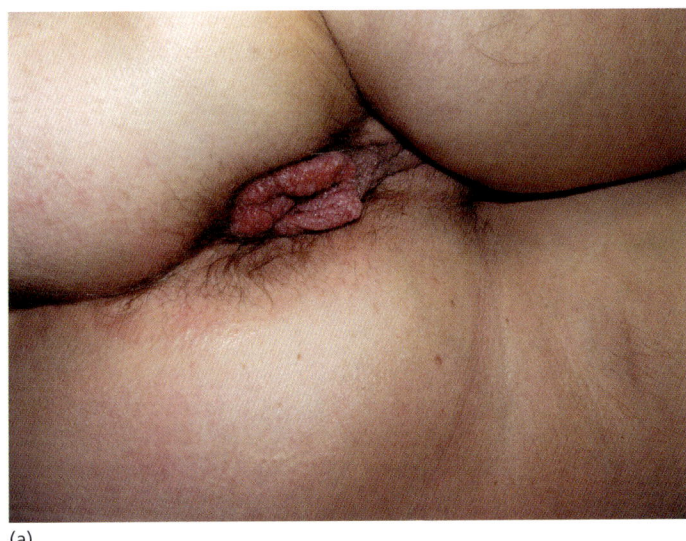

(a)

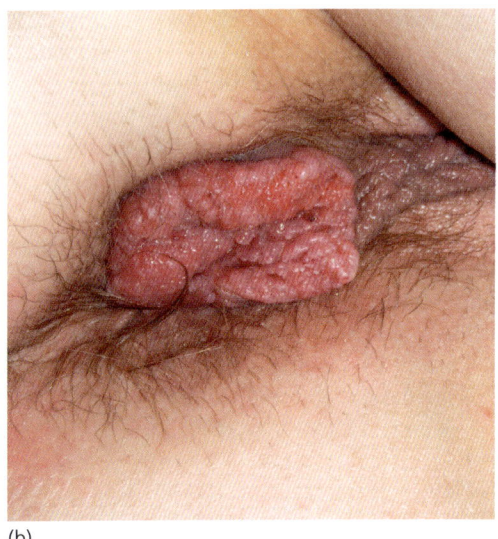

(b)

Figure 111.30 (a) Large polypoid mass of perianal carcinoma in a 56-year-old female. (b) Close-up view of the same carcinoma.

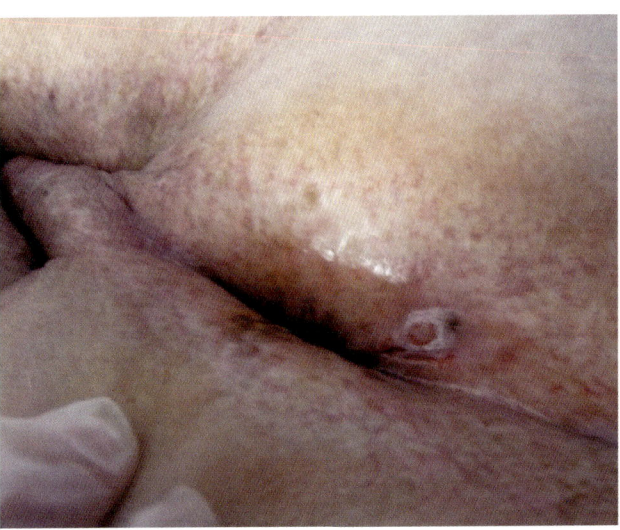

Figure 111.31 Poorly differentiated, eroded, perianal nodule of squamous cell carcinoma present at the anal margin occurring in a 50-year-old HIV-negative man within the radiotherapy treatment field 10 years after treatment of anal carcinoma with chemoradiotherapy. The patient subsequently had an abdomino-perineal resection and perineal reconstruction for the recurrent disease.

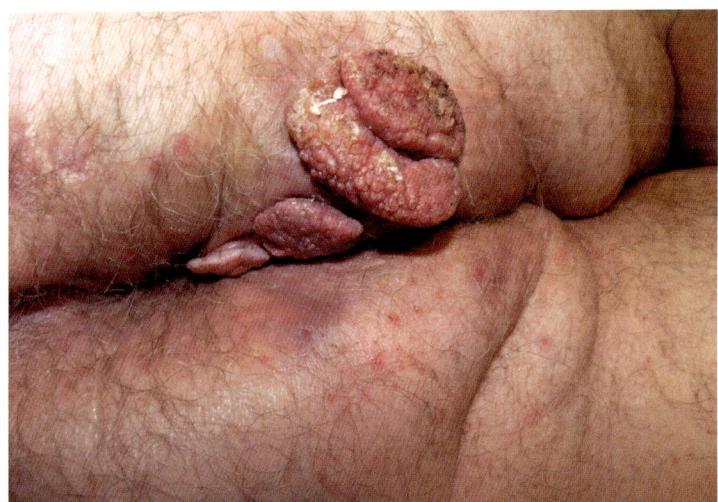

Figure 111.32 Buschke–Löwenstein tumour affecting the perianal skin of a 56-year-old male.

Clinical variants

Buschke–Löwenstein tumour (also called giant condyloma acuminatum or verrucous carcinoma) is a rare, slow-growing, cauliflower-like exophytic tumour of the ano-genital region caused by HPV and characterised by invasive growth (Figure 111.32). HPV-6 and -11 are the most common HPV genotypes identified. HPV-16 and -18 can also be detected, especially in cases with foci of invasive SCC. The histological features are similar to those of condyloma acuminatum. The Buschke–Löwenstein tumour is thought to exhibit intermediate biological behaviour towards malignancy. Wide local excision or abdomino-perineal resection is considered the treatment of choice. Adjuvant chemoradiotherapy may be necessary if there is an invasive component. Malignant transformation to SCC can occur in 40–60% of cases.

Differential diagnosis

Anal carcinoma should be considered in all nodulo-ulcerative anal and perianal disease, including when there is a history of perianal chronic inflammatory skin disease such as lichen planus, lichen sclerosus, hidradenitis suppurativa or a background of immuno-deficiency. The diagnosis of anal cancer is often delayed and is mistaken for benign disease such as haemorrhoids or anal tags.

Classification of severity

Anal and perianal SCC can be staged according to the American Joint Committee on Cancer TNM classification, which includes assessment of the tumour, lymph nodes and distant metastasis [11].

Disease course and prognosis

Tumour size (≥5 cm), nodal involvement and male sex are associated with a less favourable prognosis. Anal margin tumours have a better prognosis. Overall 5-year survival rates for localised disease, disease with regional lymph node involvement and disease with distant metastases are 80%, 58% and 31%, respectively [12]. Chemoradiation leads to complete tumour regression in 80–90% of patients. HIV-positive patients on highly active antiretroviral therapy have been shown to have similar clinical response and tolerability to chemoradiation as HIV-negative patients [13].

Anal margin SCC has a slightly better prognosis.

Investigations

Histological diagnosis is required and imaging undertaken for tumour staging. MRI of the pelvis and endoanal ultrasound enable assessment including of tumour size and anal sphincter involvement. Distant metastatic spread is assessed by computed tomography of the thorax, abdomen and pelvis.

Management

A multidisciplinary approach is essential including involvement of an ano-rectal surgeon, radiotherapist and medical oncologist.

The aim of treatment is to achieve cure with preservation of faecal continence. Chemoradiotherapy using a combination of 5-fluorouracil and mitomycin C has been established as first line treatment for invasive anal canal disease [10]. Small, well-differentiated anal margin tumours without nodal involvement can be treated with wide local excision if anal sphincter function can be preserved.

The main role for surgery in anal cancer is for residual or recurrent disease after failure of chemoradiotherapy and is referred to as salvage surgery. Abdomino-perineal resection with perineal reconstruction is the most frequently performed operation. This operation involves resection of the anus and rectum, end colostomy formation and reconstruction of the perineum.

Miscellaneous malignancies

Extramammary Paget disease (EMPD). EMPD is a rare but important diagnosis. Primary EMPD is an intraepithelial adenocarcinoma arising possibly from intraepidermal cells of the apocrine gland ducts or from pluripotent keratinocyte stem cells and is the commonest form of EMPD [1]. Secondary EMPD arises from an underlying malignancy in a dermal adnexal gland or a local organ with contiguous epithelium. Perianal EMPD represents approximately 20% of cases of extramammary disease [2]. The association between EMPD and malignancy is variable, ranging from 38% to 70% [2]. The commonest tumours are ano-rectal adenocarcinoma and adenocarcinoma of the bladder or urethra, but distant tumours including breast may be responsible. Perianal EMPD is strongly associated with ano-rectal adenocarcinoma, with up to 80% of patients having an underlying ano-rectal adenocarcinoma [1,2].

Common symptoms are pruritus ani and perianal bleeding [3]. Lesions are typically red plaques or erosions that are moist or hyperkeratotic. Perianal lesions can extend into the anal canal.

Management of primary disease is tailored to the extent of the EMPD and can include imiquimod cream, surgery (including Mohs micrographic surgery) or photodynamic therapy. Recurrence is common. Management of secondary disease is primarily directed towards the associated malignancy.

Basal cell carcinoma. This very common non-melanoma skin cancer rarely affects the ano-genital area. Predisposing factors include radiation, trauma or burns [4].

Melanoma. Anal margin melanoma is rare, accounting for 2–4% of all ano-rectal malignancies [4].

Langerhans cell histiocytosis. This condition can cause perianal ulceration.

Carcinoma erysipeloides. Infiltration of the skin with neoplastic cells produces the clinical appearance of cellulitis or erysipelas. Infiltrative papules can be seen on close inspection. It has been reported in the perineum and on the thigh in carcinoma of the bladder and prostate [5] and in the genito-crural region secondary to adenocarcinoma of the colon (Figure 111.33) (E. Mallon, personal observation).

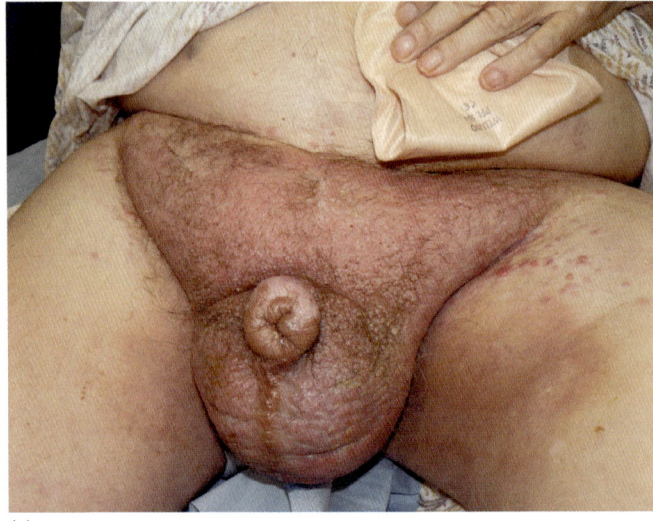
(a)

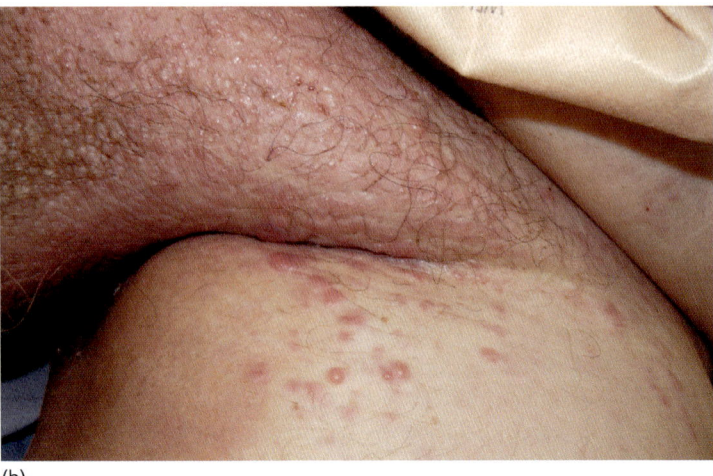
(b)

Figure 111.33 (a) Infiltrative carcinoma erysipeloides affecting the genito-crural region and lower abdomen in a man with adenocarcinoma of the colon. A colostomy bag is visible. (b) Close-up view showing a cellulitis-like appearance and infiltrated papules of cutaneous metastatic adenocarcinoma.

CONDITIONS BEST MANAGED IN COLLABORATION WITH AN ANO-RECTAL SPECIALIST SURGEON

Pilonidal sinus

Definition and nomenclature
Pilonidal sinus is an acquired midline sinus due to entrapment of hairs in the pilosebaceous unit of the sacrococcygeal region.

Synonyms and inclusions
- Pilonidal disease
- Sacrococcygeal pilonidal disease
- Pilonidal cyst
- Jeep driver's disease

Introduction and general description
Pilonidal disease is commonest in the sacrococcygeal region but can also occur on the pubis, anterior perineum or on the hands of people with certain occupations such as dog groomers or hairdressers. The word pilonidal is derived from the latin pilus (hair) and nidus (nest).

Epidemiology
Incidence and prevalence
The incidence was determined to be 26 per 100 000 in a study from Norway [1].

Age
The peak is in the second to third decades.

Sex
The male to female ratio is 2.2 : 1 [1].

Associated diseases
Other diseases involving follicular occlusion, namely hidradenitis suppurativa, dissecting cellulitis and acne conglobate, are associated.

Pathophysiology
Predisposing factors
The disease was previously thought to be congenital due to failure of fusion in the dorsal midline resulting in entrapment of hair follicles in the sacrococcygeal region, but is currently considered an acquired disorder [2].

Trauma, obesity, hirsutism, sedentary lifestyle and family history are predisposing factors. Hair follicles altered by pressure and maceration become occluded and hairs continue to grow beneath the surface, leading to a foreign body inflammatory reaction.

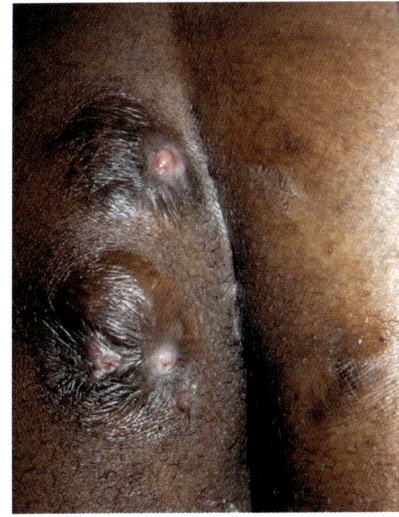

(a)

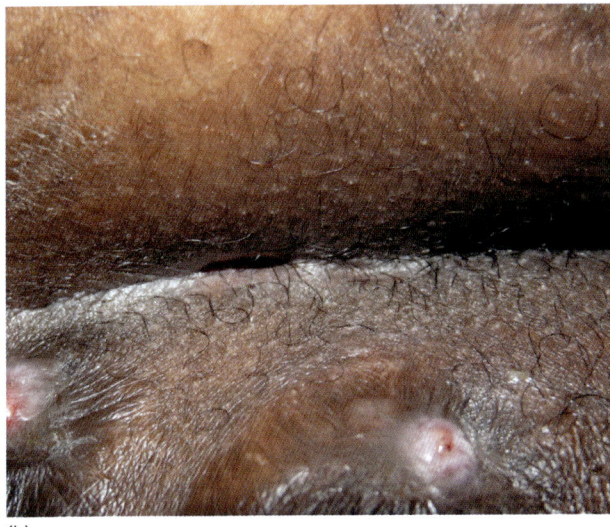

(b)

Figure 111.34 (a) Pilonidal sinuses in a natal cleft with buttock abscesses. (b) Close-up view of the same pilonidal sinus.

Clinical features
History
Symptoms include itch, pain (including coccygodynia), recurrent abscess, purulent discharge and persistent nodules in the natal cleft. It may be asymptomatic.

Presentation
A midline pit/sinus may be visible in the natal cleft (Figure 111.34) but may be obscured by a suppurative discharging nodule. Hairs may protrude from the sinuses. The sinus may extend to the sacrum. Secondary tracks and sinuses may develop off the midline in chronic disease (Figure 111.35).

Differential diagnosis
Perianal abscess, perianal fistula, Crohn disease and hidradenitis suppurativa should all be considered.

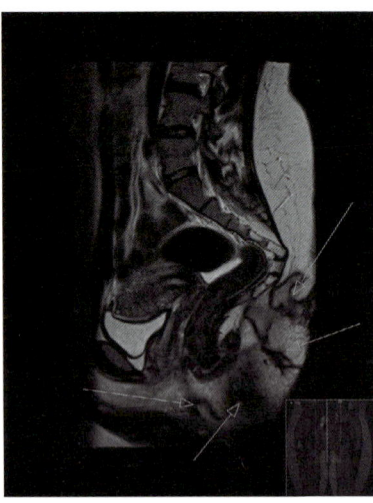

Figure 111.35 MRI scan of the patient with sacrococcygeal pilonidal disease shown in Figure 111.34. A sagittal T_2-weighted small field of view image showing multiple sinus tracks (arrows) extending from the natal cleft and buttock skin into the subcutaneous tissue, almost reaching the coccyx. Courtesy of Dr John Rendle, Department of Imaging, Croydon University Hospital, UK.

Complications and co-morbidities
Chronic inflammation over many years can lead to SCC.

Investigations
An MRI scan of the pelvis can define the sinus tracks (Figure 111.35).

Management
Depilation of hair in the natal cleft (e.g. by shaving) has been advocated [2]. The treatment of symptomatic disease is surgical. Various procedures ranging from excision, incision and marsupialisation or phenol injections to complex flaps to remove the natal cleft have been described. Asymptomatic pits do not require treatment [3].

Crohn disease

Definition and nomenclature
Crohn disease is an idiopathic, chronic, granulomatous, inflammatory disease that can affect any part of the gastrointestinal tract from mouth to anus. Perianal abscesses and fistulae are a common occurrence in Crohn disease.

Synonyms and inclusions
- Regional enteritis

Introduction and general description
Mucocutaneous manifestations of Crohn disease occur in up to 44% of patients [1] and can be categorised as granulomatous (contiguous or non-contiguous with the gastrointestinal tract), non-granulomatous reactive (e.g. pyoderma gangrenosum) or nutritional. Granulomatous disease non-contiguous with the gastrointestinal tract is referred to as metastatic Crohn disease. Crohn disease affects the perianal skin in 20–30% of cases, with the majority of patients having fistulae or abscesses. Patients with rectal or distal colonic disease are at a higher risk of developing perianal disease.

Epidemiology
Incidence and prevalence
Prevalence in the UK is estimated to be 50–100 per 100 000.

Age
The peak age of onset is the second to fourth decades.

Sex
It is commoner in females.

Pathophysiology
Predisposing factors
The aetiology is unknown. Smoking and a diet high in fatty foods may be risk factors.

Pathology
Histology is of non-caseating granulomas.

Clinical features
History
Perianal symptoms include pruritus ani, discharge and pain. Symptoms of inflammatory bowel disease include diarrhoea, abdominal pain and ano-rectal bleeding.

Presentation
Approximately 25% of patients with large or small bowel disease have perianal manifestations [2]. Perianal disease can precede symptoms of intestinal disease. The perianal manifestations are listed in Box 111.4.

Box 111.4 Perianal features of Crohn disease

- Pruritus ani
- Maceration
- Erosions
- Ulceration
- Fissures
- Abscesses
- Fistulae
- Secondary infection
- Skin tags
- Anal stenosis
- Metastatic granulomatous ulcers, nodules or plaques

The commonest perianal lesions are ulcers, anal fissures, abscesses and fistulae (Figure 111.36) [2]. Up to 50% of patients with Crohn disease develop fistulae [3], of which 54% are perianal [4]. The fistulae are often complex and multiple with severe impairment of quality of life.

Metastatic Crohn disease is rare. Lesions may present as ulcers, nodules or plaques and have been reported to occur on the face, retroauricular area, limbs, inframammary area, abdomen and genital skin.

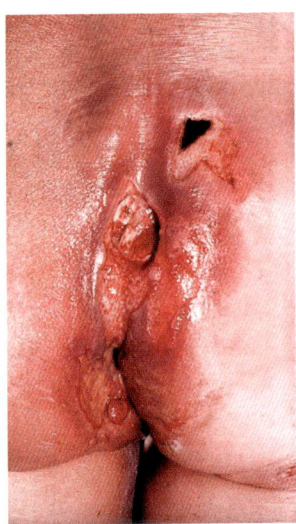

Figure 111.36 Crohn disease: perianal and buttock involvement. Courtesy of Dr D. I. McCallum, Inverness, UK.

Cutaneous disease activity does not correlate consistently with intestinal activity. Mucocutaneous manifestations of Crohn disease are listed in Box 111.5.

Box 111.5 Mucocutaneous features of Crohn disease

- Erythema nodosum
- Pyoderma gangrenosum
- Polyarteritis nodosa
- Granulomatous cheilitis
- Oral apthous ulceration
- Anal and perianal lesions (Box 111.4)
- Epidermolysis bullosa aquisita
- Genital disease including balanitis, chronic penile or vulval lymphoedema and contiguous granulomatous disease of the vulva
- Erosions and ulceration around ileostomies and colostomies
- Metastatic Crohn disease
- Ulceration of the perineum and buttocks after colectomy
- Skin changes secondary to malabsorption including pallor

Differential diagnosis

This includes the causes of pruritus ani, anal fissures, fistulae and perianal ulceration. Other possible diagnoses include ulcerative colitis, diverticulitis, hidradenitis suppurativa, pyoderma gangrenosum, HIV infection, tuberculosis and sexually transmitted disease including syphilis.

Granulomatous nodules, with or without ulceration, create a differential diagnosis that includes sarcoidoisis, tuberculosis, atypical mycobacterial infection, deep fungal infection, foreign body reaction, granuloma inguinale, lymphogranuloma venereum, chanchroid, amoebiasis and syphilis.

Complications and co-morbidities

These include fissures, anal skin tags, perianal ulceration, ano-rectal strictures, rectovaginal and anovaginal fistulae, faecal incontinence and anal carcinoma.

Disease course and prognosis

The course can be chronic and relapsing. Prognosis is variable.

Investigations

Endoscopic visualisation and biopsy are needed. Histological confirmation of non-caseating granulomas of both the skin and bowel should be sought. Endoanal ultrasound and MRI will assist in defining the anatomy of fistula tracks.

Management

A multidisciplinary approach is required, with gastroenterology being the main specialty likely to lead treatment. Management options include topical and intralesional steroids, oral prednisolone, oral antibiotics, sulfasalazine and immunosuppressive therapy including antitumour necrosis factor (anti-TNF) agents such as infliximab or adalimumab [5]. Surgical intervention may be required including for management of fistulae and drainage of abscesses.

First line

Local measures include soaks with potassium permanganate and the use of an antiseptic soap substitute. Potent or very potent topical steroid/antibiotic combinations and oral antibiotics (as for hidradenitis suppurativa) may be effective for localised perianal disease.

Anti-TNF agents should be considered as first line treatment in patients with fistulae [6] and can lead to clinical remission of trans-, supra- and extrasphincteric fistulae [2].

Resources

Further information

Crohn's and Colitis UK: www.crohnsandcolitis.org.uk (last accessed May 2022).

Anal abscess

Definition and nomenclature

Anal abscess is a form of ano-rectal sepsis. Pus formation occurs in the connective tissue around the anus and rectum.

Synonyms and inclusions

- Perianal abscess
- Ano-rectal abscess

Introduction and general description

Anal abscesses are common in healthy individuals but may occur in patients with inflammatory bowel disease including Crohn disease. Anal abscesses are classified based on their location in relation to the anal sphincters and anatomical spaces of the ano-rectal region (Figure 111.37).

PART 10: SPECIFIC SITES, SEX & AGE

Epidemiology

Incidence and prevalence
They are common.

Sex
Anal abscesses are twice as common in men as in women [1].

Age
Anal abscess is primarily a disease of the young to middle-aged.

Pathophysiology

Predisposing factors
Anal gland infection in the intersphincteric space is the likely cause secondary to impaction with faecal debris (cryptoglandular hypothesis). Anal glands tend to atrophy with age, perhaps explaining why anal abscesses are less common in the elderly. Predisposing factors include trauma (e.g. impacted fish bone), constipation, sedentary occupation, immunodeficiency (including leukaemia and HIV infection), diabetes and anal cancer.

Clinical features

History
Symptoms include pain, swelling, discharge, fever and malaise.

Presentation
Perianal abscesses are common and superficial infections that extend between the internal and external sphincter and reach the anal verge (Figure 111.37). If the abscess penetrates the external anal sphincter, it becomes an ischio-rectal abscess. Intersphincteric abscesses develop in the space between the internal and external sphincters [1].

Perianal abscess may cause an eythematous, fluctuant, tender, indurated swelling.

Clinical variants
See Figure 111.37.

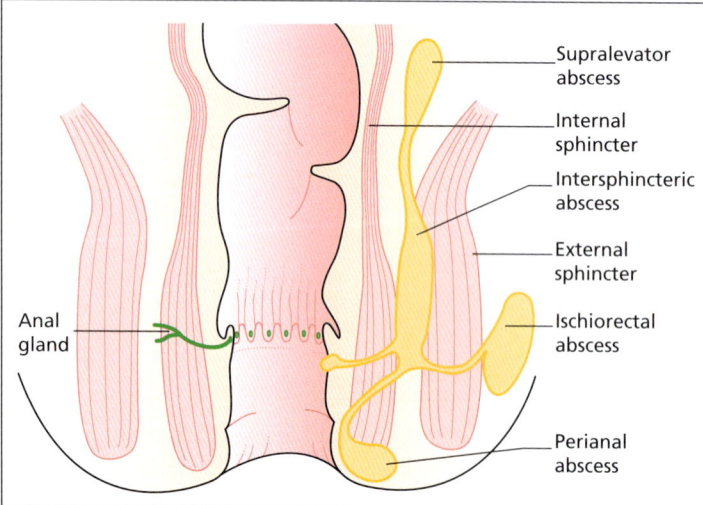

Figure 111.37 Classification of ano-rectal abscesses based on the relation of the abscess to the internal and external anal sphincters.

Labels in figure:
- Supralevator abscess
- Internal sphincter
- Intersphincteric abscess
- External sphincter
- Ischiorectal abscess
- Perianal abscess
- Anal gland

Differential diagnosis
Crohn disease, hidradenitis suppurativa, tuberculosis, thrombosed external haemorrhoids, perianal cellulitis, threadworm infection and malignancy should all be considered.

Complications and co-morbidities
Fistula formation following perianal abscess occurs in 26–37% of cases [2].

Disease course and prognosis
Risk factors for recurrence include diabetes, Crohn disease, immunosuppression and ischio-anal location.

Management
Incision and drainage are required.

First line
Antibiotics are not required unless there are signs of cellulitis or the patient is at risk from underlying co-morbidities such as diabetes or immunosuppression. Antibiotic therapy after surgical drainage does not seem to protect against fistula formation [3].

Anal fistula

Definition and nomenclature
A fistula is an abnormal communication between two epithelial surfaces. An anal fistula is a communication between the ano-rectal canal and perianal skin that is lined with granulation tissue.

Synonyms and inclusions
- Fistula-in-ano
- Ano-rectal fistula

Introduction and general description
Anal fistula is part of the spectrum of perianal sepsis. An anal fistula may present *de novo* or after an acute ano-rectal abscess. A high index of suspicion of anal fistula is necessary when examining patients with a perianal abscess.

Epidemiology

Incidence and prevalence
The prevalence of anal fistulae is 1–2 per 10 000 of population in European studies [1]. This may be an underestimate as many patients do not seek medical advice because of embarrassment.

Age
It most commonly presents at around 40 years.

Sex
Men are twice as likely to be affected.

Associated diseases
See Box 111.6.

Box 111.6 Conditions associated with anal fistulae

- Crohn disease
- Tuberculosis
- Hidradenitis suppurativa
- Pilonidal disease
- HIV infection
- Trauma: obstetric or ano-rectal
- Foreign bodies
- Surgery
- Radiotherapy
- Malignancy
- Lymphogranuloma venereum
- Perianal actinomycosis
- Bridging of anal fissure
- Sacrococcygeal teratoma
- Ano-rectal duplication
- Presacral dermoid cysts

Pathophysiology

Predisposing factors

Approximately 90% of anal fistulae are idiopathic [2]. Infection of anal glands in the intersphincteric space of the anal canal is thought to underlie both acute ano-rectal abscesses and anal fistulae [2,3]. This is called the cryptoglandular hypothesis (Figure 111.38).

It is not clear why certain cases of perianal sepsis are limited to abscess formation whereas others are associated with fistula track formation. The rate of formation of fistula following perianal abscess is 26–37% [4].

See Box 111.6 for diseases associated with anal fistulae. The prevalence of fistulae in patients with Crohn disease is up to 50% [5], of which most are perianal (Figure 111.36). The transmural inflammation characteristic of Crohn disease predisposes patients to fistula formation. Fistulae in Crohn disease are often complex and multiple.

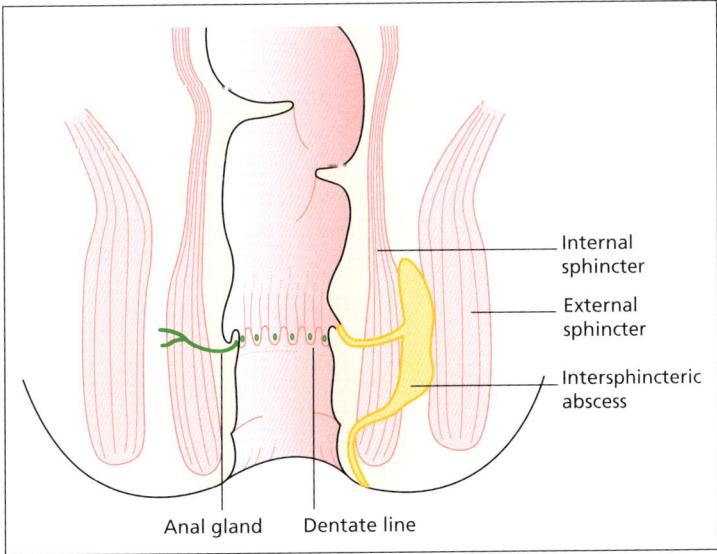

Figure 111.38 Cryptoglandular hypothesis of the development of an intersphincteric fistula.

Internal sphincter
External sphincter
Intersphincteric abscess
Anal gland   Dentate line

Clinical features

History

Patients may complain of pruritus ani, discharge, pain and constipation. In severe cases faecal material may pass through the fistula, leading to soiling of underwear and skin irritation. There is often a history of an abscess that failed to heal after surgical drainage or recurred at the same site.

Presentation

An anal fistula may appear as a pit in the skin with a surrounding rim of granulation tissue, and discharge may be noted. Surrounding skin may be indurated and tender and there may be scarring from previous abscess formation.

Fistulae have a primary track but there may be secondary extensions. Most occur on the midline posteriorly, but there may be multiple openings. The fistula may harbour chronic infection that may discharge onto the skin. Intermittent discharge is usually caused by cyclical accumulation of an abscess with associated discomfort and pain before some relief from discharge [2].

Differential diagnosis

Underlying diseases associated with anal fistula should be considered, including Crohn disease and infections such as tuberculosis (Box 111.6). Tuberculosis should always be suspected and excluded, especially in patients who fail to respond to treatment or who have recurrent disease.

Classification of severity

Fistulae are classified based on their relation to the anal sphincter complex and whether the track is low or high. A low fistula track passes through few or no sphincter muscle fibres and is relatively close to the skin. A high fistula describes a track that passes through or above large amounts of muscle (Figure 111.39).

After considering whether a fistula track is low or high, additional complexity arises from the presence of secondary tracks or residual abscess cavities.

Complications and co-morbidities

Squamous cell carcinoma is a rare complication that may arise in chronic complex fistulae.

Disease course and prognosis

Anal fistulae will not heal without intervention and if left untreated are at risk of recurrent perianal abscess and development of a complex fistula network [2]. The consequences may include chronic pain, bleeding, incontinence, cellulitis and systemic sepsis. In some cases, treatment may require stoma formation.

Investigations

Endoanal ultrasound and MRI improve the characterisation of the fistula anatomy and are the most useful imaging techniques in complex cases [6].

Management

Referral to a colorectal specialist is required. The aims of management are to eradicate the fistula and prevent recurrence whilst

PART 10: SPECIFIC SITES, SEX & AGE

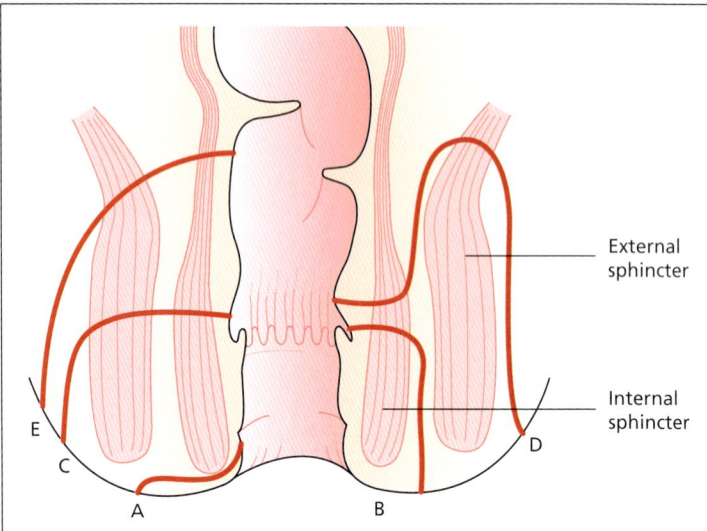

Figure 111.39 Parks classification of anal fistulae. A: superficial fistula track beneath the internal and external sphincters. B: intersphincteric fistula track between the internal and external sphincters in the intersphincteric space. C: transsphincteric fistula track crossing both the external and internal anal sphincters. D: suprasphincteric fistula passing outside the internal and external anal sphincters over the top of the puborectalis muscle and penetrating the levator muscle before tracking down to the skin. E: extrasphincteric fistula tracking outside the external anal sphincter and penetrating the levator muscle into the rectum. Adapted from Parks *et al.* 1976 [3].

maintaining continence. Successful management of an anal fistula requires that all primary and secondary tracks are drained and eradicated [2]. Antibiotics are not usually effective in treating perianal abscess or infection associated with anal fistula but are recommended in patients who have cellulitis [3].

First line
Surgical procedures performed by a colorectal specialist include fistulotomy and seton insertion (see later) [7]. Fistulotomy entails the division of superficial tissue to lay open the fistula track and is an effective way to treat low fistulae. Fistulotomy should be avoided where there is significant anal sphincter involvement to avoid the risk of postoperative faecal incontinence. A seton is a thread (usually a non-absorbable suture or vascular sling) placed through the fistula track and tied to form a continuous ring between the internal and external openings of the fistula. Setons maintain the patency of the fistula track, acting as a wick and allowing the drainage of pus and healing to occur. Secondary treatment is usually required to close the track.

Second line
Fibrin glue can be injected into the fistula track and is a sphincter-sparing technique.

Third line
Other surgical options include the insertion of a fistula plug derived from porcine small intestine and an endo-rectal advancement flap. Formation of a colostomy is considered a last resort in non-healing anal fistulae [2]. Defunctioning colostomy is more frequently utilised in Crohn disease where wound healing is poor following other surgical procedures.

Resources

Further information
Crohn's and Colitis UK: www.crohnsandcolitis.org.uk (last accessed May 2022).

Anal fissure

Definition and nomenclature
An anal fissure is a longitudinal ulcer occurring in the squamous epithelium of the anal canal located distal to the dentate line.

Synonyms and inclusions
• Fissure-in-ano

Introduction and general description
Primary anal fissures are idiopathic and usually affect the posterior midline. Secondary anal fissures usually occur in the lateral aspect of the anal canal and are associated with underlying diseases such as Crohn disease.

Epidemiology
Incidence and prevalence
The exact incidence is unknown and probably underreported as it is likely that many patients do not seek medical advice as the fissure heals without intervention. It has been suggested that the lifetime incidence is 11% [1].

Age
Anal fissures are commonly encountered in young adults but may affect extremes of age [2].

Sex
There is an equal prevalence in males and females.

Associated diseases
Atypical fissures (large, irregular, multiple and non-midline) are associated with underlying disease such as Crohn disease, HIV infection, syphilis, tuberculosis and malignancy.

Pathophysiology
Predisposing factors
The aetiology is poorly understood. Trauma causing pressure or necrosis by the passage of hard stools is thought to be an initiating factor. Pregnancy-associated anal fissures are thought to arise due to shearing forces during labour.

Pathology
Histology in idiopathic cases is of non-specific ulceration. In secondary anal fissures, specific pathology such as anal carcinoma or Crohn disease will be identified.

Clinical features
History
Painful defecation occurs, often described as a tearing sensation. Blood may be present on the surface of the stool. Other symptoms

include mucous discharge and constipation. Anal fissures result in significant morbidity and reduction of quality of life [3].

Presentation

The tear can usually be visualised in the distal anal canal [2]. Acute fissures are typically superficial with well-delineated mucosal edges and granulation tissue at the base. Chronic fissures may have a fibrotic rolled edge, sentinel tag at the anal pole of the fissure and visible transverse fibres of the internal anal sphincter.

Fissures are normally single and occur in the posterior midline in 80–90% of cases [2]. Anterior midline fissures are usually found in women. Fissures occurring in patients older than 65 are typically secondary and appropriate investigations are required to exclude underlying disease.

Clinical variants

Although not true anal fissures, erosions and fissures may occur in the sulcus beneath odematous haemorrhoids or in any area of perianal skin disease including the natal cleft. These fissures, which are secondary to inflammatory skin disease such as psoriasis or lichen simplex, or to trauma, are sometimes referred to as anal rhagades. The presence of even a small fissure in an area of cutaneous inflammation maintains the pruritus and may predispose to infection.

Differential diagnosis

Sexually transmitted diseases including primary syphilis, Crohn disease, tuberculous and HIV infection should be considered and excluded by appropriate investigations. Trauma is also a possible cause. Behçet disease occasionally presents with multiple shallow ulcers and fissures of the perianal skin.

Complications and co-morbidities

Constipation is frequently found. Perianal tags may result when an anal fissure has healed. Squamous cell carcinoma is a rare complication of chronic anal fissure.

Disease course and prognosis

More than 50% of acute fissures heal spontaneously with conservative management [2]. Only 10% of chronic fissures will heal spontaneously and either surgical or medical intervention is required to achieve healing.

Investigations

Proctoscopy and histological assessment are mandatory if the aetiology is in doubt.

Management

Management is the domain of the ano-rectal specialist. Conservative management, including advice on a high-fibre diet, is advisable. Warm sitz baths (a shallow bath used for cleansing the perineal and perianal skin) can help with symptomatic relief [4]. The aim of management of chronic fissures is to treat the triad of anal pain, spasm and ischaemia. Medical treatment should be pursued prior to surgical intervention.

First line

The use of topical nitrate (e.g. glyceryl trinitrate 0.4% ointment) may be considered. Topical calcium channel blockers (e.g. diltiazem 2% gel) can be tried in patients unresponsive to topical nitrates.

Second line

Surgery is the mainstay of treatment for chronic anal fissures unresponsive to first line measures. Lateral internal sphincterotomy results in cure rates of up to 98% but may compromise anal continence in up to 30% [2].

The relatively high risk of anal incontinence following surgical intervention has led to the search for medical therapy to reduce anal pressure. Options that may be tried prior to surgery include oral calcium channel blockers (e.g. nifedipine) or injection of botulinum neurotoxin A into the internal anal sphincter.

Third line

Fissurectomy and endoanal advancement flap are surgical options [2].

Haemorrhoids

Definition and nomenclature

Haemorrhoids are dilatations in the venous system draining the anus.

> **Synonyms and inclusions**
> - Piles (Latin *pila*, a ball)
> - Varicose veins of the anus

Introduction and general description

Internal haemorrhoids typically develop from three anal cushions present in the anal canal (Figure 111.40). Anatomically, an internal haemorrhoid is a fold of mucous membrane and submucosa containing a varicosed tributary of the superior rectal vein and a terminal branch of the superior rectal artery (Figure 111.41). Internal haemorrhoids are proximal to the dentate line and have visceral innervation with an absence of pain fibres. External haemorrhoids are varicosities of tributaries of the inferior rectal vein and are located below the dentate line in the distal third of the anal canal (Figure 111.42). They are covered by squamous epithelium and have somatic pain fibre innervation. External haemorrhoids are commonly associated with internal haemorrhoids.

Epidemiology

Incidence and prevalence

Symptomatic haemorrhoids affect up to 36% of the population [1].

Age

Prevalence increases with age.

Sex

They are common in both men and women.

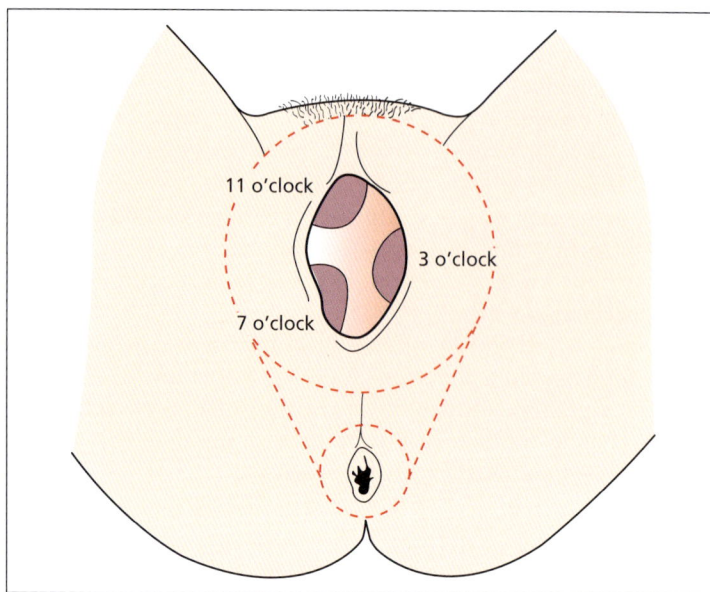

Figure 111.40 Typical positions of development of internal haemorrhoids in the anal canal at 3, 7 and 11 o'clock seen with the patient in the dorsal lithotomy position. The anal column blood vessels are largest at the left lateral, right posterior and right anterior quadrants of the anal canal where the subepithelial tissues expand to form three anal cushions. The cushions help to seal the anal canal to maintain continence to faeces and flatus, and are also important in the pathogenesis of internal haemorrhoids. Adapted from Snell 2012 [4]. Reproduced with permission of Lippincott Williams & Wilkins/Wolters Kluwer.

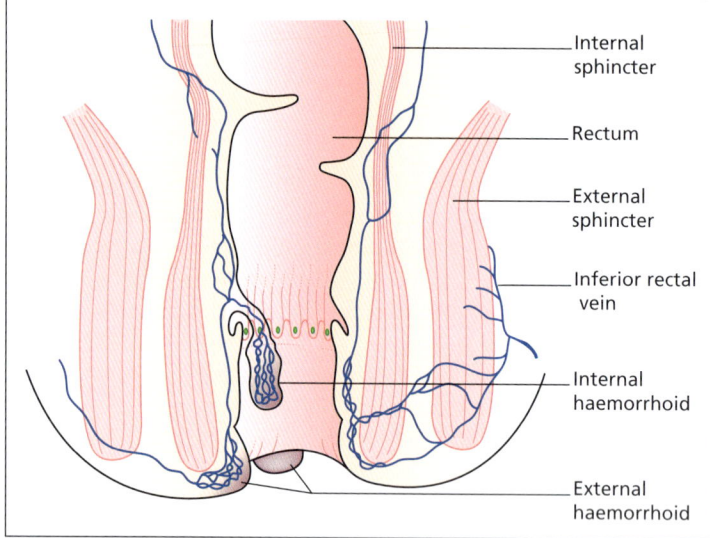

Figure 111.41 Origin of internal and external haemorrhoids. Adapted from Snell 2012 [4]. Reproduced with permission of Lippincott Williams & Wilkins/Wolters Kluwer.

Pathophysiology
Predisposing factors
Factors that increase intra-abdominal pressure, including pregnancy, obesity and straining at stool due to constipation, contribute to the incidence of haemorrhoids. Other predisposing factors include portal hypertension due to liver cirrhosis and malignancy causing compression of the superior rectal vein. Haemorrhoids are often familial and there may be a family history of leg varicose

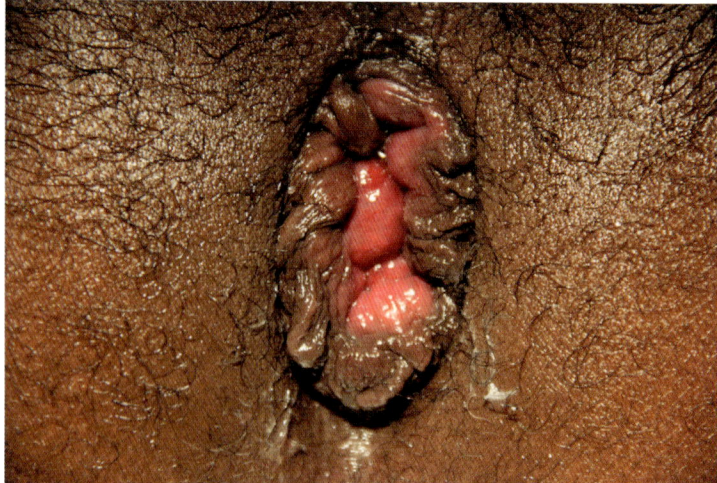

Figure 111.42 Second-degree prolapsed internal haemorrhoids with surrounding anal tags. Courtesy of Mr M. Abulafi, Croydon University Hospital, UK.

veins. Age-related loss of anal canal muscle support may explain the increase in prevalence with age [2].

Clinical features
History
Symptoms are bleeding, mucous or faecal discharge, pruritus ani and the sensation or awareness of prolapse. Typically, uncomplicated internal haemorrhoids cause painless bleeding. Pain may arise if thrombosis, ulceration or infection occurs. External haemorrhoids are more likely to cause pain. Haemorrhoidal bleeding consists of bright red blood on the stool or toilet paper or dripping into the toilet. The symptoms of haemorrhoidal disease do not correlate with the size of the haemorrhoids.

Presentation
Prolapsed internal haemorrhoids with an overlying columnar mucosal surface may be visible on inspection of the perianal skin (Figure 111.42). External thrombosed haemorrhoids can be differentiated as they are covered by squamous epithelium. A perianal dermatitis may occur secondary to skin irritation resulting from faecal leakage or a contact dermatitis (irritant or allergic) secondary to overwashing or medicaments. Examination should include digital rectal examination to exclude the presence of a mass and proctocopy to evaluate if there is any other ano-rectal pathology.

Clinical variants
Perianal skin tags (anal tags) can result from thrombosed external haemorrhoids and are common (Figure 111.43). In contrast to external haemorrhoids, perianal skin tags do not swell with blood when the patient strains or reduce with pressure. Perianal tags are usually asymptomatic but large or multiple lesions can interfere with perianal hygiene and predispose to perianal dermatitis.

Perianal haematoma (perianal thrombosis) is caused by the rupture of tributaries of the inferior rectal vein as a result of coughing or straining, with the appearance of a haematoma affecting perianal skin (incorrectly called a thrombosed haemorrhoid). The history is of sudden onset of pain and swelling. A blue-black nodule that can be multilocular can be seen on inspection of the anal margin

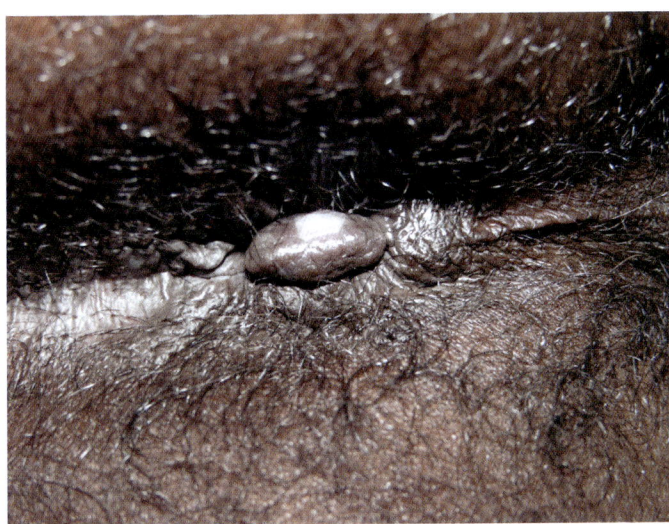

Figure 111.43 Perianal skin tag.

Table 111.3 Classification of haemorrhoid severity.

Severity	Definition
First degree	Contained within the anal canal
Second degree	Prolapse on straining and defecation but reduce spontaneously
Third degree	Prolapse on straining but remain outside the anus and require manual reduction
Fourth degree	Prolapsed and incarcerated

region. If the overlying skin perforates, a clot of blood is extruded leading to pain relief. A perianal skin tag can result when the haematoma resolves. Many perianal haematomas are associated with haemorrhoids.

Differential diagnosis
The differential diagnosis includes ano-rectal malignancy, Crohn disease, perianal metastases and Kaposi sarcoma.

Classification of severity
See Table 111.3.

Complications and co-morbidities
The complications of haemorrhoids include pain, thrombosis, strangulation, ulceration, fibrosis, infection and abscess and incarceration of a prolapsed haemorrhoid.

Management
Management of symptomatic haemorrhoids is the domain of the ano-rectal specialist. First- and second-degree disease (Table 111.3) can usually be treated conservatively without the need for operative intervention. The aims of management include addressing any predisposing factors such as constipation or diarrhoea. Symptomatic relief for perianal symptoms can be achieved with topical agents including lubricants and mild topical steroids. Dietary fibre should be increased and there should be adequate water intake.

Third-degree haemorrhoids usually require surgical intervention. First line options include injection sclerotherapy, rubber band ligation, infrared coagulation and cryotherapy. These techniques result in tissue destruction, subsequent fibrosis and resultant resolution of the haemorrhoid.

Fourth-degree haemorrhoids require urgent surgical intervention. Surgical procedures include excisional haemorrhoidectomy, stapled haemorrhoidopexy and Doppler-guided transanal haemorrhoid devascularisation [3].

Resources

Further information
https://patient.info/doctor/haemorrhoids-piles-pro (last accessed May 2022).

Key references

The full list of references can be found in the online version at https://www.wiley.com/rooksdermatology10e

Introduction
1 Standring S, ed. in chief. *Grays Anatomy. The Anatomical Basis of Clinical Practice*, 40th edn. London: Churchill Livingstone, Elsevier, 2008.

Perianal sensory disturbances
Pruritus ani
2 Markell KW, Billingham R. Pruritus ani: etiology and management. *Surg Clin North Am* 2010;90:125–35.

Other diseases and infections
Sexually transmitted diseases
1 Singhrao T, Higham E, French P. Lymphogranuloma venereum presenting as perianal ulceration: an emerging clinical presentation? *Sex Transm Infect* 2011;87:123–4.

Human immunodeficiency virus infection
1 Barrett W, Callahan T, Orkin B. Perianal manifestations of human immunodeficiency virus infection: experience with 260 patients. *Dis Colon Rectum* 1998;41:606–11.
3 Yuhan R, Orsay C, Del Pino A *et al*. Anorectal disease in HIV-infected patients. *Dis Colon Rectum* 1998;41:1367–70.

Human papillomavirus infection
2 Giuliana A, Nyitray A, Kreimer A *et al*. EUROGIN 2014 roadmap: differences in human papillomavirus infection, natural history, transmission and human papillomavirus-related cancer incidence by gender and anatomic site of infection. *Int J Cancer* 2015;136:2752–60.
4 Stanley M. Epithelial cell responses to infection with human papillomavirus. *Clin Microbiol Rev* 2012;25:215–22.
11 Yang J, Pu YG, Zeng ZM, Yu ZJ, Huang N, Deng QW. Interferon for the treatment of genital warts: a systematic review. *BMC Infect Dis* 2009;9:156.

Anal intraepithelial neoplasia
8 Palefsky J, Giuliano A, Goldstone S *et al*. HPV vaccine against anal HPV infection and anal intraepithelial neoplasia. *N Eng J Med* 2011;365:1576–85.
9 Brogden D, Walsh U, Pellini G *et al*. Evaluating the efficacy of treatment options for anal intraepithelial neoplasia: a systematic review. *Int J Colorectal Dis* 2021;36:213–26.

Anal and perianal malignancy
6 Sunesen K, Norgaard M, Thorlacius-Ussing O *et al*. Immunosuppressive disorders and risk of anal squamous cell carcinoma: a nationwide cohort study in Denmark, 1978–2005. *Int J Cancer* 2009;127:675–84.
8 Hillman R, Garland S, Gunathilake M *et al*. Human papillomavirus (HPV) genotypes in an Australian sample of anal cancers. *Int J Cancer* 2014;135:996–1001.
9 Newlin H, Zlotecki R, Morris C *et al*. Squamous cell carcinoma of the anal margin. *J Surg Oncol* 2004;86:55–62.

CHAPTER 112

Cutaneous Complications of Stomas and Fistulae

Calum Lyon

York Hospital NHS Trust, York, UK; Salford Royal Hospital NHS Trust, Salford, UK

Introduction

An abdominal stoma (ostomy) is a surgically created opening from the gastrointestinal or urinary tract onto the skin in order to drain the effluent from that system. Ostomies are inherently incontinent so this typically involves a collection device worn on the skin, usually held in place by an adhesive material. Each year in the UK approximately 21 000 people have an abdominal stoma formed with a large proportion intended as temporary or palliative procedures rather than a long-term therapeutic solution. There are no exact figures available and, although estimates vary, at any one time there are probably over 100 000 people in the UK with a chronic abdominal stoma. Skin problems are the commonest longer term complications and while estimates vary, figures from several studies would suggest that between one-third and two-thirds will experience a skin problem around their stoma at some time that will interfere with normal appliance use [1,2]. In theory, most dermatoses could affect peristomal skin but in practice the majority fall into one or more of a few groups that are predictable because of the occluded nature of the peristomal skin, prolonged contact with the appliance and any medicaments or cleansers, leakage of urine or faeces onto the skin and the underlying abdominal disease itself. The common cutaneous complications are (in order of prevalence): irritant reactions (including dermatoses exacerbated by trauma), common generalised inflammatory dermatoses (e.g. psoriasis and pemphigoid), disorders associated with the reason for surgery especially Crohn disease, infections and allergic reaction [3].

Types of stoma and appliances

Most ostomates (a person who has an ostomy) use modern stoma appliances that consist of a polythene or vinyl bag attached to a firm thermoplastic armature which is itself fixed to an adhesive system that is intended to contact the abdominal skin (Figure 112.1) [4]. Patients with a short or buried stoma may use an appliance with a convex skin barrier to effectively lengthen the stoma spout. The types of stomas covered in this chapter and the appliances used are described in Table 112.1.

Assessment of the patient

The involvement of an experienced stoma nurse specialist is invaluable, particularly as they may know the patient well. The stoma nurse can advise the patient on how to manage their stoma, including advice on appliance modifications and the use of accessory adhesives, filler pastes, etc. In this way many irritant reactions can be resolved without further dermatological input. It is important that the dermatologist examines the peristomal skin as this will quickly identify common conditions (e.g. psoriasis or seborrhoeic warts) and rarer conditions such as skin cancers as the cause of the skin problems. Specific points to consider when assessing a stoma patient in addition to a general dermatological consultation are listed in Table 112.2.

General aspects of treatment for stomas

Inflammatory dermatoses can usually be managed with topical therapies as at other body sites, but topical therapies need to be chosen carefully, particularly with regard to the vehicles used in order to minimise greasiness that would interfere with appliance adhesion (Table 112.3). Progression to systemic therapy should be considered earlier for more severe inflammatory dermatoses such as psoriasis or pemphigoid as such disorders themselves will diminish adhesion and the resulting leakage may worsen the skin disease. The avoidance of irritants or allergens are dealt with in the sections on allergic contact dermatitis and irritant reactions and in Table 112.1 [5].

Rook's Textbook of Dermatology, Tenth Edition. Edited by Christopher Griffiths, Jonathan Barker, Tanya Bleiker, Walayat Hussain and Rosalind Simpson.
© 2024 John Wiley & Sons Ltd. Published 2024 by John Wiley & Sons Ltd.

PART 10: SPECIFIC SITES, SEX & AGE

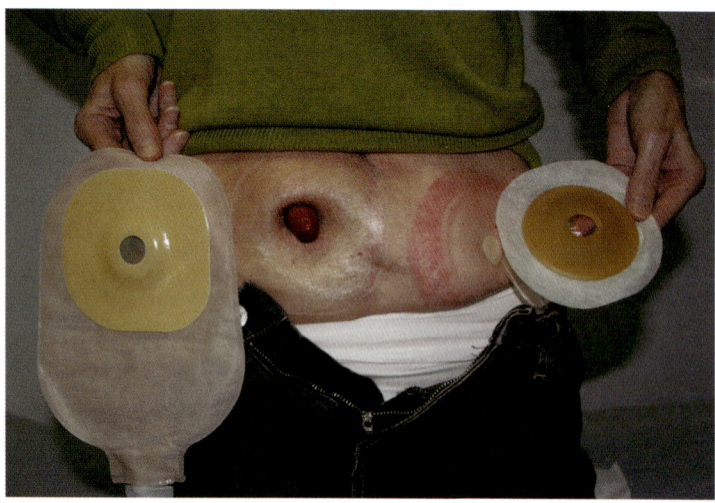

(a)

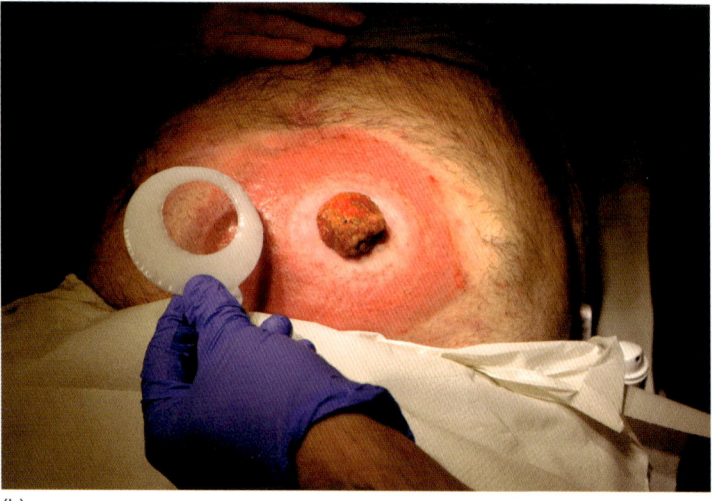

(b)

Figure 112.1 (a) Patient with a urostomy for bladder carcinoma who has reacted to the tape border of a two-piece appliance on a 5-day skin test (right of picture). She has not reacted to the hydrocolloid central portion or the all-hydrocolloid one-piece appliance on the left. The product on the left is a typical drainable urostomy bag with a nylon tap at the bottom of the device. Similar bags with different drain systems are used by ileostomy patients and some with colostomies of the ascending colon. (b) Patient with a colostomy who has clearly reacted to a component of the appliance adhesive as the central hydrocolloid washer prevents the reaction.

Irritant skin reactions

- ICD-10: L24.8
- BAD: RE800, RE801, RE802, C7210, C7211, C7212

Introduction

Irritant reactions are a common cause of skin problems in patients with a stoma.

Epidemiology

Irritant reactions account for more than 50% of the skin problems experienced by stoma patients [1,2].

Pathophysiology

See Chapter 128 for pathogenetic information on irritant contact dermatitis.

Damage to the skin barrier producing irritant reactions can result from physical trauma (e.g. pressure and skin stripping) but the reactions are most commonly due to repeated exposure to the stoma contents which may be corrosive in the case of faeces. Most stoma effluent is of neutral pH or above and ammonia from the urea in urine will also increase skin pH thus impairing barrier function. Repeated microscopic skin stripping at appliance changes may also contribute to faecal or urine dermatitis reactions [3]. When all potential causes of peristomal dermatitis have been excluded (including allergy, infection and psoriasis, etc.) there remain approximately 10% of stoma patients with what is regarded as idiopathic dermatitis [2].

Clinical features

Irritant reactions may present with a dermatitis or one of a range of distinctive papular reactions [4]. In most cases the patient's stoma nurse specialist will have diagnosed the problem and arranged effective management, usually by modification of the appliance system to prevent leaks or adhesive reactions. The causes and types of these disorders are detailed in Tables 112.1 and 112.2. Most patients presenting to dermatologists will therefore be those who require further investigations or treatments that cannot be undertaken or prescribed by the nurse.

Faecal or urinary irritant dermatitis may result from wearing an appliance that is too large so that it exposes skin to effluent because the stoma is buried or in a skin fold (Figure 112.2), or because the stoma is too short (Figure 112.3) so that faeces inevitably track under the barrier. Occasionally, ileostomies or urostomies are very contractile such that they spasmodically shorten with the same results (Figure 112.4). In this situation, the injection of botulinum toxin into the stoma musculature can be highly effective as it preferentially paralyses the longitudinal muscle thus maintaining a longer spout. It does not work with colostomies [5]. Some patients develop persistent reactions to portions of the adhesive barrier with no demonstrable allergic component. This is particularly the case with adhesive tape borders similar to the dressings used for patch testing (Figures 112.1a and 112.6). A proportion of patients (up to 10%) have persistent or recurrent dermatitis affecting the whole of the occluded skin for which no cause can be found (Figure 112.6).

Three patterns of papular reaction deserve particular mention. All are the probable consequences of exposure to stoma effluent:

1 Hypergranulating polyps or 'granulomas'. These occur particularly around colostomies as cherry red papules at the mucocutaneous junction; these may proliferate into normal skin if it is exposed to faeces (Figure 112.7) [6]. A similar process can affect an ileostomy where it presents as a flatter, red, bleeding area in which bowel metaplasia of the skin is relatively common (Figure 112.8). In either case they may be symptomatic as they bleed and cause leaks. Occasionally they are painful (Figure 112.9). The metaplastic lesions may very rarely develop primary adenocarcinoma [7]. Exceptionally, this metaplastic process may affect urostomies (Figure 112.10).

Table 112.1 Types of stoma and appliance.[a]

Type of stoma	Description	Indications	Appliance types used	Specific associated skin problems
Ileostomy	Placed usually in right iliac fossa with an ideal spout of at least 2 cm. Produces liquid output which increases in inverse proportion to the amount of functioning ileum remaining; as does the pH of effluent which ranges from 6.5 to 7.5	Inflammatory bowel disease (IBD) either as a permanent or temporary end ileostomy. Loop ileostomies (double-barrelled) intended to protect the distal bowel pending re-anastomosis or pouch formation. Other indications include bowel carcinoma and ischaemic bowel	One-piece and occasionally two-piece drainable pouches changed every 2–3 days	Irritant reactions particularly with high-output stomas. Short or imperfectly placed stomas (e.g. in an abdominal fold) and loop ileostomies are especially prone to leakage onto skin. Disorders associated with the underlying bowel pathology
Colostomy	Placed typically in the left iliac fossa with a minimal spout	Large bowel carcinoma, IBD including temporary stomas to rest diseased distal bowel or perineum	One-piece closed appliance changed daily or more frequently depending on output	Irritant reactions are relatively uncommon unless stool is not formed. Bleeding overgranulating papules
Urostomy (ileal conduit)	A length of ileum with a spout similar to an ileostomy into which one or usually both ureters drain. Can be on right or left	Bladder carcinoma, incontinence and iatrogenic damage to urological tract either due to radiotherapy or surgical trauma	One- or two-piece drainable appliances changed every 2–3 days	Irritant reactions particularly with short or poorly positioned stomas
Abdominal fistula	Opening of an abdominal viscus directly onto the skin	Usually results from dehiscence of a surgical abdominal wound especially in IBD, fistulating diverticular disease or carcinoma	A variety of appliances together with dressings may be used	Irritant reactions
Others	Gastrostomy is placed in left upper quadrant and nephrostomy on either flank	Gastrostomy is typically for nutritional support. Nephrostomy is usually temporary and used to divert urine from a distal obstruction often secondary to carcinoma	A drainable appliance is used for a nephrostomy	Nephrostomies are occasionally associated with irritant reactions. Gastrosomies develop exuberant granulation tissue that can bleed and be painful

[a] The appliances attach to the skin usually by means of a hydrocolloid material. These are commonly composed of polyisobutylene (PIB), which provides 'dry tack' adhesion to the skin, and a mixture of carboxymethylcellulose and fruit pectins, which serve to preserve the acidic pH of the skin and to absorb water thereby maintaining the dry skin adhesion. Newer products incorporate additional materials such as addition buffers, ceramide and aloe vera. In addition, silicon gel-based adhesive barriers are increasingly used. The polymer's adhesion is not optimal until warmed so most barriers incorporate an immediate adhesive tackifier on the surface. This is traditionally rosin based (pentaerythritol ester of rosin) but increasingly non-allergenic, synthetic hydrocarbon materials are used. A range of accessories may be used including belts, additional adhesive tapes, cleansers, adhesive removers, deodorisers and barrier preparations including acrylic adhesive materials.

Table 112.2 Dermatological assessment: aspects specific to peristomal skin.

Aspect	Problems	Actions
Patient's technique	Appliance may no longer be appropriate size or shape. Patient may be inappropriately rough when cleaning the skin or using inappropriate accessory products or medicaments	Stoma nurse input is essential
Patient anxiety or acceptance of the stoma	Usually fear of leaks or noise leads patients to change appliances too frequently, wear excessively tight belts or use unnecessary additional adhesive tapes	Stoma nurse input is essential
The stoma itself	The stoma may be short, in the wrong place or contractile, causing it to shorten and leak. Parastomal hernias are common (up to 34% of patients [2]) and cause bag failures	Stoma nurse input may help but surgical referral may be necessary
Bowel contents	Liquid motions are more likely to cause leaks and short bowel stomas, especially jejunostomies, will have effluent with a high pH	Consider codeine phosphate, loperamide or omeprazole
Infection	Local skin infection may not present in the typical manner under occlusion and broken skin may become secondarily infected	Always swab rashes and consider *Candida* infection
Underlying bowel disease	Extraintestinal manifestations of Crohn disease and metastatic Crohn disease. Complications of antineoplastic therapy	Consider biopsy early
Other skin diseases	These may present atypically under occlusion, for example bullae in localised pemphigoid may not be apparent	Consider biopsy early

Table 112.3 Topical corticosteroids useful for inflammatory peristomal skin diseases.[a]

Active ingredients	Trade name	Other ingredients
Betamethasone valerate 0.1%: scalp lotion	Betnovate™; GlaxoSmithKline	Carbomer, sodium hydroxide and water
Betamethasone dipropionate 0.05%: scalp lotion	Diprosone™; Schering-Plough	Carbomer, sodium hydroxide and water
Clobetasol propionate 0.05%: scalp lotion	Dermovate™; GlaxoSmithKline	Carbomer, sodium hydroxide and water
Fluocinolone 0.025%: scalp gel	Synalar™; GP Pharma	Benzoates and propylene glycol
Betamethasone and calcipotriol: scalp gel	Dovobet™; Leo Laboratories	Paraffin, liquid polyoxypropylene 15, stearyl ether, castor oil and butylhydroxytoluene (E321)
Beclometasone dipropionate 200 µg: metered dose asthma inhaler	Clenil modulate™; Chiesi	None
Fludroxycortide 4 µg/cm²: tape	Generic	None
Betamethasone valerate: plaster	Betesil™; Derma UK	None

[a] There is no perfect preparation applicable to stomas that is available 'off the shelf' and getting medicaments manufactured can be problematic and expensive. The table details some preparations that can be used. Lotions containing oils should be avoided and the patient should be warned that preparations containing propylene glycol and Dovobet™ gel should be left to dry for 10 min before placing their bag. Alcoholic scalp lotions can sting when applied to broken skin and can be applied to the bag directly and left to dry before fitting. The potency of the steroid is increased under occlusion. Continuous daily treatment should be for no more than 4 weeks and thereafter no more than three times per week to avoid skin atrophy. Haelan tape is useful for small ulcerated lesions, particularly pyoderma gangrenosum.

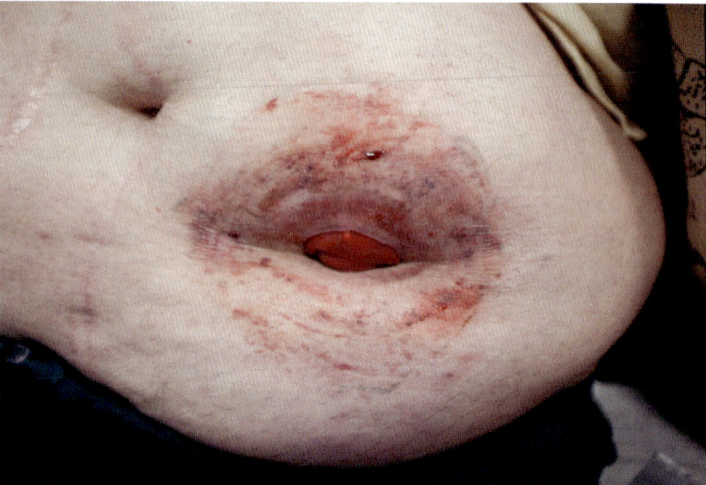

(a)

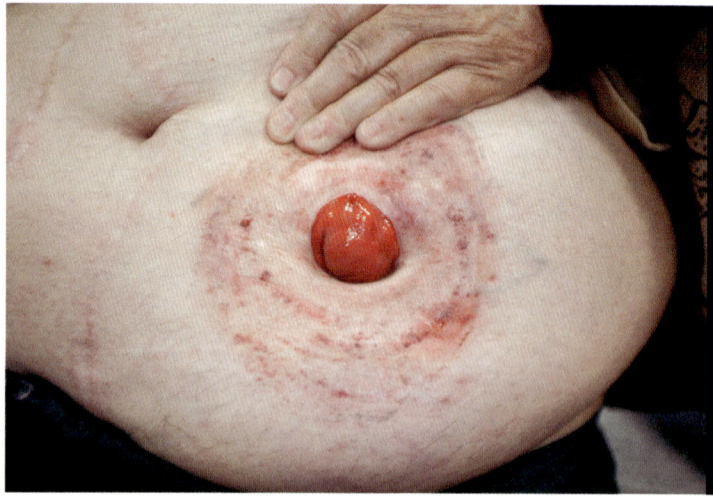

(b)

Figure 112.2 (a, b) A short colostomy that leaks onto the skin because it is in a skin fold. This results in leakage and an eroded faecal dermatitis.

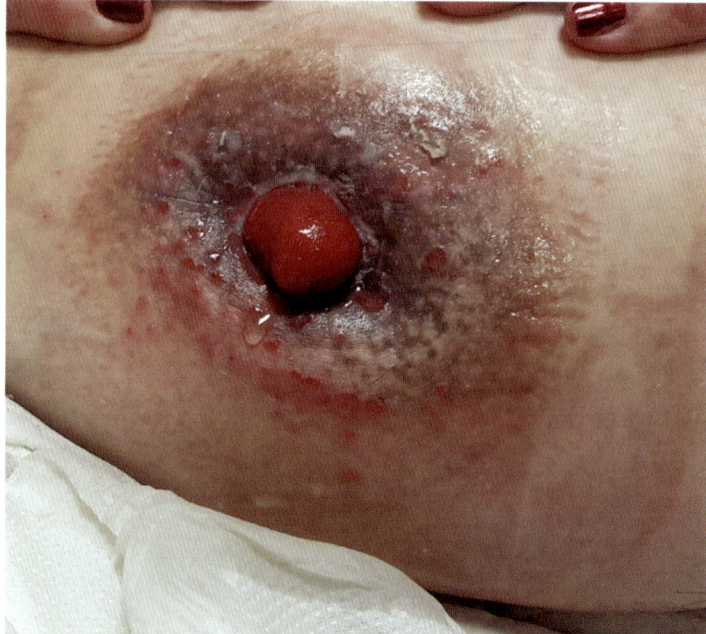

Figure 112.3 A short ileostomy that has become shortened after surgery and is fixed with its opening pointing to the skin at the 6 o'clock position. Leaks are inevitable and this will require surgery. The eroded dermatitis is due to the corrosive faecal contents.

2 Multiple hyperkeratotic and acanthotic papules. These occur around short ileostomies and particularly abdominal fistulae (Figure 112.11)

3 Chronic papillomatous dermatitis (CPD). This is a term used by Bergman *et al.* [8] to describe a distinctive hyperkeratotic irritant skin reaction affecting leaking urostomies. The term has been used by subsequent authors to refer to lesions near ileostomies but is probably best reserved for urostomies as the clinical presentation is distinct (Figure 112.12). Small hyperkeratotic papules can lead to massive and progressive hyperkeratotic plaques that may impinge on the stoma, resulting in stenosis in some cases if the leaking onto the skin is not corrected.

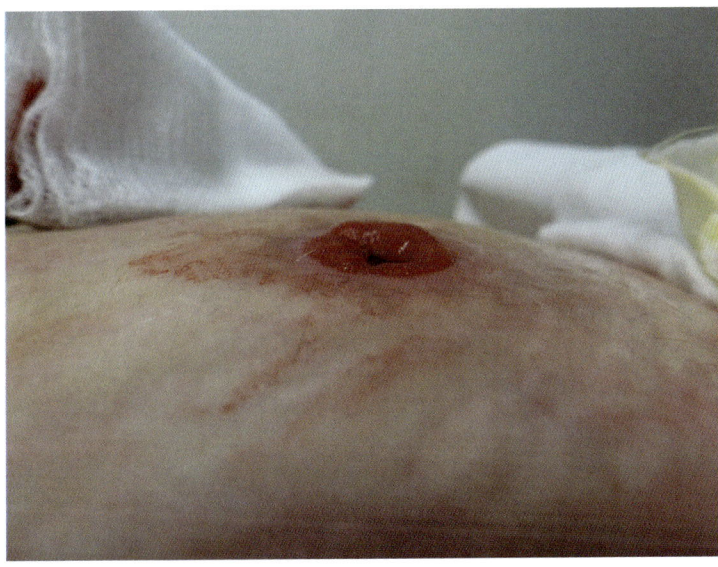

Figure 112.4 A highly contractile ileostomy that varies in length from flush (pictured) to 3 cm long. This type of stoma can respond to intramuscular botulinum toxin.

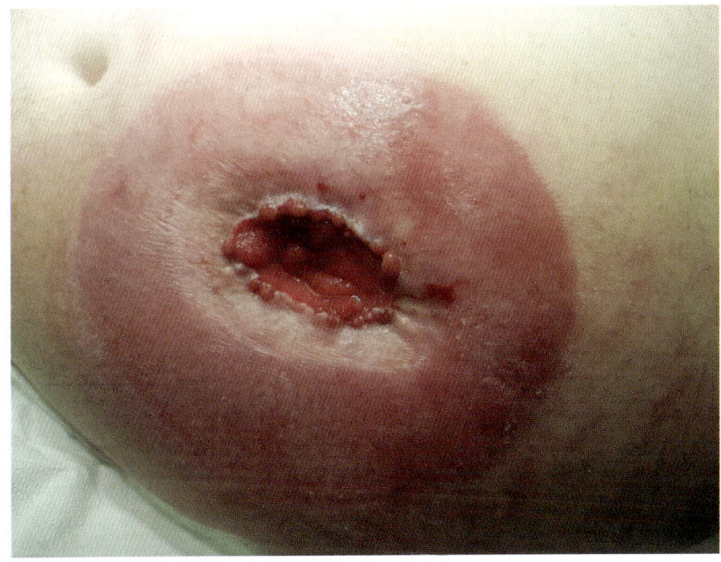

(a)

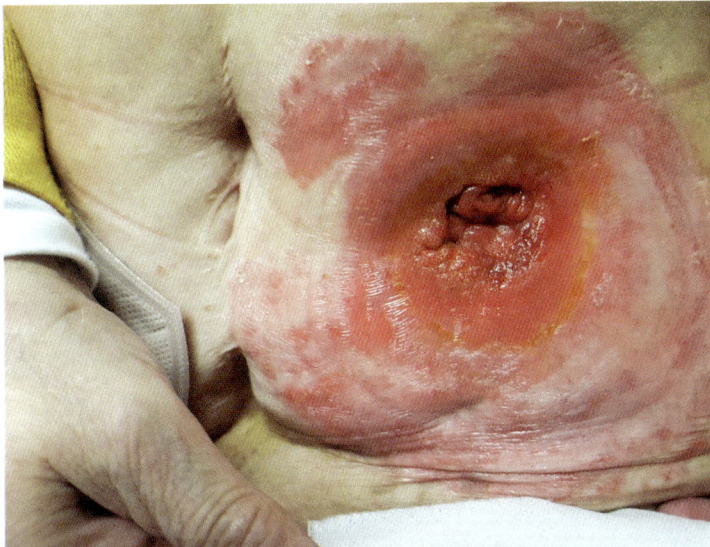

Figure 112.5 A short colostomy in a fold demonstrating severe faecal dermatitis resulting from frequent leaks.

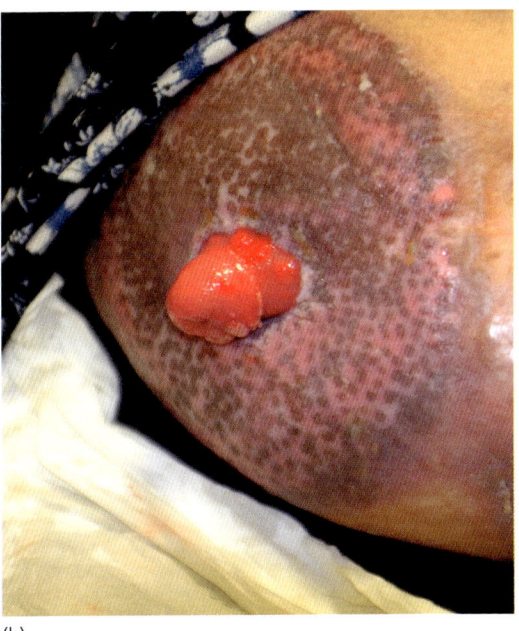

(b)

Figure 112.6 Idiopathic dermatitis affecting the whole skin covered by the stoma barrier. The patients did not develop a reaction to the appliance when worn for 7 days on a normal piece of skin. (a) A patient with a colostomy for bowel carcinoma. (b) A patient with darker skin and an ileostomy for Crohn disease. Mottled, postinflammatory hyperpigmentation occasionally occurs.

Investigations

In most cases the diagnosis is clinically obvious and measures taken to prevent further skin damage will confirm the underlying irritancy. A biopsy may be undertaken in the remaining cases to look for other diagnoses (see the section on other diseases later in this chapter). The histological features of all the irritant reactions including an idiopathic dermatitis are essentially the same, comprising various degrees of acanthosis, hyperkeratosis, erosion, mixed inflammatory infiltrate and capillary dilatation. Patients with longstanding stomas, usually ileostomies for ulcerative colitis, may very rarely develop carcinoma in the surrounding skin such that a biopsy is indicated for any unusual or persistent lesions.

Management

The general management for all irritant reactions is to prevent exposure to the irritant wherever possible. It is therefore essential to liaise with a stoma nurse specialist in the management of these patients. CPD in particular responds rapidly to measures to prevent leaks. Patients presenting to a dermatologist will, in most cases, have already seen their nurse and will require specific dermatological intervention as well. Where the stoma is short, suboptimally placed or associated with a hernia, surgical refashioning might

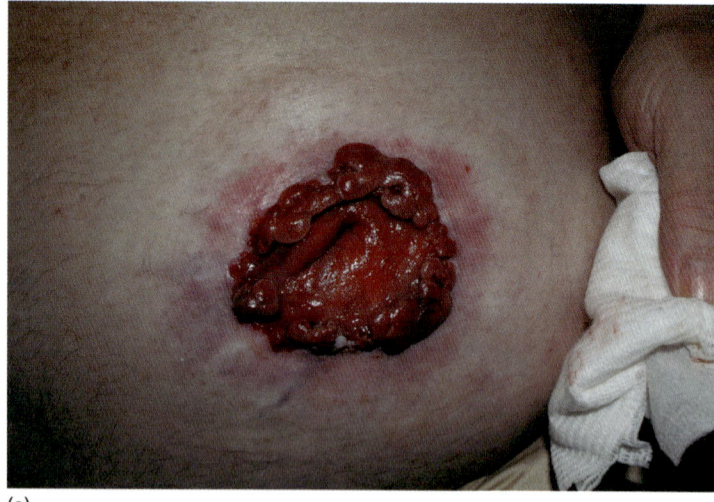

(a)

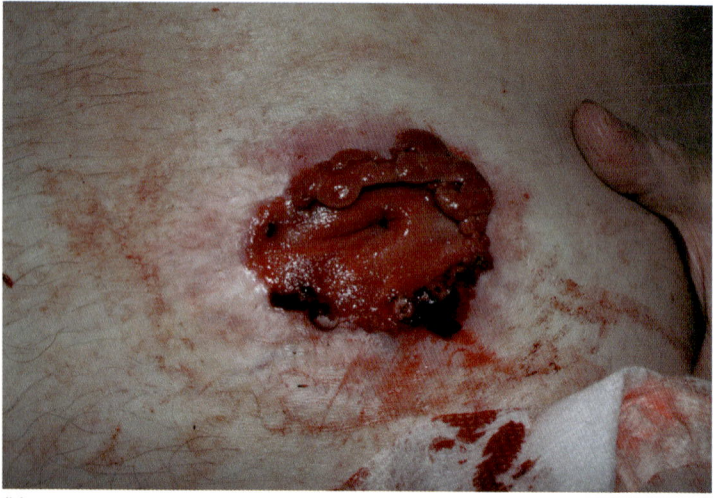

(b)

Figure 112.7 (a) Inflammatory polyps affecting a colostomy where the skin has been exposed to faeces. (b) Where these bleed, proliferate, cause pain or otherwise result in appliance failures they can be removed under local anaesthetic by curettage and cautery.

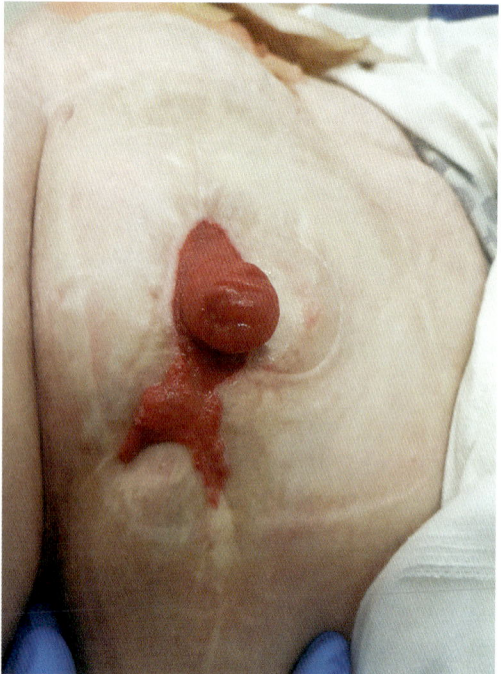

Figure 112.8 Granulation tissue with bowel metaplasia affecting an ileostomy. In this case the affected area is in a scar/fold that channels leakage onto the skin, which may be the triggering factor. These lesions cause further bag failures especially by bleeding. Because of this and in particular in the presence of metaplasia, the skin should be resurfaced under local anaesthetic with light cautery or, if available, laser.

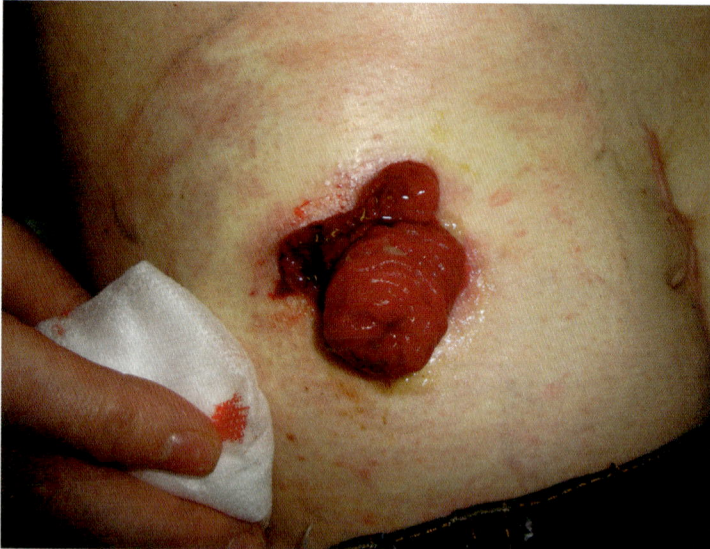

Figure 112.9 Pain is occasionally prominent and sometimes severe as in this woman with an ileostomy for Crohn disease. There are typical 'granulomas' beneath the stoma but a very painful and more vascular one at the 3 o'clock position. Treatment is as for Figure 112.8.

seem the most appropriate step, however surgical considerations such as the amount of available remaining bowel or medical considerations such as anaesthetic risk may make this too hazardous for the patient.

For dermatitis a short-term topical corticosteroid is usually all that is needed in order to settle the inflammation and to enhance appliance adhesion (Table 112.3). This may be required intermittently for a longer period, particularly for idiopathic dermatitis.

CPD responds very well to the prevention of urine leakage. This is typically more achievable than for leaking ileostomies, colostomies or fistulae. One effective additional measure for early CPD is to apply 50% domestic vinegar (diluted in tap water) to the skin for 10 min a day after cleaning [9,10]. This is best achieved using soaked gauze. It probably works by reducing the corrosive effects of ammonia produced by urea-splitting bacteria as well as maintaining the physiological pH of the skin. Papular irritant reactions that do not respond to the prevention of leaks can be removed under local anaesthetic, usually by cautery with or without prior

curettage or shaving off of the lesions (see Figures 112.7–112.11 and 112.12). This may need to be repeated periodically as often as every 3–4 months in the case of granulomas as they tend to recur. Cryotherapy with liquid nitrogen can be effective for small papular lesions even in CPD [11]. Botulinum neurotoxin A can also be an

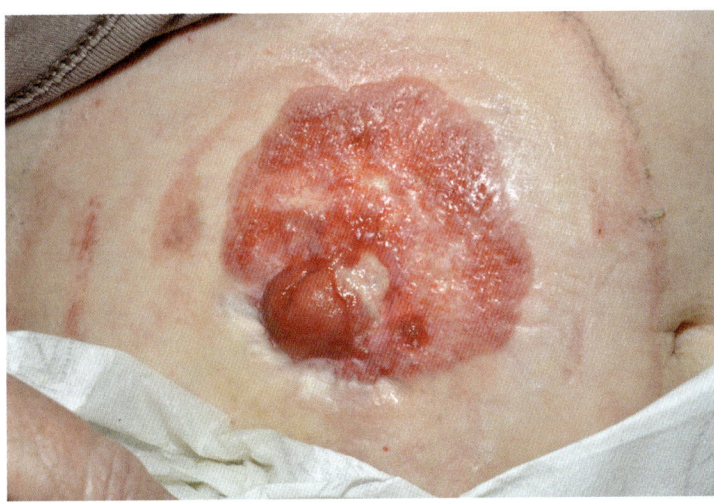

Figure 112.10 Ileal metaplasia affecting a longstanding urostomy and covering a wide area of skin. This was treated with laser resurfacing.

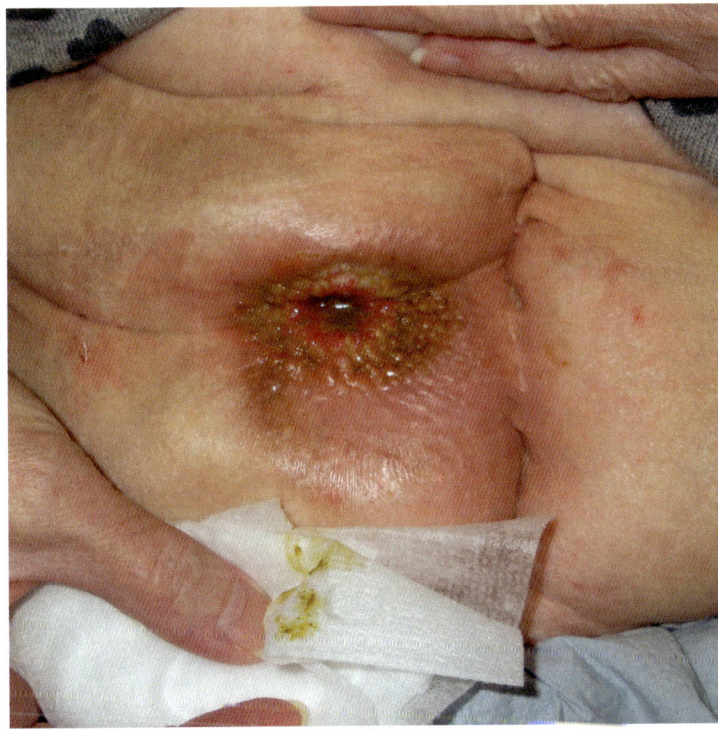

Figure 112.11 A short and buried ileostomy where leaks are inevitable. The mottled appearance of the hyperkeratotic papules is typical.

effective treatment for irritant dermatitis caused by ostomy leaks in patients with retractile stomas [12].

Occasionally patients present with bleeding granulomas which are not irritant in nature but are vascular lesions due to portal hypertension. This is almost exclusively in ulcerative colitis patients with liver disease (Figure 112.13). These granulomas will bleed profusely if approached surgically as one would with irritant granulomas and should be left, with the patient being referred for a hepatology opinion.

Allergic contact dermatitis

- ICD-10: L23
- BAD: C6zzzz

Introduction
Allergic contact dermatitis (ACD) affecting the skin can occur around stomas.

Epidemiology
Allergic contact dermatitis around stomas is uncommon, occurring in less than 1% of the skin problems seen in almost 1000 patients attending a dedicated dermatology and joint stoma care clinic [1]. Despite this many patients and stoma nurses suspect allergy to a stoma appliance as the cause of an otherwise unexplained dermatitis before considering any other aetiology. This can be partly explained by the numbers of individual case reports published in the last 30 years detailing sensitivities to individual components many of which, such as epoxy resin systems, are no longer used in appliance manufacture. These reports have been eloquently summarised by Martin *et al.* [2]. Where ACD occurs, it is usually to biocides in cleansers, fragrances in deodorisers or resin systems in pastes used to fill irregularities in the peristomal skin (Gantrez™ PMV/MA co-polymers).

Pathophysiology
See Chapter 127 for pathogenetic information on ACD.

Clinical features
The symptoms and clinical appearances of ACD and irritant dermatitis are similar in the occluded peristomal environment and are therefore difficult to distinguish on clinical grounds alone. The patient experiences an itchy, sometimes burning, eczematous rash affecting the skin in contact with the material responsible and spreading out from that area.

Investigations
Patch testing (Chapter 127) is carried out to a standard series, specific stoma series (Table 112.4) and samples of the appliance and any accessory products used (e.g. aloe vera). It is also useful for the patient to undertake a usage test. This involves applying a stoma bag together with accessories such as additional hydrocolloid washers or skin pastes to the non-stoma side of the abdomen. The appliances are changed at the same time as that on their stoma and it is important that they continue this for 5–7 days. However, occasionally patients have a severe reaction before 5 days and should stop the test and if possible photograph the reaction. The test, if positive (see Figure 112.1), can confirm which part of an appliance or which accessory product is likely to be causing the skin reaction although this may or may not be an allergic reaction. Consideration of the distribution of the dermatitis is important in identifying potential allergens. For example, patients may use fragranced deodorisers placed in the pouch. These can penetrate the plastic and contact the skin causing reactions even below the inguinal crease [3].

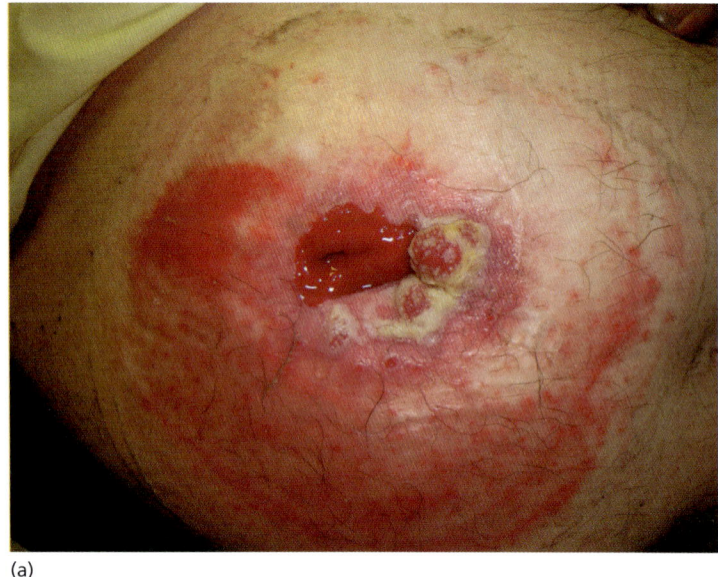

(a)

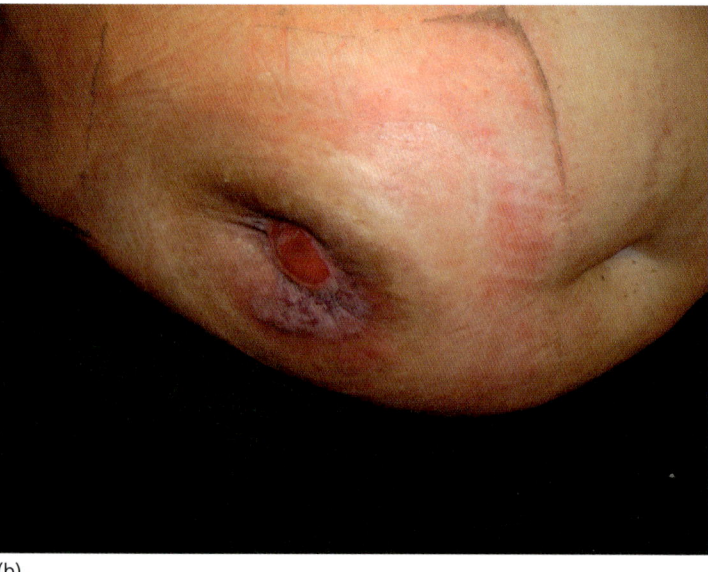

(b)

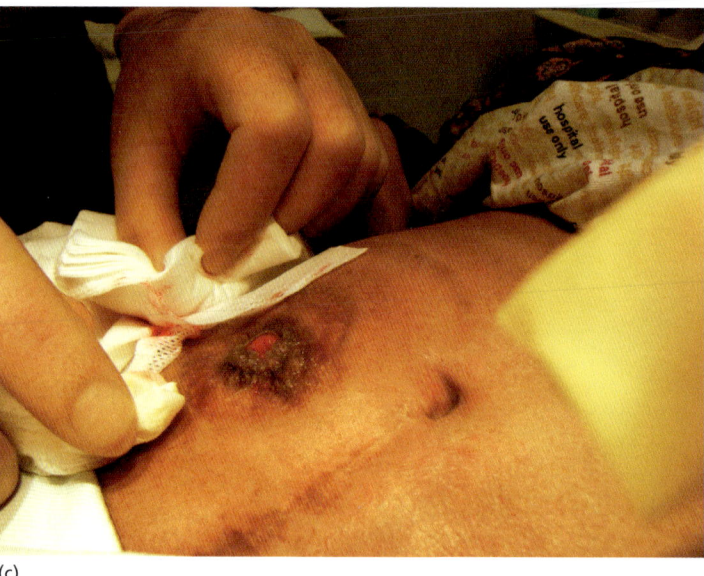

(c)

Figure 112.12 (a) Chronic papillomatous dermatitis (CPD) and irritant dermatitis associated with a leaking urostomy. The papules are typical. (b) These may proliferate and are occasionally blue due to bacterial degradation of tryptophan in the urine to produce an indigo-like substance. (c) These hyperkeratotic papules can encroach on the urostomy as in this Asian woman with a urostomy for neurological incontinence. Squamous epithelium encroaching onto the urostomy mucosa is seen in severe cases. Surgical removal under local anaesthetic may be necessary, as in this case, to prevent stoma stenosis.

Management

As confirmation of the allergy requires clearance of ACD on avoidance of the culprit product, further management is usually unnecessary. Topical corticosteroid is, however, useful to relieve symptoms and to speed resolution of the dermatitis.

Infections

Introduction

The moist occluded environment of the peristomal skin is ideal for microbiological growth.

Epidemiology

Despite the environment created by a stoma, significant infections are relatively uncommon, accounting for approximately 7% of patients that seek help for skin problems [1]. The most frequent infections are *Candida* overgrowth (Figure 112.14) and folliculitis (staphylococcal), usually from shaving or plucking the hairs with bag adhesive. Secondary bacterial infection, particularly cellulitis affecting ulcerating conditions, occurs occasionally (Figure 112.15). Synergic gangrene (Figure 112.16) and other serious infections are rare, as surprisingly is tinea corporis.

Pathophysiology

See chapters on specific infections (Chapters 26 and 32).

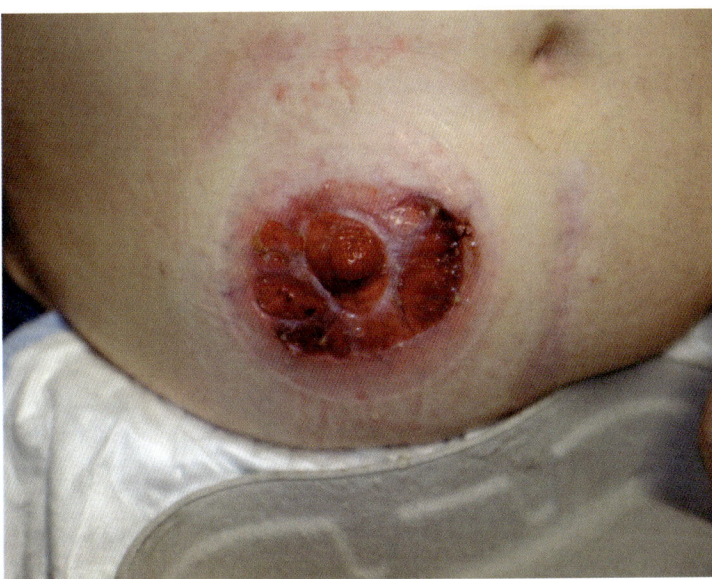

Figure 112.13 A patient with an ileostomy for ulcerative colitis with associated liver disease. Portal hypertension is affecting the peristomal skin, effectively caput medusa.

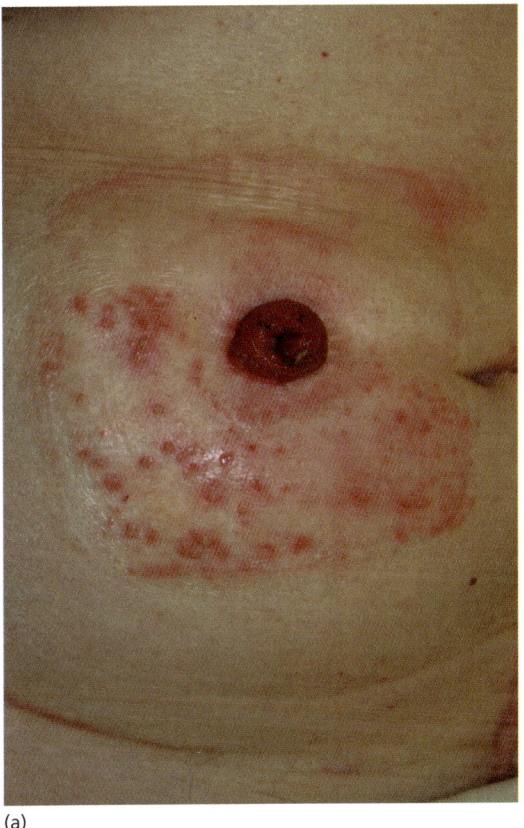

(a)

Table 112.4 Suggested stoma patch test series

No.	Agent	No.	Agent
1	Cinnamyl alcohol	20	1,6-Hexanediol diacrylate
2	Cinnamaldehyde	21	Tetrahydrofurfuryl methacrylate
3	Eugenol	22	Tetraethyleneglycol dimethacrylate
4	Alpha-amyl-cinnamaldehyde	23	N,N-dimethylaminoethyl methacrylate
5	Hydroxycitronellal	24	Ethyl cyanoacrylate
6	Geraniol	25	Diazolidinyl urea
7	Isoeugenol	26	Propylene glycol 20% in aqueous
8	Oak moss absolute	27	Chlorhexidine digluconate 0.5% in aqueous
9	Sorbitan sesquioleate	28	2-Ethylhexyl acrylate 0.1% in petrolatum
10	Methyl methacrylate	29	Isopropyl alcohol 10% in aqueous
11	n-Butyl methacrylate	30	Cetrimide 0.1% in aqueous
12	2-Hydroxypropyl methacrylate	31	Polyvinyl pyrrolidone 1% in aqueous
13	2-Hydroxyethyl methacrylate	32	Gantrez™ ES225/Gantrez ES425
14	Ethyleneglycol dimethacrylate	33	Cavilon foam applicator
15	Triethyleneglycol dimethacrylate	34	Karaya 10% in aqueous
16	1,4-Butanediol dimethacrylate	35	Benzoyl peroxide
17	Urethane dimethacrylate	36	1H-benzotriazole 1% in petolatum
18	BIS-MA (bisphenol A dimethacrylate)	37	D-Limonene 10% in petrolatum
19	BIS-GMA (bisphenol A glycerolate dimethacrylate)	38	Propyl gallate 1% in petrolatum

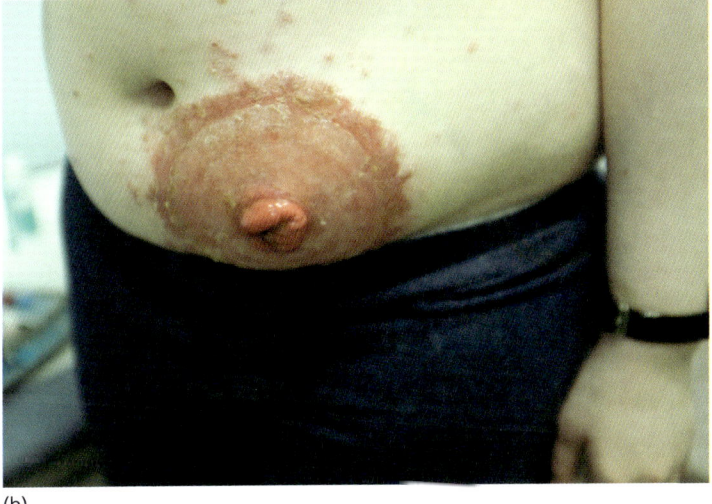

(b)

Figure 112.14 (a) Candida infection presenting as an itchy, non-follicular pustular rash affecting an immunosuppressed woman with an ileostomy for Crohn disease. (b) Psoriasis (confirmed histologically) in a young woman with Crohn disease. There are small satellite lesions, some presenting as deroofed pustules representing a significant Candida infection confirmed on mycology.

Clinical features

Bacterial infection presents either as a typical folliculitis or a patchy dermatitis with moist, superficial erosions. The latter is non-specific with psoriasiform or eczematous features and can occur with a variety of pathogens [1]. A swab should therefore be taken in all cases of unexplained rash. Bacterial cellulitis presents typically and can complicate pre-existing skin disorders (Figure 112.15). Synergic gangrene occurs in the weeks after surgery usually following surgical wound breakdown (mucocutaneous separation [2]).

Investigations

A swab should be taken from all rashes for bacteriology and skin scrapings where appropriate for mycology.

Management

Antibiotic prescribing should be guided by microbiology findings. Systemic treatment is preferable as topical creams interfere with

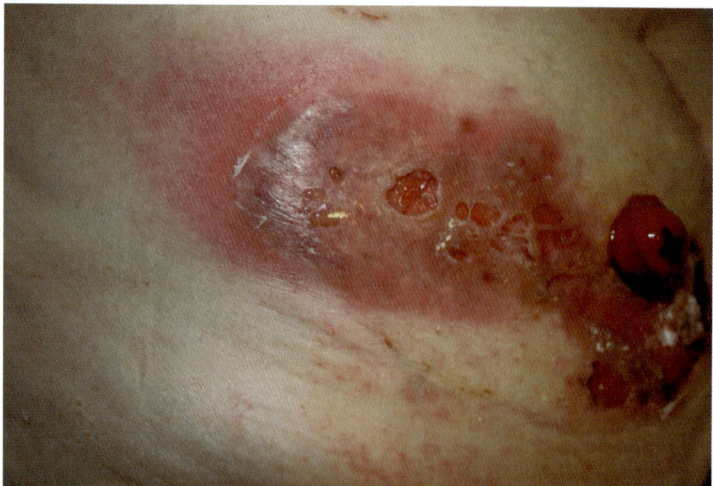

Figure 112.15 Streptococcal cellulitis complicating healing pyoderma gangrenosum in a 65-year-old woman with irritant bowel disease.

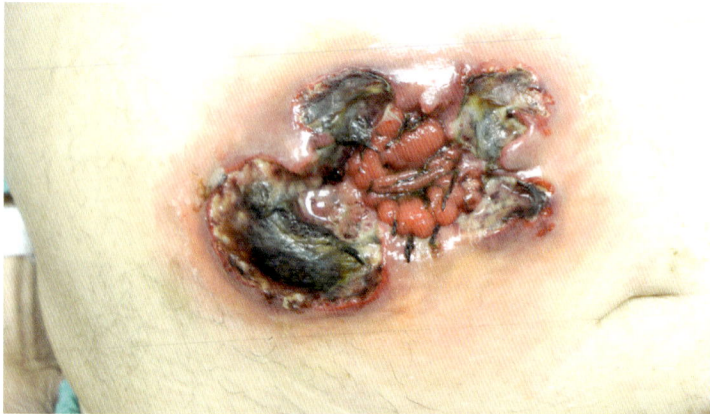

Figure 112.16 Synergic gangrene affecting a recently formed ileostomy. The patient required surgical debridement in addition to systemic antibiotics.

appliance adhesion. Patients who shave their abdomen are advised to do this no more than weekly. An adhesive remover spray is helpful if strong adhesion is causing hair plucking.

Other skin conditions presenting near stomas

Psoriasis:
- ICD-10: L40.0
- BAD: D10

Localised pemphigoid:
- ICD-10: L12.0
- BAD: ME201

Lichen sclerosus, localised extragenital:
- ICD-10: L90.0
- BAD: M412

Introduction

Theoretically almost any dermatosis could involve the peristomal skin and a dermatologist will be able to diagnose such disorders

based upon the features both locally and beyond the stoma. In practice a few skin diseases warrant special mention either because they are more common than expected or because they can present atypically. The isomorphic (Koebner) phenomenon might be expected to make certain disorders more likely in the potentially traumatised peristomal skin.

Epidemiology

Although conditions such as pemphigus vulgaris have been reported [1], in the author's experience with the exception of psoriasis [2] these are uncommon. Psoriasis is more than twice as common in patients with irritable bowel disease (IBD) compared with the population as a whole [1] and is the most frequent generalised dermatosis seen around stomas as a result of this and probably also the Koebner phenomenon [3]. Around stomas it presents like flexural psoriasis (Figure 112.17a). Features of psoriasis elsewhere may be limited and subtle (Figure 112.17b) so that diagnosis may not be immediately obvious.

Lichen sclerosus has been described involving peristomal skin [4,5] where it can present acutely with features similar to active genital lichen sclerosus (Figure 112.18). It particularly affects urostomies and can appear without associated genital involvement [6,7].

The anti-anginal nitrate drug nicorandil is known to cause oral aphthous ulceration [8], perianal ulcers [9], peristomal ulceration (Figure 112.19) [10] and bowel perforation [11] or fistula formation particularly in patients with diverticular disease [12,13]. It accounts for up to 2% of referrals to a specialist stoma care/dermatology clinic [10]. This drug is rarely used in the Americas and is now restricted in the UK because of these complications. Cases are therefore now rare.

Localised bullous pemphigoid occasionally involves peristomal skin (Figure 112.20) and can cause diagnostic confusion as the typical blisters are not seen having been deroofed by the action of the appliance adhesive [14].

Other congenital or acquired bullous, xerotic or hyperkeratotic disorders are surprisingly rare around abdominal stomas.

Pathophysiology

See chapters on specific diseases (Chapters 110 and 111).

Clinical features

Psoriasis presents typically outside the area covered by the appliance and will only cause diagnostic confusion if the features of psoriasis elsewhere are scant or subtle (Figure 112.17a, b). Under an appliance it has the features of flexural psoriasis.

Lichen sclerosus (Figure 112.18) may present as an asymptomatic, papery, atrophic plaque of typical extragenital lichen sclerosus but more usually presents as painful, purpuric plaques often associated with ulceration.

Localised pemphigoid affecting stomas (Figure 112.20a) presents as painful and often itchy denuded areas.

Investigations

For all these conditions a skin biopsy is indicated if there is any doubt about the diagnosis. Histological features are typical (Chapters 110 and 111).

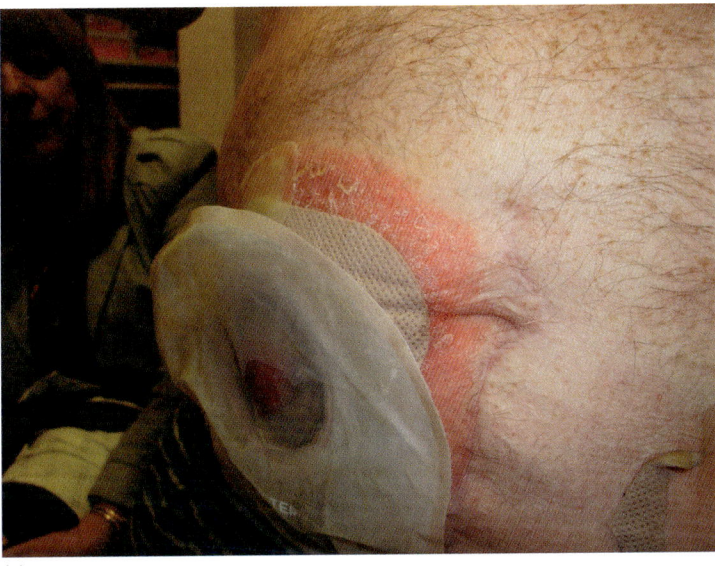

(a)

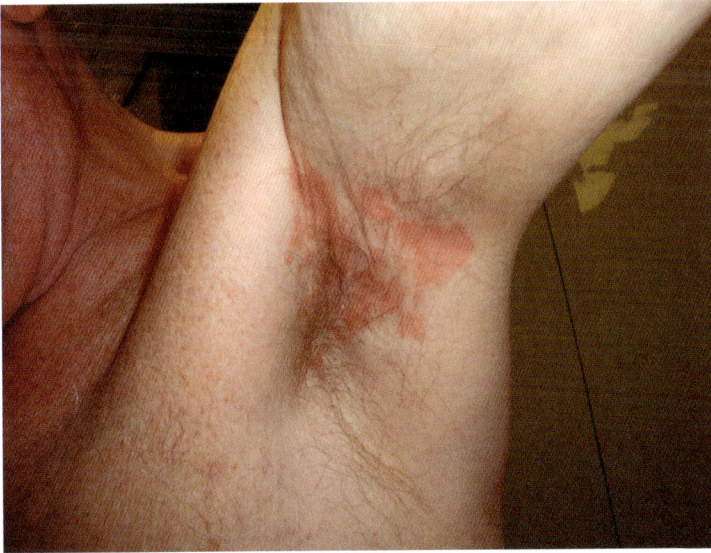

(b)

Figure 112.17 (a) Typical psoriasis affecting the abdominal skin around the stoma appliance in a man with Crohn disease. The skin beneath the adhesive plate was mildly red but asymptomatic. (b) The patient had mild flexural psoriasis elsewhere in the axillae and natal cleft.

Management
The principles of topical corticosteroid treatments are detailed in Table 112.3.

Topical treatment alone is usually effective for psoriasis. If the patient is not using a mostly or wholly hydrocolloid barrier it is worth changing to one as the psoriasis may clear under occlusion with a hydrocolloid but not a thin fabric dressing [4,15]. Ultraviolet (UV) phototherapy can be used: the patient should hold a cardboard tube (from a toilet roll or similar) filled with gauze over the stoma to protect it from UV exposure and leakage. Systemic treatment may be required early because the psoriasis reduces bag adhesion and irritation from leaks can exacerbate the dermatosis. The clinician should be aware that the nephrotoxic effects of

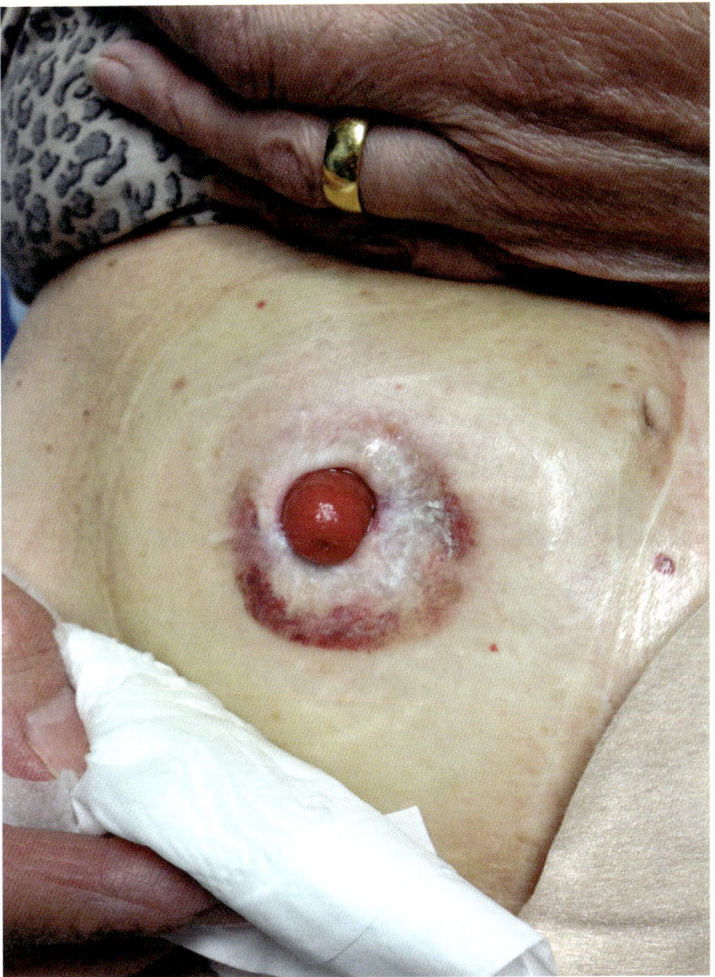

(a)

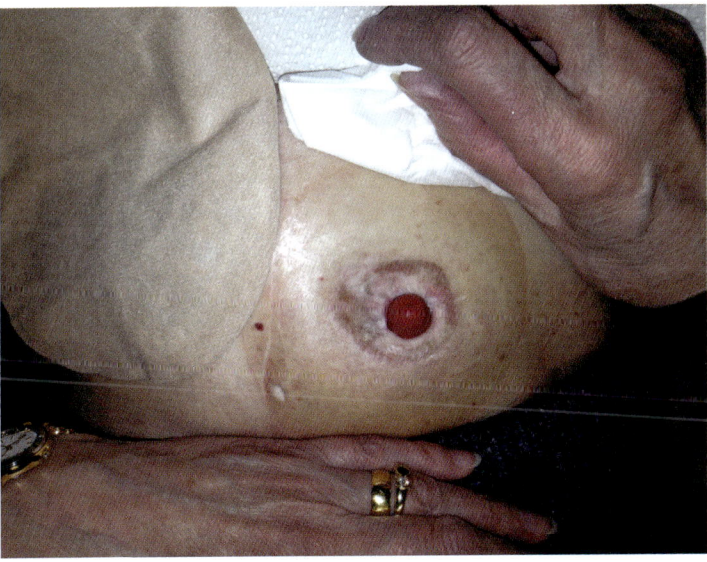

(b)

Figure 112.18 (a) Lichen sclerosus affecting a urostomy in a woman with a history of genital lichen sclerosus presenting some years prior to stoma formation for bladder carcinoma. (b) The inflammation settles rapidly within 1 month after administration of triamcinolone acetonide 20 mg intralesionally.

PART 10: SPECIFIC SITES, SEX & AGE

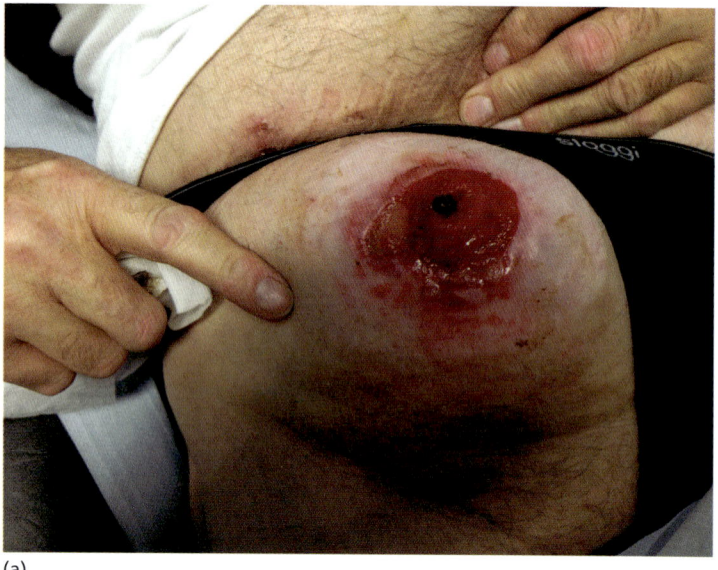

(a)

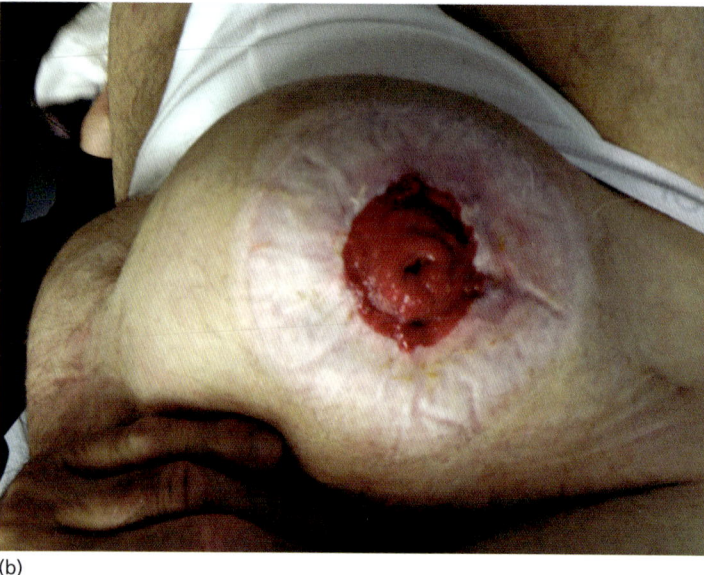

(b)

Figure 112.19 (a) Nicorandil ulceration affecting an ileostomy for ulcerative colitis. (b) This healed completely (B) within 6 weeks of stopping the drug.

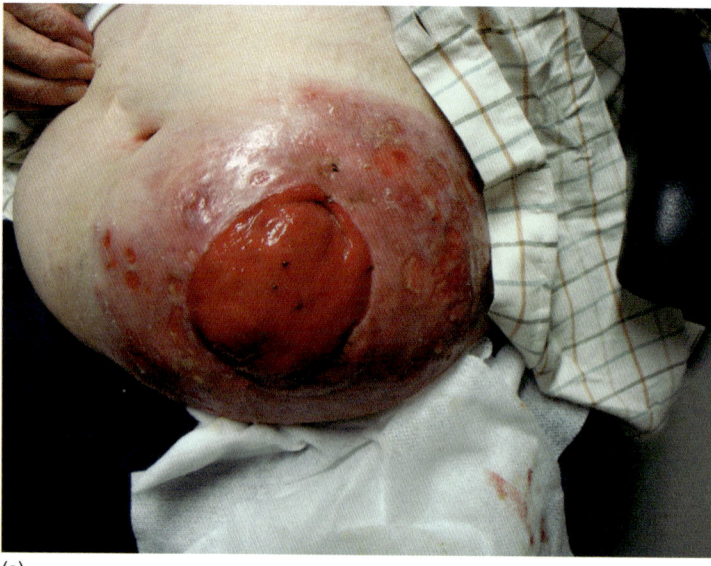

(a)

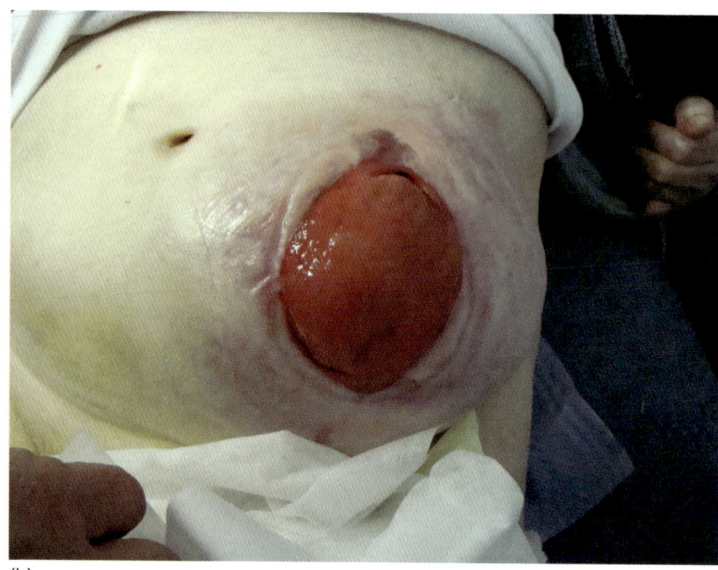

(b)

Figure 112.20 Localised bullous pemphigoid affecting a large colostomy in a 90-year-old man. (a) At presentation denuded areas of skin but no obvious blisters are seen. (b) The skin has healed 1 month later on a reducing dose of oral prednisolone (average 20 mg per day).

certain drugs, particularly ciclosporin, can be enhanced by the haemodynamic changes that result from even moderate-output ileostomies.

Lichen sclerosus, particularly if ulcerated, usually requires an intralesional corticosteroid to gain control (e.g. triamcinolone acetonide 20 mg).

Nicorandil ulceration around stomas responds to cessation of the drug. This can usually be stopped immediately and the nitrate effect replaced by an increased dose of an alternative such as isosorbide mononitrate.

Bullous pemphigoid and pemphigus vulgaris respond to the usual treatments and although topical treatments may suffice (Table 112.3), systemic treatments may be required at an earlier stage (Chapter 50).

Dermatoses associated with underlying bowel disease

Pyoderma gangrenosum:
- ICD-10: y88.3
- BAD: FA7F

Crohn disease of the skin:
- BAD: E9

Introduction

Superficial ulceration secondary to trauma is relatively common near stomas particularly if there is an associated parastomal hernia.

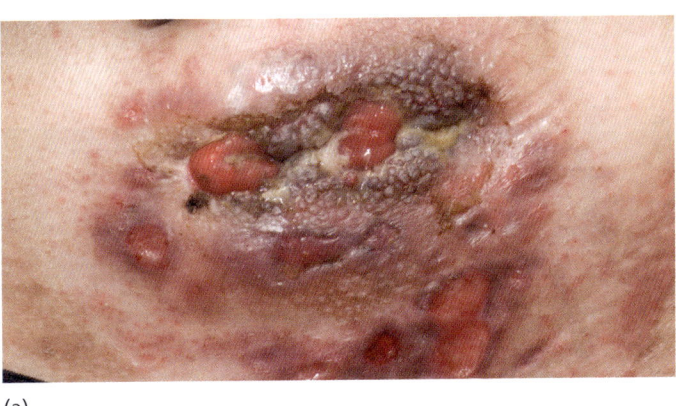
(a)

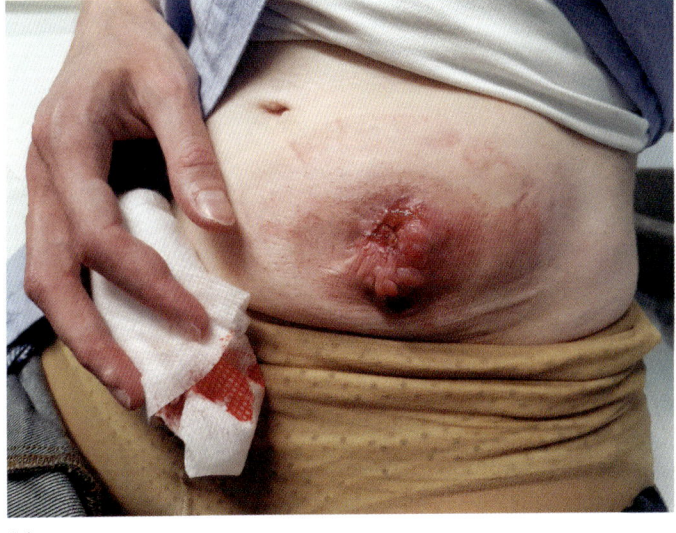
(b)

Figure 112.21 (a) Fistulating Crohn disease affecting an ileostomy in a teenage girl. The original stoma on the left has been partly destroyed by the inflammatory process and faeces emerges from this and three other fistulous openings. There is associated irritant dermatitis in which papule formation is prominent. (b) Histologically confirmed Crohn disease affecting a colostomy. There is a fistula beneath the papules and the stoma itself has been destroyed by the inflammation.

Such ulcers typically settle rapidly with conservative treatment from the stoma nurse specialist. Where they persist or worsen one should consider other diagnoses and the possibility of secondary infection or progression to pyoderma gangrenosum (PG) via the pathergy phenomenon.

Epidemiology

In the author's speciality clinics, perineal and genital Crohn disease are common referrals, while Crohn disease affecting peristomal skin is rare. Where it does occur, it is usually contiguous with the stoma itself and may be associated with fistulation (Figure 112.21). As a result, most patients require gastro-enterological and/or colo-rectal surgical management.

PG by contrast is commoner than expected. Whereas an average dermatologist might be expected to see no more than two new cases per year, PG accounts for between 1% and 4% of the patients presenting with peristomal skin problems [1,2]. This high prevalence is partly explained by the association with IBD, but PG occurs in stoma patients with no IBD and can also affect urostomies suggesting some other pathogenic mechanisms may be involved. It has been suggested that peristomal PG may be overdiagnosed [3] and there is certainly a wide differential warranting careful evaluation of each patient (Chapter 49). In the author's experience of ostomy patients these are usually Crohn patients with non-healing scars and traumatic small wounds

Pathophysiology

See Chapter 49 for pathogenetic information on PG and Chapters 111 and 153 for Crohn disease of the skin.

There is some evidence that PG is more likely where the underlying IBD is currently active [3–6] but this is not universal [7] and PG should not be considered an indication for further bowel resection unless it is otherwise indicated.

Pathergy, for example from skin stripping on appliance removal, probably contributes to the prevalence of peristomal PG. Convex appliances (see Figure 112.1) put pressure on the peristomal skin and are associated with PG. In the author's experience, in the early 2000s 14% of our stoma patients were using convex appliances. Of those with a first episode of PG, 30% were using these appliances and in patients with recurrent episodes the figure rose to 74%.

Clinical features

The clinical features of ulcers due to Crohn disease near a stoma are similar to PG and a biopsy may be necessary to distinguish them if there is no mucosal involvement. PG itself almost never involves the stoma mucosa (Figure 112.22).

The clinical features of peristomal PG are essentially the same as for PG elsewhere (Chapter 49) although patients may not recall a pustular or papular stage and this is only occasionally observed by the clinician. The ulceration is typically very painful (Figure 112.23) and this is worsened by stoma leaks. Some ulcers are not painful at all because of surgical damage to local sensory nerves. Figure 112.24 demonstrates the typical features of an overhanging, purple and perforated edge that results in cribriform scarring. Irregular scarring itself will impair appliance adhesion. Although some stoma patients have concurrent PG at more typical sites like the leg [8], the great majority in the author's experience are restricted to the peristomal area.

Investigations

A biopsy is required to differentiate an ulcer due to Crohn disease from a PG ulcer if there are no other features of Crohn disease.

Investigations for peristomal PG are the same as for PG elsewhere, and are directed at finding a potential underlying disease and ruling out other differential diagnoses. An ulcer biopsy is usually recommended for this purpose. However, because of the

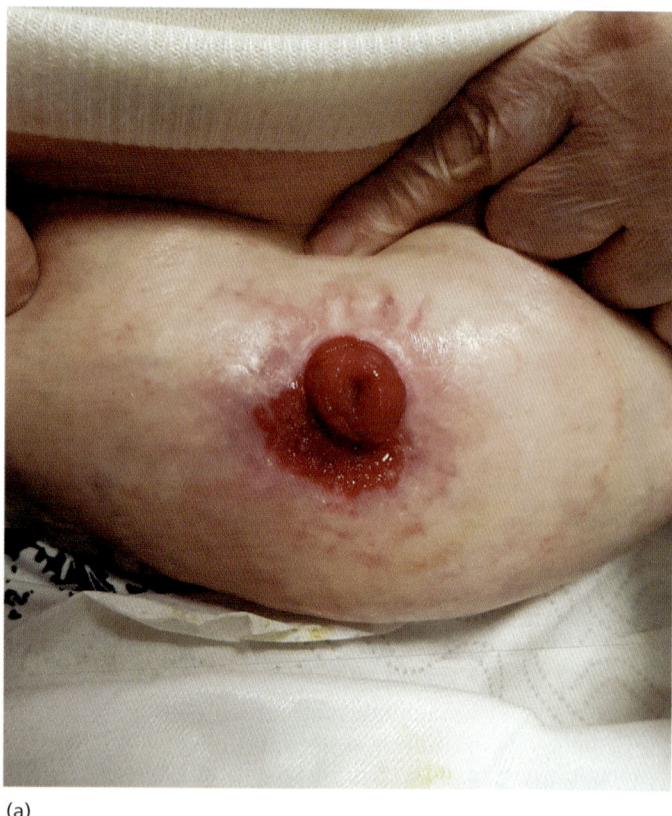

(a)

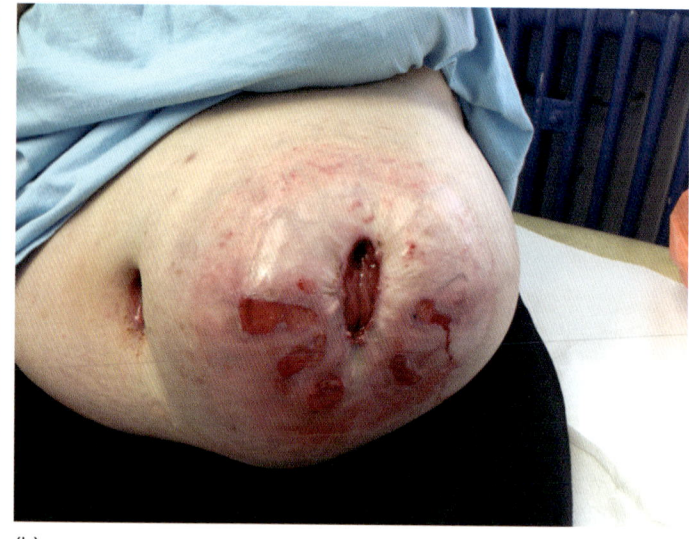

(b)

Figure 112.22 (a) Crohn ulceration beneath an ileostomy in a woman with active intestinal disease. The presentation is non-specific and requires histological confirmation. (b) Crohn ulceration affecting a colostomy site. A biopsy from the umbilical ulceration also demonstrated the granulomatous inflammation of Crohn disease.

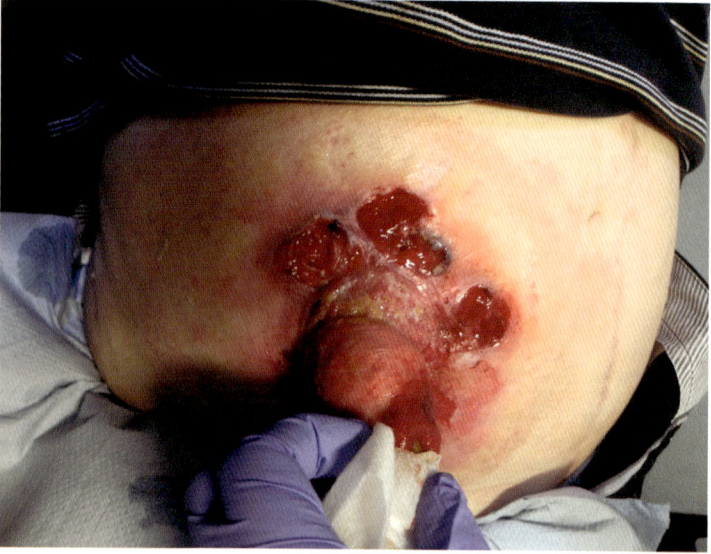

Figure 112.23 Pyoderma gangrenosum (PG) affecting an ileostomy in a man with recent surgery for Crohn disease. There are painful, typical ulcers above the stoma and some ragged scarring at the 9 o'clock position. Note the inflammation at the base of the stoma that has resulted from leaks as the PG ulcers reduce bag adherence. There is also partial squamous epithelialisation of the proximal stoma which is a rare occurrence that can cause stenosis.

risk of worsening the ulceration via pathergy, the typical peristomal clinical picture and the association with underlying bowel disease, this author recommends a trial of topical treatment for up to 2 weeks before considering a skin biopsy. The possibility of infection causing or complicating the ulcerative processes on the occluded peristomal skin should be borne in mind and a biopsy for microbiological examination as well as histology may be indicated.

Management

For both PG and the much rarer Crohn disease ulcer, the deleterious effect on normal stoma appliance use of both the active disease and the resultant scarring warrants the early introduction of effective treatments. The majority of cases respond satisfactorily to topical therapy alone [2,9]; corticosteroid preparations that can be used are detailed in Table 112.3. There is no perfect preparation applicable to stomas that is available off the shelf and obtaining medicaments manufactured can be problematic and expensive. If one of the topical corticosteroid preparations is not effective or well tolerated within 14 days in the author's service we move to tacrolimus 0.3% in Orabase™ paste applied once daily for up to 1 month. The addition of fludroxycortide tape applied over the paste reduces healing time and appears to minimise the overgranulation that can occur during healing [10]. If topical treatments are ineffective or PG is very severe at presentation (Figure 112.25) the systemic treatment approach is as for PG in general (Chapter 49). Systemic steroids are indicated first line in this clinical situation [11]. In patients with any active IBD, particularly Crohn disease, anti-tumour nuclear factor (anti-TNF) therapy with infliximab [12] or other anti-TNFs is usually highly effective.

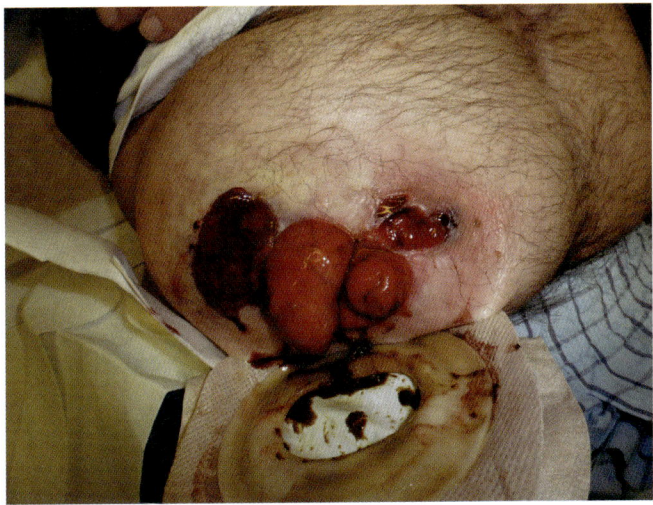

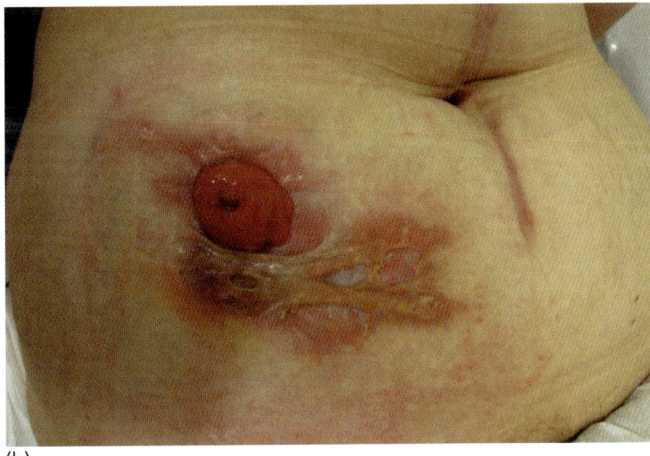

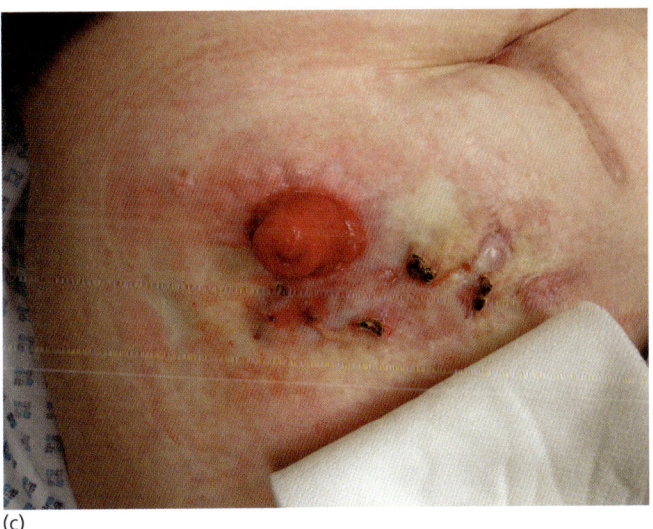

Figure 112.24 (a) Pyoderma gangrenosum (PG) affecting a temporary loop ileostomy in a man with a history of ulcerative colitis. The perforated, purple edge is typical and results, in severe cases, in very irregular cribriform scarring which can interfere with appliance adhesion. Note the exuberant granulation tissue at the 9 o'clock position where a recent PG ulcer has been treated with topical tacrolimus. (b) This shows an example in 30-year-old woman with Crohn disease where the PG has healed. (c) The skin bridging was removed under local anaesthetic to prevent trauma and maceration to the underlying skin that could have triggered further PG. This minor surgery should be delayed until after PG has healed completely to minimise the risk of further ulceration via the pathergy phenomenon.

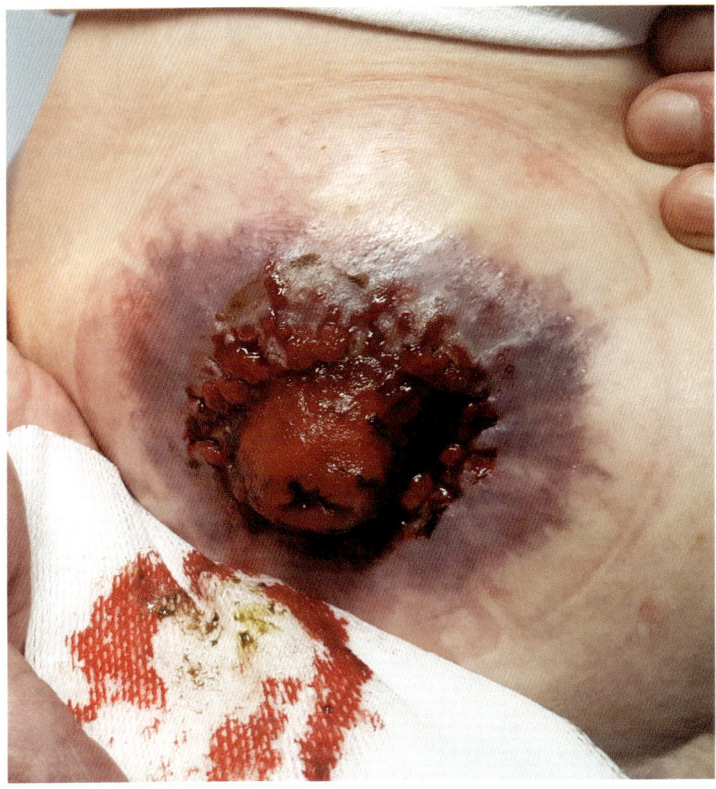

Figure 112.25 Severe pyoderma gangrenosum in a middle-aged man with Crohn disease. The ulceration failed to respond to topical or systemic treatments but resolved spontaneously a few weeks after a completion proctectomy. This is a recognised but not universal phenomenon.

Key references

The full list of references can be found in the online version at https://www.wiley.com/rooksdermatology10e

Introduction

1 Jemec GB, Nybaek H. Peristomal skin problems account for more than one in three visits to ostomy nurses. *Br J Dermatol* 2008;159:1211–12.
2 Pearson R,Knight SR, Ng JCK, Robertson I, McKenzie C, MacDonald AM. Stoma related complications following ostomy surgery in 3 acute care hospitals. *J Wound Ostomy Continence Nurs* 2020;47:32–8.
3 Lyon CC, Smith AJ, Griffiths CE, Beck MH. The spectrum of skin disorders in abdominal stoma patients. *Br J Dermatol* 2000;143:1248–60.
4 Al-Niaimi F, Almaani N, Samarasinghe V, Williams J, Lyon C. The relevance of patch testing in peristomal dermatitis. *Br J Dermatol* 2012;167:103–9.

Irritant reactions

1 Herlufsen P, Olsen AG, Carlsen B *et al.* Study of peristomal skin disorders in patients with permanent stomas. *Br J Nurs* 2006;15:854–62.
5 Bhoyrul B, Ondhia D, Lyon C. Botulinum neurotoxin A is an effective treatment for irritant dermatitis caused by ostomy leaks in patients with retractile stomas. *Br J Dermatol* 2019;181:629–31.
8 Bergman BFK, Lincoln K, Lowhagen GB, Mobacken H, Wahlen P. Chronic papillomatous dermatitis as a peristomal complication in conduit urinary diversion. *Scand J Urol Nephrol* 1979;13:201–14.

Allergic contact dermatitis

1 Al-Niaimi F, Almaani N, Samarasinghe V, Williams J, Lyon C. The relevance of patch testing in peristomal dermatitis. *Br J Dermatol* 2012;167:103–9.

PART 10: SPECIFIC SITES, SEX & AGE

Infections

1 Lyon CC, Smith AD, Griffiths CE, Beck MH. The spectrum of skin disorders in abdominal stoma patients. *Br J Dermatol* 2000;143:1248–60.

Other skin conditions presenting near stomas

3 Yates VM, Watkinson G, Kelman A. Further evidence for an association between psoriasis, Crohn's disease and ulcerative colitis. *Br J Dermatol* 1982;106:323–30.

4 Lyon CC, Smith AJ, Griffiths CE, Beck MH. The spectrum of skin disorders in abdominal stoma patients. *Br J Dermatol* 2000;143:1248–60.

5 Weng AA, Charles-Holmes R. Peristomal lichen sclerosus affecting colostomy sites. *Br J Dermatol* 2000;142:177–8.

Dermatoses associated with underlying bowel disease

2 Toh JWT, Young CJ, Rickard MJFX, Keshava A, Stewart P, Whiteley I. Peristomal pyoderma gangrenosum: 12 year experience in a single tertiary referral centre. *ANZ J Surg* 2018;88:E693–7.

10 Lyon CC, Stapleton M, Smith AJ, Mendelsohn S, Beck MH, Griffiths CE. Topical tacrolimus in the management of peristomal pyoderma gangrenosum. *J Dermatolog Treat* 2001;12:13–17.

CHAPTER 113

Dermatoses of Pregnancy

Amy Stanway

Bethlehem Skin Clinic, Tauranga, New Zealand

Physiological skin changes in pregnancy

During pregnancy there are marked changes in the sex hormones, immune system and cardiovascular system, which can lead to profound changes in the skin. It is important to recognise these physiological skin changes and to distinguish them from true skin disease (Box 113.1).

Pigmentation

Most women notice a generalised increase in skin pigmentation during pregnancy, most marked on the areolae, genitals and midline of the abdominal wall (linea nigra) (Figure 113.1). It is more marked in women with darker skin types [1]. This pigmentation usually fades after delivery, but seldom to its previous level.

In approximately 70% of women, especially those with skin of colour, melasma (or chloasma) pigmentation also develops during the second half of pregnancy. Irregular, sharply marginated areas of pigmentation develop in a symmetrical pattern, either on the forehead and temples or on the central part of the face (Figure 113.2). Melasma usually fades completely after parturition but may persist and require treatment post-delivery. Prevention includes counselling on sun protection. Azelaic acid is generally considered safe during pregnancy. Less is known about hydroquinone safety and it is generally not recommended. Patients can also develop new or worsening acanthosis nigricans lesions [2].

Hair and nail changes

Hair growth on the scalp often increases during pregnancy. In the third trimester, the proportion of hair follicles retained in the anagen phase rises, with a compensatory shedding of hair postpartum (telogen effluvium) [1]. Spontaneous recovery within 6–12 months is usual. Mild frontoparietal recession may also occur [3]. Minor degrees of hypertrichosis are not uncommon, particularly along the midline suprapubic area. New, soft, fine hairs may disappear around 6 months postpartum, but coarse hair typically persists [2].

Hirsutism, acne and rarely other evidence of virilisation occur more commonly in women with darker hair, usually during the second half of pregnancy. This may indicate an androgen-secreting tumour, luteoma, lutein cysts or polycystic ovary disease [1,4] and must be thoroughly investigated. In the absence of a tumour that can be eradicated, the problem tends to recur in subsequent pregnancies. Hirsutism may regress between pregnancies, but this is not always complete.

Multiple nail changes have been reported in pregnancy [2]. Single or multiple nail longitudinal melanonychia is recognised. Uniform, symmetrical hyperpigmentation of multiple nails due to melanocyte activation is reported during pregnancy with fading postpartum [5]; however, irregular pigmentation with cuticle involvement should prompt investigation of possible melanoma.

Rook's Textbook of Dermatology, Tenth Edition. Edited by Christopher Griffiths, Jonathan Barker, Tanya Bleiker, Walayat Hussain and Rosalind Simpson.
© 2024 John Wiley & Sons Ltd. Published 2024 by John Wiley & Sons Ltd.

PART 10: SPECIFIC SITES, SEX & AGE

Box 113.1 Physiological skin changes in pregnancy

Pigmentation
- Areola and nipple
- Linea nigra
- Genitals
- Melasma

Hair changes
- Hypertrichosis
- Postpartum telogen effluvium
- Postpartum androgenetic alopecia (rare, typically male-pattern balding)

Nail changes
- Increased brittleness
- Distal onycholysis
- Subungual hyperkeratosis
- Transverse grooving
- Longitudinal melanonychia
- Ingrown toenails
- Uniform hyperpigmentation of all nails

Glandular function
- Increased eccrine gland activity
- Increased sebaceous gland activity
- Decreased apocrine gland activity

Vascular changes
- Peripheral oedema
- Varicosities
- Spider naevi/angioma
- Palmar erythema
- Gingival hyperaemia and oedema
- Pregnancy epulis
- Pyogenic granuloma

Striae distensae
- Abdomen, thighs and buttocks

Eccrine, apocrine and sebaceous gland activity

Eccrine and sebaceous gland activity typically increases during pregnancy and apocrine gland activity decreases [6]. Increased eccrine gland activity occurs throughout the body except on the palms and may present clinically as hyperhidrosis and miliaria. The

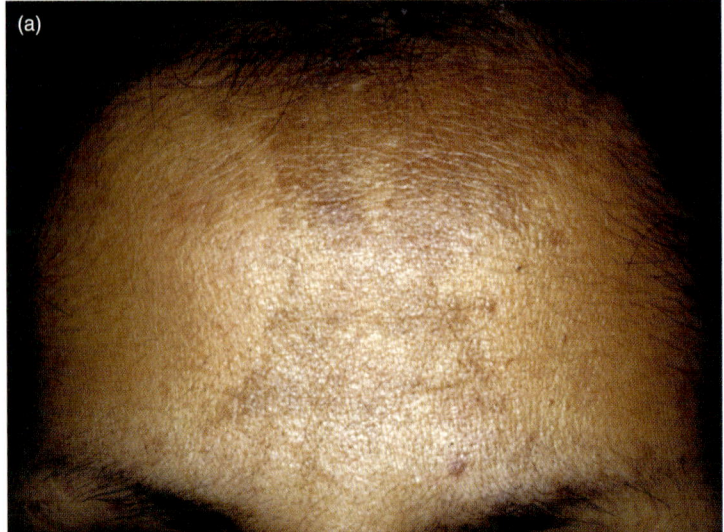

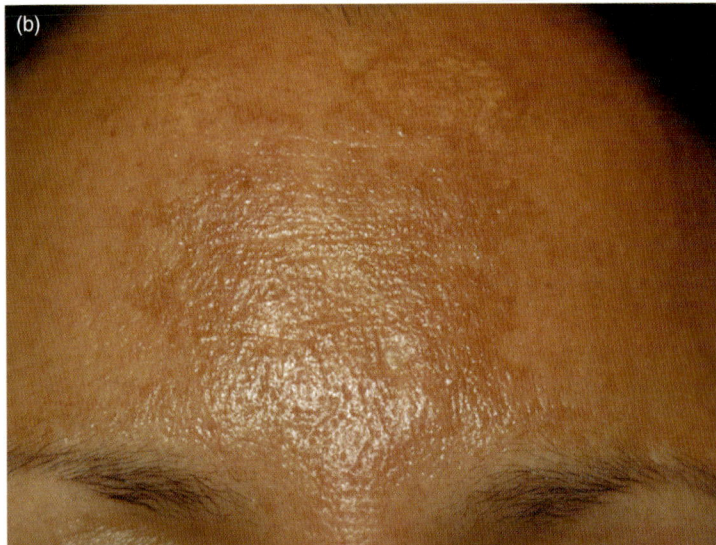

Figure 113.2 Melasma on the forehead. Courtesy of Associate Professor Amanda Oakley, Hamilton, New Zealand.

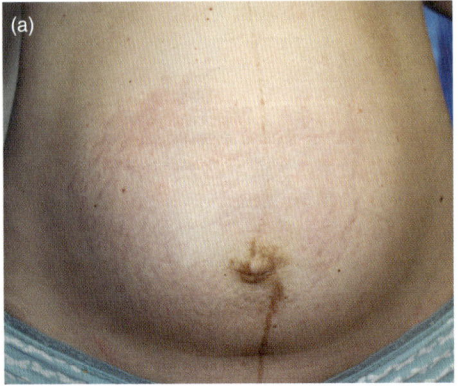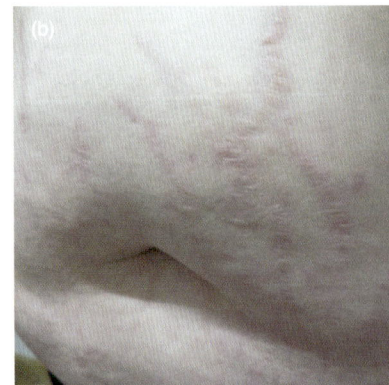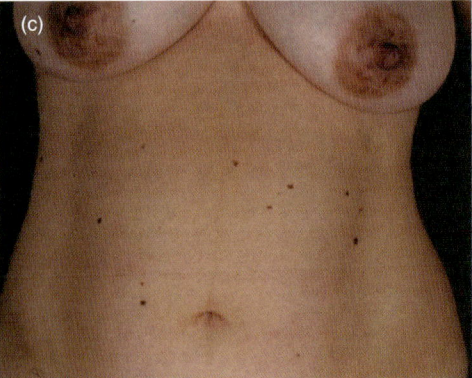

Figure 113.1 Physiological skin changes in pregnancy showing striae distensae (a, b), prominent linea nigra (a, c) and hyperpigmented areolae (c). (b, c) Courtesy of Dr Louise Reiche, Kauri Healthcare, Palmerston North, New Zealand.

rate of sebum excretion tends to increase during pregnancy and returns to normal after delivery due to rising maternal progesterone and androgen levels in the third trimester [7]. Heightened sebaceous gland activity promotes the enlargement of Montgomery tubercles, which are small papules on the areolae that provide lubrication to the nipples and areolae for breastfeeding. This can be distinguished from pregnancy-associated hyperkeratosis of the nipple and areola which appears as bilateral, yellow-to-tan, hyperkeratotic and/or warty papules that typically involve the top of the nipple [2]. Fox–Fordyce disease usually improves in pregnancy.

Vascular changes

The vascular changes of pregnancy are similar to those in hyperthyroidism or cirrhosis. All are thought to be due to sustained high levels of circulating oestrogen. Vascular 'spider naevi' are common in pregnancy in areas that are drained by the superior vena cava (face, neck, upper chest and arms) (Figure 113.3) and usually disappear postpartum. Palmar redness is also common (Figure 113.3) [2].

Less commonly, pregnant women develop small haemangiomas or pyogenic granulomas. These can occur in approximately 5% of pregnancies and often present on the head, neck or digits [1]. They may also occur on the oral and vulvovaginal mucosa (Figure 113.3). Varicose veins of the legs, haemorrhoids and vulvar varicosities are frequent complications of pregnancy. A rarer but more serious event is the development of deep vein thrombosis, which can lead to permanent damage to the veins of the legs and, occasionally, death from pulmonary embolism. Eighty per cent of pregnant women develop some gingival oedema and redness [8]. This can become painful and ulcerative, especially if oral hygiene is poor. In approximately 2%, the gingival changes are associated with the appearance of a small vascular lesion on the oral mucosa similar to a pyogenic granuloma, known as a pregnancy epulis or granuloma gravidarum [1]. In most women, gum changes resolve after parturition.

Increased venous hydrostatic pressure can result in a non-pitting oedema in up to 50% of normal pregnancies. This most commonly affects the lower extremities, but involvement of the face and hands has also been described. This benign oedema can be relieved by bed rest, leg elevation, compression stockings or sleeping in the left lateral decubitus position. Persistent oedema, particularly of the face and hands, can be a sign of pre-eclampsia [2].

Striae distensae

Striae distensae are extremely common in the second and third trimesters of pregnancy and can arise in up to 90% of pregnant women. They are linear, pink or purple atrophic bands that develop at right angles to the skin tension lines on the abdomen, breasts, thighs and buttocks (Figure 113.1). There is some evidence that creams with *Centella asiatica* extract (a medicinal herb that is thought to increase the production of collagen and elastic fibres) and a daily massage may prevent the development of striae. Postpartum treatment of existing striae includes tretinoin cream and non-ablative fractional lasers. Microdermabrasion and microneedling are newer modalities which show some success [9,10].

Immune system changes

A switch from cell-mediated to humoral immunity (T-helper cell 1 (Th1) to Th2 shift) during gestation plays a key role in placental

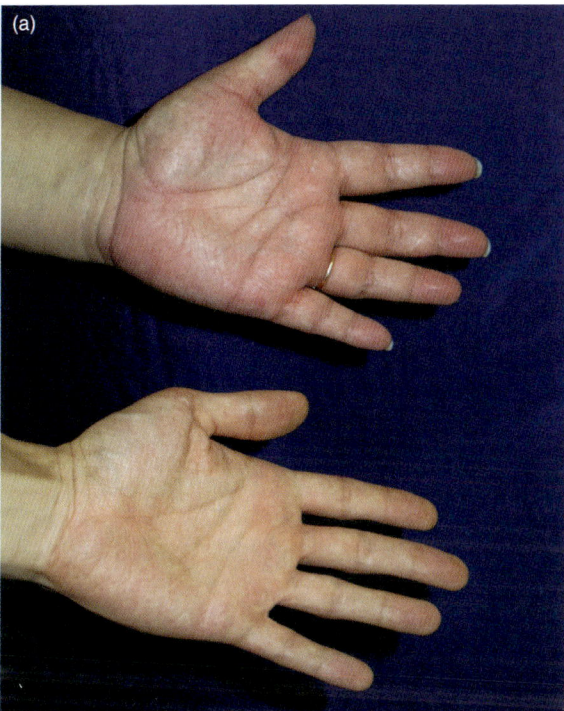
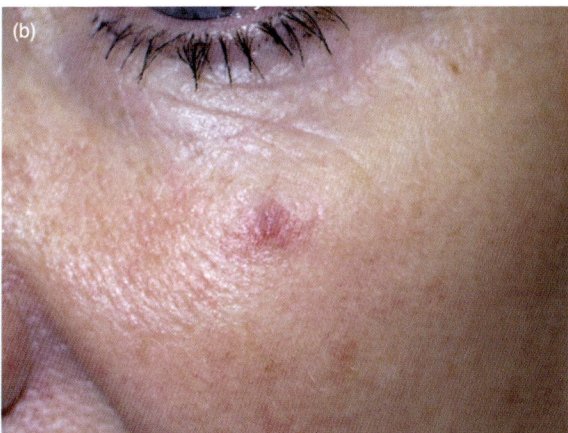
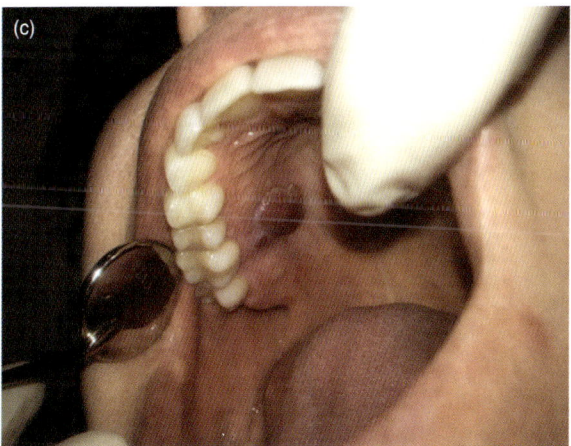

Figure 113.3 Vascular changes in pregnancy: (a) palmar redness (superior) contrasting with a normal palm (inferior); (b) spider angioma; and (c) oral pyogenic granuloma. (a, b) Courtesy of Associate Professor Amanda Oakley, Hamilton, New Zealand. (c) Courtesy of Mr David Chrisp, Tauranga Oral and Maxillofacial Surgery, Tauranga, New Zealand.

immune tolerance. This influences a woman's susceptibility to skin disease, increasing autoimmune disease and reducing cell-mediated immunity. Diseases that are Th1-driven, such as psoriasis, tend to improve, while Th2-driven diseases, such as atopic eczema and systemic lupus erythematosus, are exacerbated [11]. Reduced cell-mediated immunity during normal pregnancy probably accounts for the increased frequency and severity of certain infections such as candidiasis, herpes simplex and varicella zoster [11]. *Candida* infection, genital warts and herpes simplex virus (HSV) can all be transmitted to the baby during childbirth.

SKIN INFECTIONS AND INFESTATIONS

Human papillomavirus infection

Synonyms and inclusions
• Condyloma acuminata

Condyloma acuminata (due to human papillomavirus (HPV) infection; Chapter 25) can dramatically worsen during pregnancy, growing very rapidly particularly in the second trimester and occasionally obstructing the birth canal (Figure 113.4). Some studies have suggested that HPV infection in the mother can result in increased complications during early pregnancy; however a recent large retrospective cohort study of 15 000 women did not show an increased risk of adverse pregnancy events in HPV-positive women [1–5]. Infants born through an infected cervix are at increased risk for laryngeal papillomatosis, usually associated with HPV types 6 and 11. Therefore, genital HPV infections should be treated during pregnancy. It is still unclear whether a caesarean section reduces the risk of vertical transmission [6,7].

Management
Podophyllin, imiquimod and 5-fluorouracil should never be used in the treatment of warts during pregnancy because of potential maternal and fetal toxicity; physical treatments such as cryotherapy or electrocautery are preferable [8]. The introduction of vaccines against HPV types 16 and 18 and a quadrivalent vaccine (Gardasil®) containing HPV types 6, 11, 16 and 18 has resulted in significantly reduced risks of cervical intraepithelial neoplasia of grade 2 or 3 (CIN2 or CIN3) and adenocarcinoma in situ associated with HPV-16/18 [9]. A French study found that 88% of young men and women with genital warts had one of the HPV genotypes in the quadrivalent vaccine [10] which is consistent with the dramatic decline in prevalence of genital warts in post-HPV vaccination studies [11,12]. The occurrence of severe adverse events or adverse pregnancy outcomes was not significantly higher in recipients of HPV vaccines than in women included in control arms [9,13].

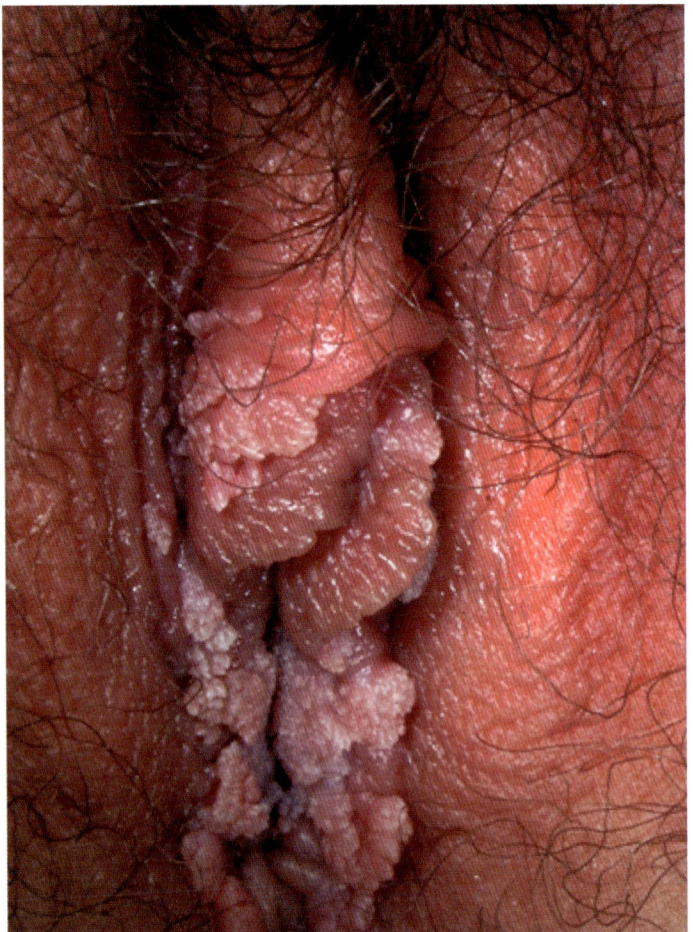

Figure 113.4 Extensive condyloma acuminata obstructing the vaginal entrance. Courtesy of Associate Professor Amanda Oakley, Hamilton, New Zealand.

Treatment ladder for human papillomavirus infection in pregnancy

First line
• Cryotherapy
• Electrocautery

Avoid
• Podophyllin
• Imiquimod
• 5-fluorouracil

Herpes simplex virus infection

Primary herpetic infection (HSV-1 or HSV-2) occurs in 2% of pregnancies and is often more severe than in the non-pregnant state. In babies of very low birth weight, infection with herpes simplex can be life threatening [14] (Chapter 25). Primary or recurrent genital HSV infection during pregnancy is an indication for drug therapy. Caesarean section is recommended when active lesions are present at term. The risk of vertical transmission to the fetus or neonate is higher in women who have a primary first episode infection (30–60%), as compared with 1% in women with a recurrent infection [15].

Systemic aciclovir is considered safe in pregnancy as it has been used extensively without adverse effects. In the case of a first or recurrent episode of genital HSV infection occurring during pregnancy, current guidance is to treat at the time of infection with 400 mg oral aciclovir three times daily for 7–10 days. Treatment should be recommended from 36 weeks' gestation (or continued if the first episode occurs after 36 weeks' gestation) with a suppressive dose of 400 mg of aciclovir three times daily until delivery to suppress viral load and reduce the likelihood of active genital lesions and caesarean section. Routine prophylaxis is not recommended for women with a history of genital herpes but no recurrence during pregnancy [15–17].

Management

> **Treatment ladder for herpes simplex infection in pregnancy**
>
> **First or recurrent episode of genital HSV occurring during pregnancy**
> - 400 mg oral aciclovir three times daily for 7–10 days for initial episode
> - Prophylactic aciclovir 400 mg three times daily from 36 weeks' gestation until after delivery

Varicella zoster virus infection

Reactivation of latent varicella zoster virus (VZV) infection (Chapter 25) in pregnancy is not associated with viraemia and therefore does not put the fetus at risk. Primary VZV infections occur in up to 1 in 2000 pregnancies and may put both mother and child at risk of pneumonia and encephalitis. Infections during weeks 1–20 (highest risk from weeks 13 to 20) can lead to fetal (congenital) varicella syndrome in 1–2% of cases, with significant neurological and growth defects. Perinatal VZV infections pose considerable risk for the development of neonatal varicella, particularly if the infant is exposed to infection at or just after birth (Box 113.2). The infant will then develop widespread cutaneous and visceral disease, usually with severe pneumonia and a 30% mortality rate [18].

Management

Passive immunisation with varicella zoster immunoglobulin to seronegative mothers within 72 h post exposure may prevent or ameliorate maternal infection. Confirmed primary varicella complications should be treated early with aciclovir either orally or intravenously.

> **Box 113.2 Potential complications of varicella zoster infection**
>
> **Fetal varicella syndrome**
> - Neurological defects
> - Growth defects
> - Pneumonia
> - Encephalitis
>
> **Maternal varicella infection**
> - Pneumonia
> - Encephalitis

> **Treatment ladder for varicella zoster virus infection in pregnancy**
>
> **VZV in seronegative mothers**
> - Immunisation with VZV immunoglobulin within 72 h of exposure
> - Confirmed infections treated early with oral aciclovir 800 mg five times daily for 7–10 days (severe cases may require intravenous aciclovir)
>
> **VZV in neonates**
> - Intravenous aciclovir is usually required
> - VZV immunoglobulin should be given to neonates whose mothers develop varicella within the period from 7 days before to 7 days after delivery
>
> **VZV in previously exposed mothers (shingles)**
> - No viraemia occurs, no prophylaxis is required and treatment is as per non-pregnant women

Scabies

Infestation with scabies (caused by *Sarcoptes scabiei*) is common during pregnancy and this diagnosis should always be considered when assessing a pregnant woman with an itchy skin eruption (Chapter 34).

Management

First line treatment should be topical 5% permethrin and second line treatment benzoyl benzoate 25% [19]. It is important to repeat the treatment after a week to kill eggs and persistent mites as cell-mediated immunity is reduced. All potentially infectious close contacts should be treated. Antihistamines and mild to moderately potent topical steroids may be needed to control the marked irritant dermatitis that often results when the mites are destroyed in the skin. Oral ivermectin is not safe to use during pregnancy.

Treatment ladder for scabies in pregnancy

First line
- Topical permethrin 5%
- Antihistamines to reduce itch, e.g. chlorphenamine, loratadine, cetirizine

Second line
- Benzoyl benzoate 25%

Avoid
- Ivermectin

Leprosy

Immune alterations in pregnancy may have an adverse effect on leprosy (Chapter 28). Leprosy reactional states are more common and the decline in immune reactivity may also lead to an increase in drug resistance [20]. Paucibacillary leprosy in remission may reactivate in the third trimester. There are limited studies on leprosy in pregnancy and it is unclear if there is vertical transmission [21,22]. The benefit of caesarean section in mothers affected with leprosy is not established. Erythema nodosum leprosum in pregnancy is associated with an early loss of nerve function and disability compared with non-pregnant individuals, so regular neurological examinations must be carried out and early treatment given.

Management

Dapsone, clofazimine and rifampicin are considered safe in pregnancy. Thalidomide is not a treatment option. Leprosy reactions can be treated with prednisolone 40–60 mg daily for 2 weeks followed by a steady reduction in the dose.

Treatment ladder for leprosy in pregnancy

First line
- Dapsone *and* clofazimine *and* rifampicin

Second line
- Prednisolone for reactional states

Syphilis

Treponema pallidum causes syphilis via sexual exposure or vertical transmission during pregnancy. Syphilis causes several hundred thousand stillbirths and neonatal deaths every year in developing nations. Consideration of syphilis in the differential diagnosis of rashes occurring during pregnancy is therefore of high importance.

The risk of mother to child transmission is highest in primary and secondary stages, followed by early latent syphilis. However, transmission risk remains high during the first 4 years after exposure, after which vertical transmission risk declines over time. The rate of fetal infection depends on the stage of maternal infection, with approximately 30% of pregnancies resulting in fetal death *in utero* or death shortly after delivery. Infants born to infected mothers are often preterm, of low birth weight or with clinical signs that mimic neonatal sepsis. Syphilis is now the second leading cause of preventable stillbirths worldwide, following malaria. The greatest burden of maternal syphilis occurs in Africa, representing >60% of the global estimate [23]. Heterosexual spread of syphilis has declined in the general population in moderate to high income countries but remains problematic in some high-risk subpopulations, such as female sex workers and their male clients.

Adverse birth outcomes caused by fetal exposure to syphilis are preventable if women are screened for syphilis and treated before the end of the second trimester of pregnancy. Many countries have routine screening for syphilis in place, but vigilance is required as higher-risk populations may not take up antenatal care.

Management

Penicillin is the only antibiotic known to be effective in treating syphilis in pregnancy and in preventing adverse birth outcomes. Doxycycline is contraindicated in pregnancy, and macrolides such as azithromycin and erythromycin do not cross the placenta well, therefore there are few alternatives to penicillin for the treatment of pregnant women with syphilis who are allergic to penicillin. Desensitisation is recommended for those who are allergic to penicillin.

Treatment ladder for syphilis in pregnancy

First line
- Penicillin

Pityriasis rosea

Pityriasis rosea is a common inflammatory skin condition that typically presents in adolescents and young adults and can present during pregnancy. It has been associated with human herpesvirus (HHV-6 and HHV-7) infection and some studies support a response to aciclovir [24,25]. Syphilis needs to be excluded. A small case series of pityriasis rosea (76 patients) in pregnancy has suggested that pityriasis rosea in early pregnancy is associated with a high risk of pregnancy complications [26]. An earlier case study of 38 of these patients suggested that fetal loss occurred in over half the women who developed pityriasis rosea in the first 15 weeks of pregnancy [27].

Management

Treatment has traditionally been conservative as the rash fades rapidly within a few weeks in most cases. However, a recent

Cochrane review did find some support for the use of aciclovir in reducing the duration of the rash and possibly improving itch for pityriasis rosea [28]. Aciclovir is safe in pregnancy and if the risk of fetal loss in early pregnancy is confirmed this may become the recommended treatment in early pregnancy or in particularly severe cases with systemic symptoms.

Treatment ladder for pityriasis rosea in pregnancy

First line
- Bland emollients and soap substitutes
- Consider oral aciclovir in early pregnancy or severe symptoms

Second line
- Oral erythromycin
- Topical steroid
- Ultraviolet B phototherapy

YEAST AND FUNGAL INFECTIONS

Candidiasis

Pregnancy can result in increased incidence of vulvovaginal candidiasis with a prevalence of 25–60% of women affected. Several studies suggest that *Candida* infections in pregnancy increase the risk of premature rupture of membranes (PROM). Systemic treatments for candidiasis are not recommended in pregnancy, but use of topical treatment is effective in most cases and may reduce the risk of PROM and neonatal candidiasis [1–6].

Management

Treatment ladder for candidiasis in pregnancy

First line
- Topical nystatin

Second line
- Topical clotrimazole
- Topical miconazole

Dermatophyte infections

Most dermatophyte infections are not life threatening and do not appear to result in complications of pregnancy. If topical antifungal treatments are not effective, then delaying use of systemic treatment until after pregnancy is prudent.

Management

Treatment ladder for dermatophyte infections in pregnancy

First line
- Topical miconazole
- Topical ketoconazole shampoo

Second line
- If there is no response to topical treatments, or if there is extensive skin surface involvement, wait until after delivery and use a systemic agent

---

AUTOIMMUNE SKIN DISEASES

Systemic lupus erythematosus

Approximately 60% of women with pre-existing systemic lupus erythematosus (SLE) will have a flare during pregnancy or the puerperium compared with 40% of non-pregnant women over the same period [1] (Chapter 51). Cutaneous flares are the most common, followed by joint symptoms. SLE in pregnancy can cause spontaneous abortion, fetal loss, pre-eclampsia, preterm delivery and intrauterine growth restriction (Box 113.3) [2]. Risk factors for adverse pregnancy outcome include the presence of antiphospholipid antibodies, lupus nephritis, Raynaud phenomenon, hypertension and either active disease at the time of conception or a first presentation of SLE during pregnancy [3].

Box 113.3 Potential complications of systemic lupus erythematosus in pregnancy

- Flare of SLE activity (60%)
- Spontaneous abortion
- Fetal loss
- Antiphospholipid syndrome – venous thromboembolism
- Pre-eclampsia
- Preterm delivery
- Intrauterine growth restriction
- Neonatal lupus erythematosus – annular rash face and scalp
- Congenital heart block (2–3%)

Neonatal lupus erythematosus

About 30% of women with SLE have anti-Ro antibodies. They are most common with subacute cutaneous lupus erythematosus and Sjögren syndrome. These antibodies cross the placenta and can cause neonatal lupus erythematosus, which presents with a scaly, annular eruption on the face and scalp, and heart block. Twenty per cent of affected babies will die in the early neonatal period, and 70% of those who survive will need a permanent pacemaker [4,5]. The risk of neonatal lupus in women with positive Ro antibodies is approximately 2% for the first pregnancy, but if there is a history of a previous pregnancy complicated by neonatal lupus, the risk increases to 13–18%. Despite efforts to prospectively monitor fetuses at risk and treat heart block immediately upon identification, sustained reversal of third-degree blocks has never been achieved [6].

Management

Family planning should be discussed as early as possible after the diagnosis of lupus. Most women can have successful pregnancies and measures can be taken to reduce the risks of adverse maternal or fetal outcomes. Risk stratification includes disease activity, autoantibody profile, previous vascular and pregnancy morbidity, hypertension and medication use. Hydroxychloroquine is recommended for women with SLE preconceptionally and throughout pregnancy. Several retrospective studies support the beneficial role of hydroxychloroquine in controlling SLE disease activity and preventing flare-ups during pregnancy. Discontinuation of hydroxychloroquine is related to an increased risk for SLE exacerbations during pregnancy. A recent prospective study has confirmed a beneficial effect of hydroxychloroquine in Ro-positive mothers with a history of previous pregnancy complicated by neonatal lupus: 400 mg of hydroxychloroquine daily started before 10 weeks' gestation was safe and resulted in a 50% reduction in the incidence of congenital heart block and a reduction in neonatal mortality from 22% to 0% [7]. Hydroxychloroquine may work by inhibiting complement activation in the placenta [8]. Flares of SLE during pregnancy should be treated as usual; corticosteroids are first line agents. Uncontrolled studies suggest an acceptable benefit : risk ratio of oral glucocorticoids, azathioprine and calcineurin inhibitors (ciclosporin, tacrolimus) in controlling SLE activity during pregnancy. In moderate to severe flares, additional modalities can be considered, such as high-dose glucocorticoids (including pulsed intravenous therapy), intravenous immunoglobulin and plasmapheresis [9–11].

Treatment ladder for systemic lupus erythematosus in pregnancy

First line for SLE flares during pregnancy
- Topical corticosteroids
- Hydroxychloroquine
- Prednisolone

Second line for SLE flares during pregnancy
- Azathioprine

General recommendations
- Obtain good disease control before conceiving
- Involve a rheumatologist and obstetrician early in the pregnancy
- All pregnant women with SLE should be on aspirin to prevent thromboembolic complications
- Hydroxychloroquine is recommended preconception when possible in women with SLE
- All women with a previous pregnancy complicated by neonatal lupus should start hydroxychloroquine 400 mg daily before 10 weeks' gestation and continue for the duration of pregnancy

---

Pemphigus vulgaris and foliaceus

There is limited literature on pemphigus in pregnancy. Pemphigus vulgaris and foliaceus can both develop or worsen during pregnancy. Exacerbations occur more commonly in the first and second trimesters and may improve in the third trimester due to maternal immunosuppression. Pemphigus in pregnancy is considered as high risk due to potential adverse outcomes for the mother and fetus (Box 113.4). In one review, maternal pemphigus was associated with a 12% rate of stillbirth, spontaneous abortion or neonatal mortality and was transmitted to the fetus in approximately 50% of pregnancies (more commonly with vulgaris than foliaceus) [12]. Two reviews combining the results of 41 and 47 case reports (respectively) found that approximately 60% of women with pre-existing pemphigus had infants with neonatal pemphigus, compared with 35% of women who developed pemphigus during pregnancy [13,**14**]. The clinical presentation in the mother is the same as in non-pregnant individuals (Figure 113.5). The blistering and erosions can be very similar to pemphigoid gestationis so a skin biopsy including direct immunofluorescence is required for an accurate diagnosis. Enzyme-linked immunosorbent assay (ELISA) using recombinant desmoglein 3 can also confirm the diagnosis [**14**]. Fetal skin shares the same desmoglein 3 profile as adult oral mucosa, so neonatal pemphigus is more likely to occur if the mother has oral disease. There is no direct correlation between the severity of the mother's disease and the extent of neonatal involvement. Neonatal skin lesions appear to resolve within 4 weeks postpartum [12].

Box 113.4 Potential complications of pemphigus vulgaris in pregnancy

- Spontaneous abortion
- Exacerbation of disease (Th-2 mediated)
- Stillbirth
- Caesarean section needed if there is severe vulvovaginal disease
- Neonatal pemphigus with transient blistering
- Perinatal mortality of 12% with placental dysfunction

Management

Treatment with immunosuppressant therapy is normally required. Treatment of pregnant women is aimed at managing maternal disease but also preventing neonatal pemphigus and adverse pregnancy outcomes such as preterm birth, low-birth-weight pre-eclampsia, stillbirth and spontaneous abortion [12,15]. The optimal treatment regimen is expert guided rather than evidence based as there is a lack of controlled trials. Wherever possible, pregnancy is planned so that medications such as methotrexate, cyclophosphamide and mycophenolate can be replaced with more appropriate immunosuppression. Consideration should be given to pre-treatment with rituximab at least 6 months before conception to induce stable remission, as this medication cannot be given during pregnancy. When exacerbations occur during pregnancy, oral corticosteroids are first line agents [12,16,17].

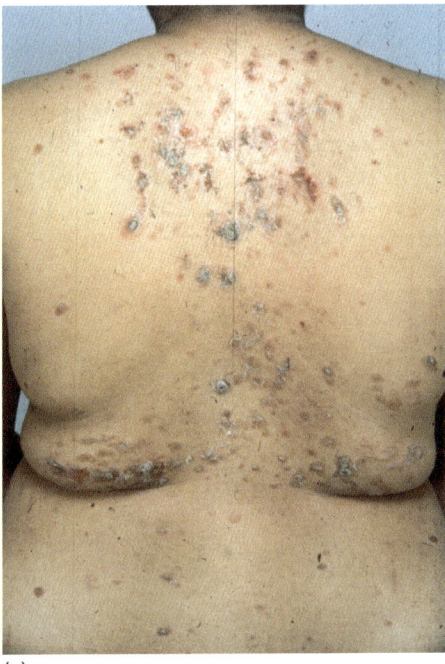

(a)

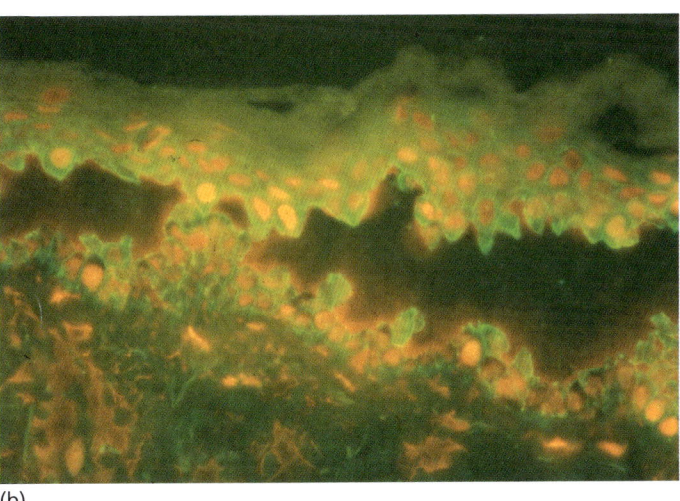

(b)

Figure 113.5 Pemphigus vulgaris. (a) New disease onset in the second trimester showing pink scaly plaques and erosions on the back. (b) Indirect immunofluorescence using the patient's serum and showing intercellular immunoglobulin G with intraepidermal split.

Treatment ladder for pemphigus vulgaris and foliaceus in pregnancy

First line
- Prednisolone

Second line
- Azathioprine

Third line
- Intravenous immunoglobulin
- Plasma exchange
- Plasmapheresis

Other connective tissue disorders

Women with Ehlers–Danlos syndrome types I and IV often have major problems during pregnancy, including bleeding, uterine lacerations and wound dehiscence. Some patients with pseudoxanthoma elasticum have suffered major gastrointestinal bleeds necessitating blood transfusion [18]. The diagnosis of Ehlers–Danlos syndrome in women of child-bearing age should prompt counselling regarding risks during pregnancy to ensure the correct specialist care is sought when required.

SKIN TUMOURS

Benign melanocytic naevi

Changes in the moles of pregnant women have frequently been attributed to pregnancy in the past, but recent studies suggest that pregnancy does not induce significant physiological changes in naevi. It is common for naevi on the breasts and abdomen to grow with skin expansion, but studies that have examined melanocytic naevi on the back or lower extremities have found no significant changes in size during pregnancy. Several studies have also investigated the belief that moles darken during pregnancy and have found insufficient evidence to support this. However, dermoscopically, transient changes have been identified during pregnancy, such as new dot formation, thickening of the pigment network, darkening of globules and increasing numbers of vessels, and have been described as the pregnancy-related nevus pattern. These changes are subtle and not suggestive of melanoma [1,2]. Any clinical or histopathological features consistent with melanoma should be viewed as suspicious and not attributed to pregnancy. Prompt excisional biopsy should be performed on any concerning skin lesion. Cutaneous surgery can be performed safely during pregnancy and should not be delayed until after pregnancy [1].

Malignant melanoma

The incidence of melanoma during pregnancy varies depending on the population studied. Melanoma was the most common malignancy during pregnancy in large population studies from Sweden [3] and Australia [4] and the third most common cancer during pregnancy in a US study [5]. Early reports suggesting a worse prognosis for melanoma diagnosed in pregnancy have not been supported by more recent larger studies, but this remains controversial. The discrepancy may reflect an historical diagnostic and therapeutic delay. While the effect of oestrogen and progesterone on melanoma is under investigation, it is generally accepted that oral contraceptive use is not contraindicated after a diagnosis of melanoma in pregnancy. A subsequent pregnancy should be delayed for 2–3 years after a diagnosis of a high-risk melanoma [6].

After staging is complete, systemic therapy may be needed in advanced melanoma. Immunotherapy or target therapy (with BRAF (proto-oncogene B-Raf or v-Raf murine sarcoma viral oncogene homolog B) and MEK (mitogen-activated protein kinase) inhibitors) is not recommended during pregnancy and lactation. Drugs used in immunotherapy act on the PD-1 (programmed death 1) pathway (e.g. nivolumab and pembrolizumab) or the cytotoxic T-lymphocyte-associated protein 4 (CTLA-4) pathway (e.g. ipilimumab) and reduce the natural regulatory mechanisms on immune response. This could reduce maternal tolerance for the fetus, therefore increasing the risk of spontaneous abortions and developmental defects [7]. Among BRAF inhibitors, dabrafenib is clearly teratogenic but animal studies suggest that although vemurafenib can cross the placenta there are no associated teratogenic effects. Animal reproduction studies demonstrated that MEK inhibitors trametinib and cobimetinib can harm the fetus. Good outcomes without apparent harm to the newborn have been reported for ipilimumab alone [7].

Box 113.5 Guidance for the management of melanoma in pregnancy

- Most studies show no adverse effect of pregnancy on prognosis
- Pigmented lesions should be evaluated as for non-pregnant patients; changes suggestive of melanoma cannot be attributed to pregnancy
- Primary excisional biopsy should be performed under local anaesthetic without delay as for non-pregnant patients (with respect for judicious dose of local anaesthetic)
- If surgery requires general anaesthesia and cannot be deferred, the second trimester is the safest time to perform it
- Staging should be performed as necessary but ultrasonography and magnetic resonance imaging are considered the safest techniques Computed tomography could be considered if the benefits clearly outweigh the risks
- The sentinel lymph node provides prognostic information only and is difficult to justify during pregnancy. If considered essential for treatment planning, technetium 99m alone should be used as a marker
- Adjuvant treatment of metastatic melanoma during pregnancy is difficult since traditional agents such as dacarbazine and interferon α, as well as targeted therapy (BRAF and MEK inhibitors) and immunotherapy, are contraindicated. Vemurafenib and ipilimumab are the agents less likely to cause harm to the fetus
- In high-risk patients a multidisciplinary tailored approach is preferred, if available, and adequate counselling and involvement of the mother in decisions are necessary

---

Metastatic pregnancy-associated melanoma (MPAM) is associated with a very poor outcome for the mother. Termination of pregnancy should be discussed with women with advanced disease in the first or second trimester, to gain more therapeutic possibilities. MPAM can involve the placenta in exceptional cases and the fetus in even rarer circumstances. Careful macroscopic and histopathological examination of the fetal adnexa with appropriate immunohistochemical staining is recommended after delivery in women with known or suspected metastatic melanoma in pregnancy. If there is no placental involvement, fetal metastasis can be reasonably excluded [7]. If there is evidence of placental involvement, thorough examination of the newborn should be performed, including skin inspection, chest radiography, abdominal ultrasound, liver enzymes and lactate dehydrogenase testing, since approximately 22% of neonates can also show clinical evidence of disease [7]. Apparently healthy neonates delivered with concomitant placental metastasis represent a high-risk population and should be followed up for at least 24 months [5,8].

Box 113.5 lists some important aspects of the management of melanoma during pregnancy.

INFLAMMATORY SKIN DISEASES

Psoriasis and generalised pustular psoriasis

Psoriasis typically improves during pregnancy but worsens in up to 10–20% of women, requiring increased treatment [1]. Severe psoriasis may be associated with a slight increased risk of complications such as low birth weight and premature delivery, but mild to moderate disease is not associated with any adverse outcomes of pregnancy [2–4]. With the increased use of biologic treatment for psoriasis many women may already be on a biologic agent when they become pregnant, or it may be considered as a treatment option for disease not controlled with other medications. There are no large, controlled trials on which to base treatment decisions, but expert opinion is concordant [3,5–7]: topical treatments are used in mild disease with the addition of ultraviolet B (UVB) in moderate to severe disease. When these fail biologics are considered preferable to ciclosporine. Biologics may act like maternal antibodies and cross the placenta to a varying extent, especially in the second and third trimesters. Certolizumab crosses the placenta less than other biologics and has been recommended as the preferred biologic in pregnancy. Neonates who have been exposed to biologics *in utero* in the third trimester should not be given live vaccines for the first 6 months of life due to persistence of biologic antibodies in the neonate.

Generalised pustular psoriasis can present in pregnancy. This is also known as impetigo herpetiformis, but the term is best avoided since the pustules are sterile and there is no evidence of viral or bacterial infection. Pustular psoriasis in pregnancy tends to occur in the early part of the third trimester of pregnancy and usually resolves after parturition. This can be severe, presenting with flexural and periumbilical redness and pustules, which rapidly desquamate and coalesce, spreading in a centrifugal manner (Figure 113.6). It may be associated with erythroderma, fever, tetany and hypocalcaemia. Recurrence in subsequent pregnancies is characteristic with earlier onset and increased severity. It must be differentiated from acute generalised exanthematous pustulosis which is typically drug related. Systemic treatment is usually required and case reports support the use of moderate- to high-dose corticosteroids, narrow-band UVB and ciclosporin [4,8–11]. Ciclosporin is becoming the preferred first line agent by many experts [12]. Infliximab is an option for resistant disease. Treatment can usually be quickly tapered postpartum.

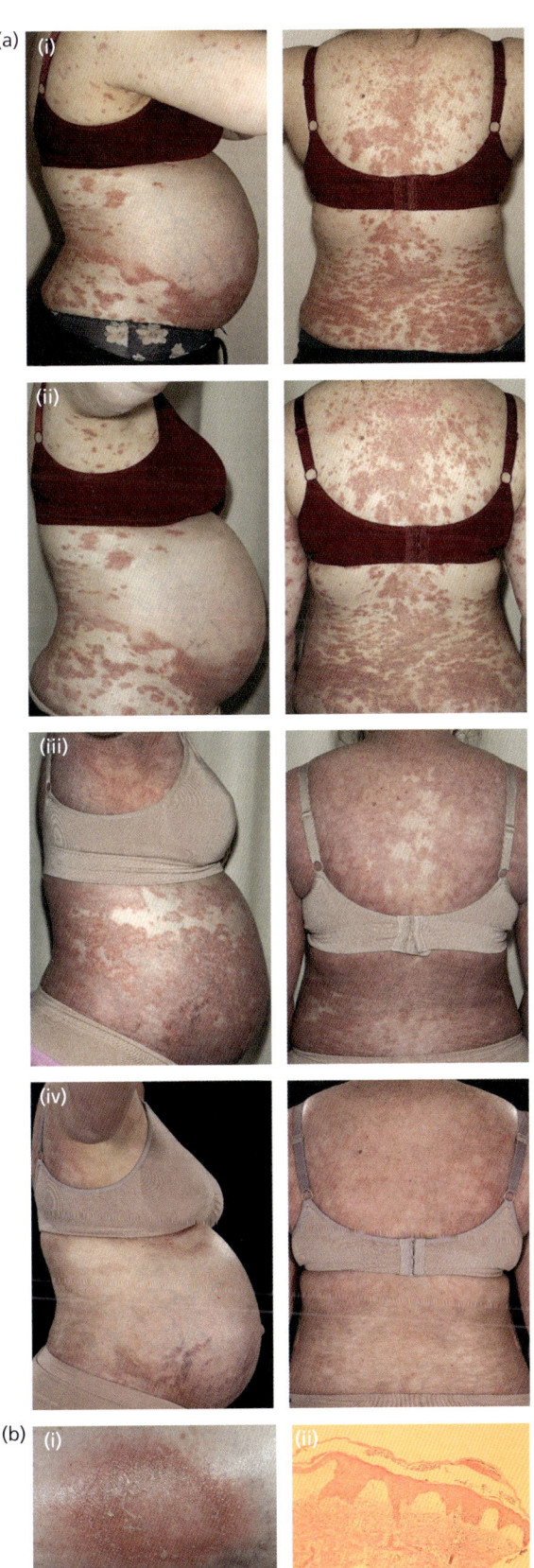

Figure 113.6 (a) Evolution of pustular psoriasis of pregnancy; the patient was treated with prednisone and ciclosporin (i, ii) and was then commenced on infliximab (iii) with good results 1 week later (iv). (b) Plaque of pustular psoriasis of pregnancy (i) and histology of pustular psoriasis of pregnancy (ii). Courtesy of Dr Caroline Mahon and Dr Julia Zhu, Department of Dermatology, Christchurch Hospital, New Zealand.

Management

> ### Treatment ladder for psoriasis in pregnancy
>
> **First line**
> - Emollients
> - Topical corticosteroids (low to mid potency)
>
> **Second line or first line for moderate to severe disease**
> - Narrow-band UVB (TL-01)
>   *Or*
> - Broad-band UVB
>
> **Third line**
> - Certolizumab is the preferred biologic agent; etanercept is an alternative
> - Ciclosporin

> ### Treatment ladder for generalised pustular psoriasis in pregnancy
>
> - Ciclosporin
> - Oral corticosteroids
> - Narrow-band UVB
> - Infliximab

Acne vulgaris and rosacea

Acne vulgaris (Chapter 88) often improves in early pregnancy but worsens in the third trimester as maternal androgen levels increase. In patients with skin of colour the sequelae of postinflammatory hyperpigmentation (PIH), keloids and severe scarring are common [13]. Early and aggressive control of the disease process is necessary in at-risk groups. Patient education is important to prevent excoriation of acne lesions and to avoid harsh skin regimens and cultural skin and hair care practices that can aggravate acne or cause PIH or scarring. All treatments during pregnancy should be kept to short courses of the lowest effective dose. Topical agents are preferred for mild to moderate acne. Systemic and topical retinoids should be avoided because of their known teratogenic potential [14]. Oral erythromycin and azithromycin appear safe (after the first trimester). Severe acne conglobata may require treatment with systemic corticosteroids in addition to oral antibiotics. Narrow-band UVB can be used as second line therapy for more severe acne vulgaris during pregnancy [15]. There is interest in light and laser treatments for acne, but further information is needed to assess safety.

Acne neonatorum may occur due to passive transfer of maternal androgens across the placenta during the third trimester. This is usually a transient eruption in the young infant that does not require ongoing treatment.

Rosacea (Chapter 89) often worsens during pregnancy and may require systemic treatment. Rosacea fulminans is a rare, severe variant of rosacea that may flare significantly in pregnancy. This is characterised by numerous pustules, marked facial redness, cystic swellings and coalescing sinuses. Rosacea fulminans normally requires treatment with oral antibiotics and oral corticosteroids, and early treatment is necessary to prevent scarring. Azithromycin is the preferred first line antibiotic [16].

Management

> #### Treatment ladder for acne vulgaris in pregnancy
>
> **First line**
> - Benzoyl peroxide gel 2.5–10%
> - Topical clindamycin
> - Topical erythromycin
>
> **Second line**
> - Oral azithromycin
> - Oral erythromycin (avoid in first trimester)
> - Topical salicylic acid
>
> **Third line/severe disease**
> - Narrow-band UVB (TL-01)
> - Prednisolone (can be combined with oral antibiotic therapy)

> #### Treatment ladder for rosacea in pregnancy
>
> **First line**
> - Topical azelaic acid 10–15%
> - Topical metronidazole
>
> **Second line**
> - Oral azithromycin (preferred over erythromycin for rosacea)
> - Oral erythromycin (avoid in first trimester)
>
> **Third line/severe disease**
> - Prednisolone (can be combined with oral antibiotic therapy)
>
> **Ocular rosacea**
> - Artificial tears and lubricating ointment
> - Eyelid hygiene morning and evening
> - If above is insufficient add in topical fusidic acid or ciclosporin ophthalmic emulsion (most likely to be implemented by ophthalmologists)

Urticaria

Urticaria can mimic other pregnancy dermatoses, particularly the pre-bullous phase of pemphigoid gestationis or polymorphic eruption of pregnancy. Urticaria presents frequently during pregnancy and can be difficult to control effectively (Chapter 42).

Management

Oral antihistamines are the treatment of choice; the second-generation antihistamines loratadine and cetirizine are safe to use from the second trimester onwards. Omalizumab is likely to become the preferred second line option for urticaria unresponsive to antihistamines as reports emerge of large cohorts of patients taking omalizumab during pregnancy (predominantly for asthma, with small series of patients with urticaria), with no apparent increased risks of poor pregnancy outcomes [17–19]. Data registries have been established to provide further information on the safety of omalizumab in pregnancy.

> #### Treatment ladder for urticaria in pregnancy
>
> **First line**
> - Topical emollients: aqueous cream + 1–2% menthol
> - Oral antihistamines: loratadine and cetirizine
>
> **Second line**
> - Omalizumab
>
> **Third line**
> - Prednisolone
> - Ciclosporin

Erythema nodosum

Erythema nodosum (Chapter 97) is a reactive inflammation of the subcutaneous fat, secondary to a wide variety of underlying conditions including streptococcal infections, tuberculosis, leprosy, sarcoidosis and inflammatory bowel disease. Pregnancy and oral contraceptive therapy can also trigger this eruption, which presents with tender red nodules or plaques over the anterior lower legs. Fever, malaise and arthralgia often occur, and the eruption typically lasts up to 6–8 weeks. Supportive treatment is normally all that is required – rest, leg elevation, compression hosiery and analgesia can all help to improve symptoms. It is important to exclude non-pregnancy-related causes of erythema nodosum.

Management

> #### Treatment ladder for erythema nodosum in pregnancy
>
> **First line**
> - Rest and leg elevation
> - Compression hosiery
> - Analgesia
>
> **Second line**
> - Short course of prednisolone

PREGNANCY-SPECIFIC DERMATOSES AND ITCHING

Introduction and classification

Itch is common in pregnant women and more common in multiple pregnancies. One-third of affected women will have either a specific dermatosis of pregnancy (atopic eruption of pregnancy, polymorphic eruption of pregnancy or pemphigoid gestationis) or a specific illness (including intrahepatic cholestasis of pregnancy) to explain the pruritus [1]. Two-thirds of women will have no specific diagnosis for the itch and this group is termed as having pruritus gravidarum.

Most pruritus during pregnancy is of symptomatic significance only but some conditions, such as pemphigoid gestationis and intrahepatic cholestasis of pregnancy, are associated with adverse outcomes for the fetus and need to be identified and managed early to reduce perinatal morbidity and mortality. The dermatosis of concern can usually be identified on clinical grounds, but specific investigations may be required (Table 113.1). Atopic eruption of pregnancy has the earliest onset during pregnancy, usually in the first or second trimester, in a patient with atopic tendencies. Pemphigoid gestationis may occasionally also occur in early pregnancy (but usually later), often involves the periumbilical region and eventually progresses to bullous lesions. Polymorphic eruption of pregnancy and intrahepatic cholestasis of pregnancy usually occur in the third trimester. Polymorphic eruption of pregnancy starts in the striae gravidarum and typically spares the periumbilical region and the palms. Pruritus gravidarum and intrahepatic cholestasis of pregnancy have no primary skin lesions and may produce intense itching of the palms.

The specific dermatoses of pregnancy have been renamed and reclassified many times over the years, with several names for each disease, which has led to confusion. There is considerable overlap in clinical presentation and histopathology between pregnant women with atopic eczema, prurigo of pregnancy and pruritic folliculitis of pregnancy. These conditions are now grouped together as 'atopic eruption of pregnancy' [2,3]. Table 113.2 gives the most up-to-date classification, with previous synonyms included.

Table 113.2 Classification of the specific dermatoses and itch of pregnancy.

Classification	Synonyms
Pemphigoid gestationis	Herpes gestationis Gestational pemphigoid
Polymorphic eruption of pregnancy (PEP)[a]	Pruritic urticarial papules and plaques of pregnancy (PUPPP) Toxaemic rash of pregnancy Late-onset prurigo of pregnancy Toxic erythema of pregnancy
Intrahepatic cholestasis of pregnancy	Cholestasis of pregnancy Pruritus/prurigo gravidarum Obstetric cholestasis Jaundice of pregnancy
Atopic eruption of pregnancy	Prurigo of pregnancy[a] Prurigo gestationis Early-onset prurigo of pregnancy Papular dermatitis of pregnancy Pruritic folliculitis of pregnancy[a] Eczema in pregnancy

[a] Previous classification by Holmes and Black, 1983 [4].

Pruritus gravidarum and intrahepatic cholestasis of pregnancy

Introduction and general description

Pruritus gravidarum is considered by most to be a mild variant of intrahepatic cholestasis of pregnancy occurring in approximately 0.03–3% of pregnancies [1,2]. There is poor correlation of severity of itch and serum bile salts [3]. The accuracy of serum bile salts in diagnosing intrahepatic cholestasis of pregnancy is not clear according to a Cochrane review and this may explain the large number of women presenting with the typical pruritus of intrahepatic cholestasis without the corresponding laboratory findings [4]. Therefore, some authors classify pruritus gravidarum as with or without cholestasis.

Table 113.1 Clinical features of the specific dermatoses and itch of pregnancy.

	Presentation in early pregnancy	Presentation in late pregnancy	Risk to fetus	Specific clinical features	Prognosis postpartum	Recurrence with subsequent pregnancy
Atopic eruption of pregnancy	✓	Less common	✗	Eczematous changes	Improvement	✓
Pruritus gravidarum without cholestasis	✗	✓	✗	Secondary excoriation only, itchy palms, bile salts <40 µmol/L	Spontaneous resolution within days to weeks	✓
Intrahepatic cholestasis of pregnancy (pruritus gravidarum with cholestasis)	✗	✓	✓	Secondary excoriation only, itchy palms, serum bile salts >40 µmol/L	Spontaneous resolution within days to weeks	✓
Polymorphic eruption of pregnancy	✗	✓	✗	Redness, urticated papules, plaques, small vesicles	May flare peripartum then resolves spontaneously	✗ May recur in multiple pregnancies
Pemphigoid gestationis	Less common	✓	✓	Initially redness, papules and plaques; eventually bullae	May persist for months; systemic treatment usually required	✓ May also recur with contraception, menstruation

Source: Dr Amy Stanway.

Pathophysiology

Intrahepatic cholestasis of pregnancy is a reversible form of hormonally triggered cholestasis that typically develops in genetically predisposed individuals in late pregnancy. The cause is thought to be multifactorial [5].

Clinical features

Presentation

Itching begins in the second or third trimester and is often localised to the abdomen, or the palms and soles, although it may also be widespread. In about 10% of cases the patient may be mildly jaundiced. Secondary skin lesions develop due to scratching and range from subtle excoriations to severe prurigo nodules as pruritus persists (Figure 113.7).

Disease course and prognosis

The prognosis for the mother is generally good. After delivery, pruritus disappears spontaneously within days to weeks, but may recur with subsequent pregnancies and oral contraception [6,7,8]. Pruritus gravidarum with serum bile salts <40 μmol/L does not seem to be associated with a poor perinatal outcome and symptomatic

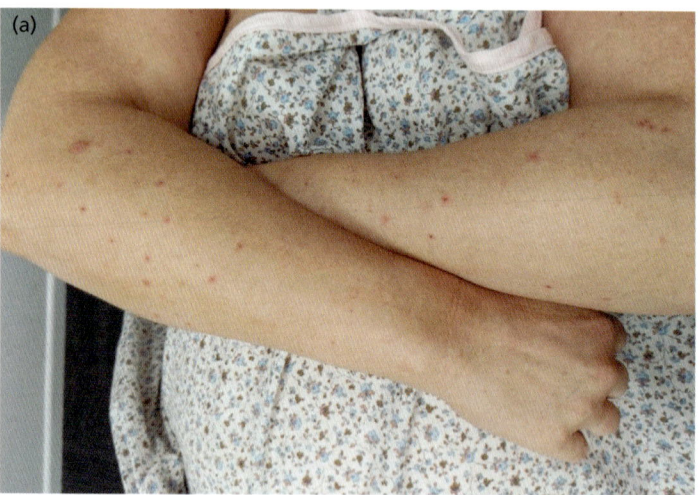

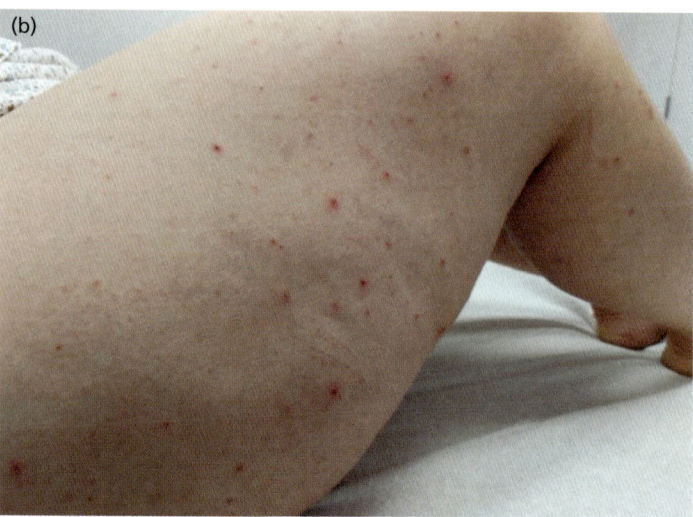

Figure 113.7 Excoriations with no background eczematous features in pruritus gravidarum (normal serum bile salts).

treatment only is required [3]. If jaundice or high serum bile salts are present, patients are at risk of developing steatorrhea with malabsorption of fat-soluble vitamins, including vitamin K, which might lead to bleeding complications and cholelithiasis [6]. Fetal prognosis may be impaired with an increased risk of prematurity, fetal distress and stillbirth [3,6]. Therefore, prompt diagnosis, specific therapy, close obstetric monitoring and maternal counselling are essential.

Investigations

Liver function tests are usually normal (alkaline phosphatase may be raised but this is a normal finding in pregnancy due to placental production) [4]. Serum bile salts may be raised. In healthy pregnancies, total serum bile acid levels may increase up to 11.0 μmol/L in the third trimester. Serum bile salts >40 μmol/L are associated with increased preterm delivery, meconium staining of amniotic fluid and asphyxial events [3].

Management

Ursodeoxycholic acid (UDCA) has been the treatment of choice based on small studies suggesting that this improved maternal itch and reduced fetal morbidity and mortality [9]. Later larger studies did not confirm this finding [10,11]. Recent Cochrane reviews showed a small benefit for maternal pruritus with UDCA but no reduction in fetal death or spontaneous preterm delivery [4,12]. Studies are needed to determine if there is a benefit in the higher-risk group with serum bile salts >40 μmol/L. There do not appear to be any safety concerns with the use of UDCA in pregnancy and it would seem reasonable to trial it in symptomatic women. There is little evidence to support the use of activated charcoal, S-adenosyl-L-methionine, dexamethasone or cholestyramine. Of note, cholestyramine and other bile acid exchange resins may contribute to the malabsorption of vitamin K with possible bleeding complications and should therefore be avoided [13]. Close obstetric surveillance is indicated in women with bile salts >40 μmol/L. Stillbirth is a sudden occurrence and there is no evidence that weekly fetal cardiac monitoring prevents this, but regular obstetric review may pick up growth retardation and early fetal distress.

Treatment ladder for pruritus gravidarum and intrahepatic cholestasis of pregnancy

First line
- Topical emollients: aqueous cream + 1–2% menthol
- Oral antihistamines: loratadine and cetirizine
- Oral UDCA 1 g per day

Second line
- S-adenosyl-L-methionine
- Dexamethasone
- Cholestyramine

Other recommendations
- Weekly fetal cardiotocography to monitor fetal heart rate and detect early signs of fetal distress if bile salts >40 μmol/L
- Maternal vitamin K replacement (if jaundice is present)
- Early delivery (36–37 weeks) if bile salts >40 μmol/L
- Dexamethasone may be needed for fetal lung maturity

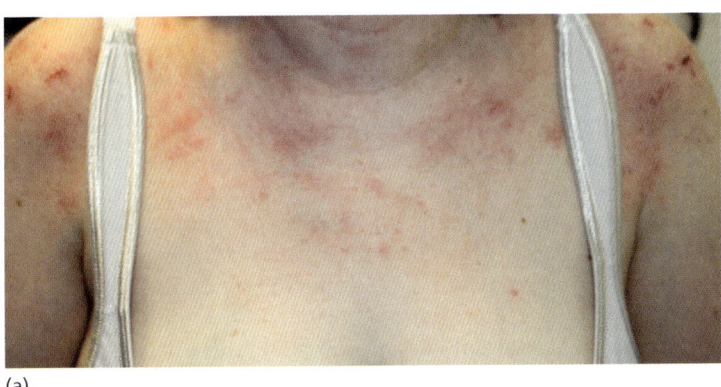

(a)

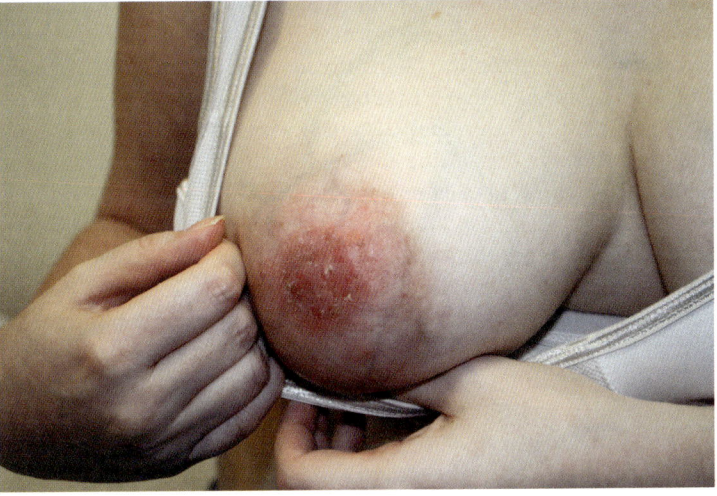

(b)

Figure 113.8 E-type atopic eruption of pregnancy: (a) on the upper trunk and shoulders in the second trimester and (b) with nipple eczema.

Atopic eruption of pregnancy

Introduction and general description

Atopic eruption of pregnancy (AEP) is the most common specific dermatosis of pregnancy, accounting for 50% of patients. It is a benign pruritic disorder of pregnancy that includes eczematous and/or papular lesions in patients with an atopic diathesis. Other dermatoses of pregnancy must be excluded (Chapter 41). It usually starts early on in pregnancy, with 75% of cases presenting before the third trimester, and tends to recur in subsequent pregnancies [1].

Pathophysiology

The pathogenesis of AEP is thought to be triggered by pregnancy-specific immunological changes: increased Th2 cytokines (interleukin 4 (IL-4), IL-10) and a reduced cellular immunity and reduced production of Th1 cytokines (IL-2, interferon γ, IL-12) [2].

Clinical features

Presentation

Twenty per cent of patients suffer from an exacerbation of pre-existing atopic eczema with a typical clinical picture. The remaining 80% experience atopic skin changes for the first time ever or after a long remission (for example, since childhood). Two-thirds of patients present with widespread eczematous changes often affecting typical atopic sites such as the face, neck, décolleté and flexural surfaces of the limbs (so-called E-type AEP; Figure 113.8). One-third of patients have papular lesions (P-type AEP; Figure 113.9) [1] which are characterised by small red papules disseminated on the trunk and limbs as well as typical prurigo nodules, mostly located on the shins and arms. A key feature is severe dryness of the skin and frequent Hanifin and Rajka atopic 'minor' features [3].

Disease course and prognosis

Maternal prognosis is good even in severe cases as skin lesions usually respond quickly to therapy. Recurrence in subsequent pregnancies is common. Fetal prognosis is unaffected.

Investigations

Histopathology is non-specific and varies with the clinical type and stage of the disease. Direct and indirect immunofluorescence are both negative. Elevated serum IgE levels are found in 20–70% of patients [1].

Management

Basic treatment with emollients and topical corticosteroids for several days will usually lead to quick improvement of skin lesions. Severe cases may require a short course of systemic corticosteroids and antihistamines. Phototherapy (UVB) is useful for severe cases in early pregnancy.

Treatment ladder for atopic eruption of pregnancy

First line
- Topical emollients
- Topical corticosteroids
- Oral antihistamines: loratadine and cetirizine

Second line
- Narrow-band UVB phototherapy

Third line
- Prednisolone
- Azathioprine

Resource

EADV (European Academy of Dermatology and Venerology). *Atopic Eruption of Pregnancy (AEP)*. https://www.eadv.org/cms-admin/showfile/EADV%20Pregnancy%20TF_%20Atopic%20Eruption%20of%20pregnancy%20%28AEP%29.pdf (last accessed February 2022).

PART 10: SPECIFIC SITES, SEX & AGE

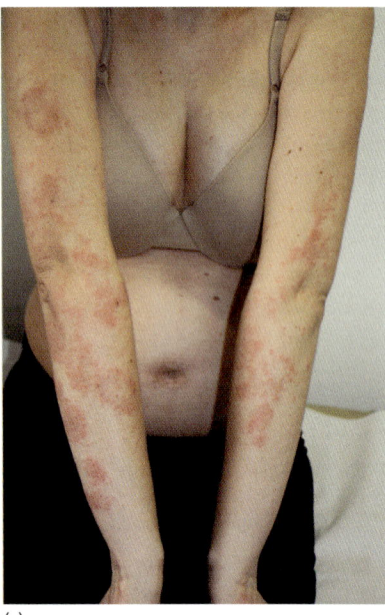

(a)

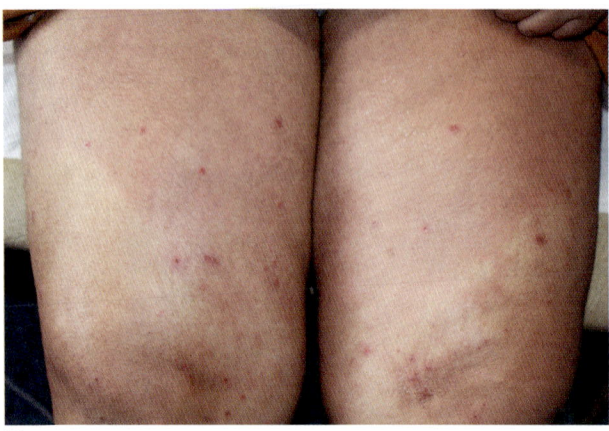

(b)

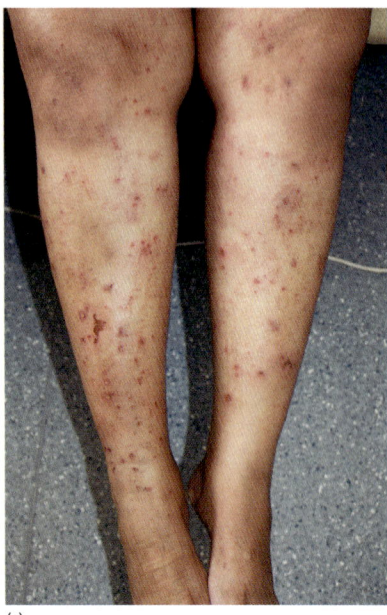

(c)

Figure 113.9 P-type atopic eruption of pregnancy showing (a) excoriated red patches on the arms; (b) excoriated papules, redness and dry skin on the upper thighs; and (c) excoriated prurigo lesions on the lower legs (all in the second trimester).

Polymorphic eruption of pregnancy

Introduction and general description
Polymorphic eruption of pregnancy (PEP) is a specific dermatosis of pregnancy also known as 'pruritic urticarial papules and plaques of pregnancy'. It is a benign, self-limited skin disorder. Key features include an increased prevalence in primigravidas, onset in the third trimester or immediately postpartum (15% of cases [1]), remission near the time of delivery, and association with multiple gestation pregnancy and maternal weight gain [1,2]. There are no associated maternal or fetal risks, and treatment is symptomatic [3].

Pathophysiology
The pathogenesis of PEP remains unclear. The main theories focus on abdominal distension and hormonal and immunological factors, but supportive evidence is insufficient for all current hypotheses [1,4,5]. The fact that PEP starts within striae distensae at the time of greatest abdominal distension may suggest that damage to the connective tissue due to overstretching plays a central role. An increase of CD1a cells in the cutaneous inflammatory infiltrate could confirm the theory that previously inert structures develop an antigenic character, thus triggering the inflammatory process. The phenomenon of peripheral microchimerism in pregnancy has also been hypothesised to play a role in triggering the inflammation [6]. Serum cortisol levels were found to be low in one study of women with PEP, while human chorionic gonadotrophin (hCG) and oestradiol were normal [5]. Unlike pemphigoid gestationis, there is no human leukocyte antigen (HLA) association [7].

Clinical features
The clinical features are crucial to diagnosis. PEP typically starts on the abdomen, often within the striae, and classically spares the umbilical area, palms, soles and face. The sparing of the umbilical area helps to differentiate PEP from pemphigoid gestationis since clinical features can be very similar early in the course of disease. The striae first become itchy, then red, and finally urticarial. The rash spreads to the buttocks and proximal thighs, coalescing into plaques (Figure 113.10). Patients are very uncomfortable, and the pruritus often interferes with sleep. The lesions are rarely excoriated [3]. Later, the morphology becomes more polymorphic; vesicles (1–2 mm in size; never frank bullae as in pemphigoid gestationis), widespread non-urticated red patches, and targetoid and eczematous lesions develop in half of patients. The rash usually resolves within 4–6 weeks, independently of delivery [6].

Disease course and fetal prognosis
There is no suggestion that PEP has any adverse effect on the outcome of the pregnancy or the newborn [5,7]. Lesions are self-limiting and the disease tends not to recur; the exception being in a multiple pregnancy when earlier presentation in pregnancy may occur.

Investigations
The histopathology of this condition is non-specific and there are many similarities with the early pre-bullous phase of pemphigoid gestationis. Most biopsies show epidermal and upper dermal oedema, with a perivascular infiltrate of lymphocytes and histiocytes. There may be a striking number of eosinophils (as there may

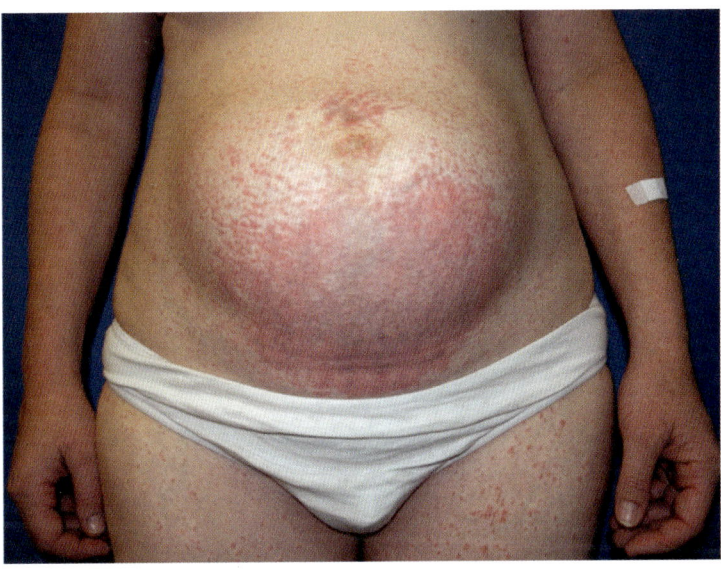

Figure 113.10 Polymorphic eruption of pregnancy showing papules and urticarial lesions on the abdomen and thighs. Note sparing of the umbilical area. Courtesy of Associate Professor Amanda Oakley, Hamilton, New Zealand.

be in pemphigoid gestationis). Spongiotic vesicles, hyperkeratosis and patchy parakeratosis are seen [7].

Direct immunofluorescence is generally negative, even by immunoelectron microscopy, and this provides the best means of distinguishing this disorder from pemphigoid gestationis should there be any diagnostic doubt [8]. There are occasional reports of equivocal direct immunofluorescence findings in PEP, including minimal C3 deposition on the basement membrane, in the epidermis and perivascularly [7]. In these rare situations of equivocal immunofluoresence, a BP180 NC16a ELISA has been shown to be highly sensitive and specific in distinguishing pemphigoid gestationis from PEP [9]. Indirect immunofluorescence is also negative [5].

Management

Symptomatic treatment with topical corticosteroids and emollients, with or without antihistamines, is usually sufficient to control pruritus and skin lesions, with relief in 24–72 h [3]. In severe generalised cases, a short course of systemic corticosteroids (prednisolone starting at 40–60 mg/day and tapering to zero over a few weeks) may be necessary and is usually very effective [2]. Early induction of labour can also be considered if the patient is close to term.

Treatment ladder for polymorphic eruption of pregnancy

First line
- Topical emollients: aqueous cream + 1–2% menthol
- Topical corticosteroids
- Oral antihistamines: loratadine and cetirizine

Second line
- Prednisolone
  Consider early induction of labour if patient is close to term

---

Pemphigoid gestationis

Introduction and general description

Pemphigoid gestationis (PG) is a rare, autoimmune, bullous disorder that presents mainly in late pregnancy or the immediate postpartum period (Chapter 50). It may occur earlier in multigravida pregnancies [1]. It also rarely presents in association with trophoblastic tumours (choriocarcinoma, hydatidiform mole) [2,3]. The incidence varies from 1 : 2000 to 1 : 50 000–60 000 pregnancies [4]. PG has a strong association with maternal major histocompatibility complex (MHC) class II antigens haplotypes HLA-DR3 (human leukocyte antigens DR3) and HLA-DR4 [5,6]. There is also an increased risk of developing other organ-specific autoimmune diseases, in particular Graves disease [6].

Pathophysiology

Circulating complement-fixing IgG antibodies of the subclass IgG1 (formerly known as herpes gestationis factor) bind to a 180 kDa protein BP-180 (or bullous pemphigoid antigen 2) in the hemidesmosomes of the dermal–epidermal junction, leading to tissue damage and blister formation [1,5]. The immune response is highly restricted to the NC16A domain [1]. Of interest, the primary site of autoimmunity seems not to be the skin, but in the placenta, as antibodies bind not only to the basement membrane zone of the epidermis but also to that of chorionic and amniotic epithelia, both of ectodermal origin. Aberrant expression of MHC class II molecules on the chorionic villi suggests that an allogenic immune reaction to a placental matrix antigen may be pathogenic [7].

Clinical features

Presentation

Pemphigoid gestationis presents with intense pruritus that may precede skin lesions. Typically, urticated red papules and plaques develop on the abdomen, characteristically involving the periumbilical region, but may spread to the entire skin surface (Figure 113.11). Extremities are involved in all cases, but face and mucous membranes are usually spared [4,8]. In the pre-bullous stage, differentiation between PG and PEP is almost impossible, both clinically and histopathologically. Whilst small vesicles (1–2 mm) may occur in PEP, tense bullae develop only in PG (Figure 113.12).

Disease course and fetal prognosis

The natural course of PG is characterised by exacerbations and remissions during pregnancy, with frequent improvement in late pregnancy followed by a flare-up at the time of delivery (75% of patients). After delivery, the lesions usually resolve within weeks to months but may recur with menstruation and hormonal contraception. Rarely, PG can persist over several years. A systematic review found that approximately 80% of women were in complete remission around 9 months postpartum, half of whom were off therapy [9].

Maternal autoantibodies can be transferred to the newborn and around 5–13% of newborns may develop mild skin lesions (neonatal PG) which resolve spontaneously within days to weeks [4,8,9,10,11]. In almost all cases, conservative management is all

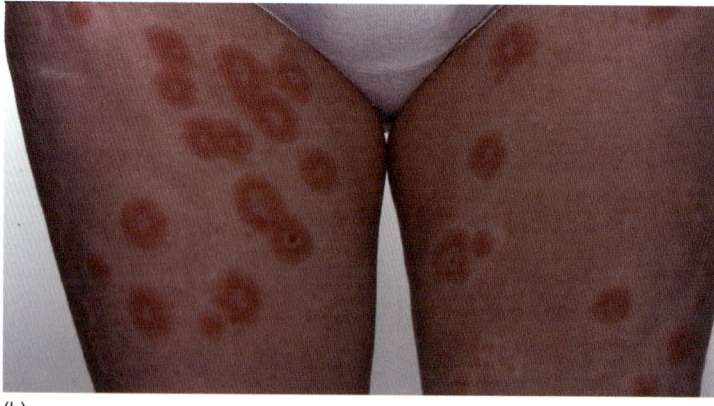

(b)

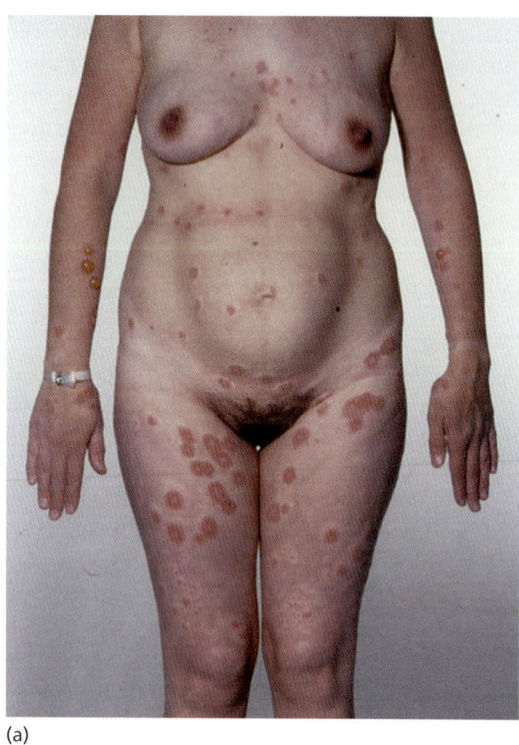

(a)

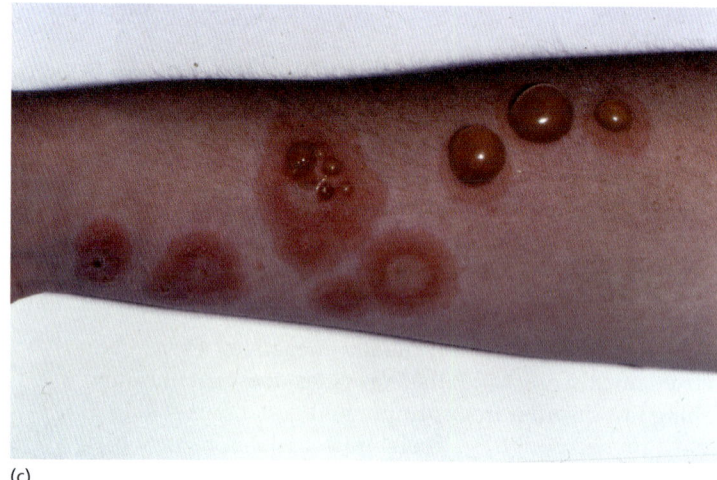

(c)

Figure 113.11 Pemphigoid gestationis that erupted 3 days postpartum. (a) Widespread red urticated plaques on the trunk and limbs with early blistering. (b) Close-up view of urticated targetoid plaques on the upper thighs. (c) Close-up view showing tense intact blisters on the forearms on a background of urticated red plaques.

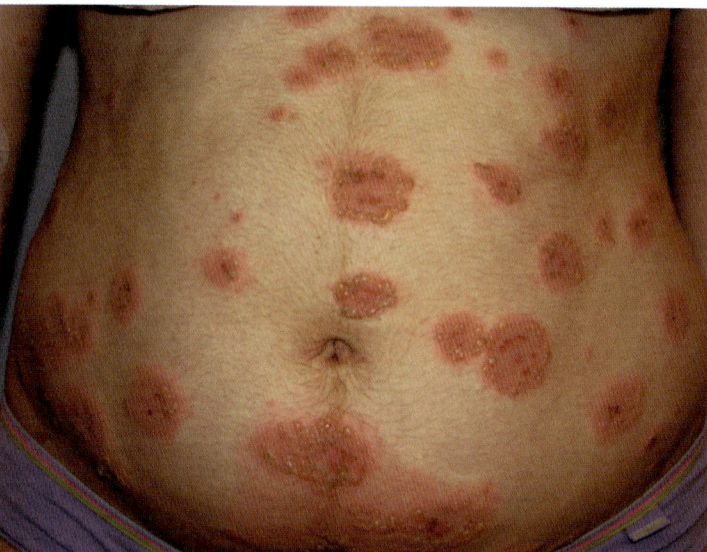

Figure 113.12 More advanced blister formation in pemphigoid gestationis. Courtesy of Associate Professor Amanda Oakley, Hamilton, New Zealand.

that is required until maternal antibodies are cleared from the fetal circulation [12]. Fetal prognosis is generally good but there is an increase in prematurity and small-for-date babies [8–11]. It has been shown that this risk correlates with disease severity, as represented by early onset and blister formation, and not with corticosteroid treatment [13]. PG commonly recurs in subsequent pregnancies, with usually earlier onset and increasing severity [11,14].

Investigations

Histopathological findings from lesional skin depend on the stage and severity of the disease. The pre-bullous stage is characterised by oedema of the upper and middle dermis accompanied by a predominantly perivascular inflammatory infiltrate, composed of lymphocytes, histiocytes and a variable number of eosinophils. Histopathology of the bullous stage demonstrates subepidermal blistering located at the lamina lucida of the dermal–epidermal junction [4].

Linear C3 deposition along the dermal–epidermal junction is present in 100% of cases and additional IgG deposition in 30% of cases [1,8,11]. Circulating serum IgG antibodies may be detected by indirect immunofluorescence, binding to the epidermal side of an artificial split on salt-split skin. Antibody levels may also be monitored using ELISA and immunoblot techniques and show a good correlation with disease activity [4,15].

Management

Treatment depends on the stage and severity of the disease and aims to control pruritus and to prevent blister formation. Topical corticosteroids with or without oral antihistamines may be sufficient in cases of mild pre-bullous pemphigoid [4,8,**9**]. All other cases require systemic prednisolone, usually started at a dose of 0.5–1 mg/kg/day [**9**]. When the disease improves, the dose can typically be reduced, but should be increased in time to prevent the flare postpartum. Cases unresponsive to systemic corticosteroid treatment may benefit from third line treatments including azathioprine, intravenous immunoglobulins and plasma exchange [12,16,17]. Ultraviolet light therapy is relatively contraindicated as it may promote new blister formation [6]. After delivery, if necessary, a greater range of immunosuppressive treatment may then be administered. If associated with gestational trophoblastic disease, treatment of this may result in remission [12].

Treatment ladder for pemphigoid gestationis in pregnancy

First line
- Topical emollients: aqueous cream + 1–2% menthol
- Potent topical steroids (see section on general treatment guidance)
- Oral antihistamines: loratadine and cetirizine

Second line
- Prednisolone

Third line
- Azathioprine
- Plasma exchange
- Intravenous immunoglobulins

General guidance on safe treatments in pregnancy, lactation and male fertility

All topical, injected, physical and systemic agents need to be carefully considered during pregnancy and lactation due to potential for harm to the fetus/infant. Pregnant and lactating women are usually excluded from controlled trials and information regarding safety of medications in pregnancy and lactation is often through case series or data registries. Inadvertent exposure to medications during pregnancy may necessitate consideration of therapeutic abortion, but in most circumstances the caution is due to an unknown risk and close monitoring of the pregnancy may be all that is required. The benefit of treating severe disease often outweighs the potential risk of treatment and many therapeutic agents commonly used in dermatology have sufficient accumulative data to support safe use in pregnancy and lactation if necessary. Treatments for mild disease and cosmetic treatments are best avoided if possible. The effect of medications on male fertility has not been well studied.

In 2015 the US Food and Drug Administration (FDA) updated the risk categories on prescription and biologic drug labelling to make them more meaningful to both patients and health care providers. The A, B, C, D and X risk categories, in use since 1979, are now replaced with individual descriptions of drugs and post-marketing information. Subsections include *Pregnancy*, *Lactation* and *Females and males of reproductive potential*. These provide information about dosing and potential risks, and registry information that collects and maintains data on how pregnant and lactating women and males of reproductive potential are potentially affected.

The following recommendations are based on the current available data and expert opinion for common dermatological treatments, but clinical judgement is still required on a case-by-case basis (Tables 113.3 and 113.4) [**1**,2–4].

Topical therapies

Topical corticosteroids
A Cochrane review on the safety of topical corticosteroids during pregnancy found no associations between mothers' use of topical steroids of any potency and type of delivery, birth defects, premature births or low Apgar score [5]. There was some evidence indicating a relation between low birth weight and maternal use of potent or very potent topical steroids, especially when high doses are used in pregnancy, but maternal use of mild or moderate topical corticosteroids is not related to low birth weight. The review also found that mild or moderately potent topical steroids protect against fetal death, but this was not seen when the mothers used potent or very potent topical steroids. This finding needs further examination. This review confirms that, if required, use of topical steroids is safe but, as in the non-pregnant patient, should be limited to the minimum potency required and for a restricted period. Topical steroid use during pregnancy will increase the likelihood of striae distensae.

Systemic therapies

Systemic corticosteroids
There is a small increased risk of cleft palate when oral corticosteroids are used in the first trimester. Prednisone may also result in premature delivery, premature membrane rupture, intrauterine growth retardation, gestational diabetes, hypertension, pre-eclampsia and eclampsia [1]. Prednisolone is the systemic corticosteroid of choice in pregnancy. Cortisol, prednisone and prednisolone are inactivated enzymatically in the placenta, but betamethasone and dexamethasone are not. Total daily doses should be kept to less than 20 mg/day and prolonged use should be limited to doses of 7.5 mg/day if possible [1]. In treating pregnancy dermatoses, corticosteroids are usually used as a short-term therapy (<4 weeks) so that side effects are minimised. In rare cases with high-dose therapy over many weeks, fetal growth should be monitored by ultrasound. Should this therapy be continued up to delivery, possible adrenal insufficiency of the newborn must be kept in mind and treated accordingly. Systemic corticosteroids are excreted in breast milk and it is recommended to delay nursing until 4 h after high doses to minimise the effect on the infant.

Systemic antihistamines
If systemic antihistamines are needed during pregnancy, the first-generation antihistamine chlorphenamine is preferable due to the greater experience with its use. This is especially valid for the first trimester. If a non-sedating antihistamine is required, then the second-generation antihistamines loratadine and cetirizine can be administered in the second and third trimesters [6,7].

PART 10: SPECIFIC SITES, SEX & AGE

Table 113.3 Topical and locally injected preparations used in pregnancy, lactation and male fertility.

Treatment		Pregnancy	Lactation	Male fertility	Notes
Anti-inflammatory and itch treatments	Topical corticosteroids	Considered appropriate in pregnancy on small surface area	Compatible, avoid nipple area	Limited data. No known adverse effect	See text
	Calcipotriene	Considered appropriate in pregnancy on small surface areas	Compatible in small doses, avoid nipple area	Limited data. No known adverse effect	
	Topical calcineurin inhibitors	Considered appropriate in pregnancy on small surface areas	Compatible in small doses, avoid nipple area	Limited data. High-dose oral tacrolimus associated with decreased sperm function in rodents, but limited systemic absorption with topical agents	High molecular size results in low systemic absorption
	Coal tar	Avoid but intermittent exposure in small doses is low risk	Avoid	Limited data. No known adverse effect	
	Tazarotene	Avoid but intermittent exposure in small doses is low risk	Caution if used over 20% body surface area	Limited data	Highly bound to plasma protein and maternal plasma concentration is low
Acne treatment (also see topical antibiotics)	Benzoyl peroxide	Considered appropriate in pregnancy on small surface areas	Compatible.	Limited data. No known adverse effect	5% Benzoyl peroxide absorbed through skin but lower exposure than from food (food preservative)
	Azelaic acid	Considered appropriate in pregnancy on small surface areas	Low risk of significant excretion in breast milk	No known adverse effect	Low risk – use if no better alternative
	2% Salicylic acid	Considered appropriate in pregnancy on small surface areas	Compatible	No known adverse effect	Low risk – use if no better alternative
	Topical retinoids	Best avoided but intermittent exposure in small doses is low risk	Low risk of significant excretion in breast milk	No known adverse effect	
Scabies treatment	Topical permethrin	Compatible	Compatible	No known adverse effect	
	Topical sulphur (2–10% precipitate in petroleum base)	Limited data, probably safe	Limited data, probably safe	Limited data	
	Topical ivermectin	Best avoided but intermittent exposure in small doses is low risk	Limited data	Limited data. Likely low risk	
	Malathion	Avoid but intermittent exposure in small doses is low risk	Avoid	Avoid	
Topical antifungal agents	Nystatin	Considered appropriate in pregnancy on small surface areas	Compatible	Limited data	Treatment of choice for superficial *Candida* infections in pregnancy
	Clotrimazole	Considered appropriate in pregnancy on small surface areas	Compatible	No known adverse effect	Best studied in lactation: first line
	Miconazole	Considered appropriate in pregnancy on small surface areas	Limited data	Limited data	
	Ketoconazole shampoo	Considered appropriate in pregnancy on small surface areas	Low risk of significant excretion in breast milk	Limited data	No known abnormality in fetus due to lack of systemic absorption
	Selenium sulphide	Considered appropriate in pregnancy on small surface areas	Compatible	Limited data	Limit time period
	Topical terbinafine	Avoid but intermittent exposure in small doses is low risk	Low risk of significant excretion in breast milk	No known adverse effect	
	Ciclopirox	Avoid but intermittent exposure in small doses is low risk	Low risk of significant excretion in breast milk	No known adverse effect	

(continued)

Table 113.3 (continued)

Treatment		Pregnancy	Lactation	Male fertility	Notes
Wart treatment	Trichloroacetic acid	Considered appropriate in pregnancy on small surface areas	Limited data	Limited data	Second line for genital warts in pregnancy (liquid nitrogen is preferred option). Avoid use as a cosmetic peel
	Salicylic acid	Considered appropriate in pregnancy on small surface areas	Compatible	No known adverse effect	Small surface area for limited time periods (liquid nitrogen is preferred option)
	Podophyllin	Avoid	Avoid	Limited data. No known adverse effect	
	Cantharidin	Avoid	Avoid	Limited data	
	Imiquimod	Avoid	Limited data	Limited data. No known adverse effect	
Topical antibiotics	Erythromycin	Compatible	Compatible	No known adverse effect	
	Clindamycin	Compatible	Compatible	No known adverse effect	
	Mupirocin	Considered appropriate in pregnancy on small surface areas	Compatible	Limited data. No known adverse effect	Topical antibacterial of choice in lactation
	Metronidazole	Considered appropriate in pregnancy on small surface areas	Compatible	Limited data. High-dose oral metronidazole caused infertility in rats	
Topical cosmetic treatments	Lactic acid peels	Considered appropriate in pregnancy on small surface areas	Compatible	Limited data	
	Glycolic acid peels	Considered appropriate in pregnancy on small surface areas	Compatible	Limited data	
	Minoxidil	Avoid	Compatible	Limited data	
	Hydroquinone	Avoid	Avoid	Limited data	High transcutaneous absorption and retained in breast milk, no known toxicity
	Jessner peel	Avoid	Avoid	Limited data	
	Salicylic acid peels	Avoid	Compatible. Avoid large surface areas and frequent treatments	No known adverse effect	
Locally injected agents	Local anaesthetic	Considered appropriate in pregnancy in small doses	Compatible	Limited data	Lignocaine preferred in pregnancy, use of adrenaline acceptable
	Intralesional steroids	Considered appropriate in pregnancy in small doses	Compatible.	No known adverse effect	
	Botulinum toxin	Avoid, but likely low risk	Limited data, likely low risk	Limited data, likely low risk in dermatological cosmetic applications	
	Sclerotherapy	Avoid	Avoid	Used commonly for varicocele with no negative effect on fertility	
	Cosmetic fillers	Avoid, but likely low risk	Limited data	Limited data	

Biologics

With increasing overall use, more women of child-bearing age are on biologic agents. If the benefits of continuing treatment are compelling, tumour necrosis factor α (TNF-α) inhibitors are preferred over IL-12/23 and IL-17 inhibitors due to greater safety data. Etanercept is preferred over adalimumab and infliximab due to less placental transfer. Discontinuing the TNF-α inhibitor in the third trimester is recommended to minimise risk of disseminated infection from live vaccines in exposed neonates. Certolizumab has minimal active placental and breast milk transfer and could be considered the preferred biologic agent during pregnancy. Dupilumab has limited safety data but is expected to cross the placenta [8–11].

Other therapies

Ultraviolet light therapy

Ultraviolet B phototherapy is considered a safe option for inflammatory skin conditions during pregnancy. However, folate

Table 113.4 Systemic therapies in pregnancy, lactation and male fertility.

Treatment		Pregnancy	Lactation	Male fertility	Notes
Systemic corticosteroids (see text)	Prednisolone	Compatible	Compatible. Delay nursing until 3–4 h after taking high doses	No known negative effect	
	Prednisone	Use with caution, limit dose and duration	Compatible. Delay nursing until 3–4 h after taking high doses	Limited data	
	Cortisol	Use with caution, limit dose and duration	Compatible. Delay nursing until 3–4 h after taking high doses	Limited data	
	Betamethasone	Avoid	Compatible. Delay nursing until 3–4 h after taking high doses	Limited data	
	Dexamethasone	Avoid	Compatible. Delay nursing until 3–4 h after taking high doses	Limited data	
Systemic antihistamines (see text)	Chlorphenamine	Considered safe in pregnancy	Caution: observe infants for sedation, tachycardia, dry mouth	Limited data	Preferred antihistamine in pregnancy
	Loratadine	Use with caution, limit dose and duration	Caution: observe infants for sedation, tachycardia, dry mouth	Limited data	Preferred non-sedating antihistamine in second and third trimesters
	Cetirizine	Use with caution, limit dose and duration	Caution: observe infants for sedation, tachycardia, dry mouth	Limited data	Second and third trimesters only
Biologics (see text)	Certolizumab	Use with caution, limit dose and duration, discontinue in third trimester if possible; biologic of choice	Compatible, biologic of choice, minimal excretion in breast milk	No known negative effect	Avoid live vaccines in infants for 6 months if exposed in third trimester
	Etanercept	Use with caution, limit dose and duration, discontinue in third trimester if possible	Compatible, minimal excretion in breast milk	No known negative effect	Avoid live vaccines in infants for 6 months if exposed in third trimester
	Adalimumab	Use with caution, limit dose and duration, discontinue in third trimester if possible	Compatible, minimal excretion in breast milk	No known negative effect	Avoid live vaccines in infants for 6 months if exposed in third trimester
	Infliximab	Use with caution, limit dose and duration, discontinue in third trimester if possible	Compatible, minimal excretion in breast milk	No known negative effect	Avoid live vaccines in infants for 6 months if exposed in third trimester
	Ustekinumab	Avoid	Avoid	Avoid	Limited data
	Secukinumab	Avoid	Avoid	Avoid	Limited data
	Omalizumab	Use with caution, limit dose and duration	Limited data	Limited data. No known adverse effect	
	Rituximab	Avoid	Avoid	Limited data. No known adverse effect	Delay conception in females for at least 12 months after discontinuation
	Dupilumab	Avoid	Limited data	Limited data	
Immunomodulators and retinoids	Hydroxychloroquine	Compatible	Compatible	Limited data	Possible toxic accumulation in neonate due to slow elimination rate, but low concentrations in breast milk
	Intravenous immunoglobulin	Compatible	Probably compatible but excreted in breast milk	No known adverse effect	
	Ciclosporin	Use with caution, limit dose and duration	Caution: monitor fetus as per usual ciclosporin guidelines	No known negative effect	May cause low birth weight, prematurity and maternal hypertension
	Dapsone	Use with caution, limit dose and duration	Caution: monitor fetus as per usual dapsone guidelines	Limited data	May cause neonatal hyperbilirubinaemia and haemolytic anaemia, avoid nursing infants with known G6PD deficiency
	Azathioprine	Use with caution, limit dose and duration	Compatible, wait 4 h after taking medication before nursing	No known negative effect	Associated with low birth weight, prematurity, sporadic birth defects and neonatal haematological toxicity. Possibly reduces efficiency of intrauterine coil contraception devices

Table 113.4 (continued)

Treatment		Pregnancy	Lactation	Male fertility	Notes
	Methotrexate	Avoid	Avoid	Avoid	Conflicting reports, recommend delay in conception (male and female) for 3 months after discontinuing methotrexate. May reduce sperm count in males but unlikely mutagenic
	Mycophenolate mofetil	Avoid	Avoid	Avoid	Delay conception in males for 3 months after discontinuing mycophenolate. Use non-hormonal contraception in females for 6 weeks after discontinuing, mycophenolate mofetil compromises efficacy of hormonal contraception
	Acitretin	Avoid	Avoid, but low risk of toxicity	No known negative effect	Avoid conception in females for 3 years after discontinuation
	Isotretinoin	Avoid	Avoid	No known negative effect	Avoid conception in females for 1 month after discontinuation
	Hydroxyurea	Avoid	Avoid	Avoid	Potentially irreversible decreased fertility in males
	Apremilast	Avoid	Avoid	No known negative effect	
	Doxepin	Avoid	Avoid	Limited data	
	Cyclophosphamide	Avoid	Avoid	Avoid	Risk of permanent infertility in males and females
	Thalidomide	Avoid	Avoid	Limited data	Avoid conception in females for 1 month after discontinuation
Antiandrogen medication	Spironolactone	Avoid in first trimester	Caution	Avoid	May suppress lactation in nursing mothers and fertility in males
	Cyproterone acetate	Avoid	Caution	Avoid	Excreted in small amounts in breast milk, unknown effect on neonate and lactation
	Finasteride	Avoid	Limited data	Avoid	Small exposure to pregnant women from male semen, mild reversible effects on male fertility
	Minoxidil	Avoid	Compatible	Limited data, avoid	
Antimicrobials	Penicillins	Compatible	Compatible, but may cause infant hypersensitivity and gastrointestinal symptoms	Caution	First line treatment in pregnancy. Loose stools and rash in some nursing infants. Some effect on male fertility at high doses
	Cephalosporins	Compatible	Compatible	No known negative effect	First line treatment
	Erythromycin	Compatible. Avoid estolate	Compatible, avoid long-term use	No known negative effect	Second line; erythromycin base or ethylsuccinate is preferred: risk of maternal hepatotoxicity with erythromycin estolate
	Clindamycin	Compatible	Compatible	No known negative effect	
	Rifampicin	Compatible	Compatible	Limited data	Treatment of choice in tuberculosis; administer vitamin K to neonate exposed in later pregnancy
	Clofazimine	Compatible	Caution	Limited data	Excreted in breast milk, may cause skin discoloration in infant

Table 113.4 (*continued*)

Treatment		Pregnancy	Lactation	Male fertility	Notes
	Quinolones	Use with caution, limit dose and duration	Compatible, watch for diarrhoea in infants	Caution	Animal studies show effect on developing cartilage in fetus and decreased male fertility, not reported in humans
	Sulphonamides/ trimethoprim	Avoid	Caution: excreted in breast milk, avoid in premature neonates, hyperbilirubinaemia or G6PD deficiency	Caution	Conflicting study results in male fertility
	Tetracyclines	Avoid after 15 weeks' gestation	Avoid, but low risk if used for <3 weeks	Avoid	Avoid breastfeeding for >3 weeks after discontinuation to avoid dental staining in infant
	Ketoconazole	Avoid	Compatible	Avoid	
	Fluconazole	Avoid	Caution: fluconazole is excreted in breast milk but low risk to infant	Limited data	
	Terbinafine	Avoid	Avoid	No known adverse effects	
	Itraconazole	Avoid	Avoid	No known adverse effects	
	Griseofulvin	Avoid	Avoid	Avoid	Avoid for 6 months prior to conception
	Ivermectin	Avoid	Low risk, use if topical treatment fails	Limited data	
Antivirals	Aciclovir	Compatible	Compatible	Limited data	Antiviral of choice in pregnancy and lactation
	Valaciclovir	Compatible	Compatible	No known negative effect	Second line antiviral in pregnancy and lactation
	Famciclovir	Compatible	Avoid	Caution: testicular toxicity in animal studies, no effect in human studies	

G6PD, glucose-6-phosphate dehydrogenase.

supplementation is necessary in the first trimester due to photodegradation of folic acid with light therapy. Currently, there is no consensus on the appropriate folate supplementation during phototherapy and patients who are at high risk may require up to 5 mg daily. Of note, vitamin B_{12} deficiency must be ruled out if a patient takes more than 1 mg folic acid per day because vitamin B_{12} deficiency and high serum folate are associated with an increased risk of cognitive impairment and anaemia in adults [12]. Pregnant women are at higher risk of melasma (especially women of skin of colour) so photoprotection of the face is important during light therapy [13]. Psoralen and UVA (PUVA) treatment is best avoided.

Surgery

Limited local anaesthetic surgery with small volumes of lignocaine or prilocaine with or without epinephrine for essential procedures is considered safe in pregnancy. Mepivacaine and bupivacaine are best avoided. Care should be taken to avoid accidental arterial injection. Topical lidocaine or prilocaine may be used with caution. Topical benzocaine should be avoided. Tetracaine has a limited use, for ocular surfaces only, if a topical anaesthetic is essential. Large volume local anaesthetic surgery such as tumescent anaesthesia is not recommended [12]. Electrocautery in short bursts is considered safe. Scars may widen in areas prone to change in size such as the abdomen and breast during pregnancy. Pregnancy-related oedema

may adversely affect the healing process. Non-essential surgical procedures should be deferred until at least the second trimester of the pregnancy. The left lateral decubitus position is the recommended positioning during lengthy surgery because it ensures optimum dynamics of the blood circulation [12].

Cosmetic treatments

Botulinum toxin is probably safe due to low systemic absorption, but the general recommendation is to avoid this for cosmetic procedures. It has been used without complication for medical indications. Glycolic and lactic acid peels are considered safe in pregnancy due to low systemic absorption, but trichloroacetic acid and salicylic acid peels are not recommended. Laser and light therapies are considered safe for medical treatment of small lesions (e.g. warts, vascular lesions, acne lesions) but cosmetic treatment of larger areas such as for facial rejuvenation or hair removal procedures is best avoided due to lack of safety data. Electrolysis should be avoided because theoretically the current could be transferred to the amniotic fluid. It does not appear that there are any additional risks of cosmetic fillers in the pregnant population other than the risk of adrenaline injected intra-arterially, but there are insufficient studies to support its safe use during pregnancy. Sclerotherapy agents can cross the placenta and should be avoided in pregnancy, although there are some small studies suggesting no adverse outcomes [12].

Key references

The full list of references can be found in the online version at https://www.wiley.com/rooksdermatology10e

Physiological changes in pregnancy

2 Motosko C, Bieber A, Pomeranz M *et al*. Physiologic changes of pregnancy: a review of the literature. *Int J Womens Dermatol* 2017;3:219–24.

Autoimmune skin diseases

7 Izmirly P, Kim M, Friedman D. Hydroxychloroquine to prevent recurrent congenital heart block in fetuses of anti-SSA/Ro-positive mothers. *J Am Coll Cardiol* 2020;76:292–302.

14 Genovese G, Derlino F, Berti E *et al*. Treatment of autoimmune bullous diseases during pregnancy and lactation: a review focusing on pemphigus and pemphigoid gestationis. *Front Pharmacol* 2020;11:583354.

Skin tumours

7 Zelin E, Conforti C, Giuffrida R *et al*. Melanoma in pregnancy: certainties unborn. *Melanoma Manag* 2020;7:MMT48.

Inflammatory skin diseases

5 Kaushik S, Lebwohl M. Psoriasis: which therapy for which patient: focus on special populations and chronic infections. *J Am Acad Dermatol* 2019;80:43–53.

12 Trivedi M, Vaughn A, Murase J. Pustular psoriasis of pregnancy: current perspectives. *Int J Womens Health* 2018;10:109–15.

Pruritis gravidarum and intrahepatic cholestasis of pregnancy

6 Lammert F, Marschall H, Glantz A *et al*. Intrahepatic cholestasis of pregnancy: molecular pathogenesis, diagnosis and management. *J Hepatol* 2000;33:1012–21.

10 Chappell L, Bell J, Smith A *et al*. Ursodeoxycholic acid versus placebo in women with intrahepatic cholestasis of pregnancy (PITCHES): a randomised controlled trial. *Lancet* 2019;394:849–60.

Pemphigoid gestationis

9 Genovese G, Derlino F, Cerri A *et al*. A systematic review of treatment options and clinical outcomes in pemphigoid gestationis. *Front Med (Lausanne)* 2020;7:604945.

General guidance on safe treatments in pregnancy

1 Murase J, Heller M, Butler D. Safety of dermatologic medications in pregnancy and lactation: Part I. Pregnancy. *J Am Acad Dermatol* 2014;70(3):401.e1–14.

PART 10: SPECIFIC SITES, SEX & AGE

CHAPTER 114

Dermatoses of the Neonate

Timothy H. Clayton[1,2] *and Jennifer C. Harrison Sharif*[2]

[1]Royal Manchester Children's Hospital, Manchester, UK
[2]Salford Royal NHS Foundation Trust, Manchester, UK

Introduction

Nomenclature

- Neonatal period: first 4 weeks of extrauterine life.
- Infancy: first 1 year of extrauterine life.
- Premature (preterm): born before the 37th week of gestation.
- Full term: born in weeks 37–42 of gestation.
- Postmature: born after the 42nd week of gestation.
- Low birth weight: born under 2500 g.
- Intrauterine growth retardation: birth weight low for gestational age (small for dates).

Skin function in the neonate

Barrier function

From the moment of birth, the skin of a newborn begins a period of adaptation. During this period various skin manifestations occur that may be transient or markers of underlying disease [1]. In the first few hours of life newborn skin undergoes adaptive changes to accommodate the transition from the wet, aseptic, thermoregulated uterine environment to a dry atmosphere with temperature oscillation as well as being surrounded by microorganisms.

The skin of the newborn performs several vital functions, including (i) being a barrier to water loss, light and irritants; (ii) infection

Rook's Textbook of Dermatology, Tenth Edition. Edited by Christopher Griffiths, Jonathan Barker, Tanya Bleiker, Walayat Hussain and Rosalind Simpson.
© 2024 John Wiley & Sons Ltd. Published 2024 by John Wiley & Sons Ltd.

control and immunosurveillance; (iii) resilience to mechanical trauma; (iv) sensation and tactile discrimination; and (v) thermal regulation. The skin's barrier function is mainly due to the stratum corneum. Histological analysis suggests that epidermal development becomes completely neutral at approximately 34 gestation weeks but will only become functional in the first week of life [2].

Neonates born before 30 weeks have reduced cornified layers and they are at risk of increased permeability to exogenous materials, additional skin damage, delayed barrier maturation and infection [3–5,**6**]. The thickness of the protective epidermal barrier is a potential marker of pregnancy dating [7].

Term infants have a thicker stratum corneum than adults as the epidermis is not adequately sloughed *in utero*, as it is in postnatal life. It can take about 2 weeks for a preterm infant to develop skin that resembles that of a term infant. This process can take even longer in ultralow-birth-weight infants who are extremely preterm [**8**]. The preterm dermis is deficient in structural proteins, and has reduced mechanical properties and increased fragility.

Post-term infants are often observed to have significant xerosis and desquamation, particularly if they have been found to have low amounts of vernix at birth. Age-related transepidermal water loss (TEWL) studies indicate that infant skin barrier function at birth [**6**] or very soon thereafter (within 2–4 weeks) is in the same range as that of healthy adults.

Toxicity resulting from percutaneous absorption in the full-term neonate appears less dependent on impaired barrier function but is more often related to one or more of the following:

1 The greatly increased ratio of surface area to volume.
2 The frequent presence of occlusive conditions, such as exist under waterproof nappies.
3 High ambient temperatures and humidity.

Percutaneous absorption is increased in preterm infants where there is evidence of impaired barrier function. Absorption correlates inversely with gestational age, but barrier function appears to improve rapidly after birth in the preterm infant and will generally be normal by the end of the second or third week after birth [4,5,9].

Preterm newborns with a gestational age >37weeks have a very thin epidermis and a less developed functional barrier than full-term newborns [10]. Preterm neonates nursed in humidified incubators have lower fluid requirements, improved electrolyte balance, higher urine output and increased growth velocity [11]. In the neonatal intensive care unit (NICU) the following interventions have been shown to be beneficial in preterm neonates: short-term application of non-adhesive polyethylene wraps within 10 minutes of birth, placement in humidified incubators, longer-term application of semipermeable, transparent dressings and air-drying the stump of the umbilical cord rather than cleansing with antiseptics [**8**].

The risk of toxicity via percutaneous absorption in the neonate, particularly in preterm babies, is high. Evidence for toxicity has been reported for aniline dyes [12], hexachlorophene and related antiseptics [13], alcohol [14–16] and corticosteroids [17]. A number of other substances should always be avoided in neonates and especially in preterm neonates; these include neomycin [18], boric acid [19], resorcinol (in Castellani paint) [20], γ-benzene hexachloride [21], benzyl alcohol [22], urea [23] and salicylic acid [24]. Antiseptics such as chlorhexidine [25] and iodine [26,27] should be used with caution

and alcohol-based products should be avoided in view of the risk of 'chemical burns' [28].

However, low-dose (0.25%) aqueous chlorhexidine applied to term babies has been shown to decrease mortality from sepsis in a community-based study of 17 500 low-birth-weight neonates from Nepal, but no differences were seen in those with birth weights over 2500 g [29].

Multiple studies show an increased risk of sepsis with the application of petrolatum ointment to preterm neonates [30]. Sunflower seed oil has been shown to reduce the incidence of nosocomial infections and to improve skin condition in studies conducted in Bangladesh and other developing countries [31,32]. The use of virgin coconut oil has been studied in 2294 preterm infants and was observed to reduce the incidence of hypothermia and apnoea. Skin maturity was noted to be improved with a better neurodevelopmental outcome [33]. No data yet exist on the use of emollients in preterm infants with severe skin disease, such as Netherton syndrome or harlequin ichthyosis, where nosocomial infection is a common problem and often lethal [34].

TEWL is greatly increased in preterm compared with full-term babies [4,35]. A recent study was undertaken to establish normal values for TEWL in early life using data gathered from the Cork BASELINE Birth Cohort Study [36,37].

The resulting outward passage of water can lead to high rates of heat loss by evaporation, which may even exceed the baby's resting rate of heat production. These losses can be reduced by increasing the ambient humidity [35,38] (although this leads to an increased risk of infection) by covering the child with a plastic bubble blanket [39] or a Perspex shield [36], or by applying a lipid barrier [40,41].

It is possible that immaturity of the skin also predisposes the premature neonate to penetration of the skin by microorganisms, leading to systemic infection. This may be the reason that the premature infant with congenital cutaneous candidiasis is at greater risk of disseminated candidiasis [42].

There is very little scientific evidence on which to base recommendations for parents on routine neonatal skin care in terms of cleansing and/or moisturising, and advice varies considerably between doctors, health visitors and midwives. In view of the risks of percutaneous absorption, it is of concern that a study undertaken in the USA several years ago revealed that parents had applied over 48 different chemicals in over-the-counter preparations to the skin of their 1-month-old babies [43].

A recent study looking at cleansers suggested there was no difference between using plain water and a commercially available wash product for babies, so this at least allows parents some choice. The same group has also shown that olive oil (often used in neonatal units or for baby massage) can damage the skin barrier in adults so probably should be avoided in neonates [44–46]. The sunflower oil used in the latter study did not show the same deleterious effect but sunflower oils vary considerably in composition and some are indeed harmful. As commercially available sunflower oils are not 'product labelled' they cannot be recommended for neonatal skin.

Bacterial colonisation of the umbilical stump may result in invasive pathogenic infection and represents a major cause of neonatal morbidity and mortality worldwide. Since 1998, the World Health Organization (WHO) has advocated the use of dry umbilical cord care in high-resource settings [47]. This includes keeping the cord clean and exposed to air. If it does become soiled the cord should be cleaned with soap and sterile water or chlorhexidine. A meta-analysis provided no evidence for antiseptic treatment of the cord with chlorhexidine [48].

It is clear that more studies are needed to provide basic recommendations for parents and health care professionals on routine basic neonatal skin care.

Eccrine sweating

By the 28th week of gestation a full complement of anatomically normal eccrine sweat glands is present. These appear to be functionally immature in neonates born before the 36th week in terms of their responses to intradermal injection of acetylcholine and epinephrine (adrenaline), and to thermal stress [1,2]. However, responsiveness usually develops in such babies by 2 weeks after birth. Neonates born after the 36th week of gestation sweat in response to thermal stress from birth, although such sweating is initially relatively inefficient as a thermoregulatory mechanism [3]. Care must therefore be taken not to overheat any neonate, particularly the preterm neonate, and although severe overheating leading to hyperpyrexia is probably rare, lesser degrees of iatrogenic overheating appear to be common and may even induce apnoeic attacks [4–7].

The forehead appears to be the principal site of thermally induced sweating in the neonate. The palms and soles, however, are sites of 'emotional' sweating, occurring in response to arousal, which appears to be well developed at birth in full-term but not preterm neonates.

Skin conductance measurements (as a measure of increased sweating) may be helpful in assessing pain levels in neonates [**8**].

Sebaceous gland secretion

The secretions of the fetal sebaceous glands make a significant contribution to the vernix caseosa [1]. Vernix caseosa acts as a naturally occurring 'barrier cream' that also contains antimicrobial peptides and is formed from week 24 of gestation [2,3]. The presence of vernix at birth is associated with better hydration of the epidermis. One group has even studied it as a 'natural' barrier cream to aid healing in a controlled wound model [4,5]. Sebum secretion rates are high in neonates compared with older preadolescent children, and it is assumed that this sebaceous gland activity reflects stimulation by placentally transferred maternal androgen, particularly by dehydroepiandrosterone [6]. Sebaceous gland activity decreases from about the end of the first month to reach a stable level by the end of the first year [6,7].

Appearance of neonatal skin

Full-term neonate

A variety of skin lesions commonly seen in the newborn are regarded as 'physiological'. Their frequency has been studied by several authors, and varies somewhat in different racial groups [1,2,**3**,4].

Vernix caseosa. At birth the skin is covered with a whitish, greasy film, the vernix caseosa. This is an acidic lipid mantle produced by fetal sebaceous glands and is composed of water (81%), lipids (19%) and protein (10%) naturally adhered to the skin [5]. Vernix may cover the entire skin surface, or it may be present only in body folds such as the groins. It usually dries rapidly and starts to flake off within a few hours of birth. The vernix also contains antimicrobial peptides so it may play some role in keeping the skin hydrated and innate immunity [6,7]. Its colour may reflect intrauterine problems, such as haemolytic disease of the newborn and postmaturity, both of which result in golden yellow staining. Fetal distress *in utero* may lead to staining of the vernix by the bile pigments present in meconium.

Peripheral cyanosis. Peripheral cyanosis (or acrocyanosis) is a feature of the newborn, particularly the full-term newborn, and is usually particularly marked on the palms and soles and around the mouth. In the absence of cyanosis of warm central parts such as the tongue, this may be regarded as normal during the first 48 h or so. It is made more obvious by hypothermia, and is improved by warming [8].

Erythema neonatorum. A few hours after birth, many babies develop a striking, generalised hyperaemia usually known as erythema neonatorum, which fades spontaneously within 24–48 h.

Harlequin colour change. Up to 15% of neonates show a vivid colour difference along the midline at some time during the first week of life. This phenomenon occurs when the baby is lying on its side: the upper half of the body is pale, the lower half a deep red colour [9,10]. The duration of the attack is highly variable, but generally is between 30 s and 20 min. If the baby is turned on the other side, the colour change may reverse. An individual neonate may have only a single episode, or it may recur on several occasions. This curious phenomenon, called harlequin colour change, appears to have no pathological significance in the great majority of cases, and is considered to reflect immaturity of the hypothalamic centres responsible for the control of peripheral vascular tone. If it persists beyond the end of the fourth week, it may be associated with hypoxia due to cardiovascular anomalies [11].

Cutis marmorata. Newborn infants who are subjected to cooling will show distinct marbling of the skin. Although this more or less disappears on rewarming, many normal neonates demonstrate faint marbling, even under optimal environmental conditions. The marbling comprises a reticulate blue vascular pattern, which has often been called cutis marmorata [12]. This response is a physiological one, and may be seen throughout infancy. Cutis marmorata telangiectatica congenita is a distinct vascular developmental disorder, and is easily distinguished as it is fixed (Chapter 71) and may be associated with a variety of other abnormalities, for example of limb growth or renal anomalies [13,14].

Desquamation. Rather superficial cutaneous desquamation (physiological scaling of the newborn) occurs in up to 75% of normal neonates [15]. This usually first appears around the ankles on the first day of life, and is more or less confined to the hands and feet. It may remain localised or may gradually become widespread, usually reaching its maximum extent and intensity by the eighth day. It tends always to be more severe in neonates who are small for dates, whatever their gestational age.

Mild variants of ichthyosis such as ichthyosis vulgaris may be hard to distinguish from pronounced physiological scaling. It should be borne in mind that X-linked hypohidrotic ectodermal dysplasia may present with scaling of the skin in the neonatal period [16].

Suction blisters. These small blisters or erosions may be present in 0.5% of newborns. They typically affect the back of their hands, fingers, arms and lips and are believed to be caused by vigorous oral suction *in utero*; hence the term sucking blister. The blisters heal rapidly without sequelae [17,18].

Neonatal occipital alopecia. The scalp hair is shed synchronously during the fifth month of fetal life. After regrowing, the hair then enters a telogen phase in wave from front to back, starting about 12 weeks before term. After shedding of the telogen hairs from the frontal and parietal areas, the roots again enter the anagen phase in a similar wave from front to back [19,20]. The roots in the occipital area do not enter telogen until term, and as a result alopecia may appear at this site at birth or within the first 2 months (neonatal occipital alopecia). Trauma from lying on this area may also contribute [21]. Neonatal alopecia has been reported to occur due to birth trauma. Trichoscopy elucidates purple dots that correspond to blood extravasation and follicular ostia [22].

Hair shedding in infancy. There appear to be two phases of hair loss and regrowth from front to back during early infancy, but by the end of the first year the typical mosaic pattern of hair growth is established [23]. In some babies, there is unusually synchronous hair loss during the neonatal period, resulting in obvious diffuse alopecia (telogen effluvium of the newborn), but, by 6 months of life, most babies have a full head of hair. At this stage, the hairline often extends to the lateral ends of the eyebrows, but the terminal hairs comprising this extension gradually convert to vellus hairs during the remainder of the first year of life, causing the hairline to recede to its characteristic childhood position.

Sebaceous gland hypertrophy/milia. Sebaceous gland hyperplasia is a physiological event in the newborn, reflecting the influence of maternal androgens. It is visible to the naked eye in the great majority of infants as multiple, uniform, pinpoint, yellowish papules that are most prominent on the nose, cheeks, upper lip and forehead, but may also be visible on the upper trunk, especially the areolae, genitalia and limbs. The phenomenon is associated in about 40% of infants with milia, which represent minute follicular epidermal cysts [24]. The numbers of milia may vary from one or two to many hundreds. They comprise 1–3 mm diameter, white, globular papules, which occur at the same sites as sebaceous gland hyperplasia. Rather larger and usually single milia, often termed pearls, are seen sometimes on the areolae, scrotum and labia majora. Both the sebaceous gland hyperplasia and the milia tend to disappear spontaneously during the first weeks of life, although a few may persist longer. Milia that are exceptionally extensive or persistent, or whose distribution is atypical, may be features of the oro-facio-digital syndrome type I (Chapters 65 and 66), Marie–Unna-type congenital hypotrichosis (Chapter 66) or the X-linked Bazex–Dupré–Christol syndrome, which features hypotrichosis and milia (Chapter 140).

'Miniature puberty'. The influence on the fetus of maternal and placental hormones may give rise to a number of features [25]: an enlarged clitoris; mucoid vaginal discharge; enlarged well-developed genitalia (boys and girls); hypertrophy of the mammary glands (boys and girls), which resolves in 2–4 weeks; desquamation of the hyperplastic vaginal epithelium (a few days after birth); frank withdrawal bleeding, which may occur from the uterus on day 3/4, usually lasting for 2 or 3 days; and lactation ('witch's milk') on day 2/3 – if persistent this can predispose to mastitis/breast abscess in girls.

Hyperpigmentary disorders. A linea alba occurs in 8% of babies and may persist for 2–3 months. Mongolian blue spots occur in up to 85% of Chinese babies [26], are common in black babies but only occur in about 3% of white babies [27]. Hyperpigmentation of the scrotum may occur especially in Chinese babies (up to 30%) [26]. Linear/reticulate pigmentary anomalies have been described in black newborns [28].

Oral findings. Epstein pearls are 1–2 mm diameter, yellowish white, keratinous cysts seen in the mouths of up to 85% of all neonates, along the alveolar ridges and/or in the midline at the junction of the hard and soft palate [29,30]. These generally disappear without treatment within a few weeks. Succulent gums, analogous to the hypertrophic gingivitis often seen in pregnant women, are common in neonates. A whitish hue to the oral mucosa ('leukoedema') is also common. This is probably synonymous with what other authors have called 'suckling pads' [29,30].

Preterm neonate

The skin of the preterm neonate tends to have a rather translucent, gelatinous quality, and the so-called miniature puberty features are much less prominent. Cutaneous vessels are easily visible [1,2]. Preterm infants are often covered in lanugo hairs, which tend to be most dense on the face, limbs and trunk. This hair would normally be shed *in utero* about 1 month before term, to be replaced by a second coat of shorter lanugo, which is present at birth in full-term infants. Like the terminal scalp hair, this downy lanugo is shed during the first months of life and is itself replaced by vellus hair [1].

Small-for-dates and postmature neonates

The small-for-dates or dysmature neonate presents a characteristic appearance due to relative prenatal malnutrition. The baby is small and, from the dermatological point of view, the most striking feature is the lack of subcutaneous fat, which causes the baby to look thin and wrinkled. Vernix is absent in the extremely immature infant, but may be profuse nearer to term. The skin and vernix are often stained yellowish green by meconium. After birth, the skin dries quickly and becomes 'crazed' with long transverse splits on the trunk. It then peels off to reveal more normal-appearing skin beneath. The fingernails are often long. The postmature infant is longer but of otherwise similar appearance to the small-for-dates neonate, having also experienced intrauterine malnutrition due to placental insufficiency. Vernix is often absent [1].

SKIN DISORDERS IN THE NEONATE

Toxic erythema of the newborn

Definition and nomenclature
Toxic erythema of the newborn is a common, transient, blotchy, red macular rash (sometimes with small pustules) seen in the first few days of life. The most widely used term for this condition is inappropriate in view of the complete absence of any evidence of a toxic cause [1].

Synonyms and inclusions
- Erythema toxicum neonatorum

Epidemiology
Incidence and prevalence
A degree of toxic erythema develops in 30–50% of children. It is hardly ever seen in preterm infants or those weighing less than 2.5 kg. A high prevalence of this dermatosis is found in higher-birth-weight newborns. It is also found to occur more frequently during the summer [2,3].

Age
It usually appears in the first 24–48 h of life.

Sex
There is equal prevalence in most studies.

Ethnicity
It occurs in all racial groups.

Associated diseases
Blood eosinophilia is associated.

Pathophysiology
The cause is unknown. There is frequently an associated blood eosinophilia. This probably does not reflect an allergic response as tissue eosinophilia is a non-specific feature of inflammatory responses in neonates [1]. The intrafollicular location of mature pustules has led to the suggestion that the inflammatory response is elicited by some component of sebum [4]. Scanning electron microscopy of neonatal skin shows that colonisation of hair follicle epithelium by staphylococci is common in early life. Furthermore, the accumulation of tryptase-expressing mast cells around the hair follicles in lesional skin has been recently demonstrated but its relation to the staphylococci and its significance in toxic erythema remain unclear [5,6].

Predisposing factors
No predisposing factors are known.

Pathology
Histologically, the macular redness shows oedema in the upper dermis, associated with a sparse and largely perivascular inflammatory infiltrate composed principally of eosinophils. Papular lesions are characterised, in addition, by eosinophil infiltration of the outer root sheath of one or more hair follicles, above the point of entry of the sebaceous duct. Pustular lesions show intrafollicular accumulation of eosinophils immediately below the stratum corneum. Smears of the pustule contents demonstrate inflammatory cells, more than 90% of which are eosinophils [4,7–10].

There is an associated blood eosinophilia of up to 20% of the white cell count in around half the cases, and this is generally more marked when there is a prominent pustular element to the eruption.

Causative organisms
No pathogenic bacteria have been isolated from pustules.

Environmental factors
No environmental factors have been demonstrated.

Clinical features
History
Some degree of toxic erythema will manifest in 30–50% of full-term infants of all racial types during the first few days of life. In most cases the onset is during the first 48 h after birth, but it may occur at any time until about the fourth day. It very rarely presents at birth [7,10–12].

Presentation
Most commonly, the eruption initially takes the form of a blotchy, macular redness, the number of individual lesions varying from one or two to several hundred. They are most profuse on the trunk, particularly the anterior trunk (Figure 114.1), but also commonly appear on the face and proximal parts of the limbs, especially the thighs. Lesions have been recorded, however, at almost any site except the palms and soles. In the mildest cases, these macules fade within a day [13–18].

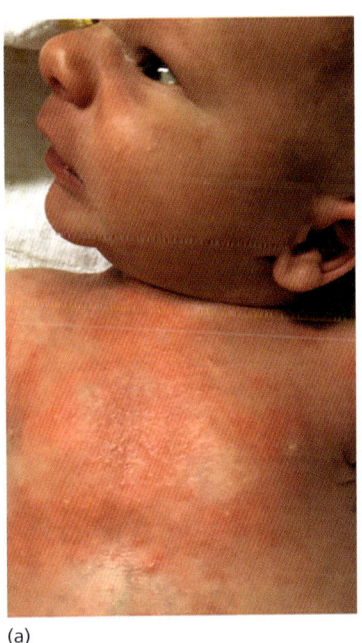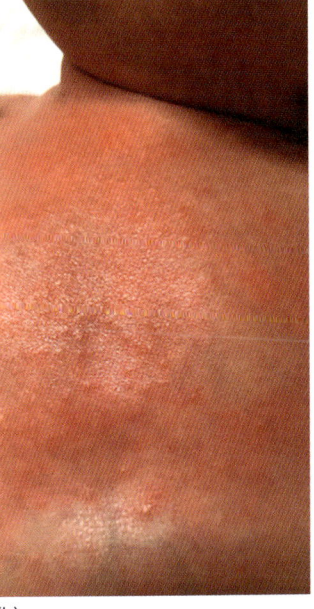

(a)   (b)

Figure 114.1 (a) Eruption on the trunk of toxic erythema of the newborn. (b) Close-up of the eruption on the trunk.

Clinical variants

In more severe cases, urticarial papules arise within the red areas or, occasionally, independently of them (particularly on the back and buttocks). These papules are, in about 10% of cases, surmounted by small pustules 1–2 mm in diameter. Presentation with scrotal pustules present at birth has been reported more recently [19].

Differential diagnosis

Toxic erythema of the newborn has to be distinguished from several other disorders featuring pustular lesions during the neonatal period, particularly miliaria, transient neonatal pustular melanosis, incontinentia pigmenti and, most importantly, herpes simplex virus (HSV) infection, varicella, impetigo neonatorum and *Malassezia furfur* pustulosis. Of these, perhaps pustular miliaria is the one most often confused clinically with toxic erythema.

Classification of severity

No classification exists but more severe cases have papules and pustules.

Complications and co-morbidities

The infant appears well, and unperturbed by the eruption. There are no complications.

Disease course and prognosis

Spontaneous recovery occurs rapidly, usually within 3 days, but recurrences are occasionally seen and have been reported as late as the sixth week of life.

Investigations

Investigations are rarely needed as it is a clinical diagnosis. If there is any diagnostic doubt, toxic erythema can be rapidly diagnosed by microscopic examination of a smear of pustule contents (stained with Giemsa) to show the eosinophils and by negative bacterial and viral cultures.

Management

No treatment is needed.

Resources

Further information

Medscape, toxic erythema of the newborn: https://emedicine.medscape.com/article/1110731-overview (last accessed June 2023).

Miliaria

Definition and nomenclature

Miliaria crystallina is a self-limiting eccrine gland disorder due to blockage of sweat glands resulting in rapidly evolving non-inflammatory vesicles that easily break (Chapter 92). It can be subdivided into three subtypes depending on the level of blockage: miliaria crystallina (stratum corneum), miliaria rubra (mid-epidermal) and miliaria profunda (dermal–epidermal junction) [1,2].

Synonyms and inclusions
- Prickly heat (for miliaria rubra)

Epidemiology

Incidence and prevalence

Miliaria occurs in about 3–8% of neonates.

Age

Miliaria may occur at any age but malaria rubra and miliaria crystallina are common in neonates.

Sex

There is an equal sex prevalence.

Ethnicity

It occurs in all racial groups.

Associated diseases

Very rarely hypernatraemia or hyperaldosteronism is associated.

Pathophysiology

Predisposing factors

Immature sweat ducts are an important factor in neonates although high levels of heat and humidity are important at any age. Occlusive clothing is probably more relevant to adults. Hypernatraemia and/or hyperaldosteronism is a very rare underlying factor.

Pathology

Miliaria crystallina is characterised by the presence of intracorneal or subcorneal vesicles in communication with the sweat ducts. In miliaria rubra, focal areas of spongiosis and spongiotic vesicle formation are seen in close proximity to the sweat ducts, which often contain an amorphous, periodic acid–Schiff (PAS) stain-positive plug [3,4–7].

Causative organisms

There is a possible link with *Staphylococcus epidermidis* and *S. aureus*.

Environmental factors

Associated factors include heat, humidity, occlusive clothes and plastic sheets.

Clinical features

History

Milaria in the neonate usually presents with a rash in the first few weeks of life.

Presentation

Miliaria crystallina presents as crops of clear, thin-walled, superficial vesicles 1–2 mm in diameter, without associated redness, resembling drops of water (Figure 114.2). These are exceedingly delicate and generally rupture within 24 h, and are followed by bran-like desquamation. Lesions are asymptomatic. They arise most frequently during the first 2 weeks of life, and are particularly likely to be seen on the forehead, scalp, neck and upper trunk. Although rare during the first 4 days, congenital cases have been reported [7–12].

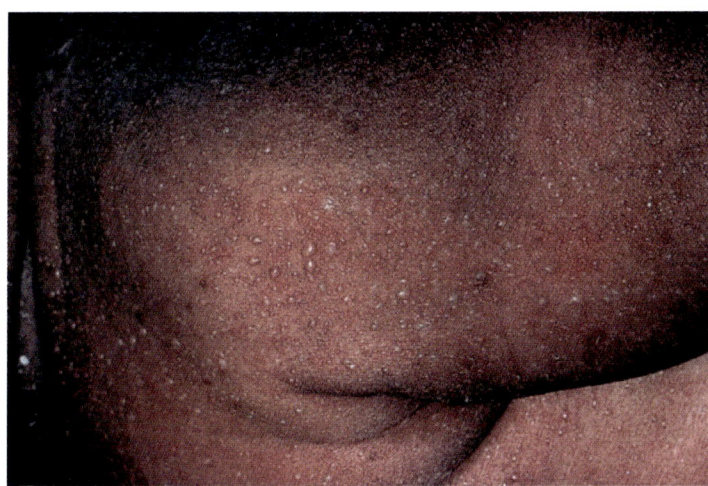

Figure 114.2 Miliaria crystallina on the upper arm of a 7-day-old infant.

Miliaria rubra ('prickly heat') comprises red papules and papulovesicles about 1–4 mm in diameter, on a background of macular redness. Sometimes, quite large, weal-like lesions occur. Frequently, some of the lesions are pustular (miliaria pustulosa), but this does not necessarily indicate secondary infection. Nevertheless, staphylococcal secondary infection of miliaria (periporitis) is not infrequent, and may lead to sweat gland abscesses. Miliaria rubra is common and, although it may be seen throughout infancy, it probably occurs most frequently during the neonatal period. Crops of lesions arise fairly symmetrically, most often in flexural areas, especially around the neck and in the groins and axillae. The face, scalp and upper trunk are also frequently affected. It may also occur rather locally at sites that have been occluded, for example where there has been direct contact between the skin and a plastic mattress cover or plastic pants. Lesions can be itchy or sore. Where the eruption is profuse, the child may be restless and distressed. Each crop of lesions will subside within 2–3 days, but recurrences are common unless the provocative environmental conditions are modified.

Recurrent bouts of miliaria pustulosa are a common finding in type 1 pseudohypoaldosteronism [13,14].

Miliaria profunda is very uncommon in neonates as it usually occurs in adults where there have been repeated episodes of miliaria rubra. However, a granulomatous variant of giant centrifugal miliaria profunda was recently described in two 3-month-old babies [15]. This presents with papules and geographic and annular plaques over the extensor aspects of the limbs and the trunk.

Clinical variants
There are three clinical variants: miliaria crystallina, miliaria rubra and miliaria profunda (granulomatous giant centrifugal variant).

Differential diagnosis
Miliaria crystallina is distinguishable from viral infections of the skin (e.g. herpes simplex) by the lack of background redness, and by the absence of inflammatory cells or giant keratinocytes on cytological examination of vesicle contents. When it occurs during the first few days of life, miliaria rubra is often confused with toxic erythema, especially if it has become pustular. However, miliaria rubra can generally be distinguished by its flexural predominance,

by the frequent presence of vesicular lesions and by its tendency to recur. If in doubt, a smear of a vesicle/pustule will show an absence of eosinophils (large numbers are seen in toxic erythema). Miliaria pustulosa may also be confused with infantile acne or folliculitis, but the lesions are not follicular.

Complications and co-morbidities
Staphylococcal infection and sweat gland abscess rarely occur.

Disease course and prognosis
Miliaria crystallina improves spontaneously as the sweat ducts mature. Milaria rubra improves if the predisposing aetiological factors (high heat/humidity and occlusion) are removed.

Investigations
The diagnosis is usually clinical. Occasionally, a smear from a vesicle or pustule is useful to exclude HSV infection or toxic erythema.

Management
Milaria crystallina spontaneously improves without therapy over a few weeks as the sweat ducts mature.

First line
Miliaria rubra will improve in a few weeks without medical treatment if the child is removed from conditions of high heat/humidity and any occlusive clothing or bedding is removed.

Second line
Antibiotics may be needed if staphylococcal infection occurs but this is rare.

Resources

Further information
Medscape, dermatological manifestations of miliaria: https://emedicine.medscape .com/article/1070840-overview (last accessed June 2023).

Transient pustular melanosis

Synonyms and inclusions
- Transient neonatal pustular melanosis

Despite transient pustular melanosis having first been described more than 40 years ago [1], its aetiology remains unknown. It was first reported in black Americans, and appears to be commoner in, but not confined to, black neonates (4.4% in black US neonates against 0.6% in white US neonates). It has been suggested that it is merely an early-onset variant of toxic erythema of the newborn [1,2].

Lesions are usually present at birth. The most characteristic component of the eruption is 1–3 mm flaccid, superficial, fragile pustules, with no surrounding redness. These pustules may occur at any site, but favour the chin, neck, forehead, back and buttocks [3–7,**8**,9]. Sites where they have ruptured are marked initially by a detachable brown crust, and subsequently by a small collarette of scale, which may surmount a pigmented macule. Sometimes, pigmented macules are already present at birth. The pigmented macules are a prominent element in black infants, and are seen more rarely in other races [5]. The pigmentation may persist for about 3 months. Affected infants are otherwise entirely well. Diagnosis can usually be made on clinical grounds without the need for a biopsy or smear.

A skin biopsy of a pustule shows intra- or subcorneal collections of neutrophils and a few eosinophils [1]. The underlying dermis may show no abnormality, or a sparse perivascular and perifollicular inflammatory infiltrate, also mainly of neutrophils with a few eosinophils. The pigmented macules demonstrate basal and suprabasal increases in pigmentation only, apparently without pigmentary incontinence. Smears of pustular contents show predominantly neutrophils, and bacterial culture is negative.

No treatment is needed for this self-resolving condition. The differential diagnoses of neonatal pustular eruptions are given in Box 114.1.

Box 114.1 Pustular eruptions in the neonate

- Congenital or neonatal candidiasis
- Congenital syphilis
- Eosinophilic pustulosis
- Herpes simplex virus infection
- Impetigo
- Infantile acropustulosis
- Langerhans cell histiocytosis
- *Malassezia* pustulosis
- Miliaria
- Neonatal acne
- Neonatal listeriosis
- Neonatal pustulosis of transient myeloproliferative disorder
- Pustular psoriasis
- Scabies
- Toxic erythema of the newborn
- Transient pustular melanosis

Infantile acropustulosis

Infantile acropustulosis is an uncommon disorder of unknown aetiology. It occurs in all races [1] although it was first described in black infants [2]. It has been suggested that eosinophilic pustular folliculitis and infantile acropustulosis may be different manifestations of the same disease [3]. It has also been suggested that, at least in some cases, infantile acropustulosis occurs following successful treatment of scabies [4–6]. It has been reported in siblings [7] and in only one of a pair of identical twins [8].

Infantile acropustulosis presents with recurrent crops of intensely itchy, 1–4 mm vesicopustules that appear principally on the soles and sides of the feet, and on the palms, but may also occur on the dorsa of the feet, hands and fingers, and on the ankles, wrists and forearms. Scattered lesions may also be seen on the face, scalp and trunk, but a predominantly acral distribution is characteristic.

Mucosal lesions do not occur [2,7,9,10]. Individual lesions appear to start as tiny, red papules, which evolve into vesicles and then pustules over about 24 h. Excoriation results in erosions and then crusts. Healing is frequently succeeded by macular postinflammatory hyperpigmentation.

In the majority of cases, the onset is in the first year of life, particularly during the first 6 months [7]. Lesions rarely present at birth. Each crop lasts for 7–14 days. They tend to occur at intervals of 2–4 weeks in most cases, often being more frequent and more numerous in the summer months.

The predilection for the palms and soles and the recurrent attacks differentiate this disorder from most other pustular eruptions seen in the neonatal period, particularly toxic erythema, miliaria and transient pustular melanosis. Scabies may initially be extremely difficult to exclude, and where there is any doubt a therapeutic trial of an appropriate acaricide is justified. Diagnosis is usually clinical. Skin biopsy of a pustule will show well-circumscribed subcorneal or intraepidermal aggregations of neutrophils, with a sparse perivascular lymphohistiocytic infiltrate in the underlying papillary dermis [9,11]. Biopsy of a pre-pustular lesion shows focal intraepidermal vesiculation with keratinocyte necrosis. This intraepidermal vesicle is subsequently invaded by neutrophils and/or eosinophils. The pustule starts its life deep in the epidermis, but does not become clinically fully developed until it reaches a subcorneal location. Direct and indirect immunofluorescence studies are negative. Stained smears of pustule contents generally show a predominance of neutrophils, but there may be a preponderance of eosinophils early in the course of the disorder. Sometimes peripheral blood eosinophilia is present [12–14].

Treatment is with potent topical corticosteroids with or without occlusion [7,9]. Dapsone has been used in a few severe cases [2] as has topical maxacalcitol [15]. The attacks occur with gradually diminishing numbers of lesions, and with decreasing frequency, until they cease altogether, usually within 2 years of the onset.

Neonatal pustulosis of transient myeloproliferative disorder

There have been several reports of neonates with trisomy 21 (and mosaic trisomy 21) developing pustules and vesicles (on a reddish background), predominantly on the face, as part of congenital leukaemia or transient myeloproliferative disorder (TMD) [**1,2**,3–5]. They may pustulate at sites of trauma, such as venepuncture sites or under adhesive tape. The patients may also have hepatosplenomegaly. There is an associated high white blood cell count, often with the presence of blasts. Skin biopsy shows intraepidermal pustules with a perivascular dermal infiltrate of neutrophils, eosinophils and atypical mononuclear cells. The lesions often resolve spontaneously over a few weeks paralleled by a decreasing white cell count.

Mutations in the transcription factor GATA1 seem to underlie TMD but a second genetic hit is needed to develop leukaemia [6]. Up to 20% of patients with TMD will go on to develop an acute megakaryoblastic leukaemia within the first 4 years of life so follow-up is mandatory.

Congenital erosive and vesicular dermatosis healing with reticulated supple scarring

Definition and nomenclature

Congenital erosive and vesicular dermatosis (CEVD) presents in neonates as erosions, ulcerations, vesicles and red skin affecting around 75% of skin surface area, which heal to leave distinctive reticulate scarring. To date, there are fewer than 40 cases reported in the literature [1–8,9].

Synonyms and inclusions
• Extensive congenital erosions and vesicles healing with reticulate scarring

Introduction and general description

This is a rare, self-limiting, blistering disorder of unknown aetiology first described in 1985 by Cohen *et al.* [1].

Epidemiology
Incidence and prevalence
It is very rare.

Age
It occurs at birth and the majority of affected infants have been premature.

Sex
Occurrence is greater in boys than in girls.

Pathophysiology
Pathology
Biopsies of vesicular areas have shown spongiosis or epidermal necrosis with dermal haemorrhage and inflammation [1–6]. In one report, an eroded area showed loss of the epidermis with a superficial and deep dermal inflammatory infiltrate comprising mostly neutrophils [4]. Parakeratotic scale may be present. Scarred areas have shown an increased density of dermal collagen, and absence of eccrine sweat glands. Direct immunofluorescence does not show any specific pattern of deposition of immunoglobulins, C3 or fibrin. Electron microscopy and immunohistochemical mapping of perilesional skin have shown nothing to suggest that this is a variant of epidermolysis bullosa [5].

Clinical features
History
The condition presents at birth with blistering and erosions which heal with soft scars.

Presentation
There are extensive, superficial erosions, with scattered vesicles and bullae, affecting up to 75% of the body surface. These erosions may extend in the first few days. The trunk and limbs tend to be more severely affected than the face and scalp. Hands and feet may be spared [10–12]. Patients are prone to infection prior to the skin healing. Bacterial, fungal and HSV infections have been described [13].

The blisters/erosions heal fairly quickly within the first few weeks of life, leaving rather characteristic soft, reticulated scarring. Following healing of the skin lesions, there may be residual loss of eccrine sweating in the scarred areas, with the potential for hyperthermia under appropriate conditions, patchy alopecia, partial loss of eyelashes and the absence or hypoplasia of nails. Teeth are normal. Mild, localised, recurrent vesiculation may occur.

The largest published review of 18 cases revealed the following associations: preterm birth (79%), nail dystrophies (46%), hyperthermia/hypophidrosis (46%), maternal chorioamnionitis (43%), neurological disorders (microcephaly, convulsions, developmental delay) and ophthalmological complications (lacrimal duct obstruction, macular or corneal scars) (36% each) and tongue atrophy (29%) [10].

Differential diagnosis

This includes infective blisters (e.g. herpes simplex), epidermolysis bullosa, bullous ichthyosiform erythroderma, incontinentia pigmenti, aplasia cutis congenita, focal dermal hypoplasia and staphylococcal scalded skin syndrome.

Complications and co-morbidities

Postnatal infection is a risk. It is unclear if the disease associations are caused by congenital erosive and vesicular dermatosis itself or by prematurity or an unidentified intrauterine pathology.

Disease course and prognosis

Spontaneous healing occurs within 2 weeks to 3 months.

Investigations

Skin swabs and blood culture are needed to investigate for infections (viral, bacterial and fungal). Skin biopsy may be useful.

Management

The baby will need to be nursed on an appropriate neonatal unit for the management of fluid balance, temperature control and any infection if this develops. Non-adhesive dressings (e.g. silicone dressings) will be needed for the first few weeks of life until healing occurs [10–12]. There is no specific treatment for this condition.

COMPLICATIONS OF PREMATURITY

Anetoderma of prematurity

Introduction and general description

Anetoderma is characterised by focal loss of elastic tissue in the mid-dermis, resulting in localised areas of macular depressions or pouch-like herniations. Anetoderma may occur in preterm babies appearing at, or soon after, birth [1,2,3]. Its early onset differentiates it from anetoderma of prematurity caused by electrocardiogram (ECG) electrodes [4].

Epidemiology

Incidence and prevalence
Its incidence is unknown but it is very rare.

Age
It is found in extremely premature babies (<29 weeks).

Sex
There is equal sex incidence.

Pathophysiology
The underlying cause is unknown although it is found in premature babies. A skin biopsy of a lesion shows reduced or absent elastic tissue, consistent with anetoderma [1,2,3,4]. There may be an underlying genetic predisposition. Anetoderma has been described in two identical premature twins but all other cases have been sporadic [3].

Clinical features

History
Anetoderma presenting in extremely premature babies was first described by Prizant *et al.* in 1996 [1].

Presentation
Anetoderma of prematurity presents with nummular areas of cutaneous atrophy appearing on the trunk and/or proximal limbs within a few weeks of birth [1,2,3]. All patients have been born between the 24th and 29th weeks of gestation and in almost all cases the lesions first appeared while the child was still in the neonatal intensive care unit. Rarely, anetoderma may be present at birth. Cases that present later at 2–3 months of age are more likely a consequence of trauma from gel ECG electrodes [4,5].

Differential diagnosis
These include anetoderma from trauma and aplasia cutis congenita type 5.

Complications and co-morbidities
Patients have the co-morbidities of extreme prematurity.

Disease course and prognosis
It is non-progressive and persistent.

Investigations
Skin biopsy should be done.

Management
There is no known treatment for anetoderma.

COMPLICATIONS OF MEDICAL PROCEDURES ON THE FETUS AND NEONATE

Antenatal procedures
Antenatal procedures and amniocentesis can lead to a range of problems arising in the fetus (Table 114.1).

Table 114.1 Complications arising from some antenatal procedures.

Procedure	Cutaneous complication or disorder
Amniocentesis needles	Punctate scars and dimples (prevalence decreased with real-time ultrasound) [1–5]
Antenatal biopsies (skin, liver, tumours)	
Intrauterine red cell transfusion (used in haemolytic disease/rhesus incompatibility)	Gangrene abdominal wall [6]
Scalp electrodes (used for monitoring fetal heart rate)	Scarring alopecia/cephalohaematoma [7,8]
	Neonatal HSV at the site of electrodes (cutaneous blisters/encephalitis) [9–12]
Scalp blood sampling (monitoring acid–base balance)	Scalp abscess (in 4% of neonates; rarely deep tissue infections) [13–17]
Forceps delivery	Subcutaneous fat necrosis
Scalpel injury during caesarean section	Lacerations/scars
Ventouse extraction	Scarring alopecia (usually after severe caput succedaneum) (very rare) [18]
	Annular blisters of the scalp ('vesicular eruption of vacuum-assisted delivery') can be traumatic or due to HSV [19]

HSV, herpes simplex virus.

Table 114.2 Complications arising from some neonatal medical procedures.

Procedure	Cutaneous complication
Umbilical artery catheterisation [**1**,2–6]	Aortic thrombosis/spasm, arterial embolism (lower limb ischaemia/gangrene)
Transcutaneous oxygen monitoring (heated electrode) [7–10]	Superficial burn (redness/vesiculation) – less risk with unheated pulse oximetry
Electrocardiograph electrodes [11,12]	Anetoderma secondary to trauma (may be purpuric initially)
Transillumination (more common if infrared filters are switched off) [13]	Blisters: 2–4 mm in diameter, often at acral sites
Extravasation intravenous medication [14–17]	Cutaneous necrosis
Heel pricks [18–20]	Cutaneous calcification (localised)
Extravasation with calcium-containing solutions [21–23]	
Scalp electroencephalograph electrodes (calcium chloride-containing paste) [24]	
Needle insertions (repeated)/chest drain insertions [17]	Punctate white scars (speckled scarring)
Chemical burns from antiseptics/alcohol-based cleansers [**25**,26–30]	Cutaneous necrosis (often on the back or buttocks where the cleanser has pooled)

Neonatal medical procedures
Adverse consequences of medical procedures on the neonate are more common if the baby is premature (Table 114.2).

Phototherapy
Phototherapy is mostly used for neonatal jaundice and can lead to various complications (Table 114.3) [21].

Table 114.3 Phototherapy-induced rashes.

Cutaneous complication	Cause
Red rash	Macular red rash (as bilirubin falls) [1]
	Ultraviolet-induced redness ('burn') [2]
Hyperpigmentation	Skin tanning (especially type VI skin) [3]
	Bronze baby syndrome (underlying hepatic disease) [4–10]
	(Differential diagnosis: central cyanosis, 'carbon baby' and 'grey baby' syndrome [11,12])
Bullous eruptions	Drug phototoxicity (furosemide, methylene blue) [13,14]
	Congenital porphyrias [15–17]
Epidermolysis bullosa-like eruptions	Transient porphyrinaemia (after repeated transfusions for severe haemolytic disease of the newborn) [18]
Localised purpura on 'exposed' sites	Transient porphyrinaemia (secondary to transfusions) [19,20]

ATROPHIC LESIONS OF NEONATES

There are a number of causes of atrophic lesions in neonates (Box 114.2). Some are covered elsewhere in this chapter.

Box 114.2 Causes of atrophic lesions in neonates

- Morphoea
- Atrophic dermatofibrosarcoma protuberans
- Cutis marmorata telangiectatica congenita
- Aplasia cutis congenita
- Anetoderma of prematurity
- Congenital erosive and vesicular dermatosis healing with reticulated supple scarring
- Medallion-like dermal dendrocyte hamartoma
- Congenital infection (HSV and VZV; may be zosteriform)
- Focal dermal hypoplasia of Goltz
- Neonatal lupus erythematosus

HSV, herpes simplex virus; VZV, varicella zoster virus.

Medallion-like dermal dendrocyte hamartoma

Introduction and general description
Medallion-like dermal dendrocyte hamartoma is a benign atrophic lesion presenting at birth and was first described in 2004 in female neonates [1,2–6].

Epidemiology
Incidence and prevalence
It is very rare with fewer than 15 cases described.

Age
There is congenital presentation.

Sex
It is more common in females.

Pathophysiology
The underlying cause is unknown.

Pathology
It shows epidermal atrophy, spindle cell proliferation in the dermis and to a lesser degree the subcutis, and reduced adnexal structures. Spindle cells stain positive for CD34, factor X111a, vimentin and fascin, suggesting a dermal dendritic origin. Atrophic dermatofibrosarcoma protuberans is also CD34 positive, but is factor X111a negative [1,2,3].

Clinical features
Presentation
This rare condition presents with a reddish brown, slightly indurated, congenital, atrophic lesion of the skin often on the side of the neck or on the upper trunk. Lesions are typically round or oval, measure 2–6 cm across and persist unaltered into adulthood. They may show a slight increase in hair growth and visible underlying blood vessels beneath a wrinkled epidermis [1,2–5]. Histology and immunohistochemistry help differentiate this disorder from other causes of neonatal cutaneous atrophy.

Differential diagnosis
Differential diagnoses include congenital dermatofibrosarcoma protuberans, aplasia cutis congenita, anetoderma of prematurity, neurofibroma (atrophic blue-red macule variant) and cutis marmorata telangiectatica congenita. There appears to be some overlap with fibroblastic connective tissue naevi, which also presents as CD34-positive solitary painless plaques or nodules.

Disease course and prognosis
The course is persistent but there is no recorded case of malignant transformation.

Investigations
Skin biopsy and immunostaining are useful.

Management
There is no known medical therapy. Lesions can be safely left or excised (usually by a plastic surgeon, depending on the size).

DISORDERS CAUSED BY TRANSPLACENTAL TRANSFER/MATERNAL MILK

Transplacental transfer of maternal autoantibodies

Clinical manifestations in the neonate have now been reported in a number of maternal disorders that are believed to be induced by circulating autoantibodies. These include pemphigus vulgaris, pemphigus foliaceus, herpes gestationis and lupus erythematosus.

Because immunoglobulin A (IgA), IgM and IgE antibodies do not cross the placenta in significant amounts, this phenomenon is restricted to diseases caused by autoantibodies of IgG class. Placental transfer of IgG is a mechanism for protecting the neonate while their immune system is immature and ineffective. Where complement is also involved in pathogenesis, this must be provided by the fetus as it does not pass across the placenta. Complement can be detected in the fetus from about the 11th week of gestation. Maternal IgG is catabolised more or less completely within the first 3–6 months of life, and antibody-mediated transplacental diseases can be expected to remit spontaneously within this period.

Neonatal pemphigus vulgaris

Pemphigus vulgaris is unusual in pregnancy because it is largely a disease of an older age group and because affected individuals receiving systemic treatment rarely become pregnant. Nevertheless, several cases of transplacentally transmitted pemphigus vulgaris have been reported [1–7,**8**,9] (Chapter 50). Not all mothers have had clinically apparent disease during pregnancy [10]; in other cases the disease has been mild [11]. It is rare that pregnancy is considered as a triggering factor for pemphigus [12].

Affected infants have had cutaneous and/or mucosal erosions or bullae; several have been stillborn [1–6]. Approximately one-third of neonates born to mothers with pemphigus are unaffected at birth [13]. Direct immunofluorescence has been positive in skin biopsies from all affected infants, and circulating IgG pemphigus antibodies have been found in the majority. There are no cases of infants born to mothers with pemphigus requiring treatment. Lesions have resolved spontaneously within about 3 weeks and no new lesions have occurred after birth. Circulating IgG antibodies become undetectable by the end of the second month of life.

Transplacental transmission of pemphigus foliaceus has been similarly described [14,15].

Transplacental pemphigoid gestationis

Cutaneous lesions occur in about 10% of infants born to mothers with pemphigoid gestationis, although maternal IgG antibasement membrane autoantibody can be found in all infants of affected mothers [1,2] (Chapter 113). The lesions may be present at birth or they may appear at any time up to the third day of life [3]. These lesions may vary from evanescent, non-specific, red or urticarial papules to fully developed bullae [4]. Lesions in the infant may be extensive [5]. Spontaneous regression of lesions within 3 weeks is the rule. Direct immunofluorescence is normal by the end of the first month, and circulating IgG antibasement membrane zone antibody can no longer be found.

The risk of fetal and infant morbidity and mortality in mothers with pemphigoid gestationis is debated [6] and has not been confirmed [7–9], although there are some reports of fetal growth restriction and pre-eclampsia [**10**,11]. However, there does appear to be an increased risk of premature delivery [8,9,**10**,11]. The risk of adrenal insufficiency should be considered in neonates whose mothers have required long-term oral prednisolone treatment.

Neonatal lupus erythematosus

Introduction and general description

Neonatal lupus erythematosus (LE) is a rare syndrome comprising transient skin lesions resembling subacute cutaneous LE and/or congenital heart block (Chapter 51). Neonatal LE occurs in the babies of mothers with clinical or subclinical autoimmune connective tissue disease, and is associated with the transplacental passage of maternal autoantibodies to the ribonucleoproteins (RNPs) Ro-SSA (>90%), La-SSB or rarely U_1-RNP [1].

Epidemiology
Incidence and prevalence
Only 1–2% of Ro-positive/La-positive mothers will have babies with neonatal LE, but babies from subsequent pregnancies have a 20–25% risk of skin or cardiac disease [2–4].

Age
It occurs in neonates up to 3 months old.

Sex
There is an equal sex incidence.

Ethnicity
It is described in all racial groups.

Associated diseases
The risk of connective tissue disease later in life is increased.

Pathophysiology
It is now accepted that this disease is provoked in the fetus or newborn infant by maternal IgG autoantibodies that have crossed the placenta [5,6]. In 95% of cases, these are of IgG1 class and are directed against the Ro RNP antigen [7–9]. These antibodies are relatively prevalent in young women, and often appear to be compatible with apparently normal health. Anti-La, anti-native DNA, anticardiolipin or antinuclear antibodies, or rheumatoid factor may be present in addition to Ro antibodies [9]. A small proportion of affected infants do not have detectable Ro antibodies but do have La and U_1-RNP antibodies [10].

The presence of Ro and La antigens has been demonstrated in fetal skin and cardiac conducting tissue [11,12]. Up to 60% of the mothers of infants with neonatal LE have no clinical evidence of connective tissue disease at the time of birth [5,9,13]. However, there is a substantial risk of a subsequent development of symptoms of autoimmune connective tissue disease. About 40% of mothers have signs or symptoms of systemic LE, subacute cutaneous LE or the sicca syndrome [14–17], although these may be minimal. More recently, it has been recognised that about 5% of women of child-bearing age who present with leukocytoclastic vasculitis will have Ro antibodies [18], and it is probable that about 5% of babies with neonatal LE have mothers with leukocytoclastic vasculitis [19].

Predisposing factors

There appears to be a genetic predisposition to develop the cardiac complications of neonatal LE.

Pathology

Skin biopsy specimens from infants with cutaneous lesions generally demonstrate the features of LE: epidermal atrophy, liquefaction degeneration of basal keratinocytes, colloid bodies and a perivascular and periappendageal lymphohistiocytic inflammatory infiltrate in the dermis [14,20]. Direct immunofluorescence is positive in about 50% of cases, showing dermal–epidermal junction and perivascular deposition of IgG, IgM and C3.

Environmental factors

Sunlight may induce skin lesions.

Clinical features

Presentation

Most infants with neonatal LE have either skin lesions (90%) or cardiac lesions (1%); approximately 8% have both [2,21,22]. In about two-thirds of those infants who develop cutaneous lesions, these are already present at birth. In the remainder, the lesions appear during the first 2–3 months (sometimes sun-induced), although their appearance may be delayed for as long as 5 months.

The skin lesions of neonatal LE generally take the form of well-defined areas of macular or slightly elevated redness, frequently annular, occurring predominantly on the face, particularly the forehead, temples and upper cheeks, and on the scalp and neck (Figure 114.3). A 'spectacle-like' distribution of lesions around the eyes is especially characteristic. The chest, back or limbs may also be affected [20,21,22–24]. Provocation or exacerbation of lesions by sun exposure has been reported in some cases.

Follicular plugging is not prominent, but scaling is a common early feature. A degree of atrophy and/or telangiectasia are frequent long-term sequelae. Permanent hair loss may occur.

In most cases, the skin lesions have resolved within the first year, but areas of atrophy and/or telangiectasia may be more persistent [25]. Longstanding depressions have followed subcutaneous lesions. The most frequent sites for such lesions are the temples and scalp [26].

Clinical variants

Less commonly, lesions take the form of annular patches of redness without an epidermal component; this type of presentation has predominantly been reported in Japanese infants [23]. Subcutaneous lesions have also been described [26].

Occasionally, neonatal LE presents as extensive reticulate redness with atrophy, closely resembling cutis marmorata telangiectatica congenita [27,28]. Depigmentation may be very prominent in infants with skin of colour [29]. Lesions resembling morphoea have been reported [30].

Differential diagnosis

The lesions of congenital rubella or cytomegalovirus infection may need to be considered, although these are of purplish colour and purpura is generally prominent. Congenital syphilis may also need to be excluded, but whereas mucosal, periorificial and palmar and

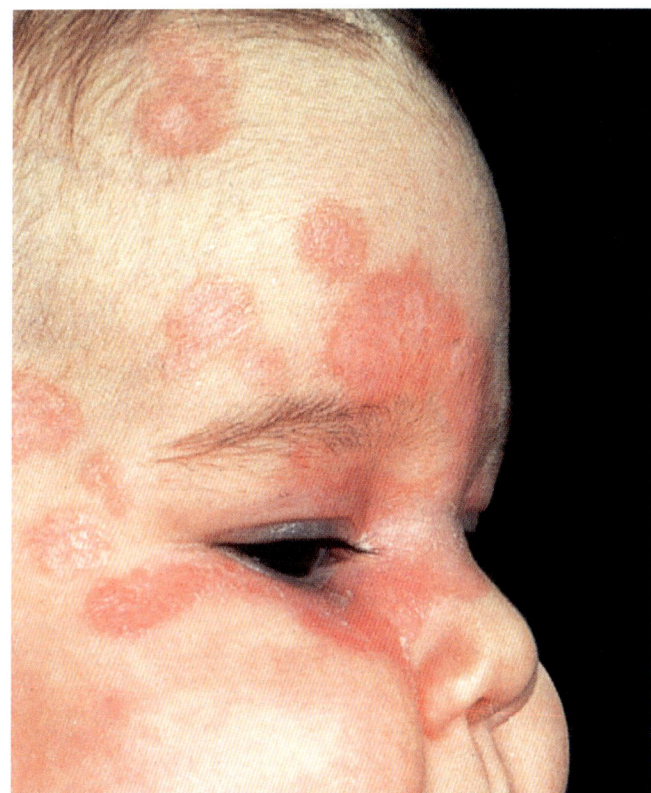

Figure 114.3 Neonatal lupus erythematosus showing fading facial lesions in a characteristic periorbital distribution, with residual atrophy, in a 4-month-old infant.

plantar lesions are common in congenital syphilis, these features are rare in neonatal LE. Confusion may be caused by the false positive antibody tests that are as much a feature of neonatal as of acquired LE.

Atrophy and telangiectasia of the cheeks is seen with photosensitivity in Bloom syndrome (Chapter 77), and without photosensitivity (in most cases) in the Rothmund–Thomson syndrome (Chapter 75). In these disorders, skin lesions are not present at birth and generally appear later than in neonatal LE.

Complications and co-morbidities

Systemic features are detectable in over half of all affected infants, of which cardiac involvement is the commonest. Congenital heart block (due to fibrosis of the conducting tissue) occurs in about 1–2% of Ro-positive pregnancies, probably due to genetic susceptibility [2,31–35]. In these families it will recur in 20% of subsequent pregnancies [3]. Anti-Ro antibodies can bind to cardiac conduction cells during mid to late fetal development, leading to altered membrane repolarisation and selective damage to the atrioventricular node. Congenital heart block can be detected as early as the 18th week of gestation by ultrasound or electrocardiography [34]. The block is generally permanent, and is not associated with structural cardiac abnormalities such as septal defects. About a half of affected infants require pacemakers [33,34].

A smaller proportion of infants have combinations of hepatomegaly, splenomegaly, lymphadenopathy and pneumonitis, which are generally mild in degree and fairly transient.

Autoimmune haemolytic anaemia and thrombocytopenia are seen in a small proportion of affected infants [36].

The central nervous system may be involved in neonatal LE and this can cause an asymptomatic vasculopathy or a more serious cerebral vasculitis [37,38].

Disease course and prognosis

Infants with skin lesions alone, or with skin lesions and systemic features other than heart block, generally show little sign of residual disease after the age of 1 year [38,39]. However, their long-term prognosis must remain slightly at risk in the light of reports of the later development by some of full-blown connective tissue disease [33,40,41]. Conduction defects of the heart tend to be permanent, and when severe are associated with a significant mortality [2,33,42].

The risk of recurrence in further pregnancies appears to be about 20–25% [2,3]. Spontaneous abortion and stillbirth do not appear to be more frequent in further pregnancies of mothers who have had a previous child with neonatal LE [2].

Neonatal LE antibodies disappear from the infant's serum within about 6 months.

Investigations

A skin biopsy will usually allow an accurate diagnosis of neonatal LE, particularly if combined with direct immunofluorescence studies, and tests for the appropriate circulating autoantibodies in both the mother and the child.

Management

The skin lesions of neonatal LE require no treatment, but sun protection is essential. Occasionally, thrombocytopenia, haemolytic anaemia or hepatitis may warrant systemic steroid therapy [43]. Up to 50% of infants with cardiac involvement will require a pacemaker [23].

The pregnancy of a woman who has Ro, La or U_1-RNP antibodies should be monitored to detect a slow fetal heart rate [44,45]. Treatment with high-dose systemic steroids may be indicated for fetal bradycardia where there are signs of heart failure [46].

Transplacental transfer of maternal malignant disease

Transplacental transfer of maternal malignant disease is fortunately extremely rare, despite the fact that malignancy occurs in 1 in 1000 pregnancies [1,2], and it is well established that maternal cells regularly reach the fetus.

Melanoma accounts for approximately 90% of transplacentally transferred malignant disease, although this particular malignancy accounts for only about 8% of those occurring in pregnant women [3]. Melanoma transmitted in this way may result in the appearance of nodular skin deposits in the neonate. Fetal melanoma metastasis is reported in mothers already known to have metastatic melanoma, and there was placental involvement in all cases [4]. Placental involvement does not always signify metastatic disease in the neonate. Although the prognosis is generally poor, spontaneous regression of transplacentally transferred melanoma has

been reported [5,6]. In cases where placental metastasis is detected with no evidence of fetal metastasis the infant should be monitored until 24 months with skin examination, imaging (chest X-ray and liver ultrasound) and blood monitoring (lactate dehydrogenase and liver enzymes).

Transplacental transmission of acute monocytic leukaemia [7], natural killer cell lymphoma [8] and choriocarcinoma [9] has also been reported.

Checking the maternal origin of a tumour in a neonate can be done quickly by a quantitative polymerase chain reaction (PCR) technique [10,11].

Transfer of toxic substances in maternal milk

When considering the cause of any rash in a young infant, the possibility that it reflects exposure of the mother to a toxic substance that has been transferred in her milk needs to be borne in mind. A good example is provided by two reports of bromoderma occurring in neonates whose mothers had taken bromide medicinally [1] or had been accidentally exposed in a photographic laboratory [2].

DISORDERS OF SUBCUTANEOUS FAT

Four separate conditions are described – cold panniculitis, neonatal cold injury, subcutaneous fat necrosis of the newborn and sclerema neonatorum – but there is some clinical and pathological overlap.

Cold panniculitis

Cold panniculitis is a distinctive form of panniculitis provoked directly by cold exposure, to which infants appear particularly predisposed. The fat of the newborn appears to be more highly saturated than that of older children and adults, with the effect that it solidifies at a higher temperature [1,2]. Applying ice for 50 s causes panniculitis in all newborn infants, in only 40% of 6-month-old infants and almost never in 9-month-old infants [3].

Cold panniculitis in infancy has most often followed exposure of the cheeks to (i) extremely cold air [4]; (ii) ice bags applied as a therapy for supraventricular tachycardia [5–7]; or (iii) frozen lollies (popsicles) [8,9]. Indurated, warm, red, subcutaneous plaques and nodules appear within hours or days of appropriate cold exposure. Skin biopsy is not usually needed but if done early it shows a lymphohistiocytic infiltrate around blood vessels at the junction of the dermis and subcutaneous fat [10]. After a few days, lipocyte rupture leads to the formation of cystic cavities surrounded by areas of marked infiltration by lymphocytes and histiocytes, with a few neutrophils and eosinophils. The induration resolves over a period of a week or so, often leaving some residual postinflammatory hyperpigmentation. No treatment is required.

Neonatal cold injury

Neonatal cold injury is a disorder, now rare in developed countries, in which cold exposure of a small-for-dates neonate causes hypothermia associated with lethargy and generalised pitting oedema of the skin, clinically and pathologically distinct from sclerema neonatorum. A low environmental temperature has been the principal cause of virtually all reported cases of this disorder [1–4]. Other factors that appear to have predisposed babies to this complication of cold exposure include intrauterine growth retardation, which results in a relatively thin panniculus, and tight wrappings, which restrict muscular activity.

The infant is usually a full-term neonate, born at home, but small for gestational age. In the great majority of cases, presentation is within the first 4 days of life, and usually during the first 24 h. The most striking features are intense redness or cyanosis of the face and extremities, and firm, pitting oedema beginning at the extremities and spreading centrally, and becoming progressively more indurated in a proportion of cases [1–4]. Petechiae have occasionally been observed. The skin feels cold, and the baby is usually hypothermic with a low core temperature. Associated non-cutaneous features of cold injury are generally present, and may occur in the absence of skin changes. These include immobility, drowsiness, poor feeding, vomiting, oliguria and gastrointestinal bleeding with vomiting of altered blood or melaena.

Skin biopsy shows a thin panniculus; otherwise there is little obvious abnormality apart from dilatation of the dermal blood vessels [5]. Profuse exudation of clear fluid from the cut surface at postmortem suggests that the induration is due to oedema.

The mortality rate of historical cases was about 25% (usually due to massive pulmonary haemorrhage). Fortunately, the condition seems to be much less common in the UK now than it was 40 years ago, probably because of improved heating in homes, reduced frequency of home delivery and abandonment of the previous habit of bathing babies at birth.

Care should be taken when rewarming in cases of accidental hypothermia as rapid rewarming in prolonged hypothermia is associated with fatal thrombocytopenia [6].

Subcutaneous fat necrosis of the newborn

Definition

Subcutaneous fat necrosis of the newborn (SCFN) is a rare and usually transient form of panniculitis which mostly affects full-term infants usually within the first few weeks of life [1,2].

Epidemiology

Incidence and prevalence

The incidence is unknown but the disease is rare.

Age

It generally occurs in full-term or post-term infants of normal birth weight during the first 6 weeks of life [3].

Sex

There is an equal sex incidence.

Ethnicity

This is an unknown influence.

Associated diseases

Maternal pre-eclampsia, diabetes, perinatal asphyxia and hypothermia, including therapeutic whole body cooling, may be associated [1,2,4–10,**11**].

Pathophysiology

Predisposing factors

The precise cause is unestablished, but a variety of insults appear to have contributed in individual cases. These have included birth asphyxia, maternal pre-eclampsia, maternal diabetes, obstetric trauma, hypothermia and hypothermic cardiac surgery [1,2,4–10]. The most important predisposing factors appear to be the combination of local tissue hypoxia and cold injury. This might explain the predominant location of lesions on the shoulders and buttocks, cutaneous areas where mechanical pressure might compromise the circulation and contribute to hypoxia. A primary abnormality in brown fat has also been postulated [12].

Pathology

It is characterised by granulomatous reaction, lobular panniculitis and multinucleated giant cells found on histology. The composition of neonatal fat with increased saturated fatty acids and its higher melting point compared with adult fat have been associated with the tendency for solidification and crystallisation [1,13–15]. Both the fat cells and the giant cells contain needle-shaped clefts, which may be radially arranged. Fibrotic obliteration of small arterioles has also been observed. Calcium deposits are commonly found in the necrotic fat.

Ultrastructural examination has shown parallel aggregations of electron-lucent, needle-shaped spaces within the adipocytes [13,14]. Similar changes in visceral adipose tissue have been reported in postmortem studies of affected infants [4]. Widespread calcium deposition in internal organs has also been shown in postmortem specimens from hypercalcaemic cases and nephrocalcinosis has been observed in such infants during life [16].

Environmental factors

Hypoxia, cold and trauma all seem to play a role.

Clinical features

Presentation

Infants who develop subcutaneous fat necrosis are generally full-term or post-term neonates of normal weight [1,2,4,8–10]. There is an association with perinatal asphyxia, therapeutic hypothermia, meconium aspiration and obstetric trauma. It is generally felt that some form of neonatal distress can reduce the blood supply to neonatal fatty tissue, resulting in necrosis in an attempt to shunt blood from the skin and adipose tissue to the vital organs [17].

Nodular thickening of the subcutaneous tissues is usually first detected between the 2nd and 21st days of life. Sometimes, the

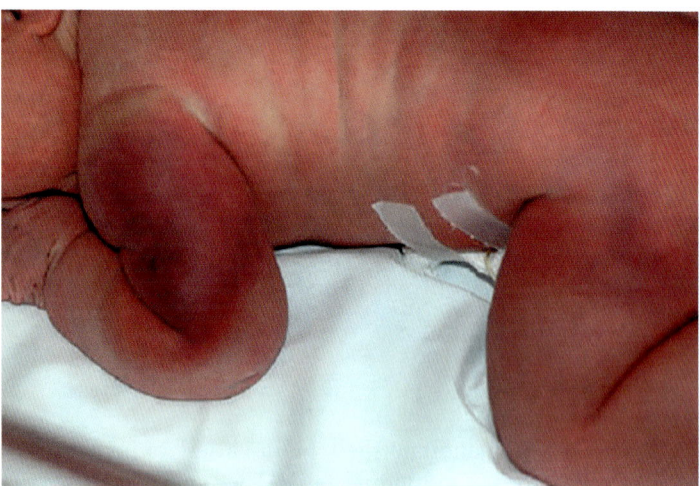

Figure 114.4 Subcutaneous fat necrosis of the newborn showing red and violaceous plaques involving the shoulders, arms and buttocks. Courtesy of Dr Luis Requena.

changes are present at birth and, rarely, they may appear as late as the sixth week. The nodules tend to be symmetrically distributed and show a predilection for the buttocks, thighs, shoulders, back, cheeks and arms (Figure 114.4). Lesions may be single or multiple, rounded or oval, and pea-sized or many centimetres in diameter. They are initially discrete, but may fuse to form large plaques. The overlying skin is often red or bluish red. The nodules feel rubbery or hard, and are not attached to deeper structures. The lesions may be painful [18]. New nodules may continue to develop for a week or more. There has been a single report of subcutaneous fat necrosis being complicated by a haematoma, requiring surgical debridement [19].

In most cases, the child's health is not substantially impaired, and within a few months the nodules disappear. Where calcium deposition is marked, the lesions may take rather longer to resolve. Usually no trace of the nodules remains but there may be slight atrophy. Rarely, the nodules may ulcerate, discharge their fatty contents and leave scars.

The condition has occasionally been fatal, particularly when visceral fat has been involved [4], or where there has been complicating hypercalcaemia which may result in gastrointestinal disorders, and neurological and cardiac life-threatening complications [20–24].

Clinical variants

There have been several reports of the occurrence of lesions analogous to those of SCFN in children who have had hypothermic cardiac surgery [7–9]. The cutaneous application of ice to induce hypothermia, trauma and/or hypoxia may all have contributed. It is noteworthy that these children appear to have developed lesions of subcutaneous fat necrosis rather than cold panniculitis. The ages of the children at the time of surgery varied from 12 days to 20 months. Lesions appeared between 14 and 30 days later, principally at the sites subjected to the greatest cold exposure. The lesions resolve within a few weeks and no treatment is usually required.

Differential diagnosis

Neonates delivered by forceps may develop subcutaneous nodules where the forceps were applied, presumably as a result of traumatic fat necrosis. SCFN was in the past frequently confused with sclerema neonatorum. Occasionally, the two conditions may occur simultaneously [25].

Complications and co-morbidities

Subcutaneous fat necrosis of the newborn may be associated with hypercalcaemia, which tends to occur in around a quarter of all cases, appears more frequently in infants with extensive disease, and almost exclusively when the trunk is affected [19–24].

The cause of the hypercalcaemia is unknown. It may be due to increased calcium absorption due to extrarenal production of 1,25-dihydroxyvitamin D [22,23], which has been observed in other granulomatous disorders including sarcoidosis. The finding of increased urinary excretion of prostaglandin E_1 led to the suggestion that increased bone calcium resorption might be responsible [24].

Transient thrombocytopenia has been reported during the period of initial development of the lesions, possibly due to sequestration of platelets [26]. Plasma lipid abnormalities have been reported in a neonate with subcutaneous fat necrosis, but their relevance was unclear [27].

All infants who have experienced subcutaneous fat necrosis should have their serum calcium measured on presentation and every 2–3 weeks for up to 3 months as the increase in calcium can be delayed. If hypercalcaemia is present, its cause requires thorough investigation to exclude disorders such as primary hyperparathyroidism and vitamin D intoxication. Nephrocalcinosis is a common persistent finding even in those children who have undergone treatment for hypercalcaemia, but fortunately renal impairment is very rare.

Disease course and prognosis

The skin condition resolves over several weeks although the hypercalcaemia can persist for a few months.

Investigations

Skin biopsy is required to confirm the diagnosis (see Chapter 97 for histopathological images and description). Serum calcium needs to be monitored for 3 months.

Management

No treatment is generally required as the condition spontaneously resolves over several weeks. Analgesia may occasionally be required.

Hypercalcaemia should be treated aggressively to prevent soft-tissue calcification. Treatments include diuretics, dietary restriction of calcium and vitamin D, and sometimes oral corticosteroids [10,18,20]. In resistant cases bisphosphonates can be used [28,29], and a case of hypercalcaemia treated with calcitonin has been reported [30]. These measures should be instituted as early as possible with maintenance of adequate hydration with intravenous normal saline. Furosemide has been used to achieve increased calcium excretion by inhibiting calcium reabsorption, but a risk of dehydration and consequent worsening of hypercalcaemia exists. Prednisolone interferes with the metabolism of vitamin D to its active form and also inhibits the production of 1,25-dihydroxyvitamin D_3 by the macrophages involved in the inflammatory process.

Resources

Further information

Medscape, subcutaneous fat necrosis of the newborn: https://emedicine.medscape.com/article/1081910-overview (last accessed June 2023).

Sclerema neonatorum

Introduction and general description

Sclerema neonatorum is an uncommon panniculitis with an invariably high mortality [1]. It predominantly affects gravely ill, preterm neonates in the first week of life. It manifests as diffuse hardening of skin and subcutaneous adipose tissue to such an extent that it hinders feeding and respiration, and usually culminates in death [2,3].

Epidemiology
Incidence and prevalence

It is very rare and its prevalence is unknown.

Age

Sclerema neonatorum almost always appears during the first week of life, although it has occasionally been recorded later in infants born preterm.

Sex

There is an equal sex incidence.

Associated diseases

There is underlying severe illness.

Pathophysiology
Predisposing factors

Prematurity and smallness for dates appear to be frequent predisposing factors [3]. It has been recorded as already present at birth in infants subjected to placental insufficiency [4]. The disorder does not seem to occur in otherwise healthy infants, and most characteristically develops during the course of one of a wide variety of severe illnesses, particularly serious infections, congenital heart disease and other major developmental defects [3]. A proportion of these infants have been hypothermic, and occasionally sclerema has been described as a complication of neonatal cold injury [5]. Nevertheless, cold does not appear to be an important aetiological factor in the majority of cases.

Lipolytic mechanisms are poorly developed in the newborn, particularly in those born preterm [6]. The maturation of these enzyme systems might be further compromised by major infection or hypoxia. It has been suggested that sclerema might reflect defective lipolysis within adipose tissue, which would result in failure of fat mobilisation and an impaired capacity to maintain body temperature. It has been reported that the ratio of saturated to unsaturated fatty acids is relatively high in the adipose tissue of all neonates, and that this ratio was even higher in an infant with sclerema [7]. This would lead to a raised melting point, and it is possible that the induration of subcutaneous fat, which is the major clinical feature of sclerema, might reflect its solidification due to a fall in the temperature of the adipose tissue during peripheral circulatory collapse.

Pathology

In most cases the subcutaneous fat layer appears to be thickened due to an increased size of the individual lipocytes and to an increased width of the intersecting bands of connective tissue, probably due to oedema [7,8]. There is very little evidence of fat necrosis and, generally, only the slightest indication of inflammation. The most characteristic histological feature of sclerema neonatorum is the presence of radially arranged, needle-shaped clefts in adipocytes and, occasionally, in multinucleate giant cells, reflecting the presence of crystals prior to processing (see Chapter 97 for histopathological images and description).

Environmental factors

These are unclear.

Clinical features
History

Sclerema neonatorum was first described by Underwood in 1784 and was called 'skinbound disease' [2]. In 1817, Alibert introduced the term sclerema, derived from the Greek word *skleros*, meaning hard.

Presentation

Sclerema neonatorum is a very rare disorder that almost always appears during the first 1–2 weeks of life [2–4]. It predominantly affects preterm neonates, although there are some case reports of term babies with this presentation [9]. It has generally been considered a non-specific sign of severe illness and has been associated with a mortality ranging from 82% to 98% [1]. The affected infant is generally very ill at the time of onset of sclerema. Woody induration of the skin starts on the buttocks, thighs or calves and extends rapidly and symmetrically to involve almost the whole surface (Figure 114.5), with the exception of the palms, soles and genitalia.

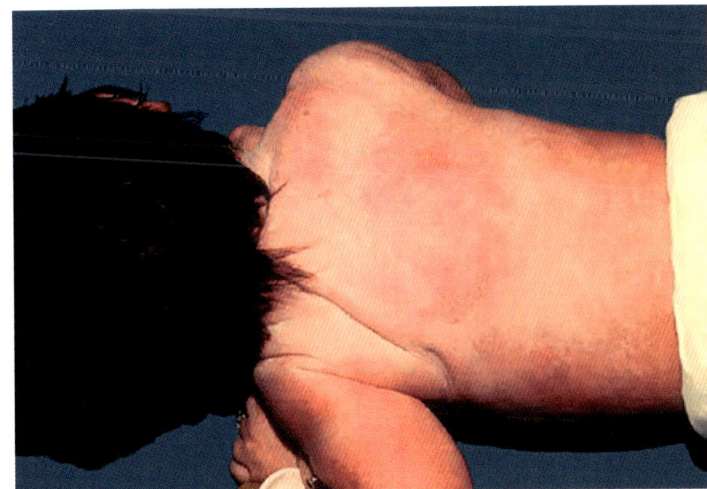

Figure 114.5 Sclerema neonatorum in a newborn with generalised woody induration of the skin. Courtesy of Dr Luis Requena.

Table 114.4 Distinctions between neonatal cold injury, sclerema and subcutaneous fat necrosis.

	Neonatal cold injury	Sclerema	Subcutaneous fat necrosis
Frequency	Previously common, now rare	Rare, usually seen in neonatal intensive care units	Uncommon
Patient	Full-term neonates, often small for dates, born at home	Usually severely ill neonates, often preterm or small for dates or post-term	Healthy infants, usually full-term
Onset	During the first week	Almost always during the first week	1–6 weeks
Sites	Extremities, spreading centrally	Lower limbs initially, becoming generalised	Trunk, buttocks, thighs, arms, face
Appearance	Pitting oedema initially with redness or cyanosis of the face and extremities	Diffuse, yellow-white, woody induration with immobility of limbs	Firm, reddish violet, subcutaneous nodules
Histology	Thin panniculus	Subtle; thickened connective tissue trabeculae, radial needle-like clefts	Granulomatous inflammation, fat necrosis
Prognosis	Mortality around 25%	Poor; mortality greater than 50% in past	Generally excellent

The skin is bound to adjacent subcutaneous tissue including muscle and bone and therefore it cannot be pitted by pressure or pinched into a fold. This skin is hard and cold to touch, and yellowish white in colour, often with purplish mottling. Mobility is limited and this can result in a typical facial appearance.

Differential diagnosis

The main area of diagnostic confusion has been between sclerema and subcutaneous fat necrosis [10,11]. It is now clear that the two disorders are distinct pathologically and clinically, although rarely they can occur together. Table 114.4 outlines their distinguishing features.

Scleredema has been reported in an infant at 2 weeks of age, and was distinguished from sclerema principally on histological grounds [12]. Turner syndrome is often recognisable at birth by the presence in a female of firm, non-pitting lymphoedema of the dorsa of the hands and feet, associated with low birth weight and loose folds of skin around the neck. Where primary lymphoedema occurs in neonates, it will already be clinically evident at birth. The condition may be familial, and generally first affects the legs, particularly the lower legs. The presence of oedema at birth, and its very slow progression in an otherwise healthy neonate, distinguishes primary lymphoedema from sclerema.

Complications and co-morbidities

Respiratory insufficiency occurs due to restricted movement of the chest wall.

Disease course and prognosis

The prognosis is poor, and is largely determined by the nature of the underlying disease. In spite of advances in the treatment of many of the predisposing disorders, particularly sepsis, the mortality probably remains in excess of 50%. In infants who survive, the appearance of the skin returns to normal without long-term complications such as calcification.

Investigations

Skin biopsy is the most useful test.

Management
First line

Treatment of the underlying medical condition(s) in a neonatal unit is the key to survival.

Second line

Systemic corticosteroids [13] are probably not effective but there is evidence that repeated exchange transfusions [14,15] and intravenous immunoglobulin [16] may be helpful in some cases.

Resources

Further information

Medscape, sclerema neonatorum: https://emedicine.medscape.com/article/1112191-overview (last accessed June 2023).

MISCELLANEOUS DISORDERS

Raised linear bands of infancy

Definition and nomenclature

These are raised bands found on the skin, usually of the legs, in the first few months after birth.

> **Synonyms and inclusions**
> - Persistent linear bands of infancy
> - Acquired raised bands of infancy

Introduction and general description

Raised linear bands of infancy was first described in 2002 in two premature babies [1]. Thirteen cases have since been described in both premature and term babies [2–7].

Epidemiology
Incidence and prevalence

Its incidence is unknown but it is very rare.

Age

The onset is usually at 1–2 months of age.

Sex

There is a female to male ratio of 8 : 5.

Associated diseases

In a few cases amniotic band syndrome may be present with potential limb defects obvious from birth.

Pathophysiology

The cause is unknown but various theories have been postulated revolving around the possibility of an abnormal reaction to pressure on the skin [5,6]. In the first four cases described, three of the children were born prematurely (28–31 weeks) and there was documented evidence of amniotic bands or placental abruption/placental tears [1–4]. Short toes and a club foot were described in two of these children. It was therefore suggested that either amniotic bands or some undetermined prenatal insult was the cause. However of the 13 cases described, 9 were in term children with no documented evidence of amniotic bands or limb constriction/defects. Marque *et al.* postulated in their three cases [5] that the lesions arose exactly under where tight socks had been worn and the pressure effect of clothing may be relevant [6]. However, lesions have been described on the trunk, the buttocks and much higher up the leg where it seems less likely that occlusive clothing is an aetiological factor [3,4].

Pathology

Skin biopsy is usually unremarkable. There may be a little oedema in the dermis and fat, but the collagen and elastin are normal [1–4]. There are no signs of smooth muscle or lipomatous naevus. One author has described a dermal infiltrate of adipocytes along blood vessels and eccrine ducts in two cases and suggested a similar aetiology to post-traumatic piezogenic pedal papules [5].

Genetics

It is not known if there is an underlying genetic cause. Two familial cases have been described (brother and sister) but no consanguinity has been recorded.

Clinical features

History

The raised bands typically present in the first few months of life. They are often multiple and can be symmetrical. They are common on the legs but may be found on the upper limbs and rarely the trunk. They vary from 1 to 3 mm across.

Presentation

The lesions are palpable and firm but not hard.

Differential diagnosis

This includes amniotic band syndrome/congenital pseudoainhum. While in a few cases amniotic bands have been suggested as a potential cause for raised linear bands of infancy, the amniotic band syndrome is a separate, more severe entity presenting with constrictions at birth. These may lead to limb malformations, lymphoedema and even ischaemia and autoamputation (congenital pseudoainhum). Constriction bands may also occur in other conditions such as Michelin tyre baby syndrome. If the amniotic band syndrome occurs early *in utero* malformations tend to be more extensive and include alopecia, aplasia cutis, neural tube defects and cranio-facial defects as well as limb constriction bands. Ultrasound and Doppler are used to assess limbs. Treatment is difficult in this condition and is by fetoscopic surgery when possible [7–9].

Classification of severity

It is a benign, non-progressive but persistent condition.

Disease course and prognosis

The condition persisted in all but one case (longest follow-up to date is 18 years [5]).

Investigations

Most cases can be diagnosed clinically but a skin biopsy (which is essentially normal) may occasionally be required to exclude other conditions like Michelin tyre baby syndrome. The finding of adipocyte infiltrates along blood vessels by one author needs to be confirmed in other cases.

Management

Reassurance is usually all that is required and explaining that the lesions will probably persist lifelong. One case failed to respond to oral antihistamines. One case was treated with topical antihistamines and the lesions resolved within 3 months. This case was not biopsied and had some atypical features in that it presented late, at 6 months (much later than the usual 1–3 months), in a child with marked dermographism [10]. Also, the clinical pictures showed more urticated and wider lesions than typical limb bands.

Neonatal adnexal polyp

Solitary, self-healing, polypoid lesions have been observed in some 4% of neonates in a Japanese survey [1,2]; their occurrence in other racial groups has yet to be documented. These lesions are firm, pink, polypoid nodules, about 1 mm in diameter, usually found close and medial to one or other nipple. They have also been reported to occur on the scrotum, labia majora, cheeks, chin and arms [3].

Histology shows a normal epidermis, a vascular dermis containing prominent hair follicles with vestigial sebaceous glands and well-developed eccrine glands. These lesions generally separate from the skin spontaneously after a few days but they may persist in early life [4–6].

Collodion baby

Introduction and general description

Collodion baby is a descriptive term that refers to an infant who is born encased in a tight shiny membrane. It may represent the first expression of some forms of ichthyosis, the commonest of which are the autosomal recessive ichthyoses [1,2].

Epidemiology

Incidence and prevalence

The incidence of collodion baby is approximately 1 per 100 000 deliveries [3].

Age

It presents at birth.

Sex

There is a slight predominance in males.

Ethnicity

There is an equal distribution.

Associated diseases

Up to 10% of babies born with a collodion membrane will later develop entirely normal skin. This is one end of the spectrum for this heterogeneous disorder and may be referred to as a 'self-healing' collodion baby. Almost 90% will, however, go on to develop a severe form of autosomal recessive ichthyosis in the first few weeks of life: lamellar ichthyosis and non-bullous ichthyosiform erythroderma (synonym congenital ichthyosiform erythroderma) are the most common (Chapter 63) [1,2]. It is difficult to predict which children will go on to have normal skin or later develop a variant of ichthyosis. The collodion baby phenotype is also reported in the rarer autosomal dominant form of lamellar ichthyosis [4] and in bathing suit ichthyosis [5]; it is also characteristic of the trichothiodystrophy–ichthyosis syndrome [6,7].

There are other ichthyoses in which an initial collodion baby phase has occasionally been reported. These include the Netherton syndrome [1], neutral lipid storage disease [8], loricrin keratoderma (syn. Camisa keratoderma) [9] and Sjögren–Larsson syndrome [1], but the great majority of neonates with these disorders do not demonstrate the collodion baby phenotype. A transient collodion membrane has also been reported in Gaucher disease [10].

In about 10% of cases, the collodion baby phase is followed by a relatively mild ichthyosis of lamellar type or indeed normal skin (self-healing ichthyosis) [11,12].

Pathophysiology

Predisposing factors

Underlying genetic mutations predispose to this condition.

Pathology

Skin biopsy is not necessary for this clinical diagnosis. Indeed histopathology does not help predict the outcome. Histologically the membrane is a compact, thickened, orthokeratotic stratum corneum; the epidermis and dermis are both relatively normal [1,13,14].

Genetics

As the collodion baby is not a disease entity but is the first expression of some forms of ichthyosis, early genetic testing is not advised. An underlying ichthyosis phenotype will usually reveal itself over the first few weeks of life after the collodion membrane has shed. At that point specific genetic testing can help confirm a diagnosis.

Clinical features

Presentation

In severe presentations the baby will appear erythrodermic and encased in a rigid, shiny, glistening, yellowish, translucent covering resembling clear plastic film [1,2,15]. The tightness of the membrane may cause the eyelids to turn out revealing the pink inner lid; a condition called ectropion. Eclabium, the turning out of the lips due to the tightness of the membrane, may accompany ectropion, and may interfere with feeding. The nostrils may also be blocked. Restriction of the skin over the fingers, hands, toes and feet may result in immobility and could interfere with blood flow, occasionally resulting in the loss of parts of the digits [16]. Surgery may be required in cases of acute ischaemia to free the constrictive bands responsible. In the absence of surgery, the constrictive bands can lead to amputation (pseudoainhum) [16].

Within a few hours of birth, the membrane usually dries and cracks, and bleeding may occur along the resulting fissures. Within 1 or 2 days, it starts to shed, either in extensive sheets or as large, light brown scales, but it may reform several times. The shedding will generally be more or less complete within 4 weeks. Subsequently, the typical features of one of several varieties of ichthyosis will be revealed over the next few weeks or months.

During the first day or two, tightness of the skin on the thorax may impede respiration, and very occasionally respiratory distress may also be induced by nasal obstruction.

Clinical variants

Rarely, the collodion phenotype may be confined to acral sites only. This usually heals spontaneously ('acral self-healing collodion baby') [12].

Differential diagnosis

The appearance of the collodion baby is unmistakable. However, a baby with a severe collodion phenotype (marked ectropion and eclabium) may be confused with harlequin ichthyosis as the facial appearances can be similar (Chapter 63). However, a child with harlequin ichthyosis has much thicker skin, which typically encases the baby like a suit of armour with deep fissures. Harlequin ichthyosis shows almost fusion of the fingers and toes with thick palmoplantar skin. Finally, the ears are usually bound down to the scalp in harlequin ichthyosis whereas they are normally 'free' in collodion babies. Restrictive dermopathy also results in a neonate with tight and immobilising skin, but in this condition the skin appears thin and transparent, with prominent underlying blood vessels. The mouth is also open, but ectropion is not present. The skin does not dry out and come away. Death occurs rapidly as a consequence of respiratory failure. Neonates with the lethal autosomal recessive Neu–Laxova syndrome may have skin changes closely resembling a collodion membrane. The condition is characterised by intrauterine growth retardation, and central nervous system, skeletal and cranial abnormalities.

Complications and co-morbidities

The collodion baby is at risk, largely because of the consequences of losing the skin barrier function [17]. This results in the following:
- Impaired temperature regulation.
- Increased insensible water loss, hypernatraemic dehydration and acute renal failure [18,19].
- Septicaemia (bacterial, *Candida*).
- Percutaneous toxicity from topical medicaments (increased absorption).
- Respiratory failure. Respiration may be impaired as a result of intrapartum aspiration of squamous debris shed into the amniotic fluid. Immobility of the chest may also compromise respiratory function, and predispose to pneumonia [20].

With good neonatal care mortality figures have fallen from 50% in the 1960s to less than 5% today in the western world.

Disease course and prognosis

The longer-term outlook depends on which type of ichthyosis develops, and it is important to be aware that there is no correlation between initial severity in a collodion baby and the gravity of the ichthyosis that follows. While advances in genetics should soon allow routine genetic screening of collodion babies, the genotype does not always correlate well with phenotype, so a 'wait and see' policy is still required.

Investigations

Genetic analysis, if available, should be used.

Management

The most important element in treatment is an awareness of the possible medical complications from skin barrier failure. The baby should be nursed in an incubator in a high-humidity atmosphere, with careful monitoring of body temperature (overheating can also be an issue). Great attention needs to be given to fluid and electrolyte balance [21]. In severe cases fluid therapy should be given intravenously, but in less severe cases oral or nasogastric fluid supplementation will suffice. Peritoneal dialysis may be indicated if renal failure occurs. Fluid loss is significantly reduced by frequent applications of lipid; a 50%/50% mixture of white soft paraffin and liquid paraffin is ideal for this purpose. Frequent oiling of the skin increases mobility and comfort, accelerates healing of fissures and may reduce the risk of infection [22]. Supplemental feeds may be needed via a naso-gastric tube. Avoid topical products that contain active compounds (e.g. urea or salicylic acid) as toxicity is a real risk due to absorption.

Prevention of infection is of the greatest importance in saving these babies. Great attention should be paid to this aspect of care. Skin punctures should be kept to a minimum, and vascular access should be avoided as far as possible. Deeper fissures are more likely to become infected especially if inflamed, so regular swabs should be done for bacteria and *Candida* as septicaemia is a common complication [21].

Bands of tight skin constricting the digits, hands or feet may occasionally require surgical division.

'Blueberry muffin' baby (dermal erythropoiesis)

This term has been used to describe a characteristic eruption in neonates, often present at birth, comprising widespread, purple-red, oval or circular macules, papules and nodules reflecting dermal erythropoiesis.

The 'blueberry muffin' type of lesion has been recorded in a number of congenital infections, congenital haematological disorders and neonatal neoplastic conditions (Table 114.5).

There may be frank petechiae on the surface of some of the lesions. Favoured sites include the trunk, head and neck. The lesions generally fade into light brown macules within a few weeks of birth.

Table 114.5 Causes of 'blueberry muffin' baby.

Underlying disease process	Specific examples
Congenital infections	Rubella, cytomegalovirus, coxsackie B2, syphilis, toxoplasmosis [2–10]
Haematological	Hereditary spherocytosis, rhesus haemolytic anaemia, ABO blood group incompatibility, twin–twin transfusion syndrome, severe maternal anaemia [11–14]
Drug induced	Erythropoietin [15]
Neoplasia[a]	Congenital leukaemia, neuroblastoma, congenital rhabdomyosarcoma, Langerhans cell histiocytosis [16–27]
Inflammatory[a]	Neonatal lupus erythematosus
Lysosomal storage disease	Gaucher disease [28,29]

[a] Shows 'blueberry muffin-like' lesions but dermal erythropoeisis is not always present histologically.

Periorbital swelling can be observed in neuroblastoma, and less frequently in congenital leukaemia [1].

Histologically the lesions show foci of dermal erythropoiesis. The reticular dermis contains aggregates of nucleated and non-nucleated erythrocyte precursors, but generally no cells of myeloid or megakaryocytic type. It is possible that this process represents persistence and exaggeration of the dermal erythropoiesis that is a normal occurrence in early fetal development.

Neonatal purpura fulminans

Neonatal purpura fulminans is a rare but potentially lethal disorder characterised by a rapidly progressive haemorrhagic necrosis of the skin associated with cutaneous vascular thrombosis. It is probably best referred to as a form of disseminated intravascular coagulation (DIC) with associated purpura and haemorrhagic infarction function of the skin [1].

It may result from genetically transmitted thrombophilic disorder, most commonly homozygous deficiency of protein C or, less frequently, protein S [2–8,9,10,11]. Protein C resistance has also been reported due to mutations in the factor V gene [12,13]. In the older child, purpura fulminans is a highly characteristic feature of meningococcal septicaemia, where it results from acquired deficiency of protein C or S. It may also occur as a result of acquired conditions (DIC, antiphospholipid antibodies, galactosaemia, severe congenital heart disease, warfarin therapy) [14].

Neonatal purpura fulminans can also rarely occur due to infection, such as with group B *Streptococcus*, meticillin-resistant *Staphylococcus aureus*, varicella, measles, *Klebsiella*, *Enterobacter* and *Citrobacter* [15–22].

The earliest cutaneous changes are redness and ecchymosis, which typically appear within the first 12 h of life but their initial development may occasionally be delayed. The lesions rapidly progress into more or less symmetrical and well-defined 'lakes' of confluent ecchymosis, without petechiae [2–8,9,10–15]. The lesions occur most often on the limbs, particularly at sites of pressure, but may also appear on the trunk and on the face and scalp. The onset is sudden, and the lesions enlarge rapidly, with coalescence and the development of haemorrhagic bullae and central necrosis. There is surrounding redness and the lesions are tender. The patient is frequently febrile. These infants are also at risk of thrombosis in the central nervous system and in the retinal vessels. There is a substantial danger of internal haemorrhage, shock and death.

Treatment should be carried out in a specialist neonatal unit [7,13,15]. The early institution of extracorporeal membrane oxygenation (ECMO) with aggressive intensive care management has led to improved outcomes [23]. Initially, fresh frozen plasma should be given urgently in a dose of 10–15 mL/kg/12 h. If protein C deficiency is confirmed, onward therapy with protein C concentrate should continue until the skin lesions have healed [24]. Longer-term treatment is with oral anticoagulants. Liver transplantation can be curative. Any concomitant infection needs to be treated as well.

INFECTIONS

Although infectious diseases affecting the skin are described in detail elsewhere in this book, the clinical features of some of the more important infections affecting the skin during the neonatal period will be briefly considered here because of their importance in the differential diagnosis of other dermatoses.

VIRAL INFECTIONS

Neonatal herpes simplex

Herpes simplex virus infection in the newborn is generally a serious disease with a high mortality (Chapter 25). The worldwide incidence is estimated at about 10/100 000 live births and up to 40% of such infants are premature [1,2]. The majority of infections are a result of peripartum transmission of HSV type 1 (20%) and HSV type 2 (80%) through contact with an infected genital tract during delivery [1–4].

However, intrauterine HSV infection occurs rarely (5% of all neonatal HSV infections) [5], due either to transmission across the placenta or to ascending infection related to prolonged rupture of the fetal membranes. Intrauterine HSV is usually due to HSV type 2 and the risk is higher when HSV is a primary and/or disseminated infection in the mother. Infection may also occur postnatally by contact with non-genital sites, both maternal and non-maternal [6].

Most infants with neonatal HSV infection are born to mothers who have no previous history of genital HSV and who show no overt clinical signs of herpes at delivery. Up to two-thirds of women who acquire genital HSV during pregnancy manifest no symptoms or develop non-specific symptoms [2]. Over 70% of all infants with neonatal HSV infection have skin or mucosal lesions [7–9], but only in about 10–20% of cases will the disease be confined to the skin or mucous membranes. The skin lesions appear between days 2 and 20, unless intrauterine infection has occurred, in which case they will generally already be present at birth [5,10].

Isolated or grouped vesicles are the most common type of lesion, and the scalp and face are the most commonly affected sites, although lesions can occur at virtually any site (Figure 114.6). Occasionally, the eruption may be generalised and bullous, and

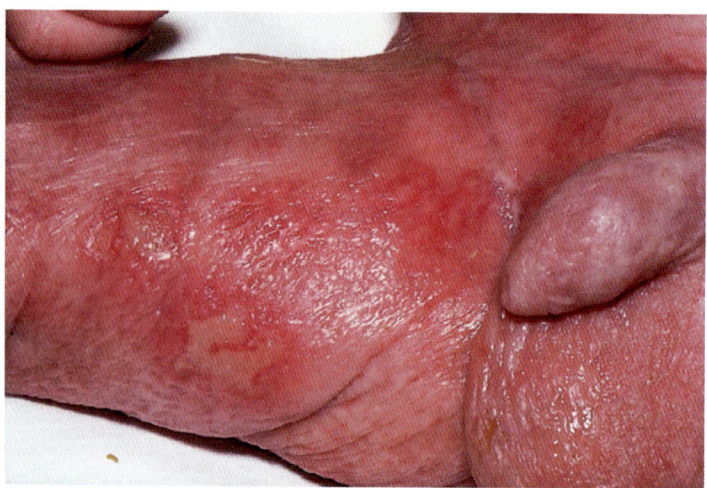

Figure 114.6 Neonatal herpes simplex showing congenital ulceration and scarring at 10 days. This infant responded rapidly to aciclovir therapy and is now entirely healthy apart from residual atrophy.

widespread erosions may occur without obvious vesicles or bullae, mimicking epidermolysis bullosa [10]. When infection is acquired during birth, the initial lesions have a predilection for the scalp in vertex presentations, and the perianal area in breech presentations. Lesions may also be localised to areas of intrauterine or intrapartum skin damage [9,11], such as the area in which a fetal scalp electrode was sited. Areas of cutaneous atrophy or scarring are not infrequent in the intrauterine form, and vesicular lesions may continue to appear within or at the periphery of these areas [5,12]. A zosteriform pattern has also been described and, in some cases [13,14], localised or generalised non-vesicular red macules. Congenital cutaneous calcification has been reported in a child with intrauterine HSV infection [15]. Oral lesions are also frequent, and take the form of erosions on the tongue, palate, gingivae and buccal mucosa. It may also present with widespread aplasia cutis [16].

A fatal outcome is unusual when infection is limited but mortality is high in disseminated or central nervous system infections even with appropriate therapy. Mortality is also higher with HSV type 2 infection [3]. Early recognition and adequate early treatment with aciclovir appear to protect infants from dissemination of infection where this is initially confined to the skin [11,12,17].

HSV infection in premature infants is even more severe in terms of clinical outcomes. In one study, 9 of 12 infants died and the other 3 had neurological sequelae [18]. It is also more difficult to diagnose as vesicular lesions are found in less than half of cases. It often presents with respiratory distress and thrombocytopenia. Non-specific signs such as lethargy, hypotension, raised aspartate transaminase and fits have also been observed. Diagnosis is by culture/PCR but treatment with intravenous aciclovir should not be delayed if HSV is suspected.

Ganciclovir (need to monitor for neutropenia) and foscarnet have also occasionally been used in treatment [19]. There is insufficient evidence to suggest that aciclovir prophylaxis in the third trimester of high-risk pregnancies affects the incidence of neonatal HSV although it will lessen the need for caesarean section [20].

Fetal varicella syndrome

Approximately 90% of adults are seropositive for the varicella-zoster virus (VZV) antibody. If a woman is seronegative, she may develop chickenpox during pregnancy (Chapter 25); this occurs in up to 10 per 10 000 pregnancies [1]. The infection may be transmitted to the fetus in about 25% of cases. Such transmission of VZV to the fetus is very rare in mothers who develop herpes zoster (shingles) during pregnancy [2].

When a mother develops varicella between the 7th and 20th week of pregnancy, spontaneous abortion may follow, or the child may be born with a variety of abnormalities considered characteristic of fetal varicella syndrome (FVS) (Box 114.3) [3–6]. This appears to occur most frequently when maternal infection has occurred between weeks 13 and 20 [1]. However, most children of such mothers are born with no detectable abnormality, despite laboratory confirmation of intrauterine infection. FVS therefore appears to be a relatively rare complication of maternal varicella early in pregnancy, with a fetal risk of approximately 2% [2,5,7]. Some authors have argued that occasionally FVS can occur as late as 28 weeks into the pregnancy [7,8].

Box 114.3 Principal clinical features of the fetal varicella syndrome

- Low birth weight
- Cutaneous lesions:
  - Localised absence of skin, usually on a limb
  - Scars, often of dermatomal outline
  - Papular lesions resembling connective tissue naevi
- Hypoplasia of one or more limbs (usually the limb affected by localised absence of skin or scarring) and/or malformed digits
- Ocular anomalies, including chorioretinitis, cataracts, microphthalmia, Horner syndrome
- Central nervous system abnormalities, including seizures, mental retardation, hydrocephalus, cortical atrophy, encephalitis, encephalomyelitis, dorsal radiculitis

---

Localised scarring, presumed to be the sequel to intrauterine ulceration, is the most common cutaneous feature of FVS. The larger single lesions characteristically occur on a limb, and have frequently been associated with hypoplasia of that limb; these lesions have generally followed infections occurring in early pregnancy [3,7–13]. Their segmental outline may be a direct consequence of damage to the fetal nervous system [4,9], as VZV is known to be strongly neurotropic, or to fetal herpes zoster [11]. The occurrence of larger numbers of smaller lesions appears to result mainly from varicella later in the pregnancy; their antecedents seem likely to be vesicular lesions, essentially the same as those occurring in postnatal varicella. If fetal infection has occurred in the last trimester, these smaller skin lesions, reflecting fetal varicella, may still be ulcerated at birth [14].

Areas of congenital localised absence of skin, without associated limb hypoplasia or other neurological abnormalities, have been a less well-recognised consequence of intrauterine varicella [15–17] and may reflect fetal herpes zoster infection later in gestation.

Skin-coloured papular lesions [18] and more verrucous lesions [19] have also been described in children with FVS.

If a child is born with 'full-blown FVS' the mortality is about 25% in the first 3 months of life [1].

Herpes zoster infection in early infancy is likely to indicate that the child has been infected with VZV *in utero* [20].

Pregnant women who are not immune (on the basis of history and, preferably, serology), and who experience exposure to VZV, should be given varicella-zoster immune globulin (VZIg) [21,22]. Although this can prevent or modify clinical varicella if given up to 3 days after contact, there is no definite evidence that it prevents fetal infection or damage [2]. Giving VZIg to neonates of mothers who have chickenpox at the time of delivery does not appear to reduce the incidence of clinical infection but may reduce its severity [**23**]. But, as the risk of fetal damage is small, termination of pregnancy is not indicated. Ultrasound examinations can be performed to detect some of the abnormalities that occur in the cardiovascular system, but several of the important ocular and neurological sequelae cannot be diagnosed in this way.

There are no reports that establish a role for aciclovir therapy in the prevention of FVS. Therefore, the decision whether to treat the mother should be based solely on the severity of her illness [21].

A potentially dangerous situation relates to maternal development of varicella in the 4 days either side of delivery [24]. In this case, neonatal varicella may also occur, but, in the absence of the protection offered by the maternal immune system, mortality may be as high as 30%. Where maternal infection occurs at this time, VZIg is recommended for the newborn. If overt varicella develops in the child, intravenous aciclovir should be added to the VZIg [25].

Congenital rubella

Rubella contracted by the fetus before the 20th week of gestation may result in disseminated infection, causing intrauterine growth retardation, microcephaly, microphthalmia and a wide variety of other abnormalities [**1**,**2**] (Chapter 25). Cutaneous lesions are among the most prominent clinical features of congenital rubella [3–7]. The typical lesions are present at birth, or make their appearance during the first 48 h. They comprise discrete, rounded, red or purple infiltrated macules, 3–8 mm in diameter. Although such lesions may be seen at any site, they generally occur in the largest numbers on the face, scalp, back of the neck and trunk. Occasionally, the lesions are slightly raised. They tend to fade over a period of weeks. These lesions have often been described as 'purpuric' and have generally been attributed to thrombocytopenia, which is another common feature of congenital rubella [4]. However, histological examination has shown them to comprise foci of dermal erythropoiesis [3,8]. Such lesions have frequently been described as 'blueberry muffin' lesions. Genuine thrombocytopenic purpura is probably rather uncommon.

Other reported skin manifestations of congenital rubella have included cutis marmorata, seborrhoea and hyperpigmentation of the forehead, cheeks and umbilical area [9], and discrete deep dimples over bony prominences, particularly the patellae [10].

Fewer cases are seen today and comprehensive vaccination programmes should allow for eradication of this condition [11].

Human immunodeficiency virus infection

Human immunodeficiency virus (HIV) infection may be transmitted to the infant *in utero*, during delivery or through breastfeeding (Chapter 31). Because most infections are probably transmitted around the time of birth, clinical manifestations are not commonly seen for the first few months, and some infected infants will remain asymptomatic for many years before manifestations first appear.

Mucocutaneous manifestations are common in infant HIV infection and frequently have an infective aetiology [1–3]. In a study in Ethiopia up to 75% of HIV-positive children had one or more mucocutaneous disorders – again showing infection to be more common than inflammatory disorders [4]. Studies in Tanzania [5] and Thailand [6] have shown similar results. Skin disease is more prevalent when there is a higher degree of immuosuppression.

Persistent mucocutaneous candidiasis is the commonest of all. In addition to infection of the oral and nappy areas, there may be extensive cutaneous involvement. Dermatophyte fungal infections are also characteristic, and infection with more unusual fungi may occur, including *Aspergillus* [7]. Bacterial infections include unusually severe or recurring impetigo, folliculitis, cellulitis and abscesses. Problems with viruses include atypical chickenpox, herpes zoster, herpes simplex and unusually severe molluscum and human papillomavirus infections. Norwegian scabies may present in infancy.

A wide variety of non-infectious manifestations of HIV infection may also occur. In a study of Ethiopian children [4], 'papular pruritic eruption of HIV' was the most common inflammatory disorder, seen in 30% of cases. Seborrhoeic dermatitis (sometimes severe) was also common, affecting 8% of children.

Drug eruptions are more frequent, especially with trimethoprim–sulfamethoxazole.

BACTERIAL INFECTIONS

As in older children and adults, *Staphylococcus aureus* causes a wide variety of cutaneous lesions in neonates. Other bacterial sources are important too, such as streptococci, *Listeria monocytogenes*, *Pseudomonas aeruginosa* and *Neisseria meningitidis*.

infection is acquired in hospital following delivery, the lesions do not generally appear until the second week of life, when the child will usually have left hospital.

The perineum, periumbilical area and neck creases are predilection sites for the initial lesions. Rapidly enlarging bullae with thin, delicate walls and a narrow, red areola contain clear fluid at first, which may later become turbid or frankly purulent. The condition may remain localised or become widespread. Untreated generalised bullous impetigo in the neonate is associated with a significant mortality; serious complications including lung abscess, staphylococcal pneumonia and osteomyelitis have been reported, even in cases treated with antibiotics [8,9].

The differential diagnoses of bullae and erosions in the neonate are given in Box 114.4.

Box 114.4 Differential diagnoses of bullae and/or erosions in the neonate [10]

More common disorders
- Miliaria crystallina
- Bullous impetigo
- Thermal or chemical burns
- Sucking blisters

Rare disorders
- Mastocytosis
- Infections: neonatal herpes simplex, fetal varicella syndrome, herpes zoster, congenital syphilis
- Passively transferred: pemphigus vulgaris, pemphigoid gestationis
- Bullous pemphigoid
- Porphyrias: congenital erythropoietic porphyria, transient porphyrinaemia
- Transient myeloproliferative disorder (Down syndrome)
- Congenital absence of skin
- Langerhans cell histiocytosis
- Extensive congenital erosions and vesicles healing with reticulate scarring
- Genodermatoses: epidermolysis bullosa, AEC syndrome, Weary–Kindler syndrome, ectodermal dysplasia–skin fragility syndrome (plakophilin-1 deficiency), bullous ichthyosiform erythroderma, incontinentia pigmenti

AEC, ankyloblepharon/ectodermal dysplasia/cleft lip and palate.

Bullous impetigo

The neonate is peculiarly liable to the development of bullous impetigo, which is most often caused by phage group II strains of *S. aureus* [1]; meticillin-resistant *S. aureus* has been reported as a causative organism [2] (Chapter 26). The disorder in neonates differs in no significant way from that in older children and adults, although it was formerly distinguished by the rather confusing term pemphigus neonatorum. Epidemics of bullous impetigo, in which some infants may develop staphylococcal scalded skin syndrome, have occurred in neonates due to transmission of infection in the nursery principally via nursing or medical staff [3–7]. Although the

Staphylococcal scalded skin syndrome

The staphylococcal scalded skin syndrome (SSSS) was first described in neonates by a German, Ritter von Rittershain [1]. It is caused by epidermolytic toxins A and/or B, which are elaborated by certain strains of *S. aureus*, most commonly of phage group II, particularly strains 71 and 55 [2,3] (Chapter 26). These toxins reach the skin via the circulation from a distant focus of infection, usually in the umbilicus, breast, conjunctiva or site of circumcision or herniorrhaphy. Transmission of the causative toxin through human milk has been reported [4]. Both these toxins attack desmoglein 1 (a desmosomal protein), so mucosal involvement does not occur (this is analogous to pemphigus foliaceus, which has the same target antigen) [5,6].

The disorder is most often seen in young children, particularly in neonates. The very much greater incidence of this condition in neonates is believed to reflect less efficient metabolism and excretion of the toxin. Multiple cases can occur in a neonatal unit [6]. Cases occurring in later childhood tend to be associated with underlying disease, especially immunosuppression and renal failure [7].

It does not present at birth, although it may appear within the first few hours thereafter [8]. The first sign of the disease is a faint, macular, orange-red, scarlatiniform eruption [3,4]. The eruption generally becomes more extensive, and over the next 24–48 h turns to a more confluent, deep redness with oedema. The surface then becomes wrinkled before starting to separate, leaving raw, red erosions. Sites of predilection for the development of erosions are the central part of the face, the axillae and the groins. It can result in widespread skin denudation.

Extreme tenderness of the skin is an early feature, and may occur at a stage where cutaneous signs are not yet striking. The child is pyrexial and distressed. These features can lead to a suspicion that the child has arthritis or an acute abdomen. The presence of impetiginous crusting around the nose and mouth can be diagnostically helpful. Recovery is usually rapid, even without antibiotic therapy, although infants occasionally die in spite of such treatment. Healing occurs without scarring.

The scalded appearance of the skin differentiates the disease from bullous impetigo, and the rapid onset with marked cutaneous tenderness distinguishes it from most of the other causes of erythroderma in infancy. The rarity of clinically apparent bullae and the confluent nature of the rash help differentiate it from those bullous disorders likely to be seen in young children.

Milder forms of SSSS have been described where the same toxin-producing *S. aureus* is isolated but where clinically the rash starts as impetigo on the face followed by an exanthem with peeling mostly confined to the skin folds [9]. The children have mild pyrexia but no shock or fluid disturbance.

The main differential diagnosis is toxic epidermal necrolysis but this condition shows mucosal involvement. If there is any doubt, the two conditions may be distinguished by histology; a frozen section provides rapid differentiation. The level of split in toxic epidermal necrolysis is lower at the subepidermal level, but is intraepidermal in SSSS.

Treatment is with either a penicillinase-resistant penicillin analogue, such as co-amoxiclav, or with a cephalosporin or sodium fusidate [10,11]. A recent study found that SSSS-associated isolates demonstrated significantly higher rates of clindamycin resistance and lower rates of nestling resistance compared with overall staphylococcal infections. Clindamycin, a ribosomal inhibitor, is frequently recommended as a first line agent in SSSS to reduce toxin production. Cephalosporins are now favoured for empirical therapy [12]. If the attack is severe, the drug should initially be given intravenously. Systemic corticosteroids are contraindicated as they aggravate the disease [13,14]. Appropriate compensation must be made for heat and fluid losses and hyponatraemia. Pain will also require treatment, and affected infants will generally be much more comfortable if the lesions are dressed rather than left open [15]. In severe cases, it may occasionally be justifiable to ventilate

the patient in order to obtain adequate relief of pain. Pneumonia itself can be a complication.

Even with treatment mortality is 2–10% in children, but this usually reflects late diagnosis.

Periporitis staphylogenes and sweat gland abscesses

Periporitis staphylogenes is the term applied to pustular lesions appearing in neonatal skin as a result of secondary infection of miliaria by *S. aureus* [1–4]. Such lesions may progress to sweat gland abscesses, although it is not clear whether sweat gland abscesses are always a complication of miliaria. These disorders have in the past been incorrectly called 'folliculitis and furunculosis of the newborn'. Sweat gland abscesses are distinguished from furuncles clinically by a lack of any tendency to 'point', 'coldness' and the absence of tenderness. Outbreaks caused by medical staff in neonatal units have been described [5].

Periporitis must be distinguished from miliaria pustulosa, which is not an infective disorder, and from bacterial folliculitis, which in the neonate is usually caused by *S. aureus*. *Candida albicans* and *Malassezia furfur* may also cause pustulosis in the neonate, and a number of non-infective conditions may cause confusion such as eosinophilic pustulosis.

Mastitis and breast abscesses

Infection of the breast is common and is usually associated with *S. aureus*, but a variety of other bacteria may be responsible including *Acinotobacter buamannii* and *Foeniculum vulgare* [1–3]. It is almost always unilateral; it occurs within the first 8 weeks of life, most commonly in the second or third week of life. It occurs more often in girls than boys, and only very rarely in the preterm infant. The affected breast is swollen and often red and hot. Systemic toxicity is usually absent. Fluctuation implies abscess formation, which will require surgical drainage [4]. Colour flow Doppler ultrasound helps distinguish mastitis from an abscess [5,6]. The development of a breast abscess may lead to the loss of breast tissue in the longer term [4,7].

Neonatal staphylococcal cold abscesses of the large folds

A number of neonates have been described presenting with 'cold' abscesses in the skin folds (groins and axillae) shortly after birth [1]. These children are well with no associated fever or malaise although the lesions may fistulate. Lesions have also been seen in occipital, submandibular and supraclavicular areas. There may be an associated omphalitis. Culture of pus from these lesions grows *S. aureus*. Treatment with oral antibiotics is usually sufficient and leads to rapid resolution of the lesions, although some children may require an incision and drainage procedure [2].

PART 10: SPECIFIC SITES, SEX & AGE

Omphalitis

Omphalitis is rare in the developed world (0.7% of births) but is more of a problem for developing countries (up to 6% of births). The mean age of development is 3.2 days [1]. It is characterised by redness, oedema and discharge of the umbilical 'stump'. Cases can progress to cellulitis and deeper tissue infection. It is more common in protracted labour, non-sterile delivery and cord care, prematurity, low birth weight and some cultural practices such as the application of tobacco ash [2].

The umbilical cord may become colonised by a variety of potentially pathogenic bacteria, and an equally wide variety of topical antiseptics and antibiotics have been used in an attempt to reduce this colonisation. The use of hexachlorophane was popular until it became apparent that this could lead to serious neurotoxicity, particularly in the preterm infant [3]. The best substitute may be chlorhexidine, applied as a dusting powder or aqueous solution rather than as an alcoholic solution [4]. In developing countries, 4% chlorhexidine has been shown to reduce omphalitis and to reduce neonatal mortality [5–8]. Since 1998, the World Health Organization has advocated the use of dry umbilical cord care where possible [9]. A recent meta-analysis provided no evidence for antiseptic treatment of the cord with chlorhexidine [8].

Occasionally, infection of the umbilical cord becomes disseminated, either by bloodstream invasion or by direct extension via the umbilical vessels to the peritoneal cavity. Tetanus, diphtheria and necrotising fasciitis [10] may also occur as complications of umbilical infection. Such infections are still responsible for a high proportion of deaths in the neonatal period in developing countries.

Preorbital and orbital cellulitis

Preorbital cellulitis is restricted to the part of the orbit anterior to the orbital septum and is manifest by eyelid swelling. Orbital cellulitis involves the structures deep to the septum and presents with painful proptosis, eyelid oedema and conjunctival redness [1]. A variety of bacteria can cause these infections, such as S. aureus, including meticillin resistant strains [2,3], and group A and other streptococci. One should always be alert to the possibility of group B Streptococcus as a rare cause of periorbital cellulitis or any form of cellulitis in a neonate in view of the high risk of septicaemia with this organism [4,5]. Treatment is with intravenous antibiotics and occasionally surgery.

Necrotising fasciitis

This name is given to a distinctive form of cellulitis in which infection tracks along the fascial planes, causing thrombosis of the blood vessels running through the fascia with resulting necrosis of the skin, subcutaneous fat and even muscle [1,2] (Chapter 26). In neonates, it may arise spontaneously, but most often is a complication of physical birth trauma, omphalitis, breast abscess or iatrogenic skin wounds such as result from scalp electrodes [3,4] or

circumcision [5]. The mother's genital tract may also be the source of the infection [6,7].

Initially, the infant develops what appears to be straightforward cellulitis, usually affecting the abdominal wall. However, the child becomes disproportionately toxic, and the area affected becomes indurated, discoloured and extends progressively [2,8–10]. The surface may show a peau d'orange appearance. Purpura and, occasionally, bullae may develop in the centre of the indurated area, often followed quite rapidly by frank necrosis. The destruction of superficial nerves results in local cutaneous anaesthesia. Gas and crepitation may be clinically apparent, or may be seen radiologically. Fever is not invariably present.

A wide variety of bacteria have been associated with necrotising fasciitis, most commonly group A streptococci, but also group B streptococci, Staphylococcus aureus and Escherichia coli [7–9]. In many cases, a synergistic infection by aerobic and anaerobic organisms appears to be responsible. Occasionally, fungi have been responsible. Antibiotic (and antifungal) therapy appears to be of limited value in this potentially lethal situation. The most important aspect of treatment is early surgical excision of the necrotic tissue [9,10]. This 'gold standard' of treatment has been challenged by some authors who advise a more conservative approach [11,12], but most doctors would still advise early surgical debridement. Cultured epidermal autografts have also been used successfully [13].

Neonatal listeriosis

Listeriosis during the neonatal period is uncommon, but dangerous. The responsible organism, Listeria monocytogenes, may be transmitted to humans principally through contaminated foods [1]. In pregnancy, it causes a non-specific, mild, influenza-like illness in the mother [2,3], but it may lead to transplacental infection of the fetus. Maternal HIV infection may predispose to neonatal listeriosis [2]. Adult listeriosis has increased in a number of European countries during the early 21st century, but mostly in the elderly and not as yet in pregnancy-related cases [4]. Attention to food hygiene and recall of contaminated products have reduced the prevalence of neonatal listeriosis by 44% in the USA. Products made with unpasteurised milk are a common source of infection. A large epidemic of L. monocytogenes occurred in South Africa in 2017; epidemic neonatal listeriosis was associated with a predominance of bacteraemic, early-onset disease. Listeriosis-associated mortality rates were higher than previously published [5].

Clinically, there are early-onset and late-onset forms of neonatal listeriosis [6–11]. The early-onset form results from the development of miliary granulomas following blood-borne dissemination of infection. Severely affected babies tend to be born prematurely and there is a high mortality. Postmortem studies reveal miliary granulomas in many organs. A few infants will have analogous miliary skin lesions during life, manifest as scattered, discrete, grey or white papules or pustules about 1–2 mm in diameter, with a red margin, which will provide a source of organisms for culture. The back appears to be the site of predilection for such lesions, which are also seen in the mouth and on the conjunctiva. Other cutaneous lesions have been described in such babies, including purpura and morbilliform rashes. However, in the majority of cases the skin is not involved in the initial clinical presentation [12].

The late form of the disease is commoner, taking the form of meningitis, occurring a week or two after birth.

Diagnosis is by culturing the organism from a variety of sites, including cerebrospinal fluid, blood, urine and from biopsy material, including the skin. Treatment is usually with a combination of parenteral ampicillin with gentamicin or tobramicin, followed by a prolonged 3–4-week course of oral ampicillin.

Ecthyma gangrenosum

Pseudomonas aeruginosa is common in the hospital environment and infections are encouraged by the widespread use of broad-spectrum antibiotics (Chapter 26). A weak mechanical defense barrier and underdeveloped cellular or humoral immunity increase the risk of infection from this pathogen in newborns. Most, but not all, neonates who develop the skin lesions of ecthyma gangrenosum have *P. aeruginosa* septicaemia, usually in the context of predisposing factors that include prematurity, renal failure, neutropenia and other immunodeficiencies, necrotising enterocolitis and bowel surgery [1–3,4]. Occasionally, the lesions develop at the site of direct inoculation of the causative organism. Other bacteria have been implicated such as *E. coli* and *Klebsiella* [4,5,6].

Histologically, the presence of vasculitis, due to bacterial infiltration of the vessel walls, is characteristic, together with haemorrhage and necrosis [7]. For this reason skin biopsy can be very helpful in diagnosis.

Clinically, lesions initially take the form of painful macular red skin or purple ecchymosis [1–3,4,8,9]. The centre then generally develops either vesicles (or less commonly bullae) or pustules, which rapidly ulcerate. Subsequently one or more ulcers occur, each with a depressed, necrotic, often black, crusted centre and a raised edge. The perioral and perianal areas may show grouped lesions.

This infection is potentially dangerous when it occurs in the setting of septicaemia. Appropriate parenterally administered combination antibiotic therapy will be required. Awareness of this presentation in neonates is critical since its presence prompts the need for early treatment, as *Pseudomonas* infections carry a high mortality rate [9].

Noma neonatorum (cancrum oris/oro-facial gangrene)

Noma neonatorum is a gangrenous disorder. The primary site of involvement is the oral cavity. Other sites have included the nose, eyelids, umbilicus, scrotum and groin [1–3]. Reported onset is from the third postnatal day to 120 days of age. Noma neonatorum occurs in low-birth-weight and/or premature neonates, almost exclusively in developing countries [1–3]. It is frequently caused by *P. aeruginosa* and is almost invariably lethal in the absence of appropriate

antibiotic treatment. A similar condition may be seen in older children and adults in the context of poor nutrition, delayed growth and immunodeficiency [4,5]. It was also seen in concentration camp victims in the Second World War.

Treatment is with parenteral antibiotics and often requires plastic surgery later to repair large facial defects. Surgical repair is generally delayed for 1 year post resolution [6].

Purpura fulminans

Although in the newborn this condition is most often a reflection of genetically transmitted thrombophilic disorder, it may be caused by acute infections, particularly with endotoxin-associated, Gram-negative bacteria such as *Neisseria meningitidis* [1,2].

Congenital syphilis

Congenital syphilis is described in detail in Chapter 29, but its cutaneous manifestations in the neonate will be considered here briefly because of their importance in differential diagnosis [1]. About 15% of children born to mothers with untreated syphilis will contract congenital syphilis, but fetal loss/stillbirth occurs in about 20% of such pregnancies.

The skin is clinically affected in about 40% of neonates with congenital syphilis [1,2]. In such cases, the skin is usually of normal appearance at birth, the initial lesions occurring between the second and eighth week, and occasionally later. Sites of predilection are the ano-genital area, the face and the palms and soles. The lesions themselves are reddish brown in colour; they may be macular or papular, and tend to be larger and firmer than those seen in acquired secondary syphilis (Figure 114.7). In about 3% of cases the lesions are bullous; keratoderma and desquamation of the extremities have been described [3,4]. Paronychia is commonly present. Small, round, moist, papular lesions, traditionally termed mucous patches,

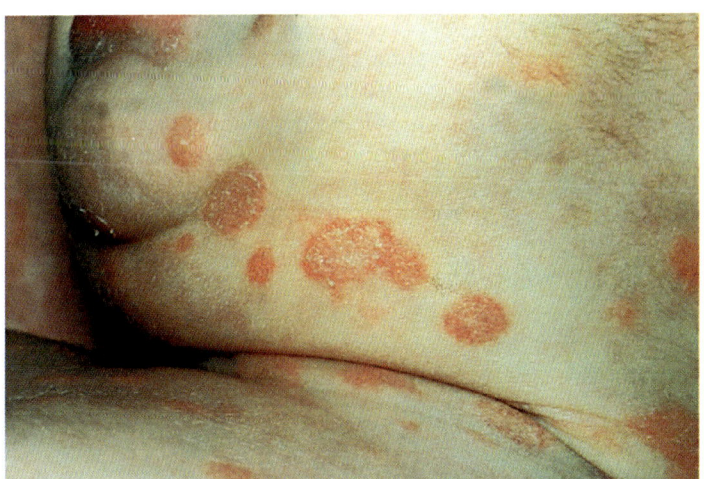

Figure 114.7 Congenital syphilis showing nummular erythematosquamous lesions in a 4-week-old infant.

are frequently present in the mouth and on other mucosal surfaces. Condylomata lata may be present in the ano-genital flexures or at other flexural sites, for example between the toes or in the angles of the mouth.

Birth weight is below 2500 g in approximately 50% of affected infants. Apart from the cutaneous features, the most frequent clinical manifestations of congenital syphilis in the newborn are hepatomegaly, splenomegaly, jaundice, pneumonia and rhinitis, often with a blood-stained discharge.

The recent resurgence in the incidence of syphilis in many countries may lead to an increase in cases of congenital disease, especially where antenatal care is poor [2,5,6].

Congenital tuberculosis

Tuberculosis in the newborn due to transmission of infection *in utero* is relatively rare (Chapter 27). The lungs and/or liver tend to be the predominant sites of involvement, and skin manifestations are unusual. However, cutaneous lesions have occasionally occurred, in the form of small numbers of discrete, umbilicated, red papules up to 4 mm in diameter [1]. Congenital tuberculosis has a high mortality rate. In a recent retrospective review from China the mortality rate was 43.48% [2].

FUNGAL INFECTIONS

Both *Candida* and *Malassezia* species can cause neonatal fungal disease. There are two distinct forms of neonatal candidiasis, present at birth or seen in the first weeks of life.

Neonatal candidiasis

This is a relatively common disorder that occurs in the early weeks after birth, in the form of oral candidiasis with or without candidiasis in the nappy area (Chapter 32). The rash is usually focused in the perianal area and is a deep 'beefy' red colour, with a moist appearance, often with pustules at the periphery, which is often scalloped in outline. Just beyond the margin, in as yet unaffected skin, there may be punctate red lesions, sometimes pustular ('satellite' lesions).

It is assumed that the infection is acquired during delivery from the mother's genital tract, and it should be borne in mind that the frequency of vaginal candidiasis at the time of delivery is between 20% and 25% [1].

Occasionally, the rash may become more generalised. The occurrence of localised palmar pustules in an infant with neonatal oral candidiasis was believed to reflect the inoculation of *Candida* from the mouth into the skin as a result of sucking [2].

Treatment is with topical anticandidal creams and oral gels. Systemic neonatal candidiasis is a particular problem for preterm babies on intensive care units where it can cause septicaemia and death. Often there are no associated skin lesions. Treatment is with intravenous antifungal therapy.

Congenital candidiasis

This is a rarer condition, seen at birth, which is generally believed to reflect maternal *Candida* chorioamnionitis resulting from ascending infection from the genital tract [1–4,5,6,7]. A total of 10–35% of women suffer from candidal vaginitis during pregnancy, but less than 1% of them develop candidal chorioamnionitis that can affect the fetus [8]. It appears that *Candida* is, however, able to find its way into the amniotic fluid without prior rupture of membranes. Foreign bodies in the uterus or the cervix increase the risk, particularly intrauterine contraceptive devices [9]. There is no evidence that maternal antibiotic therapy or immunodeficiency in the infant plays a role in predisposition [6,10].

An extensive eruption of scattered pinkish red macules and papules is present at birth or appears within a few hours. The lesions generally progress to a vesicular phase, and then either to a pustular or a bullous phase, over a period of 1–3 days. More or less any part of the skin surface may be affected, including the nails, palms and soles. In fact, palmar and plantar pustules are regarded as a hallmark of congenital cutaneous candidiasis. Paronychia may occur and isolated involvement of the nail plates has been described [11]. Oral involvement is usually absent, and the nappy area tends to be spared, at least initially.

Very low-birth-weight infants may have a scalded appearance, and are particularly at risk of systemic infection.

When infection is confined to the skin, affected infants are generally well, and the rash clears within a week with appropriate topical antifungal therapy, for example with topical ketoconazole. Usually there is prominent postinflammatory desquamation.

Skin and mucosal involvement may be complicated by systemic candidiasis, particularly in the premature baby [2,12]. The lungs may be affected [13]; hepatosplenomegaly and abnormal liver function have also been recorded [6]. Candidal meningitis is another potential complication [14]. Criteria have been proposed that indicate a high risk of systemic involvement. Systemic antifungal therapy should be considered in at-risk infants [9]; amphotericin B is probably the drug of choice [9,12].

Studies have shown that intravenous fluconazole prophylaxis in very low-birth-weight infants can reduce both invasive candidiasis and mortality rates [15–17], but a Cochrane review using oral antifungal prophylaxis in preterm infants has not shown a definitive benefit [18].

Malassezia pustulosis

Colonisation of the skin by *Malassezia furfur* starts soon after birth and progresses until the age of about 3 months, probably reflecting the activity of the sebaceous glands during this period [1,2]. This yeast has been a cause of systemic infections in infants receiving intravenous lipids, and it is presumed that the source of organisms in such cases is the skin [3].

It is now believed that *M. furfur* and *M. sympodialis* may be a frequent cause of red papulopustular eruptions occurring on the face and scalp in neonates, a condition now widely termed neonatal cephalic pustulosis [2,4,5], although not all neonates with this clinical presentation had detectable *Malassezia* in the lesions [6]. This type of rash was reported to have a frequency of 10% in neonates seen as out-patients in a paediatric dermatology department [5], with pustule contents showing *M. furfur* yeasts in over half of these. A good therapeutic response to the topical application of 2% ketoconazole cream for 15 days was seen in almost every case. A frequency of 66% was reported in one study, with 62% being culture positive for *Malassezia* [6].

Differential diagnosis includes eosinophilic pustulosis of the scalp, transient pustular melanosis, scabies, neonatal acne and infections with *Candida* or *Staphylococcus aureus* [7].

Key references

The full list of references can be found in the online version at https://www.wiley.com/rooksdermatology10e

Introduction
Skin function in the neonate
Barrier function
6 Raone B, Raboni R, Rizzo N *et al*. Transepidermal water loss in newborns within the first 24 hours of life: baseline values and comparison with adults. *Pediatr Dermatol* 2014;31:191–5.
8 Kusari A, Han AM, Virgen CA *et al*. Evidence-based skin care in preterm infants. *Pediatr Dermatol* 2019;36:16–23.

Eccrine sweating
8 Munsters J, Wallström L, Agren J *et al*. Skin conductance measurements as pain assessment in newborn infants born at 22–27 weeks gestational age at different postnatal age. *Early Hum Dev* 2012;88:21–6.

Sebaceous gland secretion
4 Visscher MO, Utturkar R, Pickens WL *et al*. Neonatal skin maturation – vernix caseosa and free amino acids. *Pediatr Dermatol* 2011;28:122–32.

Appearance of neonatal skin
Full-term neonate
3 Rivers JK, Frederiksen PC, Dibdin C. A prevalence survey of dermatoses in the Australian neonate. *J Am Acad Dermatol* 1990;23:77–81.

Skin disorders in the neonate
Toxic erythema of the newborn
5 Marchini G, Nelson A, Edner J *et al*. Erythema toxicum neonatorum is an innate immune response to commensal microbes penetrated into the skin of the newborn infant. *Pediatr Res* 2005;58:613–16.

Miliaria
3 Mowad CM, McGinley KJ, Foglia A *et al*. The role of extracellular polysaccharide substance produced by Staphylococcus epidermidis in miliaria. *J Am Acad Dermatol* 1995;33:729–33.

Transient pustular melanosis
8 Chia PS, Leung C, Hsu YL *et al*. An infant with transient neonatal pustular melanosis presenting as pustules. *Pediatr Neonatol* 2010;51:356–8.

Infantile acropustulosis
7 Dromy R, Raz A, Metzker A. Infantile acropustulosis. *Pediatr Dermatol* 1991;8:284–7.

Neonatal pustulosis of transient myeloproliferative disorder
1 Burch JM, Weston WL, Rogers M *et al*. Cutaneous pustular leukemoid reactions in trisomy 21. *Pediatr Dermatol* 2003;20:232–7.

2 Viros A, Garcia-Patos V, Aparicio G *et al*. Sterile neonatal pustulosis associated with transient myeloproliferative disorder in twins. *Arch Dermatol* 2005;141:1053–4.

Congenital erosive and vesicular dermatosis healing with reticulated supple scarring
9 Nemazi L, Cuddy L, Clayton TH. Congenital erosive and vesicular dermatosis with reticulated scarring in twins, associated with oesophageal atresia. *Clin Exp Dermatol* 2022;47:809–11.

Complications of prematurity
Anetoderma of prematurity
2 Wain EM, Mellerio JE, Robson A *et al*. Congenital anetoderma in a preterm infant. *Pediatr Dermatol* 2008;25:626–9.

Complications of medical procedures on the fetus and neonate
Neonatal medical procedures
1 Cutler VE, Stretcher GS. Cutaneous complications of central umbilical artery catheterization. *Arch Dermatol* 1977;113:61–3.
25 Harpin VA, Rutter N. Percutaneous alcohol absorption and skin necrosis in a premature infant. *Arch Dis Child* 1982;57:477–9.

Atrophic lesions of neonates
Medallion-like dermal dendrocyte hamartoma
1 Rodriguez-Jurado R, Palacios C, Duran-McKinster C *et al*. Medallion-like dermal dendrocyte hamartoma: a new clinically and histopathologically distinct lesion. *J Am Acad Dermatol* 2004;51:359–63.

Disorders caused by transplacental transfer/maternal milk
Neonatal pemphigus vulgaris
8 Mallory L, Foster BS, Spaulding RT *et al*. Neonatal pemphigus vulgaris. *JAMA* 2021;157:220.

Transplacental pemphigoid gestationis
10 Cohen S, Strowd LC, Pichardo RO. Pemphigoid gestationis: a case series and review of the literature. *J Dermatol Treat* 2018;29:815–18.

Neonatal lupus erythematosus
21 Porcel Chacón R, Tapia Ceballos L, Díaz Cabrera R *et al*. Neonatal lupus erythematosus: a five-year case review. *Reumatol Clin* 2014;10:170–3.

Disorders of subcutaneous fat
Subcutaneous fat necrosis of the newborn
11 Muzy G, Mayor S, Lellis R. Subcutaneous fat necrosis of the newborn: clinical and histopathological correlation. *An Bras Dermatol* 2018;93:412–14.

Miscellaneous disorders
'Blueberry muffin' baby (dermal erythropoiesis)
1 Karmegaraj B, Vijayakumar S, Ramanathan R *et al*. Extramedullary haematopoiesis resembling a blueberry muffin, in a neonate. *BMJ Case Rep* 2015;2015:bcr2014208473.

Neonatal purpura fulminans
9 Sharma S, Anbazhagan J, Plakkal N. Neonatal purpura fulminans due to protein C deficiency. *Arch Dis Child Fetal Neonatal Ed* 2015;100:F453.

Infections
Viral infections
Fetal varicella syndrome
23 Miller E, Cradock-Watson JE, Ridehalgh MK. Outcome in newborn babies given anti-varicella-zoster immunoglobulin after perinatal maternal infection with varicella-zoster virus. *Lancet* 1989;2:371–3.

Congenital rubella
1 Karthikeyan K, Venkatesh C, Soundararajan P. Congenital rubella syndrome: a continuing conundrum. *Lancet* 2012;379:2022.

2 Freij BJ, South MA, Sever JL. Maternal rubella and the congenital rubella syndrome. *Clin Perinatol* 1988;15:247–57.

Bacterial infections
Staphylococcal scalded skin syndrome
1 Ritter von Rittershain G. Die exfoliative Dermatitis jungerer Sauglinge. *Central Zeitung Kinderheilk* 1878;2:3–23.

Omphalitis
1 Fahmy M. Omphalitis. In: *Umbilicus and Umbilical Cord*. Cham: Springer, 2018: 119–31.

Ecthyma gangrenosum
4 Prindaville B, Nopper A, Lawrence H *et al*. Chronic granulomatous disease presenting with ecthyma gangrenosum in a neonate. *JAAD Online* 2014;71:e44–5.
8 Biddeci G, Cutrone M, Mattei I *et al*. Ecthyma gangrenosum of the cheek in a 6-month-old infant. *Arch Dis Child* 2015;100:55–6.

Fungal infections
Congenital candidiasis
5 Darmstadt GL, Dinulos JG, Miller Z. Congenital cutaneous candidiasis: clinical presentation, pathogenesis and management guidelines. *Pediatrics* 2000;105:438–44.

CHAPTER 115
Dermatoses of Infancy

Lea Solman and Mary T. Glover

Great Ormond Street Hospital for Children NHS Foundation Trust, London, UK

Introduction

No hard and fast definition of infancy exists, so for the purposes of this chapter the infant period is regarded as from 4 weeks to 18 months, with emphasis on the first year of life. An overview of the most common or important dermatoses presenting in this age group is discussed, but the list is not exhaustive.

INFLAMMATORY CONDITIONS

Cradle cap

Although cradle cap may be seen in the neonate, the condition is most common between the ages of 4 and 16 weeks, and is estimated to affect up to 41.7% of infants [1]. It can occur in isolation or in association with seborrhoeic dermatitis (see the next disorder).

Large flakes of yellowish scale are seen on the scalp, especially over the vertex and frontal regions, and may become matted into large plaques of crust (Figure 115.1). There is usually minimal inflammation. Mild cases are very common. The condition is asymptomatic and the infant is always well. In extensive cases, Langerhans cell histiocytosis (LCH) should be considered. Most cases of cradle cap resolve spontaneously after a few weeks. An emollient will help lift the scale, and may be used in combination with a mild shampoo [2]. A topical non-steroidal cream may be therapeutically beneficial [3].

Seborrhoeic dermatitis

Infantile seborrhoeic dermatitis (ISD) is distinct from seborrhoeic dermatitis in later life (Chapter 40). Typically, ISD occurs between the ages of 4 and 12 weeks, but most commonly before the age of 2 months (64%) with 28% occurring later, between 2 and 4 months [4]. Characteristically, in addition to redness and scale on the scalp and eyebrows, macerated redness occurs in the skin folds, especially the neck (Figure 115.2) and the inguinal regions. Yeasts,

PART 10: SPECIFIC SITES, SEX & AGE

Rook's Textbook of Dermatology, Tenth Edition. Edited by Christopher Griffiths, Jonathan Barker, Tanya Bleiker, Walayat Hussain and Rosalind Simpson.
© 2024 John Wiley & Sons Ltd. Published 2024 by John Wiley & Sons Ltd.

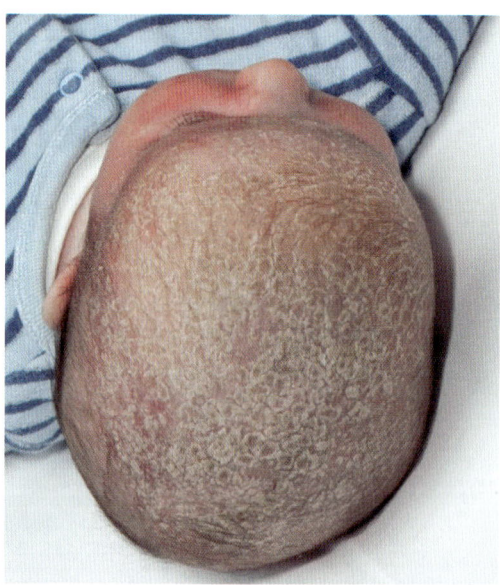

Figure 115.1 Cradle cap: adherent yellow scale on the scalp of an 8-week-old infant.

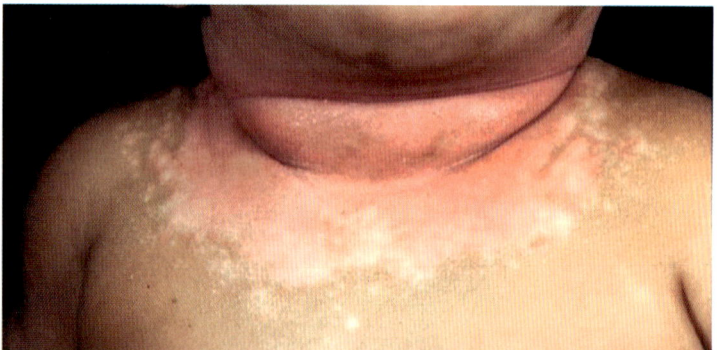

Figure 115.2 Seborrhoeic dermatitis showing macerated erythema in the neck folds of a 3-month-old girl associated with some postinflammatory hypopigmentation.

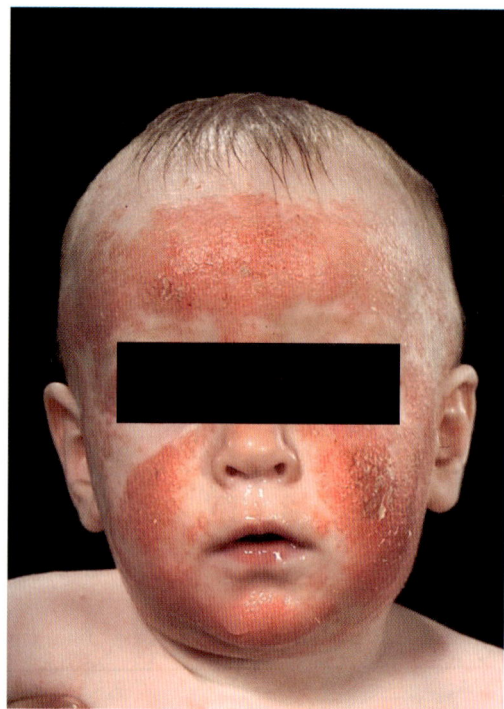

Figure 115.3 Atopic eczema showing facial involvement in a 5-month-old infant.

particularly *Malassezia* species, may be isolated from intertriginous areas and colonisation with yeasts is significantly greater in infants with ISD than in their healthy counterparts [5].

The child is healthy and often well above the median centile for weight. ISD is rarely symptomatic. Typically, the inflammation resolves with transient hypopigmentation, which can be very pronounced in children with darker skin colour. Repigmentation generally occurs within a few weeks.

Differential diagnosis includes irritant napkin dermatitis, atopic eczema and LCH. If the onset is very acute, the infant is febrile or there is significant desquamation, Kawasaki disease should be considered.

In mild cases, treatment with emollient alone has been shown to be as effective as a weak topical steroid [6]. Combination steroid–antifungal creams are often employed in cases where inflammation is marked, but should only be used for short periods.

Some infants may go on to develop atopic eczema and the two conditions can merge. It is estimated that 34% of infants with ISD go on to develop atopic eczema at an average time interval of 6 months [7].

Atopic eczema

Atopic eczema (AE) is very common in developed countries and is the most frequent reason for infants to be referred to a dermatologist (Chapter 41). Mutations in the filaggrin encoding gene (*FLG*) have been shown to be a major factor in susceptibility to AE, through the disruption of the epidermal barrier function [8]. A European cohort study has estimated that the cumulative prevalence of AE in the first 2 years of life is 21.5% [9]. Prevalence peaks at 10% at 18 months [10], slightly earlier for boys than girls [11]. Epidemiological studies have shown that the prevalence of AE among black children born in the UK or USA is significantly higher than in their white peers [12,13], and that being born abroad appears to confer protection from atopic disease for at least a decade after migration [13].

In infants, AE characteristically begins on the face (Figure 115.3) [11]. Some children show a nummular (discoid) pattern, predominantly on the back and legs (Figure 115.4), and most commonly in winter. However, evidence of flexural involvement in infancy has the highest predictive value of AE persisting at age 3 years [11]. Although secondary infection is a common component of AE, early colonisation with *Staphylococcus aureus* is not associated with persistence of AE [14].

Infantile eczema present at 1 month of age is associated with a cord blood eosinophilia and a higher rate of wheezing and subsequent AE [15]. Infants with AE who are exclusively breastfed are also significantly more likely to be sensitised to common foodstuffs, particularly if the disease is severe, possibly through epidermal barrier dysfunction [16]. However, there is a lower incidence of AE in infants who were born extremely prematurely (<29 weeks'

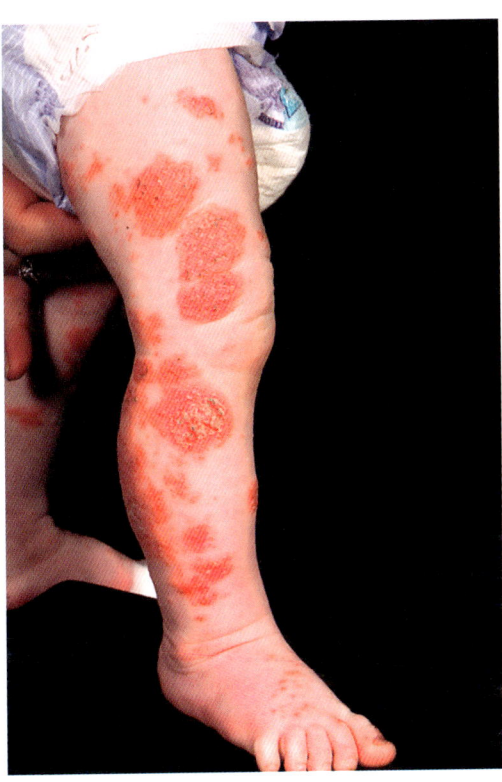

Figure 115.4 Nummular, discoid pattern on the legs of a 5-month-old infant.

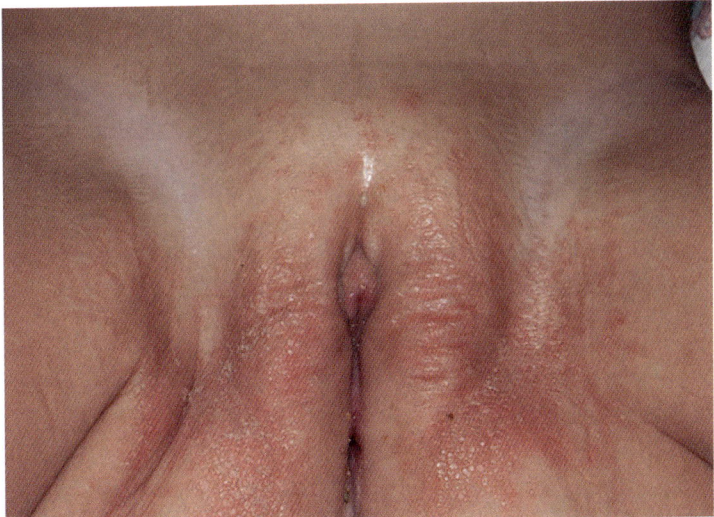

Figure 115.5 Napkin dermatitis showing redness, with relative sparing of the skin folds.

gestation) [17], and duration of neonatal intensive care exposure is associated with a decreased risk of atopic eczema [18].

Of children presenting early in infancy, 43.2% are in complete remission by age 3 years [9]; 38.3% have intermittent disease, but 18.7% have evidence of symptoms every year [9]. A history of early AE is associated with asthma at school age [9]. However, estimate of total IgE at 6 months is the best predictor of the persistence of AE [19]. Certain *FLG* mutations have also been found to predict persistent symptoms [20]. The management of infantile atopic eczema for the most part is with topical treatments, and is aimed at restoring skin barrier function [21,22], reducing inflammation, treating secondary infection and providing parental education and support (Chapter 41).

Food allergy is reported in 10–30% of children with AE, most commonly arising from allergen presentation through eczematous skin [23]. Prompt and effective treatment at this age can prevent the development of chronic eczema.

Topical therapy is the cornerstone of management of infants with AE and dietary interventions if clinical features indicate possible food-related exacerbation [24]. Dietary intervention should be undertaken in an informed and evidence-based manner to ensure it is appropriate and that the essential nutrition, growth and development of the infant are maintained.

Napkin dermatitis

Napkin (diaper) dermatitis has become less frequent since the advent of modern disposable nappies, which are more absorbent than cloth [25]. Traditional cloth nappies are still in widespread use in some parts of the world, associated with levels of napkin dermatitis as high as 50–70% [26]. Prolonged contact with urine induces an irritant redness, which may break down to form erosions if untreated. Transepidermal water loss and pH are higher in infants with napkin dermatitis than those without [26].

Involved areas are those in contact with the irritant (e.g. the buttocks), while the skin folds may be spared (Figure 115.5), in contrast to seborrhoeic dermatitis and infantile psoriasis.

Treatment is aimed at keeping the skin dry and using barrier creams or emollients. Topical steroids should only be used in the short term and only if inflammation is severe; secondary infection should be treated appropriately.

Punched-out ulcers may be seen in persistent cases of napkin dermatitis. They are thought to be due to the irritant effect of urine compounded by secondary infection and are considered to be part of the spectrum of presentation of napkin dermatitis, along with infantile gluteal granuloma [27]. Jacquet dermatitis, characterised by erosive lesions with elevated borders, is rare nowadays due to the improved absorbency of modern nappies.

Infantile gluteal granuloma

Overuse of potent, especially fluorinated, steroids under occlusion in infants with napkin dermatitis has been thought to be the cause of a granulomatous inflammatory reaction, characterised by reddish brown nodules on the buttocks [27]. Treatment requires avoidance of further topical steroids and the use of emollients to restore the epidermal barrier.

Infantile psoriasis

Estimates of the frequency of psoriasis in children are 3–4% [28,29], but the prevalence appears to be increasing [28,30]. Of children affected, 27% present before the age of 2 years [31] (Chapter 35).

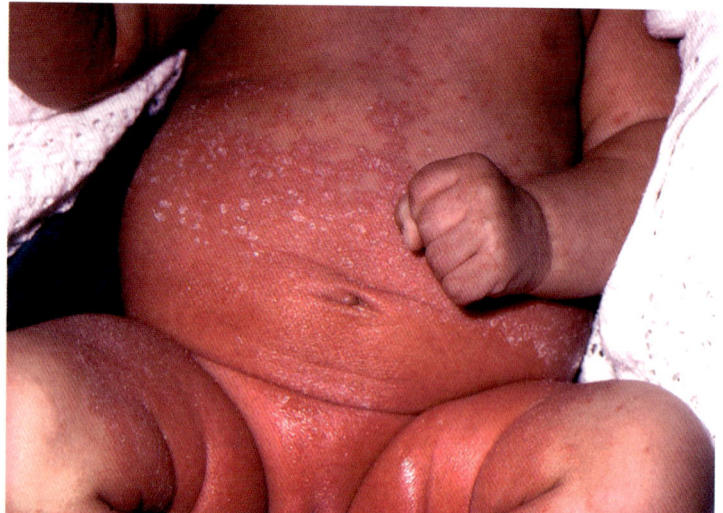

Figure 115.6 Infantile psoriasis.

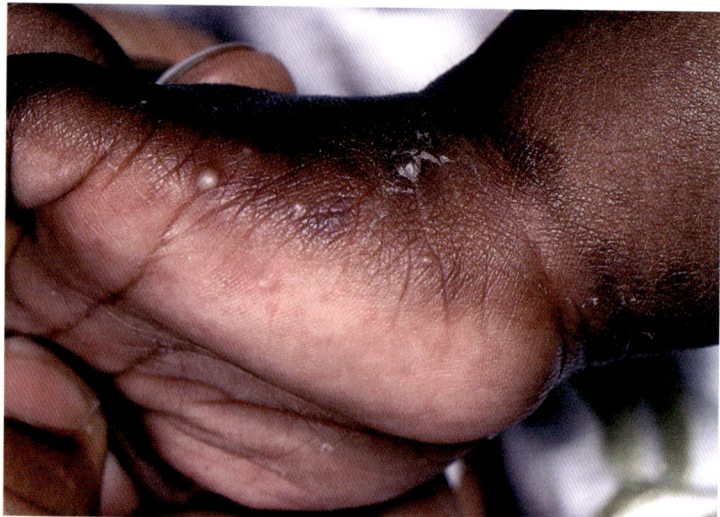

Figure 115.7 Infantile acropustulosis showing discrete pustules along the medial border of the foot of an 11-month-old boy.

Involvement of the nappy area is the most common presentation in infants (Figure 115.6) [31].

Although some authors consider infantile psoriasis to be a self-limiting disease [32], it may be a prelude to more typical chronic plaque psoriasis in later life [33]. All patterns of psoriasis have been described in children: guttate, chronic plaque, pustular and erythrodermic [29,32], but severe disease and joint involvement are relatively rare [34].

Treatment is determined by the extent and severity of disease. In the majority of infants, emollients and mild topical steroids, often in combination with an anticandidal agent, is sufficient [33].

Parakeratosis pustulosa is a localised inflammatory condition involving the distal phalanx. Usually a solitary digit is involved – fingers more frequently than toes. Characteristically, the thumb, index finger or great toe is affected. The skin signs are very characteristic [35,36], with sharply demarcated redness and scale of the skin adjacent to the nail fold, with accompanying nail dystrophy, resembling the changes seen in Hallopeau psoriasis. Pustulation is seen in 25% [35], but swabs are sterile and mycology is negative. The nail may be shed.

The condition is fairly resistant to treatment, but usually resolves over the course of 12–18 months. Potent steroids and antibiotics may be of some benefit. There may be a family history of psoriasis, and the condition may be a prelude to psoriasis in later life [35].

Infantile acropustulosis

Synonyms and inclusions
- Acrodermatitis pustulosa

Infantile acropustulosis is a rare disorder characteristically affecting children between the ages of 1 and 2 years [37]. It appears more frequent in boys. Crops of itchy vesicopustules, 2–4 mm in diameter, appear along the borders of the feet, particularly around the heel (Figure 115.7). Occasionally, similar changes occur on the palm.

The pathogenesis is not well understood. The differential diagnosis is scabies infestation and sometimes the condition is seen to follow a genuine scabies infection, as a persistent, reactive, postinflammatory phenomenon.

Topical steroids are rarely of benefit. The condition tends to resolve spontaneously over 6–12 months.

Pityriasis alba

Transient, hypopigmented areas on the face, associated in some cases with fine scale, are common in school-aged children, but less frequent in infants. When pityriasis alba does occur in infants, it may be more extensive [38]. It tends to be more common in boys [39]. It appears most frequently on the cheeks. Lesions are often ovoid, with indistinct margins. It is asymptomatic.

Individual lesions resolve over a few weeks, but can be recurrent. The condition is considered to be part of the atopic spectrum [39,40] (85% of affected infants have an atopic history [40]). Emollients can help reduce the scale and mild topical corticosteroids or calcineurin inhibitors may speed resolution [38], but are rarely required.

Infantile acne

Infantile acne is rare. The majority of infants affected (75%) are male and most do not have a family history of acne [41]. The mean age of onset is 6 months (range 0–21 months) [42]. The cheeks are the most commonly affected area [42].

Most infants have mild or moderate disease with inflammatory papules (Figure 115.8), but 17% have comedones and in 14% the disease is classified as severe [41]. Scarring is estimated to occur in 17% of infants with acne [41]. No underlying endocrinopathy was found in infants [41,43], in contrast to older children presenting with

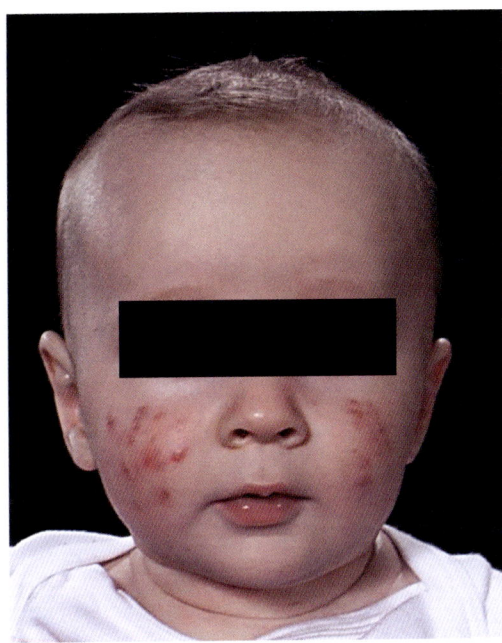

Figure 115.8 Infantile acne showing papules, pustules and comedones in a 6-month-old boy.

preadolescent acne, in whom more detailed investigation may be merited.

Treatment may be topical (benzoyl peroxide, erythromycin or retinoids) in mild cases [41]. More extensive disease may require oral erythromycin. Trimethoprim can be used in cases of erythromycin resistance [41]. Prolonged treatment may be required (18–24 months) [41]. In severe disease, oral isotretinoin, typically 0.5 mg/kg/day, with cumulative doses of up to 60–162.5 mg/kg, has been shown to be safe and effective in infants, without evidence of adverse effects on bone development [42].

Urticaria

Urticaria in infancy differs from urticaria in adults in that it presents more frequently with haemorrhagic lesions and angio-oedema [44] (Chapter 42). Anaphylactic shock is very rare in the first year of life [45,46]. Approximately half of infants presenting with urticaria have a personal or family history of atopy [44].

Infection, usually viral, with or without drug intake, appears to be the cause of urticaria in the majority of cases [44]. Foods appear to be responsible in fewer than 10% of cases. In the first year of life, cow's milk, hen's eggs and wheat are the most common allergens. In the second and third year of life the top three food allergens are hen's eggs, cow's milk and peanuts [47].

Chronic or recurrent urticaria is reported to occur in 30% of cases [44]. Physical factors are more likely to be implicated in chronic urticaria [48]. Cholinergic urticaria, precipitated by exercise, emotion and heat, is common. Cold may be a trigger in up to 8% of cases [49].

Urticaria in infancy may be a feature of systemic disease including systemic lupus erythematosus, juvenile rheumatoid arthritis, mastocytosis and Kawasaki disease [50], but is very rarely the only presenting feature. Urticaria is associated with attacks of fever, musculoskeletal and sensorineural inflammation and high levels of acute phase reactants in the cryopyrin-associated periodic syndromes including the Muckle–Wells syndrome and NOMID/CINCA (neonatal-onset multisystem inflammatory disease/chronic infantile neurological, cutaneous and articular syndrome), arising from gain-of-function mutations in the *NLRP3* gene, leading to excessive interleukin 1 (IL-1) signalling [51–53].

INFECTIVE CONDITIONS

COVID-19/SARS-CoV-2 (SEVERE ACUTE RESPIRATORY SYNDROME CORONAVIRUS 2)

Urticarial [1], papulovesicular, morbilliform and purpuric eruptions, and acral pernio-like lesions [2] have been reported in infants infected with Covid-19, although less commonly than in older children and adults (Chapter 25).

Paediatric inflammatory multisystem syndrome, temporally associated with SARS-CoV-2 (PIMS-TS), also known as multisystem inflammatory syndrome (in children) (MIS(-C)) is also less common in infants than older children. Cutaneous features have most frequently been described as morbilliform or erythrodermic, with features similar to those of Kawasaki disease (see later) [3].

VIRAL EXANTHEMS

Many viral infections are associated with a transient rash, which may be macular, maculopapular (with or without petechiae), urticarial or vesicular [1,2]. Often this is non-specific and harmless [1], but some viral infections have very characteristic features that allow a diagnosis to be made. Atypical exanthems present more of a challenge [2]. A detailed account of viral infections appears in Chapter 25, but the most frequent or important infections seen in children are highlighted here. Viral exanthems account for the most common presentation to a paediatric emergency department [3]. Differentiation from exanthems due to other causes (drugs, bacterial toxins, autoimmune disease) must be made [1,2]. Overall, petechial changes are much more likely to occur in exanthems associated with infections, particularly of viral origin (although meningococcal septicaemia should always be considered) [2]. A declining rate of vaccinations in some countries requires a high level of expertise for the clinical diagnosis of both classic and atypical presentations of viral exanthems. The spectrum of viral causes of exanthems has widened with emergence of novel viruses and advances in laboratory diagnostic methods [4].

Roseola infantum

Synonyms and inclusions
- Exanthema subitum

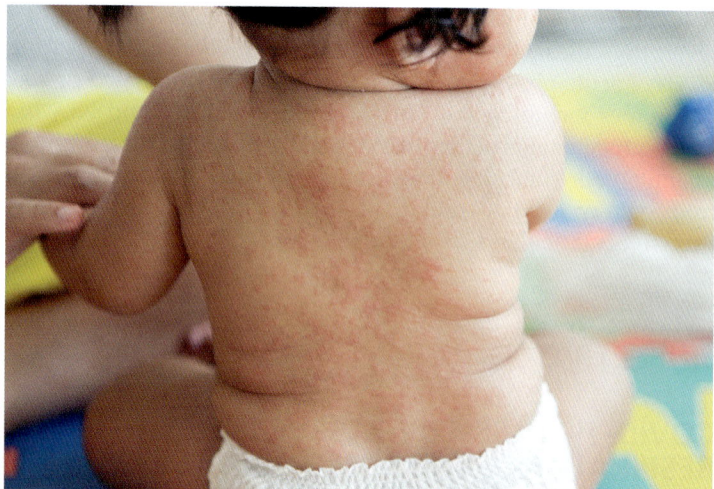

Figure 115.9 Fine, lacy rash on the back of the infant. Source: phadungsak sawasdee/Shutterstock.com.

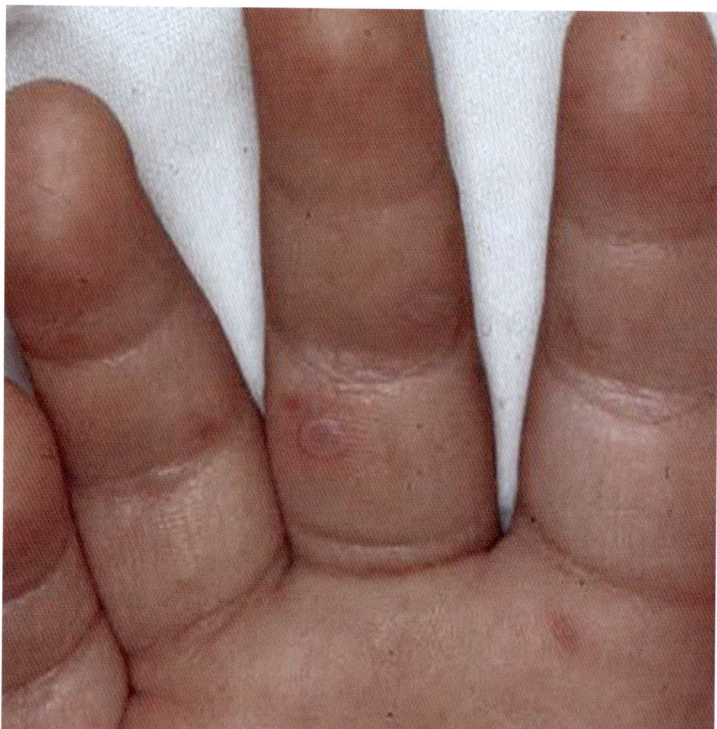

Figure 115.10 Hand, foot and mouth disease showing small vesicles with surrounding redness on the palmar aspect of the fingers.

Roseola infantum has a peak prevalence between 6 and 12 months of age with 90% of cases occurring in children younger than 2 years. It occurs equally in boys and girls [5]. It is characterised by a high fever lasting for 3–5 days and may rarely be associated with febrile convulsions [6]. As pyrexia subsides, a fine, lacy, macular redness appears, which may be accompanied by occipital or cervical lymphadenopathy (Figure 115.9). The rash fades over 48 h without desquamation. The incubation period is 5–14 days. Although initially associated with human herpesvirus 6 (HHV-6) infection [7], cases due to HHV-7 are now also reported [8].

Fifth disease

Infection is due to parvovirus B19 [7] and the incubation period is 7–14 days. Infection occurs in epidemics, predominantly in the spring. The sudden onset of a rash on the face, with hot, bright red cheeks, gives rise to the typical 'slapped cheek' appearance. A more reticulate rash then appears on the limbs and body, and palmoplantar redness is common. The eruption fades over 7 days, but recrudescences are not infrequent, particularly if the child gets hot (e.g. in sunlight, after a bath or exertion).

European studies estimate seroprevalence to be 20% in children aged 1–3 years, and rising with age [9]. Older individuals may develop a papulopruritic eruption in a glove and stocking distribution with parvovirus B19 infection [10], but this pattern is rarely seen in infants. The virus may lead to serious cytopenia in children with malignancy [11].

Hand, foot and mouth disease

This is a common infection in young children, affecting the oral cavity and extremities. Vesicles, which may be very painful, develop in the mouth and may ulcerate. Small, tense blisters, with a surrounding rim of redness, occur on the palms (Figure 115.10) and soles and fade within 3 days. It is most commonly associated with Coxsackie A viral infection, most usually A16 [12], but infection with A6 [13], Coxsackie B [12] and enterovirus 71 [12] have also been described. Spread is by droplets or faecal contamination and the incubation period is 7 days. However, virus may be present in the faeces for several weeks after infection, making isolation impractical [12]. Symptomatic treatment only is required, but it is highly contagious and widespread outbreaks are common.

Varicella

Varicella is still common in the UK, where vaccination is not routine. The incubation period is 14–21 days. The onset of the rash may be preceded by 1–2 days of malaise and fever. Skin lesions begin as small red macules which rapidly evolve into papules followed by characteristic vesicles. Lesions occur in crops, crusting over as they resolve, and lesions in different stages of evolution are evident. The eruption may become widespread but retains a centripetal pattern. The child should be isolated until the lesions have crusted over. The majority of cases are self-limiting and can be managed in the community. Severe cases, or chickenpox occurring in immunosuppressed children, should be treated with aciclovir. Encephalitis may occur, but is rare in infants younger than 12 months. The prevalence of complications in infants is inversely proportional to the level of antivaricella zoster virus maternal antibodies and varicella severity [14]. Passively acquired maternal immunity persists for about 4 months, but then rapidly declines after the neonatal period [15]. The incidence of complications from varicella among infants with severe disease hospitalised for infection rises from 10% in babies younger than 1 month of age to over 70% at 5 months [14].

Measles

The decline in uptake of MMR vaccination in the UK over recent years has been associated with a resurgence of measles infections due to loss of herd immunity. In an outbreak in northwest England, 22% of cases were younger than 13 months [16]. At this age, children would not usually have received their initial vaccination in the UK, but herd immunity would have conferred protection. Encouragingly, recent public health campaigns and immunisation programmes in schools seem to be increasing uptake again [17].

Measles is caused by an RNA paramyxovirus. The infection is spread by droplets and the incubation period is 7–14 days. An initial prodrome of fever and coryzal symptoms is followed after 3 days by the development of small, white Koplik spots on the buccal mucosa. On the fourth day of the illness the rash appears, initially on the forehead, spreading caudally down the face onto the trunk and limbs. Complications can be serious and include bronchiolitis, otitis media and encephalitis. Treatment is supportive, but children remain infectious for 7 days after the onset of the rash.

OTHER INFECTIONS AND INFESTATIONS

Impetigo

Impetigo is a very common, highly contagious cutaneous infection, occurring in children worldwide [1]. The usual causal organism is *Staphylococcus aureus*, but *Streptococcus pyogenes* may also be implicated (Chapter 26). Honey-coloured crusts appear on a background of redness. The child is usually well. Children aged 2–5 years are most frequently affected, but as the condition is so highly infectious, spread within families, including to infants, is common.

Bullous and non-bullous forms exist. Non-bullous impetigo most typically occurs on the face (Figure 115.11), whereas bullous impetigo is more often seen in intertriginous areas such as the napkin area, axilla or neck folds. Bullae arise as a result of production of staphylococcal exotoxins specific for desmoglein 1 [2]. Affected areas are painful and become eroded. The bullous form is more frequent in the autumn [2]. The choice between topical or oral antibiotics depends on the severity and extent of involvement. Antibiotic resistance is increasing [3]. Topical disinfectants can help reduce colonisation [3].

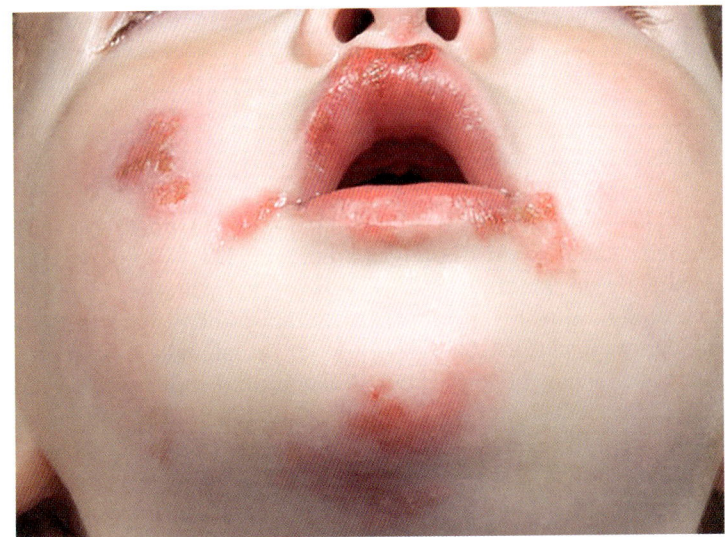

Figure 115.11 Impetigo showing multiple lesions on the cheeks, lip and chin of a 10-month-old infant.

Staphylococcal scalded skin syndrome

The estimated incidence of staphylococcal scalded skin syndrome (SSSS) is 0.56 cases/million population per year, with a median age of 2 years, males and females being equally affected [2] (Chapter 26). There is a seasonal peak in the autumn [2]. Several exfoliative toxins have been identified [2], but exfoliative toxin B is more likely to be associated with SSSS and exfoliative toxin A with bullous impetigo [4]. Isolating the causal organism can be difficult.

Following a prodrome of fever, irritability and malaise, tender redness appears with subsequent development of superficial flaccid blisters, typically around the flexures and perioral region, progressing to peeling and erosions (Figure 115.12). Pain is a prominent feature and affected infants resist movement or touch.

Management is with intravenous antibiotics and supportive care with liberal emollients, attention to fluid balance and adequate analgesia. Differentiation from Stevens–Johnson syndrome/toxic epidermal necrolysis should be made clinically, due to sparing of the

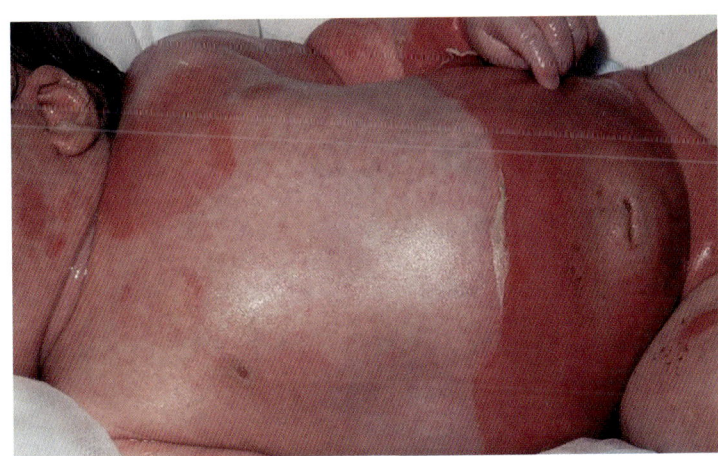

Figure 115.12 Staphylococcal scalded skin syndrome showing widespread peeling and erosions in a 2-month-old infant.

mucous membranes. Resolution over 2–3 weeks is usual and mortality is low in otherwise healthy infants. Recurrence is very rare [5].

Blistering distal dactylitis

Typically, large acral bullae, oval in shape and up to 1–3 cm in diameter, develop on the finger pulps, but may also occur more proximally on the digits and even occasionally on the palms. The condition is due to infection with Gram-positive bacteria, most frequently *Staphylococcus aureus* [6], but occasionally β-haemolytic *Streptococcus* may be implicated. When multiple bullae are present, *Staphylococcus* is the more likely culprit organism, and the condition is considered to be a localised bullous impetigo.

Infants should be swabbed to look for bacterial colonisation of the nares, conjunctiva and anus [6]. The differential diagnosis includes epidermolysis bullosa simplex and sucking blisters. Management is by deflating the blisters, dressing eroded areas and using appropriate antibiotics. Resolution is usually rapid.

Perianal streptococcal dermatitis

This presents as a beefy redness with oedema in a circumferential and well-demarcated distribution 2–3 cm around the anal margin [7] (Figure 115.13). Pain can be severe and blood may be seen in the stool. The condition is due to β-haemolytic streptococcal infection. It responds rapidly to appropriate oral antibiotics and rarely recurs unless an intrafamilial reservoir of *Streptococcus* is responsible for its transmission.

Cutaneous *Candida* infection

Transient oral candidiasis is common in infants, infection probably having been acquired during delivery [8]. Colonisation of eroded

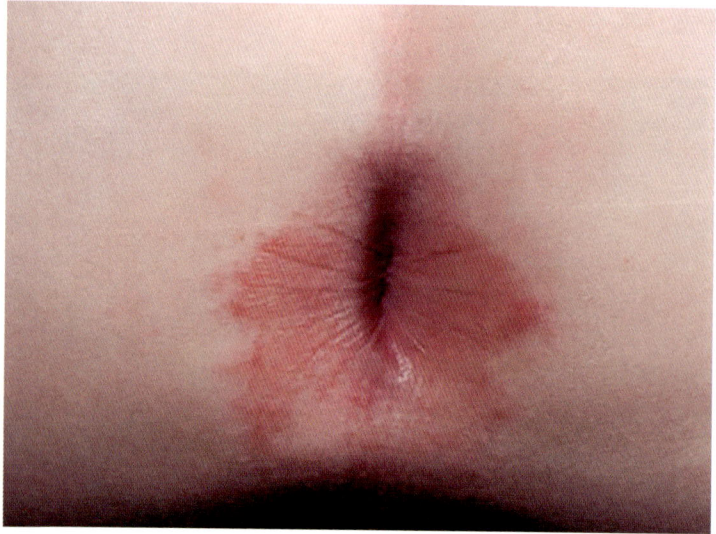

Figure 115.13 Perianal streptococcal dermatitis showing well-demarcated redness.

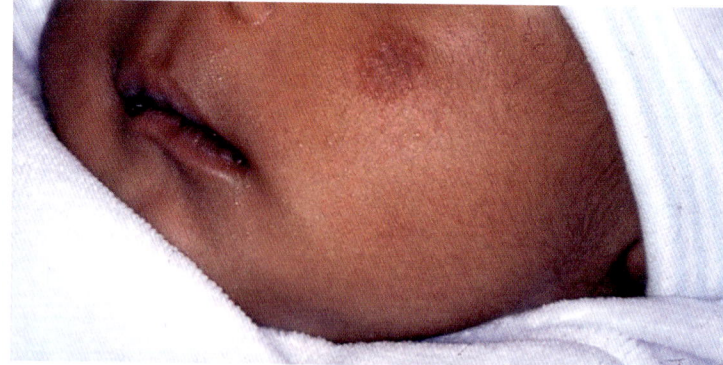

Figure 115.14 Tinea faciei in a 4-week-old baby inoculated from an older sibling with tinea capitis.

or macerated skin in intertriginous areas, especially the napkin region [9], is less common. Satellite pustules are characteristic.

Topical treatment will usually suffice and resistance is rare [9]. Recurrent, persistent or extensive infections should prompt investigation for an underlying immunodeficiency.

Tinea corporis

Tinea infections in children younger than 1 year of age are relatively unusual, and nearly always acquired from an older child [10] (Chapter 32). In very young infants, the face is the most common site of inoculation (Figure 115.14) [10]. In the UK, infection with *Trichophyton tonsurans* is predominant, especially in urban areas, but occasional sporadic cases of *Microsporum canis* or *M. audouinii* may occur. In cases of *T. tonsurans* tinea corporis, the reservoir of infection is always an infected scalp, so if an infant is seen with tinea faciei, their own scalp, but particularly those of their older siblings, should be screened for tinea capitis.

Annular, inflammatory lesions, which clear from the centre, most usually occur on the cheek in infants. Lesions may occasionally be vesicular and often resolve with postinflammatory hyperpigmentation. Treatment for purely cutaneous lesions is with a topical antifungal agent for 2 weeks, but if scalp involvement is suspected or proven, oral therapy will be required.

Tinea capitis

Scalp ringworm due to *T. tonsurans* has reached epidemic proportions in urban areas of the UK and USA in recent decades (Chapter 32). Spread through nurseries and day care facilities is common [11,12]. Tinea capitis in infants may be mistaken for seborrhoeic dermatitis. In rural areas, sporadic cases of animal ringworm may occasionally occur, but are exceedingly rare in this age group. In Europe, *M. canis* still predominates, but patterns of infection are changing with wider migration [13].

The presentation and clinical signs vary and include patchy or localised alopecia, diffuse scale and black dots due to swollen, broken-off hairs. Pustules, or a focal inflammatory kerion, may also occur. Cervical lymphadenopathy is common. Mycological confirmation is always recommended, as treatment schedules vary depending on the causal fungus [11]. Oral therapy is the gold standard [11], and although griseofulvin remains the only licensed treatment for tinea capitis in children in the UK, worldwide practice has demonstrated that in cases of *T. tonsurans*, oral terbinifine and itraconazole are preferred for their greater efficacy and are well tolerated in young children. Itraconazole has the advantage of being available in a liquid formulation, so is preferred in infants. All family contacts should be screened to try and minimise reinfection [13].

Scabies

Extreme pruritus characterises infestation with the mite *Sarcoptes scabei*. The condition is highly contagious. Estimates of prevalence in children range from 4.8% in parts of Europe [14] to 21.5% in India [15], but worldwide it is very common and has a significant impact on global health [16] (Chapter 34). In infants, burrows may be seen on the palms and soles more characteristically than in the finger webs. The wrists are commonly involved. Burrows can appear inflamed, with surrounding secondary eczematous changes. Nodular lesions develop in the axillae and genital region if the infection is untreated.

Eradication requires treatment of the individual and all close contacts using a topical scabecidal lotion or cream, in two applications 7 days apart. In recalcitrant cases, ivermectin has been shown to be safe and well tolerated in infants [17]. Post-scabetic pruritus may be prolonged.

Molluscum contagiosum

This is an extremely common cutaneous viral infection characterised by discrete, pearly, umbilicated papules 2–5 mm in diameter (Figure 115.15). Lesions usually occur in the axilla or groin, but may be widespread, especially in children with atopic eczema [18]. Spread between siblings is frequent. The condition is more prevalent in tropical climates [19]. The condition generally resolves spontaneously within 12 months [19]. Ablative treatments such as cryotherapy or laser, and topical treatments with hydrogen peroxide creams or commercially available potassium hydroxide, may destroy individual lesions but do not appear to reduce the overall duration of infection.

REACTIVE CONDITIONS

Acute haemorrhagic oedema in infancy

Acute haemorrhagic oedema is a benign, cutaneous, leukocytoclastic vasculitis, arising after respiratory infection, medication administration or immunisation in approximately 75% of cases [1]. It is thought likely to be an immune complex-mediated vasculitis.

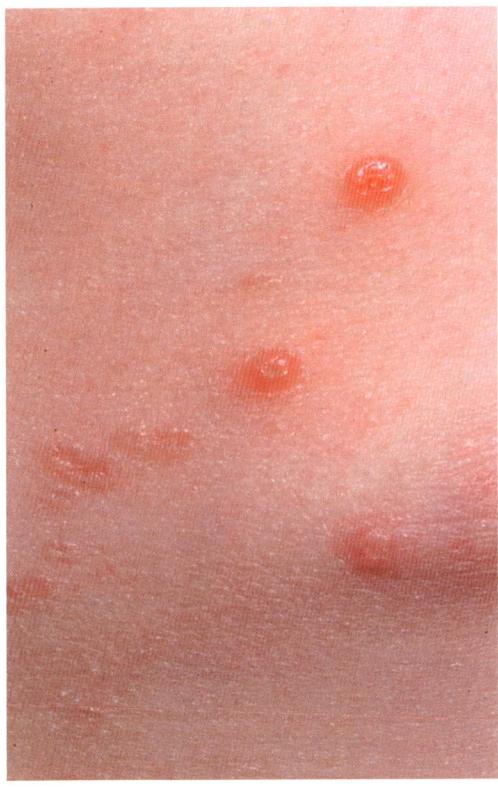

Figure 115.15 Molluscum contagiosum: typical pearly umbilicated papules on the trunk of a 12-month-old infant.

Although histopathology typically shows leukocytoclastic vasculitis with fibrinoid necrosis and erythrocyte extravasation [2], in some cases fibrinoid necrosis is not evident [1]. Perivascular IgA deposits have been found in about one-third of cases [2].

The condition affects children between the ages of 4 months and 2 years, with males being affected twice as frequently as females. Fever is mild and systemic disturbance is minor. The limbs and face are the most commonly affected areas. Lesions are discrete or confluent with purpura often appearing in a targetoid or cockade pattern (Figure 115.16). Oedema mainly affects the eyelids, face and extremities. Visceral and joint involvement is not typical. Some cases may show features of Henoch–Schönlein purpura [1]. The differential diagnosis includes purpura fulminans, erythema multiforme, urticarial disease and Kawasaki disease, but in all these conditions the child appears unwell. Resolution of acute haemorrhagic oedema in infancy occurs within 3 weeks, and recurrences are not a feature. Treatment is not required

Kawasaki disease

Kawasaki disease is a febrile illness with systemic vasculitis, first described in Japan four decades ago, but now recognised worldwide [3] (Chapter 100). It typically affects children aged 3–6 years, but can be seen in infants. It is estimated that about 17% of cases occur in children under 1 year of age, with a median age of 7 months.

Recognition of the clinical signs is imperative, as early diagnosis and treatment are central to preventing complications, such as

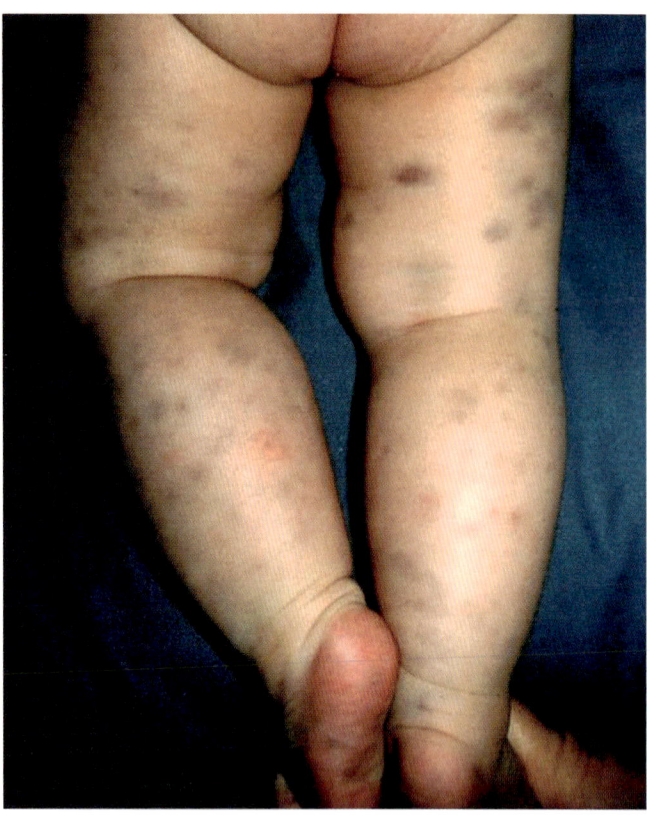

Figure 115.16 Multiple eccymotic and purpuric areas on the legs of a 10-month-old infant with acute haemorrhagic oedema in infancy.

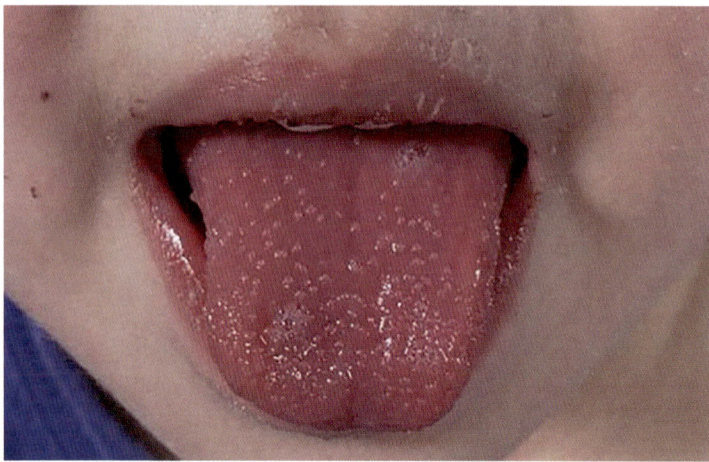

Figure 115.17 Cracked lips and strawberry tongue in a 15-month-old infant with Kawasaki disease.

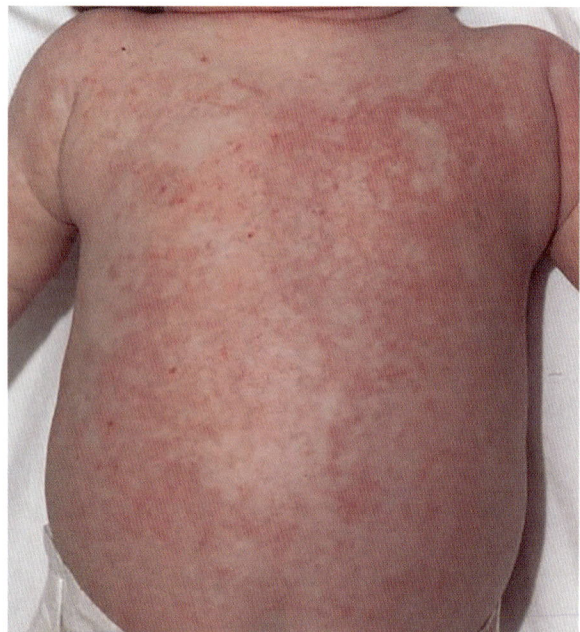

Figure 115.18 Generalised morbilliform rash on a 12-month-old infant with Kawasaki disease.

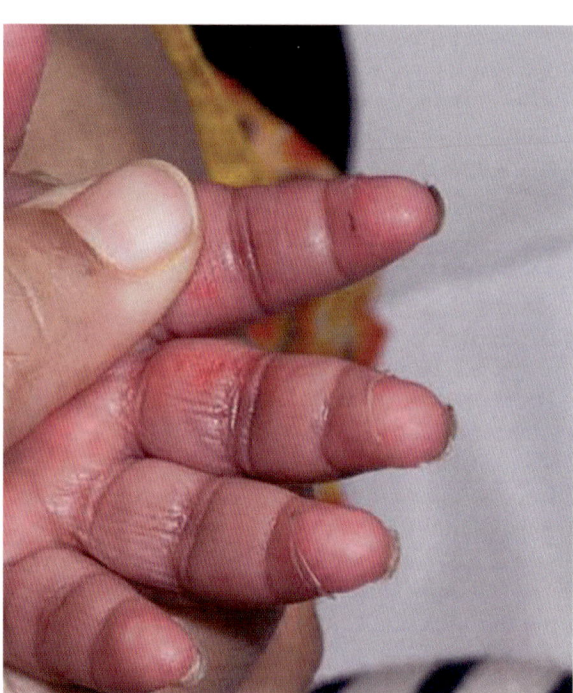

Figure 115.19 Swelling and distal desquamation of the fingers of a 13-month-old infant with Kawasaki disease.

coronary artery aneurysms. Kawasaki disease in infants is more likely to be atypical (the rash and conjunctivitis may be much less prominent), and treatment instituted late, resulting in a higher risk of complications and poorer outcome [4,5]. Kawasaki disease should be considered in all infants younger than 6 months of age with unexplained, persistent fever, as presentation is often incomplete [3].

High fever lasting up to 8 days, associated with conjunctival injection, red, cracked lips and strawberry tongue (Figure 115.17),

is followed by the development of a generalised maculopapular rash (Figure 115.18) with prominent swelling and redness of the hands and feet, which then desquamate (Figure 115.19). Cervical lymphadenopathy may be pronounced.

Leukocytosis, thrombocytosis and high erythrocyte sedimentation rate are characteristic. Echocardiography may contribute diagnostically in infants with atypical presentation [4]. Management comprises the early administration of intravenous immunoglobulin, as soon as the diagnosis is suspected, plus supportive measures.

Linear IgA disease

Synonyms
- Chronic bullous disease of childhood

Linear IgA disease (LAD) (Chapter 50) is a non-familial, autoimmune, blistering disease that occurs in prepubertal children and is characterised by linear IgA staining of the basement membrane zone on direct immunofluorescence [6]. The disease is often idiopathic but may be triggered by infections, drugs, vaccinations, ultraviolet radiation or malignancy [7]. The production of an IgA autoantibody suggests either that a cross-reacting antigen enters via the mucosa or that an IgA diathesis exists in affected patients [8]. Autoantibodies are most commonly directed against proteolytic fragments of collagen XVII.

LAD is often initially diagnosed as bullous impetigo and may even temporarily improve with a course of antibiotics. Children present with the abrupt onset of tense, clear or haemorrhagic vesicles and bullae on normal or red skin. New lesions often arise around resolving lesions, and these arciform or annular bullae surrounding a central crust have been described as being in a string of pearls, cluster of jewels or rosette pattern (Figure 115.20). The eruption occurs on the face, trunk and extremities. There is a predilection for the lower trunk, genital area and medial thighs; disease onset in the perineum has been mistaken for sexual abuse [9]. On the face, lesions tend to occur in a perioral pattern. Younger children more often have the classic distribution of facial and perineal lesions.

The disease is associated with significant morbidity and usually requires systemic therapy, most frequently with dapsone. Treatment is aimed at controlling blistering while avoiding adverse reactions. Controlled or comparative studies are lacking [10]. Spontaneous resolution usually occurs in a matter of months or years.

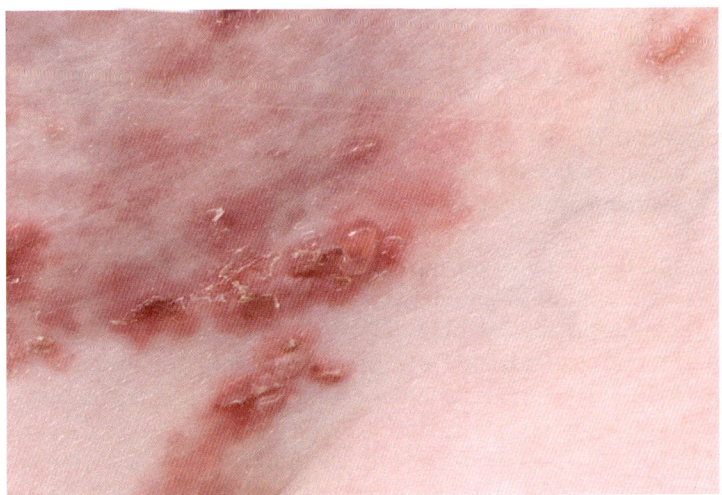

Figure 115.20 Clusters of small bullae in the groin of a child with linear IgA disease.

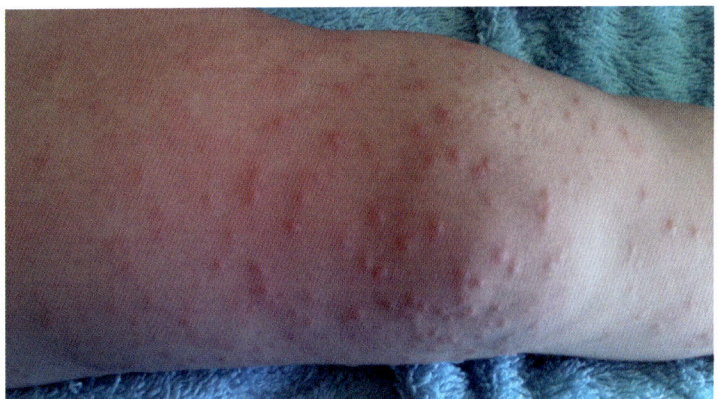

Figure 115.21 Gianotti–Crosti syndrome. Multiple monomorphic papules over the knees developed 2 weeks after an upper respiratory tract infection in this 1-year-old infant.

Gianotti–Crosti syndrome

Synonyms and inclusions
- Papular acrodermatitis
- Infantile papular acrodermatitis

Early reports of this distinctive red papular eruption on the face, buttocks and extremities showed a strong association with hepatitis B infection [11]. However, since the introduction of vaccination against hepatitis B this is now rare as a cause and it has become clear that the eruption may be associated with a variety of viruses [12], including Epstein–Barr virus [13], herpesvirus 6 [14] and Coxsackie virus [15], as well as with immunisation [16,17].

The rash appears as monomorphic, flat-topped, pink to red-brown papules or papulovesicles in a symmetrical distribution favouring the cheeks and extensor surfaces of the limbs and buttocks, often preceded by a minor illness (Figure 115.21). Lesions may sometimes be found on the trunk and flexor surfaces [18,19]. Particularly in infancy, lesions may be oedematous. Constitutional symptoms are usually mild. The presence of lymphadenopathy and hepatitis is no longer required to make the diagnosis [20]. The rash lasts for a minimum of 10 days and may persist for up to 8 weeks. Recurrences are unusual.

Histopathology is not specific [21] and there is no specific treatment.

Papular urticaria

Papular urticaria arises as a result of a hypersensitivity reaction to insect bites, usually appearing as crops of more or less symmetrically distributed, itchy papules and papulovesicles, most frequently on exposed areas of the extremities. They are often heavily excoriated and secondary bacterial infection is common.

It tends to occur more in the summer months, when blood-feeding insects are most plentiful [22], but can occur at any time of year,

PART 10: SPECIFIC SITES, SEX & AGE

particularly if caused by insects that breed in a domestic environment, such as cat fleas and bedbugs. The elapsed time between an insect bite and the formation of a firm, intensely itching papule begins to lengthen as children have increased exposure to these allergens. This delay can make it hard for parents to accept that insects are the cause of the eruption [23]. Diagnosis may also be complicated by reactivation of old lesions by new bites at a different site [23], thought to arise from circulating insect antigen-stimulating cutaneous T cells in previously sensitised sites [24].

Histopathological findings in papular urticaria vary with the particular insect, age of the lesion and sensitivity of the patient. The characteristic urticarial lesions will demonstrate prominent papillary dermal oedema and perivascular lymphocytes, eosinophils and mast cells; there may be superficial and deep perivascular and interstitial infiltrate with a variable density of lymphocytes and eosinophils. Chronic lesions may demonstrate pseudoepitheliomatous hyperplasia and atypical dermal infiltrates [23,25].

The treatment of papular urticaria includes topical steroids and systemic antihistamines, but response is usually limited, and the condition will only be controlled if insect bites can be avoided. Children eventually outgrow this disease, probably through desensitisation after multiple arthropod exposures [26].

Eosinophilic pustular folliculitis

Synonyms and inclusions
- Eosinophilic pustulosis

Eosinophilic pustular folliculitis in infants is an uncommon condition, which appears to be distinct from the condition encountered in adults and older children [27,28]. As lesions are not always truly follicular [29], the term eosinophilic pustulosis is sometimes preferred. It is more common in males than females (4:1), and usually presents before the age of 14 months and clears by the age of 3 years [30]. The cause is unknown. Theories include a hypersensitivity response to microorganisms or dust mites [31], and a possible role for neuronal nitric oxide synthetase [32].

Histopathology of scalp lesions usually shows a perifollicular and periapendigeal infiltrate in the upper and mid dermis composed mainly of eosinophils, with neutrophils and mononuclear cells. Interstitial eosinophilic flame figures may be seen between collagen bundles [27,33]. There are some histopathological similarities to erythema toxicum neonatorum, which has led to the suggestion that they may be related conditions [33].

The condition is characterised by recurrent outbreaks of groups of very itchy papulopustules on a red base, most commonly on the scalp, but also on the trunk and limbs, including the hands and feet (Figure 115.22) [33]. These may resolve in 1 or 2 weeks, to be followed by further crops every few weeks. Spontaneous resolution usually occurs by 3 years of age. Affected infants are well.

During exacerbations there is peripheral blood eosinophilia and leukocytosis. Abundant eosinophils can be seen on Wright's stained smear of pustular contents. The differential diagnosis includes

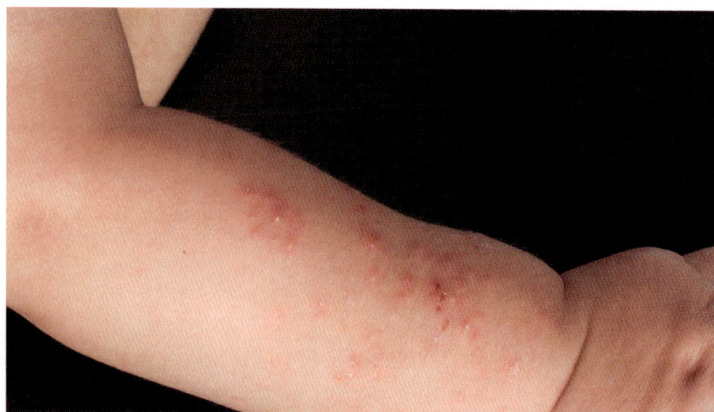

Figure 115.22 Eosinophilic pustulosis showing crops of small itchy pustules on the arm of a male infant.

staphylococcal folliculitis, scabies, herpes simplex, infantile acropustulosis and LCH.

Because of the self-limiting nature of the condition, and lack of controlled trials, it is difficult to make specific recommendations for treatment. Benefit has been reported with cetirizine dihydrochloride [34], mid- to high-potency topical steroids [28,33] and topical calcineurin inhibitors [35].

DEVELOPMENTAL/GENETIC CONDITIONS

Dermoid cysts

Dermoid cysts arise from skin trapped within embryonic fusion lines. They may contain adnexal structures such as hair or eccrine glands, and very rarely bone and teeth. They occur most commonly on the head, presenting as firm subcutaneous nodules (Figure 115.23), particularly in the area of the anterolateral frontozygomatic suture [1], but also the parieto-occipital scalp and nose. They may connect to underlying structures, including the central nervous system if lying over the midline [2].

Preauricular cysts and sinuses

Preauricular cysts and sinuses are thought to arise from a failure of fusion of the auditory component of the first two branchial arches. They usually present as very small pits just anterior to the upper anterior helix. When bilateral they may be transmitted as an autosomal dominant trait. They may be associated with deafness and with other anomalies, as in branchio-oto-renal syndrome and branchio-otic syndrome [3,4]. Auditory testing and renal ultrasound are indicated if a preauricular pit is associated with dysmorphic features or another anomaly, or with a family history of deafness [5].

Preauricular sinuses are usually asymptomatic in infancy, but may occasionally become infected. Surgery requires complete excision of the sinus tract and associated cysts [6].

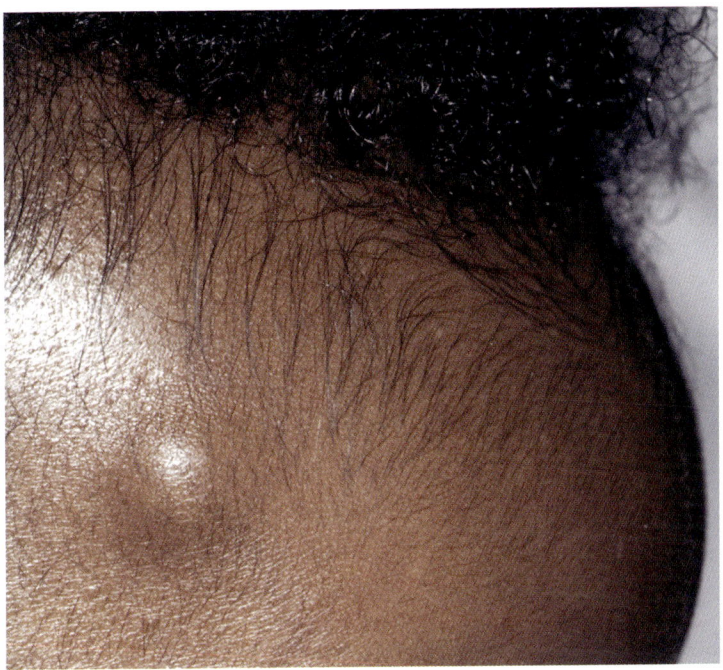

Figure 115.23 A dermoid cyst of the right temple.

Pigmentary mosaicism

Pigmentary mosaicism is a general term used to describe a wide range of phenotypes that include genetically determined variation of skin pigmentation [7] (Chapter 68). It often presents as streaks and whorls of hypo- or hyperpigmentation following the lines of Blaschko (Figure 115.24), with midline demarcation, determined by the embryonal migration paths from the neural crest of clones with different pigment-producing potential [8]. Pigmentary mosaicism may also manifest as patches, flag-like, leaf-like (phylloid) [9] or chequerboard shapes, or as patchy variation without midline demarcation. It may arise from a very wide variety of cytogenetic abnormalities [10] and may therefore be found in association with a broad range of associated clinical features, most frequently neurological and musculoskeletal. Infants with pigmentary mosaicism should be thoroughly assessed with particular attention to development, the internal organs and skeletal and ophthalmological abnormalities.

Linear morphoea

Morphoea develops less commonly in infancy than in early school-aged children [11], and most commonly presents in the linear form [11,12] (Chapter 55). The cause remains unknown. Triggers may include vaccination [13], infections, including with Epstein–Barr virus [14] and *Borrelia burgdorferi* [15], autoimmune processes [12] and genetic factors [16]. Linear morphoea follows the lines of Blaschko, suggesting that susceptible cells may be present in a mosaic state [17].

Linear morphoea tends to progress faster than plaque-type morphoea and is more likely to involve muscle and bone [18], which

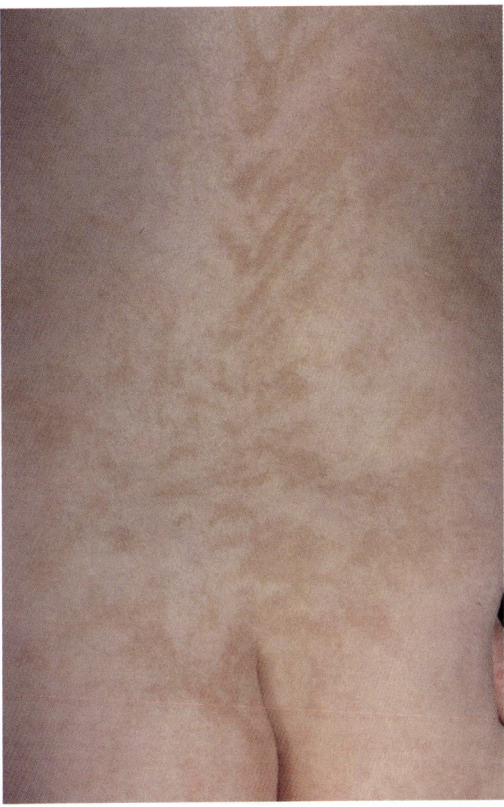

Figure 115.24 Whorls of hyperpigmentation following the lines of Blaschko on the back.

may lead to facial hemiatrophy [19]. It may present with macular redness, sometimes leading to misdiagnosis as a vascular malformation [20]. When on the head (so-called 'en coup de sabre'), scarring alopecia and partial loss of the brow or lashes are characteristic. Up to 13% of children with linear morphoea en coup de sabre have seizures [21].

Proposed minimum standards of care for children with linear morphoea on the face or scalp include brain magnetic resonance imaging (MRI), screening for uveitis and dental assessment [22]. Disease activity is difficult to determine clinically. Scanning laser Doppler imaging may be useful in predicting disease progression [23].

There is lack of consensus on optimal treatment [24], but first line treatment is usually with combined systemic steroids and methotrexate, and maintenance with methotrexate alone for at least 3 years [25].

MISCELLANEOUS CONDITIONS

Milia

Small, firm, white papules, predominantly occurring on the face of newborn babies and infants, are common and harmless (Figure 115.25). Lesions should not be confused with sebaceous hyperplasia or the more florid milia associated with bullous disorders. Infantile milia may occasionally be associated with oral lesions

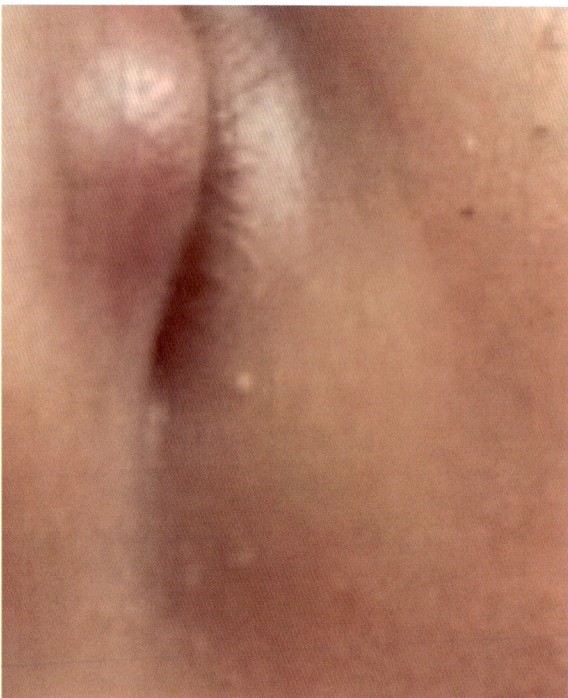

Figure 115.25 Milia on the right cheek of a 6-week-old male.

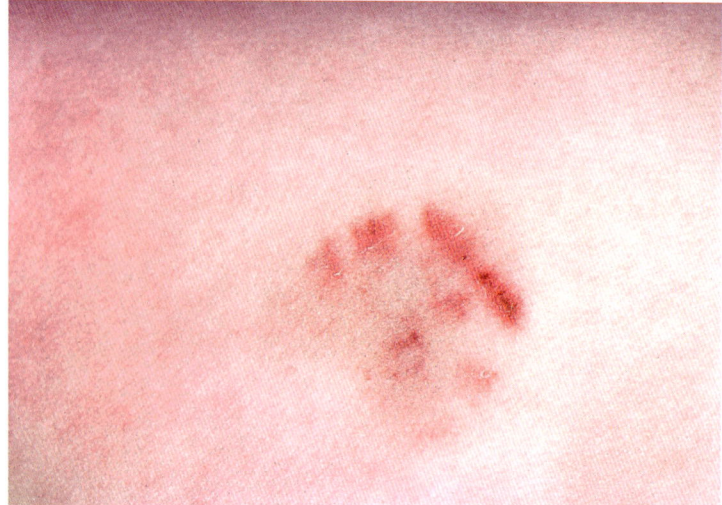

Figure 115.26 A bite mark on the upper limb of a 10-month-old infant (inflicted by his 4-year-old brother).

on the gingivae or palate. The estimated prevalence is 16% and the majority of lesions occur on the cheeks, forehead or chin [1]. Milia are more common in white children, but less frequent in children born prematurely or of low gestational weight [1].

Koilonychia

The nail plate of infants is very soft and malleable. Transient concavity of the nail plate is not uncommon [2] and not usually a manifestation of iron deficiency. The condition is self-resolving, growing out normally over time.

Non-accidental injury

Sadly, non-accidental injury (NAI) is still a widespread problem, especially among infants and toddlers. Injuries can take many forms [3] but all health care professionals, nursery workers and social service agencies should be fully aware of possible signs of NAI and the mechanisms for reporting and safeguarding children at risk.

Subconjunctival haemorrhages in an infant should arouse suspicion that the child is a victim of shaken baby syndrome. Toddlers and older children frequently have genuine accidents, but these are less likely in infants who are not yet mobile [3,4]. In children with multiple attendances at A&E, delayed attendance after an injury or unexplained injuries, the concern of NAI should be raised, and investigating clinicians must consider undertaking a skeletal

survey and CT scan of the head. Bites, burns, signs of neglect or sexual abuse may all form part of the spectrum [3,4]. Emotional abuse may coexist or occur in isolation. A young child becoming withdrawn, or wary of adults, should arouse suspicion and appropriate measures to investigate be taken.

Bite injuries

Bite injuries in infants are not infrequent. Establishing the source of the bite is imperative. Animal bites are usually clear-cut, in that they present rapidly to A&E with a clear history, but the wounds can be deep and ragged and usually require antibiotics to treat infection and expert plastic surgery to minimise scarring.

Human bites may simply leave bruising or purpura, rather than puncture marks. However, it is essential to establish whether the injury has been inflicted by an adult or another child by assessing the size of the dentition from the marks on the skin. Bites inflicted by adults are indicative of NAI and need to be managed accordingly. Bites perpetrated by children may reflect sibling rivalry/jealousy over a new arrival in the home (Figure 115.26) [5] and can usually be managed with temporary support for the family.

Pedal papules of infancy

Symmetrical, painless, flesh-coloured nodules, characteristically on the medial aspect of the heels in infants, may be present at birth, but are usually not apparent until infancy [6]. Although once thought to be uncommon, recent surveys suggest that they may occur in up to 40% of infants [6]. They may be solitary (Figure 115.27), but unlike piezogenic papules in adults, tend to be larger and asymptomatic [7].

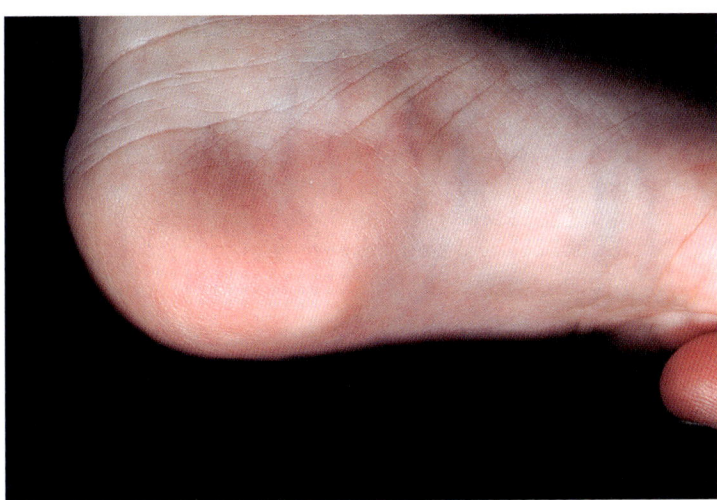

Figure 115.27 Pedal papule of infancy showing a soft swelling on the medial aspect of the heel.

Calcified cutaneous nodules of the heels

Small firm, calcified dermal lesions have been described on the heels of infants who have been on neonatal intensive care units and subjected to multiple heel pricks for venesection [8]. Histologically, the lesions appear to have features of epidermal cysts and so are believed to arise from epidermal implantation through trauma, with subsequent calcification of the cyst, rather than dystrophic calcification per se [9]. Natural resolution over the course of 18 months is the norm, but if slow to resolve they may cause pain on pressure when walking in older children [8].

Hair loss in infancy

Shedding of hair occurs during the seventh to eighth month *in utero* in all areas except the occiput, where shedding is delayed until 2–3 months postpartum [10], leading to the normal occipital alopecia in this age group.

Absent or diffusely sparse hair in infancy can arise from abnormalities of initiation of growth, hair shaft abnormalities and abnormal cycling.

Alopecia areata is relatively rare in the first year of life [11] and early onset tends to indicate a poor prognosis. It is important to distinguish rarer causes of extensive hair loss in infancy, including vitamin D-resistant rickets [12].

Telogen effluvium is less common in infants than in adults, and is more likely to be related to a sudden and transient illness than to drugs or hormonal fluctuations.

Loose anagen syndrome refers to a condition seen in children, usually girls, who have sparse hair with easily extracted anagen hairs, with misshapen bulbs, absent root sheaths and ruffled cuticles [13].

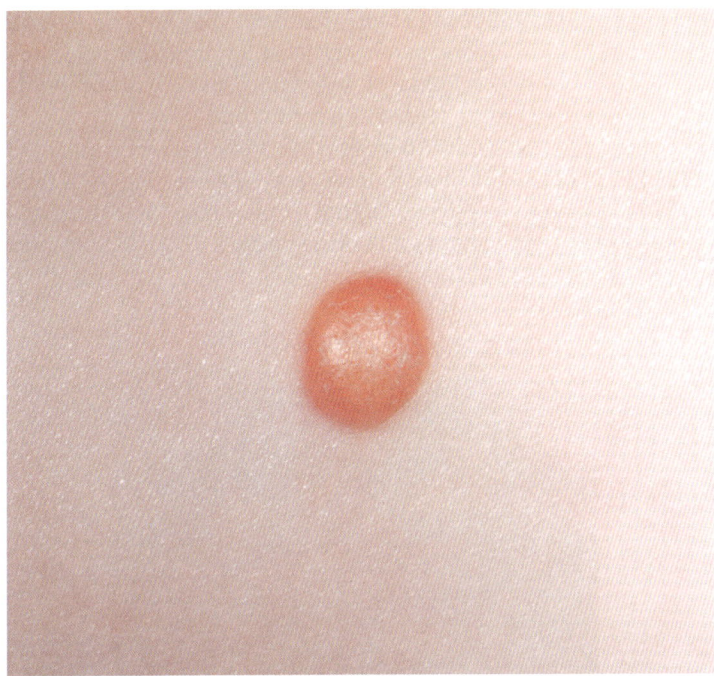

Figure 115.28 Juvenile xanthogranuloma showing a well-circumscribed yellowish nodule with a red margin on the upper back of a 6-month-old infant.

Juvenile xanthogranuloma

Juvenile xanthogranuloma (JXG) often presents in the first year of life, and is more common in boys than girls [14]. Lesions generally start as red-brown papules that become orange (Figure 115.28), occurring most frequently on the face and scalp and upper torso. The eye is involved in 0.4% of cases under the age of 2 years [15], and may lead to spontaneous hyphema, glaucoma, cataract and uveitis [16]. Localised cutaneous JXG heals spontaneously, sometimes leaving atrophic scars.

Benign cephalic histiocytosis has many similarities to JXG and may be the same disease [17]. It usually presents in the first or second year of life as multiple, small, yellow-red macules and papules, initially on the head, but sometimes spreading to other sites [18]. The lesions heal spontaneously without scarring.

Langerhans cell histiocytosis

LCH is the commonest of the histiocytic disorders in childhood, most frequently presenting in infants under the age of 1 year [19], with boys affected twice as often as girls [20] (Chapter 135). The cause of LCH is unknown. *BRAF V600E* mutations have been demonstrated in a number of cases [21], but the clinical significance of this mutation is unclear [22].

LCH can be divided into (i) an acute, disseminated form (formerly Letterer–Siwe disease); (ii) a chronic, localised form (eosinophilic granuloma); (iii) a progressive, multifocal, chronic form (Hand–Schüller–Christian disease); and (iv) a benign, self-healing form (congenital self-healing reticulohistiocytosis or Hashimoto–Pritzker disease). In practice these tend to overlap and are therefore best regarded as a continuum.

Because the cutaneous features are very variable, including seborrhoeic dermatitis-like redness and scaling (Figure 115.29), papules, pustules, vesicles, nodules, petechiae and ulceration (Figure 115.30), the diagnosis is often delayed [23]. The prognosis depends on the extent of the disease. Truly single-system disease has almost 100% survival [24], but up to 56% of infants presenting with skin-only disease may progress to multisystem disease [25].

Non-Langerhans cell histiocytoses are rare in infancy and may be related predominantly to the dendritic cell line (the juvenile xanthogranuloma group) or to the macrophage line (reticulo-histiocytoma, cutaneous Rosai–Dorfman disease, multicentric reticulohistiocytosis and sinus histiocytosis).

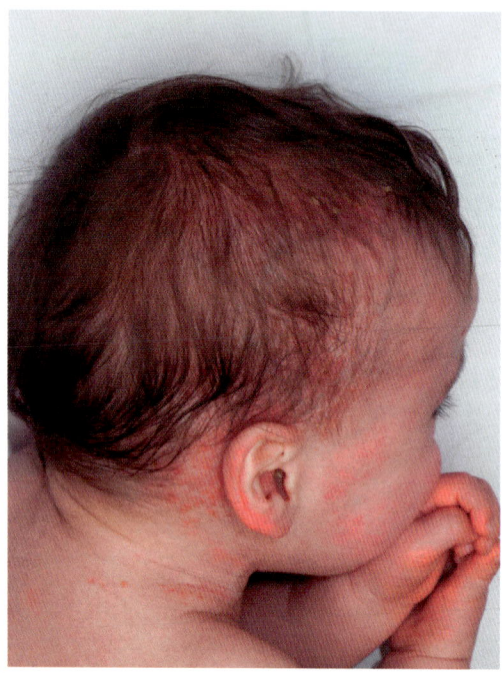

Figure 115.29 Infant with Langerhans cell histiocytosis, resembling seborrhoeic dermatitis.

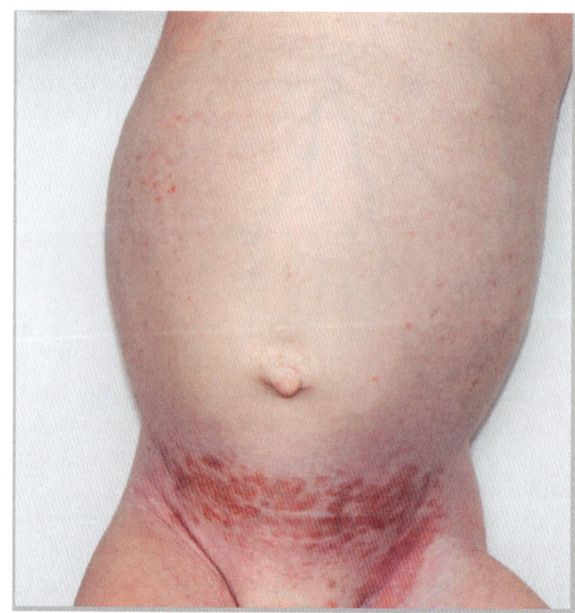

Figure 115.30 Infant with Langerhans cell histiocytosis with red and eroded areas in the groin area, resembling diaper dermatitis. Note the distended abdomen.

Mastocytosis

Mastocytosis in infancy is usually limited to the skin, with three distinct clinical presentations: maculopapular (formerly urticaria pigmentosa) (Figure 115.31), diffuse cutaneous mastocytosis and solitary mastocytoma (Figure 115.32). Somatic activating mutations in the *KIT* gene, which encodes a tyrosine kinase receptor that induces mast cell growth and maturation, play a central role in the pathogenesis of mastocytosis [26]. Unlike adults, a wider variety of *KIT* mutations occur in patients with childhood-onset mastocytosis: codon 816 in ~35–40%; exons 8–11 in ~35–40%; and no detectable mutation in ~15–20% of those with complete *KIT* sequencing of a lesional skin sample [27–30]. Serum tryptase is the best marker for mast cell burden in infants, and, at baseline, correlates well with the severity of symptoms [31]. While in adults mastocytosis is considered systemic until proved otherwise (Chapter 46), in infants this is not the case [32] as systemic mastocytosis is extremely rare in children and is usually indolent [33].

Parents of infants with extensive skin involvement should be given advice on the avoidance of factors known to stimulate mast cell degranulation, including aspirin, non-steroidal anti-inflammatory drugs, codeine, opiates, polymyxin B and intravenous radiograph contrast fluids and MRI contrast media [34]. Symptomatic therapy, usually consisting of an H_1 receptor blocker, may help control itch, blistering, flushing and urtication [35], plus

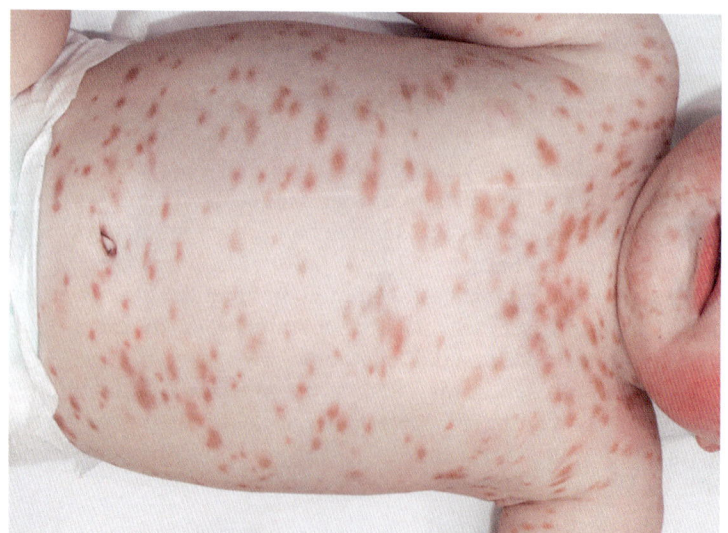

Figure 115.31 Maculopapular mastocytosis in a 7-month-old infant.

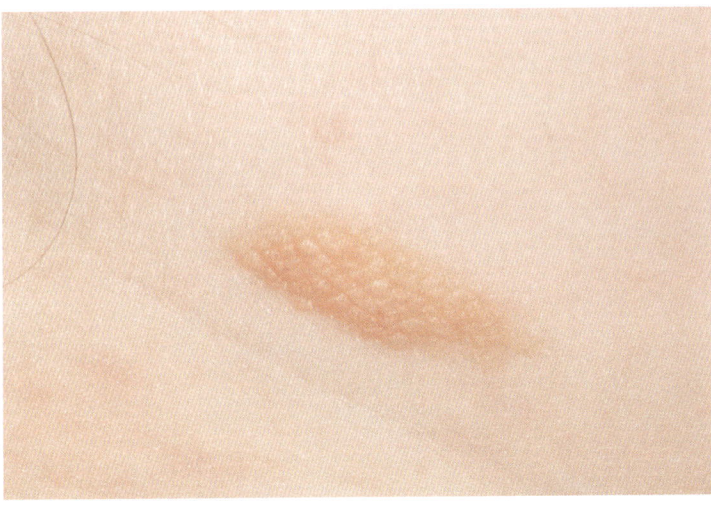

(a)

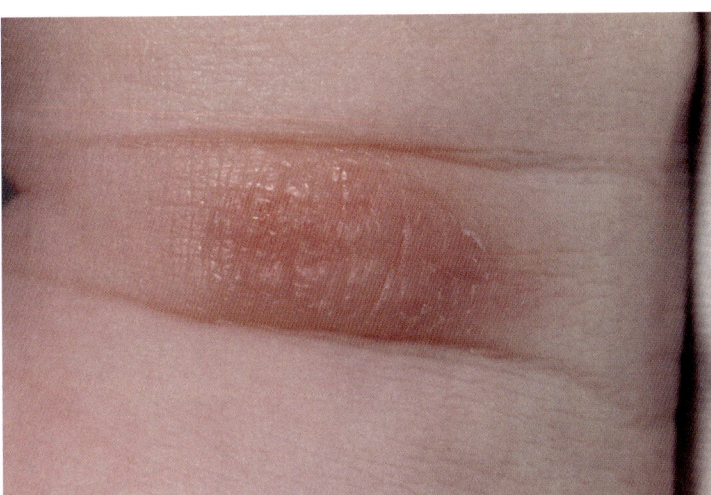

(b)

Figure 115.32 Solitary mastocytoma: (a) before rubbing; (b) urticated after rubbing showing Darier sign.

an H$_2$ blocker if there are symptoms of hyperacidity or ulceration [36], with or without oral sodium cromoglycate for diarrhoea [37,38]. Prescription of an epinephrine autoinjector is often recommended for paediatric mastocytosis patients with extensive skin involvement, a history of anaphylaxis or other severe symptoms, and/or elevated serum tryptase levels [39,40].

Key references

The full list of references can be found in the online version at https://www.wiley.com/rooksdermatology10e

Inflammatory conditions

7 Alexopoulos A, Kakourou T, Orfanou I, Xaidara A, Chrousos G. Retrospective analysis of the relationship between infantile seborrheic dermatitis and atopic dermatitis. *Pediatr Dermatol* 2014;31:125–30.

19 Kawamoto N, Fukao T, Kaneko H *et al*. Total IgE at 6 months predicts remittance or persistence of atopic dermatitis at 14 months. *Allergy Asthma Proc* 2013;34:362–9.

26 Liu N, Wang X, Odio M. Frequency and severity of diaper dermatitis with use of traditional Chinese cloth diapers: observations in 3- to 9-month-old children. *Pediatr Dermatol* 2011;28:380–6.

28 Tollefson MM, Crowson CS, McEvoy MT, Maradit Kremers H. Incidence of psoriasis in children: a population-based study. *J Am Acad Dermatol* 2010;62:979–87.

41 Cunliffe WJ, Baron SE, Coulson IH. A clinical and therapeutic study of 29 patients with infantile acne. *Br J Dermatol* 2001;145:463–6.

44 Mortureux P, Leaute-Labreze C, Legrain-Lifermann V, Lamireau T, Sarlangue J, Taieb A. Acute urticaria in infancy and early childhood: a prospective study. *Arch Dermatol* 1998;134:319–23.

Infective conditions
Viral exanthems

2 Drago F, Paolino S, Rebora A *et al*. The challenge of diagnosing atypical exanthems: a clinico-laboratory study. *J Am Acad Dermatol* 2012;67:1282–8.

14 Pinquier D, Lecuyer A, Levy C *et al*. Inverse correlation between varicella severity and level of anti-Varicella Zoster Virus maternal antibodies in infants below one year of age. *Hum Vaccin* 2011;7:534–8.

Other infections and infestations

2 Lamand V, Dauwalder O, Tristan A *et al*. Epidemiological data of staphylococcal scalded skin syndrome in France from 1997 to 2007 and microbiological characteristics of Staphylococcus aureus associated strains. *Clin Microbiol Infect* 2012;18:514–21.

11 Michaels BD, Del Rosso JQ. Tinea capitis in infants: recognition, evaluation, and management suggestions. *J Clin Aesthet Dermatol* 2012;5:49–59.

Reactive conditions

1 Legrain V, Lejean S, Taieb A, Guillard JM, Battin J, Maleville J. Infantile acute hemorrhagic edema of the skin: study of ten cases. *J Am Acad Dermatol* 1991;24:17–22.

5 Chang FY, Hwang B, Chen SJ, Lee PC, Meng CC, Lu JH. Characteristics of Kawasaki disease in infants younger than six months of age. *Pediatr Infect Dis J* 2006;25:241–4.

6 Mintz EM, Morel KD. Clinical features, diagnosis, and pathogenesis of chronic bullous disease of childhood. *Dermatol Clin* 2011;29:459–62.

19 Chuh AA. Diagnostic criteria for Gianotti-Crosti syndrome: a prospective case-control study for validity assessment. *Cutis* 2001;68:207–13.

30 Hernandez-Martin A, Nuno-Gonzalez A, Colmenero I, Torrelo A. Eosinophilic pustular folliculitis of infancy: a series of 15 cases and review of the literature. *J Am Acad Dermatol* 2013;68:150–5.

Developmental/genetic conditions

7 Happle R. Mosaicism in human skin. Understanding the patterns and mechanisms. *Arch Dermatol* 1993;129:1460–70.

Miscellaneous conditions

3 Maguire S. Which injuries may indicate child abuse? *Arch Dis Child Educ Pract Ed* 2010;95:170–7.

25 Lau L, Krafchik B, Trebo MM, Weitzman S. Cutaneous Langerhans cell histiocytosis in children under one year. *Pediatr Blood Cancer* 2006;46:66–71.

26 Schaffer JV. Pediatric mastocytosis: recognition and management. *Am J Clin Dermatol* 2021;22:205–20.

CHAPTER 116

Haemangiomas and Other Non-malignant Tumours of Infancy

Lea Solman and Mary T. Glover

Great Ormond Street Hospital for Children NHS Foundation Trust, London, UK

Infantile haemangioma

Definition and nomenclature

Infantile haemangiomas are common, benign, vascular tumours that develop in early infancy and undergo spontaneous involution thereafter.

Synonyms and inclusions

- Haemangioma of infancy
- Terms such as strawberry naevus, capillary haemangioma and cavernous haemangioma have contributed to the diagnostic confusion in the field of vascular anomalies, and are best avoided

Introduction and general description

Infantile haemangiomas are by far the most common benign vascular tumours encountered in infancy. The natural history is of proliferation in the first few months of life, and involution over a matter of years. Most resolve spontaneously without sequelae, but treatment is indicated for those causing, or likely to cause, impairment of function, permanent disfigurement or ulceration.

Segmental infantile haemangiomas of the head and neck and of the lumbo-sacral region may be associated with structural anomalies. Multifocal infantile haemangiomas are usually asymptomatic but may occasionally be associated with extensive visceral involvement. Rapidly involuting congenital haemangiomas (RICH), non-involuting congenital haemangiomas (NICH) and partially involuting congenital haemangiomas (PICH) are clinically distinct from infantile haemangiomas and appear to have completed their proliferative phase *in utero*.

The classification approved at the April 2014 General Assembly of the International Society for the Study of Vascular Anomalies (ISSVA), and revised in 2018 [1], divides vascular anomalies into tumours (including infantile haemangiomas and congenital haemangiomas) and malformations (Table 116.1). The distinction between infantile haemangiomas and vascular malformations is often straightforward on the basis of history and examination, but occasionally investigations such as ultrasound, histopathology and immunohistochemistry are required (Table 116.2).

Table 116.1 Benign vascular tumours and vascular malformations: simplified classification.

Benign vascular tumours	Vascular malformations
Infantile haemangioma (IH):	High flow:
Hepatic haemangioma (HH)	Arteriovenous
Multifocal IH:	Low flow:
Without systemic involvement	Capillary
With systemic involvement	Venous
Congenital haemangiomas:	Lymphatic
Rapidly involuting (RICH)	Mixed (for example):
Non-involuting (NICH)	
Partially involuting (PICH)	Capillary venous
Tufted angioma	Capillary lymphatic venous
Spindle cell haemangioma	Capillary arteriovenous
Epithelioid haemangioma	
Pyogenic granuloma	

Table 116.2 Distinction between infantile haemangiomas and vascular malformations.

	Infantile haemangioma	Vascular malformation
Clinical features	Usually evident within the first few weeks of life	Usually present at birth
	Proliferate rapidly	Proportionate growth
	Involute over a number of years	Do not involute
Epidemiology	More common in girls and low-birth-weight infants	No gender or birth-weight bias
Immunohistochemistry	GLUT-1 positive	GLUT-1 negative

Rook's Textbook of Dermatology, Tenth Edition. Edited by Christopher Griffiths, Jonathan Barker, Tanya Bleiker, Walayat Hussain and Rosalind Simpson.
© 2024 John Wiley & Sons Ltd. Published 2024 by John Wiley & Sons Ltd.

PART 10: SPECIFIC SITES, SEX & AGE

Table 116.3 Anomalies associated with segmental infantile haemangiomas (IHs).

Facial segmental haemangioma	Lower body segmental haemangioma
Posterior fossa malformations, haemangiomas, arterial anomalies, cardiac anomalies, eye abnormalities, sternal pit and supraumbilical raphe (PHACES syndrome)	Lower body IH, uro-genital anomalies, ulceration, myelopathy, bony deformities, ano-rectal malformations, arterial anomalies, renal anomalies (LUMBAR syndrome)
	Spinal dysraphism, ano-genital anomalies, cutaneous anomalies, renal and urological anomalies, lumbo-sacral IH (SACRAL syndrome)
	Perineal IH, external genitalia, malformations, lipomyelomeningocele, vesico-renal abnormalities, imperforate anus (PELVIS syndrome)

Adapted from International Society for the Study of Vascular Anomalies (ISSVA) 2014 [1].

Infantile haemangiomas can be classified morphologically as:
- Superficial.
- Deep.
- Mixed (superficial and deep).
- Reticular, abortive or minimal growth.
  These can exist in different patterns:
    - Focal.
    - Multifocal.
    - Segmental.
    - Indeterminate.

Infantile haemangiomas can also occur with or without associated lesions (Table 116.3) [1].

Epidemiology

Infantile haemangiomas are the most common tumours of infancy, occurring in up to 10% of infants, more commonly in girls than boys [2]. Most cases are sporadic. Amniocentesis, *in vitro* fertilisation, breech presentation, being first born and low birth weight (<2500 g) appear to be independently associated with the development of infantile haemangioma [2].

Pathophysiology
Pathogenesis

The aetiology of infantile haemangioma remains unclear [3]. Endothelial cells are characterised by the surface marker GLUT-1, an erythrocyte-type glucose transporter protein, which is also expressed on the placental vasculature. It has been proposed that this placental phenotype may be the result of embolisation of placental endothelial cells to the fetal circulation [4]. Against this theory is the lack of evidence of maternal–fetal chimerism [5]).

An autosomal dominant inheritance pattern and a linkage to 5q have been reported in a small number of families [6], as well as a twofold increased relative risk for the disorder among siblings of an affected proband [7]. Somatic mutations leading to uncontrolled proliferation of haemangioma cells have been proposed. In support of this theory, clonality of endothelial cells from haemangioma lesions has been shown in a small subset of infantile haemangiomas [7]. Mutations in the integrin-like receptor tumour endothelial marker 8, and in *VEGFR2*, have been identified in

a subpopulation of haemangioma-derived endothelial cells and corresponding blood samples from patients with infantile haemangioma [8]. There is evidence that hypoxia may contribute to pathogenesis [9].

Pathology

The diagnosis is nearly always clinical, and biopsy is rarely required to distinguish infantile haemangioma from other vascular anomalies or malignancy. During the early phase of growth the haemangiomas consist of solid groups of cells with few lumina. The endothelial cells flatten out as the lumina develop. The cells are surrounded by a thickened basement membrane. During the process of involution a more lobular appearance develops, with islands of fibrous and fatty tissue between the lobules. Mast cells are evident at all phases. Immunohistochemistry is positive for factor VIII, CD31 and von Willebrand factor. Glucose 1 transporter protein (GLUT-1) positivity can be useful in differentiating infantile haemangiomas from other vascular lesions, such as congenital haemangiomas, but it may also be positive in verrucous vascular malformations.

Clinical features
Presentation

Haemangiomas may be evident shortly after birth as a faint telangiectatic patch or an area of pallor (Figure 116.1), or as a flat pink mark, which rapidly becomes red and raised (Figure 116.2). Superficial types of infantile haemangioma show their most rapid growth between 5.5 and 7.5 weeks of age (Figure 116.3) [10]. Deep haemangiomas, which develop in the lower dermis and subcutis, tend to appear blue or purple, may have no overlying skin changes (Figure 116.4), often present later and continue to grow for longer than superficial haemangiomas. Most infantile haemangiomas reach 80% of their final size by 3 months of age [11]. Mixed infantile haemangiomas, sharing features of both the superficial and deep types, are common (Figures 116.5 and 116.6). A minority of infantile haemangiomas, sometimes referred to as abortive infantile haemangioma, show relatively little proliferation, remaining as a patch of telangiectatic vessels. Airway infantile haemangiomas most commonly occur in patients with segmental infantile haemangiomas in the so-called beard distribution (S3 segment), which includes the preauricular skin, mandible, lower lip, chin and/or anterior neck [12]. Affected infants will develop stridor, hoarseness and respiratory failure between 4 and 12 weeks of age due to rapid growth of infantile haemangioma.

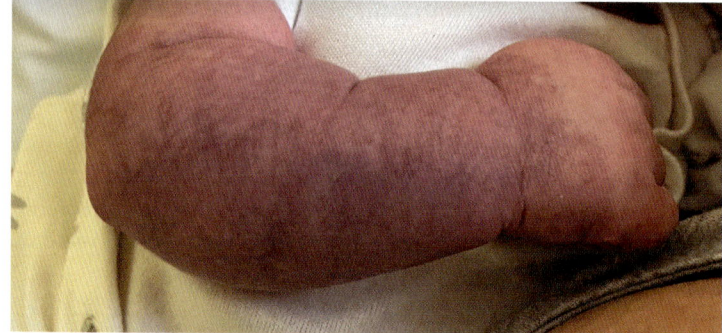

Figure 116.1 Haemangioma precursor.

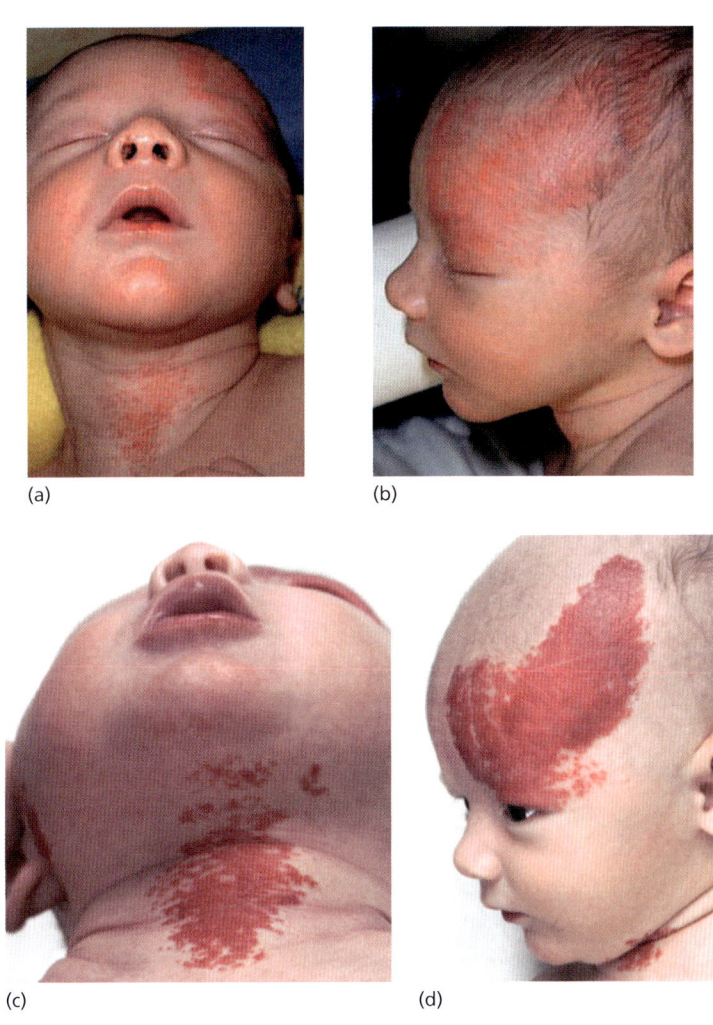

(a)   (b)

(c)   (d)

Figure 116.2 Evolution of facial and neck plaque-type haemangiomas from day 1 (a, b) to day 10 (c, d).

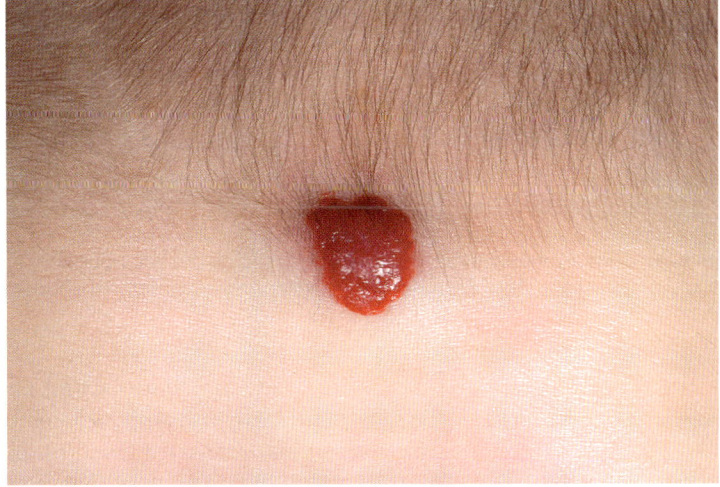

Figure 116.3 A small capillary haemangioma in the proliferative phase on the forehead of a 3-month old infant.

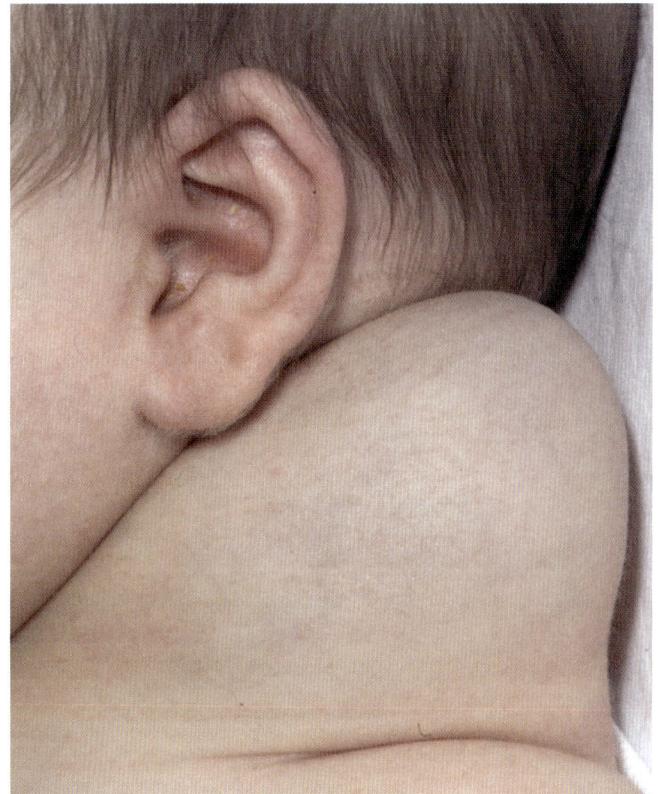

Figure 116.4 An 8-week-old infant with a deep infantile haemangioma involving the lateral neck.

During the proliferative phase, infantile haemangiomas are firm. With involution they become softer. Superficial haemangiomas develop islands of greying within the redness, with some flattening of the surface. In untreated lesions, involution of superficial haemangiomas is complete at a median age of 3 years, and most cases cease to improve substantially after 3.5 years of age [13]. Therefore, surgical reconstruction, if indicated, may be best undertaken at this age, as further aesthetically beneficial, spontaneous improvement is unlikely to occur. Permanent changes – most frequently telangiectases, atrophy and residual bulk in the form of fibrofatty tissue (Figure 116.5c) – have been reported to remain in up to 69% of untreated haemangiomas [14]. Atrophic scars frequently follow ulceration.

Clinical variants

Segmental infantile haemangioma. A proportion of infantile haemangiomas, referred to as segmental or plaque-like, involve a broad anatomical region, thought to reflect embryological metameres [15]. Segmental infantile haemangioma of the face (Figure 116.7) and of the lumbo-sacral region (Figure 116.8) may be associated with underlying structural anomalies (Table 116.3). Up to 30% of large segmental facial infantile haemangiomas are associated with the PHACES syndrome (posterior fossa malformations, haemangiomas, arterial anomalies, cardiac anomalies, eye abnormalities, sternal pit and supraumbilical raphe) [16]. Segmental infantile haemangiomas of the frontotemporal or mandibular regions are at the highest risk, but rare cases of PHACES syndrome have been reported without facial involvement [17]. Abnormalities

PART 10: SPECIFIC SITES, SEX & AGE

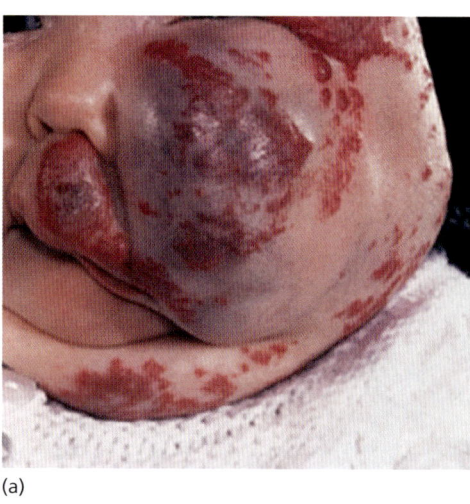

(a)

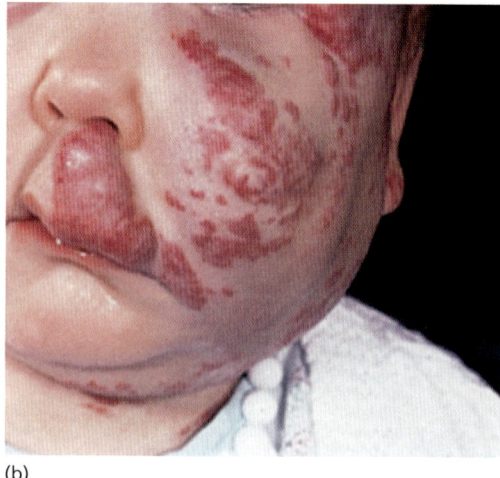

(b)

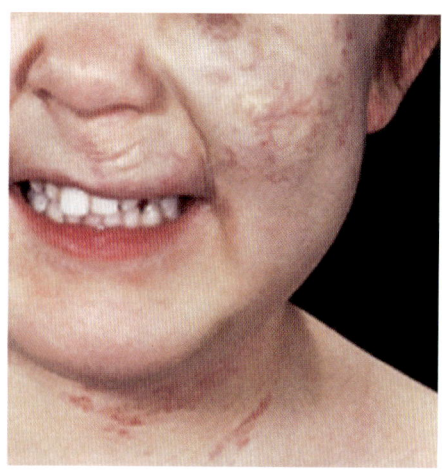

(c)

Figure 116.5 Large, mixed infantile haemangioma at (a) 3 months, (b) 16 months and (c) 3 years.

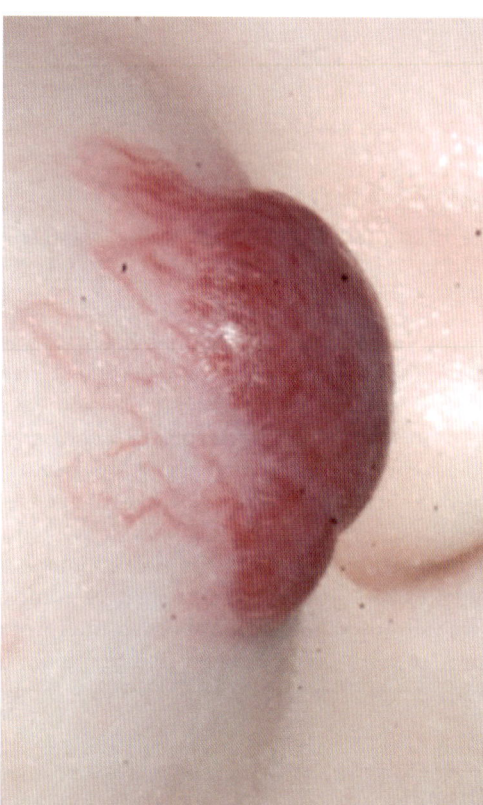

Figure 116.6 Lateral view of an infantile haemangioma on the face of a 7-week-old infant showing both superficial and deep components (mixed form).

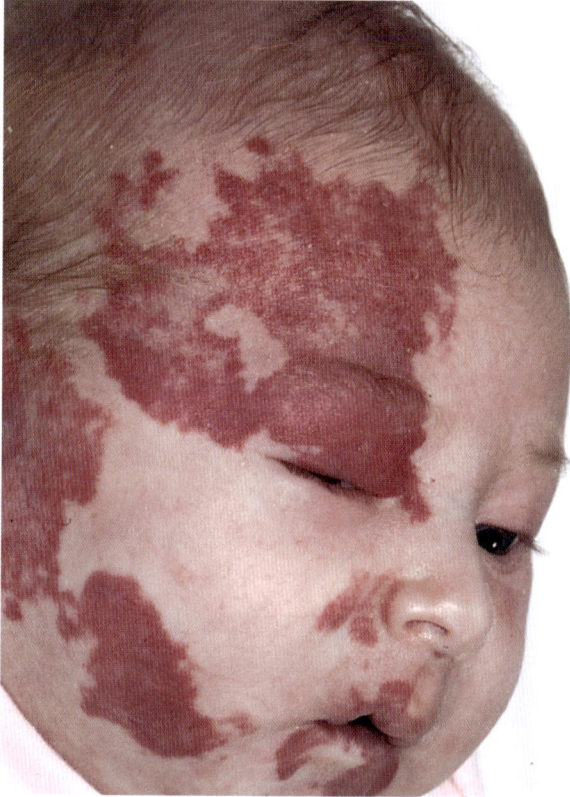

Figure 116.7 Female infant aged 4 weeks with facial segmental infantile haemangioma associated with dilatation of the right internal carotid, proximal middle cerebral and posterior communicating arteries, right III nerve palsy, and vascular ring arising from a right-sided aortic arch, retro-oesophageal left subclavian artery and patent left ductus arteriosus.

of the cerebral vasculature and coarctation of the aorta are the most common extracutaneous findings [18]. Head and neck magnetic resonance angiography (MRA), echocardiogram and ophthalmological examination are recommended for patients with large segmental facial infantile haemangiomas.

Segmental infantile haemangiomas in the beard region, especially if bilateral, may be associated with airway haemangiomas. Otolaryngological advice should be sought for such infants, even in the absence of overt respiratory symptoms.

Segmental infantile haemangioma in the lumbo-sacral and perineal regions may be associated with spinal dysraphism, uro-genital abnormalities, ano-rectal malformations, arterial anomalies and renal abnormalities [19]. For infants under the age of 3 months, spinal ultrasound may be useful for the initial assessment, but spinal magnetic resonance imaging (MRI) with contrast is advisable.

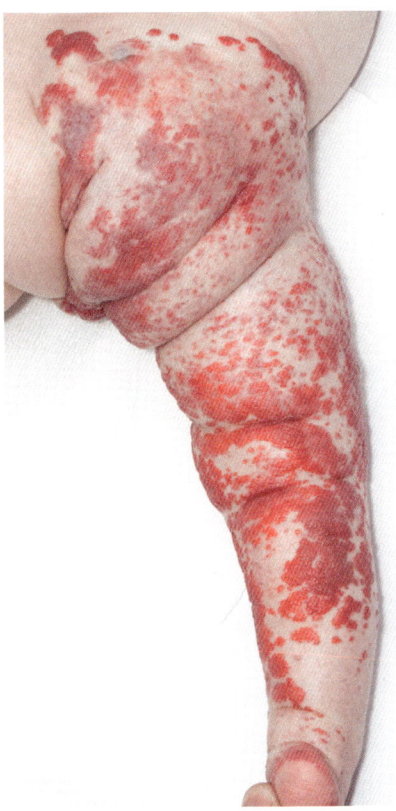

Figure 116.8 Male infant aged 6 weeks with segmental infantile haemangioma associated with complex spinal dysraphism.

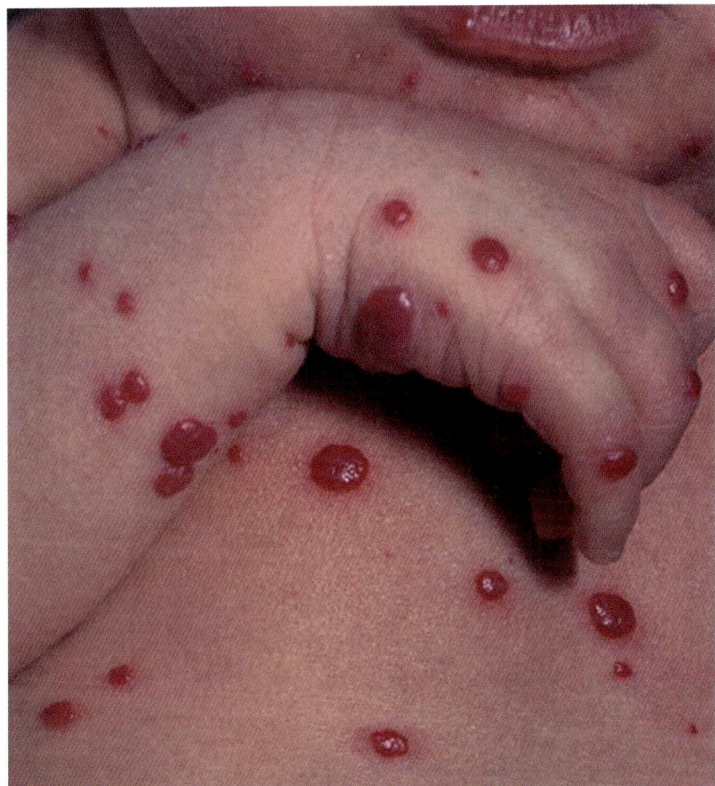

Figure 116.9 Multifocal cutaneous infantile haemangioma.

Multifocal cutaneous infantile haemangioma with and without extracutaneous involvement. Historically the term haemangiomatosis – qualified variously as diffuse, miliary or disseminated – has been used to refer to multiple haemangiomas, with or without visceral involvement. Further confusion has arisen from inclusion under this term of GLUT-1 negative conditions such as multifocal lymphangioendotheliomatosis. In this text the terms multifocal infantile haemangioma, with or without extracutaneous involvement, will be used.

Multifocal haemangiomas may range in number from a few to hundreds, and are usually small (Figure 116.9). They are histologically and immunohistochemically identical to solitary cutaneous infantile haemangiomas. Most affected infants follow an uncomplicated course [20], but some have symptomatic visceral lesions, with liver involvement being the most common.

Hepatic haemangioma. Hepatic haemangioma (HH) may occur with or without cutaneous infantile haemangioma. Many HHs are asymptomatic, and those that become symptomatic usually do so within the first 3 months of life [20,21] presenting with hepatomegaly and high-output cardiac failure. HHs may be focal, multifocal or diffuse [22]. Focal HHs may be evident on antenatal ultrasound, are usually GLUT-1 negative, occur without cutaneous lesions, regress rapidly and probably represent rapidly involuting congenital haemangioma of the liver.

Multifocal HHs are usually associated with multiple, small, cutaneous infantile haemangiomas, and are GLUT-1 positive [23].

Most HH in this group are asymptomatic and do not require treatment [20,24].

Diffuse HH is a term that has been used to describe massive involvement of the liver, often with symptomatic arteriovenous shunting and high-output cardiac failure. It is possible that historically the morbidity of HH may have been overestimated as a result of the misinterpretation of multifocal lymphangioendotheliomatosis and multifocal kaposiform haemangioendothelioma as HH.

Complications and co-morbidities

The main complications of infantile haemangiomas are ulceration, disfigurement and functional impairment.

- Ulceration is common, the risk being greatest between 4 and 6 months of age. Ulceration is more likely in large infantile haemangiomas (Figure 116.10), segmental morphology and location on the neck, ano-genital area or lip where there is exposure to friction and moisture. Early grey or white discoloration of the haemangioma surface in infants younger than 3 months might be an early sign of ulceration [25]. Ulcerated infantile haemangiomas are very painful and place the infant at risk of secondary bacterial infection and bleeding. Before the widespread use of β-blockers, ulceration occurred in up to 20% cases, almost always resulting in scarring [25].
- The risk of disfigurement depends on the location, morphological subtype and size. Even relatively small infantile haemangiomas on the central face, lips and nose (Figure 116.11), particularly those with a dermal component, can lead to permanent distortion [25]. Persistent cutaneous dysaesthesia in involuted infantile haemangiomas have been reported [26].

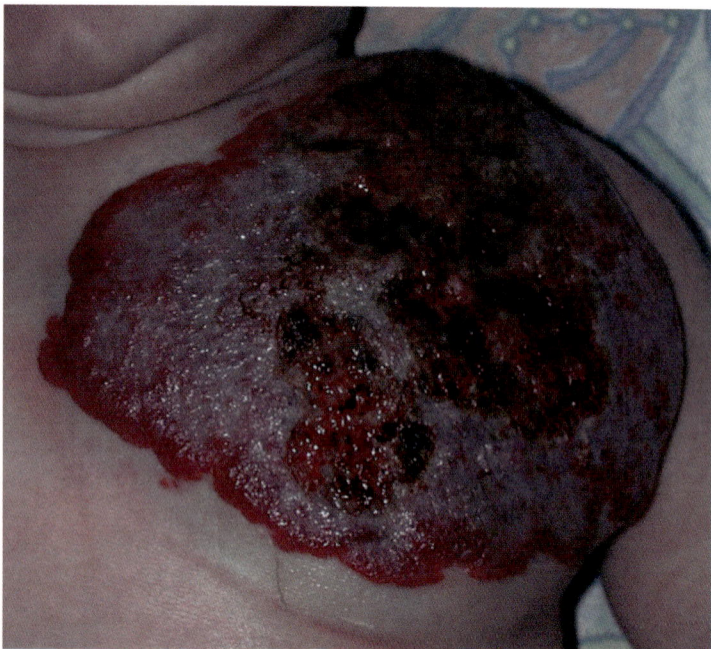

Figure 116.10 Large segmental ulcerated infantile haemangioma.

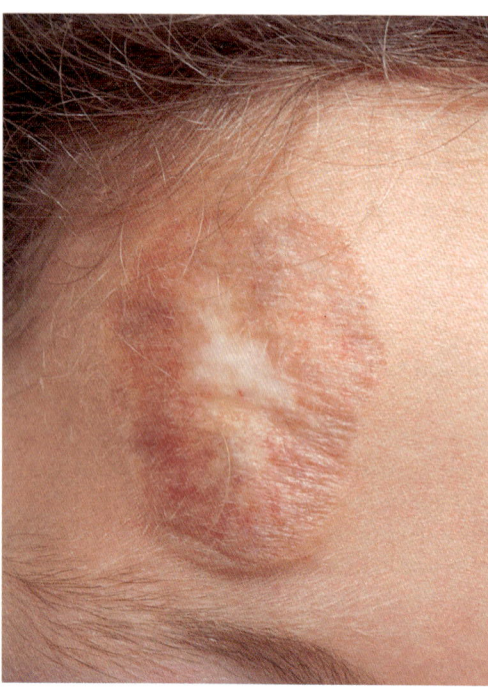

Figure 116.11 Residuum from a forehead haemangioma with residual textural change and central scarring after involution of ulcerated infantile haemangioma in an 8-year-old child.

- Impairment of function is most commonly encountered with periocular infantile haemangiomas (Figure 116.12), which may cause astigmatism, visual axis obstruction and strabismus, which in turn can lead to amblyopia and the risk of permanent visual loss [27]. Haemangiomas involving the airway and the nose can endanger breathing, and those on the lip may interfere with feeding.

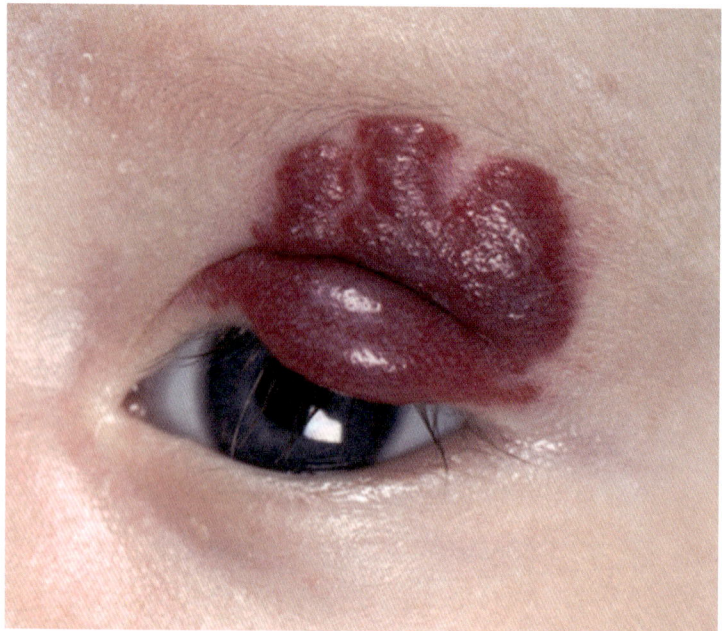

Figure 116.12 Eyelid haemangioma in the line of vision.

Disease course and prognosis

Most infantile haemangiomas follow a predictable course, appearing shortly after birth, usually achieving 80% of their growth by 3 months, and completion of growth by about 9 months. Approximately 3% of infantile haemangiomas, mainly deep ones, may show growth for longer. Involution occurs over a matter of years.

The prognosis is excellent without treatment for small infantile haemangiomas. Prognosis is also excellent for larger haemangiomas if there is no functional impairment, and if it is not at an aesthetically important site. If appropriate treatment with β-blockers is started in a timely fashion, prognosis is also good for infantile haemangiomas causing (or likely to cause) functional or aesthetic impairment.

Investigations

Investigation is rarely required as the diagnosis is usually clinical. Occasionally, ultrasound may be required to distinguish infantile haemangiomas from other soft-tissue masses or vascular malformations. Investigation may also be indicated for plaque-type infantile haemangiomas on the face and lower trunk and before treatment with β-blockers.

Management

Treatment will depend on the location, morphology and stage of evolution, impact on function, risk of disfigurement and co-morbidities [28]. Active non-intervention is appropriate if there is no impairment of function, no ulceration and it is considered that spontaneous regression will produce an excellent outcome. In the early stages parents are often very concerned about aesthetic issues, and require detailed explanation of the natural history of infantile haemangioma, supported with serial photography illustrating examples from the time of maximum proliferation until complete resolution.

Until 2008, treatment for infantile haemangiomas causing, or likely to cause, impairment of function or permanent disfigurement included systemic and intralesional corticosteroids and α-interferon. All of these treatments were associated with significant adverse effects. In 2008, the first report of the successful use of propranolol radically changed the therapeutic approach to infantile haemangioma, and propranolol is now the first line treatment (Figure 116.13) [29]. Propranolol has been shown to induce a better and faster response than systemic steroids, and is associated with fewer and less concerning adverse effects [30,31–33,34,35]. Treatment before the completion of the proliferative phase, which in most cases occurs by 5 months of age, may prevent poor outcomes [10,36].

Recommendations for pre-treatment investigation, dosage and monitoring schedules have varied, but most protocols emphasise particular care when treating very small infants and those with co-morbidities (Figure 116.13) [34,37,38,39]. Treatment of infant haemangiomas should extend beyond the proliferative period to avoid rebound growth; in the majority of patients, the treatment can be stopped at 12–14 months of age.

Systemic corticosteroids remain a treatment option in patients with severe or life-threatening infantile haemangiomas if β-blockers are contraindicated or in conjunction with β-blockers in patients not responding well to treatment with β-blockers alone. Treatment needs to be started in conjunction with paediatricians due to the risk of adrenal suppression.

Although the efficacy of topical propranolol 1% twice daily for superficial infantile haemangioma has been reported [40], there is far greater experience with timolol maleate, usually as a gel forming solution, with benefit reported particularly for very small superficial lesions [41]. Despite widespread use there are few data on percutaneous absorption, with estimates of equivalence with oral propranolol varying widely [42,43].

Although β-blockers may be helpful for the treatment of ulcerated infantile haemangioma, worsening of ulceration can occur, perhaps reflecting reduced blood flow. Most ulcerated infantile haemangiomas respond well to protective non-adherent dressings and topical or systemic antimicrobial treatment based on sensitivities on culture of swabs. The specific mechanism of action of β-blockers remains largely unknown, but it appears that clinical improvement may occur through the induction of vasoconstriction and the decreased expression of proangiogenic factors [44].

Pulsed-dye laser (PDL) can be helpful for the treatment of ulceration [45] and may be required for residual telangiectases post-involution. Use of PDL in the early proliferative phase of non-ulcerated infantile haemangiomas does not appear to improve long-term outcomes, the evidence indicating that treated lesions are more likely to show atrophy or hypopigmentation [46,47–50].

Surgery may very occasionally be required for infantile haemangioma in the proliferative phase if functional impairment or ulceration cannot be managed medically. In the involuting phase, surgery may be indicated provided the size and appearance of the scar is likely to be superior to the result from surgery when involution has ceased. In the involuted phase, indications for plastic surgery or laser resurfacing include abnormal contour due to a fibrofatty residuum and distortion of an important anatomical structure [51,52].

Treatment ladder for infantile haemangiomas

First line
- Watch and wait: for small infantile haemangiomas on the body without ulceration and no risk of disfigurement

Second line
- Topical β-blocker: for small superficial infantile haemangiomas without risk of functional obstruction and/or disfigurement, mainly for those located on the face or nappy area

Third line
- Oral β-blocker: for infantile haemangiomas on the periorbital area, nose, lip, auditory canal and airway, and for ulcerated haemangiomas, risk of disfigurement, spinal cord compression and selected liver infantile haemangiomas

Fourth line
- Oral β-blocker and oral corticosteroid: oral steroid can be added to treatment with oral β-blockers when there is an inadequate response to propranolol monotherapy

Congenital haemangioma

Congenital haemangiomas are benign vascular tumours that proliferate *in utero*, and do not show further proliferation postnatally [1]. They may be evident as early as 12 weeks of gestation by prenatal ultrasound studies [2]. They either regress within 1–2 years (RICH) or not at all (NICH). An uncommon intermediate type is also recognised, presenting with early features similar to a RICH, but showing only partial involution, and referred to as partially involuting congenital haemangioma or PICH [3]. All three types are GLUT-1 negative.

Congenital haemangiomas occur equally in male and female infants, and usually arise on the head or the extremities. The pathogenesis is unknown.

Rapidly involuting congenital haemangiomas typically present as blue or purple tumours, often with telangiectases and peripheral pallor (Figure 116.14), and sometimes with a central ulcer, scar or depression. The rapid regression may leave pronounced atrophy. Ultrasonography demonstrates a uniform hypoechoic mass with centrilobular draining channels [4]. Histology shows small lobules of capillaries with plump endothelium peripherally, and more thin-walled vessels with surrounding fibrous tissue centrally [5]. RICH may be associated with transient thrombocytopenia, which usually resolves spontaneously [6]. Large lesions may cause haemodynamic instability.

Embolisation or excision may need to be considered for RICHs that are ulcerated, bleeding or causing haemodynamic instability. There is no evidence that β-blockers accelerate the involution of RICHs. Sclerotherapy may be indicated for prominent veins in areas of atrophy following involution.

Non-involuting congenital haemangiomas present as violaceous plaques or tumours with coarse telangiectases and peripheral pallor

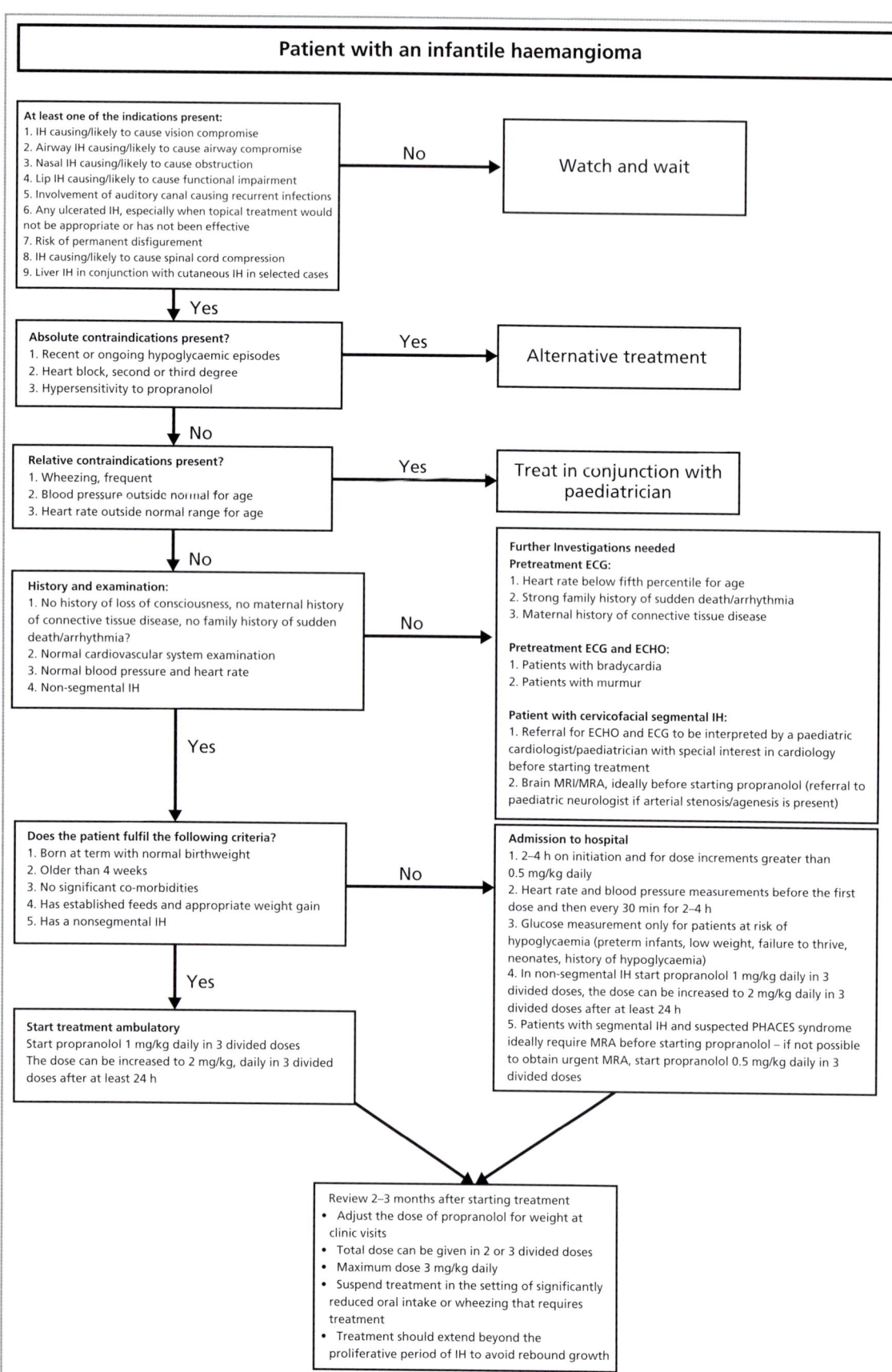

Patient with an infantile haemangioma

At least one of the indications present:
1. IH causing/likely to cause vision compromise
2. Airway IH causing/likely to cause airway compromise
3. Nasal IH causing/likely to cause obstruction
4. Lip IH causing/likely to cause functional impairment
5. Involvement of auditory canal causing recurrent infections
6. Any ulcerated IH, especially when topical treatment would not be appropriate or has not been effective
7. Risk of permanent disfigurement
8. IH causing/likely to cause spinal cord compression
9. Liver IH in conjunction with cutaneous IH in selected cases

No → **Watch and wait**

Yes

Absolute contraindications present?
1. Recent or ongoing hypoglycaemic episodes
2. Heart block, second or third degree
3. Hypersensitivity to propranolol

Yes → **Alternative treatment**

No

Relative contraindications present?
1. Wheezing, frequent
2. Blood pressure outside normal for age
3. Heart rate outside normal range for age

Yes → **Treat in conjunction with paediatrician**

No

History and examination:
1. No history of loss of consciousness, no maternal history of connective tissue disease, no family history of sudden death/arrhythmia?
2. Normal cardiovascular system examination
3. Normal blood pressure and heart rate
4. Non-segmental IH

No →

Further Investigations needed
Pretreatment ECG:
1. Heart rate below fifth percentile for age
2. Strong family history of sudden death/arrhythmia
3. Maternal history of connective tissue disease

Pretreatment ECG and ECHO:
1. Patients with bradycardia
2. Patients with murmur

Patient with cervicofacial segmental IH:
1. Referral for ECHO and ECG to be interpreted by a paediatric cardiologist/paediatrician with special interest in cardiology before starting treatment
2. Brain MRI/MRA, ideally before starting propranolol (referral to paediatric neurologist if arterial stenosis/agenesis is present)

Yes

Does the patient fulfil the following criteria?
1. Born at term with normal birthweight
2. Older than 4 weeks
3. No significant co-morbidities
4. Has established feeds and appropriate weight gain
5. Has a nonsegmental IH

No →

Admission to hospital
1. 2–4 h on initiation and for dose increments greater than 0.5 mg/kg daily
2. Heart rate and blood pressure measurements before the first dose and then every 30 min for 2–4 h
3. Glucose measurement only for patients at risk of hypoglycaemia (preterm infants, low weight, failure to thrive, neonates, history of hypoglycaemia)
4. In non-segmental IH start propranolol 1 mg/kg daily in 3 divided doses, the dose can be increased to 2 mg/kg daily in 3 divided doses after at least 24 h
5. Patients with segmental IH and suspected PHACES syndrome ideally require MRA before starting propranolol – if not possible to obtain urgent MRA, start propranolol 0.5 mg/kg daily in 3 divided doses

Yes

Start treatment ambulatory
Start propranolol 1 mg/kg daily in 3 divided doses
The dose can be increased to 2 mg/kg, daily in 3 divided doses after at least 24 h

Review 2–3 months after starting treatment
- Adjust the dose of propranolol for weight at clinic visits
- Total dose can be given in 2 or 3 divided doses
- Maximum dose 3 mg/kg daily
- Suspend treatment in the setting of significantly reduced oral intake or wheezing that requires treatment
- Treatment should extend beyond the proliferative period of IH to avoid rebound growth

Figure 116.13 Protocol for the use of propranolol in treating infantile haemangiomas. Reproduced from Solman 2018 [39] with permission of John Wiley & Sons. ECG, electrocardiogram; ECHO, echocardiogram; IH, infantile haemangioma; MRA, magnetic resonance angiography; MRI, magnetic resonance imaging; PHACES, posterior fossa malformations, haemangiomas, arterial anomalies, cardiac abnormalities, eye abnormalities, sternal cleft and supraumbilical raphe.

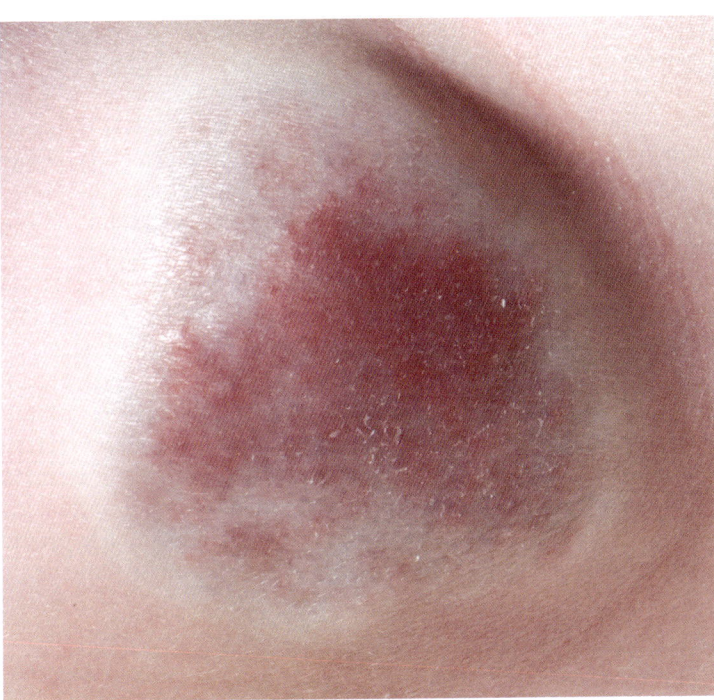

Figure 116.14 Rapidly involuting congenital haemangioma on the leg of a 6-week-old male, showing peripheral pallor.

(Figure 116.15), and may be warm to touch. They grow in proportion with the affected individual, but never regress. On ultrasound, NICHs often show prominent arterial flow. Histology shows large lobules of small vessels in a stroma of fibrous tissue containing abnormal appearing arteries and veins [5].

For NICH requiring treatment, surgery is the preferred option [7].

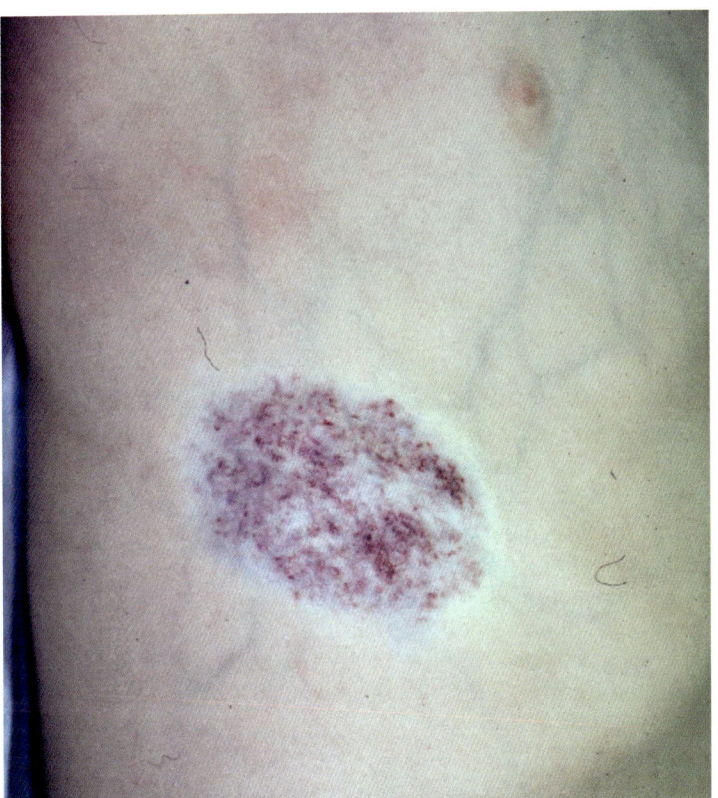

Figure 116.15 Non-involuting congenital haemangioma in an 11-year-old child.

Kaposiform haemangioendothelioma

Introduction and general description

Kaposiform haemangioendothelioma (KHE) is a rare, locally aggressive tumour named for its histological resemblance to Kaposi sarcoma. It may be present at birth or develop in early childhood, but rare cases have also been reported in adults [1]. It presents as a slightly raised, subcutaneous mass with a purpuric, bruised appearance, with occasional overlying telangiectasias (Figure 116.16) [2]. KHE is usually unifocal and most commonly involves the extremities, followed by trunk and cervico-facial region [1]. Approximately 10% of KHEs do not involve the skin [3]. Although the mechanism of tumorigenesis has not been fully defined, somatic activating *GNA14* mutations have been identified in some KHEs and have been found to induce changes in cellular morphology and increased cell growth via mitogen-activated protein kinase (MAPK) activation [4].

Pathophysiology

Histologically, KHE is marked by irregular sheets of spindle-shaped endothelial cells and characteristic slit-like vascular channels [5] with positive immunohistochemical staining for lymphatic markers, D2-40, LYVE1 and Prox-1,8, and negative for GLUT-1, the marker for infantile haemangioma [6].

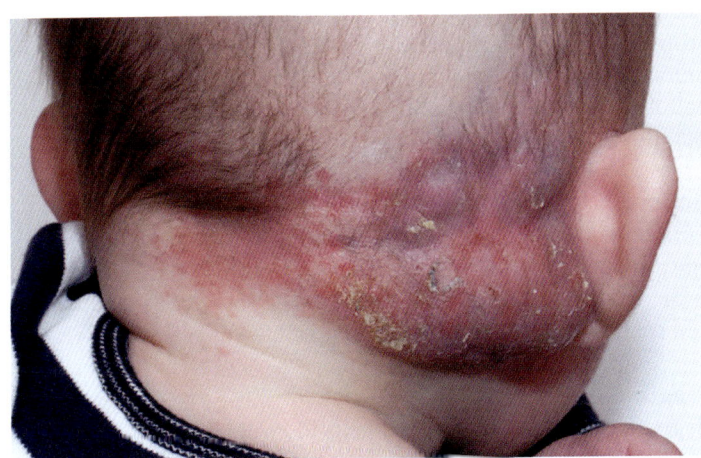

Figure 116.16 Kaposiform haemangioendothelioma on the neck of a 6-month-old infant.

Kasabach–Merritt phenomenon

Approximately 50–70% of patients with KHE develop the Kasabach–Merritt phenomenon (KMP) [7], a potentially life-threatening disorder characterised by severe thrombocytopenia, hypofibrinogenaemia, microangiopathic haemolytic anaemia and consumptive coagulopathy. For decades, KMP was thought to be a complication of infantile haemangiomas, however it is now understood to be specific to KHE and tufted angioma [8]. The mechanism is not completely clear, but it is thought that abnormal endothelium and architecture of the tumour promote platelet adhesion and trapping [9]. The presenting sign of KMP is rapid enlargement of the

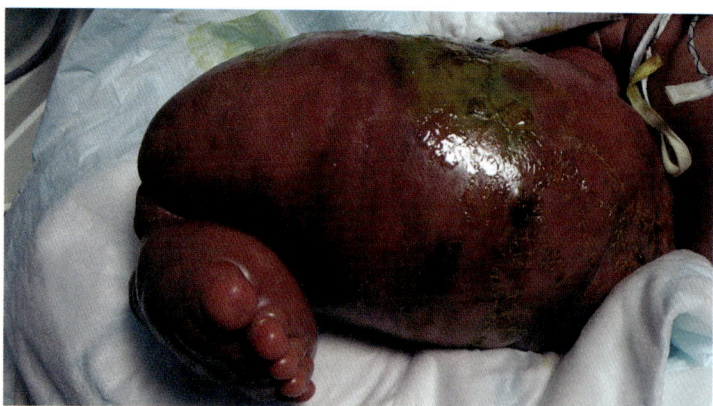

Figure 116.17 Massive kaposiform haemangioendothelioma of a newborn with severe Kasabach–Merritt phenomenon.

KHE, which becomes tense, purpuric or ecchymotic (Figure 116.17). KHE can exhibit dramatic episodes of tumour growth in response to infection or trauma [2]. These changes are accompanied by a fall in the platelet count (platelets can drop to $3–5 \times 10^9/L$) and fibrinogen (often below 1 g/L). D-dimers are almost always elevated. Despite profound thrombocytopenia, severe haemorrhage is rare.

Investigations
Blood tests
When KHE is suspected, full blood count and clotting, including fibrinogen, prothrombin time (PT), activated partial thromboplastin time (aPTT) and D-dimers, should be obtained. The detection of severe thrombocytopenia with hypofibrinogenaemia and elevated D-dimers suggest the diagnosis of KMP, however other vascular tumours of infancy (such as congenital haemangioma) and vascular malformations can also be associated with thrombocytopenia and coagulopathy [10].

Biopsy
If possible, the diagnosis of KHE should be confirmed histopathologically as long-term treatment is often required. The biopsy should be carried out in a specialist centre, as high vascularity and associated coagulopathy lead to a high risk of bleeding.

Imaging
Magnetic resonance imaging is helpful in delineating the extent of the disease and assessing the response to treatment, especially in KHE that does not involve the skin.

Management
The approach to management must be individualised, based on the size, location and severity of the coagulopathy. Although platelets can be dramatically low, life-threatening haemorrhage is rare. Platelet transfusion should not be given unless in preparation for procedures or if the patient is actively bleeding. The transfusion of platelets tends to worsen the condition, as the KHE will rapidly sequester and consume platelets, leading to increase in size and increase in the systemic bleeding risk. Fresh frozen plasma or cryoprecipitate can be given for correction of hypofibrinogenaemia if there is active bleeding, before surgical procedures or if fibrinogen is below 1 g/L. Cryoprecipitate is highly concentrated and should be

considered in patients with high-output heart failure. Symptomatic anaemia can be treated with the transfusion of red blood cells.

In the past, KHE was treated with surgical excision, however due to the risks of high vascularity, coagulopathy and size increase with trauma, pharmacological treatment is preferred. Vincristine and systemic steroids were primarily used as first line therapy for the treatment of KHE with KMP. However, more recently, several studies have demonstrated rapid normalisation of the platelet count and softening of the tumour within days of initiation of treatment with sirolimus [11–14]. Sirolimus is an oral medication and, unlike vincristine, does not require a central line.

Embolisation may be an alternative to surgery if a single feeding vessel is demonstrated, which is infrequent; necrosis and superinfection are common. Propranolol is not beneficial for KHE. Multidisciplinary team collaboration with a paediatric dermatologist, neonatal/paediatric intensivist, interventional radiologist, plastic surgeon and haematologist/oncologist is essential to provide comprehensive and individualised treatment for these patients.

Tufted angioma

Tufted angioma (TA) is so-called because of its histological appearance, which reveals groups of dermal capillary tufts. It shares several histopathological features with KHE and they are thought to be a part of a spectrum [1,2]. Most cases are present in childhood, but it can also manifest in adulthood [3].

TAs are characterised by multiple, discrete lobules of tightly packed capillaries (tufts) scattered in the dermis and sometimes in the subcutis in a so-called 'cannonball' pattern [4]. These capillary tufts are surrounded by cleft-like, semilunar, empty vascular spaces. Thin-walled lymphatic spaces may be seen throughout the dermis [4].

Lesions are usually located on the limbs or trunk and rarely on the face [5]. The size can vary from a few to 20 centimetres. A TA is usually pink, red, violaceous or blue in colour and overlying hypertrichosis and hyperhidrosis is common (Figure 116.18). Over time, the tumour can thicken; induration and fibrosis can affect limb and joint function [6]. TAs can also be painful. Only about 10% of TAs develop KMP [7].

The treatment of TA depends on size, location, impaired function, pain and presence of KMP. Observation without intervention is a reasonable option in some cases. Surgical intervention can be used for smaller lesions. TA with KMP should be treated the same way as KHE.

Pyogenic granuloma

Pyogenic granuloma (PG; acquired eruptive lobular capillary haemangioma) is a common, benign, acquired vascular lesion of the skin and mucous membranes. PG can occur at any age, but is more common in children and young adults [1].

A PG starts as a small, bright red papule that grows rapidly over weeks to months. It can be sessile or slightly pedunculated. Most PGs are less than 1 cm in size. In children, they are most common

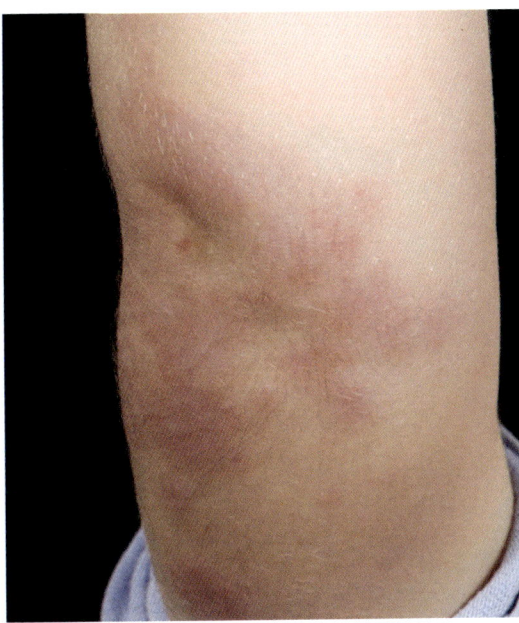

Figure 116.18 Tufted angioma on the elbow of a 6-year-old child with overlying hypertrichosis.

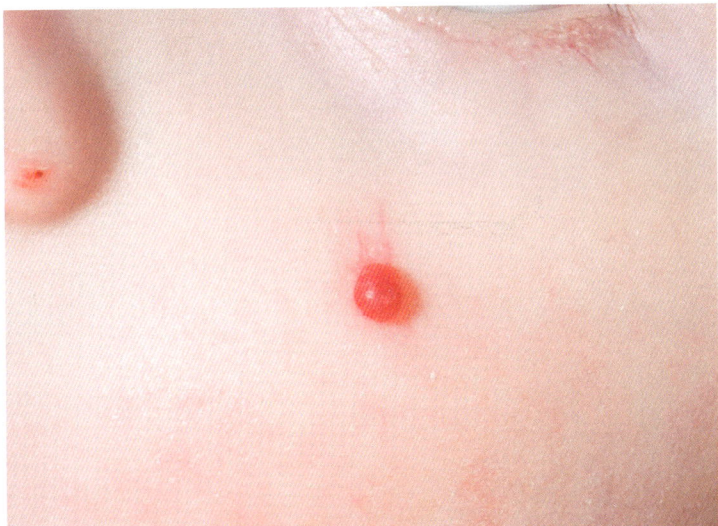

Figure 116.19 Pyogenic granuloma on the face of a 5-month-old infant.

on the face and neck (Figure 116.19), and in adults on the trunk and limbs [1]. Trauma has been suggested as a trigger, but only 7–23% of patients with PG report a preceding injury at the site [2,3]. PGs are usually solitary, but may be multiple and agminated, as seen in association with pre-existing capillary malformations [4].

Angiogenic growth factors, such as vascular endothelial growth factor (VEGF) [5], transcription factors (pATF2 and pSTAT3) [6] and MAPK signal transduction pathway proteins [7], are overexpressed in PG, although their role is not clear. A whole exome sequencing study of 40 PG lesions found *HRAS* somatic mutations in four tumours, supporting a role for the RAS-MAPK pathway in the development of PG [8].

PGs are often mistaken for infantile haemangiomas, but they rarely manifest before 4 months of age and infantile haemangiomas appear a few weeks after birth. The surface of the PG is very friable

and they bleed profusely after even minor trauma. Bleeding can be recurrent and difficult to control. In infantile haemangiomas, bleeding is uncommon and usually easily controlled with pressure.

Treatment of a PG is usually surgical, either elliptical excision or shave/scoop excision with electrodesiccation and healing by granulation. PDL or carbon dioxide laser can be effective, but more than one session may be required and is no better than surgery. Topical β-blockers, such as timolol, have been used with favourable results in some patients [9]. Treatment with salt has been regularly used in umbilical granulomas and a recent case report has shown it might be beneficial in the treatment of PG [10].

Resources

Patient resources

Birthmark Support Group: www.birthmarksupportgroup.org.uk
Changing Faces: https://www.changingfaces.org.uk
Great Ormond Street Hospital, haemangioma information: https://www.gosh.nhs.uk/conditions-and-treatments/conditions-we-treat/haemangiomas/ (All last accessed February 2023)

Key references

The full list of references can be found in the online version at https://www.wiley.com/rooksdermatology10e

Infantile haemangiomas

1 International Society for the Study of Vascular Anomalies (ISSVA). *ISSVA Classification for Vascular Anomalies 2014*. https://www.issva.org/UserFiles/file/Classifications-2014-Final.pdf (last accessed February 2023).

16 Metry D, Heyer G, Hess C *et al.* Consensus statement on diagnostic criteria for PHACE syndrome. *Pediatrics* 2009;124:1447–56.

20 Mahon C, McHugh K, Alband N *et al.* Routine liver ultrasound screening does not alter clinical management in a cohort study of multiple cutaneous infantile haemangioma. *Br J Dermatol* 2021;184:340–1.

29 Leaute-Labreze C, Dumas de la Roque E, Hubiche T, Boralevi F, Thambo JB, Taieb A. Propranolol for severe hemangiomas of infancy. *N Engl J Med* 2008;358:2649–51.

30 Marqueling AL, Oza V, Frieden IJ, Puttgen KB. Propranolol and infantile hemangiomas four years later: a systematic review. *Pediatr Dermatol* 2013;30:182–91.

34 Metry D, Frieden IJ, Hess C *et al.* Propranolol use in PHACE syndrome with cervical and intracranial arterial anomalies: collective experience in 32 infants. *Pediatr Dermatol* 2013;30:71–89.

37 Solman L, Murabit A, Gnarra M, Harper JI, Syed SB, Glover M. Propranolol for infantile haemangiomas: single centre experience of 250 cases and proposed therapeutic protocol. *Arch Dis Child* 2014;99:1132–6.

46 Batta K, Goodyear HM, Moss C, Williams HC, Hiller L, Waters R. Randomised controlled study of early pulsed dye laser treatment of uncomplicated childhood haemangiomas: results of a 1-year analysis. *Lancet* 2002;360:521–7.

Congenital haemangiomas

6 Baselga E, Cordisco MR, Garzon M, Lee MT, Alomar A, Blei F. Rapidly involuting congenital haemangioma associated with transient thrombocytopenia and coagulopathy: a case series. *Br J Dermatol* 2008;158:1363–70.

Kaposiform haemangioendothelioma

8 Sarkar M, Mulliken JB, Kozakewich HP, Robertson RL, Burrows PE. Thrombocytopenic coagulopathy (Kasabach–Merritt phenomenon) is associated with kaposiform hemangioendothelioma and not with common infantile hemangioma. *Plast Reconstr Surg* 1997;100:1377–86.

PART 10: SPECIFIC SITES, SEX & AGE

Index

Note: Page numbers in *italics* refer to figures and those in **bold** refer to tables and boxes, where they fall outside the main text range. References are to pages within chapters, thus 58.10 is page 10 of Chapter 58.

Rook's Textbook of Dermatology, Tenth Edition. Edited by Christopher Griffiths, Jonathan Barker, Tanya Bleiker, Walayat Hussain and Rosalind Simpson.
© 2024 John Wiley & Sons Ltd. Published 2024 by John Wiley & Sons Ltd.